UNDERSTANDING
Medical
Surgical
Nursing

Linda S. Williams, MSN, RN
Professor of Nursing
Jackson College
Jackson, Michigan

Paula D. Hopper, MSN, RN, CNE
Professor of Nursing
Jackson College
Jackson, Michigan

FIFTH EDITION

F.A. Davis Company • Philadelphia

Your guide to
UNDERSTANDING
Medical Surgical Nursing
FIFTH EDITION

Get the most out of your textbook and resources online at **DavisPlus.com** to prepare for class, clinical, and professional success.

Preview what you'll learn.

Learning Outcomes guide your focus. Revisit the section after you complete the chapter to assess your progress.

Key Terms show you how to pronounce the important terms you'll be learning in each chapter.

4

Cultural Influences on Nursing Care

BOBBI M. MARTIN

LEARNING OUTCOMES

1. Define common concepts related to culture and ethnicity.
2. List examples of cultural characteristics, values, beliefs, and practices.
3. Describe attributes of culturally diverse patients and their families and how they affect nursing care.
4. Identify data should you collect from culturally diverse patients and their families.
5. Apply a holistic approach to patient care that respects cultural characteristics and attributes.

KEY TERMS

acculturation (uh-KUL-chur-AY-shun)
beliefs (bee-LEEFS)
cultural (KUL-chur-uhl)
cultural assimilation (KUL-chur-uhl uh-SIM-ih-LAY-shun)
cultural awareness (KUL-chur-uhl a-WEAR-ness)
cultural competence (KUL-chur-uhl KOM-pe-tents)
cultural conflict (KUL-chur-uhl KON-flikt)
cultural diversity (KUL-chur-uhl dih-VER-sih-tee)
cultural sensitivity (KUL-chur-uhl SEN-sih-TIV-ih-tee)
cultural shock (KUL-chur-uhl SHOK)
culture (KUL-chur)
customs (KUS-tums)
ethnic (ETH-nick)
ethnocentrism (ETH-noh-SEN-trizm)
generalizations (JEN-er-al-ih-ZAY-shuns)
stereotype (STARE-ee-oh-TIGHP)
traditions (tra-DISH-uns)
values (VAL-yooz)
worldview (WERLD-vyoo)

Prepare for the real world of nursing practice.

Critical Thinking Case Studies

help you practice and understand what you're learning.

Patient Perspectives give you a patient's eye-view of the disease or condition you're studying.

Learning, Nursing Care, & Safety Tips provide

helpful advice to achieve best patient outcomes.

NEW! Safe and Effective Care Competencies.

Cultural Considerations, Gerontological Issues, Nutrition Notes & Home Health Hints

prepare you for clinical practice in the areas that will do the most to assure your professional success.

Build your confidence.

Evidence-based practice boxes offer an in-depth look at research that supports best practices.

NCLEX-style end-of-chapter questions develop your clinical judgment.

Nursing Care Plans are easy to read and clearly present the rationale for each action.

EVIDENCE-BASED PRACTICE

Clinical Question
Does use of information technology in the form of an Interactive Preventive Health Record (IPHR) increase the use of preventative health services?

Evidence
4500 patients were randomly invited to use an IPHR that provided personal health records, education, and reminders. Use of preventative services significantly increased by 2.3% in those using the IPHR over those who were not. Furthermore, the number of patients who were up to date on all recommended preventative services was double in the IPHR group.

Implications for Nursing Practice
Encouraging the use of patient-centered interactive technology might help improve patient health.

REFERENCES
Krist, A. H., Woolf, S. H., Rothemich, S. F, Johnson, R. E., Peele, J. E., Cunningham, T. D., Longo, D. R., Bello, G. A., Matzke, G. R. (2012). Interactive preventive health record to enhance delivery of recommended care: A randomized trial. *Annals of Family Medicine, 10*, 312–319.

NURSING CARE PLAN for the Postoperative Patient

Nursing Diagnosis: Ineffective Airway Clearance related to ineffective cough and secretion retention

Expected Outcomes: Patient will maintain a patent airway at all times. Breath sounds remain clear at all times.

Evaluation of Outcomes: Is patient able to clear own secretions? Are breath sounds clear?

Interventions Monitor breath sounds. **Rationale** Abnormal breath sounds such as crackles or wheezes can indicate retained secretions. **Evaluation** Are breath sounds clear?

Interventions Encourage deep breathing and coughing and use of incentive spirometer hourly while awake. **Rationale** Lung expansion helps prevent atelectasis and keeps lungs clear of secretions. **Evaluation** Does patient perform deep breathing and coughing and use incentive spirometer?

Interventions Ensure that patient's pain is relieved before activity. **Rationale** Movement can cause or increase pain. **Evaluation** Does patient state pain is controlled before activity?

Interventions Encourage movement by turning every 2 hours and ambulating as able. **Rationale** Movement promotes lung expansion and movement of secretions. **Evaluation** Is patient moving?

Nursing Diagnosis: Pain related to surgery, nausea, and vomiting

Expected Outcomes: Patient will report that pain management relieves pain satisfactorily within 30 minutes of report of pain. Patient will describe pain management plan by first postoperative day.

Evaluation of Outcomes: Does patient report satisfactory pain relief? Is patient able to describe pain management plan?

Continued

Expand your knowledge.

Explore MORE at 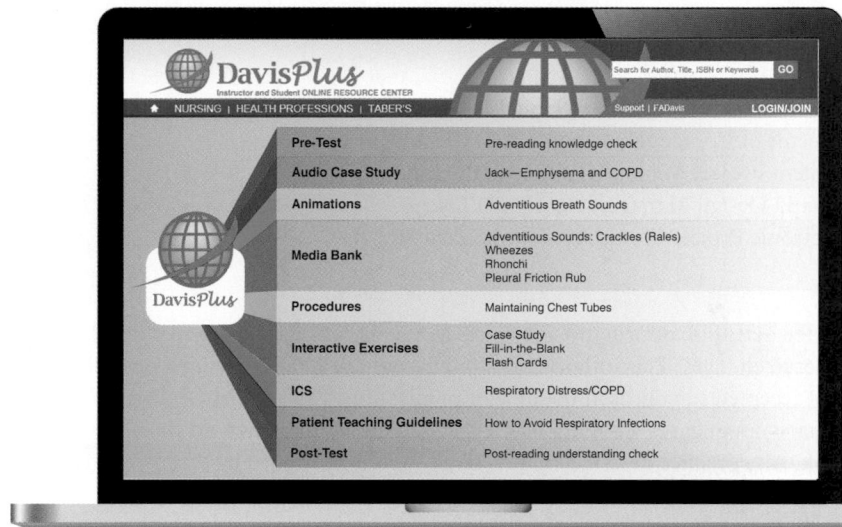 DavisPlus

Gain access to your complete text online with the Davis Digital Version.
Redeem your *Plus* Code to access these Davis*Plus* Premium Resources.

- Davis Digital Version
- **NEW!** Interactive Clinical Scenarios
- **UPDATED!** Audio Case Studies with Discussion Questions
- Animations
- Interactive Exercises
- **EXPANDED!** Test Bank
- Heart, Lung, Bowel, & Blood pressure sounds
- Patient Teaching Guidelines
- Pre- and Post Tests
- Dosage Calculation Quizzes
- Concept Map Generator
- **NEW!** Concept Maps for Concept Based Learning
- Chapter Resource Maps
- And much more!

Chapter Resource Maps outline chapter-specific online resources, as well as exercises from the student workbook.

Visit **Davis*Plus*.com** today!

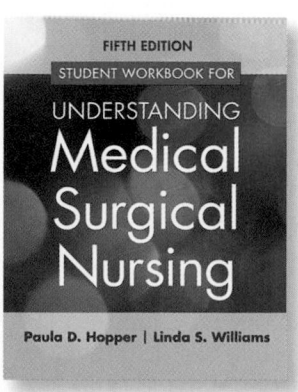

Student Workbook
Enhance your skills with critical-thinking exercises, basic matching and true/false tests, evidence-based practice exercises, and NCLEX-PN® style questions. Learn more at **www.FADavis.com.**

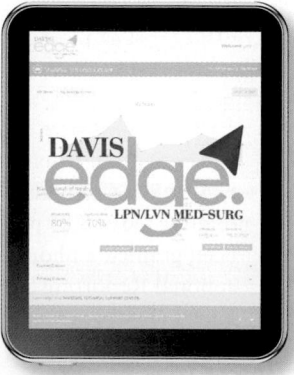

Davis Edge for LPN/LVN Med-Surg
Exam success starts here. Classroom. NCLEX. Master course content & develop your critical-thinking skills, and prepare for the NCLEX-PN® with this adaptive, online Q&A platform. Learn more at **www.DavisEdge.com.**

F.A. Davis Company
1915 Arch Street
Philadelphia, PA 19103
www.fadavis.com

Printed in the United States of America

Last digit indicates print number: 10 9 8 7 6 5 4 3 2 1

Acquisitions Editor: Lisa B. Houck
Director of Content Development: Darlene D. Pedersen
Content Project Manager II: Elizabeth Hart
Art and Design Manager: Carolyn O'Brien
Electronic Project Manager: Sandra Glennie

As new scientific information becomes available through basic and clinical research, recommended treatments and drug therapies undergo changes. The author(s) and publisher have done everything possible to make this book accurate, up to date, and in accord with accepted standards at the time of publication. The author(s), editors, and publisher are not responsible for errors or omissions or for consequences from application of the book, and make no warranty, expressed or implied, in regard to the contents of the book. Any practice described in this book should be applied by the reader in accordance with professional standards of care used in regard to the unique circumstances that may apply in each situation. The reader is advised always to check product information (package inserts) for changes and new information regarding dose and contraindications before administering any drug. Caution is especially urged when using new or infrequently ordered drugs.

ISBN 13: 978-0-8036-4068-9

Library of Congress Cataloging-in-Publication Data

Understanding medical surgical nursing / [edited by] Linda S. Williams, Paula D. Hopper. – Fifth edition.
     p. ; cm.
Includes bibliographical references and index.
ISBN 978-0-8036-4068-9 – ISBN 0-8036-4068-4
I. Williams, Linda S. (Linda Sue), 1954- , editor. II. Hopper, Paula D., editor.
[DNLM: 1. Nursing Care. 2. Evidence-Based Nursing. 3. Nursing Process. WY 100.1]

RT41
610.73—dc23

2014032848

*For practical and vocational nursing
students: you are valuable members
of the health care team.
We trust this text will help you
learn to think like nurses and become
safe practitioners.*

*To Dimitri, our angel, always in our hearts.
—Linda
And for Dave, who tried really hard to
cook and manage the household while
I worked on this edition.
—Paula*

Preface

Welcome to the fifth edition of *Understanding Medical Surgical Nursing*! We have fully updated the material and have added exciting new information on evidence-based practice, safety, and more. Boxed materials throughout the text present actual evidence-based care guidelines.

We continue to work hard to provide a text written at an understandable level, with features that help students understand, apply, and practice the challenging content required to function as practical/vocational nurses. We are thankful to the many students who tell us they find the book very readable, and actually enjoyable. We have been overjoyed to hear from several nursing programs that their NCLEX scores soared after adopting this textbook. We welcome and value your comments on this edition.

We continue to emphasize understanding, critical thinking, and the ability to make sound clinical judgments. We believe that a student who learns to think critically will be better able to apply information to new situations. We hope both students and instructors find this fifth edition a practical tool for learning and understanding the principles of medical-surgical nursing.

Features of the Book

We have kept our most popular features from the first four editions along with new ones based on reader input.
Newly Added:

- Learning Outcomes to guide reading and studying.
- An exciting new way to review anatomy and physiology with more images and less text in each function and assessment chapter.
- A Diagnostic Tests Appendix with explanations of common tests for easy reference.
- Updated design for easier readability of tables and care plans.

Based on feedback, we have kept and expanded the following:

- Web links in the text to help students do further research on topics of interest. Every effort was made to use only major, established Web sites that are unlikely to change in the near future.
- One of our most popular features, Critical Thinking Exercises. These exercises help students practice and think about what they are learning.
- Review questions at the end of each chapter. Questions have been updated and include application- and analysis-level questions, and alternate format items to reflect the NCLEX-PN.
- Suggested Answers for the Critical Thinking Exercises and Review Questions. Research supports the importance of immediate feedback to reinforce learning, so we feel strongly that students should have access to correct answers

while they are studying, without having to wait for their next instructor contact. Because there can be many answers to some of the critical thinking questions, we have provided sample answers to help stimulate students' thinking.
- Nursing Care Tips, Be Safe!, and Learning Tips help make learning easy. The Joint Commission's National Patient Safety Goals are reflected in many of the safety tips.
- Pronunciation keys for new words at the beginning of each chapter.
- Word-building footnotes throughout the chapters.
- Nursing care plans with gerontological considerations. These have been updated to reflect current practice.
- Boxed presentations of Cultural Considerations, Evidence-Based Practice, Gerontological Issues, Home Health Hints, and Nutrition Notes. Additional boxes have been added where needed.
- A comprehensive, updated glossary of new words is included in the appendix.

To Students: How to Use This Book

Learning outcomes are provided for each chapter. Review them before reading and then go back and check to be sure you understand them.

You will find a list of new words and their pronunciations at the beginning of each chapter. These words appear in bold at either their first use or most relevant use in a chapter, and they also appear in the glossary at the end of the book. By learning the meanings of these words as you encounter them, you will increase your understanding of the material. Many of these words are also broken down where they are used, so you can see how the parts of each word make up the whole.

You also will find learning tips to increase your understanding and retention of the material. You may want to develop your own memory techniques in addition to those provided. (If you think of a good one, send it to us and you may find it in the next edition!) Many of the learning tips have been developed and used in our own classrooms. We find them helpful in fostering understanding of complex concepts or as memory aids. However, we want to stress that memorization is not the primary focus of the text but rather a foundation for understanding and thinking about more complex information. Understanding and application will serve you far better than memorization when dealing with new situations.

Each chapter includes brief critical thinking case studies designed to help you apply material that has been presented. A series of questions related to the case will help you integrate the material with what you already know. These questions emphasize critical thinking, which is based on a foundation of recall and understanding of material. To enhance your learning, try to answer the questions before checking the answers.

Generic medication names are a must for you to know for NCLEX-PN. We continue to provide both the generic and trade names for medications to help you prepare for both the NCLEX and nursing practice.

Review questions appear at the end of each chapter to help you prepare for chapter tests, and also for the NCLEX-PN. Again, to assess your learning, try to answer the questions before looking up the answers at the back of the book.

Chapter reference lists provide sources for additional reading material. Websites have been included in many chapters. We believe it is important for you to interact with current technology to expand your information resources.

The following appendices are included for easy reference:

- Normal adult reference laboratory values
- Answers with rationales to chapter review questions

- Common medical abbreviations
- Common prefixes and suffixes to help learn word-building techniques
- Glossary of new words
- Common diagnostic tests

Student Resources

There is an abundance of additional student resources for this edition of *Understanding Medical Surgical Nursing* from the exercises in the accompanying Student Workbook to the digital assets found on Davis*Plus* (access code is available on the inside front cover of your book). The **Chapter Resource Guide** found on Davis*Plus* provides colorful and informative maps for each chapter outlining the specific resources.

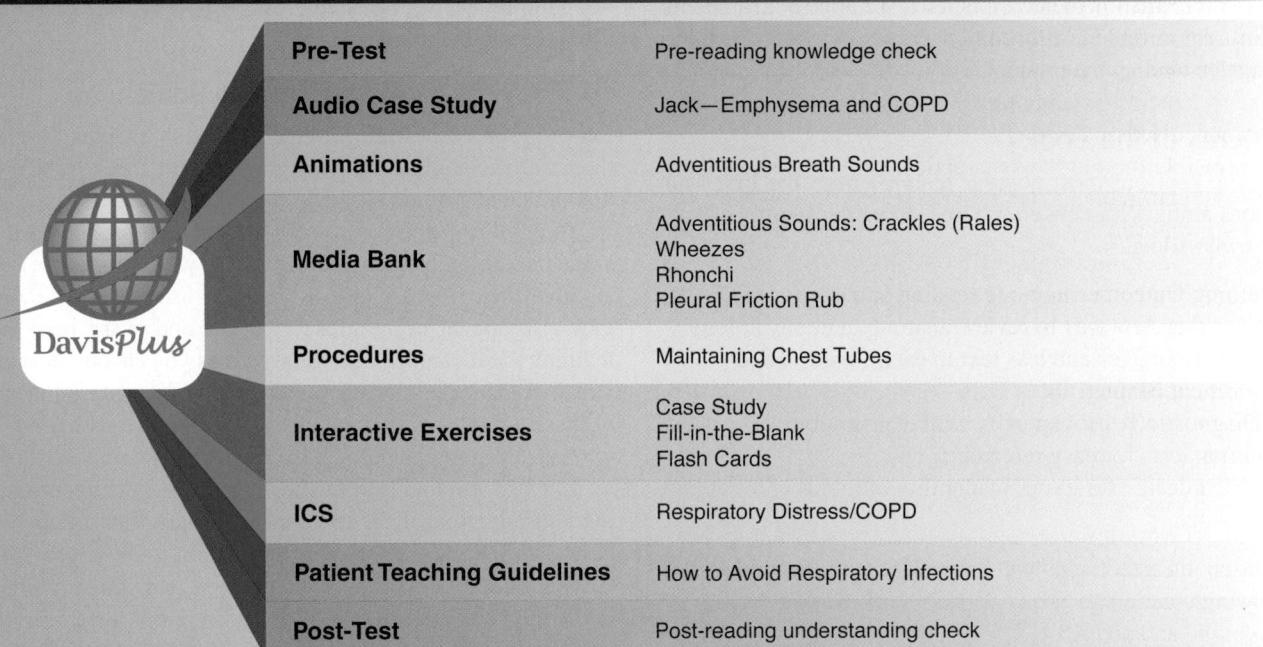

CHAPTER RESOURCE GUIDE
Chapter 31: Nursing Care of Patients With Lower Respiratory Tract Disorders

Pre-Test	Pre-reading knowledge check
Audio Case Study	Jack—Emphysema and COPD
Animations	Adventitious Breath Sounds
Media Bank	Adventitious Sounds: Crackles (Rales) Wheezes Rhonchi Pleural Friction Rub
Procedures	Maintaining Chest Tubes
Interactive Exercises	Case Study Fill-in-the-Blank Flash Cards
ICS	Respiratory Distress/COPD
Patient Teaching Guidelines	How to Avoid Respiratory Infections
Post-Test	Post-reading understanding check

DavisPlus

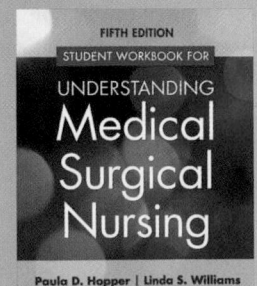

FIFTH EDITION
STUDENT WORKBOOK FOR
UNDERSTANDING
Medical Surgical Nursing
Paula D. Hopper | Linda S. Williams

Vocabulary
Respiratory Medications
Critical Thinking
Review Questions

Materials will be posted by type of resource as well as by chapter. Since topics are covered across multiple chapters you may find resources in multiple chapters. Take some time to click around Davis*Plus* and see all that is offered.

- **Pre-test and Post-test.** Do a pre-reading knowledge check with the pre-test and a post-reading understanding check with the post-test. The tests have the same questions so you can gauge your progress from start to finish. *Included for every chapter.*
- **Audio Case Study with Questions.** Chapter topic case scenarios in audio format with critical thinking questions for thought and discussion. *Included for every chapter.*
- **Animations & Media Bank.** Visual and audio enhancement of topics and concepts. *Included in relevant chapters and posted by resource.*
- **Procedures.** Selected LPN skills for you to review. *Included in relevant chapters and posted by resource.*
- **Interactive Exercises: Case Study, Fill-in-the-Blank, Flash Cards.** *Included for every chapter.* **Picture Match** is included for relevant chapters.
- **Interactive Clinical Scenarios (ICS).** Hone your critical thinking skills and make decisions for your patient based on the scenarios presented. Topics include dementia, chest pain, respiratory distress, and others. *Included in relevant chapters and posted by resource.*
- **Patient Teaching Guidelines.** Sample guidelines for disorders discussed throughout the text. These guidelines are printable for you to use in patient care settings while teaching your patients. *Included in relevant chapters and posted by resource.*
- **Student Question Bank.** NCLEX-PN–style review questions for each chapter. These questions have been reviewed and revised by an item-writing expert. *Posted by resource.*
- **Additional Bibliographic Resources.** Additional resources to enhance your learning of the chapter. *Included in relevant chapters.*

In addition you'll also find the following resources to help you as you work through the chapters: audio glossary, concept map generator, medications and calculations problems, dosage calculation quizzes, syringe exercises, sample clinical simulation, and an NCLEX prep guide.

A paperback Student Workbook is available to provide additional practice with the material. Each chapter includes vocabulary practice, objective exercises, a case study or other critical thinking practice exercises, and review questions written in NCLEX-PN format. These questions have been updated by an item-writing expert. Workbook answers are posted to the instructor's Davis*Plus* site. Ask your instructor(s) for the answers as appropriate.

Instructor Resources

Instructors have access to all student resources as well as materials specifically available to them to aid in the instruction of the material.

- **Instructor's Guide.** Each chapter has a chapter outline with suggested classroom strategies and activities. Also included are student activities for printing and using for individual practice or for collaborative learning activities. These activities help the student to interact with the material, understand it, and apply it. Many of the activities are based on real patient cases and have been used with our own nursing students. Feedback from students has helped to refine the exercises. We believe the use of collaborative learning has greatly enhanced our students' success in achieving their educational and licensure goals. Another benefit is the sense of community the students develop as a result of working in groups. A brief introduction and guidelines for using collaborative learning techniques is included.
- **PowerPoint Presentations.** For the instructor's convenience there is a comprehensive *PowerPoint* program for classroom presentations. Images from the text are included in the presentations. Review questions have been added to the end of the presentations for a quick in-class knowledge check. Each presentation can be modified, reduced, or expanded by individual instructors to suit their needs.
- **Electronic Test Bank.** Test questions for each chapter and topic that assist students to prepare for the NCLEX-PN. These questions have been updated, enhanced, and expanded by an item-writing expert for this edition. As outlined in the NCLEX-PN test plan, the questions are in multiple choice and alternate formats, and they test understanding, application, and analysis of material. The program allows instructors to choose and modify the questions that best suit their classroom needs.
- We include a **PowerPoint tutorial** and **NCLEX-style item-writing tutorial** to help you individualize our resources to your own needs.
- **Audio Case Study Q&A.** Discussion questions with suggested answers for the Audio Case Studies. *Instructors can access the audio in the Student Resources.*
- **Ethical Considerations.** Ethical scenarios with discussion questions and answers to use as case studies for classroom discussion.
- **Student Workbook.** Workbook answers are posted on the instructor's Davis*Plus* site. Provide answers to students as appropriate.

In addition to all of these great resources for students and instructors, you'll also each have access to a Davis Digital Version of the text so you can "take it on the go!"

Acknowledgments

Many people helped us make this book a reality. First and foremost are the students, who provide us with the inspiration to undertake this project. We hope that students everywhere continue to find this text worth reading.

The F.A. Davis Company is an exceptional publishing partner. We feel fortunate to have had their continued enthusiasm and confidence in our book. The staff at F.A. Davis has guided us through this project for five editions to help us create a student-friendly book that truly promotes understanding of medical-surgical nursing.

Lisa Houck, Robin Richman, Elizabeth Hart, and many others have been extremely patient and kind as we worked hard to provide a quality text.

Contributors from across the United States, including many well-known experts in their fields, brought expertise and diversity to the content. Their hard work is much appreciated.

Many of our coworkers have contributed to this book and given us ongoing encouragement and validation of the worthiness of this project. Betty Ackley, Marina Martinez-Kratz, Carroll Lutz, Erin Mazur, Sharon Nowak, and Barbara Berkeypile were especially helpful in providing material, advice, and encouragement.

We also thank several educators who have graciously provided input when we have needed it: Peggy Flener, Penny Snyder, and Terri Waisanen. Dawna Martich was a godsend as our item-writing expert for this edition. Finally, we are thankful to Gay Alcenius, PharmD, for her expertise in updating all medication materials.

We wish to thank everyone who played a role, however large or small, in helping us to provide a tool to help students realize their dreams of becoming LPN/LVNs. We hope this book will help educate nurses who can provide safe and expert care because we have helped them to learn to think critically and make sound clinical judgments.

Contributors

Betty Ackley, BSN, MSN, EdS, RN
Professor Emeritus
Jackson College
Jackson, Michigan

Gay Alcenius, PharmD
Pharmacist
Allegiance Health
Jackson, Michigan

Cynthia Barrere, PhD, RN
Associate Professor
Quinnipiac University
Hamden, Connecticut

Kathy Berchem, MSN, RN, FNP-BC
Assistant Professor
Lake Superior State University
Sault Ste. Marie, Michigan

Terri Blevins, BSN, MSEd, RN
Practical Nursing Director—Retired
Tennessee Technology Center at Elizabethton
Elizabethton, Tennessee

Michelle Block, MS, RN
Associate Professor
Purdue University Calumet
Hammond, Indiana

Janice L. Bradford, MS
Assistant Professor
Jackson College
Jackson, Michigan

Lucy L. Colo, MSN, RN
Faculty
Huron School of Nursing
East Cleveland, Ohio

Colleen Delaney, PhD, RN, AHN-BC
Associate Professor
University of Connecticut
Storrs, Connecticut

Sharon Gordon, MSN, RN, CNOR(E)
Practical Nursing Program Director
Pennsylvania State University Lehigh Valley
Allentown, Pennsylvania

Paula D. Hopper, MSN, RN, CNE
Professor of Nursing
Jackson College
Jackson, Michigan

Michelle Johnson, MSN, RN, CNE
Professor
Northern Michigan University
Marquette, Michigan

Marty Kohn, BSN, MS, RN, FNP, CWOCN
Nurse Practitioner
Wound Care Center, Allegiance Health
Jackson, Michigan

Carroll A. Lutz, MA, RN
Associate Professor Emerita
Jackson College
Jackson, Michigan

Bobbi M. Martin, MSN, RN, CNE
Dean of Nursing
Fortis College
Largo, Florida

Marina Martinez-Kratz, BSN, MS, RN, CNE
Professor
Jackson College
Jackson, Michigan

Erin Mazur, MSN, RN, FNP-BC
Assistant Professor
Jackson College
Jackson, Michigan

Laura L. McCully, MS, RN, CNM
Certified Nurse Midwife
Women First Health Services
Jackson, Michigan

Maureen McDonald, MS, RN
Professor
Massasoit Community College
Brockton, Massachusetts

Kelly McManigle, BSN, MSN, RN
Assistant Professor
State College of Florida
Bradenton, Florida

Betsy Murphy, MSN, RN, FNP, CHPN
Business Relations
Capital Hospice
Fairfax, Virginia

Sharon M. Nowak, MSN, EdD (ABD), RN
Associate Professor
Jackson College
Jackson, Michigan

Lazette V. Nowicki, BA, MSN, RN
Assistant Professor
American River College
Sacramento, California

Maryanne Pietraniec-Shannon, PhD, APRN-BC
Professor
Sault Ste. Marie, Michigan

Deb Richardson, MS, RN, CNS
President/Owner, Independent Educational Consultant
Deb Richardson & Associates
Houston, Texas

Sheria Grice Robinson, MSN, MHA, RN, CHPN
PhD Candidate
Wayne State University
Detroit, Michigan

James Shannon, BSN, JD, MHSA, RN
Attorney
Ann Arbor, Michigan

Rita Bolek Trofino, MNEd, RN
Associate Academic Dean
Chairperson, AD Nursing Program
Mount Aloysius College
Cresson, Pennsylvania

April Hazard Vallerand, PhD, RN, FAAN
College of Nursing Alumni Endowed Professor
Wayne State University College of Nursing
Detroit, Michigan

Patrice Wade, DNP, RN
Research Associate
Wayne State University
Detroit, Michigan

Deborah L. Weaver, PhD, RN
Associate Professor
Valdosta State University
Valdosta, Georgia

Linda S. Williams, MSN, RN
Professor of Nursing
Jackson College
Jackson, Michigan

Bruce K. Wilson, PhD, RN, CNS
Volunteer, American Red Cross
Lapeer, Michigan

CONTRIBUTORS TO PREVIOUS EDITIONS
We would like to acknowledge and thank the following individuals for their contributions to previous editions. All contributions have helped to make *Understanding Medical Surgical Nursing* what it has evolved into today.

Nancy Ahern, PhD, RN

Karen P. Hall, RN-C, MSHSA, NE-BC

Wendy Hockley, BS, MA, LPN

Diane Mayo, MSN, RN

Kelly Ann Morris, DNP, RN

Debra Perry-Philo, BSN, MSN, RN

Lynn D. Phillips, MSN, RN, CRNI

John Sturtevant, MSN, RN

Reviewers

Melissa Adams, MSN, RN
Director of Nursing Education, Practical Nursing
St. Louis College of Health Careers
Fenton, Missouri

Alice Alexander, MS, MSN, RN
Instructor, Practical Nursing
Southeast Community College
Beatrice, Nebraska

Kim Amos, PhD, RN, CNE
Practical Nurse Education Instructor
Isothermal Community College
Spindale, North Carolina

Janice Ankenmann, MSN, RN, CCRN, FNP-C
Coordinator Vocational Nursing Program
Napa Valley College
Napa, California

Mary Bailey, MSN
Nursing Instructor
Eastern Iowa Community College, Scott
Bettendorf, Iowa

Susan Bedwell
Instructor of Practical Nursing
Pearl River Community College
Hattiesburg, Mississippi

Robbin Bell, BSN, MS, RN
Director of Nursing
ECPI University
Virginia Beach, Virginia

Terri Blevins, BSN, MSEd, RN
Practical Nursing Director—Retired
Tennessee Technology Center at Elizabethton
Elizabethton, Tennessee

Joey Cagle, BSN
Assistant Professor of Licensed Practical Nursing
Dalton State College
Dalton, Georgia

Juanita Carlile, BSN, MEd, MSN, RN
Practical Nursing Instructor
Northeast Technology Center
Kansas, Oklahoma

Tonya Chapin, MSN, RN
Assistant Professor of Nursing
Colorado Mesa University
Grand Junction, Colorado

Marie Colucci, MN, EdD, RN
Associate Professor, Nursing
Riverside City College
Riverside, California

Sherri Comfort
Practical Nursing Department Chair
Holmes Community College, Goodman
Goodman, Mississippi

Winifred Critchlow
Teacher, Allied Health
Twin Rivers Adult School
McClellan, California

Lisa J. Davies, MSN
Practical Nursing Program Instructor/Trainer
Hutchinson Community College
McPherson, Kansas

Mary Davis, MSN
Practical Nursing Instructor
Wiregrass Georgia Technical College
Valdosta, Georgia

Judy Ennis, MSN
Nursing Instructor
Chattahoochee Valley Community College
Phenix City, Alabama

Debra Graves, RN
Practical Nursing Instructor
Tennessee College of Applied Technology, Covington
Covington, Tennessee

Lynne S. Hancock, MSN, RN
Director, Practical Nursing Program Head
Montgomery Community College
Troy, North Carolina

Evadne A. Harrison-Madu, PhD, MSN, RRT, RN
Acting Chairperson/Assistant Professor
Essex County College
Newark, New Jersey

Lori Henderson, RN
Technical Instructor, Practical Nursing
Okefenokee Technical College
Waycross, Georgia

Shari Herzfeld, MSN
Health Deputy Sector Navigator (HWI Director)
Rio Hondo College
Whittier, California

Jean Higgs, MSN, RN
Faculty
Shawsheen Valley School of Practical Nursing
Billerica, Massachusetts

Leeanne Humiston, MSN, RNC
Nursing Instructor
Southeastern Community College
Keokuk, Iowa

Connie Hunt, MS, RN
Practical Nursing Instructor
Indian Capital Technology Center, Stilwell
Stilwell, Oklahoma

Nora James, MSN, RN
Faculty, LVN Nursing
Lee College
Baytown, Texas

Donna Johnson, BSN, RN
Practical Nursing Program Administrator
Cape Girardeau Career & Technology Center
Cape Girardeau, Missouri

Ethel Jones, EdS, DSN, RN, CNE
Nursing Instructor
H. Councill Trenholm State Technical College
Montgomery, Alabama

Laura Jane Kuncaitis, RN
Instructor, Practical Nursing
Central Georgia Technical College
Macon, Georgia

Cathe Ledford, MSN
Adjunct Professor of ASPIRE
Simpson University
Redding, California

Susan R. Leferson, BSN, MSBA, COHC, RN
Nurse Educator
Medical Careers Institute, College of Health Sciences
of ECPI University
Manassas, Virginia

Selina LeMay-Kippel, DC, RN
Associate Professor of Nursing
North Country Community College, Ticonderoga
Ticonderoga, New York

Nancy Lyons, BSN, RN
Practical Nursing Instructor
Holy Name Medical Center School of Nursing
Teaneck, New Jersey

Janelle Martin, BSN, MHSA
Coordinator, Part-time PN Program, McPherson
Hutchinson Community College
McPherson, Kansas

Jamie Mathews, MSN
Nursing Instructor
Northwest College
Powell, Wyoming

Barbara Michalski, MSN, RN
Practical Nursing Instructor
Tulsa Technology Center
Tulsa, Oklahoma

Amanda Mohr, BSN, MSN, RN
Nursing Instructor
Southwestern Community College
Creston, Iowa

Nancy Morris, MSN, RN
Practical Nursing Instructor
North Georgia Technical College
Clarkesville, Georgia

John Nezbeth, BS, BA, MSN
Nursing Professor
Community College of Denver
Denver, Colorado

Danielle Nicastro, MSN, RN
Assistant Director Practical Nursing
Cumberland County College
Vineland, New Jersey

Janis Noel, BSN, RN
LPN Instructor
Tennessee College of Applied Technology, Paris
Paris, Tennessee

Patricia Noonan, MSN, RN
LPN Program Coordinator
Shawsheen Valley School of Practical Nursing
Billerica, Massachusetts

Barbara Overman, MSN
Coordinator and Instructor, Practical Nursing
Rhodes State College
Lina, Ohio

JoAnne Pearce, MS, RNC, APRN-BC
Director of Nursing Programs, Practical Nursing
Nursing Education Consultant
Idaho State University
Pocatello, Idaho

Brenda Pomerenke, BAN, RN
Nursing Faculty, PN Program
Minnesota West Community and Technical College
Worthington, Minnesota

Karen Potts, BC, MSN, RN, CDE
LPN Refresher Instructor
Delaware Skills Center
Wilmington, Delaware

Nancy Redenius
Department Chair, Health Science Education
Fort Myers Institute of Technology (FMIT)
Fort Myers, Florida

LuAnn Reicks, RNC
Professor
Iowa Central Community College
Fort Dodge, Iowa

Maria Relosa, ADN, RN, DND
Faculty
Preferred College of Nursing, Los Angeles
Los Angeles, California

Patrice Rimbey
Practical Nursing Program Coordinator
Penn State University, Hazleton
Hazleton, Pennsylvania

Carla Scheer, MSN, RN
Assistant Professor, Nursing
Massbay Community College
Framingham, Massachusetts

Elizabeth Scott, MSN, RN
ECPI University
Manassas, Virginia

Sue Smith, MS
Associate Professor—Nursing
Iowa Western Community College
Council Bluffs, Iowa

Kimmela Steed, BSN
Assistant Professor, Nursing
College of the Mainland
Texas City, Texas

Susan Thielemier
Instructor/Licensed Practical Nurse Nursing
Ozarka College
Melbourne, Arkansas

Carolyn R. Thomas, MS, RN
Health Programs Coordinator
Erie 1 BOCES
West Seneca, New York

Dora Thomas, MSN
Program Coordinator
Elizabethtown Community and Technical College
Elizabethtown, Kentucky

Kathleen Voeltzke, MSN, RN
Allied Health Coordinator
Tennessee College of Applied Technology, Nashville
Nashville, Tennessee

Jill Waletich, BSN, MA
Practical Nursing Instructor
Hennepin Technical College
Eden Prairie, Minnesota

Susan W. Whitley, MSN, RN, CNE
Practical Nursing Program Chair/Instructor
Lenoir Community College
Kinston, North Carolina

Christina Wilson, BAN, RN, CMSRN, PHN
Nursing Faculty
Anoka Technical College
Anoka, Minnesota

Contents

UNIT THREE
Understanding Life Span Influences on Health and Illness   261

xxxii   Contents

Contents in Brief

unit ONE

Understanding Health Care Issues

1

Critical Thinking and the Nursing Process

PAULA D. HOPPER AND
LINDA S. WILLIAMS

KEY TERMS

assessment (ah-SESS-ment)
clinical reasoning (KLIN-ih-kull REE-zon-ing)
collaborative (koh-LAB-rah-tiv)
critical thinking (KRIT-ih-kull THING-king)
data (DAY-tuh)
evaluation (e-VAL-yoo-AY-shun)
evidence-based practice (EHV-ah-dense baste PRACK-tis)
intervention (in-ter-VEN-shun)
nursing diagnosis (NER-sing DYE-ag-NOH-sis)
nursing process (NER-sing PRAH-sess)
objective data (ob-JEK-tiv DAY-tuh)
subjective data (sub-JEK-tiv DAY-tuh)
vigilance (VIJ-eh-lents)

LEARNING OUTCOMES

1. Explain why good critical thinking is important in nursing.
2. Describe attitudes and skills that promote good critical thinking.
3. Describe the thinking that occurs in each step of the nursing process.
4. Identify the role of a licensed practical nurse/licensed vocational nurse in using the nursing process.
5. Differentiate between objective and subjective data.
6. Document objective and subjective data.
7. Prioritize patient care activities based on Maslow's hierarchy of human needs.

Excellence in the delivery of nursing care requires good thinking. Each day nurses make many decisions that affect the care of their patients. For those decisions to be effective, the thinking behind them must be sound.

 ## CRITICAL THINKING

Nursing students must learn to think critically; in other words, to think like a nurse. This means they must use their knowledge and skills to make the best decisions possible in patient care situations. Halpern (1996) says that, "**critical thinking** is the use of those cognitive [knowledge] skills or strategies that increase the probability of a desirable outcome" (p. 5). Good thinking in nursing care has also been called **clinical reasoning**. Hawkins et al (2010) define clinical reasoning as "thinking through the various aspects of patient care to arrive at a reasonable decision regarding the prevention, diagnosis, or treatment of a clinical problem in a specific patient." Good thinking requires critical thinking attitudes and skills, which are described in this section. It also requires a good knowledge base, so your thinking is based on correct factual material. Our goal in this text is to provide you with solid medical-surgical knowledge on which to base good decisions.

Critical Thinking Traits

It is important for nurses to possess an attitude that promotes good thinking. Researchers have identified attitudes or traits associated with good critical thinking. The Foundation for Critical Thinking (2013) identifies seven traits: (1) intellectual humility, (2) intellectual courage, (3) intellectual empathy, (4) intellectual integrity, (5) intellectual perseverance, (6) faith in reason, and (7) fair-mindedness. We summarize these next.

Intellectual Humility

Have you ever known people who think they know it all? They do not have intellectual humility. People with intellectual humility have the ability to say, "I'm not sure about that . . . . I need more information." Certainly, we want our patients to think we are smart and know what we are doing, but patients also respect nurses who can say, "I don't know, but I'll find out." It is unsafe to care for patients when you are unsure of what you need to do.

Intellectual Courage

Intellectual courage allows you to look at other points of view even when you may not agree with them at first. Maybe you really believe that 8-hour shifts are best for nurses, and you have a lot of good reasons for your belief. But if you have intellectual courage, you will be willing to really listen to the arguments for 12-hour shifts. Maybe you will even be convinced. Sometimes you have to have the courage to say, "Okay, I see you were right after all."

Intellectual Empathy

Consider the patient who snaps as you enter her room, "I've been waiting all morning for my bath. If you don't help me with it right now I'm going to call your supervisor." The first response that comes into your head is, "I have five other patients; you're lucky I am here!" If you have intellectual empathy, however, you will be able to think, "If I were this patient, who is in chronic pain and is tired of being in the hospital, how would I feel?" Such thinking might change how you respond.

Intellectual Integrity

One of your patients asks a hundred questions when you bring her a medication that has been newly prescribed for her high blood pressure. But later you notice she is taking an herbal remedy from her purse. It is good that she asks a lot of questions about her drug, which has been tested extensively by the Food and Drug Administration (FDA). Herbal remedies, however, are not held to the same standards as medications in the United States. Someone with intellectual integrity would want the same level of proof applied to both medications and herbal remedies to determine if they are safe and effective before using them.

Intellectual Perseverance

Perseverance means you do not give up. Consider this scenario: You have concerns about some side effects you noticed after giving a new drug to a patient. You mention it to the health care provider, who says not to worry about it, but you are still concerned. If you have intellectual perseverance, you might do some research on the Internet, then go to your supervisor or the pharmacist to further discuss your concerns.

Faith in Reason

If you have faith in reason, you believe in your heart that good clinical reasoning will result in the best outcomes for your patients. And if you really believe, you will be more likely to attend a seminar or read an article on developing your clinical reasoning skills.

Fair-Mindedness

One of your coworkers wants to change the medication administration schedule on your unit. She says it will be better for the patients, but you think it might be because it is a better fit for her coffee-break schedule. If you have an intellectual sense of justice, you will be sure that your thinking is not biased by something that you just want for yourself, as seems to be happening with your coworker. You should examine your own motives as well as those of others when you are making decisions.

So what does all this mean to you as a nursing student? The term *metacognition* means to "think about thinking." It is important for you to try to develop the attitudes of a critical thinker and to learn to think clearly and critically about your patient care. To do that, you need to constantly reflect on how you are thinking. Are you practicing intellectual humility? Are you trying to be courageous and empathetic? These attitudes create an excellent base on which to build nursing knowledge and develop further thinking skills.

LEARNING TIP

Each time you exit a patient's room, do a mini critical thinking assessment. Think, "Did I ask the right questions? Was my thinking clear and logical? Is there anything I could have done better?" This 1-minute metacognition exercise will help you develop as a great thinker!

Nursing Knowledge Base

Nurses must have a solid knowledge base to safely care for patients. You would not drive a car without first learning the basics of how a car works and the rules of the road. In the same way, you must understand the human body in health and illness before you can understand how to take care of an ill patient. This is the reason you are going to school and studying this book.

Information is found in many places; some information is good, and some is not as good. For example, health information found on a website may have been put there by a major university medical school or other reputable source, or it may have been put there by a patient who has a particular disorder. You may learn about a patient's experience by reading his or her website, but you certainly would not base your patient care on someone's personal story.

The best knowledge on which to base your practice comes from research. Nurse researchers try new methods of caring for patients and compare them with traditional methods to determine what works best. For example, for many years, nurses were taught to massage patients' reddened bony prominences to prevent pressure ulcers. Through research, we now know that this practice should be avoided because it can further harm the damaged tissue. When nursing care is based on good, well-designed research studies, it is called **evidence-based practice**. You will read more about evidence-based practice in Chapter 2.

Critical Thinking Skills
Problem Solving

Problem solving is another way to think about clinical reasoning. Nurses solve problems every day. However, a problem can be handled in a way that may or may not help the patient. For instance, consider Mr. Frank, who is in pain and asks for pain medication. You check the medication record and find that his analgesic is not due for another 40 minutes. You can choose to manage this problem in several ways. One approach is to tell Mr. Frank that it is not time for the pain medication and that he will have to wait. This may solve your problem (you can move on to the next patient), but it does not solve the problem in an acceptable way for Mr. Frank. He is still in pain! Another approach is to use a standard problem-solving method: (1) gather data, (2) identify the problem, (3) decide what outcome is desirable,

(4) plan what to do, (5) implement the interventions in your plan, and (6) evaluate the plan of care.

1. Gather **data**, or factual information, to help you think critically about Mr. Frank's request for pain medication. As a good critical thinker, you can use intellectual empathy as well as your knowledge base about pain to decide what data you need. You decide to use a pain-rating scale on which the patient rates pain on a scale of 0 (no pain) to 10 (the greatest pain possible). Mr. Frank says that the pain is in his back and rates it as an 8 on a 10-point scale. You check his history and find that he has spinal compression fractures. Your empathetic attitude tells you that waiting for 40 minutes to relieve his pain is not acceptable. You next go to the medication record and find that he has no alternative pain medications ordered.
2. Identify the problem. Here you use your knowledge base about compression fractures, pain, and medication administration to draw the conclusion that Mr. Frank is in acute pain, and the current medication orders are not sufficient to provide pain relief.
3. Decide what outcome (sometimes called a goal) is desirable. The outcome should be determined by you (the nurse) and the patient working together. The patient is intimately involved in this situation and deserves to be consulted. You may also collaborate with the RN or health care provider. In this case, you talk to Mr. Frank and determine that he needs pain relief now; he cannot wait until the next scheduled dose of medication. He states that he can tolerate a pain rating of 3 or less on a 10-point scale.
4. Plan what to do. Formulate and consider some alternate solutions. For example, you can decide to tell Mr. Frank that he has to wait 40 minutes; however, this will not help him reach his desired outcome of pain control. You could give the medication early, but this would not be following the health care provider's orders and may have harmful effects for Mr. Frank. You could decide to try some nondrug pain-control methods, such as relaxation, distraction, or imagery. These might be helpful, but you recall from pharmacology class that complementary methods should be used in conjunction with, not in place of, medications. Another option is to report to the registered nurse (RN) or health care provider that Mr. Frank's pain is not controlled with the current pain-control regimen. Once you have several alternative courses of action, decide which will best help the patient. Then you can discuss those options with the RN and together decide the best thing to do; in this case, you might decide to have the RN contact the health care provider while you work with the patient on relaxation exercises. You might decide

to ask Mr. Frank if he would like to listen to some of the music his wife brought for him. You should also tell Mr. Frank that the health care provider is being contacted. This would assure him that his pain is being taken seriously.

5. Implement the **interventions** in your plan. The RN enters the room and informs you and the patient that the health care provider has changed the analgesic orders. You obtain and administer the first dose of the new analgesic, being sure to explain its effects and side effects to Mr. Frank. The RN also informs Mr. Frank that the health care provider has ordered a consultation with the pain clinic.

6. Evaluate the plan of care. Did the plan work? As you reassess Mr. Frank 30 minutes later, he rates his pain level at 2 on the 10-point scale. He smiles and thanks you for your attentiveness to his needs. You think back to the desired outcome, compare it with the current data collected, and determine that your interventions were successful.

Can you see how using good thinking attitudes, a good knowledge base, and the problem-solving process led to a better outcome than simply choosing the first obvious option? You were able to achieve a desirable outcome: assisting Mr. Frank in relieving his pain. And you have earned Mr. Frank's trust in the process. Problem solving is how nurses make decisions on a daily basis. You may already know this method as the *nursing process.*

Other Critical Thinking Skills

Problem solving is just one critical thinking skill. Another way you can use critical thinking in patient care is by anticipating what might go wrong, watching carefully for signs that a problem might be occurring, and then preventing it or notifying the RN or health care provider in time to intervene. Nurses save many lives each year by anticipating and preventing problems. Sometimes this is called **vigilance.** An example would be knowing the signs and symptoms of low blood glucose (because of an excellent knowledge base) and watching for them carefully (being vigilant) in a patient taking medication for diabetes. If early symptoms occur, you can intervene before the problem becomes severe. In addition, you could teach the patient and family about low blood glucose and how to prevent it, further reducing the risk to the patient.

BE SAFE!

BE VIGILANT! Always ask yourself as you prepare for patient care each day, "What is the worst thing that could happen to this patient today? What are early signs I should recognize? What will I do if they occur?" Plan ahead to be vigilant and you can prevent many patient care disasters!

There are many other thinking skills that are beyond the scope of this book. A few questions follow that you can ask yourself as you continue to develop your thinking skills. These are not in any order, nor would they all be asked for in a given situation. They are just some ideas to get you started.

- Have I thought this through?
- What information do I need?
- How do I know?
- Is someone influencing my thinking in ways I am not aware of?
- What conclusions can I draw from the information I have?
- Am I basing this decision on assumptions that may or may not be true?
- Am I thinking creatively about this, or am I in a rut?
- What do I need to watch for in order to prevent complications?
- Is there an expert I can consult who can help me think this through?
- Is there any supporting research or evidence that this is true?
- Am I too stressed or tired to think carefully about this right now?

NURSING PROCESS

You have just used the nursing process to solve a real problem. The **nursing process** is an organizing framework that links the process of thinking with actions in nursing practice. The nursing process is used to assess patient needs, formulate nursing diagnoses, and plan, implement, and evaluate care. As a nursing student, you consciously apply the nursing process to each patient problem. With experience, you will internalize the nursing process and use it without as much conscious effort.

Role of the Licensed Practical Nurse/Licensed Vocational Nurse

The licensed practical nurse (LPN) or licensed vocational nurse (LVN) carries out a specific role in the nursing process, as described in Table 1.1. The role of the LPN/LVN is to provide direct patient care. The LPN/LVN often spends more time at the bedside than the RN, which allows the LPN/LVN to develop a therapeutic relationship and understand the patient's needs. The LPN/LVN and the RN collaborate to analyze data and develop, implement, and evaluate the plan of care (Fig. 1.1).

Data Collection

The first step in the nursing process is data collection. This **assessment** is a way to evaluate a patient's condition. The LPN/LVN assists the RN in collecting data from a variety of sources. Data are divided into two types: subjective data and objective data.

Subjective Data

Information provided verbally by the patient is called **subjective data.** Symptoms are subjective data. Anxiety or pain

TABLE 1.1 ROLE OF THE LPN/LVN IN THE NURSING PROCESS

Steps of the Process	Role of the LPN/LVN
Assessment	Assists RN in collecting data.
Nursing Diagnosis	Assists RN in choosing appropriate nursing diagnoses.
Planning Care	Assists RN in planning care and developing outcomes to meet patient needs.
Implementation	Carries out portions of the plan of care that are within the LPN/LVN's scope of practice.
Evaluation	Assists RN in evaluation and revision of the plan of care.

Note: There may be slight variations by state.

Box 1-1 WHAT'S UP? Guide to Symptom Assessment

W—Where is it?

H—How does it feel? Describe the quality. (For example, is it dull, sharp, stabbing?)

A—Aggravating and alleviating factors. What makes it worse? What makes it better?

T—Timing. When did it start? How long does it last?

S—Severity. How bad is it? This can often be rated on a scale of 0 to 10.

U—Useful other data. What other symptoms are present that might be related?

P—Patient's perception of the problem. The patient often has an idea about what the problem is, or the cause, but may not believe that his or her thoughts are important to share unless specifically asked.

FIGURE 1.1 The nursing care team collaborating on a nursing care plan.

would be considered subjective data because only the patient can feel them. A nurse cannot objectively observe them. Often, subjective information is placed in quotes, such as "I have a headache" or "I feel out of breath." You must listen carefully to the patient and understand that only the patient truly knows how he or she feels.

When collecting subjective data, start with the patient's main concern. Focus on the reason the patient is seeking health care. Try asking, "What happened that brought you to the hospital (clinic, office)?"

Once the patient has identified the main concern, further questioning can reveal more pertinent information. Use the phrase **"WHAT'S UP?"** as a handy way to remember questions to ask the patient (Box 1-1). Asking the right questions can help you obtain better data with which to make the best decisions.

Next, obtain a patient history. Do this by asking the patient and family questions about the patient's past and present health problems, including specific questions about each body system, family health problems, and risk factors for health problems. The patient's medical record may also be consulted for background history information.

 LEARNING TIP

Practice assessing a symptom on a classmate. Ask the **WHAT'S UP?** questions.

In addition to assessment of physiological function, ask the patient about personal habits that relate to health, such as exercise, diet, and the presence of stressors, according to institutional assessment guidelines. Finally, assess the patient's family role, support systems, and cultural and spiritual beliefs.

Objective Data

Objective data are pieces of factual information obtained through physical assessment and diagnostic tests that are observable or knowable through the five senses. For example, a rash can be observed with the eyes and palpated with the fingers. Objective data are sometimes called *signs*. Examples of objective data include the following:

• 3-cm red lesion
• Respiratory rate 36 per minute
• Blood glucose 326 mg/dL
• Patient is moaning

These are all observable or measurable by a nurse and do not need explanation by the patient.

Objective data are gathered through physical assessment. Inspection, palpation, percussion, and auscultation techniques are used to collect objective data (Fig. 1.2). You can find more on these techniques, as well as how to obtain a complete history, in a nursing assessment text. Give special attention to areas that the patient has identified as potential problems.

Documentation of Data

Collected data are documented in the patient's medical record. If you identify any significant problem, change in the patient's status, or variation from normal, report it immediately to an RN or health care provider and then document it. Recorded data should be accurate and concise.

When documenting subjective data, use what was stated by the patient or significant other. Use direct quotations whenever possible, such as, "I feel sad." Quotes accurately represent the patient's view and are least open to mistaken interpretation.

When documenting objective data, include exactly what you observed. Avoid interpreting the data and using words that have vague meanings. For example, "nailbed color is pink" gives clearer information than "nailbed color is normal." "Normal" is an interpretation of data, rather than true data. "Capillary refill is 2 seconds" is more precise than "capillary refill is good." The statement "the wound looks better" is not meaningful unless the reader has previously observed the wound. Stating that "the wound is 1 by 2 inches, red, with no drainage or odor" provides data with which to compare the future status of the wound and determine whether it is responding to treatment.

LEARNING TIP

Beginners may be tempted to search for elaborate phrases or words to document, when simple, direct words are best. Simply stating exactly what you saw or heard provides the most clear and accurate information.

FIGURE 1.2 Nurse auscultating a patient's chest.

Nursing Diagnosis

Once data have been collected, the LPN/LVN assists the RN to compare the findings with what is considered "normal." Data are then grouped, or clustered, into sets of related information that identify problems. Problems are then labeled as nursing diagnoses.

According to the North American Nursing Diagnosis Association (NANDA-I), a **nursing diagnosis** is a "clinical judgment about actual or potential individual, family, or community responses to health problems or life processes. A nursing diagnosis provides the basis for selection of nursing interventions to achieve outcomes for which the nurse has accountability" (NANDA-I, 2013). Nursing diagnoses are standardized labels that make an identified problem understandable to all nurses. A list of NANDA-I–approved nursing diagnoses can be found in Appendix A of this book.

A diagnosis is considered "medical" when the health care provider directs most of the care. A diagnosis is considered "nursing" if the interventions needed to treat the problem are mainly independent nursing functions.

One example of a NANDA-I nursing diagnosis is *Acute Pain*. In Mr. Frank's example, the nurse identified that pain was a problem, and a plan of care was developed to manage the pain. The health care provider was contacted for analgesic orders, but independent nursing actions were also used, including relaxation and distraction. These independent nursing actions did not require a health care provider's order.

A well-written nursing diagnosis helps guide development of a plan of care. The three parts of a diagnosis follow:

- Problem—the nursing diagnosis label from the NANDA-I list
- Etiology—the cause or related factor (usually preceded by the words "related to")
- Signs and symptoms—the subjective or objective data that provide evidence that this is a valid diagnosis (often preceded by the words "as evidenced by").

The statement of problem, etiology, and signs and symptoms is called the *PES format*. Look again at the case study of Mr. Frank. A diagnosis using this format might read: "*Acute Pain* related to muscle spasms and nerve compression as evidenced by patient's pain rating of 8 on a 10-point scale." Note how the complete diagnosis gives you more helpful information than simply the label "pain." This additional information helps determine an appropriate outcome and guides the selection of interventions.

Many patient problems are **collaborative**—that is, the nurse, health care provider, and other members of the health team all work together to reach the desired outcome. For example, a patient with pneumonia (a medical diagnosis) has many needs that depend on health care provider orders, such as respiratory treatments and antibiotics. The role of the LPN/LVN is to collect important data on the patient's respiratory status and to provide nursing measures such as encouraging fluid intake, coughing, and deep breathing.

CRITICAL THINKING

Nursing Diagnosis

■ Which of the following are NANDA-I nursing diagnoses? Which are medical diagnoses? (Hint: Check Appendix A for help figuring these out!)

1. Impaired Physical Mobility
2. Ineffective Coping
3. Herniated Disk
4. Fractured Femur
5. Diabetes
6. Impaired Gas Exchange
7. Appendicitis
8. Activity Intolerance

Suggested answers are at the end of the chapter.

Planning Care

Once nursing diagnoses have been identified, an individualized plan of care is designed to help meet the patient's care needs. Planning involves setting priorities, establishing outcomes, and identifying interventions that will help the patient meet the outcomes. It is important to include the patient in the development of the plan of care. The plan will be most successful if the patient agrees with and understands the interventions.

Prioritize Care

Once you know what problems need to be addressed, you must decide which problem or intervention should be taken care of first. Because care should always be *patient-centered,* with the patient at the center of the health team, such decisions should involve the patient as well as the RN and LPN/LVN. Maslow's hierarchy of human needs is one commonly used system that can be used as a basis for determining priorities (Fig. 1.3). According to Maslow, humans must meet their most basic needs (those at the bottom of the triangle) first. They can then move up the hierarchy to meet higher level needs.

Physiological needs are the most basic. For example, a person who is short of breath cannot attend to higher level needs because the physiological need for oxygen is not being met. Once physiological needs are met, the patient can concentrate on meeting safety and security needs. Love, belonging, and self-esteem needs are next; self-actualization needs are generally the last priority when planning care.

Throughout life, people move up and down Maslow's hierarchy in response to life events. If a need occurs on a level below the patient's current level, the patient will move down to the level of that need. Once the need is fulfilled, the person can move upward on the hierarchy again.

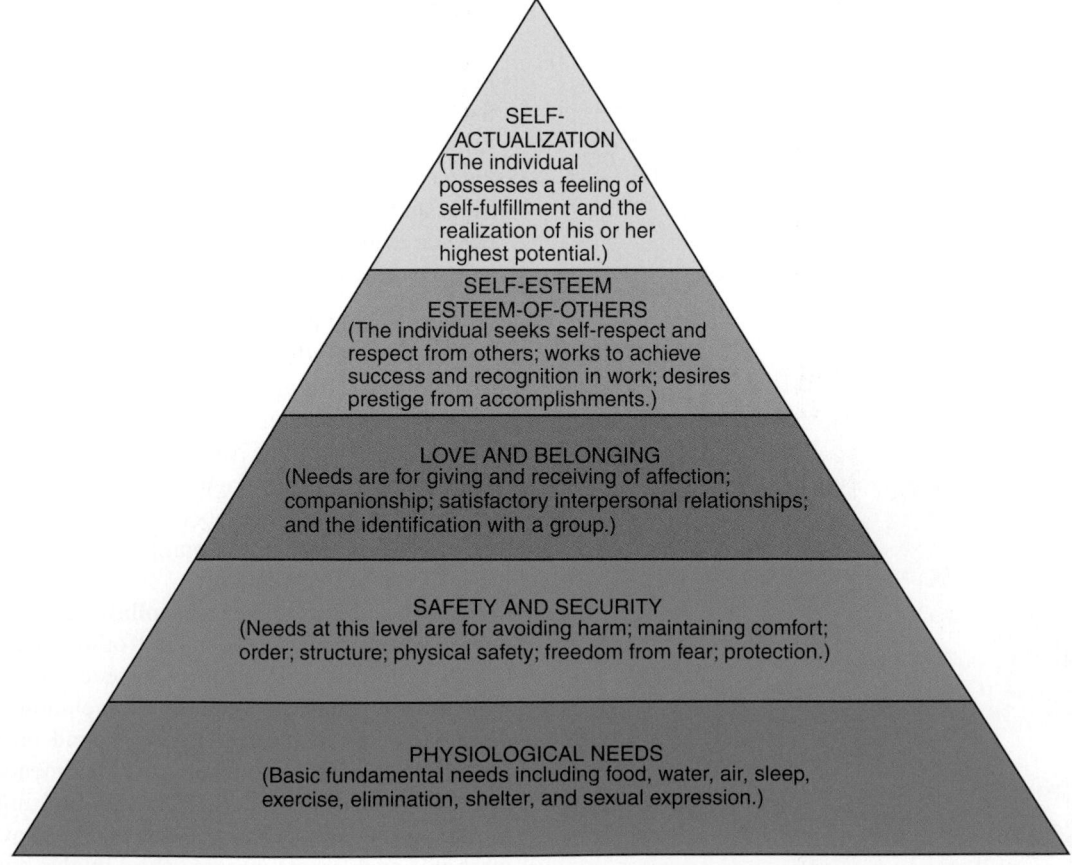

FIGURE 1.3 Maslow's hierarchy of human needs.

In a nursing plan of care, the patient's most urgent problem is listed first. This usually involves a physiological need such as oxygen or water because these are life-sustaining needs. If several physiological needs are present, life-threatening needs are ranked first, health-threatening needs are second, and health-promoting needs, although important, are last.

LEARNING TIP

If you are stuck wondering which physiological need should take priority, ask yourself, "Which problem is most threatening to my patient's life?" ABCs should also be considered: **A**irway is most emergent, then **B**reathing, and then **C**irculation.

Once physiological needs have been met, needs related to the next level of the hierarchy, safety and security, can be addressed. Remaining diagnoses are listed in order of urgency as they relate to the hierarchy. Needs can occur simultaneously on different levels and must be addressed in a holistic manner, with prioritization guiding the care provided.

LEARNING TIP

If you are developing a plan of care for a patient with complex needs and are not sure where to start, go back to the assessment phase. Often, additional information can help you better understand the patient's needs and develop a plan of care individualized to the patient's specific problem areas.

CRITICAL THINKING

Prioritizing Care

■ Based on Maslow's hierarchy of needs, list the following nursing diagnoses in order from highest (1) to lowest (5) priority. Give rationales for your decisions.

_____ *Deficient Knowledge*

_____ *Constipation*

_____ *Disabled Family Coping*

_____ *Readiness for Enhanced Self-Concept*

_____ *Ineffective Airway Clearance*

Suggested answers are at the end of the chapter.

Establish Outcomes

An outcome is a statement that describes the patient's desired goal for a problem area. It should be measurable, be realistic for the patient, and have an appropriate time frame for achievement. *Measurable* means that the outcome is objective, or can be observed. It should not be vague or open to interpretation, with the use of subjective words such as *normal, large, small,* or *moderate.* Consider, for example, two outcomes:

1. The patient's shortness of breath will improve.
2. The patient will be less short of breath within 15 minutes as evidenced by the patient rating the shortness of breath at less than 3 on a scale of 0 to 10, respiratory rate between 16 and 20 per minute, and relaxed appearance.

Although the first outcome seems appropriate, in reality it is difficult to know when it has been met. There is nothing to objectively indicate when the problem has been resolved. The second outcome is objective. You can see that when the patient rates his or her shortness of breath at less than 3, is breathing at a rate of 16 to 20 per minute, and appears relaxed, the desired outcome will have been met. The outcome is realistic, and the 15-minute time frame ensures that the patient's distress is minimized. If the plan of care does not achieve the desired outcome in the given time frame, it should be evaluated and revised as needed.

When determining criteria for a measurable outcome, look at the signs and symptoms portion of the nursing diagnosis. The resolution of signs and symptoms identified in the NANDA-I nursing diagnoses is evidence that nursing interventions were effective. If the desired outcome is not achieved, the problem and interventions need reevaluation. Look at another outcome example to see how criteria are used for measurement:

> **Nursing diagnosis**—*Ineffective Airway Clearance* related to excess secretions as evidenced by coarse crackles and nonproductive cough
>
> **Outcome**—Patient will have effective airway clearance within 8 hours, as evidenced by clear lung sounds and productive cough.

Identify Interventions

Interventions are the actions you take to help a patient meet a desired outcome. Therefore, interventions should be *goal-directed.* Any intervention that does not contribute to meeting the outcome should not be part of the plan of care.

One way to create a care plan is to include interventions that can be categorized as "take, treat, and teach." In the first intervention category, "take," or identify, data related to the problem that should be routinely collected. Next, "treat" the problem by identifying deliberate actions to help reach the outcome. Last, identify what to "teach" the patient and family for the patient to learn to care for himself or herself.

Look again at the nursing diagnosis of *Ineffective Airway Clearance.* A plan of care for this problem using the take, treat, and teach method might look like this:

> **Take:**   Auscultate lung sounds every 4 hours and as needed.
>
> Assess respiratory rate every 4 hours and as needed.

Treat: Provide 2 L of fluids every 24 hours.
Offer expectorant as ordered.
Provide cool mist vaporizer in room.

Teach: Teach the patient the importance of fluid intake.
Teach the patient to cough and deep breathe every 1 to 2 hours.

In addition to identifying interventions, it is important to understand how and why they will work. The "why" is called a *rationale*. For example, you should assess lung sounds and respiratory rate every 4 hours *because increased crackles and respiratory rate indicate retained secretions.* Fluids are provided *to minimize mucosal drying and ease secretion removal.* Sound rationales that are evidence based (research based) should guide the selection of each nursing intervention. You will find rationales with interventions throughout this book to help you understand why interventions will be effective.

Like nursing diagnoses, nursing interventions can be either independent or collaborative. Independent nursing actions can be initiated by the nurse. Examples of independent nursing actions include teaching the patient deep-breathing exercises, turning a patient every 2 hours, teaching about medications, and giving a back rub for comfort. Collaborative actions require a health care provider's order to perform. Examples of collaborative interventions include giving prescribed medications, applying elastic stockings, requesting a referral to physical therapy, and inserting a urinary catheter.

Implement Interventions

Once the plan of care has been identified, it must be communicated to the patient, family, and health team members and then implemented. One way a plan of care is communicated is by writing it as a nursing care plan. The nursing care plan is documented on the patient's medical record, to communicate to all nurses the patient's priority problems, the desired outcomes, and the plan for meeting the outcomes. Many institutions have standardized care plans that are individualized for each patient by the nurse.

Implementation of the plan of care involves performing the interventions. The patient's response to each intervention is noted and documented. This documentation provides the basis for evaluation and revision of the plan of care.

Evaluate Outcomes

The last step of the nursing process is **evaluation**. The nurse continuously evaluates the patient's progress toward the desired outcomes and the effectiveness of each intervention. If the outcomes are not reached within the given time frame or if the interventions are ineffective, the plan of care is revised. Any part of the plan of care can be revised, from the diagnosis or desired outcome to the interventions. Acute care institutions require routine review and updating of the plan of care.

SUGGESTED ANSWERS TO

CRITICAL THINKING

■ *Nursing Diagnosis*
1. Impaired Physical Mobility = nursing
2. Ineffective Coping = nursing
3. Herniated Disk = medical
4. Fractured Femur = medical
5. Diabetes = medical
6. Impaired Gas Exchange = nursing
7. Appendicitis = medical
8. Activity Intolerance = nursing

■ *Prioritizing Care*
1. *Ineffective Airway Clearance*—physiological need that can be life threatening
2. *Constipation*—physiological need that can be health threatening
3. *Deficient Knowledge*—safety and security need
4. *Disabled Family Coping*—love and belonging need
5. *Readiness for Enhanced Self-Concept*—self-esteem need

REVIEW QUESTIONS

1. In which of the following ways is critical thinking useful to the nursing process?
   1. It highlights the solution to a problem.
   2. It can lead to a better outcome for the patient.
   3. It simplifies the process.
   4. It helps the nurse arrive at a solution more quickly.

2. Which nurse is exhibiting intellectual humility?
   1. The nurse who is an expert at wound care.
   2. The nurse who reports an error to the supervisor.
   3. The nurse who tries to empathize with the patient.
   4. The nurse who asks a coworker about a new procedure.

3. Which of the following pieces of information is considered objective data?
   1. The patient's respiratory rate is 28.
   2. The patient states, "I feel short of breath."
   3. The patient is short of breath.
   4. The patient is feeling panicky.

4. An LPN/LVN is collecting data on a newly admitted patient who has an ulcerated area on his left hip. It is 2 inches in diameter and 1 inch deep, with yellow exudate. Which of the following statements best documents the findings in the patient's database?
   1. Wound on left hip, 2 inches diameter, 1 inch deep, infected
   2. Left hip wound is large, deep, and has yellow drainage
   3. Pressure ulcer on left hip, yellow drainage
   4. Wound on left hip, 2 inches in diameter, 1 inch deep, yellow exudate

5. A 34-year-old mother of three children is admitted to a respiratory unit with pneumonia. She has all the following problems. Based on Maslow's hierarchy of needs, which problem should the nurse address first?
   1. Frontal headache related to stress of hospital admission
   2. Anxiety related to concern about leaving children
   3. Shortness of breath related to newly diagnosed pneumonia
   4. Deficient knowledge related to treatment plan

6. Place the steps of the nursing process in correct chronological order of use. Use all options.
   1. Nursing diagnosis
   2. Evaluation
   3. Assessment
   4. Planning care
   5. Implementation

7. Which of the following parts of the nursing process can be carried out by an LPN/LVN?
   1. Implementation of interventions
   2. Nursing diagnosis
   3. Analysis of data
   4. Evaluation of outcomes

8. Which of the following is a nursing diagnosis?
   1. Stroke
   2. Renal Failure
   3. Fracture
   4. Acute Pain

9. A nurse teaches a patient the importance of stopping smoking. Which of the following patient responses provides the best evidence that the teaching was effective?
   1. "I have a brother who died of lung cancer. I know smoking is bad."
   2. "I tried to quit 5 years ago, and I really would like to, but it is very hard."
   3. "Thank you for the information. I will call the Smoke Stoppers organization today."
   4. "I know you are right; I should stop smoking."

Answers can be found in Appendix C.

References

Foundation for Critical Thinking. (2013). Valuable intellectual traits. Retrieved May 13, 2013, from www.criticalthinking.org/pages/valuable-intellectual-traits/528

Halpern, D. (1996). *Thought and knowledge: An introduction to critical thinking* (3rd ed.). Mahwah, NJ: Lawrence Erlbaum Associates.

Hawkins, D., Elder, L., Paul, R. (2010). *The thinker's guide to clinical reasoning.* Tomales, CA: Foundation for Critical Thinking Press (www.criticalthinking.org).

North American Nursing Diagnosis Association (NANDA-I). (n.d.). Glossary of terms. Retrieved May 16, 2013, from www.nanda.org/nanda-international-glossary-of-terms.html

 For additional resources and information visit **davispl.us/medsurg5**

2

Evidence-Based Practice

BETTY ACKLEY

KEY TERMS

evidence-based practice (EH-va-dense based PRACK-tis)
randomized controlled trial (RAN-dumb-eyesd cun-TROLLD TRY-ull)
research (re-SURCH)
systematic review (SISS-tem-AT-ick re-VIEW)

LEARNING OUTCOMES

1. Define evidence-based practice (EBP).
2. Discuss why EBP should be used.
3. Explain how to identify nursing evidence that should be put into practice.
4. Describe the EBP process.
5. List the six steps of EBP.
6. Identify the best method for oral care.
7. Identify who should give evidence-based nursing care, including when and where care should be given.
8. Describe how the Quality and Safety Education for Nurses (QSEN) project can promote safe patient care.

Amanda, an LPN, is caring for residents on Unit 4 in an extended care agency. One of the residents, Mr. Samuel, had a right-sided stroke and currently has a gastrostomy tube through which a formula is administered 12 hours per day. He has halitosis, and his teeth look fuzzy. He currently receives oral care twice daily with oral foam swabs. Let's explore with Amanda what the evidence says should be done for oral care for Mr. Samuel. (See discussion and answers throughout the chapter.)

Evidence-based practice (EBP) is a systematic process that employs current evidence to make decisions about patient care. It includes evaluation of the quality and applicability of existing research, patient preferences, costs, clinical expertise, and clinical settings (Melnyk et al, 2010). Evidence gives assurance that nursing practice will be effective. Using evidence-based nursing practice will increase your power to give the best nursing care possible.

EBP involves much more than simply evaluating **research** (scientific study, investigation, or experimentation) to determine which results apply to nursing care. Clinical reality can be very different from a research setting. It could be unsafe to apply a research study that was done in a controlled laboratory environment to the very different environment found in an actual clinical situation. Or it could be unsafe to apply research results obtained on people of one age or medical diagnosis to those of another age or with multiple diagnoses. The context in which the evidence will be used must be considered. This includes the health care environment, the patient involved, the nurse's expertise, and the cost. Using EBP is a complex process, but it is an important way to ensure quality care and optimal patient outcomes.

 ## REASONS FOR USING EBP

The use of EBP allows nurses to give patients the best care possible, which is the goal of all caring nurses. The reasons given for nursing care used to be "This is how it was taught in nursing school," "This is what they told us in orientation," or "That's the way it is done here." Now the rationale behind the best nursing care is "Nursing care is based on evidence and how it applies to an individual patient in a specific setting." EBP is considered the gold standard of health care.

Evidence-based outcome measurement is built into the EBP process as a way to measure and confirm the value of a change in nursing practice. For example, nurses are measuring the number of new pressure ulcers, new cases of pneumonia, and new urinary tract infections in health care settings. Measuring outcomes as a part of EBP reenergizes nursing by helping nurses see the results of their nursing care. Measured outcomes show nurses that they are giving the best care possible, based on the evidence available at the time.

Evidence comes from multiple sources. Medical research and research from many other professions such as psychology, gerontology, and social work are utilized, in addition to nursing research to develop EBP nursing care guidelines.

 ## IDENTIFYING NURSING EVIDENCE

How do you identify nursing evidence that should be put into practice? It depends in part on the strength of the evidence. Evidence ranges from strong to weak, and levels can be assigned to rate its strength and quality. The rating scale used to label the quality of evidence ranges from Level I to Level IV (Table 2.1). Level I is the best evidence. It includes **systematic reviews** and analysis of many high-quality **randomized controlled trials** (studies designed to assess the effects of a variable by randomly assigning subjects to experimental, placebo, or control groups). Level IV evidence is the weakest and includes the non–research-based opinions of experts or published but non–research-based clinical articles. Two of the best known sources for Level I evidence are the Cochrane Reviews (www.cochrane.org/reviews) for medical evidence and the

TABLE 2.1   LEVELS OF EVIDENCE

Level	Type of Evidence
Level I	**Systematic reviews, such as Cochrane Reviews and Joanna Briggs Best Evidence Guidelines** Evidence from a systematic review of all relevant randomized clinical trials or evidence-based clinical practice guidelines that are based on systematic reviews of randomized controlled trials. Three or more randomized controlled trials of good quality that have similar results also have been considered Level I evidence.
Level II	**Randomized controlled trials** Evidence obtained from at least one well-designed randomized controlled trial. These are true experimental studies in which as many factors as possible that could falsely change the results are controlled.
Level III	**Quasi-experimental studies** Evidence obtained from quasi-experimental research studies. These studies do not control factors that could falsely change the results and, as a result, are less predictive of effectiveness of nursing care.
Level IV	**Expert opinion** Evidence from the opinion of authorities and/or reports of expert committees. Also nursing journal articles that are opinion based, not research based.

Joanna Briggs Best Practice reviews (www.joannabriggslibrary .org/) for nursing practice.

THE EBP PROCESS

Evidence that guides nursing care can be used in two ways, generally based on whether the evidence is a dependent or an independent nursing intervention. Dependent nursing interventions are those that are delegated by a health care provider. Here any change in practice must go through a committee, such as the policy and procedure committee, to determine if it is appropriate for adoption. If the intervention is independent, however, the nurse can implement an evidence-based change based on personal knowledge of the value of the intervention, as long as the change is safe and cannot harm the patient. An example is the intervention of reality orientation. Excellent research shows that the use of reality orientation can improve thinking ability in patients with dementia and delirium. The nurse can implement this intervention independently because it does not require an order. Other intervention examples include the use of hand massage, music therapy, and other anxiety-relieving interventions.

A simplified version of the EBP process is discussed next and shown in Figure 2.1. The acronym "ASKMME!"

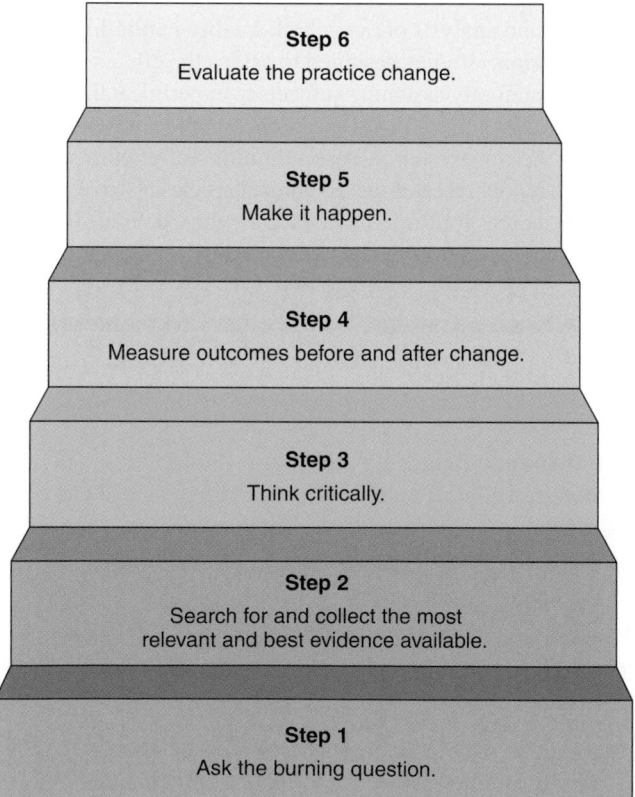

FIGURE 2.1 The six steps of the evidence-based practice process. (*Source:* Ackley, B. J., Ladwig, G. B., Swan, B. A., & Tucker, S. J. (2008). *Evidence-based nursing care guidelines: Medical-surgical interventions.* Philadelphia: Elsevier, with permission.)

is designed to help you remember the six essential steps: **A**sk, **S**earch, thin**K**, **M**easure, **M**ake it happen, and **E**valuate (Ackley et al, 2008).

Step 1: Ask the Burning Question

EBP begins with questioning the status quo, trying to solve a problem, or learning about new evidence that should be used in nursing practice. The initial question nurses often ask is, "Why do we do it that way?" or "How could we do this better?" Questioning the existing way of doing things is part of critical thinking. It helps ensure that the patient receives the best care possible. As a student nurse, you can do this as well.

For Mr. Samuel, in the case study at the start of the chapter, Amanda was motivated to find the best way to give oral care, because her instincts told her the current care was not effective. Amanda took her clinical question to the policy and procedure committee and, working with members, they began the evidence-based process to find the best way to give oral care to all tube-fed patients at their agency.

Step 2: Search for and Collect the Most Relevant and Best Evidence Available

A thorough search of the literature in the subject area needs to be conducted. As a student nurse, you will find medical librarians most helpful. It is important that you learn basic computer skills so that you also have the ability to search the nursing and medical literature. Several databases can help you find journal articles and reviews.

For nursing literature, the best known database is CINAHL, which stands for Cumulative Index to Nursing and Allied Health Literature (www.ebscohost.com/cinahl). CINAHL is available through college and hospital libraries. Evidence-based care sheets are available on CINAHL. These sheets summarize current best practice on a specific topic. For best practice nursing reviews, visit the Joanna Briggs Best Practices website, which may be available at the nearest nursing library.

For medical literature, the comprehensive Medline/ PubMed database can be accessed at www.ncbi.nlm.nih.gov. Cochrane Reviews are available at www.cochrane.org /reviews. An easy way to find Cochrane Reviews is to type in "Cochrane" when searching for a topic.

Amanda worked with a medical librarian and other members of her agency's policy and procedure committee to conduct an EBP search on oral care. They then summarized the research articles they found in this area (Table 2.2).

Step 3: Think Critically

Always appraise the evidence you find for validity, relevance to the situation, and applicability. First, evaluate the quality of the evidence you find. It is helpful to determine the level of the evidence to make sure you have the best information available (see Table 2.1). Then, using critical thinking, evaluate the evidence as it applies to the individual patient or patient population, the clinical expertise of the nurse(s) involved, the values in the situation, and agency policies that affect making a change in practice.

TABLE 2.2 ORAL CARE FOR PATIENTS WHO ARE BEING TUBE FED

Study	Population	Interventions	Key Findings
Pearson, L. S., & Hutton, J. L. (2002). A controlled trial to compare the ability of oral foam swabs and toothbrushes to remove dental plaque. *Journal of Advanced Nursing, 39*(5), 480–489.	34 volunteers	Group 1 received oral care in the a.m. using a toothbrush. Group 2 received oral care in the a.m. using oral foam swabs.	Use of toothbrushes for oral care was much more effective than foam swabs in removing plaque from the teeth.
Leibovitz, A., Plotnikov, G., Habot, B., et al (2003). Pathogenic colonization of oral flora in frail elderly patients fed by nasogastric tube or percutaneous enterogastric tube. Journal of Gerontology Series A: *Biological Sciences and Medical Sciences, 58*(1), 52–55.	215 subjects (patients in long-term care facilities)	Group 1: Patients fed via nasogastric (NG) tube had 81% pathogenic bacteria in mouth. Group 2: Patients fed by percutaneous enterogastric (PEG) tube had 51% pathogenic bacteria in mouth. Group 3: Patients fed orally had 17.5% pathogenic bacteria in mouth.	Patients fed by NG tube had more pathogenic bacteria in their mouths than those fed by PEG tube or those fed orally. If oral secretions are aspirated, the risk of pneumonia increases.
Adachi, M., Ishihara, K., Abe, S., et al (2007). Professional oral health care by dental hygienists reduced respiratory infections in older adults requiring nursing care. *International Journal of Dental Hygiene, 5*(2), 69–74.	190 subjects	Experimental group received professional oral health care by dental hygienists. Control group received regular oral care.	Oral care reduced pathogenic organisms in mouth, reduced fever above 103.5°F (37.9°C), reduced onset of influenza, and reduced fatal pneumonia.
Panchabhai, T. S., Dangayach, N. S., Krishnan, A., et al (2009). Oropharyngeal cleansing with 0.2% chlorhexidine for prevention of nosocomial pneumonia in critically ill patients. *Chest, 135*(5), 1150–1156.	512 subjects	Experimental group received oral care with chlorhexidine. Control group received oral care with 0.2% potassium permanganate.	Both experimental group and control group had greatly decreased incidence of pneumonia as compared with "usual" oral care.
Yakiwchuk, C., Bertone, M., Ghiabi, E., Brown, S., Liarakso, M., Brothwell, D. (2013). Suction toothbrush use for dependent adults with dysphagia: A pilot examiner blind randomized clinical trial. *Canadian Journal of Dental Hygiene, 47*(1), 15–23.	22 dysphagic subjects	Experimental group received oral care using a suction toothbrush. Control group received oral care using a manual toothbrush.	Both the experimental and control group demonstrated less plaque, decreased calculus, and improved gingival health after 1 month. Both groups also demonstrated a decreased incidence of pneumonia as compared with the usual rate of pneumonia in long-term care patients.

Amanda found many research articles on the value of oral care, and the results were exciting. When the research was analyzed, it became obvious that tube-fed patients should have oral care with a soft bristle toothbrush and toothpaste. Because Mr. Samuels had trouble swallowing, it was also important that suction be readily available as oral care was given. Amanda discovered that there are suction toothbrushes and oral swabs for patients such as Mr. Samuels (Figure 2.2). The studies also found that inadequate oral care resulted in more than just halitosis and fuzzy teeth; it could result in pneumonia. Amanda felt a renewed sense of purpose.

Step 4: Measure Outcomes Before and After Change

Next, determine the patient outcomes that are likely to occur as a result of a change in nursing care. Usually, a small pilot study is done within the agency before any widespread change in practice is made. That way, it can be determined if the change will be effective, as intended, when the change is implemented across the agency.

The committee members decided to measure the number of new pneumonia cases in their agency, which is an important patient outcome.

Step 5: Make It Happen

Institute the desired change in nursing practice based on evidence. This is done through education and by setting up quality systems to ensure that the desired change is actually happening.

The policy and procedure committee developed an evidence-based procedure guideline for oral care of all patients, with a separate policy for tube-fed patients. The new policy and procedure was introduced and became a care requirement for all patients at the agency. A quality audit was then done at intervals on selected patients to ensure the appropriate oral care was being given.

FIGURE 2.2 Oral suction toothbrush kit with thumb ports. *(Courtesy of Sage Products, Cary, Illinois.)*

Step 6: Evaluate the Practice Change

Evaluation is the process used to determine if the change made a significant difference. What were the results of the initial small study? Was the change in practice effective in improving patient outcomes? If it did make a difference, was the difference worth the extra cost or time it required?

Wow! Because of Amanda's concern about oral care, a change had been made that improved the care for every patient. Also, after making the change in oral care and evaluating the outcome, it was clear that Amanda's agency had a decrease in new-onset pneumonia. This was exciting and reinforcing to the committee, and especially to Amanda.

WHO SHOULD PROVIDE EVIDENCE-BASED NURSING CARE?

All nursing care should be based on use of appropriate evidence, including care provided by nursing assistive personnel such as Competency Evaluated Nursing Assistants (CENAs). Evidence-based care should be given at all times, if possible, and in all settings where nursing care is given. A good way to ensure that evidence-based care is provided by CENAs is to explain why the care should be given when the care is delegated. For example, when Amanda asks a CENA to give thorough oral care to a tube-fed patient with a toothbrush, she explains that research studies have shown that toothbrushing can help reduce the incidence of pneumonia in older adults. With this knowledge the CENA understands the importance of giving effective oral care.

EBP, QUALITY, AND SAFETY: THEY BELONG TOGETHER!

Multiple quality initiatives are currently having a positive impact on health care. Insurance companies, businesses, patients, and the government are demanding quality care. All quality initiatives require collection of data, which is greatly facilitated by the health care agency having an EBP framework. Some quality initiatives are required, such as those of the Joint Commission that accredits health care agencies. Others are voluntary but desirable for the agency's well-being. All quality initiatives should begin with a literature search to determine the most effective interventions.

Quality and Safety Education for Nurses Project

The Quality and Safety Education for Nurses (QSEN) project focuses on nursing education that promotes the continual improvement of quality and safety in patient care. The goal is for students to develop understanding, attitudes, skills, and the desire to continually improve the quality and safety of patient care. Information on the QSEN project can be found at http://qsen.org.

The development of teaching strategies for nursing students involves six areas of focus:

1. *Evidence-based practice:* Look for Evidence-Based Practice boxes throughout the book.

2. *Safety:* We all want our patients to be safe! Many interventions are available that can help us reach this goal. Look for Be Safe! throughout the chapters and the section on safety in Chapter 3.

3. *Teamwork and collaboration:* These are important aspects of providing safe, quality care. In Chapter 3, you are introduced to members of the health care team with whom you may work and collaborate. For example, you may talk with the pharmacist if you have a question about a patient's medication to ensure it is given safely, or you might alert the registered nurse to a change in a patient's vital signs so that the physician can be informed for treatment orders. This illustrates teamwork to ensure that the patient receives safe, high-quality care.

4. *Patient-centered care:* When collaborating on the development of nursing care plans, it is important to individualize interventions to provide patient-centered care. As nursing interventions are performed, they should meet the patient's needs and preferred schedules rather than those of the institution or caregiver. You will find Nursing Care Plans throughout the chapters, but always remember that no plan fits all patients. You will always evaluate each suggested intervention to see if it fits your patient and then individualize it to the patient's needs.

5. *Quality improvement:* Quality improvement (QI) is an ongoing process to improve patient care (see Fig. 3.3). You might participate in a QI project by collecting data, which is one aspect of a QI project.

6. *Informatics:* Informatics is a growing area in health care because of the increasing use of technology to provide safer care. Examples you may use include computerized medical records, medication dispensing systems, medication barcoding systems, or computerized resources.

Concern for Patient Safety

Safety is on everyone's mind. Many people know of someone who has been affected by a medical error or who has been unhappy with his or her care. As a result, guidelines to reduce errors in health care and improve patient outcomes have been developed and based on evidence when available. The Joint Commission's 2014 National Patient Safety Goals can be found at www.jointcommission.org. As you will see at the website, these goals address care in various types of health care settings.

 BE SAFE!

One important safety goal is to **use at least two ways to identify patients**—but not the patient's room number or location—when providing care, treatment, or services. This is because wrong-patient errors occur in virtually all stages of diagnosis and treatment. The intent for this goal is twofold: first, to reliably identify the patient as the person for whom the service or treatment is intended; second, to match the service or treatment to that patient (© The Joint Commission, 2013. Reprinted with permission.).

You will find other 2014 Joint Commission national patient safety goals in the Be Safe! feature throughout the text of this book. These goals are included to increase your awareness and understanding of patient safety. They address important areas of concern, such as administering medications safely, identifying patients correctly, identifying operative sites correctly, improving communication, reducing fall injuries, and reducing the risk of infection in institutionalized older persons, to name a few. You will want to become familiar with them and to look for updates at the Joint Commission website. Of course, it takes critical thinking to use them at the right times and in the right circumstances. Using them appropriately helps you provide safer care with fewer errors. EBP is critical thinking at its finest, working to determine the best care for the patient based on the evidence. The evidence provides core information to direct safe, quality-driven, excellent patient care.

REVIEW QUESTIONS

1. The nurse requests the CENA to provide oral care to a patient. Which of the following methods of request by the nurse would be most appropriate to achieve evidence-based care?
   1. Request that oral care be given with use of a toothbrush and toothpaste.
   2. Instruct the CENA to give oral care using oral swabs to clean the teeth and mouth.
   3. Ask the CENA to have the patient use a mouthwash rinse for daily oral care.
   4. Explain that use of a toothbrush and toothpaste decreases pneumonia in older adults.

2. The nurse is contributing to the plan of care for a patient. In considering appropriate care, the nurse bases the care on which of the following to provide excellent care?
   1. Content taught throughout a nursing educational program.
   2. Orientation to the health care agency for new employees.
   3. A nurse's personal judgment of what is best for each patient.
   4. Evidence that is evaluated for the health care agency and each patient.

3. A policy and procedure committee is reviewing evidence for a new policy. When considering the evidence, which of the following sources would generally be safest for a health care agency to implement?
   1. A Joanna Briggs Best Practices Guideline.
   2. One randomized controlled trial.
   3. Four quasi-experimental studies that show similar results.
   4. The opinion of a national nursing expert on the subject.

4. The nurse reads about a research study that affects nursing care and could lead to decreased wound infections. Which of the following actions should the nurse take regarding the information in the study?
   1. Put the information into practice while performing wound care.
   2. Discuss the research with a trusted coworker and, if the coworker agrees, put the information into practice at work.
   3. Present the proposed practice change to the policy and procedure committee at work for evaluation and possible adoption.
   4. Do a journal search to look for similar studies, and if three similar studies are found, incorporate the information into practice.

5. A policy and procedure committee is revising the nursing intervention of insertion of a urinary catheter. Where should the committee begin looking for evidence to write an effective policy and procedure on this intervention?
   1. In current nursing skills textbooks.
   2. In nursing articles written by national nursing experts based on opinion.
   3. In research articles, preferably systematic reviews of randomized controlled trials.
   4. In the policies and procedures of other nursing facilities.

6. A nurse is preparing to give oral care to a patient who is receiving a tube feeding. Which of the following is the best evidence-based method to give oral care?
   1. Use oral foam swabs with mouthwash and then swab the teeth and the mouth.
   2. Use a soft toothbrush and toothpaste to brush the teeth.
   3. Use a tongue scraper to remove debris from the tongue twice daily.
   4. No oral care is needed for a patient who is receiving tube feedings.

Answers can be found in Appendix C.

References

Ackley, B. J., Ladwig, G. B., Swan, B. A., & Tucker, S. J. (2008). *Evidence-based nursing care guidelines: Medical-surgical interventions.* Philadelphia: Elsevier.

Joint Commission. (2013). Joint Commission's 2014 National Patient Safety Goals. Retrieved July 6, 2013, from www .jointcommission.org/standards_information/npsgs.aspx

Melnyk B. M., Fineout-Overholt, E., Stillwell S. B., Williamson, K. M. (2010). Evidence-based practice: Step by step. The seven steps of evidence-based practice: following this progressive, sequential approach will lead to improved health care and patient outcomes. *American Journal of Nursing, 110*(1), 51–53.

 Davis*Plus* | For additional resources and information visit **davispl.us/medsurg5**

Issues in Nursing Practice

LINDA S. WILLIAMS, MICHELLE BLOCK, AND JAMES SHANNON

LEARNING OUTCOMES

1. Identify factors influencing changes in the health care delivery system.
2. Describe safe health care practices.
3. Explain the significance of hospital-acquired conditions.
4. Describe four leadership styles.
5. Discuss the LPN/LVNs role in leadership and delegation.
6. Describe the importance of ethics in health care.
7. Explain the steps of the ethical decision-making model.
8. Discuss moral distress and its effect on nursing care.
9. Identify where the regulation of nursing practice is defined.
10. Define the Health Insurance Portability and Accountability Act (HIPAA) of 1996.
11. Describe guidelines for professional use of social media.
12. Discuss how to provide quality care and limit liability.

KEY TERMS

administrative laws (ad-MIN-i-STRAY-tive LAWZ)
autocratic leadership (AW-tuh-KRAT-ik LEE-der-ship)
autonomy (aw-TAWN-uh-MEE)
beneficence (buh-NEF-i-sens)
civil law (SIH-vil LAW)
code of ethics (KOHD OF ETH-icks)
confidentiality (KON-fi-den-she-AL-i-tee)
criminal law (KRIM-i-nuhl LAW)
delegation (DELL-a-GAY-shun)
democratic leadership (DEM-ah-KRAT-ik LEE-der-ship)
deontology (DEE-on-TOL-o-gee)
diagnosis-related groups (DYE-ag-NOH-sis ree-LAY-ted GROOPS)
electronic medical record (e-LECK-tron-ick MED-ick-uhl WRECK-ord)
ethics (ETH-icks)
fidelity (FAH-dell-eh-tee)
informatics (IN-for-mat-icks)
justice (JUSS-tiss)
laissez-faire leadership (LAYS-ay-FAIR LEE-der-ship)
leadership (LEE-der-ship)
liability (LYE-uh-BIL-i-tee)
limitation of liability (LIM-i-TAY-shun OF LYE-uh-BIL-i-tee)
maleficence (ma-LEF-i-cence)
malpractice (mal-PRAK-tiss)
morality (moh-RAL-i-tee)
moral distress (moh-Ral DIS-tress)
negligence (NEG-la-ghunt)
nonmaleficence (NON-muh-LEF-i-sens)
paternalism (puh-TER-nuhl-izm)
principles (PRIN-sih-pulz)
respondeat superior (res-POND-ee-et sue-PEER-ee-or)
standard of best interest (STAN-derd OF BEST IN-ter-est)
summons (SUH-muns)
therapeutic privilege (Ther-uh-PU-tik PRIV-uh-lej)
torts (TORTS)
utilitarian (yoo-TILL-ih-TAR-ee-en)
values (VAL-yooz)
veracity (VER-ah-sit-tee)

The author acknowledges the contributions to this chapter by Maryanne Pietraniec-Shannon RN, PhD for the "Correctional Nursing" section.

HEALTH CARE DELIVERY

Health–Illness Continuum

The term *health–illness continuum* describes the continually shifting levels of health experienced by each person. One end of the continuum represents high-level health. The other end represents poor health and impending death. We all move about the continuum throughout our lives.

Health Care Delivery Systems

A focus on prevention and providing services from birth to death under one integrated system is being used by many health care systems. Hospital consolidations led to health care systems that can cover large geographic areas. Hospitals provide the integrated care delivery network for the system (Fig. 3.1).

Factors Influencing Health Care Change

Do you like change? Well, today's health care delivery is being influenced by many evolving changes, which will have an impact on your career. Some examples of these changes include the 2010 Patient Protection and Affordable Care Act (discussed later); the expanding role of technology in health care including **electronic medical records**; mobile health with tablets, smartphones, and digital apps; telehealth with telephones and online video; remote patient monitoring; robotics; the use of evidence to guide practice (see Chapter 2); and antibiotic-resistant infectious organisms that continue to emerge. Nursing **informatics** is a specialty area that deals with the study and use of information technology within nursing practice. There are educational programs with majors in informatics to consider as you continue your education. The changing characteristics of the American population are also influencing health care delivery with increases in the size of the population, number of older adults, and population's

cultural diversity (U.S. Census Bureau, 2010). These and other changes make learning a constant need in today's health care environment. We hope that you will be flexible and embrace change throughout your career!

 EVIDENCE-BASED PRACTICE

Clinical Question
Does use of information technology in the form of an Interactive Preventive Health Record (IPHR) increase the use of preventative health services?

Evidence
4500 patients were randomly invited to use an IPHR that provided personal health records, education, and reminders. Use of preventative services significantly increased by 2.3% in those using the IPHR over those who were not. Furthermore, the number of patients who were up to date on all recommended preventative services was double in the IPHR group.

Implications for Nursing Practice
Encouraging the use of patient-centered interactive technology might help improve patient health.

REFERENCES
Krist, A. H., Woolf, S. H., Rothemich, S. F, Johnson, R. E., Peele, J. E., Cunningham, T. D., Longo, D. R., Bello, G. A., Matzke, G. R. (2012). Interactive preventive health record to enhance delivery of recommended care: A randomized trial. *Annals of Family Medicine, 10,* 312–319.

Safe Practice

Preventing harmful adverse events is a concern of several organizations that promote safe health care practices. A culture of safety should exist within the health care system and nursing. The Joint Commission's National Patient Safety Goals are updated annually, and sentinel events identify safety concerns and the interventions for them (www.jointcommission.org). Examples of sentinel events are surgery on the wrong body part or death/loss of function associated with a fall within a facility.

The National Quality Forum (NQF) (2011) has identified "serious reportable events" (SRE). These 29 events that should not occur in various health care settings are found at www.qualityforum.org/Topics/SREs/List_of_SREs.aspx.

Medication errors are of primary concern, and interventions to prevent them are being researched and implemented. The Institute for Safe Medication Practices has interventions to reduce medication errors such as the Error-Prone Abbreviations List, Do Not Crush List, Drug Names Written With Tallman Letters, Letters to Distinguish between Similar Looking Drug Names to Prevent Giving the Wrong Drug, and High Alert Medications (http://ismp.org/default.asp). No

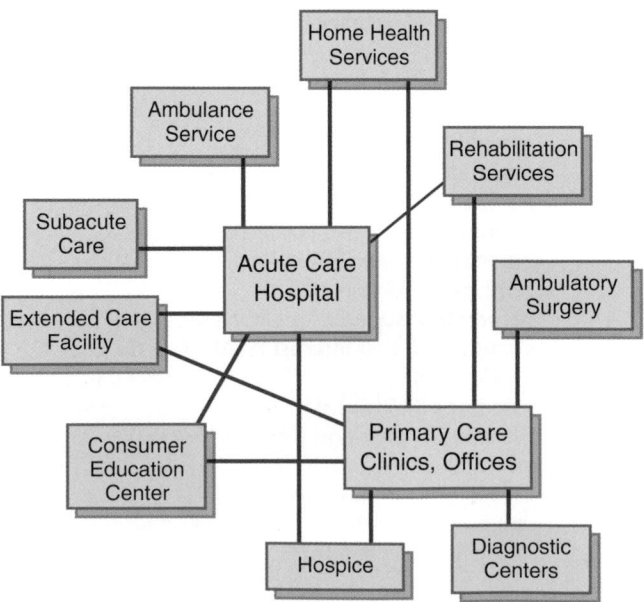

FIGURE 3.1 An integrated health care system.

interruption zones with brightly color tape or wearing bright color vests/sashes as an alert to avoid distractions are used at some agencies with great results. Distractions during medication administration can increase errors, so you should always stay focused and avoid interruptions during this time. Promote a culture of safety and ask your coworkers to avoid interrupting others during medication administration. Reducing errors requires everyone to be engaged and vigilant at all times during patient care.

 LEARNING TIP

To learn more about safe health care practices, visit the Institute for Healthcare Improvement website at www.ihi.org/IHI/Programs/IHIOpenSchool.
    Did you know that a drug made for one type of administration route, such as intravenous (IV), cannot be safely given by another route such as by NG or PEG tube? Serious effects, including death, can occur because the drug dosages or drug makeup is specific to the route. Get a new order for an alternate route if needed to obtain the proper drug form. This website shows examples of adverse effects when drugs were given incorrectly. Keep your patients safe!

ECONOMIC ISSUES

Patient Protection and Affordable Care Act

Known in brief as the Affordable Care Act, the 2010 Patient Protection and Affordable Care Act's phase-in continues through 2020 (Fig. 3.2). Its purpose is to provide insurance reforms that protect consumers from insurance industry abuses, reduce the cost of health care, increase the quality of health care, and increase health insurance availability for more Americans. Key changes of the act are listed in Table 3.1. For more information, visit www.hhs.gov/healthcare.

Medicare and Diagnosis-Related Groups

Medicare was created in 1965 to provide health insurance as part of the Social Security Act. It is run by the U.S. government and covers all people aged 65 and older and people younger than age 65 who have disabilities and are eligible for Social Security. It is funded by a deduction from every person's paycheck that is matched by the government. Several Medicare plan options are offered, including Original Medicare, Medicare Health Plans, and prescription drug coverage for everyone with Medicare. There are two parts of coverage in the Original Medicare plan. Part A covers inpatient hospital care, skilled nursing facilities, hospice services, and some home care. There is no premium or deductible for Part A. Part B is medical insurance that covers physician costs, outpatient services, some

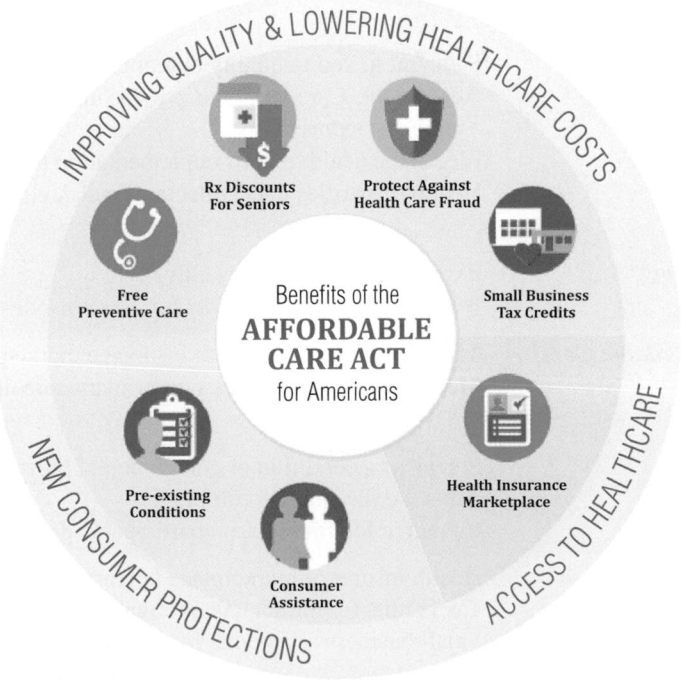

Benefits for Women
Providing insurance options, covering preventive services, and lowering costs.

Young Adult Coverage
Coverage available to children up to age 26.

Strengthening Medicare
Yearly wellness visit and many free preventive services for some seniors with Medicare.

Holding Insurance Companies Accountable
Insurers must justify any premium increase of 10% or more before the rate takes effect.

TIMELINE

October	January	March	Future
Open enrollment begins	Coverage begins	Open enrollment closes	All Americans have access to affordable health care

FIGURE 3.2 Key features of the Affordable Care Act. *(From the U. S. Department of Health and Human Services, 2013.)*

TABLE 3.1 AFFORDABLE CARE ACT OVERVIEW

Year	Key Changes
2010 *Consumer Protection*	Patient Bill of Rights for protection from insurance abuses Prevention of child preexisting condition denial Prevention of coverage rescinding No lifetime benefit dollar limits
Quality and Cost Lowering	Small business tax credits for insurance premiums Medicare prescription drug relief Free preventive services Disease prevention funding programs Fraud reduction
Increased Access to Affordable Care	Coverage for preexisting conditions Young adult coverage until age 26 under parents' plan Early retiree coverage Education funding to increase number of health care providers Insurance premium hike justification Medicaid funding increase Rural care payment increases Community health center expansion
2011 *Quality and Cost Lowering*	Medicare free preventive services Innovation center for quality and efficiency Community Care Transitions Program for hospital-discharged seniors Innovations to reduce Medicare costs
Increased Access to Affordable Care	Community First Choice Option to serve the disabled with home and community services via Medicaid
Insurance Company Accountability	Health care premium guidelines and containment
2012 *Quality and Cost Lowering*	Payment linked to quality outcomes for hospitals Accountable Care Programs provide incentives for physicians to provide quality care and reduce costs Electronic health record implementation to reduce paperwork Health disparities data collection: racial, ethnic, and language
2013 *Quality and Cost Lowering*	Expanded Medicaid preventive care Bundling flat rate payments for care episode to incent efficiency and quality
Increased Access to Affordable Care	Open enrollment for health insurance marketplace starts Medicaid payment increase to primary care doctors
2014 *Consumer Protection*	Preexisting condition or gender denial prevented Annual dollar limits prohibited Coverage for clinical trial participants protected
Quality and Cost Lowering	Health insurance marketplace begins Tax credits for middle class to make insurance affordable Small business tax credits for insurance premiums increases
Increased Access to Affordable Care	Medicaid eligibility (earn less than 133% of poverty level) increases Individuals required to obtain insurance or pay a fee unless exempt
2015 *Quality and Cost Lowering*	Physician payment based on quality of care provided

Adapted from U.S. Department of Health & Human Services key features of the Affordable Care Act by year. Retrieved September 3, 2013, from www.hhs.gov/healthcare/facts/timeline/timeline-text.html#2010

home care, supplies, and other things not covered by Part A. Some preventive services might also be covered. A monthly premium and yearly deductible are paid for Part B coverage. For more information, visit www.medicare.gov.

Congress created the **diagnosis-related group** (DRG) payment system in 1983 for 470 diagnostic categories to help control costs in the Medicare program, which previously had no reimbursement limits. All hospitals were paid the same fee for patients in the same diagnostic category regardless of length of stay and supply costs. The original DRG system has undergone modifications through the years, and today several DRG systems are in use that take into consideration all populations, complications, and comorbidities. Hospitals lose money if the patient's costs exceed the DRG payment and make money if the costs are less than the payment.

Hospital-Acquired Conditions and Present-on-Admission Reporting

In 2008, the Centers for Medicare and Medicaid Services implemented a change for Medicare Severity DRG payments to acute inpatient prospective payment system hospitals. This policy is called the Hospital-Acquired Conditions (HAC) and Present on Admission (POA) Indicator Reporting. Box 3-1 shows the 11 categories of HACs (for updates, see www.cms.gov/Medicare/Medicare-Fee-for-Service-Payment /HospitalAcqCond/Hospital-Acquired_Conditions.html). At discharge, if certain conditions are not POA, hospitals do not receive additional reimbursement for those conditions. For example, if a patient was admitted with a stroke (primary diagnosis) and then developed a pressure ulcer that was not present on admission (secondary diagnosis) that could have been prevented, the hospital would receive reimbursement only for the primary diagnosis of stroke. The hospital would have to absorb the cost of care for the pressure ulcer.

With this requirement, nurses must carefully assess and document patient conditions that are POA to show that they did not occur during the hospitalization. Providing safe, quality care and educating patients to prevent complications, such as the need to do leg exercises, turn every 2 hours, or ambulate, are essential to prevent these conditions. Documenting interventions, education provided, and the patient's refusal to participate (if applicable) are essential to help ensure reimbursement for secondary diagnoses.

Medicaid

The Medicaid payment system was also created in 1965 to provide health insurance as part of the Social Security Act for low-income or disabled persons younger than age 65 and their dependent children. Some low-income people older than age 65 can also qualify. Medicaid funding comes from federal, state, and local taxes. Benefits for Medicaid vary from state to state.

Managed Health Care

Health maintenance organizations (HMOs) deliver health care services to individuals who enroll in this type of prepaid

---

Box 3-1 Categories of Hospital-Acquired Conditions

The Centers for Medicare and Medicaid Services identified the following 11 categories of hospital-acquired conditions as those that increase health care costs or that could have been prevented by using evidence-based guidelines:

Foreign Object Retained After Surgery
Air Embolism
Blood Incompatibility
Stage III and IV Pressure Ulcers
Falls and Trauma
  • Fractures
  • Dislocations
  • Intracranial Injuries
  • Crushing Injuries
  • Burns
  • Other Injuries
Manifestations of Poor Glycemic Control
  • Diabetic Ketoacidosis
  • Nonketotic Hyperosmolar Coma
  • Hypoglycemic Coma
  • Secondary Diabetes With Ketoacidosis
  • Secondary Diabetes With Hyperosmolarity
Catheter-Associated Urinary Tract Infection
Vascular Catheter-Associated Infection
Surgical Site Infection After:
  • Coronary Artery Bypass Graft—Mediastinitis
  • Bariatric Surgery for Obesity
    • Laparoscopic Gastric Bypass
    • Gastroenterostomy
    • Laparoscopic Gastric Restrictive Surgery
  • Certain Orthopedic Procedures
    • Spine
    • Neck
    • Shoulder
    • Elbow
  • Cardiac Implantable Electronic Device
Deep Vein Thrombosis/Pulmonary Embolism
  • Total Knee Replacement
  • Hip Replacement
Iatrogenic Pneumothorax With Venous Catheterization

Source: Centers for Medicare & Medicaid Services. (2013). *Hospital-acquired conditions.* Retrieved July 12, 2013, from www.cms.gov/Medicare /Medicare-Fee-for-Service-Payment/HospitalAcqCond/Hospital -Acquired_Conditions.html

---

group practice health program. The purpose of an HMO is to reduce overlapping services and provide quality and cost-effective care. Healthy patients require fewer services, so preventive care is promoted. Preferred provider organizations (PPOs) are networks of providers who offer care to plan members at set discounted rates. PPOs are designed to reduce costs to businesses that insure employees. Hospitals and physicians develop a contract with employers to provide services at a negotiated fee.

LEARNING TIP

To understand what the term *managed care* means, reverse the words: *care management.*

Managed care has led to fewer hospitalizations and shorter lengths of stay. Patients are using home health care for more complex needs. Case management is helping to ensure that the best patient outcome is achieved while controlling costs.

 NURSING AND THE HEALTH CARE TEAM

Nursing is an integral part of the health care network. Nurses work as licensed practical nurses (LPNs) or *licensed vocational nurses* (LVNs), *registered nurses* (RNs), or registered nurses with advanced education and practice skills, which includes *certified registered nurse practitioners* (CRNPs), *clinical nurse specialists* (CNSs), *certified nurse midwives* (CNMs), *certified registered nurse anesthetists* (CRNAs), and *doctors of nursing practice* (DNP). Certified nursing assistants (CNAs) are trained to assist nurses in providing health care.

Collaborative Care

Nurses work in collaboration with other members of the health care team:

- Licensed *physicians* provide medical care to patients after graduating from a college of medicine (MD) or osteopathic medicine (DO).
- *Physician assistants* (PA-C [certified]), after graduating from a physician's assistant program, work under the supervision of a physician and perform certain physician duties, such as history taking, physical examinations, and suturing of wounds.
- Licensed *pharmacists* complete 5 or 6 years of college and dispense medications from prescriptions, consult with physicians, and provide medication information to patients.
- *Social workers* usually have a master's degree in social work (MSW), can be licensed clinical social workers (LCSW), and treat patients and their families with psychosocial issues.
- *Dietitians* provide nutrition information, analyze nutritional needs, and calculate special dietary needs.
- Licensed *physical therapists* complete a college physical therapy program and assist patients in reducing physical disability, bodily malfunction, movement dysfunction, and pain through evaluation, education, and treatment.
- *Physical therapy assistants,* whose educational requirements vary, might complete 2 years of education and be licensed and then work under the supervision of a physical therapist.

- *Occupational therapists* complete a bachelor's or master's program, can be registered (OTR), and assist patients in restoring self-care, work, and leisure skills that have been diminished as a result of developmental deficits or injury.
- *Speech and language pathologists* typically complete a master's program. They provide direct clinical services to those with communication or swallowing problems.
- *Respiratory therapists* have a 2-year college degree, can be registered (RRT), and work with patients who have respiratory problems.
- *Respiratory therapy technicians* have 1 year of education, can be certified (CRTT), and work under the supervision of a respiratory therapist to provide respiratory care.
- *Health unit secretaries* manage clerical work.
- *Student nurses* are enrolled in a nursing program and work under the supervision of nursing faculty in the clinical setting.

 LEADERSHIP IN NURSING PRACTICE

A leader seeks to influence, motivate, and enable others to achieve goals. **Leadership** skills are necessary for the LPN/LVN to effectively guide patient care and achieve patient care goals.

Effective leaders in a health care setting must be knowledgeable about management and supervisory processes. They must use critical thinking and be able to make decisions. They should be role models and an inspiration to others. A positive attitude and the use of humor are valuable assets of good leaders. Ultimately, leaders must earn the respect of their coworkers to be successful. To prepare for a leadership role, learning and applying the following principles of leadership, supervision, and management is helpful.

Leadership Styles

There are three traditional leadership styles: (1) autocratic, (2) democratic, and (3) laissez-faire. A fourth style called coaching is also used in health care settings.

Autocratic (Authoritarian) Leadership

An autocratic leader has a high degree of control. Almost no control is given to others. In **autocratic leadership**, the leader determines the goals and plans for achieving the goals. Others are instructed on what to do and are not asked to provide input. The group usually achieves high-quality outcomes under this style of leadership. This is an efficient leadership style for emergency situations when decisions must be made quickly, such as when evacuating a building or responding to a cardiac arrest.

Democratic (Participative) Leadership

A democratic leader has a moderate degree of control. Others are given some control and freedom. In **democratic leadership**, participation is encouraged in determining goals and plans for achieving the goals (Fig. 3.3). Decisions are made within the group. The leader assists the group by steering and teaching rather than dominating. The leader shares responsibility with

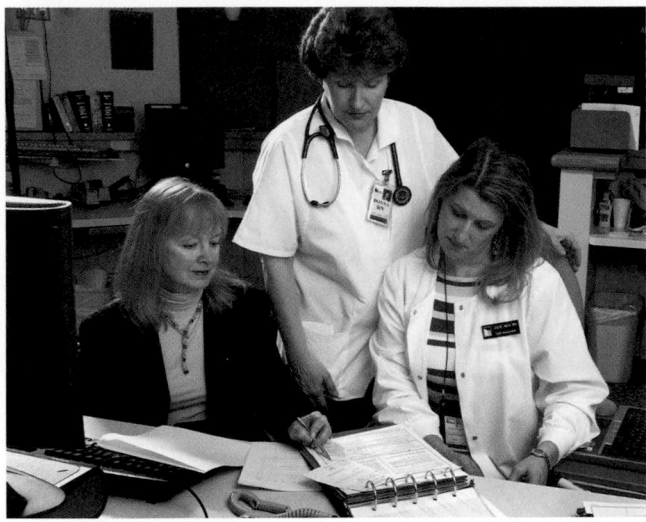

FIGURE 3.3 Group participation in decision making.

the group. The group usually achieves high-quality outcomes and is more creative under this style of leadership. This is an efficient leadership style for most situations. With this type of leadership, group members have greater satisfaction and are motivated to achieve goals because they are active participants.

Laissez-Faire (Delegative) Leadership

A laissez-faire leader exerts no control over the group, which is given complete freedom for decision making. With **laissez-faire leadership**, no one is responsible for determining goals and plans for achieving the goals. This can produce a feeling of chaos. Little is accomplished under this leadership style, and the quality of outcomes is often poor.

Coaching Leadership

By emphasizing active listening, clear communication, support, and accountability, coaching leaders work with others to develop problem-solving skills that facilitate critical thinking, prioritization, and effective communication. This leadership style helps direct-care employees feel more empowered, valued, and respected.

Management Functions

The five major components in the management process are (1) planning, (2) organizing, (3) directing, (4) coordinating, and (5) controlling.

Planning

In the first step of the management process, a plan must be developed to ensure that desired patient care outcomes are achieved. To formulate the plan, desired outcomes or problems are identified and data about them are collected. Alternatives or solutions are considered using the collected data and input from others. A decision is then made about the best option or course of action. The leader should ensure that the choice is realistic and can be implemented. Involving others in the planning and decision-making process from beginning to end can increase acceptance at the time of implementation.

Organizing

The purpose of organizing, the second step in the management process, is to provide an orderly environment that promotes cooperation and goal achievement. Providing a framework for goals and the activities that accomplish them is the initial step in organization. Policies and procedures provide this framework as well as guidance for those carrying out tasks designed to accomplish the organization's goals.

Directing

Making assignments is the primary function of directing. One person, usually the nurse in charge or the team leader, makes the assignments for patient care. The nurse practice act in each state defines who can make assignments and delegate care. Communication is important in directing. Assignments must be clearly and specifically stated. The person making assignments must be sure that each assignment is correctly understood and should seek out the receiving person for clarification. Effective directing can be accomplished by providing verbal and written assignment information, making requests rather than giving orders, and giving instructions as needed.

Coordinating

Coordination is the process of looking at a situation to ensure that it is being handled in the most effective way for the organization or coordinating services for a patient. The nurse might assess a particular activity or issues related to patient care assignments. In a long-term care facility, for example, the nurse might want to review skin assessment and care throughout the facility to see if it is being done consistently and uniformly. If a concern is found, problem-solving techniques are used.

Controlling

The final phase of the management process is controlling to evaluate the accomplishment of the organization's goals. Continuous quality improvement is linked with controlling. If the organization's efficiency or ability to reach its goals is impaired, the use of the continuous quality improvement model can facilitate correction of the concern (Fig. 3.4).

Leadership and Delegation for the LPN/LVN

LPN/LVNs are leaders and managers of care for the patients to whom they are assigned, under the supervision of an RN, health care provider (HCP), or a dentist as specified by each state nursing practice act. Beyond this application of a leader and manager role for the LPN/LVN, state nurse practice acts specify if the LPN/LVN can assume other leader or manager roles. Within this dependent role, some aspect of delegation may be allowed.

 LEARNING TIP

Review your state's nurse practice act. Does your state allow LPN/LVNs to delegate? If so, to whom and what can be delegated?

FIGURE 3.4 A continuous quality improvement (CQI) model.

FIGURE 3.5 Communication of the patient's status by a team leader when transferring the patient's care to another team leader.

Delegation is the act of empowering another person to act. Delegation occurs in a downward manner. RNs delegate to LPN/LVNs and unlicensed assistive personnel (UAP). LPN/LVNs, in certain circumstances, delegate to LPN/LVNs and UAPs (as discussed later). When delegation occurs, responsibility for care is transferred to the delegatee, but accountability for the care remains with the delegator. Guidelines for delegating can be found at www.ncsbn.org/1625.htm.

The LPN/LVN might function as a team leader or charge nurse mainly in the long-term care setting, requiring some use of delegation to UAPs. When the LPN/LVN acts as a team leader or charge nurse, an RN delegates the authority to provide supervision and delegation of tasks. Team leaders are responsible for the coordination and delivery of care to each of the patients assigned to the team. They assess the patients assigned to the team to plan appropriate care and contribute to the nursing care plan. Team leaders receive information from team members and communicate patients' needs to appropriate individuals. Because team leaders guide patient care provided by the team, they must be knowledgeable about safety policies, patients' rights, and the accountability of being a team leader.

All patients are entitled to quality care and treatment with dignity and respect. The team leader is accountable for all care provided by the team. Supervision involves initial direction for the task and then monitoring of the task and outcome at intervals. At the end of the team's work shift, team leaders are responsible for transferring patient care to the oncoming team in a way that prevents communication breakdowns that result in patient harm. This hand-off communication is accomplished by reporting the patient's condition, status, and needs to the oncoming team leader (Fig. 3.5). Institutional policy specifies whether the RN or LPN/LVN communicates the report.

Within the leadership role, the LPN/LVN must decide when delegation would most benefit the situation and the patient. All nurses must follow the state practice act and the scope of practice when making any decisions regarding delegation. Consult the charge nurse, team leader, and nurse practice act for your state when deciding if delegation is appropriate. Ultimately, you must ask several important questions to determine when delegation would best benefit the situation. These questions include the following:

• Does the state practice act allow for delegation in this situation?
• Does the person to whom I am delegating have the knowledge and education to perform this skill, and is it documented for me to make the decisions regarding delegation?
• Would it benefit the patient if I delegated this skill to the support person?

Delegation Process

Delegation is a complex process. In each case, take the following steps, which encompass the decision to delegate, what to delegate, and to whom delegation can be made:

1. Know your state practice act rules for delegation. The LPN/LVN scope of practice usually does not provide legal authority for an LPN/LVN to delegate. However, some state board rules allow LPN/LVNs to delegate tasks that are within the LPN/LVNs scope of practice as long as the RN has given the LPN/LVN authority to delegate the tasks.
2. Identify the skills of the person to whom you might delegate to determine if he or she has the knowledge and ability to carry out the task. When selecting a team member to delegate tasks to, consider if there is potential for harm to the patient during the task, whether it is a complex task that will require problem solving, how predictable the outcome is, and how much interaction with the patient is needed.

Match the skills and talents of the team member to the task being delegated. Remember, nursing judgment can never be delegated.

3. Use the National Council of State Boards of Nursing's (1995) five rights of delegation. Following these guidelines provides a framework for your decision-making process and comfort in knowing you used them to make good choices:
   • Right task—is it appropriate to delegate?
   • Right circumstances—is this situation safe and appropriate for delegating?
   • Right person—is this delegatee the appropriate person for the task and this patient's needs?
   • Right communication—is there clear understanding between you and the delegatee for terms used, communication, and reporting needs?
   • Right supervision—is it defined how and when direct supervision will occur?

Delegation requires trust. You should be comfortable with which tasks can be delegated and the team member to whom you are delegating the tasks. Also, it is important to know and understand each other's methods of communicating so that miscommunications do not occur.

When you first begin your career, the process of delegating can seem difficult. As with any skill, it takes practice to feel confident in carrying out the process.

EDUCATIONAL AND CAREER OPPORTUNITIES FOR LPN/LVNS

LPN/LVNs might seek additional education. Many schools provide for an accelerated educational tract for LPN/LVNs seeking to become RNs. Advanced educational opportunities include a master's degree or a doctoral degree. Check with colleges/universities to see which program would best meet your needs for continuing your education. Post licensure certification for the LPN in pharmacology, long-term care, or IV therapy is offered by National Association for Practical Nurse Education and Service (NAPNES) and National Federation for Licensed Practical Nurses (NFLPN).

Because of the health care needs of the increasing older adult population and an increased need overall for health care services, the need for LPN/LVNs is expected to grow 25% between 2012 to 2022, which is faster than the average for other occupations (Bureau of Labor Statistics, 2014–15). LPN/LVNs work in child day-care centers, clinics, corrections, home care, hospitals, long-term care, HCP offices, dentist offices, and schools, among other health care settings. Employment of LPN/LVNs is declining in hospitals, but it is growing in settings outside of hospitals.

Correctional Nursing

A growing clinical setting for the LPN to work in is correctional nursing. Local, regional, and state regional facilities are interested in hiring LPNs to care for inmates and handle worksite wellness programs for correctional officers and other staff. Key in this practice area is the ability for the nurse to appropriately apply professional theory, practice, and **ethics** within the correctional setting. Correctional nurses must possess good physical and mental health and retain sufficient stamina, agility, and visual/auditory acuity necessary to perform all duties associated with LPN practice. In this setting, the LPN must be able to:

• Independently implement the nursing process with inmates/residents in following HCP orders regarding diet, medication and treatments
• Utilize knowledge of current medications (actions, interactions, uses, and side effects)
• Utilize knowledge of medical, therapeutic, and psychiatric nursing interventions
• Appropriately apply quality standards, procedures, and protocols as directed
• Be knowledgeable about and sensitive to cultural and socioeconomic differences among the populace as they relate to health and behaviors
• Demonstrate an interpersonal skill set that includes high quality oral and written communication skills to facilitate cooperation, pride, trust, and commitment to quality health/medical team communication
• Maintain institutional records and provide required institutional reports
• Consistently demonstrate medical team professionalism in assessing and providing inmate health care delivery as directed by the HCP
• Interview, listen, and provide empathetic assistance to inmates in meeting their needs by carrying out prescribed treatments within the LPN scope of practice
• Respond to emergencies as a part of the health care team
• Appropriately respond to and seek supervision as needed
• Observe, monitor, analyze, and evaluate appropriate quality nursing care, teaching, and treatment
• Provide precertification for and coordination of inmates admitted to and discharged from acute care facilities by contributing to and implementing their nursing care plans and routine health tests
• Work effectively and efficiently when exposed to difficult or challenging working conditions/situations related to incarcerated patients

ETHICS AND VALUES

Ethics is a code of values which guide our choices and actions and determine the purpose and course of our lives.
AYN RAND, RUSSIAN-BORN AMERICAN NOVELIST AND PHILOSOPHER (1905–1982)

The study and practice of ethics is grounded in philosophy and dates back to the time of Hippocrates. Ethics is a systematic approach not only to understanding an ethical dilemma but also to examining the best outcome for each situation (Butts & Rich, 2013). Bioethics is a branch of ethics that studies moral values in the biomedical sciences and has come to be most closely associated with health care. Today more than ever, nurses are confronted with new technological advances mixed in with the challenges of a changing economic climate. These variables often create ethical dilemmas in health care.

Morals or **morality** are also related to ethics, and although the terms *ethics* and *morals* are often used interchangeably, *morals* refers more specifically to personally derived values, beliefs, and behaviors we tend to think of as "right and wrong" or "good and bad" (Butts & Rich, 2013).

Values are unwritten standards, ideals, or concepts that give meaning to a person's life and that often serve as a guide for making decisions and setting priorities in daily life. Although values are commonly derived from societal norms, religion, and family traditions, they can change when a person experiences life-changing events. Value conflicts often occur in everyday life, and people make decisions based on their values. For example, a nurse who values both her career and her family might be forced to decide between going to work or staying home with a sick child.

Values exist on many levels. Individuals have personal values that govern their lives and actions. Many groups and organizations have values that represent the group as a whole but may or may not be identical to personal values. When a person becomes a member of a group or organization, he or she agrees to accept the values of the group. Examples of groups include clubs, churches, political parties, and professions. Society as a whole has values. As a member of a society or country, an individual accepts the values of that culture. The values of a profession are usually outlined in a **code of ethics**. This code is a comprehensive set of guidelines that outlines the behavioral expectations for the profession.

Ethical issues surround us throughout our lifetime. Bioethical issues are particularly prevalent in our professional lives for several reasons. To begin with, advances in technology and new treatment options both offer prolonging or saving life. However, in doing so, questions arise related to medical futility such as: Who should receive treatment? How long should treatment continue? Should a patient receive a treatment because it is available, or because it will be effective? How many health care resources should be utilized for the treatment of terminal illnesses? Does quantity or length of life matter more than quality of life? Therefore, it becomes both difficult and important to decide how and when resources will be allocated.

Not all bioethical issues make headline news. In fact, many ethical dilemmas are regular occurrences in the clinical setting. Research shows that many ethical dilemmas arise related to situations such as inadequate staffing protection of patients' rights, unethical practices of HCPs, end-of-life decision making, and breeches in confidentiality (Ulrich et al, 2010). Nurses are involved in decision making every day based on the traditional ethical principles of autonomy, beneficence, **maleficence**, and justice. Have you experienced any of these examples? You are asked to consistently work on a unit that is understaffed. Your charge nurse asks you to "sign her in for the shift" on a regular basis. A patient asks you to keep his prognosis from his spouse. You overhear a coworker who is on break discussing a patient's status on the telephone,

but you do not know who is on the line. Each of these examples prompts questions such as the following: What should be done? What ethical principles are involved? Whose wishes should be honored?

An ethical dilemma is a situation in which a person must choose between two options that will affect the outcome of the case. Although each option can be justified as "good," both have pros and cons. Therefore, when one option is selected or implemented, it creates uncertainty in the outcome of the case (Butts & Rich, 2013).

Decision making in the acute care setting is a complex process involving many members of the health care team. As a result of carrying out orders, nurses must handle consequences that arise from clinical problems. In addition, there is no one-size-fits-all solution for ethical problems. Even if dilemmas share a common thread, each has individual influences that make it unique.

Potential solutions can appear to be equally good or, worse, equally risky: a promise cannot be kept; information

EVIDENCE-BASED PRACTICE

Clinical Question
How do nurses working in hospital environments experience moral distress?

Evidence
A systematic review of qualitative literature, using the Joanna Briggs method, found that nurses who experience moral distress experience a wide array of biological, psychological, and stress reactions. In addition, it was found that nurses feel the need to advocate for their patients despite being met with institutional constraints. Finally, it was found that the unequal power structure in institutions contributed to nurses not being able to practice nursing without having their professional values challenged.

Implications for Nursing Practice
Moral distress is present in clinical practice and has a direct impact on job satisfaction. Institutions should design structures of support for nurses to help lessen the effects of moral distress as well as provide an environment in which nurses can practice that does not violate their core professional values. Education on the effects of moral distress, as well as providing nurses with a way to express ethical concerns would also be helpful.

REFERENCE
Huffman, D., Rittenmeyer, L. (2012). How professional nurses working in hospital environments experience moral distress: A systematic review. *Critical Care Nursing Clinics of North America, 24*(1), 91–100.

cannot remain confidential; DNR (do not resuscitate) orders might not be acceptable for some people. Not all patients should receive CPR, even those who are young. When patients are conscious, their choices are usually respected, but on occasion, even that premise can be difficult to apply. Often, groups of individuals must work together to resolve a conflict if there is disagreement between an HCP and families, nurses and other HCPs, or among family members. Nurses can experience **moral distress** as a result of being an integral part of this team. Moral distress can be defined as distress experienced when knowing the right thing to do but being unable to carry it out because of institutional constraints (Jameton, 1984). More recently, moral distress has been associated with job satisfaction and is one of the reasons that nurses leave nursing (de Veer et al, 2013). In response to increasing ethical and moral conflicts in the clinical setting, many hospitals and facilities have created an ethics committee that helps address especially difficult cases. The multidisciplinary committee might include nurses, other HCPs such as therapists, social workers, and an ethicist.

A basic mastery of several elements enhances your ability to perform competently when bioethical issues arise and decision making is the focus. Understanding the ethical component of your nursing role is the first step. Discovering how your personal value set influences your nursing practice is another. Acquiring knowledge about relevant ethical material is also essential. An ethical decision-making process is a useful tool for examining ethical dilemmas. Together these elements provide a foundation from which you can begin to explore the meaning of bioethics in nursing practice today. For more information about bioethics, visit the Center for Bioethics and Human Dignity at www.cbhd.org.

Ethical Obligations and Nursing

As a nurse, you are an invaluable member of the health care team, contributing to patient care according to your educational preparation and assigned responsibilities. You are guided by the law and the standards set forth by the profession. A professional code of ethics provides a framework. In addition to practicing within the law, nurses have ethical obligations related to the law. First, if the law is considered unethical or has serious limitations, a basic moral obligation of the nurse is to make an effort to change that law. This might be done individually or through political activism guided by professional organizations. Becoming involved in a professional organization is one way to help change the laws that govern health care and nursing.

Nursing Code of Ethics

Some of the major ethical obligations of nursing practice are addressed in a nursing code of ethics. A code of ethics should provide guidance for appropriate decision making based on current laws and professional standards. A code of ethics not only provides a base for professional self-evaluation and reflection but also acts as a tool by which the public can hold the profession accountable. As a professional guide for ethical practice, NFLPN has practice standards that include ethical practice and conduct. See www.nflpn.org/practice-standards4web.pdf. NAPNES also has standards of practice for LP/VNs at www.napnes.org.

A code does not dictate a particular action, nor is it a legal document, although the code should not be in conflict with the law. The code is not enforced by any organization, and no punishment exists if a nurse fails to adhere to it. A code must be interpreted because it usually contains broad statements, but it does serve as a general guideline for professional ethical issues. Ethical codes are updated to reflect current practice, responsibilities, and obligations set forth by the profession.

Building Blocks of Ethics

The discipline of ethics, especially health care ethics, provides us with useful tools and knowledge that can assist us when we encounter difficult situations. An understanding of basic concepts, presented here in the form of ethical principles and ethical theories, helps specifically target the ethical components of the problem. Principles and theories offer frameworks for ethical problem solving. However, knowledge about ethics cannot in itself provide all of the answers to a problem or dilemma. What such knowledge does do is assist us in focusing on the ethical aspects of each case and possibly prevents escalating arguments about issues not related to the ethics of the case.

Ethical Principles

Ethical **principles** derive from moral theory and have two purposes. The first is to provide some framework for society's moral conduct. The second is to help us take consistent positions and approaches to moral dilemmas. Ethical principles can be found in many professional codes of conduct and are key components of ethical decision making. The ethical principles widely used when examining bioethical and health care dilemmas include autonomy, beneficence, nonmaleficence, fidelity, veracity, and justice. Given the prominence of these ethical principles in the bioethical literature, a basic understanding of them is necessary.

AUTONOMY. According to ethicists (and behaviorists, social scientists, and psychologists), what makes human beings different from nonhumans is that people have dignity based on their ability to choose freely what they will do with their lives. **Autonomy** is the right of self-determination, independence, and freedom founded on the notion that humans have value, worth, and moral dignity. Autonomy in health care applies to all people capable of and competent in making health care decisions for themselves. HCPs do not need to agree with another person's decisions, but must respect the autonomy of the person making the choice. **Paternalism** occurs when an HCP tries to prevent patients from making autonomous decisions or decides what is best for patients without regard for their preferences. Autonomy also encompasses the professional's self-determination and freedom.

There are limitations to autonomy. Typically, these limitations arise when a person's autonomy interferes with the rights, health, or well-being of self or others. For example, patients generally have an autonomous right to make decisions regarding their care and level of independence. This autonomous right is guaranteed by federal legislation known as the Patient Self-Determination Act, which can be found at www.nrc-pad.org/images/stories/PDFs/fedaddirectives2a.pdf. However, if a person is no longer capable of self-care upon discharge, a request to live independently will not be granted. A person unable to adequately care for himself cannot live alone at the expense of his health and well-being. Thus the principle of autonomy cannot be upheld.

BENEFICENCE. The principle of **beneficence** proposes that actions taken and treatments provided will benefit a person and promote welfare (Butts & Rich, 2013). The provision of good care not only means the provision of technologically competent care but also care that respects the patient's beliefs, feelings, and wishes, as well as those of their family and significant others. A common problem encountered when applying this principle is deciding what is good for someone else.

NONMALEFICENCE.   Nonmaleficence is one of the oldest obligations in health care, dating back to the Hippocratic oath (400 B.C.). **Nonmaleficence** is the obligations to "do no harm" (Butts & Rich, 2013). It is common to hear beneficence and maleficence talked about as being "two sides of the same coin."

HCPs are required to do no harm to their patients either *intentionally* or *unintentionally*. In current health care practice, the principle of nonmaleficence may be intentionally violated to produce a greater good in the patient's long-term treatment. For example, a patient might undergo a painful and debilitating or disfiguring surgery to remove a cancerous growth, thereby avoiding death and prolonging life.

By extension, the principle of nonmaleficence also requires a nurse to protect from harm those who are considered vulnerable. Vulnerable groups include children, older adults, and those who are mentally incompetent, unconscious, or too weak or debilitated to protect themselves.

FIDELITY.   **Fidelity** is the obligation to be faithful to commitments made to self and others. In health care, fidelity includes faithfulness or loyalty to agreements and responsibilities accepted as part of the practice of nursing. It also means not promising a patient something that one cannot deliver or control. Fidelity is the main support for the concept of accountability, although conflicts in fidelity might arise because of obligations owed to different individuals or groups. For example, nurses have an obligation of fidelity to the patients they care for to provide the highest quality care possible, as well as an obligation of fidelity to their employing institution to follow its rules and policies. Nurses can have an ethical dilemma when a hospital's policy on staffing creates a situation that does not allow nurses to provide the quality of care they feel is needed.

Maintaining a patient's privacy and **confidentiality** is related to fidelity (Fig. 3.6). Privacy and confidentiality may or may not be explicit promises. Nurses are obligated to discuss the patient only under circumstances in which it is necessary to deliver high-quality holistic health care, such as:

• When given specific instructions to do so by the patient
• When there is the grave possibility of harm to either the patient or others
• When legally mandated to do so

Maintaining confidentiality also applies to the necessary communication of information through the posting of unit censuses and various schedules for tests, procedures, or special examinations (operating room, physical therapy, radiology), storage and access of patient information in computers, and the transmission of patient information via fax machines. Many people other than direct caregivers have legitimate access to a patient's chart: faculty members in the course of making student assignments, accrediting agencies, risk managers, quality assurance personnel, insurance companies, and researchers. Each is obligated to maintain patient confidentiality to the extent that concealing information:

• Does not compromise mandated reports (communicable diseases or gunshot wounds).
• Considers various releases already granted by the patient (such as when insurance information was obtained).
• Ensures gathering data in the aggregate without identifying specific patients (research or institutional statistics).

Other forms of necessary communication include shift-change reporting and case conferences. Care must be taken to hold these information-sharing events in settings where the discussion remains private.

FIGURE 3.6 Maintaining privacy is a patient right and conveys caring to the patient.

• WORD • BUILDING •
nonmaleficence: non—not + maleficentia—evil doing

VERACITY. **Veracity** is the virtue of truthfulness. Within health care, it requires HCPs, whenever possible, to tell the truth and not intentionally deceive or mislead patients. As with other rights and obligations, there are limitations to this virtue. The primary limitation occurs when telling patients the truth would seriously harm their ability to recover or when the truth can produce greater illness. This is known as **therapeutic privilege** and is exercised by HCPs in cases when (1) they are trying to protect patients from heartbreaking news, as in the initial stages of treatment; (2) they do not know the facts, making it better not to answer rather than instill false hope; and (3) they state what is true rather than state what is not true (Butts & Rich, 2013). An example of this is when there is a new or experimental treatment. HCPs can say that in certain clinical trials, patients benefitted in specific ways, but they might not be able to cite all of the possible side effects because the treatment has not yet been widely used.

Another difficult situation can be created in relation to diagnostic information. Although giving diagnostic information is the responsibility of the HCP or RN, LPN/LVNs sometimes find themselves in situations in which they must deal with patients' questions. If LPN/LVNs feel uncomfortable about reinforcing explanations given by the HCP or the RN, they might avoid answering patients' questions directly. However, patients do have a right to know this information. The LPN should inform the HCP or RN of the patient's request for information, and agency policy on patient information sharing should be followed.

JUSTICE. **Justice** is based on fairness and equality (Butts & Rich, 2013). Concerns for justice can focus on how we treat individuals and groups in society (psychologically, socially, legally, and politically), and how we equitably distribute material resources such as health care (distributive justice) and burdens (taxes) and the appropriate compensation to those who have been harmed. When a patient makes an appointment for 0900 at an outpatient clinic, the patient expects to be seen by the HCP at the designated time unless an emergency occurs. Unequal treatment would result if a walk-in patient who has no pressing problem is seen by the HCP in place of the patient with the 0900 appointment, forcing subsequent appointments to be delayed. Distribution of material resources can be complex because it involves not only benefits (what we receive), but also burdens (what we may be taxed for but then do not receive). Burdens are not just monetary but also include such factors as the unequal participation of individuals in medical research and the sacrifices family members make when caring for individuals with disabilities in the home.

USE OF PRINCIPLES. One of the most serious limitations of these principles is the lack of any built-in priority when applying them to an ethical dilemma. Autonomy is not automatically prioritized over justice or beneficence over nonmaleficence. However, these principles are helpful in categorizing various preferences and positions when examining a dilemma to clarify positions within it. Working with principles moves the discussion to a focus on ethics rather than on a particular personal viewpoint or feeling. Such a strategy can also avoid a power struggle between those who simply want to win the argument.

Here is an example of an ethical dilemma. A nurse attempts to support a patient's refusal of surgery, whereas the surgeon claims that the patient must have surgery to avoid losing a foot. When you shift your thinking to realize that the nurse is arguing the case from the perspective of the patient's autonomy (self-determination) and the surgeon's actions are motivated by beneficence (to act in a way that benefits the patient), the discussion becomes one based on conflicting principles, rather than conflict between individuals. Consequently, the discussion can focus on autonomy and beneficence and their respective rationales. This strategy does not resolve the dilemma but makes it less personal and forces participants to develop sound, ethical rationales for their solution.

Ethical Theories

Ethical theories are concepts that are more complete than principles for analyzing ethical dilemmas. Theories are used to explain variables, guide inquiry, and provide a foundation with which to conduct decision making. A brief description of two of the major bioethics theories—utilitarianism and deontology—is provided here. Other theoretical approaches to ethical decision making exist, and theories are often combined to address ethical dilemmas. This section also explores the relationship of theology or religion to bioethics.

UTILITARIANISM. **Utilitarian** theory is grounded in the premise that actions are judged right or wrong based purely on their consequences, and therefore, outcomes are the most important elements to consider when making decisions. Right actions are morally preferred if they produce more happiness or greater benefits than unhappiness or burdens, and in utilitarianism, each person's happiness is equally important. This approach can be used by institutions and organizations under the guise of cost–benefit ratios. A hospital responsible for the care for hundreds of patients is not as concerned with the individual patient who unfortunately is caught in the bureaucracy of its functioning. This is not to say that all institutions operate on this theory at all times, but, in general, rules, policies, and procedures are developed with the majority in mind.

There are several major criticisms of the utilitarian theory. One is that an individual is often sacrificed for the good of the majority (often seen in wartime). The second is that it can be difficult to predict outcomes, especially when human nature is involved.

DEONTOLOGY. **Deontology** is a philosophical theory requiring human actions and attitudes to be based on duty, and the moral worth of an action (the result) should not be judged only in terms of its consequences. For example, HCPs might operate by a rule indicating that a moral person never lies. No matter how much the truth might hurt, the truth is revealed. Another rule might be to never use people as a means to an end. Translated, this means that regardless of the benefits, individuals cannot be forced to participate in medical research studies to benefit others. An individual's right to voluntarily participate in research must be respected. Research does not have to benefit the individual participant as long as this is understood by the individual. However, the individual cannot be used simply to meet the investigator's needs. Acting morally only because one has a duty to do so, without any consideration of the outcome, is a serious limitation of this theory.

THEOLOGICAL PERSPECTIVES. Theological perspectives include the many religious traditions represented in our culture. Religious teachings are key concepts for ethical decision making for some people. In fact, many consider these teachings a divine source of values and morals. Jehovah's Witnesses' rejection of blood transfusions is a common example of how religious beliefs affect health care decision making. This religious group has collected a large amount of information about blood substitutes and alternative therapies. Leaders of Jehovah's Witnesses are prepared to provide education for HCPs about their beliefs and acceptable interventions.

In another area, a number of religious traditions oppose abortion, which affects both HCPs and patients. Euthanasia is another issue addressed by numerous organized religious groups, which in turn can affect how patients make decisions regarding end-of-life issues. One of the difficulties with religious traditions is that it is not simply the official church teaching that is involved but also the individual member's interpretation of that teaching. Assessment of the importance of this dimension of the patient's life is important in an ethical analysis.

Ethical Decision Making

A variety of models and frameworks are available for ethical decision making. The steps listed in this section are a combination of several ideas that have been suggested. In its simplest form, ethical decision making is an informed logical problem-solving process. Similar to the nursing process, as discussed in Chapter 1, the steps described in this section take the user through a set of strategies that assist in approaching a problem in an organized and systematic manner. Nurses applying the steps of the nursing process use critical thinking skills to be as logical and objective as possible. Ethical decision making is a similar process. The goal is to have a balanced perspective that respects emotions but does not let them overshadow the process or the outcome.

Addressing ethical dilemmas is not a simple or easy process. However, the final decision can be more acceptable if the nurse feels the situation was thoroughly examined and all viable options weighed before the decision was made. To illustrate the process, a sample case is examined using each step.

Sample Ethical Dilemma

The Smith family was in an automobile accident out of state. The family was on their way home from vacation. Mrs. Smith is in critical condition, Mr. Smith was pronounced dead in the emergency department, and their 12-year-old daughter, Melissa, is in critical condition. Mrs. Smith is still able to speak and asks you, the nurse, how her husband and daughter are doing. What should you do?

STEP 1: IDENTIFY THE ETHICAL DILEMMA. The initial step is to identify the ethical dilemma. What makes it a true dilemma? Separating the ethical and nonethical aspects facilitates the decision-making process. A conflict can arise because of gaps in communication rather than a conflict of ethical principles. Ethical dilemmas are different from clinical problems that have clear interventions and rationales.

Our sample case is an ethical dilemma because there is no obvious right answer. Do you tell the mother that her spouse is dead and her child is critically injured?

STEP 2: IDENTIFY THE STAKEHOLDERS AND THEIR VALUES. The values, beliefs, and traditions of all participants are important because they will all influence the decision-making process. The patient is at the center of the process. Therefore, the patient's autonomy is important to the steps of the process. An advance directive or a living will can often help guide the decision-making process when the patient no longer has autonomy (the ability to express his or her own wishes). Even if there is a preexisting advance directive, it might not match the wishes of the family for clinical decision making.

In our sample case, who are the stakeholders? Obviously, family members are all stakeholders, as well as the health care team of nurses, HCPs, therapists, and others. The mother is the patient and at the center of the process. We will keep in mind that the daughter is also a patient, but her role in this situation is not the ethical dilemma. So what is the autonomy of the patient? At present, the patient is not fully autonomous because she suffered head trauma.

STEP 3: GATHER AND VERIFY THE INFORMATION. All facets of the dilemma need to be examined. Besides knowing who is involved, the context of the problem must be fully explored. How did the situation arise? Are there objective data to support various parts of the decision-making process? For example, determining competency can be an involved and frustrating process, especially when there are competing parties involved (such as a family disagreement about the competency of a parent). However, objective data such as a mental evaluation can support this fact and ease family disagreements. Both the medical record and the HCP can provide clinically relevant data. In addition, health care records from previous hospitalizations and from other institutions might also be needed. The law, facility policies and procedures, and available resources also have an impact on the overall context of the problem. Therefore, it is necessary to be comprehensive in examining all of these areas.

In our sample case, what do we know? The objective data tell us the following: (1) The spouse is dead; (2) the daughter, who is 12 years old, is in critical condition; (3) the family is from out of state; and (4) on assessment, we find that the mother experienced head trauma, and although she is asking about her spouse and daughter, her vital signs are unstable and her condition is also critical. So in considering the objective information, we must also gather more information. What comes to mind? Does Mrs. Smith or her daughter have any significant health history or take medications that the health care team should know about? What are the policies regarding contacting family in such an emergency? What resources or departments need to be called to assist in this case?

STEP 4: EXAMINE POSSIBLE ACTIONS AND THE CONSEQUENCES OF EACH ACTION. Bringing perspective to an ethical dilemma requires the development of a comprehensive set of all possible actions. In turn, each of the proposed actions should have identified consequences, both positive and negative. This makes the process more transparent and allows anyone to analyze each action by weighing the risks and benefits of implementing that action.

In our sample case, what are all of the possible actions or alternatives to resolve the dilemma? If you consider the extremes, the choices appear clear: You either tell Mrs. Smith about her husband and child, or you do not. If you tell Mrs. Smith that her husband is dead and her child is in critical condition, what are the positive and negative consequences of this action? Conversely, if you do not tell Mrs. Smith about her spouse and child, what are the consequences, both positive and negative? These are considered the extremes in the case, but there are other options. For example, we could calm Mrs. Smith by saying that her husband and daughter are both still being evaluated, or we could call a chaplain to assist the staff in telling her the truth. Even if partial truths seem unacceptable at first glance, they should be added to the list of possible actions.

So, as you can see, each proposed action should have corresponding consequences that allow those involved to ultimately choose the best action to be implemented. Can you think of any more actions appropriate for this scenario? What are the consequences for these actions?

STEP 5: DETERMINE THE ETHICAL FOUNDATION FOR EACH ACTION. Each action should be based on ethical values, principles, or theories. In addition, the code of ethics can lend support as an ethical rationale. One strategy that is proposed for an incompetent or unconscious patient is the **standard of best interest**. This standard involves determination of the best outcome for the patient, given the information known about the patient and the context of the situation. Typically, family members together with HCPs make this determination. Ideally, the decision is made in an objective manner, setting aside any special interests of the family or HCPs.

In our sample case, if we revisit the actions proposed in the previous section, we can see that telling the truth supports veracity but can also violate the principle of beneficence, while also supporting maleficence. In contrast, by not telling the truth, we violate the principle of veracity but uphold beneficence. Lastly, if we entertain the idea of only telling part of the truth, once again we are violating veracity, but the difference is that we are striving to meet the principle of beneficence. We realize that by telling the whole truth, Mrs. Smith's condition can worsen from the stress of the situation.

STEP 6: DETERMINE THE BEST ACTION WITH THE STRONGEST ETHICAL SUPPORT. Each action is judged based on its risks, benefits, and supporting rationale. The actions are then ranked in priority order. Strong ethical support for the first priority is required, as well as a reasonable potential for the action to be implemented.

In our sample case, what do you think is the best outcome? Everyone needs to examine the actions and their respective consequences and supporting ethical principles before making a final decision.

Utilitarians and deontologists might disagree about the important principles in decision making. However, do not assume that different theoretical positions cannot reach a mutually agreeable decision. Although their rationales for the decision can differ, the final solutions each proposes may be identical.

STEP 7: IMPLEMENT THE ACTION. The selected action needs to be implemented in a logical way. Responsibilities for carrying out the plan can be assigned, especially if there are multiple steps in the process. In addition, a well-implemented plan can ensure that the plan is fully operationalized and also increases the potential for success.

In our sample case, each person must implement a plan based on the stakeholders, the chosen action, and the underlying ethical principles. How would you implement your action? What resources would you need? Which members of the health care team would you work with?

STEP 8: EVALUATE THE OUTCOME. The evaluative process is most effective when the details of the care are still fresh. The resolution of an ethical dilemma, whether it has been successful or not, provides us with knowledge and experience to address the next ethical dilemma. Although each dilemma is unique in many ways, similarities between cases can provide insight into the best way to approach the decision-making process when a comparable case arises.

In our sample case, the outcome can be evaluated only after an action is implemented.

CRITICAL THINKING

Ethical Decisions

Identify a health care–related ethical dilemma you have encountered as a student. How did you solve the dilemma? What expert resources did you use?

Apply the ethical decision-making model to your ethical dilemma. How are your decision-making process and proposed actions different when using the model?

LEGAL CONCEPTS

To promote harmony, safety, and productivity as members of a society, we create rules. The rules of society can be informal or formal. An informal social rule, for example, is opening a door for someone when entering a building. Criminal statutes (law) are examples of formal rules of society. These social rules, or codes, promote our individual well-being. It would be unsafe to live in a community that existed without rules, and all societies require minimum standards of conduct for their members. Laws exist to define individuals' duties to themselves, their neighbors, and their government.

Regulation of Nursing Practice

Nursing is a licensed health care profession that is regulated by individual states. Nurses must be licensed by their state to practice nursing. The rationale for state licensure is to improve the quality of health care services and to protect the health, safety, and well-being of the general public residing in that state. As such, state governments have licensing boards that establish the requirements for nurses entering the nursing profession. Also, these state licensing boards are charged with defining the scope of practice for nurses already licensed by the state. State laws that regulate nursing practice can be found within an individual state's nurse practice act, as well as within regulations created by a state's licensing agency.

A state's nurse practice laws, including all attendant nursing regulations, establish the parameters of nursing practice. Nurses must practice within these parameters to maintain a license in good standing. These laws are commonly referred to as **administrative laws**. Violating these laws can be the basis for disciplinary actions by a state licensing body. And a nurse's failure to adhere to the regulatory mandates of a state's licensing body can result in the loss of his or her privilege to practice nursing in that state. Unprofessional conduct and conviction of a crime are two circumstances that can give rise to a nurse licensing body finding cause to revoke a nurse's license to practice.

Health Insurance Portability and Accountability Act of 1996

Since 1996, the federal government has protected the distribution of personal health information (PHI). All health care workers including students are required to follow the requirements established by the Health Insurance Portability and Accountability Act of 1996 (HIPAA). This act creates both civil and criminal liability for HCPs who wrongfully disclose a patient's health information. Developed by the U.S. Department of Health and Human Services, this privacy rule was the first of its kind to establish federal protection of PHI.

HCPs must be sensitive to the legalities concerning the dissemination of PHI, because HIPAA establishes stringent guidelines. Depending on the seriousness of the violation of HIPAA standards, an individual can be fined and/or sentenced to up to 10 years in prison, be personally sued, and face employer's disciplinary action including termination. Stay informed by reviewing your employer's HIPAA compliance policies and then adhere to them. For more information on HIPAA and its impact on health care information and HCPs, see www.hhs.gov/ocr/hipaa.

Social Media and HIPAA

With the explosion of social media use, health care organizations have heightened their oversight of PHI to protect against its improper dissemination. HIPAA is a serious law with serious consequences. It can be violated in a variety of ways by health care employees such as accessing patient medical records without authorization or a need to know, taking photos in patient settings on personal devices, posting patient information including images such as photos or x-rays on social media sites, and making personal postings on a social media site in which identifiable patient information is included. Responsible use of social media to avoid violation of HIPAA is essential for all members of the health care team.

It is safest to keep one's professional and personal life separate when using social media. Discussing your nursing shift on Facebook is not a safe practice, even if you do not use patient names. It can be a violation of HIPAA. Also be aware that employers might review social media sites as part of the hiring process. See www.ncsbn.org/Social_media _guidelines.pdf for more information and examples on safely using social media as a professional. Patient confidentiality and privacy in all settings must always be maintained.

Nursing Liability and the Law

Laws establish **liability**, or responsibility, for wrongful actions. Following the law is a major part of the practice of nursing. Administrative laws establish the licensing authority of the state to create, license, and regulate the practice of nursing. Criminal law regulates behaviors for citizens within this country. Civil law provides the rules by which individuals seek to protect their personal and property rights.

Criminal and Civil Law

Criminal laws establish rules for social behavior and define the punishment for breaking those rules. Violation of criminal laws typically results in imprisonment and/or monetary fines. Everyone, regardless of occupation, is required to obey a government's criminal laws.

Criminal law differs from civil law in two ways: (1) in criminal law, society, as a whole, is the party wronged by the criminal act, and (2) violating a criminal law can result in imprisonment. Breaking a criminal law can result in both criminal punishment and civil liability. For example, an intoxicated driver can go to jail for a crime, but that same driver can also be held liable in a civil action for any personal injury to others (an individual or multiple parties, not society) that resulted from the criminal behavior. Examples of criminal acts are assault, battery, rape, murder, and larceny. **Civil law**, generally, concerns disputes among individuals, including companies. Actions that result in violations of civil law typically do not give rise to criminal behavior; however, liability for violating civil laws can still result in stiff penalties meant to deter future violations.

For HCPs, civil liability is a constant concern. Most civil claims against HCPs arise from patient care. Civil law allows patients and families to monetarily recover for injuries received at the hands of a HCP. Patients and families must show causation between the HCP's action and the patient's injury to recover. Showing causation requires an injured party to demonstrate that an HCP's action or failure to act—an omission—directly and proximately caused the underlying injury. An injury can be physical, emotional, and financial in nature. Lawsuits involving personal injury are called **torts**.

A civil liability suit begins with the filing of a complaint with a court. Court rules require that a copy of the complaint be given, or served, on a defendant by the plaintiff. The person claiming a civil cause of action and injury is the plaintiff, and the person alleged to have caused the injury is the defendant. A **summons** (notice to defendant(s) of the lawsuit) should be attached to the complaint. The complaint describes the claim being made by the plaintiff, and the summons instructs the defendant(s) regarding the time in which to answer the complaint, usually 20 to 30 days.

Nurses served with a work-related summons should notify their employers. Summons and complaints are serious. A nurse who receives a summons must ensure that the summons is answered. If the employer does not answer the summons, the nurse must seek legal counsel to answer the summons within the specified time. Failure to answer the summons and complaint can result in a default judgment (an acknowledgment of liability).

The institution that employs the worker can also be liable for the acts or omissions of its employed HCP. This theory of liability is called *respondeat superior*. Here, it is important for employees to understand that their work can result in civil liability for their employers, too.

Malpractice is defined as a breach of the duty that arises from the practitioner–patient relationship. This term includes liability arising from either intentional or unintentional acts (torts), or both. Intentional torts concern lawsuits wherein the defendant is accused of intentionally injuring to the plaintiff (Table 3.2). On the other hand, unintentional torts concern **negligence**. Negligence occurs when one's failure to exercise due care results in an injury to another. Societal rules require

that we exercise due care when acting in the presence of others. The failure to exercise due care is referred to as a breach of duty. Professionals must uphold a duty of care when interacting with their patients. Malpractice occurs when a HCP fails to uphold this underlying duty, causing injury to a patient as a result. Malpractice is professional negligence (Box 3-2). All HCPs, including LPN/LVNs, are responsible for the actions they undertake at the bedside, no matter whether those actions are intentional or negligent.

Limitation of Liability

All professions are concerned with the **limitation of liability,** or limiting the amount of monetary damages that a defendant must pay to an injured plaintiff. Ways to limit liability include ensuring patient rights, accurately documenting in the patient record, following institutional policies, acquiring individual malpractice or liability insurance, pursuing continuing education, and practicing in accordance with the current standards of the nursing profession. Some states have enacted tort reform legislation. Much of this legislation is directed at limiting liability for HCPs and provider institutions. Examples of this reform legislation include things such as limitations on the monetary value that can be awarded to a plaintiff.

Patient Rights

All patients are entitled to quality care and to be treated with dignity and respect. To provide quality care and limit liability, understand and provide the rights your patient is entitled to and question directions that are controversial, given verbally, concern situations of high liability, or involve a discrepancy between the direction and standard policy. Rights are defined as something due to an individual according to just claims, legal guarantees, or moral and ethical principles. Welfare rights, also called legal rights, are rights that are based on a legal entitlement to some good or benefit. These rights are guaranteed by laws such as the Bill of Rights and, if violated, can come under the powers of the legal system. For example,

TABLE 3.2 INTENTIONAL TORTS

Assault	Unlawful conduct that places another in immediate fear of an unlawful touching or battery; real threat of bodily harm
Battery	Unlawful touching of another
Defamation	Wrongful injury to another's reputation or standing in a community; may be written (libel) or spoken (slander)
False imprisonment	Unlawful restriction of a person's freedom
Outrage	Extreme and outrageous conduct by a defendant in the care of the patient or the body of a deceased individual
Invasion of privacy and wrongful disclosure of confidential information	Liability when a patient's privacy is invaded physically or when records are released without authority

Box 3-2 Components Needed for a Finding of Negligence

- A duty of care owed to patients
- A breach of the duty of care
- Injury and damages occurring from the breach (of the duty of care)
- Causation (a showing that the injury was caused *directly* and *proximately* by breaching of the duty of care). Must have both:

  Direct cause = The injury resulted from the breach of duty.

  Proximate cause = The injury was a foreseeable consequence of the breach of duty.

citizens of the United States have a right to equal access to employment regardless of race, sex, or religion. The type of treatment and care a patient has the right to expect is outlined in the Patient Care Partnership (www.aha.org/content/00-10/pcp_english_030730.pdf). Stay informed about the status of patient rights' legislation because you will be expected to follow it. Knocking before entering a patient's room and introducing oneself to the patient are examples of a patient's rights.

The Importance of Documentation

Documentation is a legal record of your actions. Document nursing actions based on orders given, including the name and title of the person who gave the direction, especially if the directive was verbal. Documentation must be clear, honest, and accurate. Always document in the manner that is generally accepted by the nursing profession and your institution. Review and use your agency's documentation guidelines. Failure to maintain acceptable documentation standards can create potential liability for both you and the health care institution.

A Note on Malpractice Insurance

Some employers do not provide malpractice insurance for their nursing employees. Ask your employer exactly who is covered under the employer's liability insurance and whether those covered parties include you. If nursing employees are covered, the employer's insurance provides coverage from liability only as long as the employee follows the employer's work policies and was acting within the scope of employment. For this reason, employer-provided liability insurance is not personal liability insurance. LPN/LVNs often carry personal liability insurance.

HEALTH CARE SYSTEM AND THE LPN/LVN

The LPN/LVN of today must be equipped with knowledge and skills to function successfully in a health care delivery system. An understanding of leadership, delegation, career opportunities, and ethical and legal considerations will provide a basis to begin your journey in practicing as a LPN/LVN. We wish you well on your journey!

REVIEW QUESTIONS

1. The nurse is preparing a presentation on factors influencing health care changes. Which of the following would be a factor to include in the presentation?
   1. Decreasing use of evidence
   2. Increasing older adult population
   3. Decreasing cultural diversity
   4. Decreasing population size in the United States

2. Which of the following actions should the nurse take during admission and throughout a patient's hospitalization to help ensure reimbursement for a secondary diagnosis occurrence? **Select all that apply.**
   1. Document patient education related to complication prevention.
   2. Photograph wounds that are present on admission.
   3. Educate patients about methods used to prevent complications.
   4. Document interventions, such as turning and ambulating patients.
   5. Explain to patient that participation in preventive interventions is optional.

3. Which of these actions would the nurse correctly interpret as falling within the scope of practice of the LPN/LVN?
   1. Performing a physical assessment on admission for a critical care patient.
   2. Administering IV push morphine.
   3. Ambulating a 1-day postoperative patient.
   4. Developing the plan of care for a newly admitted surgical patient.

4. The nurse would like to suggest a new method for documenting intake and output to the nurse manager, who uses the autocratic leadership style. In approaching the manager, the nurse should understand that the autocratic leader makes decisions in which of the following ways?
   1. Seeks information from all staff members.
   2. Uses own knowledge to decide.
   3. Forms focus groups to gather information.
   4. Forms a staff committee to provide input.

5. During orientation, the newly hired LPN/LVN reviews the agency job description for an LPN/LVN. Which of these situations would be an appropriate example of a leadership role for the LPN/LVN within the job description?
   1. Consulting with an RN to modify care for assigned patient.
   2. Performing an annual employee evaluation for a nursing assistant.
   3. Supervising the RN and LPN/LVN staff on a surgical unit.
   4. Interviewing a new graduate RN for a staff position.

6. The nurse is caring for an adult patient admitted for an appendectomy who asks the nurse not to disclose any personal health information including a positive human immunodeficiency virus (HIV) status. The patient's mother arrives to visit and asks the nurse to explain why her daughter has to take so many medications. Which of the following responses applies the principle of veracity?
   1. "You will have to talk to the HCP."
   2. "The medications are for recovery after a surgical procedure."
   3. "The medications are to treat an infection."
   4. "You will need to ask the patient directly about the medications."

7. A patient with cancer who is having chemotherapy has decided to stop receiving it because the patient has accepted mortality. What is the most ethical response by the nurse to address this situation?
   1. Explain to the patient that it would be silly to stop with only eight more treatments left.
   2. Explain you are going to call a family member to report this decision.
   3. Ensure the patient understands the consequences of discontinuing treatment.
   4. Ensure that the patient knows that without treatment, death will occur.

8. A patient with terminal cancer has an advance directive indicating that a feeding tube is not to be inserted. After the patient becomes unconscious, the patient's family requests that a feeding tube be inserted. Based on a deontological perspective and supporting the patient's autonomy, what action would the nurse anticipate the HCP will take?
   1. Withhold the feeding tube.
   2. Insert the feeding tube.
   3. Order an electroencephalogram (EEG) to determine if the patient will wake up to be asked about the feeding tube.
   4. Place a Do Not Resuscitate (DNR) bracelet on the patient's wrist.

9. The nurse is assisting in the health clinic offering immunizations for school children. A mother asks the nurse why her children need to be immunized for communicable diseases. The nurse explains that when more children are immunized more people are protected from the communicable diseases. This line of thinking supports which ethical theory?
   1. Deontological perspective
   2. Utilitarian perspective
   3. Theological perspective
   4. Autonomy perspective

10. A patient in an extended care facility states that her family does not visit very often. She asks the nurse to give her extra medication so she can die. She states that she's old and no one will mind anyway. What is the nurse's best response?
    1. "Now that is just silly! Go to the activity room; they are playing bingo."
    2. "I'm sorry, but I cannot do that. Do you want to talk about how you are feeling?"
    3. "I can give extra sleeping medicine with lunch so that you can relax more."
    4. "My kids don't visit me often either, I understand how you feel."

11. Nurses must abide by which of the following practice guidelines to ensure they deliver appropriate patient care? **Select all that apply.**
    1. Institutional policies
    2. An organization's code of ethics
    3. State practice laws for nurses
    4. National association nursing standards
    5. Locality nursing standards

12. In providing professional nursing care, the nurse understands that the law of negligence requires which of the following to create liability? **Select all that apply.**
    1. A duty of care owed
    2. Assault
    3. Ethical violations
    4. A breach of duty
    5. Injury and damages
    6. A crime

13. The Health Insurance Portability and Accountability Act of 1996 (HIPAA) requires the nurse to do which of the following?
    1. Maintain continuing nursing education credit hours.
    2. Protect the privacy of an individual's personal health information.
    3. Limit nursing work hours to no more than 35 per week.
    4. Avoid membership in any union or collective bargaining agreement unit.

Answers can be found in Appendix C.

References

Bureau of Labor Statistics, U.S. Department of Labor. *Occupational outlook handbook, 2014–15 edition, licensed practical and licensed vocational nurses.* Retrieved March 3, 2014, from www.bls.gov/ooh/healthcare/licensed-practical-and-licensed-vocational-nurses.htm.

Butts, J. B., Rich, K. L. (2013). *Nursing ethics across the curriculum and into practice* (3rd ed.). Burlington, MA: Jones and Bartlett.

de Veer, A. J. E., Fracke, A. L., Struijs, A., Willems, D. L. (2013). Determinants of moral distress in daily nursing practice: A cross sectional correlational questionnaire survey. *International Journal of Nursing Studies, 50,* 100–108.

Jameton, A. (1984). *Nursing practice: The ethical issues.* Englewood Cliffs, NJ: Prentice-Hall.

National Quality Forum (NQF). (2011). Serious reportable events in healthcare—Update: A Consensus Report. Retrieved July 15, 2013, from www.qualityforum.org/Topics/SREs/List_of_SREs .aspx

Ulrich, C. M., Taylor, C., Soeken, K., O'Donnell, P., Farrar, A., Danis, M., Grady, C. (2010). Everyday ethics: ethical issues and stress in nursing practice. *Journal of Advanced Nursing,* 66(11), 2510–2519.

U.S. Census Bureau. (2010). 2010 Census Data. Retrieved July 20, 2013, from www.census.gov/2010census/data

Resources

• National Association for Practical Nurse Education and Service, Inc., P.O. Box 25647, Alexandria, VA 22313 (www.napnes.org)
• National Federation of Licensed Practical Nurses, Inc., 605 Poole Dr., Garner, NC 27529 (www.nflpn.org)
• Nursing Ethics Network provides a host of links to information on ethical decision making for health care professionals at http://jmrileyrn.tripod.com/nen/nen.html.
• U.S. Department of Health and Human Services. (May, 2003). OCR Privacy Brief: Summary of the HIPAA Privacy Rule. Online. www.hhs.gov/ocr/privacy/hipaa/understanding/summary /privacysummary.pdf

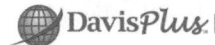 For additional resources and information visit **davispl.us/medsurg5**

Cultural Influences on Nursing Care

BOBBI M. MARTIN

LEARNING OUTCOMES

1. Define common concepts related to culture and ethnicity.
2. List examples of cultural characteristics, values, beliefs, and practices.
3. Describe attributes of culturally diverse patients and their families and how they affect nursing care.
4. Identify data you should collect from culturally diverse patients and their families.
5. Apply a holistic approach to patient care that respects cultural characteristics and attributes.

KEY TERMS

acculturation (uh-KUL-chur-AY-shun)
beliefs (bee-LEEFS)
cultural (KUL-chur-uhl)
cultural assimilation (KUL-chur-uhl uh-SIM-ih-LAY-shun)
cultural awareness (KUL-chur-uhl a-WEAR-ness)
cultural competence (KUL-chur-uhl KOM-pe-tents)
cultural conflict (KUL-chur-uhl KON-flikt)
cultural diversity (KUL-chur-uhl dih-VER-sih-tee)
cultural sensitivity (KUL-chur-uhl SEN-sih-TIV-ih-tee)
cultural shock (KUL-chur-uhl SHOK)
culture (KUL-chur)
customs (KUS-tums)
ethnic (ETH-nick)
ethnocentrism (ETH-noh-SEN-trizm)
generalizations (JEN-er-al-ih-ZAY-shuns)
stereotype (STARE-ee-oh-TIGHP)
traditions (tra-DISH-uns)
values (VAL-yooz)
worldview (WERLD-vyoo)

Your clinical instructor has assigned you to provide care to Mary Waters, a 72-year-old African American woman. Ms. Waters has diabetes and hypertension (high blood pressure). She was admitted to the hospital for gangrene of her left foot. When you enter her room, you find Ms. Waters anxious and crying. She tells you that she is scheduled for surgery later in the day. When asked about her foot, she tells you that she has been applying a poultice to draw out the germs, but it has not worked yet. She adds that she has been praying for the cure that she knows will come. As you are collecting history information about her diabetes, Ms. Waters admits that her doctor told her to attend diabetes classes years ago, but she stopped going because she didn't like what she heard. She quickly changes the subject, wanting to talk about nothing but her grandchildren. Your attempts to complete preoperative teaching are unsuccessful.

Can you think of examples of cultural practices you have seen in your experience that were unique or different from your own? Cultural diversity in the United States is increasing. According to the U.S. Census Bureau, 50.4% of our nation's population younger than age 1 as of July 1, 2011, were minorities (Bernstein, 2012). Immigration from Spanish-speaking and Asian countries has resulted in dramatic shifts in census numbers. Figure 4.1 illustrates the changes and projections in racial and ethnic makeup in the United States by 2050. As a result, **cultural** and **ethnic** differences between nurses and their patients are becoming more evident and must be recognized. More than ever, nurses must develop cultural awareness and apply cultural competence to practice. This chapter provides you with the basics of culture and its impact on health promotion and wellness.

CONCEPTS RELATED TO CULTURE

Culture refers to the socially transmitted behavior patterns, beliefs, values, customs, arts, and all other characteristics of people that guide their view of the world (**worldview**). Cultural beliefs, values, **customs**, and **traditions** are primarily learned within the family on an unconscious level. They can also be learned from the communities in which we live, from religious organizations, and in schools.

As you try to understand more about culture, keep in mind that it contains a number of characteristics (Box 4-1). All individuals and groups have the right to maintain cultural practices that they feel are appropriate, as long as they don't infringe on rights of others. However, as you will learn from this chapter, nurses must be aware of cultural health practices that can cause physical harm and require nursing intervention. Culture has strong influences on a patient's understanding of health and how he or she will respond to nursing care. You must understand how culture influences health behaviors to better meet the needs of your patients (Fig. 4.2). As you learn more about ethnic and cultural groups, you will be challenged to look at the differences and similarities across cultures.

Consider our patient, Ms. Waters. Did she behave as you would have in a similar situation? How do you think the characteristics of her culture affected her behavior? Can you think of how you could have used the information she shared to engage her in learning more about her upcoming surgery?

Although the terms *cultural sensitivity, cultural awareness,* and *cultural competence* are similar, they have different meanings. **Cultural sensitivity** is knowing politically correct language and not making statements that may offend another person's cultural beliefs. **Cultural awareness** focuses on history and ancestry and emphasizes an appreciation for and attention to arts, music, crafts, celebrations, foods, and traditional clothing. **Cultural competence** includes the skills and knowledge required to provide effective nursing care. To be culturally competent, you need to:

• Have an awareness of your own culture and not let it have an undue influence on your patient care.

Percent of the Population, by Race and Hispanic Origin: 1990, 2000, 2025, and 2050
(Middle-series projections)

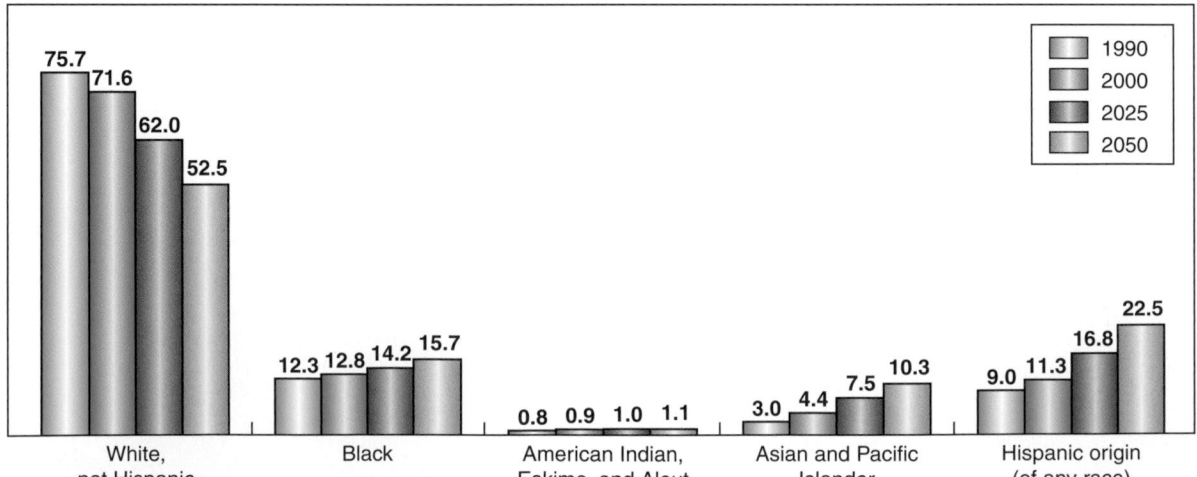

FIGURE 4.1 Percent of the population of the United States, by race and Hispanic origin. (*Source: U.S. Census Bureau, Population Division; retrieved August 15, 2009, from www.census.gov/population/www/pop-profile/natproj.html.*)

Box 4-1 Characteristics of Culture

- *Culture is learned.* Learning occurs through life experiences shared with other members of the culture.
- *Culture is taught.* Cultural values, beliefs, and traditions are passed down from generation to generation either formally (e.g., in schools) or informally (e.g., in families)
- *Culture is shared by its members.* Cultural norms are shared through teachings and social interactions.
- *Culture is dynamic and adaptive.* Cultural customs, beliefs, and practices are not static but change over time and at different rates. Cultural change occurs with adaptation in response to the environment.
- *Culture is complex.* Cultural assumptions and habits are unconscious, which may make them difficult for members of the culture to explain to others.
- *Culture is diverse.* Culture demonstrates the variety that exists between groups and among members of a particular group.
- *Culture exists at many levels.* Culture exists at material (e.g., art, dress, or artifacts) and nonmaterial (as language, traditions, customs, beliefs, and practices) levels.
- *Culture has common beliefs and practices.* Members of a culture share the same beliefs, traditions, customs, and practices as long as they continue to be adaptive and satisfy their needs. Some members do not always follow all of these, but many do.
- *Culture is all encompassing.* Culture can affect everything its members think and do.
- *Culture provides identity.* Cultural beliefs provide identity for members as long as there is no conflict with the dominant culture or lack of gratification by its members.

- Have specific knowledge about your patient's culture.
- Accept and respect cultural differences.
- Adapt your nursing care (when appropriate) to your patient's culture.

We will discuss more about cultural competence later in the chapter.

Although you may have knowledge about another culture, barriers such as ethnocentrism and stereotyping can keep you from appreciating cultural differences. **Ethnocentrism** is the tendency for humans to think that their ways of thinking, acting, and believing are the only right, proper, and natural ways. Ethnocentrism perpetuates an attitude that beliefs that differ greatly from your own are strange or bizarre and therefore wrong. Additionally, you must be careful not to stereotype your patient. A **stereotype** is an opinion or belief about a group of people that is ascribed to an individual. For example, the statement "All Chinese people prefer traditional Chinese medicine" is a stereotype. This stereotype is not true. Although many Chinese people may prefer traditional Chinese medicine for some health conditions, not all Chinese people prefer traditional Chinese medicine. However, you can still make **generalizations** about an ethnic person without stereotyping. Although a generalization or assumption may be true for the group, it does not necessarily fit every individual. Therefore, you must seek additional information to determine whether the generalization fits the individual. The challenge is for you to understand the patient's cultural perspective. If you have specific cultural knowledge, you can improve therapeutic interventions by becoming a coparticipant with patients and their families. To do this, it is important that you develop a personal, open style of communication and be receptive to learning from patients from cultures other than your own (Fig. 4.3).

A few additional terms important for your understanding of culture relate to the socialization process of those who are learning to become a member of a society or group. When

FIGURE 4.2 The nurse must assess patients' unique needs related to their cultural backgrounds.

FIGURE 4.3 Health care providers and patients may come from a variety of cultural backgrounds.

people immigrate to a new country, many gradually accept the new culture through a learning process. They learn to accept their own beliefs as well as those of their new country. This is known as **acculturation**. Acculturation is commonly seen in second-generation immigrants because they not only understand the necessity of learning their new culture, but also see the value of it. Learning the new culture helps individuals survive, and more importantly, thrive in their new environment. **Cultural assimilation** occurs when a new member takes on the dominant culture's values, beliefs, and practices, sometimes at the cost of losing some of his or her cultural heritage. This process is often viewed as negative.

Imagine for a moment that you have moved to China. At first you eat the food and try to understand the language of your new country. Over time, you may learn to cook the food, speak the language, and perhaps blend some of the Chinese beliefs, traditions, and practices with your own. This is acculturation. However, this process is not always smooth. When one's own culture conflicts with a new culture, **cultural conflict** occurs. Worse than that, **cultural shock** can happen when values, beliefs, and practices sanctioned by the new culture are very different from the ones of the native culture.

Let's look at another example. Ling Chi is a 4-year-old boy who is a recent immigrant enrolled in a new school. He is alone and afraid, although he is surrounded by other boys and girls his age. It is lunchtime, and while his teacher is trying to help him with his food, he starts crying. The fork and spoon are foreign to him. At home he is used to eating his lunch with chopsticks. In addition, he does not understand the words spoken to him. Ling Chi is experiencing cultural shock.

HEALTH CARE VALUES, BELIEFS, AND PRACTICES

Cultural values, beliefs, and practices about the nature of disease and the human body are central in the delivery of health services, treatments, and preventive interventions (Office of Minority Health, 2010). A **value** can be defined as a principle or standard that has meaning or worth to an individual (Purnell & Paulanka, 2008). Values can help shape one's beliefs and practices. Do you know what your values are regarding health and illness? "Cleanliness" is an example of a value. A **belief** is something that a person accepts as true (e.g., "I believe that germs cause illness and disease"). A *practice* is a set of behaviors that one follows—for example, washing hands before eating. It is important for you to understand the differences between these terms because we will be discussing them as they relate to cultural groups.

Consider our patient Mrs. Waters again. Can you think of cultural values, beliefs, or practices she has that may influence why she may not want to attend diabetes classes or learn more about her upcoming surgery?

To provide culturally competent care, you need to know how the people you encounter define health and illness. In general, people follow one of three major health belief systems: scientific (Western medicine or biomedical), spiritual, or holistic. You are already familiar with the scientific health system, which dominates health care in Western societies. Belief in supernatural forces dominates the spiritual system, which is considered by many to be an alternative health care system. (Some experts call this magico-religious, but this is an offensive term to some religious persons.) The holistic belief system focuses on the need for balance and harmony of the body and spirit with nature.

Health care typically focuses on health promotion, the prevention of illness, and acute illness care while considering traditional, religious, and biomedical (scientific) beliefs. Additionally, individual responsibility for health, self-medicating practices, views toward mental illness, response to pain, and the sick role are shaped by one's culture. Most societies combine biomedical health care with traditional, folk, and religious practices such as praying for good health or wearing charms or amulets to ward off illness. There are many examples of folk practices for curing or treating specific illnesses. Think for a minute about such practices that you may perform. What do you do for a fever or a sore throat? Does chicken noodle soup come to mind? Many times folk therapies are handed down from family members and may have their roots in religious beliefs. Examples of folk therapies include covering a boil with axle grease or wearing copper bracelets for arthritic pain. As you will see in Chapter 5, many people use complementary therapies such as acupressure or herbal remedies in addition to traditional Western therapies.

Often folk practices are not harmful and can be added to the patient's plan of care. However, some therapies may conflict with prescription medications, or cause a toxic effect. Other folk practices may actually cause physical harm to a patient. It is essential to inquire about the full range of therapies being used by your patients, such as food items, teas, herbal remedies, nonfood substances, over-the-counter (OTC) medications, medications prescribed by others, and medications borrowed from others.

If patients sense that you do not accept their beliefs and practices, they may be less open to sharing information and less adherent to prescribed treatment. Your goal is to try to encourage your patients' practices that could be helpful and discourage those that may be harmful. Before encouraging or discouraging such practices, you will need to discuss them with the appropriate health care team member.

Think about Ms. Waters. Does she use any folk practices? Where can you find more information about her specific folk practices? How would you address this specific situation?

Before moving on, we need to discuss the subjects of mental illness and cultural responses to pain and the sick role. Mental illness may be seen by some as being unimportant compared with physical illness. Mental illness is culture bound. What may be perceived as a mental illness in one society may not be considered a mental illness in another society. Among some cultures, having a mental illness or an emotional difficulty is considered a disgrace and is taboo. As a result, a family is likely to keep a person who is mentally ill at home as long as they possibly can.

Cultural responses to pain and the sick role can vary among cultures. For example, some people are expected to openly express their pain. Others are expected to suffer their pain in silence. For some, the sick role is readily accepted, and any excuse is accepted for not fulfilling daily obligations. Others minimize their illness and make extended efforts to fulfill their obligations despite being ill.

Nursing Assessment

To begin your assessment of your patient's health beliefs, ask the following questions:

- What do you usually do to maintain your health?
- What do you usually do when you are sick?
- What kind of home treatments do you use when you are sick?
- Who is the first person you see when you are sick?
- What do you do when you have pain?
- Do you wear charms or bracelets to ward off illness?
- Do you take herbs or drink special teas when you are sick? If so, what are they?
- Do you practice special rituals or prayers to maintain your health?

 ## CHARACTERISTICS OF CULTURAL DIVERSITY

Primary and secondary characteristics of diversity affect how people view their culture. Primary characteristics of **cultural diversity** include nationality, race, skin color, gender, age, and religious affiliation. Secondary characteristics include socioeconomic status, education, occupation, military experience, political beliefs, length of time away from the country of origin, urban versus rural residence, marital status, parental status, physical characteristics, sexual orientation, and gender issues.

Culturally appropriate care needs to take into account eight cultural phenomena that may vary with use but can be seen in all cultural groups:

1. communication styles
2. space
3. time orientation
4. social organization
5. environmental control/health beliefs
6. choice of health care providers (HCPs)
7. biological variations
8. death and dying issues.

Communication Styles

Communication occurs both verbally and nonverbally. Verbal communication includes spoken language, dialects, and voice volume. Dialects are variations in grammar, word meanings, and pronunciation of spoken language. Nonverbal communication includes the use and degree of eye contact, the perception of time, and physical closeness when talking with peers and perceived superiors. In some societies, people are expected to maintain eye contact without staring, which shows

that they are listening and can be trusted. However, in other societies, as a sign of respect, people should not maintain eye contact with superiors such as teachers and those in positions of higher status.

Nursing Assessment and Strategies

Ask the following questions:

- By what name do you prefer to be called?
- What language do you speak at home?
- Are you able to read and write in English?
- If not, what language is preferred?

Be sure to do the following:

- Take cues from the patient for voice volume.
- Be an active listener, and become comfortable with silence.
- Avoid appearing rushed.
- Be formal with greetings until told to do otherwise.
- Take greeting cues from the patient.
- Speak slowly and clearly. Do not speak loudly or with exaggerated mouthing.
- Explain why you are asking specific questions.
- Give reasons for treatments.
- Repeat questions if needed.
- Provide written instructions in the patient's preferred language.
- Obtain an interpreter if needed.

HCPs should refrain from relying on untrained individuals to interpret, especially family members (see "Evidence-Based Practice"). Although it may seem logical that a patient's best advocate is his or her family, it is risky to rely on family members to interpret medical or health information for the following reasons:

- Family members may not be proficient in medical terminology.
- They may not possess the skills needed to interpret.
- They may unintentionally or intentionally omit or alter important information.
- Using family members to interpret may raise privacy issues protected by the Health Insurance Portability and Accountability Act of 1996 (HIPAA).
- If children are used, they may not be emotionally mature enough to handle the information being conveyed.

 ## EVIDENCE-BASED PRACTICE

Clinical Question
Do patients with limited English proficiency who have professional interpreters experience improved clinical care over those who use ad hoc or family member interpreters?

Evidence
The likelihood of medical errors is significantly reduced by the use of professional interpreters

versus not using interpreters or the use of ad hoc interpreters. Ad hoc interpreters were much more likely to make errors that led to serious medical problems than professionally trained interpreters (Flores, Abreu, Barone, Bachur, & Lin, 2012).

Implications for Nursing Practice

National Standards on Culturally and Linguistically Appropriate Services recommends that cultural and linguistic appropriate services should be integrated throughout an organization (Office of Minority Health, 2012). Additionally, organizations are required by law to provide language access services to individuals with limited English proficiency (Joint Commission, 2008). Addressing communication barriers is an important task for nurses as caregivers and patient advocates. Nurses can be aware of the populations they serve and have interpreters available to facilitate communication. This is done through face-to-face interpretation, via phone, or via video. Nurses can also ensure there are written materials in the patients' native language, especially for discharge instructions. The Joint Commission provides direction and support for HCPs to use health information technology to bridge the cultural gap between HCPs and patients. They note that caregivers who have access to health information technology systems provide better care with improved outcomes (Lopez, Green, Tan-McGrory, King, & Betancourt, 2011).

Tips for Using Interpreters

Address the patient, not the interpreter.
Do not interrupt the patient and the
    interpreter.
Ask the interpreter to give you exact
    translations.
Avoid using medical jargon.

REFERENCES

Flores, G., Abreu, M., Barone, C. P., Bachur, R., & Lin, H. (2012). Errors of medical interpretation and their potential clinical consequences: A comparison of professional versus as hoc versus no interpreters. *Annals of Emergency Medicine, 50*, 545–553.

Joint Commission. (2008). Promoting effective communication: Language access services in health care. *Joint Commission Perspectives, 28*, 811. Retrieved March 24, 2009, from www.jointcommission.org/NR/rdonlyres /ACAFA57F-5F50-427A-BB98-73431D68A5E4/0 /Perspectives_Article_Feb_2008.pdf

López, L., Green, A. R., Tan-McGrory, A., King, R., & Betancourt, J. R. (2011). Bridging the digital divide in health care: The role of health information technology in addressing racial and ethnic disparities. *Joint Commission Journal on Quality and Patient Safety, 37*, 437–445.

Office of Minority Health, U.S. Department of Health and Human Services. (2012). National Standards for Culturally and Linguistically Appropriate Services (CLAS) in Health and Health Care. Retrieved May 15, 2013 from www .thinkculturalhealth.hhs.gov/pdfs/EnhancedNational CLASStandards.pdf

Space

Space refers to one's "personal space." Are you aware of your comfort zone? In other words, how close can someone get to you before you feel less safe and secure? Like you, most people have such a comfort zone. Personal space tends to be different when speaking with close friends versus strangers, and it also differs across cultures. For example, people from the Middle East tend to stand close together when talking, whereas those from European countries, such as Germany, require a much larger space. The need for space is important for the patient's privacy, autonomy, security, and self-identity. Understanding what space means for your patients can be important when you are trying to assess, treat, and teach them.

Nursing Assessment and Strategies

Ask the following questions:

• Are you comfortable?
• Do you have any concerns you would like to discuss?

    Be sure to do the following:

• Make sure your patients are comfortable before you interview them.
• Maintain appropriate physical distance (observe for cues).
• Be aware of cultural differences.
• Be aware of physical objects that may be a barrier to comfort.
• Make sure that the patient's physical environment is arranged to ensure safety, security, and familiarity.

Time Orientation

Time orientation can vary among people from different cultures. The perception of time has two dimensions. The first dimension is related to clock time versus social time. For example, some cultures have a flexible orientation to time and events, and appointments take place when the person arrives. An event scheduled for 1400 may not begin until 1430 or when a majority of the participants arrive. For others, time is less flexible, and appointments and social events are expected to start at the agreed-on time. For many, social events may be flexible, whereas medical appointments and business engagements start on time.

The second dimension of time relates to whether the culture is predominantly concerned with the past, present, or future. Past-oriented individuals maintain traditions that were meaningful in the past and may worship ancestors. Present-oriented people accept the day as it comes, with little regard for the past; the future is unpredictable. Future-oriented people anticipate a bigger and better future and place a high value on change. Some people balance all three views—they respect the past, enjoy living in the present, and plan for the future.

Hospitals, clinics, and HCPs' offices maintain a tight time schedule. It is therefore important that you understand patients' time orientation so you can prepare them for the timing of appointments, tests, and treatments. In addition, it is important that you assess their usual routines so that you can incorporate these as much as possible into their daily care.

Nursing Assessment and Strategies

Ask the following questions to understand your patients' time orientation:

- Are you normally on time for appointments?
- Are there any routines that you need to follow?
- What time do you usually eat your meals? Take your bath?

Be sure to do the following:

- Have a clock in the patient's room.
- Assess for orientation, and reorient to time as needed.
- Prepare patients before a procedure or test.
- Give time options when appropriate. ("Would you like to take a walk now or in an hour?")

Social Organization

Family organization includes the perceived head of the household, gender roles, and roles of the older and extended family members. The household may be patriarchal (male dominated), matriarchal (female dominated), or egalitarian (shared equally between men and women). An awareness of the family dominance pattern is important for determining which family member to speak to when health care decisions have to be made. Confidentiality issues can complicate this issue. Be sure to follow your institution's policies when communicating with family members. You may need to obtain the patient's permission before planning care with family members.

In some cultures, specific roles are outlined for men and women. Men are expected to protect and provide for the family, manage finances, and deal with the outside world. Women are expected to maintain the home environment, including child care and household tasks. You must accept that not all societies share or even desire an egalitarian family structure.

Roles for older adults and extended family vary among culturally diverse groups. In some cultures, older adults are seen as being wise, are deferred to for making decisions, and are held in high esteem. Their children are expected to provide for them when they are no longer able to care for themselves. In other cultures, although older people may be loved by family members, they may not be given such high regard and may be cared for outside the home when self-care becomes a concern.

The extended family is very important in some groups, and a single household may include several generations living together out of desire rather than out of necessity. The extended family may include both blood-related and non–blood-related persons who are given family status. In other families, each generation lives in a separate home or living space.

You can assist your patients with their treatment plans when you have a better understanding of their family dynamics. It is important to know whom to include for planning of care, discharge planning, and patient teaching.

Nursing Assessment and Strategies

Ask the following questions:

- Who makes the decisions in your household?
- Who takes care of money matters, does the cooking, or is responsible for child care?
- Who decides when it is time to see a HCP?
- Who lives in your household? Are they all blood related?

Be sure to do the following:

- Observe the use of touch between family members.
- Let family members decide where they want to stand or sit for comfort.

Environmental Control

Environmental control consists of three major concepts: people's perception of their ability to control what happens to them and their health, their beliefs about health and illness, and their beliefs in alternative health care therapies such as folk medicine. For example, if a person does not believe he has control of his health, he may not be receptive to nursing interventions that require self-confidence, such as self-administration of insulin. Regarding health beliefs, if a person believes that illness is due to a spiritual cause and not bacteria, he or she may not understand the need to take antibiotics. Third, many people put great faith in folk healing practices. Nurses need to consider their patient's cultural values and beliefs, especially if they are different from the dominant Western health care view.

Distinctions are made between health and illness and what people do to promote or maintain health and to prevent and treat illnesses. Not all of your patients will turn to a Western health care system or provider. Many people try some form of alternative therapy before seeking treatment. People also use alternative therapies and religious systems such as prayer in combination with the scientific medical system. Religious beliefs and practices may be important to patients (Fig. 4.4).

Nursing Assessment and Strategies

Ask the following questions:

- How do you define health? Illness?
- Do you have any special beliefs about health and illness?
- What do you do to keep well?
- When you feel ill, what is the first thing you do to get better?
- How do you deal with pain?
- How do you and your family express grief?
- Are there any cultural beliefs or practices that I need to know about to plan your care?

FIGURE 4.4 Religious artifacts are central to many people's health and illness practices.

Be sure to do the following:

• Be aware of possible cultural beliefs and practices.
• Never stereotype based on what you know about different cultures; always ask for specific information.
• Perform a cultural assessment on all of your patients.
• Ask if patients have received treatments of any kind for their illness.
• Ask about religious beliefs and practices.
• Encourage helpful practices and discourage those that are harmful.

Health Care Providers

HCP choices are made based on the patient's perceived status and previous use of traditional, religious, and biomedical HCPs. In Western societies, educated HCPs are treated with great respect. However, some people prefer traditional healers because they are known to the patient, family, and community.

It is important to respect differences in gender relationships when providing care. Some people may be especially modest because of their religion, seeking out same-gender nurses and HCPs for intimate care. Respect these patients' modesty by providing privacy and assigning a same-gender care provider when possible.

Nursing Assessment and Strategies

Ask the following questions of your patients:

• What HCPs besides physicians and nurses do you see when you are ill?
• Do you object to male or female HCPs giving physical care to you?

Be sure to do the following:

• Observe for alternative care providers who may visit the patient in the health care facility.

Biological Variations

The term *biological variations* refers to ways in which people are different from one another physiologically and genetically. These differences can make them more susceptible to certain illnesses and diseases and may also influence the effectiveness of different medications. Biological variations can include differences in (1) body build and structure, (2) skin color, (3) vital

signs, (4) laboratory values, (5) susceptibility to disease, and (6) nutrition. Darker skin color can challenge you to be more observant when you are assessing the skin color of your patient. Laboratory test results can also be different in a number of cultures. For example, American Indians and Hispanic Americans may have higher blood glucose levels than whites.

The term *biological variations* also refers to differences in nutritional practices. Nutritional practices are currently being scrutinized in our society. These practices include the personal meaning of food, food choices and rituals, food taboos, and how food and food substances are used for health promotion and wellness. Cultural beliefs influence what people eat or avoid. In addition to being important for survival, food offers security and acceptance, plays a significant role in socialization, and can serve as an expression of love.

Culturally congruent dietary counseling, such as adapting preparation practices and including ethnic food choices, can reduce health risks. Whenever possible, you should determine a patient's current dietary practices. Culturally diverse patients may refuse to eat on a schedule of American mealtimes or to eat American foods. Counseling about food group requirements or dietary restrictions must respect an individual's cultural background. Most cultures have their own nutritional practices for health promotion and disease prevention. For many, a balance of different types of foods is important for maintaining health and preventing illness. A thorough history and assessment of dietary practices can be an important diagnostic tool to guide health promotion.

Nursing Assessment and Strategies

Ask the following questions of your patients:

• Are you at risk for any diseases or genetic disorders related to your cultural background?
• Are you satisfied with your weight?
• Are you active? What is your normal exercise pattern?
• Do you protect your eyes and skin from the sun? From possible injuries?
• Do you have any drug or food allergies?
• Has anyone in your family had any major illnesses?
• What do you eat to stay healthy?
• What do you eat when you are ill?
• Are there certain foods that you do not eat? Why?
• Do certain foods cause you to become ill? What are they?
• Who purchases the food in your household?
• Who prepares the food in your household?

Be sure to do the following:

• Teach about biological variations that may pertain to your patient.
• Determine and respect usual eating patterns whenever possible.
• Teach good nutrition habits, taking into account patient preferences. Refer to a dietitian if appropriate.

Death and Dying and End-of-Life Issues

Death rituals of cultural groups are the least likely to change over time. To avoid cultural taboos, you must become knowledgeable about rituals surrounding death and bereavement. For some, the body should be buried whole. Therefore, an amputated limb may be buried in the amputee's future gravesite, and organ donation would probably not be acceptable. Cremation may be preferred for some, whereas for others, it is taboo and burial is the preferred practice. Views on autopsy vary. Some cultural groups have elaborate ceremonies that last for days in commemoration of the dead. To some these rituals appear to be a celebration, and in a sense, they are a celebration of the person's life rather than a mourning of the person's death. If you are uncertain, find out from the family if there is anything that the health care team can do to facilitate cultural practices.

The expression of grief in response to death varies within and among cultural and ethnic groups. For example, in some cultures, loved ones are expected to suffer the grief of death in silence, with little display of emotion. In other cultures, loved ones are expected to display elaborate emotions to show that they cared for the deceased. These variations in the grieving process may cause confusion if you perceive some people as overreacting and others as not caring. You must accept that culturally diverse behaviors are associated with the grieving process. Bereavement support strategies include being physically present, encouraging reality orientation, openly acknowledging the family's right to grieve as they need to, helping the family express their feelings, encouraging interpersonal relationships, promoting interest in a new life, and making referrals to other staff and spiritual leaders as appropriate.

At times you may be involved with end-of-life decisions. Some of these may include advance directives, resuscitation status, and organ transplantation. Collaborate with the RN or HCP to ensure cultural preferences are respected.

Nursing Assessment and Strategies

Ask the following questions of your patients:

- What are the usual burial practices in your family?
- What are your feelings about autopsy?

Be sure to do the following:

- Observe expressions of grief. Support the family in their expression of grief.
- Observe for differences in the expression of grief among family members.
- Offer to obtain a religious counselor/spiritual leader if the family wishes.

 ETHNIC AND CULTURAL GROUPS IN THE UNITED STATES

This section describes selected attributes of some of the cultural groups in the U.S. These groups include European American (white), Spanish/Hispanic/Latino, African American (black), American Indian/Alaskan Native, Arab American, Asian American, and Native Hawaiian or Other Pacific Islander. The groups described here by no means represent all the cultural groups in North America; they do, however, represent the largest

population percentages in the United States. As of the 2010 census, the U.S. federal government initiated new terminology for classifying people of diverse racial and ethnic backgrounds. This terminology is used in this section.

Attributes presented for each group include communication styles, space, time orientation, social organization, environmental control, biological variation, health care beliefs, traditional HCPs, and death and dying issues. Racial and ethnic biological variations, susceptibility to disease, and genetic diseases are covered to a greater extent elsewhere in this textbook (see "Gerontological Issues").

Gerontological Issues

Aging, Ethnicity, Health, and Illness

Compared with white or European American older adults, ethnic minorities are more likely to:
- Live in poverty
- Experience debilitating disease processes or functional disability at a higher rate and at an earlier age
- Have greater difficulty accessing health care services
- Be underserved for physical and mental health problems.

By 2030, the number of older adults will double. The largest growth will be among minorities. Remember that to provide culturally competent care older adults need to be assessed within their personal cultural context. Avoid generalizing cultural practices to individuals or families without first assessing whether this practice or belief is true for the individual. For example, it would be wrong to assume that an older Mexican American woman who lives with her extended family will receive the family's support for assistance with bathing and other activities of daily living. If an older Chinese woman uses herbs and folk treatments for common complaints, it does not mean that she will not use the services, treatments, or medications of Western medicine. Always assess individual and family preferences.

European American

European American is the term used to describe people living in the United States whose heritage is from western, southern, and northern Europe. European American groups include the white ethnic groups. Many of the descendants of these original European immigrants practice the unique attributes of the subcultures from which they originate. There is much diversity in the primary and secondary characteristics of diversity within this cultural group.

Many European Americans maintain the value of individualism over group norms and are activity-oriented. Most European Americans practice Western medicine, which values advanced technology and evidence-based practice (Table 4.1).

(Text continued on page 53)

TABLE 4.1 HEALTH CARE CONSIDERATIONS FOR SPECIFIC CULTURAL GROUPS IN THE U.S.*

	European American (White)	Spanish/ Hispanics/ Latino	African American (Black)	American Indian/ Alaskan Native	Arab American	Asian Americans	Native Hawaiian/ Pacific Islander
Communication	Primary language is usually English; often speak own national language. Eye contact should be maintained, without staring. Loud voice volume is the norm. Readily shares personal information.	Primary language English, Spanish, or Portuguese (many dialects). Dramatic body language. Some believe direct eye contact can cause illness ("evil eye").	Primary language is usually English. May speak "black English" occasionally depending on the situation. Usually loud voice volume. Nonverbal communication important; direct eye contact may be interpreted as aggression.	English, tribal languages. Talking loudly may be considered rude. Use body language. Avoid eye contact. Comfortable with long periods of silence. Information should be given over time, allowing adequate time to process information.	Primary language is Arabic. Most speak some English. May use spirited, loud voice. May be reluctant to disclose personal information. Maintain intense eye contact.	English (may prefer national language and specific to each country); many dialects. Loud talking is considered rude. Silence is acceptable. Avoid eye contact. Avoid use of "no."	English (may prefer national language); many dialects Prefer indirect communication style (feelings such as disappointment or anger may not be appropriate for expression). Do not use first names unless invited. It is appropriate to express ignorance about their culture and show concern for a meaningful interaction. A simple greeting in the native language goes a long way to open the relationship.
Space	Depends on area; tend to avoid physical closeness. Handshake proper.	Value physical closeness and touching.	Close personal space. Touch frequently with friends, less so with strangers. Touching another's hair considered improper.	Space very important; has no boundaries. Touch is not acceptable from strangers. Pointing and direct eye contact may be considered rude.	Stand very close when talking. Touch only between same gender.	Avoid physical closeness and touching.	Avoid physical closeness and touching.

Time Orientation	Future over present.	Present.	Present over future.	Usually present.	Present or future.	Present.	Present.
Social Organization	Nuclear family basic, extended family important. Man dominant figure. Judeo-Christian religions. Community social organizations important. Many concerned with status.	Nuclear family basic, extended family highly valued. Man is decision maker; woman is homemaker. Catholicism.	Many female single-parent families, often matriarchal. Large, extended families important. Strong social and church affiliations. Protestant (often Baptist).	Extended family basic unit. Very family oriented. Elders honored. Strong community affiliations. Sacred myths and legends.	Patriarchal household, with well-defined gender roles. Elders respected and cared for by family. Extended family important; may live in close proximity to each other. May be Christian, Jewish, or Muslim.	High value on immediate and extended family. Hierarchical family structure. Family honor and loyalty honored. Tradition important. Male has power; woman is obedient. High value placed on children and education. Christianity, Buddhism, Taoism, and Islamic religions.	High emphasis on group and the hierarchy within the group. Rights of the group outweigh rights of the individual. Always demonstrate respect as elders are revered. Elders will defer to their adult children to make health-related decisions or judgments.
Environmental Control/Health Beliefs **HCPs**	Rely mainly on modern health care system. Value individual responsibility for health. Believe humans can control nature. Have strong belief and value in technology. Most use alternative remedies or OTCs before seeing an HCP. Use prayers and religious symbols for good health.	Traditional health and illness beliefs. Folk medicine traditions. Health beliefs are strongly affected by religion, believing in God's will. May have shrines or statues in the home to pray for good health. Theory of hot and cold foods used for health maintenance and treatment of disease.	Traditional health and illness beliefs. General distrust of health care professionals, providers, and the health care system. Folk medicine tradition. May believe that serious illness sent from God. Use prayers for prevention and health recovery. Pain is seen as a sign of illness.	Traditional health and illness beliefs. Folk medicine traditions. Promote harmony with nature. Inanimate objects ward off evil spirits. Older adults may request same-gender direct-care provider. Pain is something to be endured. Sick role not usually supported.	Focus on acute care over prevention. Illness may be considered punishment for sins. May pray five times a day for health. Acceptable to purchase organs for transplantation. Sick role supported. Food is eaten with the right hand, which is considered "clean." May fast while hospitalized.	Traditional health and illness beliefs. Traditional medicine traditions. Good health is a gift from ancestors. Imbalances in the yin and yang cause illness. Believe blood is the source of life and is not replenished. Amulets worn to ward off disease.	Traditional health and illness beliefs. Some societies have great respect for physicians. Physician visits are infrequent; it may be difficult to gain compliance with follow up care for chronic illness.

Continued

TABLE 4.1 HEALTH CARE CONSIDERATIONS FOR SPECIFIC CULTURAL GROUPS IN THE U.S.*—cont'd

	European American (White)	Spanish/Hispanics/Latino	African American (Black)	American Indian/Alaskan Native	Arab American	Asian Americans	Native Hawaiian/Pacific Islander
	Have controlled expression of pain but need little encouragement to accept pain relief. Sick role not well accepted except with a major illness. Traditional healers: Western-educated HCPs; recent trend to use complementary therapists.	Expressive with pain. Easily enter the sick role. Traditional healers: curandero, espiritista, patera, señora.	Sick role not seen as a burden. Folk healers. A respected older adult female community member commonly sought for initial health care. Traditional healers: spiritualists, voodoo priest or priestess, root doctor.	Traditional healers: shamans, medicine man, diviners, crystal gazers.	Eating and drinking at the same time is considered unhealthy. Traditional healers: Western-educated HCPs; may prefer same sex caregivers.	Traditional healers: doctors, herbalists, acupuncturists who use such therapies as acupuncture, acumassage, coining, and cupping.	Older patients from specific Pacific regions my use cultural guides or clan leaders such as a "Kahuna lapa'au" (priest who heals with medicines). A belief illness is due to an imbalance in physical, mental/emotional, and spiritual.
Biological Variations	Nutritional preferences include meats (especially red) and carbohydrates. Diets tend to be high in fat and sodium. Eating and drinking may be social rituals. Culture stresses thinness as attractive.	Nutritional preferences include spicy and fried foods, beans, and rice. Important for food to be served warm. May subscribe to hot and cold theory of illness (e.g., caused when body is exposed to imbalance of hot/cold substances).	Nutritional preferences include fried foods, barbecued foods, greens, legumes. Diet commonly high in fat and sodium. Food selections may vary according to socioeconomic status and rural versus urban residence. Being overweight is seen as positive.	Nutritional preferences vary greatly depending on location and tribe. Nontraditional diets tend to be high in fat and commonly lack fruits and vegetables. Herbs used to cleanse the body of evil spirits and poison.	Nutritional preferences include fresh meats and vegetables; may avoid pork and alcohol (Islam). Less likely than general population to smoke, drink alcohol, or use illicit drugs. High risk for diabetes, hypertension, hypercholesterolemia.	Nutritional preferences include raw fish and rice. Foods are balanced between yin and yang. Diet is high in salt. Food is fundamental form of socialization. Susceptibility: lactose intolerance, thalassemia, liver and stomach cancer, hypertension, coccidioidomycosis.	Nutritional preferences include tubers, fruit, fish and coconut. Susceptibility includes: obesity, type 2 diabetes, hypertension and their resulting cardiovascular and cerebrovascular diseases. Heart valve disorders may be present as rheumatic fever and rheumatic heart

	Susceptibility: heart disease, breast cancer, diabetes mellitus, thalassemia, Tay-Sachs disease (Eastern European Jewish).	Susceptibility: keloid formation, lactose intolerance, sickle cell anemia, glucose-6-phosphate dehydrogenase deficiency, thalassemia, sarcoidosis, hypertension, coccidioidomycosis, esophageal and stomach cancers.	Food choices vary by specific country. Being overweight may be considered healthy. Susceptibility: lactose intolerance, diabetes mellitus, parasites, coccidioidomycosis, gout.	Food is seen as a symbol of health and wealth. Susceptibility: heart disease, alcoholism, liver disease, diabetes mellitus, tuberculosis, arthritis, glaucoma.	...disease continue to remain problems in the Pacific Islands. Alcohol and drug abuse is prevalent.	
Death and Dying Issues	Autopsy and burial or cremation usually connected with religious practices or individual preferences. Have varied expressions of grief. Men are expected to be in more control during grief than women.	Burial is the usual practice, rarely cremation; many resist autopsy, the body should be buried whole. May have elaborate ceremonial burial. Women very expressive with grief; men are expected to maintain control.	Believe body should go into the afterlife whole. Some engage in a cleansing ceremony after touching a dead body. Tribal laws may dictate cremation versus burial. Openly express grief. Death does not end connection between people; body is kept intact after death; prefer no autopsy. Relatives may communicate with the dead person.	Believe death is God's will. At time of death, bed should face the holy city of Mecca (for Muslims). May perform ritual washing of the body after death. Cremation or autopsy not acceptable. May weep with grief, but limited.	Autopsy not understood by many. Cremation acceptable, but burial also common. Extended grieving time (7 to 30 days) for the more traditional. Expression of grief is highly varied between men and women and among specific countries.	Adapt to change and death is seen as a part of life. There is a belief of a combined body, mind, and spiritual existence.

TABLE 4.1   HEALTH CARE CONSIDERATIONS FOR SPECIFIC CULTURAL GROUPS IN THE U.S.*—cont'd

	European American (White)	Spanish/ Hispanics/ Latino	African American (Black)	American Indian/ Alaskan Native	Arab American	Asian Americans	Native Hawaiian/ Pacific Islander
			Offer eulogy at burial with religious songs. Usually prefer burial. Express grief openly.				
Nursing Considerations	Respect personal space. Encourage health screening and preventive health care strategies. Encourage low-fat, low-cholesterol, high-fiber diet.	Ask who makes decisions for the family. Reinforce need to be on time for appointments. Collaborate on decision of what is an acceptable weight.	Negotiate acceptable weight. When possible, encourage participation of similar ethnic minorities in planning care and to promote healthy interactions.	Incorporate time for processing information. Use silence therapeutically. Monitor body language.	Respect nutritional requests, and try to obtain specific dietary requests. Attempt to provide same-sex caregiver. Screen for domestic violence.	Monitor for cues of expression and body language. Inquire in a nonjudgmental manner regarding use of traditional medicine. Provide same-sex care provider when possible.	Treat elders with respect. Rank is very important. Pacific Islanders may not understand the concept of triage as the severity of illness is less important than the rank of the patient. Engage family members and traditional healers in management of chronic illness since this population tends to accept chronic illness even when treatment to manage the illness is available.

*Although many other cultural groups are represented in the United States, the most common are presented here.
Source: Bernstein, 2008.

Spanish/Hispanic/Latino

The term *Spanish/Hispanic/Latino* is used to describe people whose cultural heritage has a strong Spanish influence. However, many people in this group prefer to identify themselves as Chicano or with terms that provide a country of origin, such as Mexican, Peruvian, Puerto Rican, and Cuban (Purnell & Paulanka, 2008). The population breakdown of Spanish/Hispanic/Latino populations in the U. S. is Mexican Americans (63%), Puerto Rican (9.2%), Central and South Americans (13.4%), Cuban (3.5%), and other groups, including the Dominican Republic (23.3%; U.S. Census, 2011). Hispanics immigrate from any number of Central and South American countries, the Caribbean, and other Spanish-speaking countries. Thus, there is much diversity in this population in the United States.

Some Spanish/Hispanics/Latinos speak only Spanish, only English, or both Spanish and English, whereas others speak neither Spanish nor English but rather an Indian dialect. The spoken language depends on individual circumstances and the length of time spent in the United States. Spanish is the second most commonly spoken language in the United States.

Spanish/Hispanics/Latinos comprise approximately 17% of the U.S. population (U.S. Census Bureau, 2011); they recently became the majority minority population. They live in all 50 states with more than 90% living in and around cities. Four of every five Spanish/Hispanics/Latinos are born and raised in the United States. Many of these individuals have come from poverty and have few opportunities for advancement. They sacrifice for their basic needs (Figs. 4.5 and 4.6).

Most Spanish/Hispanics/Latinos practice adaptations of the Roman Catholic religion. Their close relationship with God makes it acceptable for people to have visions and dreams in which God or the saints speak directly to them. Thus, HCPs must be careful not to attribute these culture-bound visions to

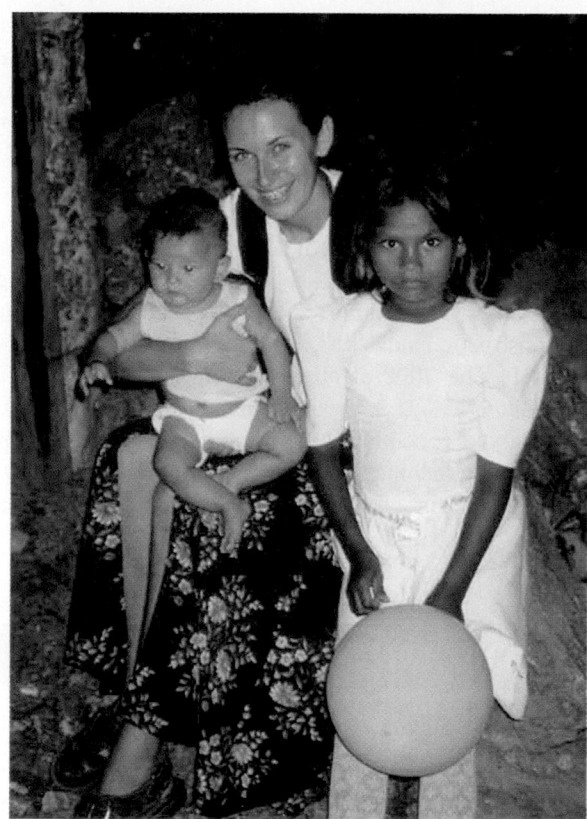

FIGURE 4.6 Many mission workers have helped with health care needs in Central and South American countries.

hallucinations that indicate a need for psychiatric services (see Table 4.1)

African American/Black

African Americans/blacks are the third largest ethnic group in the United States and represent more than 100 racial strains. They make up 13% of the population (U.S. Census Bureau, 2011). Although African Americans/blacks live in all 50 states, more than half live in the South. It is important to understand that not all people with dark skin identify themselves as African American. Many black-skinned people from the Caribbean use terms more specific to their identity, such as *Haitian, Jamaican,* or *West Indian.*

African Americans/blacks have been called by many names. Their ancient African name is Nehesu or Nubian. During slavery days in America, they were called *Negro,* a Spanish-Portuguese word meaning "black." After emancipation in 1863, they were called *colored,* a term adopted by the First Colored Men's Convention in the United States in 1831. The U.S. Bureau of the Census adopted the word *Negro* in 1880. During the civil rights movements in the 1960s, the term *black* was used to signify a philosophy of life instead of color. In the 1970s, these ethnic peoples referred to themselves as African Americans because they were proud of both their African and American heritages. In 1988, the term *African American* was widely adopted in the United States by those

FIGURE 4.5 Honduran couples wait to get married until they can afford a celebration—at 100 years young in this case.

whose ancestry originated from Africa. These terms continue to cause confusion when people try to use the "politically correct" term in this country. Additionally, titles such as the National Black Nurses Association and the National Association for the Advancement of Colored People (NAACP) still exist.

African Americans/blacks are underrepresented in colleges and universities, managerial and administrative positions, and the health care professions. They are overrepresented in high-risk, hazardous occupations such as the steel and tire industries, construction industries, and high-pollution factories (see Table 4.1) The 2008 election of Barack Obama, the first African American U.S. president, and his reelection in 2012, brought about education initiatives including outreach programs for low-income families and increased availability of advance placement classes nationwide. This will likely have an impact on such issues in the future.

CRITICAL THINKING

Ms. Waters

■ Now that you have learned more about culture, let's look at Ms. Waters again. Review Table 4.1 and answer the following questions:

1. What does your interaction with Ms. Waters tell you about her time orientation?
2. What is evident about her social organization?
3. What biological variations may Ms. Waters demonstrate that are likely part of her culture?
4. Who might you involve in discussions with Ms. Waters about her health? About her upcoming surgery?
5. Where might you learn more about the unique health practices Ms. Waters uses to address her health concerns?

Suggested answers are at the end of the chapter.

American Indian/Alaskan Native

There are more than 400 American Indian/Alaskan Native tribes in the United States, totaling 1.7% of the population (U.S. Census Bureau, 2011). Although there are similarities among American Indians, each tribe has its own unique perspective on health and illness. The preference of American Indians is to be referred to by their tribal names, but if the tribal name is not known, the term *American Indian* or *Native American* is acceptable.

Many traditional American Indians/Alaskan Natives live on reservations; others live in urban areas and practice few of their traditions. Many American Indians/Alaskan Natives have a strong belief that illness is caused by an imbalance with nature and the universe. Tribal identity is maintained through powwows, ceremonial events, and arts and crafts that are taught to children at a young age. Communicating with nature is important for maintaining life forces. American Indians/Alaskan Natives are the original inhabitants of North America.

American Indians/Alaskan Natives are underrepresented in all of the health professions. They are consistently identified as the most underrepresented minority group in institutions of higher learning (Bernstein, 2008). (See Table 4.1, *Cultural Considerations.*)

Arab American

Arab Americans are a large and diverse population, with more than 3,000,000 in the United States. Some common bonds include the Arabic language and the Islamic religion. Arab Americans include people from Morocco, Algeria, Tunisia, Libya, Sudan, Egypt and the western Asian countries of Lebanon, occupied Palestine, Syria, Jordan, Iraq, Iran, Kuwait, Bahrain, Qatar, United Arab Emirates, Saudi Arabia, Oman, and Yemen. Many early Arab immigrants were Christians from Lebanon and Syria.

Although many Arab Americans favor professional occupations, they are often underemployed. Others have their own businesses or work in a variety of other occupations. Arab Americans, whether born in the United States or in Arab countries, are more educated than the average American. They are more likely to be in managerial and professional specialty occupations than any other ethnic group in America. However, a significant number of primarily foreign-born Arab Americans are unemployed and live in poverty.

Asian American

This large group is far from homogeneous. The term *Asian,* as used in most references, includes 32 groups and refers to a person having origins in the Far East, Southeast Asia, or the Indian subcontinent. These groups include Asians, Indochinese, and other Asian groups. Asians include people from Korea, Japan, and 54 ethnic groups from China; Polynesians; Filipinos; Malaysians; and Guamanians. Indochinese populations include Cambodian, Vietnamese, Hmong, and Laotian. Other Asian groups include Asian Indian, Pakistani, and Thai. Although it is difficult to determine exact numbers of Asians from specific countries because of the method of keeping population statistics, they are a significant and fast-growing population in the United States.

It is important for many Asian patients to "save face." Individual shame is shared with the family and community. Most Asians see the nurse as an authority figure. Although known by different names, most Asian cultures practice the *yin* and *yang* balance of forces for illness prevention and maintaining health. Yin is considered female and represents cold and weakness. Yang is considered male and represents strength and warmth. Foods and all forces are classified as yin or yang and must be balanced or illness occurs. Yin and yang forces are major components of traditional Chinese medicine, which includes acupressure, acupuncture, and cupping (see Table 4.1).

Native Hawaiian/Pacific Islander

Native Hawaiian or Other Pacific Islander refers to a person having origins in Hawaii, Guam, Samoa, or other Pacific Islands. The majority of the Native Hawaiian/Pacific Islander population resides in Hawaii and California. In American homes, there are at least 39 Pacific Island languages spoken as a second language; 14% of Native Hawaiian and Pacific Islanders have limited English proficiency compared with the general population.

Native Hawaiian and Pacific Islanders have multiple health concerns. Native Hawaiians are more likely to have diabetes and have higher death rates due to cancer. Pacific Islander children have the highest rates of being overweight among all children. Together, both have the second highest rate of HIV infection and the second shortest AIDS survival rate of all Americans. Poverty remains a problem among this population with almost 20% living in poverty and 18% living below poverty (White House Initiative on Asian Americans and Pacific Islanders, 2010; Wergowske & Blanchetter, 2010).

 ## CULTURALLY COMPETENT CARE

The American Nurses Association (2013) supports the need for nurses to understand cultural diversity and to become culturally competent. However, there is no real agreement as to how your knowledge, skills, and attitudes will best help these diverse populations. You certainly cannot achieve cultural competence overnight; it is a developmental process. Each time you care for a patient from a different culture, you learn more, become more aware and sensitive to individual needs, and move toward becoming culturally competent.

The following strategies for providing culturally competent care may be helpful:

- Consider each of your patients as unique, influenced but not defined by his or her culture.
- Know your own cultural values, beliefs, and practices, and appreciate how they may be different from those of others.
- Never let your own biases about people and groups stand in the way of culturally competent care.
- Learn as much as you can about cultural groups in your community.
- Make an effort to include beliefs and practices from other cultures into your care when appropriate.
- Try to encourage helpful cultural practices and discourage harmful ones.
- Be aware of how you communicate with others; be aware of verbal and nonverbal patterns.
- Respect your patients regardless of their cultural backgrounds.
- Learn from your mistakes.

This list does not include everything you can do. Can you think of other strategies?

 ## LEARNING TIP

Take a trip to BALI:
    Be aware of your own cultural heritage.
    Appreciate that your patient is unique; influenced but not defined by his or her culture.
    Learn about your patients' cultural groups.
    Incorporate your patients' cultural values, beliefs, and practices into their plan of care.

CRITICAL THINKING

The Lopez Family

■ Jose, age 23, and his wife, Louisa, age 19, immigrated to the United States 3 years ago from Mexico. They have two children, Maria, 3 years old, and Jesus, 6 months old. The young couple has brought the children to the emergency room for the treatment of ear infections. Jose informs you that Maria has a sore throat and ear pain and Jesus is "fussy" and not eating. He states that he has been to his *curandero,* but neither child has improved. You also notice that the children are dressed in heavy clothing, although it is quite warm outside. When you question the parents, Louisa responds that they are "cold."

Jesus is admitted to the hospital for dehydration. As you are admitting the infant to your unit, you are aware that Jose is answering all of your questions and making decisions for Jesus's care. He states that they will all need to spend the night with Jesus. Jose further adds that Jesus needs more clothes on and that the temperature in the room needs to be increased. The parents refuse the warmed bottle of formula for Jesus but ask for it to be chilled. Louisa sits in the corner of the room chanting, crying, and rubbing some beads.

What nonverbal communication characteristics do these parents display that are common among people of Spanish descent?

1. Why do you think the children are dressed inappropriately for the weather?
2. Do Jose's demands mean that he is uncooperative and trying to control the care of his son?
3. Why do you think Jose refused his son's warm bottle?
4. What is the significance of Louisa's behavior?
5. What might you do to improve Jesus' care?
6. How will you handle the father's request for the entire family to stay in your patient's room?
7. How can you become more culturally competent in this situation?
8. Are there other members of the health team that might be helpful in this situation?

Suggested answers are at the end of the chapter.

REFLECTIONS ON MS. WATERS

After learning more about culture, how do you think the characteristics of Ms. Waters' culture affected her behavior? At her age, it is evident that she has learned many of her beliefs and practices about health and illness from others. Although many of her behaviors can be explained by fear and denial, it is probable that other things are going on in this situation. Ms. Waters may feel more comfortable with people of her own culture, at least when it comes to asking for health information. She may not trust biomedical or Western medicine treatments. She may be more comfortable with the practices and healers that she knows better. Can you think of other explanations?

Rarely do practicing nurses have the luxury to assess each patient comprehensively on a first encounter. The essentials for culturally competent care are obtained as needed over time. As you meet patients from other cultures, continue to learn about these new cultures. Astute observations, openness to diversity, and willingness to learn from patients are essential for effective cross-cultural competence in clinical practice. Cultural competence is not a luxury; it is a necessity.

Home Health Hints

- The effects of a patient's cultural beliefs and practices related to health care are more evident when care is provided in the home. The nurse must adapt care to the patient's environment rather than the patient adapting to the nurse's hospital environment. The nurse is a guest in the patient's home.
- When scheduling a home visit, it is important to find out the primary language spoken in the home. It is also helpful to carry a translation book when the language is known. If necessary, arrange to have an interpreter available to ensure understanding of what is discussed.
- If you have a personal digital assistant (PDA), you can also download a language translator to have available to assist with communication.
- Be aware of the cultural significance of family hierarchy. Avoid having children translate for parents.

SUGGESTED ANSWERS TO

CRITICAL THINKING

■ *Ms. Waters*

1. African Americans may be present-oriented. Her seeming lack of concern about her diabetes may reflect hesitance to worry about a future that is not here yet.

2. Family is important. She prays for healing.

3. We do not know Ms. Waters's weight, but overweight may be seen as positive in her culture, and excess weight is a risk factor for diabetes and hypertension.

4. Involving family members, both younger and older, might be helpful with Mrs. Waters's permission. You might want to ask if there is a religious person whom she might want to include in discussions and decision making.

5. Most institutions have resources for cultural assessment and practices. If you are using Internet-based resources, be sure they are credible resources and that your facility approves of the information obtained.

■ *The Lopez Family*

1. Jose's behavior indicates that he is the primary decision maker and in charge of this situation. Louisa's crying is normal. She is most likely praying.

2. This may relate to the couple's beliefs in the hot and cold theory.

3. His role as father may dictate that he should maintain control. He probably does not mean to be uncooperative.

4. Again, this may be related to hot and cold beliefs about treatment of diseases.

5. Louisa's culture-bound role dictates that she not assume control of the situation. She is upset and praying.

6. Attempt to incorporate the family's cultural beliefs and practices when possible.

7. Explain that it would not be good for Maria to remain in the hospital because she will be at greater risk for exposure to infection. Ask if there are other relatives who can care for Maria. Find out if the parents can divide their time with their son.

8. Be aware of your own cultural beliefs, appreciate your patient's culture, learn more about the Lopez family's culture (ask questions), and include their beliefs and practices when possible. Explain if there are practices that cannot be followed. Ask for alternatives.

9. Many hospitals have identified health care personnel from specific cultural backgrounds who are recommended as consultants to provide guidance to nurses. Review your hospital resources and locate additional resources if necessary. Find out whether your facility has a cultural competence task force or committee that you can become a part of, or develop one if this does not exist.

REVIEW QUESTIONS

1. Which of the following characteristics is exhibited by a nurse who assumes that all patients have the same cultural beliefs as his or her own?
   1. Cultural stereotyping
   2. Ethnocentrism
   3. Cultural sensitivity
   4. Cultural dominance

2. A 12-year-old Mexican American child is admitted for an appendectomy. His parents bring in the priest from their church to pray over the child. The prayers are continuing when it is time to take the child to surgery. How should the nurse respond?
   1. Gently tell the parents that they must stop praying so the child can be taken to surgery.
   2. Give the parents and priest as much time as they need for prayers before surgery.
   3. Tell the parents that the child could die from a ruptured appendix if surgery is delayed.
   4. Permit the parents and priest to stay and pray as the child goes into surgery.

3. An Osage American Indian woman is slow at giving responses and does not maintain eye contact with the nurse when her admission interview is being conducted. Which of the following interpretations of her behavior is most likely accurate?
   1. Direct eye contact may be interpreted as rude in her culture.
   2. She does not want to answer personal questions.
   3. She does not understand the nurse.
   4. She does not want to talk with a nurse and prefers a physician.

4. An Arab American man is refusing his dinner tray, which consists of potatoes with cheese, a slice of ham, and green beans. What knowledge should guide the nurse's data collection related to this incident?
   1. Arabs do not like foods from different sources on the same plate.
   2. Some Arabs do not eat dairy products.
   3. Islamic Arabs may not eat pork.
   4. Arabs typically do not eat vegetables.

5. A Puerto Rican man has been admitted for reconstructive orthopedic surgery on his knee. His wife brings jars of special blends of spices that he wants to put on his food because the hospital food is too bland. He is on a general diet. What action should the nurse take?
   1. Check to be sure they do not interact with his medications and let him use them.
   2. Carefully explain that family cannot bring food items to the hospital.
   3. Have the dietitian provide spices from the hospital food services.
   4. Report the situation to the HCP.

Answers can be found in Appendix C.

References

American Nurses Association. (2013). Diversity awareness. Retrieved June 12, 2013, from nursingworld.org/MainMenu Categories/ThePracticeofProfessionalNursing/Improving -Your-Practice/Diversity-Awareness

Bernstein, R. (2008). *Hispanic population surpasses 45 million. Now 15 percent of total.* Washington, DC: U.S. Census Bureau and U.S. Department of Commerce. Retrieved June 12, 2013, from www.census.gov/newsroom/releases/archives/population /cb08-67.html

Bernstein, R. (2012). Most children younger than age 1 are minorities, Census Bureau reports. Washington, DC: U.S. Census Bureau and U.S. Department of Commerce. Retrieved May 16, 2013, from www.census.gov/newsroom/releases/archives /population/cb12-90.html

Office of Minority Health, U.S. Department of Health and Human Services (2010). *Health Equity & Culturally and Linguistically Appropriate Services (CLAS): How Are They Connected?* Retrieved from www.thinkculturalhealth.hhs.gov/Content /clas.asp

Purnell, L., & Paulanka, B. (Eds.). (2008). *Transcultural health care: A culturally competent approach.* Philadelphia: F.A. Davis Company.

U.S. Census Bureau (2011). State and county quick facts. U.S. Department of Commerce. Retrieved May 16, 2013 from http:// quickfacts.census.gov/qfd/states/00000.html

Wergowske, G., & Blanchetter, P. L. (2010). Health and health care of elders from Native Hawaiian and other Pacific Islander backgrounds. Retrieved May 16, 2013, from www.stanford .edu/group/ethnoger/nativehawaiian.html

White House Initiative on Asian Americans and Pacific Islanders. (2010). Retrieved May 16, 2012, from www.whitehouse.gov /administration/eop/aapi

 DavisPlus | For additional resources and information visit **davispl.us/medsurg5**

5

Complementary and Alternative Modalities

CYNTHIA BARRERE AND
COLLEEN DELANEY

KEY TERMS

acupuncture (ak-yoo-PUNGK-chur)
allopathic (AL-oh-PATH-ik)
Ayurvedic (AY-YUR-VAY-dik)
chiropractic (ky-roh-PRAK-tik)
homeopathy (HO-mee-AH-pa-thee)
naturopathy (NAY-chur-AH-pa-thee)
osteopathic (AHS-tee-ah-PATH-ik)

LEARNING OUTCOMES

1. Explain the difference between complementary and an alternative modalities.
2. Describe selected systems of health care that have contributed to the development of new modalities.
3. Identify how the different types of modalities are classified.
4. Identify safety issues associated with complementary and alternative modalities.
5. Describe the role of the licensed practical nurse/licensed vocational nurse (LPN/LVN) in assisting a patient with complementary and alternative modalities.

Health care in the 21st century requires that nurses recognize the shift toward the inclusion of complementary and alternative approaches in care. Nurses at all levels and in every area of practice are answering the call to use new methods to care for those who are ill and enhance the health of those who are well.

Holistic nursing was a precursor to many of the now popular complementary and alternative modalities. It was introduced in the 1970s and has been growing ever since. Holistic nursing is simply defined as caring for the whole person—body, mind, and spirit—in a constantly changing environment.

 ## COMPLEMENTARY OR ALTERNATIVE: WHAT'S THE DIFFERENCE?

The words *complementary* and *alternative* are sometimes used interchangeably, but they are not the same. *Complementary therapy* refers to a therapy used in addition to a conventional therapy. For example, a nurse might suggest guided imagery, music, and relaxation techniques for pain control in addition to prescribed drug therapy. *Alternative therapy,* sometimes called unconventional therapy, refers to a therapy used instead of conventional or mainstream therapy. An example is using acupuncture instead of analgesics for pain. The terms *therapy, modality,* and *medicine* are used interchangeably. For consistency, this chapter uses the term *modality.*

A good resource for current information about complementary and alternative modalities is the National Center for Complementary and Alternative Medicine (NCCAM) at www.nccam.nih.gov. To learn about holistic nursing and complementary modalities, visit the American Holistic Nurses Association at www.ahna.org.

 ## INTRODUCTION OF NEW SYSTEMS INTO TRADITIONAL WESTERN HEALTH CARE

There are many new and different philosophies within the scope of expanded medical and nursing practice. These systems reflect cultures and attitudes in healing that range from East to West and from ancient to modern. In a landmark study, Eisenberg et al (1993) reported that unconventional therapy use in the United States far exceeded previous estimates. Of the 1539 adults interviewed, one in three (34%) reported using at least one unconventional modality during the previous year. More recent findings confirm that this trend is increasing, indicating a need for health care providers (HCPs) to ask patients about their use of complementary and alternative modalities (Tindle, Davis, Phillips, & Eisenberg, 2005). NCCAM conducted a survey in 2007 that indicated that approximately 38% of adults in the United States and about 12% of children used some form of complementary or alternative medicine (CAM) (www.nccam.nih.gov).

In the United States, the primary system of medicine is just called *medicine,* although some people refer to it as **allopathic** medicine. A number of other schools of thought

Gerontological Issues

Alternative Therapies

About 88% of older adults use some form of alternative therapy, but most are unlikely to report the use of these therapies to their physician. Alternative therapies are commonly used to treat arthritis, back pain, heart disease, allergies, and diabetes. Personal beliefs and lifestyle are motivating factors for those who chose to use alternative therapies (Cuellar, Rogers, & Hisghman, 2007).

and philosophies are also being increasingly used. The most frequently seen new systems include Ayurvedic, Chinese, chiropractic, naturopathic, American Indian, and osteopathic medicine. Each philosophical system can stand alone or, as in most instances in the United States, may be used in combination with other systems. Most of these recently introduced systems use complementary and alternative modalities.

Allopathic/Western Medicine

The most common name for allopathic medicine is *Western medicine.* Other commonly used terms for Western medicine are *conventional medicine* and *mainstream medicine.* Many people have not heard the term *allopathic* because most doctors and nurses do not refer to their modality of practice by this name. Allopathy is a method of treating disease with remedies that produce effects different from those caused by the disease itself. For example, when a patient has a bacterial infection, a Western medical practitioner prescribes an antibiotic to eliminate the invading pathogen.

Practitioners of Western medicine are medical doctors, nurses, and allied health personnel. This system of medicine uses scientific data to determine the validity of a diagnosis and the effectiveness of treatment; this is called *evidence-based medicine* (see Chapter 2). Peer-reviewed medical literature is very important. In scientific investigations, results can be verified and reproduced through various types of studies and statistical analyses. Practitioners use a variety of therapies, including drugs, surgery, and radiation therapy. Western medicine practitioners have made most of the significant advances and developments in modern medicine.

Ayurvedic Medicine

Ayurveda is the ancient Hindu system of medicine, which originated in India. **Ayurvedic** medicine's main goals are to maintain the health of well people and cure the illnesses of sick people. Ayurveda maintains that illness is the result of falling out of balance with nature. Diagnosis is based on three metabolic body types called *doshas.* An Ayurvedic doctor determines which *dosha* type is most appropriate for the patient: *vata, pitta,* or *kapha.* Treatment usually involves

• **WORD** • **BUILDING** •
allopathic: allos—other + pathic—disease or suffering
Ayurvedic: ayu—life + veda—knowledge or science

prescribing a diet, herbal remedies, breath work, physical exercise, yoga, meditation, massage, and a rejuvenation or detoxification program.

Ayurveda is rapidly becoming more popular in America. The books and videos of Deepak Chopra are examples of this increasingly popular system of therapy. An introduction to Ayurveda can be found at http://nccam.nih.gov /health/ayurveda/introduction.htm.

Traditional Chinese Medicine

Traditional Chinese medicine is thousands of years old and involves such practices as acupuncture, acupressure, herbs, massage, and qi gong. Chinese medicine involves diagnosis and treatment of disturbances of qi (pronounced "chee"), or vital energy.

Acupuncturists, one type of traditional Chinese medicine practitioners, claim to be able to tell much about a patient's state of health by checking pulses, looking at the color of the tongue, checking facial color, assessing voice and smell, and asking a variety of questions. To treat patients with **acupuncture**, practitioners insert one or more needles along the meridians (pathways) where qi flows (Fig. 5.1). Many acupuncturists prescribe herbal remedies

as well. Find information on how acupuncture is being integrated into Western medicine at http://nccam.nih.gov /health/acupuncture.

Chiropractic Medicine

Have you ever been to a chiropractor? Daniel David Palmer founded chiropractic therapy in 1895. **Chiropractic** medicine is based on the belief that illness is a result of neuromusculoskeletal dysfunction. The main treatment modality of chiropractors is manual adjustment and manipulation of the vertebral column and the limbs. They use direct hand contact and mechanical and electrical treatment methods to manipulate joints. The goal is to remove interference with nerve function so the body can heal itself. Chiropractors do not perform surgery, nor do they prescribe drugs. Review the American Chiropractic Association website at www.acatoday.org/level1_css.cfm?T1ID=42 for additional information.

• WORD • BUILDING •

acupuncture: acus—needle + punctura—puncture
chiropractic: cheir—hand + pracktos—to do

Bladder
Conception vessel
Gallbladder
Governing vessel
Heart
Kidney
Large intestine
Liver
Lung
Pericardium
Small intestine
Spleen
Stomach
Triple warmer

FIGURE 5.1 Qi meridians are used in the Chinese medicine techniques of acupressure and acupuncture.

Homeopathic Medicine

Homeopathy was developed by Samuel Hahnemann in Germany in the early 19th century. Homeopathy is based on Hahnemann's principle that "like cures like," meaning that tiny doses of a substance that create the symptoms of disease in a healthy person will relieve those symptoms in a sick person.

Although schools and courses do exist for training homeopaths, no diploma or certificate from any school or program is a license to practice homeopathy in the United States. Medical doctors and doctors of osteopathy are granted national certificates of competency by the Council for Homeopathic Certification to practice homeopathy. Other health care practitioners may be allowed to use homeopathy within the scope of their state licenses.

Visit the National Center for Homeopathy website at www.nationalcenterforhomeopathy.org. This site has a research section with annotated listings from the medical literature discussing the value of homeopathy. In addition, the site has a good review of licensing laws regarding homeopathy.

Naturopathic Medicine

Naturopathy primarily uses natural therapies such as nutrition, botanical medicine (herbs), hydrotherapy (water-based therapy), counseling, physical medicine, and homeopathy to treat disease, promote healing, and prevent illness. Naturopathic physicians have a doctor of naturopathy (ND) degree and can be licensed in 17 states. There are three schools of naturopathic medicine in the United States. For more information about naturopathy, visit www.naturopathic.org.

American Indian Medicine

American Indian medical practices vary from tribe to tribe. In general, American Indian medicine is a community-based system with rituals and practices such as the sweat lodge, herbal remedies, the medicine wheel, the sacred hoop, the "sing," and shamanistic healing. For example, an ill person may be placed in a small, enclosed sweat lodge while singing or chanting is done outside the lodge. It is believed that toxic substances are drawn out in the sweat of the person inside the lodge. After the ceremony, the ill person may be placed on a cot outside and be prayed over. Learn more about American Indian medicine at the Association of American Indian Physicians' website at www.aaip.org.

Osteopathic Medicine

Osteopathic medicine was founded in the United States in 1874 by Andrew Taylor Still, a frontier physician who was dissatisfied with the state of medicine at that time. This practice of medicine emphasizes the interrelationship of the body's nerves, muscles, bones, and organs. The osteopathic philosophy involves treating the whole person, recognizes the body's ability to heal itself, and stresses the importance of diet, exercise, and fitness with a focus on prevention. For more information about osteopathy, visit the American Osteopathic Association website at www.osteopathic.org.

COMPLEMENTARY AND ALTERNATIVE MODALITIES

Discussion of all complementary and alternative modalities is beyond the scope of this text. Table 5.1 summarizes the most commonly used modalities.

TABLE 5.1 CATEGORIES AND TYPES OF COMPLEMENTARY AND ALTERNATIVE MODALITIES

Category of Therapy	Types of Individual Therapies
Biologically based modalities	Herbal medicine Nutrition and special diet therapies Nutritional supplements
Mind–body modalities	Art therapy Dance therapy Guided imagery Hypnosis and hypnotherapy Meditation and relaxation Music/sound therapies Prayer Tai chi and qi gong Yoga
Manipulative and body-based modalities	Acupressure Chiropractic Massage and related massage therapies Osteopathic manipulation
Energetic modalities	Biofeedback Healing touch Magnet therapy Polarity therapy Reiki Spiritual healing Therapeutic touch
Miscellaneous therapies	Aquatherapy/hydrotherapy Aromatherapy Chanting Chelation therapy Colon therapy Kinesiology Light therapy Pet therapy

• WORD • BUILDING •
homeopathy: homeo—like + pathos—disease
naturopathy: naturo—nature + pathy—disease
osteopathic: osteo—bone + pathy—disease

Herbal Therapy

Have you ever tried herbs for healing? Herbs should only be taken under the supervision of a HCP. Herbs can aid in healing, but they also can do harm. Some of the more common herbs are described in Table 5.2. Figure 5.2 shows echinacea, an herb commonly prepared for use as an immune system booster.

It is important to note that herbal remedies are not foods. They have potent medicinal effects and can interact with prescribed medications and even complicate surgery. This can be problematic, both because herbs are readily available in health food stores and drugstores and because many patients do not tell their doctors or nurses about their herb use. For example, three common herbs, garlic, ginkgo, and ginseng, can each increase the risk of bleeding when taken with anticoagulant or antiplatelet medications. Another popular herb is St. John's wort, widely used for depression. It can interact adversely with many drugs, including other antidepressant agents. Be sure to assess patients' use of herbs and supplements and educate them about the need to inform HCPs, including their pharmacists, when using herbs.

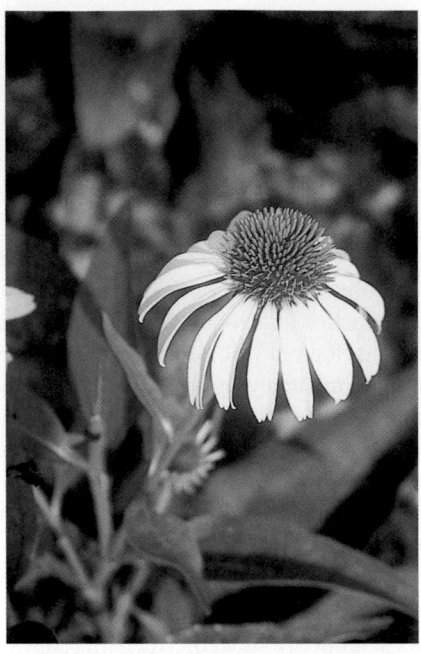

FIGURE 5.2 Echinacea is an herb commonly used for colds and flu.

TABLE 5.2 COMMON HERBS AND THEIR INTENDED USES

Herb	Purported Uses
Aloe vera	Soothing agent, used for skin lesions May absorb toxins
Bee pollen	May increase energy, stamina, and strength
Black cohosh	May ease menopausal symptoms
Capsaicin	May ease tenderness and pain of osteoarthritis, fibromyalgia, diabetic neuropathy, and shingles
Chamomile	May decrease anxiety, stomach distress, and infant colic
Echinacea	Has antiviral properties; may be effective for colds, flu, and other infections
Feverfew	Has anti-inflammatory properties; may help treat migraine headaches, stimulate appetite, promote menstruation, eliminate worms, suppress fever
Garlic	Reduces low-density lipoprotein and raises high-density lipoprotein cholesterol May reduce blood pressure Suppresses platelet aggregation, increases arterial elasticity, and decreases atherosclerotic plaque formation
Ginger	May reduce nausea and vomiting, hypertension, and high cholesterol
Ginkgo biloba	May improve memory and help cognitive function in Alzheimer's disease
Ginseng	May reduce stress and increase alertness Numerous other claims, such as lowering cholesterol, balancing blood glucose levels, slowing the aging process, treating memory loss, treating erectile dysfunction
Kava	May be effective for anxiety, insomnia, low energy, muscle tension
Red yeast rice	May reduce cholesterol and triglycerides
St. John's wort	May help mild to moderate depression; may be effective against viral infections, including HIV and herpes

Warning: Herbs may have many side effects and may interact with many prescribed and over-the-counter medications. Urge patients to consult HCPs before self-prescribing.

A great website for you and your patients is www .mayoclinic.org. Just type in the common herb you want to know about in the search window for up-to-date information. It even has an Evidence section that grades the evidence of the herb's effectiveness for each disorder it is supposed to treat. Grades range from A, which indicates strong research evidence for the herb's use, to F, which indicates strong evidence against its use.

Relaxation Therapies
Progressive Muscle Relaxation

Progressive muscle relaxation is a simple technique to learn. It involves the process of alternately tensing and relaxing muscle groups. Often this process is performed in a systematic manner, such as from toes to head. The purpose of the technique is to help the participant identify subtle levels of mental and physical tension that accompany mental and emotional stress. When our conscious awareness of the tensions increases, we can learn to relax and thus reduce the effects of stress and tension.

 LEARNING TIP

Try using progressive muscle relaxation the next time you are anxious during a nursing examination.

Guided Imagery

Guided imagery is another example of a complementary therapy that many nurses use. Guided imagery involves using mental images to promote physical healing or changes in attitudes or behaviors. Practitioners may lead patients through visualization exercises or offer instruction in using imagery as a self-help tool. Guided imagery is often used to alleviate stress and to treat stress-related conditions such as insomnia and high blood pressure. People with cancer, AIDS, chronic fatigue syndrome, and other disorders can use specific images to boost the immune system.

A common guided imagery technique begins with a general relaxation process. For those new to the process, it is good to begin with the progressive muscle relaxation as explained earlier in the chapter. Guided imagery works best when all of the senses are used. The exercise in Box 5-1 is very basic but gives an idea of how the technique works. When used for healing, many more steps are involved. It is important to note that appropriate training and skills are needed before using complementary and alternative modalities with patients. Find more on guided imagery at www.nccam.nih.gov; type "guided imagery" into the search window.

 LEARNING TIP

When you are stumped on a test question, close your eyes and imagine yourself asking the question of your favorite instructor. Imagine what his or her answer would be.

Box 5-1 **Guided Imagery**

Assist your patient to progress through the following steps:

- Assume a comfortable position in a quiet environment.
- Close your eyes and keep them closed until the exercise is completed.
- Breathe in and out deeply to the count of four, repeating this step four times.
- When relaxed, think of a favorite peaceful place and prepare to take an imaginary journey there.
- Picture what this place looks like and how comfortable you feel being there.
- Listen to all the sounds; feel the gentle, clean air; and smell the pleasant aromas.
- Continue to breathe deeply and appreciate the feeling of being in this special place.
- Feel the sense of deep relaxation and peace of this place.
- As you continue to breathe deeply, slowly and gently bring your consciousness back to the setting in this room.
- Slowly and gently open your eyes, stretch, and think about how relaxed you feel.

Biofeedback

Biofeedback could be considered the third tier of learning progressive relaxation. This technique is used especially for conditions that are aggravated by stress such as asthma, migraines, insomnia, and high blood pressure. Biofeedback is a way of monitoring and controlling tiny metabolic changes in one's body with the aid of sensitive machines that provide feedback ("Patient Perspective").

 Patient Perspective

I'm scared to death of flying. The minute I get on an airplane, I feel jittery, my heart races, and I can't calm down until we're safely back on the ground. Several years ago, I decided to try biofeedback therapy to overcome this fear.

My therapist was wonderful. She immediately put me at ease and assured me I wasn't a crazy person to be afraid to fly. She listened to my fears and responses throughout all our sessions. At each practice session, she put a temperature sensor on my finger (my hands were usually pretty cold). In her calm, soft voice, she guided me through a relaxation exercise using imagery and progressive muscle relaxation. By the time we were finished, my hands would be several degrees warmer than when we started! This showed my vessels were dilating, a sign that my sympathetic nervous system was slowing down its activity. So I felt calmer. The sensor gave me feedback that told me when my relaxation was working well. We did this every week for a couple of months, until I got really good at warming my hands and relaxing.

Now when I fly, I close my eyes, imagine a peaceful scene and use my relaxation techniques. I still don't like flying much, but at least I feel a bit calmer!

Massage Therapy

Massage is the use of touch to achieve therapeutic results and can include pressure, friction, and kneading of the body. Massage can be used to relax muscles, reduce anxiety, increase circulation, and reduce pain.

Massage also provides a caring form of touch. In the past, a back massage was a nightly routine for hospitalized patients, helping them relax for sleep. Sadly, patients today are often not touched except during technical procedures.

You can learn basic massage techniques in nursing school. You may also choose to obtain formal massage therapy education to practice more advanced techniques. Try giving your patient an old-fashioned back massage, and see how delighted he or she is!

BE SAFE!

Do not use firm massage on a patient taking an anticoagulant or a patient with a low platelet level. Tissue injury could cause bleeding. Check with the HCP before providing deep massage for any patient.

Aquatherapy

Sitting in a warm tub can feel good as aching, tired muscles relax and mental stress is decreased. People who suffer from arthritis or other chronic pain understand how warm water can ease their discomfort. Relaxing in water feels good for three reasons: warmth, water movement causing massage, and buoyancy.

Long before analgesics were developed, the human body relied on its own naturally occurring, internally generated, pain-killing chemicals called endorphins. Endorphins are released in response to both acute and chronic pain. Through research we now know that warm water also stimulates the release of endorphins.

The most recognized methods to release endogenous (naturally occurring) endorphins are physical exercise, acupuncture, and electrical nerve stimulation. Any type of skin stimulation (even the mechanical impact of water) can cause the release of endorphins. However, pain reduction is only part of the healing process. Ultimately, blood flow is what brings nutrients to damaged cells and facilitates healing. When the body is immersed in warm water, the blood vessels nearest the skin relax, allowing more blood to flow. The results are faster tissue repair and relief of pain and fatigue.

Heat and Cold Application

Local application of heat or cold provides additional skin stimulation. A warm compress can soothe sore muscles and dilate vessels in a defined area, bringing healing circulation as well as endorphin release. Ice or a cold gel pack can help numb an area. Cold can also cause overdilated vessels to constrict, yielding relief from pain and throbbing of overstimulated nerve endings. Ice can be helpful on an acute injury and for some types of headaches. Check institution policy before applying heat or cold; a physician's order may be required.

Probiotics

Probiotics are considered beneficial bacteria, and their use is increasing in popularity. The Food and Drug Administration has not approved any health claims related to probiotics. Common reasons for taking probiotics are to aid in healthy digestion or to treat constipation or infectious diarrhea. Increased stress, unhealthy eating patterns, and hectic schedules can disrupt balanced digestion in individuals. Nurses need to caution individuals to discuss plans to take probiotics with their HCPs. It is important to review the research available on a particular product because there are many strains available. Also, it is essential to consider where the research was published (preferably in a peer-reviewed journal) and examine the findings on how safe the product is. Additional information on probiotics can be found at www.nccam.nih.gov.

SAFETY AND EFFECTIVENESS OF ALTERNATIVE MODALITIES

Safety generally means that the benefits outweigh the risks of a treatment or therapy. If a patient is interested in using complementary and alternative modalities, the nurse first needs to counsel the patient to talk with the primary care provider. The patient also should ask the practitioner of the therapy about its safety and effectiveness. Patients should tell their primary care providers and alternative practitioners about all therapies they are using because this information may be important to consider in the safety of their entire treatment plan.

The patient should be as informed as possible and continue gathering information even after a practitioner or therapy has been selected (Box 5-2).

ROLE OF THE LPN/LVN

Patients may ask you about the use of a complementary or alternative modality. Because the safety and effectiveness of many therapies is still unknown, advising patients presents a challenge. The following steps are suggestions for helping to advise patients regarding the use of these kinds of therapies:

1. Advise the patient to take a close look at the background, qualifications, and competence of the proposed practitioner. Check credentials with a state or local regulatory agency with authority over the area of practice in which the patient is interested. Is the practitioner licensed or certified? By whom?

Box 5-2 Questions Patients Should Ask Before Starting a Complementary or Alternative Modality

1. What will this modality do for me?
2. What are its advantages?
3. What are its disadvantages?
4. What are its side effects?
5. What are its risks?
6. How much will it cost? Will my insurance cover the cost?
7. How long will it take? How many treatments will I need?
8. How will it interact with my other therapies and medications?
9. What research has been done on this modality?

2. Suggest that the patient visit the practitioner's office, clinic, or hospital and evaluate the conditions of the setting.
3. Advise that the patient talk with others who have used this practitioner.
4. Consider the costs. Are the treatments covered by insurance, or is it direct pay?
5. The patient should discuss use of the modality with his or her primary care provider.

NURSING APPLICATIONS

There are ways to gain confidence with complementary and alternative modalities:

• Begin by trying one or two of these modalities yourself. Start by choosing a basic therapy such as massage, music, or guided imagery. Follow the guidelines listed in Box 5-2 to make sure it is a safe strategy. Not only will you encounter the possible benefits firsthand, you will also come away with a better understanding of what your patients experience with a given modality.
• Ask your patients if they use any complementary or alternative modalities and what their responses to them have been. Try to eliminate any preconceived notions you might have. Your patients will feel more comfortable mentioning them to you if they feel you understand the treatment and why they decided to use it.
• If you decide to become involved, get instruction in the therapies before you administer them. Many universities and agencies offer continuing education courses on these therapies, and some nursing schools incorporate complementary and alternative modalities in their skills courses. Of course, you will also want to discuss the therapy with your workplace before trying it on a patient!

Before incorporating complementary and alternative modalities into practice, be sure to check your state's nurse practice act for any regulations. Discuss these therapies with the patient and his or her primary care provider before using them. If you work for a hospital or other health care institution, also check institutional policy. See "Evidence-Based Practice" for ways nurses are implementing various modalities in practice.

As the public learns more about complementary and alternative modalities, there is likely to be an even greater demand for them. Nurses have been in the forefront of developing the holistic philosophy that has now become an accepted standard of care.

CRITICAL THINKING

Mr. Jones

■ Mr. Jones asks you whether he should stop his chemotherapy and try magnet therapy for his prostate cancer. How do you respond? What other health care team members might you collaborate with in helping Mr. Jones?

Suggested answers are at the end of the chapter.

Home Health Hints

• When taking a health history, ask the patient or caregiver about the use of complementary and alternative modalities because these may influence the effects or side effects of some prescription medications.
• Be mindful of the importance of complementary and alternative modalities to the patient's health care belief system.
• Consider the alternative practitioner as part of the patient's health care team.
• Discuss concerns regarding potential interactions with the registered nurse or HCP.

EVIDENCE-BASED PRACTICE

Clinical Question
How are complementary and alternative modalities used by nurses to improve health outcomes?

Evidence
The following are examples of how complementary and alternative modalities have been used by nurses to enhance health outcomes in various patient populations.

• In a recent study by Ayan et al (2013), aromatherapy with rose essential oil was found to help reduce pain in patients with renal colic when used in addition to conventional therapies.

- In a randomized controlled trial of community-dwelling older people experiencing depression, music therapy was found to be effective in reducing depression and improving quality of life (Chan, Wong, Onishi, & Naidu, 2012).
- Chung, Brooks, Rai, Balk, and Rai (2012) conducted a study that demonstrated meditation was effective in improving quality of life and decreasing anxiety and blood pressure.
- Spiritual nursing interventions, such as active listening, creating a trusting environment, and praying with or for another were found to be effective in improving outcomes of older adults with dementia (Ennis & Kazer, 2012).
- Patients with fibromyalgia experienced less pain after an animal-assisted dog therapy visit (Marcus et al, 2013).
- A study by Yao, Giordani, Algase, You, and Alexander (2013) found a tai chi program decreased the fall risk status of persons diagnosed with Alzheimer's disease.

Implications for Nursing Practice

Complementary and alternative modalities such as music, aromatherapy, spiritual nurse interventions, animal-assisted therapy, tai chi, and meditation can improve health outcomes in diverse patient populations. After learning these healing modalities, nurses can easily implement them in a variety of patient settings. Be sure to work within your institution's policies and procedures.

REFERENCES

Ayan, M., Tas, U., Sogut, E., Suren, M., Gurbuzler, L., & Koyuncu, F. (2013). Investing the effect of aromatherapy in patients with renal colic. *Journal of Complementary and Alternative Medicine, 19, 329–333.*

Chan, M. F., Wong, Z. Y., Onishi, H. T., & Naidu, V. (2012). Effects of music on depression in older people: A randomized controlled trial. *Journal of Clinical Nursing, 21, 776–783.*

Chung, S.-C., Brooks, M. M., Rai, M., Balk, J. L., & Rai, S. (2012). Effect of Sahaja yoga meditation on quality of life, anxiety, and blood pressure control. *Journal of Alternative & Complementary Medicine, 18, 589–596.*

Cuellar N. G., Rogers A. E., Hisghman V. (2007). Evidence based research of complementary and alternative medicine (CAM) for sleep in the community dwelling older adult. *Geriatric Nursing, 28, 46–52.*

Ennis, E. M. & Kazer, M. W. (2012). The role of spiritual nursing interventions on improved outcomes in older adults with dementia. *Holistic Nursing Practice, 27, 106–113.*

Marcus, D. A., Bernstein, C. D., Constantin, J. M., Kunkel, F. A., Breuer, P., & Hanlon, R. B. (2013). Impact of animal-assisted therapy for outpatients with fibromyalgia. *Pain Medicine, 14, 43–51.*

Yao, L., Giordani, B. J., Algase, D. L., You, M., & Alexander, N. B. (2013). Fall risk-relevant functional mobility outcomes in dementia following dyadic tai chi exercise. *Western Journal of Nursing Research, 35, 281–296.*

SUGGESTED ANSWERS TO

CRITICAL THINKING

■ *Mr. Jones*

As with all medical treatments, it is important to support the established therapy the HCP has prescribed. Therefore, a good response might be the following: "Mr. Jones, chemotherapy is an established medical treatment for your condition. There is a lot of evidence for its effectiveness in the medical literature. If you want to supplement your therapy, there may be some other treatments you can add. I suggest that you discuss your feelings about seeking some additional treatments with your oncologist. If he agrees, then your RN and I can share some information with you about how to stay safe while trying new things."

REVIEW QUESTIONS

1. Which of the following statements best defines a complementary modality?
   1. An alternative treatment that is used in place of a conventional treatment.
   2. A treatment that may be dangerous and should be avoided.
   3. A treatment that can be used in addition to a conventional treatment.
   4. A treatment that is used after conventional treatments have failed.

2. Which of the following therapies is most likely to use research-based interventions?
   1. Naturopathy
   2. Osteopathy
   3. Allopathy
   4. Homeopathy

3. A patient who has high blood pressure tells his nurse he has been taking a ginger supplement in addition to his prescribed medications at home. What is the best response by the nurse?
   1. "Nonprescription supplements can interact with prescription medications. You should not take it any longer."
   2. "Ginger can be effective for hypertension. Be sure to monitor your blood pressure while you are taking it."
   3. "Ginger is a safe supplement because it is a food. It should not interact with your medications."
   4. "You should check with your HCP to make sure the ginger doesn't interact with your other medications before you continue to take it."

4. Which of the following complementary modalities are considered relaxation therapies? **Select all that apply.**
   1. Progressive muscle relaxation
   2. Tai chi
   3. Biofeedback
   4. Homeopathic therapies
   5. Guided imagery

5. Which of the following statements best describes the most important role of the LPN in complementary and alternative modalities?
   1. The LPN should become familiar enough to recommend at least one complementary or alternative modality.
   2. The LPN should become adept at collecting and reporting data related to patients' use of complementary or alternative modalities.
   3. The LPN should discourage use of complementary or alternative modalities because they can interact negatively with conventional therapies.
   4. The LPN does not need to become involved in complementary and alternative modalities.

Answers can be found in Appendix C.

References

Eisenberg, D. M., Kessler, R. C., Foster, C., Norlock, F. E., Calkins, D. R., & Delbanco, T. L. (1993). Unconventional medicine in the United States—Prevalence, costs, patterns of use. *New England Journal of Medicine, 328*(4), 246–252.

Tindle, H. A., Davis, R. B., Phillips, R. S., & Eisenberg, D. M. (2005). Trends in use of complementary and alternative medicine by U.S. adults: 1997–2002. *Alternative Therapies in Health and Medicine, 11,* 42–49.

 DavisPlus | For additional resources and information visit **davispl.us/medsurg5**

unit TWO

Understanding Health and Illness

6 Nursing Care of Patients With Fluid, Electrolyte, and Acid–Base Imbalances

KEY TERMS

acidosis (as-ih-DOH-sis)
alkalosis (al-kah-LOH-sis)
anion (AN-eye-on)
antidiuretic (AN-tee-DYE-yuh-RET-ik)
cation (KAT-eye-on)
dehydration (DEE-hye-DRAY-shun)
diffusion (dih-FEW-zhun)
dysrhythmia (dis-RITH-mee-yah)
edema (eh-DEE-mah)
electrolytes (ee-LEK-troh-lites)
extracellular (EX-trah-SELL-yoo-lar)
filtration (fill-TRAY-shun)
hydrostatic (HYE-droh-STAT-ik)
hypercalcemia (HYE-per-kal-SEE-mee-ah)
hyperkalemia (HYE-per-kuh-LEE-mee-ah)
hypermagnesemia (HYE-per-MAG-nuh-SEE-mee-ah)
hypernatremia (HYE-per-nuh-TREE-mee-ah)
hypertonic (HYE-per-TAWN-ik)
hyperventilation (HYE-per-VEN-tih-LAY-shun)
hypervolemia (HYE-per-voh-LEE-mee-ah)
hypocalcemia (HYE-poh-kal-SEE-mee-ah)
hypokalemia (HYE-poh-kuh-LEE-mee-ah)
hypomagnesemia (HYE-poh-MAG-nuh-SEE-mee-ah)
hyponatremia (HYE-poh-nuh-TREE-mee-ah)
hypotonic (HYE-poh-TAWN-ik)
hypovolemia (HYE-poh-voh-LEE-mee-ah)
interstitial (IN-tur-STISH-uhl)
intracellular (IN-trah-SELL-yoo-ler)
intracranial (IN-trah-KRAY-nee-uhl)
intravascular (IN-trah-VAS-kyoo-ler)
isotonic (EYE-so-TAWN-ik)
osmolarity (OZ-moh-LAR-it-ee)
osmosis (ahs-MOH-sis)
osteoporosis (AHS-tee-oh-por-OH-sis)
semipermeable (SEM-ee-PER-mee-uh-bull)
transcellular (trans-SELL-yoo-lar)

BRUCE K. WILSON

LEARNING OUTCOMES

1. Identify the purposes of fluids and electrolytes in the body.
2. List the signs and symptoms of common fluid imbalances.
3. Predict patients who are at the highest risk for dehydration and fluid excess.
4. Identify data to collect in patients with fluid and electrolyte imbalances.
5. Describe therapeutic measures for patients with fluid and electrolyte disturbances.
6. Identify the education needs of patients with fluid imbalances.
7. Categorize common causes, signs and symptoms, and treatments for sodium, potassium, calcium, and magnesium imbalances.
8. Identify foods that have high sodium, potassium, and calcium contents.
9. Give examples of common causes of acidosis and alkalosis.
10. Compare how arterial blood gases change for each type of acid–base imbalance.

Have you ever wondered why you get thirsty? The body is continually changing, and water supports these changes. Approximately 60% of a young adult's body weight is water. Older people are less than 50% water, and infants are between 70% and 80% water. Fat cells do not contain water, so people with a higher percentage of fat cells have a lower percentage of water.

In addition to water, body fluids also contain solid substances that dissolve, called solutes. Some solutes are **electrolytes** and some are nonelectrolytes. Electrolytes are chemicals that can conduct electricity when dissolved in water. Examples of electrolytes are sodium, potassium, calcium, magnesium, acids, and bases; these are discussed later in this chapter. Nonelectrolytes do not conduct electricity; examples include glucose and urea.

FLUID BALANCE

Fluids are located in various compartments within the body. Fluid inside the cells is referred to as **intracellular** fluid (ICF), and fluid outside the cells is called **extracellular** fluid (ECF). ECF can be further divided into three types: interstitial fluid, intravascular fluid, and transcellular fluid (Fig. 6.1).

Interstitial fluid is the water that surrounds the body's cells and includes lymph. **Intravascular** fluid, or blood plasma, is the fluid within arteries, veins, and capillaries. Fluids and electrolytes move between the interstitial fluid and the intravascular fluid. **Transcellular** fluids are those in specific compartments of the body, such as cerebrospinal fluid, digestive juices, and synovial fluid in joints.

Control of Fluid Balance

The primary control of water in the body is through pressure sensors in the vascular system that stimulate or inhibit the release of **antidiuretic** hormone (ADH) from the pituitary

gland. A diuretic is a substance that causes the kidneys to excrete more fluid. ADH works in just the opposite way. ADH causes the kidneys to retain fluid. If fluid pressures within the vascular system decrease, more ADH is released, and water is retained. If fluid pressures increase, less ADH is released, and the kidneys eliminate more water.

Movement of Fluids and Electrolytes in the Body

Fluids and electrolytes move in the body by active and passive transport systems. Active transport depends on the presence of adequate cellular adenosine triphosphate (ATP) for energy. The most common examples of active transport are the sodium-potassium pumps. These pumps, located in the cell membranes, cause sodium to move out of the cells and potassium to move into the cells when needed.

In passive transport, no energy is expended specifically to move the substances. General body movements aid passive transport. The three passive transport systems are diffusion, filtration, and osmosis.

Diffusion is the movement of a substance from an area of higher concentration to an area of lower concentration. If you pour cream into a cup of coffee, the movement of the molecules will eventually cause the cream to be dispersed throughout the beverage. If you stir the coffee, this process occurs at a faster rate. Body movement assists passive transport, like stirring the coffee. It causes diffusion to occur at a faster rate.

Filtration is the movement of both water and smaller molecules through a semipermeable membrane. A **semipermeable** membrane works like a screen that keeps larger substances on one side and permits only smaller molecules to filter to the other side of the membrane. Filtration is promoted by hydrostatic pressure differences between areas.

Hydrostatic pressure, sometimes called water-pushing pressure, is the force that water exerts. In the body, filtration is important for the movement of water, nutrients, and waste products in the capillaries. The capillaries serve as semipermeable membranes allowing water and smaller substances to move from the vascular system to the interstitial fluid, but larger molecules and red blood cells remain inside the capillary walls.

Osmosis is the movement of water from an area of lower substance concentration to an area of higher concentration.

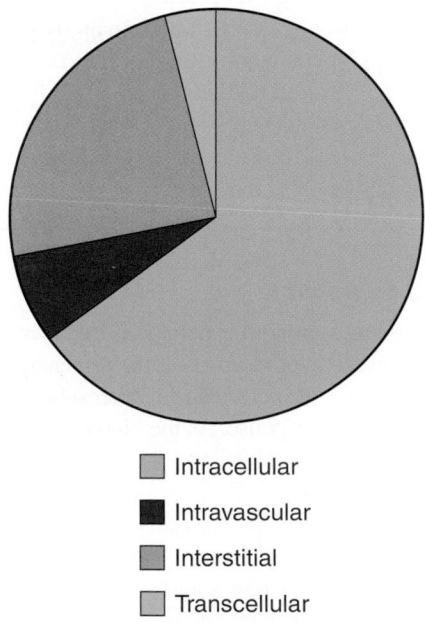

- Intracellular
- Intravascular
- Interstitial
- Transcellular

FIGURE 6.1 Normal distribution of total body water.

• WORD • BUILDING •
electrolyte: electro—electricity + lyte—dissolve
intracellular: intra—within + cellular—cell
extracellular: extra—outside of + cellular—cell
interstitial: inter—between + stitial—tissue
intravascular: intra—within + vascular—blood vessel
transcellular: trans—across + cellular—cell
antidiuretic: anti—against + diuretic—urination
diffusion: diffuse—spread, scattered
filtration: filter—strain through
semipermeable: semi—half or part of + permeable—passing through
hydrostatic: hydro—water + static—standing
osmosis: osmo—impulse + osis—condition

The substances exert an osmotic pressure sometimes called water-pulling pressure. The term **osmolarity** refers to the concentration of the substances in body fluids. The normal osmolarity of blood is between 270 and 300 milliosmoles per liter (mOsm/L).

Another term for osmolarity is *tonicity*. Fluids or solutions can be classified as isotonic, hypotonic, or hypertonic. A fluid that has the same osmolarity as the blood is called **isotonic**. For example, a 0.9% (normal) saline solution is isotonic to the blood and is often used as a solution for intravenous (IV) therapy. A solution that has a lower osmolarity than blood is called **hypotonic**. When a hypotonic solution is given to a patient, the water in the solution leaves the blood and other ECF areas and enters the cells. **Hypertonic** solutions exert greater osmotic pressure than blood. When a hypertonic solution is given to a patient, water leaves the cells and enters the bloodstream and other ECF spaces.

Fluid Gains and Fluid Losses

Water is very important to the body for cellular metabolism, blood volume, body temperature regulation, and solute transport. Although people can survive without food for several weeks, they can survive only a few days without water. Thirst is the major indicator that a healthy adult needs more water.

Water is gained and lost from the body every day. In addition to liquid intake, some fluid is obtained from solid foods. When too much fluid is lost, the brain's thirst mechanism tells the individual that more fluid intake is needed. Older adults are more prone to fluid deficits because they have a diminished thirst reflex and their kidneys do not function as effectively. An adult loses as much as 2500 mL of sensible and insensible fluid each day. Sensible losses are those of which the person is aware, such as urination. Insensible losses may occur without the person recognizing the loss. Perspiration and water lost through respiration and elimination of feces are examples of insensible losses.

FLUID IMBALANCES

Fluid imbalances are common in all clinical settings. Older people are at the highest risk for life-threatening complications that can result from either fluid deficit, more commonly called **dehydration**, or fluid excess. Infants are at risk for fluid deficit because they take in and excrete a large proportion of their total body water each day.

Dehydration

Although there are several types of dehydration, only the most common type is discussed in this chapter. Dehydration occurs when there is not enough fluid in the body, especially in the blood (intravascular area).

Pathophysiology and Etiology

The most common form of dehydration results from loss of fluid from the body, resulting in decreased blood volume. This decrease is referred to as **hypovolemia**. Hypovolemia occurs when the patient is hemorrhaging or when fluids from other parts of the body are lost. For example, severe vomiting and diarrhea, severely draining wounds, and profuse diaphoresis (sweating) can cause dehydration (Box 6-1).

Hypovolemia can also occur when fluid from the intravascular space moves into the interstitial fluid space. This process is called third spacing. Examples of conditions in which third spacing is common include burns, liver cirrhosis, and extensive trauma.

As described previously in this chapter, the body initially attempts to compensate for fluid loss by a number of mechanisms. If the cause of dehydration is not resolved or the patient is not able to replace the fluid, a state of dehydration occurs.

Prevention

You can help prevent dehydration by identifying patients who have the highest risk for developing this condition and intervening quickly to correct the cause. High-risk patients include older adults, infants, children, and any patient with one of the conditions listed in Box 6-1. Also see "Gerontological Issues—Dehydration."

Adequate hydration is another important intervention to help prevent dehydration. You should encourage patients to drink adequate fluids. Adults need 30 mL/kg/day of fluids. If a patient is unable to take enough fluid by mouth, alternate routes may be necessary.

Gerontological Issues

Dehydration

As a person ages, total body water decreases from 60% to 50% of total body weight. The age-related decrease in total body water is secondary to an increase in body fat and a decrease in thirst sensation. These factors increase the risk of developing dehydration.

Manifestations of dehydration in an older adult are different from typical manifestations in a younger person and may include altered mental status, lightheadedness, and syncope. These occur because a patient with hypovolemia has an inadequate circulatory volume and, therefore, oxygen supply to the brain.

Signs and Symptoms

Thirst is the initial symptom experienced by otherwise healthy adults in response to hypovolemia. As the percentage of water in the blood goes down, the percentage of other substances goes up, resulting in the thirst response. As the blood volume decreases,

---

• **WORD** • **BUILDING** •

isotonic: iso—equal + tonic—strength
hypotonic: hypo—less than + tonic—strength
hypertonic: hyper—more than + tonic—strength
dehydration: de—down + hydration—water
hypovolemia: hypo—less than + vol—volume + emia—blood

Box 6-1 Common Causes of Dehydration

Cecostomy
Diabetes insipidus
Diarrhea
Diuretic therapy
Draining abscesses
Draining fistulas
Fever
Frequent enemas
Gastrointestinal suction
Hemorrhage
Ileostomy
Long-term nothing-by-mouth (NPO) status
Profuse diaphoresis (sweating)
Severely draining wounds
Systemic infection
Vomiting

the heart pumps the remaining blood faster but not as powerfully, resulting in a rapid, weak pulse and low blood pressure. The body pulls water into the vascular system from other areas, resulting in decreased tear formation, dry skin, and dry mucous membranes.

A dehydrated person will have poor *skin turgor*. Turgor is considered to be poor if the skin is pinched and a small "tent" or wrinkle remains (called *tenting*). A dehydrated person's temperature increases because the body is less able to cool itself through perspiration. Temperature may not appear elevated in an older person because an older adult's normal body temperature is often lower than a younger person's. Urine output decreases and the urine becomes more concentrated as water is conserved. Dehydration should be considered in any adult with a urine output of less than 30 mL per hour. The urine may appear darker because it is less diluted. The patient becomes constipated as the intestines absorb more water from the feces. A major method of evaluating dehydration is weight loss. A pint of water (16 ounces) weighs approximately 1 pound. Symptoms of dehydration in older persons may be atypical (see "Gerontological Issues—Dehydration").

LEARNING TIP

Do you remember your grandmother saying, "A pint's a pound the world around"? It's a great way to remember how much fluid loss is represented by each lost pound.

Complications

If dehydration is not treated, lack of sufficient blood volume causes organ function to decrease and eventually fail. The brain, kidneys, and heart must be adequately supplied with blood (perfused) to function properly. The body protects these organs by decreasing blood flow to other areas. When these organs no longer receive their minimum requirements, death results.

LEARNING TIP

The magic fluid number is 30: healthy adults should drink approximately 30 mL of fluid per kilogram of body weight per day, and they should urinate at least 30 mL per hour. This is just a basic rule of thumb and will vary based on individual circumstances.

Diagnostic Tests

A patient with dehydration usually has an elevated blood urea nitrogen (BUN) level and elevated hematocrit. Both values are increased because there is less water in proportion to the solid substances being measured. The specific gravity of the urine also increases as the kidneys attempt to conserve water, resulting in a more concentrated urine.

Therapeutic Measures

The goals of therapeutic measures are to replace fluids and resolve the cause of dehydration. In a patient with moderate or severe dehydration, IV therapy is used. Isotonic fluids that have the same osmolarity as blood, such as normal saline, are typically administered.

BE SAFE!

BE VIGILANT! Use at least two ways to identify patients. For example, use the patient's name and date of birth. This is done to make sure that each patient gets the correct medicine and treatment (© The Joint Commission, 2013. Reprinted with permission.).

Note: The patient's room number or physical location is not used as an identifier.

Nursing Process for the Patient Experiencing Dehydration

Nurses can play a major role in identifying and caring for patients who are dehydrated.

DATA COLLECTION. Assess the patient for signs and symptoms of dehydration. All the classic signs and symptoms may not be present.

When assessing an older patient for skin turgor (tenting), assess the skin over the forehead or sternum. The skin over these areas usually retains elasticity and is therefore a more reliable indicator of skin turgor. Also check mucous membranes, which should be moist.

Weight is the most reliable indicator of fluid loss or gain. A loss of 1 to 2 pounds or more per day suggests water loss rather than fat loss. The patient in the hospital setting should be weighed every day. The patient in the nursing home or home setting should be weighed at least three times a week if the patient is at risk for fluid imbalance. Weigh the patient before breakfast using the same scale each time. Intake and output (I&O) are also typically measured (see "Cultural Considerations").

NURSING DIAGNOSES, PLANNING, AND IMPLEMENTATION. The primary nursing diagnosis and interventions for the patient with dehydration may include:

Risk for Deficient Fluid Volume or Deficient Fluid Volume related to fluid loss or inadequate fluid intake.

EXPECTED OUTCOME: The patient will be adequately hydrated as evidenced by stable weight, moist mucous membranes, and elastic skin turgor.

- Monitor daily weights and I&O *so problems can be detected and corrected early.*
- Plan with the patient and other members of the health care team the type and timing of fluid intake. *Planning with the patient increases the likelihood that the plan will be followed.*
- Offer fluids often to the confused patient *since he or she may not drink independently.*
- Correct the underlying cause of the fluid deficit, *so it does not recur.*
- Be careful not to overhydrate the patient, *so fluid excess does not occur.*

See Box 6-2 for best practices for maintaining oral hydration in older people.

EVALUATION. The patient who is adequately hydrated will have elastic skin turgor, moist mucous membranes, and stable weight.

Patient Education

The patient, family, and significant others need to be taught the importance of reporting early signs and symptoms of dehydration to a physician or other health care provider (HCP). At home or in the nursing home, infections often cause fever and sepsis, a serious condition in which the infection invades the bloodstream. The body attempts to decrease the temperature through perspiration. The patient becomes dehydrated as a result and can become increasingly ill.

CRITICAL THINKING

Mrs. Levitt

■ Mrs. Levitt is a 92-year-old widow who has been living in the nursing home where you work for 4 years. Today she mentions that her urine smells bad and that her heart feels like it is beating faster than usual. You suspect that she is becoming dehydrated. You check her urine and find that it is a dark amber color and has a strong odor. Her heart rate is 98 beats per minute, blood pressure 126/74 mm Hg, respiratory rate 20 per minute, and temperature 99.2°F (37.3°C).

1. What other data should you collect, and what results do you expect?
2. Which interventions should you provide at this time?
3. How should you document your findings?
4. What other team members should be informed of your plan for Mrs. Levitt?
5. How will you know if she is improving?

Suggested answers are at the end of the chapter.

Fluid Excess

Fluid excess, sometimes called overhydration, is a condition in which a patient has too much fluid in the body. Most of the problems related to fluid excess result from too much fluid in the bloodstream or from dilution of electrolytes and red blood cells.

Pathophysiology and Etiology

The most common result of fluid excess is **hypervolemia** in which there is excess fluid in the intravascular space. Healthy

• WORD • BUILDING •

hypervolemia: hyper—more than + vol—volume + emia—blood

Cultural Considerations

Muslims who celebrate Ramadan fast for 1 month from sunup to sundown. Although the ill are not required to fast, ill Muslims may still wish to do so. Fasting may include not taking fluids and medications during daylight hours. Therefore, the nurse may need to alter times for medication administration, including intramuscular medication. Special precautions may need to be taken to prevent dehydration in Muslim patients.

Box 6-2 Best Practice Recommendations for Maintaining Oral Hydration in Older People

- A fluid intake sheet is the best method of monitoring daily fluid intake.
- Urine specific gravity may be the simplest, most accurate method to determine patient hydration status.
- Evidence of a dry furrowed tongue and mucous membranes, sunken eyes, confusion, and upper body muscle weakness may indicate dehydration.
- Regular presentation of fluids to bedridden older people can maintain adequate hydration status.
- Owing to the observation that medication time can be an important source of fluids, fluids should be encouraged at this time.

Source: Adapted from *Joanna Briggs Best Practice Recommendations: Maintaining Oral Hydration in Older People,* 5:6, 2001. Retrieved June 15, 2013, from http://connect.jbiconnectplus.org /ViewSourceFile.aspx?0=4319

adult kidneys can compensate for mild to moderate hypervolemia. The kidneys increase urinary output to rid the body of the extra fluid. Sometimes, however, the kidneys cannot keep up with the excess fluid.

Conditions that can cause excessive fluid intake are poorly controlled IV therapy, excessive irrigation of wounds or body cavities, and excessive ingestion of water. Conditions that can result in inadequate excretion of fluid include renal (kidney) failure, heart failure, and the syndrome of inappropriate antidiuretic hormone. These conditions are discussed elsewhere in this book.

Prevention

One of the best ways to prevent fluid excess is to avoid excessive fluid intake. For example, you should monitor the patient receiving IV therapy for signs and symptoms of fluid excess. In at-risk patients, an electronic infusion pump or a quantity-limiting device, such as a burette, should be used to control the rate of infusion.

Also monitor the amount of fluid used for irrigations. For example, when a patient's stomach is being irrigated (gastric lavage), be sure an excessive amount of fluid is not absorbed.

Signs and Symptoms

The vital sign changes seen in the patient with fluid excess are the opposite of those found in patients with dehydration. The blood pressure is elevated, pulse is bounding, and respirations are increased and shallow. The neck veins may become distended, and pitting **edema** (excess water in tissues)

• WORD • BUILDING •
edema: swelling

in the feet and legs may be present. The skin is pale and cool. The kidneys increase urine output, and the urine appears diluted, almost like water. The patient rapidly gains weight. In severe fluid excess, the patient develops moist crackles in the lungs, dyspnea, and ascites (excess peritoneal fluid).

Complications

Acute fluid excess typically results in congestive heart failure. As the fluid builds up in the heart, the heart is not able to properly function as a pump. The fluid then backs up into the lungs, causing a condition known as pulmonary edema. Other major organs of the body cannot receive adequate oxygen, and organ failure can lead to death.

Diagnostic Tests

In the patient experiencing fluid excess, BUN and hematocrit levels tend to decrease from hemodilution. The plasma content of the blood is proportionately increased compared with the solid substances. The specific gravity of the urine also diminishes as the urinary output increases.

Therapeutic Measures

Once the patient's breathing has been supported, the goal of treatment is to rid the body of excessive fluid and resolve the underlying cause of the excess. Drug therapy and diet therapy are commonly used to decrease fluid retention.

POSITIONING. To facilitate ease in breathing, the head of the patient's bed should be in semi-Fowler's or high Fowler's position (Fig. 6.2). These positions allow greater lung expansion and thus aid respiratory effort. Once the patient has been properly positioned, oxygen therapy may be necessary.

OXYGEN THERAPY. Oxygen therapy is typically used to ensure adequate perfusion of major organs and to minimize dyspnea. If the patient has a history of chronic obstructive pulmonary disease, such as emphysema or chronic bronchitis,

FIGURE 6.2 Patient in high Fowler's position with oxygen.

be cautious if you need to administer more than 2 L per minute of oxygen. At higher oxygen doses, the patient may lose the stimulus to breathe and may suffer respiratory arrest. Monitor pulse oximetry and respiratory rate carefully.

DRUG THERAPY. Diuretics are commonly administered to rapidly rid the body of excess water. A diuretic is a drug that increases elimination by the kidneys. The drug of choice for fluid excess when the patient has adequately functioning kidneys is usually a loop diuretic such as furosemide (Lasix). Loop diuretics cause the kidneys to excrete sodium and water. Sodium (Na^+) and water tend to move together in the body. Potassium (K^+), another electrolyte, is also lost, which can lead to a potassium deficit, which is discussed later in this chapter.

Furosemide may be given by the oral, intramuscular, or IV route. The oral route is used most commonly for mild fluid excess. IV furosemide is administered by a registered nurse (RN) or HCP for severe fluid excess. The patient should begin diuresis within 30 minutes after receiving IV furosemide. If not, another dose is given. Strict I&O should be monitored, as well as daily weight, when a patient is receiving IV furosemide.

DIET THERAPY. Mild to moderate fluid restriction may be necessary, as well as a sodium-restricted diet. In collaboration with the dietitian, a HCP prescribes the specific restriction necessary, usually a 1- to 2-g sodium restriction for severe excess. Different diuretics result in differing electrolyte elimination. Specific diet therapy depends on the medications the patient is receiving and the patient's underlying medical problems.

Nursing Process for the Patient Experiencing Fluid Excess

The nurse plays a pivotal role in the care of a patient with fluid excess. Prompt action is needed to prevent life-threatening complications.

DATA COLLECTION. Observe a patient who is at high risk for fluid excess and monitor fluid I&O carefully. If the patient is drinking adequate amounts of fluid (1500 mL per day or more) but is voiding in small amounts, the fluid is being retained by the body.

Assess for edema; if it is pitting, a finger pressed against the skin over a bony area such as the tibia leaves a temporary indentation. For patients in bed, check the sacrum for edema. For patients in the sitting position, check the feet and legs. Also assess lung sounds because excess fluid accumulation in the lungs can cause crackles (see Chapter 29).

As mentioned earlier, weight is the most reliable indicator of fluid gain. Weigh at-risk patients daily. A gain of 1 to 2 pounds or more per day indicates fluid retention even though other signs and symptoms may not be present.

NURSING DIAGNOSES, PLANNING, AND IMPLEMENTATION.

Excess Fluid Volume related to excessive fluid intake or inadequate excretion of body fluid

EXPECTED OUTCOME: Patient will return to a normal hydration status as evidenced by return to weight that

is normal for patient, absence of edema, and clear lung sounds.

- Report any increase in weight to the HCP. *Increased weight indicates fluid retention.*
- Implement fluid restriction as ordered *to reduce excess intake.* Work with the patient and RN to determine how it should be implemented. For example, if a patient is on a 1000 mL per day fluid restriction, you might plan for 150 mL with each meal, 450 mL to be given to the patient to use as he or she likes during the day and 100 mL to be used during the night. Be sure to include the patient in your planning, and remember to reserve enough fluid for swallowing medications. Post a sign in the patient's room so other caregivers know how much fluid the patient can have.
- Administer diuretics as ordered, and monitor patient response. Be sure to monitor potassium in patients receiving potassium-losing loop or thiazide diuretics. *Diuretics promote diuresis.*
- Report urinary output below 30 mL per hour to the HCP or RN *because this may signify increasing renal complications.*

EVALUATION. If interventions have been effective, the patient will return to his or her normal weight with clear lung sounds and no edema. Many patients must remain on drug and diet therapy after hospital discharge to prevent the problem from recurring.

Patient Education

In collaboration with the dietitian, instruct the patient, family, or other caregiver about any fluid or sodium restrictions to prevent further problems (see "Nutrition Notes"). High-sodium foods to avoid are listed in Table 6.1.

Nutrition Notes

Reducing Sodium Intake

Many foods, such as dairy products, grain products, and some vegetables, are naturally high in sodium, but the major sources of dietary sodium are salted and processed foods, including baked goods and condiments. For example, American cheese has more sodium than cheddar, and cured ham has more than fresh pork.

Drinking water may contain significant amounts of sodium, particularly if it is softened or mineral water. Because of the numerous hidden sources of sodium, patients on low-sodium diets benefit from education by a dietitian.

The adequate intake (AI) of sodium is
- 1.5 g daily for adults through age 49
- 1.3 g daily for those aged 50 to 70
- 1.2 g daily for those aged 71 and older

The upper tolerable intake level (UL) for sodium is 2.3 g daily, which is contained in slightly more than a teaspoon of salt. None of these amounts applies to those losing large amounts of sweat daily or to unacclimatized persons exercising in a hot environment.

Specific definitions for reduced-sodium food products have been adopted. Note that serving size is an important variable.

- Salt or sodium free: <5 mg sodium per serving
- Very low sodium: <35 mg sodium per serving (per 100 g if main dish)
- Low sodium: <140 mg sodium per serving (per 100 g if main dish)

Teaching about diuretic therapy is essential to prevent electrolyte imbalances. If a potassium-losing diuretic is prescribed, teach the patient to eat foods that are high in potassium (Table 6.2). The patient's serum potassium level must be periodically monitored by a HCP or home care nurse. If it becomes too low, an oral potassium supplement is needed.

The patient or caregiver also needs to be taught common signs and symptoms of fluid excess that should be reported to a physician or other HCP. Of special importance is weight gain. A patient at high risk for fluid excess should be weighed at least three times a week in the home or nursing home, at the same time each day, and on the same scale. Weight gain should be reported.

TABLE 6.1 COMMON FOOD SOURCES OF SODIUM*

Food Group	Serving Size	Range (mg)
Frozen vegetables	1 oz	95–210
Frozen pizza, plain, cheese	4 oz	450–1200
Frozen vegetables, all types	1/2 cup	2–160
Salad dressing, regular fat, all types	2 tbsp	110–505
Salsa	2 tbsp	150–240
Soup (tomato), reconstituted	8 oz	700–1260
Tomato juice	8 oz (1 cup)	340–1040
Potato chips†	1 oz (28.4 g)	120–180
Tortilla chips†	1 oz (28.4 g)	105–160
Pretzels†	1 oz (28.4 g)	290–560

*Ranges of sodium content are for selected foods available in the retail market. This table is provided to exemplify the importance of reading the food label to determine the sodium content of food, which can vary by several hundreds of milligrams in similar foods.

†All snack foods are regular flavor, salted.

Note: None of the examples provided was labeled "low sodium."

Source: Agricultural Research Service Nutrient Database for Standard Reference, Release 17, and recent manufacturers' label data from retail market surveys. Serving sizes were standardized to be comparable among brands within a food. Pizza and bread slices vary in size and weight across brands.

TABLE 6.2 FOOD SOURCES OF POTASSIUM*

Food, Standard Amount	Potassium (mg)	Calories
Sweet potato, baked, 1 potato (146 g)	694	131
Beet greens, cooked, 1/2 cup	655	9
Potato, baked, flesh, 1 potato (156 g)	610	145
Yogurt, plain, nonfat, 8-oz container	579	127
Prune juice, 3/4 cup	530	136
Soybeans, green, cooked, 1/2 cup	485	127
Bananas, 1 medium	422	105
Spinach, cooked, 1/2 cup	419	21
Tomato juice, 3/4 cup	417	31
Tomato sauce, 1/2 cup	405	39
Milk, nonfat, 1 cup	382	83
Pork chop, center loin, cooked, 3 oz	382	197
Apricots, dried, uncooked, 1/4 cup	378	78
Cantaloupe, 1/4 medium	368	47
1% or 2% milk, 1 cup	366	102–122
Kidney beans, cooked, 1/2 cup	358	112
Orange juice, 3/4 cup	355	85
Split peas, cooked, 1/2 cup	355	116

*Food sources of potassium ranked by milligrams of potassium per standard amount, also showing calories in the standard amount. (The adequate intake for adults is 4700 mg/day of potassium.)

Source: Nutrient values from Agricultural Research Service (ARS) Nutrient Database for Standard Reference, Release 17. Foods are from ARS single nutrient reports, sorted in descending order by nutrient content in terms of common household measures. Food items and weights in the single nutrient reports are adapted from those in the 2002 revision of U.S. Department of Agriculture Home and Garden Bulletin No. 72, *Nutritive Value of Foods.* Mixed dishes and multiple preparations of the same food item have been omitted from this table.

CRITICAL THINKING

Mr. Peters

■ Mr. Peters is a 32-year-old man with a congenital heart problem. He has been recovering from congestive heart failure and fluid excess. Today his blood pressure is higher than usual, and his pulse is bounding. He is having trouble breathing and presses the call light for your assistance.

1. What should you do first when you assess Mr. Peters's condition?
2. What questions should you ask him?
3. What objective data should you collect?
4. What should you do with your findings?

Suggested answers are at the end of the chapter.

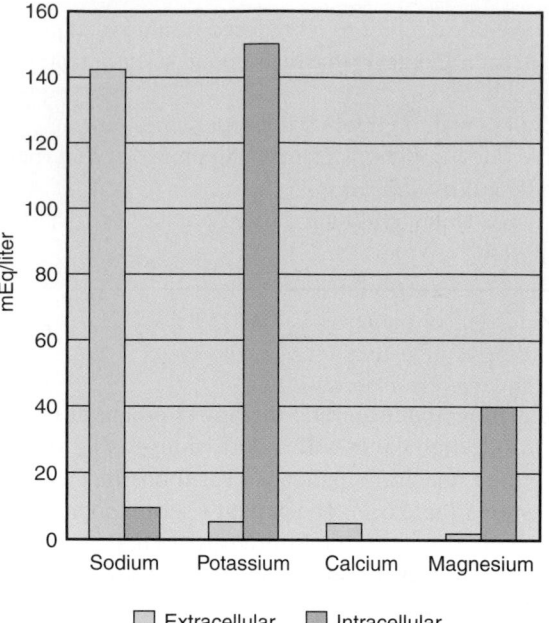

FIGURE 6.3 Extracellular and intracellular electrolytes.

ELECTROLYTE BALANCE

Natural minerals in food become electrolytes or ions in the body through digestion and metabolism. Electrolytes are usually measured in milliequivalents per liter (mEq/L) or in milligrams per deciliter (mg/dL).

Electrolytes are one of two types: **cations**, which carry a positive electrical charge, and **anions**, which carry a negative electrical charge. Although there are many electrolytes in the body, this chapter discusses the most important ones, including sodium (Na^+), potassium (K^+), calcium (Ca^{2+}), and magnesium (Mg^{2+}). These electrolytes are maintained in different concentrations inside the cell and outside the cell because of pumps in the cell wall (Fig. 6.3).

ELECTROLYTE IMBALANCES

At times, a patient may experience problems because of too much or too little of an electrolyte. In general, if a patient experiences a deficit of an electrolyte, the electrolyte is replaced either orally or intravenously. If the patient experiences an excess of an electrolyte, treatment focuses on getting rid of the excess, often via the kidneys. The underlying cause of the imbalance must also be treated.

The most important aspects of nursing care are preventing and assessing electrolyte imbalances. You must be vigilant in watching for signs of imbalance in high-risk patients. Serum electrolytes are measured on a regular basis. As a general rule, patients should be checked for electrolyte imbalance when there is a change in their mental state (either increased irritability or decreased responsiveness) or when muscle function changes. Patient education is another important nursing role.

Sodium Imbalances

The normal level of serum sodium is 135 to 145 mEq/L. Because sodium is the major cation in the blood, it helps maintain serum osmolarity. Therefore, sodium imbalances are often associated with fluid imbalances, described earlier in this chapter. Sodium is also important for cell function, especially in the central nervous system. The two sodium imbalances are **hyponatremia** (sodium deficit) and **hypernatremia** (sodium excess).

Hyponatremia

Hyponatremia occurs when the serum sodium level is less than 135 mEq/L.

PATHOPHYSIOLOGY AND ETIOLOGY. Many conditions can lead to either an actual or a relative decrease in sodium. In an actual decrease, the patient has inadequate intake of sodium or excessive sodium loss from the body. As the percentage of sodium in the ECF decreases, water is pulled by osmotic pressure into the cells. In a relative decrease, the sodium is not lost from the body but may leave the intravascular space and move into the interstitial tissues (third spacing). Another cause of a relative decrease occurs when the plasma volume increases (fluid excess), causing a dilutional effect. The percentage of sodium compared with the fluid is diminished.

PREVENTION. Additional sodium is commonly administered to patients at high risk for hyponatremia (Box 6-3), usually by the IV route. Individuals who have high fevers or who engage in strenuous exercise or physical labor, especially in the

• WORD • BUILDING •

cation: cat—descending + ion—carrying
anion: an—without + ion—carrying
hyponatremia: hypo—less than + natr—sodium + emia—blood
hypernatremia: hyper—more than + natr—sodium + emia—blood

Box 6-3 Conditions that Place Patients at High Risk for Hyponatremia

Nothing by mouth (NPO)
Excessive diaphoresis (sweating)
Diuretics
Gastrointestinal suction
Syndrome of inappropriate antidiuretic hormone
Excessive ingestion of hypotonic fluids
Freshwater near-drowning
Decreased aldosterone

heat, need to replace both sodium and water. Hyponatremia is especially dangerous for the older patient.

SIGNS AND SYMPTOMS. Unfortunately, the signs and symptoms of hyponatremia are vague and depend somewhat on whether a fluid imbalance accompanies the hyponatremia. The patient with sodium and fluid deficits has signs and symptoms of dehydration (discussed previously). The patient with a sodium deficit and relative fluid excess has signs and symptoms associated with fluid excess.

With more severe sodium deficit, the patient experiences mental status changes, including disorientation, confusion, and personality changes. This occurs because the low sodium and decrease in osmolarity cause more "water-pushing pressure," which causes water to collect in and around the brain and increase pressure (cerebral edema). Weakness, nausea, vomiting, and diarrhea may also occur. See "Gerontological Issues—Confusion."

Gerontological Issues

Confusion

Often older clients who experience a change in their electrolyte levels will present with sudden unexplained confusion. By referring the situation to the RN or HCP as soon as the situation occurs, blood work for an electrolyte panel can be conducted and the older patient can be provided the needed electrolytes via IV therapy, which may quickly relieve the confused state. Because older patients' cardiovascular systems are very sensitive to quick fluid shifts, IV infusions should only be provided at the rate prescribed by the HCP.

COMPLICATIONS. In severe hyponatremia, respiratory arrest or coma can lead to death. The patient who also has fluid excess may develop pulmonary edema, another life-threatening complication.

DIAGNOSTIC TESTS. The primary diagnostic test is a serum sodium level, which is lower than the normal value when hyponatremia is present. The serum osmolarity also decreases in patients with hyponatremia. Other laboratory results may be affected if the patient experiences an accompanying fluid imbalance. Serum chloride (Cl^-), an anion, is often depleted when sodium decreases because these two electrolytes commonly combine as NaCl (salt in solution, or saline).

THERAPEUTIC MEASURES. Therapeutic measures focus on resolving the underlying cause of hyponatremia and replacing the lost sodium. The HCP orders IV saline for patients who have hyponatremia without fluid excess.

For patients who have a fluid excess, a fluid restriction is often ordered. Diuretics that rid the body of fluid but do not cause sodium loss may also be used. For patients with cerebral edema, steroids may be prescribed to reduce **intracranial** swelling. I&O are strictly monitored, and the patient is weighed daily. Also implement interventions to keep the patient safe if mental status is affected.

Hypernatremia

Hypernatremia occurs when the serum sodium level is above 145 mEq/L.

PATHOPHYSIOLOGY AND ETIOLOGY. A serum sodium increase may be an actual increase or a relative increase. In an actual increase, the patient receives too much sodium or is unable to excrete sodium, as seen in renal failure. In a relative increase, the amount of sodium does not change, but the amount of fluid in the intravascular space decreases. Therefore, the percentage of sodium (solid) is increased in relationship to the amount of plasma (water).

In mild hypernatremia, most excitable tissues, such as muscle and neurons of the brain, become more stimulated. The patient becomes irritable and has tremors. In severe cases, these tissues fail to respond.

PREVENTION. Prevention of hypernatremia is not as simple as prevention of hyponatremia. Most patients have a sodium excess as a result of an acute or chronic illness. Patients with a potential for electrolyte imbalance must always have their IV fluids carefully regulated.

SIGNS AND SYMPTOMS. Thirst is usually one of the first symptoms to appear. If you eat salty foods, such as potato chips, the amount of sodium in the body increases, and you become thirsty. Other signs and symptoms of hypernatremia are vague and nonspecific until severe excess is present. Like the patient with a sodium deficit, the patient experiencing sodium excess has mental status changes, such as agitation, confusion, and personality changes—but this time, the cause is too little fluid in the brain tissues. Seizures may also occur.

• WORD • BUILDING •

intracranial: intra—within + cranial—cranium (skull)

At first, muscle twitches and unusual contractions may be present. Later, skeletal muscle weakness occurs that can lead to respiratory failure if it affects the diaphragm. If fluid deficit or fluid excess accompanies the hypernatremic state, the patient also has signs and symptoms associated with these imbalances.

COMPLICATIONS. A patient with severe hypernatremia may become comatose or have respiratory arrest as skeletal muscles weaken.

DIAGNOSTIC TESTS. The most reliable diagnostic test is the serum sodium level, which indicates an increase above the normal level. Serum osmolarity may also increase. If the patient has a fluid imbalance, other laboratory values, such as BUN, hematocrit, and urine specific gravity, are also affected (see earlier discussion).

THERAPEUTIC MEASURES. If a fluid imbalance accompanies hypernatremia, it is treated first. For example, fluid replacement without sodium in a patient with dehydration should correct a relative sodium excess. If the kidneys are not excreting adequate amounts of sodium, diuretics may help if the kidneys are functional. If the kidneys are not functioning properly, dialysis may be ordered (see Chapter 37). I&O and daily weights are strictly monitored.

The cause of hypernatremia is also treated in an attempt to prevent further episodes of this imbalance. For some patients, a sodium-restricted diet is prescribed.

Potassium Imbalances

Potassium is the most common electrolyte in the ICF compartment. Therefore, only a small amount, 3.5 to 5 mEq/L, is found in the bloodstream. Small changes in this laboratory value cause major changes in the body.

Potassium is especially important for cardiac muscle, skeletal muscle, and smooth muscle function. If the serum potassium level falls, the body attempts to compensate by moving potassium from the cells into the bloodstream.

The two potassium imbalances are **hypokalemia** (potassium deficit) and **hyperkalemia** (potassium excess). Hypokalemia is the most commonly occurring imbalance.

Hypokalemia

Hypokalemia occurs when the serum potassium level falls below 3.5 mEq/L.

PATHOPHYSIOLOGY AND ETIOLOGY. Most cases of hypokalemia result from inadequate intake of potassium or excessive loss of potassium through the kidneys. Hypokalemia most often occurs as a result of medications. Potassium-losing diuretics (e.g., furosemide [Lasix]), digitalis preparations (e.g., digoxin [Lanoxin]), and corticosteroids (e.g., prednisone [Deltasone]) are examples of drugs that cause increased excretion of potassium from the body. Potassium may also be lost through the gastrointestinal (GI) tract, which is rich in potassium and other electrolytes. Severe vomiting, diarrhea, and prolonged GI suction cause hypokalemia (see "Patient Perspective"). Major surgery and hemorrhage can also lead to potassium deficit.

Patient Perspective

Patricia

I take hydrochlorothiazide for my high blood pressure. Since it can make me lose potassium, I also take a potassium supplement. So I thought I was all set. But recently I ate something that did not agree with me, and I had diarrhea for a couple of days. One morning as I was driving to work, I felt so weak it made me frightened. I drove back home and asked my husband to drive me to work. I arrived safely, but as I walked down the hallway, I again felt so weak I had to sit down. I felt like I could not put one foot in front of the other. I kept thinking, "This is all in my head." I decided maybe I was dehydrated from the diarrhea, so I drank a bottle of Gatorade and a glass of orange juice. Slowly I began to feel a bit better, and I made it through the day. After work I had to take my daughter to the doctor, so I asked about my symptoms. I was sent to the lab where I had my potassium level checked, and it was 3.1! Normal is 3.5 to 5 mEq/L. Mine must have been even lower before I drank the juice and Gatorade. I learned that I probably lost a lot of potassium because of the diarrhea. I also learned that low potassium made my muscles weak and could have affected my heart function. Next time I have diarrhea, I plan to call my doctor.

PREVENTION. Most patients having major surgery receive potassium supplements in their IV fluids to prevent hypokalemia. For patients receiving drugs known to cause hypokalemia, foods high in potassium may prevent a deficit (see Table 6.2). Patients receiving digitalis must be closely monitored because digitalis can cause hypokalemia, which in turn can enhance the action of digitalis and cause digitalis toxicity.

SIGNS AND SYMPTOMS. Many body systems are affected by a potassium imbalance. Muscle cramping or muscle fatigue can occur with either a deficit or an excess of potassium. Vital signs change because the respiratory and cardiovascular systems need potassium to function properly. Diminished skeletal muscle activity results in shallow, ineffective respirations. The pulse is typically weak, irregular, and thready because the heart muscle is depleted of potassium. A major danger is an irregular heartbeat (**dysrhythmia**), which can lead to cardiac arrest. Orthostatic (postural) hypotension may also be present.

• **WORD • BUILDING •**

hypokalemia: hypo—less than + kal—potassium + emia—blood
hyperkalemia: hyper—more than + kal—potassium + emia—blood
dysrhythmia: dys—bad or disordered + rhythmia—measured motion

The nervous system is usually affected as well. The patient experiences changes in mental status followed by lethargy. The motility of the GI system is slowed, causing nausea, vomiting, abdominal distention, and constipation. Vomiting may further increase potassium loss.

COMPLICATIONS. If not corrected, hypokalemia can result in death from dysrhythmia, respiratory failure and arrest, or coma. The patient must be treated promptly before these complications occur.

DIAGNOSTIC TESTS. The primary laboratory test is to obtain a serum potassium level. The patient's electrocardiogram (ECG) may show cardiac dysrhythmias associated with potassium deficit. In addition to a decrease in the serum potassium level, the patient may have an acid–base imbalance known as metabolic **alkalosis**, which commonly accompanies hypokalemia. In metabolic alkalosis, the serum pH of the blood increases (>7.45) so that the blood is more alkaline than usual. Acid–base imbalances are discussed later in this chapter.

THERAPEUTIC MEASURES. The goal of treatment is to replace potassium in the body and resolve the underlying cause of the imbalance. For mild to moderate hypokalemia, oral potassium supplements are given.

For severe hypokalemia, IV potassium supplements are given. Because the kidneys eliminate excess potassium, potassium should be administered only after the patient has voided. Potassium is a potentially dangerous drug, especially when administered intravenously. In too high a concentration, it causes cardiac arrest. Only IV solutions that are premixed and carefully labeled should be used. Potassium is never given by IV push. The patient's laboratory values must be monitored carefully to prevent giving too much potassium.

Teach the patient about the side effects of oral potassium and precautions associated with potassium administration. Box 6-4 summarizes the precautions the patient should be aware of when taking oral potassium supplements.

Hyperkalemia

Hyperkalemia is a condition in which the serum potassium level exceeds 5 mEq/L. It is rare in a person with healthy kidneys.

PATHOPHYSIOLOGY AND ETIOLOGY. Hyperkalemia may result from an actual increase in the amount of total body potassium or from the movement of intracellular potassium into the blood. Overuse of potassium-based salt substitutes or excessive intake of oral or IV potassium supplements can cause hyperkalemia. Use of potassium-sparing diuretics (e.g., spironolactone [Aldactone]) may also contribute to hyperkalemia. Patients with renal failure are at risk for hyperkalemia because the kidneys cannot excrete potassium.

Movement of potassium from the cells into the blood and other ECF is common in massive tissue trauma and metabolic acidosis. Metabolic **acidosis** is an acid–base imbalance commonly seen in patients with uncontrolled diabetes mellitus. Acid–base imbalances are discussed later in this chapter.

Box 6-4 Tips for Patients Taking Oral Potassium Supplements

- Do not substitute one potassium supplement for another.
- Dilute powders and liquids in juice or other desired liquid to improve taste and to prevent gastrointestinal irritation. Follow manufacturer's recommendations for the amount of fluid to use for dilution, most commonly 4 oz per 20 mEq of potassium.
- Do not drink diluted solutions until mixed thoroughly.
- Do not crush potassium tablets, such as Slow-K or K-tab tablets. Read manufacturer's directions regarding which tablets can be crushed.
- Take slow-release tablets with 8 oz of water to help them dissolve.
- Do not take potassium supplements if taking potassium-sparing diuretics such as spironolactone or triamterene.
- Do not use salt substitutes containing potassium unless prescribed by the HCP.
- Take potassium supplements with meals.
- Report adverse effects, such as nausea, vomiting, diarrhea, and abdominal cramping, to the HCP.
- Have frequent laboratory testing for potassium levels as recommended by the HCP.

Source: Adapted from Lee, C. A., Barrett, C. A., & Ignatavicius, D. D. (1996). *Fluids and electrolytes: A practical approach* (4th ed.). Philadelphia: F. A. Davis.

PREVENTION. For patients receiving potassium supplements, hyperkalemia can be prevented by monitoring serum electrolyte values and the patient's signs and symptoms and adjusting the dose accordingly.

SIGNS AND SYMPTOMS. Most cases of hyperkalemia occur in patients who are hospitalized or those undergoing therapeutic measures for a chronic condition. The classic manifestations are muscle twitches and cramps, later followed by profound muscular weakness; increased GI motility (diarrhea); slow, irregular heart rate; and decreased blood pressure.

COMPLICATIONS. Cardiac dysrhythmias and respiratory failure can occur in severe hyperkalemia, causing death.

DIAGNOSTIC TESTS. In addition to an elevated serum potassium level, an irregular ECG is associated with hyperkalemia. If the patient also has metabolic acidosis, the serum pH falls below 7.35.

THERAPEUTIC MEASURES. For mild, chronic hyperkalemia, dietary limitation of potassium-rich foods may be helpful.

• WORD • BUILDING •
alkalosis: alkal—alkaline + osis—condition
acidosis: acid—acidic + osis—condition

Potassium supplements are discontinued, and potassium-losing diuretics are given to patients with healthy kidneys. For patients with renal problems, a cation exchange resin, such as sodium polystyrene sulfonate (Kayexalate), is administered either orally or rectally. This drug releases sodium and absorbs potassium for excretion through the feces and out of the body.

In cases in which cellular potassium has moved into the bloodstream, administration of glucose and insulin can facilitate the movement of potassium back into the cells. During treatment of moderate to severe hyperkalemia, the patient should be in the hospital on a cardiac monitor.

Calcium Imbalances

Calcium is a mineral that is primarily stored in bones and teeth. A small amount is found in ECF. The normal value for serum calcium is 9 to 11 mg/dL, or 4.5 to 5.5 mEq/L. Minimal changes in serum calcium levels can have major negative effects in the body.

Calcium is needed for the proper function of excitable tissues, especially cardiac muscle. The two calcium imbalances are **hypocalcemia** and **hypercalcemia**.

Hypocalcemia

Hypocalcemia occurs when the serum calcium level falls below 9 mg/dL, or 4.5 mEq/L.

PATHOPHYSIOLOGY AND ETIOLOGY. Although calcium deficit can be acute or chronic, most patients develop hypocalcemia slowly as a result of chronic disease or poor intake. The woman who is postmenopausal is most at risk for hypocalcemia. As a woman ages, calcium intake typically declines. The parathyroid glands recognize this decrease and stimulate bone to release some of its stored calcium into the blood for replacement. The result is a condition known as **osteoporosis**, in which bones become porous and brittle and fracture easily. The woman who is postmenopausal has a decreased level of estrogens, hormones that help prevent bone loss in the younger woman. Immobility or decreased mobility also contributes to bone loss in many patients. The patients at highest risk for osteoporosis are thin, petite, Caucasian women.

Hypocalcemia can also result from inadequate absorption of calcium from the intestines, as seen in patients with Crohn's disease, a chronic inflammatory bowel disease. Insufficient intake of vitamin D prevents calcium absorption as well. Conditions that interfere with the production of parathyroid hormone, such as partial or complete surgical removal of the thyroid or parathyroids, can also cause hypocalcemia.

Finally, patients with hyperphosphatemia (usually those with renal failure) often experience hypocalcemia. Calcium and phosphate have an inverse relationship. When one of these electrolytes increases, the other tends to decrease and vice versa.

• WORD • BUILDING •

hypocalcemia: hypo—less than + calc—calcium + emia—blood
hypercalcemia: hyper—more than + calc—calcium + emia—blood
osteoporosis: osteo—bone + porosis—porous

PREVENTION. In the United States, the typical daily calcium intake is less than 550 mg. The AI of calcium for adults ages 19 to 50 is 1000 mg; the AI for adults over age 50 is 1200 mg.

Hypocalcemia can be prevented by consuming calcium-rich foods and by taking calcium supplements. These supplements can be purchased over the counter in any pharmacy or large food store. An inexpensive source of calcium for patients who do not require vitamin D supplementation is calcium carbonate (Tums), which provides 240 mg of elemental calcium in each tablet. Patients should be cautioned not to routinely take high doses of calcium without checking with their primary care provider (see "Evidence-Based Practice").

EVIDENCE-BASED PRACTICE

Clinical Question
Are there problems associated with taking too much supplemental calcium?

Evidence
Studies conducted in Sweden discovered that women who had long-term calcium intakes from all sources above 1400 mg/day had higher death rates from all causes (Michaëlsson, Melhus, Lemming, Wolk, & Byberg, 2013).

Implications for Nursing Practice
When patients take calcium supplements, teach them how to calculate their total calcium intake and that too much calcium can be as harmful as too little calcium. Teach patients to consult with their providers before beginning calcium supplements.

REFERENCE
Michaëlsson, K., Melhus, H., Lemming, E., Wolk, A., & Byberg, L. (2013). Long term calcium intake and rates of all cause and cardiovascular mortality: Community based prospective longitudinal cohort study. *The British Journal of Medicine, 346*, f228.

Vitamin D supplementation may be required in addition to calcium for patients whose sun exposure is limited. The sun's ultraviolet light causes the skin to manufacture vitamin D.

SIGNS AND SYMPTOMS. Chronic hypocalcemia is usually not diagnosed until the patient breaks a bone, usually a hip. Acute hypocalcemia, which can occur after surgery or in patients with acute pancreatitis, has several signs and symptoms. These include increased and irregular heart rate, mental status changes, hyperactive deep tendon reflexes, and increased GI motility, including diarrhea and abdominal cramping. Two classic signs that can be used to assess for hypocalcemia are Trousseau's sign and Chvostek's sign.

To test for Trousseau's sign, inflate a blood pressure cuff around the patient's upper arm for 1 to 4 minutes. In a patient with hypocalcemia, the hand and fingers become spastic and go into palmar flexion (Fig. 6.4). A positive Chvostek's sign

FIGURE 6.4 Trousseau's sign.

test also indicates calcium deficit. To test for this sign, tap the face just below and in front of the ear. Facial twitching on that side of the face indicates a positive test (Fig. 6.5). The Trousseau's sign is more specific for hypocalcemia than Chvostek's sign.

 LEARNING TIP

You can remember which sign is **CH**vostek's sign because it causes spasm near the **CH**eek.

COMPLICATIONS. In severe hypocalcemia, neuromuscular irritability can lead to tetany, or continuous muscle contraction. The patient may have a sudden laryngospasm that will stop air from entering the lungs. Seizures, respiratory failure, or cardiac failure can occur and lead to death if not aggressively treated.

FIGURE 6.5 Chvostek's sign.

DIAGNOSTIC TESTS. The patient with hypocalcemia has a lowered serum calcium level and an abnormal ECG. The parathyroid hormone level may be increased as it attempts to stimulate bone to release more calcium into the blood.

THERAPEUTIC MEASURES. In addition to treating the cause of hypocalcemia, calcium is replaced. For mild or chronic hypocalcemia, oral calcium supplements with or without vitamin D are given. Calcium supplements should be administered 1 to 2 hours after meals to increase intestinal absorption. Be sure to check compatibility when administering calcium with other medications.

For patients with acute or severe hypocalcemia, IV calcium gluconate or calcium chloride is given. When a patient has had thyroid or parathyroid surgery, there is a danger that parathyroid hormone will be decreased, causing serum calcium to drop. IV calcium must be readily available for emergency use if signs of hypocalcemia occur.

For patients with hyperphosphatemia, usually those with renal failure, aluminum hydroxide is used to bind the excess phosphate for elimination via the GI tract. As the phosphate decreases, the serum calcium level begins to approach normal levels.

Diet therapy is an important part of treatment. Teach the patient, family, or other caregiver which foods are high in calcium (Table 6.3). Many foods today are fortified with calcium. Vitamin D foods are also encouraged, especially milk and other dairy products. For patients experiencing difficulty digesting dairy products and those who choose not to use dairy products, special attention must be paid to including other dietary calcium sources in the diet.

CRITICAL THINKING

Mrs. Wright

■ Mrs. Wright is a 77-year-old petite Caucasian woman who lives alone at home. She is on a fixed income and rarely eats calcium-rich foods. She recently fell and broke her hip. After surgery, she returned home under the care of a home health agency.

1. What made the patient at high risk for a fracture?
2. What would you expect her serum calcium level to have been before the fall?
3. What patient teaching related to diet and calcium supplements should the home health nurse include during his or her home visits?
4. In addition to a nurse, what other home health team members might be helpful for Mrs. Wright?

Suggested answers are at the end of the chapter.

Hypercalcemia

Hypercalcemia occurs when the serum calcium is above 11 mg/dL, or 5.5 mEq/L.

TABLE 6.3   FOOD SOURCES OF CALCIUM*

Food, Standard Amount	Calcium (mg)	Calories
Fortified ready-to-eat cereals (various), 1 oz	236–1043	88–106
Soy beverage, calcium fortified, 1 cup	368	98
Tofu, firm, prepared with nigiri†, 1/2 cup	253	88
Pink salmon, canned, with bone, 3 oz	181	118
Collards, cooked from frozen, 1/2 cup	178	31
Spinach, cooked from frozen, 1/2 cup	146	30
Turnip greens, cooked from frozen, 1/2 cup	124	24
Ocean perch, Atlantic, cooked, 3 oz	116	103
Oatmeal, plain and flavored, instant, fortified, 1 packet prepared	99–110	97–157
Okra, cooked from frozen, 1/2 cup	88	26
Pak choy (bok choy), Chinese cabbage, cooked from fresh, 1/2 cup	79	10
Dandelion greens, cooked from fresh, 1/2 cup	74	17
Rainbow trout, farmed, cooked, 3 oz	73	144
Dairy Sources	Calcium (mg)	Calories
Plain yogurt, low-fat (12 g protein/8 oz), 8-oz container	415	143
Fruit yogurt, low-fat (10 g protein/8 oz), 8-oz container	345	232
Swiss cheese, 1.5 oz	336	162
Mozzarella cheese, part-skim, 1.5 oz	311	129
Cheddar cheese, 1.5 oz	307	171
Fat-free (skim) milk, 1 cup	306	83
2% reduced fat milk, 1 cup	285	122
Whole milk, 1 cup	276	146

*Both calcium content and bioavailability should be considered when selecting dietary sources of calcium. Some plant foods have calcium that is well absorbed, but the large quantity of plant foods that would be needed to provide as much calcium as in a glass of milk may be unachievable for many. Many other calcium-fortified foods are available, but the percentage of calcium that can be absorbed is unavailable for many of them.

†Calcium sulfate and magnesium chloride.

Source: Nutrient values from Agricultural Research Service (ARS) Nutrient Database for Standard Reference, Release 17. Foods are from ARS single nutrient reports, sorted in descending order by nutrient content in terms of common household measures. Food items and weights in the single nutrient reports are adapted from those in the 2002 revision of USDA Home and Garden Bulletin No. 72, *Nutritive Value of Foods.* Mixed dishes and multiple preparations of the same food item have been omitted from this table.

PATHOPHYSIOLOGY AND ETIOLOGY. Chronic hypercalcemia can result from excessive intake of calcium or vitamin D, renal failure, hyperparathyroidism, cancers, and overuse or prolonged use of thiazide diuretics, such as hydrochlorothiazide (HydroDIURIL). Acute hypercalcemia can occur as an emergency in patients with invasive or metastatic cancers, especially cancers of the blood or bone.

PREVENTION. Although many causes of increased calcium cannot be prevented, a person receiving calcium supplements should be monitored carefully. Some patients believe that if two or three tablets a day are helpful, consuming twice that much will help even more. The result can be serum calcium

excess. Educating the public about the proper amount of calcium needed each day and the danger of too much calcium is very important.

SIGNS AND SYMPTOMS. Patients who have mild hypercalcemia or a slowly progressing calcium increase may have no obvious signs and symptoms. However, acute hypercalcemia is associated with increased heart rate and blood pressure, skeletal muscle weakness, and decreased GI motility.

COMPLICATIONS. In some cases, the patient may experience renal or urinary calculi (stones) resulting from the buildup of calcium. In more severe cases of acute hypercalcemia, the patient may experience respiratory failure caused by profound muscle weakness or heart failure caused by dysrhythmias.

THERAPEUTIC MEASURES. Patients with severe hypercalcemia should be hospitalized and placed on a cardiac monitor. Unless contraindicated by other conditions, the primary treatment is to give large amounts of fluids and promote diuresis. Saline infusions are the most useful solutions to promote renal excretion of calcium.

The HCP also discontinues thiazide diuretics if the patient was receiving them and prescribes diuretics that promote calcium excretion, such as furosemide (Lasix). Drugs that slow calcium movement from bones to the blood may also be used, such as pamidronate (Aredia), zoledronic acid (Zometa), or calcitonin.

If hypercalcemia is so severe that cardiac problems are present, hemodialysis, peritoneal dialysis, or ultrafiltration may be necessary to cleanse the blood of excess calcium. (See Chapter 37 for discussion of these procedures.)

Magnesium Imbalances

Magnesium and calcium work together for the proper functioning of excitable cells, such as cardiac muscle and nerve cells. Therefore, an imbalance of magnesium is usually accompanied by an imbalance of calcium.

The normal value for serum magnesium is 1.5 to 2.5 mEq/L. The magnesium imbalances are called **hypomagnesemia** and **hypermagnesemia**.

Hypomagnesemia

Hypomagnesemia occurs when the serum magnesium level falls below 1.5 mEq/L. It results from either a decreased intake or an excessive loss of magnesium. Causes of inadequate intake include malnutrition and starvation diets. Patients with severe diarrhea and Crohn's disease are unable to absorb magnesium in the intestines.

One of the major causes of hypomagnesemia is alcoholism, which causes both a decreased intake and an increased renal excretion of magnesium. Certain drugs, such as loop and osmotic diuretics, aminoglycosides (e.g., gentamicin), and some anticancer agents (e.g., cisplatin), can increase renal excretion of magnesium.

The signs and symptoms of hypomagnesemia are similar to those for hypocalcemia, including positive Trousseau's and Chvostek's signs, described earlier in this chapter.

The goal of management is to treat the underlying cause and replace magnesium in the body. Magnesium sulfate is administered intravenously. If the serum calcium is also low, calcium replacement is prescribed. The patient is placed on a cardiac monitor because of magnesium's effect on the heart. Life-threatening dysrhythmias can lead to cardiac failure and arrest.

• **WORD** • **BUILDING** •

hypomagnesemia: hypo—less than + magnes—magnesium + emia—blood

hypermagnesemia: hyper—more than + magnes—magnesium + emia—blood

Hypermagnesemia

Hypermagnesemia results when the serum magnesium level increases above 2.5 mEq/L. The most common cause of hypermagnesemia is increased intake coupled with decreased renal excretion caused by renal failure.

Signs and symptoms are usually not apparent until the serum level is greater than 4 mEq/L. Then the signs and symptoms include bradycardia and other dysrhythmias, hypotension, lethargy or drowsiness, and skeletal muscle weakness. If not treated, the patient experiences coma, respiratory failure, or cardiac failure.

When kidneys are functioning properly, loop diuretics such as furosemide (Lasix) and IV fluids can help increase magnesium excretion. For patients with renal failure, dialysis may be the only option.

ACID–BASE BALANCE

The cells of the body function best when the body fluids and electrolytes are within a narrow range. Hydrogen (H^+) is another ion that must stay within its normal limits. The amount of hydrogen determines whether a fluid is an acid or base.

An acid is a substance that releases a hydrogen ion. The stronger the acid, the more hydrogen ions are released. A common acid in the body is hydrochloric acid (HCl), which is found in the stomach. A base is a substance that binds hydrogen. A common base in the body is bicarbonate (HCO_3^-). Alkali is another word for base.

Sources of Acids and Bases

Acids and bases are formed in the body as part of normal metabolic processes. Acids are formed as end products of glucose, fat, and protein metabolism. These are called fixed acids because they do not change once they are formed. A weak acid, carbonic acid, can be formed when the carbon dioxide resulting from cellular metabolism combines with water. This acid can change to bicarbonate (a base) and hydrogen and therefore is not a fixed acid.

The ECF maintains a delicate balance between acids and bases. The strength of the acids and bases can be measured by pH. The pH of a solution can vary from 0 to 14, with 7 being neutral, 0 to 6.99 being acid, and 7.01 to 14 being base, also called alkaline. The normal serum pH level is 7.35 to 7.45, which is slightly alkaline. It must remain in an extremely narrow range to sustain life. An arterial pH lower than 6.9 or higher than 7.8 is usually fatal.

 LEARNING TIP

The word "acid" has fewer letters and lower numbers (<7.35). "Alkaline" has more letters and higher numbers (>7.45).

Control of Acid–Base Balance

As discussed in the sections on fluid and electrolyte balance, the body has several ways in which it tries to compensate for changes in the serum pH. Three major mechanisms are used: cellular buffers, the lungs, and the kidneys.

Cellular buffers are the first to attempt a return of the pH to its normal range. Examples of cellular buffers are proteins, hemoglobin, bicarbonate, and phosphates. These buffers act as a type of sponge to "soak up" extra hydrogen ions if there are too many (too acidic) or release hydrogen ions if there are not enough (too alkaline).

The lungs are the second line of defense to restore normal pH. When the blood is too acidic (pH is decreased), the lungs "blow off" additional carbon dioxide through rapid, deep breathing. This reduces the amount of carbon dioxide available to make carbonic acid in the body. If the blood is too alkaline (pH is increased), the lungs try to conserve carbon dioxide through shallow respirations.

The kidneys are the slowest to respond to changes in serum pH, taking as long as 24 to 48 hours to assist with compensation. The kidneys help in a number of ways, including regulating the amount of bicarbonate (base) that is kept in the body. If the serum pH lowers and becomes too acidic, the kidneys reabsorb additional bicarbonate rather than excreting it so that it can help neutralize the acid. If the serum pH increases and becomes too alkaline, the kidneys excrete additional bicarbonate to get rid of the extra base. The kidneys also buffer pH by forming acids and ammonium (a base).

Acidosis or alkalosis that is corrected for by the body is referred to as *compensated.* The pH is returned to normal or near normal, but the gases that monitor acid–base balance (PCO_2 and HCO_3^-) are abnormal.

ACID–BASE IMBALANCES

Acid–base imbalances are caused by a number of acute and chronic illnesses or conditions. The primary treatment for each of the imbalances is to manage the underlying cause, which corrects the imbalance. The role of the nurse is to identify patients at risk and monitor laboratory test values for significant changes.

The laboratory tests that are used to evaluate acid–base balance are called arterial blood gases (ABGs). As the name implies, the blood sample that is analyzed must be from an artery rather than a vein. The femoral, brachial, and radial arteries are most often used to obtain the sample. Table 6.4 lists ABG values and what they indicate.

The two broad types of acid–base imbalance are acidosis and alkalosis. Each of these imbalances can occur suddenly, which is called an acute imbalance, or develop over a long period, referred to as a chronic imbalance.

When the serum pH level falls below 7.35, the patient has acidosis because the blood becomes more acidic than normal. Too much acid or too little base in the body causes acidosis. Acidosis can be divided into two types: respiratory and metabolic. Respiratory acidosis is caused by problems occurring

TABLE 6.4 ARTERIAL BLOOD GAS VALUES AND CHANGES IN ACID–BASE IMBALANCES

	pH 7.35–7.45	PCO_2 32–45 mm Hg	HCO_3^- 20–26 mEq/L
Normal values	7.35–7.45	32–45 mm Hg	20–26 mEq/L
Respiratory acidosis	↓	↑	Normal
Respiratory acidosis with compensation	Nearly normal	↑	↑
Respiratory alkalosis	↑	↓	Normal
Respiratory alkalosis with compensation	Nearly normal	↓	↓
Metabolic acidosis	↓	Normal	↓
Metabolic acidosis with compensation	Nearly normal	↓	↓
Metabolic alkalosis	↑	Normal	↑
Metabolic alkalosis with compensation	Nearly normal	↑	↑

in the respiratory system. Metabolic acidosis is the result of problems in the rest of the body.

When the serum pH level increases above 7.45, the patient has alkalosis because the blood becomes more alkaline or basic. Alkalosis is caused by too little acid in the body or too much base. It can also be divided into two types: respiratory alkalosis and metabolic alkalosis.

Respiratory Acidosis

As the name indicates, the primary cause of this type of acidosis is respiratory problems. Carbon dioxide is not adequately blown off during expiration, causing a buildup of carbon dioxide in the blood. As mentioned earlier, carbon dioxide mixes with water to create a weak acid in the body, thus increasing the acidity of the blood.

Acute respiratory acidosis is caused by hypoventilation, usually as a result of an acute flare-up of chronic respiratory disease, drugs, or neurologic problems that depress breathing. Patients with chronic respiratory disease such as emphysema or chronic bronchitis may have chronic respiratory acidosis.

The signs and symptoms of respiratory acidosis involve the central nervous system and the musculoskeletal system. As carbon dioxide increases, mental status is altered, progressing from confusion and lethargy to stupor and coma if not treated. The lungs are not able to get rid of excess carbon dioxide. Instead respirations become more depressed and shallow as muscle weakness worsens.

Treatment of respiratory acidosis is aggressive management of the underlying respiratory problem, discussed in the respiratory unit (Unit Seven) of this text.

Metabolic Acidosis

Metabolic acidosis can result from too much acid in the body (usually fixed acids) or too little bicarbonate in the body. Uncontrolled diabetes mellitus and end-stage renal failure are the two most common causes of metabolic acidosis resulting from increased fixed acids.

The GI tract is rich in bicarbonate. Patients experiencing severe diarrhea or prolonged intestinal suction are at high risk for metabolic acidosis as a result of bicarbonate (base) loss. The serum pH decreases as the bicarbonate level decreases (see Table 6.4). As mentioned earlier in the discussion on hyperkalemia, serum potassium tends to increase in the presence of metabolic acidosis. Excess hydrogen in the ECF moves into the cells in exchange for potassium, which leaves the cells and enters the blood. In a sense, this is a way of compensating for the acidotic state.

The signs and symptoms are similar to those associated with respiratory acidosis, with the exception of the respiratory pattern. To help compensate for the acidotic state, the lungs get rid of extra carbon dioxide through Kussmaul's respirations. Kussmaul's respirations are deep and rapid and can occur only in patients with healthy lungs.

The treatment for the patient with metabolic acidosis is management of the underlying disease or condition. Information about disease management, such as management of diabetes, is found elsewhere in this book.

Respiratory Alkalosis

Respiratory alkalosis occurs when there is excessive loss of carbon dioxide through **hyperventilation**. Patients may hyperventilate when they are severely anxious or fearful. Patients who hyperventilate have rapid shallow respirations,

are lightheaded, and may become confused. The heart rate increases and the pulse becomes weak and thready. The serum pH is increased and the $PaCO_2$ is very low. Mechanical ventilation can also cause respiratory alkalosis, and it can occur as a result of being at high altitudes. You may have experienced this while deep breathing during a pulmonary examination.

Respiratory alkalosis is treated by having patients slow their breathing, breathe through pursed lips, or cover the mouth and one nostril to reduce airflow. The underlying cause must also be treated.

Metabolic Alkalosis

Metabolic alkalosis results from excessive ingestion of bicarbonate or other bases into the body or loss of acids from the body. Overuse or abuse of antacids or baking soda (sodium bicarbonate) can lead to metabolic alkalosis. Because the stomach contains HCL, prolonged vomiting or gastric suction can cause loss of acid and also lead to metabolic alkalosis.

The serum pH is increased, as is bicarbonate. As discussed under potassium imbalances, the serum potassium decreases. Hydrogen from the ICF moves into the blood in exchange for potassium, which moves from the blood into the cells. This is one way that the body works to keep an acid–base balance. Hypocalcemia may also accompany hypokalemia.

The signs and symptoms of metabolic alkalosis are related to hypokalemia and hypocalcemia rather than the alkalotic state itself. Treatment involves identifying the underlying cause and managing it as quickly as possible.

Compensation

If the respiratory system is compensating for metabolic acidosis, the PCO_2 will be decreased to return the pH level to normal or near normal. In a similar fashion, if there is metabolic alkalosis, the breathing pattern will change to conserve CO_2 and restore the pH level. In chronic respiratory conditions, the kidneys conserve HCO_3^- to buffer in the case of respiratory acidosis and excrete HCO_3^- in cases of chronic respiratory alkalosis.

• **WORD** • **BUILDING** •

hyperventilation: hyper—more than + ventilation—air

SUGGESTED ANSWERS TO

CRITICAL THINKING

■ *Mrs. Levitt*

1. Check her weight and compare it with her previous weights. Dehydration is associated with weight loss. Monitor mental status for disorientation. Check skin turgor for tenting. Continue to monitor vital signs.

2. Encourage increased fluid intake; notify the RN or HCP if Mrs. Levitt is unable to take in additional fluids or if the fluids do not normalize assessment findings.

3. S: "My urine smells bad, and my heart is beating fast."
   O: Pt's urine is dark amber and strong smelling. Weight 112# (baseline 116#); skin tenting present. VS: P 98 beats per minute, BP 126/74 mm Hg, RR 20 per minute, T 99.2. Fluids encouraged. RN notified.

4. Notify the RN but also the nursing assistant, who can help with encouraging fluids during and between meals as well as monitoring skin condition. Contact the dietary department to obtain beverages she prefers that do not contain caffeine.

Continued

SUGGESTED ANSWERS TO—cont'd

5. Watch for her weight to return to her normal, for her skin to feel more elastic, and for her urine to appear more dilute. Vital signs should also return to baseline.

■ *Mr. Peters*

1. Raise the head of the bed to assist breathing.
2. Using the **WHAT'S UP?** format as a guide, ask the following questions: How are you feeling? Did anything aggravate your symptoms? When did your symptoms begin? On a scale of 0 to 10, how difficult is your breathing? Are you having any problems besides shortness of breath? What do you think might be happening? (If the patient is too dyspneic to answer, do not ask many questions.)
3. Check breath sounds for crackles, observe for dependent edema and ascites, observe for distended neck veins, assess skin for color and temperature, check weight and compare with previous weight, and monitor I&O. Continue to monitor vital signs.
4. Notify RN or HCP of your findings.

■ *Mrs. Wright*

1. The patient is at high risk for osteoporosis, and thus fracture, because she is an older, petite, Caucasian woman. In addition, she does not get much calcium in her diet.
2. Her serum calcium levels would be low or low normal because the body will mobilize calcium in the bones in an attempt to maintain serum calcium levels.
3. Teach her about consuming foods high in calcium, the need to be compliant with taking her calcium supplements, and to take the supplements 1 to 2 hours after meals for best absorption by the body.
4. She would benefit from physical therapy for ambulation and strengthening, occupational therapy for an evaluation of her home environment and possible assistive devices, and a dietitian for dietary counseling. Caution her to avoid taking excessive calcium supplements because that can also be harmful.

REVIEW QUESTIONS

1. Which of the following are functions of sodium in the body? **Select all that apply.**
   1. Maintenance of serum osmolarity
   2. Formation of bones and teeth
   3. Control of bronchodilation
   4. Control of serum glucose
   5. Maintenance of cellular function

2. A 93-year-old patient with diarrhea and dehydration is admitted to the hospital from an extended care facility. For which of the following symptoms of dehydration should the nurse assess?
   1. Pale-colored urine, bradycardia
   2. Disorientation, poor skin turgor
   3. Decreased hematocrit, hypothermia
   4. Lung congestion, abdominal discomfort

3. Which patient is most at risk for fluid excess?
   1. An infant with pneumonia
   2. A teen with multiple injuries following an automobile accident
   3. A middle-aged man who has just had surgery
   4. An older adult patient receiving IV therapy

4. What is the most reliable way to monitor a patient's fluid status?
   1. Intake and output
   2. Skin turgor
   3. Daily weights
   4. Lung sounds

5. When caring for a patient with fluid excess, which of the following interventions will best help relieve respiratory distress?
   1. Elevate the head of the bed.
   2. Encourage the patient to cough and deep breathe.
   3. Increase fluids to promote urine output.
   4. Perform percussion and postural drainage.

6. A patient is being discharged following hospitalization for fluid imbalance. Which instruction by the nurse should take priority?
   1. "Weigh yourself at the same time every day and report changes."
   2. "Call your doctor immediately if you feel weak or fatigued."
   3. "Drink eight glasses of water a day."
   4. "Measure everything you drink, and measure how much you urinate each day."

7. A patient is being treated for hypokalemia. When evaluating response to potassium replacement therapy, which of the following assessment findings should the nurse observe for?
   1. Improving visual acuity
   2. Worsening constipation
   3. Decreasing serum glucose
   4. Increasing muscle strength

8. A patient is being placed on a potassium-losing diuretic. Which foods are high in potassium and should be recommended to the patient by the nurse? **Select all that apply.**
   1. Bread
   2. Potato
   3. Tomato juice
   4. Banana
   5. Gelatin

9. Which patient is at risk for respiratory acidosis?
   1. The patient with uncontrolled diabetes mellitus
   2. The patient with chronic pulmonary disease
   3. The patient who is very anxious
   4. The patient who overuses antacids

10. Which pH value represents acidosis?
    1. 7.26
    2. 7.35
    3. 7.4
    4. 7.49

Answers can be found in Appendix C.

Reference

Joint Commission. (2013). *2014 Hospital National Patient Safety Goals*. Retrieved June 15, 2013 from www.jointcommission.org

 DavisPlus | For additional resources and information visit **davispl.us/medsurg5**

7

Nursing Care of Patients Receiving Intravenous Therapy

LYNN D. PHILLIPS AND
DEB RICHARDSON

KEY TERMS

cannula (KAN-yoo-lah)
extravasation (eks-TRAH-vah-ZAY-shun)
hematoma (HEE-muh-TOH-mah)
infiltration (in-fil-TRAY-shun)
intravenous (IN-trah-VEE-nuss)
macrodrop (MACK-roh-DROP)
microdrop (MIKE-roh-DROP)
parenteral (pah-REN-ter-ul)
phlebitis (fla-BYE-tis)

LEARNING OUTCOMES

1. Discuss how the practice of intravenous (IV) therapy is regulated.
2. List indications for IV therapy.
3. Identify common veins used for peripheral IV (PIV) therapy.
4. Describe factors that influence the condition, size, and long-term use of veins.
5. List the steps in the procedure for inserting an IV cannula.
6. Describe methods for locating and/or visualizing difficult veins.
7. Plan nursing interventions to prevent IV therapy complications.
8. Identify common complications associated with IV therapy.
9. Calculate flow and drip rates for IV solutions.
10. Differentiate characteristics of isotonic, hypertonic, and hypotonic solutions.
11. Explain the differences between peripheral and central venous access devices.
12. Describe various types of central venous access devices.

Mrs. Brown, 85 years old, is admitted to the hospital with weight loss of 6% of her total body weight due to gastroenteritis and diarrhea. Her blood pressure is 102/80, pulse is 96 beats per minute, and respirations are 14 per minute. Her physical assessment shows decreased skin turgor over the sternum; dry, cracked lips; and a weak, thready pulse. The health care provider (HCP) has ordered an IV of 5% dextrose and 0.45% sodium chloride to be started at 100 mL per hour. As you read this chapter, reflect on the challenges of fluid volume deficit in older adults and initiation of infusion therapy.

Intravenous (IV) therapy is the administration of fluids or medication via a needle or catheter (also called a **cannula**) directly into the bloodstream. Each state's nurse practice act governs the practice of IV therapy in that state. Some states' nurse practice acts now include IV therapy within the licensed practical nurse/licensed vocational nurse (LPN/LVN) role.

Various national and specialty organizations have established and published guidelines or standards of practice related to infusion therapy. The Infusion Nurses Society (INS, www.ins1.org) is recognized as a global authority in infusion nursing and publishes standards of practice for infusion therapy. The INS (2011) standards of practice address the infusion-related scope of practice for LPNs and LVNs. The Centers for Disease Control and Prevention (CDC, www.cdc.gov, 2002) provides guidelines for isolation precautions, hand hygiene, and prevention of intravascular catheter-related infections. The Institute for Healthcare Improvement (IHI, www.ihi.org) provides information related to central line care. The National Institute for Occupational Safety and Health (NIOSH, www.cdc.gov/NIOSH) oversees workplace safety, including safety issues related to IV therapy, and the American Society for Parenteral and Enteral Nutrition (ASPEN, www.nutritioncare.org) provides resources related to IV nutrition.

LEARNING TIP

National organizations provide guidelines, but you must follow your state Nurse Practice Act to decide which of those guidelines apply to you!

INDICATIONS FOR INTRAVENOUS THERAPY

A variety of substances can be administered via IV therapy, including fluids, electrolytes, nutrients, blood products, and medications. The solutions and/or medications can be given as a continuous or intermittent infusion (see "Types of Infusions"). Why do patients receive IV therapy? Many medications are faster acting and more effective when given via the IV route. The IV route also allows rapid delivery of medication in an emergency. Other medications can be administered continuously via IV to maintain a therapeutic blood level. Patients with anemia or blood loss can receive lifesaving IV blood transfusions. Patients can receive life-sustaining

fluids, electrolytes, and nutrition via an IV when they are unable to eat or drink adequate amounts. Patients who are unable to eat for an extended period can have their nutritional needs met with peripheral parenteral nutrition (PPN) or total parenteral nutrition (TPN). The term **parenteral** refers to any medication route other than the digestive tract.

When a patient needs intermittent rather than continuous IV therapy, access to the bloodstream can be provided by a short peripheral vascular access device, sometimes called a *saline lock,* in which an IV cannula is inserted and covered with a sterile needleless cap or valve that seals after each use. (See "Intermittent Infusion" later in this chapter.) This provides access to the bloodstream for the prescribed intermittent or emergency medications, without the need for a continuous fluid infusion.

TYPES OF INFUSIONS

There are four primary administration modes for IV medications: (1) continuous, (2) intermittent, (3) direct injection, and (4) patient-controlled analgesia.

Continuous Infusion

A continuous infusion is a large-volume infusion of solution or medications (typically 250 to 1000 mL) administered over 2 to 24 hours. For a continuous infusion, the prescriber orders the infusion in milliliters to be delivered over a specific amount of time, such as 100 mL per hour or 1000 mL over 8 hours. The infusion is kept running at the prescribed rate until ordered to be discontinued.

BE SAFE!

BE VIGILANT! Always verify that orders are complete and understandable. If you have any questions, contact the RN, prescriber, or pharmacist.

Continuous infusions are used when a medication must be highly diluted, a constant plasma concentration of a drug must be maintained, or a large volume of fluids and electrolytes must be administered. Rate control is important in the delivery of continuous infusions and can be achieved by using an electronic infusion device (EID), mechanical controller, or roller clamp.

Intermittent Infusion
Primary Intermittent Infusion

These medications/solutions are delivered using a primary intermittent administration set that is connected and disconnected with each use.

• WORD • BUILDING •
intravenous: intra—within + venous—vein
cannula: tube or sheath
parenteral: para—beside + enteral—intestines

BE SAFE!

BE VIGILANT! Each time the primary intermittent set is disconnected the tip of the tubing must be kept sterile using a sterile end cap. The intermittent needle is flushed with saline or heparin to keep it patent while it is not in use.

BE SAFE!

BE VIGILANT! The medication in the piggyback must be compatible with any other solution that is in the primary IV tubing. (Check with your pharmacy for compatibilities.)

Piggyback/Secondary Infusion

Some IV medications, such as antibiotics, need to be infused over a short period of time. For example, an antibiotic may be mixed with 50 mL of 5% dextrose or 0.9% sodium chloride solution and infused over 30 minutes. This is often done as an intermittent infusion. As with any IV therapy, the prescriber orders must specify route, drug, dose, and amount to be infused over a specified time. If the patient already has a primary continuous IV infusing, the antibiotic (secondary) infusion can be "piggybacked" into the primary IV line. This piggyback set is left attached to the primary administration set. For the piggyback medication to infuse, it must hang higher than the primary infusion (Fig. 7.1). Piggyback medications can be infused using a mechanical controller, roller clamp, or an electronic infusion device.

NEEDLELESS CONNECTORS. Needleless connectors are devices that allow connection to IV catheters (such as piggybacking into a primary IV line), administration sets, and syringes without using a needle. They are important for avoiding needle stick injuries in nurses. Needleless connector is the current recommended terminology by the INS (2011) and best describes all such devices. Other terms are used as well, such as injection cap, port, or injection valve.

The hub or extension set of a peripheral cannula that is covered with a needleless connector is sometimes called a saline lock (Fig. 7.2). Intermittent IV lines can be "capped off" with a needleless connector; this makes them available for intermittent or emergency access. In addition, because the needleless connector does not have to be removed to allow access, a sterile closed infusion system is maintained. Intermittent infusions are small volumes of fluid or medication administered over 15 minutes to 2 hours by IV push or infusion through the needleless connector.

BE SAFE!

BE VIGILANT! SCRUB THE HUB for 10 to 15 seconds using friction before EACH access to prevent infection!

The patency (unobstructed flow) of an intermittent cannula must be maintained by flushing at periodic intervals based on institution flushing policy and procedure. Always check for patency of an intermittent device before administering a

FIGURE 7.1 Gravity drip setup with piggyback infusion.

FIGURE 7.2 Peripheral IV with needleless connector attached to extension tubing. *(Courtesy of Deb Richardson & Associates.)*

medication. Do this by first scrubbing the hub; attach the syringe and draw back to check for backflow of blood; if blood is seen in the syringe, the needle is patent. Once patency is confirmed, flush with normal saline (0.9% sodium chloride). To maintain patency of a cannula, flush the cannula after each use, or every 12 hours if not in use or according to institution policy. In addition to ensuring patency, flushing with saline also prevents the mixing of incompatible medications and solutions. The INS recommends the use of sodium chloride for maintaining peripheral intermittent devices, whereas heparin, an anticoagulant, is recommended for flushing central venous access devices (CVADs). Remember that heparin is a medication and may be incompatible with other medications. Check your institution's policy for specific guidelines.

Positive pressure must be maintained in the lumen of the cannula during the administration of the flush solution to prevent a backflow of blood into the cannula lumen, which could lead to occlusion of the lumen with a blood clot. The technique to maintain positive pressure is based on the type of needleless connector that is being used (Hadaway & Richardson, 2010):

• Negative fluid displacement—flush, clamp, then disconnect
• Positive fluid displacement—flush, disconnect, then clamp
• Neutral—no clamping technique required

 BE SAFE!

BE VIGILANT! Always be aware of the type of needleless connector you are using, as well as manufacturer guidelines for its use.

If resistance is met while a cannula is being flushed, a clot may be occluding the cannula. Do not exert pressure on the syringe plunger in an attempt to restore patency because doing so may dislodge the clot into the vascular system or rupture the cannula.

 BE SAFE!

BE VIGILANT! Always check for cannula patency and follow manufacturer's guidelines for use before injecting any substance into the circulatory system. Forced flushing could cause a clot to dislodge from the cannula into the patient's circulatory system.

Note: Some states require that registered nurses (RNs) administer medications given by the IV route; be sure to check your state's nurse practice act regarding the role of the LVN/LPN in administering IV therapy.

Direct Injection/IV Push

An IV push, IVP, or direct injection medication is injected slowly via a syringe into an IV site or port. It is sometimes referred to as a *bolus,* which means "all at once." IVP provides a rapid effect because it is delivered directly into the patient's bloodstream. IV push drugs can be dangerous if they are given incorrectly, and a drug reference should always be checked to determine the safe amount of time over which the drug can be injected. IVP drugs are usually administered by RNs and are not within the scope of practice of the LPN/LVN in some states. However, you should be aware of the drugs being given so you can assist in observing the patient for desired or adverse effects.

Patient-Controlled Analgesia (PCA)

PCA is used to deliver analgesic or pain medications. An electronic infusion device (EID) or pump is used to deliver the analgesic drug. The EID is programmed to administer the prescribed amount to the patient when the patient presses a button. PCA administrations are usually done by RNs and may not be within the scope of practice for LPN/LVN. Verify with the state nurse practice act to determine whether PCA administration is within the LPN/LVN scope of practice. Again, you should be aware of the drugs being given so you can assist in observing the patient for desired or adverse effects.

METHODS OF INFUSION

Gravity Drip

Gravity can be used to administer a solution into a vein (see Fig. 7.1). The solution is positioned about 3 feet above the infusion site. If it is positioned too high above the patient, the infusion may run too fast. If positioned too low, it may run too slowly. Flow is controlled with a roller, screw, or slide clamp. A mechanical flow device can be added to achieve accurate delivery of fluid with minimal deviation.

Calculating Administration Rates

When using a gravity set, you must calculate the infusion rate and/or the drops (i.e., gtt, L. *guttae*) required per minute to deliver fluid at the ordered rate. Commercial parenteral administration sets vary in the number of drops delivering 1 mL of fluid. Sets typically deliver 10, 15, 20, or 60 drops per milliliter of fluid. For example, to deliver 100 mL per hour using a set with 10-drop factor tubing, a flow rate of 17 drops per minute is needed. To administer the same amount using a set with 15-drop factor tubing, a flow rate of 25 drops per minute is needed. Check the label on the administration set to determine how many drops per milliliter (drop factor) are delivered by the set. Sets delivering 10, 15, or 20 drops per milliliter are called **macrodrop** sets and are used for fluids that need to be infused more quickly. Sets delivering 60 drops per milliliter are called **microdrop** or minidrop sets and are used for solutions that need to be infused more slowly.

To determine drops per minute for IV solution delivery, the nurse needs to know the amount of fluid to be given in a specified time interval and the drop factor of the administration set

• WORD • BUILDING •

macrodrop: macro—large + drop
microdrop: micro—small + drop

to be used. The formula for determining drops per minute is as follows:

$$\frac{mL}{hr \text{ or } hrs} \mid \frac{1 \text{ hr}}{60 \text{ min}} \mid \frac{gtt}{1 \text{ mL}} = gtt \text{ per minute}$$

LEARNING TIP

Always round to the nearest whole number when calculating drops per minute. You can't deliver a fraction of a drop!

The formula for determining milliliters per hour is as follows:

$$\frac{\text{Total \# of mL}}{\text{Total number of hr}} = mL \text{ per hour}$$

SAMPLE PROBLEMS. **Order:** 125 mL of 5% dextrose and 0.45% sodium chloride per hour
Drop factor: 15 gtt/mL

$$\frac{125 \text{ mL}}{1 \text{ hr}} \mid \frac{1 \text{ hr}}{60 \text{ min}} \mid \frac{15 \text{ gtt}}{1 \text{ mL}} = 31 \text{ gtt per minute}$$

Order: Normal saline 1000 mL over 8 hours

$$\frac{1000 \text{ mL}}{8 \text{ hours}} = 125 \text{ mL per hour}$$

LEARNING TIP

If you are having trouble with IV and drug calculations, check out the *Calculating Drug Doses* tutorial on your Student CD!

Factors Affecting Flow Rates of Gravity Infusions

CHANGE IN CANNULA POSITION. A change in the position of the cannula's tip can affect the infusion flow rate. If the bevel is against the wall of the vein, the flow rate will decrease; if it is away from the wall of the vein the flow rate can increase. Placement of a PIV in a joint area (wrist or elbow) can cause a kink in the cannula or change the tip position, which can cause a change in the flow rate. Careful cannula securement and avoiding areas of joint flexion will minimize this problem. Patients may need to be reminded to keep flexion to a minimum when an IV is placed near a joint.

BE SAFE!

BE VIGILANT! If the only useable vein is in an area of flexion, secure PIV appropriately; remind patients to keep flexion to minimum; closely monitor PIV site and flow rate.

HEIGHT OF THE SOLUTION. Because infusions flow by gravity, a change in the height of the infusion bag or bottle or a change in the level of the bed can increase or decrease the flow rate. The flow rate increases as the distance between the solution and the patient increases. A patient may inadvertently alter the flow rate greatly simply by standing up. The ideal height for a solution is 3 feet above the level of the patient's heart.

PATENCY OF THE CANNULA. A small clot or fibrin sheath can occlude the cannula lumen and decrease the flow rate or stop the flow completely. A fibrin sheath begins developing within the first twenty-four hours of the cannula insertion. Clot formation can result from irritation, vein wall injury from the insertion or tip position, increased venous pressure, or backup of blood into the cannula. Avoid use of a blood pressure cuff on the affected limb because of the resulting transient increase in venous pressure. A regular flush schedule helps maintain patency.

BE SAFE!

BE VIGILANT! NEVER exert pressure with a saline or heparin flush in an attempt to restore patency; doing so could dislodge a clot into the vascular system or rupture the cannula.

Mechanical and Electronic Infusion Devices

Flow-control devices, such as electronic infusion devices (EIDs) and mechanical controllers regulate the rate of infusion and are used in all healthcare settings (Fig. 7.3). Mechanical controllers measure the amount of solution delivered and depend on gravity to deliver the infusion. Electronic infusion devices, sometimes called pumps, use positive pressure to deliver the solution.

Pumps and controllers are used for infusing precise volumes and rates of solution. Institution policy often dictates use of controllers for infusion of potent medications, such as

FIGURE 7.3 Infusion pump.

heparin, concentrated morphine, and chemotherapy solutions, and for very fast or slow rates. Some electronic infusion devices are portable and designed to be worn on the body. These are called ambulatory infusion devices. It is important to know the type of pump being used and to follow its manufacturer's guidelines.

Filters

Filters can either be add-on devices to administration sets or built into the set during manufacturing. Various types of filters are available. The INS standards (2011) address the use of inline filters to remove bacteria, fungi, particulate matter, air, and some endotoxins from IV fluids.

A 0.22-micron filter that removes air, bacteria, fungi, and particulate matter from IV fluids is to be used for nonlipid solutions. Blood infusions generally use a standard 170-micron filter, which is built into the Y-administration set. Leukocyte-depleting filters are available for blood administration sets when concern for febrile reactions to leukocytes is anticipated (INS 2011; Roback, Combs, Grossman, & Hillyer, 2008). Other types of filters (i.e., 1.2-micron) are used for nutritional products such as parenteral nutrition and fat emulsions. Check institution policy and manufacturers' guidelines for use of filters.

 ## TYPES OF FLUIDS

There are three basic types of IV solutions: isotonic, hypotonic, and hypertonic (see Chapter 6). Fluids and electrolytes administered intravenously pass directly into the plasma space of the extracellular fluid compartment. They are then absorbed based on the characteristics of the fluid and the hydration status of the patient. The most commonly infused fluids are dextrose and sodium solutions. These are called crystalloid solutions.

Crystalloid Solutions
Dextrose Solutions

Dextrose in water is available in many concentrations (2.5%, 5%, 10%) and is typically used for continuous peripheral infusions. Concentrations exceeding 10% and above must be infused via a central line into a large vein.

Advantages of dextrose solutions are as follows:

- Dextrose solutions provide carbohydrates in a readily usable form and calories for energy, reducing breakdown of glycogen and catabolism of protein to help prevent negative nitrogen balance.
- They are nonelectrolyte and well metabolized by all tissues.
- High concentrations can be used for treating hypoglycemia or in combination with TPN because they supply a large number of calories.

Disadvantages of dextrose solutions are as follows:

- Vein irritation, damage, and thrombosis may result when hypertonic dextrose solutions are administered in a peripheral vein.

Sodium Chloride Solutions

Sodium chloride solutions are available in concentrations of 0.25%, 0.33%, 0.45%, 0.9% (normal saline), 3%, and 5%. Sodium chloride 0.9% and 0.45% solutions are used most commonly.

Advantages of sodium chloride solutions are as follows:

- Sodium chloride solutions are used for fluid replacement; treatment of shock, hyponatremia, and metabolic acidosis; as a primer for blood transfusions and during resuscitation after trauma. According to the American Association of Blood Banks, blood component administration sets can be primed only with 0.9% sodium chloride solution (Roback et al, 2008).
- Combination dextrose and sodium chloride solutions, such as 5% dextrose with 0.45% sodium chloride (often referred to as "D$_5$ and a half"), are commonly used for hydration and to check for kidney function before administration of potassium replacement therapy.

Disadvantages of sodium chloride solutions are as follows:

- They can cause circulatory overload if the prescribed rate is not monitored.
- If the patient is unable to excrete excess sodium (due to kidney disease or hormonal imbalance, for example) hypernatremia can result.

Balanced Electrolyte Solutions

Electrolyte solutions are used to replace lost fluids and electrolytes. A variety of balanced electrolyte solutions are available commercially. Maintenance electrolyte solutions, such as lactated Ringer's solution, approximate normal body electrolyte needs. Balanced solutions often contain lactate or acetate (yielding bicarbonate), which helps combat acidosis and provide a truly balanced solution. Potassium is an electrolyte that is commonly added to balanced solutions to replace potassium deficits. The patient must be monitored for signs and symptoms related to potassium imbalance (see Chapter 6).

 ### BE SAFE!

BE VIGILANT! Be sure to review institution guidelines for potassium administration before administration of any potassium-containing solution. An inappropriate rate or amount can cause a life-threatening cardiac dysrhythmia!

Osmolarity of IV Solutions

The osmolarity of an IV solution refers to its osmotic activity. As noted previously, IV fluids may be classified as isotonic, hypotonic, or hypertonic. (See Chapter 6 to review these concepts.) Isotonic fluids have the same concentration of solutes to water as body fluids. Hypertonic solutions have more solutes (are more concentrated) than body fluids. Hypotonic solutions have fewer solutes (are less concentrated) than body fluids. Water moves from areas of lesser concentration to areas of greater concentration. Therefore, hypotonic solutions send water into areas of greater concentration (cells), and hypertonic solutions pull water from the more highly concentrated cells.

Isotonic Solutions

Normal saline (0.9% sodium chloride) solution is an isotonic solution that has the same tonicity as body fluid. When administered to patients requiring water, it neither enters cells nor pulls water from cells; it therefore expands the extracellular fluid volume. A solution of 5% dextrose in water (D_5W) is also isotonic when infused, but the dextrose is quickly metabolized, making the solution hypotonic. Lactated Ringer's and 5% albumin are other examples of isotonic solutions.

BE SAFE!

BE VIGILANT! Since isotonic solutions expand the extracellular fluid volume be vigilant for signs of fluid overload.

Hypotonic Solutions

Hypotonic fluids are used when fluid is needed to enter the cells, as in the patient with cellular dehydration. They are also used as fluid maintenance therapy. Examples of hypotonic solutions are Dextrose 2.5% water and 0.33% or 0.45% sodium chloride solution.

BE SAFE!

BE VIGILANT! Hypotonic solutions, because they enter cells, can cause cardiovascular collapse and increase intracranial pressure (ICP).

Hypertonic Solutions

Examples of hypertonic solutions include 5% dextrose in 0.9% sodium chloride, 3% sodium chloride, calcium chloride 10%, and 5% dextrose in lactated Ringer's solution. Hypertonic solutions are used to expand the plasma volume, for example, in a hypovolemic patient. They are also used to replace electrolytes.

BE SAFE!

Monitor the patient receiving a hypertonic solution for circulatory overload.

 INTRAVENOUS ACCESS

IV therapy can be administered into the systemic circulation via the peripheral or central veins. Peripheral veins lie beneath the epidermis, dermis, and subcutaneous tissue of the skin. They usually provide easy access to the venous system.

Central veins are deeper and located closer to the heart. Special catheters with a tip that ends in a large vessel (i.e., superior vena cava) near the heart are CVADs. This chapter primarily focuses on short peripheral catheters. The definitions of the various types of CVADs are discussed briefly at the end of the chapter.

INITIATING PERIPHERAL INTRAVENOUS THERAPY

Starting a Peripheral (Short-Cannula) Infusion (Phillips, 2010)

The following steps are adapted from: Phillips, L. D. (2010). *Manual of IV therapeutics* (5th ed.). Philadelphia: F.A. Davis.

Precannulation (Steps 1–5)

STEP 1: CHECK AUTHORIZED PRESCRIBER'S ORDER. A physician or authorized prescriber's order is needed to start IV therapy. The order should include patient identification, solution and type, dosage, volume, rate, route, frequency, and anything requiring significant attention.

STEP 2: PERFORM HAND HYGIENE. Hand hygiene has been shown to significantly decrease the risk of contamination. Before beginning the procedure, wash your hands for a minimum of 15 to 20 seconds with antimicrobial soap and running water or alcohol-based hand rub.

STEP 3: GATHER, INSPECT, AND PREPARE EQUIPMENT.
• Clean gloves
• Skin prepping solution (i.e., 70% isopropyl alcohol, chlorhexidine gluconate, or chlorhexidine gluconate/alcohol combination)
• Sterile 2" × 2" gauze pads
• Towel or drape to place under selected IV site
• Alcohol prep pads
• Securement device
• Prefilled saline syringe (10 mL) or normal saline vial with 10-mL syringe and 20-gauge needle
• Sterile extension set to attach to cannula hub
• Dressing material
• Disposable nonlatex, single-use tourniquet
• PIV cannulas (over-the-needle sizes 18, 20, 22, and 24 are the most common)
• Appropriate administration set, if indicated
• IV solution, if indicated (Inspect and gently squeeze soft plastic bags for puncture holes or breaks; check expiration date; inspect solution for visible contamination or particles; ensure that outer wrap is dry.)
• Needleless connector
• IV pole, if needed
• Infusion pump, if needed

Some institutions have IV start kits that contain supplies needed.

STEP 4: IDENTIFY, ASSESS, AND PREPARE THE PATIENT.

Patient Identification. The 2014 National Patient Safety Goals established by the Joint Commission (© The Joint Commission, 2013. Reprinted with permission) specify that two patient identifiers should be used when administering medications, blood, or blood components. The patient's room number or physical location should not be used as an identifier.

Patient Assessment. Several factors must be considered before venipuncture: type of solution to be infused, condition of vein, duration of therapy, cannula size needed, patient age, patient activity, presence of disease or previous surgery, presence of a dialysis shunt or graft, medications being taken by the patient (such as anticoagulants), allergies, and patient preference for site. In addition, be sure to assess specific needs related to the patient's culture (see "Cultural Considerations").

Psychological Preparation. Provide privacy, explain the procedure and the reason why the IV is needed, and evaluate the patient's knowledge of the procedure before assessing the patient's arms for suitable venipuncture sites. Ask if the patient has had experience with infusions before and if he or she experienced any difficulties with venipuncture or the infusion. Make sure the patient is comfortable. Distraction techniques or music therapy may assist in reducing anxiety.

STEP 5: SELECT SITE AND DILATE VEIN.

Site Selection. Proper vein/site selection is crucial to the success of the procedure and the infusion treatment (INS 2011; Box 7-1). Avoid use of an arm on the side where the patient has had a mastectomy, has a dialysis access site, or is scheduled for a surgical procedure. The patient's condition and diagnosis; age; vein condition, size, and location; type/duration of therapy; and experience of the inserter should be considered before starting IV therapy (Box 7-2). The PIV cannula selected should be the least invasive with the smallest gauge and length needed to accommodate the ordered therapy (INS, 2011).

The first cannula should be started in the most distal site that supports therapy. This allows each successive venipuncture to be made proximal to the site of the previous one, which eliminates the passage of irritating fluids through a previously injured vein and minimizes leakage through old puncture sites. Hand veins can be used successfully for most hydrating

---

Box 7-1 Considerations for Vein Selection

- Age of patient
- Availability of sites
- Size of cannula to be used
- Purpose of infusion therapy
- Osmolarity and pH of solution to be infused
- Volume, rate, and length of infusion
- Degree of mobility desired

Box 7-2 General Considerations for Initiating IV Therapy

1. Use veins in the upper extremities. Avoid lower extremity veins in adults.
2. When multiple sticks are anticipated, make the first venipuncture distally and work proximally with subsequent punctures. Make no more than two attempts at venipuncture before getting help.
3. Use only one cannula per cannulation attempt.
4. If therapy will be prescribed for longer than 6 days, a peripherally inserted central catheter (PICC) or other type of CVAD should be considered.
5. Avoid using venipunctures in affected arms of patients with radical mastectomy or a dialysis access site.
6. If possible, avoid taking a blood pressure on the arm receiving an infusion because the cuff interferes with blood flow and forces blood back into the cannula. This may cause a clot or cause the vein or cannula to rupture.
7. Select the smallest cannula in gauge and length that supports prescribed therapy. All cannulas should be radiopaque.
8. All peripheral cannulas should be stabilized with a stabilization device to preserve the integrity of the access device and prevent migration.

---

solutions, but they are best avoided when irritating solutions of potassium or antibiotics are anticipated.

Vein size must also be considered. Small veins do not tolerate large volumes of fluid, high infusion rates, or irritating solutions.

Cultural Considerations

Among the Vietnamese, the head is considered sacred. Thus, the practice of starting IV lines in the scalp may cause a Vietnamese patient significant anxiety. Consider other sites first. If the patient must have an IV line in the scalp, carefully explain why it is needed.

Large veins should be used for these purposes. Figure 7.4 shows peripheral veins that can be used for IV therapy.

BE SAFE!

BE VIGILANT! Pay attention to the vein when choosing a cannula size. A smaller gauge cannula takes up less space within the vein, allows for better blood flow around the cannula, and decreases trauma to the vein wall.

Vein Dilation. If veins are constricted, venipuncture is more difficult. Fever, anxiety, and cold temperatures can cause veins to constrict. Smoking before the insertion of an IV line also causes veins to constrict.

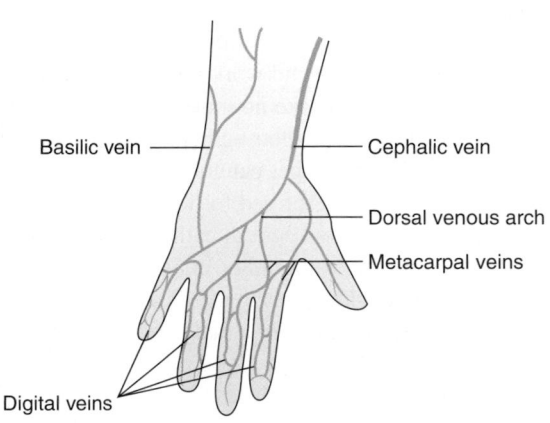

- Basilic vein
- Cephalic vein
- Dorsal venous arch
- Metacarpal veins
- Digital veins

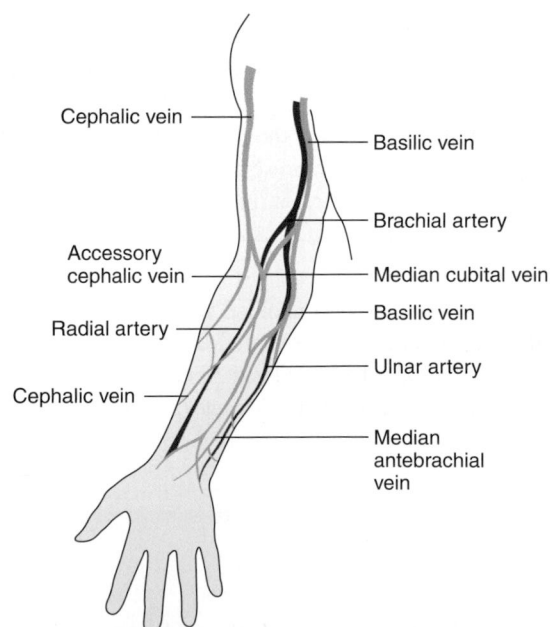

- Cephalic vein
- Basilic vein
- Brachial artery
- Accessory cephalic vein
- Median cubital vein
- Basilic vein
- Radial artery
- Ulnar artery
- Cephalic vein
- Median antebrachial vein

FIGURE 7.4 Peripheral veins used for IV therapy. (Modified from Phillips, L. D. [2010]. Manual of IV therapeutics [5th ed.]. Philadelphia: F.A. Davis.)

A tourniquet helps to dilate and stabilize the vein, easing venipuncture and threading of the cannula. Place the tourniquet 6 to 8 inches above the insertion site. If the tourniquet is too close to the insertion site, it can create too much pressure and cause a **hematoma**, which is a localized collection of blood in the subcutaneous tissue. The tourniquet should be tight enough to impede venous flow while maintaining arterial flow. A tourniquet should be at least 1 inch wide and should not be left on for more than 3 minutes to prevent impaired blood flow to the extremity. Use a nonlatex, single-use tourniquet. Tourniquets should be applied loosely or not used at all in patients with fragile veins or who bruise easily.

NURSING CARE TIP

Many patients know from experience whether their veins are difficult to access. Asking a patient to indicate his or her "best vein" may decrease the number of attempts before successful IV cannulation. When selecting a hand vein, avoid the patient's dominant hand, if at all possible, to avert accidental removal of the IV by the patient.

Occasionally, additional techniques are needed to distend a vein. Placing the arm in a dependent position or placing a warm towel over the site for several minutes before applying the tourniquet helps to dilate a vein. The whole extremity must be warmed to improve blood flow to the area. Opening and closing the fist pumps blood to the extremity and increases blood flow to help dilate the vein. Lightly stroking downward on the vein may also help. A blood pressure cuff inflated to 30 mm Hg is another appropriate method for vein dilation, especially with fragile veins in older adults. Box 7-3 lists additional tips for difficult-to-find veins.

BE SAFE!

Use a tourniquet only once to avoid cross-contamination between patients. Tourniquets may also be sources of latex exposure; use a nonlatex tourniquet or blood pressure cuff technique for patients whenever appropriate.

Cannulation (Steps 6–10)

STEP 6: SELECT CANNULA. Needles have been largely replaced with flexible plastic catheters (cannulas) that are inserted over a needle (Fig. 7.5). The needle (or stylet) is removed or retracted after the cannula is in place.

• **WORD** • **BUILDING** •
hematoma: hemat—blood + oma—tumor

BE SAFE!

PIV technology has been designed to prevent or decrease the risk of needlestick injury and blood exposure. Safety (passive or active) PIVs provide protection against needlestick injury (see Fig. 7.5). Other safety PIV devices have been designed not only to prevent needlestick injury but to control or prevent blood leakage, spill, or splatter at the time of insertion and/or maintenance.

Box 7-3 Techniques for Patients With Difficult Venous Access

Impaired skin integrity related to lesions, burns, or disease process

- Use light directed toward the side of the patient's extremity (tangential lighting) to illuminate blue veins. (This technique can also be used on dark-skinned people.)
- Do not flatten veins or cause damage to skin.
- Use a vein illumination device, which uses technology that shines a special light to identify veins beneath the surface of the skin.

Hard sclerosed vessels related to disease process, personal misuse, frequent drug therapy

- Assess for collateral circulation.
- Use multiple tourniquet technique to increase oncotic pressure inside the tissue, forcing small vessels of periphery to be visualized:
  - Place one tourniquet high on arm for 2 minutes and leave in place; stroke downward toward hand.
  - After 2 minutes, place a second tourniquet at midarm just below the antecubital fossa; leave along with first tourniquet for 2 minutes.
  - This should bring peripheral veins into view; if needed, place a third tourniquet at wrist.
  - Do not leave on for more than 6 minutes total.
- Use a vein illumination device.

Obesity or edema

- Use a 2-inch cannula.
- Use multiple tourniquet technique.
- Press down on tissue to displace edema to side to visualize veins.

Source: Phillips, L. D. (2010). *Manual of IV therapeutics* (5th ed.). Philadelphia: F.A. Davis.

FIGURE 7.5 (A) Insyte Autoguard. (B) BD Nexiva Closed IV Catheter System. (C) BD Insyte Autoguard BC Shielded IV Catheter. (D) BD SAF-T-EZ set. *(Courtesy and © Becton, Dickinson and Company. Reprinted with permission.)*

For patient comfort, choose the smallest gauge cannula that will work for the intended purpose. Use smaller gauge cannulas (22–24 gauges) for fluids and slow infusion rates. Use larger cannulas (18–20 gauges) for rapid fluid administration and viscous solutions such as blood. Also consider vein size when choosing a cannula gauge. Refer to institution policy and equipment stock for specific recommendations. For adult and pediatric patients, the INS (2011) recommends that short peripheral cannulas be removed only when clinically indicated and immediately upon suspected contamination. INS also instructs clinicians to replace or remove any PIV cannula placed in an emergency situation within 48 hours of the insertion or as soon as possible (INS, 2011).

STEP 7: PUT ON GLOVES. The INS (2011) and the Occupational Safety and Health Administration (2009) recommend following standard precautions whenever exposure to blood or body fluids is likely: wear clean latex or vinyl gloves to provide basic minimal protection from blood and body fluids. Remove gloves after contact with a patient, using proper technique to prevent hand and environmental contamination; wash hands after glove removal.

STEP 8: PREPARE THE SITE. Some agency policies allow the use of a local anesthetic agent before insertion of a peripheral IV cannula to minimize pain during the insertion. Be sure to check your agency's policy. Local anesthetic agents include lidocaine, iontophoresis low-frequency ultrasonification, pressure-accelerated lidocaine, and topical transdermal agents.

Clean the insertion site with an antiseptic/antimicrobial solution before cannula placement. If the patient's skin is visibly dirty, wash it with soap and water before applying the solution. If the patient has excess hair, it can be clipped with scissors or disposable-head surgical clippers. Avoid using a razor, which can cause skin irritation. Acceptable solutions include, but are not limited to, 70% alcohol or alcohol/chlorhexidine gluconate combination (A & CHG). CHG is the preferred prep solution of choice based on scientific evidence (O'Grady et al, 2011, INS, 2011). Avoid using alcohol after an antimicrobial preparation because alcohol negates the antimicrobial action of the skin prep agent.

Follow manufacturers' instructions for your chosen solution. Typically alcohol and povidone-iodine (PI) are applied in a circular motion, starting at the intended site and working outward to clean an area 2 to 3 inches in diameter. A & CHG combination solution is applied using a back-and-forth technique. Regardless of antiseptic solution used, it should be applied with friction for at least 30 seconds. Blotting of excess solution at the insertion site is not recommended. Let the solution air dry completely before inserting the PIV cannula.

 BE SAFE!

BE VIGILANT!

1. It is important to allow the skin prep to dry completely. This allows the prep to do its job, which is to kill off as much skin

bacteria as possible. It also decreases the risk of tracking the solution into the vein during insertion, which can lead to phlebitis.
2. Do not repalpate the site after prepping it. If you need to repalpate after cleaning, you must change to sterile gloves to perform this step (INS, 2011).

STEP 9: INSERT THE CANNULA. Make sure you have good lighting to visualize the vein. Venipuncture can be performed using a direct (one-step) or indirect (two-step) approach. For the direct approach, the cannula enters the skin directly above the vein. Small, fragile veins can be bruised more easily with the direct method. In the indirect approach, the cannula is inserted through the skin, the vein is located and the cannula is then inserted into the vein. This method is useful when cannulating small, fragile veins as bruising is less likely to occur.

Hold the cannula with the bevel (slanted opening) of the needle facing up. With the tourniquet in place, pull down on the skin to help stabilize the vein and then enter the skin/vein at a 10- to 30-degree angle using either the direct or indirect approach (Fig. 7.6).

 NURSING CARE TIP

Use traction (a downward pulling motion that makes the skin taut below the puncture site) to stabilize the skin and prevent the vein from rolling during venipuncture (Fig. 7.7).

Once the skin is punctured, lower the needle angle and locate and puncture the vein. Depending on the type of device used, a small flash of blood may be seen in the tubing or at

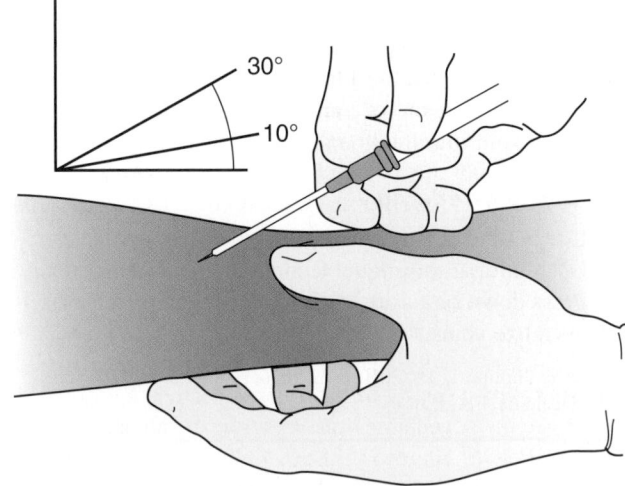

FIGURE 7.6 Insert the needle of choice bevel up at a 10- to 30-degree angle, depending on the vein location and catheter.

FIGURE 7.7 Pull skin below the intended puncture site using a downward motion to stabilize the skin and prevent the vein from rolling.

the hub of the cannula when the needle is in the vein. With the angle of the needle lowered so that it is parallel with the skin, thread it into the lumen of the vein. If a cannula-over-needle device is used, advance the cannula device 1/16th of an inch and then advance the cannula gently into the vein for its remaining length. Once the cannula is threaded into the vein, engage the safety mechanism according to device instructions to withdraw the needle out of the plastic cannula.

Once the cannula is in place, release the tourniquet and connect the preflushed extension set and needleless connector to the cannula hub. Blood may ooze from the hub at this time, so be sure to follow precautions against exposure. Clean the needleless connector and check for patency by aspirating for a blood return and flushing the cannula with 0.9% sodium chloride solution. A smooth, easy flush and good blood return along with no signs of infiltration or pain indicate that the cannula is patent and that the prescribed solution can be administered. If an IV solution is to be infused, clean the needleless connector, connect the IV tubing and initiate the infusion. Box 7-4 lists troubleshooting tips for peripheral cannula insertions.

STEP 10: STABILIZE THE CANNULA AND DRESS THE SITE. The purpose of cannula stabilization is to (1) preserve the integrity of the access device, (2) prevent cannula movement, and (3) decrease potential complications such as phlebitis, infiltration, or loss of the device. The stabilization technique should not interfere with visualization and evaluation of the insertion site or affect circulation. Several methods may be used to stabilize the cannula hub, including transparent dressings, tape, and specialized securement devices.

A transparent semipermeable membrane (TSM) dressing allows the venipuncture site to be monitored for redness or swelling and provides an occlusive dressing for the site. Other choices include sterile gauze or hydrocolloidal dressings. The dressing choice should be based on the patient's needs. Band-Aids® are not acceptable dressings over cannulas.

Arm boards, finger splints, or limb splints can be used to stabilize cannulas that are placed near joints. These devices should only be used to assist in the delivery of the infusion and to decrease the risk of complications. However, if a

---

Box 7-4 Troubleshooting Tips for Peripheral IV Therapy

Common reasons for failure of venipuncture include:

- Failure to release the tourniquet promptly when the vein has been successfully cannulated
- Use of a "stop and start" technique by beginners who lack confidence—a tentative approach that can injure the vein, causing a hematoma
- Inadequate vein stabilization, as can occur when traction is not used to hold the vein, causing the stylet to push the vein aside
- Failure to recognize that the cannula has gone through the opposite vein wall
- Stopping too soon after insertion of only the stylet so that the cannula does not enter the lumen of the vein (causing blood return to disappear when the stylet is removed because the cannula is not in the lumen of the vein)
- Attempting to insert the cannula too close to a bifurcation
- Inserting the cannula too deep, below the vein
- Failure to penetrate the vein wall because of improper insertion angle (too steep or not steep enough), causing the cannula to ride on top of or below the vein
- Poor venous access

Source: Phillips, L. D. (2010). Manual of IV therapeutics (5th ed.). Philadelphia: F.A. Davis.

---

confused patient places the IV site in danger, the extremity can be immobilized as a last resort; this requires a HCP's order.

If a joint stabilization device is used, make sure the insertion site and vein path can be seen and that placement of the device does not affect circulation or cause skin or nerve damage.

 NURSING CARE TIP

Dressing changes for PIV catheters are only done if the dressing is dirty or no longer intact. CVAD dressings should be changed every 2 days for a gauze dressing and every 5 to 7 days for a transparent semipermeable membrane dressing—sooner if it is dirty or no longer intact or if bleeding, drainage, or infection is noted (INS, 2011).

Post-Cannulation (Steps 11–15)

STEP 11: LABEL THE SITE. The IV setup should be labeled in three areas: the insertion site, the tubing, and the solution container. Once the venipuncture procedure is completed, label the insertion site dressing with the date, time, cannula type/size and length, and your initials; label tubing and solution (if applicable) with date, time, and initials.

STEP 12: DISPOSE OF EQUIPMENT AND PERFORM HAND HYGIENE. Equipment disposal should follow CDC guidelines and INS standards of practice for biohazards. All needles, cannulas, and blood-contaminated equipment should be disposed of according to institution policy in tamper-proof, nonpermeable, biohazard waste containers. Remove gloves and wash your hands.

STEP 13: EDUCATE THE PATIENT. Patients have the right to receive information on all aspects of their care in a manner they can understand. They also have the right to accept or refuse treatment. The following information should be included in education and documentation:

• Reason IV is needed and for how long.
• Limitations on mobility that result from the IV placement.
• Medications ordered and why; side effects to report.
• Meaning of alarms if an electronic infusion device is used.
• How to call for assistance if the venipuncture site becomes tender or sore or if redness or swelling develops.

STEP 14: CALCULATE DRIP RATE. All IV infusions should be monitored frequently for accurate flow rates and complications associated with infusion therapy. See the section on calculating drip rates earlier in this chapter.

STEP 15: DOCUMENT. After implementation of infusion therapy, the procedure must be documented in the medical record. Document your actions and the patient's response according to institution policy. All IV solutions are also documented on the medication administration record. Include the following:

• Date and time of insertion
• Manufacturer's brand name and style of device
• Gauge and length of the device
• Location of the accessed vein
• Presence of good blood return and patency of device
• Solution infusing and rate of flow
• Application of stabilization technique and dressing applied
• Method of infusion (gravity or pump)
• Flush solution-heparin or saline and amount used, if applicable
• Number of attempts needed for a successful IV start
• Patient's response and specific comments related to the procedure
• Patient education related to the procedure
• Signature

CRITICAL THINKING

Mrs. Green

■ Mrs. Green is admitted with a diagnosis of symptomatic anemia and has an atrioventricular (AV) dialysis shunt in her left arm. An IV line is ordered for administration of 2 units of packed red blood cells. What must be taken into consideration when assessing Mrs. Green for an appropriate venipuncture site?

Suggested answers are at the end of the chapter.

NURSING PROCESS FOR THE PATIENT RECEIVING IV THERAPY

IV therapy is a medical intervention, and the nurse is responsible for appropriate assessment, monitoring, documentation, and reporting related to the therapeutic goals.

Data Collection

Some institutions require assessment as often as every hour. An INS Position Paper (Gorski et al, 2012) provides some guidance on frequency of site assessment including the following recommendations:

• At least every 4 hours for patients not getting an irritant or vesicant and who are alert and oriented
• Every 2 hours for critically ill patients and adult patients with cognitive sensory deficits; receiving sedative medications or unable to notify the nurse of any problems; or if IV is placed in a joint area or external jugular vein
• Every hour for pediatric or neonatal patients

Assessment should be systematic and thorough and include physiological and psychosocial data, critical laboratory values, allergies and environmental issues, and presence of adverse reactions or complications related to infusion therapy. Older adults are at increased risk for complications, making careful assessment essential (see "Gerontological Issues").

Gerontological Issues

Care of the Older Adult Receiving Intravenous Therapy

When an older patient is receiving IV fluids, the nurse must regularly assess the patient for potential fluid volume excess. Symptoms of fluid volume excess include the following:
• Elevated blood pressure
• Increasing weight
• Full bounding pulse
• Shallow, rapid respirations
• Jugular venous distention
• Increased urine output
• Development of moist crackles in the lungs.
If these signs are present:
• Immediately notify the RN or turn down the IV to a minimum drip rate (1 mL per minute); do not discontinue the IV because the HCP may want to order IV diuretics.
• Position the patient to maximize lung expansion.
• Check peripheral oxygen saturation with an oximeter.
• Apply oxygen by mask or nasal cannula if indicated and per institution guidelines.
• Closely monitor patient's vital signs, level of consciousness, and oxygen saturation along with fluid output.
• Assist the HCP or RN with IV push administration of diuretic medication such as furosemide if ordered.

Physical assessments such as daily weights and measurement of intake and output (I&O) help determine whether the patient is retaining too much fluid. Skin turgor, mucous membrane moisture, vital signs, and level of consciousness also indicate hydration status. New onset of fine crackles in the lungs can indicate fluid retention. Table 7.1 lists other symptoms of complications, along with prevention and treatment strategies.

TABLE 7.1   COMPLICATIONS OF PERIPHERAL IV THERAPY

Complication	Signs and Symptoms	Prevention	Treatment
Local Complications of IV Therapy			
Hematoma	• Ecchymoses • Swelling • Inability to advance cannula • Resistance during flushing	Use indirect method of venipuncture. Choose smallest cannula appropriate. Apply tourniquet just before venipuncture.	Remove cannula. Apply pressure with 2" × 2" gauze. Elevate extremity.
Thrombosis	• Slowed or stopped infusion • Fever/malaise • Inability to flush or aspirate cannula	Use an electronic infusion device (EID). Choose microdrop sets with gravity flow if rate is less than 50 mL/hr. Avoid use of flexion areas for insertion site.	Discontinue cannula. Apply cold compress to site. Assess for circulatory impairment. Insert new cannula at another site.
Phlebitis	• Redness/warmth at site • Local swelling • Pain • Palpable cord • Sluggish infusion rate	Use larger veins for hypertonic solutions. Choose smallest cannula appropriate. Use good hand hygiene. Add buffer to irritating solutions. Change solutions and containers every 24 hours. Assess PIV site per institution policy. Remove cannula when clinically indicated.	Discontinue cannula. Apply cold compress initially; then warm. Consult RN or provider if severe.
Infiltration or Extravasation	• Coolness of skin at site • Taut skin • Dependent edema • Absent backflow of blood • Sluggish infusion rate • Pain or burning (depending on solution used)	Place cannula in appropriate site. Avoid antecubital fossa. Stabilize cannula carefully. Monitor PIV site per policy. Instruct patient to notify nurse immediately if any pain, burning or swelling occurs.	Discontinue cannula. Apply cool compress if appropriate. Elevate extremity slightly. Notify RN/provider. Follow agency infiltration/extravasation guidelines. Have antidote available (if medication extravasates).
Local Infection	• Redness and swelling at site • Possible exudate • Elevated white blood cell (WBC) count • Elevated T lymphocytes	Inspect all solutions. Use sterile technique during venipuncture and site maintenance.	Discontinue cannula. Culture site and cannula. Apply sterile dressing over site. Notify RN/HCP. Administer antibiotics if ordered.

Continued

TABLE 7.1   COMPLICATIONS OF PERIPHERAL IV THERAPY—cont'd

Complication	Signs and Symptoms	Prevention	Treatment
Venous Spasm	• Sharp pain at site • Sluggish infusion	Take thorough history. Verify allergies. Use proper patient identification. Reduce infusion rate. Warm solutions with appropriate warming device if appropriate.	Apply warm compress to site. Restart infusion in new site if spasm continues. Notify RN.
Systemic Complications of Peripheral IV Therapy			
Septicemia	• Fluctuating temperature • Profuse sweating • Nausea/vomiting • Diarrhea • Abdominal pain • Tachycardia • Hypotension • Altered mental status	Use good hand hygiene. Use aseptic techniques for insertion/maintenance of cannula, needleless connector, IV tubing and solutions. Carefully inspect fluids. Use Luer-Lok devices. Cover infusion sites with appropriate dressings. Follow standards of practice related to assessment and monitoring of PIV and hang time of infusions/IV tubing. Use appropriate preparation solutions.	Restart new IV system. Obtain cultures. Notify RN/HCP. Initiate antimicrobial therapy as ordered. Monitor patient closely.
Circulatory Overload	• Weight gain • Puffy eyelids • Edema • Hypertension • Changes in input and output (I&O) • Rise in central venous pressure (CVP) • Shortness of breath • Crackles in lungs • Distended neck veins	Monitor infusion. Maintain flow at prescribed rate. Monitor I&O. Know patient's cardiovascular history. Do not "catch up" infusion if behind schedule. Be alert that older patients are more prone to this and monitor closely.	Decrease IV flow rate. Place patient in high Fowler's position. Keep patient warm. Monitor vital signs. Administer oxygen. Use a microdrop set or an EID. Notify RN/provider.
Venous Air Embolism	• Lightheadedness • Dyspnea, cyanosis, tachypnea, expiratory wheezes, cough • Mill wheel murmur, chest pain, hypotension • Changes in mental status	Remove all air from administration sets. Use Luer-Loks. Attach piggyback to appropriate port.	**CALL FOR HELP!** Place patient in Trendelenburg position on left side. Administer oxygen. Monitor vital signs. Notify RN/HCP.
Speed Shock	• Dizziness • Facial flushing • Headache • Tightness in chest • Hypotension • Irregular pulse • Progression of shock	Reduce the size of drops by using microdrop set. Use an EID. Monitor infusion sites. Dilute IV push mediations if possible; give slowly.	**CALL FOR HELP!** Notify RN/HCP. Give antidote or resuscitation medications as ordered.

Source: Adapted from Phillips, L. D. (2010). *Manual of IV therapeutics* (5th ed.). Philadelphia: F.A. Davis.

CRITICAL THINKING

Mr. Rick

■ Mr. Rick's IV has blood backed up in the tubing. When you open the clamp to increase the flow, nothing happens. What should you do?

Suggested answer is at the end of the chapter.

Inspect the insertion site for redness or swelling, evaluate the integrity of the dressing, and document your findings. Inspect the tubing to ensure tight connections and the absence of kinks or defects. Inspect the solution container and compare it with the HCP's order for type, amount, and rate. Report abnormal findings to the RN or HCP.

Nursing Diagnoses, Planning, and Implementation

Priority nursing diagnoses for IV-related issues may include the following.

Fear related to insertion of IV cannula

EXPECTED OUTCOME: The patient will have minimal fear as evidenced by cooperation with the procedure and verbalizing minimal fear.

- Explain the IV therapy (rationale for therapy, insertion procedure, care of the IV, and importance of reporting pain, swelling, or pump alarm) to the patient. *Lack of knowledge is associated with fear.*
- Use techniques to minimize discomfort. *Pain may increase fear.*

Impaired Physical Mobility related to placement and maintenance of IV cannula

EXPECTED OUTCOME: The patient will maintain mobility as evidenced by full range of motion and avoidance of complications related to immobility.

- Avoid insertion site close to joints if at all possible. *Joint areas are mobile, making it difficult to maintain an intact site.*
- If you must use a mobile site, such as the antecubital fossa or wrist area, immobilize the joint with arm board or other immobilizer *to reduce cannula movement. (Remember to get an order for this.)*
- If site must be wrapped to protect from movement, be sure to leave insertion site visible or remove wrapping to view site according to agency policy. *The site must still be visualized for complications even if it is covered.*
- Assist patient with activities of daily living (ADLs). *The patient may have difficulty with ADLs if movement is limited.*

Risk for Infection related to broken skin or traumatized tissue

EXPECTED OUTCOME: The patient will be free from infection as evidenced by no redness, swelling, or purulence at IV insertion site, no fever, and normal white cell count.

- Watch for signs of infection *so the IV can be removed and/or site rotated and infection treated quickly if it occurs.*
- Use good hand hygiene and strict aseptic techniques during cannula insertion and maintenance care *to prevent introduction of pathogens.*
- Change tubing, and solutions regularly according to agency policy *to prevent growth of microorganisms.*
- Change or remove cannula when clinically indicated *to reduce prolonged risk.*

Evaluation

The RN is responsible for evaluation of outcomes and thus monitors the patient for evidence that the goals of therapy are being met and that complications are avoided. The LPN/LVN collects data that contribute to the evaluation. For example, if antibiotic therapy is administered, monitor the patient's temperature and other signs that the infection is resolving. If IV therapy is ordered to correct dehydration, monitor daily weights, skin turgor, vital signs, and other appropriate signs of improved fluid balance. Document all findings and report them to the RN.

COMPLICATIONS OF IV THERAPY

Complications of infusion therapy fall into two categories: local and systemic. Any complication or unusual incident should be reported to the RN or HCP, and a quality improvement report should be prepared according to institution policy.

The most common peripheral local complications are hematoma, **phlebitis**, **infiltration/extravasation**, and nerve injury. Systemic complications can be serious and include circulatory overload, septicemia, venous air embolism, and speed shock (a sudden reaction due to medication that is delivered too quickly). The nurse delivering infusion therapy must be knowledgeable in preventing, recognizing, and treating all complications of IV therapy (INS, 2011) See Table 7.1 for complications, prevention, and related care.

CRITICAL THINKING

Mrs. Gonzalez

■ Mrs. Gonzalez is receiving 5% dextrose in water at 83 mL per hour. One hour after the infusion starts, she reports pain at the site. The site is cool to the touch and swollen, and the infusion rate is sluggish.

1. What might be happening?
2. What additional data should you collect?
3. What action should you take?
4. How should you document your findings?
5. What other team members could be consulted to help in this situation?

Suggested answers are at the end of the chapter.

• WORD • BUILDING •

phlebitis: phleb—vein + itis—inflammation
infiltration: in—inside + filtrate—to strain through + tion—condition
extravasation: extra—outside + vas—vessel + tion—condition

CENTRAL VENOUS ACCESS DEVICES

The role of the LPN/LVN in CVA care in most states is limited to assisting the RN with assessments. Therefore, it is important for you to be familiar with the different CVADs so you can recognize and report problems.

Central venous catheter tips terminate in the superior vena cava near the heart (Fig. 7.8). They are used when peripheral sites are inadequate. CVADs can be used to deliver all types of solutions, medications, blood, or blood products when continuous infusion is required. They are also beneficial when irritant or vesicant medication must be given into a large vein. CVADs include tunneled and nontunneled catheters, peripherally inserted central catheters (PICCs), and implanted ports. These devices can have one, two, or three lumens in the catheter or one or more port chambers. Each lumen of a multilumen device exits the site in a separate line, called a tail. Multilumen devices allow simultaneous administration of solutions while preventing mixing of incompatible solutions.

Be careful not to confuse a central catheter with a dialysis catheter. Dialysis catheters should be used only for dialysis and not for IV therapy and should be accessed only by HCPs or specially trained dialysis nurses. If you are not sure what type of catheter your patient has, be sure to ask the RN or provider.

Nontunneled Central Catheter

A nontunneled CVAD is inserted by a physician or licensed independent practitioner into the jugular, subclavian, or femoral vein. After insertion, correct placement is determined by x-ray before the catheter is used. These short-term CVADs may remain in place up to several weeks, but placement time is typically about 7 days. A nontunneled CVAD can be inserted at the bedside or in an outpatient setting and are cost effective for short-term CAV. Nontunneled CVADs can be used for many purposes and can be easily exchanged. However, there are disadvantages, such as ongoing maintenance care and body image issues.

Tunneled Catheters

Tunneled catheters are used when venous access is needed for months to years. These catheters are typically composed of polymeric silicone with a Dacron polyester cuff that not only anchors the catheter in place subcutaneously but also provides a barrier to prevent bacteria from migrating to the tip of the catheter. The catheter tip is commonly placed in the superior vena cava (see Fig. 7.8C).

Advantages of a tunneled catheter are that a break or tear in a catheter is easy to repair, and they can be used for many purposes. Disadvantages include such concerns as weekly site care, cost of maintenance supplies, and the effect on the patient's body image.

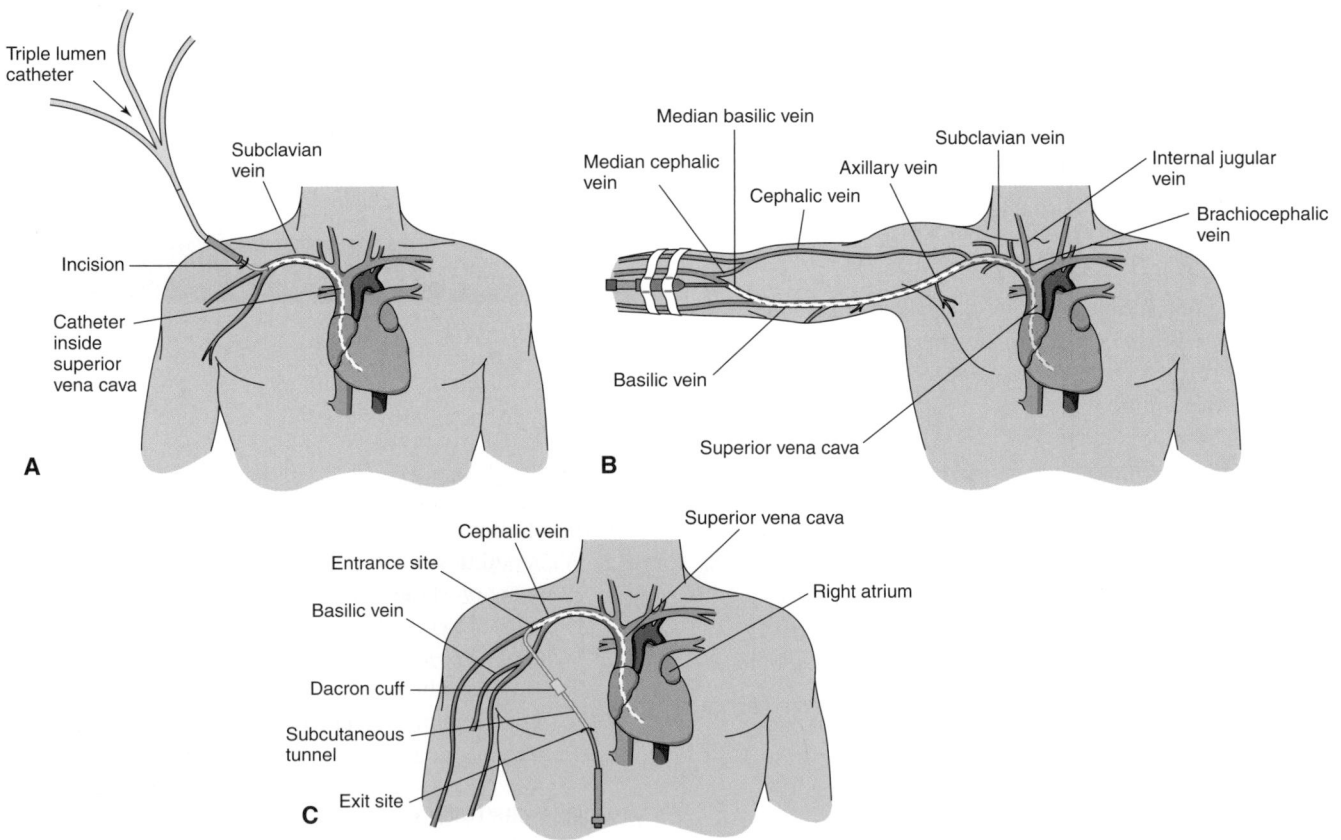

FIGURE 7.8 Central lines. (A) Triple-lumen subclavian catheter. (B) PICC line. (C) Tunneled catheter. *(B and C modified from Phillips, L. D. [2010]. Manual of IV therapeutics [5th ed.]. Philadelphia: F.A. Davis.)*

Peripherally Inserted Central Catheter

A PICC is a long catheter that is inserted in the arm and terminates in the central vasculature (see Fig. 7.8B). A PICC can be tunneled or nontunneled. This device is used when therapy will last more than 2 weeks or the medication is too caustic for peripheral administration. Specially trained RNs can insert PICC lines. They can be left in place for long periods, minimizing the trauma of frequent IV insertions. Consult with the HCP for a PICC order if long-term therapy is anticipated.

It is important to follow the manufacturer's recommended guidelines for flushing the catheter and to be aware of your institution's PICC policy. A trained RN removes the PICC catheter when therapy is terminated. An LPN/LVN may assist the RN with this procedure if the state nursing practice act permits.

Ports

A port is a reservoir that is surgically implanted into a pocket created under the skin, usually in the upper chest; a catheter is attached to the reservoir and is tunneled under the skin into a central vein such as the superior vena cava. An advantage of a port is that when not in use, a dressing is not required, and it can be flushed and left unused for long periods. When the port not in use, the patient can swim and shower without risk of contaminating the site.

Ports come in a variety of sizes and styles and are now being placed in many areas of the body. Ports are suitable for long-term therapy and can be used to administer all types of medications, including chemotherapeutic agents and antibiotics that are toxic to tissues. In addition, power injectable ports can be used for radiology imaging and procedures. Ports are usually accessed only by specially trained RNs and require the use of noncoring needles that are specifically designed for port access and infusions.

BE SAFE!

BE VIGILANT! Implement evidence-based practices to prevent central line–associated bloodstream infections. This requirement covers short- and long-term central venous catheters and PICC lines (2013 National Patient Safety Goals, www.jointcommission.org). Vascular catheter–related infections are considered "never events" because they can be prevented and should never occur. Hospitals will not be paid by Medicare for such infections acquired during hospitalization.

OTHER THERAPIES

Nutritional Support

Total parenteral nutrition (TPN) is complete IV nutrition that is administered to patients who cannot take adequate nutrients via the enteral route (by mouth or tube feeding). TPN may be used to promote nutrition for wound healing, to help a patient achieve optimal weight before surgery, or to avoid malnutrition from chronic disease or after surgery. Patients with ulcerative colitis, trauma, or cancer cachexia (wasting syndrome) are candidates for TPN. Every effort should be made to return a patient on TPN to oral or tube feedings as soon as possible.

TPN provides and maintains the essential nutrients required by the body. Solutions contain carbohydrates, amino acids, lipid emulsions, electrolytes, trace elements, and vitamins in varied amounts according to the patient's needs. Parenteral nutrition requires filtration and an electronic infusion device for administration. In the home setting, an ambulatory infusion device is used to allow the patient more mobility.

Initial assessment includes the patient's height, daily weight, nutritional status, and current laboratory values. Because of the high glucose concentration of TPN, the patient is at risk for infection and blood glucose disturbances. Insulin therapy may be necessary during TPN administration. Ongoing assessments include blood glucose levels according to institution policy and monitoring for signs and symptoms of infection, hyperglycemia, and hypoglycemia. When TPN therapy is begun, the rate is increased gradually to the prescribed rate to help prevent hyperglycemia. When it ends, the rate is gradually decreased to prevent hypoglycemia.

When nutritional solutions contain final concentrations exceeding 10% dextrose or 5% protein, they must be administered via a CVAD. When final concentrations are less than 10% dextrose or 5% protein, they may be administered through a peripheral vein. This is referred to as peripheral parenteral nutrition (PPN). PPN is a short-term intervention because it does not provide adequate nutrition over an extended period. Some states allow LVN/LPNs to initiate PPN.

The entire health care team must be involved in TPN or PPN therapy. The pharmacist, dietitian, HCP, and nurse communicate in a team conference to discuss the assessment, plan, and outcome criteria. Many institutions have nutrition teams that assess the appropriateness of TPN or PPN for individual patients.

Home Intravenous Therapy

As health care costs continue to rise, patients are using more alternatives to hospitalization. Subacute care, skilled nursing care in long-term care facilities, and home health care are growing. Home IV therapy allows many patients the benefit of early discharge and the ability to accomplish health care in the privacy and comfort of their own homes. Some home health agencies employ nurses to instruct patients and their families in the administration of home IV therapy (see "Home Health Hints").

Home IV antibiotic therapy is becoming the method of choice in the long-term treatment of a number of infections, including bacterial endocarditis, osteomyelitis, and septic arthritis. Other patients with various diseases may choose to receive TPN, chemotherapy, or IV pain medications at home. The health team can assess patients and their families for their ability to manage home IV therapy.

Home Health Hints

Before discharge:

- If IV therapy is to be continued after hospital discharge, assist the RN in teaching the patient and caregiver the skills to oversee the IV therapy.
- Obtain a referral for a home care nurse to continue monitoring and teaching after discharge.
- Teach the patient and caregiver the effects and side effects of any medication, along with signs and symptoms to report to the home care nurse or HCP.
- Provide resource and contact information to patient and caregiver.
- Work with the RN or case manager to determine supplies and equipment needed for home IV therapy.
  At home:
- Instruct the patient to refrain from smoking for at least 30 minutes before IV insertion to prevent vasoconstriction and ensure successful venipuncture.
- Instruct the patient to keep the IV site dry. If showering is permitted, instruct the patient to cover the IV with plastic (such as a grocery bag) and seal with tape on both ends to prevent water from entering the site.
- Assist the patient and caregiver to identify a safe place to store supplies. Note that some solutions or medications require refrigeration.
- Provide a biohazard container. The nurse is responsible for returning filled boxes to the home health agency for disposal.

REFLECTIONS ON MRS. BROWN

Think again about Mrs. Brown from the beginning of the chapter. She will need monitoring of I&O, daily weights, and close monitoring of her IV infusion. You should anticipate that serum electrolytes, BUN, and creatinine laboratory studies will be ordered. When initiating the infusion, use care in application of a tourniquet because older skin is thin and bruising can occur. Choose a number 20- or 22-gauge cannula to start the infusion. Once it is started, continue to monitor weights and lung sounds because older patients can quickly go from fluid depletion to fluid overload (see "Gerontological Issues").

SUGGESTED ANSWERS TO

CRITICAL THINKING

■ Mrs. Green

Consider the following when assessing the patient for an appropriate venipuncture site:

1. An 18-gauge cannula should be used for blood administration whenever possible.
2. The cannula should not be inserted in the arm that has the dialysis access site.
3. The cannula should be placed in the forearm. Hand veins are too small to accommodate the delivery of blood.

■ Mr. Rick

Your patient's IV line is likely clotted. If it has been so for a long time, it will not be salvageable. Do not flush it because doing so can dislodge the clot into the circulation. Discontinue the IV and insert a new cannula.

■ Mrs. Gonzalez

1. The IV fluid may be leaking at the insertion site and flowing into the subcutaneous tissue, a problem known as infiltration or **extravasation**, depending on the type of drug infusing.
2. Consider whether the pain could be caused by the buildup of fluid under the skin. Compare the insertion site with the opposite limb.
3. If the IV solution has infiltrated, stop the infusion, discontinue the cannula, and restart the cannula in a new site.
4. "Patient reports pain at IV site in right arm; area is cool to touch and edematous in 4.5-cm area around site. Flow rate sluggish. Infusion discontinued; IV restarted in left arm with 22-gauge cannula with good blood return. Infusing well with no signs of infiltration."
5. The RN or IV therapy nurse would be good resources.

REVIEW QUESTIONS

1. Which is the best resource for the nurse who has a question about the process and implementation of IV therapy for a specific patient?
   1. An experienced nurse
   2. Institution policy
   3. The physician
   4. INS standards of practice

2. Which patients have a need for IV therapy? **Select all that apply.**
   1. An 88-year-old man admitted to the hospital with dehydration
   2. A 21-year-old woman with an eating disorder and severe weight loss
   3. A 58-year-old woman with pneumonia who has been unresponsive to oral antibiotics
   4. A 37-year-old man recovering from a fall and broken arm
   5. A 4-year-old brought to the emergency room because of prolonged vomiting
   6. A patient with fluid overload who requires fast-acting diuretic therapy

3. A patient requests that an IV not be initiated in his hand. Which site is the next best choice?
   1. Forearm
   2. Antecubital fossa
   3. Upper arm
   4. Lower extremity

4. Place the steps for insertion of a peripheral IV cannula in chronological order. Use all of the options.
   1. Put on gloves
   2. Check HCP's order.
   3. Prepare insertion site.
   4. Label the dressing.
   5. Perform hand hygiene.
   6. Dilate the vein.
   7. Document the procedure.
   8. Insert the cannula.
   9. Stabilize the site with tape.

5. The nurse must initiate an infusion on a 21-year-old man who has a history of sclerosed veins due to IV drug abuse or misuse, and multiple tattoos over both his arms. What would be the best approach to be able to visualize and initiate a peripheral IV?
   1. Place the arm in a dependent position.
   2. Use a blood pressure cuff.
   3. Use the multiple tourniquet technique.
   4. Have another nurse hold the patient's arm.

6. A patient receiving IV therapy via a central line develops hypotension, cyanosis, and dyspnea. The nurse notes a crack in the IV tubing. Which of the following actions should the nurse take first?
   1. Have the RN call the HCP.
   2. Clamp the tubing and administer oxygen.
   3. Raise the head of the bed.
   4. Slow the infusion and lay the patient flat.

7. Which of the following solutions can be administered with a blood component?
   1. Lactated Ringer's solution
   2. $D_5/0.2\%$ NS
   3. $D_5/0.45\%$ NS
   4. 0.9% NS

8. While assessing a patient, the nurse notes a silicone catheter taped to his chest and can feel the catheter under the skin. This type of catheter would be a:
   1. Peripherally inserted central catheter
   2. Implanted port
   3. Tunneled catheter
   4. Nontunneled catheter

9. The HCP orders 5% dextrose in water at 100 mL per hour. What is the drip rate using tubing with a drop factor of 20? Round to the nearest whole number.
   Answer: ___ gtt per minute

10. A patient is to receive 1000 mL normal saline over 12 hours. How many milliliters per hour should be set on the EID?
    Answer: ___ mL per hour

Answers can be found in Appendix C.

References

Centers for Disease Control and Prevention. (2002). Guidelines for hand hygiene in health-care settings. Recommendations of the Healthcare Infection Control Practices Advisory Committee and the HICPAC/SHEA/APIC/IDSA Hand Hygiene Task Force. Retrieved April 17, 2013, from www.cdc.gov/mmwr/PDF/rr/rr5115.pdf

Gorski, L., Hallock, D., Kuehn, S., Morris, P., Russell, J., & Skala, L. (2012). Recommendations for the Frequency of Assessment of the Short Peripheral Catheter Site (Infusion Nurses Society Position Paper). Retrieved April 12, 2013, from www.ins1.org/files/public/07_05_12_Assessment_Position_Paper_BOD_FINAL.pdf

Hadaway, L., & Richardson, D. (2010). Needleless connectors: A primer on terminology. *Journal of Infusion Nursing, 33,* 22–31.

Infusion Nurses Society. (2011). *Infusion nursing standards of practice. Journal of Infusion Nursing, 34*(Suppl. 1). S1–S110.

Institute for Healthcare Improvement. (n.d.). *Pursuing perfection. Report from HealthPartners' Regions Hospital on reducing hospital-acquired infection: Ventilator-associated pneumonia and catheter-related bloodstream infection.* Retrieved March 2, 2009, from www.ihi.org.

Joint Commission. (2013). *2014 National Patient Safety Goals.* Retrieved June 18, 2013, from www.jointcommission.org/assets/1/6/2014_CAH_NPSG_E.pdf

Occupational Safety & Health Administration. (2009). Blood-borne Pathogen Standard 2009 (OSHA Compliance Directive CPL 02-0269D/29CFR1910.1030(d)). Retrieved April 10, 2013, from www.osha.gov/SLTC/bbp

O'Grady, N. P., Alexander, M., Burns, L., Dellinger, E. P., Garland, J., Heard, S. O., . . . Saint, S., and the Healthcare Infection Control Practices Advisory Committee. (2011). *Guidelines for the prevention of intravascular catheter-related infections.* Centers for Disease Control and Prevention. Retrieved from www.ncbi.nlm.nih.gov/pmc/articles/PMC3106269

Phillips, L. D. (2010). *Manual of IV therapeutics* (5th ed.). Philadelphia: F.A. Davis.

Roback, J. D., Combs, M. R., Grossman, B. J., & Hillyer, C. D. (2008). *American Association of Blood Banks technical manual* (16th ed.). Bethesda, MD: American Association of Blood Banks Press.

 DavisPlus | For additional resources and information visit **davispl.us/medsurg5**

8

Nursing Care of Patients With Infections

LINDA S. WILLIAMS

LEARNING OUTCOMES

1. List the links in the chain of infection.
2. Explain how to interrupt the routes of transmission for infections.
3. Describe the body's defense mechanisms to fight infection.
4. Describe the principles of anti-infective medication administration.
5. Plan nursing care for a patient with an infection.
6. Describe nursing care that has been effective for an infection.

KEY TERMS

aerobic (air-OH-bick)
anaerobic (ann-er-OH-bick)
antibodies (AN-ti-baw-dees)
antigens (AN-tih-jenz)
asepsis (ah-SEP-sis)
bacteria (back-TEER-ee-ah)
Clostridium difficile (klo-STRIH-dee-um dih-fih-SEEL)
colonization (coll-in-ih-ZAY-shun)
dormant (DOOR-mant)
fungi (FUNG-guy)
hand hygiene (HAND HY-jeen)
host (HOE-st)
morbidity (more-BIH-dih-tee)
mortality (more-TAH-lih-tee)
pathogen (PATH-o-jen)
personal protective equipment (PUR-sun-al pro-TEK-tiv i-KWIP-ment)
phagocytosis (fay-go-sy-TOH-sis)
probiotic (pro-buy-AH-tick)
protozoa (pro-tow-ZOH-ah)
reservoir (REZ-er-vwar)
rickettsiae (rah-KET-see-ah)
sepsis (SEP-sis)
standard precautions (STAN-derd pre-KAW-shuns)
Staphylococcus (staff-il-oh-KOCK-us)
trichinosis (TRICK-in-OH-sis)
vector (VECK-tur)
virulence (VEER-you-lence)
viruses (VIGH-rus-iz)

THE INFECTION PROCESS

A **pathogen** is an organism that causes disease in a **host** (an infected person). **Colonization** occurs when pathogenic microbes are present in the body without causing symptoms or a detectable immune response. Infection occurs when a microbe multiplies in a host. Infection with only an immune response (increased antibody level for the microbe) and no symptoms is a *subclinical infection*. An infectious disease causes signs, symptoms, and injury to the host.

To prevent infection, the links in the chain of events leading to infection must be broken (Fig. 8.1). However, if an infection does occur, treatment focuses on breaking the chain of infection to prevent its spread to others.

Reservoir

A **reservoir** is the place in the environment where infectious agents live, multiply, and reproduce so they can be transmitted to a susceptible host. A reservoir can be animate (e.g., people, insects, animals, and plants) or inanimate (e.g., water, soil, or medical devices).

Causative Agents

Microorganisms that cause infection include bacteria, viruses, fungi, protozoa, helminths, and prions (Table 8.1). The organisms that occur naturally in or on a particular body part are known as normal flora. They are usually harmless, or nonpathogenic, because they do not normally produce disease in a healthy person.

Normal flora are helpful to the human host. For example, intestinal flora (i.e. bacteria) assist in vitamin K production, a nutrient needed for normal blood clotting. However, if these same bacteria get into another area of the body, such as the blood, they may produce disease and are then referred to as pathogens.

Bacteria

Bacteria are single-celled organisms. They may depend on a host or live and reproduce outside a host. Most bacteria produce cell walls that are susceptible to antibiotic effects. However, bacteria can mutate to survive.

Bacteria are named according to their shape (spherical [coccus], rod [bacillus], and spiral [spirillum]) and classified according to their staining properties (Gram's method, acid-fast staining). Bacteria respond to stains in one of three ways: Gram-positive bacteria stain purple; Gram-negative bacteria lose purple stain when exposed to alcohol but stain pink with a second dye; and acid-fast bacteria keep purple stain when an acid is applied.

Bacterial growth depends on oxygen, nutrition, light, temperature, and humidity. **Aerobic** bacteria, such as those found on the skin, need oxygen to live. **Anaerobic** bacteria, such as bacteria in the gastrointestinal (GI) tract, live without oxygen. Most bacteria that inhabit humans grow best at body temperature, 98.6°F (37°C).

Rod-shaped bacteria form spores that are thick walled and hard to kill. Spores remain in a resting state until

• WORD • BUILDING •
pathogen: pathos—suffering + genes—producer of

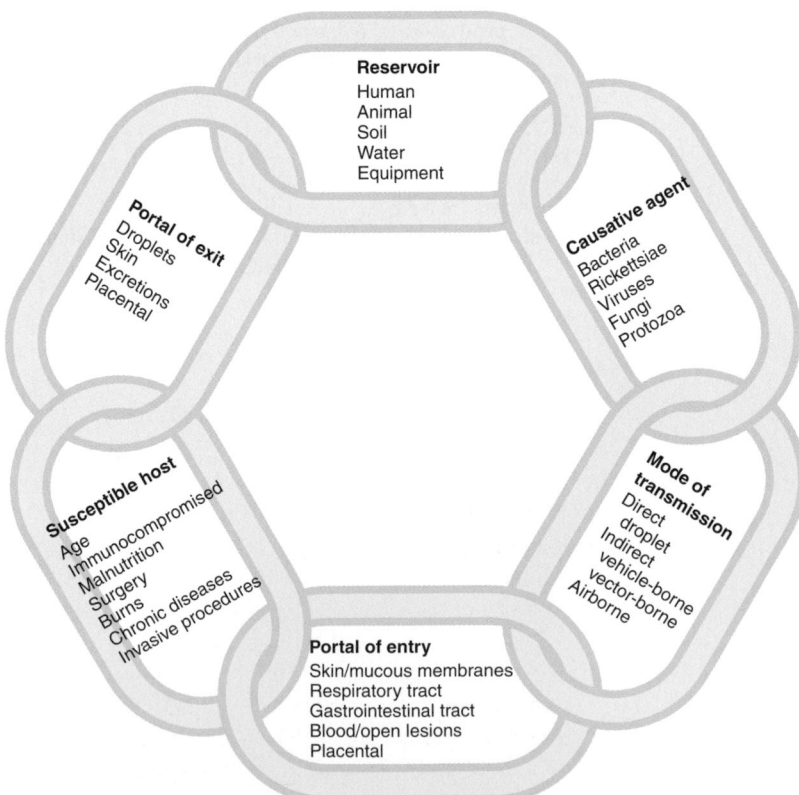

FIGURE 8.1 Chain of events in the infection process.

TABLE 8.1 COMMON INFECTIONS

Microorganism	Type or Site of Infection
Gram-Positive Bacteria	
Staphylococcus aureus	Pneumonia, cellulitis, peritonitis, toxic shock
Staphylococcus epidermidis	Postoperative bone/joints, IV line–related phlebitis
Staphylococcus pneumoniae	Pneumonia, meningitis, otitis media, sinusitis, bacteremia
Gram-Negative Bacteria	
Escherichia coli	Urinary tract, pyelonephritis, bacteremia, gastroenteritis
Klebsiella pneumoniae	Pneumonia and wounds
Legionella pneumophila	Pneumonia
Neisseria gonorrhoeae	Gonorrhea
Pseudomonas aeruginosa	Wounds, urinary tract, pneumonia, IV lines
Salmonella enteritidis	Gastroenteritis, food poisoning
Viruses	
Herpes virus group	Cold sores/fever blisters, genital herpes
Epstein-Barr	Infectious mononucleosis
Varicella zoster	Skin (chickenpox and shingles)
Hepatitis (A, B, C, D, E)	Liver
Human immunodeficiency virus	Acquired immunodeficiency syndrome
Influenza (A, B, C)	Bronchiolitis, pneumonia
Rubella	German measles
Rubeola	Measles
Fungi	
Candida albicans	Nailbed, thrush, vaginitis
Histoplasma capsulatum	Pneumonia
Protozoa	
Giardia lamblia	Gastroenteritis
Trichomonas vaginalis	Trichomoniasis
Dientamoeba fragilis	Diarrhea, fever
Entamoeba histolytica	Amebic dysentery
Toxoplasma gondii	Toxoplasmosis
Plasmodium falciparum	Malaria

EVIDENCE-BASED PRACTICE

Clinical Question
How can disinfection of *C. difficile* isolation (CDI) rooms be improved?

Evidence
Over a 21-month timeframe, a standardized process of three interventions used for room cleaning by a dedicated daily disinfection team was shown by culture to significantly enhance disinfection in CDI rooms. The interventions included fluorescent markers on high-touch surfaces to provide feedback on thoroughness of cleaning, use of an automated ultraviolet radiation device, and supervisory assessment and clearance after cleaning of CDI rooms.

Implications for Nursing Practice
Promoting evidence-based practice to prevent transmission of infectious organisms and reduce infections is a priority for all health care workers.

REFERENCE

Sitzlar, B., Deshpande, A., Fertelli, D., Kundrapu, S., Sethi, A. K., & Donskey, C. J. (2013). An environmental disinfection odyssey: Evaluation of sequential interventions to improve disinfection of *Clostridium difficile* isolation rooms. *Infection Control and Hospital Epidemiology, 34,* 459–465.

RICKETTSIAE. Rickettsiae are a type of bacteria that must be inside living cells to reproduce. Rickettsiae **vectors** (living organisms that transmit disease) are infected fleas, ticks, mites, and lice that bite humans. Several diseases are caused by rickettsiae. Rocky Mountain spotted fever, caused by *Rickettsia rickettsii,* whose reservoirs (the places in nature where the organism usually lives and multiplies without causing disease) are rodents and dogs, is transmitted to humans by a tick bite.

Viruses

Viruses are organisms smaller than bacteria that depend on host cells to live and reproduce (see Table 8.1). Invaded host cells make more of the virus material. The new viral particles are then released either by destroying the host cell or by forming small buds that break away to infect other cells.

When a virus enters a cell, it may immediately trigger disease or remain **dormant** (inactive) for years without causing illness. An example of this is *human herpesvirus 3* (varicella zoster virus), which can cause disease quickly (chickenpox) or remain dormant for years, eventually erupting in the disease called shingles. Antibiotics are not effective against viruses. Antiviral drugs are used to decrease symptoms caused by viruses and to decrease the viral load (the number of viral cells in the patient's blood).

favorable conditions exist that allow the organism to resume normal function. Prolonged exposure to high temperature destroys spores on surgical equipment. Bleach is used in patient rooms to kill spores from **Clostridium difficile** (*C. difficile*).

Fungi

Fungi are a group of organisms that includes yeasts, molds, and mushrooms and can produce highly resistant spores (see Table 8.1). Because fungi do not contain chlorophyll, they must obtain food from living organisms or dead organic matter. Normal flora of the mouth, skin, vagina, and intestinal tract include many fungi. Most fungi are not pathogenic, and serious fungal infections are rare. Antifungal medications treat fungal infections.

Protozoa

Protozoa are single-celled parasitic organisms with flexible membranes that live in the soil and obtain nourishment from dead or decaying organic material (see Table 8.1). Protozoa infect humans through fecal–oral contamination or through ingestion of food or water contaminated with cysts or spores, through host-to-host contact, or by the bite of a mosquito or other insect that has previously bitten an infected person.

Helminths

Helminths are wormlike parasitic animals: roundworms, flatworms, tapeworms, pinworms, hookworms, and flukes. Disease transmission occurs through skin penetration of larvae or ingestion of helminth eggs. **Trichinosis** (caused by the roundworm *Trichinella spiralis*) is a disease caused by eating raw or undercooked meat of pigs or wild animals that contain *Trichinella* larvae.

Prions

Prions are transmissible pathogenic agents. They cause abnormal folding of normal cellular proteins known as prion proteins. These prion proteins are found mainly in the brain. Brain damage results from the abnormal folding of prion proteins. Prion diseases have long incubation periods, cause no inflammatory response, progress rapidly, and are fatal. In humans, they include classic and variant *Creutzfeldt-Jakob disease, and in animals, bovine spongiform encephalopathy (so-called mad cow disease) and chronic wasting disease.*

Mode of Transmission

Once the causative agent exits the reservoir, a means of transfer to a susceptible host is needed. Transmission of microorganisms occurs through direct contact, indirect contact, or through the air. Understanding the modes of transmission of a particular disease allows you to use the appropriate means of personal protection without using unnecessary supplies that increase costs.

Direct Contact

Direct transmission occurs through touching, kissing, sexual contact, biting, or droplet spray into the eyes or on mucous membranes through sneezing, coughing, spitting, singing, or talking. Droplet spread is usually limited to 3 feet or less. Illnesses spread by direct transmission may include influenza,

impetigo, scabies, conjunctivitis, pediculosis, herpes, *C. difficile,* and all sexually transmitted infections, including human immunodeficiency virus (HIV). Protect yourself and your patients from direct transmission with hand hygiene, aseptic technique, and use of **personal protective equipment** (PPE) such as gloves, surgical masks, goggles, gowns, and booties. PPE is selected and used based on the task to be performed and the applicable isolation precautions (standard precautions and/or transmission-based precautions; see the Infection Prevention Guidelines discussion later in the chapter).

Indirect Contact

Indirect transmission is either vehicleborne or vectorborne. Vehicleborne transmission is the spread of an infectious organism by contact with a contaminated object, such as a toy, soiled bedding, dressings from a wound, surgical instruments, water, food, and biological products such as blood, serum, plasma, tissues, and organs. Vehicleborne illnesses include conjunctivitis, trichinosis, HIV, and hepatitis A, B, C, D, and E. Vehicle transmission can be avoided through proper hand hygiene, thorough cleaning of the patient environment, and provision of clean water and food supplies.

Vectorborne transmission is the spread of infectious organisms through a living source other than humans, such as an insect, flea, mouse, or rat. Diseases spread through vectors include malaria, plague, and Lyme disease. Vector transmission can be reduced with insect repellants, avoidance of infested areas, and rodent control.

Airborne

Airborne transmission is different from droplet transmission (see direct contact discussed earlier) because the particles floating in the air are much smaller, remain suspended in the air for a long time, and may travel large distances. Airborne organisms can be inhaled or deposited on the mucous membrane of a susceptible host. Measles, chickenpox, and tuberculosis (TB) are transmitted by airborne transmission. Airborne transmission is prevented with the use of high-efficiency particulate air (HEPA) respirators (also known as a TB mask). HEPA respirators filter the tiniest particles from the air, unlike surgical masks, which can allow such particles to pass into the respiratory system of a host. Institutions provide individual-fit testing and training for HEPA respirator use for each health care worker.

 BE SAFE!

If you provide care for patients with suspected or confirmed diseases that are spread through airborne transmission, such as TB, be sure you have your own fit-tested HEPA mask to wear. Do not use other masks because they do not provide adequate protection. If you cannot obtain your own fit-tested mask, you should never enter the patient's room.

• WORD • BUILDING •

protozoa: proto—first + zoon—animal

Multiple Modes of Transmission

Many diseases have multiple modes of transmission requiring a variety of protective techniques. For example, chickenpox is transmitted by direct contact, indirect contact, and airborne transmission. It is no wonder that 80% to 90% of susceptible persons exposed to it develop the disease.

Portal of Entry

To produce disease, organisms must gain entry into a susceptible host. Routes of entry into a susceptible host include the respiratory tract, skin (usually nonintact), mucous membranes, GI tract, genitourinary tract, and placenta. Once the organism enters the host, it may lead to disease, depending on the condition of the host and many other factors, such as the **virulence** (ability to produce infection) of the organism.

Susceptible Host

The body has many defense mechanisms to prevent infection. A breakdown in these defenses increases the possibility of infection. Factors that increase susceptibility to infection are very young age, old age, malnourishment, immunocompromised, chronic disease, stress, burns, and invasive procedures (see "Gerontological Issues").

Portal of Exit

The portal of exit is the route through which the infectious agent leaves the host, who has become a reservoir for infection: respiratory tract, skin, mucous membranes, GI tract, genitourinary tract, blood, open lesions, or placenta.

THE HUMAN BODY'S DEFENSE MECHANISMS

Skin and Mucous Membranes

Intact skin and mucous membranes are the body's first line of defense against infection. Preventing skin dryness and cracking with lotion keeps the skin intact so organisms do

not have an entry point. Oral mucous membranes have many layers, making it difficult for organisms to enter the body. The skin has acidic (pH <7) properties that render some organisms unable to produce disease. For example, many bacteria prefer an alkaline (pH >7) environment for reproduction. The body also has an abundance of normal flora that impairs the growth of pathogens both on the skin and in the GI tract.

Cilia

Cilia are hairlike structures lining the upper respiratory tract mucous membranes that protect the lungs. Cilia trap mucus, pus, dust, and foreign particles to prevent them from entering the lungs. Then the cilia push the trapped particles up to the pharynx with wavelike movements for expectoration.

Gastric Juices

Gastric juices inside the stomach are very acidic (pH 1 to 5). This acidic environment destroys most organisms that enter the stomach.

Immunoglobulins

Immunoglobulins are proteins found in serum and body fluids. They may act as antibodies to destroy invading organisms and prevent the development of infection. **Antibodies** are the proteins produced by B lymphocytes when foreign antigens of invading cells are detected. **Antigens** are markers on the surface of cells that identify cells as being the body's own cells (autoantigens) or as being foreign cells (foreign antigens). Antibodies combine with specific foreign antigens on the surface of the invading organisms, such as bacteria or viruses, to control or destroy them. Antigens are neutralized or destroyed by antibodies in several ways. Antibodies can initiate destruction of the antigen, neutralize toxins released by bacteria, promote antigen clumping with the antibody, or prevent the antigen from adhering to host cells.

Leukocytes and Macrophages

Leukocytes (white blood cells [WBCs]) are the primary cells that protect against infection and tissue damage. There are five types of leukocytes:

- Neutrophils are phagocytic cells that focus on bacteria and small particles.
- Monocytes become macrophages and are mainly phagocytic on tissue debris and large particles.
- Lymphocyte functions include antigen recognition and antibody production.
- Basophils respond to inflammation from injury.
- Eosinophils destroy parasites and respond in allergic reactions.

After recognizing a foreign antigen, neutrophils and macrophages engulf and digest it, a process known as **phagocytosis**. The macrophages move the antigen fragments to

Gerontological Issues

Infection and Older Adults

Fever is not a common sign of an infection for an older adult. This difference among older adults may cause significant delay in providing appropriate treatment and care. Be alert for the following signs of infection in older patients:

- Behavioral change, such as pacing or irritability
- Masking of the symptoms of infection by a noncommunicable disease (For example, the inflammation and pain of degenerative joint disease may make it difficult for a patient to recognize an infection in an affected joint.)

• WORD • BUILDING •
phagocytosis: phagein—to eat + cytos—cell + osis—condition

their surface to be recognized by T lymphocytes to further stimulate action of the immune system. Phagocytes ingest and destroy bacteria, damaged or dead cells, cellular debris, and foreign substances.

Lysozymes

Lysozymes are bactericidal enzymes present in WBCs and most body fluids such as tears, saliva, and sweat. These enzymes dissolve the walls of bacteria, destroying them.

Interferon

If an invading organism is a virus, WBCs and fibroblasts release interferon (a group of antiviral proteins). Interferon helps destroy infected cells and inhibits production of the virus within infected cells. Tumor cell growth may also be inhibited by interferon.

Inflammatory Response

The inflammatory response occurs with any injury to the body. This response can be caused by pathogens, trauma, or other events causing injury to tissues. Infection may or may not be present.

Vascular Response

The first step of the inflammatory process is local vasodilation, which increases blood flow to the injured area. Pathogenic organisms can trigger the first step of the inflammatory process. Increased blood flow creates redness and heat at the injury. The increase in blood flow brings more plasma to the area to nourish tissue and carry waste and debris away.

Inflammatory Exudate

The second step of the inflammatory process is increased permeability of the blood vessels, which allows plasma to move out of the capillaries and into the tissues. Swelling occurs, resulting in pain from pressure on nearby nerve endings.

Phagocytosis and Purulent Exudate

The final step of the inflammatory process is the destruction of pathogenic organisms and their toxins by leukocytes. During this process, a purulent exudate (pus) may form that contains protein, cellular debris, and dead leukocytes.

Immune System

The immune system is the body's final line of defense against infection (see Chapter 18). Immune cells and lymphoid tissue work with the body's other defense mechanisms. The immune system is a finely tuned network of specialized parts that function together to protect the body from invasion by pathogenic organisms. When this network breaks down, infection can result.

 INFECTIOUS DISEASE

Localized Infection

Localized infection is caused by an increase of microbes in one area that triggers the inflammatory response. Manifestations of a local infection include pain, redness, swelling, and warmth at the site. Pain is most severe when the infection occurs in closed cavities. Redness and swelling are seen when surface structures are involved. Warmth may be felt at the site. Body temperature may rise to produce an antimicrobial effect.

Sepsis

Sepsis is an immune system response to a serious infection. It can be fatal due to the systemic inflammatory response syndrome (SIRS) that occurs from chemicals that are released to fight the infection. This inflammation can damage organ systems and cause them to fail. Septic shock occurs with decreased blood pressure (see Chapter 9). Visit www.survivingsepsis.org or www.ihi.org/explore/Sepsis.

Laboratory Assessment

A Gram stain, using gentian violet, helps bacteria be better viewed under a microscopic for identification. Gram-positive bacteria turn purple, and Gram-negative bacteria become pink. A culture and sensitivity (C&S) identifies an illness-causing organism and determines which antibiotic would be most effective for treatment. Organisms in the culture specimen are grown on a laboratory plate and identified within 24 to 48 hours. The organism is then exposed to several antibiotics to determine to which antibiotics the organism is sensitive.

A serum antibody test measures the reaction to a certain antigen. A positive result for this test does not always mean that an active infection is present. It can simply mean there has been an exposure to the antigen, so it is not as accurate as a culture.

A complete blood cell count with differential (CBC with diff) is usually obtained when an infection disease is suspected. The levels of the five leukocytes are measured. Elevations in specific leukocytes occur based on the type and severity of the pathogen.

Erythrocyte sedimentation rate (ESR, sed rate) is an early screening test for inflammation but not a definitive test for infection. During the inflammatory process, red blood cells (RBCs) become heavier. The ESR measures in millimeters per hour the speed at which the RBCs settle in a tube. The faster the settling (due to heavier RBCs), the greater the inflammation.

Other tests such as x-rays, computed tomography (CT), and magnetic resonance imaging (MRI) are helpful in identifying abscesses (walled-off infections). Skin tests diagnose infections. For example, the purified protein derivative (PPD) skin test screens for TB (see Chapter 31).

Immunity

Immunity is the ability of the body to protect itself from disease (see Chapter 18). There are several types of immunity:

• Natural immunity occurs in species and prevents one species from contracting illnesses found in another species.

- Innate immunity is genetic; hereditary immunity is that which a person is born with.
- Acquired immunity is obtained either actively or passively through exposure to an organism, from a vaccine, or from an injection of immunoglobulins (antibodies) or is passed from mother to baby. Visit www.cdc.gov/vaccines to view vaccine schedules.

Types of Infectious Diseases

Communicable diseases are discussed in the chapters related to the body system they affect. For HIV, see Chapter 20; for respiratory diseases, see Chapter 31; for hepatitis, see Chapter 35.

Infectious Mononucleosis (Epstein-Barr Virus)

Infectious mononucleosis (IM) is caused by the Epstein-Barr virus (EBV), a herpes virus. EBV is spread through intimate contact with saliva of an infected person. IM is mainly diagnosed in adolescences or young adults. Most adults become infected with EBV and develop antibodies to it. EBV remains in the body for a lifetime.

The incubation period for IM is 4 to 6 weeks. Symptoms include fever, severe sore throat, generalized lymphadenopathy (enlarged lymph nodes in two different sites other than inguinal nodes) that last 1 to 4 weeks. The spleen enlarges 50% of the time. Occasionally, a rash develops that is similar to the rash seen with measles. Signs and symptoms, as well as diagnostic tests, confirm IM. Lymphocyte levels are elevated and positive mono spot and heterophile antibody tests confirm IM.

No specific treatment is needed for IM. Antiviral drugs are not effective. Symptoms are treated as needed with supportive care. Fatigue may last for months, and rest is important. Complications are rare.

 INFECTION CONTROL IN THE COMMUNITY

Many levels of organizations work closely together to control communicable diseases. The World Health Organization (WHO) and the Centers for Disease Control and Prevention (CDC) teach standards to prevent and control diseases and monitor disease outbreaks. Local health departments teach how to prevent and control the spread of disease. Community immunization programs have helped reduce communicable diseases.

Although requirements vary from state to state, most elementary schools require some proof of childhood immunization. Many colleges also require or recommend immunization to help control the outbreak of diseases such as measles and meningitis. In addition, educating the public about the importance of **hand hygiene**, the CDC's respiratory hygiene/cough etiquette measures, immunization, clean water, safe food handling techniques, and safer sex precautions in preventing the spread of disease is essential.

 NURSING CARE TIP

For infection control, teach the CDC's *Cover Your Cough* campaign instructions to patients and family members who have a cough, congestion, rhinorrhea, or increased respiratory secretions:

- Cover your mouth and nose with a tissue when you cough or sneeze.
- Put your used tissue in the wastebasket.
- If you don't have a tissue, cough or sneeze into your upper sleeve, not your hands.
- Wash hands frequently with soap and water for 20 seconds, or use an alcohol-based hand cleaner.
- If asked, put on a facemask to protect others.

Source: Centers for Disease Control and Prevention. (2010). Cover your cough. Retrieved November 18, 2013, from www.cdc.gov/flu/protect /covercough.htm.

Both hospital and home health care nurses provide infection control teaching for the patient with an infection and his or her family. Techniques used should be specific to the interruption of the transmission of the particular disease. This may include the use of disposable dishes, utensils, and gloves, and proper disposal of contaminated items.

 INFECTION CONTROL IN HEALTH CARE AGENCIES

If upon admission to a hospital or health care agency a patient already has an infection, it is referred to as a community-acquired infection. An infection that develops as a result of a patient's stay in the hospital is called a hospital-acquired infection (HAI). The host's condition plays a major role in whether an infection is acquired. Patients in the hospital are commonly debilitated, malnourished, or immunocompromised. Multiple antibiotic therapy also increases susceptibility to other types of infection and promotes the resistance of pathogens to antibiotics. Therefore, the risk of developing a HAI is high. Some areas within an institution tend to have an increased number of HAIs, such as intensive care, neonatal, dialysis, oncology, and burn units. Patients in these areas tend to undergo more invasive procedures and are debilitated, increasing susceptibility to infection.

Several pathogens are commonly responsible for causing HAIs:

- *Escherichia coli (E. coli)* is the most common pathogen causing hospital-acquired urinary tract infections (UTIs). *E. coli* normally lives in the healthy intestinal tract of humans. *E. coli* can be spread by the patient, by the unwashed hands of a health care worker, or through contaminated food and water.

- *Staphylococcus aureus* (known as staph) is the most common pathogen causing hospital-acquired surgical wound infections. Staph usually lives in the nose and on the skin of healthy people.
- *Pseudomonas aeruginosa* is the most common pathogen in hospital-acquired pneumonia. It is found in soil, around water, and in the health care setting around sinks, water, irrigating solutions, and nebulizers on respiratory equipment.

Hand Hygiene

What is the single most effective way to prevent and control the spread of infection? Effective hand hygiene! This easily removes the transient organisms that cause most HAIs that result from cross-transmission. Most of these organisms are transmitted via the hands of health care providers (HCPs). Hands must be cleansed before and after every patient contact to help prevent the direct transmission of organisms (Fig. 8.2). The use of gloves decreases the transmission of organisms, but CDC guidelines also require hand washing before and after glove use because hands may still become contaminated. Did you know that patients may also transmit organisms with inadequate hand hygiene? Teach them the importance of hand hygiene after handling their own secretions. Offer your patients hand hygiene at meals and throughout the day!

FIGURE 8.2 Frequent hand washing by health care workers helps reduce the spread of microorganisms.

BE SAFE!

The Joint Commission's 2014 National Patient Safety Goal for preventing infection is as follows: Use the hand cleaning guidelines from the Centers for Disease Control and Prevention or the World Health Organization. Set goals for improving hand cleaning. Use the goals to improve hand cleaning (© The Joint Commission, 2013. Reprinted with permission.).

You are responsible for using appropriate hand hygiene in the health care setting. Hand hygiene can include either the use of hand washing or an alcohol-based hand rub, although soap and water are needed to remove C. difficile. For visibly soiled hands, wash with soap and water. Using alcohol-based hand rubs is preferred to kill bacteria in many cases and may increase adherence to protocols by saving time and reducing dry skin from the washing. For an informative presentation, visit www.cdc.gov/handhygiene/download/hand _hygiene_supplement_minus_notes.pdf or www.cdc.gov/features/handhygiene.

Hand Washing
Proper hand washing requires wetting the hands with warm—not hot—water, soaping, and lathering, with at least 20 seconds of rubbing your hands together (sing "Happy Birthday" song twice), covering all surfaces. Interlace your fingers to cleanse between them, rub your nails against your palms to clean under the nails, and then rinse your hands with fingertips pointed downward under running water. Dry your hands with clean disposable paper towels. Use the paper towel to turn off the faucet. Use only facility-supplied lotions because others may reduce the effectiveness of soap or break down latex gloves (water-based lotion only). Apply lotion to your hands to prevent drying and cracking in which infection could develop (CDC, 2013).

Alcohol-Based Hand Rubs
Apply specified amount of the hand rub to the palm of one hand. Rub both hands together, covering all surfaces until the hands are completely dry to ensure the alcohol has evaporated. Do not wash off hand rub.

Asepsis

The concept of **asepsis** (freedom from organisms) is important for all health care workers who have direct or indirect patient contact. For hospitalized patients, the most common sites for infection are the genitourinary tract, respiratory tract, bloodstream, and surgical wounds. Be aware of patients at risk of developing infections and protect them with aseptic techniques.

CRITICAL THINKING

Mrs. Sampson

■ Mrs. Sampson has neutropenia from chemotherapy treatments.

1. Why is hand hygiene the most important intervention you can do to help prevent infection for Mrs. Sampson?
2. What would be a priority nursing diagnosis for Mrs. Sampson?
3. What type of isolation could be beneficial to Mrs. Sampson?

Suggested answers are at the end of the chapter.

Medical Asepsis

Medical asepsis is commonly referred to as clean technique. The goal is to reduce the number of pathogens or prevent the transmission of pathogens from one person to another. Frequent, proper hand hygiene is one of the best ways to achieve this goal. The use of gowns, gloves, masks, and protective eyewear or rooms with special ventilation may also be helpful (Fig. 8.3). Disinfectants and precautions as defined by the CDC are also crucial tools. Techniques used should be appropriate to interrupt the spread of the known pathogen. As part of medical asepsis, you should keep your own body and

clothing clean to prevent spread of infection to patients, yourself, and your family (Box 8-1).

Surgical Asepsis

Surgical asepsis (sterile technique) refers to an item or area that is free of all microorganisms and spores. Surgical asepsis is used in surgery and to sterilize equipment. Items can be subjected to intense heat or chemical disinfectants to destroy all organisms. The use of pressurized steam sterilizers, called autoclaves, kills even the most powerful organisms. Some equipment cannot be exposed to moist heat, so gas sterilizers are used instead. After these items are sterilized, they are dated, packaged, and sealed. Once a package is opened or outdated, it is no longer considered sterile.

Infection Prevention Guidelines

CDC guidelines for infection control and isolation precautions are used in hospital and health care agency policies. CDC and agency guidelines are continuously updated and should be followed for your patients' and your own protection. Current CDC guidelines for isolation precautions in hospitals include two tiers of precautions: standard precautions and transmission-based precautions (Table 8.2). Visit www.cdc.gov/hicpac/2007IP/2007 isolationPrecautions.html for more details.

FIGURE 8.3 Gloves, gown, mask, goggles, and face shield help prevent the spread of infection to health care workers and patients.

Box 8-1 Guidelines to Prevent the Spread of Infection to Patients, Self, and Family

- Bathe daily and wear a clean uniform/clothing every day.
- Keep your natural fingernail tips less than 1/4 inch long, and do not wear artificial nails. Studies have shown that long fingernails and artificial nails harbor harmful bacteria and have transmitted infections to patients that have sometimes resulted in death.
- Avoid wearing rings and bracelets at work because they harbor organisms.
- Cleanse your stethoscope at least daily and in between patient use with alcohol. Vancomycin-resistant *Enterococcus* bacteria have been cultured from stethoscopes in a hospital setting.
- Use hand hygiene between each patient contact. The use of an alcohol-based hand gel or hand washing is recognized as the single most important action to take to prevent spread of infection.
- Follow prescribed isolation precautions for your protection, as well as that of the patient.
- Perform hand hygiene before going home to prevent transfer of bacteria to your home.
- Remove your uniform in a contained area of your home to launder it, and bathe/shower when you come home from work. This will decrease the spread of antibiotic-resistant bacteria to your home and your family. Keep your nursing shoes clean and stored away from the rest of the family.

TABLE 8.2   STANDARD PRECAUTIONS AND TRANSMISSION-BASED PRECAUTIONS

Standard Precautions
Use standard precautions for all patient care. Combine standard precautions with transmission-based precautions as needed based on the patient's illness.

Hand hygiene	Use alcohol-based hand rub or wash hands with non-microbial soap unless specifically contraindicated before and after using gloves, between patients, and between procedures on the same patient.
Gloves	Wear gloves before contact with any body fluids or substances. Change gloves after each use.
Mask, eye protection, face shield	Use personal protective equipment for patient care if splashes or sprays of blood or body fluids are likely.
Gown	Wear gown to protect skin/prevent soiling of clothing for patient care if splashes or sprays of blood or body fluids are likely.
Occupational health and bloodborne pathogens	Dispose of sharps properly. Do not recap needles.
Patient care equipment	Clean reusable equipment before reuse. Dispose of single-use items properly.
Linen	Handle linen to avoid clothing contamination.
Patient placement	Use private room for infectious patients.

Transmission-Based Precautions
Airborne Precautions
Examples: measles, tuberculosis, varicella (chickenpox, shingles)

Patient placement	Provide private room with regulated airflow. Keep door closed.
Respiratory protection	Do not enter room if susceptible to measles or chickenpox unless no caregivers who are immune are available. If susceptible, wear a fit-tested (N95) disposable respirator. Do not enter room of patient with tuberculosis (TB) unless wearing a fit-tested (N95) disposable respirator. Have patient with TB also wear surgical mask during times that care is performed. Offer visitors an N95 respirator per agency policy. Teach patient respiratory hygiene/cough etiquette.
Patient transport	Limit patient transport to essential purposes. Place surgical mask on patient (may not contain all TB organisms)

Droplet Precautions
Examples: adenovirus, diphtheria (pharyngeal), *Haemophilus influenzae* (epiglottitis, meningitis, pneumonia), influenza, mumps, mycoplasma pneumonia, *Neisseria meningitidis* (meningitis, pneumonia, pertussis, pneumonic plague, rubella, group A streptococcus.

Patient placement	Provide private room or separation greater than 3 feet between the infected patient and other patients and close privacy curtain.
Respiratory protection	Wear mask upon entering patient area. Teach patient respiratory hygiene/cough etiquette.

TABLE 8.2   STANDARD PRECAUTIONS AND TRANSMISSION-BASED PRECAUTIONS—cont'd

Transmission-Based Precautions	
Patient transport	Limit patient transport to essential purposes. Place surgical mask on patient.

Contact Precautions
Examples: cellulitis, *Clostridium difficile,* skin infections (diphtheria, herpes simplex virus, impetigo, pediculosis, scabies, conjunctivitis, viral hemorrhagic infections (Ebola, Lassa, or Marburg), herpes zoster

Patient placement	Provide private room or place with patient with same infection and no other infection.
Hand washing, gloves, gown	Protect self and others from contaminated items.
Patient transport	Limit patient transport.
Patient care equipment	Dedicate the use of noncritical patient care equipment to a single patient.

Source: Data from Siegel, J. D., Rhinehart, E., Jackson, M., Chiarello, L., and the Healthcare Infection Control Practices Advisory Committee. (2007). *2007 guideline for isolation precautions: Preventing transmission of infectious agents in healthcare settings.* Atlanta, GA: Centers for Disease Control and Prevention. Retrieved November 17, 2013, from www.cdc.gov/ncidod/dhqp/pdf/guidelines/Isolation2007.pdf

Standard Precautions

Standard precautions are used in the care of all patients. These precautions require you to assume that all patients are infectious regardless of their diagnosis and to use personal protective equipment (PPE). Standard precautions apply to blood, secretions, excretions, open skin, mucous membranes, and all body fluids, excluding sweat. All patients with draining wounds or secretions of body fluids are considered infectious until an infection is confirmed or ruled out. Using PPE such as gloves, gowns, masks, goggles, face shields, along with hand hygiene helps prevent the spread of infection to health care workers and other patients.

CRITICAL THINKING

Who Is at Greatest Risk of Infection?

■ Which of the following patients is at greatest risk for infection and why?

1. Mr. Ashland, age 55, is hospitalized for a hernia repair. He is overweight and has adult-onset diabetes.
2. Mrs. Burrows, age 72, is hospitalized for a broken hip. She is thin, frail, has dementia, and has undergone placement of a urinary catheter.
3. Jackson Dunn, age 22, is hospitalized for a major surgery. Jackson is thin and small.

Suggested answers are at the end of the chapter.

Transmission-Based Precautions

Transmission-based precautions are used for patients with specific communicable diseases that can be transmitted

to others. These precautions add an additional layer of protection to the standard precautions.

Prevention of Respiratory Tract Infections

Hospital-acquired pneumonia has been linked with the highest infection mortality rate. Patients who are at highest risk for pneumonia are those with endotracheal, nasotracheal, or tracheostomy tubes because these invasive tubes bypass the normal defenses of the upper respiratory tract. Strategies to prevent infections such as ventilator-associated pneumonia (VAP) are "bundled" together so nurses remember to use these strategies. For more information on VAP bundles, visit www.cdc.gov/HAI/vap/vap.html.

Prevention of Genitourinary Tract Infections

The most common HAI is a UTI. Patients with urinary catheters are at greatest risk for this. The urinary tract is sterile, but insertion of a catheter into the bladder may allow organisms to enter it. Institutional policies on appropriate use of urinary catheters differ, so follow your agency's policy. Appropriate reasons for use of a urinary catheter may include urinary obstruction, a neurogenic bladder condition, shock, and palliative care.

Indwelling urinary catheters should be removed as soon as possible. For patients who need long-term catheter use, intermittent catheterization is preferred because it significantly reduces the risk of infection. Using strict aseptic technique while inserting and caring for the catheter in the health care agency is imperative. The catheter tubing must be securely anchored to the patient's leg, according to agency protocol, so it does not move in and out of the urethra. This is because movement can encourage organisms to enter the sterile urinary tract.

The closed urinary drainage system seal should never be opened. (If intermittent irrigation is ordered, sterile technique must be used to protect both ends of the system from contamination.) The drainage bag should be positioned so that it is never higher than the level of the bladder to prevent backflow of urine into the bladder, which could contaminate the sterile urinary tract. If an indwelling urinary catheter and a drainage system are used long term, the catheter and the entire system should be changed regularly using sterile technique. All long-term indwelling urinary catheters are considered colonized. Standards in home care differ from institutional care because patients are generally at lower risk of infection within their own environment.

Remember that the most crucial point at which bacteria may enter the patient is during insertion of the catheter, so excellent sterile technique is required. The urinary tract is highly vascular (many blood vessels close to the surface), so that an infection in this tract can easily result in bacteremia (bacteria in the blood), which can then progress to sepsis (systemic inflammatory response to infection), a potentially life-threatening condition. For more information on prevention of UTIs in adults, visit www.kidney.niddk.nih .gov/kudiseases/pubs/utiadult/index.htm.

 BE SAFE!

Catheters should be used only when necessary because of the **morbidity** (sickness) and **mortality** (death) associated with infections that can develop from them. The continued need for an indwelling catheter should be monitored daily, and the catheter should be discontinued as quickly as it is no longer needed.

CRITICAL THINKING

Mr. Carson

■ While working in an extended care facility, you see Mrs. Brandt, nursing assistant, wheeling Mr. Carson to activities. He has a long-term urinary catheter. The urine bag is hung on the arm of the wheelchair. What is your responsibility in this situation as a team member?

Suggested answers are at the end of the chapter.

Prevention of Surgical Wound Infections

The initial dressing for surgical wounds is applied in the operating room using sterile aseptic technique. Postoperative orders indicate when to change the dressing. Monitor the wound with each dressing change for signs of infection.

ANTIBIOTIC-RESISTANT INFECTIONS

Antibiotic-resistant infections, such as methicillin-resistant *Staphylococcus aureus* (MRSA) and vancomycin-resistant enterococci (VRE), are an urgent worldwide health concern. It is up to each of us to understand how to prevent antibiotic resistance. The CDC's *Get Smart: Know When Antibiotics Work* campaign aims to educate prescribers and individuals on the appropriate use of antibiotics (www.cdc.gov/getsmart/index .html). This education explains that most upper respiratory infections do not require antibiotic treatment, so avoiding the use of antibiotics for viral infections (common cold or flu) is important. Teaching patients to take all prescribed medications exactly as ordered is also vital. Resistant organisms are difficult to treat, can spread easily to others and may result in death. So preventing resistance is a major concern for HCPs.

 LEARNING TIP

Do you know what antibiotics kill? Bacteria, not viruses! See the **b** in anti<u>b</u>iotics and <u>b</u>acteria? That is how you can remember it. Antibiotics are not effective against viral infections such as colds or the flu. Taking antibiotics to treat viral infections increases the risk for antibiotic-resistant "superbugs." Nurses play a vital role in educating people about this growing problem so that no one requests antibiotics for viral infections.

Methicillin-Resistant Staphylococcus Aureus

A serious antibiotic-resistant infection, MRSA, is difficult to treat and has a high mortality rate. It affects mainly older adults and the chronically ill. Vancomycin HCL is an IV antibiotic used to treat MRSA. However, experts fear that the *S. aureus* bacterium will further mutate and become resistant to all antibiotics. A few isolated cases of this mutation have been documented worldwide. The risk that resistant organisms will spread is real, which will return us to preantibiotic days when *S. aureus* was a killer.

Vancomycin-Resistant Enterococci

Vancomycin-resistant enterococci (VRE) infections are common. Although enterococci are normal flora in the GI and female genital tracts, VRE are a pathogenic strain. VRE are transmitted via direct or indirect contact. Patients at risk for VRE infections include those with indwelling urinary or central venous catheters, the immunocompromised or critically ill, those receiving multiple antibiotics or vancomycin therapy, surgical patients, and those with extended hospital stays. Preventive VRE measures focus on proper hand hygiene, education of HCPs, aggressive infection control methods, and restricting use of vancomycin. Patients with VRE should be isolated, and CDC and agency isolation policies strictly followed. Treatment involves combination antibiotic therapy.

THERAPEUTIC MEASURES FOR INFECTIOUS DISEASES

Once an infecting causing organism and the affected body system have been identified, the appropriate medication can be selected and treatment begun (Table 8.3). The drug of choice must be able to destroy (or control) the pathogen:

- Antibiotics treat bacterial infections, not viruses, fungi, helminths, or prions.
- Antiviral medications treat viral infections, but their use is aimed at symptom control rather than cure.
- Antifungal drugs are available for fungal infections, but cure may require extended use.

Cost effectiveness is another concern when selecting a medication. Newer anti-infectives can be very expensive.

Antibiotics can be classified as either bactericidal or bacteriostatic. Bactericidal agents kill bacteria, whereas bacteriostatic agents inhibit or retard bacterial growth, leaving the final destruction of the bacteria up to the infected host's immune system. Bacteriostatic agents may be less helpful for the patient who is immunocompromised.

BE SAFE!

Whenever preparing to give an antibiotic, especially for the first time, ask what allergies a patient may have. Patients may have allergies to one antibiotic group that prevents the use of chemically similar drugs. Therefore, all allergies should be reported to the HCP.

Many antibiotics are metabolized by the liver and excreted by the kidneys. Disorders of these organs may require lower doses. Antibiotic levels fluctuate greatly depending on organ function, age, sex, health, and other factors. Antibiotic serum peak and trough levels (highest and lowest blood levels) may need to be monitored according to agency protocol to ensure therapeutic levels and to prevent toxicity.

Antibiotic-Associated Diarrhea

Antibiotic therapy may cause antibiotic-associated diarrhea (AAD) because antibiotics upset the delicate balance of natural microbiota normally found in the intestine. Any antibiotic can cause AAD, but ampicillin, cephalosporins, and clindamycin are the most common. Antibiotics destroy helpful bacteria along with harmful bacteria. With fewer good bacteria to keep potentially harmful bacteria in check, the harmful bacteria that are resistant to the antibiotic used increase in number. These bacteria can produce toxins that harm the intestinal wall and cause inflammation. Watery bowel movements result. When AAD occurs, the antibiotic therapy may be stopped, and the diarrhea usually resolves. For severe diarrhea, colitis (colon inflammation), or pseudomembranous colitis, metronidazole (Flagyl) or

vancomycin (Vancocin) is given. A **probiotic** (a substance with health-promoting effects, such as yogurt in this case) may help prevent AAD.

Clostridium Difficile

C. difficile is a Gram-positive bacterium, sometimes found normally in the intestine, that can cause infection. It can be one of the most serious causes of AAD and is a growing concern for the CDC. When normal gut microbiota has been destroyed, *C. difficile* can overgrow and release toxins that cause diarrhea of 20 or more stools daily, fever, bloating, and abdominal pain. Healthy people typically do not have *C. difficile* overgrowth. It can occur after antibiotic therapy, usually in those who are hospitalized or in nursing homes, with older adults being at greatest risk (see "Evidence-Based Practice"). *C. difficile* overgrowth can lead to pseudomembranous colitis, a serious and sometimes life-threatening condition with fever, diarrhea, and abdominal pain. The bacteria are transmitted by the fecal-oral route from touching feces-contaminated surfaces. Lidless toilets increase the risk of *C. difficile* environmental contamination by spraying organisms during flushing, so their use is discouraged (Best, Sandoe, & Wilcox, 2012). Hand washing is essential to reduce its spread, as alcohol based rubs are not effective. To treat diarrhea caused by *C. difficile* infection (CDI), the antibiotic treatment is stopped, and metronidazole (Flagyl) or vancomycin (Vancocin) given. Reoccurrence of the infection can occur.

EVIDENCE-BASED PRACTICE

Clinical Question
Are probiotics effective in preventing *C. difficile*?

Evidence
A systematic review and meta-analysis of 23 randomized controlled trials that included 4213 patients, moderate-quality evidence suggests that probiotics are both safe and effective for preventing *C. difficile*–associated diarrhea by 64% in patients who are not immunocompromised or severely debilitated.

Implications for Nursing Practice
Probiotics can be useful in preventing *C. difficile*. Nurses can encourage patients who are prescribed antibiotic therapy to consult an HCP, pharmacist, or dietitian about the use and appropriate dosage of probiotics.

REFERENCES
Goldenberg, J. Z., Ma, S. S. Y., Saxton, J. D., Martzen, M. R., Vandvik, P. O., Thorlund, K., . . . Johnston, B. C. (2013). *Probiotics for the prevention of Clostridium difficile-associated diarrhea in adults and children. Cochrane Database of Systematic Reviews, 5,* CD006095.

• WORD • BUILDING •
probiotic: pro—for + biotic—life

TABLE **8.3** MEDICATIONS USED TO TREAT INFECTIONS

Medication Class, Action	Examples	Nursing Implications
Bactericidal Antibiotics ***Penicillins*** • Most effective against Gram-positive organisms	amoxicillin (Amoxil), ticarcillin (Ticar), penicillin G, ampicillin (Omnipen)	Review signs of allergic reactions with patient. Monitor patient for allergic reaction (rash, hives, itching) or anaphylactic shock (fever, chills, dyspnea, low blood pressure, tight throat, wheezing). For signs of allergic reaction, with parenteral drug, stop infusion. Notify HCP immediately. Keep epinephrine available. Teach patient and family to hold drug and call HCP if allergy signs occur, oral white patches appear, or vaginal irritation occurs.
Carbapenems • Broad-spectrum antibacterial agents treat moderate to severe infection	doripenem (Doribax), ertapenem (Invanz), imipenem and cilastatin (Primaxin), meropenem (Merrem)	Ertapenem: Check for lidocaine (intramuscular diluent) allergy. Monitor patient for seizures and, if applicable, serum valproic acid level.
Cephalosporins • First-generation drugs are most effective against Gram-positive organisms • Second- and third-generation drugs are more effective against Gram-negative organisms	cephalothin (Keflin), cefazolin (Ancef), cefaclor (Ceclor), ceftriaxone (Rocephin)	Patients with penicillin allergy can have 10% risk of cross-allergy to cephalosporins. *Teaching:* Take drug on empty stomach, 1 hr before or 2 hr after meals, to increase absorption. Take drug at specified intervals during 24-hr period. Monitor blood urea nitrogen, creatinine, lactic dehydrogenase, aspartate aminotransferase, and alanine aminotransferase to detect kidney or liver damage.
Aminoglycosides • Treat Gram-negative organisms	amikacin (Amikin), gentamicin (Garamycin), tobramycin (Nebcin)	Check for and report elevated creatinine levels before giving this nephrotoxic agent. Monitor peak/trough levels to keep drug in therapeutic range. Teach patient to report signs of allergy, tinnitus, vertigo, or hearing loss.
Fluoroquinolones • Treats variety of infections, such as bronchitis, bone and joint infection, pneumonia, TB, sexually transmitted infections (STIs), and UTIs	moxifloxacin (Avelox), ciprofloxacin (Cipro), levofloxacin (Levaquin), norfloxacin (Noroxin), ofloxacin (Floxin)	*Teaching:* Take drug on an empty stomach and with a full glass of water. Do not take with antacids that contain aluminum, calcium, or magnesium. Monitor liver function, and report signs of dysfunction (fatal hepatitis can occur). Encourage fluids.

TABLE 8.3 MEDICATIONS USED TO TREAT INFECTIONS—cont'd

Medication Class, Action	Examples	Nursing Implications
		Explain side effects, and advise sun protection. Teach patient to report joint or muscle pain immediately. Monitor for rare but serious tendon rupture.
Nitroimidazoles • Treats anaerobic bacterial and parasitic infections	metronidazole (Flagyl)	May be taken with or without food. Tell patient to avoid alcohol use.
Glycopeptides • Treat serious Gram-positive infections. Orally for pseudomembranous colitis	vancomycin	Administer IV over 1 hr to prevent red man syndrome (flushing, rash on upper body, neck, head). Monitor peak/trough levels. Monitor IV site for thrombophlebitis.
Bacteriostatic Antibiotics *Tetracyclines* • Treats most Gram-positive and Gram-negative organisms	tetracycline HCl, doxycycline (Vibramycin), minocycline HCl (Minocin)	Give 1 hr before or 2 hr after meals. Do not give with milk, milk products, or antacids as absorption impaired. Suggest eating crackers and juice (but not a full meal) to reduce GI upset. *Teaching:* avoid prolonged sun exposure during therapy.
Macrolides • Broad-spectrum antibiotics used effectively against many Gram-negative and Gram-positive organisms	azithromycin (Zithromax)	Give with a full glass of water. Capsules must be taken on an empty stomach. Do not give with aluminum or magnesium antacids within 2 hr before or after. *Teaching:* avoid sun exposure.
	clarithromycin	Give with a full glass of water. May be taken with or without food except for time-release capsules.
	erythromycin (E-mycin, EES)	Administer IV slowly to decrease vein irritation. Give orally on an empty stomach, 1 hr before or 2 hr after meals. Give with a full glass of water (not with acidic fruit juices, such as orange juice or grapefruit juice). *Teaching:* Take drug around the clock. Complete entire course of treatment. Explain that gastric distress is common but not a reason to stop the drug. Contact HCP if side effects are intolerable.
Treats C. Difficile only.	fidaxomicin (DIFICID)	*Teaching:* take tablets with or without food.

Continued

TABLE 8.3   MEDICATIONS USED TO TREAT INFECTIONS—cont'd

Medication Class, Action	Examples	Nursing Implications
Lincomycins • Treats serious anaerobic bacterial infections, acne, methicillin-resistant *Staphylococcus aureus,* and some protozoal infections	clindamycin (Cleocin)	Monitor and report foul-odor diarrhea, fever, and abdominal pain indicating possible *C. difficile* infection.
Streptogramins • Treats vancomycin-resistant *Enterococcus faecium* bacteremia and severe skin infections. • Combination drugs are bactericidal.	quinupristin/dalfopristin (Synercid)	After infusion, flush with 5% dextrose in water solution to minimize vein irritation (incompatible with saline or heparin).
Sulfonamides • Effective against most Gram-positive and many Gram-negative organisms • Commonly used for UTIs, *Pneumocystis jiroveci* pneumonia, and otitis media	trimethoprim sulfamethoxazole (Bactrim, Septra)	IV drug given over 1 hr. Monitor intake and output. Fluid intake should be at least 1500 mL daily. *Teaching:* Take oral drug on empty stomach 1 hr before or 2 hr after meals with a full glass of water. Avoid prolonged exposure to the sun. Stop drug and call HCP if signs of allergic reaction or bleeding occur.
Oxazolidinones • Treats complicated infections caused by Gram-negative microorganisms	linezolid (Zyvox)	Before IV use, check compatibilities. Oral form may be taken with or without food. *Teaching:* avoid tyramine found, for example, in aged cheeses, smoked foods, tap beer, red wine, soy sauce, sauerkraut.
Antifungals **Amphotericin B** • Interferes with the cell wall structure of the fungus, causing it to die; treats life-threatening fungal infections		Teaching: purpose of treatment and need for long-term IV therapy, side effects and possible discomfort at IV site. Monitor patient during first hour of infusion for febrile reaction. Monitor injection site often because drug is very irritating to tissues. Monitor intake and output, blood urea nitrogen (BUN), and creatinine levels for signs of kidney damage. Obtain daily weight because fluid retention follows kidney damage. Encourage 2000–3000 mL of fluid daily to help flush drug through kidneys.
Triazoles • Treats yeast or fungus infections	fluconazole (Diflucan), itraconazole (Sporanox), posaconazole (Noxafil), voriconazole (Vfend)	Obtain cultures before giving drug. Monitor BUN and creatinine levels and liver function.

TABLE 8.3 MEDICATIONS USED TO TREAT INFECTIONS—cont'd

Medication Class, Action	Examples	Nursing Implications
		Teaching: notify HCP at the first sign of yellow skin, dark urine, or pale stools (signs of liver damage). Vfend causes blurry vision about 20 minutes after dose and patient should not drive.
Echinocandins • Disrupt fungal cell wall integrity • Treats candidal infection	caspofungin (Cancidas), micafungin (Mycamine), anidulafungin (Eraxis)	Monitor patient's liver function.

Fecal Microbiota Transplantation

Fecal transplant (fecal microbiota transplantation) is a treatment that is growing in usage for treating *C. difficile* infection (CDI), primarily when other treatments have failed. The purpose of fecal transplant is to restore the missing healthy bacteria in the intestine and restore balance to gut health. It has shown dramatic results in restoring health and quality of life to those with CDI, often rapidly. Patients who have been gravely ill from recurrent CDI can be infection-free within days after the treatment. Understanding the role the gut microbiota play in our health is leading to the exploration of other uses for fecal transplant. Conditions such as Crohn's disease, ulcerative colitis, inflammatory bowel syndrome, and even rheumatoid arthritis are being explored for this treatment.

Donated feces from a healthy person, often a family member, is transplanted into a patient via colonoscopy, nasogastric or nasojejunal tube, retention enema, or oral capsules. The multilayered capsules contain only the bacteria processed from the feces that dissolve in the small intestine. A stool substitute, made from purified intestinal bacterial cultures, is being studied for use in recurrent CDI. This synthetic stool bacterial mixture, *RePOOPulate*, has been shown to be effective and is more acceptable to patients.

Nursing Care

Nurses are responsible for administering medications correctly and for teaching patients the importance of taking these medications properly (Box 8-2). Follow these general guidelines and consult drug references for further information before giving anti-infectives:

• Note all patient allergies, and inform the HCP.
• Obtain ordered samples for culturing before starting ordered anti-infectives, so culture accuracy is not affected.
• Monitor and report to HCP any side effects or signs of allergic response, especially anaphylactic reactions, and peak and trough results.
• Observe and report to HCP any signs of superinfection (one that occurs as a result of antibiotic use). For example, oral thrush (white raised lesions on tongue) may develop because antibiotics disrupt the normal GI tract flora.

Box 8-2 **Patient Teaching**

Anti-Infective Medications

• Stress to the patient and family the need to take all of the medication exactly as prescribed.
• Explain that stopping treatment before the prescription is finished, even if the patient feels better, increases the risk of relapse and the growth of antibiotic-resistant organisms.
• Explain the signs and symptoms of side effects (allergic and nonallergic) to watch for and what to do about them.
• Explain when to call the primary care provider to report signs and symptoms.

 BE SAFE!

Always review medication doses and compare them with the normal dose of the medications before giving them to keep your patient safe and protect your nursing license. You are responsible for any medication you give, even if the dose was ordered incorrectly and you were following the order. If the dose is outside the normal range, do not give the drug. Consult with the registered nurse, pharmacist, or your supervisor, who should contact the ordering HCP for clarification.

NURSING PROCESS FOR THE PATIENT WITH AN INFECTION

General Infections
Data Collection

Early detection of signs and symptoms can help provide early treatment to prevent major complications and reduce costs. Providing emotional support to the patient is also important (see "Patient Perspective"). Patients who are prone to infection because of immunosuppression should take special precautions to prevent infection (Box 8-3).

Patient Perspective

Jeff: Emotions Experienced With Chronic Infection

It was back! I wasn't sure I could deal with it one more time. I've been hospitalized four times with this same infection (cellulitis) in my leg. It feels like I've lost my life. I can't count on being able to do anything or go anywhere because the infection just keeps coming back.

My left leg is now all swollen, red, discolored, and very painful. I can tell when I'm infected by more than the pain in the leg. I feel weak, kind of spacey, and once I passed out. I'm so sick of going to the emergency room—waiting forever to get admitted, having all the IV starts and blood draws. With these infections, I've had a PICC (peripherally inserted central catheter) line twice. I've been sent home on IV antibiotics, sometimes for weeks at a time. I've learned how to hang my own IV antibiotics; in fact, I've learned much more than I ever wanted to know.

My cellulitis is associated with chronic lymphedema, causing swelling in my legs. I'm working hard to keep the swelling down so the infection doesn't recur. Wish me luck and keep giving me psychosocial support during your nursing care. I'm not sure how I will be able to deal with this much longer.

Box 8-3 Patient Education

Prevention of Infection in Older, Debilitated, or Immunocompromised Patients

- Wash your hands often, using proper technique.
- Avoid crowds or anyone with an infection.
- Stay well nourished because food helps keep the immune system healthy.
- Have a flu shot yearly and a pneumonia shot as recommended by your primary care provider.
- Wash raw fruits and vegetables thoroughly, cook food thoroughly, and store food safely to prevent food poisoning. (*Note:* If you are severely immunocompromised, raw foods, soft cheeses, and yogurt may be contraindicated because of the risk of bacterial infection.)
- If your immune system is depressed, notify your primary care provider if you have an elevated temperature, even if you have no other symptoms. People with depressed immune function cannot mount the usual immune response to infection, and a low-grade fever may be the only sign of infection.

CRITICAL THINKING

Mr. Cheevers

■ Mr. Cheevers is admitted to the hospital for IV antibiotic therapy. He states that he has no allergies. One hour after the infusion begins, you happen to meet the nursing assistant coming down the hall with a blanket. He casually says, "Mr. Cheevers is very cold. I'm taking him a blanket. He is also restless and a bit short of breath." What is your responsibility in this situation?

Suggested answers are at the end of the chapter.

Nursing Diagnoses, Planning, and Implementation

Risk for Infection related to external factors

EXPECTED OUTCOME: The patient will remain free from symptoms of infection.

- Follow current hand hygiene guidelines *to reduce spread of infection.*
- Use standard precautions and transmission-based precautions *to prevent the transmission of organisms.*
- Observe and report signs of infection such as redness, warmth, and fever promptly, especially for neutropenic patients *because they do not have normal inflammatory response and low-grade fever is often the only sign.*
- Monitor laboratory values of WBC counts and cultures *because they correlate to patient's immune function for planning care.*

Evaluation

If interventions have been successful, the patient remains free from symptoms of infection.

Imbalanced Nutrition: Less Than Body Requirements related to problems eating or digesting food

EXPECTED OUTCOME: The patient will maintain ideal body weight for height and weight and eat a balanced diet.

- Identify and provide foods patient enjoys with pleasant presentation *because patient will be more likely to try eating enjoyable foods in a clean, odor-free environment.*
- Explain and ensure that a balanced diet with protein, fatty acids, and vitamins is available and should be eaten. *These nutrients are needed for healthy immune system function.*
- Monitor and document patient intake *to provide accurate nutritional assessment.*
- Provide antiemetics, as ordered, *to control nausea and vomiting and improve nutritional intake.*

Evaluation

If interventions have been effective, patient's body weight will be maintained within ideal body weight range and patient will eat a balanced diet.

Deficient Knowledge *related to disease process and treatment*

EXPECTED OUTCOME: *The patient will describe therapy and carry out treatment.*

• Explain infection and how to prevent infection. *Patients' understanding of how infections occur helps them in controlling their risk of infection.*
• Recommend responsible use of antibiotics *to prevent resistant organisms.*
• Explain medications, side effects, and symptoms to report *to promote adherence to treatment and safe medication use.*
• Teach patients how to participate in their own care and have them assist in the development of their plan of care *to promote adherence to treatment.*

Evaluation

If interventions have been effective, the patient will state understanding of therapy and plan and carry out treatment plan.

Respiratory Tract Infection
Data Collection

Patients with respiratory tract infections may have a cough, a congested or runny nose, a sore throat, chest congestion, or chest pain. The throat may be reddened, or there may be white patches in the back of the throat. Lung sounds can include crackles, rhonchi, or wheezing. Ask patients if they have a productive cough and the amount, frequency, and color of the sputum. A sputum culture is obtained to identify the presence of pathogenic organisms for appropriate treatment.

Nursing Diagnoses, Planning, and Implementation
Risk for Infection *related to external factors*

EXPECTED OUTCOME: *The patient will remain free from symptoms of infection.*

• Encourage coughing and deep breathing *to keep airways clear and prevent atelectasis.*
• Provide oral care with toothbrush or suction-type toothbrush (see Chapter 2) and fluoride toothpaste regularly *to remove plaque, which has been found to contribute to pneumonia development.* (Toothettes do not remove plaque.)
• Encourage fluids if not contraindicated. *Dehydration is associated with dry, sticky secretions that are difficult to cough up.*
• Provide pain relief *so patient will take deep breaths.*
• Elevate head of bed 30 degrees or more when a tube feeding is infusing *to prevent aspiration pneumonia.*
• Use sterile water rather than tap water from faucet for oral care for immunocompromised patients *to prevent hospital-acquired pneumonia.*

Evaluation

If interventions have been effective, oxygen saturation will be above 90%, with report of decreased dyspnea. Respirations will not be labored, and patient will be free of signs and symptoms of infection.

Gastrointestinal Tract Infection
Data Collection

The symptoms of GI tract infections may include nausea, vomiting, diarrhea, cramping, and anorexia. Signs of dehydration from fluid loss are reported. Stool cultures may be ordered.

Nursing Diagnoses, Planning, and Implementation
Risk for Infection *related to external factors*

EXPECTED OUTCOME: *The patient will remain free from symptoms of infection.*

• Encourage fluid intake *to replace fluid lost during fever, vomiting, and diarrhea.*
• Follow standard precautions, especially for older and immunocompromised patients, *to prevent the spread of* C. difficile, *which usually does not cause infection in healthy adults.*
• Teach hand hygiene with antimicrobial soap and water if contact with C. difficile spores is likely *because alcohols, chlorhexidine, iodophors, and other antiseptic agents are not effective in destroying* C. difficile *spores.*

Evaluation

Patient will be free of infection and nausea, vomiting, diarrhea, cramping, anorexia, and dehydration if interventions have been successful.

Genitourinary Tract Infection
Data Collection

Symptoms of a UTI include voiding urgency, frequency, burning, flank pain, change in urine color, foul urine odor, and confusion or change in mental status in older adults. Monitor frequency, amount, color, and odor of the urine. Urinalysis and urine cultures may be ordered.

Nursing Diagnoses, Planning, and Implementation
Risk for Infection *related to external factors*

EXPECTED OUTCOME: *The patient will remain free from symptoms of infection.*

• Do not request and avoid use of urinary catheters unless no other options are available *because patients are more likely to develop a UTI.*
• Use sterile technique for inserting urinary catheters *to prevent HAIs.*
• Avoid contamination when emptying urinary catheter bags *to prevent health care–acquired infections.*

Evaluation

If interventions have been effective, the patient will have normal urine output without symptoms of UTI.

SUGGESTED ANSWERS TO

CRITICAL THINKING

■ *Mrs. Sampson*

1. Hand hygiene reduces the microorganisms on the nurse's hands to help reduce their transmission from patient to patient. This helps prevent exposure to pathogens and infection.
2. *Risk for infection.*
3. Reverse isolation, the goal of which is to protect the patient from exposure to organisms rather than to protect others from exposure to the patient.

■ *Who Is at Greatest Risk of Infection?*

1. Mr. Ashland has two risk factors: chronic disease and probably stress.
2. Mrs. Burrows has many risk factors, including older age, debilitated condition, probable malnourishment, probable stress, and an invasive procedure. This patient is at greatest risk.
3. Jackson has three risk factors: probable stress, possible malnourishment, and an invasive procedure.

■ *Mr. Carson*

1. Ask the nursing assistant about the urinary bag placed above the patient's bladder. Explain that the bag should always stay below the level of the bladder both for proper drainage and for infection control.
2. Assist the nursing assistant in repositioning the bag properly.
3. Let Mr. Carson's primary nurse knows about the potential backflow of urine so that he can be assessed in the next few days for signs of a bladder infection.

■ *Mr. Cheevers*

Mr. Cheevers may be experiencing signs of allergic reaction to the medication. The fact that he has no history of allergy is no guarantee that he is not experiencing one now. If allergy is suspected, the IV should be stopped. He needs to be evaluated immediately and the primary care provider notified. Epinephrine should be on hand to treat the patient for anaphylaxis. The primary nurse needs to be alerted to the situation in the event that it worsens. Later, the nursing assistant can be instructed about the signs of an allergic response.

REVIEW QUESTIONS

1. Place the links in the chain of infection in their proper order of occurrence in causing an infection.
   1. Portal of entry
   2. Causative agents
   3. Mode of transmission
   4. Portal of exit
   5. Reservoir
   6. Susceptible host

2. The nurse prepares to bathe a patient. Which of the following is the MOST important technique for the nurse to use during patient care to prevent infection transmission?
   1. Wear gloves.
   2. Wear a gown.
   3. Wash hands.
   4. Wear a mask.

3. The nurse is caring for a patient who is on bed rest. Which of the following nursing actions should the nurse include in the plan of care to help maintain the body's first line of defense against infection?
   1. Help the patient cough and deep-breathe.
   2. Apply lotion to clean skin.
   3. Give an antibiotic as ordered.
   4. Help the patient void.

4. The LPN/LVN has taken patient temperatures. Which of the following patient temperature readings would be the PRIORITY for the LPN/LVN to report to the RN?
   1. Temperature 97°F (36.1°C) for an older patient with hypertension
   2. Temperature 98.9°F (37°C) for a first-day post-operative patient
   3. Temperature 99.6°F (37.5°C) for a patient with neutropenia
   4. Temperature 100°F (37.7°C) for a patient with appendicitis

5. The nurse is to give a newly ordered antibiotic to a patient with a wound infection. Which of the following is ESSENTIAL to do before giving the medication?
   1. Check all patient allergies.
   2. Check the patient's temperature.
   3. Change dressing and note wound appearance.
   4. Give antibiotic before mealtime.

6. The nurse is caring for a patient with an indwelling urinary catheter. Which of the following is the MOST important action for the nurse to use to prevent a hospital-acquired UTI from developing in this patient?
   1. Ensure an adequate intake of IV and oral fluids.
   2. Use clean technique for catheter insertion.
   3. Position the drainage bag higher than bladder level.
   4. Maintain a closed urinary drainage system.

7. The nurse is caring for a patient receiving an antibiotic. Which of the following statements indicates to the nurse that the patient understands the general principles of appropriate antibiotic use?
   1. "I'll take this until I start feeling better."
   2. "I have pills left over from the last time I had this infection."
   3. "I'll take all of this as it says to on the medication label."
   4. "I take only half of a pill to reduce the cost of the pills."

Answers can be found in Appendix C.

References

Best, E., Sandoe, J., & Wilcox, M. (2012). Potential for aerosolization of *Clostridium difficile* after flushing toilets: The role of toilet lids in reducing environmental contamination risk, *Journal of Hospital Infection, 80,* 1–5.

Centers for Disease Control and Prevention. (2002). Guideline for Hand Hygiene in Health-Care Settings. *MMWR 51*(RR16):1–44. Retrieved December 2, 2013, from www.cdc.gov/handhygiene /Guidelines.html

Joint Commission. (2013). *2014 national patient safety goals.* Retrieved December 2, 2013, from www.jointcommission.org /standards_information/npsgs.aspx

WHO guidelines on hand hygiene in health care. (2009). Retrieved December 2, 2013, from whqlibdoc.who.int/publications/ 2009/9789241597906_eng.pdf

 DavisPlus | For additional resources and information visit **davispl.us/medsurg5**

9

Nursing Care of Patients in Shock

BOBBI M. MARTIN

KEY TERMS

acidosis (AS-ih-DOH-sis)

acute pulmonary hypertension (ah-KEWT PULL-muh-NAIR-ee HY-per-TEN-shun)

anaerobic (AN-air-ROH-bick)

anaphylaxis (AN-uh-fih-LAK-sis)

bronchospasm (BRONG-koh-spazm)

cardiac output (KAR-dee-ack OWT-put)

cardiogenic (KAR-dee-oh-JEN-ick)

cyanosis (SY-uh-NOH-sis)

distributive (diss-TRIB-yoo-tiv)

dysrhythmia (diss-RITH-mee-yah)

epinephrine (EP-ih-NEFF-rin)

extracardiac (EX-trah-KAR-dee-ack)

hypoperfusion (HY-poh-per-FEW-shun)

hypotension (HY-poh-TEN-shun)

hypovolemic (HY-poh-voh-LEE-mick)

ischemia (iss-KEY-mee-ah)

lactic acid (LAK-tik AS-id)

laryngeal edema (lah-RIN-jee-uhl eh-DEE-muh)

myocarditis (MY-oh-kar-DYE-tiss)

myocardium (MY-oh-KAR-dee-um)

neurogenic (NEW-roh-JEN-ick)

norepinephrine (NOR-ep-ih-NEFF-rin)

perfusion (per-FEW-zhun)

pericardial tamponade (PER-ih-KAR-dee-uhl TAM-pon-AID)

sepsis (SEP-sis)

tachycardia (TAK-ih-KAR-dee-yah)

tachypnea (TAK-ip-NEE-ah)

tension pneumothorax (TEN-shun NEW-moh-THOR-raks)

thrombi (THROM-bye)

toxemia (tock-SEE-me-ah)

trauma (TRAW-mah)

urticaria (UR-ti-CARE-ee-ah)

LEARNING OUTCOMES

1. Explain the pathophysiology of shock and compensatory mechanisms.
2. Identify the etiology, signs, and symptoms for each of the four categories of shock.
3. Describe therapeutic measures for shock.
4. List data to collect when caring for patients in shock.
5. Plan nursing care for patients in shock.
6. Prioritize care for a client in shock.
7. Identify findings that demonstrate a positive response to therapeutic measures for shock.

132

Shock is a life-threatening medical emergency that requires rapid intervention by the health care team. A person in shock is in a state of circulatory collapse. Without immediate treatment, organ damage and death occur.

Shock is defined as inadequate tissue **perfusion** in which there is insufficient delivery of oxygen and nutrients to the body's tissues and inadequate removal of waste products from these tissues or, more simply, an imbalance between oxygen supply and demand. The decrease in tissue perfusion leads to impaired cellular metabolism, which in turn leads to tissue hypoxia. Tissue hypoxia results in **hypoperfusion** of vital organs and cell death. All body systems are affected by reduced oxygen supplies. The resulting injury to the body can be treated in the early stages of shock, but if shock is prolonged, it leads to irreversible cell damage and death. By the time blood pressure drops, cellular and tissue damage have already occurred. Therefore, it is important to identify patients at risk for shock and carefully monitor them to detect early signs and symptoms.

PATHOPHYSIOLOGY OF SHOCK

Tissue perfusion and blood pressure are maintained in the body by three mechanisms: (1) adequate blood volume, (2) an effective cardiac pump, and (3) effective blood vessels. The body is able to compensate for failure of one of these mechanisms by making a change in one or both of the other two. Shock occurs when compensatory mechanisms fail, resulting in inadequate tissue perfusion. Common causes of shock include inadequate **cardiac output** caused by heart failure, a sudden loss of blood volume resulting from hemorrhage, or a sudden decrease in peripheral vascular resistance caused by **anaphylaxis** (a life-threatening allergic reaction); **sepsis** (an infection that has spread to the bloodstream); or neurologic alterations.

Metabolic and Hemodynamic Changes in Shock

When blood pressure falls, the body responds by activating the sympathetic nervous system. **Epinephrine** and **norepinephrine** are released from the adrenal medulla and increase cardiac output by causing the heart to beat faster and stronger. Blood is shunted away from the skin, kidneys, and intestines to preserve blood flow to the brain, liver, and heart. Epinephrine, cortisol, and glucagon raise blood glucose levels to supply cells with fuel. Stimulation of the renin-angiotensin-aldosterone system from decreased cardiac output causes vasoconstriction and retention of sodium and water to decrease further fluid loss. Respiratory rate increases to deliver more oxygen to the tissues. Together these compensatory responses produce the classic signs and symptoms of the initial stage of shock: **tachycardia**, **tachypnea**, restlessness, anxiety, and cool, clammy skin with pallor. If oxygen delivery remains inadequate, signs and symptoms of progressive and irreversible shock are seen (Table 9.1).

TABLE 9.1   CHARACTERISTICS OF SHOCK STAGES

Characteristics	Stages		
	• *Compensated* • *Able to maintain blood pressure and tissue perfusion*	• *Progressive* • *Compensatory mechanisms start to fail*	• *Irreversible* • *No response to treatment* • *Death is imminent*
Heart rate	Tachycardia	Tachycardia Greater than 150 beats/min	Slowing
Pulses	Bounding	Weak, thready	Absent
Systolic blood pressure	Normal	Below 90 mm Hg In hypertensive patient, 25% below baseline	Below 60 mm Hg
Diastolic blood pressure	Normal	Decreased	Decreasing to 0
Respirations	Increased rate, deep	Tachypnea, crackles, shallow	Slowing, irregular, shallow
Temperature	Varies	Decreased, can rise in septic shock	Decreasing
Level of consciousness	Anxious, restless, irritable, alert, oriented, sense of impending doom	Confused, lethargic	Unconscious, comatose

Continued

TABLE 9.1 CHARACTERISTICS OF SHOCK STAGES—cont'd

Characteristics		Stages	
Skin and mucous membranes	Cool, clammy, pale	Moist, cold, clammy, pale	Cyanosis, mottled, cold, clammy
Urine output	Normal	Decreasing to less than 20 mL/hr	15 mL/hr, decreasing to anuria
Bowel sounds	Normal	Decreasing	Absent

CRITICAL THINKING

Classic Signs of Shock

■ What is the cause and compensatory purpose of each of the classic signs of shock: tachycardia, tachypnea, **oliguria**, pallor, and cool, clammy skin?

Suggested answers are at the end of the chapter.

 LEARNING TIP

Tachycardia is a compensatory mechanism that is usually the first sign of shock. When a patient develops sustained tachycardia, it is a signal that the patient's condition is changing. Older patients cannot tolerate tachycardia very long because their ability to adapt to stress is reduced.

Consider the cause of the tachycardia. For example, a surgical patient who develops tachycardia can be hemorrhaging and should be assessed for bleeding. With internal hemorrhaging, there might not be any visible signs of bleeding. Changes in vital signs can be the only evidence. Provide prompt intervention, such as applying direct pressure to an area of hemorrhage, and implement the physician's orders immediately.

Inadequate tissue blood flow causes an important change in cellular metabolism. When cells are deprived of oxygen, they shift from aerobic metabolism to anaerobic metabolism to continue to receive nutrition and energy. **Anaerobic** metabolism is an inefficient form of metabolism that can supply

• **WORD • BUILDING •**

acidosis: acid—sour + osis—condition
anaerobic: an—without + aerobic—presence of oxygen
anaphylaxis: an—without + phylaxis—protection
hypoperfusion: hypo—low + perfuser—to pour over or through
oliguria: olig—few + uria—urine
tachycardia: tachy—fast + cardia—heart
tachypnea: tachy—fast + pnea—breathing

the energy needs of the cell for only a few minutes. After that, the body's metabolic rate and temperature begin to fall as a result of reduced energy production.

Anaerobic metabolism results in the production of **lactic acid** as an unwanted byproduct. Unless the lactic acid can be circulated to the liver and thus removed from the bloodstream, the blood becomes increasingly acidic. **Acidosis**, which is a decrease in blood pH below 7.35, is one of the classic signs of shock.

Effect on Organs and Organ Systems

Why would prolonged shock cause extensive damage to the organs and organ systems (Table 9.2)? It is due to the inadequate blood flow that results in tissue **ischemia** and injury. Because blood is shunted away from the kidneys early in shock to save fluid and provide oxygen to vital organs, the kidneys are commonly injured first. The kidneys can tolerate reduced blood flow for about 1 hour before cells in the kidneys die from a lack of oxygen and nutrients. If there is widespread damage to the kidneys, complete renal failure is likely. Renal failure resulting from inadequate blood flow to the kidneys can be prevented and treated by replacing lost fluids.

CRITICAL THINKING

Anaerobic Metabolism

■ Why is anaerobic metabolism necessary and helpful if it produces the complication of metabolic acidosis?

Suggested answers are at the end of the chapter.

Several organs of the gastrointestinal (GI) system can be injured early in shock. Inadequate circulation to the intestines can result in injury of the mucosa and can even cause paralytic ileus (paralysis of the intestine). **Toxemia** can result when the body absorbs normally occurring bacteria and endotoxins from inside the bowel into the circulation. The liver can be injured by both ischemia and toxins created by the shock state as blood is circulated through it for cleansing. Signs and symptoms of liver injury include decreased production of plasma proteins, abnormal clotting (because clotting factor production by the liver is impaired), and elevated serum levels of ammonia, bilirubin, and liver enzymes.

TABLE 9.2 EFFECT OF SHOCK ON ORGANS AND ORGAN SYSTEMS

Organ or Organ System	Effect
Lungs	Acute respiratory failure Acute respiratory distress syndrome
Renal system	Renal failure
Heart	Dysrhythmias Myocardial ischemia Myocardial depression
Liver	Abnormal clotting Decreased production of plasma proteins Elevated serum levels of ammonia, bilirubin, and liver enzymes
Immune system	Depletion of defense components
Gastrointestinal system	Mucosal injury Paralytic ileus Pancreatitis Absorption of endotoxins and bacteria
Central nervous system	Ischemic damage, necrosis, brain death

The immune system is also affected by shock, leaving the body vulnerable to infection. Also, if the liver has been damaged, it is unable to assist the immune system in providing defense.

The body attempts to preserve blood supply to the heart and brain because these are vital organs that require a continuous supply of oxygen. Shock places extra demands on the heart itself, creating a situation in which the heart is in extra need of oxygen at a time when oxygen supplies are already low. When the **myocardium** (the middle layer of the heart wall) receives inadequate oxygenation, cardiac output decreases, and shock worsens. The pumping ability of the heart can be further depressed by acidosis, toxins released into the blood from ischemic tissues, or ischemia-induced **dysrhythmia** (abnormal heart rhythm). If the brain is deprived of circulation for more than 4 minutes, brain cells die from a lack of oxygen and glucose. As a result, prolonged shock can result in brain death.

COMPLICATIONS FROM SHOCK

Acute respiratory distress syndrome (ARDS), disseminated intravascular coagulation (DIC), and multiple organ dysfunction syndrome (MODS) are three especially grave conditions that can follow a prolonged episode of shock. Patients with ARDS experience respiratory failure and typically require high levels of supplemental oxygen and mechanical ventilation. DIC results from ischemic damage to the endothelial lining of blood vessels. The formation of multiple tiny **thrombi** (blood clots), microscopic debris, and depletion of tissue-clotting factors cause abnormal bleeding and additional tissue damage. DIC itself can cause shock and death. MODS is a major cause of death following shock. When an organ has inadequate perfusion, it fails, which can increase the rate of failure of other organs. It usually begins with respiratory failure, followed by failure of the kidneys, heart, liver, and finally cerebral and GI function.

LEARNING TIP

To understand what *disseminated intravascular coagulation* means, define each of the words and then put the definitions together.

>   Disseminated: scattered or widespread
>   Intravascular: intra = inside + vascular = vessels
>   Coagulation: clotting

Put together, these definitions tell you that DIC is scattered, widespread clotting inside the vessels.

At first, hemorrhage does not seem likely in light of a clotting problem, but if you think about what is occurring, it makes sense. When many clots form throughout the body in response to stressors, few clotting factors remain available to form the clots needed to prevent hemorrhage. As a result, hemorrhage is a risk in DIC.

CLASSIFICATION OF SHOCK

The four types of shock are classified by their cardiovascular characteristics (Table 9.3):

- **Hypovolemic** shock is caused by a decrease in the circulating blood volume.
- **Cardiogenic** shock is caused by cardiac failure as a pump.
- **Extracardiac** obstructive shock is caused by a blockage of blood flow in the cardiovascular circuit outside the heart.
- **Distributive** shock is caused by excessive dilation of the venules and arterioles.

Most cases of clinical shock show only some components of each of these categories. However, this classification system is helpful in understanding shock. The hallmark characteristic, seen in all forms of shock, is a decrease in blood pressure usually below the level needed to provide enough blood to the tissues.

TABLE 9.3 CATEGORIES OF SHOCK

Category	Causes	Signs and Symptoms
Hypovolemic Shock	Any severe loss of body fluid, including dehydration; internal or external hemorrhage; fluid loss from burns, vomiting, or diarrhea; or loss of intravascular fluid into the interstitium	Tachycardia; tachypnea; hypotension; cyanosis; oliguria; flat, nondistended peripheral veins; decreased jugular veins; altered mental status
Cardiogenic Shock	Myocardial infarction, traumatic cardiac injury, cardiomyopathy, myocarditis, endocarditis, dysrhythmias, valvular disease	Dysrhythmias, labored respirations, hypotension, cyanosis, oliguria, altered mental status, possibly distended jugular and peripheral veins, symptoms of heart failure
Extracardiac Obstructive Shock	Any block to the cardiovascular flow, such as pericardial tamponade, tension pneumothorax, intrathoracic tumor, massive pulmonary embolus, large systemic embolus	Tachycardia, tachypnea, hypotension, cyanosis, oliguria, altered mental status, possibly distended jugular veins
Distributive Shock	Any condition causing massive vasodilation of peripheral circulation, including the subcategories anaphylactic, septic, and neurogenic shock	*See subcategories below.*
• Anaphylactic shock	Reaction to an allergen, such as an insect sting, antibiotic, anesthetic, contrast dye, or blood product	• Tachycardia, tachypnea, wheezing, hypotension, cyanosis, oliguria, altered mental status • Can have urticaria, pruritus, angioedema, laryngeal edema, and severe bronchospasm • If conscious, can be extremely apprehensive and report a metallic taste
• Septic shock	Loss of vascular autoregulatory control and loss of fluid into the interstitium caused by massive release of chemical mediators and endotoxins from bacteria, especially Gram-positive strains, fungi, protozoans, viruses	• *Early or warm phase:* blood pressure, urine output, and neck veins can be normal; skin warm and flushed with full veins; fever usually present, although temperature can be subnormal • *Late phase:* tachycardia, tachypnea, hypotension, oliguria, flat jugular and peripheral veins, and cool clammy skin; normal or subnormal temperature
• Neurogenic shock	Dysfunction or injury to the nervous system from spinal cord injury, general anesthesia, fever, metabolic disturbance, brain injury	• *Early phase:* hypotension and altered mental status, bradycardia, and skin that is warm and dry • Late phase: Tachycardia, tachypnea, and cool, clammy skin

Hypovolemic Shock

Any severe loss of body fluid can lead to hypovolemic shock. Hypovolemic shock can be caused by dehydration; internal or external hemorrhage; fluid loss from burns, vomiting, or diarrhea; or loss of intravascular fluid into the interstitial space as a result of sepsis or **trauma** (physical injury caused by an external force). Heat exhaustion or heatstroke can also cause hypovolemic shock by excessive water loss through sweating. Clinical signs and symptoms include restlessness; pale, cool, clammy skin; tachycardia; tachypnea; flat, nondistended peripheral veins; decreased jugular vein circumference; decreased urine output; and altered mental status. The body is usually able to compensate for blood loss of less than 15%, or 750 mL. The initial symptom may only be tachycardia, although there can be an initial rise in systolic blood pressure, then a fall to below 80 mm Hg. At 20% to 25% blood loss, tachycardia and mild to moderate **hypotension** are present. With a loss of 40% or greater (2000 mL), all clinical signs and symptoms of shock are present. Volume loss might not be the only contributing factor to hypovolemic shock. The patient's age, health status, and the time frame for losing the fluid can also be factors.

Cardiogenic Shock

Cardiogenic shock results when the heart fails as a pump. It is a medical emergency. Without treatment, mortality is high. Patients with cardiogenic shock have signs and symptoms similar to hypovolemic shock, except that they might also have distended jugular and peripheral veins, as well as other symptoms of heart failure, such as pulmonary edema. The presence of pulmonary edema is what differentiates cardiogenic shock from other forms of shock. Fluid therapy can contribute further to pulmonary edema, which can be life threatening. The main cause of cardiogenic shock is acute myocardial infarction (AMI) and myocardial ischemia. Examples of other causes are traumatic injury to the heart, **myocarditis**, cardiomyopathy, heart valve defects, endocarditis, or dysrhythmias.

Extracardiac Obstructive Shock

Extracardiac obstructive shock occurs when there is a blockage of blood flow in the cardiovascular circuit outside the heart. Several conditions can cause obstructive shock. **Pericardial tamponade**, which is the filling of the pericardial sac with blood, compresses the heart and limits its filling capacity. **Tension pneumothorax** is compression of the heart from an abnormal collection of air in the pleural space, which interferes with normal cardiac function. **Acute pulmonary hypertension**, a sudden abnormally elevated pressure in the pulmonary artery, increases resistance for blood flowing out the right side of the heart. All of these conditions decrease cardiac output, which can lead to shock. Tumors or a pulmonary embolism can also cause shock. Signs and symptoms of obstructive shock are similar to those of hypovolemic shock, except that jugular veins are usually distended.

Distributive Shock

Distributive shock occurs when peripheral vascular resistance is lost because of massive vasodilation of the peripheral circulation. Unlike hypovolemic shock in which there is an actual loss of blood volume, distributive shock occurs when the body's fluid distribution is abnormally altered within the body. Distributive shock includes anaphylactic, septic, and neurogenic shock.

Anaphylactic Shock

Anaphylactic shock, the most severe type of distributive shock, occurs when the body has an extreme hypersensitivity reaction to an antigen. Death from anaphylactic shock can occur in minutes but is infrequent. Medical treatment must be sought immediately. Asthma or a delay in epinephrine injections can increase risk of death. Patients must be taught allergen avoidance techniques for safety (Box 9-1). Desensitization therapy to the allergen should be discussed with the health care provider.

Anaphylaxis occurs most commonly from food allergies such shellfish or peanuts, insect stings, antibiotics (especially penicillins), anesthetics, contrast dye, and blood products. The signs and symptoms are similar to those seen in hypovolemic shock. Additionally, patients can have symptoms specific to

---

Box 9-1 **Patient Education**

Teach patients who have severe allergies and are at risk for anaphylaxis to request a prescription for an epinephrine autoinjector. The epinephrine is given subcutaneously. It is important to carry the epinephrine at all times because life-threatening reactions can occur rapidly. Medical attention must be sought immediately after use of the epinephrine. Examples of epinephrine autoinjectors can be found at www.auvi-q.com or www.adrenaclick.com.

---

allergic reactions, including **urticaria** (hives), pruritus, wheezing, **laryngeal edema** (swelling of the larynx), angioedema (edema of skin, mucous membranes, or internal organs), and severe **bronchospasm** (narrowing of bronchi in the lungs). If conscious, patients can be extremely apprehensive and short of breath, and report a metallic taste.

Septic Shock

Sepsis is a serious bloodstream infection resulting from systemic infection and inflammation. This inflammation is the body's response to serious illness and is known as the systemic inflammatory response syndrome (SIRS). Thus, sepsis is SIRS from an infection. Many cases of sepsis are caused by Gram-positive bacteria, although other bacteria, fungi, viruses, or parasites can be the cause. Septic shock, the most common type of distributive shock, results from severe sepsis. It is characterized by a low blood pressure despite fluid therapy.

Sepsis is the leading cause of death among intensive care patients. The incidence of sepsis doubled from 2000 to 2008 with a 17% mortality rate (Hall, Williams, DeFrances, & Golosinskiy, 2011). The 2012 Surviving Sepsis Campaign's goal is to reduce the mortality rate from sepsis by 25% (see "Evidence-Based Practice" and www.survivingsepsis.org). Factors contributing to sepsis include older age, chronic illness, invasive procedures and devices, being immunosuppressed (e.g., HIV, chemotherapy, corticosteroids), antimicrobial resistant organisms, burns, and malnutrition ("Gerontological Issues"). Early diagnosis and rapid response are key to increasing survival for septic shock, especially in the vulnerable older adult population.

Gerontological Issues

The older adult population has less ability to fight infections, which places them at higher risk for sepsis. The sepsis rate for those aged 85 and over was about 30 times the rate for those under age 65 (Hall et al, 2011). Early recognition of shock signs is essential for successful treatment in this high-risk population.

SIRS is diagnosed when two or more of the following signs are present: abnormal body temperature (high or low), heart rate greater than 90 beats per minute, respiratory rate greater than 20 breaths per minute, white blood cell count of less than 4000/mm^3 or greater than 12,000/mm^3, or 10% bands (immature neutrophils). The progression of sepsis to septic shock is subtle and rapid, requiring frequent monitoring and prompt treatment of susceptible patients. Left untreated, septic shock progresses to a second phase with signs and symptoms similar to hypovolemic shock: hypotension, oliguria, tachycardia, tachypnea, flat jugular and peripheral veins, and cold, clammy skin.

EVIDENCE-BASED PRACTICE

Clinical Question
What are the best ways to manage sepsis and severe septic shock?

Evidence
The International Guidelines for Management of Severe Sepsis and Septic Shock: 2012 provide evidence-based interventions (Dellinger et al, 2013). Interventions affecting nursing care include the following: Obtain blood cultures prior to antibiotic therapy; prompt imaging studies to confirm potential source of infection, give broad-spectrum antibiotics within 1 hour of septic shock diagnosis or severe sepsis without septic shock; administer ordered IV fluids, or fluid challenge; administer ordered vasopressors, elevate head of bed for mechanically ventilated patients unless contraindicated; provide ordered oral or enteral nutrition, maintain ordered glycemic control; administer ordered deep venous thrombosis and stress ulcer prophylaxis; and prevent pressure ulcers.

Implications for Nursing Practice
Nurses should recognize that careful assessment and prompt performance of any ordered intervention included in the 2012 guidelines is vital for survival when caring for patients with septic shock or sepsis.

REFERENCE
Dellinger, R. P., Levy, M. M., Rhodes, A., Annane, D., Gerlach, H., Opal, S. M., . . . Vincent, J-L., and the Surviving Sepsis Campaign Guidelines Committee including the Pediatric Subgroup. (2013). Surviving sepsis campaign: International guidelines for management of severe sepsis and septic shock: 2012. *Critical Care Medicine, 41,* 580–637.

Neurogenic Shock

Neurogenic shock occurs when dysfunction or injury to the nervous system causes extensive dilation of peripheral blood vessels. It is a rarer form of shock and results most commonly

from an injury to the spinal cord (referred to as spinal shock). It occurs because of factors that either stimulate the parasympathetic nervous system or block the sympathetic nervous system. Other causes include general anesthesia, fever, metabolic disturbances, and brain contusions and concussions. Signs and symptoms include hypotension and altered mental status and, during the early phases, bradycardia and warm, dry skin. As shock progresses, however, tachycardia and cool, clammy skin develops.

THERAPEUTIC MEASURES FOR SHOCK

Because of the life-threatening nature of shock, immediate medical treatment is needed. The exact nature of the shock must be determined while interventions such as ventilatory and circulatory support are implemented (Table 9.4). Life-threatening symptoms must be treated immediately (Table 9.5). Medications that are used in shock are listed in Table 9.6. The order of interventions and testing is guided by the stability of the patient. Intervention priorities are as follows:

1. Airway
2. Breathing and respiratory support
3. Cardiovascular support
4. Maintenance of circulatory volume
5. Control of bleeding if present
6. Assessment of neurologic status
7. Treatment of life-threatening injuries
8. Determination and treatment of the cause of shock.

NURSING CARE TIP

Trendelenburg Position
Traditionally, the Trendelenburg position, in which the body is laid flat on the back with the feet higher than the head, was used to try to increase cardiac output to increase blood pressure. The Trendelenburg position used to be first-line treatment for hypovolemic shock. However, research has shown that it is not helpful in improving cardiac output for patients in shock and can have negative effects (Makic, VonRueden, Rauen, & Chadwick (2011). Although you might still see this position used, it is important to use valid research results in practice for the best patient outcomes.

NURSING PROCESS FOR THE PATIENT IN SHOCK

Data Collection

Recognizing patients at risk for shock and being vigilant in monitoring their condition is vital. Early detection and prevention of shock in patients at risk for shock are the desired

TABLE 9.4 ASSESSMENT OF THE PATIENT IN SHOCK

Signs and Symptoms	Tachycardia, tachypnea, hypotension, oliguria, cyanosis, altered mental status
Laboratory Tests	Complete blood count, serum osmolarity, blood chemistries, prothrombin time, partial thromboplastin time, blood typing and cross-match, serum lactate, arterial blood gases, cardiac isoenzymes, urinalysis
Imaging	Chest x-ray, spinal films, computed tomography, echocardiogram
Monitoring	Electrocardiogram, arterial pressure, central venous pressure, pulmonary artery catheter, gastric pH

goals. Rapid response teams can be helpful in providing quick assessment and management of patients at risk of developing shock.

For the patient in shock, assessment must be carried out quickly and should always start with ABCD: airway, breathing, circulation, and disability.

*A*irway is checked for patency and opened as necessary. A compromised airway must be treated immediately with the head-tilt/chin-lift method, an oral or nasal airway, or endotracheal intubation.

*B*reathing is checked for rate, depth, and symmetry of chest movement. The patient is observed for use of accessory muscles. Lung sounds are auscultated. Wheezing can be present in the patient with anaphylactic shock. Crackles can be found in the patient with cardiogenic shock or in the patient who has received too much IV fluid.

*C*irculation is checked with blood pressure. A narrowing pulse pressure can be present before a drop in systolic pressure and indicates a decrease in cardiac stroke volume and peripheral vasoconstriction. Peripheral pulses are palpated. Tachycardia is the first sign of shock. However, patients on medications that block the sympathetic nervous system

TABLE 9.5 THERAPEUTIC MEASURES FOR SHOCK

Respiratory support	Oxygen (nasal cannula, face mask, partial nonrebreather mask, assisted ventilations with bag-valve-mask, mechanical ventilator) SpO_2 >95% Venous lactic acid <2.2 mmol/L
Cardiovascular support	Vasopressor medication, if fluid resuscitation not effective Revascularization of heart in cardiogenic shock via angioplasty, with or without stent or fibrinolytic therapy Antidysrhythmics Positive inotropes
Adequate circulatory volume	1–3 L of IV fluids Crystalloid fluids: normal saline (0.9% sodium chloride) or lactated Ringer's solution; 3 mL crystalloid solution for every 1 mL fluid lost Blood or blood products Urine output >30 mL/hr Hemoglobin >10 g/dL
Control of bleeding	Pressure dressings Surgical intervention
Treatment of life-threatening injuries	Surgical intervention Medications
Treatment for types of shock	Septic shock: broad spectrum antibiotic within 1 hr of diagnosis Cardiogenic shock: morphine, diuretics, nitrates, inotropics, vasopressors Anaphylactic shock: epinephrine, diphenhydramine (Benadryl), methylprednisolone (Solu-Medrol), aminophylline

TABLE 9.6 MEDICATIONS USED FOR SHOCK

Medication Class/Action	Examples	Nursing Implications
Autonomic Nervous System Agents		
Alpha- and Beta-Adrenergic Agents		
Strengthens myocardial contraction, increases systolic blood pressure, and increases cardiac output	epinephrine (Adrenalin), dopamine (Intropin), norepinephrine (Levophed)	Correct hypovolemia before giving medications. Monitor VS often. Vasopressor use should include arterial blood pressure monitoring. Monitor intake and output.
Used to bronchodilate	epinephrine (Adrenalin)	First drug given in anaphylactic shock. Give with TB syringe.
Beta-Adrenergic Agent		
Increases cardiac output in cardiogenic shock	dobutamine (Dobutrex)	Monitor VS often. Monitor intake and output.
Antihistamine		
Inhibits histamine release	diphenhydramine (Benadryl)	Monitor VS. Caution about drowsiness.
Anti-Inflammatory		
Control of severe allergic reactions	methylprednisolone (Solu-Medrol), hydrocortisone (Solu-Cortef), dexamethasone (Decadron)	Monitor patient for signs and symptoms of infection.

TB = tuberculin; VS = vital signs.

response will not exhibit tachycardia. The pulse is assessed for quality; commonly it is weak and thready in a patient with shock. As shock progresses, the peripheral pulses become bradycardic or absent. A capillary refill greater than 3 seconds indicates inadequate circulation, although it has been found to be an unreliable indicator of shock in adults, especially older adults. Other observations regarding circulation include distended neck veins; skin that can be cool, pale, and diaphoretic; presence of **cyanosis** (bluish color of the skin and mucous membranes due to decreased oxygen in the blood); mucous membranes that can be pale and dry; and thirst. Rapidly scan the entire body for evidence of bleeding or other injuries. Palpation of the abdomen can reveal signs of internal bleeding, such as a tender, distended, boardlike abdomen.

NURSING CARE TIP

There is usually a loss of peripheral pulses in the patient whose systolic blood pressure has dropped below 80. If you are able to palpate radial pulses on your patient, the systolic blood pressure is usually at least 80.

CRITICAL THINKING

Beta Blockers

■ A patient who takes a beta-blocker medication is being monitored for septic shock. What sign of shock do you understand will not be present in a patient taking a beta blocker?

Suggested answers are at the end of the chapter.

Disability is determined by the patient's level of consciousness (LOC). A decrease in LOC indicates disability. This disability can range from lethargy to coma.

All four limbs are checked for circulation, sensation, and mobility (CSM). Bilateral responses are compared for equality. Circulation is assessed by palpating pulses for presence and quality. Sensation is determined by touching the patient's hands and feet and asking what the patient feels and if there is any numbness or tingling. Mobility (motor ability) is assessed by having the patient move all four limbs and wiggle the fingers and toes. Have the patient push with his or her feet against your hands and squeeze two of your fingers to determine strength.

NURSING CARE TIP

To determine level of consciousness, see if the patient is alert by asking his or her name, the date, and the location. If the patient can answer all three questions correctly, he or she is "alert and oriented × 3 (person, place, time)."

A head-to-toe approach can follow the primary ABCD assessment. The presence, severity, and location of pain or nausea and vomiting are noted. Body temperature is determined. Bowel sounds are auscultated to determine whether they are normal, absent, hyperactive, or hypoactive. When an indwelling urinary catheter has been placed, the color of the urine and the rate of urine output are noted.

Nursing Diagnoses, Planning, Implementation, and Evaluation

See Table 9.7 for a summary of shock. Also see "Nursing Care Plan for the Patient Experiencing Shock."

CRITICAL THINKING

Mr. Hall

■ Mr. Hall, who is 58 years old, had an AMI 2 days ago. He is reporting chest pain (rated 10/10 on the pain rating scale) and difficulty breathing. Blood pressure 96/40, Pulse 110, Respirations 22. His SpO_2 is 89%. Crackles are heard on auscultation of breath sounds. The electrocardiogram shows an irregular and rapid heartbeat. He is restless and apprehensive.

1. Name three nursing priorities for Mr. Hall's care.
2. With which members of the health team does the nurse anticipate collaborating?
3. What type of IV fluid and flow rate are appropriate for Mr. Hall?
4. What signs and symptoms indicate Mr. Hall is in cardiogenic shock?

Suggested answers are at the end of the chapter.

TABLE 9.7 SHOCK SUMMARY

Signs and Symptoms	Tachycardia Tachypnea Hypotension Oliguria Cyanosis Altered mental state
Diagnostic Tests	Decreased hemoglobin Increased lactic acid Decreased hematocrit in hemorrhage Increased WBC in sepsis Decreased pH in metabolic acidosis
Therapeutic Measures	Oxygen IV fluids Vasopressor medications Treat underlying cause
Complications	Acute respiratory distress syndrome (ARDS) Disseminated intravascular coagulation (DIC) Multiple organ dysfunction syndrome (MODS)
Priority Nursing Diagnoses	Ineffective tissue perfusion (renal, cerebral, cardiopulmonary, gastrointestinal, peripheral) Decreased cardiac output Fear

NURSING CARE PLAN for the Patient Experiencing Shock

Nursing Diagnosis: *Ineffective Tissue Perfusion* (renal, cerebral, cardiopulmonary, gastrointestinal, peripheral) related to hypovolemia or inadequate cardiac output or changes in circulatory volume or inadequate vascular tone possibly evidenced by altered level of consciousness, changes in skin color/temperature, tachycardia, reduced blood pressure, and decreased urine output.

Expected Outcomes: Patient will demonstrate adequate tissue perfusion as evidenced by warm dry skin, peripheral pulses strong, vital signs within normal parameters of baseline, breath sounds without adventitious sounds, and balanced intake and output, and patient will be alert and oriented to person, place, time within specified time frame.

Evaluation of Outcomes: Is patient's skin warm/dry and peripheral pulses present/strong? Are vital signs within patient's normal range? Are lung sounds normal, intake/output balanced, edema absent, pain/discomfort absent? Is patient alert and oriented?

Intervention Maintain airway and provide oxygen as ordered. **Rationale** Ensures adequate oxygenation and tissue perfusion. **Evaluation** Is SpO_2 >95%? Are skin and mucous membranes pink? Are respirations between 12 and 20 per minute? Are lung sounds clear?

Intervention Monitor vital signs. **Rationale** Changes in vital signs, which indicate change in condition, can be detected early and treated promptly. **Evaluation** Is heart rate between 60 and 100 beats per minute? Is heart rhythm regular? Are peripheral pulses strong? Is systolic blood pressure greater than 100 mm Hg? Is patient alert and oriented × 3?

Intervention Monitor intake and output. **Rationale** Provides adequate cardiac output to perfuse tissues. Assesses renal function. Urine output is an indicator of renal function. **Evaluation** Is urinary output greater than 30 mL/hr?

Intervention Provide adequate fluid intake. **Rationale** Maintains volume. **Evaluation** Are mucous membranes moist? Is skin turgor less than 3 seconds?

Intervention Position patient appropriately (head elevated for patients with shortness of breath, increased intracranial pressure, mechanically ventilated). **Rationale** Proper positioning promotes circulation and helps prevent skin breakdown. **Evaluation** Is edema noted? Is skin breakdown noted?

Intervention Maintain body temperature with warmed IV fluids, room temperature, blankets. **Rationale** Recovery is aided by normal body temperature. **Evaluation** Is body temperature within normal limits?

Intervention Provide quiet, restful environment. **Rationale** Conserves energy and lowers tissue oxygen demands. **Evaluation** Is patient resting comfortably without anxiety?

Intervention Monitor for pain, and provide pain relief measures. **Rationale** Pain increases tissue demands for blood and oxygen. **Evaluation** Is patient pain free?

GERONTOLOGICAL
Intervention Change positions slowly. **Rationale** Age-related losses of cardiovascular reflexes can result in hypotension. **Evaluation** Is systolic blood pressure greater than 100 mm Hg?

Nursing Diagnosis: *Decreased Cardiac Output* related to reduced circulating blood volume, structural damage, or decreased myocardial contractility as evidenced by abnormal vital signs and irregular cardiac rhythm strip.

Expected Outcomes: Patient will have adequate cardiac output as evidenced by vital signs and cardiac rhythm within normal limits (WNL) within specified time frame.

Evaluation of Outcomes: Are blood pressure, heart rate, and cardiac rhythm within normal limits? Are nailbeds and/or skin pink? Is skin warm and dry?

Intervention Monitor heart rate and cardiac rhythm with electrocardiogram, and report abnormalities. **Rationale** Changes in heart rate and cardiac rhythm can be detected immediately and treated appropriately. **Evaluation** Is heart rate and rhythm normal?

NURSING CARE PLAN for the Patient Experiencing Shock—cont'd

Intervention Monitor skin/nailbed color, capillary refill, and peripheral pulses and report abnormalities. **Rationale** Inadequate perfusion is first evident in skin/nailbeds and peripheral pulses. **Evaluation** What color and temperature is the skin/nailbeds? Is capillary refill less than 3 seconds? Are peripheral pulses present?

Intervention Give cardiovascular medications and oxygen as ordered. **Rationale** Cardiac function can be supported with medications. Supplemental oxygen increases oxygenation of heart and tissues. **Evaluation** Is heart rate and rhythm normal?

Intervention Reduce myocardial oxygen demand by utilizing comfort measures to alleviate pain and anxiety, and by keeping the body at an appropriate temperature. **Rationale** Pain, anxiety, and cold all increase tissue demands for blood and oxygen, which increases the workload on the heart to supply it. **Evaluation** Is body temperature within normal limits? Is the patient free of pain and anxiety?

GERONTOLOGICAL
Intervention Monitor perfusion by methods other than capillary refill such as skin temperature. **Rationale** Capillary refill is frequently delayed in the older adult population. **Evaluation** Is the body temperature within normal limits?

Nursing Diagnosis: *Fear* related to severity of condition and unknown outcome as evidenced by verbalization of fear (e.g., "Am I going to die?")

Expected Outcome: Patient will state fear is reduced after nurse provides information related to patient's condition.

Evaluation of Outcome: Does patient state fear is decreased?

Intervention Explore patient's level of fear and knowledge of condition. Provide explanations for condition, procedures, and treatment. **Rationale** Knowledge allows a feeling of control and reduces fear. **Evaluation** Does patient state fear is reduced?

Nursing Diagnosis: *Deficient Knowledge* related to unfamiliar condition of shock as evidenced by verbalization of deficient knowledge (e.g., "I don't understand what's happening to me.")

Expected Outcome: Patient will explain shock and its treatment.

Evaluation of Outcome: Can patient explain shock and how it is treated?

Intervention Identify patient's ability to learn and barriers to learning. **Rationale** For learning, the patient must be stable and ready to learn. **Evaluation** Is patient alert and stable? Does patient indicate willingness to learn?

Intervention Provide patient-centered information on shock and treatment. **Rationale** Giving individualized information on topic meets patient's need for understanding. **Evaluation** Can patient explain shock and purpose of treatment that patient is receiving?

Intervention Allow time for questions and clarification. **Rationale** Clarification ensures accurate information is learned. **Evaluation** Does the patient state accurate information?

GERONTOLOGICAL
Intervention Speak slowly and clearly in a low tone/pitch. **Rationale** Older adults have difficulty hearing high-pitched tones. **Evaluation** Does the patient acknowledge when being spoken to?

Intervention Provide materials in large print. **Rationale** Visual changes that accompany aging can require a patient to use larger print materials. **Evaluation** Can the patient restate and/or read aloud information that has been given?

Intervention Involve family/caregivers in teaching. **Rationale** Family/caregivers can reinforce education provided. **Evaluation** Does family/caregivers verbalize understanding of material presented?

LEARNING TIP

Here is a saying to help you remember blood pressure effects in shock: If they're 90 over 60, they're getting kind of sickly. Say it again! If they're 90 over 60, they're getting kind of sickly.

CRITICAL THINKING

Mrs. Neal

■ Mrs. Neal, who is 45 years old, came to the emergency room in severe hypovolemic shock after sustaining several bleeding wounds in an automobile accident. Her shock is resolving after receiving several transfusions and surgical repair of her injuries. She has just been admitted to the surgical unit for postoperative care.

1. What postoperative nursing assessments should be performed first?
2. How can patient-centered care be promoted during treatment?
3. Mrs. Neal's family is alarmed by her condition. What interventions can be provided to decrease their anxiety?
4. What postoperative complications can develop in Mrs. Neal?
5. What documentation is appropriate for Mrs. Neal?

Suggested answers are at the end of the chapter.

SUGGESTED ANSWERS TO

CRITICAL THINKING

■ *Classic Signs of Shock*

Tachycardia is caused by decreased cardiac output and reduced tissue oxygenation. Its purpose is to increase cardiac output and oxygen delivery by causing more heartbeats to pump out blood from the heart.

Tachypnea is caused by decreased tissue oxygenation. Its purpose is to increase respirations so more oxygen is available for delivery to tissues.

Oliguria is caused by a reduced blood flow to the kidneys. Its purpose as a compensatory mechanism is to conserve as much fluid as possible to help maintain a normal blood pressure.

Pallor is caused by reduced blood volume or flow. When pallor results from compensation, it is due to peripheral vasoconstriction that occurs to shunt blood volume to the vital organs.

Cool, clammy skin is the result of decreased blood flow to the skin and the release of moisture (sweat) from the skin. The sympathetic nervous system causes these compensatory mechanisms; peripheral vasoconstriction shunts blood to the vital organs, and sweating cools the body in anticipation of the fight-or-flight response, which generates body heat when it occurs.

■ *Anaerobic Metabolism*

Anaerobic metabolism is the source of nutrition and energy for the cell that prevents cellular death when oxygen is not available. It is a short-term compensatory mechanism to save the cell until oxygen becomes available again.

■ *Beta Blockers*

Tachycardia will not be present. Beta blockers block the response of the sympathetic nervous system, which is activated in shock.

■ *Mr. Hall*

1. Nursing priorities for Mr. Hall include adequate tissue perfusion, relief of chest pain and anxiety, and stabilization of cardiac rhythm and vital signs.
2. Health care provider and case manager.
3. Because Mr. Hall's lung sounds reveal crackles, indicating fluid in the lungs, he should probably not be given IV fluids. He already has too much fluid for his heart to handle, and giving him more IV fluids could be life threatening. He should have an IV access for IV medications as needed.
4. Signs of cardiogenic shock include decreased blood pressure; increased heart and respiratory rates; cyanosis; decreased urine output; cool, pale skin; and decreased mental status.

■ *Mrs. Neal*

1. Data collection for respiratory and cardiovascular status, inspection of surgical wounds for bleeding and noting mental status and the need for pain relief should be performed first.
2. Develop a pain management plan to meet Mrs. Neal's individualized needs. Identify her normal coping techniques to support their appropriate use. Provide explanations and teach as needed to keep patient informed for decision making. Advocate for her individualized needs such as nutritional needs.

SUGGESTED ANSWERS TO—cont'd

3. Explain the cause of shock and all interventions, rationales, and desired outcomes. Keep the environment calm, provide for privacy, and answer all questions in a matter-of-fact and reassuring manner. Allow Mrs. Neal's family to visit.

4. Unrelieved pain, bleeding, infection, and respiratory complications are possible.

5. *Airway:* rate, depth, regularity of respirations; breath sounds, SpO_2. *Vital signs:* cardiac rhythm, quality of pulses, skin color, blood pressure, body temperature. *Urine output:* oral and IV intake, fluid balance. *Pain:* measures to relieve pain and evaluation of those measures. *Dressings:* any bleeding. *Bowel sounds.*

REVIEW QUESTIONS

1. The nurse is assisting with a patient experiencing shock in the emergency department. The nurse would recognize signs of compensation as resulting from which of the following mechanisms?
   1. Peripheral nervous system depression
   2. Central nervous system depression
   3. Sympathetic nervous system stimulation
   4. Parasympathetic nervous system stimulation

2. Which of the following findings would the nurse specifically anticipate during data collection for a patient experiencing anaphylactic shock? **Select all that apply.**
   1. Wheezing
   2. Hypotension
   3. Tachycardia
   4. Oliguria
   5. Urticaria
   6. Bronchospasm

3. The nurse would recognize which of the following conditions as the cause for decreased level of consciousness commonly found in patients with shock?
   1. Severe pain
   2. Endotoxins
   3. Cerebral edema
   4. Cerebral hypoxia

4. The nurse is contributing to the plan of care for an older adult patient at risk for cardiogenic shock. Which of the following interventions for *Deficient Knowledge* would the nurse include to help this older patient learn about this condition? **Select all that apply.**
   1. Involve family/caregivers in teaching.
   2. Monitor patient's vital signs frequently.
   3. Provide materials in large print.
   4. Reinforce health promotion activities with the patient.
   5. Speak slowly and clearly in a low tone/pitch.

5. A patient with septic shock is receiving large amounts of crystalloid fluids. Which of the following findings would indicate to the nurse that the treatment is effective?
   1. decreased urine output
   2. increased heart rate
   3. clammy skin
   4. increased blood pressure

6. The nurse is contributing to the plan of care for a patient experiencing shock. Which of the following nursing diagnoses is most appropriate to include in this plan?
   1. *Fatigue*
   2. *Ineffective Tissue Perfusion*
   3. *Ineffective Health Maintenance*
   4. *Hopelessness*

7. A patient who is found lying in a pool of blood from a leg incision that has opened is restless and confused. The nurse calls for help and takes vital signs. Which of the following treatments for shock would the nurse anticipate being ordered first?
   1. Crystalloid IV fluids
   2. Oxygen
   3. Vasopressor medications
   4. One unit of packed red blood cells

8. The nurse is assigned to the team caring for the following patients. Which patient would be the priority for the nurse to see first?
   1. A patient who was in a motor vehicle accident with blood pressure 140/80 mm Hg, pulse 98 beats per minute, respirations 20 per minute.
   2. A patient who has a migraine with blood pressure 108/68 mm Hg, pulse 84 beats per minute, respirations 16 per minute.
   3. A patient who slipped and fell with blood pressure 112/74 mm Hg, pulse 68 beats per minute, respirations 14 per minute.
   4. A patient who is one day post-op with blood pressure 88/58 mm Hg, pulse beats 152 per minute, respirations 24 per minute.

9. Which of the following findings would indicate to the nurse that the therapeutic measures for a patient in shock have been effective?
   1. Heart rate 110 beats per minute
   2. SpO_2 89%
   3. Systolic blood pressure 118 mm Hg
   4. Respiratory rate 22 per minute

10. The nurse is caring for a patient who is experiencing progressive shock. Place in correct order of occurrence the systolic blood pressure findings that the nurse obtained for this patient who progressed through the three stages of shock and is now in irreversible shock. Begin with compensated shock and use all options.
    1. 56 mm Hg
    2. 116 mm Hg
    3. 86 mm Hg

Answers can be found in Appendix C.

References

Dellinger, R. P., Levy, M. M., Rhodes, A., Annane, D., Gerlach, H., Opal, S. M., . . . Vincent, J-L., and the Surviving Sepsis Campaign Guidelines Committee including the Pediatric Subgroup. (2012). Surviving sepsis campaign: International guidelines for management of severe sepsis and septic shock: 2012. *Critical Care Medicine, 41,* 580–637.

Hall, M. J., Williams, S. N., DeFrances, C. J., & Golosinskiy, A. (2011). Inpatient care for septicemia or sepsis: A challenge for patients and hospitals (NCHS Data Brief, no 62). Hyattsville, MD: National Center for Health Statistics.

Makic, M., VonRueden, K., Rauen, C., & Chadwick, J. (2011). Evidence-based practice habits: Putting more sacred cows out to pasture. *Critical Care Nurse, 31,* 38–62.

 DavisPlus | For additional resources and information visit **davispl.us/medsurg5**

Nursing Care of Patients in Pain

SHERIA GRICE ROBINSON,
APRIL HAZARD VALLERAND,
AND KAREN P. HALL

LEARNING OUTCOMES

1. Describe current definitions of pain.
2. Identify common myths and barriers to the effective management of pain.
3. Differentiate among addiction, physical dependence, and tolerance.
4. Explain current understanding about the basic physiology of the pain response.
5. Differentiate between nociceptive and neuropathic pain.
6. Perform a basic pain assessment.
7. Use the World Health Organization analgesic ladder for the treatment of pain.
8. Describe the three classes of analgesics and their uses.
9. Identify commonly used pain medication treatment modalities and their appropriate use.
10. Recognize appropriate use of nonpharmacological pain management techniques.

KEY TERMS

addiction (uh-DIK-shun)
adjuvant (ad-JOO-vant)
agonist (AG-un-ist)
analgesic (AN-uhl-JEE-zik)
antagonist (an-TAG-on-ist)
breakthrough (BRAYK-THROO)
ceiling effect (SEE-ling ee-FEKT)
endorphins (en-DOOR-fins)
enkephalins (en-KEFF-e-lins)
equianalgesic (EH-kwee-AN-uhl-JEE-zik)
hyperalgesia (HYPER-al-JEE-zee-ah)
malingerer (muh-LING-gur-er)
neuropathic (NEW-roh-PATH-ik)
nociception (NOH-sih-SEP-shun)
opioid (OH-pee-OYD)
pain (PAYN)
patient-controlled analgesia (PAY-shunt kon-TROHLD AN-uhl-JEE-zee-ah)
physical dependence (FIZZ-ik-uhl dee-PEN-dense)
prostaglandins (PRAHS-tah-GLAND-ins)
pseudoaddiction (soo-doh-ah-DIK-shun)
psychological dependence (SY-ko-LAW-jik-al dee-PEN-dense)
somatic (so-MAT-ik)
suffering (SUH-fur-ing)
tolerance (TAWL-ur-ens)
transdermal (trans-DER-mal)
visceral (VISS-er-uhl)

THE PAIN PUZZLE

Have you ever been in pain? If you have, then you know that pain is unpleasant. Not only does it hurt physically, but it can also make us feel emotionally sad or angry and lead to social isolation. **Pain** is a sensory and emotional experience that can affect every aspect of the person's being and how he or she relates to the environment. Pain management is the most common reason patients seek medical advice. However, despite the widespread nature of the problem and the millions of dollars spent on care, pain often remains untreated or undertreated. Nurses can make a difference in pain management.

Nurses often worry about overmedicating patients and may think that they are "doing good" (beneficence) or "doing no harm" (nonmaleficence) by withholding medication from a patient whom they do not believe is in pain (see "Ethical Considerations—Controlling Pain" on DavisPlus). So how can we know what pain is, and how can we truly tell when others are experiencing it?

DEFINITIONS OF PAIN

According to Margo McCaffery (1968), a well-known consultant in the care of patients with pain, "Pain is whatever the experiencing person says it is, existing whenever the experiencing person says it does." This is a reminder to nurses to accept the patient's report of pain. The International Association for the Study of Pain (IASP) describes pain in a bit more detail by noting it as "an unpleasant sensory and emotional experience associated with actual or potential tissue damage or described in terms of such damage" (2011). This definition indicates that pain is complex and is not only physical but has emotional and other components as well.

Why does pain exist? It is a protective mechanism or a warning. In the presence of injury, pain may help to prevent further injury. Consider the patient who has a fracture and holds it still to prevent further damage or a child who touches a hot stove and pulls his or her hand away before a serious burn occurs.

Suffering, or feelings of continuous distress, often accompanies pain. In a study of suffering, Ferrel and Coyle (2008) concluded, "suffering is not synonymous with pain but is closely associated with it. Physical pain is closely related to psychological, social, and spiritual distress. Pain that persists without meaning becomes suffering" (p. 246). Persistent pain can diminish patients' quality of life. It can make them feel as though their health is getting worse and take away their motivation for self-care. Suffering can often be relieved if patients believe they can achieve comfort. A good assessment and individualized, culturally congruent approaches to care increase the likelihood of comfort.

RISKS OF UNCONTROLLED PAIN

Why is untreated or undertreated pain a bad thing? Complications can occur when pain is experienced. The body produces a stress response to pain that causes harmful substances to be released from injured tissue. Reactions include breakdown of tissue, increased metabolic rate, impaired immune function, and negative emotions. In addition, pain prevents the patient from participating in self-care activities such as walking, deep breathing, and coughing. Consider the patient who has had chest surgery and then has to cough and deep breathe. It hurts! Pain may make the patient want to avoid coughing, turning, or even moving. Retained pulmonary secretions and pneumonia can develop. If the patient is less active, return of bowel function is delayed, and an ileus (disruption of normal propulsive gastrointestinal [GI] activity) can result. When pain is well controlled, complications can be avoided, and patients are able to do what they need to do to get well and go home from the hospital or continue with recovery activities.

PAIN AND CULTURE

Cultural differences can affect patient responses to pain. People from various cultures have different ways of expressing pain (see "Cultural Considerations"). Some may be dramatic and emotional; others tend to be stoic and quiet. Knowledge of widely accepted information about different ethnic and cultural groups can be useful in understanding a patient's experience and what care might be considered acceptable pain responses. It is important, however, to assess a patient's pain care needs individually and pay careful attention to the ethical principles that influence patient care rather than making assumptions based on culture or ethnicity alone.

WHO'S THE BOSS IN PAIN MANAGEMENT?

The patient is at the center of the health team. Providing accurate information and offering relevant choices helps patients to maintain autonomy. Just as risks, benefits, and alternatives to surgery and anesthesia are discussed with the patient, so too should pain management options be discussed in the process of obtaining informed consent. It is important to learn as much as you can about pain and pain management so you can effectively advocate for your patients and help with patient education.

The entire health team is responsible for pain management. All must provide care in the most cost-effective manner possible while continuing to provide the best quality. Effective pain management helps to reduce costs by minimizing the side effects of opioids, preventing complications related to inadequate pain control, and reducing the length of hospital stay or period of recovery.

Various regulatory bodies have also recognized the importance of good pain management and have incorporated a review of organizational pain management practices into accreditation and review processes. These standards support the importance of appropriate and effective management of pain. They address assessment and the safe pharmacological management of pain, as well as patient and family teaching,

Cultural Considerations

The pain experience may differ between and among individuals of differing cultural, ethnic, or religious groups. Remember that people within groups vary, and not all fit the general descriptions provided here (see Chapter 4).

Culture	Expression and Meaning of Pain	Patient Preferences	Assessment	Interventions
Arab American	See pain as something to be controlled. May express pain openly to family with elaborate verbal expressions, less so with caregivers. May use terms such as *fire, hot,* and *cold.*	Intramuscular or IV usually preferred over oral medications.	Compare verbal and nonverbal characteristics of pain to determine degree of pain.	Engage family to help with distraction and relaxation techniques. Administer medication promptly.
Asian American	Chinese and Koreans tend to be stoical and describe pain in terms of diverse body symptoms instead of locally. Filipinos may view pain as a part of living an honorable life. Some view this as an opportunity to reach a fuller life and to atone for past transgressions. Frequently stoic and tolerate pain to a high degree. Some moan as an expression of pain. For Asians, bearing pain is a virtue and a matter of family honor. Some, especially older individuals, may fear addiction.	Prefer oral or IV pain medications. May like warm compresses. For Koreans, intramuscular injections may be seen as an invasion of privacy. Vietnamese maintain self-control as a means of pain relief.	Observe for nonverbal signs of pain. Vietnamese may not understand numerical scale of rating pain. Observing facial expression may provide an indicator of pain.	Incorporate traditional healing methods as much as possible. Offer and encourage pain medicines to promote healing.
African American	May openly and publicly display pain, but this is highly variable. Many, especially older adults, fear that medication may be addictive. Many believe that suffering and pain are inevitable and should be endured.	May focus on spirituality and religious beliefs to endure pain. Prayers and the laying on of hands may be believed to relieve pain if the client has enough faith.	Observe for verbal and nonverbal expressions of pain. Use of pain scales is helpful.	Offer pain medication as needed. Allow meditation and prayer along with pain medication. Support patient's spiritual practices.

Continued

Cultural Considerations—cont'd

Culture	Expression and Meaning of Pain	Patient Preferences	Assessment	Interventions
European American	Strong sense of stoicism, especially in men. Fear of being dependent may decrease use of pain medicine. Many have fear of addiction. May continue to work and carry out daily activities and minimize pain.	May prefer relaxation and distractions as means of pain control.	Observe for nonverbal signs of pain. Use visual analog or numerical pain scales to assess severity of pain.	Encourage use of pain medicine as needed.
Hispanic American	Puerto Ricans tend to be expressive of pain and discomfort. Moaning, groaning, and crying are culturally accepted ways of dealing with and reducing pain.

Mexicans may bear pain stoically because it is "God's will." Many feel that pain and suffering are a consequence of immoral behavior. For men, expressing pain shows weakness. The Spanish word for pain is *dolor.* | Prefer oral or IV medication for pain.

Heat, herbal teas, and prayer are used to manage pain. | Visual analog and numerical scales may be helpful.

Observe and compare verbal and nonverbal behaviors indicating pain. | Incorporate distraction and relaxation techniques.

Incorporate traditional practices as permitted.

For individuals who are stoic about pain, encourage pain medicine frequently. Explain that pain control can hasten healing. |
| Native American | Frequently do not request pain medicine and are undertreated. May not realize that they can ask for pain medicine. Many believe pain is something that must be endured. May describe pain in general terms such as "not feeling good." The word for *pain* varies according to the tribal language. | Many prefer traditional herbal medicines.

May mention pain to family member or visitor, who relays message to caregiver. | Frequently ask patient and family members or visitors if patient has pain.

Observe for nonverbal clues of pain. | Explain that the control of pain can promote healing. Offer pain medicine as needed.

Allow adequate time for response; silence is valued. Maintain a calm, relaxing environment.

Incorporate traditional practices for pain relief if not harmful. |

postoperative pain, management of opioid-induced side effects, discharge planning, and process improvement. Examples of these guidelines are available through the Joint Commission website at www.jointcommission.org and the Centers for Medicare and Medicaid Services (CMS) website at www.cms.gov. For more information on pain management, visit the following websites. For some sites, you may need to type "pain" in the search window.

> www.ahrq.gov
> www.ampainsoc.org
> www.cancer.org
> www.geriatricpain.org
> www.pain-topics.org

The care of patients with pain is challenging, however, with a systematic and holistic approach to assessment and treatment, good pain management can be achieved. In this chapter, the difficulties of pain assessment and treatment are discussed. Some of the tools needed to effectively deal with these challenges are presented. Common myths and barriers that continue to affect nursing practice are clarified.

MYTHS AND BARRIERS TO EFFECTIVE PAIN MANAGEMENT

A number of factors, including the nurse's personal experiences with pain, influence how patients with pain are treated. Why are some patients not believed when they report pain? Why do some nurses and other health care team members insist that patients behave a certain way before they are believed? Common myths about pain can impair the nurse's ability to be objective about pain and may create barriers to effective treatment. Because there are few objective measure for pain, many nurses rely on assumptions rather than facts. Note the following myths.

> *Myth:* A person who is laughing and talking is not in pain.
> *Fact:* A person in pain is likely to use laughing and talking as a form of distraction. This can be effective in managing pain, especially when used with appropriate drug therapies. Patients may be more easily distracted when they have visitors and may ask for pain medication as soon as their family or significant other goes home.
> *Myth:* Respiratory depression is common in patients receiving opioid pain medications.
> *Fact:* Respiratory depression is uncommon in patients receiving opioid pain medications. If patients are monitored carefully when they are at risk, such as with the first dose of an opioid or when a dose is increased, respiratory depression is preventable. A patient's respiratory status and level of sedation (LOS) should be routinely monitored using an LOS scale.
> *Myth:* Pain medication is more effective when given by injection.

> *Fact:* Oral administration is the first choice if possible, or whenever the IV route is not an option. The IV route has the most rapid onset of action and is the preferred route for postoperative administration. Intramuscular (IM) injections are not recommended because they are painful, have unreliable absorption from the muscle, and have a lag time to peak effect and rapid falloff compared with oral administration.
> *Myth:* Teenagers are more likely to become addicted than older patients.
> *Fact:* Addiction to opioids is uncommon in all age groups when taken for pain by patients without a prior drug abuse history.
> *Myth:* Pain is a normal part of aging.
> *Fact:* Although many older adults have medical conditions that cause pain, pain is not a normal or anticipated part of aging and should be treated proactively. Effective pain treatment for older people helps them to maintain their mobility longer and improve overall health.

OPIOID ADDICTION

Nurses often express concern about patients who need large amounts of pain medication or know exactly when their next dose of pain medication is due. Nurses may worry that such patients are addicted or that they are "clock watchers," but do we really know what that means? Patients are expected to be informed about their medications and involved in their care, but when they know when their medications are due, we may become suspicious. In truth, if a patient is watching the clock, the most likely reason is because he or she is in pain. The most common reason that patients ask for more pain medicine is because they have increased pain. Similarly, patients are expected to know the effects of other medications they take, such as blood pressure medications and insulin. Yet when they ask for a specific analgesic, concern that the patient is "drug seeking" is sometimes raised.

CRITICAL THINKING

Mrs. Smithers and Mr. Brown

■ Mrs. Smithers had an abdominal hysterectomy and is sitting up in bed the morning after surgery, putting on her makeup. On morning rounds she is smiling but reports that her pain is at 6 on a scale of 0 to 10. Mr. Brown has just been transferred from the surgical intensive care unit the day after surgery for multiple injuries. He is moaning and reports his pain at 6 on a scale of 0 to 10. Which of these patients is really having as much pain as they say they are? How can you make this judgment?

Suggested answers are at the end of the chapter.

It is important to understand the differences among **addiction**, **tolerance**, and **physical dependence**. When talking with patients and teaching them about their medications, it is important to help them understand these differences as well. Addiction is something many patients fear.

Tolerance is a normal biological adaptation. Exposure to a drug induces changes that result in a decrease of one or more of the drug's effects over time. Simply put, this means it takes a larger dose to provide the same level of pain relief. *Physical dependence* is a normal physiological phenomenon that most people experience after a few weeks of continuous opioid use. If an opioid is discontinued abruptly after a few weeks of use or if an opioid antagonist such as naloxone (Narcan) is administered, the patient experiences a withdrawal syndrome that includes such symptoms as sweating, tearing, runny nose, restlessness, irritability, tremors, dilated pupils, sleeplessness, nausea, vomiting, and diarrhea. These symptoms can be prevented by weaning a patient slowly from an opioid rather than stopping it suddenly.

According to the American Society of Addiction Medicine (2011), addiction or **psychological dependence** is a disease of the brain that causes the compulsive pursuance of a substance, or behavior to obtain reward or relief. Addictive behaviors are characterized by impaired control over drug use and continued use despite harm. Patients with uncontrolled pain who desire treatment are not addicts. Sadly, patients with a history of addiction are more likely to have unmet pain needs due to medication tolerance and health provider bias. Careful assessment and monitoring of treatment is essential for *all* patients receiving treatment for pain—particularly patients who are prescribed opioid analgesics.

Pseudoaddiction has been described in patients who are receiving opioid doses that are too low or spaced too far apart to relieve their pain, and certain behavioral characteristics resembling psychological dependence, such as drug-seeking behaviors, have developed. In contrast to the addicted patient, a patient with pseudoaddiction stops drug-seeking behaviors when the pain is relieved.

CRITICAL THINKING

Janet

■ Janet is hospitalized with pancreatitis and has severe abdominal pain. She has a history of IV drug abuse. She is receiving IV morphine every 3 hours. Two hours after her last dose, she puts on her call light and says she is in severe pain, which she rates as "15" on a 0 to 10 scale. You feel like you have given her enough morphine to kill a horse, yet she keeps requesting more.

1. How is it possible for Janet to be in pain when she is receiving so much morphine?
2. It's not time for more medication. What should you do?

3. You speak to the health care provider (HCP), who prescribes acetaminophen (Tylenol) 1000 mg for breakthrough pain (between morphine doses). When you take it to Janet, she rolls her eyes and says, "You must be kidding me." How do you respond?
4. What communication with Janet is important at this time?

MECHANISMS OF PAIN TRANSMISSION

Many theories of how pain is transmitted and perceived (called *nociception*) are described in the literature. The *specificity theory,* developed by Descartes in 1644, proposed that body trauma sends a message directly to the brain, causing a sort of "bell" to ring, prompting a response from the brain. In 1965, Melzack and Wall proposed the *gate control theory,* which describes the dorsal horn of the spinal cord as a gate, allowing impulses to go through when there is a pain stimulus and closing the gate when those impulses are inhibited. The gate control theory stimulated massive research on the physiology of pain and is still considered in current research. However, much more is now known about the transmission of pain.

Pain is transmitted through four distinct processes, transduction, transmission, perception, and modulation:

1. *Transduction* represents the initiation of the stimulus and conversion of that stimulus into an electrical impulse at the time of the injury. Chemical neurotransmitters are released from damaged tissue. These substances include **prostaglandins**, bradykinin, serotonin, and substance P.
2. *Transmission* is the process of moving a painful message from the peripheral nerve endings through the dorsal root ganglion and the ascending tract of the spinal cord to the brain.
3. The third process is *perception,* or actually feeling the pain. During perception, the hypothalamus activates and controls emotional input and also generates purposeful goal-directed behavior while the cerebral cortex receives the pain message.
4. Last in the process of nociception is *modulation,* or the body's attempt to interrupt pain impulses by releasing endogenous (naturally occurring) opioids. **Endorphins** are endogenous chemicals that act like opioids, inhibiting pain impulses in the spinal cord and brain. Endorphins are the chemicals that stimulate the long-distance runner's "high." Unfortunately, they degrade too quickly to be considered effective analgesics. **Enkephalins** are one type of endorphin.

• **WORD** • **BUILDING** •

pseudoaddiction: pseudo—false + addiction—psychological dependence

Pain Transmission: Nociceptive or Neuropathic?

Pain transmission can be nociceptive and neuropathic. **Nociception** refers to the body's normal reaction to noxious stimuli, such as tissue damage, with the release of pain-producing substances. Nociceptive pain may be **somatic** or **visceral**. Somatic pain is localized in the muscles or bones. Patients can often point to the exact location of pain and will describe it as throbbing or aching. Cancer patients may experience somatic pain when the cancer has spread to the bone or a tumor has invaded soft tissue. Visceral pain, or organ pain, is not well localized and is often described as cramping or pressure. Bowel obstructions and tumors in the lung can cause visceral pain symptoms. Pain may also be felt in parts of the body away from the pain source, such as the low back/flank pain that often accompanies a bladder infection. This is called *referred pain* (Fig. 10.1).

Neuropathic pain is pain associated with injury to either the peripheral or central nervous system. Unlike nociceptive pain, neuropathic pain is poorly localized and may involve other areas along the nerve pathway. Neuropathic pain is common in cancer patients following chemotherapy or radiation therapy, patients with diabetic neuropathy, and patients who have had shingles. The pain is often described as numbness, tingling, sharp, shooting, or shocklike.

TYPES OF PAIN

Acute Pain

Pain is also categorized according to the length of time it has been present. *Acute pain* is immediate and follows injury to the body, prompts an inflammatory response, and subsides as healing takes place. It is often associated with short-term, objective, physical signs, such as increased heart rate and elevated blood pressure. As pain continues, the physiological responses that accompany acute pain cannot be sustained without harm to the body. As the body adapts, vital signs return to normal. The nurse must guard against labeling such a patient a **malingerer** (pretending to be in pain) or drug seeker simply because vital signs are no longer altered. Examples of acute pain include pain related to childbirth, surgery, burns, or other trauma. Persistent acute pain may become chronic.

Chronic Pain

Chronic pain typically lasts 3 months or longer, persisting beyond the time when healing usually takes place. Examples are neck pain that continues years after an accident, pain that accompanies diseases such as arthritis, and phantom limb pain. Patients with chronic pain may have both nociceptive and neuropathic components that require a combination of medications and nonpharmacological treatments. Because of the body's ability to adapt, patients with chronic pain may not appear to be in pain.

OPTIONS FOR TREATMENT OF PAIN

There are many pharmacological and nonpharmacological treatments available for the effective management of pain. Medications that relieve pain are called **analgesics**. Analgesics make up the largest piece of the pain management puzzle and encompass three main classes of medication: opioids, nonopioids, and adjuvants. **Opioids** bind to opioid receptors in the brain, spinal cord, and other areas of the body, inhibiting the perception of pain. Nonopioids include nonsteroidal anti-inflammatory drugs (NSAIDs) and acetaminophen (e.g., Tylenol). Adjuvants are different from opioid and nonopioids in that they include categories of medications that were originally approved by the Federal Drug Administration for purposes other than pain relief (such as depression). Some patients may require a combination of opioids, adjuvants, and NSAIDs to effectively manage their pain. Nurses should have

• **WORD • BUILDING •**
nociception: noci—pain + ception—reception
neuropathic: neuro—nerves + pathy—disease, suffering
analgesic: an—not + gesia—pain

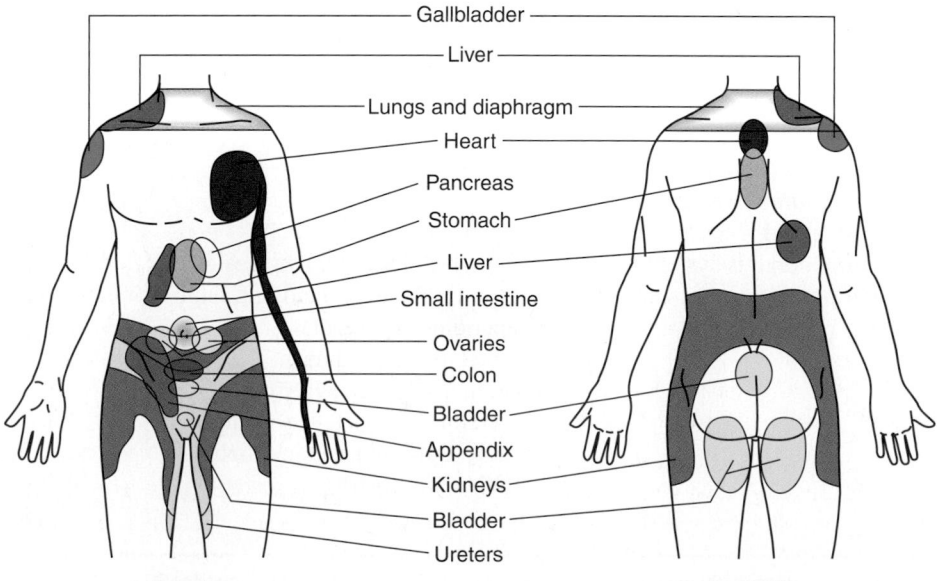

FIGURE 10.1 Sites of referred pain.   **Anterior**   **Posterior**

a good understanding of these pharmacological treatment options. Let's begin the discussion with nonopioids.

Nonopioid Analgesics

Nonopioids are typically the first class of drugs used to treat mild pain (Table 10.1). They can be useful for acute and chronic pain from a variety of causes, such as surgery, trauma, arthritis, and cancer. These drugs are limited in their use because they have a ceiling effect to analgesia. A **ceiling effect** means that there is a dose beyond which there is no improvement in the analgesic effect, but there may be an increase in adverse effects. When used with opioids, care must be taken to ensure that the nonopioid dose does not exceed the maximum safe dose for a 24-hour period. For example, if a patient receiving two Vicodin (acetaminophen and hydrocodone) tablets every 4 hours continues to experience pain, the dose cannot be increased because of the potentially toxic effects of acetaminophen at that dosage.

(See Table 10.1 for side effects and nursing implications.) Nonopioids do not produce tolerance or physical dependence. Most do have antipyretic (fever-reducing) effects.

Nonopioids work mainly peripherally, at the site of injury, rather than in the central nervous system, as opioids do. The exception in this class is acetaminophen, which is believed to act on the central nervous system. NSAIDs block the synthesis of prostaglandins, one of many chemicals needed for pain transmission. In general, it is helpful to include a nonopioid agent in any analgesic regimen, even if the pain is severe enough to require the addition of an opioid (see the section later in this chapter titled "Balanced Approach to Analgesia").

Opioid Analgesics

Opioids are drugs that have actions similar to those of morphine. Opioids are classified by how they affect receptors in the nervous system. They may be full **agonists** (stimulators), partial

TABLE 10.1 ANALGESIC AGENTS

Medication Class/Action	Examples	Nursing Implications
Salicilates		
Peripherally acting analgesics; reduce pain, fever, inflammation	aspirin	Give with food. Decrease platelet aggregation; watch for bruising or bleeding.
NSAIDs		
Peripherally acting analgesics; reduce pain, fever, inflammation	ibuprofen (Motrin) ketorolac (Toradol) naproxen (Naprosyn, Aleve)	Give with food. Decrease platelet aggregation, so watch for bleeding. Do not give ketorolac longer than 5 days.
COX-2 Inhibitors		
Reduce pain and inflammation, no effect on platelet aggregation	celecoxib (Celebrex)	Give with food.
Acetaminophen		
Relieves pain and fever; no anti-inflammatory or antiplatelet effect	acetaminophen (Tylenol)	Maximum safe dose is 4 g per day; less for those who use alcohol. Be aware of other drugs that contain acetaminophen, such as cold remedies, to prevent accidental overdose.
Opioids and Opioid Combination Agents		
Bind to opioid receptors in the central nervous system to alter perception of pain	codeine (in Tylenol 2, 3, 4)* fentanyl (Sublimaze, Duragesic) hydromorphone (Dilaudid, Exalgo) meperidine (Demerol) methadone (Dolophine) morphine (MS IR, MS Contin) oxycodone (OxyIR, OxyContin) hydrocodone and acetaminophen (Vicodin, Lortab)	May be combined with nonopioid (e.g., acetaminophen). Monitor vital signs, level of sedation, and respiratory status. Avoid fentanyl patch in patient with fever; heat increases absorption. Encourage fluids and fiber to prevent constipation. Meperidine should be avoided in older adults and those with renal dysfunction.

* Tylenol #2 = Tylenol 300 mg + codeine 15 mg; Tylenol #3 = Tylenol 300 mg + codeine 30 mg; Tylenol #4 = Tylenol 300 mg + codeine 60 mg

agonists or mixed agonists, or **antagonists** (blockers). Full agonists have a complete response at the opioid receptor site; a partial agonist has a lesser response. A mixed agonist/antagonist activates one type of opioid receptor while blocking another.

Morphine, a full agonist, is often the drug of choice for treating moderate to severe pain. It is the standard to which all other analgesics are compared (see Table 10.2 for **equianalgesic** doses of medications). Morphine is long acting (4–5 hours) and available in many forms, making it convenient and affordable for patients. It also has a slower onset than many other opioids. Other examples of opioids include controlled-release drugs such as oxycodone (OxyContin) and hydromorphone (Exalgo), which are effective for prolonged, continuous pain.

 BE SAFE!

Never crush a controlled- or time-release tablet. Because the tablet is designed to deliver a dose of medication over time, crushing it could deliver the entire dose at once, resulting in overdose.

Opioids alone have no ceiling effect to analgesia. This means that doses can safely be increased to treat worsening pain if the patient's respiratory status and level of sedation are stable. However, inappropriate prescribing can lead to **hyperalgesia**, or increased sensitivity to pain. Patients with hyperalgesia have pain at the slightest touch, such as the moving of sheets, and require further medical intervention. Institutions must have policies and procedures in place related to opioids to prevent medication errors and reduce the risk of serious side effects. It is especially important to be vigilant for side effects in patients unaccustomed to opioids, the most common of which are constipation, confusion, and fatigue, which can increase a patient's risk for falls. Although respiratory depression is not a common side effect, it is a life-threatening one, and respiratory rate should be monitored. See Table 10.1 for additional information and adverse effects of opioids.

TABLE 10.2 EQUIANALGESIC CHART

Drug	Parenteral Dose*	Oral Dose
Morphine	5 mg	15 mg
Codeine	60 mg	100 mg
Hydromorphone	1.5 mg	4 mg
Methadone	5 mg	10 mg
Meperidine	50 mg	150 mg
Oxycodone	Not applicable	10 mg

Note. Approximate doses of medications in milligrams to equal same amount of pain relief between drugs or same drug, different route. Consult pharmacist and physician before changing drugs or routes.

*Intramuscular, IV, subcutaneous.

Although opioids are extremely important in pain management, they are also on a short list of "high alert" drugs that can harm or even kill patients if they are not administered carefully (Institute for Safe Medication Practices, 2012). Institutions must have policies and procedures in place related to opioids to prevent medication errors and reduce the risk of serious side effects. It is especially important to be vigilant for side effects in patients unaccustomed to opioids. Such patients are sometimes called "opioid-naïve."

Opioids are added to nonopioids for pain that cannot be managed effectively by nonopioids alone. The use of a centrally acting opioid with a peripherally acting non-opioid can increase pain relief and reduce the amount of opioid needed.

Controlled-release opioids such as oxycodone (OxyContin) and morphine (MS Contin) are effective for prolonged, continuous pain. Whenever a controlled-release form of medication is used, it is important to have an immediate-release medication available for **breakthrough** pain (transient pain that arises during generally effective pain control), such as oral morphine solution, oxycodone immediate-release (OxyIR), or hydromorphone immediate-release (Dilaudid).

CRITICAL THINKING

Mrs. Zales

■ Mrs. Zales, a 32-year-old woman, was admitted for a hysterectomy after being treated for painful endometriosis for 12 months. After her surgery, she had a patient-controlled analgesia (PCA) pump with hydromorphone, which was effective in relieving her pain. Forty-eight hours after surgery, the surgeon discontinued the PCA pump and ordered oral hydrocodone with acetaminophen. It was ineffective, so an order was added for hydromorphone 2 mg orally every 3 to 4 hours, as needed. The nurses gave only one dose of the hydromorphone. Then, thinking that her pain should be lessening, switched Mrs. Zales back to the hydrocodone with acetaminophen. By the next morning she was in severe pain, and the on-call physician ordered IM meperidine and promethazine (Phenergan). Mrs. Zales's discharge was delayed until her pain could be controlled.

1. What do you think happened?
2. How could the delayed discharge have been avoided?
3. Who were the important team members in this scenario?

Suggested answers are at the end of the chapter.

• WORD • BUILDING •
antagonist: ant—against + agonist—stimulates receptor site
equianalgesic: equi—equal + analgesic—relieving pain

Meperidine (Demerol) was at one time a commonly used opioid, but is no longer recommended in most cases. Meperidine is an opioid agonist, and when broken down in the body, it produces a toxic metabolite called normeperidine. Normeperidine is a cerebral irritant that can cause adverse effects ranging from dysphoria and irritable mood to seizures. Normeperidine has a long half-life even in healthy patients, so those with impaired renal function are at increased risk. Meperidine use should be avoided in patients over age 65, patients with impaired renal function, and patients taking a monoamine oxidase inhibitor (MAOI) antidepressant. In general, the use of meperidine should be limited to young, healthy patients who need an opioid for a short period and to those who have unusual reactions or allergic responses to other opioids. The effective dose of oral meperidine is three to four times the parenteral dose and is never recommended.

Fentanyl (Sublimaze, Duragesic) can be given parenterally, intraspinally, or by **transdermal** patch (Duragesic). Fentanyl is commonly used IV with anesthesia for surgery. It also is used to relieve postoperative pain via the IV route, PCA pump, or epidural route (discussed later in this chapter). IV fentanyl has a short duration of action and must be given more often than other opioids to maintain an effective level of analgesia. The fentanyl patch is useful for a patient with stable cancer pain.

BE SAFE!

BE VIGILANT! It is important to monitor the patient's level of sedation and respiratory status when administering opioids. Increased sedation, decreased respiratory effort, and constricted pupils can be signs of opioid overdose. Careful monitoring and dosage adjustments of opioids can prevent opioid-induced respiratory depression.

Methadone (Dolophine) is a potent analgesic that has a longer duration of action than morphine. It has a long half-life and accumulates in the body with continued dosing. Dosing intervals may be extended after pain relief has been achieved. Methadone is well absorbed from the GI tract and is effective when given orally at doses similar to the parenteral dose.

Methadone is also used in drug treatment programs during detoxification from heroin and other opioids. Patients on methadone maintenance can present a unique challenge when admitted to the hospital. It is important to continue the maintenance dose even if additional pain medications are required after surgery or trauma. See Table 10.1 for examples of opioids.

• WORD • BUILDING •
transdermal: trans—across + dermal—skin

CRITICAL THINKING

Mrs. Shepard

■ Mrs. Shepard is 92 years old and has undergone an open cholecystectomy. Her continuous epidural infusion of analgesic is discontinued at 1400 on her second postoperative day. The physician orders oral acetaminophen with hydrocodone every 3 to 4 hours as needed for pain. At 1700 Mrs. Shepard refuses to get out of bed because her pain is 7 on a scale of 0 to 10. The nurse checks the medication administration record and notes that she has not yet received a dose of acetaminophen and hydrocodone.

1. Why is Mrs. Shepard in so much pain?
2. What complications can occur as a result of her pain?
3. Each analgesic tablet contains 500 mg of acetaminophen and 5 mg of hydrocodone. The maximum daily dose of acetaminophen is 4 g. If she takes one tablet every 3 hours, is her dose safe?
4. What can be done to relieve her pain and better prevent it in the future?

Suggested answers are at the end of the chapter.

Opioid Antagonists

Naloxone (Narcan) is a pure opioid antagonist that counteracts, or antagonizes, the effect of opioids. It is often used in emergency departments for treating the effects of opioid overdose, such as sedation and respiratory depression. Caution must be used when giving naloxone to a patient who is receiving opioids for pain control. If too much naloxone is given too fast, it can reverse not only the unwanted effects—such as respiratory depression and sedation—but the desired effect of analgesia as well.

Some antagonists are shorter acting than the opioid that is being used. If the antagonist is given because of respiratory depression, the dose may need to be repeated because its effect may wear off before the opioid wears off.

Some analgesics are classified as combined agonists and antagonists or partial agonists. These drugs bind with some opioid receptors and block others. The most commonly used drugs in this class are butorphanol (Stadol) and nalbuphine (Nubain).

How does this information translate into nursing practice? Consider, for example, a patient who receives sustained-release morphine every 12 hours to control metastatic bone pain, but the patient develops breakthrough pain between doses. You observe that butorphanol has been ordered for pain by another doctor and administer it. The butorphanol will antagonize, or counteract, some of the effects of the morphine, and the patient may experience acute pain. It is important to be informed about the actions of all drugs that are administered and to be aware of possible drug interactions that may interfere with patient care.

Analgesic Adjuvants

Adjuvants are classes of medications that are given in addition to other medications. Analgesic adjuvants can potentiate the effects of opioids or nonopioids, have analgesic activity themselves, or counteract the unwanted effects of other analgesics. They may be called *off-label* medications because they are being used in a way not specifically approved by the Food and Drug Administration; that is, they were not initially developed to treat pain. Adjuvants may have pain-relieving properties for certain conditions. Although the use of adjuvants is common, nurses must be mindful of the side effects of these medications, which often affect the central nervous system. Examples of adjuvants are corticosteroids, benzodiazepines, antidepressants, and anticonvulsants.

Corticosteroids can be used to treat a variety of painful conditions, including acute and chronic cancer-related pain. They may be used as part of actual cancer treatment because of their toxicity to some cancer cells, or they may reduce pain by decreasing inflammation and the resulting compression of healthy tissues.

Benzodiazepines such as midazolam (Versed) or diazepam (Valium) are effective for treating anxiety or muscle spasms associated with pain. These drugs do not provide pain relief alone but are effective in treating pain caused by muscle spasms. Benzodiazepines can cause sedation, which limits the amount of opioid that can be safely given at the same time.

Tricyclic antidepressants such as amitriptyline, imipramine, desipramine, and doxepin can help relieve neuropathic pain. Duloxetine (Cymbalta) is a serotonin-norepinephrine reuptake inhibitor that is also effective for nerve pain. These drugs must be taken for days to weeks before they are fully effective, and patients must be told to continue the medication even if it seems ineffective at first. Additional benefits of this class of medications may include mood elevation and improved ability to sleep, but significant side effects often limit their use.

Anticonvulsants such as carbamazepine (Tegretol) and gabapentin (Neurontin) are often used to relieve neuropathic pain. Again, these medications must be taken regularly to realize their full benefit.

Stimulants such as methylphenidate hydrochloride (Ritalin) or caffeine-containing medications may be used to counteract the sedating effects of opioids in some patients.

Balanced Approach to Analgesia

A *balanced analgesia* approach should be used, combining analgesics and adjuvants from different classes to minimize the adverse effects of opioids, such as nausea and vomiting or sedation, while maximizing pain relief. For example, an opioid and a nonopioid given together can provide pain relief with an overall lower dose of each medication than if each was given alone. Because these drugs have different mechanisms of action and different adverse effects, it is possible to safely use them together. If doses can be reduced in this manner, additional sedating medications such as antiemetics and antihistamines (to treat side effects) may not be needed.

Scheduling Options

Analgesics of any kind can be administered either as needed (prn) or on a scheduled basis. Intermittent, unpredictable pain may be best treated with as needed doses.

Pain that is predictable can be more effectively treated, or prevented, with scheduled doses of medication. Around-the-clock (ATC) dosing is an effective way to schedule doses evenly over a 24-hour period to prevent pain from becoming unbearable. It is important to use ATC dosing after surgery or trauma, with chronic pain, or in any other circumstance in which preventing pain will allow the patient to participate in daily or other recovery activities.

Patient-Controlled Analgesia

Patient-controlled analgesia (PCA) involves an opioid on an IV controller. The patient has a button on a cord that can be pushed to activate a dose of IV medication. The registered nurse (RN) programs the pump to the dose and dosing interval ordered by the HCP. A "lockout" mechanism prevents the patient from receiving the medication more often than ordered. PCA is an excellent option after surgery because it gives the patient some control over pain management. Teach the patient and family that only the patient should push the button, never the nurse or a family member. If the patient is too sedated to push the button, a dose of opioid is not likely needed and could even be dangerous.

World Health Organization Analgesic Ladder

In 1990, the World Health Organization (WHO) developed the WHO analgesic ladder to help clinicians to select appropriate medications for pain management based on pain intensity (Fig. 10.2). Although many organizations today use algorithms or flowcharts to help clinicians make appropriate medication choices, the WHO analgesic ladder remains a classic reference.

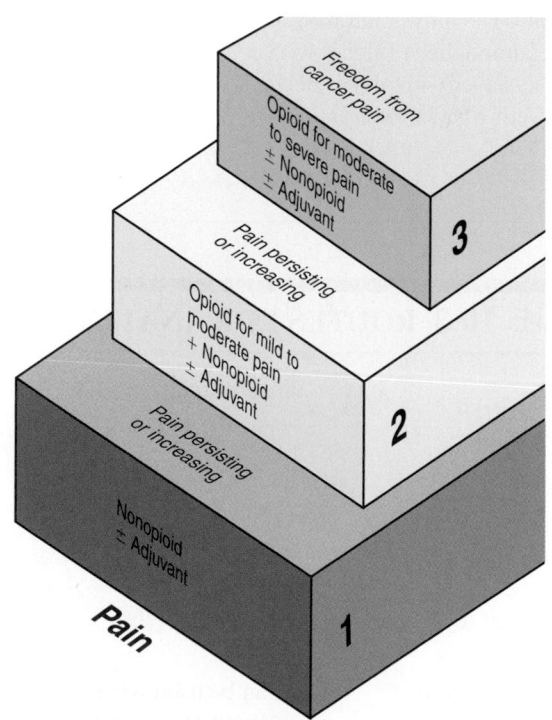

FIGURE 10.2 World Health Organization three-step analgesic ladder.

At the first level, nonopioid analgesics are recommended for mild pain (a verbal rating of 1–3). Typically, at this intensity, patients can perform usual daily activities. When pain is unrelieved by maximum ATC dosing, the treatment moves up the ladder to Level 2, moderate pain, and adds a low dose of an opioid analgesic. A patient with moderate pain (a verbal rating of 4–6) may have trouble working and staying focused. She or he may also begin to have difficulty with usual care activities such as walking, bathing, and dressing. If pain severity increases to severe pain (a verbal rating greater than 6), stronger opioids may be needed. Moderate to severe pain affects the quality of the patient's life. Addition of adjuvant agents should be considered at all levels.

Best practice mandates the scheduling of pain medications ATC to prevent breakthrough pain, especially for patients with cancer and chronic pain. For patients with surgical or traumatic pain, analgesics should be given ATC until the pain decreases to a level that allows medications to be given less often (e.g., as needed, such as before physical therapy). When using the WHO ladder, it is important to keep in mind that it is not necessary to start at Level 1 if the patient is having severe pain. Analgesics from Level 3 on the WHO ladder may be the starting point for some patients.

CRITICAL THINKING

Ms. Jackson

■ Ms. Jackson had abdominal surgery 2 days ago. She has been receiving morphine via IV PCA at an average of 2.5 mg per hour for the past 6 hours. She rates her pain at 3 on a scale of 0 to 10. She is to be discharged today. Her physician has ordered codeine 30 mg with acetaminophen (Tylenol with codeine No. 3), one or two tablets every 4 hours as needed for pain at home.

Will Ms. Jackson be comfortable at home? Why or why not?

Suggested answers are at the end of the chapter.

Other Interventions

Other pain treatments include radiation therapy or antineoplastic chemotherapy to help shrink tumors that are causing pain for a patient with cancer. Chemotherapy is also used for treating pain associated with connective tissue disorders such as rheumatoid arthritis and systemic lupus erythematosus (SLA). Topical local anesthetics such as lidocaine/prilocaine cream (EMLA) decrease the pain of procedures such as venipuncture and lumbar puncture. A lidocaine patch may be effective for patients with postherpetic or other nerve pain. In patients with osteoporosis, drugs that promote calcium uptake by the bones can aid in pain relief. These may include hormonal agents and medications that decrease calcium reabsorption from bone.

Placebos

Use of placebos involves the administration of an inactive substitute such as normal saline in place of an active medication. In the past, placebos were sometimes given in an attempt to determine whether a patient's pain was "real." This is unethical and inappropriate unless the patient has given written consent. The use of placebos is a denial of the patient's report of pain. If a placebo is ordered for a patient, discuss concerns with the physician and nurse supervisor. Placebos are only to be used in drug studies (clinical trials) to compare a new drug with an inactive substance. In this situation, patients are informed that they may be receiving a placebo.

Routes for Medication Administration

Analgesics can be administered by almost any route. The oral route is desired in most instances because it is easy and painless for the patient and can be used at home. See Table 10.3 for a comparison of the various routes.

Nonpharmacological Therapies

Nonpharmacological treatments are usually classified as either cognitive-behavioral interventions or physical agents. The goals of these two groups of treatments differ. Cognitive-behavioral interventions can help patients understand and

TABLE 10.3 ROUTES FOR ANALGESIC ADMINISTRATION

Uses	Advantages	Disadvantages	Nursing Considerations
Oral			
Preferred route in most cases	Convenient Less expensive than other forms Immediate- and controlled-release forms available	Slower onset than IV form	Can provide consistent blood levels when given around the clock. Controlled-release form recommended for long-term use in chronic pain.
Rectal			
May be used to provide local or systemic pain relief	Can be used when patient cannot take oral medication	May be difficult for patient or family to self-administer	Some oral preparations can be given rectally. (Place in empty gel cap for ease of use.) Check with HCP or pharmacist.

TABLE **10.3** ROUTES FOR ANALGESIC ADMINISTRATION—cont'd

Uses	Advantages	Disadvantages	Nursing Considerations
Transdermal Patch			
Chronic pain	Easy to apply Delivers pain relief for several days without patch change	May take up to 3 days before maximum effective drug level reached, and delay in excreting once removed. Patient must be closely monitored and alternative routes may be needed when starting and stopping therapy.	May be less effective in smokers and very thin people. Absorption may be erratic. Absorption may be increased with fever. Avoid heat application over patch. Avoid touching medication when applying patch. Keep used patches away from pets and children.
Intramuscular			
Acute pain	Rapid pain relief, although slower than IV	Painful administration Inconsistent absorption	Use only if other routes cannot be used.
IV			
Preferred route for postoperative and chronic cancer pain in patients who cannot tolerate oral route	Provides rapid relief Continuous infusion to achieve steady drug level	Difficult to use in home care setting Requires training and special equipment	Follow drug manufacturer's instructions for administration.
Patient-Controlled IV			
Allows patient some control over administration schedule	Patient pushes a button to administer a dose of opioid	Requires special training Pump must be programmed correctly	An hourly limit and lockout interval are programmed into the pump to keep the patient from receiving too much drug. Caution patient and family that only the patient should push the button.
Subcutaneous			
May be used if IV route is problematic	Can deliver effective pain relief Some opioids may be given as continuous infusion.	Injection may be painful	May be effective for treatment of chronic cancer pain.
Intraspinal (Epidural or Subarachnoid)			
Catheter into epidural or subarachnoid space used for traumatic injuries or chronic pain unrelieved by other methods May also be used for orthopedic, chest, and abdominal surgical procedures	May be able to control pain with lower doses of opioid because relief is delivered closer to site of pain Fewer systemic side effects	Requires single or continuous injection in back May be associated with intense itching Motor function must be assessed especially when local anesthetic is used	Steroids may be given with opioid to reduce pain by treating inflammation. Local anesthetic may be paired with opioid to enhance pain relief. Avoid use of anticoagulant and antiplatelet agents (including aspirin) because of risk of epidural hematoma.

cope with pain and take an active part in its assessment and control. The goals of physical agents may include providing comfort, correcting physical dysfunction, or altering physiological responses. Nonpharmacological therapies should be used in conjunction with drug therapies and are not expected to relieve pain on their own.

Cognitive-Behavioral Interventions

Included in this group are interventions such as educational information, relaxation exercises, guided imagery, distraction (e.g., music, television), and biofeedback. These treatments require extra time for detailed instruction and demonstration. The use of these modalities must be acceptable to the patient to be useful. Educating patients about what to expect and how they can participate in their own care has been shown to decrease patients' reports of postoperative pain and analgesic use.

Relaxation can be accomplished through a variety of methods. The patient may prefer a scripted relaxation exercise that can be practiced and used the same way each time or simply the use of a favorite piece of music that allows a state of muscle relaxation and freedom from anxiety. Guided imagery uses the patient's imagination to take the patient away from the pain to a favorite place, such as a beach in Tahiti. The success of guided imagery does not mean that the pain is in any way imaginary. See Chapter 5 for more information on relaxation and imagery.

As noted earlier, distraction is commonly used by patients to focus their attention on something other than the pain. They may watch a favorite television program or laugh with visitors when they are in pain. When the program is over or the visitors leave, the patient may focus on the pain again and ask for a dose of pain medication.

Biofeedback is sometimes used in chronic-pain programs to teach patients how to train their bodies to respond to different signals. Biofeedback has been very useful in patients with migraine headaches. When an aura (a warning sign) occurs before a migraine headache, patients are prompted to begin the exercise that relaxes them and may allow them to prevent the headache.

Physical Agents

Physical agents can contribute directly to the patient's comfort. Examples of physical agents include applications of heat or cold, massage, and exercise, discussed next. Additional physical interventions such as immobilization or TENS are also available.

APPLICATION OF HEAT.   The application of heat to sore muscles and joints is effective for pain relief. Heat works to increase circulation, induce muscle relaxation, and decrease inflammation when applied to a painful area. Heat can be applied using dry or moist packs or wraps, or in a bath or whirlpool. Heat is contraindicated in conditions that would be worsened by its use, such as in an area of trauma, because of the possibility of increased swelling caused by vasodilation. To prevent burns, heat should not be applied directly to skin or over areas of decreased sensation.

APPLICATION OF COLD.   Cold can reduce swelling, bleeding, and pain when used to treat a new injury. Cold can be applied by a variety of methods, such as cold wraps and cold packs, as well as localized ice massage. Patients often choose heat over cold if they have the choice, because cold can be uncomfortable. Cold may be better tolerated over a small area. Alternating heat and cold therapies is most effective if not contraindicated.

MASSAGE AND EXERCISE.   Massage and exercise are used to stretch and regain muscle and tendon length and to relax muscles. Massage pressure can be superficial or deep. It is important that massage is acceptable and not offensive to the patient. Immobilization is used after a variety of orthopedic procedures, as well as fractures and other injuries worsened by movement. Acupressure has also been shown to be beneficial for pain reduction (See "Evidence-Based Practice").

Physical agents are readily available, inexpensive, and require little preparation or instruction. But always remember, it is important to use nonpharmacological treatments to enhance appropriate drug treatments, not as a substitute.

 EVIDENCE-BASED PRACTICE

Clinical Question
Can acupressure help relieve pain and reduce the need for pharmacological analgesics?

Evidence
Fifteen small studies were reviewed to determine the effectiveness of using finger and hand pressure to stimulate acupoints and relieve pain. The studies demonstrated a reduction in menstrual, labor, low back, headache, and other types of pain in diverse populations.

Implications for Nursing Practice
"Acupressure can be efficiently conducted by health care professionals as an adjuvant therapy in general practice for pain relief" (Chen & Wang, in press).

REFERENCE
Chen, Y., & Wang, H. (In press). The effectiveness of acupuncture on relieving pain: A systematic review. *Pain Management Nursing*.

 NURSING PROCESS FOR THE PATIENT EXPERIENCING PAIN

Data Collection

Accurate assessment of pain is essential to effective treatment. Without appropriate assessment, it is not possible to intervene in a way that meets the patient's needs. Because of regulatory requirements, most organizations require detailed pain assessments of patients at admission, with any change

Patient Perspective

Terry Versus Joanne

I (Terry) have had chronic back pain for 10 years. It is very real, related to multiple herniated discs in my thoracic and lumbar spine, arthritis, and degenerative disc disease. Because I've been dealing with it for 10 years, I have adapted—I never look like I am in pain. Sometimes I limp or move around a lot to find a comfortable position, but I don't have that pained look on my face, and my blood pressure doesn't go up like some people. I have tried many, many medications over the years and have become quite educated in pain treatments. I have tried antidepressants and antiseizure medications (both are used for neuropathic pain), ice, heat, TENS, relaxation, physical therapy, more physical therapy, exercises, more exercises, massage therapy, steroid injections, and nerve blocks. I had relief once for about a month following some injections, and I kept thinking something was wrong. "Wait, where's the pain? This doesn't feel right!" Sometimes I would like a big dose of morphine, but I know that opioids for chronic pain are a one-way street to dependence. I do have a prescription for hydrocodone and acetaminophen (Vicodin) that I take a couple of times a month when I feel desperate. I ration them because I am afraid of them.

My friend Joanne also has back pain, which started 20 years ago. When it started, she was writhing in pain—I am positive her blood pressure was sky high! She couldn't move because of muscle spasms. She was also diagnosed with a herniated disc, but she was able to have surgery to fix it. She said the nerve pain relief was already evident in the recovery room. Of course, surgery causes pain, so opioids are needed for a short while. But once healing started for Joanne, no pain! She still has acute pain from time to time, when she experiences muscle spasms and can't move very easily for several days. She takes muscle relaxers and has to lay low until the spasms resolve.

Sometimes Joanne looks at me and says, "You don't look like you're in pain." At first this made me feel bad, like she was comparing her pain to mine. Then one day, I realized the difference—she experiences *acute* pain, and I have *chronic* pain. I've adapted. She is way more miserable than I am when she is in pain, but it is short-lived. My pain is not as severe, but after 10 years, it has worn me down.

When you are a nurse, please believe your patients when they say they are in pain, even if they don't look like they are. Maybe they've gotten used to it, but that doesn't mean they enjoy feeling pain. Do whatever you can to help them feel better.

in condition, and at least quarterly thereafter while in care. Nurses should verbally assess all patients under their care at least once per shift for pain and provide appropriate intervention as needed. The **WHAT'S UP?** format, introduced in Chapter 1, can help you perform a complete and effective assessment (Table 10.4). The following sections provide some additional key points for assessing pain and putting together more pieces of the pain puzzle.

Accept the Patient's Report of Pain

Pain is what the patient says it is, not what the HCP believes it is. When a member of the health care team distrusts the patient's report of pain, the patient can usually sense this. The patient may compensate by either underreporting pain or, less commonly, anxiously overreporting. Patients may try to hide their pain for fear of being thought of as complainers or drug seekers.

Obtain a Pain History

Obtain information from the patient about the pain he or she is experiencing. Letting the patient describe the pain in his or her own words helps establish a trust relationship between you and the patient. This is also the time to discover the effects the pain is having on the patient's quality of life. Does the pain prevent the patient from eating, sleeping, or participating in work or family activities? Are there adverse effects such as nausea and vomiting or constipation that need to be addressed? Also assess emotional and spiritual distress and coping abilities. Ask the patient about how he or she has coped with pain previously and what treatments have been effective and ineffective in the past. In nonverbal or cognitively impaired patients, information may be obtained from family members and the medical record. A painful diagnosis, such as arthritis, typically is a predictor of pain. A thorough history is essential so you can individualize pain interventions to fit the patient's needs.

PAIN ASSESSMENT TOOLS. Various tools are available to assist with accurate and complete pain assessment. You should become familiar with the tools used in your clinical practice, setting and use them consistently. It is of utmost importance that all health care personnel caring for a particular patient use the same pain rating scale, whether it is a numerical scale (e.g., 0–10), a visual analog scale (Fig. 10.3), or the FACES-R scale (FPS-R) (Fig. 10.4). There should also be consistent scales in place for nonverbal/cognitively impaired patients such as the PAINAD (Pain Assessment in Advanced Dementia Scale; Ward, Hurley, & Volicer, 2003; Fig. 10.5).

Whatever scale is used, it must be one that has been validated with research. The FACES-R scale was initially developed for use in children and has since been revised with faces that are more realistic for adults. The PAINAD scale was developed for patients with advanced dementia but is an effective tool for patients with cognitive and communicative barriers. Longer questionnaires are useful in meeting regulatory requirements for the completion of comprehensive pain assessments (Fig. 10.6). These scales often contain examples of verbal pain descriptors—something many patients

TABLE 10.4 WHAT'S UP? GUIDE FOR PAIN ASSESSMENT

Acronym	Key	Pain Assessment
W	Where is the pain?	Be specific. Use a drawing of the body if needed.
H	How does the pain feel?	Is the pain shooting, burning, dull, sharp, aching?
A	Aggravating and alleviating factors	What makes the pain better? What makes it worse?
T	Timing	When did the pain start? Is it intermittent? Continuous?
S	Severity	How bad is the pain on a scale of 0 to 10? Use a different tool, such as the PAINAD or FACES (see Fig. 10.4 and 10.5) scale, if needed.
U	Useful other data	Are any other symptoms associated with the pain or pain treatment? Itching, nausea, sedation, constipation? How does the pain affect lifestyle (inability to eat, sleep, work, enjoy sex, etc.)?
P	Patient perception	What is the patient's perception of what caused the pain? Is the patient experiencing suffering? Is the patient satisfied with pain control?

FIGURE 10.3 Analog pain scale.

have difficulty verbalizing. A scale should also be used to monitor the patient's level of sedation after opioid administration (Fig. 10.7). Any unexpected increase in the patient's level of sedation should be reported promptly to the RN or HCP. Finally, keeping a pain diary may help patients to document pain ratings, interventions, and responses, which can aid effective intervention.

Perform a Complete Physical Assessment

A thorough physical assessment is necessary to determine the effect of the pain and pain treatments on the body. It helps identify all of the pain sites and any medication side effects and helps prioritize the seemingly overwhelming task of helping the patient achieve acceptable pain relief and good quality of life. As discussed previously, the patient with acute pain may exhibit signs such as grimacing and moaning or elevated pulse and blood pressure. For patients with cognitive impairments, these indicators can be particularly important; however, these signs cannot be relied on to "prove" that a patient is in pain. The only reliable source of pain assessment is the patient's self-report ("Gerontological Issues"). Even patients with cognitive deficits can provide important information about pain. They can often answer simple yes or no questions regarding comfort and may demonstrate favorable changes in behavior, such as diminished calling out, when pain is effectively controlled.

Gerontological Issues

Older adults frequently have unmet pain needs. Many believe that pain is an anticipated part or aging and may be hesitant to take strong medications such as opioids for pain. NSAIDs are often contraindicated for older adults due to medication interactions and GI side effects; however, patients should be evaluated for medications on an individual basis. Patients in long-term care facilities, particularly patients with cognitive deficits, should have medications for pain scheduled ATC to ensure regular administration and effective pain control. Consider incidence of isolation, restlessness, confusion, aggression, and changes in appetite as possible signs of pain. Pulling at dressings, tugging at IV sites, and calling out can also be symptoms of discomfort. Any change in the patient's usual behavior should be considered a possible sign of discomfort. Remember to take more time when assessing pain in older patients because they may need more time to process what you are asking. Consider using the PAINAD Scale when assessing confused patients.

You can anticipate pain and provide relief measures to prevent severe pain. A trial dose of pain medication may help to determine if the patient's behavior is because of pain. Nagging achiness in hands and feet is often noted as a reason for decreased activity, inability to sleep, and altered functional ability. A hand or foot massage using lotion and gentle massage strokes is often a relaxing comfort measure.

Opioid analgesic doses may need to be decreased by 25% to 50% initially because they tend to work longer and stronger in the older patient.

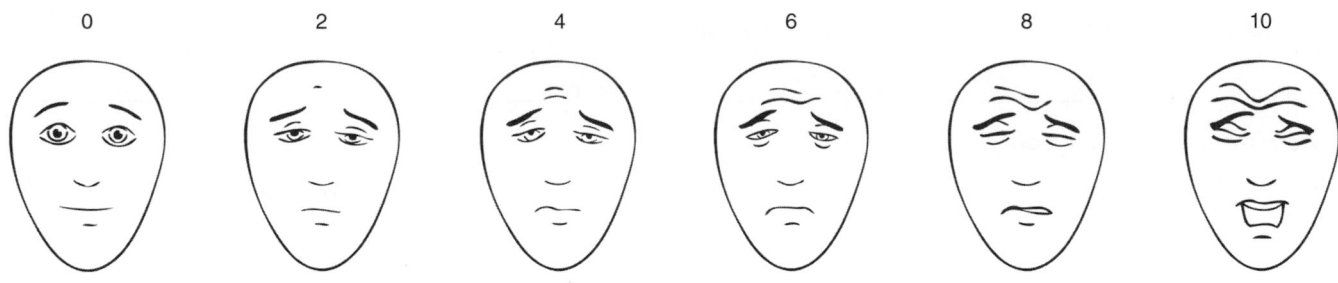

FIGURE 10.4 FACES-R Pain Scale. *(With permission from the International Association for the Study of Pain.)*

Pain Assessment in Advanced Dementia Scale (PAINAD)

Behavior	0	1	2	Score
Breathing independent of vocalization	Normal	• Occasional labored breathing • Short period of hyperventilation	• Noisy labored breathing • Long period of hyperventilation • Cheyne-Stokes respirations	
Negative vocalization	None	• Occasional moan or groan • Low level speech with a negative or disapproving quality	• Repeated troubled calling out • Loud moaning or groaning • Crying	
Facial expression	Smiling or inexpressive	• Sad • Frightened • Frown	• Facial grimacing	
Body language	Relaxed	• Tense • Distressed pacing • Fidgeting	• Rigid • Fists clenched • Knees pulled up • Pulling or pushing away • Striking out	
Consolability	No need to console	• Distracted or reassured by voice or touch	• Unable to console, distract, or reassure	
			Total*	

* Total scores range from 0 to 10 (based on a scale of 0 to 2 for five items), with a higher score indicating more severe pain (0–"no pain" to 10–"severe pain")

FIGURE 10.5 PAINAD Scale. *(From Warden, Hurley, & Volicer, 2003. The PAINAD was developed and tested by clinicians and researchers at the New England Geriatric Research Education and Clinical Center, a Department of Veterans Affairs center of excellence with divisions at EN Rogers Memorial Veterans Hospital, Bedford, MA, and VA Boston Health System. www.amda.com)*

Nursing Diagnoses, Planning, and Implementation

See the "Nursing Care Plan for the Patient in Pain." Some additional principles to consider during planning and implementation follow.

Set Goals With Patients and Caregivers

Establish a pain control goal during the planning phase. Ask the patient to determine an acceptable level of pain if complete freedom from pain is not possible. Patients with cognitive deficits should also have pain goals established that include behavioral indicators. Education is important when helping patients and caregivers set realistic pain control goals. Although a goal of 0 pain is desirable, it may not be possible or safe. On the other hand, a patient who chooses a pain goal of 6 may be unable to get out of bed and do other recovery or daily activities.

Patients should also identify activity goals. After surgery, goals may include the ability to ambulate and achieve restful sleep. For patients with chronic pain, the goals may be different. For example, a patient with terminal cancer may want to be able to eat dinner with her family in the evening. You can assist the patient in reaching that goal by teaching her to conserve energy during the day for the activity that is most important to her. Instructing both patients in optimal timing of pain medications will also assist them in reaching their desired activity goals.

Giving patients pain management options can provide autonomy and may help prevent feelings of helplessness and hopelessness. It is the nurse's responsibility to engage the patient and family in the pain management plan.

Pain Assessment Chart (For Admission and/or Follow-up)

1. Patient _____ 2. DX _____

Assessment on Admission

Date _____ / _____ / _____   Pain ☐   No Pain ☐   Date of Pain Onset _____ / _____ / _____

1. Location of Pain (indicate on drawing)

2. Description of Predominant Pain (in patient's words) _____
_____
_____

3. Intensity [Scale 0 (no pain) — 10 (most intense)] _____   Right   Left   Left   Right
_____

4. Duration and when occurs _____
_____

5. Precipitating Factors _____
_____

6. Alleviating Factors _____
_____

7. Accompanying Symptoms

    GI: Nausea ☐   Emesis ☐   Constipation ☐   Anorexia ☐

    CNS: Drowsiness ☐   Confusion ☐   Hallucinations ☐

    Psychosocial: Mood _____   Anger _____

    Anxiety _____   Depression _____

    Relationships _____
    _____

8. Other Symptoms

    Sleep _____   Fatigue _____

    Activity _____   Other _____

9. Present Medications _____
_____
_____

    Doses and times medicated last 48 hours _____

10. Breakthrough Pain _____
_____

Signature: _____

FIGURE 10.6 Pain assessment chart. *(Modified from the Purdue Frederik Company, Norwalk, CT.)*

S | 1 | 2 | 3 | 4
Normal Sleep | Awake and Alert | Occasionally Drowsy | Frequently Drowsy | Unable to Arouse

FIGURE 10.7 Level of sedation scale.

Understand That Pain Affects the Whole Family

It is important to include the whole family in the pain management plan. Understanding family dynamics helps the nurse in implementing an effective plan. Cultural influences are also important to consider (see Chapter 4 and "Cultural

---

NURSING CARE PLAN for the Patient in Pain

Nursing Diagnosis: *Pain (acute or chronic)*

Expected Outcomes: Pain will be at a level that is acceptable to the patient. Patient will be able to participate in activities that are important to him or her.

Evaluation of Outcomes: Is pain at a level that is acceptable to the patient? Is the patient able to participate in activities that he or she has identified as important?

Intervention Assess pain based on patient report. Use the **WHAT'S UP?** format. **Rationale** Patient's pain is defined as what the patient says it is, when the patient says it is occurring. **Evaluation** Does the patient verbalize his or her pain? Does the patient use verbal or nonverbal messages that imply trust in nurse's belief of pain report?

Intervention Teach the patient to use a pain rating scale. Use the same scales consistently. **Rationale** A rating scale is the most reliable method for assessing pain severity. **Evaluation** Does the patient understand the use of the scale and use it to report pain?

Intervention Have the patient or caregiver keep a pain diary, documenting time of pain, interventions, and pre- and postpain ratings. **Rationale** A diary can show patterns of pain and pain relief, and help in planning care. **Evaluation** Does the diary reveal patterns that help with planning?

Intervention Determine what is an acceptable pain level for the patient. Consider activities the patient should be able to perform. **Rationale** Only the patient can decide what pain level is acceptable. **Evaluation** Is the patient's pain at an acceptable level? Can they perform necessary activities of daily living (ADLs) with minimal pain?

Intervention Assess whether pain is nociceptive, neuropathic, or both. **Rationale** Nociceptive and neuropathic may present differently and may require different interventions. **Evaluation** Has nociceptive versus neuropathic pain been identified? Are treatments appropriate?

Intervention Assess need for and offer emotional, spiritual, and social support for the experience of pain and suffering. **Rationale** Pain, as well as disease processes, can be accompanied by feelings of powerlessness, distress, and isolation. **Evaluation** Does the patient appear emotional, angry, or withdrawn? Does the patient have difficulty making decisions? Does the patient have a support system? Is the patient-nurse relationship therapeutic?

Intervention Give analgesics before pain becomes severe. For persistent pain, give analgesics around the clock. **Rationale** Pain can be more difficult to relieve when it becomes severe. **Evaluation** Is analgesic schedule effective?

Intervention Combine opioid and nonopioid analgesics as ordered. **Rationale** Balanced analgesia provides optimum pain relief with fewer side effects. **Evaluation** Is the analgesic combination effective?

Intervention Assess for pain relief approximately 1 hr after administration of oral analgesics, or 30 min after IV analgesics. **Rationale** If pain is not relieved, additional measures will be needed. **Evaluation** Does patient report acceptable level of relief?

Intervention Observe for adverse effects of pain medication. **Rationale** Many pain medications cause nausea and fatigue. Both tend to subside after a few days. **Evaluation** Are adverse effects occurring? Can they be managed? Does medication regimen need to be adjusted?

Continued

NURSING CARE PLAN for the Patient in Pain—cont'd

Intervention If opioids and/or muscle relaxants are being used, assess for respiratory depression and level of sedation at regular intervals. **Rationale** If patient is opioid-naïve or dose is increased, monitor patient carefully for sedation. Sedation always precedes respiratory depression. **Evaluation** Is the patient's respiratory rate greater than 8 per minute or above the parameter ordered by the physician? What is the patient's level of consciousness?

Intervention Institute measures to prevent constipation: 8 to 10 glasses of noncaffeinated fluid daily (unless contraindicated), stimulant laxatives, and exercise as tolerated. **Rationale** Opioid-induced constipation is a problem of GI motility; stimulant laxatives are most effective. Caffeine can exacerbate constipation. **Evaluation** Is the patient easily passing soft feces in expected amount every 1–3 days?

Intervention Teach patient alternative (nonpharmacological) pain relief interventions, such as relaxation and distraction, to be used with medication. **Rationale** Nonpharmacological interventions can help the patient feel in control and may help reduce the perception of pain. **Evaluation** Does the patient use nonpharmacological interventions effectively?

Intervention Assess whether patient is taking pain medications appropriately, and if not, assess reasons. Discuss how interventions may be modified. **Rationale** Pain medications must be taken appropriately to be effective. **Evaluation** Is the patient able to manage the pain control regimen? Does he or she have concerns about medications? Are adjustments necessary?

Considerations"). It is difficult for family members to see loved ones in pain or in heavily sedated states. Including them in planning helps them feel that they can help make the patient more comfortable and recognizes the important role they have in the patient's care.

Pain Is Exhausting

Pain may keep the patient from sleeping well. This cycle of sleeplessness and pain must be interrupted to help the patient. Fatigue is a common problem for the patient with chronic pain and can complicate the treatment process. Although older adults do not require as much sleep as younger adults, patients must get at least 6 to 7 hours of uninterrupted sleep to be relaxed enough to break the cycle. Controlled-release opioids may help maintain pain relief throughout the night. If controlled-release medications are not used, it may be necessary to wake a patient to administer pain medication so that the pain does not get out of control. The addition of a sedative or sleep aid may be needed to allow the patient to sleep. Aromatherapy such as lavender, ensuring patient is comfortable, and limiting caffeine intake after 1500 can increase productive sleep.

A Team Approach to Pain Management

The interdisciplinary pain management team includes the patient and family, the nurse, the physician or HCP, therapists, spiritual advisers, social workers, and pharmacists. Communication among team members is essential. It is the important link that allows the team to be effective in creating a plan that works for the patient. As the nurse, you play a vital role in ensuring effective communication among team members, always remembering that the patient is at the center of the team.

Patient Education

Patients, and in some instances their family members, must be informed about the medications they are taking for pain management. This allows them to take an active role in their care. Patients who are informed about the goals of pain management and who are confident that their providers believe them are more likely to report unrelieved pain so that they can receive prompt and effective treatment. Goals include a satisfactory comfort level with minimal side effects and complications of pain and its treatment, as well as a reduced period of recovery.

The patient should be provided with information about a drug's effects, common adverse effects, frequency of the dose and duration of action, and potential drug-drug and drug-food interactions, if indicated. There are many special considerations for medications, such as controlled-release oral agents and transdermal patches; care must be taken to include these considerations in the education plan for the patient taking these drugs at home. Drug-specific instructions are found in drug handbooks or databases. Education must be presented at a level that the patient can understand. Written information should be included when appropriate. Informed patients use their medications more effectively and safely.

CRITICAL THINKING

Mr. Sebastian

■ Mr. Sebastian is a 75-year-old man who has been diagnosed with lung cancer and is anxious about leaving the hospital to return home following surgery. The nursing assessment reveals the need for home health care for dressing changes and teaching about the medications he will need at home. While in the hospital, Mr. Sebastian has required 5 mg of IV morphine every 4 hours around the clock.

1. The morphine is available in syringes prefilled with morphine grains 1/6 per mL. How many milliliters should the nurse administer while Mr. Sebastian is in the hospital?
2. What discharge instructions must be given to Mr. Sebastian and his wife before sending him home?
3. How might his pain be managed at home to prevent unnecessary readmissions to the hospital?

Suggested answers are at the end of the chapter.

NURSING CARE TIP

Many medication interventions are available for the treatment of pain. Whenever possible, administer analgesics by the mouth, by the WHO ladder, and by the clock.

Evaluation

The final phase of the nursing process is evaluation. Once the plan of care has been implemented, evaluate whether the patient's goals have been met. What is the patient's pain rating? Has the patient's identified goal for an acceptable level of pain been met? How were the pain treatments tolerated? Was the patient able to participate in activities that he or she identified as important? The plan should be continuously updated based on the evaluation.

Home Health Hints

- Emotional or spiritual distress and fear related to dependence on family caregivers may alter the patient's perception or report of pain. Some patients may feel pain more intensely because of the influence of fear, and others may underreport if they are trying to protect family members.
- Pill boxes are useful to ease in administration of medications and for nurses to track usage.
- Massage is commonly used for the treatment of chronic pain, especially musculoskeletal pain. Remember a physician's order might be necessary for this type of treatment. Discuss this option with the HCP, patient, and caregiver to help determine if this intervention is appropriate for your patient.

SUGGESTED ANSWERS TO

CRITICAL THINKING

■ Mrs. Smithers and Mr. Brown

It is important to accept both patients' pain reports. Assessment should be based on what the patient says rather than what is observed. Each patient copes with his or her pain in a unique way, and the nurse cannot judge whether one is in more pain than the other.

■ Janet

1. Remember, pain is whatever the experiencing person says it is, existing whenever the experiencing person says it does. You must assume that Janet is in pain. She has pancreatitis, which is commonly very painful. She has a history of IV drug abuse and is likely tolerant to the effects of the morphine. She may be experiencing "end-of-dose failure," when pain medication does not last as long as expected. If her vital signs are within normal limits, it should be safe to treat her pain.

2. Contact the RN or HCP and explain the problem. Making Janet wait another hour in pain is not appropriate.
3. Tylenol works differently from morphine and may offer minimal relief but is not an appropriate order for severe pain. Talk to the RN or supervisor and explain the situation.
4. Listen to Janet and let her know that you understand she is in pain. Keep her updated at all times and assure her that you will continue to advocate for her until she achieves adequate pain relief.

■ Mrs. Zales

1. Mrs. Zales may have been tolerant to opioids because of her need for medication for chronic pain during the past year. For this reason, she needed more medication than a nontolerant patient who does not usually use opioids. Also, the belief that promethazine and other phenothiazines potentiate opioids is a myth. They do cause increased levels of sedation and may limit the

Continued

SUGGESTED ANSWERS TO—cont'd

amount of opioid that can be given safely. IM injections are not recommended because they are painful, absorption is not predictable, and there is a delay between injection and relief. A more rational approach to Mrs. Zales's pain management would have been regular pain assessment with ATC treatment until the pain began to subside.

2. If her pain level had been better controlled, she might have been discharged on oral analgesics without the delay.

3. The most important team member here was Mrs. Zales—the patient should be the CENTER of the team! If she had been listened to more carefully and her history considered, she might have been kept more comfortable.

■ *Mrs. Shepard*

1. Pain medication is most effective when given on a routine schedule around the clock to avoid breakthrough pain. Mrs. Shepard's epidural infusion should continue to relieve her pain for a time, up to several hours after it is discontinued, depending on the medication used. The oral medication is most effective when given at the time the epidural is stopped so that it is taking effect as the epidural effects wear off. See "Gerontological Issues" for special considerations for the older patient.

2. Pain prevents patients from moving freely. Postoperative complications such as retained pulmonary secretions and ileus can occur when patients are immobile. Effective pain management can help prevent these complications.

3. If she takes a dose every 3 hours, then she will receive eight doses in 24 hours: 500 mg × 8 = 4000 mg or 4 g, which is the maximum safe dose. Recall that older adult patients metabolize and excrete medications more slowly than younger patients. If she will need the hydrocodone/acetaminophen for more than a few days, it would be wise to consult with the physician about giving the opioid and acetaminophen separately.

4. Mrs. Shepard should be instructed about what her role will be when her pain management regimen is altered. Does she have to ask for the pain medication, or will it just be brought to her? Patient and family education are vital to success in management of a patient's pain.

■ *Ms. Jackson*

Using an equianalgesic conversion, we can determine whether Ms. Jackson is likely to have good pain relief based on her requirement with the PCA. Her current pain level of 3 shows that the morphine has been effective. Remember that the pump keeps a history of what the patient uses, which is the best indicator of what the patient needs. Ms. Jackson has used 15 mg of morphine during the past 6 hours. An equianalgesic dose of Tylenol with codeine No. 3 would be almost 200 mg of codeine, but only 30 to 60 mg has been ordered. In addition, if Ms. Jackson takes enough Tylenol with codeine No. 3 to get 200 mg of codeine, she will receive a dangerous dose of both the codeine and the acetaminophen. The physician needs to be contacted for different analgesic orders.

■ *Mr. Sebastian*

1. $\dfrac{5 \text{ mg}}{} \left| \dfrac{1 \text{ grain}}{60 \text{ mg}} \right| \dfrac{1 \text{ mL}}{\text{grains } 1/6} = 0.5 \text{ mL}$

2. Home instruction regarding ATC administration of pain medication is indicated, as well as effects and side effects to report. He will also need to implement measures to prevent constipation.

3. MS Contin, a long-acting oral form of morphine, may be an option for Mr. Sebastian, along with an immediate-release preparation for breakthrough pain. Make sure to check an equianalgesic chart to be sure his oral dose is adequate. Also, information about what to do and whom to contact if pain becomes unmanageable is necessary to help prevent readmissions to the hospital.

REVIEW QUESTIONS

1. A patient is walking up and down the hall and visiting and laughing with other patients. When the nurse approaches, the patient reports a pain level of 6 on a scale of 0 to 10. Based on McCaffery's definition of pain, which of the following assumptions by the nurse is most likely correct?
   1. The patient is not really in pain but just wants his medication.
   2. The patient is having pain at a level of 6 on a scale of 0 to 10.
   3. The patient is in minimal pain and should receive an oral analgesic instead of an injection.
   4. The patient is in pain but does not need his pain medication yet.

2. A patient with terminal cancer has been requiring 5 mg of IV morphine every 1 to 2 hours to control pain, yet is engrossed in a movie on television and appears to be in no pain. Which of the following explanations of this behavior is most likely correct?
   1. Denial of pain is common in patients with cancer.
   2. The cancer treatment is working and the pain is improving.
   3. The patient is hiding the pain to finish watching the movie undisturbed.
   4. Distraction can be an effective treatment for pain when used with appropriate drug treatments.

3. What action should the nurse take when a patient who is in pain develops tolerance to opioid analgesics?
   1. Slowly wean the patient from opioids.
   2. Request a referral to an addiction specialist for the patient.
   3. Talk to the RN or HCP about increasing the dose of analgesic.
   4. Offer the patient nonopioid alternatives for pain control.

4. A patient has surgical site pain 24 hours after a total hip replacement. All the following medications are ordered. Which would be the most appropriate choice for the patient at this time?
   1. ibuprofen (Motrin)
   2. hydromorphone (Dilaudid)
   3. acetaminophen (Tylenol)
   4. gabapentin (Neurontin)

5. A patient is receiving duloxetine (Cymbalta) for neuropathic pain related to diabetes. For which symptoms of neuropathic pain should the nurse assess?
   1. Tingling, shocklike pain
   2. Dull aching pain
   3. Deep cramping pain
   4. Throbbing, aching pain

6. Which of the following methods is the most reliable way to assess the severity of a patient's pain?
   1. Ask the patient to describe the pain.
   2. Observe the patient for physical signs of pain such as moaning or grimacing.
   3. Ask the patient to rate his or her pain using a valid assessment scale.
   4. Ask a family member to rate the patient's pain.

7. According to the World Health Organization's analgesic ladder, at what point in a patient's pain experience is it appropriate to use adjuvant treatments? **Select all that apply.**
   1. In addition to analgesics for early, mild pain
   2. As an alternative to analgesics for mild to moderate pain
   3. As an alternative to analgesics for severe pain
   4. In addition to analgesics for pain that is persistent despite treatment
   5. In addition to analgesics for pain that is growing increasingly severe

8. A patient is hospitalized following a motor vehicle accident with multiple orthopedic injuries and reports acute pain at an 8 on a 0 to 10 scale. An order is written for morphine 6 mg IV every 4 hours as needed, as well as a nonopioid oral analgesic every 4 hours as needed. To reduce the risk of adverse effects and maintain an acceptable level of sedation and pain control, which of the following analgesic schedules will be most effective?
   1. Offer the opioid every 4 hours.
   2. Tell the patient to call when pain becomes severe, and then give the drugs immediately.
   3. Give both the IV opioid and the PO nonopioid every 4 hours around the clock.
   4. Alternate the IV analgesic with the nonopioid oral analgesic as needed.

9. An 88-year-old patient is admitted with a broken hip after a fall. An order is written for meperidine 50 to 75 mg IM every 4 hours prn (as needed) for pain. Which of the following actions should the nurse take first?
   1. Give the meperidine every 4 hours ATC.
   2. Offer the meperidine every 4 to 6 hours prn.
   3. Administer an NSAID with the meperidine for added pain relief.
   4. Discuss the order with the RN or HCP.

10. A patient is started on gabapentin (Neurontin) 300 mg by mouth three times daily for chronic low back pain related to lumbar disc herniation. Which instruction should the nurse provide?
    1. "Take the medication at the first sign of any pain, up to three times daily."
    2. "Take one capsule every 8 hours continuously to keep the pain under control."
    3. "Take the medication only when you need it, to prevent becoming addicted."
    4. "Take one capsule three times a day, then stop it when the pain is under control."

11. A nurse receives an order to administer 1 mL of sterile normal saline solution IM to a patient suspected of opioid abuse. Which response by the nurse is appropriate first?
    1. Administer the saline and carefully document the patient's response in the medical record.
    2. Administer the saline but inform the patient exactly what it is and why it was ordered.
    3. Refuse to administer the medication and inform the physician that the order is inappropriate.
    4. Share concerns about the order with the supervisor and explain why the nurse cannot in good conscience administer the saline.

12. A nurse needs to administer morphine 10 mg IM. It is supplied as grains 1/4 per mL. How many milliliters should the nurse prepare for injection?
    Answer: _____ mL

Answers can be found in Appendix C.

References

American Pain Society. (n.d.). *Definitions related to the use of opioids for the treatment of pain.* Retrieved May 30, 2009, from http://www.ampainsoc.org/advocacy/opioids2.htm

American Society of Addiction Medicine. (2011). *Public policy statement: Definition of addiction.* Retrieved October 26, 2013 from www.asam.org/for-the-public/definition-of-addiction

Institute for Safe Medication Practices. (2012). ISMP's list of high alert medications. Retrieved October 26, 2013 from http://www.ismp.org/tools/highalertmedications.pdf

International Association for the Study of Pain. (2011). *IASP taxonomy.* Retrieved October 26, 2013 from www.iasp-pain.org/Content/NavigationMenu/GeneralResourceLinks/Pain Definitions/default.htm

McCaffery, M. (1968). *Nursing practice theories related to cognition, bodily pain, and man-environment interactions.* Los Angeles: University of California at Los Angeles Students' Store.

Warden, V., Hurley, A. C., & Volicer, L. (2003). Development and psychometric evaluation of the Pain Assessment in Advanced Dementia (PAINAD) scale. *Journal of the American Medical Directors Association* 4:9–15.

 DavisP*lus* | For additional resources and information visit **davispl.us/medsurg5**

11

Nursing Care of Patients With Cancer

LUCY L. COLO AND
JANICE L. BRADFORD

LEARNING OUTCOMES

1. Explain the normal structures and functions of the cell.
2. Describe changes that occur in a cell when it becomes malignant.
3. Identify commonly used chemotherapeutic agents.
4. Discuss the special nursing needs of the patient receiving chemotherapy or radiation therapy.
5. Identify data to collect when caring for a patient with cancer.
6. Recognize common oncological emergencies and related nursing care.
7. Discuss how you will know if your nursing interventions have been effective.
8. Describe the role of hospice in providing care for patients with advanced cancer.

KEY TERMS

alopecia (AL-oh-PEE-she-ah)
anemia (uh-NEE-mee-yah)
anorexia (AN-oh-REK-see-ah)
benign (bee-NINE)
biopsy (BY-opp-see)
cancer (KAN-sir)
carcinogen (kar-SIN-oh-jen)
chemotherapy (KEE-moh-THAIR-uh-pee)
contact inhibition (kon-takt in-huh-BIH-shun)
cytotoxic (SY-toh-TOCK-sik)
desquamation (dee-skwa-MAY-shun)
in situ (in-SY-too)
leukopenia (LOO-koh-PEE-nee-ah)
malignant (muh-LIG-nunt)
metastasis (muh-TASS-tuh-sis)
mucositis (MYOO-koh-SY-tis)
nadir (NAY-dur)
neoplasm (NEE-oh-PLAZ-uhm)
neutropenia (noo-troh-PEE-nee-ah)
oncology (on-CAW-luh-gee)
oncovirus (ON-koh-VY-russ)
palliation (pal-ee-AY-shun)
radiation therapy (RAY-dee-AY-shun THAIR-uh-pee)
stomatitis (STOH-mah-TY-tis)
thrombocytopenia (THROM-boh-SY-toh-PEE-nee-ah)
tumor (TOO-merr)
vesicant (VESS-ih-kent)
xerostomia (ZEE-roh-STOH-mee-ah)

REVIEW OF NORMAL ANATOMY AND PHYSIOLOGY OF CELLS

Cells are the smallest living structural and functional subunits of the body. Although human cells vary in size, shape, and certain metabolic activities, they have many characteristics in common.

Cell Structure

Human cells have a plasma membrane, cytoplasm (cytosol, organelles), and a nucleus (Fig. 11.1). Organelles are specific in structure and function. Variations in the relative amounts of organelles and cell features allow great diversity in cells, and therefore in tissues.

Nucleus

The nucleus of a cell is its control center, containing the individual's unique deoxyribonucleic acid (DNA) sequence (Fig. 11.2). Most cells have one central nucleus, although variations exist.

DNA coding regions are called genes; a gene is the code for one protein. Not all of the genes in a particular cell are active, only those needed for the proteins required to carry out their specific functions. These proteins may be structural, such as the collagen of connective tissue, or functional, such

as the hemoglobin of red blood cells (RBCs). Important functional proteins are the enzymes that catalyze the specific reactions characteristic of each type of cell.

Genetic Code and Protein Synthesis

The genetic code of DNA is the code for the amino acid sequences needed to synthesize a cell's proteins. The assembly of amino acids into the primary structure of a protein is a two-step process: transcription and translation. Transcription makes a copy of the code needed for a protein so DNA can remain guarded in the nucleus. Translation occurs at the ribosome where the nucleotide code of nucleic acids is translated into the amino acid code of protein (see Fig. 11.3).

As with any complex process, mistakes are possible. If there is a mistake in the DNA code, the process of protein synthesis may continue, but the resulting protein will not function normally; this is the basis for genetic diseases. DNA mistakes acquired during life are called *mutations*. A mutation is any change in the DNA code. Ultraviolet rays or exposure to certain chemicals may cause structural changes in the DNA code. These changes can kill the affected cells or may irreversibly alter their function. Such altered cells can become malignant, being unable to function normally. These cells actively replicate the mutated DNA during division, creating a mass of faulty cells. This is the basis of some forms

Golgi apparatus

Centriole

Mitochondrion

Smooth endoplasmic reticulum

Rough endoplasmic reticulum

Plasma membrane: The boundary of the cell

Cilia

Nucleus: The center of the cell

Nuclear envelope

Nuclear pores

Nucleolus

Vacuole

Microfilaments

Microtubules

Cytoplasm: A gel-like substance surrounding the nucleus and packed with various organelles and molecules, each of which serves a specific function

Lysosome

FIGURE 11.1 Schematic of a typical human cell. From Thompson, G. C. (2013). *Understanding anatomy and physiology.* Philadelphia: F.A. Davis, p. 38.

A double-layered membrane called the **nuclear envelope** surrounds the nucleus.

Perforating the nuclear envelope are **nuclear pores.** These pores regulate the passage of molecules into the nucleus (such as those needed for construction of RNA and DNA), as well as out of the nucleus (such as RNA, which leaves the nucleus to perform its work in the cytoplasm).

Extending throughout the nucleoplasm (the substance filling the nucleus) are thread-like structures composed of DNA and protein called **chromatin.** When a cell begins to divide, the chromatin coils tightly into short, rod-like structures called **chromosomes**.

In the center of the nucleus is the **nucleolus.** The nucleolus manufactures components of **ribosomes**, the cell's protein producing structures.

Ribosomes

Endoplasmic reticulum (attached to nucleus)

FIGURE 11.2 The nucleus. From Thompson, G. C. (2013). *Understanding anatomy and physiology.* Philadelphia: F.A. Davis, p. 40.

Transcription

DNA double helix

mRNA strand

1 When the nucleus receives a chemical message to make a new protein, the segment of DNA with the relevant gene unwinds.

2 An RNA enzyme then assembles RNA nucleotides that would be complementary to the exposed bases. The nucleotides attach to the exposed DNA and then bind to each other to form a strand of messenger RNA (mRNA). This strand is an exact copy of the opposite side of the DNA molecule.

3 The length of mRNA actually consists of a series of three bases (triplets). Each triplet, called a codon, is the code for one amino acid.

Once formed, the mRNA separates from the DNA molecule and moves through a nuclear pore and into the cytoplasm, where it begins the process of translation.

mRNA strand

Ribosome

Translation

Waiting in the cytoplasm are tRNA molecules. Each tRNA consists of three bases (a triplet called an anticodon) that will perfectly complement a specific site (the codon) on the mRNA. Attached to the tRNA is the amino acid for that site, according to the genetic "blueprint."

Amino acid

tRNA disengages for reuse

The tRNA finds the three bases that are complementary to its own and deposits the amino acid.

The ribosome then uses enzymes to attach the lengthening chain of amino acids together with peptide bonds.

When each triplet has been filled with the correct amino acid and the peptide bonds have been formed, the protein is complete.

FIGURE 11.3 Protein synthesis. From Thompson, G. C. (2013). *Understanding anatomy and physiology.* Philadelphia: F.A. Davis, p. 49.

of cancer, which is a general term for many types of malignant growths.

Mitosis

Mitosis is cell reproduction. One cell, after its 46 chromosomes have replicated, divides into two cells, each with a complete set of chromosomes. Mitosis is necessary for the growth of the body and the replacement of dead or damaged cells. Not all cells are capable of mitosis; of those that are capable, the rate of division varies widely by tissue type. Some cells are capable of only a limited number of divisions; once that limit has been reached and the cells die, they are not replaced. Shortly after birth, almost all neurons lose their ability to divide, and muscle cells have limited mitotic capability. When such cells are lost through injury or disease, the loss of their functions in the individual is usually permanent.

Cell Cycle

The cell cycle involves a series of changes through which a cell progresses, starting from the time it develops until it reproduces itself. The duration of the cell's life, the time it takes for mitosis to occur, the growth ratio (percentage of cycling cells), the frequency of cell loss, and the doubling time (the time for a **tumor**—an abnormal mass—to double its size) are important concepts related to tumor growth and treatment strategies.

At any point in time, some cells are actively dividing, others leave the cycle after a certain point and die, and still others temporarily leave the cycle and remain inactive until reentry into the cycle. Inactive cells continue to synthesize (ribonucleic acid [RNA] and protein; Fig. 11.4).

Cells and Tissues

A tissue is a group of like cells with the same structure and function. The four categories of human tissues are epithelial, connective, muscle, and nervous. Tissues organize into organs; organs construct systems; and systems form the individual. Because of this hierarchy, if a dividing mass of cells is mutated, the abnormality will produce symptoms at the higher levels.

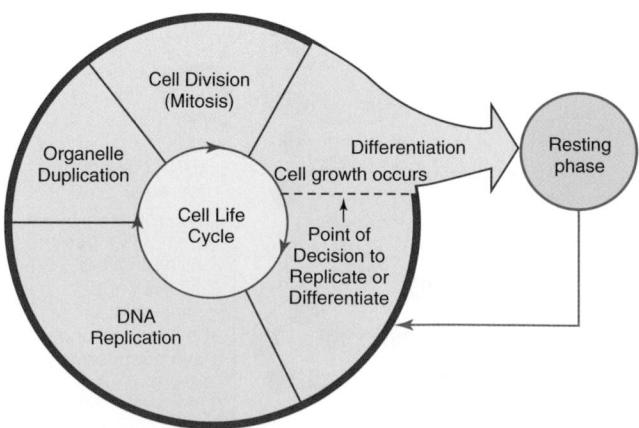

FIGURE 11.4 Cell cycle.

INTRODUCTION TO CANCER CONCEPTS

Oncology is the branch of medicine dealing with tumors. Oncology nursing is also called cancer nursing; it is an important component of medical-surgical nursing care. The National Cancer Institute (NCI) reports that an estimated 13.7 million Americans alive today have a history of cancer (American Cancer Society [ACS], 2013a). Early accounts of cancer date back to the 17th century B.C. Documentation of the benefits of early cancer detection and treatment exist from the beginning of the 19th century. Today, microscopic technology and genetic engineering provide health care providers (HCPs) with a better understanding of tumor growth and cell activity and a means for early cancer detection and intervention. Box 11-1 lists some helpful cancer resources.

Benign Tumors

Cells that reproduce abnormally result in **neoplasms**, or tumors. *Neoplasm* is a term that combines the Greek word *neo,* meaning "new," and *plasia,* meaning "form," to suggest new tissue growth. A **benign** tumor is a cluster of cells that is not normal to the body but is noncancerous. Benign tumors grow more slowly than malignant ones and have cells that are the same as the original tissue. An organ containing a benign tumor usually continues to function normally. A neoplastic growth is difficult to detect until it contains about 500 cells and is about 1 cm in diameter.

Cancer

Cancer is a group of cells that grows out of control, taking over the function of the affected organ. Cancer cells are poorly constructed, loosely formed, and disorganized. A simplistic definition is "confused cell." An organ with a cancerous tumor eventually ceases to function. **Malignant**, a term

• WORD • BUILDING •
oncology: onco—mass + logy—word, reason
neoplasm: neo—new + plasm—form

Box 11-1 **Cancer Resources**
American Cancer Society
800-4-CANCER (422-6237)
www.cancer.org
CancerCare
800-813-HOPE (4673)
www.cancercare.org
www.lungcancer.org
National Cancer Institute
301-496-8531
www.nci.nih.gov
http://cis.nci.nih.gov
Oncology Nursing Society
412-921-7373
www.ons.org

often used to describe cancer, means that the tumor resists treatment and tends to worsen and threaten life. A comparison of benign and malignant tumors is found in Table 11.1.

 NURSING CARE TIP

Teach patients and families that cancer is not contagious.

Pathophysiology

Cancer is not one disease but many diseases with different causes, manifestations, treatments, and prognoses. There are more than 100 types of cancer caused by mutation of cellular genes. Normal cells are limited to about 50 to 60 divisions before they die. Cancer cells do not have a division limit and are considered to be immortal, that is, they keep on dividing, unless they are killed or their host dies.

The progression from a normal cell to a malignant cell follows a pattern of mutation, defective division, abnormal growth cycles, and defective cell communication. Cell mutation occurs when a sudden change affects the chromosomes, causing the new cell to differ from its parent. The malignant cell's enzymes destroy the gluelike substance found between normal cells, which disrupts the transfer of information used for normal cell structure.

Cancer cells also lack **contact inhibition**. Growth-regulating signals in the cells' surrounding environment are ignored as the abnormal cell growth increases. Cells continue to divide and invade surrounding tissues.

Etiology

Cancer cell growth and reproduction involve a two-step process: initiation and promotion. The first step in cancer growth is called *initiation*. Initiation causes an alteration in the genetic structure of the cell (DNA). Cell alteration is associated with exposure to a **carcinogen**, which is a substance or agent that increases the risk of cancer. The cellular change primes the cell to become cancerous.

Promotion is the second step of cancer cell growth. It occurs after repeated exposure to carcinogens causes the initiated cells to mutate. During the promotion step, a tumor forms from mutated cell reproduction.

A healthy immune system can often destroy cancer cells before they replicate and become a tumor. It is important to remember that any substance that weakens or alters the immune system puts the individual at risk for cell mutation. Medical researchers support the theory that cancer is a symptom of a weakened immune system.

Risk Factors

Increased risk of cancer is linked to many environmental factors. An evaluation of cancer begins with assessment of well-known risk factors such as specific viruses; exposure to radiation, chemicals, and irritants; genetics; diet; hormones; and general immunity. Certain racial and ethnic groups also are at higher risk for some types of cancer (see "Cultural Considerations").

• WORD • BUILDING •
carcinogen: karkinos—cancer, crab + genesis—birth

TABLE 11.1 COMPARING BENIGN AND MALIGNANT TUMORS

	Benign	Malignant
Growth rate	Typically slow expansion	Often rapid growth; malignant cells infiltrate surrounding tissue
Cell features	Typical of the tissue of origin	Atypical in varying degrees compared with the tissue of origin; altered cell membrane; contain tumor-specific antigens
Tissue damage	Minor	Often causes necrosis and ulceration of tissue
Metastasis	Not seen; remains localized at site of origin	Often spreads to form tumors in other parts of the body
Recurrence after treatment	Seldom recurs after surgical removal	Recurrence can be seen after surgical removal and following radiation and chemotherapy
Related terminology	Hyperplasia, polyp, benign neoplasia	Cancer, malignancy, malignant neoplasia
Prognosis	Not injurious unless location causes pressure or obstruction to vital organs	Death if uncontrolled

Cultural Considerations

Many racial and ethnic groups in the United States have high rates of cancer. Although risk factors for the development of specific cancers are similar, barriers to prevention and nursing strategies to reduce risk factors vary among ethnicities.

Europeans

Foreign-born and first-generation white men from Norway, Sweden, and Germany have an increased risk of stomach cancer. This suggests an interrelation among ethnic, geographic, and dietary risk factors. Assessing for these data among these populations may assist in the diagnostic process.

Recent Eastern European immigrants may be at risk for thyroid cancer and leukemia because of the current industrial pollution and radiation exposure from the Chernobyl nuclear disaster in the former Soviet Union in 1986. Some contamination occurred in Estonia, Latvia, Lithuania, and Poland. This may constitute a health hazard and may affect both recent immigrants and visitors to these countries. It is essential for HCPs to carefully screen individuals for these cancers.

African Americans

Common cancer sites among African Americans include the prostate, breast, lung, colon, rectum, cervix, pancreas, and esophagus. Because African Americans are overrepresented in the working class, they experience increased exposure to hazardous occupations. For example, African American men are at a higher risk for developing cancer related to their work in the steel and tire industries and in factories manufacturing chemicals and pesticides. They have the highest overall cancer rate and highest overall mortality rate, and their 5-year survival rate is 30% lower than that of European Americans. In general, African Americans report later for treatment than European Americans. Colon tumors may be deeper in African Americans, making detection on digital examination more difficult. Poverty, a diet high in fat and low in fiber, and lower levels of thiamine, riboflavin, vitamins A and C, and iron may increase cancer risk among African Americans. Additionally, cigarette smoking, inner-city living with pollution, obesity, and alcohol consumption increase their risk for developing cancer.

Lack of access to medical care acts as a barrier to prevention among African Americans. Survival, not prevention, is the priority for some. Additional barriers include a lack of cancer risk teaching and detection in some African American communities, lack of health insurance, and little stigma attached to alcohol consumption and smoking. Strong family ties encourage seeking health care advice from family members before professionals.

Primary strategies for preventing cancer and increasing survival among African Americans include using African American professionals as speakers in community activities, using church-based information dissemination, providing forums in African American communities, and addressing smoking advertisements in African American communities. Additional strategies include involving "granny" healers and ministers, changing food preparation practices and amounts rather than changing cultural food habits, involving extended family members in educational campaigns, and using high-profile African American leaders in media campaigns.

Hispanics

Hispanic populations in the United States have an increased incidence for some types of cancer. Cervical cancer is increased among Central and South American women. Pancreatic, liver, and gallbladder cancer is increased among Mexican Americans. Many Mexican Americans are less aware of the early warning signs of cancer; many are more fearful of getting cancer than the general public; and many work in mining, factories using chemicals, and farming using pesticides.

Barriers to preventive health care among many Hispanics include high poverty rates, low educational rates, a preference for HCPs who understand Spanish, a preference for health care information presented in Spanish, a delay in seeking treatments for symptoms, and using lay healers as a first choice in health care. Additionally, many have a fear of surgical intervention because the body will be exposed to air, and many have decreased access to health care. For some, an undocumented immigration status creates a fear of reprisal.

Nursing approaches effective among Hispanics include educating lay healers regarding cancer prevention and early warning signs of cancer, using bilingual HCPs, using Hispanic HCPs whenever available, using respected Hispanic community leaders in educational programs, presenting videos in Spanish using Hispanic actors, educating the entire family because of close family networks, and connecting with Hispanic community churches, restaurants, and stores. Additionally, the nurse can use the 1-800-4-CANCER telephone number for Spanish translation and counseling,

Cultural Considerations—cont'd

become involved with Hispanic community movements, and provide information in community and regional Hispanic newspapers and community publications.

Asians and Pacific Islanders

Cervical, liver, lung, stomach, multiple myeloma, esophageal, pancreatic, and nasopharyngeal cancers are higher among Chinese Americans. Chinese-American women have a 20% higher rate of pancreatic cancer. High rates of stomach and liver cancer in Korea predispose recent immigrants to these conditions. Thus, the nurse needs to assess and teach newer immigrants regarding these types of cancer.

High rates of stomach, breast, colon, and rectal cancer common among Japanese people may be related to the high sodium content of the Japanese diet, a genetic predisposition, consumption of salted fish and contaminated grain, hepatitis B, cigarette smoking, vitamin A deficiency, low vitamin C intake, and chronic esophagitis. Various barriers to prevention exist: prevention models are not native to their culture; they may lack trust in Western medicine; they have decreased access to health care; some are unable to speak the English language; and for some, an undocumented immigration status creates a fear of reprisal.

Nursing approaches to improve cancer risk prevention among Asians and Pacific Islanders include education about prevention versus acute care practice, educating native healers, involvement in the community with respected native leaders, videos and literature in the native language, and incorporating native healing practices such as traditional Chinese medicine.

Arab Americans

Arab Americans are mainly at risk for lung cancer and other cancers related to smoking. Although many Arab Americans are Islamic and Islamic beliefs discourage tobacco use as well as alcohol or drug use, cigarette smoking continues to be a risk behavior among this population. Arab American women are considered very modest, and rates of breast cancer screening and cervical Pap smears are low. Arab Americans tend to lead a sedentary lifestyle with high fat intake, which places them at higher risk for cardiovascular disease as well as certain cancers.

Nursing approaches with this population include promoting awareness and primary prevention strategies. Nurses should encourage cancer screenings and smoking cessation. Because of the modesty of Arab American women, nurses should attempt to ensure that women are given same-sex caregivers to promote breast and cervical cancer screenings.

American Indians/Native Americans

American Indian populations have an increased risk for skin, pancreatic, gallbladder, liver, and prostate cancer. Risk factors for the development of cancer include obesity, a diet high in fat, high rates of alcohol consumption, and high rates of smoking. Barriers to prevention include a lack of American Indian HCPs, HCPs' unfamiliarity with American Indian cultures, lack of financial resources, and a lack of integration of American Indian healing practices into prevention practices.

Nursing approaches to decrease cancer risk prevention among American Indian populations include the following: incorporate prevention into American Indian healing practices; educate American Indian lay healers regarding cancer prevention practices; work with tribal community leaders; respect modesty, gender roles, and tribal customs; work with the Indian Health Service and Bureau of Indian Affairs; encourage traditional customs of physical fitness and exercise; and encourage dietary portion control and healthy food preparation practices instead of changing cultural food habits.

VIRUSES. Certain viruses, such as the **oncoviruses** (RNA-type viruses), are linked to cancer in humans. A retrovirus is an enzyme produced by RNA tumor viruses and is found in human leukemia cells.

The Epstein-Barr virus (EBV), which causes infectious mononucleosis, is associated with Burkitt's lymphoma. Herpes simplex virus 2 has been associated with cervical and penile cancers. Human papillomavirus (HPV) is associated with cervical cancer in women, penile cancer in men, and cancer of the anus and some head and neck cancers in both sexes. Vaccination against HPV (Gardasil®) is recommended for girls and boys age 11 to 12 (Centers for Disease Control, 2013). Chronic hepatitis B is linked with liver cancer.

• **WORD** • **BUILDING** •

oncovirus: onco—mass + virus

RADIATION. There is an increased incidence of cancer in persons exposed to prolonged or large amounts of radiation. Ionizing radiation involving ultraviolet rays such as sunlight, x-rays, and alpha, beta, and gamma rays plays a major role in promoting leukemia and skin cancers, primarily melanomas.

Persons exposed to radioactive materials in large doses, such as a radiation leak or an atomic bomb, are at risk for leukemia and breast, bone, lung, and thyroid cancer. Controlled **radiation therapy** is used to treat cancer patients by destroying rapidly dividing cancer cells, but radiation can also damage normal cells. The decision to use radiation is made after careful evaluation of the tumor's location and vulnerability to other treatments.

CHEMICALS. Chemicals are present in air, water, soil, food, drugs, and tobacco smoke. Chemical carcinogens are implicated as triggering mechanisms in malignant tumor development. Length of exposure time and degree of exposure intensity to chemical carcinogens are associated with risk for cancer development.

Smoking accounts for 90% of lung cancers in men and 80% in women (National Cancer Institute, 2012). Chemical agents, such as those in tobacco, are more toxic when used with alcohol. Alcohol and tobacco are the most frequent causes of cancers of the mouth and throat. Chemicals used in manufacturing, such as vinyl chloride, are associated with liver cancer.

IRRITANTS. Chronic irritation or inflammation caused by irritants such as snuff or pipe smoke often cause cancer in local areas. Nevi (moles) that are chronically irritated by clothing, especially clothing contaminated by chemical residue, can become malignant. Asbestos found in temperature and sound insulation has been proven to cause a particularly destructive type of lung cancer.

GENETICS. Genetics plays a large part in cancer formation. Certain breast cancers are linked to a specific gene mutation. Skin, colon, ovarian, and prostate cancers have a genetic tendency. People with Down syndrome (a chromosomal abnormality) have a higher risk of developing acute leukemia.

DIET. Diet is a major factor in both cause and prevention of malignancies. People who eat high-fat, low-fiber diets are more prone to develop colon cancers. Diets high in fiber reduce the risk of colon cancer. High-fat diets are linked to breast cancer in women and prostate cancer in men. Consumption of large amounts of pickled, smoked, and charbroiled foods has been linked with esophageal and stomach cancers. A diet low in vitamins A, C, and E is associated with cancers of the lungs, esophagus, mouth, larynx, cervix, and breast.

HORMONES. Hormonal agents that disturb the body's balance can also promote cancer. Long-term use of the female hormone estrogen is associated with cancer of the breast, uterus, ovaries, cervix, and vagina. It has been found that children born of mothers who took diethylstilbestrol (DES) during pregnancy have an increased incidence of reproductive cancers. DES is a synthetic hormone with estrogen-like properties that was used in the past to prevent miscarriage.

Tumors of the breast and uterus are tested for estrogen or progesterone influence. If a breast tumor is malignant, the tumor is tested and treatment varies depending on whether it is positive for estrogen or progesterone dependence.

IMMUNE FACTORS. A healthy immune system destroys mutant cells quickly on formation. An individual with impaired immunity is more susceptible to cancer formation when exposed to small amounts of carcinogens compared with someone with a healthy immune system. Immune system suppression allows malignant cells to develop in large numbers.

Altered immunity is noted in persons with chronic illness and stress. An increased risk of cancer follows a traumatic, stressful period in life, such as the loss of a mate or a job. Failure to decrease stress productively contributes to a higher incidence of chronic illnesses. Thus, a cycle of stress, illness, and increased cancer risk develops. People with acquired immunodeficiency syndrome (AIDS) have a compromised immune system and an increased risk for certain cancers. A decline in the immune system and increase in cancer risk is also noted as the body ages.

Cancer Classification

Cancers are identified by the tissue affected, speed of cell growth, cell appearance, and location. Neoplasms occurring in the epithelial cells are called carcinomas. *Carcinoma* is the most common type of cancer and includes cells of the skin, gastrointestinal (GI) system, and lungs (Figs. 11.5 and 11.6). Cancer cells affecting connective tissue, including fat, the sheath that contains nerves, cartilage, muscle, and bone, are called *sarcomas. Leukemia* is the term used to describe the abnormal growth of white blood cells (WBCs). Cancers involving cells of the lymphatic system, lymph nodes, and spleen are called *lymphomas.* See Table 11.2 for cancer types based on origin.

LEARNING TIP

A person's cancer risk results from the balance between exposure and susceptibility to carcinogens.

Metastasis (Spread of Cancer)

Neoplastic cells that remain in one area are considered localized, or **in situ**, cancers. These tumors may be difficult to visualize on clinical examination and are detected

• WORD • BUILDING •
in situ: in—in + situ—position

FIGURE 11.5 Adenocarcinoma of the cecum. *Photo courtesy of Dinesh Patel, MD, Medical Oncology, Internal Medicine, Zanesville, OH.*

FIGURE 11.6 Lung cancer. *Photo courtesy of Dinesh Patel, MD, Medical Oncology, Internal Medicine, Zanesville, OH.*

TABLE 11.2   TUMOR DESCRIPTIONS

Tumor Type	Character	Origin
Fibroma	Benign	Connective tissue
Lipoma	Benign	Fat tissue
Carcinoma	Cancerous	Tissue of the skin, glands, and digestive, urinary, and respiratory tract linings
Leukemia	Cancerous	Blood, plasma cells, and bone marrow
Lymphoma	Cancerous	Lymph tissue
Melanoma	Cancerous	Skin cells
Sarcoma	Cancerous	Connective tissue, including bone and muscle

through microscopic cell examination. In situ tumors are often removed surgically and may require no further treatment. **Metastasis** is the term used to describe the spread of the tumor from the primary site into separate and distant areas.

Metastasis is the stage at which cancer cells acquire invasive behavior characteristics and cause the surrounding tissue to change (Fig. 11.7). Metastasis occurs mainly because cancer cells break away more easily than normal cells and can survive for a time independently from other cells. There are three steps in the formation of a metastasis. Cancer cells are able to (1) invade blood or lymph vessels, (2) move by mechanical means, and (3) lodge and grow in a new location.

Metastatic tumors carry with them the cell characteristics of the original or primary tumor site. As a result, surgeons are able to determine the original tumor site based on metastatic cell characteristics. For example, lung tissue found in the brain suggests a primary lung tumor with metastasis to brain tissue. Common sites of metastasis are the lungs, liver, bones, and brain.

Incidence of Cancer

Cancer affects all age groups, although the incidence is higher in people aged 60 to 69 years. The second highest age group is ages 70 to 79. Men have a higher incidence of cancer than women. Cancer in people over age 60 is thought to occur from a combination of exposure to carcinogens and weakening of the body's immune system.

Some cancers, such as Wilms's tumor of the kidney and acute lymphocytic leukemia, are more common in young people. The cause of tumors in young people is not well understood, but genetic predisposition tends to be a major factor.

The most common type of cancer in adults is skin cancer; it is also considered to be the most preventable. Exposure to

• WORD • BUILDING •
metastasis: meta—beyond + stasis—stand

FIGURE 11.7 Invasive metastasis to skin area following mastectomy for breast cancer. *Photo courtesy of Dinesh Patel, MD, Medical Oncology, Internal Medicine, Zanesville, OH.*

ultraviolet radiation (sunlight) increases the risk of skin cancer. Wearing protective clothing and sunscreen can greatly reduce the risk of skin cancer.

Lung cancer has the highest of the cancer mortality rates in both men and women and also is commonly preventable. Cigarette smoking is the main cause, along with air pollution and exposure to radon and other chemicals.

Men have a high incidence of prostate cancer between ages 60 and 79. Cancer of the colon and rectum has been linked to consumption of high-fat, low-fiber diets and ranks as the third highest cancer in men.

The highest incidence of cancer in women is in the breast. Women with a family history of breast cancer have a greater risk than those with no family history. Commercial testing for the oncogene linked with breast cancer is available and marketed for high-risk women, especially those in the Ashkenazi Jewish population. Genetic testing is done through genetic counseling programs, and the cost ranges from $700 to $2400, depending on the geographic region. See Figure 11.8 for estimated new cancer cases and deaths for 2013.

Mortality Rates

Cancer survival rates have improved during the past 30 years and, since the 1990s, the number of cancer deaths has decreased for both men and women. A 5-year period is used to monitor cancer patients' progress following diagnosis and treatment. Survival statistics are based on those who live 5 years in remission. Remission is considered to have occurred when all signs and symptoms of cancer have disappeared, even though there may still be cancer in the body.

For more information about cancer incidence and mortality data, visit the National Cancer Institute website at www.cancer.gov or the American Cancer Society at www.cancer.org.

Early Detection and Prevention

Nurses play an important role in preventing and detecting cancer. You can help educate patients about risk factors, self-examination, and cancer screening programs. Early diagnosis and treatment provide time to stop the progression of cancer.

EARLY DETECTION. Regular physical examinations help HCPs detect early warning signs of cancer. The American Cancer Society recommends mammography (a special x-ray of breast tissue used to detect a mass too small for palpation) is recommended every 1 to 2 years in women after age 40 (some sources say after age 50). The U.S. Preventive Services Task Force (2009), however, recommends beginning mammography at age 50 and screening every 2 years. All women should discuss their individual risk factors and frequency of screening with their physicians. A clinical breast exam is recommended every 3 years for women in their 20s

---

Estimated New Cases*

Male

Prostate
238,590 (28%)

Lung and bronchus
118,080 (14%)

Colon and rectum
73,680 (9%)

Urinary bladder
54,610 (6%)

Melanoma of the skin
45,060 (5%)

Kidney and renal pelvis
40,430 (5%)

Non-Hodgkin lymphoma
37,600 (4%)

Oral cavity and pharynx
29,620 (3%)

Leukemia
27,880 (3%)

Pancreas
22,740 (3%)

All sites
854,790 (100%)

Female

Breast
232,340 (29%)

Lung and bronchus
110,110 (14%)

Colon and rectum
69,140 (9%)

Uterine corpus
49,560 (6%)

Thyroid
45,310 (6%)

Non-Hodgkin lymphoma
32,140 (4%)

Melanoma of the skin
31,630 (4%)

Kidney and renal pelvis
24,270 (3%)

Pancreas
22,480 (3%)

Ovary
22,240 (3%)

All sites
805,500 (100%)

Estimated Deaths

Male

Lung and bronchus
87,260 (30%)

Prostate
29,720 (10%)

Colon and rectum
26,300 (9%)

Pancreas
19,480 (6%)

Liver and intrahepatic bile duct
14,890 (5%)

Leukemia
13,660 (4%)

Esophagus
12,220 (4%)

Urinary bladder
10,820 (4%)

Non-Hodgkin lymphoma
10,590 (3%)

Kidney and renal pelvis
8,780 (3%)

All sites
306,920 (100%)

Female

Lung and bronchus
72,220 (26%)

Breast
39,620 (14%)

Colon and rectum
24,530 (9%)

Pancreas
18,980 (7%)

Ovary
14,030 (5%)

Leukemia
10,060 (4%)

Non-Hodgkin lymphoma
8,430 (3%)

Uterine corpus
8,190 (3%)

Liver and intrahepatic bile duct
6,780 (2%)

Brain and other nervous system
6,150 (2%)

All sites
273,430 (100%)

*Excludes basal and squamous cell skin cancers and in situ carcinoma except urinary bladder.

FIGURE 11.8 Leading new cancer cases and deaths—2013 estimates. *From the American Cancer Society, Cancer Facts & Figures 2013. Retrieved June 5, 2013, from www.cancer.org/acs /groups/content/@epidemiologysurveilance/documents/document/acspc-037129.pdf*

and 30s and annually after age 40 (ACS, 2013b). However, if a woman has a high risk for breast cancer because of family history, the type and frequency of screening should be discussed with her doctor.

Initial Papanicolaou testing (Pap smear) for cervical cancer is currently recommended to begin no later than age 21 and performed every 3 years up to age 29. The preferred approach for women aged 30 to 65 is to have the Pap test with an HPV test, also referred to as cotesting, every 5 years, but it is acceptable to have just the Pap test every 3 years in this age group (ACS, 2013b). After age 65, a woman who has had three normal Pap tests in a row within the past 10 years can choose to stop screening.

Some women choose not to be screened, even when they have access to health care. Barriers to screening include fear of health care personnel and testing procedures, as well as lack of knowledge. Women who fear cancer but trust their HCPs and seek information are more likely to be screened. As a nurse, you can help by developing a trusting relationship and providing information to your female patients.

The ACS considers monthly breast self-examinations to be optional for women and testicular self-examinations to be optional for men. ACS guidelines encourage everyone to be familiar with their bodies and to report changes to their HCPs. Offer men and women instruction in breast and testicular self-examinations if they are interested in doing them.

The ACS (2013b) recommends one of the following options to screen for colorectal cancer, beginning at age 50:

Tests that find polyps and cancer

• Flexible sigmoidoscopy every 5 years
• Colonoscopy every 10 years
• Double-contrast barium enema every 5 years
• Colonography (virtual colonoscopy using computed tomography) every 5 years.

Tests that mainly find cancer

• Fecal occult blood test every year
• Fecal immunochemical test every year

If any tests are positive, a colonoscopy should be done.

Before 2009, the ACS recommended annual digital rectal examination and prostate-specific antigen (PSA) blood testing for men aged older than 50 years with a life expectancy of at least 10 years and for younger men at higher risk. More recently, ACS withdrew this recommendation because routine screening has not been shown to prolong lives (ACS, 2013b). It seems reasonable, however, to still offer these tests as options to men in these populations.

GENETIC TESTING. Currently, much attention is directed toward genetic testing and identification of persons at risk for cancer. Genetic testing technology poses both legal and ethical questions concerning confidentiality and insurance cost issues. The cooperation of family members is important because genetic testing is done after a family member has been diagnosed with cancer. Family members may experience a variety of emotions surrounding the increased risk for themselves and their guilt over the role they may have played in increasing the risk for their children.

HEALTHY LIFESTYLE. Promotion of healthy lifestyles, including proper diet and exercise, helps strengthen the immune system and reduce cancer risk. Smoking is the most preventable cause of death from lung cancer, and smoking cessation is the subject of ongoing campaigns by the American Cancer Society. Secondhand smoke contributes to a significant increased risk of lung cancer in nonsmokers as well.

PROTECTANT FOODS. Much research related to diet and cancer risk is being conducted. A diet poor in folate, a B vitamin, can lead to development of cancers of the colon, rectum, and breast. Folate is best obtained by eating fruits, vegetables, and enriched grain products.

People who ingest a diet high in saturated fat are at a greater risk of obesity, which can be a risk factor for colon, prostate, and breast cancers.

A diet rich in vegetables and fruits can reduce the risk of lung, oral, esophageal, stomach, and colon cancer. The ACS recommends eating a variety of fresh fruits and vegetables daily. Because it is not known which compounds in vegetables and fruits are actually beneficial, there are no supplements that can take the place of eating whole foods. Frozen and canned foods can be healthy alternatives, but be careful to read labels for ingredients.

See www.cancer.org and "Nutrition Notes—Reducing Cancer Risk" for additional dietary recommendations.

 Nutrition Notes

Reducing Cancer Risk

Throughout life, excessive energy (calorie) intake and obesity increase cancer risk.
Proportions of meals should be:
• 2/3 (or more) vegetables, fruits, whole grains, and legumes
• 1/3 (or less) animal protein
Selections should be varied and include:
• Vitamin C rich fruits (e.g., oranges, cantaloupe, strawberries)
• Cruciferous vegetables (e.g., cabbage, broccoli, Brussels sprouts, cauliflower)
• Low-fat dairy products
Consumption of the following should be limited:
• Excessive red meat, especially when
  • processed (smoked, salted)
  • charbroiled or cooked at high temperatures
• Excessive fat, especially saturated fat
• Highly processed carbohydrates
• Recommended alcohol intake, if any, should be limited to one (women) or two (men) standard drinks per day (12 oz. of beer, 5 oz. of wine, or 1.5 oz. distilled spirits)

VACCINES. Preventive vaccines are being developed for cancers associated with specific viruses. Gardasil (a vaccine for HPV) can be given to prevent a variety of cancers, as mentioned earlier.

Most cancer vaccines are therapeutic rather than prophylactic and are used to stimulate the patient's immune system to destroy cancer cells. Currently, the only therapeutic cancer vaccine approved by the Food and Drug Administration is sipuleucel-T for the treatment of advanced prostate cancer that no longer responds to hormone therapy (ACS, 2013c). Vaccine therapy for malignant melanoma and lymphoma is being tested.

Diagnosis of Cancer

A cancer diagnosis is a frightening experience (see "Patient Perspective"). Often, people try to mask symptoms because they are so frightened of the disease. A physical examination along with careful and thorough assessment of the patient's current status, medical and surgical histories, and pertinent family history should be completed. The most conclusive information about the health of tissue is acquired by examining cell activity through biopsy.

For explanations of the following tests, see Appendix A.

Patient Perspective

I am a 43-year-old woman with three children and in the prime of my life—at least that's what I thought. That was before I was diagnosed with cancer in my left breast. I was breastfeeding at the time I felt the lump and, although I went for a biopsy, I felt sure the lump resulted from a blocked milk duct or fibroid cyst. But, unbelievably, the biopsy came back positive for cancer. My whole life flipped upside down. I was devastated.

I was scheduled for surgery within a week, and my emotions were in complete turmoil. I felt nauseated all the time, vomited almost every morning, and had diarrhea daily. My stomach felt like it had a pot of bees inside. I never cried so much in my life. Thinking about all the tests, the surgery, and the untold ways my life could be affected made me a nervous wreck. Finally, I got down on my knees and turned this whole crisis over to God. I couldn't handle it anymore, so I asked God to give me peace, and I placed all my trust and faith in Him. It worked, and I was finally able to get control and face this thing head-on.

As I went for further testing, everyone made me feel like I was the at the center of the care system because wherever I went, whatever tests I had done, there were always compassionate nurses and technicians who either directed me to others who had suffered from breast cancer in their facility or were going through the treatments and told me to come and talk to them if I ever needed help or support or just had any questions. Some actually broke down with me because they had endured this same disease. We would hold each other and then exchange phone numbers just to talk if I needed it. It was very encouraging to know these women had made it through, and I could too.

The surgery went smoothly, and I was released the next day. There wasn't much discomfort, and I felt good physically. The nerve was removed, and a scar runs from the center of my chest down under my armpit. I was able to return to work in 3 weeks. The doctor gave me a prescription for a prosthesis as soon as the drains were removed and I began healing. We went to a specialty place to be fitted, and, although the prosthesis was nothing like the real thing, I looked normal, and it helped to build my confidence.

The impact on my family was one of complete bewilderment because I had no family history of this type of cancer. Everyone tried to help with positive sentiments like "we caught it early," "breast cancer has a high cure rate," "periodic follow-up can keep you cancer free," and so on. My husband and children supported and comforted me. I tried to focus on them because I want to be there for them when they graduate, get married, etc. My mother and sister helped get me to all my appointments and filled my prescriptions.

Chemo was advised as a follow-up treatment, and I was scheduled for four rounds, one every 3 weeks. This was undoubtedly the worst thing I have ever endured. Not even giving birth can compare to the way chemo makes you feel. I had a very bad experience the first round and was extremely sick and unable to eat for 5 days. I wondered why I didn't just die from the cancer because I felt that this was killing me. Before the second round, I told the doctor how violently ill I'd been, and she adjusted the dosages of some of the drugs. I was very groggy; although I didn't vomit, I still wasn't feeling myself. For the third round, they changed a medication and I withstood the side effects a lot better—although I was still nauseated, lightheaded, fatigued, and unable to focus, eat, or taste anything. At times, it was hard just to put one foot in front of the other. They prepared me for the loss of my hair, but you really don't know how hard that is until it starts coming out in globs. Not just the loss, but then you have such a long time to wait for it to grow back. When the chemo is over, it's hard to look back and feel the way you did then, but when you look in the mirror and your hair is still gone, it's a hard reminder.

All through being diagnosed and dealing with breast cancer I have felt a tremendous outpouring of love and caring, not only from my immediate family but also from my church family. I was never so well taken care of. All the hugs, cards, calls, food, and flowers brought to the house encouraged me tremendously. It makes it a little easier to cope when you know you have so many people who care and are concerned enough to take time out of their daily lives to give you support.

I'm lucky because my sister is an RN and prepared me for many of the side effects and difficulties. She was also there to help ask questions and get information from other survivors that kept me in a positive frame of mind. I know that without her help and God's grace and peace, my recovery would not have been so easy. Looking back I can't really feel all those terrible emotions and symptoms, but I still am afraid of the unknown. It is not easy when it is you and not someone else this happens to.

Now that I'm through the worst part of this, I take positive steps every day to enjoy the little things in life. I feel that the more you keep involved in everyday activities and become educated about the disease and its treatments, the easier it is to deal with. I am taking a drug called tamoxifen now and will be for 5 years. Two of the side effects are hot flashes and sweats. If this is all I have to deal with, however, praise God. My prognosis is very good, and I am expecting a complete cure because I am a survivor.

FIGURE 11.10 Stereotactic biopsy of a brain lesion. *Photo courtesy of Dinesh Patel, MD, Medical Oncology, Internal Medicine, Zanesville, OH.*

FIGURE 11.11 Mammogram. *Photo courtesy of Dinesh Patel, MD, Medical Oncology, Internal Medicine, Zanesville, OH.*

BIOPSY. Accurate identification of a cancer can be made only by **biopsy**. Microscopic examination of a sample of suspected tissue or aspirated body fluid can confirm the presence of mutant cells. A biopsy is commonly done in an HCP's office or outpatient surgery department. See Figures 11.9 and 11.10 for two types of biopsy.

RADIOLOGICAL PROCEDURES. X-ray examination is a valuable diagnostic tool in detecting cancer of the bones and hollow organs. Chest x-ray examination is one diagnostic test used in detecting lung cancer. Mammography is a reliable and noninvasive low-radiation x-ray procedure for detecting breast masses (Fig. 11.11).

Contrast media x-ray studies are used to detect abnormalities of bone and the GI and urinary systems. Contrast media can be given by various methods. Barium is given orally for visualization of the esophagus and stomach or rectally as a barium enema for visualization of the colon. IV injection of contrast media is used for lung and brain scans.

Computed tomography (CT) scans are important in the diagnosis and staging of malignancies and can detect minor variations in tissue thickness. The use of a contrast medium enhances the accuracy of an abdominal CT scan. CT scans are also used to improve the accuracy of inserting a fine needle for biopsy.

NUCLEAR IMAGING PROCEDURES. Nuclear medicine imaging involves camera imaging of organs or tissues containing radioactive media. Radioactive compounds are given intravenously or by mouth. These studies are highly sensitive and

FIGURE 11.9 Fine-needle breast biopsy. *Photo courtesy of Dinesh Patel, MD, Medical Oncology, Internal Medicine, Zanesville, OH.*

can detect sites of abnormal cell growth months before changes are seen on an x-ray.

Positron emission tomography (PET) scanning provides information about cellular function. Patients are given biochemical compounds, and images are made of the tissue through gamma-camera tomography. PET scans have been useful in brain imaging as well as the detection of the spread of cancers of the lung, ovaries, colon, rectum, and breast.

ULTRASOUND PROCEDURES. Ultrasonography helps detect tumors of the pelvis and breast. Ultrasound also may be used to distinguish between benign and malignant breast tumors.

MAGNETIC RESONANCE IMAGING. Magnetic resonance imaging (MRI) is valuable in the detection, localization, and staging of malignant tumors in the central nervous system, spine, head, and musculoskeletal system.

ENDOSCOPIC PROCEDURES. An endoscopic examination allows the direct visualization of a body cavity or opening. Endoscopy enables the surgeon to biopsy tissue and is used to detect lesions of the throat, esophagus, stomach, colon, and lungs.

LABORATORY TESTS. For normal values for the following laboratory tests, see Appendix B. Blood, serum, and urine tests are important in establishing baseline values and general health status. An elevated white blood cell (WBC) count is expected if the patient has evidence of infection; however, an increase in WBCs without infection raises suspicion of leukemia. Fifty percent of patients with liver cancer have increased levels of bilirubin, alkaline phosphatase, and glutamic-oxaloacetic transaminase.

Bone marrow aspiration is done to learn the number, size, and shape of RBCs, WBCs, and platelets. Bone marrow aspiration is a major tool for diagnosis of leukemia. (See Chapter 27 for a description of this test and related nursing care.) Tumor markers, also called biochemical markers, are proteins, antigens, genes, hormones, and enzymes produced and secreted by tumor cells. Tumor markers help confirm a diagnosis of cancer, detect cancer origin, monitor the effect of cancer therapy, and determine cancer remission. Some examples of tumor markers are shown in Table 11.3.

CYTOLOGICAL STUDY. Cytology is the study of the formation, structure, and function of cells. Cytological diagnosis of cancer is obtained mainly through Pap smears of cells shed from a mucous membrane (e.g., cervical, anal, or oral). Test results are based on the degree of cell abnormality. Slight cellular changes are considered normal, with a possible link to abnormal cells seen in infection. Significant cellular changes reflect a higher probability of precancerous or cancerous activity.

Staging and Grading

Tumor staging is used to determine the stage of solid tumor masses, providing valuable information to guide treatment plans. The most common system used for staging is the

TABLE 11.3 TUMOR MARKERS AND ASSOCIATED CANCERS

Tumor Marker	Associated Cancer
Alpha-fetoprotein (AFP)	Hepatocellular cancer
Cancer antigen (CA) 15-3	Breast cancer (useful in monitoring patient response to therapy for metastatic breast cancer)
CA 125	Ovarian, cervical, liver, and pancreatic cancers
CA 19-9	Colorectal, pancreatic, and hepatobiliary cancers (used to aid diagnosis and evaluation)
Carcinoembryonic antigen (CEA)	Colon and rectal cancers
Prostatic acid phosphatase (PAP)	Prostate cancer
Prostate-specific antigen (PSA)	Prostate cancer

tumor-node-metastasis (TNM) system, an international system that allows comparison of statistics among cancer centers. This staging system classifies solid tumors by size and degree of spread (Table 11.4). For example, a breast cancer staged as T3 N2 MX is a large breast cancer that has spread to regional lymph nodes, but metastasis cannot be evaluated at this time.

The TNM ratings correspond with one of five stages, but stages may differ based on the type of cancer. In general, the lower the number of the stage, the less the cancer has spread. A higher number means a more serious situation exists. In this classification system, stages range from stage 0 (tumor in situ, no invasion of other tissues) to stage IV (distant metastasis to other sites).

A rating system has also been established to define the cell types of tumors. Tumors are classified according to the percentage of cells that are differentiated (mature). If the tissue of a neoplastic tumor closely resembles normal tissue, it is called *well differentiated*. A *poorly differentiated* tumor is a malignant neoplasm that contains some normal cells, but most of the cells are abnormal. The better defined or differentiated the tumor, the easier it is to treat.

Treatment for Cancer

There are three main types of treatment for cancer: surgery, radiation therapy, and chemotherapy. To find out more about cancer treatment options, visit the ACS website at www.cancer.org.

TABLE 11.4 TUMOR-NODE-METASTASIS SYSTEM FOR CANCER STAGING

Primary Tumor (T)	
TX	Primary tumor cannot be evaluated
T0	No evidence of primary tumor
Tis	Carcinoma in situ (early cancer that has not spread to neighboring tissue)
T1, T2, T3, T4	Size and/or extent of the primary tumor
Regional Lymph Nodes (N)	
NX	Regional lymph nodes cannot be evaluated
N0	No regional lymph node involvement
N1, N2, N3	Involvement of regional lymph nodes (number and location of lymph nodes)
Distant Metastasis (M)	
MX	Distant metastasis cannot be evaluated
M0	No distant metastasis
M1	Distant metastasis

Note: From the U.S. National Institutes of Health. Updated 2013. *Cancer staging.* Retrieved July 6, 2013, from www.cancer.gov/cancertopics /factsheet/detection/staging

SURGERY. Surgery can be curative when it is possible to remove the entire tumor. Skin cancers and well-defined tumors without metastasis can be removed without any additional intervention. For some tumors, as much of the tumor is removed as possible (this is called debulking), and follow-up chemotherapy or radiation is used to treat the remaining tumor cells.

Prophylactic surgery is used to remove moles or lesions that have the potential to become malignant. Colon polyps are often removed to prevent malignancies from developing, especially if the polyps are considered premalignant. An extreme example of prophylactic surgery is a woman who elects to have a mastectomy (surgical removal of the breast) because of a high incidence of breast cancer in her family.

Surgery also may be done for **palliation** (symptom control). Surgical removal of tissue to reduce the size of the tumor mass is helpful, especially if the tumor is compressing nerves or blocking the passage of body fluids. The goals of palliative surgery are to increase comfort and quality of life.

Reconstructive surgery can be done for cosmetic enhancement or for return of function of a body part. Facial reconstruction is important for a patient's self-image after removal of head or neck tumors. Women can elect to have breast reconstruction after mastectomy.

Nurses should encourage patients to express and discuss their fears. Patients with a limited understanding of cancer may fear that tissues will not heal postoperatively. Provide information about wound care, including dressing changes and drainage tubes, to increase the patient's knowledge base and sense of control. Visual aids concerning tumor site and surgical procedures are valuable teaching tools.

Patients who are undernourished are poor surgical candidates and require intervention such as enteral or parenteral nutrition before and after surgery. Patients with cancer also are at increased risk for postoperative deep venous thrombosis (DVT). Preoperative teaching includes the importance of leg movement, early ambulation, wearing antiembolism stockings, and recognizing symptoms of DVT, such as calf redness, warmth, or pain.

RADIATION. Radiation is used commonly in cancer control and palliation, and it can be curative if the disease is localized. The decision to use radiation is commonly based on cancer site and size. Radiation destroys cancer cells by affecting cell structure and the cell environment. It is used in fractionated (divided) doses to prevent destructive side effects; however, side effects can occur in the area being treated because of damage to normal cells.

Radiation can be used before surgery to decrease the size of a large tumor, making surgical intervention more effective and less dangerous, or it can be used after surgery as adjuvant treatment. Palliative radiation is used to reduce the size of a large cancerous lesion and consequently reduce pressure and pain. Radioisotopes can be inserted into cancerous tissue during surgery to help destroy cancerous cells without removing the organ. This is called brachytherapy.

Nursing Care of the Patient Receiving Radiation Treatment. Symptoms of tissue reaction to radiation can be expected about 10 to 14 days after treatment starts and continue for up to 2 to 4 weeks after treatment ends. Typical reactions and appropriate nursing interventions include the following:

- *Fatigue:* Encourage the patient to nap often and prioritize activities. Reassure the patient that the feeling will go away after the treatments are completed.
- *Nausea, vomiting, and* **anorexia**: Encourage the patient to take prescribed medication for nausea and vomiting. Anorexia can be eased by providing small amounts of high-carbohydrate, high-protein foods and avoiding foods high in fiber.
- ***Mucositis*** (*inflammation of mucous membranes, especially of the mouth and throat*): Urge the patient to avoid irritants such as smoking, alcohol, acidic food or drinks, extremely hot or cold foods and drinks, and commercial mouthwash. Advise the patient to perform mouth care before meals and every 3 to 4 hours. A neutral mouthwash can be made by using 1 ounce of diphenhydramine

• WORD • BUILDING •

anorexia: an—not + orexis—appetite
mucositis: muco—mucous (membrane) + itis—inflammation

hydrochloride (Benadryl) elixir diluted in 1 quart of water or normal saline solution. Agents that coat the mouth, such as calcium carbonate (Maalox), are sometimes used. Lidocaine hydrochloride 2% viscous has an anesthetic effect on the mouth and throat.

• *Xerostomia (dry mouth):* Encourage frequent mouth care. Saliva substitute is available over the counter and is helpful, especially at night when patients describe a choking sensation from extreme dryness.

• *Skin reactions:* These can vary from mild redness to moist **desquamation** (peeling skin) similar to a second-degree burn. Skin surfaces that are warm and moist, such as the groin, perineum, and axillae, are especially vulnerable. Prophylactic skin care includes keeping skin dry; keeping it free from irritants, such as powder, lotions, deodorants, and restrictive clothing; and protecting it from exposure to direct sunlight. Irradiated skin can be fragile during treatment. It is important to wash these areas gently with mild soap and water, rinse well, and pat dry. The skin may have markings or tattoos to delineate the treatment field. Take care not to wash off the markings.

• *Bone marrow depression:* Low blood cell counts occur with both radiation and chemotherapy because they can attack all rapidly dividing cells, not just cancer cells. Weekly blood cell counts are done to detect low levels of white blood cells, red blood cells, and platelets. Transfusions of whole blood, platelets, or other blood components may be needed.

Safety Considerations. Radiation may be administered externally or internally. External radiation is given by a trained medical specialist in a designated area in a hospital or clinic. Patients receiving external radiation therapy do not emit radioactive material and do not require any safety precautions before or after treatment.

Internal radiation is administered to patients admitted to a health care facility. Safety guidelines must be followed when caring for a patient with internal radioactive materials that have been implanted into tissue or body cavities or administered orally or intravenously, because the patient will be radioactive. Nursing responsibilities include knowledge about the following:

• Radiation source being used
• Method of administration
• Start of treatment
• Length of treatment
• Prescribed nursing precautions

Personnel involved with radiation therapy must recognize three primary factors to protect themselves: time, distance, and shielding. These three factors depend on the type of radiation used. *Time* involves the time spent administering care, *distance* involves the amount of space between the radioisotope and the nurse, and *shielding* involves the use of a barrier such as a lead apron.

You must work efficiently when caring for patients who are receiving radioisotopes that are releasing gamma rays. Your exposure to radiation is proportionate to the time spent and the distance from the radiation source. For example, you will receive less exposure standing at the foot of the bed of a patient with radioisotopes inserted into the head than if you stand at the head of the bed (Fig. 11.12). Principles of time and distance are used to protect the nurse, visitors, and other personnel.

It is important to teach the patient and family members the reason nursing care focuses on providing only essential care. Speedy nursing encounters and visitor restrictions are better

---

• WORD • BUILDING •

xerostomia: xero—dry + stoma—mouth
desquamation: de—down, from + squamation—epidermis

Nurse A   Nurse B   Nurse C
(2 feet away)   (4 feet away)   (8 feet away)

FIGURE 11.12 Radiation distancing. Nurse B receives less radiation than Nurse A, and Nurse C receives less radiation than Nurse B.

accepted and less likely to promote feelings of isolation when patients understand the reasons behind them.

Drainage from the site of a radioactive colloid injection is considered radioactive, and the HCP must be informed immediately if it occurs. Dressings contaminated with radioactive seepage must be removed with long-handled forceps. Radioactive materials must never be touched with unprotected hands; shielding is required to prevent exposure to radiation. Contamination from radioisotope applicators or interstitial implants cannot occur when the capsule is intact; contamination occurs when the capsule is broken.

BE SAFE!

BE VIGILANT! Remember to use the principles of time, distance, and shielding to protect yourself from radiation exposure.

CHEMOTHERAPY. Chemotherapy is chemical therapy that uses **cytotoxic** drugs to treat cancer. Cytotoxic drugs can be used for cure, control, or palliation of cancerous tumors. They are classified according to how they affect cell activity. Examples of specific drugs are listed in Tables 11.5 and 11.6.

The effects of chemotherapy are systemic unless used topically for skin lesions. Chemotherapy is used preoperatively to shrink tumors and postoperatively to treat residual tumors. Tumor type and genetics influence the effectiveness of chemotherapy. Age is also a consideration, but treatment should be based on physiological age rather than chronological age. That is, just because a patient might be 70 years old doesn't mean his body is the same as that of other 70-year-olds.

Combination Chemotherapy. In this kind of therapy, two or more antineoplastic agents are used together to treat the patient's cancer. This can expose a larger number of cells at

• WORD • BUILDING •
chemotherapy: chemo—chemistry + therapy—treatment
cytotoxic: cyto—cell + toxic—poison

TABLE 11.5 INJECTABLE CANCER CHEMOTHERAPY MEDICATIONS

Medication Class/Action	Examples	Nursing Implications
Antitumor Antibiotics Damage cells' DNA and the ability to make DNA and RNA.	doxorubicin (Adriamycin, Doxil)	This drug is a vesicant and should be given through a running IV or a central line if it is a continuous infusion. Turns urine red. Doxil is less irritating than Adriamycin. Monitor cardiac status. Lifetime dose is 550 mg/m^2.
Antimetabolites	cytarabine (Cytosar, Ara-C)	Check CBC before each dose. Review the signs of infection or bleeding. Instruct patient to call primary care provider for any temperature increases greater than 100.0°F (37.8°C).
	fluorouracil (5-FU)	Check CBC before the dose. Nadir occurs in 10–14 days. Instruct about mouth care.
	gemcitabine (Gemzar)	Check CBC before each dose. Premedicate with antiemetics. Instruct patient to report flu-like symptoms to primary care provider.
Alkylating Agents Cause the DNA strands to bind together and prevent the cell from dividing.	cisplatin (Platinol)	Monitor neurologic status, renal function studies. Premedicate with antiemetics. Monitor for signs of anaphylaxis. Nadir occurs in 2–3 weeks; check CBC before each dose.

Continued

TABLE 11.5 INJECTABLE CANCER CHEMOTHERAPY MEDICATIONS—cont'd

Medication Class/Action	Examples	Nursing Implications
		Ensure adequate hydration to prevent renal failure.
	cyclophosphamide (Cytoxan)	Check CBC before each dose. Monitor BUN and creatinine levels. Ensure adequate hydration to prevent renal failure. Oral form should be taken early in the morning to keep drug from building up in the bladder at night.
	ifosfamide (Ifex)	Monitor urine for blood. Given with Mesna (Mesnex) to prevent hemorrhagic cystitis. Ensure adequate hydration before and after each dose. Premedicate with antiemetics. Monitor CBC.
Antimitotic Agents Come from plant sources. Prevent mitosis from occurring in the cell and then cells cannot divide.	docetaxel (Taxotere)	Patient must take dexamethasone starting 1 day before scheduled chemotherapy to prevent hypersensitivity. Monitor CBC. Nadir occurs on day 7. Monitor weight. Assess skin for changes. Watch for changes in neurologic status from baseline.
	paclitaxel, nanoparticle albumin bound (Abraxane)	Watch for signs of hypersensitivity. Monitor CBC and platelet counts. Watch for changes in neurologic status from baseline. Teach mouth care. Monitor vital signs for changes.
	vincristine (Oncovin)	Drug is a vesicant and should be given through a running IV. Assess for neuropathies and changes in neurologic status from baseline. Monitor CBC and platelets.
	vinorelbine (Navelbine)	Drug is a vesicant. When giving through a running IV, use the port closest to the IV bag rather than the patient. Check CBC before each dose. Nadir occurs in 7–10 days. Teach signs of infection and bleeding. Monitor neurologic status and changes from baseline. Teach mouth care.
Topoisomerase Inhibitors Inhibit enzyme topoisomerase to interfere with DNA synthesis.	irinotecan (Camptosar)	Teach measures to control diarrhea, and patient to contact primary care provider if it occurs.

TABLE 11.5 INJECTABLE CANCER CHEMOTHERAPY MEDICATIONS—cont'd

Medication Class/Action	Examples	Nursing Implications
		Dose of loperamide may be higher than normal—verify with provider. Check CBC before each dose.
	topotecan (Hycamtin)	Monitor CBC. Premedicate for nausea.
Hormones Synthetic analog of luteinizing hormone-releasing hormone, causes decrease in testosterone levels.	leuprolide (Lupron)	Monitor PSA results.
Angiogenesis Inhibitors Blocks formation of new blood vessels to slow growth and spread of cancer.	bevacizumab (Avastin)	Assess for pregnancy. Avoid administration after surgery.
Monoclonal Antibodies Bind to receptor sites on cancer cells to inhibit proliferation.	alemtuzumab (Campath), trastuzumab (Herceptin), gemtuzumab (Mylotarg), cetuximab (Erbitux), ipilimumab (Yervoy)	Watch for signs of allergic reaction.

Note: BUN = blood urea nitrogen; CBC = complete blood count; DNA = deoxyribonucleic acid; PSA = prostate-specific antigen; PT = prothrombin time; WBC = white blood cell.

TABLE 11.6 ORAL CANCER CHEMOTHERAPY MEDICATIONS

Medication Class/Action	Examples	Nursing Implications
Tyrosine kinase inhibitor Targets abnormal proteins on surfaces of some cancer cells to block the signals for cells to replicate.	imatinib mesylate (Gleevec), erlotinib (Tarceva)	Supportive care for nausea, diarrhea, tumor lysis syndrome. Monitor lab studies for decrease in WBC and platelet counts. Tarceva: Should be taken on an empty stomach to prevent raising the level of the drug in the body.
Immunomodulating agent Affects immune system function. Angiogenesis effect: prevents blood vessels from growing, which prevents tumor from growing.	lenalidomide (Revlimid)	Pregnancy must be avoided due to the risk for serious birth defects. Monitor labs and electrolytes.
Alkylating agent Interferes with the ability of the cells to replicate.	temozolomide (Temodar)	Monitor labs for WBC and platelet counts routinely while on Temodar. Supportive care for nausea and diarrhea.

Continued

TABLE 11.6 ORAL CANCER CHEMOTHERAPY MEDICATIONS—cont'd

Medication Class/Action	Examples	Nursing Implications
Antimetabolite Prevents cells from making DNA and RNA. Used in metastatic breast, colon, or rectal cancer.	capecitabine (Xeloda)	Monitor labs for RBC, WBC and platelet counts. Supportive care for diarrhea, nausea and vomiting.
Hormones Antagonize effects of androgen.	exemestane (Casodex)	Monitor PSA and liver function tests.
Synthetic analog of luteinizing hormone-releasing hormone, causes decrease in testosterone levels.	leuprolide (Lupron)	Monitor PSA results.
Competes with estrogen for binding sites in breast and other tissues to reduce breast cancer recurrence.	tamoxifen (Nolvadex)	Anticoagulants increase PT. Instruct patient not to take antacids within 2 hours of tamoxifen.
Reduces amount of estrogen produced to reduce breast cancer recurrence.	anastrozole (Arimidex)	Should only be taken by postmenopausal women. Recommend regular bone density studies.
Miscellaneous Agent Work by interfering with enzyme systems or metabolic pathways in the cells.	hydroxyurea (Hydrea)	Monitor WBC count. Monitor metabolic panel for signs of tumor lysis syndrome. Monitor neurologic status and changes from baseline.

Note: Cyclophosphamide (Cytoxan) can also be administered by the oral route. PSA, prostate-specific antigen; PT, prothrombin time; RBC, red blood cell; WBC = white blood cell count.

different points in the cell cycle to chemotherapy. Combining drugs also decreases the side effects of therapy and decreases the possibility of the tumor becoming resistant to the therapy. For drugs to be combined this way, several criteria must be met. Each drug must be effective when used alone to treat the cancer, and each must have a different toxicity that would limit its use. For example, if three drugs that are all cardiotoxic are given, the patient is more likely to develop cardiotoxicity. Patients are still monitored for toxic effects from the treatment as well as improvement in their status.

Routes of Administration. Chemotherapy can be given by the oral, intramuscular, IV, or topical route. The dosage is determined by the size of the patient and the toxicities of the drug. IV administration requires specialized training and knowledge of antineoplastic drugs.

Vesicant drugs are given only by the IV route into a large vein. These drugs cause blistering of tissue that eventually leads to necrosis if they infiltrate, or leak, out of the blood vessel and into soft tissue (Fig. 11.13). Skin grafts may be needed if tissue damage is extensive.

FIGURE 11.13 Necrosis of skin tissue resulting from administration of a vesicant chemotherapy drug. *Photo courtesy of Dinesh Patel, MD, Medical Oncology, Internal Medicine, Zanesville, OH.*

• WORD • BUILDING •

vesicant: vesicate—to blister

Oral Chem Gents. The number of oral chemotherapy agents has increased in the past several years. Be aware that oral agents can be just as potent as chemotherapy administered intravenously. Nursing considerations for oral chemotherapy include proper timing of medication administration, safe storage, and side effects to assess for. Some oral agents must be given concurrently with another treatment such as radiation, so timing is important. See Table 11.6 for sample oral chemotherapy agents.

BE SAFE!

BE VIGILANT! Oral chemotherapy pills should not be stored with other oral medications and should never be crushed or broken. The nurse administering the pills should wear chemotherapy safety gloves.

Side Effects. Toxicities in patients receiving chemotherapy vary with the medications given; however, some general side effects are common to chemotherapeutic drugs because they affect all rapidly growing cells. Fast-growing epithelial cells, such as those of the hair, blood, skin, and GI tract, are usually the most affected by both chemotherapy and radiation.

Hematologic System. Chemotherapy is toxic to bone marrow, which is where blood cells are produced. The number of blood cells (especially white cells) drops after approximately 7 to 14 days of chemotherapy, depending on the drug. This period when the cell counts are lowest is called the **nadir** and is when patients are most at risk for complications. Patients may develop low WBC counts (**leukopenia**), increasing their susceptibility to infection and sepsis. Sometimes this is called **neutropenia** because neutrophils are the most plentiful white cells. A reduction in platelets (**thrombocytopenia**) increases the risk of bruising and bleeding and can require platelet transfusions. Increased risk of **anemia** occurs with the reduction of RBCs and may require blood transfusions. See Table 11.7 for medications that can be used to stimulate production of these cells.

• WORD • BUILDING •
leukopenia: leuko—white cells + penia—lack
neutropenia: neutron—neutrophils + penia—lack
thrombocytopenia: thrombo—clot + cyte—cell + penia—lack
anemia: an—not + emia—blood

TABLE 11.7   COLONY-STIMULATING FACTORS

Medication Class/Action	Examples	Nursing Implications
Granulocyte Colony-Stimulating Factor (G-CSF) Stimulates proliferation of stem cells into granulocytes (neutrophils).	filgrastim (Neupogen) pegfilgrastim (Neulasta)	Monitor CBC. Teach subcutaneous administration if drug will be given at home.
Granulocyte-Macrophage Colony-Stimulating Factor (GM-CSF) Stimulates proliferation of stem cells into neutrophils, monocytes, macrophages, and eosinophils.	sargramostim (Leukine)	Monitor vital signs and respiratory status during IV infusion. Monitor CBC. Teach subcutaneous administration if drug will be given at home.
Erythropoietin Stimulates proliferation of stem cells into red blood cells.	epoetin alfa (Epogen, Procrit) darbepoetin alpha (Aranesp)	Black box warning for heart disease risk. Monitor blood pressure and hematocrit. Teach subcutaneous administration if drug will be given at home. Aranesp is long acting.
Interleukin-11 Stimulates production of platelets.	oprelvekin (Neumega)	Watch for fluid retention. Monitor CBC, platelet count. Teach subcutaneous administration if drug will be given at home.

Note: Because these drugs are proteins, they all require refrigeration, and you cannot shake them. Many thousands of dollars have been lost because a drug was not returned to the refrigerator when it was not used. Be sure to check package instructions. CBC = complete blood count.

LEARNING TIP

When assessing patients with possible side effects of chemotherapy and radiation, use the mnemonic BITES:
B—Bleeding suggests low platelet count.
I—Infection suggests low WBC count and a risk for infection.
T—Tiredness suggests anemia.
E—Emesis places the patient at risk for altered nutrition and fluid and electrolyte imbalance.
S—Skin changes may be evidence of radiation reaction or skin breakdown.

Gastrointestinal System. Because the lining of the GI tract is made up of rapidly dividing cells, it is susceptible to the toxicity of chemotherapy drugs. Patients often experience nausea, vomiting, and diarrhea. **Stomatitis** (inflammation of the mouth) is a common complaint and is discussed under side effects of radiation. These side effects can be controlled with medication.

Hair. **Alopecia,** or hair loss, is common with many, but not all, chemotherapeutic drugs. This is a temporary condition, and growth of the new hair usually starts when the chemotherapeutic medication is stopped. Alopecia involves the entire body and includes eyebrows, eyelashes, and axillary and pubic hair. Hair that regrows may be a different color or texture than the original hair. It is not uncommon for individuals who originally had straight hair to regrow curly hair.

BE SAFE!

Some websites promote icing the scalp to cause vasoconstriction and reduce the amount of chemotherapy agent affecting hair loss. Teach patients that this practice MAY NOT BE SAFE and may leave pockets of cancer cells in the brain and scalp that are not reached by the chemotherapy.

Reproductive System. The effects of chemotherapy or radiation can cause temporary or permanent changes in the reproductive system. Chemotherapy can damage sperm and ova. Issues concerning fertility should be discussed with the patient before treatment. Measures such as freezing ova and using a sperm bank can provide options for the patient and his or her partner. Patients should also talk to their HCPs before engaging in intercourse during chemotherapy and use protection against pregnancy.

• WORD • BUILDING •
stomatitis: stoma—mouth + itis—inflammation

Neurologic System. Drugs may affect the neurologic system. An adverse reaction to vincristine (Oncovin) is neurotoxicity, which can result in tingling or numbness in the extremities and in severe cases can cause footdrop from muscle weakness.

Other Systems. Less common complications include renal toxicities, such as pain and burning on urination, and hematuria. Doxorubicin (Adriamycin) has been associated with permanent heart damage, and bleomycin can cause pulmonary fibrosis.

Severe toxic side effects can be controlled by carefully limiting the amount of medication given and constantly monitoring the patient for complications.

CYTOPROTECTIVE AGENTS. Cytoprotective agents protect healthy cells from some side effects of certain chemotherapeutic drugs. For example, dexrazoxane helps prevent cardiac damage associated with doxorubicin. Amifostine (Ethyol) helps protect the kidneys from platinum-based chemotherapy. It also protects normal cells in parts of the body against damage from radiation treatments. Mesna (Mesnex) protects the bladder against chemotherapy drugs such as cyclophosphamide (Cytoxan).

New Treatments Being Researched

New therapies for cancer are constantly being researched. For example, hyperthermia has been used with radiation and chemotherapy. It has been beneficial in some types of cancer but is usually used only in investigational studies.

Biological response modifiers (such as interferons) are drugs used to stimulate the immune system. These drugs are used commonly for specific types of cancer and have produced some beneficial results. They are also being used in many investigational studies. Go to www.cancer.gov for information on current clinical trials.

NURSING PROCESS FOR THE PATIENT WITH CANCER

Data Collection

Patients with cancer are assessed for many problems associated with the disease and its treatment. Thorough assessment will help the health team build a plan of care relevant to the patient's needs.

The nurse should monitor laboratory studies. Potential for bleeding exists when the platelet count is 50,000/mm³ or less; risk for spontaneous bleeding occurs when the count is less than 20,000/mm³. Monitor the WBC count for risk of infection and the RBC count for anemia.

Monitor the patient's weight, and note reports of nausea, changes in taste, vomiting, and diarrhea related to either the disease or treatment. Monitor the oral mucosa for lesions or inflammation. Also watch for signs of dehydration. "Nutrition Notes—Assessing the Need for Nutritional Support" presents criteria for determining whether a patient needs nutritional support.

Nutrition Notes

Assessing the Need for Nutritional Support

Intensive nutritional support may not benefit all cancer patients because the tumor interferes with the patient's utilization of nutrients. Clinical judgment is required to analyze the patient's needs and expected response. In general, if any of the following findings are present, you should talk with the dietitian or HCP about the need for nutritional support.

• Weight 5 kg (11 lb) below a healthy body weight
• Intolerance of oral/enteral feedings for more than 7 days
• Serum albumin level of less than 3 g/dL
• Location of cancer in head and neck or GI system
• Severe GI injury in patients with cured/controlled cancer

Psychosocial issues related to cancer are as varied as the persons afflicted with the disease. Help the patient explore perceptions about quality of life. Culture and age affect cancer perceptions. Assess the patient's ability to cope and coping strategies that have been effective in the past. Determine what information the patient has received and understands about his or her disease and prognosis.

Assess the roles of the patient and caregiver in the family. Be aware of whether the caregiver can be at home or whether he or she must work outside the home and also care for the patient. Isolation can be either self-imposed or imposed by friends and family as terminal illness issues are confronted. It can be very distressing to see a loved one decline with cancer; often people say they are "afraid of saying or doing the wrong thing" so they "just stay away." Listen for cues from patients expressing self-blame, anger, or depression. It is important to recognize signs of depression and suicidal tendencies.

Assess for fatigue and anxiety in a patient being treated for cancer. A decline in sexual desire is not uncommon during cancer treatment. Assess for anxiety about sexual intercourse, including fears concerning contracting cancer from the patient and fears that sexual intercourse will make the cancer worse.

Assess the patient's feelings about any actual or perceived change in appearance due to surgery, radiation, or chemotherapy.

Nursing Diagnoses, Planning, and Implementation

See the "Nursing Care Plan for the Patient With Cancer" for top nursing care priorities. Additional nursing diagnoses are presented below.

NURSING CARE PLAN for the Patient With Cancer

Nursing Diagnosis: *Risk for Ineffective Coping* related to the diagnosis and treatment of cancer as evidenced by behaviors such as denial, isolation, anxiety, and depression

Expected Outcomes: Patient will cope effectively as evidenced by identifying stressors related to illness and treatment; communicating needs, concerns, and fears; and use of appropriate resources to support coping.

Evaluation of Outcomes: Is patient able to identify stressors and communicate concerns? Does patient effectively draw on past coping mechanism? Does patient have and appropriately use support systems?

Intervention Assess effective coping mechanisms used in the past and currently available to the patient. **Rationale** Coping mechanisms that worked in the past may be helpful again, and the nurse can support appropriate choices. **Evaluation** Is the patient able to identify and draw on past coping mechanisms?

Intervention Use active listening skills to encourage the patient to express feelings and fears. **Rationale** The patient must identify fears to be able to cope effectively with them. **Evaluation** Does the patient identify fears and concerns?

Intervention Assess the meaning of quality of life to the patient. **Rationale** Once identified, the nurse can assist the patient to achieve quality-of-life goals. **Evaluation** Is the patient able to identify the meaning of quality of life? Are there ways the nurse can assist the patient to reach quality-of-life goals?

Intervention Assess for suicide risks. **Rationale** A patient who feels hopeless may be at risk for suicide. **Evaluation** Is the patient at risk? Are suicide precautions necessary?

Continued

NURSING CARE PLAN for the Patient With Cancer—cont'd

Intervention Explore outlets that promote feelings of personal achievement. **Rationale** Personal achievement promotes self-esteem. **Evaluation** Does the patient have creative outlets that promote feelings of achievement? Can the nurse assist in implementing these activities?

Intervention Consider the use of humor. **Rationale** Humor can be both distracting and therapeutic. **Evaluation** Does the patient use humor? Does it provide temporary distraction from concerns?

Nursing Diagnosis: *Acute Pain* or *Chronic Pain* related to tissue injury from disease process and treatment

Expected Outcomes: Pain will be prevented and patient will be comfortable at all times as evidenced by patient stating pain is at an acceptable level on pain scale.

Evaluation of Outcomes: Does patient state pain is controlled?

Intervention Assess the patient's pain including onset, location, duration, character, and aggravating and alleviating factors. **Rationale** Assessment provides direction for the treatment plan. **Evaluation** Is assessment complete and used to guide treatment?

Intervention Ask patient to rate pain on a scale from 0 to 10 (0 = absence of pain; 10 = worst pain). **Rationale** A pain rating should guide treatment and evaluate effectiveness of treatment. **Evaluation** Does patient use pain assessment scale effectively? Is patient in pain?

Intervention Administer analgesics as ordered, around the clock (ATC). (See "Evidence-Based Practice" box.) **Rationale** Using an ATC schedule prevents pain from becoming severe. **Evaluation** Is patient's pain kept under control at all times?

Intervention Check pain relief within 1 hour of administration of medication and every 2 to 4 hours. **Rationale** Alternative short-acting medications may be necessary for breakthrough pain. **Evaluation** Is breakthrough pain present? Does long-acting analgesic need to be increased to prevent pain?

Intervention Educate patient on use of patient-controlled anesthesia (PCA). **Rationale** PCA allows the patient to be in control of own pain relief. **Evaluation** Does PCA keep patient pain free and able to participate in desired activities?

Intervention Monitor level of sedation and respiratory status if opioid dose is increased. **Rationale** Patients who receive long-term opioid therapy develop a tolerance to the depressant effects of opioids. **Evaluation** Is patient alert with respiratory rate between 12 and 20?

Intervention Explain the use of non-pharmacological interventions such as relaxation once the pain is controlled with medications. **Rationale** Nonpharmacological interventions supplement but do not replace analgesics. **Evaluation** Does patient use non-pharmacological interventions? Do they help?

Nursing Diagnosis: *Risk for Infection* related to diminished immunity and bone marrow suppression as a result of chemotherapy or radiation

Expected Outcomes: The patient will be free and safe from infection as evidenced by being afebrile and stating self-care measures to protect from infection. Signs and symptoms of infection are identified and treated early.

Evaluation of Outcomes: Are signs and symptoms of infection absent? If present, are they reported quickly? Can the patient identify self-care measures for preventing infection?

NURSING CARE PLAN for the Patient With Cancer—cont'd

Intervention Promote good hand-washing technique before interaction with the patient. **Rationale** Appropriate hand hygiene can reduce the transmission of antimicrobial organisms. **Evaluation** Are you careful with your hand washing? Have you also instructed the patient, family, and nursing assistants about careful hand washing?

Intervention Monitor body temperature every 4 hours. **Rationale** Elevated body temperature is an early sign of infection. **Evaluation** Is body temperature within normal limits?

Intervention Monitor WBC count daily. **Rationale** For the neutropenic patient, the WBC will not be elevated. Neutropenia is a risk factor for infection. **Evaluation** Is the WBC count 5000 to 10,000/mm^3?

Intervention Assess for signs of inflammation or drainage at potential infection sites, such as old aspirate sites, venipuncture sites, oral and rectal mucosae, perineal area, axillae, incisions, pierced earlobes, under breasts, and between toes. **Rationale** Intact skin is the first line of defense against invading microorganisms. **Evaluation** Are there any sites that need special care to maintain skin integrity?

Intervention Watch for signs of respiratory infection, such as sore throat, cough, shortness of breath, and sputum production. **Rationale** Hospital-acquired pneumonia has high morbidity and mortality rates. **Evaluation** Are signs of respiratory infection present?

Intervention Assess for signs of urinary tract infection (UTI) including burning, pain, urgency, blood in urine. **Rationale** Genitourinary tract is the most common site for hospital-acquired infection. **Evaluation** Are signs of UTI present?

Intervention Teach administration of G-CSF or GM-CSF as ordered. **Rationale** These medications help the body produce more WBCs. The patient may need to administer it subcutaneously at home. **Evaluation** Does patient demonstrate correct self-administration? Is WBC count improving?

Intervention Limit visitors to only healthy adults. **Rationale** Viral infection in an immunosuppressed patient has a high mortality rate. **Evaluation** Are the patient and family aware of visiting restrictions and rationale? Is there a sign on the door reminding visitors?

Intervention Teach patient to ask HCP about avoiding unwashed, unpeeled fruits and vegetables. (See "Nutrition Notes.") **Rationale** Unwashed or unpeeled fresh fruits and vegetables can carry pathogens. **Evaluation** Are the patient and family aware of the risks of eating unwashed, unpeeled fruits and vegetables?

Intervention Keep fresh flowers and potted plants out of the patient's room. **Rationale** *Aspergillus* is a fungus found in soil and water and can cause pneumonia. **Evaluation** Is the room free from potential sources of infection?

ATC = around the clock; G-CSF = granulocyte colony-stimulating factor; GM-CSF = granulocyte macrophage colony-stimulating factor; GU = genitourinary; PCA = patient-controlled analgesia.

EVIDENCE-BASED PRACTICE

Clinical Question
Is oral morphine effective for cancer pain?

Evidence
A review of 54 studies found that various formulations of oral morphine were effective at relieving cancer pain but had unwanted side effects—primarily constipation, nausea, and vomiting (Wiffen & McQuay, 2007).

Implications for Nursing Practice
Administer oral morphine as ordered for pain. Be sure to institute preventive measures against constipation before it becomes a problem. Talk with the HCP about medications for nausea if it occurs.

REFERENCES
Wiffen, P. J., & McQuay, H. J. (2007). Oral morphine for cancer pain. *Cochrane Database of Systematic Reviews, 4,* CD003868 (doi:10.1002/14651858.CD003868.pub2).

National Cancer Institute. (Modified 2013, May 3). Basic principles of cancer pain management. Retrieved July 6, 2013 from www.cancer.gov/cancertopics/pdq/supportivecare /pain/HealthProfessional/page3

Ineffective Protection related to thrombocytopenia associated with chemotherapy and radiation

EXPECTED OUTCOME: The patient will be free of bleeding as evidenced by stable blood counts and the absence of bruising or frank bleeding.

- Monitor platelet counts. *A platelet count of less than 50,000 indicates potential for bleeding.*
- Teach self-administration of oprelvekin as ordered. *Oprelvekin stimulates production of platelets.*
- Test all urine and stool for occult blood *to detect the presence of blood.*
- Avoid giving intramuscular, subcutaneous, or rectal medications. *Medications given via invasive routes can cause bleeding.*
- Apply pressure for at least 5 minutes to venipuncture or injection sites. *Pressure for a longer time is needed at sites of invasive procedures to stop bleeding.*
- Teach the patient about gentle mouth care including no flossing, a soft toothbrush, and wearing properly fitting dentures *to help prevent trauma and bleeding.*
- Avoid trauma to rectal tissue by avoiding rectal temperatures and enemas. Teach importance of avoiding anal intercourse. *Trauma to rectal tissue can cause bleeding.*
- Instruct the patient not to take any salicylates or non-steroidal anti-inflammatory drugs *because they can interfere with platelet function and cause bleeding in the GI tract.*
- Observe for bruising, petechiae, bleeding gums, tarry stools, and black or coffee-ground appearing emesis. *These are signs of bleeding.*
- Advise the patient to use an electric razor *to decrease risk for trauma and bleeding.*
- Teach the patient to avoid forcefully blowing his or her nose or inserting objects into the nose *to reduce trauma to nasal mucosa to prevent spontaneous bleeding.*
- Teach the patient to monitor for bleeding with intercourse because of the risk of trauma to tissues.

Imbalanced Nutrition: Less Than Body Requirements related to anorexia, nausea, or vomiting associated with disease, pain, and treatment

EXPECTED OUTCOME: The patient will have caloric intake that is adequate to meet body requirements and balanced intake and output, as evidenced by stable weight and albumin level of 3 g/dL or greater.

- Monitor food and fluid intake and output every 8 hours. *This will provide objective data for the amount of nutrients and fluids taken in.*
- Weigh the patient daily. *Weight is an objective measurement to determine if intake is adequate enough to maintain weight.*
- Consult a dietitian for dietary supplements. *Dietitians can calculate the calories needed for adequate nutrition and make recommendations for supplements.*
- Consult with the primary care provider for medications to control nausea, vomiting, and diarrhea. *If these*

symptoms are controlled, then the patient is better able to eat.

- Keep the environment free of strong odors, such as disinfectants, perfumes, deodorizers, and body wastes. *Strong odors can induce nausea.*
- Provide room-temperature or cold foods and clear liquids. *These foods have fewer odors and may be more comfortable for the patient to eat.*
- Offer sour foods such as hard candy and lemon. *These can help control nausea.*
- Encourage listening to music or doing relaxation exercises. *These can provide distraction from pain and nausea.*
- Add nutmeg to foods. *Nutmeg may help slow the motility of the GI tract and decrease the risk of nausea and vomiting.*
- Provide mouth care before meals. *Oral care allows for a better taste in the mouth, and saliva is needed for digestion of food.*
- Provide small, high-calorie meals. *Eating smaller, more frequent meals prevents the patient from feeling full and nauseated.*
- Administer pain medication before meals *to help reduce the impact of pain on appetite.*
- Instruct the patient to avoid fluids with meals *to prevent premature feelings of fullness.*
- Teach the patient to avoid exercise before meals. *If the patient is fatigued, he or she will not have the energy to eat and digest food.*

See "Nutrition Notes—Treating Problems Related to Nutrition" for additional nutrition interventions.

Nutrition Notes

Treating Problems Related to Nutrition

Early Satiety and Anorexia

- Select nutrient-dense foods. For example, fortify puddings and milkshakes with dry skim milk powder.
- Encourage appropriate exercise.
- Present food attractively.
- Offer small, frequent meals.
- Encourage family to provide home-cooked food.
- If meals are not tolerated, offer 1 oz of a complete nutritional supplement every hour.

Bitter or Metallic Taste

- Provide oral hygiene before meals.
- Cook in glass containers in a microwave oven.
- Use nonmetallic utensils when eating meals.
- Serve food cold or at room temperature.
- Offer lemon-flavored beverages.
- See if the patient prefers eggs, fish, poultry, and dairy products to beef and pork.

• Experiment with sauces and seasonings. Sweet sauces and marinades may improve the palatability of meats.

Local Oral Effects

• *Ulcerations:* Offer soft, mild foods; cream sauces, gravies, and dressings for lubrication; cold foods for numbing; and straws for liquids. Avoid hot items, salty or spicy foods, and acidic juices. If an anesthetic mouthwash is prescribed, the mouth may be numb; caution the patient to chew carefully to avoid biting the lips, tongue, or cheeks.
• *Dry mouth:* Offer frequent sips of water or artificial saliva. Lubricate with gravies, butter, margarine, milk, cream, or bouillon. Sugarless hard candy, chewing gum, or popsicles may stimulate saliva production.
• *Dysphagia:* Teach the patient to make swallowing a conscious act (inhale, swallow, exhale) and to experiment with head position. Offer foods with a smooth, even consistency. Thick liquids are easier to swallow than thin. Encourage dunking breads in a beverage to soften.

Nausea and Vomiting

• Administer antiemetics on a regular prophylactic schedule.
• Suggest dry crackers.
• Offer liquids between instead of with meals to reduce stomach volume, and low-fat meals to facilitate stomach emptying.
• Remove covers from food containers away from the bedside if strong odors disturb the patient's appetite.
• Instruct the patient to chew thoroughly, eat slowly, and rest afterward.
• Arrange meal schedule to take advantage of times when patient feels better.
• Avoid serving favorite foods when the patient is nauseous to avoid an association between those foods and vomiting.

Diarrhea

• Suggest a low-fiber diet.
• Try a lactose-free diet for temporary lactose intolerance.
• Propose pectin-containing foods (apples, strawberries, citrus fruits) to absorb water in the bowel.
• Investigate the feasibility of probiotic therapy to repopulate intestine (see below).
• Consult with a dietitian about special feedings.

Altered Immune Response

• Institute protective isolation to minimize exposure to microorganisms.
• Observe strict procedures for food safety and sanitation.
• Some providers attempt to limit exposure to microorganisms by restricting unpasteurized, uncooked, and unwashed foods but the effectiveness of this dietary approach has not been substantiated with direct proof (Fox & Freifeld, 2012).

Fox, N., & Freifeld, A. G. (2012). The neutropenic diet reviewed: Moving toward a safe food handling approach. *Oncology (Williston Park), 26*, 572–575, 580, 582 passim.

Self-Care Deficit related to weakness and fatigue

EXPECTED OUTCOME: Care needs will be met at all times as evidenced by statement that needs are being met by self or caregiver.

• Assess what self-care activities the patient can do independently (bathing, grooming, feeding, toileting, ambulating). *By assessing what the patient can do independently, you can develop goals and interventions appropriate for the patient.*
• Identify and include the patient's strengths in self-care activities *to help increase the patient's independence.*
• Provide the tools needed for the patient to assist with his or her own bathing, grooming, feeding, toileting, and ambulation. Physical and occupational therapy departments may be able to help identify assistive devices. *Adaptive and assistive devices can promote independence.*
• Teach the patient about options available for when he or she is no longer able to care for his or her own needs. *Support from other sources will help the patient conserve energy. Planning ahead can help reduce anxiety.*
• Instruct family members in how to assist in daily care. *Allowing family members to assist in the daily care will promote their role as caregivers.*
• Consult home health care or hospice nurses to assist with care needs upon discharge from the acute setting. *Support from these sources will assist the patient to maintain dignity when independence is no longer possible.*

Risk for Ineffective Role Performance related to needs of patient and anticipated outcome

EXPECTED OUTCOME: The caregiver will be prepared to provide care effectively as evidenced by (1) identification of resources available to assist in providing care for the patient and (2) maintenance of caregiver's physical and emotional health.

• Observe the caregiver's ability to provide care for the patient. *The nurse needs to know if the caregiver will be able to handle the care needs.*
• Observe the quality of the relationship between the patient and caregiver. *The quality of the relationship impacts the care delivered.*
• Actively listen to the caregiver's concerns. *Doing so can assist the nurse in assessing the caregiver's ability to cope and can help in planning care.*
• Teach appropriate caregiving skills as needed. *The caregiver may not be aware of how to bathe a patient or how to provide basic or advanced care.*

- Assist the caregiver to identify available supports. *Assistance can provide a break and decrease the risk of exhaustion and depression in the caregiver.*
- Instruct the caregiver in the resources available in the community. *Support groups can help the caregiver by providing an outlet for sharing concerns and finding support.*
- Consult the multidisciplinary team to provide the services needed at time of discharge. *Preparing the caregiver for discharge needs/care with the proper resources will help the caregiver feel empowered to deliver the care.*
- Watch for signs of depression in the caregiver, and intervene to help coping. *The caregiver can develop a weakened immune system secondary to stress and depression.*
- Arrange for respite for the caregiver or encourage the caregiver to utilize this service. *Respite care can provide a break for the caregiver.*
- Encourage the caregiver to grieve over the patient. *Caregivers will grieve for the loved one's loss of function or role in the family, even before death.*
- Assist the caregiver with ways to decrease stress. *Encouraging caregivers to take time to care for themselves will leave them with the energy they need to continue providing care.*

Social Isolation related to changing relationships

EXPECTED OUTCOME: The patient will manage social isolation as evidenced by (1) ability to identify feelings of isolation and (2) ability to participate in chosen activities.

- Observe the patient for signs of barriers to social interaction, such as incontinence, lack of transportation, and inadequate money or support system. *Why a patient feels isolated can vary from one person to another, but knowing the reason can help the nurse plan appropriate interventions.*
- Discuss causes of perceived or actual isolation. *How the patient is dealing with the illness will have an impact on how he or she manages the illness.*
- Listen to the patient describe reasons for isolation. *Listening and being present are ways to show caring.*
- Promote opportunities for the patient to interact socially, such as at mealtimes or during therapy sessions. *The patient will feel less isolated if given an opportunity to participate in diversional activities.*
- Provide positive reinforcement when the patient starts conversation with others. *Positive feedback from the nurse can have an impact on the patient's confidence.*
- Provide information about support groups, and encourage the patient to contact them. *Support groups can help the patient cope better with stressful events in life.*

Ineffective Sexuality Pattern related to change in body functions

EXPECTED OUTCOME: The patient will have knowledge about limitations or changes in sexual activity during cancer treatment as evidenced by statement of understanding.

- Provide a private environment to discuss issues of sexuality. *Privacy promotes a comfort level that allows the patient to express concerns.*

- Assess what the patient understands about sexuality during cancer treatment. *This discussion can clear up any misinformation the patient and partner may have.*
- Encourage the patient to discuss concerns about sexuality with his or her partner. *Communication is a key component of emotional intimacy.*
- Stress to the patient that cancer cannot be passed from person to person through sexual intimacy. *Cancer is not contagious.*
- Instruct the patient that sexual activity is usually safe during and after cancer treatment. *Sexual activity does not necessarily hurt the patient.*
- Advise the patient to abstain from sexual intercourse while the blood count is low to prevent secondary infections and bleeding. *A low white blood cell count can raise the risk of infection, and a low platelet count can raise the risk of bleeding.*
- Advise men to ask their primary care provider about using condoms for intercourse during chemotherapy *because some chemotherapy agents can be found in semen.*
- Advise the patient to consult the primary care provider about birth control during treatment *because of chemotherapy effects on sperm and ova.*
- Discuss with the patient and partner that closeness and touching may still be desired even if sexual intercourse is not. *Closeness and touching are ways to be intimate without intercourse.*
- Instruct the patient and partner that pain during intercourse can be related to surgery or treatment, and advise taking pain medication before intercourse *to help make the patient more comfortable.*

Disturbed Body Image related to cancer and its treatment (e.g., surgical procedures such as mastectomy, ostomy, or loss of hair from chemotherapy)

EXPECTED OUTCOME: The patient will be able to accept the changes in body image as evidenced by willingness to participate in care and adjust to changes in lifestyle.

- Allow the patient to discuss feelings of anger or depression, and confirm that these feelings are normal when adjusting to body changes. *A patient may be better able to cope with body changes if he or she can talk about feelings and understand that they are normal.*
- Encourage the patient to select a wig before hair loss *so the patient can find one resembling his or her own hair color and style.*
- Provide education, and urge the patient to care for the ostomy site or surgical wound when ready *to promote independence.*
- Provide information about resources such as Reach to Recovery (www.cancer.org; type in Reach to Recovery) and Look Good . . . Feel Better support groups (www .lookgoodfeelbetter.org). *Support groups provide a forum for patients to share their experiences with others undergoing similar changes.*
- Provide information about community assistance and financial aid for programs or services. *Social workers can help with community resources that can provide equipment or supplies for the patient.*

Grieving related to diagnosis and potential disease outcome
Grieving and end-of-life care are covered in depth in Chapter 17.

Evaluation

If the interventions have been effective, the patient will have no unusual bleeding or bruising. The patient and family will be knowledgeable about risk factors for bleeding and about signs of bleeding to report promptly.

The patient will be nourished and maintain weight within normal limits. The patient will maximize the potential for self-care activities. The patient and caregiver will know about available resources to assist with self-care activities in the home setting. Caregivers will know how to provide care for the patient. The patient will be able to openly discuss feelings and be able to spend time with family and loved ones to resolve any issues.

Effective interventions will allow the caregiver to make use of resources in the community to assist with patient care and to maintain her or his own physical and psychological health while caring for the patient. The patient will be able to discuss feelings of isolation and seek out activities to participate in. The patient will maintain a healthy sexuality and be able to discuss feelings openly and honestly with her or his partner.

The patient will be able to openly discuss concerns regarding body changes and be able to maintain control of his or her body. The patient will know about community resources and support groups to assist with needs related to body image.

CRITICAL THINKING

Mrs. Jones

■ Mrs. Jones is admitted to your unit after a simple mastectomy for breast cancer. The tumor was staged as a T2, N0, M0. A bone scan was negative for metastasis. She is scheduled for four chemotherapy treatments, 3 weeks apart. The medications prescribed are high doses of doxorubicin and cyclophosphamide. A central line is inserted for chemotherapy.

1. What does the staging of Mrs. Jones's tumor mean?
2. What major side effects of her medications should you look for?
3. Why was a central line inserted?
4. What nursing diagnoses are appropriate for Mrs. Jones?

Suggested answers are at the end of the chapter.

 ## SURVIVORSHIP

Millions of people around the world are no longer dying from cancer but rather are survivors of the disease. There are an estimated 13.7 million cancer survivors in the United States alone (NCI, 2012). Cancer survivors deal with emotional and physical effects of their disease and treatment.

Survivorship begins at the time of the diagnosis and continues even after treatments have been completed. In 2011, the Commission on Cancer of the American College of Surgeons published new accreditation standards relating to care of patients with cancer. The development of a survivorship plan of care that not only documents the care provided but also addresses the improvement in the quality of life of the cancer survivor is one of the key components for accreditation. Focus is on reassessment of psychosocial needs at the time of completion of treatment to create a survivorship plan of care for continued medical follow-up as well as management of emotional and social challenges. Cancer centers around the country with strong support from their patient and family advisory councils and advocacy groups are developing survivorship programs. For further information about cancer survivorship programs, see the American College of Surgeons website: www.facs.org/cancerprogram/index.html.

HOSPICE CARE OF THE PATIENT WITH CANCER

Patients who are considered terminal and have a life expectancy of 6 months or less are eligible for hospice care, which provides humanistic care for dying people and their families. The dying person is provided care at home or in a homelike setting that promotes comfort and quality of life until death. Hospice care is offered as an inpatient or outpatient service (see "Home Health Hints").

 ## Home Health Hints

• The home health or hospice nurse helps manage cancer pain in the home. Oral, transdermal, or IV analgesics are preferred. For moderate to severe pain, doses should be given around the clock with as-needed doses for breakthrough pain. Intramuscular delivery of pain medication should be avoided because of the pain of the injections and the burden it places on the caregiver.

• The nurse should anticipate constipation from opioid administration and treat prophylactically.

• Some patients are fearful of taking prescribed pain medications. Explain the importance of taking the medications as ordered and note that it is easier to maintain pain relief than to reverse severe pain.

• Home health nurses are in key positions for making timely referrals for hospice care. Eligible patients are those who have a life expectancy of 6 months or less and who have a desire for supportive palliative care rather than continued treatments. To have hospice care in their own home, they must also have a friend or relative who is willing to coordinate the care.

Inpatient services are used for symptom control and respite care for the family. Family and pets may be allowed to stay with the patient. Hospice care assists the family in crisis and continues for up to 1 year after the patient dies, with follow-up counseling, listening, nurturing, and referrals.

Outpatient care is given in the home with family members providing the primary care. Support care is given by the hospice staff. Medications and supplies are furnished by the hospice service. At home, the patient can enjoy loved ones, pets, plants, music, and personal surroundings for as long as possible. See Chapter 17, "Nursing Care of Patients at the End of Life," for more information.

ONCOLOGICAL EMERGENCIES

Superior Vena Cava Syndrome

Superior vena cava syndrome (SVCS) occurs in patients with lung cancer or cancers of the mediastinum when the tumor or enlarged lymph nodes block circulation in the vena cava. This results in edema of the head, neck, and arms. Symptoms include shortness of breath, cough, chest pain, facial redness, and swollen neck veins. Radiation therapy can be used to shrink the tumor and allow circulation to resume naturally. Nursing interventions for the patient with SVCS include removing rings and restrictive clothing, avoiding taking blood pressure and venipunctures in the arms, and elevating the head of the bed to decrease feeling of dyspnea.

Spinal Cord Compression

Spinal cord compression occurs when a malignant growth presses on the spinal cord. This is a painful problem and requires pain management while radiation is given to relieve the symptoms. Patients may develop some motor loss when this occurs. Commonly, a myelogram or bone scan is used for diagnosis. Nursing care includes providing a safe environment, assisting with activity, and watching for changes in neurologic status as well as changes in the location or intensity of pain. Patients at risk include those with cancers that spread to the bone and spinal cord, such as lung, breast, and prostate cancer.

Hypercalcemia

In hypercalcemia, the serum calcium level exceeds 11 mg/dL. Hypercalcemia may result from the release of calcium into the blood from bone deterioration or from ectopic secretion of parathyroid hormone by a tumor. It is common in patients with bone metastasis, especially metastasis from breast cancer. It can be treated with IV medication and hydration to lower the calcium level. Nursing care includes maintaining safety and monitoring intake and output, pain control, and changes in pulse rate and rhythm.

SUGGESTED ANSWERS TO

CRITICAL THINKING

■ *Mrs. Jones*

1. Mrs. Jones's tumor is beginning to invade surrounding tissue. There is no lymph node involvement and no metastasis.

2. Doxorubicin is commonly associated with red urine and also poses a risk for cardiac toxicity. Cyclophosphamide can cause blood in the urine and a risk for hemorrhagic cystitis. Therefore, the patient should take in plenty of fluids and void often (every 2 hours). Both medications can cause nausea, vomiting, and alopecia. Both are vesicants.

3. Because the drugs are vesicants, it is important to inject them into a large vein.

4. Many diagnoses are appropriate, including *Acute Pain* related to surgical incision, *Disturbed Body Image* related to alopecia and loss of a breast, *Imbalanced Nutrition: Less Than Body Requirements* related to nausea and vomiting, *Risk for Injury* related to medication side effects, and *Deficient Knowledge* about cancer treatment and management of side effects. A thorough nursing assessment is needed to determine actual diagnoses.

REVIEW QUESTIONS

1. A patient asks, "How do malignant tumors differ from benign tumors?" Which of the following statements by the nurse are correct? **Select all that apply.**
   1. "Malignant tumors invade surrounding cells and tissues."
   2. "Malignant tumors are generally encapsulated."
   3. "Malignant tumors remain localized."
   4. "Cells in malignant tumors stop dividing prematurely."
   5. "Cells in malignant tumors lack contact inhibition."
   6. "Malignant tumors have defective cell communication."

2. A patient has received vinorelbine on day 1 of treatment. The nadir will occur in about 10 days. For which complication should the nurse be vigilant around Day 10?
   1. Infection
   2. Hair loss
   3. Diarrhea
   4. Myalgia

3. A female patient is starting on doxorubicin. Which of the following nursing interventions will be most helpful as she plans for hair loss?
   1. Obtain a prescription for a hair growth product.
   2. Massage her scalp to increase circulation and delay hair loss.
   3. Teach her to apply ice to her scalp to prevent hair loss.
   4. Help her choose a wig before her hair loss begins.

4. Which of the following nursing actions will best help the patient with cancer to control pain?
   1. Assess the patient's anxiety level.
   2. Assess the patient's understanding of the side effects of pain medication.
   3. Encourage the patient to use nonpharmacological methods for pain.
   4. Teach the use of a relaxation exercise to be used with prescribed analgesics.

5. The nurse notes that a patient undergoing treatment for bone cancer is having trouble walking. For which oncological emergency should the patient be assessed?
   1. Tumor lysis syndrome
   2. Hypercalcemia
   3. Spinal cord compression
   4. Thrombocytopenia

6. A nurse is intervening for a patient receiving radiation therapy with reddened skin over the treated area. How will the nurse know if nursing interventions have been effective?
   1. The patient will be able to describe a proper skin care regimen.
   2. The nurse will keep the skin clean and dry.
   3. The patient's skin will remain intact without breakdown or infection.
   4. The nurse will report the reddened area to the physician.

7. Which of the following patients will benefit from hospice care?
   1. A patient who has liver cancer and is expected to live 4 to 6 weeks
   2. A patient who is having multiple side effects from aggressive chemotherapy
   3. A patient who is trying to make a decision about cancer treatment
   4. A patient with uncontrolled pain related to cancer and radiation treatment

8. A patient is receiving internal radiation therapy for a gynecological malignancy. The patient expresses feelings of isolation in her private room. What intervention would be best on the part of the nurse?
   1. Encourage the patient's significant other to stay overnight.
   2. Move the patient into a semiprivate room so she can have a roommate.
   3. Instruct the patient about the safety procedures for internal radiation therapy.
   4. Plan to spend more time with the patient.

Answers can be found in Appendix C.

References

American Cancer Society. (2013a). *Cancer treatment and survivorship: Facts and figures.* Retrieved July 6, 2013, from www.cancer.org/acs/groups/content/@epidemiologysurveilance/documents/document/acspc-033876.pdf

American Cancer Society. (2013b). *American Cancer Society guidelines for the early detection of cancer.* Retrieved July 6, 2013, from www.cancer.org/healthy/findcancerearly/cancerscreeningguidelines/american-cancer-society-guidelines-for-the-early-detection-of-cancer

American Cancer Society. (2013c). *Sipuleucel-T.* Retrieved July 6, 2013, from www.cancer.org/treatment/treatmentsandsideeffects/guidetocancerdrugs/sipuleucel-t

Centers for Disease Control and Prevention. (2013). *HPV vaccine for human papillomavirus—preteen-teen-adolescent.* Atlanta: Author. Retrieved June 1, 2013, from www.cdc.gov/vaccines/who/teens/vaccines/hpv.html

Centers for Disease Control and Prevention. (2013). *Lung cancer.* Atlanta: Author. Retrieved June 1, 2013, from www.cdc.gov/cancer/lung/basic_info/risk_factors.htm

National Cancer Institute. (2012). *Cancer survivorship research.* Retrieved July 6, 2013, from http://cancercontrol.cancer.gov/ocs/prevalence

U.S. Preventive Services Task Force. (2009). Screening for breast cancer. Retrieved October 17, 2013, from www.uspreventiveservicestaskforce.org/uspstf/uspsbrca.htm

 DavisPlus | For additional resources and information visit **davispl.us/medsurg5**

12

Nursing Care of Patients Having Surgery

LINDA S. WILLIAMS

KEY TERMS

adjunct (ADD-junkt)
anesthesia (AN-es-THEE-zee-uh)
anesthesiologist (an-es-THEE-zee-uhl-la-just)
aseptic (ah-SEP-tik)
atelectasis (AT-e-LEK-tah-sis)
débridement (da-breed-MAHNT)
dehiscence (dee-HISS-ents)
evisceration (E-VIS-sir-a-shun)
hematoma (HEE-muh-TOH-mah)
hypothermia (HY-poh-THUR-mee-ah)
induction (in-DUCK-shun)
intraoperative (IN-trah-AW-pruh-tiv)
perioperative (PER-ee-AW-pruh-tiv)
postoperative (post-AW-pruh-tiv)
preoperative (pre-AW-pruh-tiv)
purulent (PURE-u-lent)
serosanguineous (SEER-oh-SANG-gwin-ee-us)
surgeon (SURGE-un)

LEARNING OUTCOMES

1. Describe factors that influence surgical outcomes.
2. Identify the LPN/LVN role in each perioperative phase.
3. Explain the LPN/LVN role in obtaining informed patient consent.
4. Develop a teaching plan to enhance learning for the older preoperative patient.
5. Identify nursing interventions used for common postoperative patient needs.
6. Describe how to evaluate effectiveness of nursing interventions.
7. List signs and symptoms of common postoperative complications.
8. List the criteria for ambulatory discharge.
9. Describe the role of the home health nurse in caring for postoperative patients.

Surgery is the use of instruments during an operation to treat injuries, diseases, and deformities. Surgical procedures are named according to (1) the involved body organ, part, or location and (2) the suffix that describes what is done during the procedure (Table 12.1). Physicians who perform surgery include **surgeons** or other physicians trained to do certain surgical procedures. Surgery is scheduled based on the urgency required for a successful outcome for the patient (Table 12.2). The reasons for surgery to be performed are listed in Table 12.2.

 TYPES OF SURGERY

Laser, scope, and robotic technologies reduce the invasiveness of surgical procedures. Minimally invasive surgery is less damaging to tissues than traditional open incision surgery. This allows a faster and less painful recovery. Laser surgery uses a laser instead of a scalpel to cut tissue. It is often used for eye surgery. An endoscope is used for minimally invasive surgery, also called keyhole surgery. Minimally

TABLE 12.1 SURGICAL PROCEDURE SUFFIXES

Suffix	Meaning	Word-Building Examples
-ectomy	Removal by cutting	crani (skull) + ectomy = craniectomy appen (appendix) + ectomy = appendectomy
-orrhaphy	Suture of or repair	colo (colon) + orrhaphy = colorrhaphy herni (hernia) + orrhaphy = herniorrhaphy
-oscopy	Looking into	colon (intestine) + oscopy = colonoscopy gastr (stomach) + oscopy = gastroscopy
-ostomy	Formation of a permanent artificial opening	ureter + ostomy = ureterostomy colo (colon) + ostomy = colostomy
-otomy	Incision or cutting into	oust (bone) + otomy = osteotomy thoro (thorax) + otomy = thoracotomy
-plasty	Formation or repair	oto (ear) + plasty = otoplasty mamm (breast) + plasty = mammoplasty

TABLE 12.2 SURGERY URGENCY LEVEL AND PURPOSE

Type	Definition	Examples
Urgency Level Emergency	Immediate surgery needed to save life or limb without delay	Ruptured aortic aneurysm or appendix, traumatic limb amputation, loss of extremity pulse from emboli
Urgent	Surgery needed within 24–30 hours	Fracture repair, infected gallbladder
Elective	Planned/scheduled, with no time requirements	Joint replacement, hernia repair, skin lesion removal
Optional	Surgery requested by the patient	Cosmetic surgery
Purposes of Surgery Aesthetic	Requested by patient for improvement	Blepharoplasty, breast augmentation
Diagnostic	To obtain tissue samples, make an incision, or use a scope to make a diagnosis	Biopsy
Exploratory	Confirmation or measurement of extent of condition	Exploratory laparotomy

Continued

TABLE 12.2 SURGERY URGENCY LEVEL AND PURPOSE—cont'd

Type	Definition	Examples
Preventive	Removal of tissue before it causes a problem	Mole or polyp removal to prevent cancer
Curative	Removal of diseased or abnormal tissue	Inflamed appendix, tumor, benign cyst, hernia
Reconstructive	Correction of defects of body parts	Scar repair, total knee replacement, face lift, mammoplasty
Palliative	Alleviation of symptoms when disease cannot be cured	Rhizotomy (cuts nerve root to relieve pain), partial tumor removal to relieve pain or pressure; gastrostomy tube to provide tube feedings for swallowing problem; colostomy for incurable bowel obstruction

invasive surgery includes laparoscopic surgery (abdominal and pelvic cavity) and thoracoscopic surgery (chest and thoracic cavity). The endoscope is a flexible tube with a light, camera, and suction attached. It is inserted through a small incision and projects an image on a screen for the surgeon to watch. Additional incisions are made for other instruments depending on the type of surgery.

Robotic surgery, which uses robots, includes minimally invasive surgery. The *da Vinci* is one type of surgical robot with three or four arms. One is a camera, two are robotic arms that act as the surgeon's hands, and the fourth arm moves obstructions out of the way (Fig. 12.1). As the surgeon moves his or her hands, the robotic arms (which are inside the patient's body) mimic the movements by cutting, suctioning, or suturing. Visit www.intuitivesurgical.com for more information and videos.

PHASES OF SURGERY

There are three phases in the surgical process: preoperative, intraoperative, and postoperative. These phases together are referred to as **perioperative**, which is the time before, during, and after surgery. Each of the perioperative surgical phases has a defined time frame in which specific events related to surgery occur (Table 12.3).

FIGURE 12.1 Operating room featuring the da Vinci Si Surgical System with surgeon at the da Vinci robotic surgery console and nurse at the vision cart. *Courtesy of Intuitive Surgical, Inc., Sunnyvale, CA.*

TABLE 12.3   PERIOPERATIVE SURGICAL PHASES

Perioperative	All three phases surrounding and during surgery
Preoperative	Begins with decision for surgery and ends with transfer to the operating room
Intraoperative	Begins with transfer to operating room and ends with admission to perianesthesia care unit (PACU)
Postoperative	Begins with admission to PACU and continues until recovery is complete

◼ PREOPERATIVE PHASE

Your primary role as a licensed practical nurse/licensed vocational nurse (LPN/LVN) in the **preoperative** phase is to:

- Assist in data collection for developing the patient's plan of care.
- Reinforce explanations and instructions given to the patient and family by the surgeon and registered nurse (RN).
- Provide emotional and psychological support for patients and their families.

You can help reduce family members' anxiety by providing explanations so that they are less anxious and able to assist the patient during recovery.

Other health team members assist in preparing the patient for surgery. The surgeon obtains a medical history, performs a physical examination, and orders diagnostic testing. RNs perform a baseline preoperative assessment, provide explanations and instructions, offer patients and families emotional and psychological support to ease anxiety, develop a plan of care, and then verify the patient's name, surgical site (along with the patient), allergies, and related information when the patient arrives in the surgical area.

Factors Influencing Surgical Outcomes

When preparing a patient for surgery and assisting in the development of a nursing care plan, the goal is to identify and implement actions that reduce surgical risk factors. Preoperative care focuses on helping the patient achieve the best possible surgical outcome by being in the healthiest possible condition for surgery.

Emotional Responses

The word *surgery* causes a common anxious emotional reaction in patients and their families. You need to be aware of

these reactions to assist the patient in coping with them. If any of the patient's fears are extreme, such as a fear of dying or not waking up after surgery, the surgeon should be informed.

Surgical patients may experience various fears related to **anesthesia** (reversible loss of sensation): possible brain damage, feeling sensation during surgery, feeling loss of control, or a fear of not waking up. The patient should discuss these concerns with the anesthesia professional. Listening to music or using guided imagery before surgery may reduce a patient's anxiety (see "Evidence-Based Practice").

It is normal for patients to be concerned about pain. During surgery, the anesthesia provider gives medications to control pain. Nurses give prescribed analgesics for pain relief after surgery. Complementary techniques can also be used to help reduce pain, such as guided imagery or focused breathing.

Changes in body image may be a great fear for some patients. The thought of disfigurement, mutilation, bleeding, or having a scar causes great anxiety for some patients. Allow them to discuss these fears.

EVIDENCE-BASED PRACTICE

Clinical Question
Does listening to music reduce preoperative anxiety for surgical patients?

Evidence
Twenty-six studies comparing music listening with standard care preoperatively (Bradt, Dileo, & Shim, 2013). Music listening was found to have a beneficial effect on preoperative anxiety. Music even reduced anxiety more effectively than a sedative in one study.

Implications for Nursing Practice
Patients can be informed to bring in favorite music to listen to before surgery to reduce anxiety.

REFERENCE

Bradt, J., Dileo, C., & Shim, M. (2013). Music interventions for preoperative anxiety. *Cochrane Database of Systematic Reviews, 6,* CD006908. DOI: 10.1002/14651858 .CD006908.pub2.

Age

Surgery can be a positive experience that promotes quality of life for many older patients. For healthy older patients, age alone does not mean that they are at greater surgical risk. Complications can occur, however, related to previous health status, immobilization occurring from surgery, normal aging changes reducing the effectiveness of deep breathing and coughing, and the effects of administered medications (see "Gerontological Issues"). Older patients may need a longer time to recover from anesthetic agents because of changes in drug metabolism and elimination related to aging.

Gerontological Issues

Surgical Considerations for the Older Adult

Older adults usually have limited physiological reserve, resulting in decreased ability to compensate for changes that occur during surgery. The risk for hemorrhage, anemia, fluid/electrolyte imbalance, and infection are increased in older adults. Increased risk for complications is secondary to age-related loss of blood vessel elasticity and decreased cardiac, respiratory, and renal reserves. Nursing interventions should be aimed at these age-related changes before, during, and after the surgical procedure to help reduce complications.

Preoperatively

- Reassure the patient and family.
- Pad bony prominences to protect against pressure ulcers and muscle and bone discomfort.
- Teach what to expect before, during, and after surgery; diet changes; description and length of surgical procedure; activities in the recovery room; pain management; coughing and deep breathing exercises; procedures; and treatments (e.g., dressings, catheters).
- Ensure preoperative screening: blood work, radiographic studies, nutritional assessments, pulmonary function tests, electrocardiogram (ECG).

Intraoperatively

- Assess patient for **hypothermia**
- Assess patient for hypoxia (older adult may exhibit restlessness).
- Assess patient for hemorrhage.
- Assess patient's output (urine, drainage, bleeding, emesis).

Postoperatively

Pain Control—Provide adequate pain relief so required postoperative activities, such as deep breathing, coughing, position changes, and exercise, can be performed more effectively.

Respiratory Function—Reduce respiratory complications by encouraging deep breathing and coughing:

- Perform after pain medication has begun to take effect to encourage deep breaths due to less pain. Assess the patient carefully when giving narcotics because they can cause respiratory depression.
- Use a pillow and instruct the patient to hold it firmly over abdominal or chest incisions to support the incision. Taking a deep breath increases chest expansion, as well as abdominal pressure, which may pull or stretch an incision.
- Older adults perform deep-breathing and coughing exercises better if the nurse performs the exercises with them. For example, say the following: "Let's take a deep breath in through the nose, hold it and count to three, then slowly blow it out completely through the mouth. When you blow the air out, shape your lips like they are going to whistle. Great, let's do it again."

Mobility—Encourage mobility through the following nursing actions and observations:

- Use pillows to support the patient's body alignment; assist the patient to ambulate as soon as possible after surgery; and regularly help the patient with passive or active range-of-motion exercises, along with flexion and extension exercises, for legs and feet.
- Monitor for unilateral swelling of the leg and calf or groin pain, which may indicate deep venous thrombosis (DVT), a risk related to venous pooling in the lower extremities. This risk is increased with postoperative inactivity.
- Assist the patient to change position at least every 2 hours. If patients lay in one position too long, pressure ulcers can develop. When tissues are compressed between bones and the bed surface, blood supply is reduced to the tissue and cells begin to die. This results in painful open wounds.

Bowel Function—Assess bowel sounds. It is common for patients to feel bloated after surgery. Increasing activity, such as walking—not just sitting in a chair—stimulates peristaltic action of the bowel. This helps expel flatus and reduce discomfort.

Urinary Function—Be aware of the following aspects of urinary function:

- Individuals often have difficulty emptying their bladder after surgery. Patients who are sleeping but restless should be evaluated for bladder distention. It is often difficult to void on a bedpan or in a urinal in a supine position.
- Older men with an enlarged prostate may have even greater difficulty voiding if they have received medications that have urinary retention side effects.
- Assisting patients to sit or stand to use urinals, use a bedside commode, or ambulate to the bathroom promotes bladder emptying and helps avoid the use of urinary catheters.
- Measure urine output that is voided or from a catheter. Note the color and odor of the urine. Older adults are prone to dehydration, and this provides an indication of their hydration status for intervention.

Delirium—Perform the following nursing actions to minimize delirium:

- Monitor level of consciousness routinely. Provide a calm environment and orient patients to their environment. Restraints should not be used because they can worsen delirium.
- Recognize that the presence of a urinary catheter can contribute to delirium, so methods to avoid the need for a catheter should be tried.

Nutrition

Patients should be well nourished to adequately heal and recover from surgery ("Nutrition Notes"). Higher levels of protein (tissue repair and healing), vitamin C (collagen formation), and zinc (tissue growth, skin integrity, and cell-mediated immunity) are required. Patients who are obese or underweight may not heal as well and may have complications. Patients who are obese have more respiratory problems and wound healing difficulties, such as delayed healing and wound *dehiscence* (opening of the incision). Patients who are emaciated may have more infections and delayed wound healing because they lack the nutrients needed for tissue healing.

Nutrition Notes

Screening and Nourishing the Preoperative Patient

Identifying and treating malnutrition before surgery may improve the patient's outcome. Unintended weight loss or a low serum albumin level should prompt further nutritional assessment. Before elective surgery, the patient may have time to correct some nutritional deficiencies. If patients are overweight they are often instructed to lose weight to reduce the risk of surgery. For anemia, an iron preparation can be administered. At least 2 to 3 weeks are required for objective evidence of the effectiveness of nutritional therapy. Before surgery on the gastrointestinal (GI) tract, a low-residue diet may be given for 2 to 3 days to minimize bowel contents.

Preoperative fasting time orders vary but the American Society of Anesthesiologists' (2011) guidelines recommend a minimum of the following time frames before anesthesia:
- Clear liquids: 2 hours
- Light meal (toast/clear liquid): 6 hours
- A meal containing meat or fat: 8 hours.

Clinical judgment is required regardless of the guidelines, which do not apply to:
- Patients with gastromotility or metabolic disorders
- Those with potential airway problems
- Women in labor

Smoking and Alcohol

Tobacco and alcohol use increases the surgical patient's risks. Smoking thickens and increases the amount of lung secretions and reduces the action of cilia that remove the secretions. Patients should be encouraged to avoid smoking for at least 24 hours before surgery or 3 to 4 weeks before surgery if they have a chronic lung disorder. Not smoking increases the action of the lungs' defense mechanisms and makes more hemoglobin available to carry oxygen during surgery. It also improves wound healing.

Long-term alcohol use may cause nutritional deficiencies and liver damage, which can create bleeding problems, fluid volume imbalances, and drug metabolism alterations. In addition, alcohol interacts with medications and should be avoided before surgery.

Chronic Disease

Chronic disorders may increase the patient's surgical risk unless they are well controlled. A medical clearance for surgery may be needed from the patient's health care practitioner (HCP).

Preadmission Surgical Patient Assessment

Nonemergent surgical patients have either an interview with the **anesthesiologist** or a preadmission telephone or face-to-face interview with RNs in the preadmission testing department under the direction of the anesthesia professional. The interview process includes a health history, identification of risk factors, patient and family teaching, discharge planning, and necessary referrals to social work, support groups, and educational programs. Patients are asked if there have been any personal or family problems with anesthesia or malignant hyperthermia. Malignant hyperthermia is a rare hereditary muscle disease that can predispose the patient to a serious life-threatening reaction to certain anesthetic agents (discussed later).

Preoperative diagnostic testing is based on the patient's age, medical history, assessment findings, and institutional protocols (see Table 12.4). A urine or serum pregnancy test as appropriate for female patients may be done to prevent fetal exposure to anesthetics. Health information and diagnostic testing results are reviewed by anesthesia providers. Abnormal test results are reported to the surgeon. Interventions are ordered for abnormalities.

TABLE 12.4 PREOPERATIVE DIAGNOSTIC TESTS

Diagnostic Test	Purpose
Chest x-ray	Detect pulmonary and cardiac abnormalities
Oxygen saturation	Obtain baseline level and detect abnormality
Serum Tests	
Arterial blood gases	Obtain baseline levels and detect pH and oxygenation abnormalities

Continued

TABLE 12.4 PREOPERATIVE DIAGNOSTIC TESTS—cont'd

Bleeding time	Detect prolonged bleeding problem
Blood urea nitrogen	Detect kidney problem
Creatinine	Detect kidney problem
Complete blood cell count	Detect anemia, infection, clotting problem
Electrolytes	Detect potassium, sodium, chloride imbalances
Fasting blood glucose	Detect abnormalities, monitor diabetes control
Pregnancy	Detect early, unknown pregnancy
Partial thromboplastin time	Detect clotting problem
International normalized ratio (INR)	Detect clotting problem, monitor warfarin therapy
Type and cross-match	Identify blood type to match blood for possible transfusion
Urine Tests Pregnancy	Detect early, unknown pregnancy
Urinalysis	Detect infection, abnormalities

Federal law says patients must be asked before surgery if they have a signed advance directive (e.g., health care durable power of attorney or living will) for their medical record (see Chapter 17). If there is no advance directive, written information on advance directives is offered.

Preoperative Teaching

Preoperative Routines

Preoperative teaching provides information about common surgical preparation procedures and routines:

- Date and time of admission and surgery
- Admission procedures, including arriving about 2 hours before surgery to allow preparation time
- Length of stay, items to bring and wear
- Recovery after surgery
- Family information, such as where to wait during surgery and who communicates patient's status to them
- Discharge criteria, including the need for a responsible adult to take the patient home after outpatient surgery.

Preoperative Instructions

To reduce the risks of pulmonary aspiration during surgery, the anesthesia professional orders fluid and food restrictions. The minimal fasting time frame guidelines of the American Society of Anesthesiologists are listed in the "Nutrition Notes." Patients may brush their teeth or rinse their mouth without swallowing. Cancellation of surgery can result if the patient has not followed instructions to stop eating or drinking as specified.

Medications the patient is to take the morning of surgery, with an ounce of water, are explained. Special preparations, such as an enema, are also described. For abdominal or intestinal surgery, enemas are ordered to empty the bowel to reduce fecal contamination preoperatively and straining or distention postoperatively.

Instructions for postoperative care are given before surgery so the patient is alert when being taught and has time to learn. Patients should be told that active participation in postoperative care aids in their recovery. Teach patients how to report their pain level using a pain rating scale so that prompt pain relief can be provided (see Chapter 10). Pain rating scales include a 0 (none) to 10 (worst possible) rating scale, a color-based rating scale, or a scale using pictures of faces showing varying degrees of frowning or smiling that indicate a certain pain level. Pain relief methods are described, such as analgesic injections, an epidural catheter, or patient-controlled analgesia (PCA). Anticipated dressings, tubes, casts, or special equipment are also described. If needed, crutches are fitted to the patient, and their proper use is explained and demonstrated.

Postoperative exercises are taught to decrease complications. They include deep breathing and coughing, use of incentive spirometry, leg exercises, turning, and how to get out of bed. After an exercise is taught, the patient should perform a return demonstration so understanding and ability to perform the exercise correctly can be evaluated.

Deep breathing helps prevent the development of **atelectasis** (collapse of the lung caused by hypoventilation or mucous obstruction preventing some alveoli from opening and being fully ventilated) by expanding and ventilating the lungs. The patient is taught to sit up, exhale fully, take in a

• **WORD** • **BUILDING** •
atelectasis: ateles—imperfect + ektasis—expansion

deep breath through the nose, hold the breath and count to three, and then exhale completely through the mouth. The patient is told to repeat this hourly while awake, in sets of five, for 24 to 48 hours postoperatively.

Incentive spirometry can also be ordered postoperatively to prevent atelectasis by increasing lung volume, alveoli expansion, and venous return (Fig. 12.2). All patients can benefit from incentive spirometry, especially the older adult and those at increased risk for lung complications. The spirometer stays at the patient's bedside for hourly use while awake (not on the window sill or in a drawer where it cannot be reached by the patient!). Offer the spirometer to the patient each hour to ensure that it is used. Teach patients to do the following:

- Sit upright, at 45° minimum, if possible.
- Take two normal breaths. Place mouthpiece of spirometer in mouth.

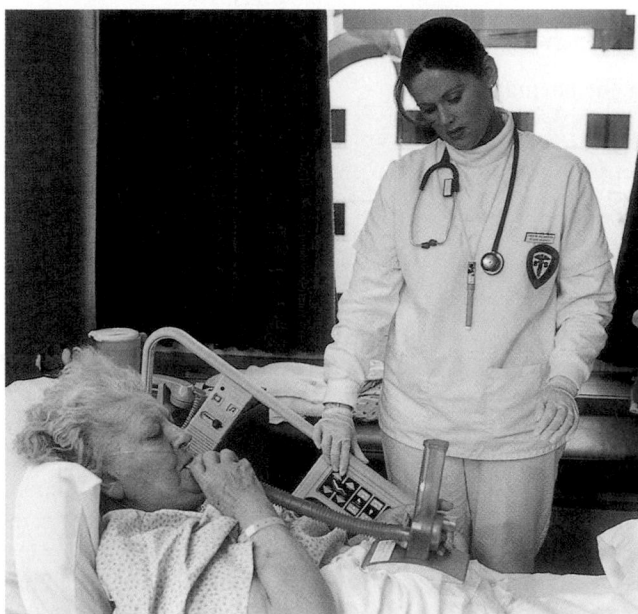

FIGURE 12.2 An incentive spirometer aids lung expansion.

- Inhale until target, designated by spirometer light or rising ball, is reached, and hold breath for 3 to 5 seconds.
- Exhale completely.
- Perform 10 sets of breaths each hour.

Coughing moves secretions to prevent pneumonia. Teach patients how to cough effectively if not contraindicated by the patient's condition (such as hernia repair or head injury; Table 12.5). Give pain medication before asking the patient to cough and offer reassurance that coughing should not harm the incision. Splinting the incision with a pillow may be comforting. Several sets of coughing are performed every 1 to 2 hours while the patient is awake.

Leg exercises and foot circles done every hour while awake, if not contraindicated, improve circulation and help prevent complications related to stasis of blood, such as emboli formation. Teach patients to do the following:

- Lie down, raise leg, and bend leg at the knee.
- Flex foot, extend leg, and lower it to the bed.
- Do sets of five for each leg.
- For foot circles, raise a leg slightly off the bed with toes pointed.
- Draw a circle in the air with the great toe.
- Rotating to the right four times, then to the left four times.
- Repeat this five times and then repeat with the other foot.

Patients are taught that turning from side to side in bed is aided by bending the leg that is to be on top and placing a pillow between the legs to support the top leg. Unless contraindicated, have patients use the bed's side rail to pull themselves over to the side. To promote comfort, patients are encouraged to deep breathe while turning instead of holding their breath.

To make it easier for patients to get out of bed and to reduce strain on the incision, instruct patient to do this:

- Turn on side without pillows between knees.
- Place hands flat against the bed.
- Push up while swinging legs out of bed into a sitting position.

TABLE 12.5 TEACHING PATIENTS COUGHING TECHNIQUES

Procedure	Rationale
Have patient sit up and lean forward.	Promotes lung expansion and ability to generate forceful cough.
Show patient how to splint incision with hands, pillow, or blanket.	Reduces incision pressure so it does not feel as if incision is opening.
Have patient inhale and exhale deeply three times through mouth.	Helps expand lungs.
Have patient take in deep breath and cough out the breath forcefully with three short coughs using diaphragmatic muscles. Take in quick deep breath through mouth, cough deeply, and deep breathe.	Generates forceful cough and expands lungs to help move secretions.

• Sit for a few minutes after changing position to avoid dizziness and falling.
• Deep breathe while sitting to expand lungs.

Nursing Process for Preoperative Patients
Data Collection

HEALTH HISTORY.   Upon admission for surgery, patient data are collected (Table 12.6). Ensure that patients use their contact lenses, glasses, or hearing aids for accurate communication. Note the patient's emotional reaction to surgery. If the patient is anxious, explore the cause of the anxiety and allow the patient to express concerns. Anxiety is a feeling of apprehension or uneasiness resulting from the uncertainties and risks associated with surgery, whereas fear, a feeling of dread from a source known to the patient, is an extreme reaction to surgery.

Medications.   All prescription and over-the-counter medications that the patient takes are reviewed, along with any herbal remedies or recreational drugs. Anticoagulants such as warfarin (Coumadin), or nonsteroidal anti-inflammatory drugs (NSAIDS) including aspirin may need to be stopped several days before surgery to avoid bleeding problems during surgery. Because herbal medicines can interfere with medications used during surgery or increase bleeding times, patients may be instructed to stop them 1 to 2 weeks before surgery.

TABLE 12.6   NURSING ASSESSMENT OF THE PREOPERATIVE PATIENT

Subjective Data: Health History Questions	
Demographic information	Name, age, marital status, occupation, roles?
Condition for which surgery is scheduled	Why are you having surgery?
Medical history	Any allergies, acute or chronic conditions, current medications, pain, or prior hospitalizations?
Surgical history	Any reactions or problems with anesthesia? Previous surgeries?
Tobacco use	How much do you smoke? Pack-year history (number of packs per day × number of years)?
Alcohol use	How often do you drink alcohol? How much?
Coping techniques	How do you usually cope with stressful situations? Support systems?
Family history	Hereditary conditions, diabetes, cardiovascular or anesthesia problems?
Female patients	Date of last menses and obstetrical information?
Physical Assessment Vital signs, oxygen saturation	
Height and weight	
Emotional status	Calm, anxious, tearful
Neurologic	Ability to follow instructions
Skin	Color, warmth, bruises, lesions, turgor, dryness, mucous membranes
Respiratory	Infection (cough; breath sounds); chronic obstructive pulmonary disease; respiratory rate, pattern, and effort; barrel chest
Cardiovascular	Angina, myocardial infarction, heart failure, hypertension, valvular heart disease, mitral valve prolapse, heart rate and rhythm, peripheral pulses, edema, jugular vein distention
Gastrointestinal	Bowel sounds, date of last bowel movement, abdominal distention, firmness, ostomy
Musculoskeletal	Deformities, weakness, decreased range of motion, crepitation, gait, artificial limbs, prostheses

Patients with diabetes who take insulin are usually instructed by anesthesia either to hold their insulin or to take half of their normal dose of insulin the day of surgery. On the day of surgery, blood glucose monitoring is done every 4 hours or as ordered to ensure that blood glucose levels are maintained within a desired range.

Patients on chronic oral steroid therapy cannot abruptly stop steroids even though they may be NPO (nothing by mouth) before or after surgery. Serious complications, such as circulatory collapse, can develop if steroids are stopped abruptly. The physician should order a patient's steroid therapy to be given by a parenteral route if the patient is NPO, so that it is not interrupted. Make sure that the steroid therapy is ordered and continued for the patient.

Patients should be asked about the use of alcohol or drugs such as cocaine, marijuana, or opioids because they can interact with anesthesia or other medications. To obtain honest, accurate information, patients should be told of this potential interaction. Information and questions should be stated in a nonjudgmental manner. For example, you should ask, "How much alcohol do you drink daily or weekly?" instead of "Do you drink alcohol?" The first statement assumes that people drink alcohol. This allows the patient who does not drink to indicate none and the patient who does to state an amount rather than having to say yes and then give an amount upon further questioning. More accurate responses are given because this approach is viewed more positively by the patient who consumes alcohol. Another example would be to ask the patient, "What roles do drugs or alcohol play in your life?"

Physical Assessment

A physical assessment of body systems is performed. This information can highlight risk factors for surgery, determine the type of anesthesia to be used, and assist in planning interventions to reduce risk factors. A cough, cold, or fever is reported to the surgeon because surgery may be delayed until the patient recovers from an acute infection. Dentures, bridges, capped teeth, and loose teeth are documented because they can become dislodged during intubation (insertion of endotracheal breathing tube) for general anesthesia, causing complications.

Nursing Diagnoses, Planning, and Interventions

Anxiety or Fear related to potential change in body image, hospitalization, pain, loss of control, and uncertainties surrounding surgery

EXPECTED OUTCOME: Patient will state reduced anxiety or fear before surgery.

- Inform patients about procedures and surgical routines, *which helps reduce anxiety.*
- Allow patients to express their concerns *to allow inaccurate information to be corrected.*
- If patients express extreme anxiety or fear, inform the surgeon *because complications or even death could result. When fear is excessive, the surgeon may reschedule the surgery until the patient is better able to cope.*

Deficient Knowledge related to lack of previous experience with surgical routines and procedures

EXPECTED OUTCOME: Patient will demonstrate understanding of surgical information and routines before surgery.

- Patient anxiety levels should be considered when providing explanations *because learning can be affected by high anxiety levels.*
- Identify knowledge deficiencies with the patient *so that he or she is motivated to learn.*
- Reinforce information provided before admission and new information to patients *to promote informed choice and increase self-care abilities. Teaching is caring in action and empowers patients to be a participant in their care.*
- Include the patient's family or caregivers in teaching sessions *so they can assist the patient through the surgical experience.*
- Use a variety of teaching methods (discussion, written materials and instructions, models, and videos) *to allow for different learning styles and to reinforce learning.*
- Individualize explanations *so the patient is not overwhelmed.*
- Use teaching methods that can be adapted to aging changes that may affect learning. "Gerontological Issues" *describes methods to provide a positive learning experience for the older patient.*
- Document teaching and patient understanding. *Documentation is essential as proof of what was explained and patient understanding.*

Gerontological Issues

Considerations for Older Patient Teaching Sessions

Environmental Considerations

- Comfortable: anxiety free, quiet, appropriate temperature
- Correctly lit: small, intense lighting with nonglare, soft white light (not fluorescent)
- Private: no distractions, no background noise, turn off pagers

Presentation Considerations

- Assess readiness to learn.
- Assess comfort and safety needs.
- Use past experience and relate to new learning.
- Base learning on assessment data and current knowledge base.
- Use simple, understandable words and avoid medical jargon.
- Use legible audiovisual materials: large print, black print on white nonglare paper.
- If using colors, remember that older adults see red, orange, and yellow best; blue, violet, and green are more difficult to see.

- Perform ongoing assessment of energy level of patient.
- Answer questions as they occur.

Presenter Considerations

- Have a positive attitude and belief in self-care promotion for older adults.
- Earn trust by being viewed as a credible, positive role model.
- Maintain a professional appearance.
- Use knowledge of aging changes in presentation.
- Speak slowly in a low tone.
- Sit near patient for best visibility.
- Ensure that prostheses are in place, such as glasses, hearing aids.
- Allow patient increased response time, and use memory aids such as pictures or diagrams.
- Use touch appropriately to convey caring.
- Teach most important information first.
- Present one idea at a time.
- Provide instruction using multiple senses (vision and hearing).
- Provide repetition.
- Ask for feedback to ensure comprehension.
- Provide feedback and positive reinforcement.

Evaluation

The goal of decreased anxiety is achieved if the patient states and demonstrates that anxiety is relieved. If the patient is able to learn during teaching sessions, anxiety is not a barrier to learning. The goal for correcting deficient knowledge is reached if the patient states understanding of the information presented and accurately performs return demonstrations of presented information.

Preoperative Consent

Before performing surgery, it is the surgeon's responsibility to obtain voluntary, written, informed consent from the patient. The consent gives legal permission for the surgery and has two purposes: It protects the patient from unauthorized procedures, and it protects the surgeon, anesthesia professional, hospital, and hospital employees from claims of performance of unauthorized procedures. A signed consent is needed for all invasive procedures, surgery, anesthesia, blood administration, and radiation or cobalt therapy. It is typically valid for 30 days after signing.

Informed consent involves three elements:

1. The surgeon must explain in terms the patient understands about the diagnosis, the proposed treatment and who will perform it, the likely outcome, possible risks and complications of treatment, alternative treatments, and the prognosis

without treatment. If the patient has questions before signing the consent, the surgeon must be contacted to provide further explanation to the patient. It is not within the nurse's scope of practice to provide this information.

2. The consent must be signed before analgesics or sedatives are given because patients must demonstrate to the witness that they are informed and understand the surgery.

3. Consent must be given voluntarily. No persuasion or threats can be used to influence the patient. The patient can withdraw consent at any time, even after the consent form has been signed.

To ensure that patients are truly informed before signing a consent form, in some institutions, patients must take and pass a knowledge quiz, which can be given verbally. If they do not pass the quiz, then further explanation is needed by the surgeon. Also, in the surgical holding area, patients verbally reconsent. They are asked, "Do you still remember what you were told about your surgery?"

It is often your role to obtain and witness the patient's or authorized person's signature on the consent form (Fig. 12.3). As the patient's advocate, you must ensure that the person signing the consent form understands its meaning and has no further questions to be directed to the HCP before it is signed and that it is being signed voluntarily. If the patient is unable to read, the entire consent must be read to the patient before it is signed. Patients are unable to give consent if they are unconscious, are mentally incompetent, are minors, or have received analgesics or drugs that alter central nervous system function within time frames specified by agency policy. Consent may be obtained in any of these cases from parents, next of kin, or legal guardians as specified by law.

FIGURE 12.3 Nurse is witnessing signature of patient on surgical consent.

NURSING CARE TIP

Witnessing a Consent

Your signature as a witness on a consent form indicates that you observed the informed patient or patient's authorized representative voluntarily sign the consent form. It does not mean that you informed the patient about the surgical procedure; that is the responsibility of the HCP.

In a medical emergency, the patient may not be able to give consent. In this case, the next of kin or legal guardian may give telephone consent, or a court order can be obtained. If time does not permit this, the surgeon documents the need for treatment in the chart as necessary to save the patient's life or avoid serious harm, according to state law and institutional policy.

Preparation for Surgery

Preoperative Preparation Checklist

A preoperative checklist is usually completed and signed by the nurse (per agency policy) before the patient is transported from the surgical unit to surgery (Fig. 12.4). The checklist provides guidance for preoperative preparation of the patient:

- An identification band is placed on the patient. A hospital gown is given to the patient to wear. Underwear is removed, depending on the type of surgery.
- Vital signs are taken and recorded as baseline information and to assess patient status.
- Makeup, nail polish, and artificial nails (if applicable) are removed to allow assessment of natural color and pulse oximetry for oxygenation status during surgery.
- Removal of hairpins, wigs, and jewelry prevents loss or injury. Rings, such as wedding rings, are taped in place if the patient does not want to take them off, except if the ring is on the operative side (arm or chest surgery), because edema may occur.
- Dentures, contact lenses, and prostheses are removed to prevent injury. Some patients are concerned about body image and do not want family members to see them without dentures or makeup. Remove dentures after the family goes to the waiting room and insert them before the family sees the patient postoperatively.
- Glasses and hearing aids go with patients to surgery if they are unable to communicate without them. Label them with the patient's name and document where they go.
- All orders, diagnostic test results, consents, and history and physical (required on the chart) are reviewed for completion and documented on the checklist.
- Patient valuables are recorded and given to a family member or locked up per institutional policy by the nurse.

- Antiembolism devices are applied if ordered.
- Patients are asked to void before sedating preoperative medications are given, unless a urinary catheter is present, to prevent injury to the bladder during surgery.

Preoperative Medications

Preoperative medications are given at the time ordered or on call to surgery (i.e., surgery calls to instruct that it is time to give the drugs; Table 12.7). If sedatives or analgesics are given, the bed rails are raised for safety and the patient is instructed not to get up alone.

BE SAFE!

National Surgical Care Improvement Project (SCIP)

Goal: Improve the safety of surgical care by reducing postoperative complications.

The Centers for Medicare and Medicaid Services, the Joint Commission, and other national organizations partnered for this quality project (www.jointcommission.org). Education for the public is provided in "Tips for Safer Surgery," which summarizes project categories for reducing surgical complications. The information encourages patients to ask their HCP and nurses questions about their surgery. Being aware of this project will help you accurately answer your patients' questions in providing safe surgical care.

Prevention: Areas covered by the SCIP include surgical site infections (SSIs), normothermia, venous thrombo event (VTE), and adverse cardiac events. Methods for preventing SSIs include the following:

- Giving prophylactic antibiotics within 1 hour before incision time and stopping them within 24 hours.
- Using electronic clippers for site hair removal, controlling perioperative serum glucose during major cardiac procedures, and removing urinary catheters by postoperative day 2.
- Maintaining core body temperature within normal range (normothermia) reduces risk (infection, impaired wound healing, MI, blood transfusion) in the perioperative period.
- VTE can be prevented by administering appropriate perioperative anticoagulants to those at risk.
- Avoiding adverse cardiac events includes giving beta blockers during the perioperative period to eligible major noncardiac surgical patients and to surgical patients who have coronary artery disease, and informing the HCP of all medications and herbs taken.

Pre-op Surgical Checklist   **Client Name**

_____ I.D. BAND ON   _____

_____ NPO AS ORDERED

_____ PRE-OP TEACHING COMPLETED

_____ INFORMED CONSENT SIGNED

_____ HISTORY AND PHYSICAL ON CHART

_____ ALLERGIES

_____ LAB RESULTS

_____   CBC: HGB _____ HCT _____ WBC _____ PLATELETS _____

_____   POTASSIUM _____

_____   URINALYSIS _____

_____   PREGNANCY TEST   SERUM _____ URINE _____

_____   PT _____ PTT _____ BLEEDING TIME _____

_____   TYPE AND SCREEN _____ CROSSMATCH _____-___ UNITS

_____ ECG ON CHART

_____ CHEST X-RAY REPORT ON CHART

_____ SHOWERED/BATHED

_____ HOSPITAL GOWN ON

_____ PREPS COMPLETED AS ORDERED

_____ ANTIEMBOLISM STOCKINGS

_____ JEWELRY TAPED/REMOVED: DISPOSITION _____

_____ VALUABLES: DISPOSITION _____

_____ DENTURES, PROSTHESIS REMOVED

_____ HAIR PINS, WIGS, MAKE UP, NAIL POLISH, ONE ACRYLIC NAIL REMOVED

_____ CONTACT LENSES REMOVED

_____ VOIDED

_____ VITAL SIGNS: T _____ P _____ R _____ BP _____

_____ PRE-OP MEDICATIONS GIVEN _____ SIDE RAILS UP _____

_____ IV STARTED _____

_____ EYE GLASSES AND HEARING AID(S) TO OR

_____ OLD CHART TO OR

_____ X-RAYS TO OR

_____ FAMILY LOCATION _____

_____ NEXT OF KIN _____

_____ CLIENT READY FOR SURGERY _____

          TIME _____   (NURSE SIGNATURE)

       COMMENTS:

FIGURE 12.4 Sample preoperative checklist form.

Transfer to Surgery Department

When the surgery department is ready, the patient is transported to the surgical holding area on a gurney (Fig. 12.5). The patient's chart, inhaler medications for those with asthma, and glasses or hearing aids to aid communication are taken with the patient. Family members can accompany the patient. During the surgery, the family waits in the surgical waiting area, which is a communication center where the family can be called via cell phone or given a beeper to be kept informed of the patient's status.

Post-Transfer to Surgery Department

After the patient goes to the surgery department, you can prepare the patient's room and necessary equipment so it is ready upon the patient's return (Table 12.8).

Patient Arrival in Surgery Department

The holding area nurse greets the patient; verifies the patient's name, age, allergies, surgeon performing the surgery, informed consent, surgical procedure (right site, especially right

TABLE 12.7 PREOPERATIVE MEDICATIONS

Class/Action	Examples	Nursing Implications
Analgesic/Antipyretic Relieves mild to moderate pain and reduces fever.	acetaminophen (OFIRMEV)	Given intravenously as 15-minute infusion. Antipyretic effect may mask fever.
Antianxiety and Sedative Hypnotics Sedation; anxiety reduction	diazepam (Valium) lorazepam (Ativan) midazolam (Versed)	Contraindicated for acute narrow-angle glaucoma. Monitor respirations.
Antiemetics Control nausea and vomiting	ondansetron (Zofran) metoclopramide (Reglan) promethazine hydrochloride (Phenergan)	Redness, pain, or burning at the site of injection. Increased drowsiness with opioids.
Antibiotics Prevention of postoperative infection	Variety of antibiotics used	Give within 30–60 minutes of incision for best effect.
Opioids Bind to opioid receptors in the central nervous system to alter perception of pain and enhance postoperative pain relief	fentanyl (Sublimaze, Duragesic) morphine sulfate meperidine (Demerol)	Monitor vital signs, level of sedation, and respiratory status. Avoid meperidine use in older adult.

or left when applicable), and medical history; answers questions; and alleviates anxiety. The patient is introduced to the anesthesiologist and certified registered nurse anesthetist (CRNA), who also verify patient information and explain the type of anesthesia that is to be used. All surgical patients have IV fluids started. The patient may also receive prophylactic antibiotics.

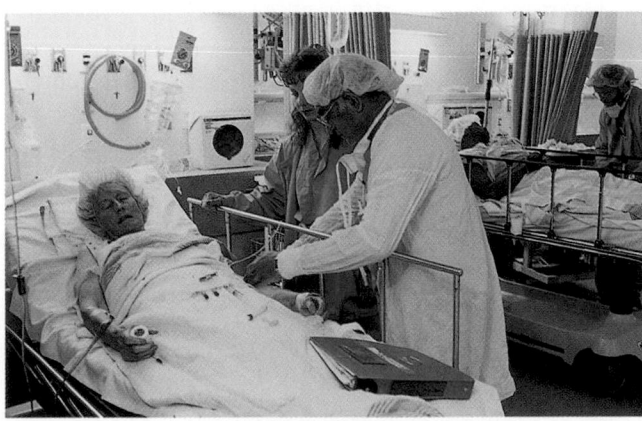

FIGURE 12.5 Surgical holding area.

Before entering the operating room (OR), the patient should be told what to expect:

• "If the room feels cool, you can request extra blankets."
• "There is a lot of equipment in the room, including a table and large, bright overhead lights."
• "Several health care team members will introduce themselves to you."
• "Your surgeon will greet you."
• "A safety checklist will be performed."

Preoperative Warming

To maintain normal body temperature (normothermia) and reduce intraoperative hypothermia, which is associated with complications, prewarming peripheral tissues or surface skin before anesthesia is helpful. Use of forced-air warming devices for 30 minutes may reduce hypothermia. Patients should be normothermic before transfer to surgery.

INTRAOPERATIVE PHASE

When the patient is transferred to the operating table, the next phase of the perioperative period, the **intraoperative** phase, begins. Surgery may take place in a hospital OR or

TABLE 12.8 POSTOPERATIVE PATIENT HOSPITAL ROOM PREPARATION

After patient transfer to surgery, prepare the patient's room for the patient's postoperative care needs on return from the perianesthesia care unit.

Preparation	Rationale
Bed	
Bed linens should be clean and are changed if used by patient before surgery.	Reduces contamination of surgical wound.
Place disposable, absorbent, waterproof pads on bottom sheet if drainage is expected.	Protects linen from wetness and soiling so a patient in pain does not have to be disturbed for linen change.
Apply lift sheet on bed of patient needing assistance with repositioning.	Makes lifting and turning easier for patient and nurse.
Have extra blankets available.	Patient may be cold.
Fanfold top cover to end of bed or to side of bed away from patient transfer side.	Readies bed to receive patient on transfer and allows covers to be easily pulled up over patient.
Obtain extra pillows as needed for positioning, elevating extremities, splinting during coughing.	Pillows help maintain position when patient is turned, or splint an incision during coughing, or elevate operative extremities for comfort and swelling reduction.
Equipment	
Have vital sign equipment available.	Promotes ability to promptly obtain vital signs.
Have intravenous (IV) pole/controller pump available.	Surgical patients have IV infusions postoperatively.
Have oxygen set up as needed.	After tracheostomy, patients wear humidified oxygen mask.
Prepare suction setup for tracheostomy, nasogastric tube, or drains as ordered.	Suction may be ordered related to surgical procedures: *Sterile suction:* tracheostomy *Nasogastric tube:* thoracic, abdominal, gastrointestinal surgery *T-tube:* cholecystectomy.
Have emesis basin at bedside.	Nausea or vomiting may occur, especially after movement during transfer.
Have tissues and washcloths in room.	Promotes comfort: washing face or a cool cloth on forehead.
Have urinal or bedpan available in room.	Patients may be unable to get out of bed for first voiding.
Obtain special equipment as indicated by the surgical procedure.	Institutional policy and surgeon orders may require specialized equipment. Examples: *Jaw surgery:* suction, wire cutters, tracheostomy tray *Tracheostomy:* suction, extra tracheostomy set, tracheostomy care supplies
Documentation Forms Place any agency postoperative documentation forms in room.	Promotes timely and accurate documentation of patient data.

BE SAFE!

Follow the Joint Commission's Universal Protocol for Preventing Wrong-Person, Wrong-Site, Wrong-Procedure Surgery.

Preprocedure Verification

Conduct a preprocedure verification process to ensure that all relevant documents, information, and equipment are available. Implement a process to mark the surgical site and involve the patient in the marking process.

Time Out

Take a time out immediately before beginning the procedure to conduct a final assessment that the correct patient, site, and procedure have been identified. No procedure (conducted in any setting) should start unless all personnel involved in the patient's care have honored the "time out" (Joint Commission's 2014 National Patient Safety Goals. © The Joint Commission, 2013. Reprinted with permission.).

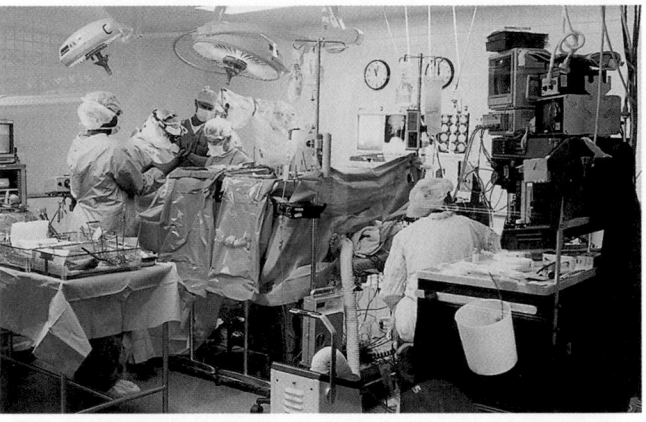

FIGURE 12.7 Operating room in use. Anesthesia equipment is on the right.

worn. If nail polish is worn, it should not be chipped and should be removed and reapplied every 4 days. Sterile gloves are then worn by the surgical team to keep the surgical field sterile.

The OR is designed to enhance **aseptic** (elimination of microorganisms) technique. Clean and contaminated areas are

freestanding ambulatory or outpatient surgical center (Figs. 12.6 and 12.7). Additionally, surgery is performed in physician's offices, cardiac catheterization laboratories, radiology centers, emergency rooms, and specialized units that perform endoscopy procedures.

The OR team members (Box 12-1) must perform a sterile surgical hand scrub to reduce the amount of microorganisms on their hands and arms. Jewelry (e.g., watches, rings, bracelets) is also removed. Fingernails are kept short and clean. Artificial nails and nail polish may harbor microorganisms and therefore are recommended not to be

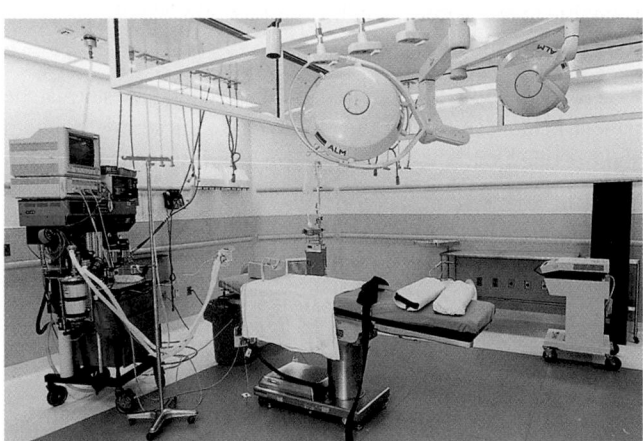

FIGURE 12.6 Operating room. Anesthesia equipment is on the left.

Box 12-1 Surgical Health Care Team Members and Roles

Members of the surgical health care team and their roles are as follows:

- Surgeon (medical doctor, doctor of osteopathy, oral surgeon, or podiatrist)
- *Surgical (first) assistant:* assists the surgeon and is another physician, a specially trained RN, or a physician's assistant
- *Anesthesiologist:* physician who specializes in administering anesthesia and supervises certified registered nurse anesthetists (CRNAs) in the operating room
- *CRNA:* an RN trained and certified in administering anesthesia, usually at the master's degree level
- *RN:* circulates in the OR; roles include being patient's advocate, planning care, protecting patient safety, monitoring patient positioning, checking vital signs and patient assessment, reducing patient's anxiety, monitoring sterility during surgery, preparing skin before incision, managing equipment such as by making sponge counts, documenting the procedure, and aiding health team communications
- *Surgical (second assistant) technician:* assists surgeon (may be an RN, LPN/LVN, or surgical technologist)

separated. Special ventilation systems control dust and prevent air from flowing into the OR from hallways. The temperature and humidity in the room are controlled to discourage bacterial growth. Ambient room temperature to reduce patient hypothermia is recommended to be 68° to 77°F (20°–25°C). Everyone entering the OR wears surgical scrubs, shoe covers, caps, masks, and goggles to protect the patient from infection and themselves from bloodborne pathogens. Traffic in and out of the OR is limited. Strong disinfectants are used to clean the OR after each surgical case, and instruments are sterilized.

Before the patient arrives in surgery, a nursing plan of care with intraoperative nursing diagnoses and expected outcomes is developed from preadmission assessment data (Box 12-2). Attention is given to the safety needs of the patient. A surgical case cart containing sterile instruments required for the patient's case is prepared ahead of time.

The patient is assisted onto the operating table, and a safety strap is carefully applied. A time-out is taken. Then monitoring equipment is applied and readings recorded. The anesthesia provider begins administering anesthesia. When the anesthesia provider gives permission, the patient is carefully positioned to prevent pressure points that could cause tissue or nerve damage. Any needed tubes that are not already in place, such as a nasogastric (NG) tube or urinary catheter, are inserted by the RN.

Patient allergies, including skin prep solutions, are rechecked. If the patient requires body hair removal, hair should be removed with electric clippers. Shaving is avoided because of the potential for microabrasions and colonization

by microorganisms. Then a skin prepping solution such as povidone-iodine is used to cleanse the skin. A large area surrounding the operative site is scrubbed to allow for extension of the incision. The scrub is completed in a circular motion from inside to outer edge. If an allergic reaction to the solution occurs, it can cause skin redness and blistering wherever the solution was used. After the skin is scrubbed, a sterile drape is applied with the incisional area left exposed.

BE SAFE!

Improve the safety of using medications. Label all medications, medication containers (e.g., syringes, medicine cups, basins), or other solutions on and off the sterile field in perioperative and other procedural settings (Joint Commission's 2014 National Patient Safety Goals. © The Joint Commission, 2013. Reprinted with permission.).

Anesthesia

Anesthesia is used during surgery to prevent pain and allow the procedure to be done safely. The type of anesthesia and the anesthetic agents are ordered by the anesthesia provider with input from the patient and surgeon.

There are two types of anesthesia: general and local (regional). General anesthesia causes the patient to lose sensation, consciousness, and reflexes. It acts directly on the central nervous system (Box 12-3). Local anesthesia blocks nerve impulses along the nerve where it is injected, resulting in the loss of sensation to a region of the body without the loss of consciousness.

General Anesthesia

General anesthesia is commonly given by IV or inhalation. It is chosen when patients are anxious or do not want local anesthesia, when the surgical procedure will take a long time and there is a need for muscle relaxation, or when the patient is unable to cooperate, as in head injury, muscle disorders, or impaired cognitive function.

INTRAVENOUS AGENTS. To begin most general anesthesia, the patient is induced (which means "to cause anesthesia") with a short-acting IV agent that provides a rapid, smooth **induction** (the period from when the anesthetic is first given until full anesthesia is reached). Because these agents last only a few minutes, they are used along with inhalation agents, which maintain anesthesia during surgery. After induction, the patient is intubated with an endotracheal (ET) tube to provide mechanical ventilation and anesthesia (Fig. 12.8).

INHALATION AGENTS. Maintenance of anesthesia is accomplished by using inhalation agents. These agents are delivered, controlled, and excreted through mechanical ventilation.

Box 12-2 Intraoperative Nursing Diagnoses and Expected Outcome

• *Risk for Injury* related to perioperative positioning, chemicals, electrical equipment, and effect of being anesthetized

  Is free from injury.

• *Risk for Impaired Skin Integrity* related to chemicals, positioning, and immobility

  Skin integrity is maintained.

• *Risk for Deficient Fluid Volume* related to NPO status and blood loss

  Maintains blood pressure, pulse, and urine output within normal limits.

• *Risk for Infection* related to incision and invasive procedures

  Is free of symptoms of infection.

• *Pain* related to positioning, incision, and surgical procedure

  Reports pain is relieved to satisfactory level.

• **WORD-BUILDING** •
induction: inductio—to lead in

Box 12-3 **Malignant Hyperthermia**

Malignant hyperthermia is a rare hereditary muscular disease that can be triggered by some types of general anesthetic agents. A history of anesthetic problems in the patient or family members detects the potential for development of this condition so that precautions can be taken. A history of heat stroke increases the risk of malignant hyperthermia. A muscle biopsy diagnoses this problem. Patients with this condition can undergo surgery safely with careful planning and choice of anesthetic agents by the anesthesia provider.

In malignant hyperthermia, metabolism in the muscles is increased, which produces a very high fever and muscle rigidity, as well as tachycardia, tachypnea, hypertension, dysrhythmias, hyperkalemia, metabolic and respiratory acidosis, and cyanosis. Malignant hyperthermia is life threatening, so immediate treatment is required to prevent death. Surgery is stopped, and anesthesia discontinued immediately. Oxygen at 100% is given. The patient must be cooled with ice and infusions of iced solutions. Dantrolene sodium (Dantrium), a muscle relaxant that relieves the muscle spasms, is the most effective medication for malignant hyperthermia. Dantrolene sodium is kept readily available in the operating room and given according to the treatment protocol of the Malignant Hyperthermia Association of the United States (www.mhaus.org).

Inhalation agents and the ET tube can be irritating to the respiratory tract. Complications that can occur from their use include laryngospasm (sudden violent contraction of the vocal cords), laryngeal edema, irritated throat, or injury to the vocal cords. When the tube is removed, the nurse should closely monitor the patient and be prepared

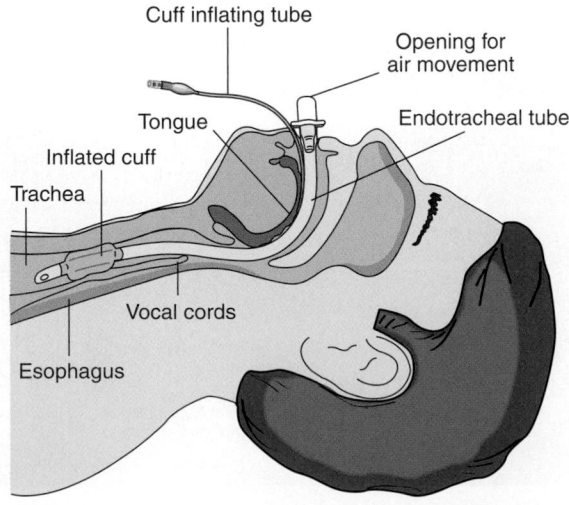

FIGURE 12.8 Endotracheal tube with cuff inflated.

to provide respiratory support and assist with reintubation if complications arise.

ADJUNCT AGENTS. An **adjunct** agent is a medication used along with the primary anesthetic agents. These medications can include opioids to control pain, muscle relaxers to avoid movement of muscles during surgery, antiemetics to control nausea or vomiting, and sedatives to supplement anesthesia.

Local (Regional) Anesthesia

Local anesthesia is selected for the patient who is not anxious, can tolerate the local agent, and is not required by the surgical procedure to be unconscious or have relaxed muscles. It is a good choice for some outpatient procedures. The anesthesia provider, or sometimes the surgeon, administers local anesthesia.

In topical administration, the agent is placed directly on the surgical area. Local infiltration is achieved by injecting the medication into the tissue where the incision is to be made. A regional block is done by injecting the local agent along a nerve that carries impulses in the region where anesthesia is desired. There are several types of regional blocks. A nerve block is the injection of a local agent into a nerve at a specific point. A Bier block is done by placing a tourniquet on an extremity to remove the blood and then injecting the local agent into the extremity. A field block is a series of injections surrounding the surgical area. Use of these blocks has risen.

SPINAL AND EPIDURAL BLOCKS. Injection of a local agent into the subarachnoid space produces spinal block (Fig. 12.9). Epidural block occurs when the local agent is injected into the epidural space. Spinal and epidural blocks are used mainly for lower extremity and lower abdominal surgery. Both motor and sensory function is blocked. The patient must be carefully monitored for complications. Hypotension results from sympathetic blockade causing vasodilation, which reduces venous return to the heart and therefore reduces cardiac output. Respiratory depression results if the block travels too far upward. As the block wears off, patients feel as if their legs are heavy and numb. This is normal, and reassurance should be offered to the patient that this type of feeling does not last after the block wears off.

Complications. A postdural puncture headache results from leakage of cerebrospinal fluid (CSF) from the needle puncture hole in the dura. This reduces pressure on the spinal cord and brain, causing a low-pressure headache, which can be severe. The use of less than 25-gauge spinal needles helps prevent headache. Nausea, dizziness, tinnitus, and vision disturbances may also be present. The headache can worsen when standing or sitting.

Conservative treatment is not usually effective. An autologous epidural blood patch can be used to block the CSF leakage. This sterile procedure is done by the anesthesiologist. To create an epidural blood patch, approximately 15 to 20 mL of the patient's blood is injected into the epidural

FIGURE 12.9 Injection of spinal anesthesia. (A) Epidural anesthesia. (B) Epidural catheter. (C) Spinal anesthesia.

space one interspace below the previous puncture site. Blood patch treatment can be repeated if needed.

Procedural Sedation and Analgesia

Procedural sedation and analgesia (formerly conscious sedation) is purposeful, minimal sedation that does not cause the complete loss of consciousness during selected painful or uncomfortable dental, diagnostic, or medical procedures. The patient may fall asleep but arouse easily and respond. Patients remain in control of their own airway, are comfortable and respond purposefully. Medications such as propofol, ketamine, midazolam, and opioids (fentanyl or morphine) are given to produce sedation. Selection of patients who are eligible for this sedation is based on the procedure, the patient's general health, and patient or physician preference. Examples of short procedures for which this type of sedation is used are dental procedures, endoscopy, cardioversion, and closed fracture reduction. Procedural sedation can be provided by anesthesia providers or ordered by a physician and given by a specially trained RN.

The patient does not eat for 6 hours before the procedure but may have clear liquids up to 2 hours before the procedure. A signed informed consent is obtained. Then an IV for medications and fluids is inserted before the procedure. Patient monitoring is done every 5 minutes to check vital signs, ECG, and oxygen saturation. Changes are reported to the physician. Oxygen may be given by nasal cannula or mask. Emergency equipment (e.g., airway suction, defibrillator, drugs) is on standby, according to advanced cardiac life support (ACLS) protocols.

After the procedure, the patient awakens easily and quickly but may remember little about the procedure. The patient is monitored about every 15 minutes for response to the procedure and medications until he or she is fully awake and stable. The patient is ready for discharge when vital signs return to baseline and are stable, oral fluids are retained, voiding has occurred (if applicable), and written and oral discharge teaching is given to both the patient and the responsible adult to whom the patient is being discharged. The responsible adult and the patient must sign the instructions. Instructions include the following: An adult must drive the patient home and provide a safe environment, and the patient must not and will not drive or operate heavy machinery or sign legal documents for 24 hours.

> ### LEARNING TIP
>
> In comparison with general anesthesia, procedural sedation and analgesia:
>
> - Is less invasive.
> - Requires less medication.
> - Causes less depression of the cardiovascular and respiratory systems.
> - Allows the patient to more quickly return to a wakeful state.

Transfer From Surgery

When surgery is completed and anesthesia stopped, the patient is stabilized for transfer. The patient is normothermic upon transfer from surgery. After local anesthesia, the patient may return directly to a nursing unit. After general and spinal anesthesia, the patient goes to the perianesthesia care unit (PACU) or, in some cases, an intensive care unit (ICU; Fig. 12.10).

FIGURE 12.10 Perianesthesia care unit (PACU).

Patient safety, which is always a priority, is an important concern at this time. The patient is never left alone. Ensuring a patent airway and preventing falls and injury from uncontrolled movements are priorities. The anesthesia provider and OR nurses transfer the patient to the PACU and monitor the patient until the perianesthesia nurse is able to receive the report and assume care of the patient to promote safe recovery from anesthesia. The family is updated on the patient's status after surgery by the surgeon.

BE SAFE!

Improve the effectiveness of communication among caregivers. Implement a standardized approach for "handing off" communications, including an opportunity to ask and respond to questions (Joint Commission's 2014 National Patient Safety Goals. © The Joint Commission, 2013. Reprinted with permission.).

POSTOPERATIVE PHASE

The **postoperative** phase, which is the final perioperative phase, begins when the patient is admitted to the PACU or a nursing unit and ends with the patient's postoperative evaluation in the surgeon's office.

Admission to the Perianesthesia Care Unit

When the patient is admitted to the PACU, an admission assessment is done. The priority areas of patient assessment are:

- Respiratory status and patency of airway
- Vital signs with temperature and Sao_2
- Exhaled end-tidal carbon dioxide ($EtCO_2$)
- Level of consciousness and responsiveness
- Surgical site incision/dressing/drainage tubes
- Pain level and pain management

Oxygen by nasal cannula or mask is given if the patient has had general anesthesia, or as ordered. Some patients who are still intubated may require mechanical ventilation. Continuous monitoring is done on all patients for ECG, vital signs, exhaled end-tidal carbon dioxide, and pulse oximetry. The surgical site incision or dressing is assessed. Drainage amount and color, and **hematoma** formation are documented and reported as needed. Tubes (urinary catheter, drains, NG) or other equipment are checked for function and patency as applicable.

The patient's temperature is measured on admission to the PACU. If the patient's temperature is normal, the temperature is monitored hourly and at discharge from PACU. Passive methods to maintain temperature are continued: room temperature at or above 75°F (24°C), head covering, and cotton blankets. If shivering due to hypothermia occurs, the temperature is retaken. For hypothermia, active warming usually

with a forced-air warming system is used. Temperature is monitored every 15 minutes until normal. Patients are taught to stay warm with a warm room, blankets, layered clothing, head coverings, or warm liquids. The patient must be normothermic before PACU discharge.

The responsibilities of perianesthesia nurses are listed in Box 12-4. It is essential for nurses to perform hand hygiene between patients in the PACU. Vital signs and assessment are done at least every 5 to 15 minutes, IV fluid infusion is maintained, and IV or PCA analgesics are given for pain as needed. Antiemetics are administered for nausea or vomiting. Deep breathing and coughing, if not contraindicated by the surgical procedure (hernia repair; eye, ear, intracranial, and jaw surgery; and plastic surgery) are encouraged. If the patient is no longer NPO, ice chips or sips of water may be offered for a dry mouth when the patient is fully awake.

Nursing Process for Postoperative Patients in PACU

Postoperative complications may occur due to the surgical procedure, anesthesia, blood and fluid loss, immobility, unrelieved pain, or other diseases the patient may have. Nursing care focuses on preventing, detecting, and caring for these complications.

Respiratory Function

DATA COLLECTION. Normal respiratory function can be altered in the immediate postoperative period by airway

---

Box 12-4 Perianesthesia Nursing Responsibilities

- Airway maintenance
- Vital signs including temperature, Sao_2, and exhaled end-tidal carbon dioxide ($EtCO_2$)
- Respiratory assessment
- Neurologic assessment
- Surgical site status
- General assessment
- Patient safety
- Monitoring anesthetic effects
- Pain relief treatment
- Accurate intake and output
- Assessing PACU discharge readiness
- Documentation
- Transfer report to receiving nurse (name, allergies, procedure, type of anesthesia, status, complications, oxygen, dressing/drains/equipment, medications, postoperative orders, pertinent history, family, opportunity to ask questions)

• **WORD-BUILDING** •

hematoma: heimatos—blood + oma—tumor

obstruction, hypoventilation, secretions, laryngospasm, or decreased swallowing and cough reflexes. Respiratory function assessment includes respiratory rate, depth, ease, and pattern. Breath sounds, chest symmetry, accessory muscle use, and sputum are also observed.

Nursing Diagnoses, Planning, and Implementation

Ineffective Breathing Pattern related to anesthesia, pain, and analgesic/sedative medications

EXPECTED OUTCOME: Patient will maintain normal $EtCO_2$ and SaO_2 levels levels at all times.

- Maintain oxygen therapy as ordered *to prevent hypoventilation, which can be an effect of anesthesia medications or analgesics, decreased level of consciousness, or an incision in the thorax causing painful respirations.*
- Encourage deep breathing *to expand the lungs.*
- Give analgesics carefully *to promote deep breathing but avoid respiratory depression.*
- Maintain continuous positive airway pressure/bilevel positive airway pressure (CPAP/BiPap) *to treat sleep apnea.* (Patients may bring their CPAP/BiPap machines with them.)
- Report respiratory depression or abnormal $EtCO_2$ to the anesthesiologist *to obtain prompt treatment.*

Ineffective Airway Clearance related to obstruction, anesthesia medications, and secretions

EXPECTED OUTCOME: Patient will have a patent airway at all times.

- Ensure that patient maintains a patent airway *because airway obstruction may result when relaxed muscles allow the tongue to block the pharynx in patients with a decreased level of consciousness.*
- Use jaw-thrust method to manually open patient's airway *if patient has snoring respirations and has not completely emerged from anesthesia.*

Risk for Aspiration related to depressed cough and gag reflexes and reduced level of consciousness

EXPECTED OUTCOME: Patient will have clear lung sounds at all times.

- Position patient onto side, unless contraindicated, *to protect the airway until fully awake.*
- Have suction equipment always available *to clear secretions or emesis.*

EVALUATION. The goal for ineffective airway clearance and aspiration is achieved if the patient's airway remains patent and lung sounds remain clear. The goal for ineffective breathing pattern is met if the patient's respiratory rate is within normal limits, no dyspnea is reported, and arterial blood gases are within normal limits.

Cardiovascular Function

DATA COLLECTION. Alterations in cardiovascular function can include hypotension, dysrhythmias, and hypertension. Hypotension can be the result of blood and fluid volume loss or cardiac abnormalities. Shock can result from the significant blood and fluid volume loss or from sepsis (see Chapter 9). Dysrhythmias can occur from hypoxia, altered potassium or magnesium levels, hypothermia, pain, stress, or cardiac disease. New-onset hypertension can develop from pain, a full bladder, or respiratory distress.

Cardiovascular function assessment includes heart rate, blood pressure, ECG, and skin temperature, color, and moistness. Vital signs are compared with baseline readings to determine if they are normal. Tachycardia, hypotension, pale skin color, cool, clammy skin, and decreased urine output indicate hypovolemic shock, which requires reporting and prompt treatment.

Nursing Diagnoses, Planning, and Implementation

Deficient Fluid Volume related to blood and fluid loss or NPO status

EXPECTED OUTCOME: Patient will maintain blood pressure, pulse, and urine output within normal limits at all times.

- Check dressings and incisions for color and amount of drainage *to detect fluid loss.*
- Maintain IV fluids at ordered rate *to replace lost fluids but avoid fluid overload.*
- Monitor intake and output (I&O) *to detect imbalances.*

EVALUATION.
The goal for deficient fluid volume is met if vital signs and urine output are within normal limits.

NURSING CARE TIP

Tachycardia: An Early Warning Sign

Tachycardia is a compensatory mechanism designed to provide adequate delivery of oxygen in times of altered function. It is usually the earliest warning sign that an abnormality is occurring. It should be an indicator to assess the patient. Ask yourself what this particular patient is likely to be experiencing that is compromising oxygenation. This will allow you to begin prompt intervention.

PATIENT CONDITION	POSSIBLE CAUSES OF COMPROMISED OXYGENATION
Postoperative patient	Hemorrhage, respiratory depression, pain
Myocardial infarction patient	Cardiogenic shock, pain
Respiratory patient	Respiratory distress
Trauma patient	Hemorrhage, severe pain

Neurologic Function

Until its effects wear off, anesthesia can alter neurologic function. Patients may arrive in the PACU awake, arousable, or sleeping. Patients who are sleeping should become more alert during their stay in the PACU. As they emerge from anesthesia, they may become agitated or act wild for a short time; this is called *emergence delirium*. During this time, it is important to provide safety measures such as side rails and restraints—following restraint protocols—to protect IV lines and keep endotracheal (ET) tubes in place. Once resolved, the patient returns to calm state and has no recollection of the episode. Movement, sensations, and perceptions may also be altered by anesthesia. Movement is the first function to return after spinal anesthesia.

For older adults, it is important to review their history to understand if they have any cognitive or neurologic deficits. Confused patients may be agitated or frightened when they awaken. It is helpful to know how caregivers normally communicate with the patient. You should understand that the patient may not be able to report pain or follow commands. If possible, it may be helpful to have a familiar relative or caregiver with the patient in the PACU to calm him or her and help with communication. You should watch for nonverbal pain cues such as moaning, grimacing, rubbing of an area, and restlessness because you recognize that postoperative patients will have pain and require pain relief even if they cannot report it. If patients have limited movements or sensations before surgery, you should know this to obtain an accurate assessment of anesthetic effects.

DATA COLLECTION. A neurologic assessment includes level of consciousness; orientation to person, place, time, and event; pupil size and reaction to light; and motor and sensory function.

Pain

DATA COLLECTION. If the patient is awake, he or she is asked to rate the presence of pain using a scale, such as the 0-to-10 scale, a color scale, or pictures that rate pain. The location and character of the pain are documented. If the patient is not fully awake, vital signs and nonverbal indications of pain should be monitored. Nonverbal indications of pain can include abnormal vital signs, restlessness, moaning, grimacing, rubbing, or pulling at specific areas or equipment.

Nursing Diagnoses, Planning, and Implementation
Pain related to tissue damage (mechanical [incision])

EXPECTED OUTCOME: The patient will report that pain is relieved at a satisfactory level within 15 to 30 minutes of the pain report.

- Monitor the patient for pain, *because pain may result from surgical procedure, movement, deep breathing, anxiety, a full bladder, positioning during surgery, NG tubes, catheters, IVs, ET tubes, or prior medical conditions, such as arthritis, cancer, or back pain.*
- Give IV opioid analgesics promptly *for their rapid onset.*
- Begin PCA as ordered, *because it is initiated in PACU.*

- Reposition the patient, provide warmth, and empty full bladder *to help alleviate pain.*
- Play music (e.g., nature sounds or classical music) in the PACU, dim lights, and reduce room noise *to help alleviate pain.*

EVALUATION. The goal for pain is met if the patient reports a satisfactory decrease in level of pain. For example, the patient reports pain of 10 on a scale of 0 to 10. You medicate the patient, and 30 minutes later, the patient rates pain as 2 on a scale of 0 to 10. The patient indicates that 2 is an acceptable pain level, so the goal is achieved.

Family Visitation

Family visitation in the PACU has been shown to be helpful to patients and their families. Allowing family visitation varies by hospital. Patients and families should be educated about the expectations for family visitation to keep it safe for the patient. During visitation, remember that the confidentiality of all patients must be ensured according to HIPAA (Health Insurance Portability and Accountability Act of 1996). For example, some patients may not want the surgical procedure revealed to their spouse or any family members.

Discharge From the Perianesthesia Care Unit

The length of stay in the PACU if the patient remains stable is normally about 1 hour. A postanesthesia recovery scale is used to score the patient's readiness to be discharged. The scale rates categories such as respiration, oxygen saturation, level of consciousness, activity, and circulation. The anesthesiologist discharges the patient for transfer to a nursing unit, or home when discharge criteria are met (Box 12-5). The patient may be transferred to the ICU if patient status and/or frequent or invasive monitoring is needed.

Box 12-5 Discharge Criteria for Perianesthesia Care Unit or Ambulatory Surgery

- Vital signs stable with temperature normal
- Patient awake or at baseline level of consciousness
- Drainage or bleeding not excessive
- Respiratory function not depressed
- Oxygen saturation above 90%

Additional Criteria for Ambulatory Surgery

- No nausea or vomiting
- No IV opioids within last 30 minutes
- Voided if required by surgical procedure or ordered
- Is ambulatory or has baseline mobility
- Understands discharge instructions
- Provides means of contact for follow-up telephone assessment
- Released to responsible adult

Transfer to Nursing Unit

The perianesthesia nurse gives a report of the patient's condition to the unit nurse when the patient is transferred to the nursing unit. The patient is moved into bed on the nursing unit with assistance to prevent dislodging of IVs, tubes, and drains. After the patient is placed in bed, the following safety interventions are performed to help prevent falls:

- The bed is placed in its lowest position, with the side rails raised.
- The nurse's call button is placed within easy patient reach and answered promptly.
- Patients are instructed that they should call for assistance with ambulation.
- When the patient gets up postoperatively, especially for the first time, he or she may be weak or dizzy. One or two health care workers should assist the patient and allow the patient to dangle before standing (Fig. 12.11).

Nursing Process for Postoperative Patients

A complete patient assessment is performed after transfer to the nursing unit. Respiratory status, vital signs (including temperature), level of consciousness, surgical site, dressings, and pain assessment are noted. IV site, patency, and IV solution and infusion rate are assessed and monitored. NG tubes are hooked to suction or clamped as ordered. Drains and catheters are positioned to promote proper functioning.

After discharge from the PACU, interventions to promote recovery include monitoring for complications (respiratory depression, hemorrhage, and shock), providing postoperative care, educating patients and their significant others, making needed referrals, and providing home health care. See the *Nursing Care Plan for the Postoperative Patient.*

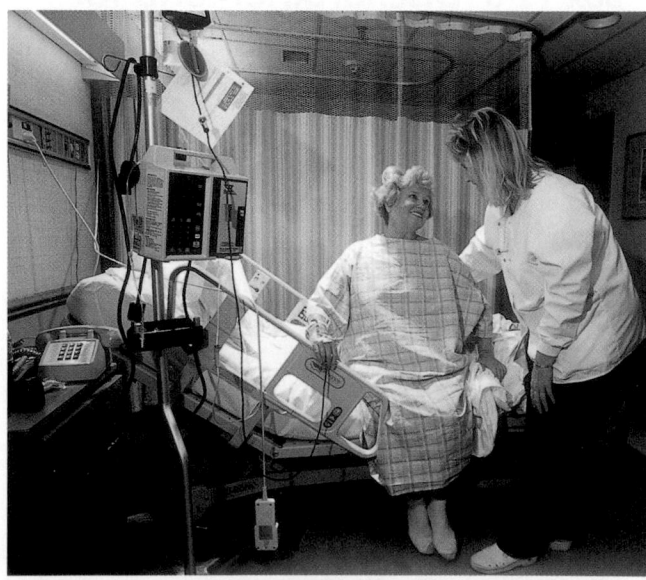

FIGURE 12.11 Postoperative patient dangling.

Respiratory Function

DATA COLLECTION. Regular monitoring of the patient's respiratory rate, depth, and effort and breath sounds as well as cough strength (if not contraindicated by the type of surgery, such as hernia repair or eye, ear, intracranial, jaw, or plastic surgery) should be done. Postoperative patients are at risk for developing atelectasis and pneumonia. They may have a weak cough as a result of being drowsy from anesthesia or analgesics. If fine crackles are heard in the lung bases, the patient should be encouraged to deep breathe or cough. Afterward you should listen again to see if the crackles have cleared. If the patient's airway is compromised, immediate action is taken to support the airway and the surgeon is notified.

Nursing Diagnoses, Planning, and Implementation

Ineffective Breathing Pattern related to pain and analgesic medications

EXPECTED OUTCOME: Patient will maintain normal Sao_2 levels and normal arterial blood gases at all times.

- Encourage deep breathing *to expand the lungs.*
- Give analgesics as needed *to promote deep breathing so the patient does not guard against deep respirations or coughing, especially if incision is near the diaphragm.*

Ineffective Airway Clearance related to ineffective cough and secretion retention

EXPECTED OUTCOME: Patient will have a patent airway and clear breath sounds at all times.

- Encourage deep breathing and coughing every hour while the patient is awake, especially through the first postoperative day, *to prevent mucous plugs that block bronchioles, causing alveoli to collapse and atelectasis or infection to develop from the stasis of mucus, resulting in pneumonia.*
- Place the incentive spirometer within patient's reach and encourage hourly use while awake *to prevent atelectasis.*
- Turn the patient at least every 2 hours *to help expand the lungs and move secretions.*
- Ambulate the patient as soon as possible *because immobility decreases movement of secretions.*

EVALUATION. If the patient's breath sounds are clear and arterial blood gases remain normal, the goals have been met.

Circulatory Function

DATA COLLECTION. Monitor the patient's circulatory status to detect and prevent hemorrhage, shock, and thrombophlebitis. Vital signs, Sao_2, and skin temperature, color, and moistness are monitored (per institutional policy) and compared with baseline data for abnormal trends. The incision or dressing is checked for drainage or hematoma formation. Drainage may leak down the patient's side and pool underneath the patient. Turn the patient if able, or while wearing gloves slide hands underneath the patient to check for bleeding. Report any signs of hemorrhage or shock promptly.

The lower extremities of surgical patients are observed. Peripheral pulses and capillary refill are checked. Tenderness or pain in the calf may be the first indication of a deep venous thrombosis (DVT). Leg swelling, warmth, and redness, as well as fever, may also be present. Bilateral calf and thigh measurements are taken daily if DVT is suspected or diagnosed.

Nursing Diagnoses, Planning, and Implementation

Deficient Fluid Volume related to blood and fluid loss or NPO status

EXPECTED OUTCOME: Patient will maintain blood pressure and pulse within normal limits at all times.

- Monitor dressings, incisions, drains, and tubes for color and amount of drainage and report bright red drainage or excessive drainage amounts immediately *to detect hemorrhage.*
- Monitor I&O *to detect imbalances.*
- Maintain IV fluids at the ordered rate *to maintain fluid volume.*

Ineffective Peripheral Tissue Perfusion related to interruption of blood flow during surgery, dehydration, and use of leg straps

EXPECTED OUTCOME: Patient will maintain normal tissue perfusion at all times.

- Encourage leg exercises hourly while the patient is awake *to prevent venous stasis and thrombosis.*
- Assist with early postoperative ambulation as ordered *to prevent thrombosis.*
- Apply thigh-length graduated compression stockings (if contraindicated, use knee-length stockings) or intermittent pneumatic compression as ordered *to help prevent stasis of blood.* Thigh-length stockings are more effective than knee-length stockings in reducing the risk of thrombophlebitis (Fig. 12.12).
- Give anticoagulants or plasma expanders such as dextran 40 and dextran 70 as ordered *to reduce clot formation.*
- Avoid pressure under the knee from pillows, rolled blankets, or prolonged bending of the knee and elevate legs *to help prevent venous stasis.*

NURSING CARE PLAN for the Postoperative Patient

Nursing Diagnosis: *Ineffective Airway Clearance* related to ineffective cough and secretion retention

Expected Outcomes: Patient will maintain a patent airway at all times. Breath sounds remain clear at all times.

Evaluation of Outcomes: Is patient able to clear own secretions? Are breath sounds clear?

Intervention Monitor breath sounds. **Rationale** Abnormal breath sounds such as crackles or wheezes can indicate retained secretions. **Evaluation** Are breath sounds clear?

Intervention Encourage deep breathing and coughing and use of incentive spirometer hourly while awake. **Rationale** Lung expansion helps prevent atelectasis and keeps lungs clear of secretions. **Evaluation** Does patient perform deep breathing and coughing and use incentive spirometer?

Intervention Ensure that patient's pain is relieved before activity. **Rationale** Movement can cause or increase pain. **Evaluation** Does patient state pain is controlled before activity?

Intervention Encourage movement by turning every 2 hours and ambulating as able. **Rationale** Movement promotes lung expansion and movement of secretions. **Evaluation** Is patient moving?

Nursing Diagnosis: *Pain* related to surgery, nausea, and vomiting

Expected Outcomes: Patient will report that pain management relieves pain satisfactorily within 30 minutes of report of pain. Patient will describe pain management plan by first postoperative day.

Evaluation of Outcomes: Does patient report satisfactory pain relief? Is patient able to describe pain management plan?

Continued

NURSING CARE PLAN for the Postoperative Patient—cont'd

Intervention Explain pain relief interventions and set goals with patient for pain management. **Rationale** Patients are partners in their pain management and need understanding of plan to collaborate on the goals. **Evaluation** Does patient understand plan and have a goal for acceptable pain level?

Intervention Assess pain using rating scale such as 0 to 10. **Rationale** Self-report is the most reliable indicator of pain. **Evaluation** Does patient report pain using scale?

Intervention Provide analgesics as needed (prn). **Rationale** Analgesics relieve pain. **Evaluation** Is patient's pain less after receiving medication?

Intervention Provide antiemetics prn. **Rationale** Antiemetics relieve nausea and vomiting. **Evaluation** Is patient's nausea and vomiting less after receiving medication?

Intervention Position patient comfortably. **Rationale** Incisions, drains, tubing, equipment, and bedrest can cause discomfort, which positioning can relieve. **Evaluation** Does patient report positioning is comfortable?

GERIATRIC
Intervention Prioritize assessment of cognitively impaired patients as high at beginning of shift and frequently throughout shift. **Rationale** Cognitively impaired patients are vulnerable to undertreatment of pain and deserve excellence in pain relief management. **Evaluation** Is priority given to cognitively impaired patient for assessment of pain and at regular intervals?

Intervention When assessing pain, speak clearly and slowly so older patient can hear. **Rationale** If older patient does not hear or misunderstands, pain may not be reported accurately, resulting in failure to ensure appropriate intervention is provided. **Evaluation** Does patient hear and report pain and relief accurately using pain scale?

Intervention Assess older patients' pain level regularly, observing nonverbal pain cues (restlessness, grimacing, moaning), especially for those who are cognitively impaired. **Rationale** The pain of older patients is often under-reported and undertreated, especially if cognitively impaired, and noting nonverbal cues can aid in pain treatment. **Evaluation** Are nonverbal pain cues present in older patients, especially those who are cognitively impaired?

Nursing Diagnosis: *Risk for Infection* related to inadequate primary defenses from surgical wound

Expected Outcome: Patient will remain free from infection at all times.

Evaluation of Outcome: Does patient remain free from infection?

Intervention Observe incision for signs and symptoms of infection. **Rationale** Redness, warmth, fever, and swelling indicate infection. **Evaluation** Are signs and symptoms of infection present?

Intervention Monitor drainage and maintain drains. **Rationale** Drains remove fluid from the surgical site to prevent infection development. **Evaluation** Are drainage amount and color normal for procedure?

Intervention Maintain sterile technique for dressing changes. **Rationale** Sterile technique reduces infection development. **Evaluation** Is incision free of signs and symptoms of infection?

FIGURE 12.12 Postoperative patient wearing A-V Impulse System foot pump. The foot pump is used to prevent deep venous thrombosis, reduce pain and edema, and enhance arterial blood flow.

EVALUATION. The goal for deficient fluid volume is met if vital signs and urine output are within normal limits. The goal for ineffective tissue perfusion is met if tissue blood flow remains normal.

Postoperative Pain

Pain is common after surgery, although each patient's pain experience varies. In addition to incisional pain, painful muscle spasms can occur. Nausea and vomiting, ambulation, coughing, deep breathing, and anxiety can cause discomfort and increase postoperative pain. Unrelieved pain has negative physiological effects. It also impairs deep breathing and coughing and hinders early ambulation, which may increase complications, length of hospital stay, and health care costs. It is important for nurses to stay informed of advances in pain management and ensure that they make pain relief a priority in providing patient care to reduce suffering and promote a quicker recovery (see Chapter 10).

DATA COLLECTION. If patients are not fully awake on transfer, vital signs and nonverbal indications of pain should be monitored ("Gerontological Issues"). Nonverbal indicators of pain may include abnormal vital signs (usually elevated blood pressure, although hypotension can occur in some patients), restlessness, moaning, grimacing, and rubbing or pulling at specific body areas or equipment. Patients who are awake are asked the location of the pain, to rate the presence of pain, and to describe the pain quality, such as sharp, aching, throbbing, or burning, which is then documented.

Gerontological Issues

Postoperative Pain

Pain is not a normal part of aging. Careful assessment of older patients' unique aging changes, chronic diseases, and pain relief needs is required to appropriately treat their postoperative pain.

Cognitively impaired adults are at risk for undertreatment of their postoperative pain. Make these patients a priority to assess and provide pain relief at the start of your shift and throughout it. Pain rating scales are available for use with those who are cognitively impaired to determine if they are experiencing pain.

CRITICAL THINKING

Mrs. Owens

■ Mrs. Owens returned from a bowel resection 2 days ago. She is receiving 1000 mL of 0.9% normal saline solution over 10 hours on an IV controller pump.

1. As you monitor the patient, you understand that the IV pump rate would be set at what rate?
2. How many milliliters should you record as intake for 12 hours?
   • Intake for 12 hours:
      • One 8-ounce (oz) cup of coffee
      • 4 oz orange juice
      • 6 oz tomato soup
      • 3/4 cup gelatin
      • Two cups of water
      • 1200 mL of 0.9% normal saline solution IV
   • Output for 12 hours:
      • 1700 mL of urine

Suggested answers are at the end of the chapter.

Nursing Diagnoses, Planning, and Implementation

Pain related to tissue damage from surgery, muscle spasms, nausea, or vomiting

EXPECTED OUTCOME: Patient will report pain relief at a satisfactory level using a pain rating scale within 30 minutes of pain report.

• Monitor pain using pain rating scale of 0 to 10 *to identify patient's needs.*
• Provide medications promptly as ordered *to relieve symptoms.*
• Understand appropriate timing intervals between IV to intramuscular (IM) doses of analgesics *so that patients do not wait and suffer needlessly after an IV analgesic.* IV analgesics usually have a shorter duration than IM analgesics.
• Reposition patient *to promote comfort.*

EVALUATION. Thirty minutes after pain medication is given, patients are asked to rate their pain level. If patients are sleeping at this time, let them sleep. When they awaken, ask them to rate their pain level. The goal for pain is met when patients report a decreased level of pain that is satisfactory to them. If a patient does not report satisfactory pain relief and additional orders are needed, the surgeon should be promptly notified of the inadequate pain relief.

 NURSING CARE TIP

- Anticipate the postoperative patient's pain by regularly assessing the pain level instead of waiting until the patient asks for the next dose of pain medication; this approach is essential to provide excellence in nursing care for pain relief.
- For the first dose of an IM analgesic after an IV analgesic dose is given, a patient in pain should not have to wait the ordered time interval of the IM dose (i.e., 3 hours if the IM order is morphine 10 mg IM every 3 hours prn). Having to wait while the IV analgesic is no longer effective can cause needless pain. Consult surgeon or pharmacist for safe time interval.
- With PCA, the patient's ability to use it, the patient's response to the medication, and the relief obtained from the medication are monitored. If PCA is not effective or if side effects occur, the surgeon is notified.
- Comfortable positioning, warming the patient, and relieving a patient's full bladder can also alleviate pain. Attention to environmental factors such as bright overhead lighting, excessive noise or visitors, and extreme room temperatures also helps promote comfort.
- Antiemetics should be given as ordered to relieve the discomfort of nausea and vomiting. If vomiting occurs, the patient should be turned onto one side to aid emesis removal and prevent aspiration.

Urinary Function

DATA COLLECTION. Monitor the patient's urinary status to ensure normal function is maintained after anesthesia administration. If the patient has a urinary catheter, the amount, color, and consistency of the urine are noted. Otherwise, watch for the patient's first postoperative voiding to prevent bladder distention. Patients should void within 8 hours of their last voiding. Patients having urinary or gynecological procedures may need to void within 4 to 6 hours to prevent increased pressure on the surgical site. Catheterization may be needed if the patient is unable to void. After

CRITICAL THINKING

Mrs. Wood

■ Mrs. Wood, age 42, returns to the surgical unit after a hysterectomy. Her postoperative vital signs and assessment findings are normal. Mrs. Wood rates her pain level at 9, and the nurse notes that she moans occasionally, repeatedly moves her legs, and pulls at her covers near her abdominal incision. She is drowsy but repeatedly says it hurts. In the PACU, she received 10 mg of morphine IV 55 minutes ago. Morphine 5 to 10 mg IM is ordered every 3 hours as needed.

1. What nonverbal pain cues does Mrs. Wood display?
2. How should the nurse document Mrs. Wood's pain?
3. What action should the nurse take to relieve Mrs. Wood's pain?
4. When should the nurse next monitor Mrs. Wood's pain level?
5. If Mrs. Wood indicates that her pain is unrelieved after 30 minutes, what action should the nurse take and with which team members will the nurse collaborate?
6. The nurse is to give Mrs. Wood morphine 8 mg IM now. Morphine 10 mg/mL is available. How many milliliters will the nurse give?

Suggested answers are at the end of the chapter.

outpatient surgery, patients may be required to void before being discharged.

If a patient reports the inability to void, the bladder is palpated for distention, or a bladder volume measurement is done, which determines the amount of urine in the bladder. You should be aware that restlessness can be caused by discomfort from a full bladder. A distended bladder requires intervention to empty it. Efforts are made to promote voiding before inserting an invasive urinary catheter because of the risk of infection.

The body's stress response to the surgical experience stimulates the sympathetic nervous system ("fight-or-flight" response), which saves fluid by reducing urine output. Therefore, initially urine output may be reduced and concentrated. Then it should gradually increase, becoming less concentrated and lighter in color.

Nursing Diagnoses, Planning, and Implementation

Urinary Retention related to surgery, pain, anesthesia, altered positioning

EXPECTED OUTCOME: Patient will completely and regularly empty bladder.

- Measure and record output on postoperative patients, especially those undergoing major procedures or urological surgery, older patients, and those with an IV or urinary catheter *to detect urinary elimination problems.*
- Report urinary output of less than 30 mL in 1 hour from the urinary catheter *because this is typically the minimum acceptable output.*

- Recognize that patients who are voiding small amounts frequently (30–50 mL every 20 to 30 minutes) or who dribble may have retention overflow and may not be emptying their bladder. This is not normal and may require catheterization *to empty the bladder and prevent complications.*
- Assist patients to the bathroom or bedside commode, and allow men to stand or sit to urinate if possible *to promote voiding.*
- Warm bedpans *to prevent reflexive sphincter tightening.*
- Use techniques to promote voiding before catheterization for the patient who is unable to void (running water, pouring warm water over a female patient's perineum, or drinking a hot beverage to stimulate voiding) *because catheterization increases the risk of infection.*
- Provide privacy after safety is ensured *to promote voiding.*
- Have patients place their feet solidly on the floor to relax the pelvic muscles *to aid voiding.*
- Notify the surgeon if the patient is uncomfortable, has a distended bladder, or has not voided within the specified time frame *to obtain treatment orders.*

EVALUATION. The goal for urinary retention is met if the patient is able to void without pain or complications.

Surgical Wound Care

A puncture wound has a small opening and is made to insert a tube or drain. An incision is a wound made by a surgeon with a sharp instrument such as a scalpel. Incisions are closed with sutures, staples (Fig. 12.13), or surgical adhesives, or adhesive strips. As the wound heals, sutures or staples are removed in 7 to 10 days.

Wounds can be clean or dirty. Clean wounds are surgical wounds that are not infected. Dirty (contaminated) wounds include accidental wounds or surgical incisions exposed to GI contents or unsterile conditions. Infected wounds and dirty wounds contain microorganisms from trauma, ruptured organs, or infection. Necrotic and infected tissue is removed before infected wounds are closed. This is known as **débridement**.

WOUND HEALING. Wound healing occurs in phases (Table 12.9). Wounds can heal by first (primary) intention, second (secondary) intention, and third (tertiary) intention (Fig. 12.14). In first-intention healing, the edges of the wound are approximated with staples or sutures. This usually results in minimal scarring. To heal by second intention, the wound is usually left open and allowed to heal by granulation. Scarring is usually extensive with prolonged healing. For healing by third intention, an infected wound is left open until there is no evidence of infection and the wound is then surgically closed.

WOUND COMPLICATIONS. Wound problems can include hematoma, infection, dehiscence, and evisceration. A hematoma occurs from bleeding in the wound and into the tissue around the wound. A clot forms from the bleeding. If the clot is large with swelling, the clot may need to be removed by the surgeon.

Infected wounds may be warm, reddened, and tender and have **purulent** drainage (pus). The drainage may have a foul odor. A fever and elevated white blood cell (WBC) count may be present. Antibiotics are used to treat the infection.

Dehiscence and evisceration are serious wound complications (Fig. 12.15). Wound **dehiscence** is the sudden bursting open of a wound's edges, which may be preceded by an increase in **serosanguineous** drainage. **Evisceration** is the viscera spilling out of the abdomen. Dehiscence and evisceration often occur with abdominal incisions in patients who are malnourished, obese, older, or who have poor wound healing. Supporting the wound during coughing and other activities that pull on the incision or applying an abdominal binder on patients who are at risk helps prevent dehiscence and evisceration. When evisceration occurs, the patient may have pain and vomiting and may report that "something let loose" or "gave way."

 BE SAFE!

If dehiscence or evisceration occurs:

- Place the patient in low Fowler's position with flexed knees.
- Cover the wound with sterile dressings or towels moistened with warm sterile normal saline.
- Notify the surgeon immediately of this surgical emergency.
- Apply gentle pressure over the wound and keep the patient still and calm.
- Monitor vital signs for evidence of shock (e.g., tachycardia, tachypnea, dyspnea, hypotension).
- Infuse IV fluids as ordered.
- Prepare the patient for immediate surgery to close the wound.

For dehisced surgical incisions that resist healing, vacuum-assisted closure (VAC) aids in healing the incision (see Chapter 54). VAC applies negative pressure to wound edges. The device can also be used on other types of wounds.

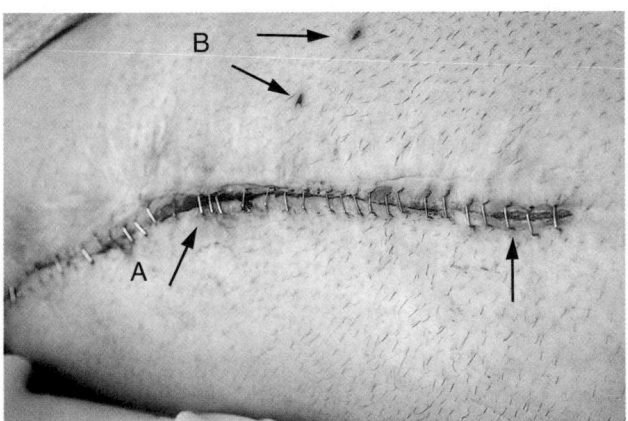

FIGURE 12.13 A stapled incision. (A) Note wound edges not approximated at arrows. (B) Arrows indicate puncture sites where drains were inserted.

• **WORD-BUILDING** •

serosanguineous: sero—whey + sanguineous—bloody
evisceration: e—out + viscera—body organs

TABLE 12.9 WOUND HEALING PHASES

Phase	Time Frame	Wound Healing	Patient Effect
I	Incision to 2nd postoperative day	Inflammatory response	Fever, malaise
II	3rd to 14th postoperative day	Granulation tissue forms	Feeling better
III	3rd to 6th postoperative week	Collagen deposited	Raised scar formed
IV	Months to 1 year	Collagen deposited	Flat, thin scar

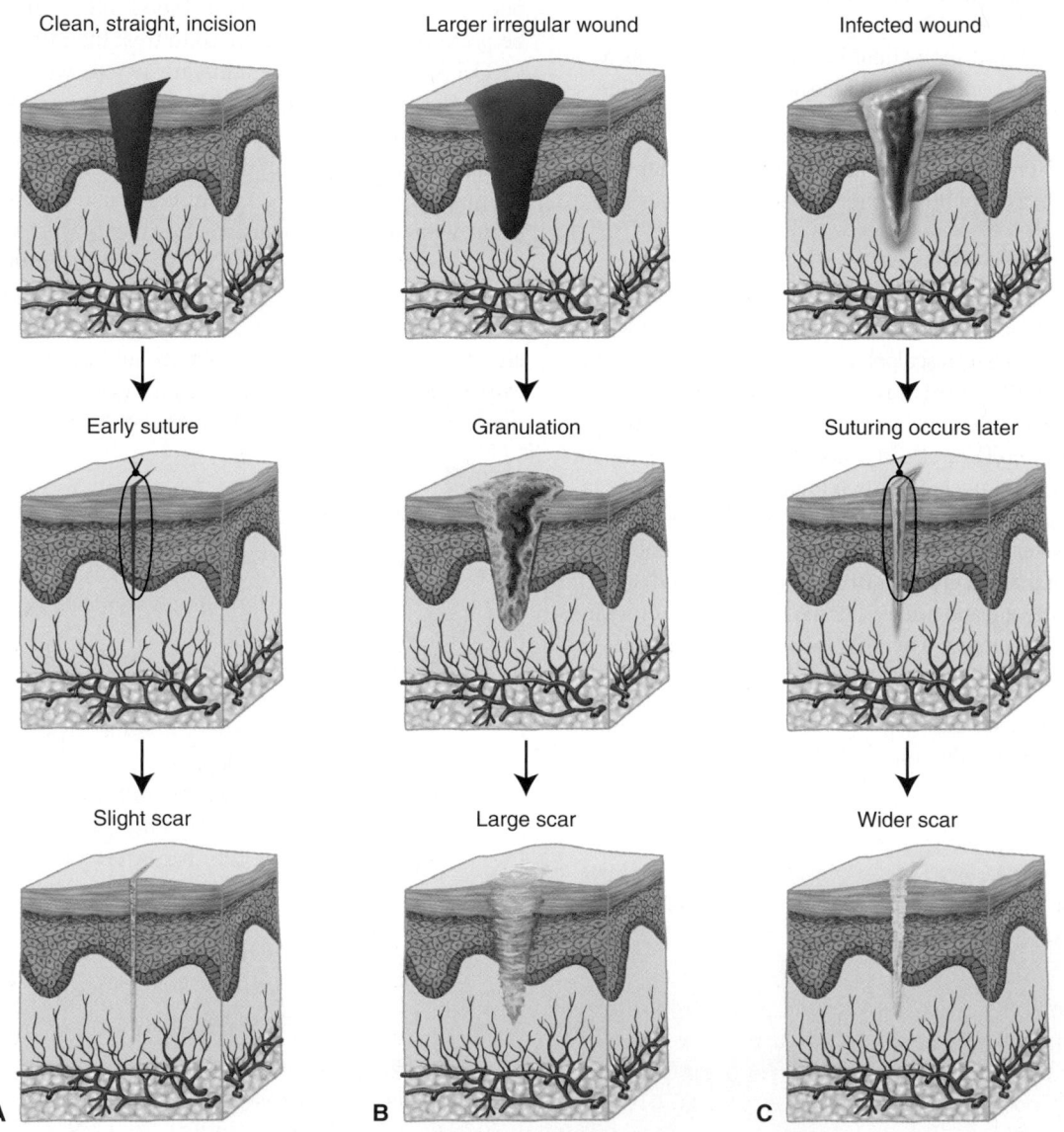

FIGURE 12.14 Wound healing. (A) Primary intention. Wound healing occurs in a clean wound, such as a surgical wound, for which edges are approximated, typically with staples or sutures. Healing occurs quickly with slight scarring. (B) Secondary intention. Large irregular or infected wounds are left open to allow healing to occur from the inside out. Pressure ulcers or chronic wounds are often treated this way. Large scarring occurs with lengthy healing time. (C) Tertiary intention. Infected or contaminated wound is left open for a brief time period until wound is clean. Granulation tissue fills in for some wound healing, and then edges are approximated and closed surgically. Wider scarring occurs.

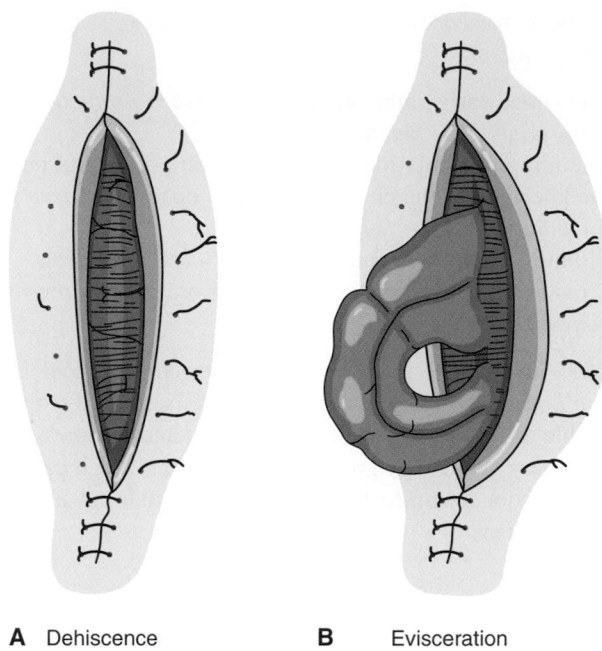

A Dehiscence   **B** Evisceration

FIGURE 12.15 (A) Wound dehiscence. (B) Wound evisceration.

DATA COLLECTION.

Drains. Drains are inserted into wounds during surgery to prevent accumulation of blood, lymph, or necrotic tissue in wounds that can lead to infection or delayed healing. Drains may work by gravity or suction. Penrose drains are soft, flat, drains that carry drainage from the wound. Moderate, pink serosanguineous (consisting of blood and serous fluid) drainage is expected from a Penrose drain and may require frequent dressing changes. Examples of drains that use suction to gently enhance drainage include the Jackson-Pratt and Hemovac (www.zimmer.com). These drains are closed systems that may require periodic emptying and reapplication of the suction by compressing the drain.

Output is recorded when the drainage is emptied. The amount of drainage expected varies with the type of surgery. Be alert for excessive amounts to report. Specialized drainage systems allow the transfusion of drainage containing blood back to the patient (autotransfusion) to maintain hemoglobin levels without the risks associated with blood transfusions, such as transfusion reactions or transmission of infections.

Dressings. Dressings protect the wound, absorb drainage, prevent contamination from body fluids, provide comfort, and apply pressure to reduce swelling or bleeding as in a pressure dressing. The initial dressing is applied in surgery and then is usually removed by the surgeon approximately 24 hours postoperatively. If drainage appears on the initial dressing, reinforce it with another dressing, according to surgeon orders or institution policy.

After the initial dressing is removed, if the wound is dry and the edges intact (approximated), the surgeon can order the wound to be left uncovered. This allows easy observation of the wound and avoidance of applying tape to the skin. Draining wounds are dressed with several layers that are changed as needed. When the old dressing is removed, it should be done carefully to prevent dislodging of tubes or drains. The condition of the wound is documented with each dressing change. It is normal for the incision to be puffy and red from the inflammatory response. The surrounding skin should be the patient's normal color and temperature. Correct tape application over the dressing is done by gently laying the tape over the dressing and applying even pressure on each side of the wound. Pressure should not be applied on top of the wound by pulling on the tape from one side of the wound to the other side.

EVIDENCE-BASED PRACTICE

Clinical Question
Do wound dressings prevent surgical site infection in people with surgical wounds healing by primary intention?

Evidence
A review of 16 randomized controlled trials of 2578 subjects looked at the use of wound dressings versus leaving postoperative surgical wounds healing by primary intention uncovered. No reduction in surgical site infection was found related to covering surgical wounds with dressings.

Implications for Nursing Practice
Dressings should be selected based on their cost and purpose, such as exudate absorption.

REFERENCES

Dumville, J. C., Walter, C. J., Sharp, C. A., Page, T. (2011). Dressings for the prevention of surgical site infection. *Cochrane Database of Systematic Reviews, 7,* CD003091. DOI: 10.1002/14651858.CD003091.pub2.

Nursing Diagnoses, Planning, and Implementation
Impaired Skin Integrity related to surgical incision

EXPECTED OUTCOME: *Patient will regain skin integrity within [specify individualized realistic time frame].*

- Monitor skin color and temperature and report changes *to detect need for treatment.*
- Monitor dressings and note drainage color, amount, and consistency. *Surgical wound drainage initially is sanguineous (red) and changes to serosanguineous (pink) and then serous (pale yellow) after a few hours to days.*
- Promptly report drainage that is bright red, remains sanguineous after a few hours, or is profuse to the surgeon *because the patient may be hemorrhaging.*

- Use standard precautions when changing dressings *to protect yourself.*

EVALUATION. The goal for impaired skin integrity is met if the patient's wound heals and skin integrity is regained without delayed healing or complications.

Gastrointestinal Function

Nutritional intake and bowel function can be affected by surgery and anesthesia. Being NPO and having bowel preparation often occur preoperatively. After abdominal surgery, peristalsis and bowel sounds, and flatus usually stop (paralytic ileus) for 24 to 72 hours. Flatus, bowel movements, and an appetite signal the return of GI function. Interventions to shorten ileus time include the following:

- Medication such as Alvimopan (Entereg) 12 mg, which is given 30 to 90 minutes before surgery and twice daily for up to 15 doses in 7 days to increase recovery of the functioning of the GI tract after partial small or large bowel resections
- Use of minimally invasive surgery
- Chewing gum
- Ambulation
- Avoidance of NG tubes when able as complications and later feeding occur
- Early feeding

DATA COLLECTION. After abdominal surgery, GI assessment includes monitoring vital signs, the return of flatus and appetite, first bowel movement, nausea or vomiting, or signs of paralytic ileus, such as distention, bloating, and cramps. The abdomen is documented to be soft or firm, and flat or distended. The patient's abdominal girth is measured if distention occurs. Abnormal findings are reported to the surgeon.

Traditionally after GI surgery, bowel sounds were monitored by the nurse, and the patient was kept NPO until flatus and bowel sounds returned. Research about this practice shows that bowel sounds are not correlated with bowel motility and a patient's ability to safely drink and eat postoperatively. In fact, patients can be hydrated and fed early to promote healing and faster recovery.

Nursing Diagnoses, Planning, and Implementation

Imbalanced Nutrition: Less Than Body Requirements related to NPO, pain, and nausea

EXPECTED OUTCOME: Patient will resume normal dietary intake and maintain weight within normal limits.

- Maintain IV fluids, total parenteral nutrition, or enteral feedings *until the patient resumes oral intake* ("Nutrition Notes").
- Try water and clear liquids at first as ordered, then advance the diet *to promote tolerance.*
- Give antiemetics as ordered *to control nausea and vomiting.*

Constipation related to decreased peristalsis, immobility, altered diet, opioid side effect

EXPECTED OUTCOME: The patient will return to normal bowel elimination patterns and report freedom from

gas pains and constipation within 3 to 4 days postoperatively.

- Encourage early ambulation and exercise *to promote restoration of GI function.*
- Encourage ambulation, have patient lie prone, and pull the knees up to the chest if gas pains occur *to relieve the pain.*
- Monitor elimination and document *to detect problems.*
- Provide stool softeners or laxatives as ordered *to prevent constipation.*

EVALUATION. The goal for the *Imbalanced Nutrition: Less Than Body* Requirements nursing diagnosis is met if patients are able to maintain their baseline weight and resume a normal dietary intake. The goal for constipation is met if patients are free from discomfort and establish a regular bowel elimination pattern.

Nutrition Notes

Nourishing the Postoperative Patient

After surgery, IV 5% glucose in water is commonly prescribed. Two liters of this solution contain only 340 calories, which is insufficient to meet the patient's energy needs but enough to prevent ketosis from breakdown of adipose tissue. Previously well-nourished adults generally have nutrient reserves for 3 to 4 days of semistarvation. To prevent excessive muscle protein from being used for energy, adequate nourishment should be delivered to the patient within 3 days. (Citrotein and Enlive can be used to supplement clear liquid diets.)

To avoid abdominal distention, oral feedings traditionally have been delayed until peristalsis returns but scientific evidence supporting this practice is lacking. Researchers are beginning to test the practice. In some situations, delaying oral intake seems to offer no advantage in preventing complications over earlier resumption of feeding.

Patients usually progress from clear liquids to a regular diet as soon as possible. If "diet as tolerated" is prescribed, the patient should be asked what sounds good. Sometimes a full dinner when the patient doesn't feel well "turns off" the appetite.

After GI surgery, oral food and fluids are deferred longer than with other surgeries to allow healing. When particular amounts are prescribed, those limits should be strictly implemented to preserve the suture lines. After surgery on the mouth and throat, no red liquids are given so that bleeding can be seen and vomitus is not mistaken for blood.

Specific nutrients necessary for healing are:
- Vitamin C for collagen formation
- Vitamin K for blood clotting

- Zinc for tissue growth, skin integrity, and cell-mediated immunity
- Protein for controlling fluid balance and edema, for manufacturing antibodies and white blood cells, and for building scar tissue

 NURSING CARE TIP

Most IV solutions do not provide enough nutrients or calories to prevent malnutrition. The primary purpose of most IV fluids is to provide hydration. A 1000-mL IV solution containing 5% dextrose provides only about 170 calories. This does not meet an adult's daily caloric needs, especially if healing is occurring. You should ensure that early consideration of other nutritional methods is made to meet the patient's dietary needs.

Mobility

DATA COLLECTION. It is important for the patient to move as much as possible to prevent complications and promote healing. Pain, incisions, tubes, drains, dressings, and other equipment may make movement difficult. You should determine the patient's ability to move in bed, to get out of bed, and to walk. Pain levels that may interfere with movement are assessed. The patient's tolerance to activity is observed. Patient understanding of how to perform exercises is noted.

Nursing Diagnoses, Planning, and Implementation

Impaired Physical Mobility related to surgery, decreased strength, and movement restriction

EXPECTED OUTCOME: Patient's goal will be to resume normal physical activity.

- Position patient in bed with pillows *to support the body in good alignment.*
- Turn at least every 2 hours, alternating from supine to side to side if not contraindicated, *to prevent complications.*
- Encourage patients to move themselves *to increase circulation and promote lung expansion.*
- If ambulation is not possible, encourage hourly exercises (deep breathing, range of motion of all joints, and isometric exercises of the abdominal, gluteal, and leg muscles) while awake *to prevent complications.*
- If patient cannot perform active range-of-motion exercises, perform passive joint range of motion *to prevent complications.*
- Raise the head of the bed slowly *to let the circulatory system adjust to the position change.*
- If patient reports dizziness or feeling faint, lower the head of the bed *to let the circulatory system adjust more slowly.*

- Dangle patient's feet on the side of the bed *to prepare for ambulation* (see Fig. 12.11).
- If dangling is tolerated, ambulate the patient. Before getting up, patient should pedal the feet to "wake up" the muscles controlling the arteries. To rise, patient should keep eyes forward and move slowly until feeling adjusted to being up. Usually the patient ambulates a short distance the first time and increases the distance as tolerated. One or two health care workers should assist the patient and use a gait (walking) belt for safety. Walkers with wheels and seats also may be used for support and for resting if the patient becomes dizzy or tired. If patient feels faint or dizzy or if vital signs change, help patient back to bed. A wheelchair may be needed for safe transport back to the room.

EVALUATION. The goal for impaired physical mobility is met if the patient can increase ambulation and resume normal activities.

Postoperative Patient Discharge

Discharge planning begins during preadmission testing and continues after admission to ensure that the patient is ready for a timely discharge. When the patient meets discharge criteria, the surgeon discharges the patient.

Ambulatory Surgery

DISCHARGE CRITERIA. Usually, a patient can be considered a candidate for discharge 1 hour after surgery if the PACU discharge scoring system or clinical discharge criteria are met (see Box 12-5). Clinical discharge criteria include stable vital signs, no bleeding, no nausea or vomiting, and controlled pain that is not severe. Depending on the type of surgical procedure, such as urological, gynecological, or hernia surgery, the patient may be required to void before discharge. The patient also should be able to sit up without dizziness before discharge. Patients meeting discharge criteria are discharged by the surgeon and released to a responsible adult. Patients are not permitted to drive themselves home because of the effects of anesthesia and medications they have received.

DISCHARGE INSTRUCTIONS. Patients and their families are given written discharge instructions before discharge. Older patients should have a caregiver participate in the discharge instruction session to understand what observations to make and what to do if complications develop. The instruction form is signed by the patient or an authorized representative to indicate understanding. Prescriptions and a copy of the instructions, to provide a reference for later, are sent with the patient. The patient is encouraged to rest for 24 to 48 hours. The patient is to avoid operating machinery, driving, drinking alcoholic beverages, and making major decisions for 24 hours because the effects of undergoing surgery can alter energy levels and thinking ability. The surgeon orders any fluid, dietary, activity, or work restrictions.

Patients are taught wound care, medication information (including side effects), and signs and symptoms of complications to report to the surgeon. Phone numbers for the surgeon, surgical facility, and emergency care are provided.

Patients are informed of the date for their follow-up visit to the surgeon and told to call and make an appointment.

Inpatient Surgery

DISCHARGE CRITERIA. The surgeon determines the patient's readiness for discharge from the hospital. Postoperative lengths of stay vary based on the surgical procedure and the patient's individual needs. Before discharge, a complete assessment of the patient is performed and documented.

DISCHARGE INSTRUCTIONS. All necessary teaching is completed before discharge (Fig. 12.16). Patients and their families or caregivers are given prescriptions and a copy of written instructions that are signed by the patient to indicate understanding before discharge. If more teaching or reinforcement is needed, a referral to a home health nurse can be requested.

The surgeon orders any fluid, dietary, activity, or work restrictions. Patients are taught wound care, medication information (including side effects), and signs and symptoms of complications to report to the surgeon. Patients are informed of the date for their follow-up visit to the surgeon.

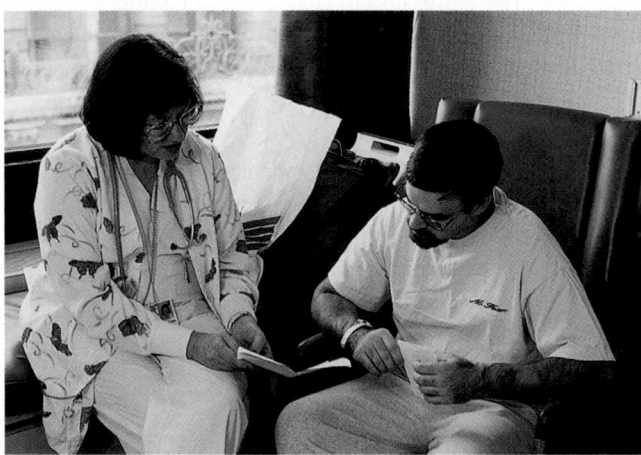

FIGURE 12.16 Nurse providing discharge teaching to patient.

Home Health Hints

A referral for a home health nurse to assist a patient in the recovery process is made when the patient needs skilled nursing care following surgery (See Chapter 16, "Nursing Care of Patients at Home," for examples of skilled care).

It is helpful for caregivers to keep a notebook in the hospital and continue it at home. Treatments, medicines, observations, procedures, HCP and nurse visits, instructions, and therapies with dates and times can be recorded. This helps prevent confusion, prepares the next caregiver, and affords better organization of time and resources for everyone. Families of patients recovering from surgery can provide items to keep the patient occupied and comfortable: talking books, electronic reading tablet, inspirational reading material, pictures, favorite pajamas, robe and slippers, and coverlet.

After a patient comes home from surgery, the home care nurse can help give direction to the family to prepare the room where the patient will be staying:
- It is helpful if the room can be on the same floor with the bathroom, kitchen, and living space.
- If an extended recovery period or illness is expected, the den or living room might be considered as the primary living space to provide room for equipment and make companionship easier. The patient can see activity in the home and be included in family activity. Also, caregivers can be more attentive to the patient's needs and save countless footsteps.

Reinforce any discharge instructions the patient and caregivers bring home with them. Although these instructions are reviewed by the surgeon and hospital nurses, frequently the patient and family are tired and anxious and can miss important details. If possible keep a copy of these instructions in the patient's home health folder in order to communicate to all members of the health care team.

Special equipment may be needed, including the following:
- For the patient on bedrest, a hospital bed with full side rails helps with a variety of position changes and better height for the caregiver.
- Draw sheets made of folded twin sheets are needed, as well as extra pillows for positioning and splinting.
- A bedside stand is needed for personal and toilet articles.
- A bedside commode can be placed near the bed if the patient cannot walk to the bathroom. A bedpan or urinal may be needed. A functional female urinal is easier to use than a bedpan.
- A flexible tube with a showerhead that connects to the bathtub faucet is convenient and allows the patient more independence in bathing.
- Installation of grab bars and tub stools and skid-proofing of a shower or tub are important safety measures to help prevent falls.
- If the patient is eligible for insurance coverage for durable medical equipment, a HCP's order must be obtained.
- If the patient is discharged on anticoagulants and/or antiembolic stockings, reinforce instructions and importance of adherence to them for prevention of deep vein thrombosis.
- Monitor nutritional status to assist with wound healing. Discuss need for supplementation with RN.
- Instruction on wound care to the patient and family includes hand hygiene before and after wound care to prevent infection. Reinforce frequently.
- If discharged on oral pain medication discuss pain management and potential side effects (See Chapter 10, "Nursing Care of Patients in Pain," for further details).

SUGGESTED ANSWERS TO

CRITICAL THINKING

■ *Mrs. Owens*

1. 100 mL per hour. IV pumps are always set to deliver the amount of milliliters per hour. Divide the total volume of 1000 mL by the total time of 10 hours = 100 mL per hour.

2. Intake = 2400 mL.
   To calculate this:
   Remember your conversions:

   30 mL = 1 oz

   1 cup = 8 oz (don't supersize the cup!)
   Calculations:

   1 8-oz cup of coffee = $1 \times 8 \times 30 = 240$ mL

   4 oz orange juice = $4 \times 30 = 120$ mL

   6 oz tomato soup = $6 \times 30 = 180$ mL

   3/4 cup gelatin = $3/4 \times 8 \times 30 = 180$ mL

   2 cups of water = $2 \times 8 \times 30 = 480$ mL

   1200 mL of 0.9 normal saline IV

   The patient's output does not affect the intake total, so it is not used for this calculation.

■ *Mrs. Wood*

1. Moaning occasionally, moving legs restlessly, and pulling covers near abdominal incision are nonverbal pain cues.

2. Document pain levels by actual observations: occasional moaning, restless leg movements, and pulling of covers near abdominal incision. By patient's statement: "It hurts." Because Mrs. Wood is too drowsy to use the pain scale, other data are used. When Mrs. Wood is more awake, explanation of the pain scale should be reinforced and used.

3. Review pain medication orders to determine if analgesics can be given. Noting that an IV analgesic was given 50 minutes ago and the IM analgesic is ordered every 3 hours, request that the surgeon or pharmacist be consulted to determine appropriate time intervals. The patient should not have to wait 3 hours to receive the next dose of pain medication. If the consultation indicates it is time to give the analgesic, verify that vital signs are still stable and then give the analgesic. Also consider other pain relief measures such as patient warmth, positioning, or environmental issues such as bright lighting, room temperature, and noise.

4. After administration of the analgesic, Mrs. Wood's pain level should be assessed in at least 30 minutes to determine pain relief. If Mrs. Wood is asleep, she should not be awakened unless it is necessary. Nonverbal cues should be observed and respirations counted and documented. If no indication of pain is noted, Mrs. Wood's pain level should be monitored at least hourly or as needed.

5. Document pain level on scale of 0 to 10. Collaborate with the surgeon for notification of inadequate pain relief and the pharmacist for safe time intervals for ordered analgesic routes. The patient should not have to wait the 3-hour interval if in pain. Consider providing other pain relief measures while the surgeon is being notified.

6. Try unit analysis for solving mathematical calculations. It is easy to understand, and our students say it is a helpful method.
   Unit Analysis Method:

$$\frac{8 \text{ mg}}{} \left| \frac{1 \text{ mL}}{10 \text{ mg}} \right| = \frac{8}{10} = 0.8 \text{ milliliter}$$

REVIEW QUESTIONS

1. The nurse is contributing to the plan of care for a preoperative patient. Which of the following nursing actions should the nurse implement to reduce surgical risk factors for the preoperative patient? **Select all that apply.**
   1. Playing music of patient's choice
   2. Avoiding discussion of fears
   3. Reinforcing pain control methods
   4. Showing use of incentive spirometer
   5. Monitoring blood glucose for a patient with diabetes
   6. Teaching to perform leg exercises hourly while awake

2. The LPN/LVN is caring for a preoperative patient. Which of the following roles can the LPN/LVN provide for the patient's care in the preoperative phase?
   1. Assisting in data collection
   2. Explaining the surgical procedure
   3. Obtaining preoperative orders
   4. Conducting the preoperative anesthesia interview

3. The LPN/LVN is caring for a patient preoperatively who is to sign consent for surgery. Which of the following is within the LPN/LVN's scope of practice related to the patient providing consent for surgery? **Select all that apply.**
   1. Witnessing minor patient's signature on the consent
   2. Providing informed consent
   3. Answering surgical procedure questions
   4. Requesting patient questions be referred to surgeon
   5. Witnessing the patient's signature on the consent
   6. Reading the consent to a patient before he or she signs it

4. The nurse is contributing to the teaching plan for an older adult. Which of the following is a teaching strategy that improves learning for the older adult?
   1. Sit near a window with bright sunlight.
   2. Use large black-on-white printed materials.
   3. Sit beside patient.
   4. Use blue and green colors for brochures.

5. The nurse is contributing to the plan of care for a patient undergoing a cholecystectomy. Which of the following interventions would help prevent atelectasis for this patient? **Select all that apply.**
   1. Coughing and deep breathing
   2. Holding breath while moving
   3. Restricting fluids
   4. Leg exercises
   5. Pain control
   6. Ambulation

6. The nurse is caring for a patient after thoracic surgery. Which of the following would the nurse evaluate as indicating that interventions to prevent respiratory complications have been effective?
   1. Pain level "2"
   2. No abdominal distention
   3. Clear lung sounds
   4. Good appetite

7. The nurse is caring for a patient who returned from surgery 3 hours ago. Which of these findings would the nurse recognize as being the most urgent to report to the surgeon?
   1. Tachycardia
   2. Polyuria
   3. Nausea
   4. Fever

8. The nurse is assisting with data collection on an ambulatory postoperative patient. Which of the following criterion would the nurse evaluate as indicating patient readiness for discharge after ambulatory?
   1. Ability to drive an automobile
   2. Ability to ambulate 50 feet
   3. Being pain free
   4. Absence of nausea or vomiting

9. What is the role of the home health nurse in caring for postoperative patients? **Fill in the blank.**

   Answer: _____

Answers can be found in Appendix C.

References

American Society of Anesthesiologists Committee. (2011). Practice guidelines for preoperative fasting and the use of pharmacologic agents to reduce the risk of pulmonary aspiration: application to healthy patients undergoing elective procedures: An updated report by the American Society of Anesthesiologists Committee on Standards and Practice Parameters. *Anesthesiology, 114*, 495–511. Retrieved February 2, 2014, at http://journals.lww.com/anesthesiology/fulltext/2011/03000

/practice_guidelines_for_preoperative_fasting_and.13.aspx#P232

Joint Commission. (2014). *2014 national patient safety goals.* Retrieved January 31, 2014, from www.jointcommission.org/patientsafety/nationalpatientsafetygoals

 DavisPlus | For additional resources and information visit **davispl.us/medsurg5**

Nursing Care of Patients With Emergent Conditions and Disaster/ Bioterrorism Response

ERIN MAZUR

LEARNING OUTCOMES

1. Explain the components of the primary survey.
2. Plan nursing interventions for a trauma victim.
3. Identify the symptoms of inhalation injury.
4. Describe the stages of hypothermia.
5. Describe the stages of hyperthermia.
6. Explain the priorities of care for poison overdose.
7. Discuss the LPN/LVN role in crisis situations and psychiatric emergencies.
8. Describe the LPN/LVN role in identifying a bioterrorist attack or disaster response.

KEY TERMS

abrasion (ah-BRAY-zhun)
amputation (am-pew-TAY-shun)
anaphylactic shock (an-uh-fah-LAK-tik SHAWK)
anaphylaxis (an-uh-fah-LAK-sis)
anthrax (AN-thracks)
asphyxia (as-FIX-ee-ah)
bioterrorism (BY-oh-TARE-UR-is-um)
botulism (BOTCH-uh-liz-um)
capillary refill (KAP-ih-lar-ee REE-fill)
cardiac tamponade (KAR-dee-ack tam-pon-AID)
cardiogenic shock (KAR-dee-oh-JEN-ick SHAWK)
distributive shock (dis-TRIB-u-tive SHAWK)
flail chest (FLAY-ul CHEST)
full-thickness burn (FUL-THICK-ness BERN)
gastric lavage (GAS-trick la-VAHJ)
heatstroke (HEET-strohk)
hypovolemic shock (HIGH-poh-voh-LEE-mick SHAWK)
laceration (lass-ur-A-shun)
obstructive shock (ub-STRUK-tive SHAWK)
partial-thickness burn (PARR-shul THICK-ness BERN)
plague (PLAYG)
shock (SHAWK)
smallpox (SMALL-pocks)
superficial burns (SOO-purr-fish-ul BERNS)
tetanus (TET-nus)
triage (TREE-ahj)

The ability to recognize an emergent condition, prioritize, and provide quick assessments and interventions is essential in nursing. Upon arrival in the emergency department (ED), most patients are triaged by a registered nurse (RN). During the triage process, the RN evaluates the patient's condition, asks appropriate questions related to the condition, and performs a rapid assessment of the patient to provide the appropriate level of care (Fig. 13.1). This chapter presents specific emergent conditions with application of the nursing process.

PRIMARY SURVEY

What do you think the nurse does first when a patient arrives in the ED? Well, to recognize life-threatening conditions and determine priorities of care, an initial assessment of the patient's airway, breathing, circulation, and disability is conducted. This process is known as the primary survey. The components of the primary survey are listed in Table 13.1.

A—Airway

The airway is the most important component of the primary survey. The neck should not be hyperextended, flexed, or

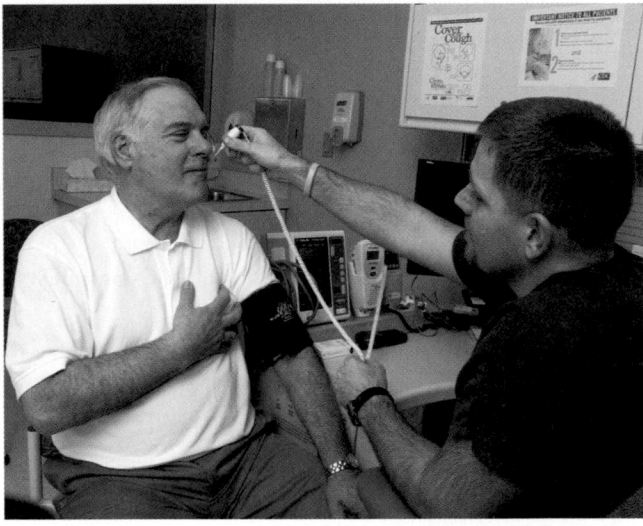

FIGURE 13.1 Triage nurse evaluating patient who has just arrived in the ED.

TABLE 13.1 COMPONENTS OF THE PRIMARY SURVEY

A	Airway
B	Breathing
C	Circulation
D	Disability/central nervous system

rotated until spinal injury is ruled out because any movement can worsen an existing cervical spine injury. During cardiopulmonary resuscitation (CPR), if there is a possible or known spinal injury, the jaw-thrust maneuver rather than the chin-lift maneuver must be used to avoid moving the head and neck (Fig. 13.2). The airway is inspected for obstruction, including loose teeth, foreign objects, bleeding, and vomitus. Next, any visible airway obstructions are removed using suction.

Airway adjuncts, such as nasopharyngeal or oropharyngeal airways, can be used to keep the airway open. When additional airway support and mechanical ventilation are required, advanced airway adjuncts, such as endotracheal intubation or cricothyroidotomy, can be performed by specially trained emergency personnel or health care providers.

B—Breathing

After the airway is opened, the patient is assessed for spontaneous breathing and respiratory rate and depth. The nurse observes whether the patient's chest rises and falls spontaneously and auscultates for breath sounds bilaterally. If the patient is not breathing, interventions are performed before proceeding. The patient can be ventilated with a mouth-to-face mask or a bag-valve face mask. Endotracheal intubation is the preferred method of maintaining an airway in an unconscious patient because it opens the airway and protects the lungs from aspiration (see Fig. 29.23).

FIGURE 13.2 (A) Chin-lift maneuver is used to open the airway. (B) Jaw-thrust maneuver is used to open the airway if the patient might have a head or neck injury.

C—Circulation

The carotid pulse is palpated for quality and rate. The skin is inspected for color and temperature. External bleeding is controlled by external pressure and elevation when possible. Any life-threatening conditions that can compromise circulation are assessed, and interventions are provided before proceeding. Other conditions that can compromise circulation include internal bleeding, shock resulting from hemorrhage, or major burns. Large-gauge IV cannulas (16 or 18 gauge) are initiated for fluid resuscitation. If the patient does not have a pulse, CPR must be initiated. If a pulse can be palpated, vital signs are taken and recorded.

D—Disability/Central Nervous System

To detect serious central nervous system injury, a brief neurologic assessment is conducted to determine the level of consciousness, which can range from alert (A) and responds to verbal stimuli (V), to responds to painful stimuli (P), or unresponsive (U). To assess response to painful stimuli, a painful stimulus is applied, such as applying periorbital pressure or applying pressure with a pen to the lateral outer aspect of the second or third interphalangeal joint. The patient is observed for the response to the pain, and the response is recorded. Movement of all extremities is also assessed.

SECONDARY SURVEY

For victims of severe trauma, a secondary survey is conducted. This assessment identifies areas of medical or injury problems that are not immediately life threatening but require treatment (see "Evidence-Based Practice"). Major body areas that can sustain serious injury, such as the head, spine, chest, abdomen, and musculoskeletal system, are quickly examined to detect additional injuries (Table 13.2). To adequately perform a head-to-toe assessment, the patient's clothing is removed. Each major body area is inspected and palpated for deformity, bruising, open wounds, bleeding, and pain.

 EVIDENCE-BASED PRACTICE

Clinical Question
What are types and causes of medication errors in the ED?

Evidence
Medication administration is one of the most common nursing interventions in health care. One study found that medication errors were the most commonly reported error in the ED with 36% of these errors occurring during the administration phase (Blank et al, 2011). One study demonstrated that, on average, the ED nurse is interrupted 3.3 times each hour, and 27.5% of these interruptions occurred during medication administration (Kosits & Jones, 2011). Other studies have demonstrated that temporary staff in emergency made more medication errors, resulting in greater harm than permanent staff members (Pham et al, 2011).

Contributing factors to the high rate of medication errors included ED overcrowding, the increased volume of medications given in the ED, increased numbers of complicated and chronically ill patients, frequency of verbal orders, time pressure, and interruptions and distractions (Blank et al, 2012).

Implications for Nursing Practice
Medication errors can result from the acute, crowded, and fast-paced nature of emergency care. Nurses and health care agencies need to be aware of the causes and types of medication errors and maintain vigilance in following interventions that can reduce the incidence of error such as following the five rights of medication administration, reducing distractions and interruptions during administration, and double checking high-risk medications with another nurse (Athanasakis, 2012).

REFERENCES
Athanasakis, E. (2012, October–December). Prevention of medication errors made by nurses in clinical practice. *Heath Science Journal*, 6, 773–780.

Blank, F., Tobin, J., Macomber, S., Jaouen, M., Dinoia, M., & Visintainer, P. (2011). A "back to basics" approach to reduce ED medication errors. *Journal of Emergency Nursing*, 37, 141–147.

Kosits, L., & Jones, K. (2011, January). Interruptions experienced by registered nurses working in the emergency department. *Journal of Emergency Nursing*, 37, 3–8.

Pham, J. C., Andrawis, M., Shore, A. D., Fahey, M., Morlock, L., & Pronovost, P. J. (2011, July). Are temporary staff associated with more severe emergency department medication errors? *Journal for Healthcare Quality*, 33, 9–18.

SHOCK

Shock is a condition of acute peripheral circulatory failure, causing inadequate and progressively decreasing blood pressure and failing tissue perfusion (see Chapter 9). There are three phases of shock: compensated, progressive, and decompensated. During the initial phase of shock, compensated, compensatory adjustments allow the body to adapt to the circulatory changes. In the second phase (progressive)

TABLE 13.2 COMPONENTS OF THE SECONDARY SURVEY

Head	Inspect for lacerations, bleeding from orifices. Check pupil size and response to light. Are pupils equal in size?
Chest	Auscultate for breath sounds in all lung fields. Inspect for lacerations, wounds, foreign bodies.
Abdomen	Auscultate for bowel sounds in all four quadrants. Palpate for areas of tenderness and rigidity. Inspect for lacerations, wounds, and foreign bodies. Inspect for ecchymosis (bruising).
Extremities	Inspect for lacerations, wounds, and foreign bodies. Inspect for injuries and deformities. Note areas of tenderness. Palpate for pulses. Evaluate temperature and capillary refill and compare the left to the right extremities.

compensatory mechanisms fail, resulting in inadequate tissue and cellular perfusion and causing cell death if left untreated. In the third and final stage, decompensated, the patient will no longer respond to treatment.

There are four types of shock: hypovolemic, cardiogenic, obstructive, and distributive. **Hypovolemic shock** signs and symptoms are caused by a decrease in the circulating blood volume. **Cardiogenic shock** signs and symptoms result from cardiac failure. **Obstructive shock** caused by a blockage of blood flow in the cardiovascular circuit outside the heart results in signs and symptoms of reduced blood flow and oxygenation. **Distributive shock** caused by excessive dilation of the venules and arterioles causes signs and symptoms of decreased blood pressure. Therapeutic interventions for shock are listed in Box 13-1.

Box 13-1 Guiding Principles for Treating Shock

- Maintain an open airway and give oxygen as ordered.
- Control external bleeding by direct pressure.
- Keep the patient supine if possible.
- Accurately record vital signs.
- Give IV fluids as ordered.
- Give the patient nothing to eat or drink until surgery is ruled out.

ANAPHYLAXIS

Anaphylaxis is a severe allergic reaction. The reaction can occur suddenly after initial contact with an allergen or after any subsequent exposure. Signs and symptoms result from a massive release of chemical mediators from mast cells and basophils throughout the body (Box 13-2). Chemical mediators lead to vasodilation and capillary leakage, which results in hypotension and eventually vascular collapse.

NURSING CARE TIP

One of the increasing causes of anaphylactic shock is latex allergy reaction. This type of allergy is on the rise among health care workers as a result of repeated exposure to health care products made with latex, such as gloves. The use of latex-free products limits exposure and reduces the risk of developing this allergy.

Pathophysiology

Anaphylactic shock is a form of distributive shock. There is no loss of blood, but excessive vasodilation occurs. Bronchi constrict, and air movement into the lungs becomes increasingly difficult. Increased fluid and mucus are secreted into the bronchial passages. Fluid in the air passages and constricted bronchi cause wheezing. The body is rapidly deprived of needed oxygen by this respiratory system reaction. Signs of severe anaphylaxis include hypotension due to vasodilation, decreased level of consciousness due to decreased oxygenation, and respiratory distress with stridor and cyanosis due to airway constriction and fluid.

• WORD • BUILDING •
anaphylaxis: an—without +phylaxis—protection

Box 13-2 Signs and Symptoms of an Allergic Reaction

- Generalized itching and flushing
- Urticaria (hives)
- Swelling of the lips, tongue, or uvula
- Dyspnea
- Bronchospasm, wheezing, and stridor
- Chest tightness and cough
- Crampy abdominal pain and vomiting
- Anxiety
- Hypotension

Nursing Process for the Patient Experiencing Shock or Anaphylaxis

Data Collection

When monitoring a patient at risk for shock, be aware of the signs and symptoms common to all types of shock (Box 13-3). It is important to note the patient's initial level of consciousness and monitor the patient for any subsequent changes. A progressive decline in level of consciousness indicates an urgent need for intervention. Pulses indicate the strength of the heart's contractions. Because a pulse is an immediate indicator of the patient's condition, it should be taken frequently during any emergency condition. Changes in blood pressure can indicate changes in blood volume. Blood pressure changes can occur rapidly but usually not as swiftly as pulse changes.

Skin temperature and color changes can occur with shock. Severe blood loss activates the "fight-or-flight" response in the sympathetic nervous system, which causes the skin to become cool and clammy. This occurs when peripheral blood vessels constrict to shunt blood to vital organs. Skin color depends on the presence of circulating blood in the vessels of the skin. Pale, white, or ashen skin indicates insufficient circulation. In patients with deeply pigmented skin, color changes can be seen in the nailbeds, conjunctiva of the eye, or mucous membranes of the mouth.

Capillary refill is checked on nailbeds to evaluate arterial circulation to an extremity. The nailbed is compressed to produce blanching (lighter color change), released, and the seconds counted until color returns to the blanched area. Normally, nailbed color should return within 3 seconds after the pressure is released. Older adults can normally have a delayed refill time. Patients in shock can have delayed or absent capillary refill.

 LEARNING TIP

Gently squeeze and release your own nailbed. Do you see the color change? Count the seconds until the color returns. That is your capillary refill time.

Box 13-3 Common Signs and Symptoms of Shock

- Restlessness and anxiety
- Weak, rapid, thready pulse
- Cold and clammy skin
- Pale skin color
- Shallow, rapid, labored breathing
- Gradually and steadily falling blood pressure
- Alteration in consciousness in severe shock state
- Thirst

Risk for Shock related to hypotension, hypovolemia, or hypoxia

EXPECTED OUTCOME: The patient will maintain vital signs within normal baseline range.

- Obtain frequent vital signs and oxygen saturation *to monitor patient status.*
- Administer oxygen *to maintain SpO₂ greater than 90%.*
- Maintain isotonic IV fluids, as ordered, *to maintain fluid volume and thus blood pressure.*
- Monitor intake and output *to monitor fluid status.*

Risk for Ineffective Peripheral Tissue Perfusion related to decreased circulating blood volume secondary to internal and/or external bleeding

EXPECTED OUTCOME: The patient's bleeding will be controlled to maintain vital signs within limits normal for the individual.

- Apply direct pressure to external bleeding site *to stop the flow of blood and allow normal coagulation to occur.*
- Elevate the bleeding limb and combine with direct pressure *to help stop bleeding.*
- When direct pressure and elevation do not control hemorrhage, pressure-point control should be attempted *to stop the bleeding* (Fig. 13.3). The chosen artery for pressure-point control must be proximal to the injury site and must be over a bony structure.
- Monitor vital signs continually, record, and report to the health care provider *to identify early changes in vital signs indicative of progressing shock.*
- Use a blanket *to help keep the patient from getting cold;* however, the patient also should not be allowed to overheat *because this causes peripheral blood vessels to dilate, which draws blood away from vital organs.*
- Monitor IV fluids as ordered *to increase circulating volume* (IV fluid contraindicated in cardiogenic shock).

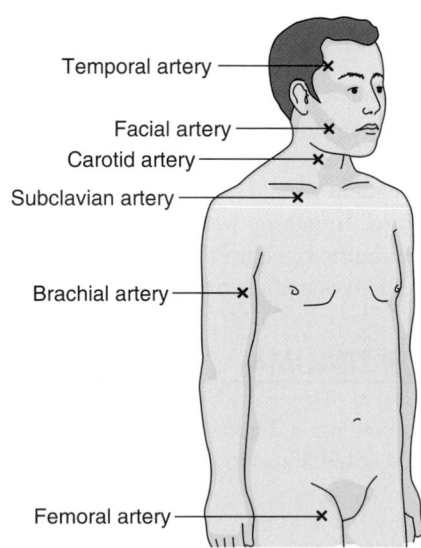

FIGURE 13.3 Arterial pressure points to control bleeding.

Risk for Allergy Response related to exaggerated immune response to substances

EXPECTED OUTCOME: The patient will implement plan to treat allergic reaction.

• Administer epinephrine (Adrenalin) intramuscularly (IM) in the vastus lateralis muscle (preferred because it provides better absorption to work faster) with a 22-gauge, 1- to 1.5-inch needle, or subcutaneously as ordered *to suppress the immune system and alleviate allergy symptoms.*
• Seek immediate medical attention *because effects of epinephrine are temporary.*

NURSING CARE TIP

• Epinephrine is given IM and should not be given IV for anaphylaxis (allergy symptoms with ABC involvement).
• Give antihistamines as second-line therapy as ordered *to control the allergic rash and pruritus.*
• Steroids are given in gradually tapered doses *to prevent return of symptoms.*

Ineffective Airway Clearance related to allergic airways

EXPECTED OUTCOME: The patient will maintain a patent airway and clear breath sounds at all times.

• Monitor breath sounds *to detect abnormal sounds such as wheezing.*
• Administer oxygen as ordered *to maintain the pulse oximetry at 95% or greater.*
• Position patient upright for optimal respiration *to allow maximal lung expansion.*
• Encourage patient to breathe deep and cough *to clear airways.*

Evaluation

If interventions have been effective, the blood pressure will improve to within normal limits for the patient and the patient will demonstrate a strong pulse; warm, dry skin; and be less anxious. The patient should show an immediate reversal of shock symptoms. Breathing becomes easy, and blood pressure and pulse return to the normal range. Breath sounds become clear, and hives and pruritus subside.

 MAJOR TRAUMA

Accidents or unintentional injury were the fifth leading cause of death in the United States in 2011 according to the Centers

for Disease Control and Prevention (CDC), mainly affecting persons under age 34 and over 70. Victims of major trauma might receive injury to an isolated vital organ or to multiple body systems.

Mechanism of Injury

When assessing a victim of major trauma, it is important to determine the mechanism of injury (see "Gerontological Issues"). Injuries are classified as either penetrating or

Gerontological Issues

Injuries and Older Adults

Older adults are at a high risk for falls that put them at risk for bruises, abrasions, cuts, and fractures. Nurses who initially assess older adults with injuries requiring treatment must ask questions and perform assessments that would identify if the patient is a victim of abuse or neglect.

Remember that the resolution of injuries occurs in a longer timeframe in the older patient when compared with the same injury resolution in a younger patient.

Injuries Caused by Falls Versus Battery or Assault

Any unexplained bruises, burns, abrasions, cuts, fractures, evidence of old injuries or bruises, burns, and cuts that are in different stages of healing suggest abuse. The pattern of an injury can also suggest abuse—for example, cigarette burns in areas covered with clothing; bruises or friction burns in a ring around the neck, ankles, or wrists; welts, burns, or bruises in the outline of a hand or belt buckle; multiple similar injuries in an area, such as whip marks across the buttocks or back of the legs; defensive injury pattern of bruising; and trauma to the hands and forearms.

Injuries related to falls have a predictable injury pattern related to the history and report of the fall. When an older adult falls, there is bruising of the hands and knees caused when the person attempts to break the fall. Additional bruising or injuries to the front of the body, arms, and head could be caused by hitting furniture or other items during the fall. Skin tears on the arms are common with a fall. Often, a friend or family member sees the older adult starting to fall and tries to steady the person by grabbing the area, tearing the skin. Ask questions to be sure that the report of the fall incident is consistent with the presenting injuries.

Any form of abuse or suspicion of abuse must be reported to the state agency that investigates reports of suspected abuse. It is not the nurse's responsibility to prove that there has been abuse or neglect, only to report incidents or cases of possible abuse.

• WORD • BUILDING •
epinephrine: epi—on +nephros—kidney
adrenalin: ad—on +renes—kidney

blunt. Penetrating, or open, injuries can be caused by any sharp object, such as broken glass or a knife, or by projectiles traveling at high speed, such as bullets or fragments from an explosion. In blunt, or closed, injuries, the skin surface is intact. An injury from blunt trauma usually extends beyond the point of impact to surrounding and underlying structures. For example, a blow to the chest can cause a fracture of several ribs that can, in turn, cause blunt trauma (such as a laceration or hematoma) to the spleen.

Damage caused by a gunshot wound and the trajectory of the bullet depends on the projectile mass, the type of tissue struck, the striking velocity, and the range. Entrance wounds are round or oval and can be surrounded by a rim of abrasion. Powder burns are visible if the firearm was discharged at close range. Documentation of these wounds should include a clear description of their appearance but should not include the words *entry* or *exit* because this is determined by trained experts. Patients with gunshot wounds near the level of the diaphragm should be evaluated for both abdominal and thoracic injuries.

Surface Trauma

Surface trauma includes any injury that does not break the skin (closed wound) and any open wound in which the skin surface is broken. Types of closed wounds include contusions (bruising) and hematomas (collection of blood under the skin). Types of open wounds include abrasions, punctures, lacerations, avulsions, and amputations.

Abrasions are a scraping away of the epidermal and dermal layers of the skin. They bleed very little but can be extremely painful because of inflamed nerve endings. Dirt can be ground into abrasions and can increase the risk of infection when large areas of skin are involved.

Puncture wounds result from sharp, narrow objects such as knives, nails, or high-velocity bullets. They can often be deceptive because the entrance wound can be small with little or no bleeding. It is difficult to estimate the extent of damage to underlying organs as a result. Puncture wounds usually do not bleed profusely unless they are located in the chest or abdomen.

Lacerations are open wounds resulting from snagging or tearing of tissue. Skin tissue can be partly or completely torn away. They vary in depth and can be irregular in shape. Lacerations can cause significant bleeding if blood vessels or arteries are involved.

Avulsions involve a full-thickness skin loss in which wound edges cannot be approximated. This type of injury is often seen in machine operators or in lawn-mower and power-tool accidents.

An **amputation** is a partial or complete severing of a body part. In cases of complete amputation, the arteries usually spasm and retract into the tissue, resulting in less bleeding than does a partial amputation, in which the lacerated arteries continue to bleed.

If the patient has sustained an amputation, bleeding is controlled with direct pressure and elevation. A tourniquet is applied only as a last resort. If a tourniquet is needed, it should be made of wide material such as a blood pressure cuff, which is less damaging to nerves and blood vessels. A dressing is applied to the amputated extremity, which is referred to as the stump. The stump is covered with sterile saline–moistened gauze followed by dry gauze, which is held in place with an elastic bandage for pressure. Amputated parts are taken to the hospital with the patient for possible reattachment. At the hospital, the amputated part is rinsed with saline solution, wrapped in sterile gauze, and placed in a sealed plastic bag, which is then placed on ice (not covered with ice or in ice water). The goal is to keep the body part cool without causing further damage from cold ice.

For a patient impaled by an object, it is imperative that the object not be removed unless it is obstructing the airway. Removing an impaled object can cause additional trauma and uncontrollable internal bleeding. Impaled objects are never cut off, broken off, or shortened unless transportation to the ED is otherwise impossible. A bulky dressing is applied around the object to stabilize it and reduce motion.

Tetanus

Tetanus is a disease caused by the bacillus *Clostridium tetani*, which enters the body through an open wound. Tetanus causes seizures, muscle spasms, stiffness of the jaw, coma, and death. Tetanus vaccinations should begin at 2 months of age and be followed by a series of pediatric immunizations until age 15. Thereafter, booster vaccinations are recommended every 10 years in the absence of an open wound.

Head Trauma

Sharp blows to the head can cause shifting of intracranial contents and lead to brain tissue contusion. The pathophysiology of head trauma can be divided into two phases. The first phase is the initial injury that occurs at the time of the accident and cannot be reversed. The second phase involves intracerebral bleeding and edema from the initial injury, which causes increased intracranial pressure (ICP). Management of head trauma is directed at the second phase and involves decreasing ICP. Early and late signs and symptoms of ICP are listed in Box 13-4.

Spinal Trauma

Spinal cord injury most often results from motor vehicle crashes, sports injuries, falls, and assaults, with most cases occurring in men ages 16 to 30. The cervical spine is especially vulnerable to traumatic injury. Patients who have sustained severe multiple injuries should be suspected of having a spinal cord injury, especially when they have signs of head trauma. All trauma patients should be treated as though they have a spinal cord injury until proven otherwise. Moving a patient with a vertebral injury can cause displacement of the injured bones and can increase damage to the spinal cord. Patients should be moved only by qualified people. Stabilization of the neck and back with a cervical collar and backboard is essential until spinal cord injury is ruled out (Fig. 13.4).

Box 13-4 Signs and Symptoms of Increased Intracranial Pressure (ICP)

Early Signs and Symptoms of Increased ICP

• Headache
• Nausea and vomiting
• Amnesia
• Altered level of consciousness
• Changes in speech
• Drowsiness

Late Signs and Symptoms of Increased ICP

• Dilated nonreactive pupils
• Unresponsiveness
• Abnormal posturing
• Widening pulse pressure
• Decreased pulse rate
• Changes in respiratory pattern

FIGURE 13.4 Immobilization of a patient suspected of having a spinal cord injury using a backboard and cervical collar.

 BE SAFE!

Do not move a patient with suspected vertebral or spinal cord injury until sufficient qualified help is available to prevent further injury to the spinal cord.

Chest Trauma

Chest trauma can damage the heart and lungs and cause life-threatening injuries, including pericardial tamponade, hemothorax, tension pneumothorax, and **flail chest**. Potentially life-threatening injuries include pulmonary and myocardial contusion, aortic and tracheobronchial disruption, and diaphragmatic rupture.

Chest trauma can result in laceration of lung tissue and cause a change in the negative intrapleural pressure. Air or blood leaking into the intrapleural space collapses the lung, resulting in a pneumothorax (air) or hemothorax (blood) and ineffective ventilation. In a tension pneumothorax, air is trapped in the pleural space during exhalation, resulting in increased pressure on the unaffected lung. The heart, great vessels, and trachea shift toward the unaffected side of the chest. As a result, blood flow to and from the heart is greatly reduced, causing a decrease in cardiac output. An uncorrected tension pneumothorax is fatal.

Chest trauma can also injure the heart and great vessels and reduce the amount of circulating blood volume. The heart can be bruised (myocardial contusion) or can sustain direct trauma. **Cardiac tamponade** occurs when blood accumulates in the pericardial sac and increases pressure around the heart. The increased pericardial pressure prevents the heart chambers from filling and contracting effectively. A patient with cardiac tamponade will have hypotension, tachycardia (rapid heart rate), and neck vein distention and requires immediate intervention to reduce the pressure in the pericardial sac and restore normal filling and contraction of the heart chambers.

Abdominal Trauma

The organs of the abdomen are vulnerable to injury because there is limited bony protection. Injury to organs such as the spleen and liver, which have a rich blood supply, can result in rapid loss of blood volume and hypovolemic shock. Abdominal organs can be injured as a result of severe blunt or penetrating trauma. If hypotension is present, intra-abdominal hemorrhage can exist. If the urinary bladder ruptures, urine leaks into the abdomen and blood can be detected at the urinary meatus or perineum. Penetrating trauma can cause lacerations to abdominal organs, resulting in rapid blood loss and hypovolemic shock.

Orthopedic Trauma

Fractured bones can result in blood loss, compromised circulation, infection, and immobility. Unstable pelvic fractures can cause injury to the genitourinary system or disrupt pelvic veins. Fractures of large bones such as the femur and tibia can cause significant blood loss. For example, a fractured femur can cause up to 1500 mL of blood loss, and a fractured tibia or humerus can cause up to 750 mL of blood loss. Joint dislocations can cause neurovascular compromise by applying pressure to the nerves and blood vessels. Delayed fracture reduction (realignment or setting) can cause avascular necrosis, which leads to death of the affected tissue and bone.

 LEARNING TIP

If a limb is fractured, splint it as it lies to prevent further damage. If the distal circulation is severely compromised, the patient needs immediate medical intervention.

• WORD • BUILDING •
tachycardia: tachy—fast +cardia—heart condition

Nursing Process for the Patient Experiencing Trauma

Data Collection

The mechanism of injury is determined to identify the extent of injury. Loss of consciousness immediately after an injury indicates that a concussion has occurred. The Glasgow Coma Scale (GCS) is used to rate a patient's level of consciousness (Fig. 13.5). The highest score is 15, indicating that the patient is alert and needs only observation. Scores lower than 13 can indicate the need for immediate treatment. It is important that nurses be adequately trained in using the scale and that all members of the health care team are consistent in their assessments. Morbidity and mortality are highest for patients with GCS scores of 8 or lower. Pupil size and reaction are monitored and recorded. Dilated or nonreactive pupils indicate increased ICP and a need for immediate intervention. Movement of extremities should also be assessed and documented. Posturing and differences between limb movement on the right and left side can indicate increased ICP.

Spinal nerves are located in the spinal cord and transmit sensory impulses to the brain and motor impulses to the body. The higher a traumatic lesion is on the spinal column, the more extensive will be the loss of muscle and sensory function (Table 13.3). A spinal cord injury at the level of C5 or above interferes with diaphragm function and respiratory effort, which must be carefully assessed. The patient's level of muscle control and ability to feel each limb are noted and recorded.

TABLE 13.3 CORRELATING SPINAL INJURY WITH IMPAIRMENT OF MOTOR FUNCTION

Injury Level	Impairment
S3–S5 or above	Patient unable to tighten anus.
L4–L5 or above	Patient unable to flex foot and extend toes.
L2–L4 or above	Patient unable to extend and flex legs.
C5–C7 or above	Patient unable to extend and flex arms.

Patients with major chest injuries can have dramatic symptoms, including classic signs of shock with cyanosis, dyspnea, and restlessness. The patient's breathing pattern and effectiveness of respirations are assessed. The rise and fall of the chest is observed, as well as symmetrical chest movement. Any bruising on the chest or upper abdomen is noted. Seat belts and restraint systems can cause significant bruising in high-impact crashes.

Vital signs are taken to detect tachycardia and hypotension from shock. The shape of the abdomen is observed to detect distention from intra-abdominal hemorrhage. Skin color, bruising, open wounds, and penetrating trauma are noted. The abdomen is auscultated for bowel sounds. The perineum is inspected for blood from the urethra.

Vital signs and pain level are assessed to detect orthopedic abnormalities. A respiratory assessment is done to detect a pulmonary embolism as a result of a long bone fracture. The injured extremity is inspected, and skin color and capillary refill time are noted. Skin integrity, protruding bone, or deformity is noted. Pulses distal to the injury are palpated to assess circulation to the area distal to the injury. Motor function and sensation are assessed to determine the extent of nerve injury.

Nursing Diagnoses, Planning, and Implementation

Acute Pain related to tissue trauma
EXPECTED OUTCOME: The patient will experience relief after measures are provided to relieve pain as evidenced by verbal and nonverbal expressions of pain relief.

- Apply ice, elevate, and immobilize the affected area *to decrease swelling and relieve pain.*
- Provide analgesics as ordered *to relieve pain.*

Impaired Skin Integrity related to tissue trauma
EXPECTED OUTCOME: The patient will demonstrate healing of impaired tissue.

- Apply direct pressure to open wounds *to control bleeding.*
- Irrigate open wounds with sterile saline solution *to thoroughly remove dirt and debris and clean exposed tissue to prevent infection.*

GLASGOW COMA SCALE	
Areas of Response	**Points**
Eye Opening	
Eyes open spontaneously	4
Eyes open in response to voice	3
Eyes open in response to pain	2
No eye opening response	1
Best Verbal Response	
Oriented (e.g., to person, place, time)	5
Confused, speaks but is disoriented	4
Inappropriate, but comprehensible words	3
Incomprehensible sounds, but no words are spoken	2
None	1
Best Motor Response	
Obeys command to move	6
Localizes painful stimulus	5
Withdraws from painful stimulus	4
Flexion, abnormal decorticate posturing	3
Extension, abnormal decerebrate posturing	2
No movement or posturing	1
Total Possible Points	**3–15**
Major Head Injury	**≤8**
Moderate Head Injury	**9–12**
Minor Head Injury	**13–15**

FIGURE 13.5 The Glasgow Coma Scale is used to determine level of consciousness. From Teasdale, G., & Jennett, B. (1974). Assessment of coma and impaired consciousness. A practical scale. *Lancet, 2,* 81–84. PMID 4136544.

Risk for Infection related to tissue trauma

EXPECTED OUTCOME: The patient's wounds will remain free of infection.

- With open wounds, give tetanus immunization as ordered if it has been more than 5 years since one was last given *to prevent tetanus infection.*
- Give antibiotics as ordered *to prevent infection.*

Risk for Ineffective Cerebral Tissue Perfusion related to cerebral edema

EXPECTED OUTCOME: The patient will maintain adequate cerebral homeostasis without cerebral edema as evidenced by a GCS score of 14 or greater.

- Give oxygen as ordered *to maintain adequate oxygenation of brain tissues and prevent cellular damage from hypoxia at the cerebral level.*
- If the patient has an altered level of consciousness or deteriorating respiratory effort, anticipate and assist with endotracheal intubation as needed *to provide respiratory support to patient.*
- Elevate the head of the patient's bed 30 to 45 degrees, if possible, *to reduce ICP.*
- Maintain the patient's head position at midline *to ensure unobstructed venous drainage to help reduce ICP.*
- Maintain IV access for fluids *to maintain hemodynamic stability and access for medications.*
- Monitor mannitol IV, an osmotic diuretic, or hypertonic saline (1.7%–29.2%) as ordered *to decrease cerebral edema.*
- If the patient is agitated, provide calming measures *because agitation increases ICP.*

Ineffective Breathing Pattern related to neck injury or unstable chest wall segment or lung collapse

EXPECTED OUTCOME: The patient will maintain effective respiratory rate and experience improved gas exchange in the lungs.

- If signs of respiratory distress are present, use the jaw-thrust or chin-lift maneuver, along with suction and airway adjuncts as needed, *to maintain patency of the airway.*
- Maintain cervical collar and backboard *to prevent further injury.*
- Give oxygen as ordered *to improve tissue oxygenation.* Advanced adjunct airway equipment, including an endotracheal tube, must be readily available.
- Administer supplemental oxygen as ordered *to promote tissue oxygenation.*
- Maintain chest tube drainage system if inserted *to help expand lung.*

Ineffective Airway Clearance related to neck injury

EXPECTED OUTCOME: The patient will maintain clear lung sounds.

- Suction the oropharynx and nasopharynx *to clear secretions and prevent aspiration of secretions into the airway.*

- If the patient vomits, log roll the patient onto one side and use suction as needed *to prevent aspiration of emesis.*

Impaired Physical Mobility related to neck injury

EXPECTED OUTCOME: The patient will maintain movement of extremities normal for patient.

- Maintain neck immobility during initial treatment of a patient with head or neck trauma *to prevent serious injury until trauma damage is identified.*

Decreased Cardiac Output related to compression of heart and great vessels

EXPECTED OUTCOME: The patient will maintain vital signs within baseline limits.

- Report unstable vital signs to physician *because patient may need immediate surgical intervention in the operating room.*
- Explain diagnostic testing to patients with stable vital signs if radiographic studies are ordered *to determine the extent of cardiac or pulmonary injury.*
- Monitor patient's vital signs and oxygen saturation continuously *to detect signs of shock.*

Deficient Fluid Volume related to hemorrhage or abdominal organ injury

EXPECTED OUTCOME: The patient will maintain vital signs within baseline limits.

- Monitor for signs of shock *to detect hypovolemic shock.*
- Maintain IV fluids as ordered by 18- or 16-gauge IV cannulas *to restore circulating volume.*
- Assist with peritoneal lavage, if performed, *to detect intra-abdominal hemorrhage.*
- Maintain nasogastric tube, if ordered, *to decompress the stomach.*
- Cover abdominal wounds with a sterile dressing *to prevent infection.*
- If abdominal organs are exposed, cover with sterile saline-soaked dressings *to prevent tissue necrosis.*
- Assist with blood and blood product administration, as ordered and per agency policy, *to maintain circulating volume and improve tissue oxygenation.*

Impaired Physical Mobility related to bone injury

EXPECTED OUTCOME: The patient will maintain movement of extremities normal for patient.

- Remove all jewelry before applying a splint *because the extremity can swell after injury.*
- Maintain extremity in a splint in the position found, unless distal circulation is severely compromised, and keep it immobilized if there is severe pain or deformity. *Splinting promotes comfort and prevents further damage to surrounding tissue by preventing movement of broken bone ends.*
- Immobilize the joints above and below the affected area using a folded towel or a pillow *to provide comfort and protection until the patient is evaluated by a health care provider.*

- Monitor skin color, temperature, distal pulses, capillary refill, movement, and sensation of the extremity after splint application *to detect abnormalities.*
- Elevate and ice extremity *to reduce edema and relieve pain.*

Evaluation

If interventions have been effective, the following results will be evident: A patient with trauma reports an acceptable pain level, and the patient's wound heals without infection; a patient with spinal injury maintains a regular rate, rhythm, and pattern of breathing, clear lung sounds, intactness of mobility, and GCS score of 14 to 15; a patient with chest trauma maintains an open airway and effective breathing pattern; a patient with abdominal trauma has effective circulating volume as evidenced by vital signs within normal limits; a patient with orthopedic trauma has strong and palpable pulses, normal blood pressure, normal skin color, skin that is warm and dry, capillary refill time of less than 3 seconds, pain controlled to a satisfactory level, and normal motor function and sensation in the extremity.

BURNS

The skin protects the body by preventing bacterial or viral invasion, enhancing temperature regulation, and conserving body fluids and electrolytes. These functions are impaired with a burn injury and can lead to multisystem alterations. Burn injuries are acutely painful and can be dramatic in appearance. Nursing care depends on the extent and depth of the burn injury and the presence of any associated factors, such as smoke inhalation, blunt trauma, or fractures. The more extensive the burn injury, the greater the potential for complications and mortality. The patient's age can contribute to the risk of mortality as well. Infants younger than age 2 and adult patients older than age 60 have the highest mortality rates from major burns. (See Chapter 55 for more on burns.)

Assessment of the burn patient begins with the ABCDs of the primary survey with exposure E and F, fluid resuscitation added to the secondary survey of burned patients. The history should include the mechanism and time of the injury and a description of the surrounding environment, including the presence of noxious chemicals and inhalation of smoke in an enclosed space. The greatest threat to life in a patient with a major burn injury is smoke or heat inhalation, which causes edema in the respiratory passages. Continuous assessment of respiratory status is essential when you observe burns or soot on the face, singed nasal hairs, a hoarse voice, coughing, or restlessness.

Burns of the face can swell rapidly and can compromise the airway. Facial burns are treated by elevating the head of the bed to 30 degrees to minimize edema. Oxygen is administered to the patient with potential pulmonary injury. Equipment for endotracheal intubation should be readily available. Because large fluid losses occur in burn injuries, an IV infusion with large-bore cannulas should be started. The patient's weight and the extent of the burn determine fluid resuscitation needs. The patient is kept warm because when skin is lost, a burn victim cannot maintain body heat. IV opioids are administered for pain.

Burn depth is described as superficial, partial thickness, or full thickness (Fig. 13.6). **Superficial burns** are confined to the epidermis. **Partial-thickness burns** are either superficial dermal (epidermis and upper dermis of the skin) or deep (entire epidermal layer and deep dermis; Fig. 13.7). **Full-thickness burns** involve destruction of all layers of the epidermis and dermis and can include muscle, fascia, and bone. Partial-thickness burns that involve a small area are cleaned with sterile saline solution, covered with a 1/8-inch layer of an anti-infective cream such as silver sulfadiazine (Silvadene, Flamazine), and then covered with dry, bulky, fluffed dressings. Major full-thickness wounds are covered with dry, sterile dressings or linen. Patients with major burns are transferred to a specialized burn unit.

FIGURE 13.6 Partial- and full-thickness burns and structures affected.

FIGURE 13.7 A blistered partial-thickness thermal burn.

BE SAFE!

BE VIGILANT! Is there anything you would want to check before applying silver sulfadiazine? Yes! Check allergies to sulfa medications. Look at the name of the medication, it contains sulfa. A patient allergic to sulfa drugs should not be given this medication!

LEARNING TIP

Over-the-counter ointments, lotions, butter, and antiseptics are never used on a major burn because they can promote infection, retain heat, and cause more pain.

CRITICAL THINKING

Mr. Smith

■ Mr. Smith is a 28-year-old man who was welding close to a natural gas line. The flame of the welder caused the gas line to explode, throwing Mr. Smith 50 feet. He landed on his back. He is brought to the ED by the rescue squad. Mr. Smith is awake, alert, and oriented. He has soot around his mouth and nose. He sustained deep partial-thickness burns to his neck, upper chest, and both forearms. He reports pain from his burns and also thoracic back and hip pain. His pulse rate is 100 beats per minute. His blood pressure is 160/90 mm Hg. His respiratory rate is 20 per minute.

1. What is the first priority of care for Mr. Smith?
2. Is Mr. Smith at risk for respiratory burns? Why?
3. Are Mr. Smith's vital signs within normal limits?
4. Would wet or dry dressings be preferable for his large areas of deep partial-thickness burns? Why?
5. Mr. Smith is wearing a neck chain and a wedding ring. Should they be removed immediately, or should you wait until Mr. Smith's wife arrives to take them off? Why?
6. Mr. Smith continues to report hip and back pain. In reviewing his mechanism of injury, what other injuries could Mr. Smith have?
7. With what members of the health team should you anticipate collaborating?

Suggested answers are at the end of the chapter.

HYPOTHERMIA

Normally the body maintains its temperature in a narrow range on either side of 98.6°F (37°C) to allow chemical reactions to work most efficiently. Body heat escapes to the environment through conduction, convection, radiation, and evaporation. Heat loss is inversely proportional to body size and body fat. Fat insulates because it has less blood flow and consequently has less ability to vasodilate and lose heat.

Hypothermia occurs when the core body temperature falls below 95°F (35°C). As the core temperature falls below 95°F, the body is less able to regulate its temperature and generate body heat, causing progressive loss of body heat to occur.

Nursing Process for the Patient With Hypothermia
Data Collection

In cases of mild hypothermia (core temperature between 90° and 95°F [32.2° and 35°C]), the patient is usually alert, shivering, and can appear clumsy, apathetic, or irritable (Table 13.4). Hypoglycemia can occur because glucose and glycogen stores are depleted by long-term shivering. Respiratory rate, heart rate, and cardiac output decrease.

TABLE 13.4 DEFINING CHARACTERISTICS AND OUTCOME CRITERIA FOR HYPOTHERMIA

Core Body Temperature	Defining Characteristics
Below 95°F (35°C)	• Skin cold to touch • Lack of coordination • Slurred speech • Vigorous shivering
Below 91.4°F (33°C)	• Cardiac dysrhythmias • Cyanosis
Below 89.6°F (32°C)	• Shivering replaced by muscle rigidity • Hypotension • Dilated pupils
Below 82.4°F (28°C)	• Absent deep tendon reflexes • Hypoventilation (3–4 breaths per minute) • Ventricular fibrillation possible
Below 80.6°F (27°C)	• Coma • Flaccid muscles • Fixed, dilated pupils • Ventricular fibrillation to cardiac standstill • Apnea

Outcome Criteria
• Core body temperature is greater than 95°F (35°C).
• Patient is alert and oriented.
• Cardiac dysrhythmias are absent.
• Acid–base balance is normal.
• Pupils react normally.

More severe hypothermia occurs between 85° and 90°F (29.4° and 32.2°C). Shivering stops and muscle activity decreases. Initially, fine muscle coordination ceases. Then, as core body temperature continues to drop, all muscle activity stops and the muscles become rigid. The patient becomes lethargic and less interested in fighting the cold environment. The patient's level of consciousness begins to markedly decrease at 89.6°F (32°C); the patient becomes lethargic and disoriented and begins to hallucinate. The pupils become dilated. As the core body temperature falls to 82°F (27.8°C), the patient becomes apneic, the pulse becomes slower and weaker, and cardiac dysrhythmias occur. The profoundly hypothermic patient has a core temperature of less than 80°F (26.7°C) and usually appears dead, with no obtainable vital signs. Determination of death should be made only after aggressive core rewarming to at least 90°F (32.2°C).

Nursing Diagnoses, Planning, and Implementation

Initial treatment of the hypothermic patient consists of rewarming the patient, stabilizing vital functions, and preventing further heat loss (see the "Nursing Care Plan for the Patient With Hypothermia"). The patient is removed from the cold environment. All wet clothing is removed to prevent further heat loss. The patient's core body temperature guides treatment. If body temperature is above 82.4°F (28°C), passive rewarming is preferred. The room temperature is set to 70° to 75°F (21.1°–23.9°C). The patient is wrapped in warm, dry blankets. Heat loss from the head is reduced by covering the head with warm towels.

If core body temperature is below 82.4°F (28°C), active rewarming is needed. A heating blanket (carbon-fiber) and radiant heat lights are used. Warm, humidified oxygen is administered. Warm IV fluids are administered. Body temperature is constantly monitored using a rectal probe. Heated **gastric lavage**, heated peritoneal lavage, or cardiopulmonary bypass can be performed for profound hypothermia. Cardiac drugs are given

sparingly because, as the body warms, peripheral vasodilation occurs. Drugs that were trapped in the peripheral circulation are then suddenly released during rewarming, leading to a bolus effect that can cause fatal dysrhythmias.

Evaluation

Desired outcome criteria for the patient with hypothermia is a core body temperature higher than 95°F (35°C), no cardiac dysrhythmias, pulse and blood pressure within normal limits, and an alert and oriented status.

 FROSTBITE

The extremities are vulnerable to cold injury. Frostnip occurs when exposed parts of the body become very cold but not frozen. This condition usually is not painful. The skin becomes pale and blanched. Contact with a warm object such as someone's hand can be all that is needed to rewarm the part. During rewarming, the affected part might tingle and become red.

Frostbite occurs when body parts become frozen. The extremities are at increased risk because blood shunts away from them to maintain core body temperature. The affected tissue feels hard and frozen. Most frostbitten parts are white, yellow-white, or blue-white. When rewarmed, the skin appears deep red, hot, and dry to touch. The severity of a cold injury is determined by the duration of the exposure, the temperature to which the body part was exposed, and the wind velocity during exposure.

Interventions for frostbite include protecting the affected area from further trauma. To prevent additional damage, the frostbitten part is handled gently and never rubbed. The injured part is loosely covered with a dry, sterile dressing. The patient is not allowed to stand or walk on a frostbitten foot. The affected extremity is elevated to heart level to minimize edema and promote blood flow.

NURSING CARE PLAN for the Patient With Hypothermia

Nursing Diagnosis: *Hypothermia* related to exposure to cold environment

Expected Outcomes: The patient's body temperature and vital signs will be within normal limits.

Evaluation of Outcomes: Is patient's body temperature greater than 95°F (35°C)? Is patient alert and oriented? Is cardiac rhythm normal?

Intervention Monitor patient's core body temperature. **Rationale** Abnormal body temperature can be detected and treated. **Evaluation** Is body temperature greater than 95°F (35°C)?

Intervention Monitor pulse and electrocardiogram (ECG) rhythm. **Rationale** Cardiac dysrhythmias can occur at temperatures below 91.4°F (33°C). **Evaluation** Is pulse rate and ECG rhythm normal?

Intervention Monitor patient's level of consciousness. **Rationale** Level of consciousness becomes markedly decreased at temperatures of 89.6°F (32°C). **Evaluation** Is the patient alert?

Intervention Institute rewarming passively or actively as ordered. **Rationale** Rewarming is necessary to return body temperature to desirable range. **Evaluation** Is body core temperature rising to normal range?

HYPERTHERMIA

The body's heat-regulating mechanisms usually work very well, allowing people to tolerate significant temperature changes. The body's most efficient mechanisms for decreasing body heat are sweating and dilation of blood vessels in the skin. When blood vessels dilate, blood comes to the skin surface to increase the rate of radiation of heat from the body. However, when these mechanisms become overwhelmed, the consequences can be disastrous and irreversible. Those at greatest risk for heat illnesses include children, older people, and patients with cardiac disease.

BE SAFE!

BE VIGILANT! Older adults are vulnerable to hyperthermia. In times of extreme summer temperatures, older people who live alone should be checked to make sure they are not experiencing hyperthermia. If they do not have fans or air-conditioning available, they should be taken to a cooler environment.

Hyperthermia results when thermoregulation breaks down because of excess heat generation, an inability to dissipate heat, overwhelming environmental heat, or a combination of these factors. Unlike a fever, in which the thermal set point is elevated, in heat illness the thermal set point remains normal and hyperthermia occurs because of an inability to dissipate heat. Antipyretics are of no use in hyperthermia and can contribute to complications.

Nursing Process for the Patient With Hyperthermia

Data Collection

Illness from heat exposure can take three forms: heat cramps, heat exhaustion, and heatstroke (Box 13-5). As heat illness progresses, circulating blood volume decreases, causing dehydration. Fluid intake is crucial in the prevention of heat illness.

HEAT CRAMPS. Heat cramps, the mildest form of heat illness, involve painful muscle spasms, usually in the legs or abdomen, that occur after strenuous exercise. Large amounts of salt and water can be lost as a result of excessive sweating, causing stressed muscles to spasm. With adequate rest and fluid replacement, the body adjusts the distribution of electrolytes and the cramps disappear.

HEAT EXHAUSTION. Heat exhaustion occurs when the body loses so much water and electrolytes through heavy sweating that hypovolemia occurs. Heat exhaustion is largely a manifestation of the strain placed on the cardiovascular system as it tries to maintain normothermia. Cerebral function is

---

Box 13-5 Defining Characteristics and Outcome Criteria for Environmental Hyperthermia

Defining Characteristics

Early Signs
- Core body temperature 100.4° to 102.2°F (38°–39°C)
- Diaphoresis
- Cool, clammy skin
- Dizziness
- Pulse rate greater than 100

Late Signs
- Increasing body core temperature of 106°F (41.1°C) or higher
- Hot, dry, flushed skin
- Altered mental status
- Coma or seizures possible
- Hypotension

Outcome Criteria
- Core body temperature less than 101°F (38.3°C)
- Patient alert and oriented
- Skin warm and dry to touch

---

unimpaired, although the patient can show minor irritability and poor judgment. The ability to sweat remains. The skin is usually cold and clammy and the face gray. Sodium and water loss cause the patient to become dehydrated. The body temperature is usually normal or slightly elevated: from 100.4° to 102.2°F (38°–39°C). The patient might report feeling dizzy, weak, or faint, with nausea or a headache. Vomiting and diarrhea can also be present.

HEATSTROKE. If symptoms of heat exhaustion are not treated, **heatstroke** can develop. Altered mental status and an inability to sweat are key symptoms in heatstroke. Some patients show confusion, irrational behavior, or psychosis; others develop seizures or go into a coma. Because the sweating mechanism has been overwhelmed, many heatstroke victims have hot, dry, flushed skin. The body temperature rises rapidly to 106°F (41.1°C) or higher, and level of consciousness decreases. If heatstroke is not treated, death results.

Patients with heatstroke are admitted to the intensive care unit because late complications can appear suddenly and require immediate management. Relatively common occurrences include seizures, cerebral ischemia, renal failure, late cardiac decompensation, and gastrointestinal (GI) bleeding. Long-term prognosis varies with the patient's previous state of health and length of time under heat stress.

Nursing Diagnoses, Planning, and Implementation

Hyperthermia related to exposure to hot environment
EXPECTED OUTCOME: The patient will maintain body temperature within normal limits.

- For heat cramps, remove the patient from the hot environment *to allow cooling to begin.*
- Have patient sit or lie down until muscle cramps subside *to prevent further injury.*
- Remove patient from the hot environment and undress patient *to allow patient to cool rapidly.*
- Mist-spray tepid water over the patient while maintaining a strong continual breeze from electric fans *because evaporative cooling is the most efficient method of cooling.*

Deficient Fluid Volume related to hypervolemia
EXPECTED OUTCOME: The patient will maintain blood pressure within normal limits of baseline.

- Give patient oral fluids, water, or a diluted (half-strength) balanced electrolyte solution if patient is fully alert *to replace lost fluids.*
- If patient is hypotensive, maintain IV fluids as ordered *to restore volume.*

Evaluation

Interventions have been successful if the hyperthermic patient has a core body temperature below 101°F (38.3°C), warm and dry skin, a strong pulse, blood pressure within normal limits, and is alert and oriented.

POISONING AND DRUG OVERDOSE

Poisons are introduced into the body by ingestion, inhalation, injection, absorption, or venomous bites. Poisons act by changing cellular metabolism, causing damage to structures, or disturbing function. Many toxins and poisons alter the patient's mental status, making it difficult to obtain an accurate history.

Nursing Process for the Patient With Ingested Poisoning

Data Collection

The primary nursing responsibility is to recognize that a poisoning has occurred and then try to determine the nature of the poison. The method of exposure is established so that removal or interruption of the toxin can begin. Most ingested poisons are drugs, but about one-third of poisonings are caused by cleaners, soaps, insecticides, acids, or alkalis. Many household plants are poisonous if they are accidentally ingested. Some plants cause local irritation of the skin, and others can affect the circulatory system, GI tract, or central nervous system.

Empty medication bottles, scattered pills, and relevant chemicals should be examined by emergency medical personnel at the scene to help identify the poisonous substance. The patient's physical appearance also can give a clue to the type of substance ingested. IV needle tracks, burns,

erythema, and flushed skin can help identify the poison or toxic exposure.

Nursing Diagnoses, Planning, and Implementation

Risk for Injury related to absorption of poisoning agent
EXPECTED OUTCOME: The patient will maintain normal vital signs and be free of injury.

- Contact a poison control center *to access information concerning virtually all poisonous substances, available antidotes, and appropriate emergency treatment.*

NURSING CARE TIP

- Syrup of ipecac is NOT recommended for at-home treatment of accidental overdose because evidence shows that its use does not improve patient outcomes. For example, giving it to a person who had swallowed a caustic chemical results in greater tissue damage from the vomiting of the chemical, or after being given syrup of ipecac, a person who was poisoned may vomit the necessary antidote.
- Gastric decontamination, activated charcoal, and gastric lavage are no longer routinely recommended and should be reserved for the most severe cases.

Evaluation

Interventions have been successful if the patient remains free from injury and has vital signs within normal limits.

Inhaled Poisons

Inhaled poisons include natural gas, pesticides, carbon monoxide, chlorine, and other gases. Carbon monoxide is odorless and can produce profound hypoxia by combining with hemoglobin molecules and displacing oxygen in red blood cells. The patient's carboxyhemoglobin level is monitored to direct appropriate therapy. Inhalation of chlorine is irritating to the respiratory system and can produce airway obstruction and pulmonary edema.

When an inhalation injury from a poison occurs, the patient must be moved into fresh air and away from the toxin. Supplemental oxygen is given as ordered. A patient exposed to prolonged inhalation of a poison can experience lung damage. Respiratory status must be closely monitored to detect complications.

Injected Poisons

Injected poisons pose compelling problems because they are difficult to remove or dilute. Usually they result from drug overdose, but they can also result from the bites and stings of insects or animals. Local swelling and tissue destruction can occur at the injection site. All jewelry is removed because swelling can occur. A cold pack is applied to decrease local pain and swelling around the injection site. The identity of the injected drug or toxin must be established so that adverse effects can be anticipated and managed.

Insect Stings or Bites

Insect stings or bites cause anaphylaxis in a small percentage of people (only 5%–10% among adults). Symptoms in most people are limited to localized pain, swelling, heat, and redness. Potentially dangerous stings or bites can come from bees, wasps, yellow jackets, hornets, certain ants, scorpions, and some spiders. Treatment involves applying ice to the site and elevating the affected part. Cellulitis can occur hours later and can require medical treatment.

When a patient has sustained a bee or wasp sting, examine the area for the stinger and remove it by gently scraping it off the skin. Tweezers or forceps are not used to remove the stinger because squeezing the stinger can inject more venom into the patient. Placing ice over the injury site can help slow the rate of toxin absorption.

Two types of spiders, the black widow and the brown recluse, can inflict serious and sometimes life-threatening bites. Both species are found throughout the United States. Antivenin (an antitoxin that counteracts a specific venom) for treating the toxic effects of both is available. Black widow spiders are glossy black and have a distinctive, bright red-orange marking in the shape of an hourglass on the abdomen. They are found in dry, dim places around buildings, in woodpiles, and among debris. Their venom is neurotoxic and causes systemic symptoms, including cramping of large muscle groups, dyspnea, weakness, sweating, nausea, vomiting, and rash. Death is uncommon, and symptoms typically subside in 48 hours.

The brown recluse spider is dull brown and has a dark violin-shaped mark on its back. It tends to live in dark areas, under rocks, in woodpiles, and in old abandoned buildings. The venom of the brown recluse causes severe local tissue damage. The area becomes red, swollen, and tender and develops a pale, mottled, cyanotic center. A large ulcer can develop within 48 hours if not treated promptly. Systemic symptoms include fever, chills, nausea, vomiting, arthralgia, and weakness. Death is not common.

Snakebites

Only a small percentage of snakebites are caused by poisonous snakes. The most prevalent poisonous snakes are the coral snake and the pit vipers, which include rattlesnakes, copperheads, and cottonmouth moccasins. Envenomation occurs when the snake's hollow fangs puncture the skin and inject venom, which is stored in sacs located at the back of the snake's head. A poisonous snakebite leaves two small puncture wounds with surrounding discoloration, swelling, and pain. Envenomation by any of the pit viper snakes produces burning pain at the site of the injury. Swelling and discoloration occur within 5 to 10 minutes after the bite.

Interventions are focused on decreasing the circulation of venom throughout the patient's system by keeping the patient calm and immobilizing the affected part. The affected extremity should be positioned below the level of the heart. The site of the bite is cleaned with soap and water but should not be irrigated or flushed. The wound should be covered with loose, clean dressing. Ice should not be applied to the bite. The patient is kept calm until antivenin can be given. Medical treatment of the patient with a poisonous snakebite should be directed by an experienced toxicologist.

■ NEAR-DROWNING

Drowning is death from **asphyxia** (insufficient oxygen intake) after submersion in water. *Near-drowning* is used to describe submersion with at least temporary survival of the victim. Life-threatening complications of near-drowning are respiratory failure and ischemic neurologic injury from hypoxia and acidosis. When submersion occurs, conscious victims hold their breath until reflex inspiratory efforts override breath holding. As water is aspirated, laryngospasm occurs, producing severe hypoxia. In wet drowning, the laryngospasm is less prolonged and fluid enters the lungs after the vocal cords relax. In dry drowning, cold water causes laryngospasm and vagal stimulation, which leads to asphyxiation. Most successfully resuscitated victims experience dry drowning. Risk factors for drowning include inability to swim, diving accidents, use of alcohol and drugs before swimming, exhaustion, and hypothermia.

If a person survives submersion, acute respiratory failure can follow. The incidence of serious pulmonary complications is high in this group. Symptoms of impaired gas exchange (known as secondary near-drowning) can be delayed as long as 72 hours after the incident. Contaminants in the water can irritate the pulmonary system and cause inflammatory reactions and impaired surfactant functioning. Metabolic acidosis is usually present, leading to tissue anoxia and dysrhythmias. Hypoxemia and hypothermia predispose the patient to arrhythmias. Neurologically, there is neuronal damage and cerebral edema.

Aggressive resuscitative efforts should be used on victims of cold-water drowning when submersion time is 1 hour or less. Hypothermia can decrease the metabolic needs of the brain and contribute to neurologic recovery even after prolonged submersion. Resuscitation should not be stopped until the body temperature is at least greater than 32°C.

Nursing Process for the Near-Drowning Patient

Data Collection

Most near-drowning victims have mild dyspnea, a deathlike appearance with blue or gray skin color, apnea or tachypnea (abnormally fast breathing), hypotension, slow heart rate (possibly less than 10 beats per minute), cold skin temperature, dilated pupils, hypothermia, and vomiting. Vital

• WORD • BUILDING •
tachypnea: tachy—fast +pnea—breathing

signs are assessed to detect abnormal readings. Respiratory rate and pattern are observed. Any dyspnea or signs of airway obstruction are noted. Skin color or cyanosis is noted. The patient's level of consciousness can be altered from anoxia.

Nursing Diagnoses, Planning, and Implementation
Ineffective Tissue Perfusion related to severe anoxia
EXPECTED OUTCOME: The patient will maintain level of consciousness and vital signs within normal range, with clear breath sounds that are equal bilaterally.

• Conduct ABCDs of the primary survey, which always begin resuscitative efforts, *to determine patient's status.*
• Give supplemental oxygen as ordered *to increase tissue oxygenation.*
• Ensure that adjunct airway equipment is available *because endotracheal intubation and insertion of a nasogastric tube to decompress the stomach can be needed.*

Evaluation

Factors that influence the outcome of near-drowning include the temperature of the water, length of time submerged, cleanliness of the water, and age of the victim. The younger the patient, the better the chance of survival. Interventions have been successful if the patient has normal respiratory rate and pattern and vital signs, is alert and oriented, and skin that is warm and dry to touch with a capillary refill time of less than 3 seconds.

 PSYCHIATRIC EMERGENCIES

A psychiatric emergency occurs when a person no longer has the coping skills needed to maintain the usual level of functioning. The patient's moods, thoughts, or actions can be so disordered that the patient could harm self or others if the situation is not quickly controlled. If acute psychiatric episodes are not managed, they can result in life-threatening, suicidal, violent, or psychologically damaging behavior. If an emotional trauma is not managed successfully, a condition known as posttraumatic stress disorder can result, in which tension, anxiety, guilt, and fear concerning the traumatic event produce cognitive, affective, and behavioral responses to memories of the event long after the event has passed.

A crisis occurs when people enter a sudden state of emotional turmoil and are unable to resolve the situation with their own resources. Common emotional or behavioral manifestations of psychiatric crises include responses to stressful events, anxiety, depression, psychosis, and mania. Anxiety can range in severity from mild to a state of panic. Panic evolves into complete disorganization and loss of control. A patient in panic is terrified and needs external controls to avoid harm.

Depression is an affective disorder most commonly characterized by physical ailments and somatizations. Antidepressants and certain forms of therapy are used to restore the balance of brain neurochemicals and diminish the symptoms of depression.

Psychotic patients experience impaired thought processes and thought content characterized by hallucinations, delusions, ideas of reference, thought broadcasting, and thought insertion. Psychotic thinking and abnormal speech patterns interfere with the patient's attempt to communicate rationally.

Manic behavior is most commonly the result of manic-depressive (bipolar) disorder. Manic persons typically exhibit bizarre, extreme, and hyperactive behaviors. Manic persons are also at high risk for injuring themselves or others.

Nursing Process for the Patient With a Psychiatric Emergency
Data Collection

Causes of psychiatric emergency symptoms are varied and require thorough assessment of the patient's history and mental status. Information from the patient's medical history can produce possible organic causes contributing to the patient's presenting symptoms. Endocrine dysfunction, electrolyte abnormalities, and head trauma are examples of medical conditions that can cause changes in mental status. A medication history is obtained to determine compliance with medication regimens and any recent changes in medications. Information regarding recent use of alcohol or illicit drugs should be obtained because these substances can heighten psychiatric emergencies. A brief mental status examination is conducted. Determining a person's suicide risk is very important. The patient's appearance, behavior, cognitive function, thought content, and thought processes are noted. The nurse determines whether the patient is having problems concentrating, following instructions, or recalling his or her medical history.

The nurse's role is to keep the patient free from harm. To do this, the nurse needs to establish a trusting relationship with the patient. Ways to accomplish this include being respectful and truthful, listening carefully, and providing a safe and calm environment for the patient.

Nursing Diagnoses, Planning, and Implementation
Anxiety related to situational stress
EXPECTED OUTCOME: The patient will state reduced anxiety.

• Establish an atmosphere of trust *so the patient feels free to discuss problems.*
• Use active listening *to acknowledge patient's physical and emotional concerns.*
• Speak directly and truthfully to the patient *to gain patient trust,* and do not promise unachievable things.
• Trusted supportive members of the patient's family can be involved *to calm the person and encourage cooperation.*
• Do not allow bystanders or adversarial family members to visit the patient *because they could create further upset for the patient.*
• Speak compassionately with the patient and refrain from laughing or joking *to show respect for the patient.*

Risk for Injury related to impaired judgment
EXPECTED OUTCOME: The patient will remain free from injury.

• Do not threaten, challenge, or argue with a disturbed patient *to prevent injury.*
• Make sure the environment is safe and that external sources of stimulation are reduced *to prevent injury.*
• Be firm but unthreatening *to help patient feel safe.*
• Administer antipsychotic medications as ordered, *to reduce psychosis,* and monitor the patient to determine their effect.
• Follow agency policy for use and documentation of physical restraints, if needed and ordered by health care provider, *to ensure patient safety.*
• Monitor patient and check pulses and capillary refill after restraints have been applied *to prevent patient harm or restriction of circulation.*

Evaluation

Interventions are successful if the patient reports reduced anxiety and remains free from injury.

 ## DISASTER RESPONSE

A *disaster* is defined as any event that overwhelms existing personnel, facilities, equipment, and capabilities of a responding agency, institution, or community. Potential sources of disaster include internal events such as fires and explosions; external events such as floods, storms, fires, earthquakes, and tornadoes; and created events such as motor vehicle accidents, plane crashes, and acts of terrorism.

External disasters involve a community-wide response of several agencies, including emergency medical system (EMS) providers, fire agencies, law enforcement (all first responders), and hospitals. These agencies work together to coordinate search, rescue, transportation, communication, and treatment of multiple victims. Hospitals serve as the major treatment area for victims of a disaster, referred to as *casualties* who have been injured. When a disaster occurs, the hospital activates its disaster plan, which outlines specific duties for each nursing unit and the staff for each nonnursing department as well. Typically, each nursing unit prepares for the influx of casualties by calling all available off-duty staff to report to work and by discharging noncritical patients. In a hospital disaster plan, each nursing unit is usually designated to receive specific types of casualties, such as major trauma, burns, medical, pediatric, or psychiatric. The ED serves as the **triage** (sorting for the purpose of assigning priorities) and stabilization area for casualties. To facilitate the triage, stabilization, and transportation of numerous casualties, the hospital disaster plan can assign one or more staff from each nursing unit and each nonnursing department to a specific area or task within the ED, such as first aid, critical care, burn treatment area, family room, or transportation.

During a disaster, decision making and prioritization of patient care are guided by the resources and personnel available. Patients who are seriously injured and have the greatest chance of full recovery are treated first. Each hospital and agency involved in responding to a disaster follows a disaster response plan that outlines the roles and responsibilities of the staff and the procedures to follow when interacting with the media, families, other agencies, and casualties. Disaster drills are conducted on a regular basis to evaluate and rework plans. You should be familiar with your agency's disaster plans and policies and know your role and responsibilities during a disaster.

 ## BIOTERRORISM

Recognition of Potential Bioterrorism Agents

The CDC evaluates and prioritizes bacteria, viruses, and toxins on their risk for use in a **bioterrorism** attack (see www.bt.cdc.gov and Table 13.5). As in naturally occurring outbreaks, early recognition of a bioterrorism attack is critical for rapid implementation of preventive measures, treatment, and public

TABLE 13.5 BIOLOGICAL AGENTS RISK CATEGORIES

Category	Agent/Disease
A High-priority agents	Anthrax *(Bacillus anthracis)* Botulism *(Clostridium botulinum toxin)* Plague *(Yersinia pestis)* Smallpox *(Variola major)* Tularemia *(Francisella tularensis)* Viral hemorrhagic fevers (filoviruses; Ebola and arenaviruses; Lassa)
B Second-priority agents	Brucellosis *(Brucella* species)* Epsilon toxin of *Clostridium perfringens* Food safety threats *(Salmonella, Escherichia, Shigella)* Glanders *(Burkholderia mallei)* Melioidosis *(Burkholderia pseudomallei)* Staphylococcal enterotoxin B Psittacosis *(Chlamydia psittaci)* Q fever *(Coxiella burnetii)* Ricin toxin from *Ricinus communis* (castor beans) Typhus fever *(Rickettsia prowazekii)* Viral encephalitis (alphaviruses) Water safety threats *(Vibrio cholerae, Cryptosporidium parvum)*
C Third-priority agents	Emerging infectious diseases such as Nipah virus and hantavirus

Adapted from Centers for Disease Control and Prevention (n.d.), *Bioterrorism Agents/Diseases (by Category).* Retrieved March 13, 2014, from www.bt.cdc.gov/agent/agentlist-category.asp

communication. Early recognition can be challenging, however, because patients presenting for medical care after exposure to a biological agent can initially have nonspecific symptoms or symptoms that differ from typical natural infections.

Smallpox/Variola Major

Smallpox is caused by the variola virus, an orthopoxvirus unique to humans. This virus is not known to be transmitted by animals or insects. Smallpox was declared eradicated in 1980, three years after the last naturally occurring case was reported. Smallpox is stable and highly infectious in the aerosol form. The risk for a smallpox attack currently is considered low but not zero.

Smallpox has an average fatality rate of 30%. The incubation period is 7 to 17 days. Symptoms of the initial phase include the acute onset of high fever, malaise, headache, backache, and prostration. Other prominent symptoms include vomiting and abdominal pain. The characteristic rash occurs 2 to 3 days later, appearing first as small red spots on the tongue and in the mouth. The rash will then appear on the face and extremities and spread to all parts of the body within 24 hours. The rash progresses slowly, from macules to papules to vesicles and pustules and finally to scabs, with each stage lasting 1 to 2 days. The lesions are firm, discrete vesicles or pustules (4–6 mm in diameter) deeply embedded in the dermis. Fever is present throughout the evolution of the rash, which can become painful as pustules enlarge. A second fever spike 5 to 8 days after onset of the rash can signify a secondary bacterial infection. Pustules remain for 5 to 8 days, after which crusting occurs. Pustules are more concentrated on the face and distal limbs than on the trunk and can involve the palms and soles. Scarring occurs with scab separation from destruction of sebaceous glands.

Complications of smallpox include fluid and electrolyte disturbances, extensive skin loss that resembles burns, bronchitis and pneumonitis, blindness due to eye infection, arthritis, and encephalitis.

Diagnosis

A suspected case of smallpox is a public health emergency. Local and state health authorities, the hospital epidemiologist, and other members of a hospital response team for biological emergencies should be notified immediately if smallpox is suspected.

The differential diagnosis of smallpox includes other illnesses that can cause fever and a rash. Severe varicella (chickenpox) is the disease most likely to be confused with smallpox. However, familiarity with the clinical features of the two diseases, particularly the rash, should help differentiate them. Additional information that can be useful in differentiating smallpox from chickenpox includes a history of exposure to persons with chickenpox, a personal history of chickenpox, a history of vaccination against varicella or smallpox, and the clinical course of illness.

Infection Control and Postexposure Isolation

In the event of a limited outbreak, patients should be admitted to the hospital and confined to rooms that are under negative atmospheric pressure and equipped with high-efficiency particulate air (HEPA) filtration. Standard, contact, and airborne precautions, including use of gloves, gowns, and masks, should be strictly observed. Unvaccinated staff caring for patients suspected of having smallpox should wear fit-tested N95 or higher quality respirators. Patients should wear a surgical mask and be wrapped in a gown or sheet to cover the rash when they are not in a negative-airflow room.

All laundry and waste should be placed in biohazard bags and autoclaved before being laundered or incinerated. Surfaces that can be contaminated with smallpox virus can be decontaminated with disinfectants that are used for standard hospital infection control, such as hypochlorite and quaternary ammonia.

Anthrax

Anthrax is a disease caused by the spore-forming bacterium *Bacillus anthracis.* The organism is found worldwide in soil. Animals become infected through grazing in contaminated areas. Under natural conditions, humans contract the disease after close contact with infected animals or contaminated animal products such as hides, wool, or meat. On exposure to the tissues or blood of an animal or an infected human, the spores germinate.

Classification and Epidemiology

Anthrax occurs in three clinical forms in humans: inhalational, cutaneous, and GI. In a biological attack, aerosol exposure to anthrax spores would be most likely. Before 2001, exposure to powdered anthrax spores in an envelope or package was not thought to be an efficient means of causing inhalational disease. However, exposure to anthrax spores sent through the U.S. mail in the 2001 anthrax attack resulted in cases of inhalational anthrax and cutaneous disease.

Cutaneous anthrax is the most likely way to develop anthrax. It results from inoculation of spores subcutaneously through a cut or abrasion. GI and oropharyngeal anthrax occur in rural parts of the world where anthrax is endemic. They result from ingestion of meat contaminated with spores.

Inhalational Anthrax

CLINICAL PRESENTATION AND DIAGNOSIS. Clinical symptoms develop rapidly after germination of anthrax spores. The incubation period for inhalational disease is most commonly reported as 1 to 6 days but can be prolonged by antibiotic administration.

Inhalational anthrax is a two-stage disease. The initial stage is a nonspecific, flu-like illness lasting from several hours to a few days. The early clinical presentation includes some combination of fever, myalgia, headache, cough, mild chest discomfort, weakness, abdominal pain, and chest pain. Profound malaise, fever, and drenching sweats are prominent symptoms, and nausea and vomiting are frequent. Classically, the initial stage is followed 1 to 3 days later, sometimes after brief improvement, by the rapidly progressive second stage, characterized by fever, dyspnea, diaphoresis, cyanosis, and shock.

There is no rapid screening test to diagnose inhalational anthrax in its early stages. In persons with a compatible clinical illness for whom there is a heightened suspicion of anthrax based on clinical and epidemiological data, the appropriate initial diagnostic tests are a chest x-ray or chest computed tomographic (CT) scan, or both, and culture and smear of peripheral blood. Pleural fluid and cerebrospinal fluid, as well as biopsy specimens taken from the pleura and lung, are also potentially useful for culture and other testing when disease is present in these sites, whereas sputum culture and Gram stain are unlikely to be useful.

THERAPEUTIC INTERVENTION. Early IV antibiotic treatment can improve survival in inhalational anthrax. Aggressive supportive care, including attention to fluid, electrolyte, and acid–base disturbances and drainage of pleural effusions, also play an important role in treatment. At present, IV ciprofloxacin or doxycycline plus one or two additional antimicrobials are recommended (CDC, 2008).

Cutaneous Anthrax

After an incubation period of approximately 7 days (range: 1–12 days), the primary lesion of cutaneous anthrax appears as a nondescript, painless, pruritic papule, usually on an exposed area such as the face, head, neck, or upper extremity (Fig. 13.8). The papule enlarges and develops a central vesicle or bulla with surrounding brawny, nonpitting edema. The central vesicle enlarges and ulcerates over 1 to 2 days, becoming hemorrhagic, depressed, and necrotic and leading to a central black eschar. Satellite vesicles can be present. The eschar dries and falls off over the next 1 to 2 weeks (Fig. 13.9). Tender regional lymphadenopathy, fever, chills, and fatigue can occur. Systemic disease has been reported to have a mortality of 20% if untreated.

INFECTION CONTROL. Person-to-person transmission of anthrax is not known to occur. Patients can be hospitalized in a standard hospital room with standard barrier isolation

FIGURE 13.9 Cutaneous anthrax in later stage of infection. *From the Centers for Disease Control and Prevention, Public Health Image Library, #1934.*

precautions. No treatment is necessary for persons who come in contact with the patient.

Plague

Plague is caused by the Gram-negative coccobacillus *Yersinia pestis.* Under natural conditions, plague is transmitted to humans by the bite of an infectious flea and, less frequently, by direct contact with the infectious body fluids or tissues of an infected animal or by inhaling infectious droplets. Plague has a long history of use and development as a biological weapon. After a biological attack, primary pneumonic plague would be most likely.

Clinical Presentation

Plague is a severe febrile illness. Pneumonic plague, the most fatal form of the infection, can develop from inhalation of plague bacilli (primary pneumonic plague).

The incubation period for pneumonic plague is typically 2 to 4 days (range: 1–6 days). Presenting symptoms typically include the acute onset of malaise, high fever, chills, headache, chest discomfort, dyspnea, and cough concomitant with or followed rapidly by clinical sepsis. Hemoptysis is a classic sign that should suggest plague in the appropriate clinical context, but sputum can be watery or purulent. GI symptoms can be prominent with pneumonic plague; these include nausea, vomiting, diarrhea, and abdominal pain. A cervical bubo (swelling of the lymph nodes) is infrequently present. The disease is rapidly progressive, with increasing dyspnea, stridor, and cyanosis. Rapidly progressive respiratory failure and sepsis within 2 to 4 days of onset of illness is typical of pneumonic plague.

Diagnosis

During a confirmed outbreak of pneumonic plague after a biological attack, a presumptive diagnosis can be made on the basis of symptoms, especially if there is a high index of

FIGURE 13.8 Cutaneous anthrax on right forearm in early stage of infection. *From the Centers for Disease Control and Prevention, Public Health Image Library, #1809.*

suspicion. However, other causes of severe pneumonia or rapidly progressive respiratory infection with or without sepsis should be considered.

Laboratory findings are consistent with the systemic inflammatory response syndrome. The leukocyte count is elevated and the differential shows a neutrophil predominance, including immature forms. Platelets can be normal or low. Coagulation abnormalities include prolongation of the international normalized ratio (INR), prothrombin time (PT), and partial thromboplastin time (PTT). Elevated liver function tests and abnormal renal function tests are seen with systemic disease.

Therapeutic Intervention

When plague is suspected, antibiotic treatment should begin before laboratory confirmation of the diagnosis. Levofloxacin (Levaquin) has been approved by the Food and Drug Administration to treat plague and reduce the risk of plague after exposure.

Botulism

Botulism is a paralytic illness caused by a potent neurotoxin produced by *Clostridium botulinum,* an anaerobic, spore-forming bacterium. Natural forms of the disease are foodborne botulism, wound botulism, and infant botulism. Foodborne botulism results from ingestion of improperly processed foodstuffs containing preformed toxin produced by *C. botulinum.* (Botox is the trade name of a toxin made by C. botulinum that is used as a cosmetic treatment to reduce facial aging lines by blocking nerve impulses to the muscles whose action causes the lines). Wound botulism results from production of botulinum toxin by *C. botulinum* organisms that contaminate wounds. Infant botulism results from the colonization of the intestinal tract of infants after ingestion of spores. (Honey can contain the bacteria, so infants under 1 year of age should not eat honey.) Botulinum toxin has been developed as a biological weapon. An aerosol attack is considered the most likely use of botulinum toxin for bioterrorism.

Botulinum toxin is the most potent lethal toxin known. The estimated toxic dose of type Abotulinum toxin is 0.001 mcg/kg of body weight. Botulinum toxin acts to block neurotransmission by binding to the presynaptic nerve terminal at the neuromuscular junction and preventing the release of acetylcholine, resulting in skeletal muscle weakness. The toxin is colorless, odorless, and presumably tasteless.

Clinical Presentation

The incubation period for foodborne botulism is 2 hours to 8 days; the typical incubation period is 12 to 72 hours. The incubation period for inhalational botulism has not been established. The neurologic features of botulism are similar. Although initial symptoms in foodborne botulism can include nausea, vomiting, abdominal cramps, and diarrhea, these symptoms are thought to result from other bacterial metabolites in contaminated food and cannot occur in inhalational botulism.

The so-called classic triad of botulism summarizes the clinical presentation: an afebrile patient, symmetrical descending flaccid paralysis with prominent bulbar palsies, and a clear mentation. Patients typically present with difficulty seeing, speaking, or swallowing. Clinical hallmarks include ptosis, blurred vision, and the so-called four Ds: diplopia, dysarthria, dysphonia, and dysphagia.

Anticholinergic symptoms are common, including dry mouth, ileus, constipation, nausea and vomiting, urine retention, and mydriasis. Other symptoms include dizziness and sore throat. Sensory findings are not present, with the exception of circumoral and peripheral paresthesias secondary to hyperventilation resulting from anxiety. Botulinum toxin does not cross the blood-brain barrier. Cranial nerve dysfunction and facial nerve weakness can make communication difficult; these symptoms can be mistaken for lethargy and signs of central nervous system involvement.

Diagnosis

Treatment with botulinum antitoxin should begin based on the clinical diagnosis and should not await laboratory confirmation. For potential foodborne botulism, samples of stool, gastric aspirate, emesis, and suspect foods should also be submitted.

The possibility of a bioterrorism attack should be considered in any outbreak of botulism. A bioterrorism attack should especially be considered when a cluster of cases occurs, when an outbreak has a common geographical location but there is no common dietary exposure (suggestive of possible aerosol exposure), when there is an outbreak of an unusual botulinum toxin type, or when multiple simultaneous outbreaks occur. A careful dietary and travel history must be taken to help identify the source. Patients should be asked if they know of others with similar symptoms.

Therapeutic Intervention

The mainstay of treatment for botulism is supportive care, including intensive care, mechanical ventilation, and parenteral nutrition. Morbidity and mortality are usually from:

- Pulmonary aspiration secondary to loss of the gag reflex and dysphagia leading to inability to control secretions
- Respiratory failure secondary to inadequate tidal volume from diaphragmatic and accessory respiratory muscle paralysis
- Airway obstruction from pharyngeal and upper airway muscle paralysis.

Careful and frequent monitoring of the gag and cough reflexes, swallowing, oxygen saturation, vital capacity, and inspiratory force are critical. Airway intubation is indicated for inability to control secretions and impending respiratory failure. Secondary infections are common and should be sought in patients who develop fever.

Trivalent (ABE) equine antitoxin is available from the CDC through state and local health departments and should be administered as soon as possible after clinical diagnosis. Antitoxin can prevent progression of disease caused by subsequent binding of toxin but does not reverse the effects of already bound toxin. For this reason, antitoxin is not useful if the patient is no longer showing progression of disease or is improving from maximum paralysis.

Transmissibility and Infection Control

Botulism is not transmitted from person to person. Botulinum toxin does not penetrate intact skin. Standard infection-control precautions are adequate. Clothes of persons exposed to an aerosol release of botulinum toxin should be removed and washed. Exposed persons should shower with soap and hot water. Exposed environmental surfaces can be decontaminated with 0.1% hypochlorite bleach solution.

SUGGESTED ANSWERS TO

CRITICAL THINKING

■ Mr. Smith

1. The airway is the first priority because edema from inhalation burns can occlude the airway.

2. You know that Mr. Smith is at risk for respiratory burns because of the soot near his mouth and nose. He should be closely monitored. Assessment should include respiratory rate and pattern and the patient's ability to speak without a hoarse voice. Abnormal breathing sounds such as wheezing indicate partial upper airway occlusion.

3. The vital signs are within normal limits.

4. Deep partial-thickness burns should be covered with dry dressings. Because the skin can no longer protect the patient, wet dressings provide a medium for bacterial invasion. Wet dressings can also cause a decrease in body temperature because the skin can no longer maintain thermoregulation.

5. Jewelry should always be removed immediately, before edema formation begins.

6. Mr. Smith was involved in an explosive incident and thrown 50 feet. He could have sustained fractures of the pelvis or back. He may also have internal organ injuries from blunt trauma.

7. The ED health care provider, registered nurse, respiratory therapist.

REVIEW QUESTIONS

1. Which of the following assessments would the nurse include in a primary survey of a multisystem trauma victim? **Select all that apply.**
   1. Airway
   2. Breathing
   3. Circulation
   4. Chronic illness
   5. Vital signs
   6. Deformity

2. The nurse is caring for a trauma patient who is hemorrhaging from a puncture wound. Which of the following interventions should the nurse use to control the arterial bleeding?
   1. Pressure at the puncture site
   2. Application of a tourniquet
   3. Pressure-point massage
   4. Pressure dressing

3. The nurse would anticipate the potential for inhalation injury in a patient who was in a house fire with which of the following assessment findings?
   1. Peripheral edema
   2. Singed nasal hairs
   3. Jugular vein distention
   4. Increased capillary refill time

4. Which of the following actions should be taken first for a patient who is found with hyperthermia?
   1. Undress the patient.
   2. Use tepid water as a mist spray.
   3. Remove patient from the hot environment.
   4. Place patient in continual breeze from electric fans.

5. For which of the following should the nurse observe the patient who has inhaled chlorine? **Select all that apply.**
   1. Airway obstruction
   2. Sacral edema
   3. Increased capillary refill time
   4. Unequal pupils
   5. Dyspnea
   6. Pulmonary edema

6. When interacting with a psychotic patient, which of the following interventions is helpful to gain the patient's trust?
   1. Play along.
   2. Show respect.
   3. Avoid eye contact.
   4. Make promises.

7. Which of the following patients should be treated first in a disaster situation?
    1. A 10-year-old with a closed leg fracture that is painful
    2. A 32-year-old with slight bleeding from a hand laceration
    3. A 45-year-old with an open head injury, no pulse or respirations
    4. A 62-year-old reporting chest pain and shortness of breath

8. Which one of the following would the nurse recognize as an immediate threat to life during acute anaphylaxis?
    1. Hypotension
    2. Generalized itching
    3. Airway obstruction
    4. Tachycardia

9. The nurse is collecting data on a patient who is hypovolemic. Which of the following signs and symptoms indicate that the patient is experiencing progressive shock?
    1. Sacral edema
    2. Jugular vein distention
    3. Decreasing blood pressure
    4. Palpable, bounding pulse

10. The nurse is to give penicillin G 500,000 units IM. The nurse has a 10-mL vial labeled "penicillin 400,000 units/mL." How many milliliters should the nurse give?
    Answer: _____ mL

Answers can be found in Appendix C.

Reference

Stern, E. J., Uhde, K. B., Shadomy, S. V., & Messonnier, N. (2008, April). Conference report on public health and clinical guidelines for anthrax. *Emerging Infectious Disease.* Retrieved August 3, 2013, at wwwnc.cdc.gov/eid/article /14/4/07-0969.htm

 DavisPlus | For additional resources and information visit **davispl.us/medsurg5**

Understanding Life Span Influences on Health and Illness

14

Developmental Considerations in the Nursing Care of Adults

LINDA S. WILLIAMS

KEY TERMS

chronic illness (KRAW-nick ILL-ness)
developmental stage (deh-vell-up-MEN-tal STAYJ)
health (HELLTH)
hopelessness (HOHP-less-ness)
illness (ILL-ness)
powerlessness (POW-er-less-ness)
reminiscence therapy (reh-meh-NISS-enss THAIR-
a-pee)
respite care (RESS-pit CARE)
spirituality (SPEER-ih-chu-AL-ih-tee)

LEARNING OUTCOMES

1. List Erikson's eight stages of psychosocial development.
2. Identify the effects of chronic illness.
3. Describe special needs that caregivers have.
4. Explain health promotion methods.
5. Plan nursing interventions for a patient who is chronically ill.

HEALTH, WELLNESS, AND ILLNESS

Health is much more than just the absence of disease. Have you ever known someone with what appears to be a small health problem who considers himself unwell or disabled, or a person with major health problems who sees himself as well? Many things play a role in a person's perception of health. One is the ability to function or perform desired or necessary tasks such as activities of daily living (ADL). Another is the ability to fulfill one's roles, such as student, parent, or employee. The quality of one's life is another component of health. A person's ability to adapt to changes in physical, psychological, social, and spiritual aspects of life is considered to plan health care. *Wellness* is a term used to describe a progression toward a higher level of functioning. Even though a person has a disabling illness, he or she may still be able to achieve a higher level of wellness.

NURSING CARE TIP

To foster understanding of how an ill patient, especially an older patient, was once healthy and active, ask family members to bring in photos showing the patient healthy at various ages or doing favorite activities. Displaying these photos in the patient's room allows caregivers to appreciate the patient in wellness roles.

The concept of illness is one of imbalance or disharmony with the environment. The physical causes of illness are most easily recognized, such as exercise that induces an asthma attack or a fall that causes a broken bone. But illness can also result from a psychological, sociological, cultural, or spiritual imbalance. After the loss of a spouse, for example, one may experience loneliness, depression, and a loss of balance in the social and psychological aspects of life.

A hospitalization may increase disharmony if cultural beliefs and practices are not understood or upheld by health care providers (HCPs). A person faced with a terminal diagnosis may lose hope and direction in life, causing anxiety and despair. So rather than being exclusive concepts, **health** and **illness** are dynamic and ever-changing states of being. A health crisis such as a myocardial infarction (MI) overwhelms a patient's ability to maintain a normal level of wellness. Two months after the MI, however, the patient could be enjoying a higher level of wellness than before the MI if he or she is following a healthy lifestyle.

THE NURSE'S ROLE IN SUPPORTING AND PROMOTING WELLNESS

The goal of nursing care is to help patients achieve their highest possible level of wellness. To do this, the patient's strengths, assets, and resources, as well as weaknesses, liabilities, and disabilities, are considered. Working together, the patient, family, and members of the health care team develop a plan of care that includes wellness goals and a plan of action to accomplish those goals. The plan of care focuses on six main areas:

• Mobilizing resources
• Providing a safe and adaptable environment
• Helping the patient learn about his or her health problem and treatment
• Performing and teaching the patient to perform health care procedures
• Anticipating problems and recognizing potential crises
• Evaluating the plan and progress toward the goals with the patient and family

Nurses assume a variety of roles in promoting the health of their patients, such as educator, advocate, caregiver, and consultant.

DEVELOPMENTAL STAGES

Understanding the patient's **developmental stage** can help the nurse more accurately assess health and health practices. The developmental stages of life focus on the balance a person must achieve for high-level wellness within that stage. Erik Erikson (1980, 1993) described eight stages of psychosocial development (Table 14.1). These stages illustrate the acquisition of a sense of trust in self and others and a sense of personal worth. Each stage must be completed before accomplishing the next. The first five stages describe the development of the child and adolescent. The last three stages relate to young adulthood, middle adulthood, and late adulthood and are discussed next.

The Young Adult

Erikson's sixth developmental stage, from ages 18 to 40, addresses intimacy versus isolation. The young adult's task is to develop relationships with a spouse, family, or friends that are warm, affectionate, and developed through fondness, understanding, caring, or love. When this stage is not successfully resolved, the person typically experiences isolation from others. Physically, growth is usually completed by age 20. Socially, young adults begin to move away from their parents to start their own families. The young adult begins to develop a place in society through school, work, and social activities. This is the stage in which intimacy or closeness develops with partners and friends. Decisions to have a pet, to marry, and to have children show the desire for intimacy. Challenges to intimacy are tasks that must be overcome in this stage. Melding one's traditions and customs with the traditions and customs of a spouse, family, and friends is a major responsibility, as is the passing on of culture to children. Values and beliefs, which arise from a person's culture or conscience, serve as guidelines for behavior for the young adult.

Common Health Concerns

The lifestyle choices of young adults may place their health at risk. Health promotion for this age group focuses on preventing

TABLE 14.1 ERIC ERIKSON'S STAGES OF PSYCHOSOCIAL DEVELOPMENT

Stage	Age Range	Developmental Task
Infancy	Birth to 18 months	Trust versus mistrust
Toddler	18 months to 3 years	Autonomy versus shame and doubt
Preschool	3 to 5 years	Initiative versus guilt
School age	5 to 12 years	Industry versus inferiority
Adolescence	12 to 18 years	Identity versus role confusion
Young adulthood	18 to 40 years	Intimacy versus isolation
Middle adulthood	40 to 65 years	Generativity versus stagnation
Late adulthood	65 years to death	Integrity versus despair

or limiting risks through teaching. Young adults should understand the importance of diet and exercise in maintaining health for themselves and their children. Lifelong positive health practices help prevent long-term health complications. Avoiding sun exposure and using sunscreen are important to avoid sunburn, permanent sun damage to the skin, and increased risk of skin cancer. Tobacco use started in the teen years is often carried on throughout young adulthood and is linked to chronic bronchitis, emphysema, and oral, throat, and lung cancer in later life. Additional preventive measures that may be taught at this stage include breast self-examination (BSE) for women and testicular self-examination (TSE) for men.

In the early part of young adulthood, the individual is in the workforce or is preparing for the work world with a college or vocational education. Being a novice in the work world and accepting new independence, freedom, and responsibilities can introduce stressors into the young adult's life. Overeating, alcohol use, drug use, cigarette smoking, and violence are risky lifestyle choices and poor coping mechanisms for stress. Young adults need to be aware of their individual stressors and be encouraged to develop positive coping mechanisms for stress. Exercise, support groups, music, and meditation are positive ways to cope with stress.

Although marriage commonly occurs during this phase, this group also has the highest rate of divorce. The blending of two people into a couple requires a lot of creative communication and loving care. When stressors overwhelm the couple's coping mechanisms or coping strategy, the relationship may be at risk.

If young adults are sexually active with multiple partners, they are at risk for sexually transmitted infections. Safer sex guidelines and information on birth control should be available for the young adult.

Pregnancy is a common health occurrence for women in this age group. Because research indicates that a mother's health practices directly affect the health of the developing fetus, nutrition, drug and alcohol use, physical health, and effective stress coping mechanisms are lifestyle issues that need to be discussed with every pregnant woman. Prenatal care should be encouraged and readily available to pregnant women.

CRITICAL THINKING

Mrs. Michaels

■ Mrs. Michaels, age 25, and her husband have been trying to start a family. Mrs. Michaels visits her physician, who confirms that she is pregnant. What information and health practices should Mrs. Michaels and her husband be taught during a prenatal health examination?

Suggested answers are at the end of the chapter.

The Middle-Aged Adult

In the middle adult years, ages 40 to 65, the psychological developmental stage is developing *generativity* versus self-absorption. Generativity includes a sense of productivity and creativity and is demonstrated by concern and support for others, along with a vision for future generations. Unresolved conflict may be seen as preoccupation with personal needs or self-absorption.

Physically, middle-aged adults start to notice signs of decreased endurance and intolerance for physical exercise if they have not maintained healthy lifestyle choices. Socially, their children are adolescents or young adults who need assistance with entering adulthood and launching their own careers and families. The term *empty nest* has been used to describe the middle-aged couple's home after their children have left.

This period is often complicated by the challenging demands of also caring for aging parents. Today's middle-aged adult generation has been labeled the *sandwich generation* because of the need to care for their children and their aging parents at the same time. Middle-aged adults look over their lives and assess accomplishments versus unrealized goals. Midlife crisis may occur as this self-inspection leads to a desire to change work, social, or family situations to try to meet unrealized goals. Planning for retirement by developing meaningful pastimes and interests outside of work and preparing for financial security is another important task during this stage.

Common Health Concerns

The need for immunizations continues into adulthood (visit www.CDC.gov). Unhealthy choices, such as smoking, use of alcohol or drugs, a sedentary lifestyle, a diet high in saturated fat, or overeating, often have serious consequences for middle adulthood. Hypertension and heart disease are major health concerns, as are chronic bronchitis, emphysema, and lung cancer. Cardiovascular disease and cancer cause most of the deaths in this age group. However, middle adulthood is not too late to begin lifestyle changes that positively affect health, such as regular exercise, not smoking, healthful eating, weight reduction, and using positive stress-coping mechanisms. Helping adults in this age group recognize the benefits of these positive lifestyle choices and empowering them to change is the major challenge for HCPs.

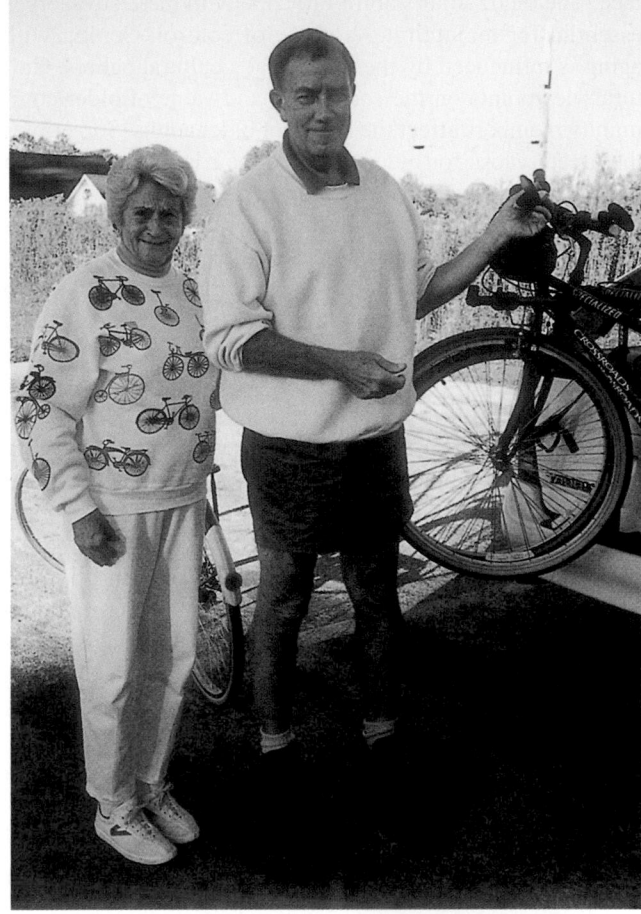

FIGURE 14.1 Socialization helps older adults maintain integrity.

> ## CRITICAL THINKING
>
> ### Mr. Paul
>
> ■ Mr. Paul, age 54, calls his HCP's office for the fourth time this month reporting severe indigestion and requesting a medication to fix it. He has refused to have an x-ray examination or other diagnostic tests because he "can't fit them" into his "busy schedule." Mr. Paul has his own insurance business. His wife quit her job to supervise their 15-year-old son, who was not going to school every day. The couple's twin daughters are both in college out of state.
>
> 1. What might be causing Mr. Paul to experience health problems?
> 2. What is affecting the developmental tasks Mr. Paul needs to perform?
>
> *Suggested answers are at the end of the chapter.*

The Older Adult

The final developmental stage affects adults from age 65 until death. *Ageism* is a term that describes stereotypical misconceptions about older adults in society. Although they are the most diverse age group, common misconceptions about older people include that they are senile, disabled, and in nursing homes. However, more positive attitudes about aging are developing, in part as a result of the growing number of older adults. Advances in living conditions and health care have allowed more people to reach old age. People are living productive, fulfilling lives into their 80s, 90s, and even 100s. Older adults are likely to be found working in their gardens, hiking, exercising, or socializing (Fig. 14.1). Some older adults continue to work beyond typical retirement age or begin a rewarding second career after retiring.

Developmental work for older adults focuses on integrity versus despair. In this stage, older adults look back and evaluate what they have done with their lives. Integrity refers to accepting responsibility for one's life so far and reflecting on it in a positive way. Reaching this stage is a sign of maturity. Failing to reach this stage is an indication of unsuccessful completion of previous stages, causing feelings of despair that life has been lived in vain, and a fear of death. **Reminiscence therapy** may be one way to assist the older adult through this stage.

Aging is associated with role changes and transitions. Some roles, such as employee, son, or daughter, are lost because of retirement, death, or illness, causing sadness or depression. New roles may arise, such as grandparent, volunteer, or widow/widower. With retirement, household management roles may need to change. If an older adult becomes ill and dependent and needs to be cared for by an adult child, the parent–child role may be reversed.

Health, relationships, lifestyle choices, and environment influence the diversity found in this age group. Physical health is often a concern for older adults. Chronic health problems that require medication and treatment often require lifestyle changes or adaptations.

Life events such as decreased physical ability, retirement, illness, or death of a spouse are challenges that older adults

• WORD • BUILDING •

reminiscence: re—backward + minisc—mind + ens—action

face. The older adult's ability to cope with these stressors is essential for maintaining a sense of control. Coping with aging is influenced by the individual's cultural beliefs. Cultural viewpoints on the social role and value of older community members affect the health of older adults. Sometimes the greatest loss for older adults is their lack of connection with the world and lack of being part of a greater purpose. However, being alone is not the same as being lonely. For some older adults, being by oneself for a time allows for reflection to better understand one's situation. Older adults who feel unwanted or unloved are more likely to develop anxiety, depression, and failure to thrive.

Common Health Concerns

The focus of care for the older adult is assistance in meeting physical, psychological, cultural, sociological, and spiritual needs. Promoting self-care and encouraging the use of community services for seniors is important. Most older adults continue to live in their own homes or apartments, but impairment in mobility and the ability to carry out instrumental activities of daily living (IADLs), such as shopping for groceries, preparing meals, and cleaning and maintaining a home, threaten their independence. Having to ask or pay others to perform tasks that they formerly were able to do themselves is seen as a significant loss by many older adults. Adding the loss of a spouse, the death of friends, or the lack of social contacts further isolates an older person and can lead to depression and a feeling of **hopelessness**. The accumulation of losses can overwhelm an older adult's resources and coping mechanisms and is related to a high rate of suicide, especially for older men. Suicide is the ultimate expression of hopelessness.

Older adults might need to be encouraged to remain active and to continue to pursue interests. Most communities have transportation services that operate to meet the needs of older adults. Senior centers offer diverse programs and services such as trips, dances and bowling leagues. Older adults can also continue to work as volunteers for schools, hospitals, nursing facilities, parks, museums, zoos, community theaters, and youth groups. Colleges and universities may offer discounted tuition for senior citizens, and there are Elderhostel programs across the country. Elderhostel offers thousands of educational travel programs, such as photography, Civil War history, nature survival, bird watching, and painting.

Chronic diseases can limit an older person's ability to be independent in ADLs and IADLs. Hypertension is common in this age group, as are heart disease and strokes. Managing these conditions and living a healthy lifestyle can help keep the older adult active.

One of the most difficult tasks for the nurse in dealing with the older adult is to distinguish normal age-related changes from pathological changes. Changes in mobility and chronic pain may limit an older person's activity and impede an active lifestyle. Pain is not normal and should be investigated rather than attributing it to aging and ignoring it.

CRITICAL THINKING

Mr. Klein

■ Mr. Klein, age 82, visits his HCP. He reports left hip pain. The HCP replies, "It can be common to experience pain as you get older." Mr. Klein thinks a minute and says, "But my right hip doesn't hurt and it's as old as my left hip!"

1. What is occurring in this situation?
2. What actions could be taken to provide patient-centered care and improve the quality of life for Mr. Klein?

Suggested answers are at the end of the chapter.

Falls are a serious concern for older adults, resulting in decreased independence and death. Osteoporosis is a bone disease common among postmenopausal women and men over age 80, causing bone weakness and fracture risk. Falls and accidents can be prevented by in-home safety assessments and altering the home environment to ensure the safety of the older adult. Bathrooms should be equipped with grab bars and nonskid mats. Bath chairs or benches make getting into a bath or shower safer. Removing clutter, throw rugs, small furniture, and electrical cords decreases the risk of falls.

Hearing and vision loss can affect physical and psychological health in the older adult. Good sensory function is needed to protect oneself from accidents, social isolation, and limitations in self-care. One of the most dramatic losses for many older adults is not being able to safely drive a car. This can be associated with a loss of independence. Sensory impairments can further isolate the patient. Impaired vision can be caused by decreased peripheral vision, macular degeneration, cataracts, or glaucoma. Many older adults continue to drive during the day but not at night because of night vision problems. Decreased hearing is also common in older adults. Loss of high-pitch discrimination and reduced ability to filter background noise causes older adults to hear the background noise more clearly than a one-to-one conversation when in a crowded room. Social stigmas related to memory changes such as forgetfulness and dementia are a serious worry for many older adults. They commonly confuse depression with memory changes and attempt to hide their symptoms rather than seek treatment.

CHRONIC ILLNESS

A major challenge facing HCPs is the management and prevention of chronic illness. A **chronic illness** is defined as an illness that is long lasting or that recurs. It usually interferes with the person's ability to perform ADLs. A chronic illness is never completely cured or prevented. The amount of disability a person has depends not only on the condition and its severity but also on the individual effects for that person. The degree of disability and altered lifestyle relate as much to the person's perception of the disease as to the disease itself. For example, both John F. Kennedy and Franklin D. Roosevelt would have been eligible for 100% disability benefits because of their chronic illnesses, but both managed to serve as presidents. The long-term effects of treatments such as radiation therapy can become chronic diseases in themselves. Radiation for a tumor can leave the person with persistent diarrhea that may cause malnourishment and exhaustion.

CRITICAL THINKING

Mrs. Riccardi

■ Mrs. Riccardi, age 87, lives alone in her small apartment. Her daughter and son are both retired and live in the same community. Mrs. Riccardi had a dizzy spell, so her daughter brought her to the hospital emergency department (ED). Upon admission, Mrs. Riccardi's blood pressure was 208/128 and she had blurred vision in the left eye that resolved after 1 hour in the ED. She was diagnosed with hypertension, which possibly contributed to a small stroke or transient ischemic attack (TIA). Mrs. Riccardi was started on metoprolol (Lopressor) 100 mg daily. She was discharged to her home with instructions to limit salt in her diet and to begin an exercise program. The plan of care addressed safety issues.

1. Why might Mrs. Riccardi be at increased risk of falling?
2. What patient-centered nursing interventions would help promote Mrs. Riccardi's independence and safety?
3. The nurse is to give metoprolol 100 mg, and 50-milligram tablets are available. How many tablets should the nurse give?

Suggested answers are at the end of the chapter.

When caring for those with chronic illnesses, the goal of nursing care is to maintain and improve the patient's quality of life. A chronic illness also affects the quality of life of the patient's family. Therefore, when planning patient care, consider the family's needs for adapting to the patient's chronic illness.

Fostering hope is an important intervention that should be a primary foundation of care planning for people who are chronically ill. A chronic illness may appear to be a hopeless situation if no cure is possible. If recovery from an illness is not possible, people might think that nothing can be done for the patient. However, whenever there is life, there is potential for growth in areas such as developmental tasks, health promotion, knowledge, or spirit. Individuals have developmental tasks to perform even as they cope with illness or prepare for a peaceful death.

Incidence of Chronic Illness

The incidence of chronic illness is rising for several reasons. First, people are living longer, in part because of better hygiene, nutrition, exercise, vaccinations, antibiotic development, and new treatment options. Fewer people are dying from acute diseases. As a result, a larger older population is living long enough to develop many chronic illnesses. Second, medical advances have resulted in reduced mortality from some chronic illnesses, so that patients live longer with these illnesses. Third, today's technology and modern lifestyles may contribute to the development of some chronic illnesses. Examples include a sedentary lifestyle; exposure to air and water pollution, chemicals, and carcinogens; substance abuse; and stress.

Types of Chronic Illnesses

Chronic illnesses have different causes (Box 14-1). These illnesses have varying degrees of severity and effect on length of life. One chronic illness can lead to development of other illnesses, such as hypertension, which then causes chronic renal failure. Chronic illnesses can begin at various ages, but with advancing age, the likelihood of developing chronic illness increases, and many older adults have several chronic illnesses at once (Box 14-2).

Gerontological Influence

As people live longer, spouses or older family members are increasingly being called on to care for a chronically ill family member. Children of older adults who themselves are reaching their 60s are being expected to care for their parents. These older caregivers may have chronic illnesses of their own. A family in this situation is at great risk for ineffective coping or further development of health

---

Box 14-1 Examples of Chronic Illnesses by Cause

Genetic
- Cystic fibrosis
- Huntington's disease
- Muscular dystrophy
- Sickle cell anemia

Congenital
- Heart defects
- Malabsorption syndromes
- Spina bifida

Acquired
- AIDS
- Arthritis
- Cancer
- Chronic obstructive pulmonary disease
- Diabetes
- Head or spinal cord injury
- Multiple sclerosis

Box 14-2 Examples of Chronic Illnesses in the Older Adult

- Arthritis
- Cerebrovascular accident
- Chronic lung disease
- Dementia
- Diabetes mellitus
- Heart failure
- Hypertension
- Orthopedic dysfunction
- Peripheral vascular disease
- Sensory losses: vision, hearing

problems. Assessment of all members of the family with older adults is essential to ensure that their health and coping needs are being met. Healthy People 2020, a national health promotion and disease prevention initiative, calls for public health surveillance and health promotion programs for people with disabilities and their caregivers (www .healthypeople.gov).

Older adults are concerned about becoming dependent on others. They may become depressed and give up hope if they feel that they are a burden to others. Establishing short-term goals or self-care activities that allow them to participate or have small successes are important nursing actions that can increase their self-esteem (see "Cultural Considerations—Traditional Appalachians").

Barriers to care for a chronically ill older patient include a lack of information about treatments, medications, or special diets and being unfamiliar with supportive services in the community such as meal programs or respite care. Develop an understanding of this information and share it, as well as a resource number for older patients and their families that they can call with questions.

Effects of Chronic Illness

When a patient lives with a chronic illness, many adjustments are usually needed. Lifelong routines and habits may need to be changed to cope with the illness. Treatment needs, such as going to therapy sessions, performing peritoneal dialysis

exchanges, or monitoring blood glucose, can interrupt daily life and require adaptation into the daily routine.

Chronic Sorrow

Chronic sorrow is a normal response felt by those affected by a chronic illness. It is an intermittently occurring sadness in response to losses caused by a chronic illness. It can be felt by the patient or the patient's significant others. The nursing diagnosis *Chronic Sorrow* may apply to those with chronic illness. When this sadness occurs, nursing care should focus on active listening to understand the loss and then on offering appropriate comfort and support. Providing information and assisting with coping strategies such as fostering support systems are great interventions to help those with chronic sorrow.

Spiritual Distress

Patients with chronic illness can experience spiritual distress when faced with the limitations of their illness. Maintaining patients' quality of life includes assisting with their spiritual needs. Religious and spiritual needs are important to most people whose lives have been disrupted by new challenges from chronic illness. Patients must be helped to find realistic hope and meaning in the illness. Interventions that address **spirituality** might need to be performed first to promote later success with the plan of care.

Several factors may make one uncomfortable in caring for a patient's spiritual needs. These factors include a lack of training, a lack of understanding of one's own spiritual needs and beliefs, and not recognizing or believing that this is your role. Develop a comfortable approach in assessing and meeting patients' spiritual needs. Examine your own spiritual needs to define a personal spiritual view. By doing this, you will develop insight into others' spiritual needs and resources, as well as gain a greater understanding of issues surrounding your patients' spiritual needs.

Many people use spirituality to cope with chronic illness. It helps give them a sense of wholeness, hope, and peace during a time filled with uncertainty and anxiety. Spirituality plays an important role in empowering patients to handle their condition. It is a source of inner strength that allows the patient to experience a sense of unity. Hospital interventions may include use of a meditation room for quiet reflection or prayer, chaplain visits, or worship services. To help meet the patient's spiritual needs, assist the patient with transportation to the meditation room or worship services.

Cultural Considerations

Traditional Appalachians

Traditional Appalachians believe that disability is natural and inevitable with aging. This belief discourages the use of rehabilitation as an option. Thus, to promote rehabilitation efforts among Appalachians, the nurse may need to stress self-help and a return to physical function.

NURSING CARE TIP

Spiritual needs should not be thought of in only religious terms. Spirituality is feeling connected with a higher power. Everyone has spiritual needs that involve hope, peace, and wholeness. Spiritual care goes beyond simply asking the patient's religion. It involves assessing the patient's perceptions of spirituality and then devising ways to help meet the person's spiritual needs.

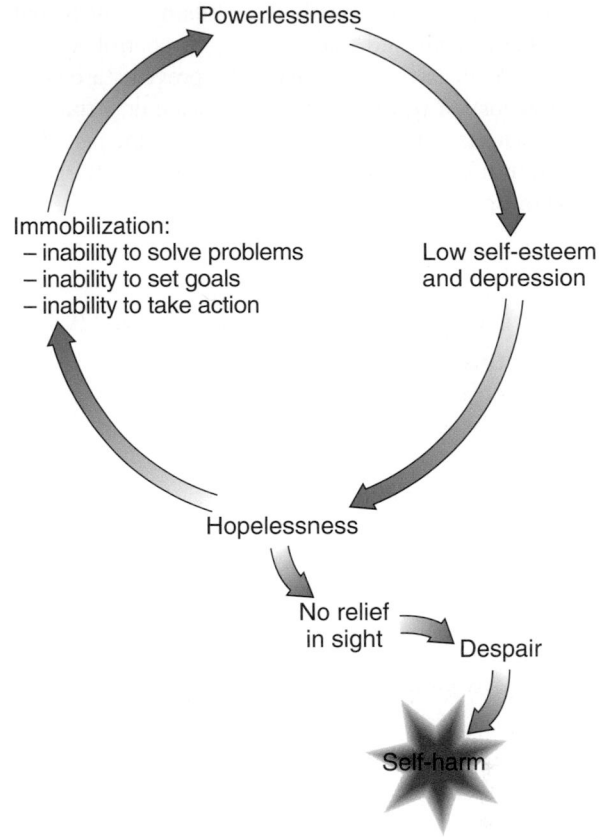

FIGURE 14.2 Powerlessness–hopelessness cycle. *Modified from Miller, J. (2000). Coping with chronic illness: Overcoming powerlessness (3rd ed., p. 526). Philadelphia: F.A. Davis.)*

Accreditation agencies require the spiritual needs of patients to be addressed and documented by nurses. Nursing diagnoses related to spiritual needs may include *Spiritual Distress, Readiness for Enhanced Spiritual Well-Being,* and *Impaired Religiosity.*

Powerlessness

A chronic illness can take an unknown course in relation to its seriousness and controllability. This leaves the patient vulnerable to the many phases of a chronic illness: the diagnosis, the instability phase, an acute illness or crisis, remissions, and a terminal phase. Treatments that the patient undergoes may be painful, frightening, and invasive. A patient who does not understand what is happening can feel overwhelmed and alone. This contributes to a feeling of **powerlessness** because the patient cannot control the outcome (Fig. 14. 2). This lack of control throughout an illness influences the patient's reactions to the illness. The nursing diagnosis *Powerlessness* can apply to chronically ill patients.

COPING. Patients can be helped to feel more in control of their illness if you remember to include them in their care; listen to their feelings, values, and goals; and explain all procedures before they occur. Avoid using complex medical language when talking with patients to increase their understanding and feeling of being included in their care instead of isolated. In addition, coping with a chronic illness can be aided if the patient develops a positive attitude toward the illness. This can be accomplished if the patient gains knowledge, uses a problem-solving approach, and becomes motivated to continue adapting to the illness.

Having a variety of coping techniques can be useful. Ask the patient's perception of the illness and coping techniques that the patient has previously used successfully. New coping resources may need to be added to help the patient effectively deal with the chronic illness. Support services in the community should be offered to the patient and family. To cope effectively, the patient should be helped to become comfortable with the newly defined person he or she is to become. The nursing diagnoses *Ineffective Coping, Compromised Family Coping, Disabled Family Coping,* and *Readiness for Enhanced Family Coping* may apply to those dealing with chronic illness.

HOPE. Before coping resources can be used, hope must be established in the patient. False hope is not beneficial and should be replaced with realistic hope. Providing patients with accurate knowledge regarding their fears helps do this. Hope should not be directed toward a cure that may not be possible but rather at living a quality life with the functional capacity that the patient has. Over the course of the illness, hope needs to be maintained for both the patient and family. Periodically assess if the patient is maintaining hope. Many studies have shown that patients adapt better when hope is high (see "Evidence-Based Practice"). The nursing diagnoses *Readiness for Enhanced Hope* or *Hopelessness* may apply to chronically ill patients.

Many nursing interventions may increase hope. The use of humor helps patients be lighthearted and hopeful. Patients should be tactfully and sensitively encouraged to live each moment to the fullest and experience the joy of being alive. Awakening the senses to appreciate the environment can bring a feeling of hope and peace. Simple things, such as the smell of baking bread, the clean scent of the air after a rain, or the scent of pine trees, can make one appreciate the beauty of nature and inspire hope. Family members need to be encouraged to help foster hope for the patient. In doing this, family members may feel hopeful as well. During times of acute illness, the patient needs to maintain as much control as possible and be told that any loss of control related to treatments is usually temporary. This prevents a continual feeling of loss of power. The use of music or inspirational reading material can reduce stress and help the patient find meaning in life. This in turn fosters hope. Hopeful patients are empowered and no longer feel powerless.

EVIDENCE-BASED PRACTICE

Clinical Question
How do older adults use hope to cope with chronic illness?

Evidence
A meta-synthesis of 20 qualitative studies (*n* = 305 people) of the hope experience for those 60 years or older with chronic illness was done. Hope was found to be a significant coping resource in all the studies. Hope resulted in positivity (feeling of control, quality of life, better future) and was used in multiple contexts (comfort, cure, loved ones).

Implications for Nursing Practice
Assess older patients' feelings of hope for their current experience with illness as it may change as their situation evolves. Encourage hope by assisting patient to maintain relationships with others and adjust to transitions and losses. Strategies that can be used include a life review, reminiscence therapy and spiritual support.

REFERENCE
Duggleby, W., Hicks, D., Nekolaichuk, C., Holtslander, L., Williams, A., Chambers, T., & Eby, J. (2012). Hope, older adults, and chronic illness: A metasynthesis of qualitative research. *Journal of Advanced Nursing, 68*, 1211–1223.

Sexuality

Chronic illness can affect a patient's sexuality, which includes femininity and masculinity as well as sexual activity. Body image changes affect the way patients view themselves and are viewed by others. If patients have a negative body image perception, they may withdraw and become depressed. When interacting with patients, be aware of your facial expressions, nonverbal cues such as appearing hurried or keeping a distance, use of or lack of touch, and amount of time spent with the patient. When patients believe they have lost their femininity or masculinity, their self-worth decreases. Interventions to enhance sexuality should be used, such as obtaining a wig for patients undergoing chemotherapy.

There are many forms of sexual expression. Sexual intimacy can include touching, hugging, or sharing time together. Provide patients with the opportunity to discuss sexuality concerns or questions. Assume a professional and

confidential approach to this topic, which is usually considered a private matter by patients. Chronically ill patients can be referred to sexuality counselors for information on ways to cope with sexual issues in relation to their illness.

CRITICAL THINKING

Mr. Soloman

■ Mr. Soloman, age 88, lives in his own home with his wife of 60 years. He is in good health except for limited vision. He grows prize-winning tomatoes each year, plays golf weekly, and walks every day to the neighborhood stores. The employees know him and cheerfully assist him.

Mr. Soloman's wife was the homemaker, and now she is in the early stages of Alzheimer's disease. She cannot perform ADLs, so he has willingly assumed the caregiver role. They complement each other's limitations because she has good vision and is helpful when she is not confused.

Over time, Mr. Soloman's wife's health declines, and she enters a long-term care facility. Mr. Soloman remains in his home alone, which concerns his family. They eventually convince him to move into senior housing. He is very reluctant to leave his home and does not actively participate in moving and selling his home. Mr. Soloman rarely leaves his apartment, sleeps 14 hours a day, and eats one daily meal. He tries to visit his wife by taking a bus but finds it difficult because of his limited vision, so he rarely sees her. A few months later, Mr. Soloman develops pneumonia and dies in his sleep.

1. Why do you think Mr. Soloman behaved the way he did after he moved?
2. What patient-centered interventions could have been used to empower Mr. Soloman?
3. Why might Mr. Soloman have developed pneumonia and died?

Suggested answers at end of chapter.

Because sexuality is a part of a person's lifelong identity, make sure that older patients' sexuality is addressed in their plans of care. Patients in long-term care facilities should be given private time with their significant other, if appropriate. Grooming methods can increase a patient's self-esteem and sexual identity. Women may get their hair and nails done; men can be shaved or get a haircut. Older patients' sexuality needs should be met just as younger patients' are.

Roles

Chronically ill patients usually are faced with altering their accustomed roles in life. Common roles that may be affected for the adult patient include that of being a spouse, grandparent, parent, provider, homemaker, or friend. Not only must the patient deal with these role alterations, the family must adapt to them as well. Family members may have to take on new roles themselves to compensate for roles the patient can no longer perform. The nursing diagnosis of *Ineffective Role Performance* should be included in the plan of care for the patient and family.

The patient is faced with giving up aspects of old roles at the same time that new roles related to being chronically ill need to be assumed. Grieving accompanies the loss of old roles. If a patient is no longer able to participate in social events such as golfing or being a committee member, grief work needs to occur to help the patient accept the loss and maintain dignity. With other roles, only certain aspects of the role may change. For example, in the parenting role, patients may still function as support systems for a child, although they can no longer be the disciplinarian. Whatever the role loss, the patient needs to be allowed to grieve the loss. The nursing diagnosis of *Grieving* may help in planning care for the patient.

New roles the patient may have to assume related to chronic illness include dependent, ongoing health care consumer, self-care agent, and chronically ill person. Patients need to learn how to cope with these new roles. They need to gather knowledge and be given understanding while they become familiar with these roles. For patients used to being independent before the illness, being dependent on others to meet ADLs can cause a loss in self-esteem. Navigating the complex health care and financial reimbursement systems can be overwhelming. Transportation needs and waiting times for medical appointments can be difficult for the patient who must deal with them on an ongoing basis. Becoming a self-care agent requires assuming responsibility for meeting one's own care needs. *Deficient Knowledge* and *Readiness for Enhanced Knowledge* are nursing diagnoses helpful for fostering learning for these new roles.

As patients live with chronic illness over time, they become experts on their own illness. However, today's health care system often tends to assume control over patients and does not respect the patient's own knowledge. Patients who are not given this respect take charge of caring for themselves by seeking knowledge and trying complementary healing methods. Being sensitive to the patient's knowledge and respecting it increases patients' self-esteem.

Family and Caregivers

Families are affected by the chronic illness of a family member in many ways. Most chronic illness care is provided in the home so that families become involved in the management of the illness (see "Home Health Hints"). Family members may have to take on new family roles or assume the role of caregiver. Decreased socialization, lost income, and increased medical expenses can increase family stress and tension.

Families must learn to cope with the stress of illness and its often unpredictable course. Most families develop ways to cope with the patient's illness the majority of the time and may become closer as a family unit. Families often deal with the illness on a day-by-day basis and take a passive approach to letting problems work themselves out. During times of exacerbation or crisis, however, the family may need coping assistance (Box 14-3).

Box 14-3 Caregiver Resources

aarp.org/caregiving
alzheimers.gov
caregiver.org
eldercare.gov

Patients are often concerned about being a burden to their families. It is important to determine both the family's and the patient's feelings about the care required by the patient. The family's ability to provide this care adequately must also be considered in care planning. If the family lacks the desire, skills, or resources to adequately care for the patient, alternative care options must be explored such as home health care, adult foster care, or long-term care.

Patients' caregivers often have certain ideas about the care that the patient should receive. This may come into conflict with the views of HCPs. Caregiver input into the patient's plan of care should be sought so that everyone has a clear understanding of goals and expectations for the patient's care.

Home Health Hints

Self-Concept/Humor

- Home care nurses can strengthen a patient's self-care capacity by (1) saying "Let me assist you" instead of "Let me do this for you," (2) being a partner in caring instead of being a caregiver, and (3) empowering the patient instead of doing it all for him or her.
- The home health nurse has an opportunity to increase a patient's self-concept by emphasizing the patient's existing abilities, joys, and talents. This can be done by observing the home environment for clues: photographs, trophies, hobby paraphernalia, flowers, or homemade items. Each clue observed can be a springboard to discussing triumphs and losses. It can help the nurse understand how the patient copes, which will assist in planning care.
- Being attentive to any of the patient's efforts or accomplishments, such as number of steps taken, shaving without help, interest in a book or TV show, or decisions on fixing up the house or cleaning, provides opportunities to offer support and praise for accomplishments.
- Using humor can be helpful during a visit, unless the patient is distraught, anxious, or angry. Comics or jokes from magazines can be read. Humor can relieve the patient's and caregiver's stress and humanize the care that must be performed. Keep in mind, however, that humor may be irritating if it is taken as downplaying the seriousness of a situation.

Continued

Resources

- Encourage the family of bed-confined patients to purchase an inexpensive portable intercom (such as a nursery monitor) to give the caregiver freedom to move about the house and hear the patient if help is needed.
- When patients have the use of only one hand or arm, provide a sponge for personal grooming instead of a washcloth; it is easier to use and hold.
- The home health social worker should be informed of any patient concerns regarding cost of medicines or equipment. Many programs are available to assist chronically ill people to obtain resources.

Cardiopulmonary Resuscitation

- Always carry a pocket mask for cardiopulmonary resuscitation (CPR).
- Encourage discussion regarding advance directives with the patient and family/caregiver early in the care process. Decisions regarding resuscitation and the use of technology to prolong life are more difficult when the patient is in crisis.
- Refer families to community CPR classes as desired. Families can be empowered and the patient may feel more secure when families are taught CPR.
- Patients and families should be taught that if an ambulance is called, they should turn on an outside light, open the door, and move furniture, if possible, to enable the emergency medical technicians to get to the patient more easily.

Respite care is designed to provide caregivers with a much-needed break from caregiving by providing someone else to assume the caregiver role. Be familiar with your community's respite care services and share that information with caregivers. Most respite care is provided by volunteers who receive training.

CRITICAL THINKING

Mrs. Burden

■ Mrs. Burden, age 64, is caring for her husband, who has Alzheimer's disease. He wanders. He gets up at night and in freezing winter weather is found walking down the street in only his pajamas. He tries to cook and burns the pans. He cannot express his needs. He disrobes frequently and is incontinent. Mrs. Burden quit her job to care for him. She no longer goes to lunch weekly with her friends. Her children live out of town. She places a chair and tin cans in front of the home's doors as an alarm in case her husband opens the doors while she tries to sleep.

1. What indicates that Mrs. Burden is experiencing stress related to caregiving?
2. What nursing diagnoses should be included in a plan of care for Mrs. Burden?
3. What nursing interventions would be beneficial for Mrs. Burden?

Suggested answers are at the end of the chapter.

Caregivers commonly experience depression, role strain, guilt, powerlessness, and grieving related to caregiving. Being aware of this will help nurses detect indications that caregivers are in need of help in dealing with these feelings. Chronic-care coaches are available who can provide caregivers with insight, encouragement, and support for caring for someone who is chronically ill. Nursing diagnoses for caregivers include *Risk for Caregiver Role Strain* and *Caregiver Role Strain.*

RESPITE CARE. When caregivers are required to provide 24-hour care for a patient, they can experience burnout, fatigue, and stress, which, if extreme, might lead to patient abuse. Caregivers may not be able to leave patients alone even briefly because of wandering behaviors, confusion, or safety issues. They may not ever be able to get a normal night's sleep and suffer from sleep deprivation because of the patient's wandering or around-the-clock treatment needs.

Caregivers must be given periodic relief from their responsibilities of caregiving to reduce the stress of always having to be responsible. Everyone requires private time for reflection or pursuing favorite hobbies or interests. Caregivers may need to get away overnight or for a weekend simply to sleep soundly and be refreshed.

Finances

Managing a chronic illness can be expensive. Income can be lost if the patient is unable to work or caregivers are forced to stay home. Insurance may not cover all of the patient's expenses. Family savings can quickly be used up and place a strain on families. This can lead to the nursing diagnoses *Compromised Family Coping, Disabled Family Coping,* or *Readiness for Enhanced Family Coping.* Nurses may need to refer patients for financial aid.

Health Promotion

Health promotion is possible and necessary at all levels of age or disability. With the increase in the older population, it is essential to understand the role of health promotion for older adults who have chronic illness. Patients with chronic illness make daily lifestyle choices that affect their health. For example, the patient with chronic lung disease who smokes can make a choice to smoke or to quit smoking. Patients with degenerative joint disease can choose whether to keep their weight within ideal weight ranges to reduce wear and tear on their joints. Those with arthritis can reduce their fatigue levels by pacing their activities and scheduling daily rest periods.

Those with chronic illness often consider health promotion important, so encourage health promotion efforts. Patients need to be helped to strive toward high-level wellness. This can be achieved by looking at the patient's strengths and weaknesses holistically to develop a plan of care. Determine the patient's risk factors to help plan methods of promoting health. Providing patients with knowledge to make informed decisions empowers them to take control of their lives and reach their greatest potential.

Nursing Care

Because of the nature of chronic illness, nurses should understand the unique needs of patients and families experiencing chronic illness. These needs differ from those of patients experiencing acute care as far as depth of knowledge needs and the compounding problems that the patient usually faces. Develop an understanding that the wishes of the patient must be respected even if you do not agree with them. Patients have the right to establish their own goals in partnership with the health care team. Patients are participating in or leading their own daily bedside rounds with the health care team in institutions. This is true patient-centered care!

Most chronic illness care occurs in the home and community rather than the acute care setting. Therefore, family members and caregivers, even more so than in acute care, must be assessed and included in the plan of care. As the numbers of those with chronic illness grow, community support for chronically ill people and their caregivers needs to continue to grow. Training programs for caregivers should be available and offered affordably.

A major focus of nursing care for the chronically ill is teaching. These patients and their families have tremendous educational needs if they are to learn to cope successfully with a long-term illness. The following are primary tasks that chronically ill patients need to perform:

- Be willing and able to carry out the medical regimen.
- Reorder time to meet demands caused by the illness, such as treatments, medication schedules, and pacing of activities.
- Understand and control symptoms.
- Prevent and manage crises.
- Adjust to changes in the disease over the course of time, whether positive or negative.

- Prevent social isolation as a result of physical limitations or an altered body image.
- Compensate for symptoms and limitations in order to be treated as normally as possible by others.

Explain individualized interventions to deal with these tasks during teaching sessions. Provide dignity and show respect to all patients ("Patient-Centered Care—Mr. Lyman"). Unique approaches are needed to positively assist chronically ill patients and their families on their long-term journey.

Patient-Centered Care

Mr. Lyman

To the nurse caring for me:
- Don't call me "sweetie" or "honey." My name is Mr. Lyman. If I want you to call me by my first name, I'll tell you.
- Be polite!
- Don't give me a huge glass of water—give me a small glass and don't fill it full. Otherwise, when I drink it, it spills all down the front of me.
- When you leave my meal tray, make sure I can reach it. Then when you take it away, don't leave a bunch of stuff on my table. There is not much room on those little tables.
- Ask how I like my blankets. Don't just do them the way you do for anyone else.
- Make sure my call light is where I can reach it.
- Make sure my overhead light is working and that I can reach it.
- Keep a wastebasket where I can reach it.
- Ask if I need anything before you leave the room.
- Try to talk quietly in the hallway, instead of being so loud.
- Thank you for preserving my dignity and showing me respect. I appreciate it!

SUGGESTED ANSWERS TO

CRITICAL THINKING

■ Mrs. Michael

Prenatal education information should be offered to Mrs. Michael and her husband. This education should include an overview of Mrs. Michael's health needs, what to expect during pregnancy, ways Mrs. Michael's husband can be supportive, and information on prenatal classes. Mrs. Michael's physical examination should include a vaginal examination, blood pressure, and blood

work. It is important to be aware of any sexually transmitted infections that may be transferred to the developing fetus or during birth. A rubella titer (a test for immunity to rubella or measles) is important because of potential birth defects if the mother has rubella while pregnant. Elevated blood glucose may be a sign of diabetes, and low red blood cell counts and low hemoglobin are related to anemia.

To prepare a woman for pregnancy, prenatal vitamins or vitamins with iron and folic acid (necessary for

Continued

SUGGESTED ANSWERS TO—cont'd

effective neural tube development in the first 3 months of pregnancy) are recommended. Because of the increased workload of the heart during pregnancy, blood pressure needs to be closely monitored. Eating a balanced diet, maintaining an exercise program, and continuing to develop effective and positive ways to deal with stress are very important for pregnant women. In preparation for pregnancy, Mrs. Michael also needs information on the negative effects that cigarette smoking, alcohol use, and drug use can have on the developing fetus.

■ Mr. Paul

1. Mr. Paul's physical health is being affected by poor diet choices, excessive stomach acid secretion or other gastrointestinal problems, and stress.

2. It is easy to recognize the psychological stress related to parenting skills when a child is in trouble. Decreased family income with increased family expenses (two children in college) can cause financial strains and more economic pressure on Mr. Paul's business. With family problems or health problems, Mr. Paul may be questioning why things are happening to him and his family, causing him spiritual distress.

■ Mr. Klein

1. Ageism, stereotypical misconceptions about older adults, is occurring. This can lead to the belief that pain is part of the aging process and, therefore, it is often not diagnosed and treated appropriately.

2. Gathering data to assist with the diagnosis of the cause of the pain and treatment for the pain would improve Mr. Klein's quality of life. Taking him seriously would also convey that Mr. Klein is a valued member of society and increase his self-esteem.

■ Mrs. Riccardi

1. Falls could be caused by environmental problems, such as throw rugs that may move or cause tripping, clutter, electrical cords in walking paths, lack of hand grips in the bathroom, or lack of nonskid mats in the shower or tub. Poor vision and altered depth perception can result in missing a stair step or obstacles. Weakness or orthostatic hypotension can cause an unsteady gait or fall.

2. It is important for the nurse to instruct the patient and family about home safety. Mrs. Riccardi may even benefit by using a cane or a walker if she is unsteady. Because Mrs. Riccardi lives alone, an emergency alert system, such as a small transmitter that is worn around the neck or wrist with a button that can be activated in emergencies, would be beneficial. When activated, the transmitter alerts an answering service to contact designated individuals to check on the patient. Safety with medications is also an important consideration. Patients who take medications that lower blood pressure must be aware of the potential for orthostatic hypotension. Orthostatic hypotension is a drop in blood pressure that happens when a person moves from a lying to sitting or sitting to standing position. It is often accompanied by dizziness or light-headedness. Some people may even faint, causing a fall.

3. Two tablets of 50 mg each.

■ Mr. Soloman

1. Mr. Soloman had lost control of his world and felt powerless. His environment, both home and outdoors, was shrinking. He had to give up his daily routines and interactions with others. His purpose in life was gone when he was no longer caring for his wife. He was separated from his loved one. His visual limitations made his new environment unfamiliar and frightening.

2. Options to keep him safely in his home could have been explored with his input. After the move, he should have been thoroughly oriented to his environment. He should have been asked to explain what he wanted his life to be like as he adapted to this new period. Hobbies and interests should have been continued. Visual support services should have been contacted for ideas. Transportation should have been arranged to allow him to visit his wife and golf. It should have been determined whether phone calls to his wife were possible.

3. He was depressed and slept from a lack of interests. His lungs were at risk for pneumonia because of his long periods of immobility. He lost hope and gave up on living, which decreased his ability to fight the pneumonia.

■ Mrs. Burden

1. Mrs. Burden is at risk for sleep deprivation, fatigue, stress, and burnout.

2. Nursing diagnoses include *Disturbed Sleep Pattern, Fatigue, Social Isolation, Risk for Caregiver Role Strain,* and *Deficient Knowledge.*

3. Beneficial nursing interventions would include teaching about Alzheimer's, a chronic-care coach, respite care referral, alarm devices for wandering, and stress management techniques.

REVIEW QUESTIONS

1. The nurse is collecting data regarding a 68-year-old patient's developmental stage and finds that the patient is retired and that the patient's spouse died 4 months ago. The nurse identifies the patient as being in which of the following developmental stages?
   1. Generativity versus self-absorption
   2. Identity versus role confusion
   3. Integrity versus despair
   4. Intimacy versus isolation

2. The nurse is planning care for a patient with heart disease. Which of the following effects should the nurse consider is most likely to occur with a chronic illness when gathering further data collection?
   1. Hopefulness
   2. Increased socialization
   3. Powerfulness
   4. Spiritual distress

3. A 70-year-old man is the primary caregiver for his wife, who has moderately severe Alzheimer's disease. He becomes angry with her for spilling her dinner on the floor. He later feels guilty and begins to cry. The home health nurse is developing a plan of care. Which of the following would be an appropriate nursing diagnosis for the nurse to include?
   1. *Caregiver Role Strain*
   2. *Hopelessness*
   3. *Powerlessness*
   4. *Risk for Caregiver Role Strain*

4. A 64-year-old woman goes to a clinic for a yearly physical. She has a history of hypertension and osteoarthritis. In contributing to the plan of care, which of the following would be a priority intervention to promote wellness in this patient who has chronic illnesses?
   1. Demonstrating how to take a blood pressure
   2. Explaining hypertension and osteoarthritis
   3. Encouraging increased socialization
   4. Evaluating progress with the patient and family

5. The nurse is providing care for a chronically ill patient. Which of the following are appropriate nursing interventions for a chronically ill patient? **Select all that apply.**
   1. Limiting educational information
   2. Encouraging visits by family members
   3. Including family members in teaching sessions
   4. Setting the goals for the patient
   5. Limiting visits from friends
   6. Obtaining patient input on plan of care

6. Which of the following nursing interventions would be most appropriate for a patient with a chronic illness who is experiencing chronic sorrow? **Select all that apply.**
   1. Provide quiet time.
   2. Make time to listen.
   3. Share information.
   4. Limit interactions.
   5. Use active listening.
   6. Encourage hope.

7. The nurse would evaluate the patient with a chronic illness as responding positively to interventions for chronic sorrow if the patient stated which of the following?
   1. "I have nothing left to accomplish."
   2. "Maybe tomorrow will be a better day."
   3. "I should not keep hoping for a cure."
   4. "There is nothing I can do."

Answers can be found in Appendix C.

References

Erikson, E. H. (1980). *Identity and the life cycle.* New York: W.W. Norton & Company.
Erikson, E. H. (1993). *Childhood and society.* New York: W.W. Norton & Company.

 Davis*Plus* | For additional resources and information visit **davispl.us/medsurg5**

15

Nursing Care of Older Adult Patients

KEY TERMS

activities of daily living (ack-TIH-vih-tees of DAY-lee LIH-ving)
arrhythmias (uh-RITH-mee-yahs)
aspiration (AS-pi-RAY-shun)
constipation (KON-sti-PAY-shun)
contractures (kon-TRACK-churs)
delirium (del-LEER-ee-um)
dementia (dee-MEN-cha)
depression (dih-PRESH-shun)
edema (eh-DEE-muh)
expectorate (eck-SPEK-tuh-RAYT)
extrinsic factors (eks-TRIN-sick FAK-ters)
holistic (hoh-LISS-tick)
homeostasis (HOH-mee-oh-STAY-siss)
intrinsic factors (in-TRIN-sick FAK-ters)
nocturia (nock-TOO-ree-ah)
optimum level of functioning (OP-tih-mum LEV-uhl of FUNK-shun-ing)
osteoporosis (AWS-tee-oh-puh-ROH-siss)
perception (per-SEP-shun)
pressure ulcer (PRESH-ur ULL-sir)
range of motion (RAINJE of MOH-shun)
reality orientation (ree-AL-ih-tee OR-ee-en-TAY-shun)
sensory deprivation (SEN-suh-ree DEP-rih-VAY-shun)
sensory overload (SEN-suh-ree OH-ver-lohd)
urinary incontinence (YOUR-ih-NARE-ee in-KON-tih-nents)

MARYANNE PIETRANIEC-SHANNON

LEARNING OUTCOMES

1. Define aging.
2. List basic physiological changes associated with advancing age.
3. Describe the psychological and cognitive changes associated with advancing age.
4. Plan nursing care for the physiological and psychological changes associated with advancing age.
5. Identify nursing practices that promote safety for the older patient.

WHAT IS AGING?

Over time, it is easy to see changes that occur in the human body. Both physical structures and body functions undergo changes and declines with advancing age. Although there is not one commonly accepted definition or theory to explain these declines, there is an understanding that aging is a universal and normal process that starts at conception and continues until death.

Older adults are continuing to increase in number. According to the 2010 U.S. Census, 40.3 million adults were older than age 65. This represents a 15.1% increase for this age group from 2000 (U.S. Census Bureau, 2010). The fastest growing segment within this group was those aged 85 to 94. For current population data and older adult information, visit www.census.gov or www.agingstats.gov.

In this chapter, *aging* is defined as a maturational process that creates the need for individual adaptation because of physical and psychological declines that occur throughout life. Even though aging truly begins at conception, the focus in this chapter is on the maturational process that is experienced after age 65 (older adult). People older than age 84 usually are the frailest, although chronological age should not be the basis for determining health issues. For some people, aging effects go unnoticed in their daily functioning; for others these effects cause varying degrees of impairment. Functional age (health, independence, and functional abilities) should be used as the basis of individual care needs. It is important to understand that most older adults function independently in the home and community. Many older people remain in the workforce by choice or financial necessity. With supportive, educative care as needed, these people are able to maintain their independent abilities. This chapter discusses aging changes and the resulting disabilities that can require more intensive nursing care than that required by older adults who are independent and healthy. About 1.3 million (3.1%) of those aged 65 or older resided in skilled-nursing agencies in 2010 (U.S. Census Bureau, 2010).

NURSING CARE TIP

Placing older adults into one category titled "old" overlooks aging as a unique experience. The concept of functional age recognizes that aging is individual and promotes individualized nursing assessment and development of plans of care for the older adult.

Although aging is universal, it remains a unique experience for each individual. Factors that contribute to this process can be grouped into two categories. **Intrinsic factors** focus on genetic theories of aging, such as the biological clock theory or programmed aging theory, and on some aspects of physiological theories of aging, such as wear-and-tear theory or stress adaptation theory. **Extrinsic factors** focus on environmental influences, such as pollutants, free-radical theory, and stress-adaptation theory.

Regardless of which factors have the greatest influence on the process of aging, **perception** and attitude also play key roles in how changes over time affect the individual. It is through the filter of perception and attitude that the individual identifies, defines, and adapts to the changes that occur in structure and function over time. These factors have implications not only for older patients but also for their families and the health care providers (HCPs) working with them.

PHYSIOLOGICAL CHANGES

Over time, cells change and do not function as efficiently as in earlier years (Table 15.1). Compared with cellular changes, the physical changes seen when looking at an older person are slight. Cellular decline in structure and function increases in severity and extent over time. Although the body works hard to maintain **homeostasis**, it is often unable to fully adapt to many of the declines that result from aging. Cells that die cannot regenerate themselves. As a result, structures are altered, and the body tries to adapt to make the revised structure meet functional demands.

Common Physical Changes in Older Patients and Their Implications for Nursing

Key Changes in the Muscular System

Age-related changes in the muscular system include the following:

- Decrease in muscle mass, so muscles look smaller
- Decrease in muscle tone, so muscles look less toned
- Slower muscle responses, so response time is increased
- Decrease in elasticity of tendons and ligaments, restricting movements.

NURSING CARE.   Changes in the muscular system have implications for movement, strength, and endurance. Restricted movements are most commonly seen in the arms, legs, and neck of the older patient, who can have limited **range of motion** (ROM) in these areas. Because muscle response abilities are slowed, it will take longer for the older patient to move. This increased response time has implications for the older person's confidence in being able to perform routine tasks.

Key Changes in the Skeletal System

Age-related changes in the skeletal system include the following:

- Eroding cartilage
- Exaggerated bony prominences
- Joint stiffening and decreased flexibility

• WORD • BUILDING •

homeostasis: homios—similar + stasis—standing

TABLE 15.1 PHYSIOLOGICAL CHANGES OF AGING

Body System	Aging Change	Effect of Change
Cardiovascular	Increased conduction time	Heart rate slows, unable to increase quickly
	Decreased cardiac output	Less oxygen delivered to tissues
	Decreased blood vessel elasticity	Increased blood pressure increases cardiac workload
	Irregular heartbeats	Poor heart oxygenation, decreased cardiac output, heart failure
	Dilated leg veins, less efficient valves	Varicose veins, fluid accumulation in tissues
Endocrine and Metabolism	Slowed basal metabolic rate	Possible weight gain
	Altered adrenal hormone production	Decreased ability to respond to stress
	Decreased insulin release	Hyperglycemia
Gastrointestinal	Reduced taste and smell	Appetite can be reduced
	Decreased saliva	Dry mouth, altered taste
	Decreased gag reflex, relaxation of lower esophageal sphincter	Increased aspiration risk
	Delayed gastric emptying	Reduced appetite
	Reduced liver enzymes	Reduced drug metabolism and detoxification
	Decreased peristalsis	Reduced appetite, constipation
Genitourinary	Kidney size decreases	Able to live with 10% renal function
	Decreased bladder size, tone, changes from pear to funnel shaped	Frequency of urination increased
	Weakened muscles	Incontinence
	Decreased ability to concentrate	Nocturia
	Less sodium saved	Risk for dehydration
	Reduced renal blood flow	Decreased renal clearance of all medications
Immunological	Decreased function	Increased infection and cancer risk
	Increased autoimmune response	Increased autoimmune diseases
Integumentary	Reduced cell replacement	Healing slower
	Water loss	Dryness of the skin
	Increased pigmentation	Aging spots
	Thinning of skin layers	Skin more fragile
	Decreased subcutaneous fat	Less insulation and protective cushioning
	Decreased sebaceous and sweat glands	Dryness and decreased temperature regulation
	Hard, dry nails	Brittle nails
	Baldness	Thinning scalp hair
	Decreased melanin	Gray hair
	Decreased skin elasticity	Wrinkle development
Musculoskeletal	Decreased muscle mass	Reduced strength
	Decreased muscle tone	Muscles look flabbier
	Decreased elasticity of tendons and ligaments	Movements are restricted
	Slowed muscle responses	Response time increased
	Bone thinning, softening	Decreasing bone density
	Joint stiffening	Decreased flexibility
	Vertebral disk water loss	Decreased height
Neurologic Central nervous system	Loss of brain cells	Able to maintain function with remaining cells
	Decreased brain blood flow	Short-term memory loss
	Decreased regulation of body temperature	Hypothermia, hyperthermia risk
	Decreased endorphins	Increased depression

TABLE 15.1   PHYSIOLOGICAL CHANGES OF AGING—cont'd

Body System	Aging Change	Effect of Change
Peripheral nervous system	Decreased sensation	Risk for injury, burns
	Increased reaction times	Slow response, injury risk
	Decreased motor coordination	Unsteady, fall risk
Respiratory	Decreased lung capacity	Dyspnea with activity
	Decreased cough and gag reflexes	Aspiration, infection risk
	Reduced lung tissue tone	Shallow, faster respirations
	Reduced lung emptying on exhalation	CO_2 retention
	Decreased fluid and ciliary action	Mucous obstruction, infection risk
Sensory		
Eye	Lens less elastic	Decreased near and peripheral vision
	Lens opaque, yellows	Cataracts
	Cornea more translucent	Blurry vision
	Smaller pupil	Decreased dark adaptation
	Decreased violet, blue, green color vision	See red, orange, yellow colors better
	Arcus senilis—milky lipid ring on iris edge that does not cover pupil	No effect on vision
Ear	Degeneration of auditory nerve	Lose high-frequency tones, deafness
	Excess bone impairs sound conduction	Deafness
Nose	Decreased smell	Decreased ability to smell substances such as smoke or gas, causing safety risk; appetite reduced
Sexuality	Availability of partner or privacy decreases	Lack of sexual expression, suppression of desires
Men	Slower sexual arousal time	Increased time needed for sexual stimulation
	Decreased erection, slower ejaculation	Psychologically causes concern
Women	Less vaginal lubrication	Painful intercourse
	Vaginal acidity reduced	Increased vaginal infection risk

- **Osteoporosis**, a thinning (decrease in density) and softening of the bone
- Shortening in height caused by water loss in the intervertebral disks of the spinal column and flexion of the spine associated with the influence of gravity over time.

NURSING CARE. Because muscles and bones work together for movement, aging skeletal changes are most obvious when the older patient is moving. **Contractures** of the fingers and hands can limit the person's ability to perform self-care tasks called **activities of daily living** (ADLs). It is important to assist the patient with ROM exercises if help is needed to prevent the long-term disabilities that contractures bring (Fig. 15.1). Performing ROM exercises in warm water helps the patient for whom movement is uncomfortable. If the person has arthritis, the administration of any prescribed anti-inflammatory

medications should be timed so their action peaks when the exercises begin. Older patients on anti-inflammatory medicines should be monitored closely for gastrointestinal (GI) upset or bleeding and taught the symptoms of bleeding to report.

Decreased bone density is influenced by diet and weight-bearing exercise, so balanced diets rich in calcium and vitamin D and safe and sensible weight-bearing exercise programs should be promoted (see "Evidence-Based Practice").

Encourage patients to ambulate whenever possible wearing supportive, sensible shoes with nonskid soles. In addition to making sure the environment is safe for walking, sturdy

• WORD • BUILDING •

osteoporosis: osteon—bone + poros—a passage + osis—condition

FIGURE 15.1 Nurse assists patient in range of motion exercises to prevent the development of contractures.

assistive devices such as handrails, canes, or walkers should be encouraged as needed. Because of the decreasing density of older bones, fractures not only can result from falls; they can cause falls as well.

EVIDENCE-BASED PRACTICE

Clinical Question
What are the most common causes of falls for residents in the nursing home setting?

Evidence
According to a 2012 Centers for Disease Control and Prevention report on nursing home falls, nursing home residents fall often and repeatedly. Consequences of falls include death or hip fractures and head injuries that can impair quality of life. Causes of these falls are complex and can include muscle weakness, gait and transfer difficulties, hazards such as wet floors, inadequate lighting, bed height too high, medications such as sedatives and antianxiety agents and the 3-day period after changes in these medications, improper shoe fit, or incorrect use of walking aids.

Implications for Nursing Practice
Fall prevention requires a commitment by the organization and multidisciplinary team to plan interventions that look at multiple causation factors including the environment and resident medical treatment and rehabilitation. Interventions can be implemented by patients, staff, multidisciplinary

team members, and the organization. Vigilance by everyone is essential to help prevent resident falls.

REFERENCE
Centers for Disease Control and Prevention. (2012, February 29). Falls in nursing homes. Retrieved June 19, 2013, from www.cdc.gov/homeandrecreationalsafety/falls/nursing.html

BE SAFE!

BE VIGILANT! Reduce the risk of harm from falls with a fall reduction program that includes monitoring of its effectiveness. Assess residents' or patients' risk for falls and establish a fall prevention plan. Assessment includes a history of falls, medication review for medications that can cause dizziness, weakness or sleepiness, alcohol use, gait and balance screening, and use of assistive aids. Educate the staff, resident/patient, and family members on the resident/patient-centered fall prevention plan (2014 National Patient Safety Goals, © The Joint Commission, 2013. Reprinted with permission.).

Key Changes in the Integumentary System

Age-related changes in the integumentary system include the following:

• Increased dryness of the skin
• Increased pigmentation, causing liver or aging spots

- Thinning of the skin layers, which makes the skin more fragile
- Decreased skin elasticity, causing wrinkles to develop
- Decreased subcutaneous fat layer, so older patients have less insulation and less protective cushioning
- Hardness and dryness of nails, making them more brittle
- Decrease in nail growth rate and strength
- Thinning of scalp hair, mainly in men
- Increased growth and coarseness of nose, ear, and facial hair
- Decrease in melanin, which results in gray hair
- Decreased sebaceous and sweat glands, which has implications for dryness and decreased temperature regulation.

NURSING CARE.   The skin is the first line of defense against infection and injury (Fig. 15.2). In the older adult, skin injuries take longer to heal, and those longer healing times are usually complicated by the fact that many older patients have multiple chronic diseases, such as diabetes and circulatory ailments.

The older patient with limited mobility is especially prone to developing **pressure ulcers** (Fig. 15.3). These ulcers are caused by ischemia, which results from continuous pressure on an area of the body. They usually develop over a bony prominence (ears, shoulders, elbows, tip of the spine, pelvic bone ridges, knees, heels, or ankles). Ischemia from unrelieved pressure can begin to develop in 20 to 40 minutes. Early signs of pressure ulcer formation are warmth, redness, tenderness, and a burning sensation at the potential ulcer site. These potential ulcer sites are aggravated by lack of activity and the weight of the body. For this reason, it is especially important to take time to assess skin integrity daily, especially in high-risk areas of the body.

BE SAFE!

BE VIGILANT! Assess and periodically reassess each resident's risk for developing a pressure ulcer and take action to address any identified risks. Educate staff on risk identification and prevention strategies for pressure ulcers (2014 National Patient Safety Goals, © The Joint Commission, 2013. Reprinted with permission.).

Skin care includes gently stimulating nonreddened, intact skin sites with massage, using moisturizing creams regularly (except between toes because too much moisture can lead to infections), refraining from use of electrical heating pads that can burn, and gentle bathing techniques, such as the towel bath or bag bath, which avoid the use of hot water, drying soap, and rubbing the skin to dry. The New York Edge Project details techniques for these types of gentle bathing at www.health.ny.gov/diseases/conditions/dementia/edge/interventions/gentle/index.htm. Patients should be taught, if they are able, to shift their weight every 15 minutes when sitting. For immobile patients, consistent repositioning is essential. Ideally, use of pressure-relieving devices or repositioning every 30 minutes is the most beneficial for high-risk patients to help prevent pressure ulcer development (see Chapter 54). Keeping bed linens clean, dry, and wrinkle-free also aids in the prevention of pressure ulcer formation.

As with skin care, nail care is important for older people. Soaking in warm water helps soften nails to ease in their trimming while encouraging blood flow to the peripheral areas of the body. Filing nails with an emery board is safer than cutting nails. To prevent accidental injury to the feet, patients should be instructed not to walk barefoot. Potential pressure points of the feet should be identified and closely monitored, and the patient should be referred to a podiatrist for treatment if there are any concerns. People with diabetes should assess their feet daily because they can have decreased sensation (neuropathy), causing lack of awareness of foot irritation or injury.

Key Changes in the Cardiovascular System

Age-related changes in the cardiovascular system include the following:

- Slowed heart rate
- Decreased cardiac output from less effective functioning of the heart and blood vessels, yielding less oxygen to body tissues

FIGURE 15.2 Thin, fragile skin of an older person.

FIGURE 15.3 Pressure ulcer. From Goldsmith, L. A., Lazarus, G. S., & Tharp, M. D. (1997). *Adult and pediatric dermatology: A color guide to diagnosis and treatment*, p. 445. Philadelphia: F.A. Davis.

BE SAFE!

BE VIGILANT! Shoes should be checked before putting them on to ensure there is nothing in them that could cause injury if it was not felt and walked on. A person with severe neuropathy wore shoes for 8 hours, into which a tiny toy had fallen and didn't even feel it. Ulceration developed in the area of the foot where the toy was walked on and hospitalization was required. Teach patients the importance of daily foot and shoe assessment for safety!

- Decreased elasticity of the blood vessels, so the circulatory system is less efficient
- Reduced ability of the heart to quickly increase its rate in response to an emergency because of thickening of the heart valves, left ventricle, and aorta (when rate does increase, the heart takes longer to return to resting rate)
- More **arrhythmias** (irregular heartbeats), which lead to poor oxygenation of the heart
- Commonly, a lack of classic symptoms of cardiac emergencies
- Increased peripheral vascular resistance in blood vessels, yielding increased blood pressure
- More visible superficial blood vessels of the legs
- Less efficient leg vein valves, creating the risk for an accumulation of excess fluids in the leg tissues.

NURSING CARE. Be a good observer when it comes to caring for older patients because many early symptoms related to circulatory problems are subtle. Cardiovascular disease, which is separate from the process of aging, accounts for half of all deaths in people older than age 65. Older adults must be educated about prevention practices that promote healthy circulation and encouraged to take prescribed medications as ordered. In addition to encouraging oral fluids to balance fluid output in older patients, the nurse must carefully monitor for the hazards of fluid overload in all older patients on intravenous therapy.

Special care should be taken to maintain good skin integrity and provide appropriate stimulation. If **edema** is present in the legs, they should be elevated to promote fluid return to the upper body; supportive, nonrestrictive stockings should be worn as ordered. Concerns regarding leg and foot circulation in the older patient must be identified and reported as early as possible so the primary care provider can order the appropriate arterial or venous therapy to address circulatory concerns before they become problems.

Because quick changes in body position can make the older patient feel weak and dizzy, it is important to stand next to older patients as they dangle their legs over the side of the bed before rising to stand. Changes in body position from lying to sitting to standing should occur gradually to accommodate the less efficient circulatory systems of older patients. Older patients might find comfort in the security of an ambulatory belt or walker if they fear unsteadiness in an upright position. Because falls continue to rank as a leading cause of accidental death in older patients (and because a history of falls remains the key indicator to predict future falls), it is important for the nurse to identify fall risk to determine which older patient might be at greater risk so preventive measures can be documented in the care plan.

Key Changes in the Respiratory System

Age-related changes in the respiratory system include the following:

- Decreased lung capacity
- Weaker cough or gag reflex, increasing the risk of upper respiratory infection
- Reduced tone of lung tissue, so respirations increase to 16 to 25 per minute and are more shallow
- Reduced tone of the diaphragm muscle
- Less complete emptying of the lungs, with greater CO_2 retention
- Decreased blood flow to the lungs, contributing to cardiac arrhythmias.

NURSING CARE. Because the respiratory system is less efficient with advancing age, older patients have a decreased tolerance for activity. Nurses should, therefore, pace activities for older patients instead of letting them confine themselves to bed. The nurse should schedule rest periods to prevent overexertion; however, rest periods should not outnumber the activity sessions planned throughout the course of the patient's day.

Cough, fatigue, and confusion can be early signs of inadequate oxygen uptake. Respiratory rates greater than 25 per minute can be an early indication of a lower respiratory tract infection. Because overall muscle strength is reduced, the older patient performs the O_2–CO_2 exchange in the less efficient upper lobes of the lung instead of the larger lower lobes specifically designed for this purpose. Because lung recoil strength is decreased, mucus can be more difficult for the older patient to **expectorate** (cough up). This situation is compounded by the fact that older people also have less effective cough and gag reflexes, which creates greater potential for lung problems.

Because of the normal changes that take place in the respiratory system with aging, it is important to include coughing, deep breathing, and position changes in an exercise program designed to stimulate all lobes of the older patient's lungs. At the prevention level, encourage the older person to receive a pneumonia vaccination and an annual flu shot. This is important because influenza and pneumonia combine to be the fourth leading cause of death in people over age 65. Be aware that lifelong habits, such as smoking and respiratory pollutant exposure in employment settings, secondhand smoke, or paints and glues used in hobbies, are cumulative over time and can contribute to respiratory sensitivity for the older patient. Nurses can help

• WORD • BUILDING •
edema: oidema—swelling
expectorate: ex—out + pectus—breast

prevent the spread of respiratory illnesses by getting flu shots, performing hand hygiene between patients, not exposing patients to any nurses' illness, and using universal precautions.

Key Changes in the Gastrointestinal System

Age-related changes in the GI system include the following:

- Changes in taste and smell, which affect the enjoyment of eating
- Decreased saliva production
- Decreased gag reflex and relaxation of lower esophageal sphincter, increasing the risk of **aspiration** (inhalation of oropharyngeal or gastric contents into the lower airways)
- Delayed gastric emptying
- No functional changes in the small intestine
- Decreased tone in the external sphincter
- Marked decline in liver enzymes, which affects drug metabolism and detoxification
- Decreased peristalsis from generalized weakness of muscle activity
- Alteration in bowel habits

NURSING CARE. Many factors can alter appetite, ingestion, digestion, and absorption of nutrients in food, regardless of age. However, the structural and functional changes that occur with advancing age put the older patient at greater risk for not obtaining the nutrients needed to sustain a healthy body system (see "Nutrition Notes—Older Adult Nutritional Needs").

Nutrition Notes

Older Adult Nutritional Needs

Three areas of nutritional concern for older adults are insufficient amounts of protein, calcium, vitamin D, and vitamin B_{12}. The Recommended Dietary Allowance (RDA) for protein is 46 grams per day for women and 56 for men, amounts found in two glasses of milk and 4.3 to 5.7 ounces of meat, fish, or poultry.

For women older than 50 years and men older than 70 years, the RDA for calcium is increased to 1200 milligrams. For adults older than 70 years, the RDA for vitamin D is increased to 800 International Units (20 micrograms). Both of those nutrients have an impact on bone integrity and can be insufficient in older persons who neither drink milk nor spend time outdoors, and even if they did, their skins are less able to synthesize the vitamin D precursor. To derive the higher RDAs for calcium and vitamin D from milk would require 4 cups of milk for the calcium and 8 cups for the vitamin D. Thus, fortified foods or supplements might be advised.

Achlorhydria (low or absent gastric acid in the stomach) can occur as a result of aging or from chronic ingestion of antacids. In either case, protein digestion and absorption of iron and vitamin B_{12} can be impaired by the lack of gastric acid and intrinsic factor required for vitamin B_{12} absorption (see "Nutrition Notes" in Chapter 28). Malabsorption of iron and vitamin B_{12} can lead to anemia; however, sources of blood loss should also be considered. Because 10% to 30% of older persons malabsorb vitamin B_{12}, its RDA for individuals older than 50 years specifies fortified foods or supplements as the main sources of the vitamin.

Decreased visual acuity and impaired dexterity can make shopping for food and preparing it difficult or even hazardous. Arthritis affects not only mobility, but also jaw movements, so chewing can be problematic. By age 65, about 26% of U.S. residents have lost all their teeth (become *edentulous*) and have to develop skill in the use of dentures. People who need dentures should learn to use them in this order:
- Drinking
- Manipulating soft foods
- Biting and chewing.

Older persons produce less saliva than younger people. The sense of taste declines in most but not all aging patients, who as a result might increase their intake of salt and sugar to the detriment of a prescribed diet plan.

Many older patients are at increased risk for food, nutrient, and drug interactions. Situations associated with these interactions are:
- The use of many drugs, including alcohol
- The need for long-term drug therapy in chronic illness
- Poor or marginal nutritional status.

Identification of any of these factors should prompt a thorough nutritional assessment or referral to a registered dietitian.

Particularly among older people, rigid application of diet rules can be inappropriate. For example, restricting fat by eliminating whole milk and eggs, which are easily eaten and relatively inexpensive, could endanger nutrition in the short term for uncertain long-term benefits.

Little can be done to change the physical alterations in the older body that make getting needed nutrients more difficult. Being knowledgeable and committed to providing the assistance needed to meet nutritional goals is important. Patients should be offered toileting before sitting down to eat. An appropriate amount of time must be provided for the older patient to accomplish the task of eating. If the patient needs help with eating, the nurse must be sensitive to the patient's pace while giving the patient as much control of the process as possible.

Eating has a strong social component. Encourage the patient to eat out of bed and with others as much as possible, while respecting the patient's right of refusal to eat in a designated social setting. Some patients might not eat as well when seated next to agitated or confused residents in a common dining hall.

Offer a calm and comfortable environment that aids digestion. Food combinations that enhance nutrient absorption should be offered together whenever possible (i.e., when a vitamin C food is taken with plant foods high in iron, vitamin C increases the iron absorption rate). Familiar seasonings can help stimulate a lagging appetite; ask family members to bring the patient's favorite seasonings in shakers so the patient can use them. Dietitians can provide other ideas to promote healthful eating for older patients.

Although many older patients wear dentures or partial plates, it is important not to assume that all older people wear dentures. Tooth loss is not a normal change of aging because, with proper dental care, teeth can last a lifetime. If an older patient does have dentures, be aware that any significant change in body weight will affect the fit and comfort of the dentures and, therefore, affect nutritional intake. Because of this, it is important to conduct regular assessments of the mouth when assisting the older patient during oral care.

Medications can cause taste disturbances or problems with dry mouth that can also affect the older patient's ability to meet nutritional needs. Some medications create problems with bowel motility, resulting in **constipation**. Constipation can also result from stress, anxiety, or a change in routine. To gain a greater understanding of the situation, talk with the patient about previous assistive procedures and establish a baseline expectation for bowel elimination. Educate the older patient about the important relationship between intake (e.g., fiber and water) and exercise in the promotion of effective bowel evacuation. Enemas, suppositories, and medications should be considered only after dietary management is found to be ineffective.

Key Changes in the Endocrine-Metabolic System

Age-related changes in the endocrine-metabolic system include the following:

- Slowing of the basal metabolic rate, requiring a 5% reduction in calorie consumption to maintain weight
- Alteration in hormone production, including changes in estrogen, progesterone, and adrenal secretions
- Decreased pancreatic insulin release and peripheral sensitivity
- Decreased glucose tolerance with advancing age.

NURSING CARE. Increased incidence of metabolic disease, such as diabetes, occurs with advancing years. Because of this, older patients should be encouraged to participate in screening programs for early detection of metabolic problems.

Because there is a notable decrease in the effectiveness and interaction of all hormones as one ages, it becomes especially difficult for the older body to respond appropriately to stressful situations. Nurses should spend time addressing the psychological needs of patients by recognizing and addressing actual and perceived stressors that affect their care. Preventive care to keep patients free from the stress of illness is also important.

Key Changes in the Genitourinary System

Age-related changes in the genitourinary system include the following:

- Decreased kidney size
- Decreased kidney function, urine output, and adaptability
- Reduced blood flow to the kidneys because of decreased cardiac output and increased peripheral resistance
- Decreased kidney filtration rate and tubular function, which cause a decrease in the renal clearance of all medications
- Decreased bladder size, shape, and tone
- Increased incidence of urinary tract infection (UTI), especially in women
- Longer correction time to address fluid and electrolyte imbalances.

NURSING CARE. Many older people have the urge to urinate at night, which is referred to as **nocturia**. Changes in the kidneys, the influence of gravity when in the recumbent position, fluid retention, and medications contribute to nocturia. About 30 minutes after lying down, many older people need to urinate. This occurs with position change, because fluid held in the legs by gravity is now circulated through the kidneys, producing more urine and the urge to void. Controlling bladder function can become more difficult with age and result in **urinary incontinence**.

 ### NURSING CARE TIP

With advancing age, older patients do not get the urge to void as early in the process as they did when younger. This aging change, accompanied with other normal aging changes in the urinary system (such as the bladder becoming funnel shaped), contributes to the older patient's voiding urgency. If the patient is not assisted to void promptly after making a request, incontinence can result. This can create a safety issue if the patient attempts to get up alone. Provide safe patient-centered care by planning for and meeting the patient's voiding needs promptly.

First and foremost, the nurse must ensure safe access for all older patients who use the toilet alone or with assistance. Pathways to the toilet must be close and uncluttered. Toilets must be easy to access, and clothing must be easy to remove. Incontinence is socially embarrassing and is one of the main reasons older people are placed in long-term care facilities by family members. Urinary incontinence in older men is most often attributed to benign prostate enlargement, whereas older women are more likely candidates because of short urethras and weakened perineal muscles. Because UTIs are more

• WORD • BUILDING •
nocturia: nocte—night + ouron—urine

common in older people (and often more dangerous), nurses must closely monitor not only the quantity of intake and output for older patients but also the quality.

Management of urinary incontinence needs to be tailored to the particular need of the patient. Bladder training programs can be effective when patients are reminded on a regular basis that it is time to urinate. If incontinence results from problems that affect the toileting task itself, such as clothing removal or distance to the bathroom, steps should be taken to eliminate obstacles that stand in the way of continence. Clothing with Velcro fasteners can replace buttons or zippers that are difficult for the patient to manipulate. Urinary briefs can help instill confidence in older patients who previously restricted their activities because of fear of urine leakage. With use of the supportive incontinence brief, assess for early signs of perineal skin breakdown and proper application of the correct type of brief to meet individual needs.

Older patients who are aware of their incontinence might try to inappropriately decrease the chance for leakage by severely limiting fluid intake. This approach often results in dehydration, which disturbs the acid-base and electrolyte balance in the body. Over time, dehydrated patients can have problems with vomiting, diarrhea, weakness, and confusion. Because fluid intake needs to be encouraged in older patients, focus educational efforts on topics such as liquid intake timing and beverage selection (teaching that caffeine and alcoholic beverages should be avoided because they increase urinary output).

In addition, it is important for the nurse to review patient medications and personal medication practices (such as taking diuretics late in the day), which then results in nighttime urination (nocturia) and possible sleep disruption. Teaching perineal muscle support exercises and techniques is successful for some. All patients with unexplained urinary incontinence should be referred to a specialist for further evaluation because it is *not* a normal condition of aging.

Key Changes in the Immunological System

Age-related changes in the immune system include the following:

- Decreased immune response
- Decreased number and function of T cells, leading to impaired ability to produce antibodies to fight disease.

NURSING CARE. Older patients tend to have more chronic diseases that can increasingly depress their immune responses over time. Although older patients have fewer colds, they are at higher risk for influenza and other complications once they get a cold. It takes longer to recover from infections, so patients and their family members need to be told that a prolonged recovery is to be expected. It is also important to screen visitors for illness before they visit a recuperating older patient.

Efforts at prevention should focus on teaching the older patient about the importance of obtaining immunizations such as the shingles (a painful, contagious rash caused by the chickenpox virus—varicella zoster) vaccine for those aged 60 and older, reducing stress, eating right, exercising, and maintaining a healthful lifestyle. Those who are immunocompromised (such

---

CRITICAL THINKING

Mr. Jones

■ Mr. Jones, age 72, lives at home and is visited by the home health nurse. His home has wood floors with throw rugs. The bathroom is located in the hall outside his bedroom. Mr. Jones has nocturia and is occasionally incontinent from urgency to void. He takes bumetanide (Bumex) 1 milligram orally daily.

1. What additional assessment data should be obtained about Mr. Jones regarding his urinary status and home environment?
2. Are safety concerns present in the home environment?
3. What nursing diagnoses should be included in Mr. Jones's nursing care plan?
4. What should be included in a teaching plan for Mr. Jones?
5. Mr. Jones is to take bumetanide 1 milligram orally now. Bumetanide 0.5-milligram tablets are available. How many tablets are required?

Suggested answers are at the end of the chapter.

---

as those who take steroids) should be aware of the need to take additional safety precautions around others who are ill. Nurses can help patients help themselves by encouraging techniques, such as proper hand hygiene, that support universal precautions.

Key Changes in the Neurologic System

Age-related changes in the neurologic system include the following:

- Progressive loss of brain cells
- Decreased blood flow to and oxygen utilization in the brain
- Decreased protein synthesis
- Decrease in sensitivity and the sensation pathways
- Increased reaction times
- Decreased motor coordination
- Decreased equilibrium
- Decreased ability of the hypothalamus to regulate body temperature
- Change in neurotransmitter secretion levels

NURSING CARE. Changes in the nervous system of the older patient can be seen in both the peripheral and central systems. These changes have significant meaning for the older person, especially in the area of safety. With normal aging, there is a slowed response to stimuli and a marked decrease in the speed of the psychomotor response to those stimuli. Because stronger stimuli are required to elicit any neurologic response, the older patient is unable to perceive early signs of danger. To protect from accidental skin burns, the thermostat on water heaters should be lowered, and electrical heating devices such as heating pads, electric blankets, and mattress pads should not be used.

Another safety issue of concern focuses on changes in balance. It is more difficult to maintain balance as one ages, especially when musculoskeletal changes are considered. Special caution should be taken to assist older patients with transferring and ambulation activities so optimum levels of safety can be maintained.

Fine tremors of the hand can be a normal finding with advancing age. These movements tend to increase when the older patient is cold, excited, hungry, or active. Assistive devices provided by an occupational therapist (such as handle grips or anchored equipment) can help eliminate the unsteadiness created when fine tremors make it more difficult to accomplish ADLs (Fig. 15.4). Accompanied by generalized muscle weakness, normal neurologic changes that arise with advancing age usually occur on both sides of the body at the same time. One-sided weakness, sensory deficits, and performance problems should always be referred for further evaluation. Coarse tremors of the finger, forearm, head, eyelids, or tongue that occur when the body part is at rest can be a sign of a neurologic problem such as Parkinson's disease. These typically occur on one side of the body first and should always be referred for further evaluation.

Key Changes in the Sensory System

Age-related changes in the sensory system include the following:

• Decreased visual perception
• Decreased elasticity of the eardrum
• Decreased sense of smell
• Decreased taste perception
• Decreased touch sensation

NURSING CARE. Sensory changes associated with advancing age tend to occur gradually. Early identification and prompt referral and treatment can sometimes minimize sensory loss, which has a strong impact on the older person's psychological health.

Normal age-related changes in the eye affect the focus ability of the lens and the maneuverability of the eye muscles to meet the needs of near and far vision. It is especially difficult for older patients to read fine print, although it is usually manageable with reading glasses or bifocal lenses. When caring for a patient who wears glasses, it is important to remind the patient to consistently wear the glasses as needed and to help the patient keep them clean and in good repair. When glasses are removed by the patient, keep them accessible and in a protective, labeled case.

The older patient has a more difficult time adjusting to changes between light and dark settings. Seeing in the dark can be enhanced with the use of a red nightlight because red lighting is more easily detected by the cones and rods in the older patient's eye. Make every effort to reduce glare from bright sunlight because sensitivity to glare is enhanced by normal changes that occur in the aging eye. The glare from car headlights can impair vision in older patients who are still driving, creating added safety issues with night driving.

Several eye disorders can affect the aging eye (see Chapter 52). Regardless of the cause, any vision loss in older

FIGURE 15.4 Assistive devices for activities of daily living. (A) Sock and stocking aid. (B) Easy-pull hairbrush. (C) Food guard. *Courtesy of Sammons Preston, Inc., Bollingbrook, IL.*

patients puts them at risk for psychological problems with disorientation, withdrawal, or self-imposed isolation caused by **sensory deprivation**.

Hearing loss is common in older adults. Although the severity of age-related hearing loss is variable, the stigma it carries is the same. For older patients, the first difficult sounds to discriminate are the high-pitched tones. Therefore, it is often more effective to whisper when communicating with an individual who has a hearing impairment because whispering decreases the pitch of the sounds. Shouting is not helpful because both volume and pitch are increased. It is best to speak to a hearing-impaired person in a moderate volume and a lower tone. It is also helpful to stand in front of hearing-impaired patients so they can see the speaker's face during communication (Box 15-1).

Two types of hearing loss, conductive or sensorineural, can occur separately or in combination in the patient with a hearing impairment (see Chapter 52). It is important to use hearing protection throughout life because noise damage to the ear is usually not reversible. New-technology hearing aids can help most people with hearing loss. Patients should be referred to an audiologist for further evaluation if hearing loss is suspected. Hearing aids are often not well accepted by older persons or their family members because they are visual signs of a loss. Because of possible sensitivity, it is important to maintain patient privacy if a referral for further evaluation is made. If the older patient has a hearing aid, it should be kept accessible to the patient at all times. The hearing aid should be kept clean with soap and water. A cotton swab removes wax buildup in tiny areas of the hearing aid. When not in use, the hearing aid should be stored in a labeled protective container and the battery turned off to conserve it. Extra batteries should be kept readily available.

As discussed in the GI section of this chapter, the senses of taste and smell work closely together. Like other sensory losses, a declining ability to taste is not a problem exclusive to the older person. Both ill-fitting dentures and poor oral care can contribute to an alteration in the sense of taste, as can certain medications, tobacco products, and oral disease.

Box 15-1 Communicating With Patients Who Have Hearing Impairments

- Ensure that hearing aids are on with working batteries, if applicable.
- Face the patient so the speaker's face is visible.
- Speak toward the patient's best side of hearing.
- Speak in a clear, moderate-volume, low-pitched tone.
- Do not shout because doing this distorts sounds.
- Recognize that high-frequency tones and consonant sounds are lost first—*s, z, sh, ch, d, g*.
- Eliminate background noise because it can distort sounds.

Because of their codependent nature, taste and smell are two senses often treated as one. Age-related losses are expected to occur gradually in the older patient. In some cases, the loss of smell can result from sinus problems, nasal obstruction, or allergies. If olfactory receptors are the primary cause for losing the sense of smell, little can be done except to teach safety issues related to the loss (e.g., use of smoke alarms and natural gas alarms at home). Because some medications have been linked to the loss of taste, a medication review and daily mouth inspections help the nurse find a source that can be treated. However, any report of sudden loss in taste or smell sensation should be reported to the HCP because it can signal other health care problems.

Nurses also need to be aware of the environment they provide for the older patient. Overstimulation produced by **sensory overload** (as in intensive care hospital settings) can create psychological and physical strain that is difficult for an older patient to cope with. As a patient advocate, be sensitive to the patient's environment and changes in the patient's health care status, identifying and minimizing overload situations early in the recuperation period.

Key Changes in Sexuality

Age-related changes in sexuality include the following:

- Chronic illnesses, which can affect sexual functioning
- Functional sexual changes in older men, commonly alteration in ability to obtain or maintain an erection and to ejaculate
- Functional sexual changes in older women, such as decreased vaginal lubrication
- Sexual problems caused by psychological factors, which are more common than physical ones in older adult patients
- Longer sexual arousal time in the older patient
- Increase in sexual activities that focus on nonintercourse intimacy behaviors, including various forms of touch.

NURSING CARE. The older patient's sexuality is an important aspect to consider when providing care. It is essential to accept that sexuality is one of the basic physiological needs identified in Maslow's hierarchy of needs for all people regardless of age. Be aware of personal attitudes and values about sexuality, sex, and aging, being careful that personal stereotypes and beliefs do not interrupt the older person's attempt to maintain sexual identity. Because privacy remains a common problem for individuals in health care settings, provide the patient some scheduled private time for sexual expression. As new sexual enhancement treatments become more available to patients, there can be a greater openness to discuss sexual expression in conversations with older patients. Still, many older patients have difficulty overcoming barriers to sexual expression because of cultural or religious beliefs, lack of a suitable partner, fear of failure, fear of consequences, illness, side effects of medications, and certain chronic diseases that can alter libido or sexual function. Because sexual discussions with these patients can be more difficult, it is important to address the sexual history section as sensitively, professionally, and completely as other sections of the patient assessment form (Box 15-2).

 COGNITIVE AND PSYCHOLOGICAL CHANGES IN THE OLDER PATIENT

Cognition

In addition to the physiological changes that occur with advancing age, older patients also experience changes that have an effect on cognition. Cognition includes abilities related to intelligence, memory, orientation, judgment, calculation, and learning. Cognition focuses on intake, storage, processing, and retrieval of information. For the most part, older patients store information without much conscious effort. If dealing with information becomes difficult, the older person can begin to worry. Unless this worry is addressed, the patient's concern can result in psychological problems and fears.

Many factors can affect cognition. Sensory changes and diseases associated with age can cause misinterpretation of information being collected. Pain from chronic diseases, such as arthritis, can limit cognition as pain takes over the body and mind. Sleep deprivation caused by worry or fear can make it more difficult to perform routine tasks. Medications that cause drowsiness as a side effect can also impair cognition.

Long-term memory retrieval is easier to accomplish in old age than short-term memory retrieval. Assist the patient having short-term memory problems by using written lists, visual cues, and other memory-enhancing systems to aid in strengthening short-term memory skills.

Intelligence does not decline as one ages if it is measured using an appropriate instrument that focuses on accuracy and not on speed of response. Although cognitive abilities do tend to slow down with advancing age, they are not lost. Most of the subtle declines that occur with information processing and retrieval do not need to interfere with the older patient's abilities in performing ADLs.

Nurses need to assist in the identification of individual problem situations and work with older patients and their families in developing strategies to better address their needs. It is common knowledge that health, good nutrition, and adequate sleep are important factors for brain functioning. These factors should be the cornerstones in planning care for the older patient.

Coping Abilities

How a person chooses to adapt to a change in functional ability over time has a significant impact on how that person will work through the entire maturational process called aging. In addition to normal aging changes, many older patients are coping with compounding changes that occur because of chronic disease. Nurses must not lose sight of the fact that in addition to changes caused by some decline in physical and cognitive functioning, older persons simultaneously work to deal with many societal and culturally perceived losses associated with advancing age. Changes in employment status and societal and family roles and shifts from independence to dependence can leave a strong psychological impact on both older patients and significant others. With such a combination of losses, an older patient's confidence level can be affected, requiring encouragement of self-care behaviors.

Personality, attitude, past life experiences, and the desire to adapt to change are all intrinsic influencing factors that help the older patient cope with changes brought on by advancing age. Extrinsic factors include things such as financial status, family support, and support provided by those who directly care for the patient. If older patients have the energy, desire, determination, and support of those who care for them, they are better able to optimize use of their cognitive functions toward health.

Depression

There are times when the psychological impact of change is too difficult to cope with, and loneliness, grief, or sadness does not easily allow the older person to cognitively focus on health. When this happens, **depression** can result, with the potential to disable the older person's mind and body. Depression is the most common psychiatric problem among older adults. This psychological condition, which includes a disturbance in mood, increases the risk for suicide, physical health complaints, and sleep disturbances.

Box 15-2 Sexuality Data Collection

As with any nursing skill, practice will increase your comfort in collecting sexuality data for the older patient so these needs are not ignored. Identification of sexuality concerns is a valuable part of data collection, and it also can lead to the discovery of other health issues. Establish rapport with the patient by collecting other data first and turning to sexuality data at the end of the history. Older patients often respond to sexuality questions but will not bring up the topic. As you collect data, be aware of problems (e.g., pain, medication side effects, mobility, dexterity, elimination, angina, surgery) identified in the history that can have an impact on sexual function.

Naturally, you should use a professional approach and manner and tell the patient that you will now ask questions about sexuality. Start with questions that are likely to be more comfortable for the patient, as follows:

• Address roles first. For example: What concerns (do you have or has your illness created) in carrying out your roles with your (spouse or sexual partner)?
• Address relationship issues next. For example: What effect on your relationship with your (spouse or sexual partner) has this (illness, symptom, chronic illness) had?
• Address body image. For example: What effect has your (illness, surgery [mastectomy, prostate, ostomy], chronic illness, age-related changes) had on your self-concept of being a (man or woman)?
• Address sexually transmitted infections. For example: Do you have any discharge or open sores (vaginal, penile)?

It is important to understand that the frequency and intensity of depression generally increase with advancing age. Depression can result from physical changes in the brain, as from a medication or a condition affecting neurotransmitters, or from psychological changes at an emotional level, such as maladaptive coping from a perceived loss. Regardless of the cause, depression has the potential to be reversed with prompt identification and treatment. It is important, therefore, to be sensitive to what the older person is and is not saying during communications. If depression is suspected, patients should be referred for treatment before maladaptive behaviors occur.

Dementia

Unlike depression, **dementia** involves a more permanent progressive deterioration of mental function. Dementia is often characterized by confusion, forgetfulness, impaired judgment, and personality changes. There are two main types of dementia: multi-infarct dementia and Alzheimer's disease.

For dementia, help the older patient maintain an **optimum level of functioning** in an atmosphere that provides physical and emotional safety. To help ground the confused patient, if appropriate, incorporate **reality orientation** or validation into all nursing interventions. Sensory overload should be decreased for confused patients. Speak calmly and slowly, and provide nonthreatening therapeutic touch if accepted by the patient.

In addition, it is important to address the education and support needs of the patient's family as they learn to deal with changes in the older patient's behavior. Refer any patient with confusion for a mental status examination to help determine whether the person has depression or dementia. It is essential that a sensory status examination be conducted before a mental status examination to help ensure the accuracy of the test results.

Delirium

Delirium reflects the patient's level of alertness and psychomotor activity and is commonly a complication of acute illness and its treatment. Although it can occur in hospitalized patients at any age, it occurs most often in hospitalized older patients and is often charted as "confusion." Although the actual mechanism through which delirium occurs is not known, it is thought to stem from changes in brain neurotransmitters that control cognitive function, mood, and behavior. Unlike depression and dementia, delirium has a sudden onset, tends to be worse at night, and can last for a few hours or a few weeks. The patient seems disturbed or frightened. Based on patient behaviors, delirium can be classified as hypoactive, hyperactive, or mixed.

Also different from depression and dementia, delirium is a cognitive state that can be easily reversed once the cause is identified and treated. For this reason, the nurse must not assume that the older patient's current mental status is his or her usual state. The nurse must be able to identify risk factors for this condition (e.g., acute illness, infection, alcohol or other drug abuse, surgery, hip fracture, metabolic disturbance) and report any patient concerns before they become problems.

Sleep and Rest Patterns

The need for sleep does not decrease with age, but the pattern in older adults usually varies from earlier times in their lives. As in any age group, lack of sleep leads to fatigue, irritability, increased sensitivity to pain, and increased likelihood of accidents. This is why it is important to obtain a baseline sleep and rest history when an older patient is admitted to a health care unit. Consider sleep patterns, bedtime rituals, rest and nap patterns, daily exercise patterns, stress level, dietary intake patterns, and lifestyle issues such as caffeine, alcohol, and nicotine intake when completing a sleep and rest assessment for an older patient.

Circulatory problems can disrupt normal sleep patterns for the older person and might be the only clue of an impending health problem. The anxious patient who is unable to sleep might be calmed with back rubs, foot rubs, a warm towel bath, warm milk, or a glass of wine, if not contraindicated, when patterned bedtime rituals prove to be unsuccessful. Sleep medications should be used only as a last resort because they can affect the quality or depth of the sleep the older person receives and can produce unwanted side effects.

Medication Management

Medication management is one of the most difficult tasks for older patients, family members, and the health care providers caring for them. Because older patients are more susceptible to drug-induced illness and adverse side effects for a variety of reasons already addressed in this chapter, nurses need to be especially aware of what the older patient is taking, how it is being taken, and its effects. The Beers Criteria updated by the American Geriatrics Society identifies potentially inappropriate medication use in older adults (The American Geriatrics Society, 2012) (Table 15.2).

Older adults often have more than one chronic illness for which they take multiple medications. Polypharmacy can result in side effects that can be dangerous or duplication of medications with similar actions. Not only do HCPs need to be aware of prescribed medicines; they also need to review all over-the-counter medicines and self-prescribed extracts, elixirs, herbal remedies, herbal teas, cultural healing substances, and other home remedies that are being used by the older adult.

HCPs not only need to be concerned about overuse and combinations of medications but also misuse of them. If an older patient crushes a large enteric-coated pill so it can be taken in food and easily swallowed, destruction of the enteric protection can inadvertently cause damage to the stomach and intestinal system. Some patients intentionally skip prescribed doses as a way to save money. When prescribed doses are not being taken as expected, problems do not clear up as quickly, and new problems can result.

Be a patient advocate by working closely with older patients and their families on medication education. Patients need to know the purpose of each prescribed medicine, the importance of adherence to medication therapy, when a medication should be taken, how it should be taken, what food–beverage–medicine combinations are not safe, and the early and late side effects of the medicine that must be reported to the physician (see "Evidence-Based Practice").

TABLE 15.2 MEDICATIONS AND GERONTOLOGICAL ISSUES

Ten Medications to Use With Caution or Avoid in Older Adults	Rationale
Caution: Nonsteroidal Anti-Inflammatory Drugs (NSAIDs) Avoid: Long-acting NSAIDS (indomethacin, piroxicam)	Increases risk of indigestion, ulcers, bleeding in stomach or colon. Increases blood pressure, worsens heart failure, impairs kidneys.
Avoid: digoxin (Lanoxin) greater than 0.125 mg	Can become toxic in older adults and those with impaired kidney function.
Avoid: glyburide (Diabeta, Micronase), chlorpropamide (Diabinese)	Can cause severe low blood sugar.
Avoid: Muscle relaxants such as cyclobenzaprine (Flexeril), methocarbamol (Robaxin), carisoprodol (Soma)	Can cause grogginess, confusion, increase fall risk, constipation, dry mouth, urination problems.
Avoid: Medications for anxiety/insomnia such as benzodiazepines, including diazepam (Valium), alprazolam (Xanax), chlordiazepoxide (Librium); sleeping pills such as zaleplon (Sonata), zolpidem (Ambien)	Increases confusion, fall risk, and prolonged grogginess and sleepiness.
Avoid: Anticholinergic drugs such as amitriptyline (Elavil), imipramine (Tofranil), trihexyphenidyl (Artane), dicyclomine (Bentyl), oxybutynin (Ditropan)	Can cause blurry vision, low blood pressure, confusion, constipation, urination problems (caution with enlarged prostate).
Avoid: Demerol	Increases risk for seizures and confusion.
Avoid: antihistamines diphenhydramine (Benadryl), chlorpheniramine (AllerChlor, Chlor-Trimeton)	Can cause blurry vision, confusion, constipation, dry mouth, urination problems (caution with enlarged prostate).
Avoid unless prescribed for psychosis: haloperidol (Haldol), risperidone (Risperdal), quetiapine (Seroquel)	Increases risk of stroke or death. Causes tremors, other side effects, increase fall risk.
Avoid: Estrogen pills and patches	Increases risk for breast cancer, blood clots, dementia.

Note. For additional information on these medications, go to www.americangeriatrics.org/files/documents/beers/FHATipMEDS.pdf. From Ten Medications Older Adults Should Avoid or Use with Caution, April 2012. Retrieved August 6, 2013, from www.americangeriatrics.org/files/documents/beers/FHATipMEDS.pdf. Used with permission from the American Geriatrics Society.

Medication use, abuse, and misuse need to be addressed regularly with older persons. Concerns need to be closely monitored and promptly addressed. Older patients can be helped to adhere consistently to a prescribed medication routine through the use of visual and verbal reminders that have meaning for the patient. Encouraging proper medication use, self-care, and supportive independence helps everyone involved in the patient's medication management.

bitter oranges used to make orange marmalade) can interfere with the enzyme activity needed to break down some drugs in the digestive system. This can result in overly high levels of some drugs that can cause serious side effects and toxicity (Dolton, Roufogalis, & McLachlan, 2012).

Implications for Nursing Practice
Because grapefruit and some bitter orange citrus fruits can interfere with safe drug absorption, they should not be used with some medications until after approval by the pharmacist.

REFERENCE
Dolton, M. J., Roufogalis, B. D., McLachlan, A. J. (2012). Fruit juices as perpetrators of drug interactions: The role of organic anion-transporting polypeptides. *Clinical Pharmacology & Therapeutics, 92,* 622.

 EVIDENCE-BASED PRACTICE

Clinical Question
Can medications be taken with grapefruit juice?

Evidence
Research studies have shown that the chemicals found in grapefruit juice and pulp (as well as some

BE SAFE!

BE VIGILANT! For medication safety:

- Document a complete list of the patient's medications on admission by actively questioning the patient and family members.
- Make sure newly prescribed medications are compatible with the patient's current medications and reviewed by a pharmacist.
- Use at least two patient identifiers other than room number, such as patient name and birth date, when giving medications.
- Before the patient goes home, provide a complete written list of medicines and doses to the patient, family members, and the next caregiver or physician.

HEALTH PROMOTIONAL ROLE IN NURSING CARE OF THE OLDER PATIENT

Before the nurse is able to focus on health promotion and disease prevention, it is important to accurately determine the present health status of the older patient. When gathering **holistic** health data, the nurse focuses on the older patient's mind, body, and spirit, separately and in combination. Care must be taken to use valid and reliable data collection tools during this process to gain a true picture of the older patient's

condition, needs, and strengths. Listening and observing are two key nursing skills required to accurately obtain information from older patients because symptom patterns often differ between younger and older patients with the same health conditions. For example, older patients can have confusion rather than chest pain during a heart attack.

Health education is the most important health promotion tool for the nurse to use in the care of older patients. Educational efforts must first focus on erasing stereotypes about aging and erroneous associations between aging and illness. (For example, although research shows that urinary incontinence is not a normal sign of aging, many still think it is inevitable with old age.) Providing evidence-based health information at the right time, in the right amount, and in the right way can empower the older patient to value a proactive approach for wellness in old age. Once a health promotion approach is accepted, the nurse can work with the older patient in health screening, immunization updates, safety program participation, and activity planning aimed at an optimal level of functioning and wellness for the older patient (Table 15.3).

Gerontological Issues

Playing Nintendo Wii games such as bowling can be an enjoyable activity for the older adult. It can provide socialization, exercise and diversion to reduce boredom and loneliness. It is being used in settings such as long-term care.

TABLE 15.3 NURSING CARE FOCUS ON SAFETY ALPHABET FOR OLDER PATIENTS

A is for ABILITIES	• Know your abilities. • Know patient's abilities. • Base nursing actions on your abilities. • Seek out assistance when needed.
B is for BODY MECHANICS AND ALIGNMENT	• Use proper body mechanics. • Use appropriate assistive devices. • Ensure patient is in proper body alignment.
C is for COMFORT	• Ensure physical and emotional comfort during care. • Use pain scale during each assessment.
D is for DELIBERATE MOVEMENTS	• Plan ahead and communicate plans to patient. • Demonstrate confidence during care. • Alert patient to planned movements by saying, "Moving on three. One, two, three." • Ensure patient assists with moves as able.
E is for ENVIRONMENT	• Always place call light within reach. • Keep environment uncluttered and safe. • Ask patient's permission before moving items. • Put items back as patient prefers.

Continued

TABLE 15.3 NURSING CARE FOCUS ON SAFETY ALPHABET FOR OLDER PATIENTS—cont'd

F is for FALLS	• Remember that falls are a primary concern for older patients. • Use interventions to prevent falls: assist patients with ambulation, use assistive devices, answer call lights promptly, provide accessible toileting facilities, use nightlights, avoid use of throw rugs.
G is for GIVING YOUR TIME	• Allow more time to perform actions. • Do not rush older patients. • Provide time for listening and observing, so concerns are addressed before becoming problems.
H is for HAND HYGIENE	• Use correct hand hygiene protocols to protect yourself and older patients. • Use standard precautions to protect yourself and older patients.

Home Health Hints

Home Visits

• Schedule therapy visits and nurse visits on the same day, if possible, to decrease the risk of fatiguing the older patient.
• Because many older patients keep their homes warm, wear layers of clothing, removing a layer as needed, rather than adjusting the heat in the home.
• Place cell phones and pagers on a silent mode, if possible, to avoid startling or confusing the older patient.
• Do not assume that the older patient will remember the health care nurses who come to the door. Each time, state your name and why you are there. Wear a large-letter photo nametag that is in clear view.
• To enhance the effectiveness of a visit, ask the older patient to talk in a quiet room of the home with the main caregiver invited in at the appropriate time. This can help the older patient stay more focused while ensuring privacy and fostering the person's ability to hear.
• Stressors in a patient's life, such as annoying visitors, chastisement by caregivers, and harassment by bill collectors, are often experienced firsthand by the home health nurse. Document and share those with the home care team, so a coordinated approach can be taken.

Home Environment

• Making a sign for the door of the home giving visitors instructions, such as ringing the doorbell several times, knocking loudly, or using another door, can be helpful to visitors of the older patient. Do not provide specific information that would put the older person at risk for victimization.
• Assess the older patient's environment for safety hazards on each visit, and promote safety. Patients can easily trip on a scatter rug or fall trying to navigate around furniture. Urge the patient and caregiver to pack away scatter rugs and unneeded furniture.
• If the home is two stories, help the patient and caregiver consider how to relocate the bedroom to the first floor. Stairs are difficult to manage, especially if patients have visual disturbances or use an assistive device.
• Assist patients in obtaining a medical alert device that can be worn around the neck and activated in case of falls or other emergencies.

Medications

• Assist patients and/or caregivers with obtaining and setting up a weekly pill dispenser. These can be purchased at the local pharmacy. For patients who are forgetful, a pill dispenser with a timer can be purchased. An audible or visual alarm will go off when it is time for them to take medications.
• It is important for the home health nurse to assess the patient's ability to follow instructions. During visits, check the medication dispenser to ensure that pills are being taken as prescribed. If there is a concern, inform the primary care provider.

Nutrition/Fluids

• One of the first signs of dehydration is tachycardia. Instruct the patient regarding adequate hydration.
• If the older patient has dentures, assess if they are worn for eating. If not, assess why they are not worn (e.g., sores, improper fit from weight loss) and discuss solutions.
• Check the refrigerator for outdated food. Many older patients are on a limited budget and have been taught not to waste food. These factors, along with a decreased sense of smell and taste, can increase the risk of food poisoning.
• Encourage the uses of spices and herbs, such as parsley, oregano, lemon, garlic, and basil, instead of salt and sugar. Suggest keeping pared apples and segments of oranges in the refrigerator for snacks.

- If a Meals-on-Wheels program is available, ask if the older patient would like to be placed on the service.
- Use a warming tray when feeding an older patient who takes a longer time to eat.
- When swallowing is difficult, freezing of liquids helps, so they can be eaten with a spoon or like a popsicle. Milkshakes, high-protein drinks, instant breakfast mix, or eggnog are thicker liquids that are easier to swallow.

Elimination

- If an older person wears perineal pads or adult briefs, ask how many are used in a 24-hour period to assess the degree of incontinency or amount of output. Have the patient keep a voiding diary to further assess the degree of incontinence.
- Suggest a bedside commode when a weakened older patient is on diuretics or has a history of falling or confusion. Placing it next to the bed at night helps reduce the risk of falls and eases caregiver burden.
- If the older patient reports constipation, review the diet and make suggestions regarding adequate fluid and fiber. A mixture of equal parts of applesauce, bran, and prune juice is often helpful to prevent or relieve constipation. Discourage the use of mineral oil because it will interfere with vitamin absorption.

Rest

- If the older patient seems fatigued early in the day, ask about sleeping patterns and things that disturb it, such as barking dogs, traffic noise, and visitors. Recommend earplugs or changing rooms to obtain a good night's rest. Check medications for insomnia listed as a side effect and suggest dosing of these medications early in the day if appropriate. A 15- to 30-minute nap in the early afternoon can be helpful.

Infection Symptom

- One of the first signs of infection in the older patient is confusion.

Education

- Suggesting that limiting visitors or not allowing persons with colds to visit can be helpful in preventing illness in the older patient.
- When auscultating lungs, ask the older patient to take deep breaths slowly in and out through the mouth. This can stimulate coughing, which is an opportune time to teach deep-breathing and coughing exercises.
- When teaching, it is important to acknowledge the patient's knowledge and life experiences. When given a chance, patients tell how they have maintained their health over the years. Use open-ended scenarios for teaching such as, "What would you do if you fell and you were alone?"
- Teaching should occur *with* patients, not *to* them. The nurse is in the patient's home, which is a personal place. Patient dignity should always remain intact during home care visits and teaching sessions.

Lab Draws

- When drawing blood from the hand of an older patient, use the smallest needle possible and a butterfly device. Hold light pressure at the injection site for at least 2 minutes after the needle is removed.
- Do not use a bandage on the fragile skin of an older patient if the bleeding has stopped with pressure.

SUGGESTED ANSWERS TO
CRITICAL THINKING

■ *Mr. Jones*

1. Does he live alone? Does he have a history of falls? If so, does he wear a safety device to signal for help? What type of nightlight is used? How far is it to the bathroom? Does he take his bumetanide (Bumex) early in the day rather than at night? Does he void before going to bed? Does he anticipate needing to void 30 minutes after lying down?

2. Wood floors that are slippery when wet from incontinence are a safety hazard. Throw rugs can slide or cause tripping. An appropriate nightlight should be available.

3. Nursing diagnoses include *Functional Urinary Incontinence* related to distance to bathroom; *Deficient Knowledge* related to safety, medication administration, and nocturia; and *Risk for Injury* related to slippery floors from incontinence, use of throw rugs, and inadequate lighting.

4. A teaching plan should include the following:
   - *Safety:* Place urinal at bedside to prevent incontinence on way to bathroom. Consider red nightlight to improve vision and prevent falls. Use easily cleaned floor covering that is secure and absorbent to avoid falls. Consider the need for wearing a device that can send a signal for help.
   - *Medication administration:* Take diuretics early in the day to avoid having to get up frequently while sleeping at night.
   - *Nocturia:* Void before lying down. Anticipate need to void after lying down by reclining in chair for 30 minutes with legs elevated before going to bed and then void on way to bed.

5. Two 0.5-mg tablets.

REVIEW QUESTIONS

1. When planning care for the older adult, the nurse understands the definition of aging as being which of the following?
   1. A disease state that results in the death of a person's body cells all at once
   2. A condition that starts for all people when they reach the age of 65
   3. A maturational process with individual adaptations for physical and psychological changes over time
   4. A state of accelerating decline in body functioning directly related to a disease process

2. The nurse is collecting data on a patient who is 77 years old and says, "I am shorter now." The nurse would recognize that which of the following commonly contributes to individuals becoming shorter with age?
   1. Contractures
   2. Bone degeneration in the legs
   3. Hyperextension of the cervical spine
   4. Water loss from the intervertebral disks of the spine

3. Which of the following interventions should the nurse perform to protect skin integrity in the older adult?
   Select all that apply.
   1. Assess skin daily
   2. Apply moisturizer between toes
   3. Use gentle bathing techniques
   4. Gently massage nonreddened, intact skin sites
   5. Use hot water for bathing

4. Which of the following is the best approach for the nurse to use with a cognitively alert older patient recently diagnosed with hypertension that would help encourage prescribed antihypertensive medication compliance?
   1. The nurse says, "It is important that you take your blood pressure pill every day. Do you understand this?"
   2. The nurse explains the medication and gives the patient a grid to record daily when the pill is taken. The nurse then asks, "How do you see this working for you?"
   3. The nurse asks the patient, "Do you have a relative or friend who can call you every day to remind you to take your blood pressure pill? It is really important that you take it and as you get older it is harder to remember things."
   4. The nurse tells the patient, "If you don't take your blood pressure pill, you will probably have a heart attack or a stroke, so you better figure out a way that you don't forget to take it everyday."

5. The nurse contributes to the plan of care for an older patient on bedrest based on the understanding that pressure ulcers occur at sites of ischemia and can begin to develop as early as which of the following time frames?
   1. 5 to 10 minutes
   2. 20 to 40 minutes
   3. 50 to 60 minutes
   4. 75 to 120 minutes

6. The nurse is planning care for an older patient at risk for aspiration. Which of the following does the nurse understand would place the older patient at greater risk for aspiration?
   1. Increased lung capacity
   2. Decreased lung capacity
   3. Decreased gag reflex
   4. Increased gag reflex

7. Which of the following actions could the nurse institute to help prevent constipation in the older adult patient?
   Select all that apply.
   1. Increase dietary fiber intake.
   2. Decrease water intake.
   3. Encourage participation in ADLs.
   4. Review medication effects.
   5. Increase daily exercise.
   6. Decrease fresh fruit intake.

Answers can be found in Appendix C.

References

Centers for Disease Control and Prevention. (2012, February 29). *Falls in nursing homes.* Retrieved September 27, 2013, from www.cdc.gov/HomeandRecreationalSafety/Falls/nursing.html

U.S. Census Bureau. (2011). *The older population: 2010.* Retrieved September 27, 2013, from www.census.gov/prod /cen2010/briefs/c2010br-09.pdf

 DavisPlus For additional resources and information visit **davispl.us/medsurg5**

Nursing Care of Patients at Home

KELLY McMANIGLE

LEARNING OUTCOMES

1. Describe how the history of home health nursing has shaped the nursing care of today.
2. List the members of the home health team and their roles.
3. Compare and contrast hospital-based nursing care and home health nursing care.
4. Explain the steps involved in making a home health visit.
5. Explain safety practices for the nurse while making home visits.
6. Identify home safety interventions for the patient.
7. Describe methods of infection control the home health nurse uses.
8. Identify what is to be included in documenting a home visit with a patient.
9. Plan nursing interventions for the home health patient and caregiver.

KEY TERMS

autonomous (awe-TAH-nah-mus)
collaborative (cull-AB-rah-tiv)
respite (RES-pit)
telenursing (tell-a-nurs-ing)

INTRODUCTION TO HOME HEALTH NURSING

What do you think home health nursing care is? It is health care conducted in the home by qualified nurses. It is an important component of patient care. The Bureau of Labor Statistics (2012) indicates that there will be a 22% increased need for licensed practical/vocational nurses (LPN/LVNs) from 2010 to 2020. This increase in need will lead the LPN to positions in home health. Part of this increase is due to the aging baby boomer population (those born between 1946 and 1964) who will develop functional disabilities, patient preference for care in the home, and technological advances that are making complex care in the home cost-effective. LPN/LVNs need to understand how care is received in the home because the home and hospital settings differ.

HISTORY OF HOME HEALTH NURSING

Home care is not a new concept. Nurses have been caring for patients in their homes for more than 100 years. In 1893, Lillian Wald set out to improve the New York community in which she lived. Health care was available only to those who could afford it. Because of limited access to health care and lack of education, the home environment that poor families and immigrants were living in was not conducive to health and wellness. With the help of fellow nurse Mary Brewster, Wald established the Henry Street Settlement in New York City. The services started by Wald and Brewster laid the groundwork for establishing home care as a nursing specialty. Because of Lillian Wald and the nurses who worked with her, families were able to receive care and education in their homes to maintain or improve their health (Friends of Mt. Hope Cemetery, n.d.).

During the early 20th century, nurses took the initiative to develop community programs to meet the needs of the patients in their care. Nurses in the 21st century can learn from this and be involved in improving the communities in which they live. Home health nurses focus not only on the patient but also on the patient's family and the community. In home health care, nursing care and its differences from medical care can be truly understood.

HOME HEALTH ELIGIBILITY

Home health care requires skilled nursing care and must be delivered by a licensed professional nurse. Physical therapy and occupational therapy may also be needed, independent of nursing. A patient who is receiving home health nursing is required to be home bound. If patients are able to drive, then it is felt they are able to transport themselves to health care services. Patients are allowed to attend special events, go to church, or go to medical appointments and still be considered homebound. If the nurse suspects a patient is driving daily, he or she needs to reinforce eligibility for home health and suggest alternative options for health care to permit the patient to maintain independence. These options can include activities such as going to a clinic to have a blood pressure reading done, attending an outpatient physical therapy or occupational program, or having skilled needs (such as dressing changes) completed in a day surgery facility. If you have concerns about a patient, discuss them with the registered nurse (RN), who can work to assist the patient in receiving the needed care.

Home health services usually are ordered for care after discharge from the hospital when there is a need for skilled care in the home. Skilled care includes those skills that patients cannot complete alone and that require the interventions of a qualified nurse (Box 16-1).

It is not uncommon, however, for a health care provider's (HCP's) office to request home health services after seeing a patient in the office. For example, a patient who is having difficulty controlling blood glucose levels could benefit from having a nurse come to the home to assess how the patient is using a glucometer and what types of food are being purchased, to monitor the glucose level, and to teach the patient appropriate diabetic management. Another

---

Box 16-1 Skilled Activities for the Home Health Nurse

According to the Centers for Medicare and Medicaid (2011), which is the agency responsible for establishing home health rules and guidelines, a visit is considered "skilled and necessary" when the patient cannot perform the needed skill, there is no family member available to perform it, and the patient's medical issues make it necessary to have a licensed professional nurse monitor and manage the situation. Examples of skilled activities include:

- Dressing changes
- Administration of IV medications
- Management and assessment of newly inserted feeding tubes and tracheostomies
- Management and assessment of a new colostomy or urostomy
- Foley insertion and maintenance
- Patient and family education
- Monitoring a patient's status following a change in medications or condition
- Blood draws (only if the patient is receiving other home health services; this is not covered as an independent skilled visit)

If a family member is present and able to perform the skill part of the time, the nurse can teach that person how to perform the skill. The nurse may still complete skilled visits to monitor patient progress and attend to the patient's needs when family members are not available. It is important to remember that a skill must be involved, as discussed earlier. If the patient can manage the care either independently or with help from a family member, the services of a home health nurse may not be required.

example would be patients who cannot easily get to the HCP's office to have their blood pressure checked weekly. If the HCP has changed the patient's medications, he or she might need to make sure the adjustment is improving the patient's health as demonstrated by stable blood pressure readings. These types of visits are usually short term with the goal of facilitating independent care by the patient and/or family.

 BE SAFE!

BE VIGILANT! *Accurately and completely reconcile medications across the continuum of care. Use a process for comparing the patient's current medications with medications ordered for the patient while under the care of the organization. When a patient is referred, transferred, or discharged to home, a complete and reconciled list of the patient's medications should be documented and communicated to the next provider of service, the primary care provider, or the original referring provider, as well as to the patient and family. The list should be explained to the patient and family (2014 National Patient Safety Goals, © The Joint Commission, 2013. Reprinted with permission.).*

 THE HOME HEALTH CARE TEAM

With what members of the home health team might you collaborate? Home care is **collaborative**, and the LPN/LVN is an important part of the health care team. Teamwork and communication play a large part in ensuring that patients and their families receive the care they need (Fig. 16.1).

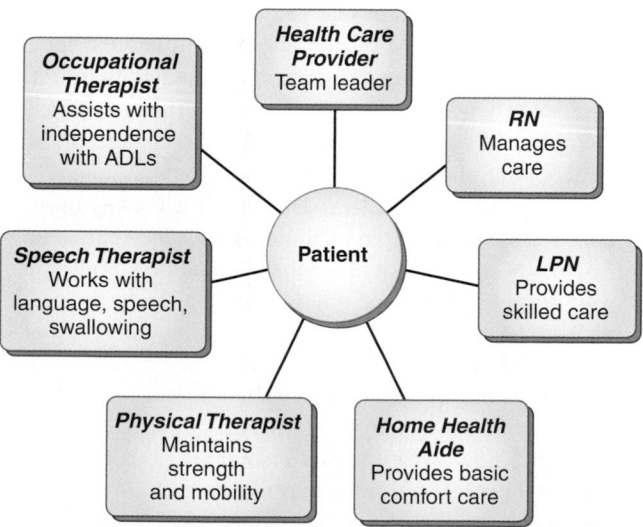

FIGURE 16.1 Home health team members and their roles.

OTHER MEMBERS OF THE HOME HEALTH TEAM

Social Services

Based on recommendations from the RN or hospital case manager, the HCP may order a social worker to evaluate community resources to assist the patient. Social services can be helpful in creating a link between the patient and resources available within the community. These resources can include meals on wheels, safety resources, or outreach programs.

Assisted Living Facilities

Home care may be provided in an assisted living facility for patients living in this type of facility. Because these facilities are not skilled nursing facilities, the facility staff is not able to perform nursing skills. Home health nurses need to understand the facility's policies when visiting a patient in assisted living and maintain communication with the facility staff regarding health care instructions (e.g., keep the dressing clean and dry).

CRITICAL THINKING

Mr. Rosa

■ Mr. Rosa, 75 years old, was just discharged from the hospital following an acute exacerbation of heart failure. You notice that he has little food in his house. It appears that the home has not been cleaned in several weeks and that the clothes he is wearing are torn and soiled. Talking with him, you learn that his wife died 6 months ago from cancer and he has had a difficult time adjusting to this loss.

1. What are some community services that might be available to Mr. Rosa?
2. What information would be important to discuss with Mr. Rosa's HCP?
3. Are there any other services that the home health agency can offer Mr. Rosa for patient centered care?

Suggested answers are at the end of the chapter.

 TRANSITION FROM HOSPITAL-BASED NURSING TO HOME HEALTH CARE

When working in the hospital, the nurse has many resources available, including resource staff such as other nurses, HCPs, respiratory therapists, and unit secretaries. Patients who enter the hospital are leaving behind the comfort of their own homes. They may be scared and isolated, trying to adjust not only to an illness but also to a new environment. The opposite is true in home health nursing. In the patient's home, the nurse is the visitor. There is no resource staff to answer questions, and the surroundings are unfamiliar. This can be a difficult adjustment for the nurse. As your confidence in being a home health nurse grows, so too will your comfort level with entering someone else's home.

Cultural Considerations

In the Hispanic culture, families may be large and their living spaces may be small. When you first enter such a home, you may have a feeling that the lack of space is unhealthy. It is important to realize, however, that this is part of the Hispanic culture. You must evaluate the overall home environment, not just its appearance. Chapter 4, *"Cultural Influences on Nursing Care,"* offers further discussion of transcultural nursing care.

It is important to remember that you have entered another person's home. Cultural issues need to be recognized and considered (see "Cultural Considerations"). Do not make quick judgments because the dishes are not done or the bed is not made. People have different values that may not always match yours. If the home is in such a state that it poses a health or safety risk, then it might be necessary to inform the RN.

Resources are not always quickly available when working in a patient's home. As such, it is important to have a good understanding of nursing skills. Home health nursing requires an ability to adapt and remain flexible because the home environment, unlike the hospital environment, can be unknown. Because of this, it is necessary to assess both the patient and his or her home setting.

Consider the patient who has been referred to home health services after a fall at home and subsequent fracture of an arm. The referral was to start physical therapy services, not skilled nursing. During the initial assessment, the nurse notes that the patient is lethargic and has extremely low blood pressure readings upon standing. Further data gathering of the home environment leads the nurse to find that the patient's wife has been giving too much of the patient's heart medication. The home health nurse can contact the supervising RN to obtain orders from the HCP to assess the patient's blood levels of this medication. This example demonstrates how nurses in the home need to evaluate the patient's case based not only on the referral diagnosis but also on what can be occurring within the home that could have contributed to that diagnosis.

Families play a large part in the care of patients in the home. Do not be surprised to walk into a home and find several anxious family members with a list of questions they would like answered. They will be very involved in your visits. This can be intimidating at first. When preparing for a visit, take the time to review and learn about an unfamiliar diagnosis or medication. Also be prepared for the unexpected. Carry extra common supplies such as various sizes of urinary catheters, sterile dressing gauze, different types of tape, and lots of alcohol wipes. This will help you feel more prepared and assist with developing a helping, trusting relationship with your patients and their families.

Because of the **autonomous**, or independent, nature of home health, most agencies require at least 1 year of medical-surgical nursing experience. This helps ensure that you have gained the basic knowledge needed to work in home care. You will continue to learn as you work in the home setting. Home health agencies also hire nurses for specialty areas such as cardiac or wound care. Nurses with a specific specialty will usually work with patients who have diagnoses within their specialty. See Box 16-2 for a review of liability issues.

THE ROLE OF THE LPN/LVN IN HOME HEALTH

The LPN/LVN's role in home health is varied and complex. Skilled care may be similar to those performed in the hospital setting, such as wound care, or medication administration (Fig. 16-2). The difference is the setting in which these skills are performed. Many factors need to be considered when

Box 16-2 Liability Issues to Consider When Working in Home Health Care

When starting in home health care, review your state's nurse practice act and your scope of practice. The National Council of State Boards of Nursing (www.NCSBN.org) lists all the state boards of nursing Web sites. This is a useful tool for any nurse.

Understanding your scope of practice will ensure that you complete care that follows your state's guidelines. When in patients' homes, they might ask you to perform a skill or request something that is outside your scope of practice. It is important that you explain to them that it is outside your scope of practice but still address their concern by contacting your agency immediately to find out how to handle their request. It is important to address their request because it could indicate a change in the status of their health.

For example, if a patient asks you if it is okay to increase a medication, you should understand that as an LPN/LVN, you cannot prescribe medications. So if you were to say it was okay, you would be altering the prescribed dose, and thus practicing outside your scope of practice because only an HCP can prescribe medications.

Always discuss your concerns with your supervisor and review your agency's guidelines, policies, and procedures. Know what you can and cannot do before you start, and never be afraid to question something that you feel or know violates your nurse practice act. Remember: It is your license, so follow your nurse practice act!

FIGURE 16.2 Patient receiving home IV therapy.

assisting patients in the home (e.g., having necessary supplies, infection control, patient education material, documenting, and personal and patient safety).

 STEPS IN THE HOME HEALTH VISIT

Preparing for the Visit

A typical day for the home nurse consists of six to seven home visits. These visits typically last 30 to 45 minutes. Most agencies try to arrange visits in the same geographical location for convenience. If your visits are focused on a specialty, such as wound care, you may have to travel long distances to visit your patients, but then you would be assigned fewer than seven visits. Agencies allow for mileage reimbursement, so be sure to keep close track of mileage from house to house.

The night before your visit, develop a plan of action for how your visits will be structured. Sometimes you will need to be at a certain place at a particular time, so factor this into your planning. Each patient needs to be contacted. Give the patient a 1- to 2-hour window for your arrival time. Remember, you cannot always anticipate what is going to happen during a visit. It is better to give your patients a time range as opposed to an exact time. If you are unsure how to locate your patient's home, ask for directions while you are arranging the visit time.

The agency will usually provide you with a form to use that reviews the patient's diagnosis, pertinent medical information, and reason for home health care. Writing directions

to the patient's home on these forms is an easy way to have the information close by. It is important for this process to be organized. If you have too many papers with information on them, it is difficult to manage both your time and the patient's needs, creating frustration for all.

 LEARNING TIP

Map sites on the Internet are a great place to find driving directions (see http://maps.google .com or www.mapquest.com). Simply type in starting and ending addresses to obtain detailed directions. Carry with you a map and cell phone—even the best of directions can be confusing once on the road. GPS apps are now available that the nurse can download to a cell phone, which will provide step-by-step instructions while driving.

If you are going to be late for any reason, contact the patient. Remember, these patients are homebound and often anxious. Arriving late can interfere with development of an effective therapeutic relationship.

Safety Considerations

Home health nurses' travels can take them to areas that are dangerous. It is important to be vigilant about personal safety. Box 16-3 lists tips on how to protect yourself before, during, and after a home health visit.

Patient safety in the home is also of importance. Stay alert to things in the home that can pose a hazard to the patient. Teaching the patient how to prevent injuries in the home is an essential intervention. Physical or occupational therapy can help the patient build strength, learn how to use assistive devices, and maintain safety. "Gerontological Issues" offers some ideas for patient safety considerations in the home.

 Gerontological Issues

Older adults make up a significant proportion of home health patients. Because of changes in their health, many items in patients' homes can become potential safety hazards. The home health nurse should always assess the patient's safety in the home. Things to look for are as follows:

• Overcrowded spaces
• Scatter/throw rugs
• Bathroom safety
• Adequate lighting
• Access to needed supplies
• Steps to enter the home
• Pets
• Electrical cords

Box 16-3 Safety Guidelines for Home Health Nurses

In general, providing home health services is a safe occupation. Most communities recognize the importance of the role of home health nurses and are receptive to their visits. It is still important to understand how you can protect yourself in case an unsafe situation arises.

Here are some tips for maintaining safety when completing a home health visit:

- Always carry a map, whistle, and cell phone.
- Keep your gas tank filled.
- Complete recommended maintenance on your car and have the tires checked regularly.
- If possible, park on the street or road in front of the house. This prevents someone from blocking you in the driveway.
- When entering a home, be aware of where the exit doors are and any windows that will allow safe evacuation from the home.
- Be aware of your outside surroundings. When leaving the home, have your supplies packed up and keys out, ready to open the car door.
- If lost in an unknown area, leave and go to a familiar place and contact the patient for directions. Call your agency if you are concerned about home safety.
- If you need to complete a visit at night, request an escort. Many communities will have a police officer accompany you to and from the home. Discuss this option with your supervisor.
- Never complete a visit if you feel concerned for your safety.

EVIDENCE-BASED PRACTICE

Patient Home Safety

Home health nurse resources for best practices for safety in the home can be found at such sites as www.champ-program.org. This information is current and relevant to home care. Topics available include toolkits with information on fall prevention, medication management, and transitioning to home care to prevent avoidable readmission to the hospital.

Infection Control

Maintaining asepsis in the patient's home may be a challenge. The home health agency will review infection control policies and procedures during in-service orientation. In the hospital, everything is available for infection control. In the home, the nurse is responsible for bringing supplies, provided by the home health agency, for safe care. Periodically go through

---

your equipment supply to make sure you have enough. It is always important to have extras of basic equipment, including the following:

- Personal protective equipment—disposable gowns, masks, goggles, and shoe covers
- Gloves, including latex-free gloves
- Biohazard bags and containers of various sizes
- Disposable underpads—can be used to provide a clean field for supplies; also used on the floor to place the home health bag
- Antibacterial soap
- Sanitizing liquid
- Disinfecting spray to clean equipment and bag after each visit
- Alcohol wipes for disinfecting thermometers and stethoscopes
- A small chemical spill kit

An important infection control measure is hand hygiene. It is important to wash your hands with soap and water before and after completing your patient care. If water is not available, use sanitizing liquid. Do not wash your hands in the patient's kitchen sink; always ask to use the bathroom for washing your hands.

Documentation

Because of reimbursement guidelines, the nurse needs to document specific things during the visit. Home health agencies receive their income based on a prospective pay system (predetermined rate), not per-visit payments. On admission, the RN fills out information that is entered into a computer system. This information is called the Outcome and Assessment Information Set, or OASIS-C. This tool is used to generate information about the home health agency and patient outcomes.

It is also used to help develop a plan of care that best meets the patient's problems. The LPN/LVN should be familiar with the general function of this form and its relevance to creating a plan of care.

For home health agencies to be reimbursed, they need to demonstrate that a skill was completed. Documenting information is based on the patient's plan of care and the corresponding skill that was completed at the visit. For example, the HCP orders skilled nursing observation and medication management for a patient. In documenting the visit for this order, the nurse needs to state that this skill was completed. Documentation would include the following:

• Patient's response to medication—vital signs, level of consciousness, or other potential side effects
• Patient's current understanding of medication regimen and the action the nurse took to improve that understanding
• Patient's response to that education and any areas in which the patient might continue to need assistance.

Home health agencies, like hospitals, have different ways of documenting. The following items are typically included in all agencies' home health documentation:

• Nurse's arrival and departure times
• Assessment findings
• Vital signs
• A narrative note
• Patient's signature verifying that the nurse was present in the home.

The documentation flow sheet is returned to the agency within an identified time frame (usually within 24 hours of a visit). Some agencies have secure drop boxes in which to leave paperwork after hours. When placing paperwork in the drop box, forms need to be neatly organized and attached together.

A folder with information is also kept at the patient's residence. It usually consists of relevant patient information and a communication form that all staff members complete at each visit. Similar to hospital charting, this documentation is important to ensure continuity of care. It is even more vital in the home setting because staff members might not cross paths for a verbal report.

 EVIDENCE-BASED PRACTICE

EBP and Documentation
OASIS-C, updated in 2012, is an assessment form that is completed by the RN during the first initial visit. Questions are related to identifying if problems exist beyond the referral diagnosis. It allows the RN to implement a plan of care that is evidence based, helping to eliminate potential complications and improve outcomes. These quality measures address the timeliness of care, care implementation, education, and prevention interventions. Indicators that can be flagged for further investigation by the RN include but are not limited to immunizations, falls, depression, pain, diabetic foot care, and heart failure. Additional information can be found at www.cms.gov.

The Agency for Healthcare Research and Quality is another resource to help guide the nurse in providing current care. A visit to www.qualitymeasures.ahrq.gov can offer information on disease specific care from the acute setting to home care. Follow links for "Measures"— "Disease and Conditions" (2013).

Patient Education

A primary responsibility of nurses in home health is educating patients about their illness and ways to effectively manage that illness at home with the intention of decreasing the need for hospitalization. Most home health agencies have handouts to help reinforce the verbal instructions the nurse provides. Many handouts are available from other sources as well, if needed.

 LEARNING TIP

An easy way to make sure you always have the handouts you need is to organize them into a three-ringed binder. Always have plenty of these handouts when making a visit. Many times, family members who do not live with the patient request copies so that they can have them at home. You can organize the information in several ways—for example, based on the diagnosis or alphabetically.

NURSING PROCESS FOR THE HOME HEALTH PATIENT

Data Collection

Monitor and document patient and family adjustment to change and illness. Perform a complete patient assessment during each visit. Assess the home environment for potential safety hazards and the need for devices to assist with care.

Nursing Diagnoses, Planning, and Implementation

***Ineffective Self Health Management** related to deficient knowledge, complexity of medical needs, and limited access to social support*
 EXPECTED OUTCOME: The patient will demonstrate changes in lifestyle needed to maintain health.

• Work with patient in developing both short- and long-term goals *to ensure patient's goals are being met.*
• Recognize small accomplishments positively *to reinforce patient's progress.*

- Educate patient on management of the health care regimen *to allow patient to carry out regimen.*
- Provide educational material in both written and verbal format *to promote understanding of complex issues.*
- Review plan of care with patient *to facilitate involvement and eventual independence.*
- Identify and work with social support systems *to meet patient's needs.*
- Help patient obtain needed supplies *to promote wellness.*
- Assess the home environment for hazards and assist patient with making needed changes *to promote safety.*
- Assess the patient for changes in health status *to detect changes that can affect progress.*

Risk for Caregiver Role Strain related to management of a chronic illness and lack of understanding of resources available

EXPECTED OUTCOME: The caregiver will identify effective ways for dealing with the complexity of a chronic illness.

- Include caregiver in the plan of care *to help develop an understanding of the management of the illness.*
- Assist caregiver with identifying community resources available such as **respite** care, Meals on Wheels, and support groups *to meet patient's needs.*
- Enlist the help of a social worker *to facilitate contact with community resources.*
- Assess caregiver's expectations of the patient's health. *Misconceptions regarding progress can foster anger and frustration toward the patient.*
- Discuss ways to help caregiver deal effectively with feelings of anger and frustration *to allow dealing with the feelings and issues causing them.*
- Acknowledge the change in roles (e.g., a child taking care of a parent) and the challenges associated with this change in family roles *to allow planning for the changes.*

Evaluation

The patient and caregiver will acknowledge acceptance and understanding of the change in health status. This is evidenced by involvement in the plan of care and participation with goal setting, use of community resources, maintenance of a safe home environment, and demonstration of ability to manage medical regimen.

 ## OTHER FORMS OF HOME HEALTH NURSING

Telenursing

Technology makes it possible to provide care in the home to patients in remote or rural areas, or after office hours. **Telenursing**, a branch of telehealth, uses information technology and telecommunication to provide nursing care. Various types of technology can be used including telephone, fax, e-mail, and video/audio conferencing. When it is time

for the nurse to visit a patient located a great distance away, the nurse connects with the patient via equipment set up in the patient's home. Because the nurse can see the patient, physical assessments can be made, including wounds. The nurse can then plan care and provide education to the patient. This form of home health care will likely grow as the aging population increases.

So far, this chapter has focused on home health care that is covered under the Medicare and Medicaid systems. The purpose of this type of home health is to assist the patient with managing health needs on an intermittent basis. Other types of home agency service work are also available for nurses, including private-duty nursing and hospice nursing (see Chapter 17).

Private Duty Nursing

Private-duty nursing consists of scheduled care to assist patients with personal and homemaking needs. These services have been called home companion services, homemaker services, and private-duty care. Many of these services focus more on companionship and respite care. Families who are taking care of a patient with complex needs, such as a patient with Alzheimer's disease, may need time away from the home to complete personal tasks. Agencies can provide both licensed and unlicensed assistive personnel (UAP) to help the patient while the family is away. These services are considered an out-of-pocket expense and are not covered by Medicare and Medicaid.

Families can contract with an agency to have a staff member spend 2 to 3 hours a day in the home. The staff can complete homemaking tasks and companion tasks, such as arts and crafts or playing cards. Nurses can work in these agencies in the role of supervisor to UAP. Nurses also may be involved in helping patients fill weekly medication dispensers. Many nurses enjoy this type of work because of the relationships that are formed with patients and families. They may be involved with the same family for months to years, as opposed to a few months, as is typical with Medicare home health patients.

 ## SUMMARY

Home health nursing is a rewarding career path. Nurses who work in the home have the unique opportunity to assist patients during times of crisis and to experience the results of their interventions. Home health nursing will continue to grow in the 21st century, and the need for qualified professionals will offer many opportunities for the LPN/LVN. Thinking back on the impact that nurses such as Lillian Wald had and her ability to change the lives of so many because of her willingness to meet those patients in their homes, one can see the importance that home health nurses have in the successful progression for patients from illness to health and wellness.

SUGGESTED ANSWERS TO

CRITICAL THINKING

■ *Mr. Rosa*

1. The loss of Mr. Rosa's wife and his subsequent health problems have affected his ability to properly care for himself. A nutritional diet is important for healing and maintenance of health. A referral to Meals on Wheels would be appropriate. This agency will deliver at least one healthy meal each weekday (usually lunch). The meal can be adapted to meet the patient's dietary guidelines.

   Many communities offer elder services to patients at a reduced cost to assist with housekeeping services. Helping the patient set up homemaker services will help him through this difficult time. Offering the patient information about grief counseling services in the community can be beneficial during this time. Once discharged from home health, the patient can begin attending counseling services. Other community resources to consider are neighborhood socials, church services if appropriate, and online communities that match the patient's values.

2. The HCP needs to be contacted about the patient's withdrawn demeanor and lack of interest in self-care. Mr. Rosa may be experiencing a situational depression because of the recent loss of his wife and his own health problems. During this time, the HCP might decide to prescribe an antidepressant to help.

3. The nurse recognizes that Mr. Rosa needs extra help at this time. Consider a referral for social services to assist with community resources and grief counseling. Because heart failure is a chronic disease that can contribute to fatigue, an occupational therapist can work with the patient in developing energy-conserving techniques for completing activities of daily living. Also the services of a home health aide can help with personal care and provide additional emotional support.

■ *Mrs. Ambani*

1. Because anemia can cause extreme fatigue, it is important for Mrs. Ambani to have safety devices in the home to prevent falls. These devices can be obtained from a medical supply store and are usually covered by Medicare. Equipment to consider includes a bath stool for the shower so the patient can sit while bathing, a detachable shower head, handrails in the shower and hallways, a bedside commode, an over-the-toilet seat, a reacher to assist with obtaining objects at a distance, a medical alert device that can be worn at all times, and, if fatigue is severe enough, a motorized wheelchair.

2. The home has many hazards. Important things to assess for include scatter/throw rugs, overcrowded spaces, sharp edges along furniture, inadequate lighting, and stairs. Instruct the patient to keep frequently used kitchen appliances and foods on shelves that are easy to reach. The same is true for the bathroom and bedroom. Assist the patient with setting up a "command center" in the living room so that favorite items are kept in proximity and the patient does not have to get up so frequently.

3. Links include checklist on assisting with fall prevention in relation to vision loss, medication safety, and general fall preventions. These checklists can be left in the home. Assessment forms that the nurse can use offer topics on orthostatic protocols and environmental safety.

REVIEW QUESTIONS

1. What impact did Lillian Wald have on the nursing profession?
   1. Allowed nurses to function as medical care providers.
   2. Demonstrated the impact nursing can have on patients' health and wellness.
   3. Made it possible for nurses to obtain prescription drugs for patients in the home.
   4. Developed the Henry Street Settlement in 1890.

2. Which of the following are members of the home health team? **Select all that apply.**
   1. LPN/LVN
   2. Health care provider
   3. Social worker
   4. Home health aide
   5. Lawyer
   6. Patient

3. A patient is being seen by home health nurses for monitoring of weight and vital signs and education about medication changes following an acute exacerbation of heart failure. The nurse must document which of the following?
   1. What the patient ate for breakfast
   2. Distance the patient was able to ambulate while working with physical therapy
   3. Education about the role of the home health aide in assisting the patient with personal care
   4. Education about how to keep a log of daily weights and when to contact the HCP about a potential problem

4. An LPN/LVN has started working for a local home health agency and is concerned about the transition to home health nursing after working in the hospital for 10 years. What are some recommendations that would ease this transition for the LPN/LVN?
   1. Explain that home health nursing is just like hospital nursing.
   2. Instruct the nurse to always be prepared, to keep paperwork organized, and spend some time the night before a visit to review patient health information to help gain confidence in the home.
   3. Allow an opportunity for exploring feelings and acknowledging that this is a hard transition.
   4. Let the nurse know it is not possible to completely adjust to home health nursing because of variability in the home.

5. What steps can the home health nurse take to ensure that a patient is not exposed to infectious materials in the home?
   1. Disinfect the home health bag after each patient visit with a germicidal spray supplied by the home health agency.
   2. Perform hand hygiene in the kitchen sink rather than the bathroom sink.
   3. Use the same red bag from patient to patient for disposing of soiled dressings.
   4. If a chemical spill occurs, contact the agency to send personnel to clean it up.

Answers can be found in Appendix C.

References

Bureau of Labor Statistics, U.S. Department of Labor. (2012). *Occupational outlook handbook, 2012–13 edition: Licensed practical and licensed vocational nurses.* Retrieved June 4, 2013, from www.bls.gov/ooh/healthcare/licensed-practical -and-licensed-vocational-nurses.htm#tab-6

Centers for Medicare and Medicaid Services. (2011). *The home health agency manual.* Retrieved June 4, 2013, from www .cms.gov/Regulations-and-Guidance/Guidance/Manuals /downloads/bp102c07.pdf

Centers for Medicare and Medicaid Services. (2012). *OASIS-C user manual.* Retrieved June 4, 2013 from www.cms.gov /Medicare/Quality-Initiatives-Patient-Assessment-Instruments /HomeHealthQualityInits/HHQIOASISUserManual.html

Collaboration for Homecare Advances in Management and Practice (CHAMP). (2009). Retrieved June 4, 2013, from www.champ-program.org

Friends of Mt. Hope Cemetery. (n.d.). *Famous women in Mt. Hope Cemetery: Lillian Wald (1867–1940).* Retrieved September 16, 2009, from www.fomh.org/Data/Documents /Lillian_Wald.pdf

Joint Commission. (2013). *2013 national patient safety goals.* Retrieved June 4, 2013, from www.jointcommission.org /patientsafety/nationalpatientsafetygoals

U.S. Department of Health and Human Services. (2013). *Measures; disease and conditions.* Retrieved June 4, 2013, from www.qualitymeasures.ahrq.gov

 DavisPlus | For additional resources and information visit **davispl.us/medsurg5**

17

Nursing Care of Patients at the End of Life

BETSY MURPHY

LEARNING OUTCOMES

1. Identify characteristics of the patient who is approaching the end of life.
2. List necessary legal documents for patients with life-limiting illness.
3. Explain choices that are available to patients at the end of life.
4. Demonstrate appropriate communication with dying patients and their families.
5. Describe physical changes to expect during the dying process.
6. Plan nursing interventions for patients at the end of life.
7. Describe postmortem care.
8. Plan nursing interventions for the grieving patient and family.
9. Discuss the role of the LPN/LVN in hospice care.

KEY TERMS

advance medical directive (ad-VANSE MED-ih-kuhl dur-EK-tiv)
advocate (ADD-vuh-ket)
artificial feeding (ART-ih-FISH-uhl FEE-ding)
artificial hydration (ART-ih-FISH-uhl hy-DRAY-shun)
do not resuscitate (DNR) (DOO not re-SUSS-ih-TATE)
durable power of attorney (DUR-uh-buhl POW-ur OV uh-TUR-nee)
hospice (HOS-pis)
living will (LIH-ving WIL)
palliative (PAH-lee-uh-tiv)
postmortem care (pohst-MOR-tum KARE)

Mr. Moran, 89 years old, resides in a long-term care facility and has been losing weight and growing weaker for the past 6 months. Despite treatment for depression, he continues to grow weaker and more dependent on his caregivers. As you read this chapter, consider what decisions his family will face and what resources are available to them in their quest to provide appropriate care for him.

A GOOD DEATH

Despite our best efforts, there will come a time when all our patients will die. Death is the expected end to a life well lived. In America, only 10% of us will die suddenly. The remaining 90% will experience a gradual decline over a period of months or years.

In the 21st century, most Americans will die from chronic and acute illnesses such as cancer, heart disease, stroke, and dementia. We have the technology to prolong life, but sometimes this longer life can carry with it profound disability and reduced quality of life. Our patients sometimes tell us that this is not what they intended for the last phase of their life. So what is the role of the nurse with patients nearing the end of life? Two priorities are (1) to help identify patients with life-limiting illnesses early so that they and their families have the opportunity to redefine their goals of care and (2) to help our patients communicate their wishes to health care providers (HCPs), both orally and in writing, to ensure that their wishes are understood.

Perhaps the most important role for nurses is to give our patients support and validation as they move through the series of losses leading to a good death. Dying is, after all, the final phase of our growth and development. The developmental tasks associated with this phase involve reflecting on our lives, saying goodbye, saying, "I'm sorry," and saying, "I love you." The goal of having a "good death" is a valid goal.

There have been multiple studies focused on identifying the needs of terminally ill patients and their families (Gardner & Kramer, 2010). The findings fit into five categories:

- Adequate pain and symptom management
- Ability to make their own decisions
- Avoidance of unnecessary life-sustaining treatment and prolongation of the dying process
- Reducing the emotional and financial burden on their families
- Ability to use remaining time to strengthen relationships with loved ones

This description of a good death helps nurses listen to what patients want and to focus on how best to help them achieve their goals. Nurses who choose to provide care for the dying will experience personal growth in their own lives. Facing the inevitability of our own mortality can force us to look more deeply at our beliefs, values, and priorities in life. This can result in a richer, more focused life.

IDENTIFYING IMPENDING DEATH

Most Americans say that they want to die at home. Home for many patients will mean the place they are most comfortable, surrounded by caregivers who understand their needs and provide attentive care. Home can be where they live independently or with their families. It can also be in a continuing care retirement community, assisted living facility, or nursing home. In the United States, 30% to 40% of older adults die in long-term care facilities. A surprising 80% of older patients die within a year of admission to a nursing home (Kelly et al, 2010). Nurses who are working in long-term care and assisted living facilities will find themselves in a position both to identify patients who are likely to die soon and also to support these patients' families in planning for a good death. Because so many patients die within months of admission to long-term care, identification of their wishes should be done soon after admission. If a frail older patient's wishes are not documented and the person becomes ill, he or he will be routinely transported to the hospital, possibly to receive unwanted treatments.

How can you identify patients who are nearing the end of their lives? Some patients die because of disease, but some patients simply show weight loss and progressive weakness as signs that they are in the final months of life. Research has shown that measuring both weight loss and increasing dependency in activities of daily living (ADLs) can help to identify patients who are dying. Weight loss is a useful marker of mortality risk in older adults (Alley et al, 2010). Weight loss caused by depression or acute illness can sometimes be reversed with aggressive treatment. But if neither depression nor acute illness is the cause of the patient's decline, he or she may be entering the final months of life. Worsening symptoms may also be an indicator of decline. One study shows that 25% of older men had pain in their final 2 years of life, and 50% to 60% of men had pain in the final months of life (Smith et al, 2010).

Older patients who are having trouble swallowing and require treatment for aspiration pneumonia are likely to die within a year. Their decreased respiratory muscle strength, lack of lung elasticity, and poor immune response make recovery unlikely. Older patients with poor renal and cardiac functions are also at high risk for dying. The final truth is that for some older patients with chronic illness, many treatments offer little benefit.

For most patients, the transition from treating an illness to allowing the patient to die is a gradual process. Figure 17.1 shows the evolving relationship between treatments intended to cure and treatments intended to comfort as the patient approaches the end of life. As curative therapies are reduced, comfort care, or **palliative** measures, are increased. This chapter explores some of the choices people need to make at the end of life and the interventions you can use to help patients during this time.

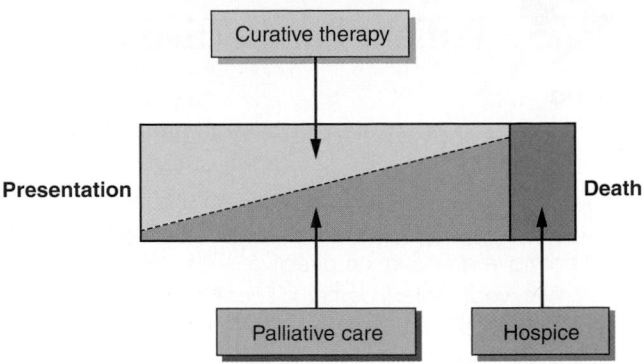

Simultaneous Care Model

FIGURE 17.1 The simultaneous care model. From Emanuel, L. L., von Gunten, C. F., & Ferris, F. D. (Eds.). (1999). *The Education for Physicians on End-of-Life Care [EPEC] Curriculum.* Chicago: The EPEC Project. Copyright Robert Wood Johnson Foundation.

ADVANCE DIRECTIVES, LIVING WILLS, AND DURABLE MEDICAL POWER OF ATTORNEY

The Patient Self-Determination Act, which took effect in 1991, ensures that every patient has the right to accept or refuse any medical treatment that is offered. The act also requires HCPs to ask patients entering a hospital if they have prepared **advance medical directives**. These include a **living will** and a **durable power of attorney** for health care. In preparing advance medical directives, patients are exercising their right to make their wishes known regarding specific medical treatments they would want—or not want—if they become unable to make decisions on their own. The directives require the signatures of two witnesses; neither can be a family member or HCP.

A living will is a document instructing HCPs about a patient's preferences (such as to withhold or withdraw life-sustaining procedures) if the patient is unable to communicate, found to be permanently unconscious, and/or has been declared "terminal." A durable power of attorney for health care specifies who will speak for a patient when he or she cannot speak. Many states provide standard forms to use and may require the patient to have both a durable power of attorney for health care and a living will to ensure the patient's wishes are followed. An attorney, although not required, may be helpful for some families.

Encourage patients not only to fill out the necessary forms but also to discuss their wishes with all family members. It is estimated that only about 20% to 30% of Americans have advance medical directives. Some patients are reluctant to complete them, concerned that they may change their minds about treatments in the future. It can be helpful to talk about advance care planning as a *process.* Patients can change their minds at any time about any treatment and write new advance directives. What matters most is that they get started and document their wishes today.

END-OF-LIFE CHOICES

Cardiopulmonary Resuscitation

During the 1960s, cardiopulmonary resuscitation (CPR) was developed as a method of rescuing healthy people who suffered a cardiac or respiratory arrest. Some of the early guidelines specified that CPR was not to be used in patients with terminal illnesses. It was intended for healthy patients with reversible conditions. Today, CPR has become standard in both hospitals and long-term care facilities. All patients receive CPR unless they have a **do not resuscitate (DNR)** order. There is also a perception that CPR can save most lives. The real statistics about CPR are presented in Table 17.1.

One reason for the low survival rates shown in Table 17.1 is that CPR must begin within 3 to 5 minutes of collapse. The most successful cases are ones in which CPR plus an automatic external defibrillator (AED) are used within 3 to 5 minutes of collapse. Patients who are not in a hospital and who survive after CPR have a 5% chance of living for 1 year (Fairbanks et al, 2007). CPR success in a hospital setting depends greatly on the patient's age. The best rate of CPR success is 10% in the 40- to 59-year age group. In patients over age 80 years, the CPR success rate declines to 3%. In patients over age 90 years, it declines further to 1% (Swor et al, 2008).

Some patients choose to have CPR because they fear that without CPR, they will be deprived of treatments that will benefit them or alleviate their distress. Most patients do not realize that their chance of survival is statistically low and also that after CPR, if they survive, their quality of life may be diminished. A small number of patients erroneously believe that CPR is a procedure that may improve their overall medical condition. A helpful way of presenting the DNR option is to talk about three issues: (1) the statistics outlined here; (2) that the choice is really whether the patient will receive aggressive comfort care as he or she is dying a natural death or CPR, which may cause distress and will likely prove futile; and (3) even if older patients receive successful CPR, their quality of life afterward is usually greatly reduced, not improved.

TABLE 17.1 SUCCESS OF CARDIOPULMONARY RESUSCITATION IN SAVING LIVES

In hospital: all patients	10%–15% survival rate
In hospital: older adult patients	Less than 5% survival rate
Out of hospital: all patients	Less than 5% survival rate
Nursing home patients	1%–2% survival rate

Do Not Resuscitate Orders

A "No Code" or DNR order is written in a hospital or long-term care facility after collaboration with the patient, family, and the HCP, usually after it has been determined that the patient will not benefit from CPR. A DNR order simply means that CPR will not be done. Patients must still decide whether they want aggressive treatment of their underlying condition, up to but not including CPR, or whether they want only comfort measures without therapeutic treatment. Some hospitals offer several options:

- DNR/Comfort Care Only
- DNR/Full Therapeutic Support
- Full Code

Outside the hospital, at home, or in most nursing facilities, patients will have fewer options for aggressive treatment. Patients can, however, choose to have a DNR order that will be recognized by emergency personnel. Many states have a Durable DNR document that, once signed, can be displayed in the patient's home to advise rescue personnel that the patient does not want CPR. These may also be called out-of-hospital or prehospital DNR orders.

Many people assume that their documented desire not to receive resuscitation in a living will is all that is needed. This is not correct. In states that have an out-of-hospital DNR policy, patients must also complete the durable DNR document or they will receive CPR regardless of their stated wishes. There is also a new document for patients with life-limiting illness called Physician Orders for Life Sustaining Treatments (POLST). This document is signed by both the patient or the patient's decision maker and the patient's physician. This is a physician's order for emergency medical services (EMS) to follow. The order can specify whether the patient wants CPR and list the patient's choice of treatments. EMS workers are trained to look for such a document, often in a bright color and hanging on the patient's refrigerator.

Some patients fear that in choosing DNR status, they will suffer and be alone at the time of their death. Patients and families may erroneously perceive DNR as withholding a treatment that could benefit the patient. It is important to tell patients that DNR does not mean *do not treat*. Patients who have a DNR/Comfort Care Only order will still receive oxygen, medications, and other comfort measures to aggressively manage their symptoms and ensure a comfortable death. A gentler way of discussing this choice may be to ask patients and families if they prefer to allow natural death. All DNR orders and discussions with families should be documented on the patient's chart (see "Patient Perspective—Anna").

Artificial Feeding and Hydration

Patients may be unable to eat or drink as a result of three conditions: an acute illness, a long illness with multiple medical problems, or simply the aging process. Otherwise, healthy patients who are unable to eat while recovering from an acute illness will probably benefit from artificial feeding. An example of this would be a cancer patient receiving total parenteral nutrition (TPN; see Chapter 7) or tube feeding to prevent weight

Patient Perspective

Anna

My mom, Anna, was diagnosed with cardiomyopathy and congestive heart failure when she was 60 years old. At that time, she was still working and had just remarried. She thought she had many years left in life. She did not have an advance directive—why would she?

Two years later, as her disease progressed, she decided she did not ever want to "live on machines." So with the help of her doctor and our family, she wrote her living will and made her new husband her durable power of attorney for health care, with me as his backup person. Because she was still functioning really well with lots of medications and occasional hospitalizations, she chose a DNR status, but with full therapeutic, aggressive interventions. She even took a tour of Europe during this time in her life, knowing she would not be able to do it later.

By age 67, she had a lot less energy to do things, and her heart failure really cramped her lifestyle. But she still enjoyed life, and her goal was to see her oldest grandson, my son, graduate from high school. She considered a heart transplant, but her doctor told her she was too old to qualify. She did have a new kind of valve surgery that was supposed to make her feel better, but it didn't help much.

Three months after my son's graduation, she was hospitalized several times with progressively worse outcomes. She weighed barely 100 pounds and could not eat much. She was only 70 years old, and still looked and acted so young! Finally, she was in a semi-coma in the hospital, and our family had to make the difficult decision to withdraw all therapeutic support. She was now a DNR, with comfort measures only. We were confident this would be what she wanted because we had talked about it with her. She was alert enough to let us know that she wanted to die at home.

She was discharged home with hospice care and died within a week. I moved in for her final days to help out, and between her husband and me, her hospice nurse (who was a godsend), and frequent visits from family and her minister, she was well cared for. We kept her comfortable with lots of attention and morphine. She was alert and able to converse much of the time. She ate what and when she wanted, which amounted to one-quarter of a cheese and tomato sandwich one day, but she enjoyed it! She could finally enjoy a glass of grapefruit juice, which she had been unable to have for years because it interacted with one of her heart medications.

At the end, she died with me holding her left hand and her husband holding her right. We were telling her we loved her. It was a good death.

CRITICAL THINKING

Mrs. Hart

■ Mrs. Hart has written a living will specifying her wishes should she become incapacitated. Because she has advanced disease, she tells you she would not want to be resuscitated if she has a cardiac arrest. She is currently hospitalized but will be discharged to her home in a few days.

1. What documents does she need to have in place to ensure she will not receive resuscitation?
2. What health team members should you collaborate with in helping Mrs. Hart through this process?

Suggested answers are at the end of the chapter.

loss while receiving a treatment such as chemotherapy or radiation that is known to cause weight loss. In contrast, patients who are losing weight because of a life-limiting illness with multiple medical problems or the aging process itself will probably not benefit from artificial feeding. Research has shown that "no strong evidence exists supporting the use of parenteral hydration/nutrition for the majority of terminally ill patients" (Dev, Dalal, & Bruera, 2012). "Terminally ill patients" includes not just patients declining from advanced cancer but also patients with life-limiting diseases such as Alzheimer's dementia, Parkinson's disease, and other conditions.

It is now widely accepted that feeding advanced dementia patients via feeding tube does not prolong their life or enhance their quality of life. Despite this fact, many patients continue to receive feeding tubes because their families are not consistently provided with evidence-based information to make good decisions (Teno et al, 2011). Providing families this evidence-based information as part of advance care planning can help families to make the best possible decisions for their loved ones. The Alzheimer's Association provides educational information for families of patients with dementia. It recommends that instead of a feeding tube, these patients receive an effective program of hand feeding (www.alz.org).

When a patient is recognized as having entered the dying phase, medical treatment should contribute to comfort. Research suggests the benefits of artificial nutrition and hydration may be limited and may not outweigh the burdens (Raijmakers et al, 2011). There are some benefits to withholding **artificial feeding** and **artificial hydration** in the final weeks of life in all actively dying patients. These benefits are:

• Fewer pharyngeal and lung secretions, which can reduce dyspnea
• Reduced swelling around tumors, which can reduce associated pain
• Less urination, resulting in dryer skin with less skin breakdown

It has been theorized that as dehydration occurs, the body produces a form of endorphin that enhances comfort. As

ketone levels rise from the breakdown of body fat, patients experience an anesthetic effect that creates a sense of well-being. Families often express concern that the patient will experience hunger or thirst. Hospice providers report observational evidence that dying patients do not report hunger but do report having a dry mouth. Mouth dryness can be easily managed with good mouth care.

The issue of feeding is emotionally difficult for families. Often their loved one has been ill a long time. Bringing favorite foods may have been one of the ways they showed love and communicated caring. Families will need support in making decisions about feeding in three important ways:

• Identifying goals of care and evaluating whether artificial feeding will help meet those goals
• Weighing the benefits and burdens of feeding
• Finding new ways (besides feeding) to communicate their love, such as skin care, mouth care, or reading to their loved one

For a different perspective on artificial feeding, see "Ethical Considerations" for Chapter 17 at davispl.us/medsurg5.

Hospitalization

A hospital is where patients go to receive aggressive medical treatment. The goal of care in a hospital is to improve the patient medically and transfer him or her to an appropriate level of care that will better meet individualized needs. There are burdens associated with hospitalization for older adult patients approaching the end of life. They may actually decline more rapidly in a hospital setting. When removed from a setting with predictable routines and known caregivers, the older patient often eats less and becomes at risk for weight loss. Research has shown that all older adult patients suffer accelerated cognitive decline after hospitalization (Wilson et al, 2012). They enter a foreign environment and are cared for by health care workers who do not know them. Patients may be physically restrained as they become agitated and fearful while away from home. Patients who are frail and have poor immunity are at risk for developing infections. They often enter the hospital with one infection and are discharged with other infections that may be resistant to antibiotics or caused by antibiotics, such as *Clostridium difficile*. There is evidence that receiving antibiotic therapy for infection may prolong survival in some patients with advanced dementia, but patients who received antibiotics had more discomfort than those who received no antibiotics (Givens, Jones, Shaffer, Kiely, & Mitchell, 2009). Helping families decide on goals for the patient's care will help with making decisions in the future. If the patient or family decides on comfort care only, then going to the hospital or receiving antibiotics may not meet their goal.

Patients living in nursing facilities with end-stage dementia who have severe cognitive impairment will benefit from having a "do not hospitalize" order. This will maintain the patient in an environment that feels safe and preserves his or her chosen quality of life. Having hospice care in place (see next section) in nursing facilities can help reduce hospitalizations (Dobbs, Meng, Hyer, & Volicer, 2012).

Hospice Care

Many people think of **hospice** as a place. It is actually a service. The service is provided in private homes or independent and assisted living facilities. It can also be provided in hospitals and nursing homes when there is a signed contract between the hospice organization and the facility. To qualify for hospice care, a patient must have an estimated prognosis of 6 months or less. Patients can receive hospice care longer than 6 months as long as their health continues to decline.

Some indicators of a 6-month or less prognosis (regardless of diagnosis) are 10% loss of weight in 6 months, functional decline, frequent hospital admissions, and recurrent infections. The goal of hospice care is holistic: to manage symptoms such as pain and nausea, to provide emotional and spiritual counseling for the patient and family, and to support the patient in achieving his or her goals of care. Each patient is assigned a multidisciplinary hospice team (Table 17.2) to assist with care.

Most health insurance companies now provide a hospice benefit. Many are modeled after the Medicare hospice benefit. The Medicare benefit pays for both routine hospice care at home and for inpatient hospice care provided in a contracted hospital, skilled nursing facility, or freestanding hospice unit. Medications, medical supplies, oxygen, and medical equipment are also covered if they are related to the terminal diagnosis.

Hospice care can help a family take care of a patient at home, but hospice nurses do not routinely provide 24-hour in-home care. (A nurse is on call for in-home visits 24 hours a day.) Nurses and other team members make regular visits to support the patient and family. In times of medical crisis, short-term inpatient hospice services or 24-hour in-home continuous nursing care may be provided under some hospice benefits.

COMMUNICATING WITH PATIENTS AND THEIR LOVED ONES

Terminal illness is a family experience. Family is defined by the patient and may include blood relatives, friends, significant others, or partners. The primary role of the nurse is to facilitate a comfortable death that honors the choices of the patient and family. The nurse, therefore, becomes the **advocate**, assuring that patient and family wishes are communicated to other members of the health care team. In addition, the nurse is often the professional caregiver and educator of the nonprofessional caregivers and family.

To successfully work with dying patients and families, you must demonstrate empathy, unconditional positive regard, trustworthiness, and critical thinking. You are part of an interdisciplinary team. The team consists of the HCP, nurse, social worker, chaplain, and others. Each discipline has expertise and can lend support to the others in providing care. As illustrated in the earlier section on end-of-life choices, patients and their loved ones need support and evidence-based information to make good decisions. All members of the team can assist with this support.

Good communication requires that you take time to listen, answer questions honestly, help identify choices, and allow verbalization of fears. Eighty percent of communication is nonverbal, such as eye contact, body language, and tone of voice. Take time to identify your own communication barriers that will affect your ability to talk with families. Do you have fears about your own mortality or lack personal experience with death? Do you fear being blamed for decisions, or disagree with decisions that were made? These barriers will affect your ability to sit with patients and families in crisis, sustain eye contact, and support them in their process. Practice attentive listening with patients and families. Allow them to talk. Be silent, don't change the

TABLE 17.2　THE HOSPICE TEAM

Physician or other HCP	Works with the patient's primary HCP, offering suggestions to improve care. Directs team activities and often will make visits to the patient's home.
Nurse	Makes routine home visits, assessing patient needs and implementing plan of care. Nurses are available 24 hours per day to make visits as needed.
Social worker	Provides emotional counseling and long-term planning, assists patients with insurance issues, and helps identify community resources.
Chaplain or minister	Provides spiritual counseling or coordinates care of spiritual issues with the patient's chosen spiritual counselor. May participate in funeral or memorial service.
Home health aide	Provides personal care, linen changes, light housekeeping.
Volunteers	Support caregivers by staying with the patient while they get out of the house. May also read to patient, run errands, etc.
Bereavement counselor	Provides counseling for family and significant others for 13 months after patient's death.

subject, and know that you do not need to have all the answers. Your role can be to help them reflect on what they are trying to communicate and to clarify their goals of care so you can better advocate for them.

Set the stage for communication by sitting down to show you are not in a hurry (Fig. 17.2). Maintain eye contact, encourage patients to speak, repeat what they say to gain clarification, and reflect on its meaning. Some things to say to facilitate good communication include the following:

- "Do you feel like talking?"
- "Tell me more about your fears of . . . . "
- Repeat back what you hear: "You mentioned you were upset by . . . . "
- Reflect: "So are you saying that . . . ?"

FIGURE 17.2 Nurses can be a comfort to patients and family members.

- "What does this mean to you?"
- "How can I help you?"

From the patient's perspective, many factors influence the content and quality of communication with you. Some patients are so afraid that they cannot hear what they have been told about their illness. It can be helpful to ask what the doctor has said to get baseline information about where they are in understanding their disease.

Patients may use denial as a mechanism to protect themselves from becoming overwhelmed by emotion. The denial is necessary to enable them to survive on a day-by-day basis. You do not need to correct their denial. Some patients remain in denial throughout the course of their illness. When patients in denial ask you a direct question about their condition, it can be an indicator that they are ready to hear the truth. It is essential that you always answer questions honestly and to the best of your knowledge. Dishonesty destroys trust and credibility.

Patients and their families may also feel angry. Allowing them to express their anger will validate it and enable them to progress emotionally. Comments such as "It is okay to be angry with God and anybody else" will encourage them to continue to talk. Patients who fully understand their prognosis will express sadness and regret. Sitting with patients as they express sadness will allow them to share their feelings and give you an opportunity to offer emotional support.

THE DYING PROCESS

This section discusses the expected changes in the days and hours before death. Assessing patients for these changes, planning and implementing treatments, and evaluating patients' responses to interventions are all important. Nursing interventions are summarized in the "Nursing Care Plan for the Patient at the End of Life."

(Text continued on page 316)

NURSING CARE PLAN for the Patient at the End of Life

Nursing Diagnosis: *Impaired Gas Exchange* related to dying heart and lungs as evidenced by dyspnea, change in respiratory rate, and SpO_2 less than 90%

Expected Outcomes: Patient will state that breathing is comfortable; respiratory rate is between 12 and 20 per minute; SpO_2 will be 90% or greater.

Evaluation of Outcomes: Is patient's breathing relaxed and rate between 12 and 20 per minute? Is SpO_2 90% or greater?

Intervention Monitor respiratory rate and effort. **Rationale** Increased rate and effort indicate distress.
Evaluation Is patient in distress? Are further interventions needed?

Intervention Administer diuretics or antibiotics as ordered. **Rationale** Diuretics or antibiotics may be given to treat dyspnea and promote comfort, not to prolong life. **Evaluation** Do diuretics or antibiotics reduce dyspnea?

Continued

NURSING CARE PLAN for the Patient at the End of Life—cont'd

Intervention Explain to the family the rationale for medical interventions. **Rationale** Blood transfusions may be given to improve oxygenation and reduce dyspnea; a thoracentesis may promote lung expansion. These are not intended to prolong life but to promote comfort. **Evaluation** Are additional interventions needed and effective? Does family understand rationale for their use?

Intervention Plan activities to conserve energy. **Rationale** Spacing rest with activity will help reduce oxygen consumption. **Evaluation** Can patient tolerate spaced activities?

Intervention Place patient in a recliner with pillows to 45 degrees. **Rationale** An upright position allows lung expansion. **Evaluation** Does positioning reduce dyspnea?

Intervention Offer alternative comfort measures, such as massage and muscle relaxation. **Rationale** Relaxation reduces anxiety and resulting dyspnea. **Evaluation** Are alternative measures effective?

Intervention Administer oxygen as ordered. **Rationale** Oxygenation raises SpO_2 and reduces dyspnea. **Evaluation** Does oxygen raise SpO_2 and relieve dyspnea?

Intervention Place a fan in room if patient desires. **Rationale** The feeling of breeze may reduce subjective feelings of dyspnea. **Evaluation** Does patient report increased comfort or appear more comfortable with fan on?

Intervention Administer low-dose morphine as ordered. **Rationale** Morphine causes peripheral vasodilation, which can reduce pulmonary edema. It can also reduce anxiety. **Evaluation** Are respirations less labored after morphine?

Intervention Explain to patient and family that small dose of morphine will help to slow breathing, so patient feels more comfortable and will work on the part of the brain that makes patient feel short of breath, reducing the sense of panic. **Rationale** The informed patient and family will be able to cooperate and assist with keeping the patient comfortable. **Evaluation** Do patient and family understand reasons for care and feel secure that patient is receiving best possible care?

Nursing Diagnosis: *Ineffective Airway Clearance* related to excessive secretions and inability to swallow as evidenced by gurgling sound, "death rattle"

Expected Outcome: The patient's airway will be free of secretions.

Evaluation of Outcome: Is patient's breathing quiet and unlabored?

Intervention Adjust the patient's head to allow secretions to move down the throat. **Rationale** This will help the patient swallow the secretions and decrease frightening noise. **Evaluation** Is breathing quieter?

Intervention Place a humidifier in the room. **Rationale** Humidified air can liquefy secretions and help the patient cough. **Evaluation** Is patient able to cough up secretions?

Intervention If secretions are copious, administer hyoscyamine or scopolamine as ordered. **Rationale** These anticholinergic medications can dry secretions. **Evaluation** Do medications help dry secretions?

Intervention Administer low-dose morphine as ordered. **Rationale** Morphine has an anticholinergic action that can help dry secretions. **Evaluation** Does morphine help quiet breathing and help patient stay calm?

Intervention Suction patient as needed. **Rationale** If secretions are not controlled by noninvasive measures, suctioning may be needed. **Evaluation** Is suctioning needed? Is it effective?

Intervention Explain to patient and family that, "Because he can no longer swallow saliva, it collects in the back of his throat. This medication will help reduce the secretions and reduce the feeling of shortness of breath." **Rationale** The informed patient and family will be able to cooperate and assist with keeping the patient comfortable. **Evaluation** Do patient and family understand reasons for care and feel secure that patient is receiving best possible care?

NURSING CARE PLAN for the Patient at the End of Life—cont'd

Nursing Diagnosis: *Imbalanced Nutrition: Less Than Body Requirements* related to inability to swallow and lack of appetite as evidenced by refusing food, weight loss

Expected Outcomes: The patient will state satisfaction with amount and types of food offered. The patient will not aspirate food or fluid.

Evaluation of Outcomes: Does patient appear content with foods and fluids offered? Does he or she swallow without aspirating?

Intervention Let the patient choose when and what to eat. Do not force the patient to eat if he or she does not wish to. **Rationale** The goal is no longer providing adequate nutrition but keeping the patient comfortable. **Evaluation** Is the patient receiving the foods and fluids he wants?

Intervention Sit the patient upright to eat or drink. **Rationale** This can help the patient swallow and prevent aspiration. **Evaluation** Does patient swallow effectively?

Intervention Explain to family, as needed, that, "He is afraid to swallow now because his swallowing is impaired and it causes him to choke. As he becomes dehydrated, his comfort will increase as the body produces naturally occurring anesthesia." **Rationale** The informed patient and family will be able to cooperate and assist with keeping the patient comfortable. **Evaluation** Do patient and family understand reasons for care and feel secure that the patient is receiving best possible care?

Nursing Diagnosis: *Impaired Oral Mucous Membrane* related to dehydration, not eating, medication side effects

Expected Outcome: The patient's mucous membranes will be clean and moist.

Evaluation of Outcome: Are mucous membranes clean and moist? Does patient indicate that his mouth is moist?

Intervention If patient is alert, offer ice chips or sips of water. **Rationale** These keep mucous membranes moist. **Evaluation** Does patient indicate mouth feels comfortable?

Intervention Provide frequent mouth care with sponge-tipped Toothettes. **Rationale** This can keep mucous membranes moist when patient is not able to drink adequate fluids. **Evaluation** Is mouth clean and moist?

Intervention Apply lanolin to lips. **Rationale** Lanolin keeps mouth and lips from becoming dry and crusty. **Evaluation** Are lips smooth and moist?

Nursing Diagnosis: *Impaired Comfort* (pain, terminal restlessness) related to disease process, dying process, medications

Expected Outcome: The patient will state that he or she feels comfortable or, if unable to speak, will appear calm and peaceful, not restless or agitated.

Evaluation of Outcome: Is patient comfortable, calm, and peaceful?

Intervention Assess for reversible causes of agitation: • Pain or other discomfort • Urine retention or fecal impaction • Medications that are no longer beneficial • SpO$_2$ <90%. **Rationale** Often, agitation is a sign of discomfort. Identifying and removing the cause of the discomfort can help calm the patient. **Evaluation** Can causes be identified? Are they removed?

Continued

NURSING CARE PLAN for the Patient at the End of Life—cont'd

Intervention Reposition in bed at least every 2 hours and as needed. **Rationale** Repositioning frequently can promote comfort and relieve pressure on bony prominences. When other medical interventions are discontinued, the patient still needs to be repositioned regularly to prevent uncomfortable complications. **Evaluation** Does repositioning promote comfort?

Intervention If Spo$_2$ is low, administer oxygen as ordered. **Rationale** Low Spo$_2$ causes dyspnea, which is not comfortable. **Evaluation** Is Spo$_2$ raised to 90%? Is patient's breathing unlabored?

Intervention Discuss with the HCP discontinuing all uncomfortable procedures, such as blood draws and finger-sticks for blood glucose. **Rationale** Many procedures provide information to the staff but are not beneficial to the patient at the end of life. They should be discontinued. **Evaluation** Are any uncomfortable procedures still being carried out that are not absolutely necessary?

Intervention If the cause of the agitation cannot be determined, try medication for pain, dyspnea, or anxiety as ordered. **Rationale** Medication may need to be administered based on objective observations if the patient is unable to communicate. **Evaluation** Does medication promote comfort?

Intervention Keep the patient safe with one-on-one monitoring and side rails up. **Rationale** A fall would increase the patient's discomfort. **Evaluation** Is patient safety maintained?

Intervention Keep perineal area clean and dry, frequently checking adult briefs. **Rationale** A wet brief is not comfortable. Unchanged briefs can also lead to skin breakdown, another source of discomfort. **Evaluation** Is patient clean and dry with intact skin?

Intervention Teach the patient and family that "Restlessness can have many causes. It can be a sign of pain, bowel or bladder problems, or a medication issue. I will work with the HCP to improve the situation." **Rationale** The informed patient and family will be able to cooperate and assist with keeping the patient comfortable. **Evaluation** Do patient and family understand reasons for care and feel secure that patient is receiving best possible care?

Nursing Diagnosis: *Hypothermia* or *Hyperthermia* related to dying central nervous system and inability to regulate body temperature

Expected Outcomes: The patient's temperature will be maintained as close to normal as possible, and discomfort from temperature extremes will be managed.

Evaluation of Outcomes: Is temperature within normal limits? If unable to control temperature, does patient appear comfortable?

Intervention Administer acetaminophen suppository as ordered. **Rationale** Acetaminophen is an antipyretic. It is given by suppository if the patient cannot swallow. **Evaluation** Does acetaminophen reduce fever?

Intervention Keep the patient clean and dry. Change gown and bed linens as needed. **Rationale** A fever can cause diaphoresis (excessive sweating), and lying in damp sheets can be uncomfortable and cause skin breakdown. **Evaluation** Is patient kept dry and comfortable?

Intervention If the patient is cold, add blankets as needed. Do not use an electric blanket or heating pad. **Rationale** Blankets will warm the patient without risking burns from electric heating devices. **Evaluation** Are blankets helpful?

Nursing Diagnosis: *Acute Confusion* related to neurologic changes

Expected Outcomes: The family will voice understanding that confusion is not uncommon and will show appropriate responses if it occurs.

Evaluation of Outcomes: Does the family respond appropriately to patient during times of confusion?

NURSING CARE PLAN for the Patient at the End of Life—cont'd

Intervention Assure families that some confusion is common. **Rationale** If family is prepared, confusion will be less disturbing. **Evaluation** Is family informed? Do they verbalize understanding of what to expect?

Intervention Do not correct the patient but instead encourage the patient to talk about what is happening. **Rationale** Sometimes patients talk about their fears in metaphor. Allowing them to express this fear will promote relaxation and decrease loneliness. **Evaluation** Is the patient less distressed after speaking?

Intervention Keep a dim light on in the room, and remind the person gently of who is present. **Rationale** Being able to see clearly helps keep the patient oriented if he or she awakens during the night. **Evaluation** Is the light on? Is patient able to orient himself or herself on awakening?

Intervention Explain to family that "Many patients don't make sense at times. It is as if they are in two worlds at the same time. The patient will be less distressed if you let him (or her) talk about what he (or she) is experiencing." **Rationale** Family members will be less distressed if they understand what is happening. **Evaluation** Does the family respond appropriately to the patient's confused statements?

Nursing Diagnosis: *Fear* related to threat of death

Expected Outcome: The patient will be treated as still present and respected, and not as though he is already gone.

Evaluation of Outcome: Is communication respectful toward the patient?

Intervention When providing care, always speak as if the patient can hear you. When conversing with family members in the room, remember that the patient also can hear what you are saying. **Rationale** Patients may be able to hear even when they appear to be nonresponsive. Always assume the patient can hear you. **Evaluation** Are caregivers and family members sensitive to the patient's presence when communicating?

Intervention When giving care, explain softly to the patient what you are doing and why. **Rationale** Knowing what is happening can reduce anxiety and increase cooperation. **Evaluation** Does patient appear calm? Does he respond to your explanations?

Intervention Explain to family that "Hearing is the last sense to go. This can be a good time to say the things you have not been able to say. He (or she) may still hear you." **Rationale** Continued communication can be comforting to both the patient and the family. **Evaluation** Is communication appropriate?

Nursing Diagnosis: *Anticipatory Grieving* related to impending death

Expected Outcome: The patient and family will be able to openly communicate their feelings to each other and say goodbye.

Evaluation of Outcome: Are patient and family able to communicate effectively and say goodbye to each other?

Intervention Be present with the patient. Just sit quietly and hold the patient's hand for a period of time. **Rationale** This can help the patient feel less alone, especially if there are no family members present. Many patients fear dying alone. **Evaluation** Is someone present with the patient as much as possible?

Intervention Show appropriate concern. **Rationale** This will promote trust and empower the family members to ask for what they need. **Evaluation** Is the family communicating openly with the providers?

Continued

NURSING CARE PLAN for the Patient at the End of Life—cont'd

Intervention Provide a quiet environment where each loved one can say goodbye in a way that will reflect their culture and values. **Rationale** These interactions will serve as valuable memories after the death and provide a feeling that all participants did what they needed to do for their loved one. **Evaluation** Do family members appear satisfied with their participation in the process?

Intervention Consult a minister or religious counselor of the family's choice. **Rationale** A minister often has special skills and training in communicating with people during difficult times. Talking about an afterlife may also be comforting to the patient and family. **Evaluation** Does the family appear to benefit from the presence of a minister or religious counselor?

Intervention Ask about the family's cultural and religious beliefs, and allow time for prayers and ceremonies. **Rationale** Providing a culturally familiar environment will reduce the patient's and family's anxieties and give them more control over the process. **Evaluation** Do family members feel free to carry out cultural and religious beliefs?

Educating family caregivers about what to expect is essential. Caregivers who anticipate the expected changes and understand the rationale behind the interventions are more successful in their caregiving and have fewer regrets or concerns after the death. The *Nursing Care Plan* includes specific communications that may help caregivers understand what is happening and how they can help.

Eating and Drinking

As our bodies move toward death, there is less desire for food and fluids. Patients are conserving energy and often do not feel hunger. The swallowing reflex can be impaired, increasing the risk of choking. Patients fear choking and may hold their mouth tightly closed when food or fluids are offered. This is normal, and the resulting dehydration will increase comfort due to endorphin production and rising ketone levels.

Changes in Breathing

About 50% to 70% of patients have dyspnea at the end of life. Patients who are alert may report dyspnea. Those who are not alert may have tachypnea (respiratory rate greater than 24 per minute), facial grimacing, and use of accessory muscles to breathe. Untreated dyspnea can lead to fear and agitation, leading to more dyspnea. Some patients also will have episodes of apnea in the days or hours before they die.

Dyspnea has many causes. Pneumonia, anemia, congestive heart failure, and pleural effusion can be successfully treated early in the course of illness. Dyspnea that occurs in the final hours of life is not treated by correcting the underlying condition but can be effectively managed and controlled (see the "Nursing Care Plan for the Patient at the End of Life" and "Evidence-Based Practice").

Oral Secretions

Saliva that the patient is now unable to swallow may collect in the back of the throat, causing a sound sometimes called a *death rattle*. This can be disconcerting for the family. See the

"Nursing Care Plan for the Patient at the End of Life" for interventions.

Temperature Changes

As the body loses its ability to control temperature, the patient may become diaphoretic or feel cold all the time. Some patients have experienced fevers as high as 105°F (40.5°C). As death approaches, the feet and legs may become cool, cyanotic, and mottled. This is often an indicator that death will occur within hours.

Bowel and Bladder Changes

Most patients will become incontinent of bowel and bladder during the course of the dying process. Urine output will decrease as dehydration occurs. Urine often will darken in color and have a strong odor.

Sleeping

In the final weeks of life, patients may be sleeping for most of the day. This is due to a change in metabolism. They also begin to emotionally detach from families as part of their preparation to leave.

 EVIDENCE-BASED PRACTICE

Clinical Question
Are opioids (morphine) effective in controlling dyspnea? Do opioids compromise the respiratory system of patients with dyspnea?

Evidence
A review of randomized controlled trials of patients with chronic obstructive pulmonary disease (COPD) showed that opioids were effective in relieving dyspnea without major adverse effect (Varkey, 2010).

The use of opioids with increasing doses in cancer patients is safe in both hospitalized and home-care patients and is not associated with reduced survival (Bengoechea, Gutierrez, Vrotsou, Onaindia, & Lopez, 2010). Finally, researchers found that there was no higher risk of respiratory depression among opioid-naive patients (patients taking opioids for the first time) than those who have been taking large doses of opioids (Clemens, Quednau, & Klaschik, 2008).

Implications for Nursing Practice
Oral and parenteral opioids are effective for dyspnea and can be safely administered to patients with COPD, cancer, and other life limiting conditions.

REFERENCES

Bengoechea, I., Gutierrez, S. G., Vrotsou, K., Onaindia, M. J., & Lopez, J. M. (2010). Opioid use at the end of life and survival in a Hospital at Home unit. *Journal of Palliative Medicine, 13,* 1079–1083.

Clemens, K. E., Quednau, I., & Klaschik, E. (2010). Is there a higher risk of respiratory depression in opioid-naïve palliative care patients during symptomatic therapy of dyspnea with strong opioids? *Journal of Palliative Medicine, 11,* 204–216.

Varkey, B. (2010). Opioids for palliation of refractory dyspnea in chronic obstructive pulmonary disease patients. *Current Opinion Pulmonary Medicine, 16,* 150–154.

Mental Status Changes

As patients go through the process of dying, they often have episodes of confusion, possibly from electrolyte imbalance or medications. Some patients will say things like, "I have to catch a train" or "I need my passport." This metaphorical communication is well documented in the hospice literature. It is almost like patients are living in two worlds (Callanan & Kelley, 1992).

Terminal Restlessness

Terminal restlessness is a syndrome observed in a significant number of patients with various diagnoses during the final days of life. The patient may be unable to concentrate or relax and may show nonpurposeful motor activities such as picking at the sheets. The patient may hallucinate or try to climb out of bed. Terminal restlessness can have many causes, including hypoxemia, metabolic abnormalities, and liver failure. Some physical causes may be reversible, so it is important to assess whether pain, urine retention, or fecal impaction may be the cause.

Restlessness may also be caused by medications. As kidney and liver functions decline, medication levels rise in the body and cause toxicity. Consult with the HCP and pharmacist to determine if all the medications the patient is receiving are beneficial or necessary. Table 17.3 reviews medications that may be helpful at the end of life.

Unconsciousness

Most patients are unconscious for hours or days before they die. Before they lose consciousness, their ability to see may

TABLE 17.3   MEDICATIONS TO INCREASE COMFORT AT THE END OF LIFE

Medication Class/Action	Examples	Nursing Implications
Opioids Bind to opioid receptors to reduce pain and dyspnea.	morphine (MS, MS-IR, MS Contin, Roxanol) hydromorphone (Dilaudid) fentanyl (Sublimaze, Actiq, Fentora)	For pain and dyspnea. Must be given routinely to be effective. Give routinely. Give short-acting analgesia for 24–72 hours until fentanyl patch takes effect. Do not cut patches before application. Wear gloves when applying or removing patch because drug may be absorbed during handling. Do not apply heat over a patch. Heat increases drug absorption and may cause overdoses. Used patches may still contain drug. Dispose of used patches to prevent accidental exposure to others, especially children and pets.

Continued

TABLE 17.3 MEDICATIONS TO INCREASE COMFORT AT THE END OF LIFE—cont'd

Medication Class/Action	Examples	Nursing Implications
Anxiolytics Depress central nervous system to reduce anxiety.	lorazepam (Ativan) alprazolam (Xanax) diazepam (Valium)	Not first-line drugs for treating dyspnea. Effective for dyspnea caused by anxiety
Neuroleptics Reduce severe agitation, terminal restlessness.	haloperidol (Haldol)	Useful in treating anxiety or agitation when lorazepam ineffective.
Anticholinergics For treating excessive pharyngeal secretions	hyoscyamine (Levsin) Atropine drops scopolamine (Transderm-Scop) glycopyrrolate (Robinul)	Works faster than scopolamine patch. For early treatment of secretions. Place patch behind the ear. Consider if hyoscyamine ineffective.

be diminished. Hearing is the final sense to be lost. It is important for you to remember as you are caring for the patient and conversing with the family that your patient likely hears everything you are saying. Encourage the family to continue talking to the patient.

CRITICAL THINKING

Mr. Johnson

■ Mr. Johnson is in the final hours of his life and has become increasingly short of breath throughout the day. With each inspiration, his respirations are moist and noisy. Currently, his respiratory rate is 30 per minute, and you notice he is using his accessory muscles to breathe.

1. What is the cause of his noisy breathing?
2. What can be done to lower his respiratory rate and decrease his dyspnea?

Suggested answers are at the end of the chapter.

CARE AT THE TIME OF DEATH AND AFTERWARD

Death has occurred when you observe the absence of heartbeat and respirations. The skin becomes pale and waxen, the eyes may remain open, and pupils are fixed. Telling the family that the patient has died should be done with sensitivity, providing

small amounts of information according to the family's level of understanding. Be sure to check and adhere to the policies in your health care setting and state regarding death pronouncement and organ donation. Document the general appearance of the body, including absent pulse and lung sounds. Your goal now is to provide a personal closure experience for the family.

After death has been pronounced, you will provide **postmortem care**. First, remove the tubes, medical supplies, and equipment. Bathing and dressing the patient and making him or her look presentable for the family shows respect. Some cultures dictate specific care of the body after death and who should provide that care (see Chapter 4 for more information). The nurse can assess and advocate for cultural practices requested by the family. Work toward providing a clean, peaceful impression of the deceased. Position the body in proper alignment, insert dentures, place dressings on leaking wounds, and use briefs as needed. Allow the family time with the body. Embalming is necessary within 12 hours. Do not remove the body from the room until the family is ready. Covering or uncovering the face at removal should be done according to the family's preference. Additional activities, such as contacting the HCP or funeral home, should be carried out according to institution policy.

 GRIEF

Grief is the emotional response to a loss. Loss is a daily experience in everyone's life. Loss can occur due to divorce, children leaving home, loss of job, loss of possessions, or other losses, including death. People express grief in their own way according to their coping skills, life experiences, and cultural norms. In end-of-life care, grief is a process that begins before the patient's death and continues through a series of tasks that the survivors move through to resolve grief. Feelings associated with grief may include anger, frustration, regret, guilt, sadness, and many others. Although each person is different, the process commonly includes three general stages (Table 17.4).

Interventions for the grieving patient are addressed in the "Nursing Care Plan for the Patient at the End of Life." The nursing process for the grieving family is addressed next.

NURSING PROCESS FOR THE GRIEVING FAMILY

Data Collection

Some things to consider when assessing grief include the following:

- Where is the family in the grief process?
- Are family members experiencing physical problems, such as shortness of breath, sweating, or skin color changes?
- Is the stress of grieving worsening medical conditions?
- What support systems are available to the family?
- What interventions can I use to facilitate their grief process?

Nursing Diagnoses, Planning, and Implementation

Although many nursing diagnoses may be appropriate, the priority diagnosis is simply *Grieving*.

Grieving related to impending death or loss of loved one.
EXPECTED OUTCOME: Family members will be able to express feelings of anger, guilt, or sadness. They will be able to think about the future and perform ADLs as needed.

- Simply be present. *Sitting with the bereaved, without having to have all the answers, is very powerful. If you don't know what to say, just be silent.*

- Actively listen, letting the bereaved talk about the loved one and their feelings about the loss. Ask open-ended questions to encourage them to continue talking. *One of the greatest needs of the bereaved is to trust someone enough to share their pain.*
- Help family members identify their support systems (religious or spiritual affiliation, friends, family) and encourage them to use them. *Support systems can help in practical ways (meals, transportation) as well as lend emotional support.*
- Consider acknowledging the event by attending the memorial service or sending a card. *This simple act of caring is very important to families.*

Evaluation

Healing takes time. If interventions have been effective, however, family members will have the support to function effectively while they grieve.

THE NURSE AND LOSS

Working with dying patients triggers awareness of your own losses and fears about death and mortality. Adapting to the care of the dying requires that you explore and experience your personal feelings toward death. Unresolved losses from your past can resurface and affect your ability to care for dying patients. You may find that you continue to think about patients who have died long after the event. Emotionally continuing to care about deceased patients takes energy away from the daily care you are providing to current patients and your own family. Unresolved grief can lead to symptoms that resemble burnout, such as insomnia, headaches, and fatigue.

If you find yourself distancing and withdrawing from your dying patients, it is an indicator that you need to attend to caring for yourself. Some nurses may find counseling helpful to effectively process losses from the past and learn healthy ways to process future losses.

TABLE 17.4 STAGES OF GRIEF

Stage	Tasks	Characteristics
Stage 1 Shock and disbelief	Acknowledge the reality of the loss. Recognize the loss.	Has difficulty with feelings of numbness, emotional outbursts, poor daily functioning, and avoidance.
Stage 2 Experiencing the loss	Work through the pain by expressing and experiencing the feelings.	Anger, bargaining, depression. May feel guilt over not preventing the death or not providing enough care. May feel angry at loved one who has "left them behind." May experience insomnia, loss of appetite, apathy, lack of interest in daily life.
Stage 3 Reintegration	Adjust to an environment without the deceased.	Finds hope in the future, participates in social events, feels more energetic.

Both formal and informal support systems should be in place to support staff through multiple losses. Informal support can be one-on-one sharing of experiences with coworkers, peers, pastoral counselors, and HCPs. Understanding and acknowledging your limitations, asking for help, and getting regular exercise and relaxation are important components. Some nurses find journal writing a helpful process; writing down feelings may allow you to release them. Formal support systems can be established in many ways:

• Preplanned gatherings where nurses can express feelings in a safe environment
• Postclinical debriefings after difficult deaths to alleviate anxiety and promote learning
• Ceremonies such as memorial services in facilities to allow both staff and residents to recognize and honor the loss of patients.

In addition, many employers offer free employee assistance programs that provide counseling.

REFLECTIONS ON MR. MORAN

Remember Mr. Moran from the beginning of the chapter? Clearly he is approaching the end of life. Determine what he and his family want to happen in the final months of his life and where he wants to be. What are the goals of care? If comfort is the goal, how can this best be achieved? If keeping him in his familiar and safe environment is the goal, then help his family weigh the benefits and burdens of CPR, hospitalization, artificial feeding, and artificial hydration.

Home Health Hints

• Allow time during your visit to sit quietly with the patient and caregiver. Sitting quietly lets the patient and caregiver know you are there to meet both physical and emotional needs.
• Encourage family involvement with care. Families need reassurance that they are not going to hurt the patient; take the time to teach them how to assist the patient with basic care.
• Prepare the family for what to expect as death approaches.
• When the patient is no longer conscious, encourage the family to continue to spend time at the bedside sharing personal thoughts and memories with the patient. For example, a spouse might talk about when they first met, or family members can play a favorite song.

SUGGESTED ANSWERS TO

CRITICAL THINKING

■ *Mrs. Hart*

1. Mrs. Hart will need a DNR order in the hospital setting and, when she goes home, she will need an out-of-hospital, prehospital, durable DNR or POLST—whatever is called for in her state of residence. In addition, her family members should be aware of her wishes.
2. Her HCP, hospital social worker, or case manager can be helpful.

■ *Mr. Johnson*

1. Mr. Johnson's noisy breathing may be caused by saliva collecting in the back of the throat or by pulmonary edema.
2. Mr. Johnson may benefit from oxygen, positioning, and suctioning oral secretions. Low-dose morphine will decrease his respiratory rate and improve his oxygenation. Morphine also has a drying effect on secretions. If morphine is unsuccessful, the addition of hyoscyamine may be helpful.

REVIEW QUESTIONS

1. A 94-year-old patient is admitted from home to the hospital with pneumonia. What factors would lead the nurse to believe the patient is nearing the end of life?
   1. Distended abdomen and yellow skin tone
   2. Fever of 101.6°F (38.7°C) and a respiratory rate of 28 per minute
   3. Difficulty swallowing and weight loss
   4. Inability to cough and bring up secretions

2. What is a durable power of attorney for health care?
   1. A document that outlines a patient's wishes at the end of life
   2. A document that gives a patient a "do not resuscitate" status
   3. A document specifying the person who will make decisions for a patient once the document is signed
   4. A document specifying the person who will make decisions for a patient when the patient is no longer able to speak for himself

3. A patient's family member says, "I heard someone say my mother could have a 'good death.' What on earth is a good death?" Which response by the nurse is best?
   1. "We consider a good death to be one that follows the patient's wishes for care, is comfortable, and allows them to die where they choose."
   2. "In reality, no death is a good death, but we do our best to make sure patients are comfortable right up until they die."
   3. "A good death is when the patient is kept sedated so they don't really know what is happening during the last days until they die."
   4. "A good death occurs when the patient is kept alive as long as possible, so she can take care of all her unfinished business first."

4. A husband whose wife has just died cries, "What am I going to do? She is all I had." What is the best response the nurse can provide?
   1. "You are going to go on with your life. You still have your work and your children."
   2. "I am sorry you lost your wife, but I know she would not want you to be sad. You have to be strong for her."
   3. "I know how you feel. I lost my grandmother recently, and it was really hard."
   4. There is no need to say anything. Just be present and listen.

5. A dying patient has excessive secretions that are causing dyspnea. Which medications will best help dry the secretions and increase comfort? **Select all that apply**.
   1. Haloperidol
   2. Scopolamine
   3. Acetaminophen
   4. Morphine
   5. Guaifenesin

6. Which of the following nursing interventions should the nurse provide at the end of life? **Select all that apply**.
   1. Position the patient to increase comfort and prevent complications.
   2. Provide comfort measures such as massage.
   3. Research experimental treatments that may help the patient find a cure.
   4. Administer medications to control symptoms.
   5. Teach the family CPR for use if the patient dies when the nurse is not present.
   6. Sit quietly with the patient and family.

7. A patient has just died, and his family is waiting to see him. What postmortem care is essential first?
   1. Document the time and circumstances of the death.
   2. Place identification on the body according to hospital policy.
   3. Clean the patient up and make him look peaceful.
   4. Cover the patient's body and face with a sheet.

8. The wife of a hospitalized patient who died an hour ago is crying and unwilling to leave the hospital room. The rest of the family is in the waiting room. The admitting department just called and wants to have the room cleaned for a new patient. Which action should the nurse take?
   1. Allow the wife to stay in the room as long as she likes.
   2. Call a taxicab for the wife and gently guide her out of the room.
   3. Sit with the wife for a few minutes, then take her to the waiting room.
   4. Tell the wife that you are sorry for her loss, but that another patient needs the room.

9. A patient who has been receiving hospice care for 3 months tells the LPN he has decided he wants to return to active treatment of his disease. What should the LPN do?
   1. Encourage the patient to discuss his desire with his HCP.
   2. Tell the patient that he cannot change his goals once hospice care has been initiated.
   3. Check his medication supply for any leftover medications he was taking during treatment.
   4. Explain to the patient that since he is terminal, treatment will not help the course of his disease.

Answers can be found in Appendix C.

References

Alley, D. E., Metter, E. J., Griswold, M. E., Harris, T. B., Simonsick, E. M., Longo, D. L., & Ferucci, L. (2010). Changes in weight at end of life: Characterizing weight loss by time to death in a cohort study of older men. *American Journal of Epidemiology, 172,* 558–565.

Dev, R., Dalal, S., & Bruera, E. (2012). Is there a role for parenteral nutrition or hydration at the end of life? *Current Opinion in Supportive and Palliative Care, 6,* 365–370.

Dobbs, D., Meng, H., Hyer, K., & Volicer, L. (2012). The influence of hospice use on nursing home and hospital use in assisted living among dual-eligible enrollees. *Journal of the American Medical Director's Association, 13,* 189.e9–189.

Fairbanks, R. J., Shah, M. N., Lerner, E. B., Ilangovan, K., Pennington, E. C., & Schneider, S. M. (2007). Epidemiology and outcomes of out-of-hospital cardiac arrest in Rochester, New York. *Resuscitation, 72,* 415–424.

Gardner, D. S., & Kramer B. J. (2010). End-of-life concerns and care preferences: Congruence among terminally ill elders and their family caregivers. *Omega (Westport), 60,* 273–297.

Givens, J. L., Jones, R. N., Shaffer, M. L., Kiely, D. K., & Mitchell, S. L. (2010). Survival and comfort after treatment of pneumonia in advanced dementia. *Archives of Internal Medicine, 170,* 1102–1107.

Kelly, A., Conell-Price, J., Covinsky, K., Cenzer, I. S., Chang, A., Boscardin, W. J., & Smith, A. K. (2010). Length of Stay for Older Adults Residing in Nursing Homes at the End of Life. *Journal of the American Geriatric Society, 58,* 1701–1706.

Raijmakers N. J. H., Zuylen L., Costantini, M., Caraceni, A., Clark J., Lundquist, G., . . . Van der Heidel A. (2011). Artificial nutrition and hydration in the last week of life in cancer patients. A systematic literature review of practices and effects. *Annals of Oncology Advance Access, 22,* 1478–1486.

Smith, A. K., Cenzer, I. S., Knight, S. J., Puntillo, K. A., Widera, E., Williams B. A., . . . Covinsky, K. E. (2010). What Can Population-Based Studies Tell Us About Pain in the Last Years of Life? *Annals of Internal Medicine, 153,* 563–569.

Swor, R. A., Jackson, R. E., Tintanalli, J. E., & Pirrallo, R. G. (2000). Does advanced age matter in outcomes after out-of-hospital cardiac arrest in community-dwelling adults? *Academic Emergency Medicine, 7,* 762–768.

Teno J. M., Mitchell, S. L., Kuo, S. K., Gozalo, P. L., Rhodes, R. L., Lima, J. C., & Mor, V. (2011). Decision-making and outcomes of feeding tube insertion: A five-state study. *Journal of the American Geriatrics Society, 59,* 881–886.

Wilson, R. S., Herbert, L. E., Scherr, P. A., Dong, X., Leurgens, S. E., & Evans, D. A. (2012). Cognitive decline after hospitalization in a community population of older persons. *Neurology, 78,* 950–956.

 Davis*Plus* | For additional resources and information visit **davispl.us/medsurg5**

unit FOUR

Understanding the Immune System

18

Immune System Function, Assessment, and Therapeutic Measures

KEY TERMS

active immunity (AK-tiv im-YOO-nih-tee)
anaphylactic (AN-uh-fih-LAK-tik)
antibody (AN-tih-baw-dee)
antigen (AN-tih-jen)
autoimmune (AW-toe-ih-mewn)
cell-mediated immunity (SELL mee-dee-ay-ted ih-MYOO-nih-tee)
humoral immunity (HYOO-mur-uhl ih-MYOO-nih-tee)
lymphocyte (LIM-fuh-site)
neutrophil (NEW-troh-fil)
passive immunity (PASS-iv ih-MYOO-nih-tee)
white blood cells (WYTE BLUHD SELLS)

SHARON M. NOWAK AND
JANICE L. BRADFORD

LEARNING OUTCOMES

1. Identify the type of immunity that is obtained with a vaccine.
2. Describe the two mechanisms of immunity.
3. Discuss the function of each class of immunoglobulin and how each behaves in a particular immune response.
4. Describe how aging affects the immune system.
5. Explain subjective data that are collected when caring for a patient with a disorder of the immune system.
6. Explain the objective data that are collected when caring for a patient with a disorder of the immune system.
7. Describe nursing care provided for patients undergoing diagnostic tests for the immune system.
8. Discuss common therapeutic measures used for disorders of the immune system.

NORMAL IMMUNE SYSTEM ANATOMY AND PHYSIOLOGY

Immunity is defined as the ability to destroy pathogens or other foreign material and to prevent further cases of infectious disease. Immunity is typically the body's response to foreign microorganisms such as bacteria, viruses, and fungi. However, immune responses can be directed toward other cells or substances that are identified by the body, correctly or incorrectly, as foreign. Malignant cells are considered foreign and are usually destroyed by the immune system after mutation but before they become malignant. Unfortunately, transplanted organs are usually perceived as foreign and are therefore rejected. Occasionally, the immune system mistakenly reacts to self (**autoimmune** disease) or to a substance that should be tolerated (allergic reaction).

The immune system consists of lymphoid organs and tissues, **lymphocytes** and other **white blood cells** (WBCs), and many chemicals that activate our own cells for the destruction of foreign antigens (Fig. 18.1). The lymphatic system includes lymph, lymphatic vessels that help return tissue fluid to the circulatory system; lymph nodes, nodules, and the spleen, where macrophages phagocytize (engulf and destroy) pathogens and B and T cells carry out immune functions; and red bone marrow and the thymus (which functions primarily in childhood and atrophies with age). Lymph flows from vessels through lymph nodes where pathogens are percolated out and destroyed. Lymph nodes are especially concentrated in the cervical, axillary, and inguinal areas. Lymph nodules, lacking encapsulation, are found under the surface of mucous membranes (e.g., tonsils).

Antigens

Antigens are chemical markers that identify cells or molecules. Human cells have their own antigens—thousands of markers that identify the cell as "self." These are the major histocompatibility complex antigens, also called human leukocyte antigens, which are genetically determined. Major histocompatibility complex antigens are tolerated by the body's immune system, whereas foreign antigens will be destroyed in one of several ways.

Lymphocytes

There are three types of lymphocytes: natural killer (NK) cells, thymus-derived lymphocytes (T cells), and bone marrow–derived lymphocytes (B cells), each with different functions.

Natural Killer Cells

NK cells are found throughout the body and are nonspecific in action, destroying a variety of foreign cells including altered self-cells. After binding with an abnormal cell, NK cells release either perforins or granzymes, which cause cytolysis. Cell fragments are then phagocytized by WBCs.

T Cells and B Cells

The lymphocytes called T cells and B cells are involved in specific immune responses; that is, each cell is programmed to respond to one kind of foreign antigen.

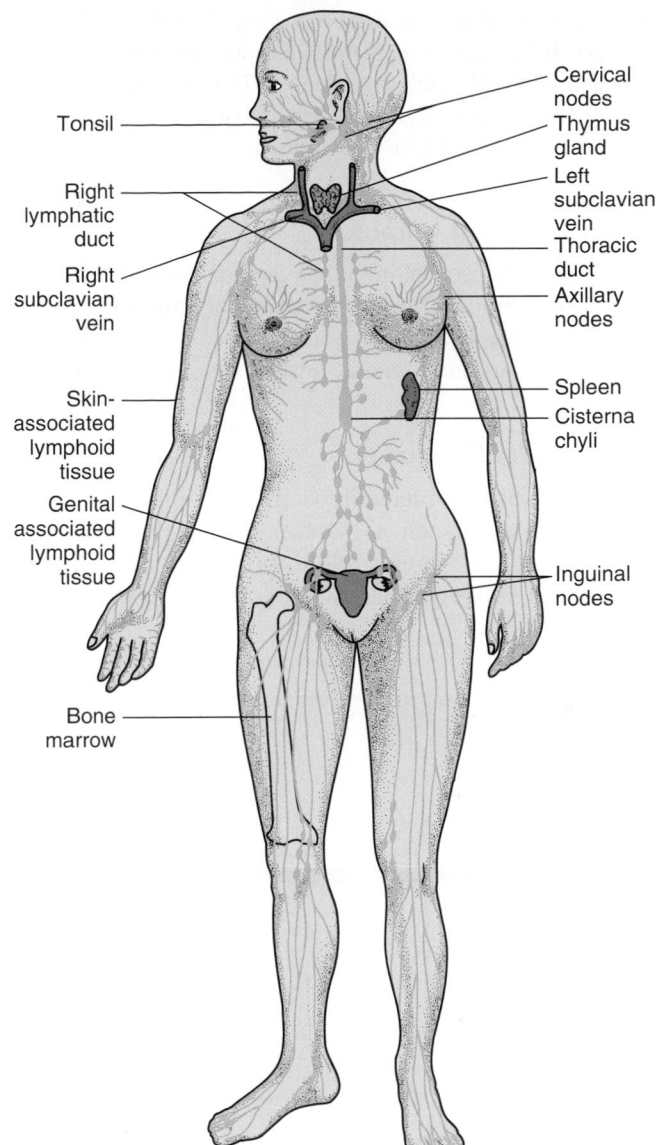

FIGURE 18.1 Immune system organs, lymph vessels, and major lymph nodes.

Both T cells and B cells arise in the red bone marrow. T cells then migrate to the thymus, where the thymic hormones bring about their maturation. From the thymus, T cells migrate to the lymph nodes and nodules and to the spleen. B cells mature in the bone marrow and migrate directly to lymphatic tissue. When activated during an immune response, T cells perform direct attack, whereas B cells differentiate into plasma cells that release antibodies for an indirect approach.

Antibodies

Antibodies are also called immunoglobulins (Ig) or gamma globulins and are glycoproteins produced by plasma cells in response to foreign antigens. Antibodies do not themselves destroy foreign antigens but rather become attached to such antigens to label

• **WORD • BUILDING** •
lymphocyte: lympho—lymph + kytos—cell
antigen: anti—against + gennan—to produce

them for destruction. Each **antibody** is specific for only one antigen, and B cells (that become plasma cells) are capable of producing millions of different antibodies. There are five classes of human antibodies, designated by letter names: IgG, IgA, IgM, IgD, and IgE (Fig. 18.2). Their functions are summarized in Table 18.1.

Mechanisms of Immunity

The two mechanisms of immunity are **cell-mediated immunity**, which involves T cells, and **humoral immunity**, which involves mainly B cells but is assisted by T cells. Although the mechanisms are different, invasion by a pathogen often triggers both.

Cell-Mediated Immunity

This mechanism of immunity is effective against intracellular pathogens (such as viruses or fungi), malignant cells, and grafts of foreign tissue. A T-cell response results in cytotoxic Ts, which attack altered cells; helper Ts, which

assist; and memory Ts, which retain knowledge of the pathogen in the event of future encounters with the same (Fig. 18.3).

Humoral Immunity

Humoral immunity is also called *antibody-mediated immunity* and involves antibody production. It is effective against extracellular pathogens, which are usually bacteria but can also be viral or fungal infections (Fig. 18.4).

Although B cells are stationary, the antibodies produced by plasma cells circulate throughout the body and bond to the antigen, forming an antigen–antibody complex. This immobilizes the bacteria; also, the antigen is now labeled for phagocytosis by macrophages or **neutrophils**. The antigen–antibody complex also activates the *complement cascade*.

• WORD • BUILDING •

neutrophil: neutro—neuter + philein—to love

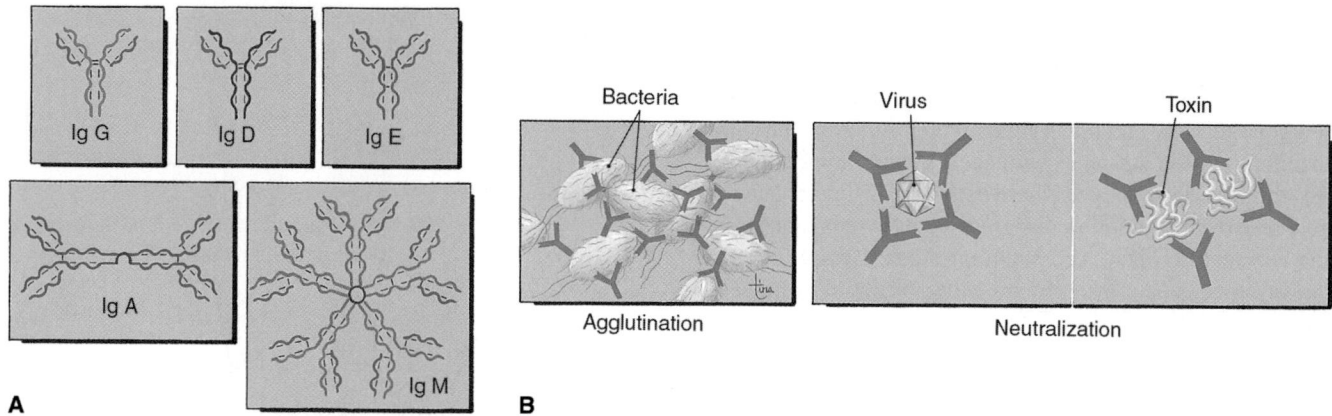

FIGURE 18.2 Antibodies. (A) Structure of the five classes of antibodies. (B) Antibody activity. Adapted from Scanlon, V., & Sanders, T. (2015). *Essentials of anatomy and physiology* (7th ed.). Philadelphia: F.A. Davis.

TABLE 18.1 CLASSES OF ANTIBODIES

Immunoglobulin (Ig)	Location	Function
IgG	Blood, extracellular fluid, lymph	Crosses the placenta to provide passive immunity in newborns. Provides long-term immunity after a vaccination or illness recovery
IgA	External secretions (e.g., tears, saliva)	Provides passive immunity for breastfed infants. Found in secretions of all mucous membranes
IgM	Blood, lymph	Produced first during an infection (IgG production follows)
IgD	B cells	Antigen-specific receptors on B lymphocytes
IgE	Mast cells or basophils	Important in allergic reactions. Mast cells release histamine

Source: Scanlon, V., & Sanders, T. (2015). *Understanding human structure and function* (7th ed.). Philadelphia: F.A. Davis.

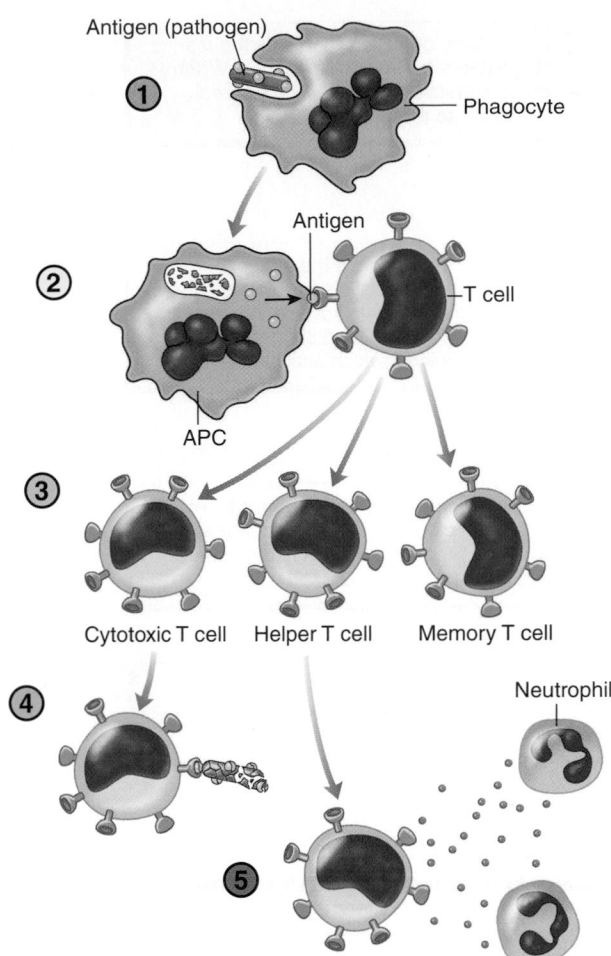

1 The immune process begins when a phagocyte (such as a macrophage, reticular cell, or B cell) ingests an antigen.

2 The phagocyte, called an **antigen-presenting cell (APC)**, displays fragments of the antigen on its surface—a process called **antigen presentation**—which alerts the immune system to the presence of a foreign antigen. When a T cell spots the foreign antigen, it binds to it.

3 This activates (or sensitizes) the T cell, which begins dividing repeatedly to form clones: identical T cells already sensitized to the antigen. Some of these T cells become effector cells (such as cytotoxic T cells and helper T cells), which will carry out the attack, while others become memory T cells.

4 The cytotoxic T cell binds to the surface of the antigen and delivers a toxic dose of chemicals that will kill it.

5 Helper T cells support the attack by secreting the chemical **interleukin**, which attracts neutrophils, natural killer cells, and macrophages. It also stimulates the production of T and B cells.

FIGURE 18.3 Cellular immunity. From Thompson, G. S. (2013). *Understanding anatomy and physiology.* Philadelphia: F.A. Davis, p. 321.

Complement is a group of more than 30 plasma proteins that circulate in the blood until activated by either the presence of foreign bacteria or by an antigen–antibody complex. The activation of complement results in the formation of a protein cascade that lyses (causes disintegration of) the cell. Other complement proteins bind to foreign antigens and serve as further labels to attract macrophages.

ANTIBODY RESPONSES

The first exposure to a foreign antigen stimulates antibody production, but the antibodies are produced too slowly to prevent the disease. However, with time, the person accumulates antibodies and memory cells specific for that pathogen. On a second exposure to the antigen, the memory cells begin rapid production of large amounts of antibody, often enough to prevent a second occurrence of the illness (Fig. 18.5). This is the basis for the protection given by vaccines. A vaccine contains an antigen that is not pathogenic. The vaccine stimulates the formation of antibodies and memory cells.

Antibodies may also neutralize viruses; that is, they attach to a virus and render it unable to enter a cell (see Fig. 18.2). Viruses cannot reproduce outside of living cells, and those coated with antibodies are phagocytized by macrophages. Interferon, another defense against viruses, is a chemical produced by cells infected with viruses. Although it does not help the infected cell, interferon protects surrounding cells by enabling them to resist viral replication.

Antibodies are also involved in allergic responses, in which the immune system responds to foreign but harmless antigens (an allergen), such as plant pollen. IgE antibodies bond to mast cells, which break down and release histamine and other chemicals that contribute to inflammation. **Anaphylactic** shock is an allergic reaction, but massive in response. It is characterized by loss of plasma from capillaries (an effect of histamine) and a sudden drop in the intravascular blood volume and blood pressure.

TYPES OF IMMUNITY

Two categories of immunity are passive immunity and active immunity. In **passive immunity**, antibodies are not produced by the person but are obtained from another source. One form

• WORD • BUILDING •
anaphylactic: ana—up + phylaxis—protection

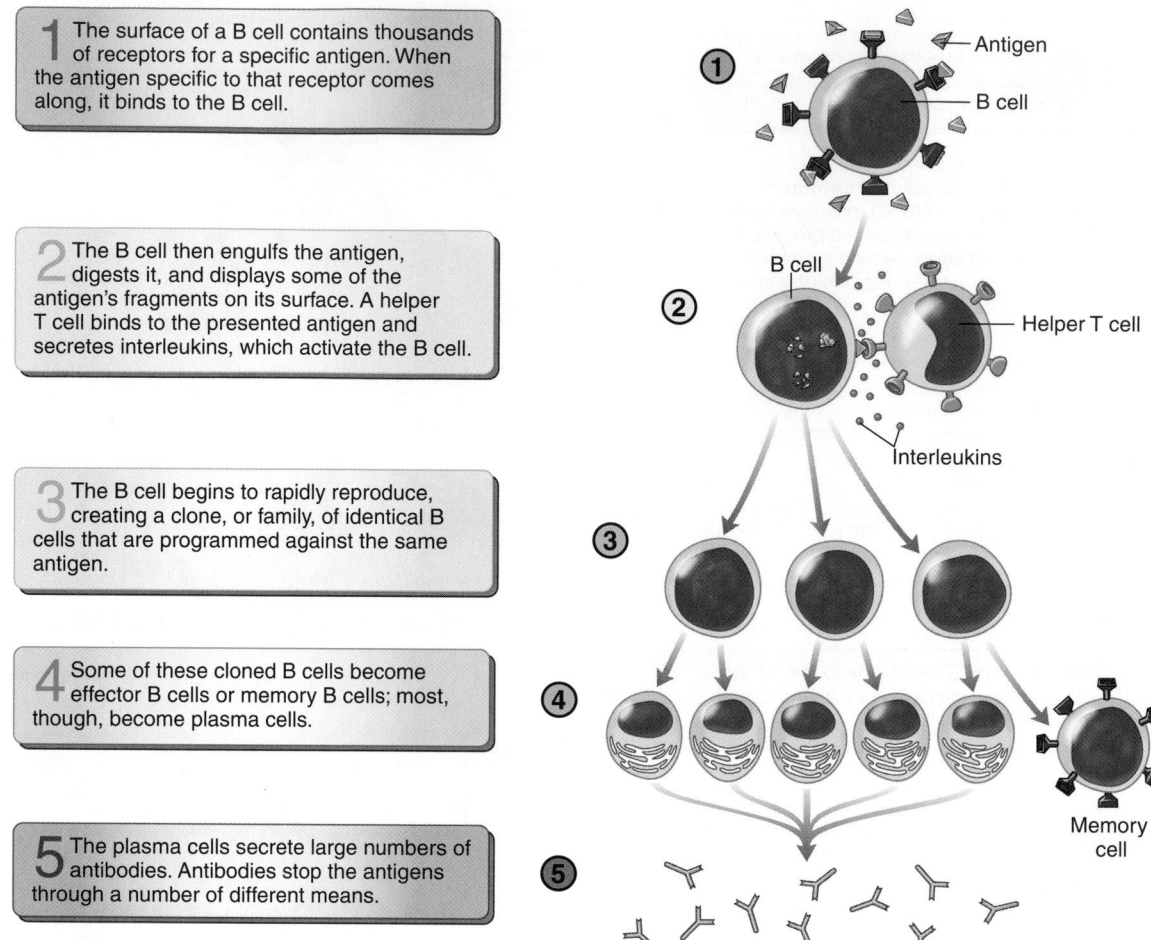

1 The surface of a B cell contains thousands of receptors for a specific antigen. When the antigen specific to that receptor comes along, it binds to the B cell.

2 The B cell then engulfs the antigen, digests it, and displays some of the antigen's fragments on its surface. A helper T cell binds to the presented antigen and secretes interleukins, which activate the B cell.

3 The B cell begins to rapidly reproduce, creating a clone, or family, of identical B cells that are programmed against the same antigen.

4 Some of these cloned B cells become effector B cells or memory B cells; most, though, become plasma cells.

5 The plasma cells secrete large numbers of antibodies. Antibodies stop the antigens through a number of different means.

FIGURE 18.4 Humoral immunity. From Thompson, G. S. (2013). *Understanding anatomy and physiology.* Philadelphia: F.A. Davis, p. 322.

of *naturally* acquired passive immunity includes placental transmission of antibodies from mother to fetus and transmission of antibodies in breast milk. *Artificially* acquired passive immunity involves injection of preformed antibodies; this may help prevent disease after exposure to a pathogen such as the hepatitis B virus. Passive immunity is always temporary, in that antibodies from another source eventually break down.

Active immunity means that the person produces his or her own antibodies. An example of naturally acquired active immunity occurs when a person recovers from an infection and then has antibodies and memory cells specific for that pathogen. Artificially acquired active immunity occurs as the result of a vaccine that stimulates production of antibodies and memory cells. The duration of active immunity depends on the particular disease or vaccine; some confer lifelong immunity, but others do not.

Aging and the Immune System

The efficiency of the immune system decreases with age (Fig. 18.6). As such, older adults are more susceptible to infections and autoimmune disorders (see "Gerontological Issues"). The incidence of cancer is also higher; malignant cells that might once have been quickly destroyed by the immune system live and proliferate.

Gerontological Issues

Significant changes occur in the immune system of the older adult. These changes are known as *immune senescence,* which refers to a decline in immune system function. Some specific changes include the following:

- Thymus gland decreases in size, increases production of immature T cells, and has a subsequent decline in response to antigens.
- Antibody response to foreign organisms decreases.
- Immunizations to support the immune responses of older adults include the following:
  - Influenza vaccine (plus H1N1 flu vaccine if recommended) yearly mid-October to mid-November, before influenza season
  - Pneumococcal vaccine once when age 65
  - Herpes zoster vaccine once when age 60
  - Tetanus, diphtheria, and pertussis booster every 10 years.

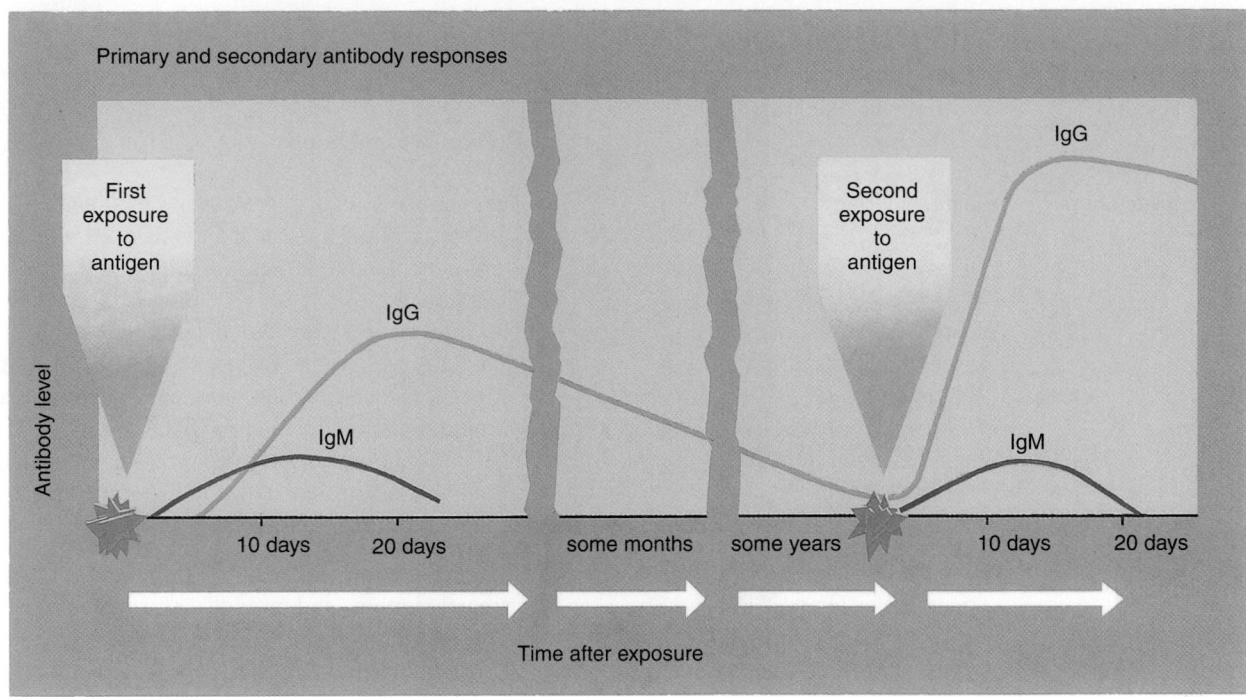

Primary and secondary antibody responses

FIGURE 18.5 Antibody responses to a first and then subsequent exposure to a pathogen. From Scanlon, V., & Sanders, T. (2015). *Essentials of anatomy and physiology* (7th ed.). Philadelphia: F.A. Davis.

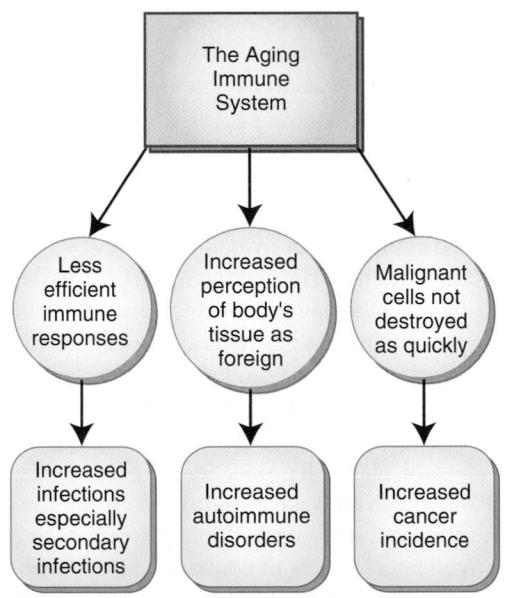

FIGURE 18.6 This concept map shows the effects the aging process has on the immune system.

NURSING ASSESSMENT OF THE IMMUNE SYSTEM

Disorders of the immune system can affect every system in the body, so it is important to collect head-to-toe data as well as a patient history (Table 18.2).

History
Demographic Data

The patient's gender and ethnicity are important to note because some diseases tend to be associated with a particular gender or ethnicity. For instance, systemic lupus erythematosus (SLE; see Chapter 19), an autoimmune disorder, affects women up to nine times more than men (Ferenkeh-Koroma, 2012). In addition, Hispanic, Native American, Asian, and African American women develop SLE two to three times more often than Caucasian women.

Health History

Assessment of the patient's past and present medical conditions should also include a family history. Many atopic (allergic) disorders, such as allergic rhinitis and asthma (see Chapter 31), and autoimmune disorders, such as ankylosing spondylitis (see Chapter 19), are thought to be either familial or have a genetic predisposition in certain ethnic or cultural groups ("Cultural Considerations"). For example, 4 new genes have been identified that are strongly associated with SLE, and 10 others are possible risk factors.

Patients' surgical history may give clues about their previous health or current condition. For example, with thymus gland removal (thymectomy), T-cell production may be altered, which affects the cell-mediated immune response. If the spleen was removed (splenectomy), lymphocyte and plasma cell production may be altered, which affects the humoral immune response.

TABLE 18.2 SUBJECTIVE DATA COLLECTION FOR THE IMMUNE SYSTEM

Category	Questions to Ask During the Health History	Rationale/Significance
Demographic Data	What is your age?	The immune system decreases in functional effectiveness as one ages, and a number of immune disorders tend to afflict individuals of particular age ranges.
	Where were you born? What is your ethnic or cultural background?	This information can aid in determining ethnic and cultural background influences. Some immune disorders tend to afflict individuals of particular cultural/ethnic groups more than others.
	Where have you lived? Where do you currently reside?	This information can aid in determining ethnic and cultural background as well as possible environmental influences.
History	Do you have allergies to any medications? Latex? Foods? Insects? Environmental allergens? If yes, have you had a recent exposure to any of these? Describe the reaction.	This information may lead to a direct cause of current symptoms and provides information regarding the status of the patient's immune system. Medication side effects are commonly inaccurately considered allergies by patients.
	Is anyone in your family allergic to medications? Latex? Foods? Insects? Environmental allergens?	If family members (especially immediate) have severe reactions to substances, the patient may be predisposed to immune reactions to the same antigen or in general.
	What medications are you currently taking?	Some medications can mask symptoms or immune responses, others can suppress immune responses.
	What illnesses or conditions are you currently being treated for? Have you been treated for?	May provide clues to patient's current condition or symptoms.
	What surgeries have you had?	Have any immune organs been removed, therefore reducing immune function? May also provide indications about overall health.
	Have you ever had a blood transfusion? If so, why?	Antibodies to various antigen markers on the blood cells may have been formed. May also provide indications regarding overall health.
	What is your occupation? Have you been exposed to hazardous chemicals, fumes, or radiation?	Many chemicals can produce local reactions, usually skin reactions or systemic immune reactions, and some can lead to bone marrow suppression in which all cell production is reduced.
	Do you engage in any form of risky behavior?	Risky behavior, such as intravenous drug use or unprotected sex with multiple partners, increases a patient's chances of contracting the human immunodeficiency virus (HIV), which leads to a reduction in the immune system function.
	Describe your overall stress level and life stressors.	Stress is known to suppress the immune system and, over prolonged periods, can lead to a variety of illnesses.
	What do you do to cope with stress?	Not all coping behaviors and mechanisms are healthy; therefore, it is important to assess what the patient's coping behaviors are to see if the patient needs education.
	What sort of support systems do you have?	Support systems can buffer the day-to-day stress as well as during crisis.

Cultural Considerations

The Navajo people have a high incidence of severe combined immunodeficiency syndrome (SCIDS), an immunodeficiency syndrome unrelated to acquired immunodeficiency syndrome (AIDS). SCIDS is a failure of the antibody response and cell-mediated immunity. Infants who survive are initially sent to tertiary care facilities. They must receive gamma globulin on a regular basis until a bone marrow transplant can be performed. Thus far, studies indicate that SCIDS is unique to the Navajo population.

For current medications, include prescription drugs, over-the-counter drugs, and herbal preparations. Corticosteroids and immunosuppressants decrease the immune response, and some anti-infectives and antineoplastics depress the bone marrow. This results in decreased production of the cells made in the bone marrow. Bone marrow depression of WBCs can alter cell-mediated and humoral immune responses. The herbal preparation licorice, which is sometimes used for its anti-inflammatory and expectorant effects, when taken with corticosteroids, increases the effects of the corticosteroids.

A patient's lifestyle may influence immune system function and should be assessed. Knowing a patient's dietary habits and supplemental vitamins gives insight into the potential reserve of the patient's immune system for fighting infection. Anaphylactic reactions can be caused by exposure to latex, which may be found in gloves and other medical products that health care workers and their patients touch. Be aware of this potentially life-threatening reaction, and know the agency's latex allergy protocol. Patients who are allergic to latex should wear medical identification jewelry or have other readily available identification and carry an epinephrine auto-injector (EpiPen).

The patient's life stressors, coping behaviors, and support systems should be explored. Stress (environmental, physical, and psychological) can depress immune system function. Coping behaviors are essential to keep stress within manageable limits to maintain optimum immune function. Support systems play an important role in coping with stress and should be encouraged and nurtured by nurses.

Current Problem

Use the **WHAT'S UP?** format to collect data about the current immune system problem. For immune disorders, ask the patient the following questions:

- Where is it? What part of the body is affected?
- How does it feel? Painful? Itching?
- Aggravating and alleviating factors?
- Timing: Was there exposure to a pathogen? Did you have a previous infection? Does it occur only in certain settings? Did you have chemotherapy or radiation therapy? How long have symptoms persisted?
- Severity. Does it affect activities of daily living (ADLs)? Work? Roles?

- Useful data for associated symptoms. Immunosuppression? Family history? Allergies?
- Perception of the patient of the problem. What do you think is wrong?

Common signs and symptoms present with immune disorders include fever, fatigue, joint pain, swollen glands, weight loss, and rash.

Physical Examination

Physical data collection begins by observing the patient's general appearance, color, posture, gait, facial expression, skin, and nailbeds (Table 18.3). Any cyanosis or erythema (redness) is noted. Rashes should be examined for size, shape, location, texture, drainage, and pruritus (itching). Visual and hearing changes can be associated with an immune disorder.

Adventitious lung sounds, such as wheezing, may indicate asthma or an allergic response. Crackles are often associated with upper respiratory infection. Lymph nodes should be inspected and then gently palpated (by the advanced practitioner; see Fig. 18.1). Normally, lymph nodes are not palpable in the adult. If enlarged, note the following characteristics: location, size, shape, tenderness, temperature, consistency, mobility, symmetry, pulsation, and if red streaks, redness, or edema are present.

LEARNING TIP

A normally functioning immune system is required to trigger an inflammatory response and production of the signs of inflammation or infection: fever, redness, pain, swelling, and warmth. If the immune system is suppressed or functioning abnormally, this normal inflammatory response may not occur. Thus, the patient may have only a low-grade fever with none of the other signs of inflammation or infection (redness, pain, swelling, and warmth).

Recognize patients with suppressed immune systems so that low-grade fevers are reported to the physician for prompt treatment. This may be the only sign of a life-threatening infection that develops because of the suppressed immune system.

TABLE 18.3   OBJECTIVE DATA COLLECTION FOR THE IMMUNE SYSTEM

Category	Physical Examination Findings	Possible Abnormal Findings/Causes
Neurologic	Alertness and orientation	Confusion or lethargy are common in later stages of systemic lupus erythematosus (SLE) and acquired immunodeficiency syndrome (AIDS).
Skin	Warm, dry, smooth, supple, even coloring, nonpruritic	Rash, urticaria, pruritus, pustules with many forms of allergic reactions. "Butterfly rash" (red rash over bridge of nose and cheek bones) occurs in less than 50% of patients with SLE. Painless purple lesions with Kaposi's sarcoma, associated with HIV and AIDS.
	Pink mucous membranes	Pale edematous mucous membranes along with rhinorrhea and "allergic shiners" (dark circles under the eyes) occur with allergic rhinitis. Pale conjunctiva is associated with anemia. Periorbital edema can indicate hypothyroidism.
	Nail attached to nailbed	Onycholysis (nail detaches from nailbed) occurs with Hashimoto's thyroiditis.
Heart Sounds	Clear S_1 and S_2	Pericardial friction rub may be heard with rheumatoid arthritis or SLE because of inflammation of the connective tissue surrounding the heart (pericardium).
Lung Sounds	Clear throughout	Pleural effusion with tachypnea and diminished sounds in lungs can be seen in SLE or rheumatoid arthritis; pleural friction rub can occur. Crackles with a dry cough may be indicative of *Pneumocystis jiroveci* pneumonia (PCP).
Lymph Nodes	Nonpalpable and nontender	Enlarged lymph nodes that are painless, firm, and fixed are associated with cancerous lesions, whereas painful enlarged lymph nodes are associated with inflammation and infection.
Gastrointestinal	Appropriate appetite without nausea or vomiting	Anorexia, nausea, and vomiting associated with immune disorders.
	Regular pattern of brown, soft, formed stools	Diarrhea or diarrhea alternating with constipation is common with irritable bowel syndrome (IBS).
Renal	An average of 30 mL per hour of clear, yellow/amber urine without presence of protein or pain	Urine output of less than 30 mL/hour, the presence of protein in urine, and edema occur with SLE or serum sickness. Transfusion reactions can cause hematuria, flank pain, or oliguria. Glomerulonephritis may cause hematuria, flank pain, or oliguria.
Musculoskeletal	Painless and nonswollen joints with full range of motion	Swollen, painful joints and limited joint range of motion occur in rheumatoid arthritis.
	Overall strength, endurance and coordination appropriate for age and physical fitness	Decreased strength and coordination occur in patients with multiple sclerosis. Patients with myasthenia gravis lose strength and endurance with repetitive movements.

CRITICAL THINKING

Mrs. Sims

■ Mrs. Sims is scheduled for a lymph node biopsy and is seen in preadmission testing before surgery. As the nurse prepares to draw blood specimens, he learns that Mrs. Sims is allergic to latex.

1. How can the nurse promote patient-centered care during this lab draw?
2. Why is this patient allergy information important?
3. What should the nurse do next?
4. What precautions should the nurse use for drawing the blood specimen?

Suggested answers are at the end of the chapter.

If enlarged, the spleen may be palpable (by an advanced practitioner) in the left upper quadrant of the abdomen with disorders in which there is an overproduction or excessive destruction of red blood cells (RBCs).

Renal impairment from an immune disorder causes a change in urinary output, flank pain, edema, weight gain, or elevated renal function studies.

A general neurologic assessment of muscle strength and coordination, changes, or abnormalities is made. Changes may be an indication of an immune-based disorder such as multiple sclerosis or myasthenia gravis.

DIAGNOSTIC TESTS FOR THE IMMUNE SYSTEM

Presenting signs and symptoms and the patient's history determine which tests and procedures may be ordered. Table 18.4 describes the most common blood tests for patients with allergic, autoimmune, or immune disorders. Table 18.5 presents common noninvasive and invasive procedures for immune disorders. Chest X-ray, magnetic resonance imaging (MRI), and computed tomography (CT) scans might also be useful.

Gene Testing

With human genome mapping data, scientists are able to test for numerous diseases, predisposition to diseases, and enzyme deficiencies that can alter immune response.

THERAPEUTIC MEASURES FOR THE IMMUNE SYSTEM

Allergies

With allergies, medical identification jewelry or other readily available identification is essential. Allergies must be verified before giving any medications or foods. All allergies, including those to food, must be taken very seriously (see "Evidence-Based Practice").

EVIDENCE-BASED PRACTICE

Clinical Question
If a patient is allergic to shellfish, is the person allergic to iodine and therefore unable to tolerate iodine in products such as Betadine, Povidone being used on the skin?

Evidence
True hypersensitivity reactions to seafood, including shellfish, arise from the group of antigens called tropomyosins, which are proteins needed for muscle contraction. These reactions are not caused by iodine in the seafood (Harrison, 2013).

Implications for Nursing Practice
Although nurses need to continue to ask patients about their allergies, there is no need to exchange the povidone-iodine solution found in procedural kits for a non-iodine-based bactericidal cleanser in patients with seafood allergies.

REFERENCES
Harrison, P. (2013, March 19). Shellfish allergy doesn't predict reaction to imaging agents. *Medscape Medical News.* Retrieved on November 15, 2013, from www.medscape.com /viewarticle/781031

TABLE 18.4   DIAGNOSTIC LABORATORY TESTS FOR IMMUNE SYSTEM

Test	Definition/Normal Value	Significance of Abnormal Findings
RBC Count	Number of RBCs per 1 mm of blood *Adult male:* $4.7–6.1 \times 10^{12}/L$ *Adult female:* $4.2–5.4 \times 10^{12}/L$	Decreased in all forms of anemia, such as pernicious anemia that develops from the autoimmune form of gastritis or idiopathic autoimmune hemolytic anemia.
Differential	Each of these tests (MCV, MCH, MCHC, RDW) provides information about RBC size, shape, color, and intracellular structure.	Can help determine the cause of anemia. Pernicious anemia can develop because of the autoimmune form of gastritis.

Continued

TABLE 18.4 DIAGNOSTIC LABORATORY TESTS FOR IMMUNE SYSTEM—cont'd

Test	Definition/Normal Value	Significance of Abnormal Findings
	Normal:	
• MCV	80–95 mm^3	
• MCH	27–31 pg	
• MCHC	32–36 g/dL	
• RDW	11.0%–14.5%	
WBC Count	Number of WBCs per 1 mm of blood *Adult:* 5–10 × 10^9/L	Increased with immunosuppression and infection.
Differential	Percentage of type of WBCs in 1 mm of blood. Or the actual numbers of specific types of WBCs if an absolute count is performed. *Normal:*	Eosinophils elevate with type I hypersensitivity reactions such as allergic rhinitis or anaphylaxis.
	% Absolute/mm^3	
• Neutrophils	55–70 2500–8000	
• Lymphocytes	20–40 1000–4000	
• Monocytes	2–8 100–700	
• Eosinophils	1–4 50–500	
• Basophils	0.5–1.0 25–100	
Erythrocyte Sedimentation Rate (ESR)	A nonspecific test for generalized inflammation. Measures the RBC descent (in millimeters) in test tube after being in normal saline solution for 1 hr (Westergren method). *Male:* Up to 15 mm/hr *Female:* Up to 20 mm/hr	False negative may result if steroids or NSAIDs are being used when test is performed.
Rheumatoid Factor (RF or RA)	An abnormal protein found in serum when IgM reacts with an abnormal IgG; found in 80% of patients with rheumatoid arthritis and other autoimmune disorders. *Normal:* Negative	Increased in rheumatoid arthritis, SLE, leukemia, tuberculosis, older age, scleroderma, infectious mononucleosis.
Antinuclear Antibody (ANA) • Anti-dsDNA (ANA subset)	Measures autoantibodies that attack the cell's nucleus. *Normal:* Negative *Normal:* <70 international units/mL *Borderline:* 70–200 international units/mL *Positive:* >200 international units/mL	Most commonly present in SLE (>95% sensitivity), leukemia, scleroderma, rheumatoid arthritis, and myasthenia gravis; many medications influence levels. Positive in 65%–80% of SLE patients.
Complement	Specific serum proteins that help mediate inflammation. Measures the amount of each of the components in the complement system. *Normal:*	Deficiencies of specific complement proteins are seen in SLE.
• Total	75–160 units/mL	
• C3	0.55–1.20 g/L	
• C4	0.2–0.5 g/L	

TABLE 18.4   DIAGNOSTIC LABORATORY TESTS FOR IMMUNE SYSTEM—cont'd

Test	Definition/Normal Value	Significance of Abnormal Findings
C-Reactive Protein (CRP)	An abnormal protein found in plasma during acute inflammatory processes; more sensitive than sedimentation rate. *Normal:* <10 mg/L	Increased in rheumatoid arthritis, cancer, SLE. Suppressed by aspirin and steroids.
Radioallergosorbent test (RAST)	Patient serum is mixed with a specific allergen, incubated with radiolabeled anti-IgE antibodies, and then the total amount of the specific IgE antibodies is measured.	A viable alternative to skin testing if the patient does not have multiple allergies.
Enzyme-Linked Immunosorbent Assay (ELISA)	Patient's blood is tested for antibodies on HIV antigen test plates.	Positive results may indicate HIV infection, but results *must* be confirmed by another test, usually the Western blot.
Western Blot	A blood test to detect the presence of any of the four major HIV antigens. Is considered positive when at least two of the four antigens are detected. Used as a confirmation test.	If being used as the confirmation test, positive results indicate HIV infection. False positives do occur in patients who have autoimmune disease, leukemia, lymphoma, or syphilis, and in people with alcoholism.
Immunoglobulin Assay or Electrophoresis	Antibodies are made up of immunoglobulins, of which there are five different classes. *Normal (mg/dL):*	
• IgG	500–1500	Increased in all types of infections, liver disease, rheumatoid arthritis, dermatological disorders. Decreased in agammaglobulinemia, lymphoid aplasia, Bence-Jones proteinuria.
• IgM	50–300	Increased in malaria, infectious mononucleosis, SLE, rheumatoid arthritis. Decreased in lymphoid aplasia, chronic lymphoblastic leukemia.
• IgA	100–490	Increased during exercise, obstructive jaundice. Decreased in familial inheritance, immunosuppressive therapy, benzene exposure.
• IgE	<100 IU/mL	Increased in allergic reactions, allergic infections.
• IgD	<3 U/mL	Decreased in agammaglobulinemia.
CD4+ Count	CD4+ T lymphocytes are counted. *Percentage:* 60%–75% *Normal count:* 600–1500/mm³	Increased in allergy-proven patients. Decreased in cancer, HIV and AIDS, and immunosuppression.
CD8 + Count	CD8+ T lymphocytes are counted. *Percentage:* 25%–30% *Normal count:* 300–1000/mm³	Increased in viral infections. Decreased in SLE.
CD4+/CD8 + Ratio	Ratio of CD4+ and CD8+ absolute counts are determined. *Normal:* >1	As HIV/AIDS progresses, the CD4+/CD8+ ratio will become smaller as the CD4+ count decreases and the CD8+ count remains relatively unchanged.

AIDS = autoimmune deficiency syndrome; HIV = human immunodeficiency virus; MCH = mean corpuscular hemoglobin; MCHC = mean corpuscular hemoglobin concentration; MCV = mean corpuscular volume; NSAIDs = nonsteroidal anti-inflammatory drugs; RBC = red blood cell; RDW = red blood cell distribution width; SLE = systemic lupus erythematosus; WBC = white blood cell.

TABLE 18.5 DIAGNOSTIC PROCEDURES FOR THE IMMUNE SYSTEM

Procedure Noninvasive	Definition/Normal Finding (if applicable)	Significance of Abnormal Findings	Nursing Management (if applicable)
Gene Testing	A sample of DNA, which can be taken as an oral or nasal swab, is examined and mapped for a variety of genetic disorders.	Abnormal findings may confirm a certain diagnosis or indicate that the patient may develop symptoms or pass on a disorder to offspring.	Assess support systems and for possible counseling referral.
Invasive			
Biopsy (of a Specific Organ)	Biopsy tissue examined microscopically to confirm a diagnosis, determine a prognosis, or evaluate treatment. Specimen can be obtained through needle aspiration, incision, excision, or gavage, and with or without endoscopy, fluoroscopy, stereotaxic, or needle localization.	Cancers, lymphomas, leukemias, transplant rejections.	Ensure informed consent obtained. Monitor vital signs and site for bleeding as organs are very vascular with a higher risk for bleeding after the biopsy.
Skin Testing	Done if immune system is intact. Testing is done for *Candida,* tetanus, tuberculosis (purified protein derivative [PPD] test), or specific allergens such as medications, food, or environmental factors.	If erythema (redness) or induration (firmness) occurs at the site within a prescribed time frame, test is positive. Indicates patient has been exposed to an organism, has an active infection, or has developed antibodies that stimulate an immune response.	Ask if patients have any allergies and the type of reaction or symptoms that occur.

Food allergies create serious management problems and have become the most common cause of anaphylaxis in the community setting, resulting in numerous deaths from anaphylactic shock ("Nutrition Notes"). The offending allergen may be present in extremely small amounts. Sometimes a food product is contaminated by a previous batch of food made with the same equipment. Occasionally, the allergen may enter the body not by ingestion but by inhalation or contact with skin or mucous membranes.

Epinephrine is the drug of choice for life-threatening anaphylactic reactions. If possible, treatment should begin immediately with administration of epinephrine until other medical care can be provided.

An epinephrine autoinjector (EpiPen) is commonly prescribed for patients with allergies to food or insect stings. It is a prepackaged, single-use device that allows the patient to self-inject a physician-ordered dose of epinephrine right through clothing. The patient must carry the EpiPen at all times when insect stings are possible. The expiration date of the EpiPen must be checked routinely and replaced as needed. The patient should be instructed that the EpiPen does not replace the need for immediate and continued medical attention because the duration of the single dose of epinephrine varies from 1 to 4 hours. Also, anaphylaxis can be biphasic, which means a relapse can occur hours after the initial improvement from the dose of epinephrine.

Nutrition Notes

Respecting Food Allergies

Allergies and Anaphylaxis

In the community, food is the most common trigger of anaphylaxis, which can be fatal (Sicherer, 2011). Epinephrine is the drug of choice for acute reactions and the only medication shown to be lifesaving when administered promptly, but it is underutilized (Chipps, 2013). An analysis of 13 anaphylactic reactions to food in children, 6 of which were fatal, illustrates the criticality of epinephrine: mean elapsed time between ingestion of the allergenic food and a dose of epinephrine was 36 minutes in the survivors and 93 minutes in the deceased. Despite histories of asthma and food allergies, *fewer than half the children had self-injectable epinephrine prescribed, and only one of the six children with a fatal reaction used a dose* (Boch, Munoz-Furlong, & Sampson, 2001). Analysis of 63 later cases of fatal anaphylaxis caused by food allergies confirmed the original findings (Boch, Munoz-Furlong, & Sampson, 2007).

Guidelines for Treating Anaphylaxis

Guidelines specify that all patients who have experienced anaphylaxis should be discharged with (1) an anaphylaxis emergency action plan, (2) an epinephrine autoinjector (2 doses), (3) a plan for monitoring autoinjector expiration dates, (4) a plan for arranging further evaluation, and (5) printed information about anaphylaxis and its treatment (Burks et al, 2011). More education at all levels—physicians, patients, families, school personnel, restaurateurs, and the public—is required to combat these potentially preventable tragedies. Food allergies deserve more respect and timely treatment.

Immunotherapy

To help desensitize a patient with anaphylactic reactions or chronic allergic symptoms, subcutaneous immunotherapy (SCIT) involves preparing an extract of the allergen and injecting small amounts of it as a vaccine. Initially, the subcutaneous injections are given once or twice weekly with a very dilute preparation. Over a 3- to 6-month period, the concentration of the allergen in the vaccine is increased until the desired hyposensitivity is reached. Once the desired allergen concentration is reached, maintenance injections may be given every few weeks, usually for up to 3 to 5 years. It is important that the patient not miss a dose. If this happens, the allergen strength may need to be reduced.

Clinical trials are ongoing in the United States using the sublingual (under the tongue) route as an alternate to subcutaneous injections. Sublingual immunotherapy (SLIT) is the use of tablets or drops containing specific allergen extracts placed under the tongue and swallowed. It is popular in Europe, South America, Asia, and Australia. It has been found to have advantages over SCIT in a few select situations, such as when older people experience allergic rhinitis from house dust mites.

When administering the allergen injection, it is important to understand that an anaphylactic reaction can occur. A physician and emergency equipment should be readily available. After the injection, the patient should be observed for about 20 to 30 minutes to detect a reaction. The patient and family should be taught that a reaction could occur up to 24 hours after the injection and how to respond if it does occur. Local inflammatory reactions are much more common than anaphylaxis and can be minimized by giving a histamine blocker before giving the vaccine.

Medications

Medications are one of the primary treatment options for immune disorders. General categories of these medications include epinephrine, corticosteroids, antihistamines, histamine (H_2) blockers, decongestants, mast cell stabilizers, antivirals, antibiotics, immunosuppressants, interferon, leukotriene antagonists, and hormone therapy (see Chapter 19).

Surgical Management

In some cases, splenectomy is needed to control symptoms of an immune disorder. It usually is done when other lines of treatment are not effective. A significant side effect of this surgery is the reduced ability of the immune system to fight infections.

Monoclonal Antibodies

Monoclonal antibodies can be produced against a variety of antigens. A monoclonal antibody is made by cloning one specific antibody and then growing unlimited amounts of it in tissue cultures. Many uses are being found for these antibodies, such as in dealing with transplant rejections.

Recombinant DNA Technology

Recombinant deoxyribonucleic acid (DNA) technology combines genes from one organism with genes from another. This therapy is used to replace an abnormal or missing gene with the goal of producing a normal gene. The normal gene can then be injected into the patient in an attempt to cure the disorder if the patient's body reproduces the normal genes. T-lymphocyte-directed gene transfer for severe combined immune deficiency has been performed successfully. Along these same lines is the research regarding injection of stem cells, the precursors to all cells, into abnormal areas to produce normal cells. Studies continue in this area for possible uses of gene therapy. Since the completion of the mapping portion of the human genome project, new discoveries in this area occur daily. For more information, visit www.nhgri.nih.gov or www.ncbi.nlm.nih.gov/guide.

SUGGESTED ANSWERS TO

CRITICAL THINKING

■ *Mrs. Sims*

1. Review the patient's history and allergies to prevent complications. Explain the procedure, and allow the patient to ask questions or verbalize concerns.

2. The patient may have an anaphylactic reaction if exposed to latex, which can result in death for some patients.

3. The nurse should follow the agency's latex allergy protocol, enter this information into the patient's medical record, notify surgery scheduling so latex precaution protocols can be planned for surgery, and ensure that the patient's health care provider is informed.

4. Following the agency's protocol, the nurse should wear nonlatex gloves and use nonlatex equipment to draw the specimens.

REVIEW QUESTIONS

1. The nurse taught a patient about vaccines. The nurse would evaluate the patient as understanding the information taught if the patient stated that a vaccine provides which of these types of immunity?
   1. "Naturally acquired passive immunity"
   2. "Artificially acquired passive immunity"
   3. "Naturally acquired active immunity"
   4. "Artificially acquired active immunity"

2. Which of the following vaccines would the nurse correctly recommend to be given annually during a teaching session on health maintenance with an older patient?
   1. Influenza
   2. Pneumovax
   3. Diphtheria tetanus
   4. Polio

3. The nurse is assisting with data collection on a patient. Which of the following past surgeries found in the patient's history would alert the nurse to possible immune system dysfunction when planning care?
   1. Splenectomy
   2. Thyroidectomy
   3. Pneumonectomy
   4. Parathyroidectomy

4. During data collection, the patient reports tenderness in the cervical lymph nodes. The nurse recognizes that enlarged and tender lymph nodes usually indicate which of the following problems?
   1. Cancer
   2. Degeneration
   3. Inflammation
   4. Arthritis

5. The nurse is caring for a patient with suspected HIV infection. The nurse anticipates that which of the following is a confirmation test that will be ordered to test for HIV antibodies?
   1. Murex SUDS
   2. Western blot
   3. Enzyme-linked immunosorbent assay
   4. p24 antigen testing

6. Biaxin 200-mg oral suspension is ordered for a patient. The nurse has 125 mg/5 mL available. How many milliliters should the nurse give? **Fill in the blank.**
   Answer: _____ mL

Answers can be found in Appendix C.

References

Boch, S. A., Munoz-Furlong, A., Sampson, H. A. (2001). Fatalities due to anaphylactic reactions to foods. *Journal of Allergy and Clinical Immunology, 107,* 191–193.

Boch, S. A., Munoz-Furlong, A., & Sampson, H. A. (2007). Further fatalities caused by anaphylactic reactions to food, 2001–2006. *Journal of Allergy and Clinical Immunology, 119,* 1016–1018.

Burks, A. W., Jones, S. M., Boyce, J. A., Sicherer, S. H., Wood, R. A., Assa'ad, A., & Sampson, H. A. (2011). NIAID-sponsored 2010 guidelines for managing food allergy: Applications in the pediatric population. *Pediatrics, 128,* 955–965.

Chipps, B. E. (2013). Update in pediatric anaphylaxis: a systematic review. *Clinical Pediatrics, 52,* 451–461.

Ferenkeh-Koroma A. (2012). Systemic lupus erythematosus: Nurse and patient education. *Nursing Standard, 26,* 49–57.

Sicherer, S. H. (2011). Food allergy. *Mount Sinai Journal of Medicine, 78,* 683–696.

 For additional resources and information visit **davispl.us/medsurg5**

Nursing Care of Patients With Immune Disorders

SHARON M. NOWAK

LEARNING OUTCOMES

1. Explain the immunological mechanism for the four types of hypersensitivities.
2. Explain the pathophysiology of disorders of the immune system.
3. Identify the etiologies, signs, and symptoms of immune system disorders.
4. Plan nursing care for patients undergoing tests for immune system disorders.
5. Describe current medical treatment for immune system disorders.
6. List data collected when caring for patients with disorders of the immune system.
7. Explain factors that alter or influence the self-recognition portion of the immune system.
8. Plan nursing care for patients with disorders of the immune system.
9. Evaluate effectiveness of nursing interventions.

KEY TERMS

anaphylaxis (AN-uh-fih-LAK-siss)
angioedema (AN-gee-oh-eh-DEE-mah)
ankylosing spondylitis (ANG-kih-LOH-sing SPON-da-LEYE-tiss)
histamine (HISS-tah-mean)
urticaria (UR-tih-KAIR-ee-ah)

Disorders of the immune system can be divided into three categories. The first category is hypersensitivity reactions, which include conditions such as anaphylaxis, hemolytic transfusion reactions, measles, and transplant rejections. Autoimmune disorders (e.g., rheumatoid arthritis, ulcerative colitis, and multiple sclerosis) are the second category. The third category includes the immune deficiencies, such as hypogammaglobulinemia and acquired immunodeficiency syndrome (AIDS; see Chapter 20).

HYPERSENSITIVITY REACTIONS

The immune system is an adaptive system that protects the body. However, sometimes this system can cause injury to the body because of its exaggerated response. One of these occasions is when a hypersensitivity reaction occurs. In 1963, Gell and Coombs developed a system of classifying hypersensitivity reactions as types I, II, III, and IV, according to the way the tissue is injured.

Type I Hypersensitivity Reaction

An anaphylactic reaction, a type I reaction, is an immediate reaction that occurs on exposure to a specific antigen (Fig. 19.1). The reaction can range from mild to severe and life threatening. The patient must have had previous exposure (sensitization) to the antigen. During this exposure, immunoglobulin E (IgE) antibodies are made and attach to mast cells throughout the body. When a subsequent exposure occurs, the antigen causes IgE to trigger mast cells to release their contents. One of the substances released is **histamine**, which causes vasodilation, changes in vascular permeability, an increase in mucous production, and contraction of various smooth muscles.

If the second antigen exposure is localized, the reaction is mild and remains local. However, if the exposure is systemic, the reaction is massive and widespread. Respiratory allergies, such as allergic rhinitis and allergic asthma, with associated disorders of atopic dermatitis, tend to be reactions of a larger scale. Anaphylaxis, urticaria, and **angioedema** are the severest forms of type I reactions.

A type I reaction occurs when the patient has a positive reaction to a scratch test. A scratch test is done to identify specific allergens to which a patient is reactive. Tiny amounts of a variety of common allergens are scratched onto the skin,

• WORD • BUILDING •
angioedema: angeion—vessel + oidema—swelling

First Exposure

Antigens

Memory cell

Plasma cell

Macrophage

Helper T cell

B cell

Antibodies (immunoglobulins)

After Exposure

Mast cell

Second Exposure

Mast cell

○ = Histamine
◐ = Prostaglandins

FIGURE 19.1 Type I hypersensitivity.

which is then observed for indications of a reaction: redness, edema, and pruritus. If these indicators occur, it is considered to be a local reaction.

Allergic Rhinitis

Allergic rhinitis is the most common form of allergy. When symptoms occur throughout the year, it is called perennial allergic rhinitis. If the symptoms occur seasonally, it is called hay fever. The causative antigens are environmental and airborne.

PATHOPHYSIOLOGY. Allergic rhinitis is the result of an antigen–antibody reaction. Ciliary action decreases and mucous secretions increase. Vasodilation and local tissue edema occur.

SIGNS AND SYMPTOMS. Signs and symptoms vary in intensity and include sneezing, nasal itching, profuse watery rhinorrhea (runny nose), and itchy red eyes. The nasal mucosa is pale, cyanotic, and edematous. Frequently there are dark circles under the eyes, called allergic shiners, caused by venous congestion in the maxillary sinuses.

DIAGNOSTIC TESTS. Skin testing may be performed to identify the specific offending allergens to allow avoidance of the allergen. However, skin testing does not always identify the allergen, and has limited usefulness for allergens that cannot be easily avoided once identified. The in vitro allergy test or radioallergosorbent test (RAST), can be a beneficial alternative to skin testing for some patients.

THERAPEUTIC MEASURES. Initial treatment involves eliminating the offending environmental stimuli. Antihistamines and nasal decongestants may be prescribed to relieve symptoms. If the symptoms are severe, corticosteroids may also be given via inhalation or nasal spray. Rinsing the sinuses can be an inexpensive and effective way to reduce nasal congestion. Key to this intervention is to avoid introducing microorganisms into the nasal passage. The saline solution must be either sterile or made from distilled water or previously boiled then cooled water.

Rhinophototherapy uses light waves to reduce the hyperimmune response seen in this disorder. The treatment is usually done three times a week for 3 weeks and relieves symptoms such as sneezing, itching, and runny nose.

Immunotherapy, referred to as allergy shots, is reserved for patients with severe or debilitating symptoms (see Chapter 18). This therapy continues until the patient no longer has symptoms when exposed to the environmental antigen.

Atopic Dermatitis (Eczema)

Atopic dermatitis, often called eczema, is a familial, chronic inflammatory skin response.

PATHOPHYSIOLOGY. These skin lesions are not typical for a type I hypersensitivity reaction, and a specific antigen cannot usually be identified as the cause. However, the pathophysiology of atopic dermatitis is believed to be a type I hypersensitivity reaction, mediated by IgE antibodies, because it is commonly found in patients with allergic rhinitis or allergic asthma.

SIGNS AND SYMPTOMS. Initially there is pruritus, edema, and extremely dry skin, which is followed by eruptions of tiny vesicles (blisters); these eventually break open, crust over, and scale off. There is decreased sweating in these areas with the skin eventually thickening (lichenification) in the areas of dermatitis.

DIAGNOSTIC TESTS. There are no tests to confirm this diagnosis. A detailed history and physical examination are used to diagnose it and to exclude other diseases with similar symptoms. Serum IgE levels will be elevated in these patients and tend to correlate with the severity of the disease. If an infection is present, culture and sensitivity tests may be ordered to determine the infecting organism and appropriate treatment.

THERAPEUTIC MEASURES. Treatment focuses on the symptoms of pruritus and dry and inflamed skin. Antipruritics are vital in reducing the itch–scratch cycle that predisposes the patient to lesion infections. Lukewarm soaks followed with application of emollients and oil-in-water lubricants such as Alpha Keri oil tend to be the most effective for dryness. Topical corticosteroids may be ordered for their anti-inflammatory properties. Topical calcineurin inhibitors such as tacrolimus and pimecrolimus also reduce the inflammatory response and relieve itching and rash when steroids are not effective. If skin lesions become infected, topical or systemic antibiotics are prescribed. Dilute bleach soaks may also be used twice a week to reduce severity of symptoms, especially those of infection. For long-term management of symptoms, it is important to identify and eliminate the triggers of the hypersensitivity, while controlling environmental temperature and humidity.

Anaphylaxis

Anaphylaxis is a severe systemic type I hypersensitivity reaction. Table 19.1 lists the numerous possible causes of anaphylaxis.

• WORD • BUILDING •
anaphylaxis: ana—up + phylaxis—protection

TABLE 19.1 SUBSTANCES THAT COMMONLY TRIGGER ANAPHYLACTIC REACTIONS

Antibiotics	Aminoglycosides
	Amphotericin B
	Cephalosporins
	Penicillins
	Sulfonamides
	Tetracyclines
Anesthetics, Antiarrhythmics	Lidocaine
	Procaine
Hormones	Adrenocorticotropic hormone
	Estradiol
	Insulin
	Vasopressin

Continued

TABLE 19.1 SUBSTANCES THAT COMMONLY TRIGGER ANAPHYLACTIC REACTIONS—cont'd

Other Medications	Barbiturates Diazepam (Valium) Phenytoin (Dilantin) Protamine Salicylates
Diagnostic Agents	Contrast dyes
Medical Products	Latex rubber
Foods	Beans Chocolate Eggs Fruits (e.g., strawberries) Grains (e.g., wheat) Nuts Shellfish
Food Additives	Bisulfites Monosodium glutamate (MSG)
Proteins	Horse serum Rabbit serum
Venoms	Bees, wasps, hornets Fire ants Snakes
Pollens	Grass Ragweed

PATHOPHYSIOLOGY. IgE antibodies produced from previous antigen sensitization are attached to mast cells throughout the body. In this reaction, the antigen is introduced at a systemic level, which causes widespread release of histamine and other chemical mediators contained within the mast cells. The most profound complications of an anaphylactic reaction are respiratory and cardiac arrest. Immediate treatment is needed to prevent death.

SIGNS AND SYMPTOMS. Anaphylaxis produces sudden and life-threatening signs and symptoms (Table 19.2). Generalized smooth muscle spasms occur, causing bronchial narrowing and creating stridor, wheezing, dyspnea, and laryngeal edema, which can lead to respiratory arrest. Cramping, diarrhea, nausea, and vomiting also result from these spasms. Capillary permeability increases, allowing fluid to shift from the vessels to the interstitium. This causes hypotension, tachycardia, and an increase in respiratory symptoms. The blood volume in the vessels decreases while the blood vessels dilate, resulting in a further decrease in circulating blood volume. The dilation also causes diffuse erythema (redness) and warmth of the skin. Neurologic changes include apprehension, drowsiness, profound restlessness, headache, and possible seizures.

TABLE 19.2 ANAPHYLAXIS SUMMARY

Signs and Symptoms	Generalized smooth-muscle spasms • Bronchial narrowing • Stridor • Wheezing • Dyspnea • Laryngeal edema • Abdominal cramping and diarrhea • Nausea and vomiting Increased capillary permeability • Fluid shifts from blood vessels to interstitium • Hypotension • Tachycardia • Increased respiratory symptoms Blood vessels dilate • Further decreasing circulating volume • Diffuse erythema (redness) • Increased skin temperature Apprehension Drowsiness Profound restlessness Headache Possible seizures
Diagnostic Tests	Testing to guide treatment • Arterial blood gases • Electrocardiogram (ECG) monitoring History and physical exam After recovery—allergen testing for prevention
Therapeutic Measures	Intravenous (IV) access Epinephrine IV Vasopressive drugs IV (dopamine) Oxygen Antihistamines (oral, IV, injection) Corticosteroids (oral, IV, injection) If severe respiratory compromise: • Tracheostomy or endotracheal intubation • Mechanical ventilation
Complications	Respiratory and cardiac arrest
Priority Nursing Diagnoses	*Impaired Gas Exchange* *Anxiety* *Ineffective Health Maintenance*

DIAGNOSTIC TESTS. There is no time for tests to be performed during an anaphylactic reaction other than those needed to guide symptom treatment, such as arterial blood gases or electrocardiogram (ECG) monitoring. Anaphylaxis is diagnosed based on physical assessment and history from the patient or significant other. After the patient's recovery, allergen testing may be considered for future prevention.

THERAPEUTIC MEASURES. Intravenous (IV) access is a priority for administration of IV epinephrine, vasopressor drugs (dopamine), and fluids to increase blood pressure. Oxygen therapy is started. If respiratory symptoms are severe, a tracheostomy or endotracheal intubation may be needed, with mechanical ventilation. Antihistamines and corticosteroids may also be given.

EVIDENCE-BASED PRACTICE

Clinical Question
What is the effectiveness of epinephrine auto-injectors in relieving symptoms during anaphylaxis when they occur in the community?

Evidence
After a review of the literature, no new recommendations could be made for the effectiveness of epinephrine auto-injectors. So the use of epinephrine auto-injectors in anaphylaxis is recommended based on the best currently available information.

Implications for Nursing Practice
Reinforce teaching to patients with prescribed epinephrine autoinjectors on the importance of carrying the epinephrine autoinjector as directed and refilling prescriptions as needed.

REFERENCE
Sheikh, A., Simons, F. E. R., Barbour, V., & Worth, A. (2012). Adrenaline auto-injectors for the treatment of anaphylaxis with and without cardiovascular collapse in the community. *Cochrane Database of Systematic Reviews, 8*, CD008935.

CRITICAL THINKING

Mrs. Barnes

■ Mrs. Barnes, a 32-year-old woman, was brought into the emergency department after having been stung multiple times by bees while gardening. She has numerous red welts over her body that she says are itchy. She is very anxious. Her temperature is 99.2°F (37.22°C), blood pressure is 102/58 mm Hg, pulse is 102 beats per minute, and respiratory rate is 26 per minute.

1. What might be causing Mrs. Barnes' symptoms?
2. What additional information is needed?

3. What should the licensed practical nurse/licensed vocational nurse (LPN/LVN) do to help Mrs. Barnes?
4. What members of the health team should the LPN/LVN anticipate collaborating with?

Suggested answers are at the end of the chapter.

Urticaria

PATHOPHYSIOLOGY AND ETIOLOGY. Urticaria (hives) is a type I hypersensitivity reaction. It is triggered by the antigen-stimulated reaction of IgE antibodies, which causes the release of mast cell contents, especially histamine. The causes of urticaria are numerous. In addition to medications and foods, cold, local heat, pressure, and stress can also cause urticaria. Many patients with underlying chronic conditions, such as systemic lupus erythematosus (SLE), lymphoma, hyperthyroidism, or cancer, are susceptible to urticaria.

SIGNS AND SYMPTOMS. The lesions of urticaria are raised, pruritic, nontender, and erythematous wheals on the skin. They tend to be concentrated on the trunk and proximal extremities.

DIAGNOSTIC TESTS. Diagnosis is based on physical examination and history.

THERAPEUTIC MEASURES. Treatment depends on the degree of symptoms. In the most severe cases, epinephrine may be given to quickly resolve the urticaria. Corticosteroids may be given orally, topically, or IV. Antihistamines and histamine (H_2) blockers may aid in resolution by blocking the release of histamine. Patients suffering with the chronic form of urticaria might require IgE monoclonal antibody therapy such as with omalizumab (Xolair). The use of acupuncture as an adjunctive measure is being studied.

Angioedema

PATHOPHYSIOLOGY AND ETIOLOGY. There are two major classifications of angioedema, acquired and hereditary. Hereditary angioedema is considered rare and consists of three types; acquired angioedema, the more common form, consists of six types. The underlying physiologic factor in the hereditary and most of the acquired types of angioedema is a defective or deficient C1inhibitor (C1-INH). This deficiency leads to a buildup of bradykinin, which leads to the symptomology. Visit the U.S. Hereditary Angioedema Association at www.haea.org for more information.

SIGNS AND SYMPTOMS. Depending on the location and extensiveness of the edema, angioedema eruptions are usually nonpruritic and painless. Unlike the epidermal eruptions of urticaria, angioedema eruptions are of the dermal and subcutaneous layers of the skin. There may also be mucous membrane edema. The eruptions usually last longer than with urticaria.

DIAGNOSTIC TESTS. A comprehensive history and physical examination confirm the diagnosis. Skin testing may be performed to determine the specific antigen.

THERAPEUTIC MEASURES. The most basic treatment involves avoiding the antigen. Symptoms may be relieved with antihistamines and corticosteroids. For long-term treatment, immunotherapy for allergen desensitization may be indicated.

Treatment modalities for acute symptoms include a number of newer Food and Drug Administration–approved medications:

- To build up the patient's C1-INH, there is Cinryze, a purified C1-INH and ecallantide (Berinert) a C1-esterase inhibitor, which prevents the breakdown of any C1 inhibitor present.
- Kalbitor, a brand of plasma kallikrein inhibitor helps symptoms.
- Icatibant (Firazyr), a selective bradykinin B2 receptor antagonist, helps symptoms.
- Infusion of fresh frozen plasma reverses the angioedema symptoms associated with angiotensin-converting enzyme inhibitor–induced angioedema, which tends to be resistant to standard treatments.
- Androgens, antifibrinolytics, and immunosuppressive therapy are useful in the long-term treatment of some of the acquired types of angioedema.

Nursing Process for the Patient With a Type I Hypersensitivity Disorder

DATA COLLECTION. Gather information about the patient's signs and symptoms. Immediately report any sudden dyspnea, shortness of breath, anxiety, restlessness, or chest or back pain. Identify any allergies the patient may have as well as signs and symptoms that occur with exposure to the allergen. Perform a thorough skin assessment, and carefully document any lesions or rashes. Note any changes in rashes or lesions or signs of infection, such as redness, warmth, and drainage. Assess the patient's knowledge of disease process, causes, treatment plan, and self-care. Note responses to treatments.

NURSING DIAGNOSES, PLANNING, AND IMPLEMENTATION.
Impaired Gas Exchange related to laryngeal edema
EXPECTED OUTCOME: The patient will maintain clear lung fields and remain free of signs of respiratory distress at all times.

- Monitor respiratory rate, depth, and effort such as use of accessory muscles, nasal flaring, or abdominal breathing *to identify problems early.*
- Monitor the patient for restlessness, changes in mentation, level of consciousness, changes in voice, or dysphagia *to identify problems and intervene early.*
- Position the patient in a high-Fowler's or semi-Fowler's position *to improve ventilation and decrease upper airway edema.*

Anxiety related to dyspnea or pruritus
EXPECTED OUTCOME: The patient will state that anxiety is controlled.

- Stay with the patient and speak calmly *to reduce fear or frustration.*
- Teach patient to visualize the absence of anxiety, itching, or dyspnea *to decrease anxiety.*

- Provide family with the information needed to distinguish between anxiety or panic and a serious physiological problem *so that they can make informed decisions regarding obtaining emergency medical care.*

Risk for Impaired Skin Integrity related to effects of allergic reaction
EXPECTED OUTCOME: The patient's skin will remain intact.

- Assess and document skin and lesions *to provide a basis for interventions and evaluation.*
- Teach patient to keep fingernails short and clean *to minimize the damage or risk for infection if scratching does occur.*
- Teach patient to apply clean, white cotton clothing (socks, gloves/mittens, undershirt) over affected area, especially at bedtime, *to minimize scratching while allowing for air movement with minimal irritation from dyes.*
- Teach patient to use gentle rubbing or pressure instead of scratching *to minimize the amount of skin trauma.*

Ineffective Health Maintenance related to lack of knowledge of methods to decrease inflammation and pruritus and reduce episodes of inflammation
EXPECTED OUTCOME: The patient or caregiver will state understanding and follow the mutually agreed-on plan of care.

- Assess patient's knowledge of disease and its causes *to provide a basis for teaching and evaluation.*
- Assess patient's values and beliefs regarding plan of care *to ensure that it corresponds to patient's ideals, thereby improving compliance.*
- Assess barriers to patient's ability to carry out plan of care and plan interventions to decrease barriers *to improve the likelihood of the patient implementing the plan of care.*
- Discuss methods of avoiding the allergen with the patient, such as wearing a mask when mowing the lawn or working outdoors, having heating ducts cleaned, covering heat registers with filters, and frequent home vacuuming and dusting *to promote an understanding of preventive methods and prevent allergen exposure and anaphylaxis.*
- Teach patient to use medical identification for allergies *so prompt medical attention can be given if the patient is unable to give information.*
- Explain need to obtain a prescription for an epinephrine autoinjector, and teach patient how to use it if antigen is environmental (e.g., insect sting or foods; see Chapter 18).
- The teaching plan for atopic dermatitis includes signs and symptoms of infection, use of humidification during the winter months *to prevent dryness,* wearing cotton clothing *to minimize irritation,* and cool soaks *to decrease pruritus.*
- Teaching for urticaria includes stress management and relaxation techniques *to relieve urticaria* and to follow therapeutic regimen including prescribed medications and their correct usage *to reduce symptoms.*
- Document teaching and patient understanding.

EVALUATION. If interventions have been effective, there will be no signs of respiratory distress, and lung fields will be clear. The patient's posture, facial expressions, gestures, and concentration will reflect no anxiety. The skin will remain intact. If there are lesions, they will be reduced and healing. The patient will express knowledge of disorder and treatment plan. The patient will verbalize no barriers to attaining treatment goals.

Type II Hypersensitivity Reaction

A type II hypersensitivity reaction involves the destruction of a cell or substance that has an antigen attached to its cell membrane, which is sensed by either immunoglobulin G (IgG) or immunoglobulin M (IgM) as being a foreign antigen (Fig. 19.2). When an antigen marker is sensed as foreign, an antibody attaches to the antigen on the cell membrane, causing lysis of the cell or accelerated phagocytosis (engulfing and ingestion). When a cell is foreign, such as a bacterium, this process is beneficial. However, sometimes antigens on the surface of a red blood cell (RBC) can be sensed as foreign for the different ABO blood types, which results in the RBC being destroyed.

Hemolytic Transfusion Reaction

PATHOPHYSIOLOGY. A hemolytic transfusion reaction is a type II hypersensitivity reaction in which incompatible surface antigens on RBCs are transfused. These antigens may be ABO or Rh incompatible. (ABO and Rh [Rhesus] are human blood group systems.) The recipient's antibodies attach to the foreign antigens on the transfused RBCs, causing rapid lysis (destruction) of the RBC. The rapid RBC lysis

results in a massive amount of cellular debris that blocks blood vessels throughout the body. This leads to ischemia and necrosis of tissue and organs and can be life threatening.

ETIOLOGY. Occasionally, antibodies form after a bacterial or viral infection. However, prior sensitization is usually from a previous blood transfusion or pregnancy. ABO and Rh blood type must be matched for transfusions. The ABO blood types are A, B, AB, and O (Fig. 19.3). People with blood type O are universal donors because they do not have A or B antigens. However, those with type O blood can receive only type O blood. People with type AB blood are universal recipients, because they do not make A or B antibodies. Those with blood types other than AB cannot receive AB blood because they have A or B antibodies.

Rh antigens are present in people who are Rh+. A person who is Rh+ has the D antigen, which is the strongest antigen of the 50 possible antigens. Rh antibodies are present in those who are Rh− after a sensitizing event. A person who is Rh− does not have the D antigen. Those who are Rh+ can receive Rh− blood, but those who are Rh− cannot receive Rh+ blood because of the formation of antibodies to the Rh+ blood. If maternal and fetal blood Rh factors (RBC surface antigens) are different, the mother becomes sensitized by the fetal Rh type, which can

FIGURE 19.2 Type II hypersensitivity.

FIGURE 19.3 ABO blood types. From Venes, D. (Ed.). (2009). *Taber's cyclopedic medical dictionary* (21st ed., p. 306). Philadelphia: F.A. Davis.

affect future fetuses. For example, an $Rh_0(D)$-negative pregnant woman becomes sensitized by a $Rh_0(D)$-positive fetus. As a result, the blood cells of future $Rh_0(D)$-positive fetuses can be destroyed by maternal antibodies crossing the placenta.

CRITICAL THINKING

Blood Types

1. Who is the universal ABO Rh recipient?
2. Who is the universal ABO Rh donor?
3. Can someone with an A Rh^- blood type safely receive O Rh^+ blood?

Suggested answers are at the end of the chapter.

SIGNS AND SYMPTOMS. A hemolytic transfusion reaction is usually accompanied by a rather sudden onset of low back (flank) or chest pain, hypotension, fever rising more than $1.8°F$ ($1°C$), chills, tachycardia, tachypnea, wheezing, dyspnea, urticaria, and anxiety (Table 19.3). The patient also may report a headache and nausea.

TABLE 19.3 HEMOLYTIC TRANSFUSION REACTION SUMMARY

Signs and Symptoms	Low back or chest pain Hypotension Fever rising more than $1.8°F$ ($1°C$) Chills Tachycardia Tachypnea, wheezing, dyspnea Urticaria Anxiety Headache Nausea
Diagnostic Tests	Direct Coombs' test • Small amount of patient's RBCs are washed • Antihuman globulin is added • If agglutination (clumping) occurs, an immune reaction is occurring
Therapeutic Measures	Depends on severity of reaction and organs affected Antihistamines Corticosteroids Epinephrine Diuretics, to assist kidneys
Complications	If severe: shock, acute renal failure
Priority Nursing Diagnoses	*Fear* *Ineffective Tissue Perfusion* *Risk for Injury*

DIAGNOSTIC TESTS. The direct Coombs' test confirms this diagnosis. In the laboratory, a small amount of the patient's RBCs is washed to remove any unattached antibodies. Antihuman globulin is added to see if agglutination (clumping) of the RBCs results. If agglutination occurs, an immune reaction such as a hemolytic transfusion reaction is taking place.

THERAPEUTIC MEASURES. To prevent production of anti-$Rh_0(D)$ antibodies, a $Rh_0(D)$ immune globulin (RhoGAM) injection is given to $Rh_0(D)$-negative patients accidentally given $Rh_0(D)$-positive blood or exposed to $Rh_0(D)$-positive fetal blood by delivery, miscarriage, abortion, amniocentesis, or intra-abdominal trauma. When antibodies do not form, then a hemolytic reaction can be prevented.

If a reaction occurs, medications are given to treat the reaction such as those listed in Table 19.4.

NURSING PROCESS FOR THE PATIENT EXPERIENCING A HEMOLYTIC TRANSFUSION REACTION.
Data Collection. Prevention of hemolytic reactions is crucial. Following strict institutional guidelines for blood transfusion administration helps ensure the patient's safety. After blood is released from the hospital blood bank, two nurses, designated per institutional policy, double-check specified data. At the bedside, transfusion guidelines include double-checking the patient's name and identification number on the chart, unit of blood, and patient's identification bracelet, as well as checking the patient's blood type in the chart, on the unit of blood, and paperwork with the unit of blood.

Agency policy is followed for taking vital signs during a blood transfusion. Minimally, vital signs are taken before the start of the blood transfusion, 15 minutes into the transfusion, and when the transfusion is completed. It takes only a small amount of blood to trigger a hemolytic transfusion reaction, so it is critical to stay with the patient at the bedside during the first 15 minutes of any blood transfusion. This enables detection of a blood transfusion reaction early for quick action to minimize cell destruction and complications, including death.

If symptoms of a reaction are noted, the blood transfusion is immediately stopped, and agency policy for a suspected transfusion reaction is followed. A normal saline infusion with new tubing is started to keep the vein patent. The health care practitioner (HCP) and blood bank are immediately notified. A nurse remains with the patient for reassurance and monitoring of symptoms and vital signs. If a blood incompatibility is suspected, the unused blood and blood tubing are returned to the blood bank for testing. A series of blood and urine specimens are collected and sent to the laboratory for analysis. The HCP's orders are followed to treat the patient's symptoms.

 BE SAFE!

Every unit of blood, even of the same blood type, is unique and can trigger a blood transfusion reaction. Careful monitoring with every transfusion is necessary.

TABLE 19.4 MEDICATIONS USED IN HEMOLYTIC TRANSFUSION REACTIONS

Medication Class/Action	Examples	Nursing Implications
Antihistamines Block histamine at histamine₁ receptors, thereby preventing or reversing the effects of histamine (capillary permeability, itching, and bronchospasms).	diphenhydramine (Benadryl)	Take with or without food. Avoid ethanol, central nervous system depressants, and over-the-counter antihistamines. Avoid prolonged exposure to sunlight. Use caution with activities requiring mental alertness.
Corticosteroids Hormones with marked anti-inflammatory effects due to inhibition of prostaglandin synthesis and accumulation of macrophages and leukocytes at site.	dexamethasone (Decadron) hydrocortisone (Solu-Cortef) methylprednisone (Solu-Medrol) prednisolone (Delta-Cortef) prednisone (Deltasone) beclomethasone (Beconase)	Take PO with food. **Never** stop taking suddenly. Monitor weight. Assess for edema, shortness of breath, jugular vein distention, and signs and symptoms of congestive heart failure. Monitor blood glucose level. Monitor for evidence of gastrointestinal bleeding.
Sympathomimetics Marked stimulation of alpha, beta₁, and beta₂ receptors, causing vasoconstriction, bronchodilation, and cardiac stimulation.	Epinephrine (Adrenalin, EpiPen)	Use only 1:1000 solution for IV; 1:100 IV will cause death. Do not expose drug to heat, light, or air. Ophthalmic and nasal preparations may sting. May elevate blood glucose level.

Nursing Diagnoses, Planning, and Implementation.
Fear related to serious threat to health status
EXPECTED OUTCOME: The patient will state reduced fear.

• Allow patients to express their concerns *to allow inaccurate information to be corrected.*
• Inform patients about procedures and treatments *to reduce fear.*
• Remain with patient and allow significant others to visit *to offer emotional support.*

Ineffective Tissue Perfusion, Cardiopulmonary and Peripheral, related to arterial/venous blood flow exchange problems
EXPECTED OUTCOME: The patient will have adequate tissue perfusion as evidenced by palpable peripheral pulses, urinary output of 30 mL per hour, and no respiratory distress.

• Assess and maintain airway, and provide oxygen *to promote oxygenation.*
• Assess for pain and provide pain relief measures *to reduce pain.*
• Monitor vital signs and intake and output *to detect changes for prompt treatment.*
• Position patient with head elevated if short of breath *to aid breathing.*

Risk for Injury related to prolonged shock resulting in multiple organ failure, death
EXPECTED OUTCOME: The patient will remain free of injury at all times.

• Use two methods to identify patient before giving blood products *to prevent incorrect identification and administration of blood product.*
• Remain with patient during first 15 minutes of transfusion and then obtain vital signs *to detect signs of reaction.*
• Give medications such as epinephrine or steroids, as ordered, *to support affected tissues and organs.*
• Give diuretics as ordered *to assist kidney excretion of cellular debris from reaction.*

Deficient Knowledge related to lack of exposure to blood transfusions
EXPECTED OUTCOME: The patient will state understanding of blood transfusion options.

• Encourage patient to discuss autologous (self) blood donation option with HCP *to avoid a transfusion reaction.* This may be an option for patients having elective surgery.
• After a hemolytic transfusion reaction, explain to patients the importance of informing future health care providers

about the reaction *to ensure that specific blood tests are performed for less common antibodies if the patient is ever typed for a blood transfusion again.*

EVALUATION. If interventions have been effective, the patient states reduced fear, has normal organ and tissue function, and reports understanding of blood transfusion options to prevent transfusion reactions.

Type III Hypersensitivity Reaction

A type III hypersensitivity reaction involves immune complexes formed by antigens and antibodies, usually of the IgG type (Fig. 19.4). The patient is sensitized with an initial exposure to the antigen, and a reaction occurs with a later exposure. The reaction is localized and evolves over several hours, with symptoms ranging from a red, edematous skin lesion to hemorrhage and necrosis. The process involves formation of antigen–antibody complexes in the blood vessels as the antigen is absorbed through the vessel wall. Neutrophils are attracted to the area and release enzymes that ultimately lead to blood vessel damage.

Serum Sickness

PATHOPHYSIOLOGY AND ETIOLOGY. Serum sickness is a type III hypersensitivity immune reaction in which antigen–antibody complexes form and lodge in small vessels, which leads to inflammation, tissue damage, and necrosis. Serum sickness occurs occasionally after administration of penicillin or sulfonamide.

SIGNS AND SYMPTOMS. The signs and symptoms usually occur 7 days to 3 weeks after the exposure. Most predominant is severe urticaria and angioedema. The patient may have a fever, malaise, muscle soreness, arthralgia, splenomegaly, and occasionally nausea, vomiting, and diarrhea. Lymphadenopathy may occur, especially in the lymph nodes closest to the antigen entry site.

DIAGNOSTIC TESTS. With serum sickness, there is often a slight elevation in the white blood cell (WBC) count, sedimentation rate, and C-reactive protein. IgG and IgM immunoglobulins increase substantially, while the complement assay decreases. Plasma cells are seen on the peripheral blood smear.

THERAPEUTIC MEASURES. Because serum sickness tends to be self-limiting within about 10 days, treatment is focused on symptoms. Antipyretics may be given for fever and analgesics and anti-inflammatories for arthralgia. Antihistamines and epinephrine may be given for urticaria and angioedema. If symptoms persist, corticosteroids may be ordered.

FIGURE 19.4 Type III hypersensitivity.

NURSING PROCESS FOR THE PATIENT WITH SERUM SICKNESS.
Data Collection. Symptoms are noted. Responses to prescribed medications are documented. The causative agent may be identified through the history-taking process and is important for the patient to determine to prevent a recurrence of the condition.

Nursing Diagnoses, Planning, and Implementation
Pain related to muscle and joint soreness
EXPECTED OUTCOME: The patient will state pain is reduced to acceptable level within 30 minutes of report of pain.

• Monitor pain using a pain rating scale of 0 to 10 *to identify need for treatment.*
• Provide analgesics as ordered *to relieve symptoms.*

Risk for Deficient Fluid Volume related to fever and gastrointestinal fluid loss
EXPECTED OUTCOME: The patient will maintain blood pressure, pulse, and urine output within normal limits.

• Observe for signs of hypovolemia, such as restlessness, weakness, muscle cramps, headaches, inability to concentrate, irritability, and postural hypotension *to detect deficiencies to report to the HCP.*
• Monitor intake and output *to detect imbalances.*
• Provide antiemetics as ordered *to relieve nausea.*
• Encourage oral replacement therapy with hypotonic glucose-electrolyte solutions, such as sports replacement drinks or ginger ale, *because they increase fluid absorption and correct deficient fluid volume.*
• Maintain IV fluids at ordered rate *to replace lost fluids, but avoid fluid overload.*

EVALUATION. Goals are met if the patient reports less pain and if vital signs and urine output are within normal limits.

Type IV Hypersensitivity Reaction

A type IV hypersensitivity reaction, also called a delayed reaction, occurs when a sensitized T lymphocyte comes in contact with the particular antigen to which it is sensitized (Fig. 19.5). The resulting necrosis is caused by the actions of macrophages and the various T lymphocytes involved in the cell-mediated immune response.

Contact Dermatitis

PATHOPHYSIOLOGY. When a substance or chemical comes in contact with the skin, it is absorbed and binds with special skin proteins called *haptens.* With the first contact, there is no reaction or symptoms, but within 7 to 10 days, T memory cells are formed. Therefore, on subsequent exposures, the T memory cells quickly become activated T cells, which secrete the chemicals that may cause symptoms.

ETIOLOGY. Poison ivy and poison oak are the most common irritants causing this reaction. Latex rubber also may cause contact dermatitis and can trigger type I anaphylactic reactions.

Latex Allergy. Latex allergy is a serious problem for those who work in health care. Anaphylactic reactions to latex can be fatal. Exposure to latex for those in health care has increased

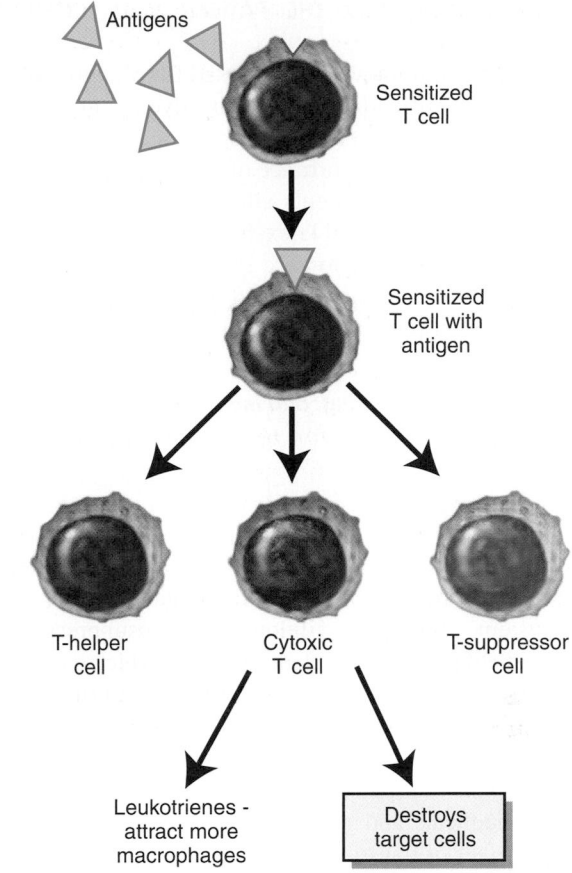

FIGURE 19.5 Type IV hypersensitivity.

dramatically since the implementation of universal precautions and the use of latex gloves began in 1987. Many times, latex gloves are worn when they are not needed, which increases exposure to the latex protein. Latex-free gloves are available. For patients who are allergic to latex, special protocols are followed using latex-free equipment. For information about latex allergy, visit the American Academy of Allergy, Asthma, and Immunology at www.aaaai.org. Also visit the U.S. Food and Drug Administration at www.fda.gov.

SIGNS AND SYMPTOMS. Within a number of hours of exposure, the area of contact becomes red and pruritic, with fragile vesicles. Secondary infections may develop. (See earlier discussion of atopic dermatitis.)

DIAGNOSTIC TESTS. Diagnosis is made by assessment of the skin and lesions through biopsy, culture or patch testing, and a detailed patient history.

THERAPEUTIC MEASURES. Treatment consists of controlling symptoms. Oral or topical antihistamines and topical drying agents may be used. Topical corticosteroids may be used and are most effective if sparingly applied after a bath or shower. If symptoms are severe, systemic corticosteroids may be prescribed. Tacrolimus (Protopic) and pimecrolimus (Abreva), which are classified as topical immunomodulators, may also be prescribed when other treatments fail.

NURSING PROCESS FOR THE PATIENT WITH CONTACT DERMATITIS.

Data Collection. Symptoms are assessed for planning of interventions. Identification of the causative agent is noted in the patient's history. Patient recognition of the cause is important to prevent a recurrence of the condition. Special protocols are used for patients allergic to latex. Some facilities may prepare special latex-free kits containing common supplies nurses use to care for patients. Ensure that latex allergy protocols are followed if a patient has a latex allergy to prevent possible development of life-threatening anaphylaxis.

Nursing Diagnoses, Planning, and Implementation.
See *Nursing Care Plan for the Patient With Contact Dermatitis.*

Transplant Rejection

PATHOPHYSIOLOGY AND ETIOLOGY. Any form of transplanted living tissue is sensed as foreign material by the immune system. This is why lifelong immunosuppression is needed to help prevent transplant rejection, which can occur at any time. Lymphocytes become sensitized during an induction phase immediately after the tissue is transplanted. If immunosuppression is not effective, the sensitized lymphocytes invade the transplanted tissue and destroy it via the release of chemicals and macrophage activity, resulting in varying degrees of transplant rejection.

SIGNS AND SYMPTOMS. Various signs and symptoms occur depending on the transplanted tissue or organ involved and the severity of the rejection (Table 19.5). Signs and symptoms reflect failure of the organ or tissue, such as renal failure for a rejected kidney.

COMPLICATIONS. A total failure and loss of the transplanted tissue or organ can occur, or the tissue or organ can be damaged from immunological reactions and not function at full capacity. The greatest cause of death following a transplant is infection. Immunosuppression therapy, which is needed to prevent tissue rejection after the transplant, is a major contributory factor for severe infection development. Because the immune system is suppressed, it is unable to effectively fight infections.

DIAGNOSTIC TESTS. Biopsy, scans, blood tests, arteriography, and ultrasonography are some tests that may be performed to aid in diagnosing a transplant rejection.

THERAPEUTIC MEASURES. Depending on the type of transplant, the body's immunological system is prepared before surgery with medications, transfusions, or radiation to minimize the risk of rejection. After the transplant, lifelong immunosuppression is needed (although studies are ongoing in which the same organ donor's bone marrow is transplanted at the same time as the organ transplant such as a kidney to reduce or elimination the need for antirejection drugs). Improved specificity of immunosuppressants has

TABLE 19.5 TRANSPLANT REJECTION SUMMARY

Signs and Symptoms	Depend on: • Involved transplanted tissue or organ • Severity of reaction Reflect failure of the organ or tissue
Diagnostic Tests	Biopsy Scans Blood tests Arteriography Ultrasonography
Therapeutic Measures	Depends on type of transplant Preventive preoperative preparation with medications, transfusions, or radiation to minimize the risk of rejection
Complications	Total failure and loss of transplanted organ or tissue Cause of death is most commonly due to infection, with immunosuppression therapy a contributory factor
Priority Nursing Diagnoses	*Grieving* (actual or anticipatory) *Fear* *Deficient Knowledge* Other diagnoses depend on which organ is failing

reduced medication side effects while improving patient outcomes. If rejection occurs, medications may be used to attempt to reverse the rejection. Supportive care is provided based on the failing organ, such as hemodialysis if a kidney rejection occurs.

NURSING CARE. Nursing care depends greatly on the type of transplant performed. Initially, the patient is in an intensive care unit under close observation and support. Observing for signs of rejection is a priority throughout the patient's hospitalization. Another consideration for nursing care is the psychological support of patient and family. Many patients wait a long time before a donor match is found. Once a matching donor is found, there is usually great elation. Yet if a donor's death made the transplant possible, the patient and family may simultaneously feel a profound sadness for the donor's family. Patients need time to verbalize feelings and understand that these feelings are normal and diminish with time. Also, the fear of transplant rejection is always present and must be discussed.

NURSING CARE PLAN for the Patient With Contact Dermatitis

Nursing Diagnosis: *Risk for Impaired Skin Integrity* related to effects of allergic reaction and pruritus

Expected Outcome: The patient's skin will remain intact.

Evaluation of Outcome: Is patient's skin intact? If not intact, is skin healing? Does patient express a plan for preventing impaired skin integrity?

Intervention Identify and document skin and lesions. **Rationale** Provides a basis for intervention planning and evaluation of healing. **Evaluation** Are lesions present? Are lesions healing?

Intervention Teach patient to keep fingernails short and clean. **Rationale** Short, clean nails cause less damage or infection if scratching occurs. **Evaluation** Does skin remain intact despite scratching?

Intervention Teach patient to apply clean, white cotton clothing (socks, gloves/mittens, undershirt) over affected area, especially at bedtime. **Rationale** Cotton allows air movement. White cloth is less irritating than those with dyes. Scratching is decreased during sleep with the use of gloves/mittens or by covering affected area. **Evaluation** Are symptoms of skin irritation reduced?

Intervention Teach patient to use gentle rubbing or pressure instead of scratching. **Rationale** Use of gentle rubbing or pressure instead of scratching causes less skin trauma. **Evaluation** Does skin remain intact despite itchy sensation?

Intervention Explain that tepid baking soda baths, colloidal oatmeal baths (e.g., Aveeno), and cool washcloths or cool baths reduce itching. **Rationale** These items help dry the vesicle and minimize the pruritus. **Evaluation** Is itching reduced?

Nursing Diagnosis: *Ineffective Health Maintenance* related to lack of knowledge of methods to decrease inflammation and reduce episodes of inflammation

Expected Outcome: The patient or caregiver will follow the mutually agreed-on plan of care.

Evaluation of Outcome: Can patient express knowledge of etiology, signs and symptoms, and treatment plan? Does patient discuss any emotional, social, financial, or material blocks to attaining treatment goals?

Intervention Identify patient's knowledge of disease and causes. **Rationale** Provides a basis for the teaching plan. **Evaluation** Does patient state baseline knowledge?

Intervention Ask patient's values and beliefs regarding plan of care. **Rationale** Patients are more compliant if their belief system fits into plan of care. **Evaluation** Does patient's belief system work with plan of care?

Intervention Identify barriers to patient's ability to carry out plan of care and plan interventions to decrease barriers. **Rationale** Barriers can prevent patient from carrying out plan of care. **Evaluation** Are barriers identified? Are solutions to barriers planned?

Intervention Teach patient to wear medical alert identification for allergen. **Rationale** With allergen identification, prompt medical care can be given in case patient is unable to give information. **Evaluation** Does patient agree to use allergen identification?

Intervention Discuss methods of avoiding allergen with patient. **Rationale** Understanding prevention methods can help prevent allergen exposure. **Evaluation** Can patient state methods to help prevent allergen exposure?

Continued

NURSING CARE PLAN for the Patient With Contact Dermatitis—cont'd

Intervention Teach patient to wash with a brown soap (e.g., Fels-Naptha) or, if unavailable, any soap when contact with the offending agent is suspected. **Rationale** This removes offending agent. **Evaluation** Does patient state understanding of need to wash off agent with exposure?

Intervention Teach patient not to scratch skin. **Rationale** Scratching can spread the dermatitis, as well as cause infection. **Evaluation** Does patient avoid scratching?

Education. Rejection can take place weeks, months, or years after a transplant (with decreasing risk). The patient and family need to be educated about specific signs and symptoms of rejection. Also, because infection is a major complication of long-term immunosuppressant medications, the patient and family need to know signs and symptoms of infection and when to notify the HCP of problems. Steroid use may mask the symptoms of infection, so small indicators such as a low-grade fever should be reported promptly. Education regarding prescribed medications is a must because the long-term success of a transplant depends on compliance with immunosuppressant therapy. Avoidance of people with colds or infections is also important to reduce the immunosuppressed patient's risk of infection.

AUTOIMMUNE DISORDERS

In autoimmune disorders, the immune system no longer recognizes the body's normal cells as self. Instead, antigens on these normal body cells are recognized as foreign material, and the body launches an immune response to destroy them.

A number of factors either cause or influence this breakdown of self-recognition, including viral infections, drugs, and cross-reactive antibodies. Some microbes stimulate production of antibodies but are so closely related to normal cell antigens that the antibodies also attack some normal cells. Hormones also may influence this breakdown of self-recognition.

Some autoimmune disorders are discussed next, whereas others are discussed in chapters related to the body system most affected. Table 19.6 lists additional autoimmune disorders and the chapters in which they are discussed.

TABLE 19.6 AUTOIMMUNE DISORDERS

Disorder	Refer to
Idiopathic thrombocytopenic purpura	Chapter 28
Multiple sclerosis	Chapter 50
Myasthenia gravis	Chapter 50
Rheumatoid arthritis	Chapter 46
Ulcerative colitis	Chapter 34

Pernicious Anemia

PATHOPHYSIOLOGY. Antibodies that destroy gastric parietal cells lead to decreased production of intrinsic factor. Other intrinsic factor antibodies (type I and type II) alter the binding sites, which ultimately decreases the ability of intrinsic factor to assist in the absorption of vitamin B_{12} in the ileum. Intrinsic factor plays a role in vitamin B_{12} absorption in the small bowel, so a vitamin B_{12} deficiency may result, causing decreased production of RBCs. Intrinsic factor is involved in most vitamin B_{12} absorption, but evidence has demonstrated that there is a route independent of intrinsic factor for some absorption of vitamin B_{12}. This has important treatment implications.

ETIOLOGY. There tends to be a familial tendency toward the autoimmune form of pernicious anemia. Causes of the acquired form of pernicious anemia (non–immune-related) include any type of gastric or small-bowel resections coupled with no or inadequate vitamin B_{12} or intrinsic factor replacement.

SIGNS AND SYMPTOMS. The patient experiences increasing weakness, loss of appetite, glossitis (inflammation or infection of the tongue), and pallor. Irritability, confusion, and numbness or tingling in the extremities (peripheral neuropathy) occur because the nervous system is affected.

DIAGNOSTIC TESTS. On microscopic examination of the patient's RBCs, macrocytic (enlarged cells) anemia is diagnosed. Macrocytic anemia and low vitamin B_{12} levels are indicators of pernicious anemia and folic acid deficiency. To determine if the diagnosis is pernicious anemia, intrinsic factor antibodies and parietal cell antibodies can be tested. Methylmalonic acid levels (when vitamin B_{12} low), and homocysteine, will be elevated, whereas serum cobalamin will be decreased.

A Schilling test can be done but is used less today than in the past because it is a complicated test. For the Schilling test, radioactive vitamin B_{12} is administered to the patient. The patient's urine is then collected for 24 hours (48 hours for patients with renal disease), and the amount of radioactive vitamin B_{12} excreted in the urine is measured. If intrinsic factor is decreased, gastric absorption of vitamin B_{12} is also decreased, so that more vitamin B_{12} is excreted in the urine. Gastric secretion analysis is done to measure levels of hydrochloric acid (HCl) because low or absent HCl may indicate pernicious anemia.

Further studies such as radioimmunoassay (RIA) or enzyme-linked immunosorbent assay (ELISA) may be performed to confirm an autoimmune etiology and specify which antibody is present, type I or type II.

THERAPEUTIC MEASURES. Corticosteroids may correct the problem if it is immunologically caused. Otherwise, vitamin B$_{12}$ therapy is needed, usually for life.

NURSING CARE. Vitamin B$_{12}$ is administered as ordered. Care related to fatigue and safety are important. Ambulation, frequent rest periods, and providing assistance with activities of daily living (ADLs) as indicated by the patient's activity tolerance are helpful for the patient with anemia.

Education. The patient and family need education regarding oral or parenteral medication therapy. If vitamin B$_{12}$ injections are prescribed, the patient must understand that this is a lifelong need to prevent the return of symptoms. Patients should not miss injections, periodic vitamin B$_{12}$ testing, or follow-up appointments.

Idiopathic Autoimmune Hemolytic Anemia

PATHOPHYSIOLOGY. In this disorder, autoantibodies, for no known reason, are produced that attach to RBCs and cause them to either lyse or agglutinate (clump). When lysis occurs, fragments of the destroyed RBCs circulate in the blood. If agglutination occurs, occlusions in the small blood vessels are followed by tissue ischemia.

SIGNS AND SYMPTOMS. Clinical manifestations vary from mild fatigue and pallor to severe hypotension, dyspnea, palpitations, headaches, and jaundice. Problems concentrating and thinking frequently occur.

DIAGNOSTIC TESTS. The RBC count, hemoglobin (Hgb), and hematocrit (Hct) are low, and microscopic examination reveals fragmented RBCs. Lactate dehydrogenase (LDH) and serum bilirubin levels are elevated because of RBC destruction and tissue ischemia.

THERAPEUTIC MEASURES. Supportive measures such as supplemental oxygen may be started. Folic acid may be prescribed to increase production of RBCs. IV immunoglobulin, immunosuppressant medications, and corticosteroids may be useful in obtaining remission. In more severe cases, blood transfusions and erythrocytapheresis (a process in which abnormal RBCs are removed and replaced with normal RBCs) may be instituted. For severe cases a splenectomy may be performed in an attempt to stop the destruction of RBCs.

NURSING CARE. The patient's signs and symptoms should be monitored and reported as needed. Frequent rest periods should be planned into the patient's daily routine to prevent fatigue. Blood products are administered as ordered to replace RBCs.

Education. The patient and family are instructed on the medical regimen, and their understanding is verified.

Hashimoto's Thyroiditis

PATHOPHYSIOLOGY. Autoantibodies for thyroid-stimulating hormone (TSH) form in Hashimoto thyroiditis. However, instead of inactivating TSH, the autoantibodies bind with hormone receptors on the thyroid gland and stimulate the thyroid gland to secrete thyroid hormones. The thyroid gland enlarges as a result of this overstimulation (hyperthyroidism). It becomes infiltrated with lymphocytes and phagocytes, causing inflammation and further enlargement. Then different autoantibodies appear that destroy thyroid cells, which slows secretion activity, causing hypothyroidism.

ETIOLOGY. The exact cause is unknown, although it occurs in females eight times more often than in males. It is also more common in people aged 30 to 50 years and patients with Down syndrome and Turner syndrome.

SIGNS AND SYMPTOMS. Initial signs and symptoms are those of hyperthyroidism, such as restlessness, tremors, chest pain, increased appetite, diarrhea, moist skin, heat intolerance, and weight loss.

These manifestations may go unrecognized and progress quickly into hypothyroidism. At this point, an enlarged thyroid gland (goiter) may be seen. Signs and symptoms may include fatigue, bradycardia, hypotension, dyspnea, anorexia, constipation, dry skin, weight gain, sensitivity to cold, facial puffiness, and a slowing of mental processes.

DIAGNOSTIC TESTS. Immunofluorescent assay, a test that detects antigens on cells using an antibody with a fluorescent tag, detects antithyroid antibodies. Serum TSH levels are elevated, whereas triiodothyronine (T$_3$) and thyroxine (T$_4$) levels are low. A thyroid scan is also done.

THERAPEUTIC MEASURES. Thyroid hormone replacement therapy of thyroxine is the primary means of treatment. Lifelong thyroid hormone therapy is needed.

NURSING CARE. If the patient has a goiter, a soft diet may be needed for comfort. Frequent rest periods may be needed, as well as slowly increasing patient activity. Antiembolic stockings may help prevent venous stasis during the low-energy, decreased-activity phase. Daily weights and monitoring intake and output when cardiac status is compromised are important to detect abnormalities such as fluid retention. Because weight gain and facial puffiness alter patients' self-image, patients need an opportunity to verbalize their feelings to help them adjust to this disease process.

Education. Patients taking thyroid hormone replacement therapy should avoid foods high in iodine. The diet should also consist of large amounts of fiber to combat constipation. During the hyperthyroidism phase, a diet high in protein and carbohydrates encourages weight gain. Education regarding prescribed medications is also needed. Cholestyramine, ferrous sulfate, sucralfate, iron-containing multivitamins, calcium carbonate and all other antacids interfere with the absorption of levothyroxine from the gastrointestinal tract. Therefore, levothyroxine should not be taken within a minimum of 4-hour period from these medications.

Lupus Erythematosus

There are four types of lupus. Neonatal is the rarest form and is passed on from a mother who has lupus to her fetus.

Drug-induced lupus erythematosus (DILE) affects approximately 10% of total lupus patients and rarely affects major organs. Research has identified about 80 prescription medications that have caused DILE (Box 19-1). A small percentage of lupus patients have the type that affects only the skin, a condition called discoid lupus erythematosus (DLE). This form is not life threatening and does not affect any internal organs. Most patients with lupus have the systemic type, which can be life threatening because it is a progressive, systemic inflammatory disease that can cause major body organ and system failure. Although this definition seems similar to the definition of rheumatoid arthritis, one distinct difference exists. Patients with systemic lupus erythematosus (SLE) typically have more body organ involvement earlier in their disease than patients with rheumatoid arthritis.

PATHOPHYSIOLOGY. SLE is an autoimmune disease characterized by spontaneous remissions and exacerbations. In SLE, the body develops abnormal antibodies (antinuclear antibodies [ANAs]) against its own tissue, leading to the formation of immune complexes. These in turn activate the complement system, resulting in negative autoimmune effects on the patient's healthy connective tissue. Many of the manifestations result from recurring injuries to the patient's vascular system. The resulting immune complexes lodge in the blood and organs, leading to inflammation, damage, and possibly death.

ETIOLOGY. The cause of SLE is unknown, but the disorder tends to occur in families. Identified chromosomal markers indicate a genetic link. Environmental factors may also play a critical role in the development of SLE. Infections, high stress levels, various hormones and drugs (especially antibiotics such as sulfa and penicillin), and ultraviolet light have all been linked to triggering SLE. Exacerbation of symptoms, also called a "flare," often occurs before the start of menstruation and during pregnancy, demonstrating the link hormones may have in triggering SLE. See Box 19-2 for a list of flare triggers.

African American, Hispanics, Native Americans, and Asians are two to three times more likely to develop SLE than others. Lupus most often affects women between ages 15 and 40 and at a rate of 9 times more often than for men. Women represent 90% of all SLE cases.

With improved therapy, the mortality rate for patients with SLE has improved greatly during the past 30 years. The leading causes of death are kidney failure, heart failure, and central nervous system involvement.

SIGNS AND SYMPTOMS. Clinical manifestations vary from mild to severe (Table 19.7). The classic feature of lupus is the characteristic reddened butterfly rash found over the bridge

---

Box 19-1 Medications Associated With Triggering Lupus Erythematosus*

- Adalimumab
- Chlorpromazine
- Diltiazem
- Etanercept
- Hydralazine
- Infliximab
- Isoniazid

- Methyldopa
- Minocycline
- Nitrofurantoin
- Phenytoin
- Procainamide
- Quinidine
- Rifampin

*Information is inconclusive and contradictory regarding some medications.

Box 19-2 Common Lupus Erythematosus Flare Triggers

- Sunlight (reflected off water and snow, glass does not fully protect)
- Fluorescent and halogen lights
- Stress
- Emotional crisis
- Overwork
- Lack of rest
- Infection
- Surgery or injuries
- Hormones

- Pregnancy and after delivery (postpartum)
- Stopping medications suddenly
- Environmental sensitivities or allergies
- Immunizations
- Certain prescription drugs
- Some over-the-counter drugs, such as cough syrups

TABLE 19.7 LUPUS ERYTHEMATOSUS SUMMARY

Signs and Symptoms	*Discoid*
	• Patchy, crusty, sharply defined skin plaques
	• Tend to occur on face or sun-exposed areas
	Drug-Induced
	• Pleuropericardial inflammation
	• Fever
	• Rash
	• Arthritis

TABLE 19.7 LUPUS ERYTHEMATOSUS SUMMARY—cont'd

Systemic
- Early symptoms are vague, then fatigue, fever
- Dermatological:
  - Butterfly rash (face), photosensitivity, mucosal ulcers, alopecia, pain, pruritus, bruising
- Musculoskeletal:
  - Arthralgia, arthritis
- Hematologic:
  - Anemia, leukocytopenia, elevated erythrocyte sedimentation rate (ESR), thrombocytopenia, false-positive venereal disease research laboratory test
- Cardiopulmonary:
  - Pericarditis, myocarditis, myocardial infarction, vasculitis, pleurisy, valvular heart disease
- Renal:
  - Renal failure, urinary tract infections, fluid and electrolyte imbalances
- Central nervous system:
  - Cranial neuropathies, cognitive impairment, mental changes, seizures
- Gastrointestinal:
  - Anorexia, ascites, pancreatitis, intestinal vasculitis
- Ophthalmological:
  - Conjunctivitis, dry eyes, glaucoma, cataracts, retinal pigmentation

Diagnostic Tests	CBC
	Antinuclear antibody (ANA)
	Anti-Sm (a highly specific immunoglobulin for SLE)
	Anti-nDNA positive in 60%–80% of SLE patients
	Anti-Ro (SSA), an immunoglobulin, positive in 30% of SLE patients
	Anti-La (SSB), an immunoglobulin, positive in 15% of SLE patients
	Complement
	ESR is nonspecific
	C-reactive protein (CRP) is nonspecific
	24-hour urine creatinine clearance
	If ruling out kidney involvement:
	    Urinalysis
	    Serum creatinine
	    Kidney biopsy

Therapeutic Measures	Symptomatic management Nonsteroidal anti-inflammatory drugs Immunosuppressants Corticosteroids Antimalarials IV immunoglobulin
Complications	Osteonecrosis Renal failure Thrombocytopenia Emboli Myocarditis Vasculitis Mesenteric or intestinal vasculitis leading to obstruction, perforation, or infarction Sepsis
Priority Nursing Diagnoses	*Acute Pain* *Disturbed Body Image* *Fatigue* *Ineffective Health Maintenance*

of the nose that extends to both cheeks, although less than half of patients develop the rash (Fig. 19.6). The rash is typically flat, not painful or pruritic and is photosensitive, worsening when exposed to ultraviolet light. Instead of the butterfly rash, some patients have discoid (coinlike) skin lesions on other parts of the body.

DIAGNOSTIC TESTS. Skin lesions can be biopsied and examined microscopically for signs of inflammation. Other tests include the erythrocyte sedimentation rate (ESR; to detect systemic inflammation) and ANA titers (to detect the presence of abnormal antibodies). There are also two subtypes of ANA: anti-ds DNA and anti-sm antibodies, which are found only in patients with SLE and can be useful in confirming a diagnosis of SLE. A blood test involving serine/arginine-rich (SR) proteins also may aid in diagnosis of SLE. Patients with SLE make antibodies against SR proteins (which are important in cell division). Seventy percent of SLE patients react positively to these anti-SR antibodies. Although no laboratory test confirms a diagnosis of SLE, the results of immunological tests may support the diagnosis.

THERAPEUTIC MEASURES. Treatment of SLE focuses on decreasing inflammation and preventing life-threatening organ damage (Table 19.8). The human monoclonal antibody belimumab (Benlysta) is the only medication directed at one of the

FIGURE 19.6 Lupus erythematosus: Red papules and plaques in butterfly pattern on face. From Goldsmith, L. A., Tharp, M., & Lazarus, G. (Eds.). (1997). *Adult and pediatric dermatology* (p. 230). Philadelphia: F.A. Davis.

TABLE 19.8 MEDICATIONS USED TO TREAT LUPUS ERYTHEMATOSUS

Medication Class/Action	Examples	Nursing Implications
Nonsteroidal Anti-inflammatory Drugs (NSAIDs) Reduces inflammation.	ibuprofen (Motrin) indomethacin (Indocin) naproxen (Naprosyn)	Take with food. Avoid taking with ethyl alcohol. Protect from ultraviolet rays. Assess for abnormal bleeding.
Antimalarials Action is not clearly understood but can significantly help reduce inflammation, decreases platelet aggregation while lowering plasma lipid levels.	chloroquine (Aralen) hydroxychloroquine sulfate (Plaquenil)	Administer before or after meals at the same time of day. Obtain a thorough assessment for a baseline, including an ophthalmic examination. May take weeks or months for effects to be noticed.
Corticosteroids Reduces inflammation and suppresses immune response.	dexamethasone (Decadron) methylprednisolone (Solu-Medrol) hydrocortisone (Solu-Cortef) prednisone (Deltasone)	**Never** stop taking suddenly. Don't miss doses. Use measures to avoid infection. Take with food or milk. Monitor for weight gain, decreased urine output, pulse irregularities, increased blood pressure, edema, and temperature. May elevate blood sugar.

TABLE 19.8   MEDICATIONS USED TO TREAT LUPUS ERYTHEMATOSUS—cont'd

Medication Class/Action	Examples	Nursing Implications
Immunosuppressants Target and damage auto-antibody-producing cells.	azathioprine (Imuran) cyclosporine (Sandimmune) methotrexate (Rheumatrex)	Monitor joints for range of motion, edema, temperature, and erythema. Protect patients from those who may carry infections. Monitor complete blood count, renal and liver function tests. Give with food if causes gastrointestinal upset. Monitor for abnormal bleeding.
Human Monoclonal Antibody Only drug aimed at one of the underlying processes of SLE: overstimulated B-lymphocytes.	belimumab (Benlysta)	May have serious side effects; careful monitoring is needed.

underlying processes of SLE, overstimulated B-lymphocytes. This medication decreases the activity of these cells, which in turn decreases the production of auto-antibodies. Many of the drugs used for SLE have serious side effects, and patients receiving them are carefully monitored.

Research is ongoing regarding the possible cause of SLE. Researchers have found more than 25 genes that are associated with or that, in combination, increase the risk for the development of lupus. These genetic discoveries are enabling researchers to develop new methods of therapy, including gene therapy.

NURSING CARE. Prevention of exacerbations (flares) is important, and therefore taking preventive measures is suggested. Minimizing exposure to the sun and artificial ultraviolet light by wearing protective clothing and 70 SPF sunscreens will help those patients who are photosensitive. Fatigue during activities of daily living can be minimized through the use of a daily personal schedule. Additionally, the patient needs a minimum of 8 hours of sleep per night with naps as needed to combat fatigue. Because most patients with SLE develop transitory arthralgia (joint pain), maintaining fitness and joint range of motion through a regular fitness program while decreasing activity during flares is vital. Warm baths may help with morning stiffness, and application of heat and cold compresses, splints, assistive devices, and physical therapy may help soreness. Eating a well-balanced diet will also influence the level of fatigue and the corticosteroid-induced weight gain, which also can affect joint soreness. Additionally, it is recommended that patients keep immunizations up to date.

Finally, but most importantly, the patient's psychological state and support systems need to be addressed. The period from the onset of symptoms to the diagnosing of lupus is usually costly in terms of time, money, and emotions. Patients may face anger, frustration, and confusion before the diagnosis. For many, there is a sense of relief at diagnosis that

may quickly be replaced with feelings of anger, fear, depression, or grief. It is here when empathy, support, hope, and, most importantly, education for the patient, family, and significant others are vital for acquiring successful long-term coping skills. In addition, local support groups and educational and self-management programs available through the Lupus Foundation of America (www.lupus.org) can provide patients with avenues for attaining more specific knowledge and skills for coping and taking control of their lives.

Education. Explain the signs of bleeding and of cardiac and vascular problems, such as myocardial infarction and thrombophlebitis. Encourage the use of a medical alert bracelet. Provide smoking cessation information to patients who smoke. Because renal disease is a major complication of SLE, patients must learn the signs of impending problems that need to be relayed to the HCP immediately. These are such findings as facial puffiness and "foamy" urine or "coke-colored" urine indicative of proteinuria and hematuria, respectively. Explain that regular ophthalmic examinations are needed for early detection and treatment of the complications that antimalarial drugs and corticosteroids can produce, such as retinal bleeding, glaucoma, and cataracts.

CRITICAL THINKING

Mr. Ellis

■ Mr. Ellis is suffering from a flare of SLE. The HCP has ordered intramuscular Solu-Cortef 80 mg to be given every 8 hours. Solu-Cortef 125 mg per 2 mL is available. How many milliliters will the nurse administer per dose?
Suggested answers are at the end of the chapter.

Ankylosing Spondylitis

PATHOPHYSIOLOGY. **Ankylosing spondylitis**, also called rheumatoid spondylitis, is a chronic progressive inflammatory disease primarily of the spine and sacroiliac area. It can also affect the large limb joints. The inflammatory process begins in the lower region of the back and progresses upward. A specific histocompatibility antigen (antigen that identifies self), human leukocyte antigen (HLA) B27, is formed that stimulates an immune response. It can result in complete fusion of the spine, causing complete rigidity in the spine, a condition known as "bamboo spine."

ETIOLOGY. There is strong evidence of a familial tendency, but no other specific causes are known. Ankylosing spondylitis tends to afflict men more than women and is usually diagnosed at ages 18 to 30.

SIGNS AND SYMPTOMS. Ankylosing spondylitis causes an insidious onset of lower back stiffness and pain, which is worse in the morning. As the disease progresses, the pain worsens and there are spasms of the back muscles. The normal curvature of the lower back (lordosis) flattens, and the curvature of the upper back increases (kyphosis). Patients may also experience fatigue, anorexia, and weight loss.

DIAGNOSTIC TESTS. Findings such as a positive family history, a positive HLA-B27 blood test, negative Rh, and radiographs of the joints showing spinal changes and fusion (although these changes are a late finding) confirm a diagnosis of ankylosing spondylitis. There are no specific immunological tests to diagnose ankylosing spondylitis.

THERAPEUTIC MEASURES. Because there is no cure for ankylosing spondylitis, treatment consists of measures to minimize the symptoms. Analgesics and muscle relaxants for pain relief, anti-inflammatory agents to decrease joint inflammation, and physical therapy to maintain muscle strength and joint range of motion are used. Biological agents such as anti-tumor necrosis factor (TNF)-α, including etanercept (Enbrel), infliximab (Remicade), and adalimumab (Humira), have shown promising results in changing the disease progression. Surgery can be done to replace fused joints. For kyphosis, cervical or lumbar osteotomy can be performed. Physiotherapy and exercise can be beneficial in managing symptoms.

Klebsiella bacterium, which is found naturally in the gut but is found in high levels in the feces of patients with ankylosing spondylitis, may be a trigger for the disease. This bacterium requires starch to grow, so it's thought that reducing starch in the diet might reduce symptoms. Visit the Spondylitis Association of America at www.spondylitis.org/main.aspx.

NURSING CARE. Nursing care focuses on patient education and administration and evaluation of prescribed medications (Box 19-3). Pain management, rest periods, assistance with ADLs, and exercise promotion are provided.

• WORD • BUILDING •
ankylosing spondylitis: anayle—stiff joint + osing—condition + spondyl—vertebrae + itis—inflammation

---

Box 19-3 Patient Education

Ankylosing Spondylitis

Help reduce pain and stiffness by:
• Providing disease information
• Explaining proper posture and range-of-motion exercises
• Teaching to change positions frequently
• Urging patients to sleep on a mattress that is firm without a pillow

---

CRITICAL THINKING

Mr. Beck

■ Mr. Beck, a truck driver who was recently diagnosed with ankylosing spondylitis, verbalizes concern about how this diagnosis will affect his ability to work.

1. How would the LPN/LVN answer his questions?
   a. "What is happening to me?"
   b. "Will I have to quit my job driving an interstate truck?"
   c. "Am I eventually going to have really bad pain?"
   d. "Am I eventually going to be dependent on someone?"
2. Mr. Beck plans to continue driving his truck and therefore has a need upon discharge for specific interventions that will help him maintain his independence. What will the nurse say to Mr. Beck on discharge about why each of the following instructions is important for him to follow?
   a. Perform range-of-motion exercises daily.
   b. Do not stay in one position too long. Stop and walk around often.
   c. Sleep on a firm mattress without a pillow.
   d. Maintain good posture, even when driving the truck.

Suggested answers are at the end of the chapter.

IMMUNE DEFICIENCIES

Immune deficiencies occur when one or more components of the immune system are either completely absent or deficient in quantities sufficient to elicit or sustain an adequate immune response to combat an infectious agent.

Hypogammaglobulinemia

PATHOPHYSIOLOGY AND ETIOLOGY. This condition is either a hereditary congenital disorder or acquired after childhood from unknown causes. It is characterized by the absence or deficiency of one or more of the five classes of immunoglobulins (IgG, IgM, IgA, IgD, and IgE) from defective B-cell function. The lack of normal function of these antibodies makes the patient prone to infections. The congenital form of this disorder affects males. Patients usually have a normal life span.

SIGNS AND SYMPTOMS. The infant is usually asymptomatic until 6 months of age, when the maternal immunoglobulins are gone. At this time, the infant begins having many recurrent infections, especially from *Staphylococcus* and *Streptococcus* organisms.

DIAGNOSIS. Until an infant is 9 months old, diagnosis is extremely difficult. At 9 months of age, immunoelectrophoresis, which measures the level of each immunoglobulin, can be performed.

THERAPEUTIC MEASURES. Treatment is aimed at minimizing infections while increasing immune system function through subcutaneous injections or IV infusions of immunoglobulin. Immunoglobulin mainly contains IgG, so fresh frozen plasma is given to replace IgM. IgA cannot be replaced, increasing the risk for frequent pulmonary infections. Gene therapy has been shown to be successful in stabilizing infant immune systems with severe combined immunodeficiency but less effective with older patients.

NURSING CARE. The infant is monitored for infections. Any break in the skin must be cleansed immediately and monitored for infection development. Genetic counseling may be recommended for parents.

Education. The family is educated about signs and symptoms of a variety of infections and the importance in seeking medical help immediately. They are taught that the infant should not be in crowds and that good nutrition, hydration, and hygiene are important in preventing infections.

Home Health Hints

Atopic Dermatitis

- Instruct patients with atopic dermatitis to use a skin moisturizer daily to help prevent dryness, which can lead to the complications of eczema. Avoid baby lotions or any lotion that contains perfumes, which can irritate the skin, and alcohol products, which can further dry the skin.
- Use of regular soaps can be drying to the skin. Urge the patient and family to use only soaps labeled for sensitive skin.
- Assist the patient with choosing an oatmeal bath product that can be helpful in relieving skin dryness.
- Use an ice pack on the irritated area to help relieve the itching of atopic dermatitis.
- Monitor for a rash, especially around the torso and abdomen. If rash develops, consider the laundry soap being used and encourage a mild soap, such as one of those used to wash baby clothes (e.g., Dreft).

Latex Allergy

- Always have latex-free gloves available.
- Use a latex-free silicone urinary catheter.

Transplants

- Teach patients who have had a transplant and are taking immune-suppressing medications to avoid those who are ill with colds or flu and public places such as stores to help prevent infection. If they do go out, suggest they wear a surgical mask to help prevent exposure to illness.
- Teach patients to take medications as prescribed especially immunosuppressant medications.

SUGGESTED ANSWERS TO

CRITICAL THINKING

■ *Mrs. Barnes*

1. Mrs. Barnes is most likely having an anaphylactic reaction to the bee stings with accompanying urticaria or even angioedema.
2. Further assessment might include identification of any previous allergies to food, medications, and environmental stimuli and what reactions occur with any allergies. Thorough respiratory assessment is needed, noting any adventitious sounds, particularly wheezing. Note any dysphagia or changes in her voice.
3. Therapeutic measures to implement include monitoring vital signs, staying with the patient, using

semi-Fowler's to high-Fowler's position, giving oxygen at 2 to 3 L per minute, and ensuring a patient IV access. Notify the registered nurse (RN) and/or HCP right away. Anticipate administration of antihistamines, epinephrine, and fluids.
4. HCP, RN, respiratory therapist

■ *Blood Types*

1. AB Rh⁺.
2. O Rh⁻.
3. No, they can safely receive only A Rh⁻ or O Rh⁻ blood.

■ *Mr. Ellis*

1.28 mL per dose.

Continued

SUGGESTED ANSWERS TO—cont'd

■ Mr. Beck

1. a. "Human leukocyte antigen B27 is formed, stimulating a chronic immune (inflammatory) response specifically in the spine, sacroiliac area, and large peripheral joints. This leads to thickening of the joints, joint pain, and stiffness."

 b. "No, you shouldn't have to quit your job, but you may need to alter the way you drive your truck."

 c. "No, you may not eventually be in severe pain, with use of medications and exercise."

 d. "No, this disease may not affect your independence, with proper treatment and rehabilitation."

2. a. "Range-of-motion exercises will help maintain joint mobility and a full range of motion and prevent contractures from forming."

 b. "Again, this frequent movement prevents stiffness and joint pain and contractures of joints."

 c. "Sleeping on a firm mattress without a pillow keeps the spine in correct alignment, which in turn helps prevent progressive changes in spine alignment (kyphosis, scoliosis) that affect various major body systems (respiratory, etc.)."

 d. "Again, good posture will aid in preventing bone deformities."

REVIEW QUESTIONS

1. A patient asks the nurse how an allergy can develop to a medication that has been taken before without problems. Which of the following is the most appropriate for the nurse to respond?
 1. "It probably is due to your age, because as we age, the body becomes more sensitive to environmental stimuli, which leads to hypersensitivities."
 2. "What have you eaten in the last 24 hours? Most medications are altered by food, thereby producing different effects in the body."
 3. "Viral illnesses and exposure to various chemicals and environmental substances can alter the immune system and its response to previously benign stimuli."
 4. "Patients who have autoimmune disorders such as lupus or arthritis tend to develop sensitivities to common medications."

2. The nurse is caring for a patient who asks what ankylosing spondylitis is. Which of the following responses from the nurse is appropriate?
 1. Chronic progressive inflammatory disease of large limb joints
 2. Autoantibodies that lyse RBCs
 3. Formation of antigen–antibody complexes leading to inflammation
 4. Production of IgE antibodies

3. The nurse is collecting data on a patient with suspected pernicious anemia. Which of these signs or symptoms would the nurse expect to find for this patient?
 1. Glossitis
 2. Itching
 3. Kyphosis
 4. Lower back spasms

4. The nurse is caring for a patient who is to have a Schilling test. What action would the nurse take for this test?
 1. Maintain on bedrest.
 2. Monitor vital signs.
 3. Collect 24-hour urine specimen.
 4. Maintain pressure dressing.

5. The nurse is caring for a patient with allergic rhinitis. Which of the following interventions should the nurse anticipate will be included in the treatment plan for this patient? **Select all that apply**.
 1. Antihistamines
 2. Avoiding environmental stimuli
 3. Immunotherapy
 4. Steroids
 5. Anticholinergics
 6. Decongestants

6. The nurse is collecting data from a patient with contact dermatitis. What data are essential for the nurse to obtain?
 1. Date of gastric surgery
 2. Appearance of skin lesions
 3. Weight gain
 4. Appetite

7. A patient is admitted with an autoimmune disease and asks the nurse what autoimmune means. Which of the following responses by the nurse would be appropriate?
 1. "Immune cells produce too many antibodies."
 2. "Immune cells grow and multiply too rapidly."
 3. "Immune cells are not produced in sufficient amounts."
 4. "Immune cells are unable to distinguish between 'self' and 'not self.'"

8. A patient who has an allergy to penicillin is receiving cefazolin (Ancef) intravenously. Fifteen minutes after the cefazolin is started, the patient reports an uneasy feeling, as well as feeling very warm. Which actions would the nurse take now? **Select all that apply.**
   1. Offer the patient ice water.
   2. Discontinue the IV.
   3. Stay with the patient.
   4. Turn off the IVPB (IV piggyback).
   5. Call for assistance.
   6. Monitor vital signs.

9. A patient who has been diagnosed with SLE is being discharged. The patient reports leaving on a 3-week tour of the Grand Canyon and going whitewater rafting in 1 week. Which of the following patient statements conveys the patient's understanding of the plan of care?
   1. "As long as I wear sunscreen, I'll be fine in the sun."
   2. "I'll wear clothing on all exposed skin and use sunscreen."
   3. "If I develop a rash, I should avoid the sun."
   4. "I should avoid the sun in the morning."

Answers can be found in Appendix C.

Reference

Gell, P. G. H., & Coombs, R. R. A. (Eds.). (1963). *Clinical aspects of immunology.* Oxford, England: Blackwell.

 DavisPlus. For additional resources and information visit **davispl.us/medsurg5**

20

Nursing Care of Patients With HIV Disease and AIDS

PATRICE WADE

KEY TERMS

acquired immunodeficiency syndrome (uh-KWHY-erd im-yoo-noh-dee-FISH-en-see SIN-drohm)
cytomegalovirus (SY-tow-MEH-guh-low-vy-russ)
human immunodeficiency virus (HYOO-man im-yoo-noh-dee-FISH-en-see VY-rus)
personal protective equipment (PUR-sun-al pra-TEK-tiv ee-KWIP-mant)
Pneumocystis pneumonia (new-moh-SISS-tiss new-MOH-nee-ah)

LEARNING OUTCOMES

1. Define human immunodeficiency virus (HIV) and acquired immunodeficiency syndrome (AIDS).
2. Explain how HIV is transmitted.
3. List how HIV is diagnosed.
4. Describe the prognosis for HIV and acquired immunodeficiency syndrome (AIDS).
5. Develop a teaching plan for prevention of an HIV infection.
6. Identify prevention measures used to decrease infection and opportunistic diseases for patients with HIV.
7. Develop a teaching plan for a patient with HIV receiving antiretroviral therapy.
8. Plan nursing care for patients with HIV/AIDS related to medications, coinfection prevention, and maintaining nutritional status.

Acquired immunodeficiency syndrome (AIDS) is the late phase of a chronic immune function disorder caused by infection with the **human immunodeficiency virus** (HIV). AIDS can develop after a long period of HIV infection and can eventually be fatal, if left untreated. The Centers for Disease Control and Prevention (CDC) specifies the criteria for determining when HIV infection has developed into AIDS (Box 20-1).

Not all HIV-infected people develop AIDS, largely because current treatments help to improve immune function and reduce the risk of opportunistic infections, which can be life threatening in these patients. The first antiretroviral (ARV) drug was introduced in 1987 and highly active antiretroviral therapy (HAART) began in 1996; both greatly reduced the death rate from AIDS. As a result, the number of people living today with HIV/AIDS is at its highest level ever (Fig. 20.1).

Box 20-1 CDC AIDS-Defining Conditions

CD4+ T-lymphocyte count below 200/mm³, or a CD4+ T-lymphocyte percentage under 14 of total lymphocytes, or the presence of one of the following specified clinical conditions:

- Candidiasis of bronchi, trachea, or lung
- Candidiasis, esophageal
- Cervical cancer, invasive
- Coccidioidomycosis, disseminated or extrapulmonary
- Cryptococcosis, extrapulmonary
- Cryptosporidiosis, chronic intestinal (greater than 1-month duration)
- Cytomegalovirus (CMV) disease (not including liver, spleen, or nodes)
- CMV retinitis with loss of vision
- Encephalopathy, HIV related
- Herpes simplex, chronic ulcers (>1 month's duration) or bronchitis, pneumonitis, or esophagitis (onset at age >1 month)
- Histoplasmosis, disseminated or extrapulmonary
- Isosporiasis, chronic intestinal (>1-month's duration)
- Kaposi's sarcoma
- Lymphoid interstitial pneumonia or pulmonary lymphoid hyperplasia complex
- Lymphoma, Burkitt
- Lymphoma, immunoblastic
- Lymphoma of the brain, primary
- *Mycobacterium avium intracellulare* complex or *Mycobacterium kansasii,* disseminated or extrapulmonary
- *Mycobacterium* tuberculosis, any site (pulmonary or extrapulmonary)
- *Mycobacterium,* other species or unidentified species, disseminated or extrapulmonary
- *Pneumocystis jiroveci* pneumonia
- Pneumonia, recurrent
- Progressive multifocal leukoencephalopathy
- Salmonella septicemia, recurrent
- Toxoplasmosis of brain
- Wasting syndrome

Note. Modified from CDC. (2008). Revised Surveillance Case Definitions for HIV Infection Among Adults, Adolescents, and Children Aged <18 Months and for HIV Infection and AIDS Among Children Aged 18 Months to <13 Years—United States, 2008. *MMWR, 57*(RR10), 1–8. Retrieved December 5, 2008, from www.cdc.gov/mmwr/preview/mmwrhtml/rr5710a1.htm

LEARNING TIP
HIV disease is no longer characterized as a life-ending illness. With ARV therapy, HIV disease is a chronic, sometimes progressive immune disorder.

NURSING CARE TIP
More than any other chronic disease in recent history, AIDS challenges nurses to call into play all of their physical, emotional, social, and spiritual care skills. As you care for patients who are HIV-positive or who have AIDS, it is important for you to understand current information. Being informed helps you to provide caring, competent, nonjudgmental care without fear (Table 20.1). Knowledge about HIV/AIDS and its treatment continues to evolve with new discoveries.

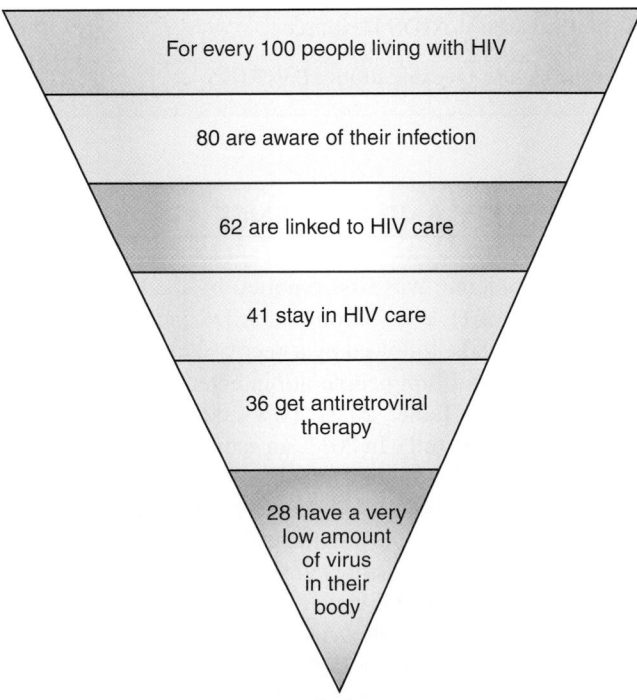
FIGURE 20.1 Living with HIV.

TABLE 20.1   STAYING CURRENT: HIV/AIDS INFORMATION RESOURCES

AIDS Education Global Information System	www.aegis.org
AIDS information from U.S. Department of Health and Human Services (in English and Spanish)	www.aidsinfo.nih.gov (800) HIV-0440
AIDS worldwide	www.avert.org
AIDS drug fact sheets	www.aidsinfonet.org
Association of Nurses in AIDS Care	www.anacnet.org (800) 260-6780
CDC (in English and Spanish)	(800) 342-2437
CDC HIV and STD test site locator	www.hivtest.org (800) CDC-INFO
CDC National AIDS Hotline (TTY service)	www.cdc.gov/hiv (800) 243-7889
CDC National Center for HIV/AIDS, Viral Hepatitis, STD, and TB Prevention	www.cdc.gov/nchhstp
CDC National Prevention Information Network	www.cdcnpin.org (800) 458-5231
Gateway to federal domestic HIV/AIDS resources	www.AIDS.gov
HIV Prevention Trials Network	www.hptn.org
HIV/AIDS Treatment Information Service (in English and Spanish)	www.hivatis.org (800) 448-0440
National HIV/AIDS Clinicians' Consultation Center Post-Exposure Prophylaxis Hotline	www.nccc.ucsf.edu/Hotlines/PEPline.html (888) 448-4911
National Library of Medicine	www.nlm.nih.gov (888) 346-3656
The Body: HIV/AIDS Resource	www.thebody.com
World Health Organization: HIV/AIDS	www.who.int/hiv

 ## HISTORY AND INCIDENCE

The HIV epidemic was first reported by the CDC in June 1981. Cases of HIV infection and AIDS increased rapidly through the 1980s, followed by a decrease in the later 1990s. More than 1.1 million people are infected with HIV in the United States (Table 20.2) (www.cdc.gov/hiv/statistics /basics/ataglance.html). In 2011, an estimated 49,273 people were newly infected in the United States, and the CDC estimated that one in six infected people were not aware of their status (www.cdc.gov/hiv/statistics/basics/ataglance.html). African Americans are estimated to have an incidence rate of new HIV infections that is eight times higher than that of Caucasians (www.cdc.gov/hiv/risk/racialEthnic/aa/facts/index .html). Women account for 25% of HIV infections (www.cdc .gov/hiv/risk/gender/women/facts/index.html).

Older adults are increasingly contracting HIV. Currently, 11% of new infections are in those aged 50 and older; patients in this age group must be educated about prevention (Brooks, 2012). Although HIV/AIDS can occur in a person of any age, this chapter focuses on adults with HIV/AIDS.

 ## PATHOPHYSIOLOGY

Infection with HIV causes destruction of immune cells. Without a normally functioning immune system, infections and cancers can take over. AIDS is the result of this immunodeficiency.

Two strains of HIV have been identified: HIV-1 and HIV-2. HIV-1 is found around the world, whereas HIV-2 is found mainly in a small area in West Africa. It is possible to

TABLE 20.2 DATA FOR U.S. ADULTS/ADOLESCENTS WITH STAGE 3 HIV (AIDS)

By Years of Age	Cumulative Estimate Through 2011
12 or younger	9521
13–14	1452
15–24	55,086
25–34	354,919
35–44	439,476
45–54	211,455
55–64	64,741
65 and older	19,143
By Ethnicity/Race	
Black	486,282
White	435,613
Hispanic	202,182
Asian/Pacific Islander	9955
American Indian/ Alaskan Native	3787

Source: Centers for Disease Control and Prevention. (2013, February). *HIV Surveillance Report, 2011;* vol. 23. Retrieved July 28, 2013, from www.cdc.gov/hiv/topics/surveillance/resources/reports.

become infected with both strains of HIV. They are transmitted in the same way, have the same symptoms, are incurable, and can progress to AIDS. Tests that are sensitive to both strains identify the type of HIV. Because HIV-1 is most common, reference to HIV in this chapter is generally to HIV-1, unless noted.

HIV is a retrovirus (which only has ribonucleic acid [RNA] for genetic material). HIV is attracted to immune cells that have a surface-attaching site referred to as a CD4 receptor. Cells with CD4 receptors include lymphocytes (called CD4+ T lymphocytes, T4 lymphocytes, or helper T lymphocytes) and macrophages (in which HIV hides). HIV begins its infection by binding to the CD4 receptor of the host cell. The CD4+ T lymphocytes are the primary targets for HIV infection. Because CD4+ T lymphocytes orchestrate all immune functions, HIV's attack on these cells results in progressive impairment of the body's immune response. The CD4+ T lymphocytes do not function normally and are too busy replicating more HIV to perform their intended immune functions.

Understanding how HIV fuses with the cell has been the focus of treatments to block fusion of HIV with a host cell.

After fusion occurs with a host cell, the HIV viral particle is taken into the cell and its covering is destroyed to expose its viral RNA. The retrovirus then uses an enzyme called reverse transcriptase to force the human cell to produce a new piece of deoxyribonucleic acid (DNA) from the viral RNA. The new DNA is then integrated into the person's cellular DNA. As a result, the human cell creates more viral particles, which spread through the lymphoid system (Fig. 20.2). Inhibitors of reverse transcriptase were the first anti-HIV medications developed and are still an essential part of current treatment.

Once the genetic material of HIV has been changed to DNA, the enzyme *integrase* integrates it into the genetic material of the host cell. The cell is then translated into viral proteins. One of these proteins is HIV protease, which is required to process other HIV proteins into their functional forms. Protease inhibitors, potent types of antiviral medications, act by blocking this critical step. Following development of the cell surface, the virus then buds from the cell and is released to infect another cell. Thus the virus can spread throughout the body. HIV can persist in a latent (inactive) state for many years. There is no cure for HIV, but it can be controlled with lifelong antiviral treatment. The ultimate challenge is to use knowledge of the HIV life cycle to develop treatments that will eradicate HIV from those who are infected and to create a protective vaccine.

After a person has been infected with HIV, other immune system components form antibodies to fight HIV. These HIV antibodies typically become present within 3 to 6 months after infection. The time between infection and developing antibodies is called the window period. Testing for these antibodies can be done to diagnose HIV. Laboratory tests are available that detect the virus directly, but these are more costly for routine HIV testing.

LEARNING TIP

Being HIV-positive means that the person has been infected with the HIV virus. It does not mean that the person has AIDS.

Progression of HIV Infection

The initial infection is followed by a relatively symptom-free period called the clinical latency stage. The virus remains in the lymph nodes, liver, and spleen and reproduces. If the infection is untreated, CD4+ T lymphocytes gradually decrease. B lymphocytes also become dysfunctional and dysregulated by the events of HIV progression. B and T cells work together for a normal healthy immune system, so this can further impair the immune system. This period, from infection to the beginning of the symptomatic stage, varies for each person and averages 8 to 12 years. During

Normal Immune System

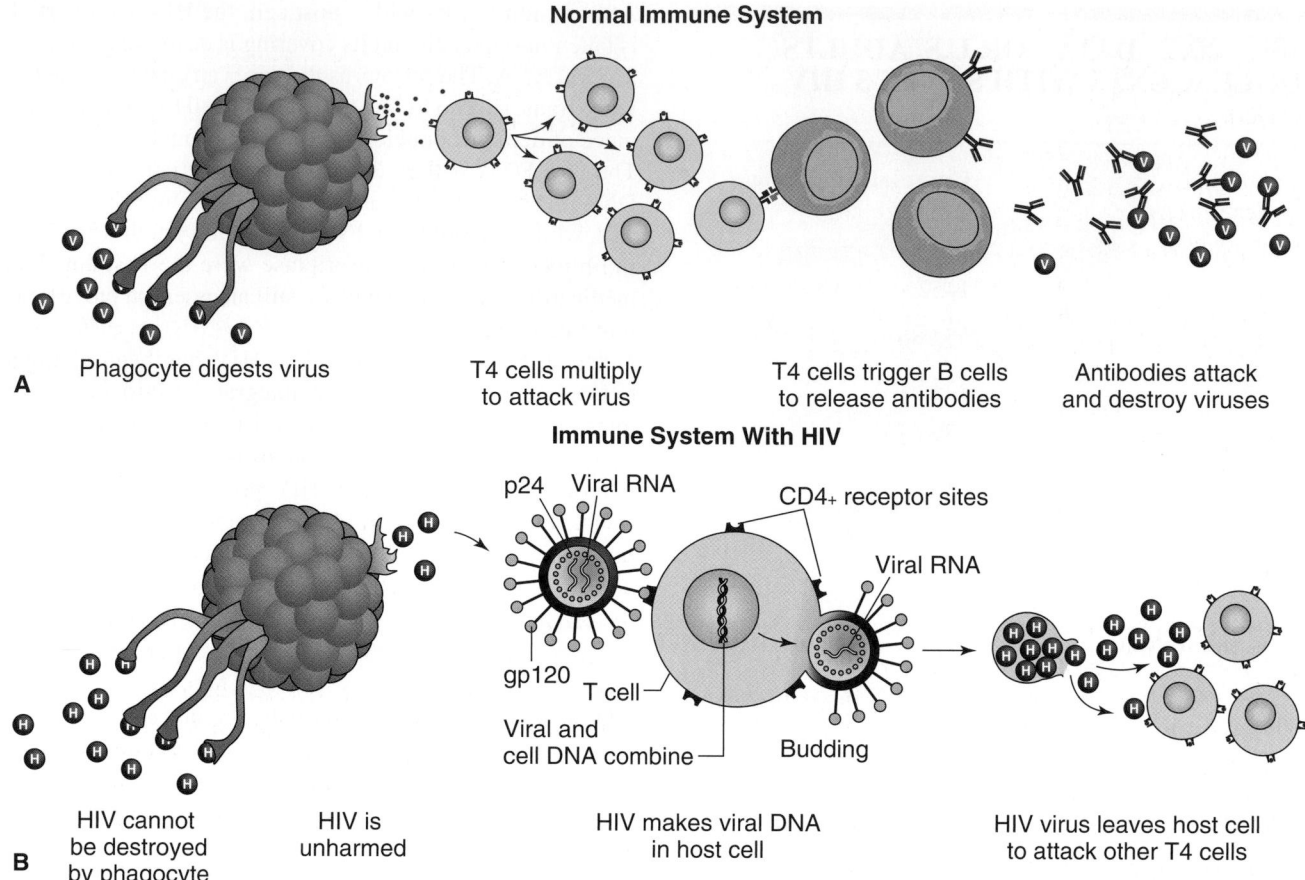

A Phagocyte digests virus | T4 cells multiply to attack virus | T4 cells trigger B cells to release antibodies | Antibodies attack and destroy viruses

Immune System With HIV

p24 Viral RNA   CD4+ receptor sites

Viral RNA

gp120   T cell

Viral and cell DNA combine   Budding

B HIV cannot be destroyed by phagocyte | HIV is unharmed | HIV makes viral DNA in host cell | HIV virus leaves host cell to attack other T4 cells

FIGURE 20.2 (A) Normal immune system. (B) HIV contains several proteins: gp 120 protein around it and viral RNA and p24 protein inside. The gp 120 proteins attach to CD4+ receptors of T lymphocytes; HIV enters the cell and makes viral DNA; the enslaved host cell produces new viruses that bud, which destroys the host cell's membrane, causing cellular death and allowing the virus to leave to attack other CD4+ T-lymphocyte cells.

this stage, the person is considered to be HIV infected. One in six persons (15.8%) do not know they are infected with the virus, causing increased rates of transmission related to uncontrolled viral loads from lack of HAART (www.cdc.gov/hiv/statistics/basics/ataglance.html). During the early symptomatic stage of HIV disease, symptoms of the weakening immune system are seen. When the immune system is severely weakened, opportunistic infections and cancers can occur (see Box 20-1).

PREVENTION

Education and prevention are the best ways to manage the HIV/AIDS epidemic ("Evidence-Based Practice"). Education regarding the disease and its transmission should begin with the older school-age child and include the general population, including older adults (www.cdc.gov) (see "Gerontological Issues"). Nurses can be advocates for this education.

 ## LEARNING TIP

Opportunistic diseases are referred to as *opportunistic* (i.e., they take advantage of the opportunity to attack) because an uncompromised immune system would be able fight off the infection. However, with HIV/AIDS, the immune system is weakened and unable to fight off the opportunistic infections.

 ## Gerontological Issues

In 2013, the CDC reported 11% of new cases and 24% of all persons living with HIV/AIDS are over age 50. Numbers will continue to rise as the older population increases, yet little attention has been given to this age group. This can be due to an ageist view of the older adult and sexual activity. It is important to understand that HIV infection can occur at any age. Older adults should be asked about their sexual and drug use history and be given preventive education and information about products that reduce transmission of HIV and sexually transmitted infections (STIs). At-risk people older than age 50 are less likely than younger at-risk adults to use condoms during sex or to be tested for HIV. In this age group, condoms are often thought of as a birth control measure. The availability of treatments for erectile dysfunction has also contributed to the number of older adults who are sexually active.

HIV/AIDS is thought of as being a disease of young, sexually active people. Many older people remain sexually active and can have multiple partners. Like their younger counterparts, older people are also contracting the virus through same-sex contact.

A decline in the older adult's immune system increases the risk for infection with HIV. Increased vaginal dryness and friability further increases an older woman's susceptibility to HIV infection. Because older adults are not usually taught HIV prevention, the rise in HIV infection among older adults is expected to continue. With AIDS death rates dropping as a result of more effective treatments, the number of older adults living with HIV will increase.

Symptoms of HIV in older adults can be confused with commonly perceived problems of aging, such as fatigue, decreased endurance, and altered cognitive status. The effect of HIV on the brain can be mistaken for Alzheimer's disease, delaying proper treatment.

REFERENCES

Padian, N., McCoy, S., Abdool Karim, S., Hasen, N., Kim, J., Bartos, M., et al (2011). HIV prevention transformed: The new prevention research agenda. *The Lancet, 378*, 269–278.

Sanchez, J., Victor, S., James, H., Baeten, J., Jonathan, F., Buchbinder, S., . . . Celum, C. (2011). Male circumcision and risk of HIV acquisition among MSM. *AIDS, 25*, 519–523.

Siegfried, N., Muller, M., Deeks, J. J., & Volmink, J. (2009, April 15). Male circumcision for prevention of heterosexual acquisition of HIV in men. *Cochrane Database of Systematic Reviews, 2*, CD003362.

Mode of Transmission

HIV is a fragile virus that is transmitted from person to person through infected blood, vaginal secretions, semen, breast milk, or body fluids containing blood. HIV is not spread casually and does not live long when outside the body. It needs a portal of entry into the body, such as a tear in a mucous membrane or nonintact skin, or access to the bloodstream or lymphatic tissue. Casual contact such as hugging, closed-mouth kissing, shaking hands, or sharing eating utensils, towels, or bathroom fixtures with an HIV-positive person does not transmit HIV. It is not transmitted in the air, water, food, or by insects. Since 1985, donated blood has been tested for HIV antibodies; donated organs are also tested, so infection is rare. Transmission within households from contact with infected blood or body secretions is also rare. Education for those living with someone infected with HIV is important (see www.cdc.gov/hiv).

Pre-exposure Prophylaxis (PrEP)

Pre-exposure prophylaxis (PrEP), with an ARV, is an effective way to prevent HIV transmission for those who are at high risk of contracting the virus. It is a daily pill and should be used along with appropriate other HIV transmission precautions.

EVIDENCE-BASED PRACTICE

Clinical Question
Does circumcision prevent HIV acquisition in heterosexual males, men who have sex with men (MSM), and females?

Evidence
Three large randomized controlled studies in Africa revealed strong evidence that male circumcision prevents men from acquiring HIV from heterosexual sex. However, in the MSM population, a randomized placebo controlled trial done in Peru and the United States reported that circumcision did not affect HIV transmission rates of 1,822 MSM over an 18-month study period. For women, there is some evidence of the benefit of male circumcision to prevent HIV transmission, but further research is needed (Padian et al, 2011; Sanchez et al, 2011; Siegfried et al, 2009).

Implications for Nursing Practice
Understanding current evidence-based HIV prevention measures is important in providing care and education to patients.

LEARNING TIP

HIV can be transmitted to others within a few days of initial infection and throughout all phases of the HIV and AIDS infection.

Counseling

Early knowledge of HIV status helps reduce the spread of HIV infection. The CDC recommends routine testing for those aged 13 to 64 years old, pregnant females, or those who have been sexually assaulted. Testing is done either confidentially or anonymously. Permission is needed to release one's test results. Posttest counseling is available to help the patient understand the test results, assist with informing sexual partners and drug needle sharers, risk-factor reduction, and care options, if needed.

Sexual Transmission

HIV can be transmitted through sexual contact with infected body fluids and mucus membranes; some sexual contact carries a higher rate of transmission. Oral and anal sex have high rates of transmission for both males and females. Anal sex has the highest risk because it often results in tearing of the mucous membrane, allowing for exposure to infected semen. Females have a greater risk for becoming infected because the vagina has a greater area of mucous membranes than the penis, and there is a greater amount of HIV found in semen compared with vaginal secretions. The presence of a STI can increase the risk of transmission through an STI-related lesion.

Research has shown that starting early ARV therapy for HIV-infected individuals can reduce HIV transmission rates to uninfected sexual partners by 96% (Cohen et al, 2011). Visit www.hptn.org/research_studies/hptn052.asp for more information. Studies are also looking at the benefits of PrEP with an ARV for non-HIV-infected people before sexual exposure to HIV. Results to date have shown effectiveness in preventing the sexual transmission of HIV (Grant et al, 2010). Visit www.cdc.gov/hiv/prevention /research/prep/index.html for more information.

Safer Sex Practices

Abstaining from sexual intercourse is the only sure way to prevent sexual exposure to HIV. A long-term, mutually monogamous sexual relationship is considered safest, when both partners have been tested and are HIV-negative. Using latex condoms correctly and regularly, limiting sexual partners, wearing latex gloves to protect hands during genital or anal contact, using condoms and dental dams (latex sheets) as a barrier for the mouth and genitals or anus and understanding safer sex techniques reduce risk of HIV transmission (Box 20-2).

Parenteral Transmission

The best way to prevent parenteral transmission of HIV is to avoid or stop injecting drugs and enroll in a substance abuse treatment program. If a person who injects drugs is unable or unwilling to stop, it is recommended that a new sterile syringe and needle, obtained from pharmacies, is used each time along with new sterile water and new or disinfected preparation equipment, and alcohol swabs to clean the injection site. Afterward, the syringe should be safely disposed of. Drug injection equipment should never be shared or reused. Syringe exchange program availability varies by location, although these programs have been shown to decrease the risk of transmission of HIV and other bloodborne pathogens. If injection equipment is reused, it should be boiled or cleansed with bleach. Additionally, sexual activity should be discouraged when judgment is impaired from drug use because protective measures, which should be taught, may not be used. Research showed that PrEP with an ARV for non-HIV-infected people

---

Box 20-2 Patient Education

Condom Use to Prevent HIV Transmission

Condoms should be:

- New for each sex act.
- Made of latex (highly effective) because other materials have large pores that allow HIV to pass.
- Undamaged and used before expiration date.
- Applied before partner is touched. (Tip of condom is held while unrolling over erect penis, allowing room at tip for semen collection.)
- Used with adequate amounts of only water-soluble lubricant. (Petroleum or oil-based lubricants such as petroleum jelly, cooking oil, shortening, or lotions can damage latex condoms.)
- Replaced if broken. (If ejaculation occurs before replacement, immediate use of a spermicide can give some protection.)
- Withdrawn from partner by holding condom against base of erect penis to avoid semen leakage.

---

who inject drugs was effective in reducing HIV exposure by 49% (Choopanya et al, 2013). This is another option for reducing HIV transmission risk.

Autologous (one's own) blood transfusion, when possible, is the safest type of blood transfusion to prevent HIV infection. There is a reported 1 in 1.8 million units chance of HIV transmission from donated blood that is infected but has not yet had time to develop antibodies.

Perinatal Transmission

Guidelines for HIV screening of pregnant women recommend that HIV counseling and testing be offered during routine prenatal care for all pregnant women and again in the third trimester for women at high risk (Branson et al, 2006). All pregnant women who are HIV-positive can reduce the risk of perinatal HIV transmission to less than 1% by taking ARV therapy (including zidovudine [AZT]) during pregnancy, labor, and delivery. At the time of labor, pregnant women who have not been tested for HIV should be offered rapid HIV tests, and therapy should be started if HIV is confirmed. After delivery, the infant of a mother with HIV is given AZT for 6 weeks.

Health Care Providers and HIV Prevention

Occupational HIV transmission is rare. Using standard precautions (see Chapter 8), performing hand hygiene after contact with body fluids, and using safety devices to prevent needlesticks (needles systems, protective covers, and not recapping used needles) or other injuries reduce the risk of HIV exposure. It is essential to understand and use these practices with all patients to protect yourself from exposure and transmission of HIV. If you are unsure of the appropriate **personal protective equipment** or isolation precautions to use, ask your instructor or the patient's nurse before providing care to the patient.

Know the occupational exposure protocol for the agency or hospital in which you are employed. If an exposure occurs, wash the exposure site with soap and water immediately. For mucous membrane exposure, flush with water and then report to the closest emergency room immediately for further assessment and possible treatment. The U.S. Public Health Service guidelines for occupational exposures can be viewed at www.jstor.org/stable/10.1086/672271.

HIV SIGNS AND SYMPTOMS

Each patient's HIV response is different. Initially after HIV infection, the patient can have no symptoms or can develop acute retroviral syndrome with symptoms of extreme fatigue, headache, fever, lymphadenopathy (enlarged lymph nodes in two sites other than inguinal nodes), diarrhea, or a sore throat (Fig. 20.3 and Table 20.3). Symptoms typically develop 6 to 12 weeks after HIV transmission and can last a few days to weeks. These symptoms are usually mild and not attributed to the HIV infection.

After an extended asymptomatic phase, untreated HIV infection usually progresses to a symptomatic stage when the virus has greatly impaired the immune system. The patient can have shortness of breath, fever, weight loss, fatigue, night sweats, persistent diarrhea, oral or vaginal candidiasis ulcers, dry skin, skin lesions, peripheral neuropathy, shingles (varicella zoster virus reactivation), seizures, or dementia. In the final stage of HIV infection, AIDS is diagnosed when the CD4+ T-lymphocyte count is below 200 or opportunistic infections and diseases, with their specific signs and symptoms, occur (see Box 20-1).

COMPLICATIONS

Complications from HIV/AIDS vary from patient to patient. With HAART, fewer complications are seen than in the past. Some, such as Kaposi's sarcoma (a connective tissue tumor), are rarely seen anymore. A few complications are discussed next.

AIDS Wasting Syndrome

AIDS wasting syndrome is defined by involuntary loss of more than 10% of baseline body weight plus chronic weakness or fever or chronic diarrhea for more than 30 days. Several factors contribute to this syndrome: decreased appetite, oral lesions, altered metabolism, malabsorption, gastrointestinal (GI) infections, diarrhea, medication side effects, and cognitive impairment. The progressive weight loss impairs the function of all body systems from malnourishment. Careful planning, intervention, and education of the patient when HIV is first diagnosed can help maintain body weight.

HIV-Associated Neurocognitive Disorder

HIV infection in the brain or other parts of the central nervous system (CNS) results in CNS conditions with varying degrees of severity. Examples include asymptomatic neurocognitive impairment, minor neurocognitive disorder, and HIV-associated dementia [HIV encephalopathy or AIDS dementia complex]. Symptoms range from mild to severe and can include memory impairment, personality changes, hallucinations, leg weakness, loss of balance, and slower responses. In advanced AIDS, with HAART, AIDS dementia complex is less common than before and minor cognitive motor disorder has become more common. When CNS changes occur, safety is an important consideration for the patient and caregiver.

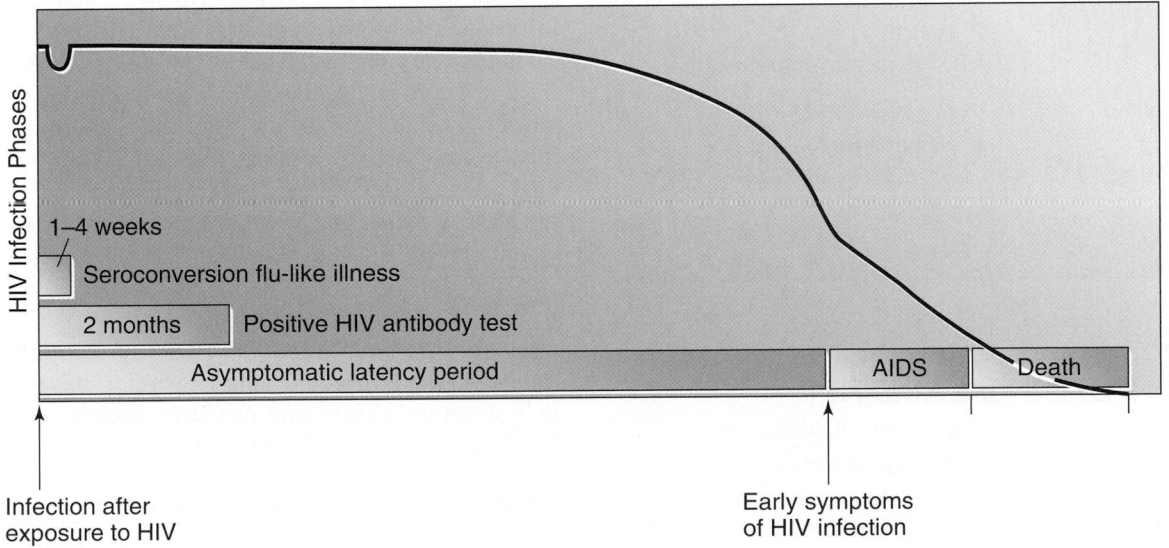

CD4+ T-lymphocyte Count During HIV Disease and AIDS

FIGURE 20.3 Typical phases of HIV infection, AIDS development, and CD4+ T-lymphocyte counts without treatment. Length of latency period varies but is usually many years. As CD4+ T-lymphocyte counts drop, symptoms, AIDS, opportunistic infections, and then death can result.

TABLE 20.3 HIV/AIDS SUMMARY

Signs and Symptoms	Initially vary; none or acute retro-viral syndrome Asymptomatic phase Immune system impairment: dyspnea, fever, weight loss, fatigue, night sweats, persistent diarrhea, oral or vaginal candidiasis ulcers, dry skin, skin lesions, peripheral neuropathy, shingles, or dementia AIDS diagnosed when CD4+ T-lymphocyte count below 200 or opportunistic infections and diseases occur.
Diagnostic Tests	HIV antibody tests RNA Tests Complete blood cell count/ lymphocyte count CD4+/CD8+ T-lymphocyte count Viral load testing Genotyping
Therapeutic Measures	Nonnucleoside reverse transcriptase inhibitors (NRTIs) Nucleoside reverse transcriptase inhibitors (NNRTIs) Protease inhibitors (PIs) Fusion inhibitors Cellular chemokine receptor (CCR5) antagonists Integrase inhibitors
Complications	AIDS wasting syndrome Opportunistic infections and cancer AIDS dementia complex
Priority Nursing Diagnoses	*Ineffective Protection* *Acute* or *Chronic Pain* *Ineffective Coping* *Risk for Injury*

NURSING CARE TIP

AIDS wasting syndrome is challenging. Do not give up! Be creative in developing interventions to help increase the patient's appetite and calorie intake. Small, frequent meals are usually helpful. A registered dietitian can be a helpful member on the care team for HIV patients.

Cancer and Opportunistic Infections

Why would a person with HIV/AIDS have increased risk for cancer and opportunistic infections? With an impaired immune system, the incidence of certain kinds of cancer rises because the immune system is not able to destroy the abnormal cells. Opportunistic infections, which a healthy immune system could fight, are also a complication of HIV/AIDS. Infections that develop even with a healthy immune system, such as tuberculosis, can also occur. Opportunistic infections can be viral, bacterial, mycobacterial, fungal, protozoal, or parasitic. They can affect many areas of the body. Some opportunistic infections can now be prevented with prophylactic treatments. Some infections are discussed here.

Candida Albicans

Candida albicans is a fungus normally found in the GI tract that does not infect a person with a healthy immune system. In AIDS, overgrowth of this fungus occurs. Candidiasis of the mouth or esophagus is common in AIDS. Signs and symptoms of candidiasis include oral or esophageal pain, dysphagia, and yellow-white plaques that look like cottage cheese in the mouth and throat. Nutrition can be affected by oral or esophageal candidiasis. Recurrent vaginal candidiasis, with severe itching and a white discharge, is common in women with AIDS.

Cytomegalovirus

Cytomegalovirus (CMV) infection can be serious for those with HIV/AIDS, especially when CD4+ T-lymphocyte counts fall below 100/mm³. It can cause retinitis, which can result in blindness. Other symptoms can include fever, fatigue, diarrhea, GI upset, and hepatitis.

Mycobacterium Avium Complex

Mycobacterium avium complex (MAC), a serious bacterial infection, can occur in those with AIDS when CD4+ T-lymphocyte counts drop below 50. MAC is found in water, food, and soil, so avoidance is difficult. Prophylactic drugs when CD4 counts fall below 50 include azithromycin, clarithromycin, or rifabutin. With infection, symptoms can include fever, night sweats, weight loss, abdominal pain, tiredness, and diarrhea. Treatment includes a combination of clarithromycin and ethambutol, and possibly rifabutin.

Pneumocystis Pneumonia

Pneumocystis pneumonia (PCP) is caused by the fungus *Pneumocystis jiroveci* in immunocompromised persons. PCP develops slowly and produces shortness of breath, fever, and dry cough. When CD4+ T-lymphocyte counts fall below 350/mm³, prophylactic oral trimethoprim-sulfamethoxazole (TMP-SMX [Bactrim, Septra, Cotrim]) is recommended. PCP is less likely to occur than in the past with TMP-SMX but remains a concern for those with HIV/AIDS. PCP can be treated with oxygen, TMP-SMX, or pentamidine isethionate. Steroids can help reduce lung inflammation.

Tuberculosis

Tuberculosis is a bacterial infection caused by the mycobacterium tuberculosis. Symptoms include dyspnea, cough, chest pain, fever, night sweats, and weight loss. A Mantoux tuberculin skin test (TST) with tuberculin purified protein derivative should be performed at least yearly in patients with HIV infection. Induration of 5 mm or more is defined as a positive result in patients with HIV infection and so defines the development of AIDS (see Chapter 31).

NURSING CARE TIP

When assessing the results of a TST, only the induration (palpable, raised, hardened area or swelling) is measured across the forearm and recorded in millimeters. If there is no induration, it is recorded as 0 mm.

DIAGNOSIS

HIV screening is recommended for people from 15 to 65 years of age at least once (Moyer, 2013). Those with increased risk outside of this age range should also be screened. For those at high risk, screening should occur more frequently.

Fingerstick blood, oral fluid (OraQuick Rapid HIV test—swab of complete upper and lower outer gums), and serum specimens can be used for HIV testing. Urine can also be tested but is slightly less accurate. Results can be available in less than 20 minutes with the Multispot HIV-1/HIV-2 Rapid Test or in 1 hour for immunoassay (IA) testing. Consumer-controlled test kits (home sample collection devices) can be purchased at drug stores; the blood sample is sent in for HIV testing, with the individual anonymously calling for results, counseling, and referral if needed.

After HIV infection, antibodies cannot be formed for 3 weeks to 3 months or longer in some cases. Early-detection HIV tests are available for detection as soon as 1 week after potential exposure.

HIV Antibody Tests

The traditional HIV-1 antibody testing pattern:

- An enzyme-linked immunosorbent assay (ELISA) test is done to detect antibodies to HIV antigen in the patient's blood using test plates.
- If positive, the ELISA test is repeated because false positives can occur (0.1%).
- If the ELISA test is again positive, the Western blot test is done to detect the presence of antibodies to four major HIV antigens. The test is positive if two antibodies are present.
- If all test results are positive, the patient is HIV-antibody positive.

- If the test is negative, the patient is said to be in the window period or HIV negative.
- Other tests can be used, especially if initial test results are not conclusive. Testing directly for the virus is available but more costly.

New testing guidelines were evaluated in 2011–2013 by the CDC to reduce missed HIV diagnoses. Third- and fourth-generation immunoassays are very sensitive and can be positive when the confirming tests are falsely negative. This false result can lead to delayed treatment and continued transmission of HIV. For a positive HIV immunoassay result and a negative antibody test result, additional testing to detect the virus directly is needed to confirm an acute HIV infection. (Visit www.cdc.gov for testing guidelines).

Complete Blood Cell Count/Lymphocyte Count

Because patients with HIV are susceptible to leukopenia, lymphopenia, anemia, and thrombocytopenia related to HIV infection and as a complication of antiretroviral therapy, a complete blood cell count (CBC) including a lymphocyte count should be obtained. The CBC should be repeated at 3- to 4-month intervals or more often if there is a change in therapy or the patient's clinical course is unstable.

CD4+/CD8+ T-Lymphocyte Count

The count of CD4+ and CD8+ (cytotoxic cells) T lymphocytes is essential for evaluating the status of the immune system. In healthy adults, CD4+ levels average 500 to 1600 cells per mm³. In HIV/AIDS, CD4+ cell levels drop but CD8+ cell levels do not. A low ratio of CD4+ cells to CD8+ cells is seen as HIV/AIDS progresses. It is recommended that CD4+/CD8+ T-lymphocyte counts be performed at 3-month intervals for most patients, especially those on ARV therapy.

Viral Load Testing

Viral load testing measures the amount of HIV RNA in plasma and is extremely important for determining the risk of disease progression if left untreated, the risk of opportunistic infections, and the response to ARV therapy. Combination ARV regimens usually produce a 50% decrease in total-body HIV levels within just a few days. Viral loads should be performed 1 month after starting new treatments and at 3-month intervals thereafter. The goal on ARV therapy is to obtain and maintain an ultrasensitive undetectable viral load.

Genotyping

Genotyping measures resistance to currently available ARV treatments. This information guides HCPs in choosing treatment regimens that will most likely be effective against that person's virus.

General Tests

Standard serological testing for syphilis is recommended annually in patients who are sexually active. Hepatitis A, B, and C serologies and liver chemistry panels are indicated in the early evaluation because of the high incidence of concurrent hepatitis coinfection for HIV-positive patients. Coinfections can influence the course of either the patient's HIV or the coinfection. It can also affect the HIV treatment options.

 THERAPEUTIC MEASURES

The goal of therapy is to prevent or delay development of opportunistic diseases. In 2013, the federal *Guidelines for the Use of Antiretroviral Agents in HIV-1 Infected Adults and Adolescents* was updated (Panel on Antiretroviral Guidelines for Adults and Adolescents, 2013). They recommend that all patients with HIV be started on HAART, independent of CD4 count. In addition, to increase life expectancy and treatment cost-effectiveness, it is recommended for patients to be prophylactically treated for opportunistic infections, especially hepatitis A and hepatitis B viruses, herpes simplex virus, *Mycobacterium avium*

complex, and *Pneumocystis jiroveci* pneumonia (Table 20.4). Other opportunistic infections are treated with appropriate medications if they occur.

ARV drugs that inhibit reproduction of the virus (but do not kill it) are used to treat HIV infection. These ARV agents have been developed to act predominantly on processes specific to the viral particle to protect the integrity of the host cell. Strategies specifically aimed at interrupting the viral life cycle include the following:

• Preventing the virus from attaching to the CD4+ receptor of the T4 lymphocyte
• Interfering with "uncoating" of the virus within the cell, the first essential step in allowing the virus to integrate into the cell's DNA
• Inhibiting reverse transcriptase, a viral enzyme specific to retroviruses, which enables the virus to make a DNA copy

TABLE 20.4 TREATMENT FOR AIDS-RELATED CONDITIONS

Opportunistic Infection/Complication	Treatment
Candidiasis	nystatin, ketoconazole (Nizoral), fluconazole (Diflucan), amphotericin B (Fungizone)
Cytomegalovirus retinitis	ganciclovir (Cytovene)
Hepatitis B virus	Hepatitis B virus vaccine when HIV infection diagnosed, unless already infected with hepatitis B
Hepatitis C virus	interferon, lamivudine, tenofovir for infection; pegylated interferon and ribavirin
Herpes simplex, herpes zoster, varicella zoster	acyclovir (Zovirax), valacyclovir, famciclovir, foscarnet
Influenza	annual influenza vaccine
Mycobacterium avium complex	azithromycin, clarithromycin, ethambutol
Pneumococcal pneumonia	pneumococcal vaccine when HIV infection diagnosed
Pneumocystis jiroveci pneumonia	trimethoprim-sulfamethoxazole (Bactrim, Septra), dapsone, atovaquone, pentamidine isethionate
Tuberculosis	TB skin test; drug therapy per CDC guidelines: pyrazinamide, isoniazid (Laniazid, Isotamine), ethambutol (Myambutol)
HIV wasting	*Patient education:* Eat frequent small high-calorie and high-protein meals with snacks daily. Eat low-residue diet for diarrhea control. Control odors if they cause nausea. Develop easy meal plan: favorite foods, meal programs, frozen dinners, cold food to control nausea. Use antiemetics, appetite stimulants, and/or testosterone. Rest, listen to music. Numb painful oral sores with ice, popsicles, or topical analgesic; avoid spicy foods. Use artificial saliva for dry mouth. Use nutritional supplements. Use food stamps, community food pantries, or free meal programs as needed. Exercise to increase muscle mass. Take medications prescribed to treat HIV wasting.

from single-stranded viral RNA before integration into cellular DNA
- Blocking viral regulatory and transactivating proteins, which are involved in the transcription and translation of viral RNA proteins from proviral DNA as the virus goes from the quiet, integrated state to active replication
- Inhibiting protease, a viral enzyme responsible for the adherence of viral proteins both before proviral integration and as the viral particles recombine into functional proteins needed for viral maturation
- Preventing viral assembly and budding out of the cell.

For more information, visit the AIDS Info quick reference guide to ARVs at http://aidsinfo.nih.gov/drugs.

ARV Therapy

Aggressive treatment with cocktails of multiple ARV drugs aim to reduce viral loads to undetectable levels in the bloodstream which increases CD4+ T lymphocyte counts, resulting in prolonged survival and quality of life. There are six drug classes of HIV treatment available. Each class affects the virus in a different stage of its life cycle. Use of these drugs in combination is referred to as antiretroviral therapy (ART). Usually at least three medications in at least two classes of treatment categories are used (Table 20.5).

The major cause of drug resistance occurs when medications are not taken as directed so teaching is important. *Adherence* is the word used to describe taking medications

TABLE 20.5 ANTIRETROVIRAL MEDICATIONS FOR HIV INFECTION

Medication Class/Action	Examples	Nursing Implications
Non-Nucleoside Reverse Transcriptase Inhibitors (NNRTIs) Prevent reverse transcriptase enzyme from working.	efavirenz (Sustiva) etravirine (Intelence) nevirapine (Viramune) rilpivirine (Edurant)	Monitor for rash (especially first month); Stevens-Johnson syndrome can occur, requiring discontinuation of the drug. Can be life threatening. Teach patient to report rash immediately. Monitor white blood cell count, liver tests, especially with history of hepatitis B or C.
	abacavir sulfate (Ziagen)* didanosine (Videx, Videx EC) emtricitabine (Emtriva) lamivudine (Epivir) stavudine (Zerit, Zerit XR) tenofovir DF, (Viread)** zidovudine (Retrovir, AZT, ZDV)	Monitor for peripheral neuropathy, bone marrow suppression, lactic acidosis, kidney and liver function. *Flu-like symptoms indicate life-threatening condition can develop. Report immediately. **Monitor for hepatomegaly with steatosis for lactic acidosis, which can be fatal, especially in women. **Take 2 hours before or 1 hour after didanosine.
Protease Inhibitors (PIs) Bind to active site of HIV protease enzyme (cuts reproduced HIV strands), interrupting formation of mature viral particles.	atazanavir (Reyataz) darunavir (Prezista) fosamprenavir (Lexiva)* indinavir (Crixivan)** lopinavir/ritonavir (Kaletra) nelfinavir (Viracept) ritonavir (Norvir) saquinavir (Invirase) tipranavir (Aptivus)	Manage GI symptoms. Monitor lab results. Watch for increased bleeding in patients with hemophilia. *Report rash. *Should not be given if patient is allergic to sulfa. **Teach about importance of hydration (at least 48 oz of liquids in 24 hours).
Fusion Inhibitors Blocks HIV-1 fusion with the CD4+ cell membrane to prevent cell entry.	enfuvirtide (Fuzeon)	Teach subcutaneous injection and injection site rotation. Teach if dizzy, do not drive.

Continued

TABLE 20.5 ANTIRETROVIRAL MEDICATIONS FOR HIV INFECTION—cont'd

Medication Class/Action	Examples	Nursing Implications
Cellular chemokine receptor (CCR5) antagonists Blocks CCR5 receptor preventing HIV-1 entry into CD4+ cells.	maraviroc (Selzentry)	Monitor for liver problems.
Integrase Inhibitor Blocks HIV from combining with its genetic code so more copies of itself cannot be made.	raltegravir (Isentress) dolutegravir (Tivicay)	Teach patient to report side effects.
Combination Agents Single tablet multiple-drug regimen.	Combivir: Lamivudine + Zidovudine Complera: Emtricitabine + Rilpivirine + Tenofovir DF Epzicom: Abacavir + Lamivudine Stribild: Elvitegravir + Cobicistat + Emtricitabine + Tenofovir Trizivir: Abacavir + Lamivudine + Zidovudine Truvada: Emtricitabine + Tenofovir DF	See individual agents above.

GI, gastrointestinal.

exactly as directed. Another increasing potential cause of drug resistance is when an infected person with resistant virus exposes another infected person to the resistant virus through unprotected sexual exposure or injected drug use.

NURSING CARE TIP

Medication Adherence Teaching

Teach patients that it is essential to take all medications as ordered. Missing just 10% of medication doses (1 of 10) decreases effectiveness to about 80%, depending on the drug. This means that if a patient is taking three to seven pills each day, missing one to two pills a week will decrease the medications' effectiveness by 20%.

Many anti-HIV drugs have side effects. If they occur, the drug regimen can be changed or interventions can be used to help control the side effects. The patient should be taught about side effects and instructed always to report them immediately, especially rashes (such as with trimethoprim-sulfamethoxazole) and abdominal pain (such as with AZT [Retrovir]); they could be serious or even life threatening.

When someone with a suppressed immune system (very low CD4/T-cell count) is started on ART, the person can experience immune reconstitution syndrome. The patient's immune system can be greatly improving, but the patient is feeling worse. This is because, when the patient's immune system was severely damaged, immune responses can have been too weak or absent to show the signs of infection. When immune function improves and the immune system begins to fight off infections that were already present in the body, such as *Pneumocystis jiroveci* pneumonia, symptoms can arise.

This can be a serious, sometimes fatal condition that can occur a few weeks after antiretroviral therapy starts. Educating the patient to report immediately any symptoms of opportunistic infections after starting therapy can allow for prompt diagnosis and treatment of the infection—and can save the person's life.

 ## NURSING PROCESS FOR THE ADULT PATIENT WITH HIV/AIDS

Data Collection

Ongoing monitoring is important for the patient with HIV/AIDS to detect problems early. Health history information is obtained (Box 20-3). Determining the patient's understanding of HIV/AIDS information is necessary for planning and teaching. A physical examination provides data on the effects of HIV/AIDS and ARTs. Monitoring the patient's level of pain is ongoing; however, many patients with HIV do not have pain related to their HIV. You should also check for signs and symptoms of opportunistic infections.

 ## LEARNING TIP

Key points to remember:

- HIV and AIDS are disease labels, not people labels.
- Each person reacts to an HIV or AIDS diagnosis differently.
- It is not the HIV that ultimately causes death; it is compromised immunity and the invasion of an opportunistic infection or disease that the patient's body is unable to successfully fight off, even with medical intervention.
- With today's successful ARTs, HIV has changed from being a life-ending infection to a chronic disease requiring constant management.

Box 20-3 Data Collection: Health History Information for HIV/AIDS

- Demographic data: gender, age, marital status, occupation, residence
- Date of diagnosis of HIV/AIDS
- Past medical history and surgeries
- Current health status and concerns
- Allergies
- Medication history of antivirals used with reason for discontinuing

- Current medications, dose, and frequency (including over-the-counter medications and supplements)
- Immunizations
- Family history
- Height/weight: weight loss
- Infections/cancers (see Box 20-1, "CDC Conditions in the AIDS Surveillance Case Definition")
- Sexually transmitted infections and treatments
- Social history, sexual practices, risk behaviors, safe sex practices
- Needle and blood exposure, injection drug use, blood transfusions/treatment for hemophilia
- Tobacco use
- Drug and alcohol use
- Exercise and sleep
- Pets
- Occupational history
- Nutrition history
- Female: gynecological history, last Pap test

Nursing Diagnoses

Nursing care is individualized to the patient's presenting symptoms. Nursing diagnoses for HIV/AIDS can include the following:

- *Ineffective Protection* related to decreased immune function
- *Impaired Gas Exchange* related to respiratory infection
- *Acute* or *Chronic Pain* related to neuropathy, cancer, infection, or dyspnea
- *Fatigue* related to HIV infection and/or side effects of treatments
- *Risk for Injury* related to weakness, fatigue, sedation, neurologic impairment
- *Imbalanced Nutrition: Less Than Body Requirements* related to anorexia, nausea and vomiting, increased caloric need, diarrhea, dysphagia, oral lesions
- *Impaired Oral Mucous Membrane* related to decreased immune function
- *Diarrhea* related to infection, medications
- *Impaired Skin Integrity* related to infection, cancer, immobility, incontinence
- *Social Isolation* related to fear of disclosure of status, infection control, transmission of virus
- *Risk for Situational Low Self-Esteem* related to body image changes
- *Deficient Knowledge* related to lack of previous experience with HIV/AIDS and treatment
- *Grieving* related to loss of function or death
- *Disabled Family Coping* related to chronic, potentially progressive disease
- *Ineffective Coping* related to chronic progressive disease
- *Ineffective Sexuality Pattern* related to fear of disease transmission.

See the *Nursing Care Plan for the Patient With AIDS.*

Planning and Implementation

HIV/AIDS can affect every system of the body and every aspect of a person's life. Nurses have the opportunity to positively influence the patient's experience with HIV/AIDS by providing a nonjudgmental approach, empathy, and psychological support.

INEFFECTIVE PROTECTION. To reduce infection risk, the patient should be taught to wash hands frequently, especially before eating and after toileting; bathe regularly; avoid sharing personal grooming items (e.g., toothbrush, toothpaste, razor); wash toothbrush; and wash all dishes between uses (Table 20.6). In addition, the patient is taught signs of infection to report to the health care provider immediately (Box 20-4, "Patient Education"). Treatment of opportunistic infections is most effective when begun early.

IMPAIRED GAS EXCHANGE. If a patient develops a condition that interferes with respiration, the goal is to maintain oxygenation within normal limits and reduce dyspnea. PCP is a potential respiratory infection with AIDS (see Table 20.4). Monitoring the patient's vital signs, including respiratory rate, depth, rhythm, and oxygen saturation, is important. Medications and oxygen therapy are given as ordered. Positioning the patient for comfort is often done by raising the head of the bed. Assisting with activities helps reduce fatigue.

TABLE 20.6 PATIENT TEACHING: PREVENTING OPPORTUNISTIC INFECTIONS

Precaution Category	Reducing Exposure Risk	To Protect From
Environmental/ occupational	Consider risk for exposure to infectious agents from the following: health care setting, correctional facilities, homeless shelters.	Tuberculosis
	Child-care settings: wash hands after diaper changing/body fluid contact.	CMV, cryptosporidiosis, hepatitis A, giardiasis
	Animal contact: exposure possible from veterinary work, pet stores, farms.	Cryptosporidiosis, toxoplasmosis, salmonellosis, campylobacteriosis
	Gardening/soil contact: avoid gardening/houseplant care/bird-roosting site, soil, cleaning chicken coops. Wear gloves and mask and wash hands after soil contact.	Cryptosporidiosis, toxoplasmosis, histoplasmosis, coccidioidomycosis
Food/water	*General measures for home or restaurants include the following:* Food handlers should practice good hand washing and hygiene. Discard food past expiration date and dented or swollen cans. Maintain adequate refrigeration and cooking temperatures. Control insects and rodents to prevent food contamination. *Foods to avoid:* Raw/undercooked eggs and foods with raw eggs, such as hollandaise sauce, Caesar dressing, mayonnaise, uncooked batters, ice cream, eggnog. Raw/undercooked poultry, meat, seafood. Unpasteurized milk/dairy products and fruit juice, raw seed sprouts. Soft cheeses, which can harbor bacteria: feta, brie, camembert, blue veined, queso fresco. Wash produce and avoid unwashed produce on salad bars. Avoid cross-contamination of foods with uncooked meat on food preparation surfaces.	Foodborne and waterborne infections caused by bacterial, viral, protozoal, or parasitic pathogens

TABLE 20.6 PATIENT TEACHING: PREVENTING OPPORTUNISTIC INFECTIONS—cont'd

Precaution Category	Reducing Exposure Risk	To Protect From
	Cook meat until internal temperature is 180°F (82.2°C) for poultry, 165°F (73.8°C) for red meats, with no trace of pink.	
	Foods to avoid or cook until steaming hot: leftovers, ready-to-eat, delicatessen foods, refrigerated pâtés, and meat spreads.	Cryptosporidiosis, giardiasis
	Water safety: Avoid public drinking fountains. Avoid drinking or swallowing water directly from lakes or rivers. Use safe water supply or boil water for 1 minute when unsure. Avoid beverages made from tap water in public places in areas where water sources are known not to be safe. Drink bottled water purified from reverse osmosis, filtration through absolute 1-micrometer filter, or distillation (only safe methods) in areas where water sources are known not to be safe. For information, contact www.bottledwater.org. Bottled or canned carbonated soft drinks, commercially packaged unrefrigerated beverages, pasteurized beverages, and beers are safe.	Hepatitis A, campylobacteriosis, *E. coli,* giardiasis, leptospirosis, norovirus, rotavirus, shigellosis
Sexual	Always use latex condom for every sex act.	STIs, herpes simplex virus, cytomegalovirus, human papillomavirus, resistant HIV strain
	Avoid oral-anal contact or use dental dams; use latex gloves for hand-anal contact; wash hands and genitals with warm soapy water after contact.	Intestinal infections: amebiasis, hepatitis A, cryptosporidiosis, shigellosis, campylobacteriosis, giardiasis
	Get hepatitis A vaccine.	Hepatitis A
	Get hepatitis B vaccine	Hepatitis B
Injection drug use	Get hepatitis A and B vaccines. Stop using injection drugs and enter substance abuse treatment. If unable to stop, never reuse or share syringes, needles, water, or drug preparation equipment. If shared, use bleach and water to clean equipment. Use sterile syringes from pharmacies or community syringe exchange programs and dispose of safely. Use clean water and equipment and new alcohol swab.	Hepatitis A, hepatitis B, hepatitis C, resistant HIV strain
Pet-related	Avoid pet feces/diarrhea; seek veterinary treatment for pet's illness. Counsel on pet contact risks but recognize emotional benefits of pets. Pets should have up-to-date immunizations.	*Cryptosporidium, Salmonella, Campylobacter* spp. infection

Continued

TABLE 20.6 PATIENT TEACHING: PREVENTING OPPORTUNISTIC INFECTIONS—cont'd

Precaution Category	Reducing Exposure Risk	To Protect From
	For new pet, avoid those younger than 6 months old (and cats younger than 1 year old); obtain pets from known sanitary source; avoid strays; wash hands after handling pets	
	Avoid exotic pets.	
	Cat ownership increases risk from litter box cleaning, scratches, bites, licking, fleas. If must clean litter box, wear mask and gloves and wash hands well afterward. Efforts should be made to keep cats indoors to avoid contact with infected prey.	Toxoplasmosis, *Bartonella* spp. infection, salmonellosis, campylobacteriosis
	Unhealthy birds can transmit infectious organisms.	*Cryptococcus neoformans, Mycobacterium avium, Histoplasma capsulatum* infection
	Avoid reptiles, turtles, chicks, and ducklings.	Salmonellosis
	Wear gloves for cleaning aquariums.	*Mycobacterium marinum* infection
Travel	Consult health care providers on travel to developing countries.	Opportunistic pathogens, foodborne and waterborne infections
	Traveler's diarrhea prophylaxis is not recommended. Carry supply of antimicrobial agent to take for diarrhea.	
	Consider prophylaxis for other types of exposures.	
	Avoid raw fruits, vegetables, raw/undercooked seafood or meat, tap water, ice from tap water, unpasteurized milk/dairy products, items from street vendors.	
	Safe items include steaming-hot foods, self-peeled fruits, bottled (especially carbonated) beverages, hot coffee/tea, beer, wine, and water boiled 1 minute.	
	Avoid soil/sand contact by wearing shoes, using beach towels.	

CMV, cytomegalovirus; STI, sexually transmitted infection.

Source: Data from U.S. Department of Health and Human Services. (2013). *USPHS/IDSA guidelines for the prevention of opportunistic infections in persons infected with human immunodeficiency virus.* Washington, DC: Author. Retrieved July, 28, 2013, from www.aidsinfo.nih.gov/contentfiles /lvguidelines/adult_oi.pdf

Box 20-4 Patient Education

Signs and Symptoms of Opportunistic Infections to Report

Teach patient to monitor temperature and to report the following symptoms to a health care provider immediately:

- New fever higher than 100°F (38.5°C) or a change in fever pattern if low-grade fevers are common
- Cough, shortness of breath, fever, or chest tightness, which can be signs of early pneumonia
- Signs of central nervous system infection, such as severe headache; stiff neck; visual changes; problems with balance, walking, or speech; weakness of an arm or leg; or changes in moods or memory

- Foul-smelling drainage or pus
- Cloudy or foul-smelling urine
- Signs of dehydration, such as a dry mouth, dark concentrated urine, or dizziness when standing
- Diarrhea lasting longer than 48 hours; more than six stools a day; watery, mucousy, or bloody stools
- Rashes (possible side effect of medication)
- Sore mouth or tongue, difficulty swallowing, white patches on tongue or back of mouth
- Worsening fatigue
- Change in vision and if floaters develop
- Unintended weight loss

PAIN. Pain can occur from a variety of causes. Treatment is focused on the cause to achieve pain control and relief. Medications can be given as ordered. Timing medication administration before planned activities is helpful in increasing ability to function. Complementary therapy can be used by patients (see Chapter 5). Measures such as heat or cold, massage, and frequent position changes can be helpful.

FATIGUE. Some patients with HIV experience fatigue. Other causes of fatigue include infections, medications, anemia, dehydration, depression, and poor nutrition. The patient can help manage fatigue by alternating periods of activity and rest. Tasks that use more energy should be planned at times when the patient is most energetic. Helping a patient prioritize activities is important in planning the best use of the energy available.

IMBALANCED NUTRITION: LESS THAN BODY REQUIREMENTS. Maintaining general health and nutrition is important for a healthy immune system. For patients with HIV, maintaining nutrition is vital (see "Nutrition Notes"). Patients with AIDS can have difficulty maintaining adequate nutrition and preventing weight loss. Many factors interfere with nutrition in HIV/AIDS (e.g., anorexia, oral lesions, nausea and vomiting, diarrhea, or wasting syndrome). The cause needs to be identified for appropriate intervention planning.

- Alter seasonings.
- Add powdered milk to mashed potatoes or puddings to increase calories and protein.
- Modify texture to accommodate chewing difficulty or oral lesions.
- Provide nutritional supplements (e.g., Boost or Ensure)

The patient's baseline weight is obtained. Then ongoing monitoring of the patient's weight, calorie intake, and intake and output is done. A dietitian is consulted to help plan nutritious and affordable meals. The patient should be on a high-calorie, high-protein diet. Small, frequent meals can be helpful. Vitamins and/or nutritional supplements can be needed to maintain adequate nutrition. Antiemetics are used to control nausea and vomiting, if present. Medications that help stimulate appetite can be helpful. Easy-to-prepare meals are helpful when energy is limited. Creative interventions and resources can be needed to ensure the patient receives adequate nutrition (see "Nutrition Notes"). Along with adequate nutrition, exercise helps maintain muscle mass, promotes relaxation, aids sleep, and gives the person a sense of control and well-being. An effective exercise program includes exercises that increase strength, flexibility, and endurance. For many, becoming physically fit is a lifestyle change that requires dedication.

IMPAIRED ORAL MUCOUS MEMBRANE. Oral or esophageal candidiasis is more common in the late stage of AIDS. The painful lesions interfere with swallowing and nutrition. In patients with AIDS who smoke, there is an increased incidence of oral thrush (candidiasis). Therefore, patients should be encouraged to quit smoking. Antifungal medication is given. Mouth care is important. A soft toothbrush promotes comfort. Xylocaine viscous (Lidocaine viscous) can be given to decrease pain during eating.

DIARRHEA. Diarrhea can occur in patients with HIV. Diarrhea can be caused by HIV infection, opportunistic infections, or ARTs. An antimotility agent can be prescribed. Consulting the dietitian can be helpful in making dietary changes that reduce diarrhea (e.g., low-residue diet, no dairy products, no spicy foods, no caffeine or alcohol). Sitz baths can be soothing. Thorough cleansing of the anal area after each stool is a must. Ointments can be applied to protect and soothe the anal area from excoriation.

IMPAIRED SKIN INTEGRITY. Many skin conditions can occur with HIV infection. Medications can cause skin infections that can be life threatening and must be reported immediately. A dermatologist can need to be consulted to help diagnose and treat skin infections.

SOCIAL ISOLATION. Unfortunately, many patients with HIV/AIDS continue to face discrimination, rejection, and isolation. The Americans With Disabilities Act (ADA) makes discrimination toward patients with HIV illegal. Even relatives, friends, and others sometimes avoid or refuse to have anything to do with the person with HIV.

Nutrition Notes

Nourishing the Patient With HIV or AIDS

Nutrition has preventive and therapeutic functions for patients with HIV infections. Well-nourished people infected with the HIV virus are better able to resist opportunistic infections and tolerate the side effects of treatment. Multiple studies have found that the use of a nutritional supplement delayed the onset of advanced disease in HIV-positive people (Botros, Somarriba, Neri, & Miller, 2012). The person infected with HIV displays reduced appetite possibly due to oral infections and diarrhea from damage to intestinal cells that interferes with absorption of nutrients. Coupled with nausea and vomiting related to medications, the clinical picture often leads to loss of weight and lean body mass. Malnutrition adds fuel to the fire by accelerating the progress of HIV infection to AIDS. An HIV-infected adult requires 10% to 15% more energy per day and approximately 50% to 100% more protein than someone not infected (Duggal, Chung & Duggal, 2012). The current World Health Organization recommendation for an intake of micronutrients at Recommended Dietary Allowance levels is a reasonable target for persons with clinically stable HIV infection (Forrester & Sztam, 2011).

Diet should be integral to the treatment plan. Every effort should be made to feed the patient orally. Strategies that can be helpful are as follows:

- Offer small, frequent feedings.
- Serve food cold or at room temperature.

NURSING CARE PLAN for the Patient With AIDS

Nursing Diagnosis: *Ineffective Protection* related to immune disorder, inadequate nutrition, intravenous (IV) therapy, and possible invasive procedures

Expected Outcomes: The patient will remain free of hospital-acquired infections. Patient will describe measures to maintain skin integrity and avoid infections.

Evaluation of Outcomes: Is patient free of hospital-acquired infections? Can patient explain and demonstrate skin maintenance techniques?

Intervention Identify patient's risk factors, such as skin condition, laboratory results, portals of entry for infections, and presence of any infections. **Rationale** Status of these assessment factors determines plan for care. **Evaluation** Does patient have intact skin or nonreddened, nonpurulent sites of interrupted integrity?

Intervention Caregivers should use standard precautions and strict aseptic technique for all patients and procedures. **Rationale** Transmission of microorganisms can occur in both directions. Many patients with HIV are not aware of their HIV status. **Evaluation** Do all caregivers use standard precautions?

Intervention Instruct visitors about techniques to avoid transmission of infection, such as hand hygiene and not visiting when they have an infection. (Use extreme caution not to divulge the patient's HIV/AIDS status to visitors/family.) The nurse with an infection, especially respiratory infection, should not care for the patient with AIDS. (If you must care for the patient, wear a mask and explain why you are wearing it.) **Rationale** The immune system is damaged by HIV. Ability to combat infections can be severely compromised. A minor infection for most people can kill a person who has AIDS. **Evaluation** Do those with infections avoid contact with patient until their infection is resolved? Do laboratory tests indicate that patient is so immunocompromised that reverse isolation can be necessary?

Intervention Promote skin integrity by frequent turning, optimum mobilization, use of protective mattress and chair pads, application of emollient to dry areas, and prompt treatment of any injuries. **Rationale** Skin is the body's first line of defense. **Evaluation** Does patient's skin remain intact and infection free?

Intervention Teach strategies for skin care and avoidance of infection to patient. **Rationale** Self-care offers a measure of control in a frequently uncontrollable situation. **Evaluation** Does patient satisfactorily explain or demonstrate good skin care and knowledge of how to avoid infection?

Nursing Diagnosis: *Risk for Injury* related to impaired mobility, weakness, fatigue, possible electrolyte imbalances, neurologic impairment, and sedative effects of pain medications

Expected Outcome: The patient's care and mobility needs will be met without injury.

Evaluation of Outcome: Does patient remain free from injury?

Intervention Identify patient's abilities and disabilities. **Rationale** Particular disabilities can increase danger to patient. **Evaluation** Does patient have deficits?

Intervention Look for potential hazards in environment (hospital or home) and eliminate as many hazards as possible. **Rationale** Awareness of hazards is necessary to decrease occurrence of accidents and injuries. **Evaluation** Are there currently any hazards in the environment?

Intervention Instruct patient about how to avoid hazards (if cognitively and physically able to comply). **Rationale** Patients can help avoid injury if they understand hazards. **Evaluation** Is patient effectively avoiding hazards, or is patient a danger to self?

NURSING CARE PLAN for the Patient With AIDS—cont'd

Intervention Encourage self-care as much as is feasible without tiring patient. **Rationale** Self-care promotes feelings of self-efficacy and can combat depression. **Evaluation** Does patient evidence satisfaction with self-care efforts?

Intervention Assist with care activities as needed. **Rationale** Varying levels of assistance with care are necessary due to the potentially debilitating nature of disease. **Evaluation** Are patient's care and mobility needs being met satisfactorily without injury?

Intervention Institute safety measures as required, such as close observation, frequent reorientation, two staff members for ambulation, use of side rails, bed motion alarm, or room near nurse's station. **Rationale** Protection of patient against inadvertent removal of tubes or equipment, falls, and other injuries can require extraordinary measures due to neurologic damage. **Evaluation** Are safety measures effective for patient? Does patient respond negatively to the protective measures? Can these be modified to be less offensive?

Nursing Diagnosis: *Ineffective Coping* related to potentially terminal disease and progressive debility

Expected Outcome: The patient will show use of effective coping skills.

Evaluation of Outcome: Does patient show use of effective coping skills?

Intervention Establish and maintain open and trusting therapeutic relationship. **Rationale** Effective communication is based on trust—*assurance of confidentiality is essential.* **Evaluation** Does patient talk about concerns with nurse?

Intervention Allow grieving to take place (keeping a journal has been effective for some patients who have AIDS). **Rationale** AIDS brings about losses of health, strength, employment, and, in many cases, friends; it threatens one's sense of security and life. Healthy grieving is a natural coping response. **Evaluation** Is grief being expressed? Is patient finishing things that matter to him or her?

Intervention Encourage patient to express feelings and concerns. Contact counselor, chaplain, or AIDS support worker if patient so desires. **Rationale** Talking about feelings and concerns helps defuse anger, clarify needs, and relieve tension. **Evaluation** How are family members, friends, and support persons interacting with patient? How is patient responding to family members, friends, and support persons?

Intervention Provide patient with desired information or refer to others who can supply information. **Rationale** Knowledge dispels unreasonable fears and helps patient prepare adequately to cope with stressors. **Evaluation** Does patient evidence enough understanding of disease to be able to cope effectively?

Intervention Ask if patient would like information about support group and arrange such. **Rationale** Social support can help patient cope. **Evaluation** Does patient show satisfaction with coping resources?

Source: Linda Hopper Cook.

Misunderstanding and fear lead to misuse of infection control procedures and increase a patient's isolation. Being knowledgeable about the transmission of HIV allows interaction with the patient to reduce feelings of isolation. Providing patient education to reduce fear of HIV transmission also decreases isolation. Taking care to maintain confidentiality is essential. It is important to be aware that many patients with HIV do not share their diagnosis with family or friends who visit when they are hospitalized.

RISK FOR SITUATIONAL LOW SELF-ESTEEM. Changes in self-esteem and self-concept occur from several of the effects of HIV infection. Patients often experience changes in their relationships with others and in day-to-day activities such as work. Major weight loss and changes in fat distribution from

ARV agents, a condition called lipodystrophy, can cause dramatic changes in appearance that alter body image and reduce self-esteem. Tesamorelin (Egrifta) is used to treat lipodystrophy. Nurses can assist patients in maintaining self-esteem and self-concept by ensuring a climate of acceptance and promoting a trusting relationship. Patients should be encouraged to express feelings, if ready, and to identify positive aspects of self. Receiving emotional and spiritual support can help improve the patient's self-esteem.

Stress has an impact on health. Having others to talk with and provide support is essential to stress management. Identifying and maintaining social networks is important. Patients should be taught a variety of relaxation strategies and techniques to reduce stress. Relaxation strategies can range from working on a favorite hobby to talking with friends. Relaxation techniques include progressive muscle relaxation and imagery to aid in relaxation. Stress management techniques are most effective when used every day, not just during times of stress.

DEFICIENT KNOWLEDGE. Extensive teaching is needed for patients to understand this chronic, potentially life-threatening disease that alters everything in their lives. (See also "Prevention" earlier in the chapter.) Teaching is evaluated for understanding and provided as the patient is ready. Understanding of adherence to treatment and medication regimens is essential to prevent resistance to treatment and reduce the risk of disease progression.

CRITICAL THINKING

Zoe Sampson

■ Zoe, 22, is diagnosed as HIV-positive. She is tearful and asks many questions.

1. How would you answer her questions?
   a. "Am I going to die?"
   b. "How is AIDS diagnosed?"
   c. "Can my boyfriend get it?"
2. What food and water safety methods would you teach her?
3. Years later, Zoe loses weight and becomes malnourished. What interventions can you use to promote adequate nutrition?

Suggested answers are at the end of the chapter.

MEDICATIONS. Nurses must stress during patient teaching that medication doses must not be missed. Using teaching aids to assist patients in remembering to take their medications is important. Encourage the patient to take medications exactly as instructed. If a dose is missed, it should be taken as soon as possible unless it is very close to the time of the next dose. Doses should not be doubled. Missing doses of medication could cause therapy failure because viral loads can increase and resistance to current treatments can develop.

Strongly encourage the patient to consult promptly with the primary care provider with any questions or side effects. Many of these medications can cause severe reactions.

FOOD AND WATER SAFETY. Food and water safety are vital to an immunocompromised patient. Bacterial, viral, protozoal, or parasitic pathogens can cause foodborne and waterborne infections. The patient must be taught methods to prevent foodborne and waterborne infections for all phases of handling (see Table 20.6). Kitchen counters and food preparation appliances (e.g., cutting boards, can openers) should be disinfected. Freezing does not kill bacteria in foods. Foods should not be thawed at room temperature. Dating and using the oldest foods first is helpful. If symptoms of foodborne or waterborne infection develop (e.g., diarrhea, nausea, vomiting, abdominal cramps, headache, fever), teach patient to report them immediately. In certain areas of the country, tap water is not safe to drink. Patients can need to be taught to boil water for drinking and making ice cubes or to drink bottled water.

RESOURCES. Financial resources can need to be addressed so that food and medications can be obtained. Treatment can be expensive, and the patient may be unable to work. However, with the new combination ARTs, many people are now able to continue working longer. The Ryan White Comprehensive AIDS Resources Emergency (CARE) Act provides funding for some services and treatment-related needs. Knowledge of local resources and referrals to financial resources and support groups are very important.

COMMUNITY AND HOME HEALTH CARE. During the course of HIV infection, the patient will be mainly at home and in the community. Luckily, hospitalization is less frequently needed in the treated patient but can be needed intermittently for acute illness. If the disease progresses, the patient can need more care from caregivers and home health nurses. The home health nurse provides physical care, establishes a therapeutic relationship with AIDS patients and their significant others and family/friends, and coordinates care with other health care team members (see "Home Health Hints").

Caregivers should be assessed for caregiver role strain. Support services should be identified, such as community AIDS organizations, Meals on Wheels, respite care services, community mental health, and Internet support groups. Respite care provides the caregiver time away from the caregiver role to reduce stress. When a patient is terminal, comfort care and emotional support for the family are essential. Hospice care can be used at this time.

Home Health Hints

• When providing patient care, perform hand hygiene and wash hands frequently, follow standard precautions, and use plastic bags to contain soiled items or clothing.

- Teach patients with AIDS and their families how to properly clean and disinfect the home to prevent infections. The least expensive recommended disinfectant is a diluted bleach mixture that contains 1 part household bleach to 10 parts water. However, this solution must be mixed daily to be effective. Many spray-type disinfectants are available and can be easier for patients/families to use.
- Wearing gloves, clean body fluid spills with soap and water.
- Flush body fluids, solid waste, and contaminated solutions down toilet.
- Use disinfectant to (1) disinfect spill areas, (2) clean toilet seats and bathroom fixtures, and (3) clean inside the refrigerator to avoid mold growth.
- Rinse clothing and then wash separately from other clothes with 1 cup of bleach if soiled with blood, urine, feces, or semen.
- Patients with HIV/AIDS do not require separate sets of dishes or silverware. Dishes and silverware are washed in hot, soapy water and rinsed thoroughly or placed in dishwasher.
- To dispose of sharps (e.g., needles, lancets, razors) provide a red biohazard container if available. If not, use a rigid labeled container such as a tin can with a sealable lid. Add 1:10 bleach solution to disinfect the sharps. Tape the lid. Place in a bag and dispose of in the trash.
- Contaminated articles are disposed of by bagging and sealing in plastic and placing in the trash.
- Teach the family of a patient with AIDS which signs and symptoms to report to the physician or nurse immediately: fever; increased dyspnea; pain; change in sputum production; upper respiratory tract infection; pneumonia; respiratory distress syndrome; diarrhea five times a day or more for 5 days; uncontrolled weight loss greater than 10 pounds in the past month; persistent headaches; falling; seizures; mental status changes, including memory loss and personality changes; rashes and skin changes; difficulty swallowing; and problems with urination.

Evaluation

Patient goals are met if the patient remains free from infection and maintains the desired quality of life and activities as long as possible. If the disease should progress, goals are met if the patient's needs are met and the patient's dignity is maintained.

SUGGESTED ANSWERS TO

CRITICAL THINKING

■ *Zoe Sampson*

1. a. There is no cure for HIV/AIDS; however, medications are available that make an HIV infection a manageable chronic illness. Research continues in the search for a cure.

   b. AIDS is diagnosed when CD4+ T-lymphocyte counts are below 200 cells per microliter, or the CD4+ T-lymphocyte percentage is under 14 of total lymphocytes, and/or an opportunistic clinical disease, as defined by the CDC, is present in an HIV-infected person.

   c. Yes, your boyfriend could become infected through exposure to your blood or vaginal secretions. You need to learn about preventive measures and discuss them with him. If you have had unprotected sex, he should be tested for HIV.

2. Food handlers must maintain good hand washing and hygiene practices. Discard food that has past the expiration date and dented or swollen cans. Ensure adequate refrigeration and cooking. Control insects and rodents to prevent food contamination. Drink purified bottled water if you live in areas with unsafe drinking water. Use a safe water supply or boil water 1 minute when unsure. Avoid unpasteurized milk, other dairy products, fruit juice, and raw seed sprouts. Avoid raw and undercooked eggs, meats, and seafood.

3. Eat three to four high-calorie, high-lean protein meals and snacks daily. Eat a low-residue diet for diarrhea control. Develop an easy meal plan. Use antiemetics, if needed. Numb painful oral sores. Avoid spicy foods. Refer for food stamps/free meal programs if necessary. Engage in regular exercise.

REVIEW QUESTIONS

1. The nurse would evaluate the patient as understanding modes of HIV transmission if the patient stated that the modes of HIV transmission include which of the following?
   1. Saliva, tears, fecal-oral contamination
   2. Close physical contact involving skin surfaces, mosquito bites
   3. Sharing towels, sharing eating utensils, skin contact
   4. Unprotected sex with HIV-infected partner, contact with infected blood products

2. The nurse is teaching a patient about HIV testing. Place traditional HIV-1 diagnostic tests in the sequential order in which they are performed.
   1. Western blot test
   2. Enzyme-linked immunosorbent assay (ELISA) test
   3. Repeated ELISA test

3. A patient who is newly diagnosed with HIV infection asks what to expect for future health status. The best response for the nurse to give is based on the understanding that HIV disease and AIDS are characterized as which of the following?
   1. An acute disease
   2. A life-ending disease
   3. A chronically managed disease
   4. A disease with remissions and exacerbations

4. The nurse is planning to teach a patient about HIV prevention. What should the nurse include in a teaching plan to prevent HIV infection? **Select all that apply.**
   1. Recapping of used needles by caregiver permitted.
   2. Abstain from sexual intercourse.
   3. Avoid injection drug use.
   4. Avoid use of male or female condoms.
   5. Plan for autologous blood transfusion.
   6. Test for HIV at time of labor.

5. The nurse is contributing to the teaching plan for a patient with HIV on reducing infection risks. Which of the following should the patient with HIV be taught to do to decrease risk of infections? **Select all that apply.**
   1. Wash hands before eating.
   2. Wash toothbrush.
   3. Reuse dishes.
   4. Buy prepared deli foods.
   5. Report signs of infection.
   6. Share razor if no visible blood.

6. The nurse would recognize that the patient needs further reinforcement of knowledge if the patient stated that one of the goals of antiretroviral therapy is which of the following?
   1. Reduce the viral load.
   2. Improve survival rates.
   3. Decrease CD4+ T lymphocytes.
   4. Delay the progression of HIV disease.

7. The nurse would recognize that the patient is having a reaction to abacavir sulfate (Ziagen) if which of the following occurred?
   1. Flu-like symptoms
   2. Edema
   3. Abdominal pain
   4. Blurred vision

Answers can be found in Appendix C.

References

Botros, D., Somarriba, G., Neri, D., & Miller, T. (2012). Interventions to address chronic disease and HIV: Strategies to promote exercise and nutrition among HIV-infected individuals. *Current HIV and AIDS Report, 9,* 351–363.

Branson, B. M., Handsfield, H. H., Lampe, M. A., Janssen, R. S., Taylor, A. W., Lyss, S. B., & Clark, J. E. (2006). Revised recommendations for HIV testing of adults, adolescents, and pregnant women in health care settings. *MMWR, 55*(RR), 1–17.

Brooks, J., Buchacz, K., Gebo, K., & Mermin, J. (2012). HIV infection and older Americans. *The Public Health Perspective, 102,* 1516–1526.

Choopanya, K., Martin, M., Suntharasamai, P., Sangkum, U., Mock, P., Leethochawalit, M., . . . Vanichseni, S., for the Bangkok Tenofovir Study Group. (2013). Antiretroviral prophylaxis for HIV infection in injecting drug users in Bangkok, Thailand (the Bangkok Tenofovir Study): A randomised, double-blind, placebo-controlled Phase 3 trial. *The Lancet, 381,* 2083–2090.

Cohen, M. S., Chen, Y. Q., McCauley, M., Gamble, T., Hosseinipour, M. C., Kumarasamy, N., . . . Fleming, T. R., for the HPTN 052 Study Team. (2011). Prevention of HIV-1 infection with early antiretroviral therapy. *New England Journal of Medicine, 365,* 493–505.

Duggal, S., Chugh, T. D., & Duggal, A. K. (2012). HIV and malnutrition: Effects on immune system. *Clinical and Developmental Immunology, 2012.*

Forrester, J. E., and Sztam, K. A. (2011). Micronutrients in HIV/AIDS: Is there evidence to change the WHO 2003 recommendations? *American Journal of Clinical Nutrition, 94,* 1683S.

Grant, R., Lama, J., Anderson, P., McMahan, V., Liu, A., Vargas, L., Goicochea, P., . . . Glidden, D. V., for the iPREx Study Team. (2010). Pre-exposure chemoprophylaxis for HIV prevention in men who have sex with men. *New England Journal of Medicine, 363,* 2587–2599.

Moyer, V. A. (2013). US Preventive Services Task Force. Screening for HIV: US Preventive Services Task Force recommendation statement. *Annals of Internal Medicine, 159,* 51–60.

Panel on Antiretroviral Guidelines for Adults and Adolescents. (2013, February 12). *Guidelines for the use of antiretroviral agents in HIV-1-infected adults and adolescents.* Washington, DC: U.S. Department of Health and Human Services. Retrieved July 20, 2013, from http://aidsinfo.nih.gov/contentfiles /lvguidelines/adultandadolescentgl.pdf

 DavisPlus | For additional resources and information visit **davispl.us/medsurg5**

Understanding the Cardiovascular System

21

Cardiovascular System Function, Assessment, and Therapeutic Measures

KEY TERMS

atherosclerosis (ATH-er-oh-skleh-ROH-siss)
bruit (brew-EE)
claudication (KLAW-dih-KAY-shun)
clubbing (KLUH-bing)
dysrhythmias (dis-RITH-mee-yahs)
Homans' sign (HOH-manz SYNE)
hypomagnesemia (HYE-poh-MAG-neh-SEE-mee-ah)
ischemic (iss-KEY-mick)
murmur (MUR-mur)
pericardial friction rub (PEAR-ih-KAR-dee-uhl FRIK-shun RUB)
poikilothermy (POY-kih-loh-THER-mee)
point of maximum impulse (POYNT OF MAKS-ih-muhm IM-puls)
preload (PREE-lohd)
pulse deficit (PULS DEF-ih-sit)
sternotomy (stir-NAW-tuh-mee)
thrill (THRILL)

LINDA S. WILLIAMS AND
JANICE L. BRADFORD

LEARNING OUTCOMES

1. Identify the normal anatomy of the cardiovascular system.

2. Explain the normal function of the cardiovascular system.

3. List data to collect when caring for a patient with a disorder of the cardiovascular system.

4. Identify diagnostic tests commonly performed to diagnose disorders of the cardiovascular system.

5. Plan nursing care for patients undergoing diagnostic tests for cardiovascular disorders.

6. Describe current therapeutic measures for disorders of the cardiovascular system.

7. Describe preoperative and postoperative care for patients undergoing cardiac surgery.

NORMAL CARDIOVASCULAR SYSTEM ANATOMY AND PHYSIOLOGY

The cardiovascular system consists of the heart, blood, and vessels (including arteries, capillaries, and veins). Its function is to distribute the blood throughout the body.

Heart

Cardiac Structure and Function

LOCATION OF THE HEART. The heart is located in the mediastinum within the thoracic cavity. It is enclosed by three membranes. The outermost is the fibrous pericardium, which forms a loose-fitting pericardial sac around the heart. The second, or middle, layer is the parietal pericardium, a serous membrane that lines the fibrous layer. The third and innermost layer, the visceral pericardium or epicardium, is a serous membrane on the surface of the heart muscle. Between the parietal and visceral layers is serous fluid, which prevents friction as the heart beats.

STRUCTURE OF THE HEART AND CORONARY BLOOD VESSELS. The walls of the four chambers of the heart are made of cardiac muscle (myocardium) and are lined with endocardium, which is smooth epithelial tissue that prevents abnormal clotting. The epithelium also covers the valves of the heart and continues into blood vessels as the endothelium. Coronary circulation provides oxygenated blood throughout the myocardium and returns deoxygenated blood to the right atrium via the coronary sinus. The two main coronary arteries are the first branches of the ascending aorta, just outside the left ventricle (Fig. 21.1).

The superior chambers of the heart are the thin-walled right and left atria, which are separated by the interatrial septum. The lower chambers are the thicker walled right and left ventricles, which are separated by the interventricular septum. Each septum is made of myocardium that forms a common wall between the two chambers.

CORONARY BLOOD FLOW. The right atrium receives deoxygenated blood from the coronary sinus, the upper body by way of the superior vena cava, and from the lower body by way of the inferior vena cava (see Fig. 21.1). This blood flows from the right atrium through the tricuspid valve into the right ventricle. Backflow during ventricular systole (contraction and emptying) is prevented by the tricuspid, or right, atrioventricular (AV) valve (Fig. 21.2). The right ventricle pumps blood through the pulmonary semilunar valve to the lungs by way of the pulmonary artery. The pulmonary semilunar valve prevents backflow of blood into the right ventricle during ventricular diastole (relaxation and filling).

The left atrium receives oxygenated blood from the lungs by way of the four pulmonary veins. This blood flows through the mitral, or left, AV valve (also called the bicuspid valve) into the left ventricle. The mitral valve prevents backflow of blood into the left atrium during ventricular systole. The left ventricle pumps blood through the aortic semilunar valve to the body by way of the aorta. The aortic valve prevents backflow of blood into the left ventricle during ventricular diastole.

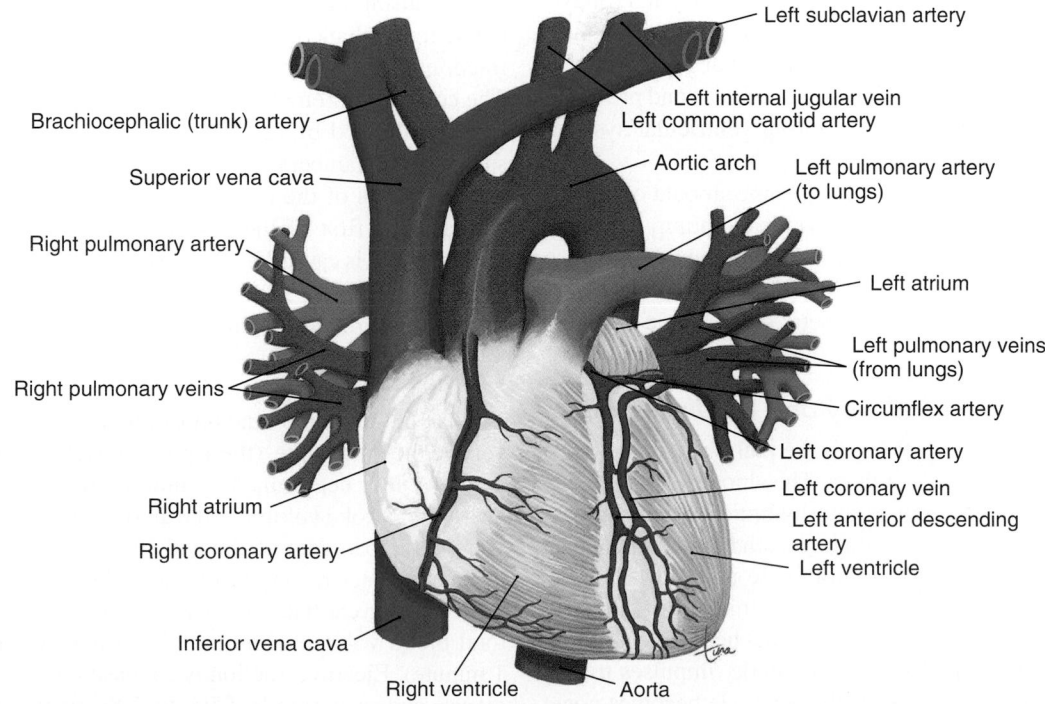

FIGURE 21.1 Anterior view of the heart and major blood vessels. From Scanlon, V., & Sanders, T. (2015). *Essentials of anatomy and physiology*, 7th ed. Philadelphia: F.A. Davis, with permission.

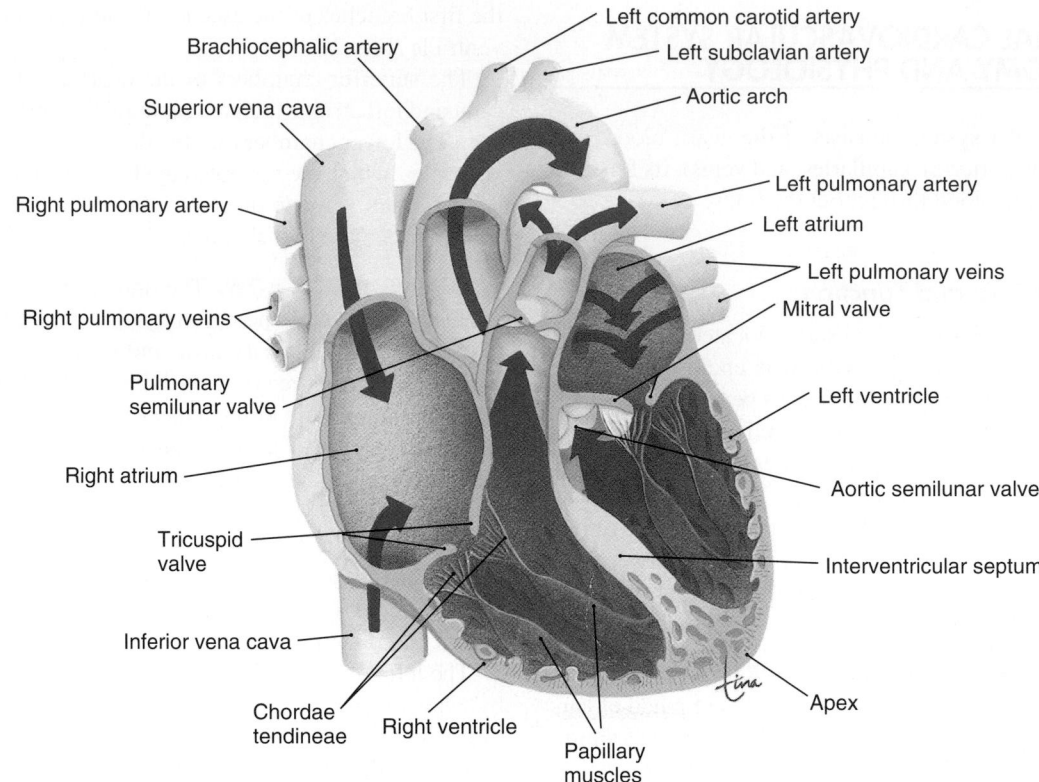

FIGURE 21.2 Frontal section of the heart showing internal structures and cardiac blood flow. From Scanlon, V., & Sanders, T. (2015). *Essentials of anatomy and physiology*, 7th ed. Philadelphia: F.A. Davis, with permission.

The tricuspid and mitral valves consist of three and two cusps, respectively. These cusps, or flaps, are connective tissue covered by endocardium and are anchored to the floor of the ventricle by the chordae tendineae and papillary muscles. The papillary muscles are columns of myocardium that contract along with the rest of the ventricular myocardium. This contraction pulls on the chordae tendineae and prevents hyperextension of the AV valves during ventricular systole (see Fig. 21.2).

Although each ventricle pumps the same amount of blood, the much thicker walls of the left ventricle pump with approximately five times the force of the right ventricle to distribute the blood throughout the body. This difference in force is reflected in the great difference between systemic and pulmonary blood pressure.

Cardiac Conduction Pathway and Cardiac Cycle

The cardiac conduction pathway is the pathway of electrical impulses that generates a heartbeat. The sinoatrial (SA) node in the wall of the right atrium is autorhythmic and depolarizes about 100 times per minute, initiating each heartbeat. (While at rest, parasympathetic fibers dominate and slow the SA node to about 75 beats per minute.) For this reason, the SA node is called the pacemaker, and a normal heartbeat is called a normal sinus rhythm. From the SA node, impulses travel on a specific path (Fig. 21.3). If the SA node becomes nonfunctional, the AV node can initiate each heartbeat, but at a slower rate of 40 to 60 beats per minute. The bundle of His is

capable of generating the beat of the ventricles, but at the much slower rate of about 20 to 35 beats per minute.

A cardiac cycle is the sequence of mechanical events that occurs during each heartbeat. Simply stated, the two atria contract simultaneously, followed by the simultaneous contraction of the two ventricles (a fraction of a second later). The contraction (emptying), or systole, of each set of chambers is followed by relaxation (filling), or diastole, of the same set of chambers.

The events of the cardiac cycle create the normal heart sounds. The first of the two major sounds (the "lubb" of "lubb-dupp") is caused by the closure of the AV valves during ventricular systole. The second sound is created by the closure of the aortic and pulmonary semilunar valves.

Cardiac Output

Cardiac output is the amount of blood ejected from the left ventricle in 1 minute (the right ventricle pumps a similar amount). It is determined by multiplying stroke volume by heart rate. Stroke volume is the amount of blood ejected by a ventricle in one contraction and averages 60 to 80 mL/beat. With an average resting heart rate of 75 beats per minute, average resting cardiac output is 5 to 6 L (approximately the total blood volume of an individual that is pumped within 1 minute). Ejection fraction is a measure of ventricular efficiency and is normally 55% to 70% of the total amount of blood within the left ventricle that is ejected with every heartbeat.

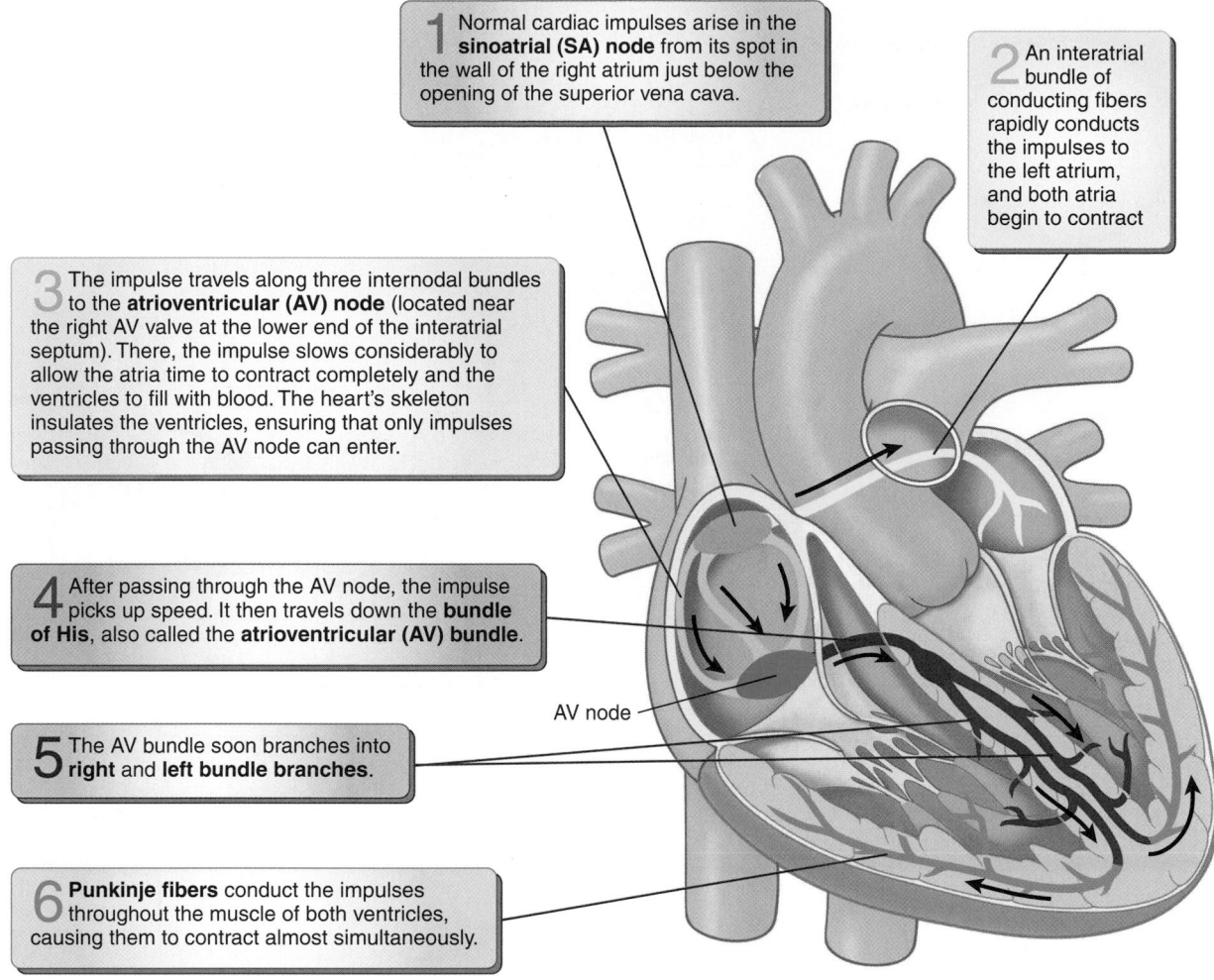

1 Normal cardiac impulses arise in the **sinoatrial (SA) node** from its spot in the wall of the right atrium just below the opening of the superior vena cava.

2 An interatrial bundle of conducting fibers rapidly conducts the impulses to the left atrium, and both atria begin to contract

3 The impulse travels along three internodal bundles to the **atrioventricular (AV) node** (located near the right AV valve at the lower end of the interatrial septum). There, the impulse slows considerably to allow the atria time to contract completely and the ventricles to fill with blood. The heart's skeleton insulates the ventricles, ensuring that only impulses passing through the AV node can enter.

4 After passing through the AV node, the impulse picks up speed. It then travels down the **bundle of His**, also called the **atrioventricular (AV) bundle**.

AV node

5 The AV bundle soon branches into **right** and **left bundle branches**.

6 **Punkinje fibers** conduct the impulses throughout the muscle of both ventricles, causing them to contract almost simultaneously.

FIGURE 21.3 Conduction pathway. From Thompson, G. S. (2013). *Understanding anatomy and physiology*. Philadelphia: F.A. Davis, p. 274.

During exercise, venous return increases and stretches the ventricular myocardium, which in response contracts more forcefully. This is known as Starling's law of the heart, and the result is an increase in stroke volume. More blood is pumped with each beat, and at the same time, the heart rate increases, causing cardiac output to increase by as much as four times the resting level, or more for fit athletes.

Regulation of Heart Rate

The heart generates its own electrical impulse, which begins at the SA node. The nervous system, however, can change the heart rate in response to environmental circumstances. In the brain, the medulla oblongata receives sensory input and alters heart function (Fig. 21.4).

Hormones and the Heart

The hormone epinephrine, secreted by the adrenal medulla in stressful situations, is sympathomimetic in that it increases the heart rate and force of contraction and dilates the coronary vessels. This in turn increases cardiac output and systolic blood pressure.

Aldosterone, a hormone produced by the adrenal cortex, is important for cardiac function because it helps regulate blood levels of sodium and potassium, both of which are needed for the electrical activity of the myocardium. The blood level of potassium is especially critical because even a small deviation impairs the rhythmic contractions of the heart.

The atria of the heart secrete a hormone of their own called atrial natriuretic peptide or atrial natriuretic hormone. As its name suggests, atrial natriuretic peptide increases the excretion of sodium by the kidneys by inhibiting secretion of aldosterone by the adrenal cortex. Atrial natriuretic peptide is secreted when a higher blood pressure or greater blood volume stretches the walls of the atria. The loss of sodium is accompanied by the increase loss of water in urine, which decreases blood volume and therefore blood pressure as well.

Blood Vessels

Arteries and Veins

Arteries and arterioles carry blood from the heart to capillaries. Their walls are relatively thick and consist of three

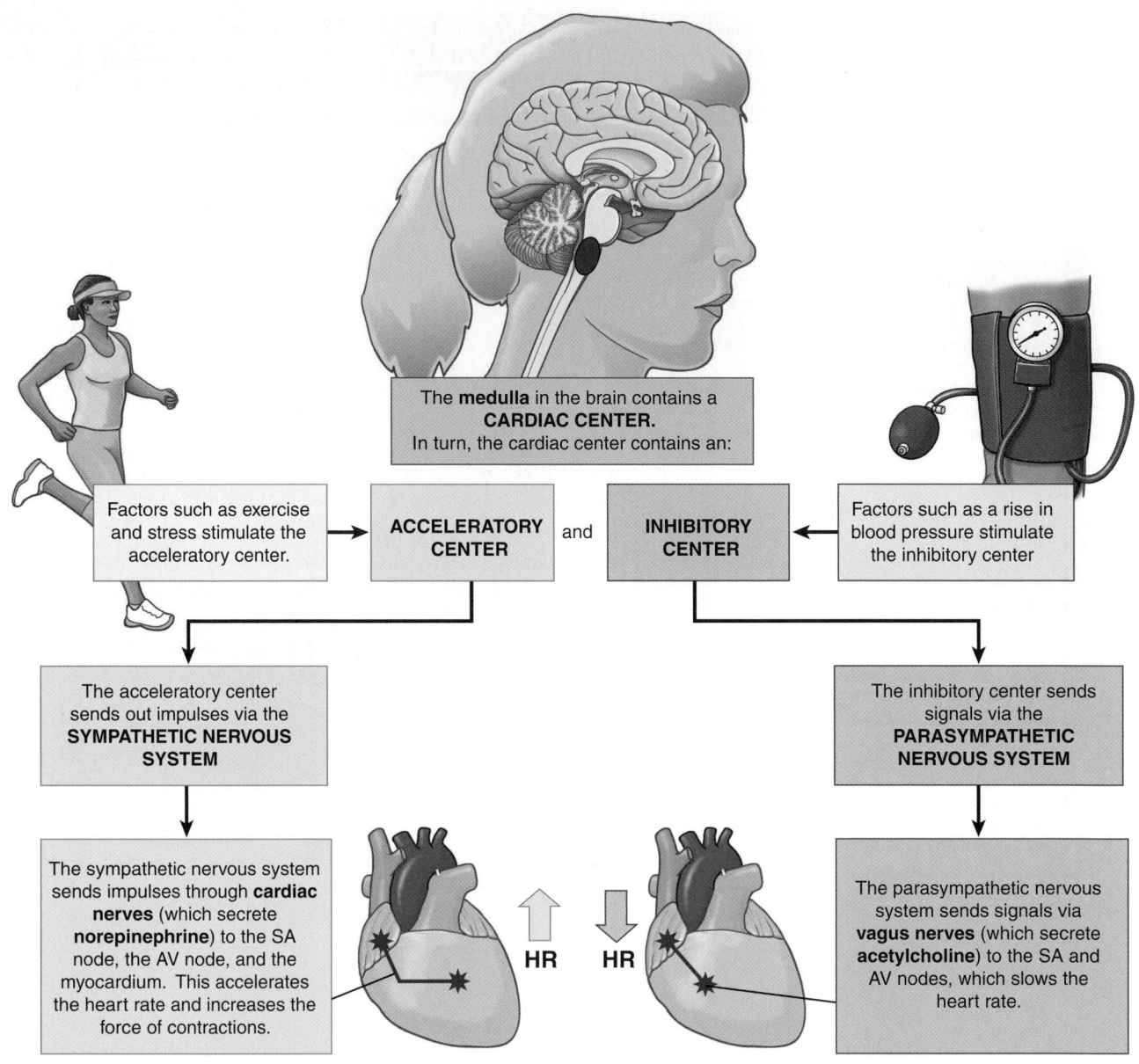

The **medulla** in the brain contains a
CARDIAC CENTER.
In turn, the cardiac center contains an:

Factors such as exercise and stress stimulate the acceleratory center.

ACCELERATORY CENTER   and   **INHIBITORY CENTER**

Factors such as a rise in blood pressure stimulate the inhibitory center

The acceleratory center sends out impulses via the **SYMPATHETIC NERVOUS SYSTEM**

The inhibitory center sends signals via the **PARASYMPATHETIC NERVOUS SYSTEM**

The sympathetic nervous system sends impulses through **cardiac nerves** (which secrete **norepinephrine**) to the SA node, the AV node, and the myocardium. This accelerates the heart rate and increases the force of contractions.

HR   HR

The parasympathetic nervous system sends signals via **vagus nerves** (which secrete **acetylcholine**) to the SA and AV nodes, which slows the heart rate.

FIGURE 21.4 Factors affecting heart rate. From Thompson, G. S. (2013). *Understanding anatomy and physiology.* Philadelphia: F.A. Davis, p. 278.

layers. Arteries carry blood under high pressure, and the outer layer of fibrous connective tissue prevents rupture of the artery. The middle layer of smooth muscle and elastic connective tissue contributes to the maintenance of normal blood pressure, especially diastolic blood pressure, by changing the diameter of the artery. The diameter of arteries is regulated primarily by the sympathetic division of the autonomic nervous system. By use of the smooth muscle, the arteries can also alter where the greatest volume of blood is directed. The inner layer or lining of the artery is simple squamous epithelium, called endothelium, which is very smooth to prevent abnormal clotting.

Veins and venules carry blood from capillaries to the heart. Their walls are relatively thin because they have less smooth muscle than arteries. Sympathetic impulses can bring about extensive constriction of veins, however, and this becomes

important in situations such as severe hemorrhage. The lining of veins is, like arteries, endothelium that prevents abnormal clotting; at intervals it is folded into valves to prevent backflow of blood. Valves are most numerous in the veins of the extremities, especially the legs, where blood must return to the heart against the force of gravity.

Capillaries

Capillaries carry blood from arterioles to venules and form extensive networks in most tissues. The exceptions are cartilage, covering/lining epithelia, and the lens and cornea of the eye. Capillary walls, a continuation of the lining of arteries and veins, are one cell thick to permit the exchanges of gases, nutrients, and waste products between the blood and tissues (Fig. 21.5). Blood flow through a capillary network is regulated by a precapillary sphincter, a smooth muscle fiber ring

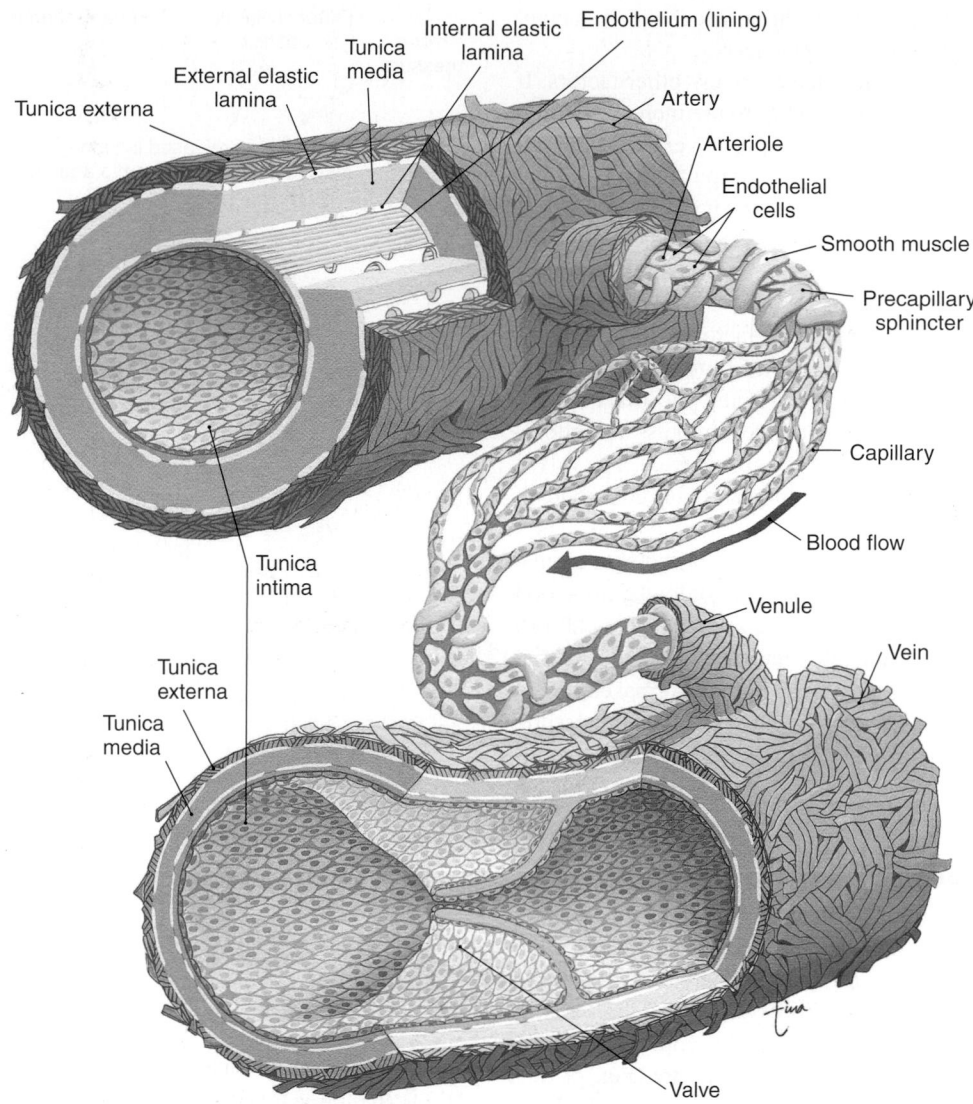

FIGURE 21.5 Structure of an artery, arteriole, capillary network, venule, and vein. From Scanlon, V., & Sanders, T. (2015). *Essentials of anatomy and physiology*, 7th ed. Philadelphia: F.A. Davis, with permission.

that contracts or relaxes in response to tissue needs. In an active tissue such as exercising skeletal muscle, for example, the rapid oxygen uptake and carbon dioxide production cause dilation of the precapillary sphincters to increase blood flow. At the same time, precapillary sphincters in less active tissues constrict to reduce blood flow. This is important because the body does not have enough blood to fill all of the capillaries at once; the fixed volume must constantly be shunted or redirected to where it is needed most.

Exchange between blood and tissue fluids occurs primarily due to diffusion and/or filtration at the capillaries. Diffusion is important to gas exchange. Filtration is a vital mechanism for homeostasis of extracellular fluids. Some of this tissue fluid returns to the capillaries, and some is collected in lymph capillaries. Lymph is returned to the blood by lymph vessels. Should blood pressure within the capillaries increase, more tissue fluid than usual is formed, too much for the lymph vessels to collect. This may result in tissue swelling, called edema.

Blood Pressure

Blood pressure is the force of the blood against the walls of the blood vessels and is measured in millimeters of mercury (mm Hg), systolic over diastolic. The normal average of systemic arterial pressure is 120/80 mm Hg. Blood pressure decreases in the arterioles and capillaries, and the systolic and diastolic pressures merge into one pressure. As blood enters the veins, blood pressure decreases further and approaches zero as it flows into the right ventricle. As mentioned previously, the blood pressure in the capillaries is of great importance, and normal blood pressure is high enough to permit filtration for nourishment of tissues but low enough to prevent rupture.

The arterioles (and veins during increased sympathetic stimulation) are usually in a state of slight constriction that helps to maintain normal blood pressure, especially diastolic pressure. This is called peripheral resistance; it is regulated by the vasomotor center in the medulla, which receives input via the glossopharyngeal and vagus nerves.

Blood pressure is also affected by many other factors. If heart rate and force increase, blood pressure increases within limits. If the heart is beating very fast, the ventricles are not filled before they contract, cardiac output decreases, and blood pressure drops. The strength of the heart's contractions depends on adequate venous return, which is the amount of blood that flows into the atria. Decreased venous return results in weaker contractions.

Venous return depends on several factors: constriction of the veins to reduce pooling, the skeletal muscle pumping to squeeze the deep veins of the legs, and the diaphragm's downward pressure during inhalation to compress the abdominal veins as the thoracic veins are decompressed. The valves in the veins prevent backflow of blood and thus contribute to the return of blood to the heart.

The elasticity of the large arteries also contributes to normal blood pressure. When the left ventricle contracts, the blood stretches the elastic walls of the large arteries, which absorb some of the force. When the left ventricle relaxes, the arterial walls recoil, exerting pressure on the blood. Normal elasticity, therefore, lowers systolic pressure, raises diastolic pressure, and maintains normal pulse pressure. Pulse pressure is the difference between the systolic and diastolic pressures. The usual ratio of systolic to diastolic to pulse pressure is 3:2:1.

Renin-Angiotensin-Aldosterone Mechanism

The kidneys are of great importance in the regulation of blood pressure. If blood flow through the kidneys decreases, renal filtration decreases and urinary output decreases to preserve blood volume. Decreased blood pressure stimulates the kidneys to secrete renin, which initiates the renin-angiotensin-aldosterone mechanism, raising blood pressure (Fig. 21.6).

Other hormones that affect blood pressure include those of the adrenal medulla, norepinephrine and epinephrine, which increase cardiac output and cause vasoconstriction in skin and viscera. Antidiuretic hormone, released from the posterior pituitary, directly increases water reabsorption by the kidneys, thus increasing blood volume and blood pressure. Atrial natriuretic peptide, secreted by the atria of the heart, inhibits aldosterone secretion and thereby increases renal excretion of sodium ions and water, which decreases blood volume and subsequently blood pressure.

Circuits of Circulation

The two circuits of circulation are pulmonary and systemic (see Fig. 21.2). Pulmonary circulation begins at the right ventricle, which pumps deoxygenated blood toward the lungs for gas exchange at the alveoli. Oxygenated blood returns to the left atrium by way of the pulmonary veins. Low pressure in the pulmonary capillaries prevents filtration in pulmonary capillaries, keeping tissue fluid from accumulating in the alveoli of the lungs, which can otherwise result in pulmonary edema.

Systemic circulation begins in the left ventricle, pumping oxygenated blood into the aorta, the many branches of which eventually give rise to capillaries within the tissues. Deoxygenated blood returns to the right atrium by way of the superior

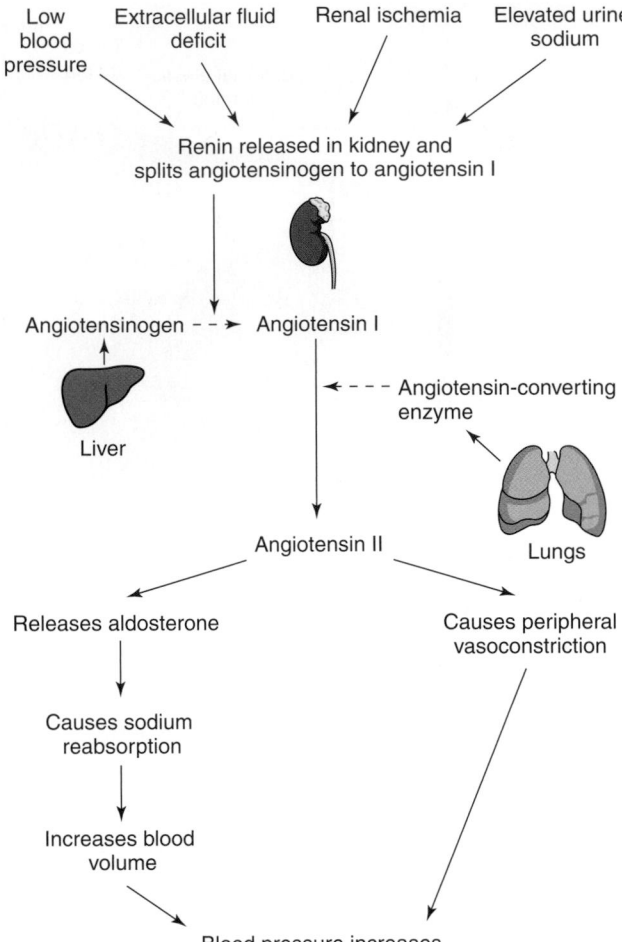

FIGURE 21.6 The renin-angiotensin-aldosterone mechanism.

and inferior vena cava and the coronary sinus. The hepatic portal circulation is a special part of the systemic circulation in which blood from the capillaries of the digestive organs and spleen flows through the portal vein and into the sinusoids in the liver before returning to the heart. This pathway permits the liver to regulate the blood levels of nutrients such as glucose, amino acids, and iron and to remove potential toxins such as alcohol or medications from circulation.

Aging and the Cardiovascular System

The aging of blood vessels, especially arteries, is believed to begin in childhood, although the effects are not apparent until later in life (Fig. 21.7). **Atherosclerosis** is the deposition of lipids in the walls of arteries over a period of years. The deposited lipids can narrow the arteries' lumens and form rough surfaces that may stimulate intravascular clot formation. Atherosclerosis decreases blood flow to the affected organ. With age, the heart muscle becomes less efficient, and maximum cardiac output and heart rate both decrease, although resting levels may be more than sufficient ("Gerontological Issues"). Valves may become thickened by fibrosis, leading to heart murmur.

• **WORD • BUILDING** •

atherosclerosis: athere—porridge + sklerosis—hardness

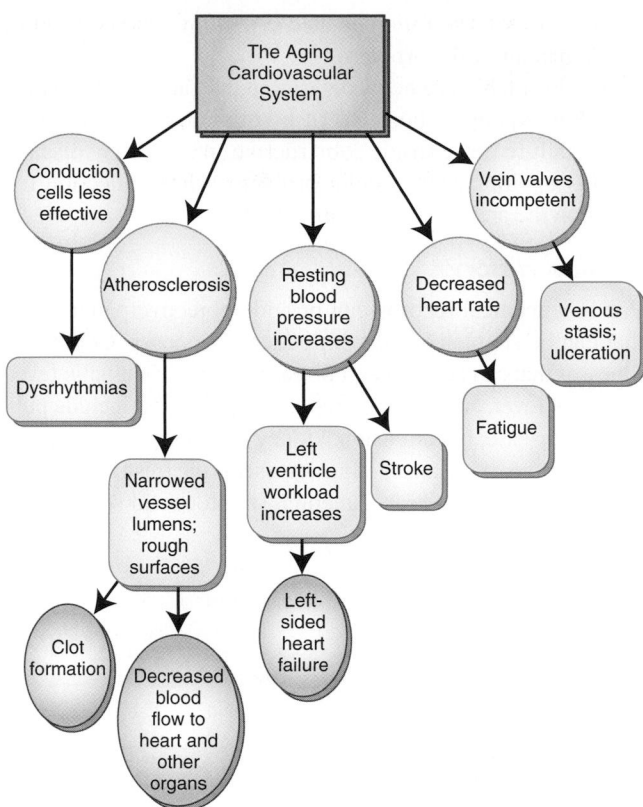

FIGURE 21.7 Aging and the cardiovascular system concept map.

Gerontological Issues

The older adult is at increased risk for developing orthostatic hypotension, which could precipitate a fall. This is often due to a combination of age-related changes, immobility, chronic illnesses, and medications.

 CARDIOVASCULAR DISEASE

In 2010, according to U.S. statistics of the American Heart Association (AHA, 2014), about one in six deaths were due to coronary heart disease; about 33% of United States adults over 19 years of age have hypertension per data from 2007 to 2010, and hypertension occurrence in African American adults is the highest in the world. For more information on cardiovascular disease statistics, visit www .americanheart.org.

In women, the greatest cause of death is cardiovascular disease. A movement called Go Red for Women gives women encouragement and tools to prevent cardiovascular disease and live healthy. For more information on Go Red for Women, visit www.goredforwomen.org.

Lifestyle plays a major role in risk factors for cardiovascular disease. The AHA recommends improving cardiovascular

health by not smoking, exercising, following a healthy diet, and maintaining normal blood pressure, blood glucose, total cholesterol levels, and weight. Exercise is essential for everyone, especially children, because Americans continue to be sedentary and eat excess calories.

 NURSING ASSESSMENT OF THE CARDIOVASCULAR SYSTEM

Nursing assessment of the cardiovascular system includes a patient health history and physical examination ("Gerontological Issues"). If the patient is experiencing an acute problem, focus on the most serious signs and symptoms and physical data until he or she is stabilized (Table 21.1). In-depth data collection can be completed when the patient is stable.

TABLE 21.1 ACUTE CARDIOVASCULAR DATA COLLECTION

History	**Significance**
Allergies	For medication administration, diagnostic dyes
Smoking history	Risk factor for cardiovascular disorders
Medications	Toxic levels; influencing symptoms
Pain: location, radiation, description	Possible angina, myocardial infarction, thrombus, embolism
Dyspnea	Left-sided heart failure; pulmonary edema or embolism
Fatigue	Decreased cardiac output
Palpitations	Dysrhythmias
Dizziness	Dysrhythmias
Weight gain	Right-sided heart failure
Physical Examination	**Possible Abnormal Findings**
Vital signs	Bradycardia, tachycardia, hypotension, hypertension, tachypnea, apnea, shock
Heart rhythm	Dysrhythmias
Edema	Right-sided heart failure
Jugular venous distention	Right-sided heart failure
Breath sounds	Crackles, wheezes with left-sided heart failure
Cough, sputum	Acute heart failure—dry cough, pink frothy sputum

Gerontological Issues

Older adults commonly have signs and symptoms that are not typical of a disorder, such as fatigue and nausea. The only symptom of myocardial infarction (MI) in an older patient may be dyspnea. Chest pain, a typical symptom, may not be present.

Health History

To understand a patient's cardiovascular problems, ask about past and current symptoms, medications, use of recreational drugs, surgeries, treatments, and risk factors such as diet, activity, tobacco use, and recent stressors. Data collection includes asking questions in the **WHAT'S UP?** format: where it is, how it feels, aggravating and alleviating factors, timing, severity, useful data for associated symptoms, and perception by the patient of the problem.

The health history helps determine the cause of the symptom. For example, shortness of breath can be the result of heart failure or chronic obstructive pulmonary disease (COPD). With cardiovascular problems, data collection focuses on the areas listed in Table 21.2.

Medical History

Previous medical records can provide objective patient data that can be supplemented with patient responses. Childhood illnesses that can lead to heart disease, such as rheumatic fever or scarlet fever, are noted. Other conditions noted include pulmonary disease, hypertension, kidney disease, cerebral vascular accident or brain attack, transient **ischemic** (restricted blood flow) attack, renal disease, anemia, streptococcal sore throat,

• WORD • BUILDING •

ischemic: ischein—hold back + haima—blood

TABLE 21.2 CARDIOVASCULAR HEALTH HISTORY

Question	Rationale
Pain: WHAT'S UP? Format	
Where is pain? Does it radiate?	Cardiac pain may radiate to shoulders, neck, jaw, arms, or back. Vascular disorders cause extremity pain.
How does it feel? Discomfort, burning, aching, indigestion, squeezing, pressure, tightness, heaviness, numbness in chest area? Fullness, heaviness, sharpness, throbbing in legs?	Pain can be associated with angina or myocardial infarction. The quality of pain varies. Venous pain is a fullness or heaviness. Arterial pain is sharp or throbbing.
Aggravating/alleviating factors that increase/relieve the pain?	Activity may cause or increase angina. Rest or medications may relieve angina. Leg activity pain, intermittent claudication, results from decreased perfusion that is aggravated by activity. Rest pain, from severe arterial occlusion, increases when lying. Dangling reduces the pain because blood flow is increased by gravity.
Timing of pain: onset, duration, frequency?	Pain may be continuous, intermittent, acute, or chronic. Arterial occlusion causes acute pain.
Severity of pain?	Rate pain on a scale of 0 to 10.
Useful data for associated symptoms?	Accompanying symptoms and their characteristics guide diagnosis and treatment.
Perception of patient about problem?	Patient's insight to problem is helpful in planning care.
Level of Consciousness (LOC)	
What is your name? What is the month? Year? Where are you now?	A lack of oxygen caused by cardiac disease can decrease LOC.
Dyspnea	
Are you short of breath? What increases your shortness of breath? What relieves your shortness of breath?	Dyspnea can be present with heart failure that reduces cardiac output, on exertion in angina pectoris or from a pulmonary embolus resulting from thrombophlebitis, heart failure, or dysrhythmias.

TABLE **21.2** CARDIOVASCULAR HEALTH HISTORY—cont'd

Question	Rationale
Palpitations Are you having palpitations or irregular heartbeat? Does your heart ever race, skip beats, or pound?	Palpitations can occur from dysrhythmias resulting from ischemia, electrolyte imbalance, or stress. Dizziness can be associated with dysrhythmias.
Fatigue Have you noticed a change in your energy level?	Fatigue occurs from reduced cardiac output resulting from heart failure.
Are you able to perform activities that you would like to?	Functional abilities can be limited from fatigue.
Edema Have you had any swelling in your feet, legs, or hands?	Right-sided heart failure can cause fluid accumulation in the tissues.
Have you gained weight?	Fluid retention causes weight gain.
Paresthesia/Paralysis Any numbness, tingling, or other abnormal sensations in extremities?	Numbness and tingling, pins and needles, and crawling sensations are paresthesia.
Can you move your extremity?	Paralysis is inability to move extremity. Reduced nerve conduction from decreased oxygen supply causes paresthesia and paralysis.

congenital heart disease, thrombophlebitis, and alcoholism. Patient allergies, previous hospitalizations, and surgeries are documented. Baseline diagnostic tests are helpful for comparison with current tests. Functional limitations that are related to cardiovascular problems, such as difficulty performing activities of daily living (ADLs), walking, climbing stairs, or completing household tasks, are also assessed.

Medication

Use of prescription drugs, over-the-counter medications such as aspirin that can prolong clotting time, and recreational drugs is noted. Patient's understanding of medications (name, dosage, reason for taking, last dose, and length of use) is documented.

Family History

A family history (parents, siblings, and grandparents) of cardiovascular conditions is noted because many cardiac problems are hereditary. For example, those who have had a parent die of sudden cardiac death before age 60 are at increased risk for sudden cardiac death.

Health Promotion

Risk factors such as diet, activity, tobacco use, and recent stressors for the patient are noted. The patient's health promotion activities are explored, especially for risk factors that are modifiable with changes in lifestyle.

Physical Examination

The patient's general appearance is observed. The patient's level of consciousness, which is an indicator of oxygenation

of the brain, is noted. Height, weight, and vital signs are recorded.

Blood Pressure

Normal blood pressure is considered less than 120/80 (see Chapter 22). Readings in both arms are done for comparison (Box 21-1). A difference in the readings is reported to the HCP. The arm with the higher reading is used for ongoing measurements. If necessary, blood pressure may be measured in the leg using a larger blood pressure cuff. The reading in the leg is normally 10 mm Hg higher than in the arm (see "Evidence-Based Practice").

 EVIDENCE-BASED PRACTICE

Clinical Question

Is blood pressure self-measurement at home more accurate for hypertension control and predictive of the risk of cardiovascular events than office blood pressure measurement?

Evidence

In a meta-analysis of studies conducted across a variety of populations, it was shown that home blood pressure recordings were a stronger predictor of long-term cardiovascular events than office blood pressure measurements. Home blood pressure monitoring overcomes the "white

Continued

coat effect" (increase in blood pressure during an office visit) of traditional office blood pressure measurement, increases accuracy, and is cost-effective.

Implications for Nursing Practice

Patients can effectively be taught to take blood pressure at home. Teaching guidelines include using an oscillometric monitor that measures blood pressure on the upper arm with proper cuff size; return demonstration of blood pressure measurement; resting for 5 minutes in the seated position; then taking three consecutive readings in the morning and at night, over a period of 1 week. Monitors should be validated periodically.

REFERENCE

Sheikh, S., Sinha, A., & Agarwal, R. (2011). Home blood pressure monitoring: How good a predictor of long-term risk? Current Hypertension Report, 13, 192–199.

Box 21-1 Taking Accurate Blood Pressure Measurements

- Instruct patient to avoid exercise, caffeine, and smoking for 30 minutes before the blood pressure measurement and to void before the reading.
- Use auscultatory method with properly calibrated and validated blood pressure instrument.
- Seat patient quietly for at least 5 minutes in a chair (not on examination table) with feet on the floor and arm supported at heart level before the blood pressure measurement.
- Use appropriate-sized cuff in which cuff bladder encircles at least 80% of arm.
- Ask patient to remain still and do not talk during measurement as motion alters reading.
- Determine the patient's baseline blood pressure by inflating the cuff and noting the reading when the radial pulse is no longer felt. When taking blood pressure, inflate the cuff to 20 numbers above the obtained baseline reading. (Overinflation may cause inaccurate reading.)
- During measurement, deflate the cuff slowly at rate of 2 mm Hg/seconds.
- Take at least two blood pressure measurements and average.
- Systolic blood pressure = first of two or more sounds heard.
- Diastolic blood pressure = disappearance of sounds.
- Provide patients, verbally and in writing, their specific blood pressure reading.

Note. Adapted from National Heart, Lung, and Blood Institute. Retrieved January 26, 2014, from www.nhlbi.nih.gov/hbp/detect/tips.htm

ORTHOSTATIC BLOOD PRESSURE. Measurements are taken with the patient lying, sitting, and standing to detect abnormal variations with postural changes. When the patient sits or stands, a drop in the systolic pressure of up to 15 mm Hg and either a drop or slight increase in the diastolic pressure of 3 to 10 mm Hg is normal. In response to the drop in blood pressure, the pulse increases 15 to 20 beats per minute to maintain cardiac output. Orthostatic hypotension (postural hypotension), is a drop in systolic blood pressure greater than 15 mm Hg, a drop or slight increase in the diastolic blood pressure greater than 10 mm Hg, and an increase in heart rate greater than 20 beats per minute in response to the drop in blood pressure. It indicates a problem that should be investigated by the health care provider (HCP) (Box 21-2). The patient often reports lightheadedness or syncope because the drop in blood pressure decreases the amount of oxygen-rich blood traveling to the brain. Factors that may cause orthostatic hypotension include deficient fluid volume, diuretics, analgesics, and pain.

Pulses

The apical pulse is auscultated for 1 minute to assess rate and rhythm. Normal heart rate is 60 to 100 beats per minute. In athletic people, the heart rate is often slower, around 50 beats per minute, because the well-conditioned heart pumps more efficiently. Apical pulse rhythm is documented as regular or irregular. The apical rate can be compared with the radial rate to assess equality. If there are fewer radial beats than apical beats, a **pulse deficit** exists and should be reported to the HCP.

Arterial pulses are palpated for volume and pressure quality. They are palpated bilaterally and compared for equality. A normal vessel feels soft and springy. A sclerotic vessel feels stiff. The quality of the pulses is described on a four-point scale as follows: 0 is absent; 1+ is weak, thready; 2+ is normal; and 3+ is bounding. An absent pulse is not palpable. A thready pulse is one that disappears when slight pressure is applied and returns when the pressure is removed. The normal pulse is easily palpable. The bounding pulse is strong and present even when slight pressure is applied. When the normal vessel is palpated, a tapping is felt. In the abnormal vessel that has a bulging or narrowed wall, a vibration is felt, which is called a **thrill**. When auscultating an abnormal vessel, a humming is heard that is caused by the turbulent blood flow through the vessel. This is referred to as a **bruit**.

BE SAFE!

Anticipate potential drops in blood pressure with position changes. Orthostatic hypotension can be found in patients of any age but is most commonly found in the older patient. The blood pressure drop increases the risk of fainting and falling. Use fall precautions such as a walking belt or two-person assist for patients at risk of or with orthostatic hypotension.

Box 21-2 Orthostatic Hypotension Assessment

To assess orthostatic hypotension:

1. Explain procedure to patient; determine if patient can safely stand.
2. Patient should not exercise, eat, or smoke 30 minutes before readings.
3. Have patient lie flat in bed at least 5 minutes before readings.
4. Use correct size blood pressure cuff.
5. Patient should not talk during readings and should sit up with legs uncrossed while sitting.
6. Take patient's lying blood pressure and heart rate.
7. Assist patient to sitting position. Ask if dizzy or light-headed with each position change. If yes, ensure safety from fainting or falling. A gait or walking belt can be used. With any position change, if patient experiences additional symptoms with the dizziness and decreased blood pressure and increased heart rate, assist the patient to lie down, take blood pressure, and notify the HCP. Consider the possible cause of the orthostatic hypotension (hemorrhaging, dehydration, diuretics) to plan patient care.
8. Wait 3 minutes, and then take patient's sitting blood pressure and heart rate. If patient is dizzy or light-headed, continue sitting position for 5 minutes if tolerated. Do not attempt to bring the patient to standing. Repeat sitting blood pressure. If blood pressure has increased and patient is no longer dizzy, assist patient to stand.
9. Assist patient to stand and take blood pressure and pulse immediately. Then take again in 3 minutes. If blood pressure drops and patient is dizzy or lightheaded, do not attempt to ambulate patient.
10. Document all heart rate and blood pressure measurements, including extremity used and patient position when reading was obtained (e.g., right arm: lying 132/78 mm Hg, sitting 118/68 mm Hg, standing 110/60 mm Hg). Also document patient tolerance, symptoms, and nursing interventions if symptomatic.
11. Report abnormal findings to HCP.

Respirations

The rate and ease of respirations are observed. Breath sounds are auscultated. Sputum characteristics such as amount, color, and consistency are noted. Pink, frothy sputum is an indicator of acute heart failure. A dry cough can occur from the irritation caused by the lung congestion resulting from heart failure.

Inspection

During the health history, inspection begins by noting shortness of breath when the patient speaks or moves. The patient's skin is noted for oxygenation status through the color of skin, mucous membranes, lips, earlobes, and nailbeds. Pallor may indicate anemia or lack of arterial blood flow. Cyanosis shows an oxygen distribution deficiency. A reddish brown discoloration (rubor) found in the lower extremities occurs from decreased arterial blood flow. A brown discoloration and cyanosis when the extremity is dependent may be seen in the presence of venous blood flow problems. Hair distribution on the extremities is observed. Decreased hair distribution, thick, brittle nails, and shiny, taut, dry skin occur from reduced arterial blood flow. Venous blood return is assessed by inspecting extremities for varicose veins, stasis ulcers, or scars around the ankles and signs of thrombophlebitis such as swelling, redness, or a hard, tender vein.

The patient's internal and external jugular neck veins are observed for distention in a 45- to 90-degree upright position. Normally, the veins are not visible in this position. Distention indicates an increase in the venous volume, often caused by right-sided heart failure.

Capillary refill time is 3 seconds or less and indicates arterial blood flow to the extremities. The patient's nailbed is briefly squeezed, causing blanching, and then released. The time that it takes for the color to return to the nailbed after release of the squeezing pressure is the capillary refill time. Longer times indicate anemia or a decrease in blood flow to the extremity.

Clubbing of the nailbeds occurs from oxygen deficiency over time. It is often caused by congenital heart defects or the long-term use of tobacco. The distal ends of the fingers and toes swell and appear clublike. With clubbing, the normal 160-degree angle formed between the base of the nail and the skin is lost, causing the nail to be flat (Fig. 21.8). Later, the nail base elevates, the angle exceeds 180 degrees, and the nail feels spongy when squeezed. To check for this, touch your index fingers together at the nailbeds and first joint. Look through the space created at the nailbeds. Do you see a diamond? If so, that is normal. If there is not a diamond, this indicates the nailbeds are clubbed and therefore filling that space. This should be reported to an HCP for follow-up.

LEARNING TIP

Six Ps characterize peripheral vascular disease:

- Pain
- Poikilothermia
- Pulselessness
- Pallor
- Paralysis
- Paresthesia (decreased sensation)

Clubbing—early

160°

Clubbing—severe

Greater than 180°

FIGURE 21.8 Clubbing of the fingers.

Palpation

In addition to palpating the arteries, the thorax can be palpated at the **point of maximum impulse**. The point of maximum impulse is palpated by placing the right hand over the apex of the heart. If palpable, a thrust is felt when the ventricle contracts. An enlarged heart may shift the pulse of maximum impulse to the left of the midclavicular line.

The temperature of the extremities is palpated bilaterally for comparison. Palpation begins proximally and moves distally along the extremity. In areas of decreased arterial blood flow, the ischemic area feels cooler than the rest of the body because it is blood that warms the body. In the absence of sufficient arterial blood flow, the area becomes the temperature of the environment **(poikilothermy)**. A warm or hot extremity indicates a venous blood flow problem.

Edema is palpated in the lower extremities or dependent areas such as the sacrum for the supine patient (Fig. 21.9). Edema can occur from right-sided heart failure, gravity, or altered venous blood return. The nurse assesses the severity of the edema by pressing with a finger for 5 seconds over a bone, the medial malleolus or tibia, in the area of edema. If the finger imprint or indentation remains, the edema is pitting. Measuring the leg circumference is an accurate method for monitoring the edema.

Homans' sign is an assessment for venous thrombosis; however, in less than 50% of patients with thrombosis, the test is not positive. A positive Homans' sign is pain in the patient's calf or behind the knee when the foot is quickly dorsiflexed with the knee in a slightly flexed position (Fig. 21.10). Homans' sign should not be performed if a positive diagnosis of thrombosis has been made because a clot could be dislodged with the movement.

Auscultation

Normal heart sounds are produced by the closing of the heart valves. Sound in blood-flowing vessels is transmitted in the direction of the blood flow. The first heart sound (S_1) is heard at the beginning of systole as "lubb" when the tricuspid and mitral (AV) valves close (Fig. 21.11). The second heart sound (S_2) is heard at the start of diastole as "dupp" when the aortic and pulmonic semilunar valves close. The diaphragm of the stethoscope is used to hear the high-pitched sounds of S_1 and S_2. Normally, no other sounds are heard between S_1 and S_2. With the bell of the stethoscope placed at the apex, a third heart sound (S_3) or a fourth heart sound (S_4) may be heard. Having patients lean forward or lie on their left side can make the heart

- WORD • BUILDING •
poikilothermy: poikilos—varied + therme—heat

FIGURE 21.9 Pitting edema. Application of pressure over a bony area displaces the excess fluid, leaving an indentation or pit.

FIGURE 21.10 Assessment of Homans' sign for venous thrombosis. The foot is quickly dorsiflexed with the knee flexed. Calf or knee pain is noted. This assessment should not be performed if a positive diagnosis of thrombosis has been made.

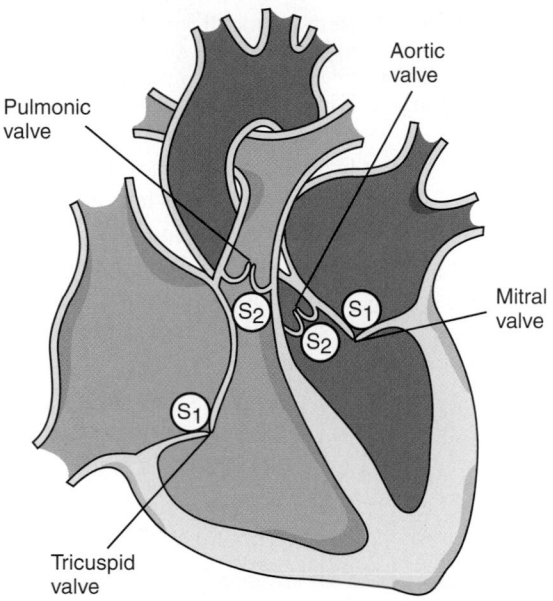

FIGURE 21.11 Heart sounds shown on electrocardiogram: S_1 is heard at the beginning of systole, and S_2 is heard at the beginning of diastole.

sounds easier to hear by bringing the area of the heart where the sound may be heard closer to the chest wall. The S_3 heart sound is normal for children and younger adults. It sounds like a gallop and is a low-pitched sound heard early in diastole. In older adults, S_3 may be heard with left-sided heart failure, fluid volume overload, and mitral valve regurgitation. The S_4 heart sound is also a low-pitched sound, similar to a gallop but heard late in diastole. It occurs with hypertension, coronary artery disease, and pulmonary stenosis.

LEARNING TIP

This sentence can help you remember the heart's auscultation points:

All	(aortic)
People	(pulmonic)
Eat	(Erb's point)
Three	(tricuspid)
Meals	(mitral)

Murmurs are caused by a narrowed valve opening or a valve that does not close tightly. A **murmur** is a prolonged, swishing sound that ranges in intensity from faint to very loud.

A **pericardial friction rub** occurs from inflammation of the pericardium. The intensity of a rub can range from faint to loud enough to be audible without a stethoscope. A rub has a grating sound like sandpaper being rubbed together that occurs when the pericardial surfaces rub together during a heartbeat. (See the Learning Tip on pericardial friction rub in Chapter 23.) Having the patient sit and lean forward allows a rub to be heard more clearly. The rub is best heard to the left of the sternum using the diaphragm of the stethoscope. A pericardial friction rub may occur after a MI or chest trauma.

CRITICAL THINKING

Mrs. Smith

■ Mrs. Smith, age 78, baseline weight 162 pounds, is admitted to the hospital with shortness of breath. Initial assessment findings are BP 152/88 mm Hg, pulse 104 beats per minute, respirations 26 per minute, temperature 99.4°F (37.2°C), shortness of breath at rest that increases with activity, ankles swollen, heart tones distant, nailbeds pale, no pain, has not eaten well for 2 weeks, 6-pound weight gain in 1 week, sleeps on three pillows, neck veins visible bilaterally. A diagnosis of acute MI with heart failure is made by her HCP.

1. Why might Mrs. Smith not be having chest pain with a diagnosis of acute MI?
2. How should swollen ankles be assessed to provide complete and measurable data?
3. What should be documented for the assessment performed on the swollen ankles and how should the assessment findings be documented?
4. How should the assessment findings be documented for the additional symptoms Mrs. Smith has?
5. What is Mrs. Smith's weight in kilograms?
6. What health care team members might provide collaborative care for Mrs. Smith?

Suggested answers are at the end of the chapter.

DIAGNOSTIC TESTS FOR THE CARDIOVASCULAR SYSTEM

Diagnostic test results are combined with the health history and physical assessment to plan care for the patient (Table 21.3).

Noninvasive Studies
Chest X-Ray Examination

A chest x-ray examination shows the size, position, contour, and structures of the heart (Fig. 21.12). It can reveal
(Text continued on page 406)

TABLE 21.3 DIAGNOSTIC PROCEDURES AND LABORATORY TESTS FOR THE CARDIOVASCULAR SYSTEM

Procedure	Definition	Significance of Abnormal Findings	Nursing Management
Noninvasive Chest x-ray film	Anterior-posterior and left lateral views of chest.	Heart enlargement, calcifications, fluid around heart	Ask females if pregnant. Remove metal items. Teaching: no discomfort.
Computed tomography scan	Evaluates heart, structures.	Plaque or calcification indicates atherosclerosis.	Kidney function checked if contrast used. If renal insufficiency, prophylaxis such as N-acetylcysteine (Mucomyst) and IV hydration with 0.45% sodium chloride hydration or a bicarbonate infusion can be given to protect kidneys.
Cardiac magnetic resonance imaging (MRI)/angiography (MRA)	Provides three-dimensional image of heart. Contrast agent given for MRA to visualize arteries.	Cardiac abnormalities	Ask if implants, non-MRI safe pacemaker, metallic items, and claustrophobia. Give antianxiety medication as ordered before MRI. Assess allergies for contrast agent. Teaching: must lie still in cylinder with loud, pounding sounds. Can talk to technician, listen to music.
Electrocardiogram (ECG)	Electrodes on skin carry electrical activity of heart from different views.	Dysrhythmias, enlarged heart chamber size, myocardial ischemia or infarction, electrolyte imbalances	Teaching: no discomfort. Explain procedure.
Holter monitor	Recording of ECG for up to 24 hours to match abnormalities with symptoms recorded in patient's diary.	Dysrhythmias, infrequent myocardial ischemia	Apply electrodes and leads. Teaching: keep accurate diary; push event button for symptoms. No showers or baths. Return visit.
Event Recorder	Worn longer time periods and can record 3 cardiac events.	Infrequent cardiac events.	Teaching: push event button for symptomatic event. Can bathe.
Echocardiogram	Sound waves bounce off heart to produce heart images and show blood flow.	Heart enlargement, coronary artery disease, valvular abnormalities, thickened cardiac walls or septum, pericardial effusion	May be done at bedside. Patient lies on left side. Teaching: no discomfort, gel applied.
Strain echocardiogram	Comprehensive assessment of the function of the heart muscle.	Useful in heart failure, cardiomyopathy, to guide treatment,	Can eat before test. Teaching: no discomfort, gel applied.

TABLE 21.3 DIAGNOSTIC PROCEDURES AND LABORATORY TESTS FOR THE CARDIOVASCULAR SYSTEM—cont'd

Procedure	Definition	Significance of Abnormal Findings	Nursing Management
		evaluate cardiac surgery or transplant	
Transesophageal echocardiogram	Probe with transducer on end inserted into esophagus.	See Echocardiogram.	Monitor vital signs and oxygen saturation. Check gag reflex before NPO status is discontinued. Suction continually during procedure. Teaching: NPO 6 hours before test. Sedation and local throat anesthetic given.
Exercise stress echocardiogram	Evaluates effects of exercise on heart and vascular circulation.	Dysrhythmias, ischemia	Monitor vital signs and ECG before, during, and after test until stable. Teaching: explain procedure, wear walking shoes and comfortable clothes.
Doppler ultrasound	Sound waves bounce off moving blood producing recordings.	Decreased blood flow in peripheral vascular disease	Teaching: explain procedure.
Radioisotopes			
Thallium imaging	IV injection of thallium-201 to evaluate cardiac blood flow. With exercise, thallium given 1 minute before end of test to circulate thallium. Scan done within 10 minutes and repeated in 2 to 4 hours for comparison.	If thallium not delivered to cardiac cells by good blood flow then see "cold spots" that show ischemia initially or infarcted areas later.	Teaching: explain procedure, inform that radioactivity is small and gone within a few hours. Light meal only between scans.
Dipyridamole thallium imaging	Dipyridamole (Persantine) IV is a vasodilator given to increase blood flow to coronary arteries; test is same as thallium imaging.	If thallium not delivered to cardiac cells by good blood flow then see "cold spots" that show ischemia initially or infarcted areas later.	Teaching: explain procedure, instruct no caffeine or aminophylline 12 hours before. Same as thallium imaging.
Technetium pyrophosphate or technetium-99m sestamibi imaging	Radioisotope given IV. Scanned 1.5 to 2 hours later.	Areas of myocardial cell damage take up the radioisotope, which appears as hot spots.	Teaching: explain procedure, inform that radioactivity is small and gone within a few hours.
Multiple-gated acquisition (MUGA) scan	Technetium-99m pertechnetate is given IV.	Studies effects of drugs, recent myocardial infarction	Teaching: explain procedure.

Continued

TABLE 21.3 DIAGNOSTIC PROCEDURES AND LABORATORY TESTS FOR THE CARDIOVASCULAR SYSTEM—cont'd

Procedure	Definition	Significance of Abnormal Findings	Nursing Management
	Serial studies are done over several hours. May be done at bedside.	(MI), and congestive heart failure.	
Positron emission tomography (PET)	Nitrogen-13 ammonia IV given and scanned for cardiac perfusion. Then fluoro-18-deoxyglucose IV given and scanned for cardiac metabolic function. Exercise may also be used.	In normal heart, scans match; in injured heart, they differ.	Patient's blood glucose must be 60 to 140 mg/dL for accuracy. Teaching: explain procedure. Must lie still during scan. If exercise used, NPO and no tobacco use.
Serum Tests Highly sensitive C-reactive protein (hs-CRP)	CRP level can indicate low-grade inflammation in coronary vessels. *CV disease risk:* Low = <1 mg/L Average = 1–3 mg/L High = >3 mg/L	Elevated levels indicate MI risk.	No special care.
Homocysteine	Amino acid in the blood. *Normal:* 7–8 micromol/L	Elevated levels linked with higher risk of coronary artery disease (CAD) and PVD.	Encourage high-risk patients to have adequate intake of folic acid and vitamin B.
Creatine kinase (CK)	Heart, brain, skeletal muscle contain CK enzymes. *Normal male:* 5–55 units/mL *Normal female:* 5–25 units/mL	Damaged cells release CK. With MI, CK elevates in 6 hours and returns to baseline in 48–72 hours.	Avoid IM injections, and take baseline CK before inserting IVs to avoid elevating CK from muscle cell damage. Serial sampling done.
CK-MB	Heart muscle contains MB isoenzyme. *Normal:* 0–7 international units/L	Rises with MI in 6 hours and returns to baseline in 72 hours.	Same as CK.
Cardiac troponin I or T	Cardiac cell protein. *Normal:* Varies by lab; very low levels	Elevated levels sensitive indicator of MI. Levels elevated up to 7 days.	No special care.
Myoglobin	Protein found in cardiac cells; 99% indicative of MI. *Normal:* 0–85 ng/mL	Rises in 1 hour after MI and peaks in 4 to 12 hours, so must be drawn within	No special care.

TABLE **21.3** **DIAGNOSTIC PROCEDURES AND LABORATORY TESTS FOR THE CARDIOVASCULAR SYSTEM—cont'd**

Procedure	Definition	Significance of Abnormal Findings	Nursing Management
		18 hours of chest pain onset.	
Magnesium	Electrolyte necessary to regulate heartbeat and blood pressure. *Normal:* 1.6 to 2.6 mg/dL	Hypomagnesemia may cause cardiac arrhythmias, hypertension, tachycardia.	No special care.
Phospholipids	May elevate in cardiovascular disease. *Normal:* 125–380 mg/dL	CAD risk	Same as triglycerides.
Lipoproteins	Electrophoresis done to separate lipoproteins: VLDL, LDL, HDL. HDL protects against CAD *Normal lipoproteins:* 400–800 mg/dL *Desirable:* LDL less than HDL (values vary with age)	Elevated LDL increases CAD risk. LDL <100 desirable HDL >60	Same as triglycerides.
Invasive Angiography	Contrast agent injected into vessels to make them visible on x-rays. Coronary: coronary arteries via cardiac catheter. Peripheral: peripheral arteries or veins.	Assesses vessel patency, injury, or aneurysm.	Precare: Informed consent. NPO 4 to 18 hours before test. Assess allergies. Teaching: sedative and local anesthesia may be used; burning sensation from dye; monitored continuously. Postcare: Monitor vital signs, hemorrhage at the injection site, pulses.
Cardiac catheterization	Catheter inserted into heart for data on oxygen saturation and chamber pressures. Contrast may be injected to visualize structures.	Cardiac disease	Precare: Same as angiography. Sensory teaching: table is hard; cool cleansing solution used; sting felt from local anesthetic; hear monitor beeping; feel pressure of catheter insertion; dye warm, burning feeling; headache; brief chest pain; hear camera; feel table move. Postcare: Monitor vital signs, circulation, mobility, sensation, catheter insertion site, for hemorrhage or hematoma every 15 minutes for 1 hour, then every 30 minutes to 1 hour. Apply insertion site pressure as needed.

Continued

TABLE 21.3 DIAGNOSTIC PROCEDURES AND LABORATORY TESTS FOR THE CARDIOVASCULAR SYSTEM—cont'd

Procedure	Definition	Significance of Abnormal Findings	Nursing Management
			Immobilize extremity for several hours as ordered.
Hemodynamic monitoring	Diagnoses and guides treatment with continuous readings compared to normal for: *Right atrial pressure:* 2–6 mm Hg *Pulmonary artery systolic/diastolic:* 20–30/0–10 *Pulmonary artery wedge pressure:* 4–12 mm Hg *Cardiac output:* 4–8 L/min SvO_2: 60%–80%	Blood pressure, cardiac and pulmonary pressure abnormalities.	Informed consent signed. Continuous monitoring. Recording of readings and monitoring of insertion site for signs of infection.
Electrophysiological studies	Assesses heart's electrical system, with electrodes inserted into the right side of the heart.	Dysrhythmias	Consent is obtained. Patient is NPO 6 to 8 hours before the test.

FIGURE 21.12 Normal chest x-ray film. Note white outline of heart borders in center. From McKinnis, L. N. [2014]. *Fundamentals of musculoskeletal imaging* [p. 287]. Philadelphia: F.A. Davis.

heart enlargement, calcifications, fluid around the heart, heart failure, and placement of pacemaker leads and pulmonary artery catheters. Fluoroscopy uses a luminescent x-ray screen to guide cardiac catheter or pacemaker lead placement. Visit www.radiologyinfo.org for more information on radiology tests.

Computed Tomography

Computed tomography (CT) for calcium scoring of calcified plaque (the body deposits calcium to harden plaques, which are not normally found in the coronary arteries) in the coronary arteries can be done.

CT angiography (view body blood vessels) and coronary CT angiography (view coronary arteries) use an iodine contrast agent. Patient kidney function (glomerular filtration rate, creatinine) must be checked before the test to help prevent contrast-induced nephropathy (Chapter 36).

Cardiac Magnetic Resonance Imaging and Angiography

Two- or three-dimensional still or moving images of the beating heart are produced with magnetic resonance imaging (MRI). Cardiac MRI is useful for identifying ischemia and heart damage as well as other conditions affecting the heart. For magnetic resonance angiography, a non–iodine-based contrast, gadolinium-DTPA, may or may not be used to view the blood vessels.

Electrocardiogram

The electrocardiogram (ECG) records electrical activity of the heart in various views. Abnormalities related to conduction, rate, rhythm, heart chamber enlargement, myocardial ischemia, MI, and electrolyte imbalances may be reflected on an ECG. When an ECG is requested, information that aids in its interpretation is provided, including the patient's sex, age, height, weight, blood pressure, and cardiac medications. There is no special preparation for the ECG, which is painless.

To obtain an ECG, electrodes are placed on the skin to transmit electrical impulses to the ECG machine for recording. The electrical impulses from the heart appear as waves on graph paper. One view of the heart using a combination of the electrodes to obtain the view is called a lead. The standard 12-lead ECG, using a combination of the electrodes, provides 12 views of the heart. Eighteen-lead ECGs can also be done.

SIGNAL-AVERAGED ECG. The signal-averaged ECG is used to diagnose whether a patient is at risk of developing ventricular tachycardia and possible sudden death. A computer records low-level signals not detected by a regular ECG. These electrical signals, referred to as late potentials, occur at the end of the QRS wave and into the ST segment (see Chapter 25). Late potentials place the patient at risk for ventricular **dysrhythmias** (abnormal heart rhythms).

HOLTER MONITORING (AMBULATORY ELECTROCARDIOGRAM). A Holter monitor, which weighs 2 pounds, continuously records an ECG in one lead for up to 48 hours as a patient goes about his or her daily activities. The patient wears loose-fitting clothing and may only sponge bathe while wearing the monitor. The patient records a diary of activities and symptoms and pushes the event button if symptoms occur. Symptoms are documented for later correlation with the ECG recordings. Dysrhythmias or myocardial ischemia that occurs infrequently can be detected. Recordings are scanned by a computer and interpreted by an HCP.

Doppler Ultrasound

In a Doppler ultrasound test, sound waves bounce off moving blood cells and return a sound frequency in relationship to the amount of blood flow. With decreased blood flow the sounds are reduced. This test requires no patient preparation, takes about 20 minutes to complete, and is painless.

Echocardiogram

An echocardiogram is an ultrasound test that records the motion of the heart structures, including the valves and chambers, as well as the heart size, shape, and position. Three-dimensional images of the heart and four-dimensional (real-time) heart imaging is possible. Color Doppler can record blood flow through the heart valves. No preparation is required. This test transmits ultrasonic sound waves across the chest wall (transthoracic) and through lung and rib tissue into the heart so that the returned echoes can be recorded. An ECG is recorded at the same time.

STRAIN ECHOCARDIOGRAM. A comprehensive assessment of the function of the heart muscle (myocardium) is obtained with a strain echocardiogram. It shows changes in the shape of the heart (deformation). It is used for heart failure, cardiomyopathy, to guide treatment, or evaluate cardiac surgery or transplant.

EXERCISE STRESS ECHOCARDIOGRAM. Coronary artery disease is diagnosed during exercise-induced cardiac ischemia by detecting cardiac wall motion abnormalities. If the patient is unable to exercise (treadmill, stationary bike), giving dobutamine for a dobutamine stress echocardiography simulates exercise while the echocardiogram is done.

TRANSESOPHAGEAL ECHOCARDIOGRAM. A transesophageal echocardiogram (TEE) provides a clearer picture than transthoracic echocardiography. Three-dimensional images of the heart and four-dimensional (real-time heart imaging) images are also possible with TEE. Images are produced by using a transducer on a probe that is placed in the esophagus. The images are clearer because lung and rib tissue does not have to be penetrated by the sound waves. The physician controls the position of the probe and takes pictures as it travels within the esophagus. Patients take nothing by mouth (NPO) for about 6 hours before the test, receive a sedative, and have their throats locally anesthetized.

 BE SAFE!

Anytime a patient's throat is anesthetized for a procedure, the patient must remain NPO until the nurse has verified (by touching the back of the throat with a cotton tip swab) that the gag reflex has returned. The patient could aspirate or choke while drinking or eating if the gag reflex is not present.

Cardiac Stress Test

The exercise stress test measures cardiac function or peripheral vascular disease during a defined exercise protocol (Fig. 21.13). It shows the heart's response to increased oxygen needs. Before the test, patients are given an explanation of the test and told not to smoke, eat, or drink for 2 to 4 hours before the test. They are also instructed to wear comfortable walking shoes, a loose top, and, for women, a supportive bra. Before the test, baseline vital signs are obtained.

Then, while the patient exercises on a treadmill, on a stationary bicycle, or by climbing stairs, vital signs, oxygen saturation, skin temperature, physical appearance, chest pain, and ECG are monitored to help ensure patient safety. The test is completed when the patient reaches his or her peak heart

FIGURE 21.13 Performance of stress test.

rate (patient's age subtracted from 220), experiences chest pain, is unable to exercise further, or develops vital sign or ECG changes. Vital signs and ECG continue to be monitored after the test until they return to baseline. After the test, patients should rest and wait to eat. They should also avoid eating or drinking stimulants such as caffeine and temperature extremes such as going out into cold weather for a few hours after the test.

The cardiac stress test is used to evaluate coronary artery disease. It aids in diagnosing ischemic heart disease, the cause of chest pain, and dysrhythmias. The functional capacity of the heart can also be measured after a cardiac event or to plan a physical fitness or rehabilitation program.

Peripheral Vascular Stress Test

In a peripheral vascular stress test, the patient walks for 5 minutes at 1.5 miles per hour on the treadmill. At certain intervals, pulse volume measurements are taken, including baseline resting, during the test, and final resting after the test. This test assesses response to activity. If intermittent **claudication** (pain in the legs with activity) occurs, the test is stopped.

Arterial Stiffness Index

Stiffness of the brachial artery is measured to determine arteriosclerosis and cardiovascular disease risk. The brachial artery correlates with the coronary arteries in regard to the extent of atherosclerosis. The arterial stiffness index test is done with a device that has a blood pressure cuff hooked to a computer that maps the waveforms during the blood pressure reading.

Tilt Table Test

The tilt table test is used to help diagnose the cause of syncope (fainting spells). Heart rate and blood pressure are monitored during a change in position from lying down to standing up.

Nuclear Radioisotope Imaging

For nuclear radioisotope imaging, small amounts of radioisotopes are given intravenously (IV). The patient is then scanned with a gamma camera to produce a radionuclide image. Radiation exposure is similar to that of other x-ray examinations. These tests can provide information about myocardial ischemia or infarction, cardiac blood flow, and ventricle size and motion.

Thallium Imaging

Thallium-201, a radioactive analog of potassium, is used to detect impaired myocardial perfusion. It is injected IV, and muscle cells absorb it. After 10 to 15 minutes, the heart is scanned to see where the thallium has concentrated. Four hours later, the scan is repeated to look for changes. Healthy myocardial cells with good blood flow take up the thallium. Areas in which the thallium is not seen are referred to as cold spots and indicate ischemia or infarction. The patency of a coronary artery graft may also be assessed with this test. This test is used often because the short half-life of thallium results in lower radiation exposure.

Exercise testing may be combined with thallium injection to detect blood flow changes with activity and after rest. The patient exercises and about 2 minutes before stopping is given thallium. Scans are taken immediately and again in 2 to 4 hours. Cold spots on initial images indicate ischemia. If the cold spots are gone in later images, exercise-induced ischemia is present. If the cold spots are still present in later images, they show scarred areas.

If patients are unable to participate in exercise for the thallium stress test, dipyridamole (Persantine) or adenosine, coronary vasodilators, can be given. These drugs simulate the increased blood flow to healthy myocardial cells that occurs with exercise.

Technetium Pyrophosphate Scan

Technetium-99m pyrophosphate is injected for this test. Areas of ischemia or myocardial cell damage take up the radioisotope, and when scanned these areas appear as hot spots. Acute MI size and location can be detected, but old MIs cannot be detected.

Technetium-99m Sestamibi

For this test, technetium-99m sestamibi is given IV and the patient is scanned 1.5 to 2 hours later. Areas of myocardial cell damage take up the radioisotope, and when scanned these areas appear as hot spots.

Multiple-Gated Acquisition Scan

In a multiple-gated acquisition scan, technetium-99m pertechnetate is injected IV and remains in the bloodstream; it is not taken up by myocardial cells. A camera follows the flow of the radioactivity, which shows ventricular function and wall motion and the ejection fraction of the heart.

Positron Emission Tomography

Positron emission tomography (PET) shows myocardial perfusion and viability with three-dimensional images. Nitrogen-13 ammonia is injected IV first and then scanned to show myocardial perfusion. Next, fluoro-18-deoxyglucose is given IV and then scanned to show myocardial metabolic function. If ischemia or heart damage is present, the two scans are different. For example, in ischemia of viable cells, blood flow is decreased but metabolism elevated. Treatment to increase blood flow improves cardiac function in this case. Before the test, the patient's blood glucose should be in the normal range, and caffeine and tobacco should be avoided for 4 hours before the test.

BE SAFE!

Improve the accuracy of patient identification:

- Use at least two ways to identify patients when providing care, treatment, and services. For example, use the patient's name and date of birth.
- Use two identifiers and label sample collection containers in the presence of the patient.
- Conduct a preprocedure verification process. Implement a preprocedure process to verify the correct procedure, for the correct patient, at the correct site (2014 National Patient Safety Goals, © The Joint Commission, 2013. Reprinted with permission.).

Blood Studies

Blood Lipids

Lipids include triglycerides, cholesterol, and phospholipids. Lipoproteins carry these lipids attached to proteins. Triglycerides are found in very low-density lipoproteins (VLDLs). Cholesterol is mainly found in low-density lipoproteins (LDLs). High-density lipoproteins (HDLs) are a mixture of one-half protein and one-half phospholipids and cholesterol.

A lipid profile can screen for increased risk of coronary artery disease. For more information, visit www.nhlbi.nih.gov/guidelines/cholesterol/atglance.pdf. Patients must fast for 12 hours and avoid alcohol for 24 hours before the test. Water is not withheld. High levels of LDLs are linked to an increase in coronary artery disease because they circulate cholesterol in the arteries. HDLs play a protective role against coronary artery disease because they carry cholesterol to the liver to be metabolized. Controlling lipids is important in reducing coronary artery disease ("Cultural Considerations").

C-Reactive Protein

C-reactive protein is an acute-phase protein that increases during the inflammatory process. A highly sensitive C-reactive protein (hs-CRP) test can predict heart attack risk. With elevated hs-CRP levels, nurses have the opportunity to help patients understand and reduce cardiac risk factors.

Homocysteine

Homocysteine is an amino acid in the blood that may damage the lining of arteries and promote blood clots. Elevated levels are associated with increased cardiovascular disease risk. Folic acid, vitamin B_6, and vitamin B_{12} break down homocysteine. Adequate dietary intake of green leafy vegetables and grains fortified with folic acid, as well as vitamin B, can help reduce homocysteine levels.

Cardiac Biomarkers

Proteins and enzymes released into the blood by damaged cardiac cells are known as cardiac biomarkers. These biomarkers help identify whether a patient is having or has had a recent MI.

CREATINE KINASE. Creatine kinase CK is an enzyme found in the brain, skeletal muscle, and heart muscle. Isoenzymes of creatine kinase contained in these tissues are CK-BB (brain), CK-MM (skeletal muscle), and CK-MB (heart muscle). CK-MB helps diagnose a MI because its level rises within 4 to 6 hours after cardiac cells are damaged, peaks in 12 to 18 hours, and returns to normal in 24 to 36 hours. Invasive procedures such as IV and intramuscular (IM) injections are avoided before drawing the first creatine kinase to prevent elevation in the creatine kinase levels from cell trauma caused by the procedure. Medications are often given IV rather than IM to prevent contributing to this elevation.

Cultural Considerations

Among French Canadians, familial chylomicronemia (hyperlipoproteinemia type I), an autosomal recessive disorder, occurs with the highest frequency worldwide. Familial chylomicronemia can lead to coronary thrombosis. Thus, the nurse can improve the health of French Canadians by encouraging early diagnostic workups for familial chylomicronemia and encouraging healthful lifestyles.

CARDIAC TROPONIN. Cardiac muscle contains proteins called troponin I and troponin T, which control the muscle fibers that contract or squeeze the heart muscle. They detect minor myocardial damage not detected by CK-MB so it is the more commonly done test to diagnose MI. Levels elevate within 4 to 6 hours of damage. These levels peak in 10 to 24 hours and remain elevated for 10 to 14 days. Troponin T appears slightly earlier than troponin I and remains elevated longer after cardiac damage.

MYOGLOBIN. Myoglobin, a protein found in skeletal and cardiac muscle, is not site specific so it can only indicate that muscle damage has occurred. However, it rises before CK-MB or troponin so it can detect a MI earlier for prompt treatment. Myoglobin levels elevate within 1 hour of an acute MI. Peak levels are reached 4 to 12 hours after a MI, and levels return to normal within 18 hours after the onset of chest pain.

Magnesium

Magnesium, an electrolyte, is important to many functions in the body. Among these is control of the heartbeat, and regulating blood pressure. A normal magnesium level is 1.6 to 2.6 mg/dL. **Hypomagnesemia**, a low level of magnesium in the blood, can cause cardiac arrhythmias, hypertension, and tachycardia. Many things can contribute to low magnesium levels, including diuretic therapy, digitalis, some antibiotics, diabetes mellitus, and MI.

BE SAFE!

Improve the effectiveness of communication among caregivers. Report critical results of tests and diagnostic procedures on a timely basis (2014 National Patient Safety Goals, © The Joint Commission, 2013. Reprinted with permission.).

Invasive Studies
Angiography

Arteriography and venography are the two types of angiography (Fig. 21.14). Arteriography examines arteries. Venography studies veins. Angiography uses dye injected into the vascular system to visualize the vessels on radiographs. This test is used to assess blood clot formation, peripheral vascular disease, and test vessels for potential grafting use.

The patient must be assessed for allergies, give informed consent, be NPO for about 4 hours before the test, and be informed that the dye produces a hot, burning feeling when injected. After the procedure the patient is assessed for several hours. Vital signs, allergic reaction signs, hemorrhage at the injection site, and pulses are monitored.

Cardiac Catheterization

Cardiac catheterization allows the heart's anatomy and physiology to be studied or therapeutic procedures to be done. As an invasive diagnostic procedure, it measures pressures in the heart

FIGURE 21.14 Coronary angiography and cardiac catheterization.

chambers, great blood vessels, and coronary arteries and provides information on cardiac output and oxygen saturation. Fluoroscopy, an x-ray procedure that produces real-time images of internal organs in motion on a video monitor, is used to guide the insertion of the catheter into the heart. Dye can be injected once the catheter is in place to visualize the heart chambers and vessels. This procedure is often done before heart surgery.

An informed consent must be obtained. The patient is assessed for allergies to contrast agents used in the procedure. IV hydration may be given before the procedure while the patient is NPO. Patients should be told that during the test they will be awake and a warm, flushing sensation may be felt when the dye is injected; the room has a lot of equipment; a movable table is used; the patient's vital signs and ECG are monitored constantly; and the length of the procedure is 2 to 3 hours.

In right-sided catheterization, a catheter with or without a fiber-optic tip is inserted into the jugular vein (neck) or the femoral vein (leg) and advanced into the vena cava. It is then moved through the right chambers of the heart and into the pulmonary artery. The catheter can be wedged momentarily in the artery by inflating the balloon at the tip of the catheter. This position provides the pulmonary artery wedge pressure, which reflects pressures in the left side of the heart. Other pressures obtained with right-sided cardiac catheterization are right atrial pressure, which reflects central venous pressure, pulmonary artery systolic and diastolic pressures, cardiac output, and mixed venous oxygen saturation (SvO_2) if a fiber-optic catheter is used.

The left side of the heart can be directly assessed by inserting a catheter into the radial artery or the femoral artery. It is advanced against the flow of blood into the aorta, through the aortic valve, and into the left ventricle. Coronary angiography, which visualizes the coronary arteries with dye, can be done with this approach. The catheter is inserted into the opening of the coronary arteries, the dye is injected, and x-ray films are

• **WORD** • **BUILDING** •
hypomagnesemia: hypo—low + magnes—magnesium + emia—in blood

taken. Coronary artery disease can be assessed with coronary angiography.

After the procedure, the catheter is removed, and firm pressure must be applied to the insertion site for several minutes to prevent hemorrhage or hematoma formation. A pressure dressing or sandbag may be applied to the site when bleeding is stopped and is removed after several hours. Vital signs are assessed according to the HCP's orders and the institution's policies. During vital sign checks, the puncture site is assessed and peripheral pulses are verified. The patient is on bed rest without moving or flexing the leg for a few hours to allow healing of the puncture site, if the groin was used. For comfort, modified positioning and use of a pillow may be used without complications as ordered. Patients can eat and are instructed to drink fluids to help eliminate the dye from the body. If the patient is stable and no significant findings are found, the patient may be discharged.

Complications of cardiac catheterization can be allergic reaction, breaking of the catheter, hemorrhage, thrombus formation, emboli of air or blood, dysrhythmias, MI, cerebrovascular accident (stroke), and puncture of the heart chambers or lungs.

Hemodynamic Monitoring

Bedside monitoring can be done to monitor the pressures in the blood vessels or heart. A catheter attached to a transducer and monitor, called an arterial line, can be inserted into the radial or femoral artery to measure continuous arterial blood pressure.

Ongoing monitoring of cardiac pressures, cardiac output, and central venous pressure can be done with either a central catheter or a pulmonary artery catheter. Central venous pressure is measured directly with a central catheter inserted into the vena cava via the brachial, femoral, subclavian, or jugular vein (Fig. 21.15). It is measured indirectly with the pulmonary artery catheter (Fig. 21.16). The right atrial pressure measurement obtained

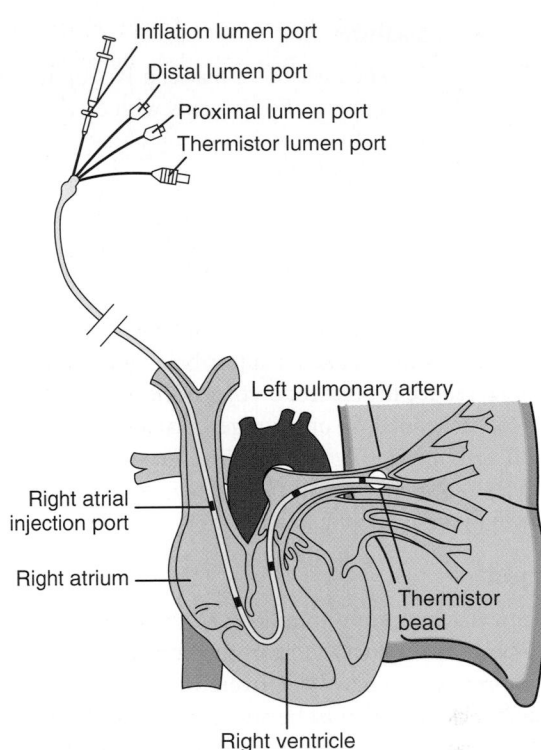

FIGURE 21.16 Pulmonary artery catheter and placement of the inflated balloon in the pulmonary artery.

from the pulmonary artery catheter reflects the pressure in the vena cava. Central venous pressure measures **preload** (pressure stretching the ventricle of the heart from fluid returned to the heart) or fluid volume status; central venous pressure readings used in fluid or diuretic therapy have been primarily replaced by pulmonary artery catheter measurements.

Electrophysiological Study

To study the heart's electrical system, one or more catheters with electrodes are inserted via the femoral vein into the right side of the heart. Two to three electrodes are usually inserted. The heart's electrical impulses are then recorded and pacing can also be done. Dysrhythmias can be triggered to help the HCP diagnose why they are occurring. A consent is obtained, and the patient is NPO 6 to 8 hours before the test.

THERAPEUTIC MEASURES FOR THE CARDIOVASCULAR SYSTEM

Exercise

A prescribed walking program helps promote blood flow by contracting the skeletal muscles and may reduce symptoms of peripheral vascular disease. For patients recovering from cardiac surgery or a MI, activity is gradually increased. Exercise is very important for optimum cardiac functioning. A cardiac rehabilitation program is usually prescribed, and individualized exercise goals are determined. After discharge from the hospital, exercise three times a week for 20 to 30 minutes is encouraged.

FIGURE 21.15 Central venous pressure measurement.

may require assistance in applying the stockings if they have impaired manual dexterity. Devices are available that aid in applying the stockings, such as the Sigvaris Doff N' Donner.

Intermittent Pneumatic Compression Devices

An intermittent pneumatic compression device consists of plastic inflatable stockings that are filled intermittently with air by an attached motor (Fig. 21.17). This device simulates the contraction of the leg muscles, promoting fluid movement, which helps to prevent thrombosis development. The compartments in the stockings inflate to 35 to 55 mm Hg of pressure, beginning in the ankle compartment and progressing next to the calf compartment and finally the thigh compartment. Monitor the device for proper pressure inflation.

Health Promotion and Lifestyle Changes

To reduce risk factors or promote recovery from cardiovascular disease, lifestyle changes are often needed. Long-standing habits are difficult to change. Support groups can offer encouragement that is helpful in promoting a healthy lifestyle. Patients should be referred to community support groups as needed.

Patients recovering from cardiac disorders are often anxious about resuming sexual activity but are embarrassed to discuss it. This is an area that is often overlooked when caring for patients. Sexual counseling should be offered to patients and their partners. Patients often have misconceptions that are unfounded but interfere with resuming sexual activity. If patients have angina, nitroglycerin can be taken prophylactically before sexual activity. After a MI, sexual activity can be resumed in 1 to 2 months or when the patient can climb two flights of stairs without symptoms, as ordered by the HCP. Patients are given information to make an informed decision on when they are ready to resume this physical activity. Referral to a sexuality counselor for information on ways to cope with sexual issues in relation to their illness can be helpful to the patient.

FIGURE 21.17 The Kendall SCD Response Compression system provides sequential personalized compression cycles that minimize stasis and maximize blood flow to prevent thrombosis and pulmonary embolus development. *Courtesy of Kendall, Mansfield, MA.*

Cardiac Surgery

As heart disease symptoms increase in severity and frequency or the disease process worsens, cardiac surgery may be used as treatment.

Preparation for Surgery

A nursing assessment is important to provide baseline data that can be used for postoperative comparison and early discharge planning. In addition to routine admission testing, patients with chronic obstructive pulmonary disease (COPD) may have pulmonary function tests and baseline arterial blood gases (ABGs) done (Box 21-3). Patients with carotid bruits have carotid studies to determine the amount of occlusion in the carotid artery. If the occlusion is significant, a carotid endarterectomy, which removes the plaque on the lining of the blocked or diseased carotid artery, is performed, usually several weeks before having cardiac surgery.

Medications that may increase bleeding or reduce fluid volume may be ordered by the HCP to be held before surgery. Drugs that increase bleeding include aspirin, often stopped 3 to 7 days preoperatively; warfarin (Coumadin), often stopped 4 to 5 days preoperatively; and heparin, usually stopped 4 hours preoperatively. During surgery, fluid volume and blood pressure may be decreased by blood loss or medications. Therefore, diuretics, which could further reduce fluid volume and blood pressure, are withheld up to 2 days before surgery. The patient usually takes nothing by mouth (NPO) 8 to 12 hours before surgery. For this reason, patients with diabetes have insulin and oral hypoglycemic agents reduced or withheld the morning of surgery with blood glucose monitoring. The anesthesiologist assesses the patient before surgery and orders preoperative medications.

Patients recover more quickly and have less postoperative stress with thorough preoperative teaching. Explanations of expected procedures and care including pain management, endotracheal tube, methods of communicating, ventilator, chest tubes, coughing and deep breathing exercises (IV lines, urinary catheter, incision care, and various equipment alarms) are provided to the patient and family. It should be emphasized that patients are not able to talk while the endotracheal tube is in place. Additionally, a preoperative family tour of the patient's postoperative unit and the waiting area helps prepare them for the surgical experience. A referral to pastoral care, if desired, can be comforting to the patient and family.

Box 21-3 Routine Admission Testing

- Twelve-lead electrocardiogram (ECG)
- Chest x-ray
- Complete blood cell count (CBC)
- Coagulation studies
- Chemistry profile
- Blood cross-match

Cardiopulmonary Bypass

Cardiac surgeries may use a cardiopulmonary bypass pump in which blood is temporarily diverted away from the heart and lungs to the special pump (Fig. 21.18). This diversion allows for a bloodless and motionless surgical field while the function of the heart and lungs is maintained by the pump (Fig. 21.19).

Before going on the pump, the patient is anticoagulated with heparin until the partial thromboplastin time (PTT) is five to six times greater than normal. Immediately before the patient comes off the pump, the effects of the heparin are reversed with protamine sulfate (antidote for heparin). Heparin is absorbed and stored in organs and tissue and can be sporadically released hours after surgery. As a result, the patient may have excessive bleeding. The risk of an air embolism is minimized by priming the pump with lactated Ringer's solution. The priming solution increases circulating volume, which then results in a shifting of fluid into the interstitial tissue and edema formation. These fluid shifts can continue up to 6 hours after surgery and can cause hypotension.

General Procedure for Cardiac Surgery

After the patient is placed on cardiopulmonary bypass, a cardioplegic solution is infused into the aortic root along with iced saline to cause cardiac standstill. When the surgery is completed, the patient's blood is warmed in the cardiopulmonary bypass circuit and the patient is slowly weaned from bypass. The heart starts beating again after it is warmed and defibrillated. Temporary pacing wires are attached to the heart before the cardiopulmonary bypass pump is discontinued, so an external temporary pacemaker can be used if bradycardia develops. Once the heart is beating, bypass is stopped. Mediastinal chest tubes are placed to drain remaining blood and fluid from the chest. The **sternotomy** is closed with wires through the sternum and then sutures for the layers of tissue and skin. While still

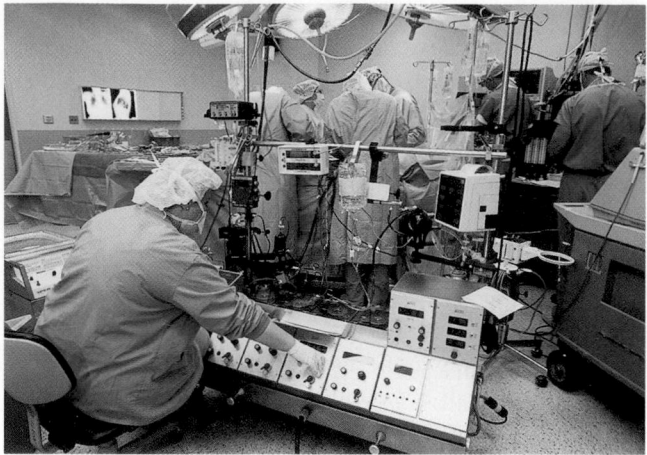

FIGURE 21.19 Cardiopulmonary bypass pump in use.

under anesthesia, the patient is transferred to a cardiac care unit. Cardiac universal beds may be used, in which patients stay in the same room during their entire hospitalization to receive care.

Minimally Invasive Cardiac Surgery

Minimally invasive direct visualization coronary artery bypass (MIDCAB) is a technique that is done without the use of cardiopulmonary bypass. Port-access coronary artery bypass combines peripheral cardiopulmonary bypass with minimally invasive heart access (see Chapter 24). Risk for complications associated with these surgeries are much lower than with the traditional procedure, and the recovery time is often weeks less.

• WORD • BUILDING •

sternotomy: stern—sternum + otomy—incision into

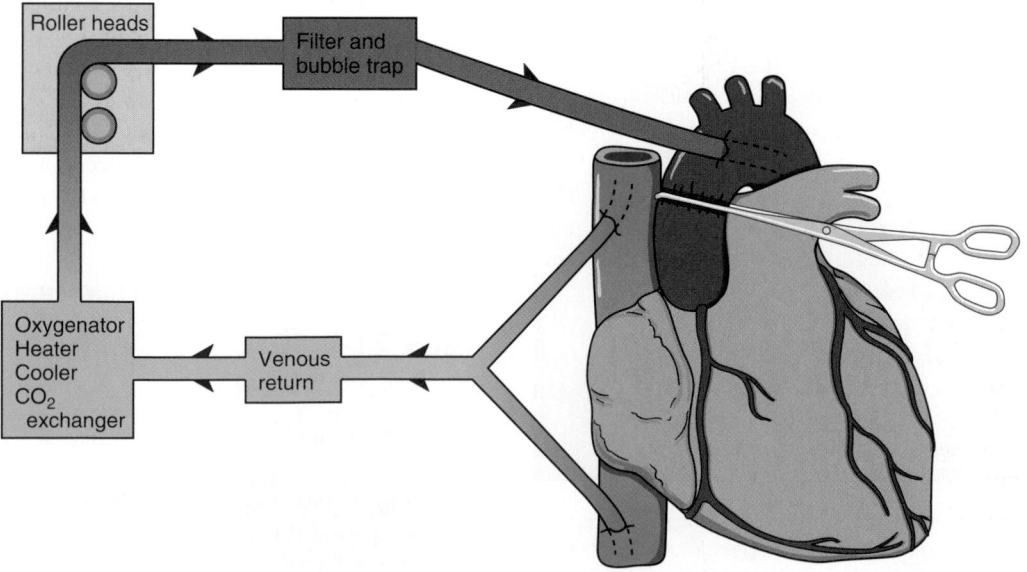

FIGURE 21.18 Cardiopulmonary bypass pump components.

SUGGESTED ANSWERS TO

CRITICAL THINKING

■ *Mrs. Smith*

1. An older patient commonly does not experience typical disorder symptoms. Chest pain is often not present in an MI because of reduced nerve sensitivity with aging. Dyspnea is the classic symptom of MI in the older patient.

2. Inspect both legs to determine edematous areas. Determine location and severity of edema by pressing finger for 5 seconds over the medial malleolus and moving up the leg along the tibia until no edema is found. Assess bilaterally. Measure leg circumference.

3. Document location of edema and whether edema is nonpitting or pitting for both legs. Documentation should state "Bilateral pitting ankle edema" with leg circumference measurement number.

4. Additional symptoms should be documented as follows: dyspnea at rest that increases with exertion, heart tones clear and distant, nailbeds pale, pain free, poor appetite for 2 weeks, 6-pound weight gain in 1 week, three-pillow orthopnea, bilateral jugular venous distention.

5. Unit analysis method:

$$\frac{162 \text{ pounds}}{} \bigg| \frac{1 \text{ kilogram}}{2.2 \text{ pounds}} = 73.6 \text{ kilograms}$$

6. HCP, nurses, pharmacist, respiratory therapist, dietician, social worker or case manager

REVIEW QUESTIONS

1. The nurse is contributing to the plan of care for a patient with heart disease. Which of the following is a modifiable cardiovascular risk factor identified during patient data collection that should be included in the teaching plan?
   1. 56 years old
   2. Male
   3. Asian
   4. Tobacco use

2. The nurse is checking capillary refill on a patient. If it takes longer than 3 seconds for the color to return when assessing capillary refill, the nurse would recognize that which of the following may be indicated?
   1. Decreased arterial flow to the extremity
   2. Increased arterial flow to the extremity
   3. Decreased venous flow from the extremity
   4. Increased venous flow from the extremity

3. The nurse is to obtain orthostatic blood pressure measurements. Which of the following is an important safety intervention that should be used during this procedure?
   1. Reality orientation
   2. Gait or walking belt
   3. Liquids at bedside
   4. Standing patient quickly

4. The nurse is caring for a patient on bed rest who is on diuretic therapy. In which area should the nurse check for the presence of edema?
   1. Arms
   2. Ankles
   3. Sternum
   4. Sacrum

5. The nurse is providing teaching for a patient undergoing a coronary angiography. Which of the following should be included in the teaching plan for a coronary angiography with femoral catheter insertion site? **Select all that apply.**
   1. Dye injection causes hot, flushing sensation.
   2. General anesthesia is administered.
   3. Claustrophobia may be experienced.
   4. Ambulation is not possible immediately after procedure.
   5. Allergies are assessed before testing.
   6. Firm pressure must be applied to the insertion site.

6. The nurse is reinforcing teaching about a high-fiber diet for a cardiac patient. The patient asks what the purpose of the diet is. Which of the following replies by the nurse would be appropriate?
   1. "To increase absorption of nutrients in your diet."
   2. "It will reduce your heart's workload."
   3. "To prevent edema from developing."
   4. "To reduce your appetite."

7. A patient is scheduled for vascular surgery. The patient is taking digoxin (Lanoxin), furosemide (Lasix), potassium, warfarin (Coumadin), and famotidine (Pepcid). Which medication would the nurse question the possible need to stop several days before surgery?
   1. Digoxin (Lanoxin)
   2. Furosemide (Lasix)
   3. Warfarin (Coumadin)
   4. Famotidine (Pepcid)

Answers can be found in Appendix C.

References

American Heart Association. (2014). *Heart disease and stroke statistics—2014 update: A report from the American Heart Association.* Dallas, TX: Author. Retrieved January 26, 2014, from http://circ.ahajournals.org/content/129/3/e28

Joint Commission. (2014). *2014 national patient safety goals.* Retrieved January 26, 2014, from www.jointcommission .org/standards_information/npsgs.aspx

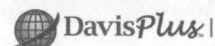 **DavisPlus** | For additional resources and information visit **davispl.us/medsurg5**

Nursing Care of Patients With Hypertension

LINDA S. WILLIAMS

LEARNING OUTCOMES

1. Explain the pathophysiology of hypertension.
2. Identify causes and risk factors for hypertension.
3. List signs and symptoms of hypertension.
4. Describe therapeutic measures for hypertension.
5. Define classifications and treatment recommendations for hypertension in adults.
6. Define hypertensive emergency.
7. List common complications of hypertension.
8. Plan nursing care for patients with hypertension.
9. Evaluate effectiveness of nursing interventions.

KEY TERMS

cardiac output (KAR-dee-yak OWT-put)
diastolic blood pressure (dy-uh-STAH-lik BLUHD PREH-shure)
essential hypertension (ee-SEN-shul HY-per-TEN-shun)
hypertension (HY-per-TEN-shun)
hypertensive emergency (HY-per-TEN-siv ee-MUR-gehn-see)
hypertensive urgency (HY-per-TEN-siv UR-gehn-see)
hypertrophy (hy-PER-truh-fee)
normotensive (nor-moe-TEN-siv)
peripheral vascular resistance (puh-RIFF-uh-ruhl VAS-kyoo-lar ree-ZIS-tense)
plaque (PLAK)
primary hypertension (PRY-mare-ee HY-per-TEN-shun)
secondary hypertension (SEK-un-DAR-ee HY-per-TEN-shun)
systolic blood pressure (siss-TALL-ik BLUHD PREH-shure)
viscosity (vis-KAW-sih-tee)

During 2011–2012, 29.9% of U.S. adults aged 18 or older had hypertension. The prevalence of those with hypertension increases with age, from 7.3% in those aged 18 to 39 to 65% in those ages 60 or older (Nwankwo, Yoon, Burt, & Gu, 2013). The highest occurrence was in non-Hispanic blacks at 42.1%, then non-Hispanic whites at 28%, followed by Hispanics at 26%. The prevalence of hypertension remains high despite effective treatments.

The 2014 Evidence-Based Guideline for the Management of High BP in Adults by the Eighth Joint National Committee (JNC 8; James et al, 2014) takes a different approach than the *Seventh Report of the Joint National Committee on Prevention, Detection, Evaluation and Treatment of High BP* (JNC 7; National Heart, Lung, and Blood Institute, 2004). JNC 8 does not define hypertension, as JNC 7 did, but rather defines pharmacologic treatment thresholds, recommends drug therapy, and supports the 2013 American Heart Association/American College of Cardiology (AHA/ACC) lifestyle modifications guidelines (James et al, 2014).

The lifestyle interventions to reduce cardiovascular risk are identified in the 2013 AHA/ACC Guideline on Lifestyle Management to Reduce Cardiovascular Risk. In general, the guidelines recommend restricting sugary foods and beverages, trans and saturated fats, and sodium; following a Dietary Approaches to Stop Hypertension (DASH)-type (see "Nutrition Notes") or Mediterranean or diet with fruits, vegetables, whole grains, nuts, low fat dairy, poultry, fish and nontropical vegetable oils; and participating in 40 minutes of moderate to vigorous aerobic activity three to four times weekly (Eckel et al, 2013).

Follow-up studies involving overweight or obese persons with above-normal BP found the DASH diet alone reduced BP by 11.2/7.5 mm Hg but the addition of exercise and weight loss to the DASH diet resulted in reductions of 16.1/9.9 mm Hg. Even the control group consuming their usual diet recorded 3.4/3.8 mm Hg reductions in the 4-month program (Blumenthal et al, 2010). In this same group, greater adherence to the DASH diet was associated with larger BP reductions independent of weight loss. African Americans were less likely to adhere to the DASH dietary eating plan compared with whites, suggesting that culturally sensitive dietary strategies might be needed to improve adherence to the DASH diet (Epstein et al, 2012).

The JNC 7 redefined normal and abnormal BPs for adults aged 18 and older (Table 22.1) www.nhlbi.nih.gov/guidelines/hypertension/express.pdf). Because they were not addressed nor eliminated by JNC 8, they remain included here.

BP MEASUREMENT

It is essential to take BP readings correctly for accurate readings. A normal BP reading is one in which systolic pressure is below 120 mm Hg and diastolic pressure is below 80 mm Hg with the patient in a seated position and the arm supported at heart level (see Chapter 21). Prehypertension is a **systolic BP** of 120 to 139 mm Hg or a **diastolic BP** of 80 to 89 mm Hg. **Hypertension**, also known

Nutrition Notes

Reducing BP With Diet

The original DASH diet reduced blood pressure (BP) significantly in **normotensive** people and produced even greater reductions in hypertensive people in an 8-week feeding trial that was designed to maintain the subjects' starting weight. Rather than emphasizing food restriction, the DASH diet increases the intake of certain commonly available, not specialty, foods. On a 2,000-calorie diet, a person following the DASH diet would consume the following:

Food Group	Number of Servings	Example of One Serving
Grains	7–8	• 1 slice of bread • 1/2 cup cooked cereal or pasta
Vegetables	4–5	• 1 cup raw leafy • 1/2 cup cooked, nonstarchy
Fruits	4–5	• 1 medium fresh • 1/2 cup canned or frozen • 1/4 cup dried
Low-fat or nonfat dairy	2–3	• 8 ounces of milk • 1 1/2 ounces of cheese
Lean meat, poultry, or fish	2 or fewer	• 3 ounces cooked
Fats and oils, preferably monounsaturated (canola, olive, peanut)	2 1/2	• 1 teaspoonful
Nuts, seeds, legumes	4–5 weekly	• 1/3 cup of nuts • 2 tablespoonfuls of seeds • 1/2 cup cooked beans

as high BP, is a condition in which the average of at least two or more readings on different dates is above prehypertension levels. For more information on hypertension, visit www.americanheart.org.

• WORD • BUILDING •

systolic: systole—concentration
diastolic: diastole—expansion
hypertension: hyper—excessive + tensio—tension

TABLE 22.1 BLOOD PRESSURE (BP) CATEGORIES AND MEASURES*

BP Category	Systolic BP (mm Hg)	Diastolic BP (mm Hg)	Recommended Follow-Up	Lifestyle Modification
Normal	Less than 120	Less than 80	2 years	Encourage
Pre-hypertension	120–139	80–89	1 year	Yes
Stage 1 hypertension	140–159	90–99	2 months	Yes
Stage 2 hypertension	160 or higher	100 or higher	1 month. For BP over 180/110 mm Hg, evaluate and seek treatment immediately; then 1 week as needed.	Yes

Note. Adapted from National Heart, Lung, and Blood Institute (2004) and James et al (2014). *Treatment is based on highest BP category.

BE SAFE!

Research studies show that stethoscopes used by all types of health care providers (HCPs), such as nurses, physicians, paramedics, and emergency medical technicians, are contaminated with bacteria. With infection rates on the rise, reduce the transmission of organisms to help keep your patients safe. Clean your stethoscope between every patient! (See "Evidence-Based Practice.")

EVIDENCE-BASED PRACTICE

Clinical Question
Are stethoscopes contaminated, and what is the best way to decontaminate them?

Evidence
An observational study of 100 nurses and their stethoscopes found high stethoscope contamination rates in the emergency department, with a low prevalence of *Staphylococcus aureus* or methicillin-resistant *S. aureus* (MRSA) and that only 8% of nurses cleaned their stethoscopes (Tang, Worster, Srigley, & Main, 2011). In a study comparing an ethanol-based cleanser (EBC) with isopropyl alcohol pads in reducing bacterial contamination of stethoscope diaphragms, 99 stethoscopes were cultured, and all were positive for bacterial growth (Lecat, Cropp, McCord, & Haller, 2009). The use of either EBC or isopropyl alcohol reduced the bacteria count significantly.

Implications for Nursing Practice
Stethoscopes become contaminated with use. To protect patients from potential organism transmission and reduce infection, stethoscopes must be cleaned between every patient by all HCPs. Stethoscopes should be cleaned as often as hands are washed using either EBC or isopropyl alcohol pads.

REFERENCES
Lecat, P., Cropp, E., McCord, G., & Haller, N. (2009). Ethanol-based cleanser versus isopropyl alcohol to decontaminate stethoscopes. *American Journal of Infection Control, 37,* 241–243.

Tang, P. H. P., Worster, A., Srigley, J. A., & Main, C. L. (2011). Examination of staphylococcal stethoscope contamination in the emergency department (pilot) study (EXSSCITED pilot study). *Canadian Journal of Emergency Medicine, 13,* 239–244.

PATHOPHYSIOLOGY OF HYPERTENSION

Normally the heart pumps blood through the body to meet the cells' needs for oxygen and nutrients. As it pumps, the heart forces blood through the blood vessels. The pressure exerted by blood on the walls of the blood vessels is measured as BP. BP is determined by **cardiac output** (CO), **peripheral vascular resistance** (PVR; the ability of the vessels to stretch), the **viscosity** (thickness) of the blood, and the amount of circulating blood volume. Decreased stretching ability of blood vessels, increased blood viscosity, and/or increased fluid volume may cause an increase in BP.

• WORD • BUILDING •
viscosity: viscous—sticky

Several processes influence BP. These include nervous system regulation, arterial baroreceptors and chemoreceptors, the renin-angiotensin-aldosterone mechanism, and the balance of body fluids. One way BP is influenced is through adjustment of the CO, which is the amount of blood that the heart pumps each minute. The heart rate rises to increase CO in response to physical or emotional activities that increase the need for oxygen in the organs and tissues. PVR also influences BP; it is the opposition that blood encounters as it flows through vessels. Anything causing blood vessels to become narrower increases PVR. Any time PVR is increased, more pressure is needed to push the blood through the vessels, so BP increases as a result. If PVR is decreased, less pressure is needed. Increased arteriolar PVR is the main mechanism that elevates BP in hypertension.

Factors that impair normal regulation of BP may lead to hypertension. Many of these factors are not well understood. Sympathetic nervous system overstimulation, which causes vasoconstriction, can contribute to hypertension. Alterations in baroreceptors and chemoreceptors may also influence the development of hypertension. For example, baroreceptors may become less sensitive from prolonged increases in vessel pressure, and subsequently fail to stimulate vasodilation through vessel stretching. Additionally, increases in hormones that cause sodium retention, such as aldosterone, lead to increased fluid retention. Changes in kidney function that alter the excretion of fluid also result in an increase in overall body fluid that may contribute to hypertension.

Types of Hypertension
Primary Hypertension

Primary, or **essential**, **hypertension** is chronic elevation of BP from an unknown cause.

Secondary Hypertension

Secondary hypertension has a known cause. In other words, it is a sign of another problem, such as a kidney abnormality, a tumor of the adrenal gland, or a congenital defect of the aorta. When the cause of secondary hypertension is treated before permanent structural changes occur, BP usually returns to normal.

Isolated Systolic Hypertension (ISH)

ISH is a systolic pressure of 140 mm Hg or greater and a diastolic pressure of 90 mm Hg or less. This type of hypertension occurs mainly in the older adult, although it can occur at any age ("Gerontological Issues"). People with a systolic pressure higher than 140 mm Hg and a diastolic pressure less than 90 mm Hg found on two separate readings should be further evaluated. Treatment of ISH is recommended to decrease cardiovascular disease, especially heart failure episodes and risk of stroke. Lifestyle modifications are usually tried first if the systolic elevation is not too severe. If lifestyle modifications fail to reduce the systolic pressure, antihypertensive medication is added.

Alcohol consumption in the older adult can aggravate age-related hypertension. Guided relaxation has been shown effective in reducing high BP in older adults.

Gerontological Issues

It is now known that after age 55, diastolic pressure falls while systolic pressure continues to rise with age. This means that it is important to control systolic BP, not just diastolic pressure, in older adults to prevent heart disease and stroke. In fact, lowering diastolic BP too much may be unhealthy.

SIGNS AND SYMPTOMS OF HYPERTENSION

Have you known someone with high BP? Did that person have signs and symptoms of hypertension? If not, it is because hypertension often causes no signs or symptoms other than elevated BP readings. As a result, hypertension is referred to as the "silent killer." Patients with hypertension are often first diagnosed when seeking health care for reasons unrelated to hypertension. In a small number of cases, a patient with hypertension may report a headache, bloody nose, severe anxiety, or shortness of breath, although it is usually impossible for a patient to correlate the absence or presence of symptoms with the degree of BP elevation (Table 22.2).

DIAGNOSIS OF HYPERTENSION

Diagnosis of hypertension considers a patient's risk factors for hypertension, a previous diagnosis of hypertension, presence of signs and symptoms, history of kidney or heart disease, and current use of medications. When the average seated BP is above prehypertensive levels of 120 to 139 systolic or 80 to 89 diastolic on two or more occasions, then hypertension is diagnosed (see Table 22.1).

The JNC 7 recommends that patients undergo various routine tests to identify damage to organs or blood vessels before beginning therapy for high BP. Tests recommended by JNC 7 include electrocardiogram (ECG), blood glucose level, hematocrit, serum potassium and calcium levels, lipoprotein profile, high-density and low-density lipoprotein cholesterol (HDL-C and LDL-C, respectively), and triglyceride level. These tests help determine if target-organ damage has been caused by elevated BP. An example of this is testing for kidney damage with a urinalysis or serum creatinine level.

RISK FACTORS FOR HYPERTENSION

A combination of genetic (nonmodifiable) and environmental (modifiable) risk factors is thought to be responsible for the development of hypertension, although the cause remains unknown. Nonmodifiable risk factors—those that cannot be changed—include a family history of hypertension, age,

TABLE 22.2 HYPERTENSION SUMMARY

Signs and Symptoms	Often none Increased BP Headache, bloody nose, severe anxiety, or shortness of breath
Diagnosis	Prehypertension is greater than systolic of 120 mm Hg and diastolic of 80 mm Hg. Hypertension is an average BP, using two or more readings on different dates, greater than a systolic of 139 mm Hg and diastolic of 89 mm Hg.
Therapeutic Measures	Lifestyle modification Medications
Complications	Heart failure, myocardial infarction, stroke, renal failure
Priority Nursing Diagnoses	*Deficient Knowledge* *Ineffective Self Health Management*

ethnicity, and diabetes mellitus. Modifiable risk factors—those that can be changed—include blood glucose level, activity level, smoking, salt and alcohol intake, and insufficient sleep (less than 5 hours per night). Managing these risk factors can help to decrease BP.

Nonmodifiable Risk Factors
Family History of Hypertension

Hypertension is more common among people with a family history of hypertension. Indeed, people with a family history have almost twice the risk of developing hypertension as those with no family history. People with a family history of hypertension should be encouraged to have their BP checked regularly.

Age

People age differently because of their genetic and environmental risk factors and lifestyle habits. Thus, the results of the aging process may be reflected in wide variations of BP among older adults. As a person ages, **plaque** builds up in the arteries, and blood vessels become stiffer and less elastic, causing the heart to work harder to force blood through the vessels. These vessel changes increase the amount of work required by the heart to maintain blood flow into the circulation and, consequently, BP increases.

Race and Ethnicity

"Cultural Considerations" discusses hypertension among various ethnic groups.

 ## Cultural Considerations

African Americans

Hypertension continues to be the most serious health problem affecting African Americans in the United States. This population suffers higher mortality and morbidity rates related to hypertension and at an earlier age than all other ethnic groups. African Americans from lower socioeconomic backgrounds have higher BP than African Americans from higher socioeconomic backgrounds. Additionally, African Americans are three to four times more likely to develop kidney failure related to hypertension than European Americans. Addressing obesity, high sodium intake, low potassium intake, and lack of physical activity is especially important for cardiovascular health in African Americans.

Hypertension among African Americans is usually caused by increased renin activity, resulting in greater sodium and fluid retention. Thus, African Americans respond better to diuretics such as furosemide (Lasix) and hydrochlorothiazide (HydroDIURIL) than to beta blockers such as propranolol (Inderal). Hypertension among European Americans is more often caused by chemical imbalances; thus, they respond better to beta blockers.

Chinese Americans

Chinese people are more sensitive than Caucasians to the effects of propranolol on heart rate and BP, requiring only half the blood level of European Americans to achieve a therapeutic effect. Propranolol is eliminated from the bodies of many Chinese people at double the rate of European Americans. They are more likely to suffer fatigue as a side effect. Thus, the nurse must carefully monitor the Chinese patient for therapeutic and side effects.

Continued

Cultural Considerations—cont'd

Japanese Americans

Hypertension among Japanese Americans is primarily related to the high sodium content of the Japanese diet, stress, and a high rate of cigarette smoking.

Korean Americans and Filipino Americans

High rates of hypertension among Koreans and Filipinos are due to the stress of immigration, salt preservatives in their foods, and the use of condiments high in sodium.

Diabetes Mellitus

Many adults who have diabetes mellitus also have hypertension. The risk of developing hypertension with a family history of diabetes and obesity is greater than when there is no family history. Lifestyle modifications and adherence to therapy are crucial to prevent the heart attacks, strokes, blindness, and kidney failure associated with high blood glucose and BP levels.

Modifiable Risk Factors: Lifestyle

JNC 8 supports patients with hypertension making lifestyle modifications. These modifications include adoption of the DASH or Mediterranean diet, reduction of dietary sodium, and increased physical activity (see "Nutrition Notes"; Eckel et al, 2013). The HCP and dietitian should be consulted to help the patient develop a healthy diet plan. Lifestyle modifications are used along with antihypertensive drugs to control hypertension.

CRITICAL THINKING

Ms. Miller

■ Ms. Miller, age 54, visits a health clinic because she has a headache every morning. The nurse collects data on Ms. Miller and finds that she is an office manager, smokes a pack of cigarettes a day, eats fast food for lunch at her desk, has two adult children, is recently divorced, and has two to three alcoholic drinks every evening. Ms. Miller has been in good health and takes two aspirin tablets for her headaches daily.

1. What are Ms. Miller's risk factors for hypertension?
2. What is the most significant patient information identified? Why?
3. Why is hypertension referred to as the "silent killer"?
4. Why should Ms. Miller be told of the need for lifelong therapy if she is diagnosed with hypertension?

Suggested answers are at the end of the chapter.

THERAPEUTIC MEASURES FOR HYPERTENSION

JCN 8 recommends therapy to achieve a BP less than 150/90 mm Hg for those 60 and older; for those aged 30 to 59, the goal is a diastolic BP less than 90 mm Hg; and a goal BP less than 140/90 mm Hg for other adults. Treatment may begin with lifestyle modifications and then consideration of drug therapy. For initial drug therapy, a thiazide diuretic, angiotensin-converting enzyme (ACE) inhibitor, angiotensin receptor blocker (ARB), or calcium channel blocker (CCB) is recommended. African Americans should receive a CCB or thiazide diuretic (if chronic kidney disease with proteinuria ACE inhibitor or ARB), and anyone with chronic kidney disease an ACE inhibitor or ARB. For those with chronic kidney disease or diabetes, the goal BP is less than 140/90. If the response does not achieve the BP goal, dosage may be increased or a second drug from a different class may be added. See Table 22.3 for examples of medications used to treat hypertension. Safe administration of medications is important, especially for older patients ("Gerontological Issues").

Gerontological Issues

Managing Antihypertensive Therapy

• For safety, teach older adults who take antihypertensive drugs to rise slowly to prevent the effects of orthostatic hypotension. Dizziness may increase the risk of falling.
• Deficiencies in fluid volume can be a common problem for older adults as well, and diuretics can contribute to them. Careful monitoring of fluid balance is important to prevent dehydration.
• Older adults may be more sensitive to medications, so monitor them carefully for adverse effects. Older patients may need lower dosages.

TABLE 22.3 MEDICATIONS USED TO TREAT HYPERTENSION

Medication Class/Action	Examples	Nursing Implications
Diuretics Increase urine output by inhibiting sodium and water reabsorption by the kidney. Several types.		Take with food to prevent GI upset. Monitor I&O and weight to determine fluid loss. Assess for improvement of edema in patients with HF, and reduced BP in hypertension. Electrolyte imbalances may occur quickly. Teach patient to take during waking hours to prevent excessive urination during sleeping hours.
Thiazide and Thiazide-Like Diuretics Increase urine output by promoting sodium, chloride, and water excretion. Causes loss of potassium, sodium, magnesium. Calcium saved. No immediate effect. Most effective in normal renal function.	*Thiazide:* hydrochlorothiazide (HydroDIURIL) chlorothiazide (Diuril) *Thiazide-like:* chlorthalidone (Hygroton) indapamide (Lozol) metolazone (Zaroxolyn)	Monitor potassium level for hypokalemia. Blood glucose may increase in diabetics. Teach patient to wear sunscreen and protective clothing to prevent photosensitivity. Hypercalcemia could be hazardous to patient on digoxin.
Loop Diuretics Act on ascending loop of Henle in kidney to cause sodium and water loss. Also causes loss of potassium, magnesium, and calcium.	bumetanide (Bumex) furosemide (Lasix) torsemide (Demadex)	Monitor potassium level for hypokalemia. Contraindicated if allergic to sulfonamides. Teach patient to use sunscreen to prevent photosensitivity. Take with food or milk to prevent GI upset.
Potassium-Sparing Diuretics Mild diuretic. Can be used as combination therapy. Promote sodium and water excretion and potassium retention by the kidney.	amiloride (Midamor) spironolactone (Aldactone)	Check potassium level for hyperkalemia. Check BP before administration. Avoid foods rich in potassium such as oranges, bananas, salt substitutes, dried fruits. Triamterene: Take after meals for GI upset; may turn urine blue.
Sympatholytics **Beta Blockers** Decrease sympathetic nervous system response, resulting in decreased BP, heart rate, contractility, cardiac output, and renin activity.	atenolol (Tenormin) metoprolol (Lopressor) metoprolol, extended release (Toprol XL) nadolol (Corgard) propranolol (Inderal) propranolol, long acting (Inderal LA)	Check heart rate and BP before administration as causes bradycardia and orthostatic hypotension. Daily I&O and weight. Monitor for bronchospasm. *Teaching:* Rise slowly. Do not stop drug abruptly to avoid rebound hypertension, angina, or dysrhythmias.

Continued

TABLE **22.3**   **MEDICATIONS USED TO TREAT HYPERTENSION—cont'd**

Medication Class/Action	Examples	Nursing Implications
		HIGH ALERT: IV vasoactive medications are inherently dangerous. Oral and parenteral doses of propranolol are not interchangeable; IV dose is 1/10 the oral dose. Patient harm or fatalities have occurred when switching from oral to IV route.
Alpha1 Blockers Block effects of sympathetic nervous system on smooth muscle of blood vessels, resulting in vasodilation and decreased BP.	prazosin (Minipress) terazosin (Hytrin)	Check heart rate and BP before administration; causes hypotension and tachycardia. *Teaching:* Rise slowly.
Combined Alpha and Beta Blockers Block alpha-adrenergic receptors, causing vasodilation and reduced BP. Decrease sympathetic nervous system response, resulting in decreased heart rate and contractility.	carvedilol (Coreg) labetalol (Normodyne)	Daily I&O and weight. Check heart rate and BP before administration as causes bradycardia and hypotension. Monitor edema, neck vein distention, lung sounds. *Teaching:* Rise slowly. Do not stop drug abruptly to avoid rebound hypertension, angina, or dysrhythmias.
Central-Acting Alpha$_2$ Agonists Block effects of sympathetic nervous system centrally.	clonidine (Catapres) guanfacine HCl (Tenex)	Check for decreased BP and edema. Suggest gum or hard candy for dry mouth. *Teaching:* Rise slowly. Do not stop drug abruptly to avoid rebound hypertension, angina, or dysrhythmias.
Angiotensin-Converting Enzyme (ACE) Inhibitors Blocks production of angiotensin II, a potent vasoconstrictor. Reduces peripheral arterial resistance and BP.	benazepril HCl (Lotensin) captopril (Capoten) enalapril (Vasotec) fosinopril (Monopril) lisinopril (Prinivil, Zestril) moexipril (Univasc) perindopril (Aceon) quinapril (Accupril) ramipril (Altace) trandolapril (Mavik)	Monitor patient for edema with HF, decreased BP with hypertension and new-onset cough. *Teaching:* Rise slowly. Tell to report new-onset cough. Use sunscreen to prevent photosensitivity. Do not stop drug abruptly to avoid rebound hypertension, angina, or dysrhythmias
Angiotensin II Receptor Antagonists (ARB) Block angiotensin II receptors, causing vasodilation and reduction in BP.	candesartan (Atacand) eprosartan (Teveten) irbesartan (Avapro) losartan (Cozaar) olmesartan (Benicar) telmisartan (Micardis) valsartan (Diovan)	Monitor patient for edema with HF and decreased BP with hypertension. *Teaching:* Tell to report new-onset cough. Use sunscreen to prevent photosensitivity.

TABLE 22.3   MEDICATIONS USED TO TREAT HYPERTENSION—cont'd

Medication Class/Action	Examples	Nursing Implications
Aldosterone Receptor Antagonist Blocks binding of aldosterone at receptor site to reduce sodium reabsorption and then BP.	eplerenone (Inspra)	Monitor potassium for hyperkalemia before and during therapy.
Calcium Channel Blockers Prevent movement of extracellular calcium into the cell which vasodilates.	amlodipine (Norvasc) diltiazem (Cardizem) felodipine (Plendil) isradipine (DynaCirc) nicardipine HCl (Cardene, Cardene SR) nifedipine (Procardia) nisoldipine (Sular) verapamil (Calan SR, Isoptin SR)	Take pulse before administration. Check BP for hypotension, heart rate, dysrhythmias, angina. May increase blood levels of digoxin.
Direct Vasodilators Relax smooth muscles of blood vessels, causing vasodilation and decreased BP.	hydralazine (Apresoline) minoxidil (Loniten)	Monitor BP for hypotension/hypertension and increasing heart rate. Treat headache with acetaminophen. Often given with diuretic to reduce edema resulting from water and sodium retention.
Combination Agents See individual agent for action.	Hyzaar = Cozaar + HCTZ, Micardis HCT = Micardis + HCTZ	

Note. GI, gastrointestinal; HF = heart failure; I&O = input and output; PO = oral; IV = intravenous.

 BE SAFE!

Clonidine, an alpha-adrenergic agonist, and clonazepam, a benzodiazepine, have lookalike and sound-alike drug names. Be aware of drug names that look alike and sound alike to prevent errors involving these drugs.

The treatment plan of lifestyle modifications and medications is effective only when patients are motivated to accept the diagnosis of hypertension and include lifelong treatment in their daily routine. Empathy and trust can increase patient motivation. Patients should be instructed that antihypertensive therapy usually must be continued for the rest of their lives. Patients should be reminded that although they may be feeling better with the modifications and medications, the hypertension is still present even if it is well controlled. Patients should be told not to stop taking their medications unless instructed to do so by their HCP.

Antihypertensive medications can have unpleasant side effects. Patients should be told what these side effects are and to report them if they occur, so that medications can be altered if possible. Erectile dysfunction can be one of the side effects of these medications. Men may be reluctant to discuss this side effect and instead choose to stop the medication. The nurse should be proactive and inform men about this side effect so they will understand that, if it occurs and is reported, the HCP can make medication changes.

 ## COMPLICATIONS OF HYPERTENSION

Common complications of hypertension include coronary artery disease, atherosclerosis, myocardial infarction (MI), heart failure (HF), stroke, and kidney or eye damage. The severity and duration of the increase in BP determine the extent of the vascular changes causing organ damage. High BP levels may also increase the size of the left ventricle, referred to as **hypertrophy**. Over time elevated BP damages the small vessels of the heart, brain, kidneys, and retina. The results are a progressive functional impairment of these organs, known as target-organ disease.

LEARNING TIP

Walking for 30 minutes is an effective way to lower BP, as is listening to 30 minutes of classical, Celtic, or raga music with slow abdominal breathing daily. Transcendental meditation also helps control high BP.

Here are additional, important lifestyle modifications arranged in an easy-to-remember mnemonic:

L—Limit salt, caffeine, and alcohol.
I—Include daily potassium and calcium.
F—Fight fat and cholesterol.
E—Exercise regularly (walking).
S—Stay on your BP regimen.
T—Try to quit smoking.
Y—Your medications are to be taken daily.
L—Lose weight.
E—End-stage complications will be avoided!

SPECIAL CONSIDERATIONS

BP should be well controlled before the patient has an invasive procedure. Hypertensive patients are at greater risk for strokes, MI, HF, kidney failure, and pulmonary edema. These patients should be instructed to continue their BP medications until the time of the procedure, unless otherwise directed by their HCP. Antihypertensive medications should be resumed as soon as possible after the procedure, as directed by the HCP.

CRITICAL THINKING

Mrs. Bell

■ Mrs. Bell, 80 years old, is seen in her physician's office. She lives a sedentary lifestyle alone in her own home with a bathroom down the hall from the bedroom. Mrs. Bell's son lives in the same city and visits her often. She has wood floors with throw rugs in the hall and a tile floor in the bathroom. She wears glasses and has a cataract. She has an unsteady gait and nocturia. She is 40 pounds overweight and has a 10-year history of hypertension for which she is taking chlorothiazide (Diuril) and propranolol (Inderal) when she remembers them.

1. What are Mrs. Bell's modifiable and nonmodifiable risk factors for hypertension?
2. Why is Mrs. Bell taking chlorothiazide and propranolol to treat her hypertension?

3. What teaching methods could be used to help ensure that Mrs. Bell will understand and follow her treatment plan?
4. Why should patient safety needs be addressed in the nursing care plan?
5. What patient-centered safety interventions should the patient and family be taught?
6. Inderal 20 mg by mouth (PO) is ordered now because Mrs. Bell forgot to take her medication. The nurse has on hand Inderal 10-mg tablets. How many tablets should the nurse give?

Suggested answers are at the end of the chapter.

HYPERTENSIVE EMERGENCY

How would you know if a patient's BP was in the dangerous range? **Hypertensive emergency** is a severe type of hypertension characterized by elevations in systolic BP greater than 180 mm Hg and diastolic BP greater than 120 mm Hg that are complicated by a risk for or progression of target-organ dysfunction (examples include MI, HF, and dissecting aortic aneurysm). Patients who are untreated, fail to adhere to antihypertensive therapy, or stop their medications abruptly are at risk for hypertensive emergency.

These patients require immediate reduction of BP to prevent or limit damage to target organs. Patients with hypertensive crises should be admitted to the critical care unit. In some cases, the BP may need to be reduced by 25% within 1 hour to prevent organ damage. If the patient is stable, BP is then decreased to 160/100 to 110 mm Hg in the next 2 to 6 hours. Gradual reduction of BP is desired to prevent decreased blood flow to the kidneys, heart, and/or brain. An intravenous (IV) medication such as nitroprusside (Nipride) may be given to quickly reduce BP during the crisis.

HYPERTENSIVE URGENCY

The JNC7 considers **hypertensive urgency** to occur in situations when BP is as elevated as in a hypertensive emergency but without progression of target-organ dysfunction. A patient with hypertensive urgency may have severe headaches, nosebleeds, shortness of breath, and severe anxiety. Patients with hypertensive urgency usually can be treated with combination oral medication and scheduled for a follow-up visit within several days.

NURSING PROCESS FOR THE PATIENT WITH HYPERTENSION

Data Collection

Data collection for a patient with hypertension includes the patient's health history, BP measurements, medications, and physical assessment (Fig. 22.1). Determining what hypertensive patients and their families know about hypertension and associated risk factors is essential for planning patient and family education and subsequent lifelong lifestyle modification needs.

Nursing Diagnoses, Planning, Interventions, and Evaluation

Possible nursing diagnoses, planning, interventions, and evaluation must be agreed on by the patient and the health care team. See the *Nursing Care Plan for the Patient With Hypertension.*

FIGURE 22.1 Nurse obtaining BP measurement. Correct size cuff use is essential for accurate reading.

NURSING CARE PLAN for the Patient With Hypertension

Nursing Diagnosis: *Deficient Knowledge* related to disease process and treatment regimen

Expected Outcome: The patient will verbalize knowledge of disease process and treatment regimen.

Evaluation of Outcome: Is patient able to discuss and explain hypertension disease process, including its risk factors, complications, and treatment regimen?

Intervention Identify patient's readiness and ability to learn. **Rationale** Patient must accept the hypertension diagnosis and be able to receive and understand information given. Determine patient's preferred method of learning. **Evaluation** Does patient verbalize acceptance of hypertension diagnosis? Does patient demonstrate ability to read, write, and retain information?

Intervention Provide patient with information concerning disease process including risk factors, complications, and treatment regimen. **Rationale** Patient will be more willing to participate in treatment regimen when able to understand need for changes in behavior. **Evaluation** Is patient able to participate in discussion concerning hypertension disease process including risk factors, complications, and treatment regimen?

Nursing Diagnosis: *Ineffective Self Health Management* related to complexity of therapy, cost of medications, lack of symptoms, side effects of medications, need to alter long-term lifestyle habits, normal BP controlled by therapy

Expected Outcome: The patient will verbalize ability and willingness to adhere to treatment.

Evaluation of Outcome: Is patient able to state how lifestyle will include therapy? Does patient identify and problem solve barriers for therapy?

Intervention Identify patient's modifiable risk factors and lifestyle modification needs. **Rationale** Identifying risk factors is the first step in planning therapy. Patient must understand the relationship of these risk factors with hypertension and complication development. **Evaluation** Can patient state rationale for modifying risk factors to prevent development of complications?

Continued

NURSING CARE PLAN for the Patient With Hypertension—cont'd

Intervention Identify factors that are barriers to patient adhering to therapy. **Rationale** Factors such as finances, transportation, aging changes, patient motivation, habits, and reading and educational level can be barriers for therapy. **Evaluation** Are barriers present for patient?

Intervention Develop plan to overcome barriers. Make referrals as needed. **Rationale** Identified barriers can be overcome with planning and intervention, such as referral to support groups or for financial assistance or prescription delivery service, and instructions provided at level of patient's learning ability. **Evaluation** Have barriers been eliminated? Is patient willing to use referrals?

Intervention Assess ability to take medications daily: financially, obtaining refills, understanding directions. **Rationale** Older adult patients may be on a fixed income, lack transportation, or lack ability to take several medications several times a day. Simplifying this process, to one medication if possible, can increase adherence to medication treatment. **Evaluation** Is patient able to obtain medications? Can patient self-administer medications accurately on daily basis?

Intervention Teach patient to take medications as prescribed and not to skip dosages. **Rationale** Older patients may skip dosages to save money, reduce side effects, or reduce need to void. **Evaluation** Does patient take dosages as prescribed? Does patient express concern over cost, side effects, or frequent voiding?

Intervention Teach patient to change positions slowly to prevent falls. **Rationale** Antihypertensive medications can cause hypotension, resulting in dizziness and weakness and possibly leading to falls. **Evaluation** Does patient understand how to change positions slowly? Does patient experience dizziness or weakness?

Home Health Hints

- Discuss medication usage with the patient and count the number of remaining pills in the patient's pill bottles, if needed, to assess compliance. Remind the patient to get refills and keep medical appointments by writing them on a calendar.
- Monitor carefully for symptoms of congestive HF if the patient takes a beta blocker. This is a side effect that needs to be caught early and reported to the HCP.
- Instruct patients to take medication as prescribed even if they are feeling well or if side effects, which they should report, are present. Medication compliance can be a challenge for the older adult patient with hypertension. If medicines are too expensive for the patient, check with the HCP and pharmacist for less expensive alternatives.
- Encourage the patient to obtain a home BP monitoring device. Instruct the patient or caregiver on proper use and logging the date, time, and reading obtained. The home health nurse should review the log on each visit.
- Teach the patient or caregiver to take the patient's pulse and to call the nurse if it is below 60 beats

per minute or the parameters defined by the HCP. Many antihypertensive medicines can cause bradycardia.
- Instruct patients to weigh themselves every morning after voiding, to wear the same amount of clothing each time, and to keep a log for the nurse to review.
- Advise patients who are leaving home for the weekend or holidays to refill medicines ahead of time to make sure they do not run out. The HCP can write a prescription for the patient to have for emergency refills.
- Discuss with the registered nurse if the DASH eating plan would be appropriate for the patient (see www .nhlbi.nih.gov/health/public/heart/hbp/dash/new _dash.pdf).
- Instruct patients and caregivers to avoid frozen dinners and deli meats because many are high in sodium.
- Teach patient to consult HCP about use of salt substitutes, which often contain potassium, because medication and electrolyte interactions can occur.
- Teach patients how to read food labels for fat and salt content. If patients are on a 2- to 3-g sodium diet, instruct them about eating breads or cereals that contain 200 mg or less of sodium per serving

or canned vegetables that contain 150 mg of sodium per serving. Fresh vegetables are better, but cost and storage must be considered. Providing written suggestions for the caregiver who does the grocery shopping increases adherence to diet therapy.
- Provide the following suggestions to help a patient decrease or stop smoking: use cinnamon mouthwash on arising; put away all ashtrays but one, and keep it in a place not normally used for

smoking; find ways to keep hands busy at times when usually holding a cigarette, such as when drinking coffee or alcohol.
- Encourage patients to put "No Smoking" signs on their door to avoid passive smoking.
- Promote home exercise if cleared by HCP. Weights for exercising can be improvised using canned goods and bags of sugar. The amount of weight being used is easily identified for documentation by the labeling on the food item.

SUGGESTED ANSWERS TO

CRITICAL THINKING

■ *Ms. Miller*

1. Risk factors include gender; age; smoking; a diet high in fat, salt, and calories; consumption of two to three alcoholic drinks per evening; and possibly her morning headaches.

2. Morning headaches. Ms. Miller may be experiencing an episode of hypertensive urgency and should be evaluated immediately by an HCP.

3. "Silent killer" refers to the fact that there are often no signs or symptoms associated with hypertension.

4. Lifelong therapy is required because there is no cure for hypertension, and complications need to be prevented.

■ *Mrs. Bell*

1. Nonmodifiable risk factors include age, gender, and history of hypertension. Modifiable risk factors include weight and adherence to antihypertensive therapy.

2. Thiazide diuretics are first-line drugs. Diuretics remove excess salt and water to decrease blood volume and lower BP. Beta blockers stop the beta receptors from receiving the message from the brain for the heart to work harder. Therefore, the heart rate and BP decrease.

3. Identify patient's reading level and primary language. Provide patient with written instructions in

large letters about medications. Include family members and enlist their support in reinforcing the importance of adhering to the treatment plan.

4. Patient is 80 years old, makes frequent trips to the bathroom related to diuretics, has vision problems, and a side effect of propranolol is weakness and fatigue.

5. Make arrangements for a bedside commode to reduce the distance and urgency to get to the bathroom. Encourage the patient and family to place nightlights in the bedroom, hall, and bathroom. Explain that throw rugs increase the risk of falling and that wood or tile floors can be slippery when wet and hard if a fall occurs. Encourage removal of throw rugs, and suggest carpeting these areas if possible. Suggest the use of safety bars in the hall and bathroom for support or other walking aids as needed. If incontinence is a concern, suggest wearing an adult brief to prevent a wet, slippery floor. Suggest discussing with the physician an exercise program to increase strength, such as lifting small, lightweight objects (e.g., soup can), squeezing a rubber ball, or riding an exercise bike if able. These exercises can be done while sitting so they are not a fall-risk activity.

6. Unit analysis method:

$$\frac{20 \text{ mg}}{} \left| \frac{1 \text{ tablet}}{10 \text{ mg}} \right. = 2 \text{ tablets}$$

REVIEW QUESTIONS

1. The nurse provides a teaching session for a newly diagnosed patient with hypertension. Which of the following statements if made by the patient would indicate the need for further teaching about the cause of primary hypertension? **Select all that apply.**
   1. It is caused by a tumor of the adrenal gland.
   2. There are no tests that can identify the cause.
   3. An arteriogram can show why hypertension is occurring.
   4. The cause is unknown.
   5. The cause can be identified with magnetic resonance imaging (MRI).

2. Which of the following would the nurse reinforce after a teaching session as the most important lifestyle modification for the patient who is age 59, 5'11", weighs 280 pounds, and is hypertensive?
   1. Reduce weight.
   2. Restrict salt intake.
   3. Increase potassium intake.
   4. Decrease alcohol intake.

3. The nurse is reinforcing teaching on hypertension for a patient. Which of the following statements if made by the patient after a teaching session would indicate understanding of what is often the only sign of hypertension?
   1. Sacral edema
   2. Elevated BP
   3. Tachycardia
   4. Jugular venous distention

4. The nurse is participating in a teaching session on diet for a patient with hypertension. Which of the following statements if made by the patient would indicate understanding of the teaching? **Select all that apply.**
   1. "Canned fruit and vegetables are best to eat."
   2. "Add salt to food during cooking."
   3. "Increase foods high in saturated fat."
   4. "Choose fresh or frozen fruits and vegetables."
   5. "Read food labels."
   6. "Watch for potassium in salt substitutes."

5. The nurse is obtaining BP readings for patients during a clinic visit. For which of the following BP readings should a 1-year follow-up visit be recommended in the patient's teaching plan?
   1. 108/66 mm Hg
   2. 116/76 mm Hg
   3. 138/84 mm Hg
   4. 142/90 mm Hg

6. During a health screening, a patient's BP is confirmed by two nurses to be 210/120 mm Hg. Which of the following actions should the nurse recommend to the patient?
   1. Take off work for the rest of the day and rest.
   2. Sit quietly while we call 911 to request an ambulance.
   3. The patient should take two doses of BP medication right now.
   4. The patient may return to work and have BP rechecked in 2 days.

7. The nurse is collecting data for a patient experiencing the complication of heart failure from hypertension. Which of the following findings would the nurse expect for this patient? **Select all that apply.**
   1. Abnormal hair growth pattern on face
   2. Distended jugular veins in semi-Fowler's position
   3. Pain in the right hand when writing
   4. Depression from taking BP medication
   5. Bilateral ankle edema

8. The nurse is reinforcing medication teaching for a patient. The nurse would include which of the following instructions to a patient receiving a diuretic?
   1. Change positions slowly.
   2. Eliminate salt in your diet.
   3. Take your medication before bed.
   4. Empty your bladder after taking the first dose.

9. The nurse is collecting data at a follow-up visit for a patient with hypertension. Which of the following data would best indicate to the nurse that the patient's BP therapy has been successful?
   1. Weight decreased by 3 pounds.
   2. Diary of dietary intake is within suggested diet.
   3. BP is less than 120/80 mm Hg.
   4. Patient reports walking 30 to 40 minutes daily.

Answers can be found in Appendix C.

References

Blumenthal, J. A., Babyak, M. A., Hinderliter, A., Watkins, L. L., Craighead, L., Lin, P. H., . . . Sherwood, A. (2010). Effects of the DASH diet alone and in combination with exercise and weight loss on BP and cardiovascular biomarkers in men and women with high BP: The ENCORE study. *Arch Intern Med, 170,* 126–135.

Eckel, R. H, Jakicic, J. M., Ard, J. D., Hubbard, V. S., de Jesus, J. M., . . . Yanovski, S. Z. (2013, November 12). 2013 AHA/ACC guideline on lifestyle management to reduce cardiovascular risk: A report of the American College of Cardiology/American Heart Association Task Force on Practice Guidelines [published online]. *Circulation.* Retrieved April 5, 2014, at http://circ .ahajournals.org/content/early/2013/11/11/01.cir.0000437740 .48606.d1.citation

Epstein, D. E., Sherwood, A., Smith, P. J., Craighead, L., Caccia, C., Lin, P. H. . . . Blumenthal, J. A. (2012). Determinants and consequences of adherence to the dietary approaches to stop hypertension diet in African-American and white adults with high BP: Results from the ENCORE trial. *Journal of the Academy of Nutrition and Dietetics, 112,* 1763–1773.

James, P. A., Oparil, S., Carter, B. L., Cushman, W. C., Dennison-Himmelfarb, C., Handler, J., . . . Ortiz, E. (2014). 2014 Evidence-based guideline for the management of high blood pressure in adults: Report from the panel members appointed to the Eighth Joint National Committee (JNC 8). *Journal of the American Medical Association, 311,* 507–520.

National Heart, Lung, and Blood Institute. (2004). *The seventh report of the Joint National Committee on Prevention, Detection, Evaluation, and Treatment of High BP.* Washington, DC: U.S. Department of Health and Human Services, National Institutes of Health. Retrieved February 17, 2014, from www.nhlbi .nih.gov/guidelines/hypertension/jnc7full.htm

Nwankwo, T., Yoon, S. S., Burt, V., & Gu, Q. (2013). Hypertension among adults in the United States: National Health and Nutrition Examination Survey, 2011–2012 (NCHS Data Brief No. 133). Hyattsville, MD: National Center for Health Statistics. Retrieved February 17, 2014, from www.cdc.gov /nchs/data/databriefs/db133.htm

 Davis*Plus* | For additional resources and information visit **davispl.us/medsurg5**

23

Nursing Care of Patients With Valvular, Inflammatory, and Infectious Cardiac or Venous Disorders

TERRI BLEVINS

KEY TERMS

annuloplasty (AN-yoo-loh-PLAS-tee)
beta-hemolytic streptococci (BAY-tuh-HEE-moh-LIT-ick STREP-toh-KOCK-eye)
cardiac tamponade (KAR-dee-yak TAM-pon-AYD)
cardiomegaly (KAR-dee-oh-MEG-ah-lee)
cardiomyopathy (KAR-dee-oh-my-AH-pah-thee)
chorea (core-REE-ah)
commissurotomy (KOM-ih-shur-AHT-oh-mee)
Dressler syndrome (DRESS-lers SIN-drohm)
emboli (EHM-boh-lye)
infective endocarditis (in-FEK-tive EN-doh-kar-DYE-tiss)
insufficiency (IN-suh-FISH-en-see)
international normalized ratio (IN-ter-NASH-uh-nul NOR-muh-lized RAY-she-oh)
murmur (MUR-mur)
myectomy (my-EK-tuh-mee)
myocarditis (MY-oh-kar-DYE-tiss)
pericardial effusion (PEAR-ih-KAR-dee-uhl ee-FYOO-zhun)
pericardial friction rub (PEAR-ih-KAR-dee-uhl FRICK-shun RUB)
pericardiectomy (PEAR-ih-kar-dee-EK-tuh-mee)
pericardiocentesis (PEAR-ih-KAR-dee-oh-sen-TEE-siss)
pericarditis (PEAR-ih-kar-DYE-tiss)
petechiae (peh-TEE-kee-eye)
regurgitation (ree-GUR-jih-TAY-shun)
rheumatic fever (roo-MAT-ick FEE-vur)
stenosis (steh-NOH-siss)
thrombophlebitis (THROM-boh-fleh-BYE-tiss)
valvotomy (val-VAW-tuh-mee)
valvuloplasty (VAL-vyoo-loh-PLASS-tee)

LEARNING OUTCOMES

1. Explain the pathophysiology, etiology, signs and symptoms, and diagnostic tests for each of the valvular disorders.

2. Plan nursing care for a patient with a valvular disorder.

3. Compare and contrast the differences between commissurotomy, annuloplasty, and valve replacement.

4. Identify postoperative complications that can occur for the two types of cardiac valve replacements.

5. Explain the pathophysiology, etiology, signs and symptoms, diagnostic tests, therapeutic measures, and nursing care for infective endocarditis, pericarditis, and myocarditis.

6. Explain the pathophysiology, etiology, signs and symptoms, complications, diagnostic tests, therapeutic measures, and nursing care for dilated, hypertrophic, and restrictive cardiomyopathy.

7. Explain the pathophysiology, etiology, signs and symptoms, complications, diagnostic tests, and therapeutic measures for thrombophlebitis.

8. List risk factors and prevention measures for thrombophlebitis.

9. Plan nursing care for thrombophlebitis.

■ CARDIAC VALVULAR DISORDERS

Within the normal heart, blood flows in one direction because of the presence of heart valves. There are four valves in the heart: mitral, tricuspid, pulmonic, and aortic (see Fig. 21.2). The chordae tendineae and papillary muscles are attachment structures for both the mitral and tricuspid valves. They ensure that these valves close tightly.

Damage to the valves or their surrounding structures can result in abnormal valvular functioning (Fig. 23.1). The valves of the left side of the heart are most commonly affected. Forward blood flow is hindered if the valve is narrowed, or stenosed, and does not open completely. If the valve does not close completely, blood backs up; this is referred to as **regurgitation** or **insufficiency**. The abnormal blood flow increases the workload of the heart and increases the pressures in the affected heart chamber. Valvular damage may result from congenital defects, **rheumatic fever**, or infections.

Rheumatic fever occurs as an autoimmune reaction to an upper respiratory (sore throat) group A **beta-hemolytic streptococci** infection. Two to 3 weeks after the streptococcal infection, rheumatic fever occurs. Although rheumatic fever can occur at any age, it typically occurs between ages 5 and 15. Rheumatic fever and subsequent rheumatic heart disease and valvular damage can be prevented by detecting and treating streptococcal infections promptly with penicillin. A throat culture is used to diagnose a streptococcal infection at the time of the infection. It is a rare complication of strep throat in the United States.

Signs and symptoms include polyarthritis, subcutaneous nodules, **chorea** (brief, rapid, uncontrolled movements), carditis, fever, arthralgia, and pneumonitis. Rheumatic heart disease may not be evident for years after rheumatic fever.

Valvular disorders are summarized in Table 23.1 and discussed in more detail in the following sections.

LEARNING TIP

The opening of a stenosed valve and an insufficient valve look very similar, and the results of extra blood building up in a chamber are the same (see Fig. 23.1). However, the pathophysiology is different. Think of what the defect is in each disorder to understand why the blood is building up in that particular chamber.

A stenosed valve does not open fully which does not allow the heart chamber to empty normally causing blood to build up in that chamber. Therefore, mitral **stenosis** does not allow the left atrium to empty easily, so blood builds up in the left atrium.

An insufficient valve does not close fully, allowing blood to flow back into the chamber that is supposed to empty. Blood continues to build up in that chamber as a result. For example, mitral insufficiency allows blood to backflow from the left ventricle into the left atrium after the left atrium has emptied, resulting in blood buildup in the left atrium.

Mitral Valve Prolapse
Pathophysiology

During ventricular systole, as pressure in the left ventricle rises, the flaps of the mitral valve normally remain closed and

---

• WORD • BUILDING •
regurgitation: re—again + gurgitare—to flood
insufficiency: in—not + sufficiens—sufficient
stenosis: stenos—narrow

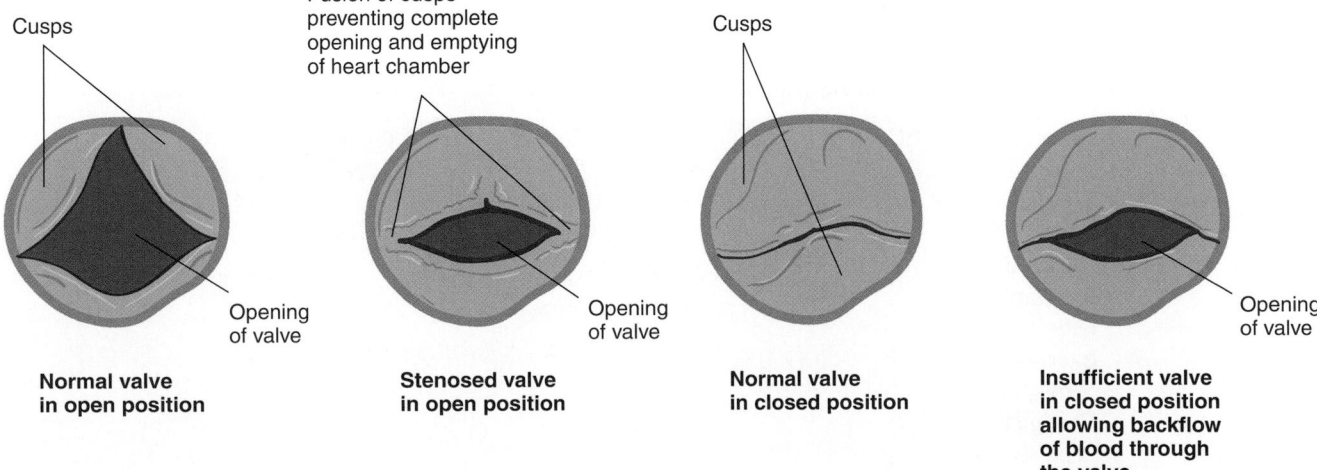

FIGURE 23.1 Openings of stenosed and insufficient valves compared with a normal valve.

TABLE 23.1 CARDIAC VALVULAR DISORDERS SUMMARY

Valve Disorder	Signs and Symptoms	Diagnostic Tests	Complications	Therapeutic Measures	Priority Nursing Diagnoses
Mitral valve prolapse	None Murmur Chest pain Palpitations Dizziness Syncope Fatigue Dyspnea	Echocardiography Cardiac catheterization	Emboli Infective endocarditis	None Beta blockers Antidysrhythmics Valvuloplasty Valve replacement	*Activity Intolerance* *Decreased Cardiac Output*
Mitral stenosis	None Murmur Chest pain Palpitations Fatigue Exertional dyspnea Cough Hemoptysis	ECG Chest x-ray Echocardiography Doppler ultrasound TEE Cardiac catheterization	Emboli Heart failure Anticoagulants	None PBV Valvuloplasty Valve replacement	*Activity Intolerance* *Decreased Cardiac Output*
Mitral regurgitation	None Murmur Chest pain Palpitations Fatigue Exertional dyspnea Cough Hemoptysis *Acute:* Pulmonary edema Shock	ECG Chest x-ray Echocardiography Doppler ultrasound TEE Cardiac MRI Cardiac catheterization	Emboli Heart failure	None ACEI Anticoagulants Valvuloplasty Valve replacement	*Activity Intolerance* *Decreased Cardiac Output*
Aortic stenosis	None Angina Murmur Syncope Heart failure	ECG Chest x-ray Echocardiography Serial echocardiogram Cardiac catheterization	Heart failure	Valve replacement: surgical or transcatheter	*Activity Intolerance* *Decreased Cardiac Output*
Aortic regurgitation	None Forceful pulse Murmur Chest pain Palpitations Fatigue Exertional dyspnea Corrigan's pulse Diaphoresis	ECG Chest x-ray Echocardiography Cardiac catheterization	Heart failure	Valve replacement Digitalis (Lanoxin) Diuretics Vasodilators	*Activity Intolerance* *Decreased Cardiac Output*

Note. ACEI = angiotensin-converting enzyme inhibitor; ECG = electrocardiogram; PBV = percutaneous balloon valvuloplasty; TEE = transesophageal endoscopy.

stay within the atrioventricular junction. In mitral valve prolapse (MVP), however, one or both flaps bulge backward into the left atrium (like a parachute) during systole. This can happen when one flap is too large or if a defect occurs in the chordae tendineae that secure the valve to the heart wall. If the bulging flaps do not fit together, blood can leak backward into the left atrium (mitral regurgitation). Increased pressure on the papillary muscles results in ischemia within the muscle, causing further dysfunction of the mitral valve.

Etiology

MVP can be due to a hereditary collagen tissue disorder, with unknown etiology, an infection damaging the mitral valve, ischemic heart disease, or cardiomyopathy. MVP is the most common form of valvular heart disease. It typically occurs in women, mainly from ages 15 to 30, who are thin and have slight chest deformities.

Signs and Symptoms

Most patients with MVP do not have symptoms, and prognosis is very good (see Table 23.1). MVP severity ranges from having a **murmur** to chordae tendineae rupture with mitral regurgitation. The murmur, which is best heard at the heart apex, begins midsystolic and becomes more intense until the end of systole. Symptoms may include atypical chest pain not related to exertion, dysrhythmias causing palpitations, dizziness or syncope, fatigue, dyspnea, or anxiety.

Complications

Rare complications include mitral regurgitation, dysrhythmias, heart failure (HF), or infective endocarditis.

Diagnostic Tests

Auscultation for a click caused by the stress on the chordae tendineae or valve leaflets when they prolapse, or a murmur (if blood is leaking backward), is the first diagnostic step for MVP. Other diagnostic tests are used when MVP is suspected (Box 23-1). A normal electrocardiogram (ECG) is usually seen with MVP, although inverted (downward) T waves (indicating ischemia) may be seen (see Fig. 25.7). A two-dimensional echocardiogram with Doppler can show valve abnormalities and identify mitral regurgitation from MVP. For more severe cases, cardiac catheterization can show the bulging flaps of the mitral valve on a coronary angiogram.

Box 23-1 Diagnostic Tests for Cardiac Valvular Disorders

- History and physical examination
- Electrocardiogram
- Chest x-ray examination
- Echocardiography
- Cardiac catheterization

Therapeutic Measures

Unless patients have severe mitral regurgitation, MVP is a benign disorder. No treatment is needed unless symptoms are present (Box 23-2). The severity of MVP and symptoms produced determine the treatment used. A healthy lifestyle, including a good diet, exercise, stress management, and avoidance of stimulants and caffeine, can be important to prevent symptoms. Beta blockers reduce the heart rate and may help relieve chest pain. Aspirin or anticoagulants may be ordered to help prevent formation of blood clots on the valve. Surgical repair or replacement of the valve can be done for severe cases of MVP. (See Box 23-2 and the surgical interventions section later in the chapter.)

CRITICAL THINKING

Mrs. Tepley

■ Mrs. Tepley, age 32, has MVP and reports palpitations whenever she experiences stress. She drinks three cups of coffee daily.

1. What might you hear when auscultating Mrs. Tepley's heart sounds?
2. Why does Mrs. Tepley experience palpitations? Would experiencing palpitations make you fearful?
3. What patient-centered information does Mrs. Tepley need to manage her MVP?

Suggested answers are at the end of the chapter.

Box 23-2 Therapeutic Measures for Cardiac Valvular Disorders

- Rheumatic fever prophylaxis
- Prophylactic antibiotic therapy per high-risk infective endocarditis criteria
- Anticoagulant therapy
- Medication therapy
  - Digitalis
  - Diuretics
  - Angiotensin-converting enzyme inhibitors
  - Beta blockers
  - Antidysrhythmics
- Percutaneous balloon valvuloplasty
- Surgery
  - Valvuloplasty
  - Closed commissurotomy
  - Open commissurotomy
  - Annuloplasty
  - Valve replacement

Mitral Stenosis
Pathophysiology

Mitral stenosis results from thickening of the mitral valve flaps and shortening of the chordae tendineae, causing narrowing of the mitral valve opening. Older patients with mitral stenosis usually have calcification and fibrosis of the mitral valve flaps. The narrowed opening obstructs blood flow from the left atrium into the left ventricle. The left atrium enlarges to hold the extra blood volume caused by the obstruction. As a result of this increased blood volume, pressure rises in the left atrium. Pressures then rise in the pulmonary circulation and the right ventricle as blood volume backs up from the left atrium. The right ventricle dilates to handle the increased volume. Eventually the right ventricle fails from this excessive workload, reducing the blood volume delivered to the left ventricle and subsequently decreasing cardiac output.

Etiology

The major cause of mitral stenosis is rheumatic fever. It often takes two to four decades after the illness for symptoms to appear. Because rheumatic fever is rare in developed nations, less mitral stenosis is being seen except in older adults who were exposed to rheumatic fever as children. Mitral stenosis is still a problem in underdeveloped areas where rheumatic fever still occurs. Less common causes include congenital defects of the mitral valve, tumors, rheumatoid arthritis, systemic lupus erythematosus, and calcium deposits.

Signs and Symptoms

Patients may be asymptomatic (see Table 23.1). A click or low-pitched murmur may be heard. This murmur is a rumbling sound over the heart apex during diastole and is more pronounced right before systole. Pulmonary symptoms, such as exertional dyspnea, cough, hemoptysis (bloody sputum), and respiratory infections can occur. Fatigue, intolerance to activity, dizziness, or syncope result from decreased cardiac output. Edema of ankles and feet may be present. Palpitations from atrial flutter or fibrillation caused by atrial enlargement and chest pain from decreased cardiac output may be experienced.

Complications

Emboli can form from the stasis of blood in the left atrium and may cause stroke and seizures. If the right ventricle fails, symptoms related to HF are seen (see Chapter 26). Pulmonary edema may develop from the backup of blood into the lungs.

Diagnostic Tests

Mitral stenosis is diagnosed with data from the patient history and physical examination and findings from diagnostic tests (see Box 23-1). The ECG shows enlargement of the left atrium and right ventricle and changes in the P waveform (see Fig. 25.2). Atrial flutter or fibrillation may be seen (see Chapter 25). A chest x-ray examination confirms enlargement of the affected heart chambers. Transthoracic two-dimensional color flow Doppler echocardiography and Doppler ultrasound are the noninvasive gold standard for evaluation of valvular disease. They show the narrowed

mitral valve opening and decreased motion of the valve. Computed tomography (CT) scan and magnetic resonance imaging (MRI) may be done. A cardiac catheterization is typically done only if needed to validate unclear echocardiography results for preoperative evaluation or postprocedure for symptom recurrence.

Therapeutic Measures

No treatment is needed if symptoms are not present. Monitoring of the stenosis is done to provide invasive treatment if needed. Anticoagulants are given to patients at risk of development of emboli from stasis of blood in the atrium. Atrial fibrillation, an irregular heart rhythm, may develop and require treatment. For HF, symptoms are treated with medications (see Chapter 26).

For less severe cases, percutaneous balloon **valvuloplasty**, which uses a balloon to dilate the stenosed heart valve, is done in a cardiac catheterization lab (Fig. 23.2). Surgical treatment can include valvular repair (valvuloplasty), but mitral valve replacement is typically needed (Fig. 23.3; see Box 23-2).

Mitral Regurgitation
Pathophysiology

Mitral regurgitation, or insufficiency, is the incomplete closure of the mitral valve leaflets. It allows backflow of blood into the left atrium with each contraction of the left ventricle. This blood is then extra volume that is added to the incoming blood from the lungs. With chronic mitral regurgitation, the increase in blood volume dilates and increases pressure in the left atrium. In response to the extra blood volume delivered by the left atrium, the left ventricle compensates by dilating. If the compensatory mechanism of dilation is inadequate, pressures rise in the pulmonary circulation and then in the right ventricle as blood volume backs up from the left atrium. The left ventricle and eventually the right ventricle may fail from this increased strain.

FIGURE 23.2 Percutaneous balloon valvuloplasty.

Mechanical mitral valve

FIGURE 23.3 Mitral valve replacement with mechanical valve.

Etiology

Causes of mitral regurgitation include rheumatic heart disease, endocarditis, rupture or dysfunction of the chordae tendineae or papillary muscle, MVP, hypertension, myocardial infarction (MI), cardiomyopathy, annulus calcification, aging, or congenital defects.

Signs and Symptoms

Initially, patients may be asymptomatic; however, symptoms may develop gradually and are similar to those of mitral stenosis (see Table 23.1). A murmur begins with S_1 (first heart sound) and continues during systole up to S_2 (second heart sound). Exertional dyspnea (shortness of breath), fatigue, syncope (feeling faint), cough, and edema may occur. Palpitations and an irregular pulse due to atrial fibrillation may result. Weakness from decreased cardiac output occurs if the left ventricle begins to fail. If acute mitral regurgitation develops, as in papillary muscle rupture following MI, pulmonary edema and shock symptoms will be exhibited.

Complications

Atrial fibrillation may develop from the enlargement of the left atrium. Pulmonary hypertension or heart failure may occur (see Chapter 26). Endocarditis is a risk due to the damaged valve.

Diagnostic Tests

A patient history and physical examination are done. The ECG shows enlargement of the left atrium and left ventricle and changes in the P waveform (see Fig. 25.2). Atrial flutter or fibrillation may be seen. A chest x-ray examination confirms hypertrophy of the affected heart chambers. Two-dimensional echocardiography with Doppler or trans-esophageal echocardiography shows left atrial enlargement

and regurgitation of blood. Cardiac MRI may be used for some people to determine treatment approaches. Cardiac catheterization further identifies regurgitation effects.

Therapeutic Measures

Without symptoms, there is no general medical treatment. Angiotensin-converting enzyme (ACE) inhibitors are often used to reduce afterload. If atrial fibrillation with rapid heart rate is present, it can be controlled with digitalis, calcium channel blockers, or beta blockers. Anticoagulants are used for emboli prevention. Symptoms of HF are treated with therapies for HF (see Chapter 26). When symptoms develop or surgery is indicated to prevent further left ventricular dysfunction, mitral valve repair or replacement is done. For acute mitral regurgitation, emergency surgery may be needed (see Box 23-2).

Aortic Stenosis

Pathophysiology

Blood flow from the left ventricle into the aorta is obstructed through the stenosed aortic valve. The opening of the aortic valve may be narrowed from thickening, scarring, calcification, or fusing of the valve's flaps. To compensate for the difficulty in ejecting blood into the aorta, the left ventricle contracts more forcefully. In chronic stenosis, the left ventricle hypertrophies to maintain normal cardiac output. As narrowing increases, the compensatory mechanisms are unable to continue and the left ventricle fails to move blood forward, resulting in decreased cardiac output and HF.

Etiology

The major causes of aortic stenosis are congenital defects or rheumatic heart disease. Calcification of the aortic valve can be related to aging and occurs after age 60. Aortic stenosis is the most commonly acquired valvular heart disease in adults. As the population ages, it is expected to increase in prevalence.

Signs and Symptoms

Many years or decades may pass before signs or symptoms of aortic stenosis are observed (see Table 23.1). When symptoms do occur, evaluation is essential because the disease can progress dramatically. If the mitral valve is also diseased, signs and symptoms can appear earlier.

Angina pectoris (chest pain) is the primary symptom that occurs as a result of a lack of oxygen to the myocardium. In the young patient, angina indicates severe obstruction.

Other signs and symptoms include a murmur, syncope from dysrhythmias or decreased cardiac output, and HF signs and symptoms. The murmur is a systolic murmur that begins just after the first heart sound, increasing in intensity till midsystole, then decreasing and ending right before the second heart sound. Orthopnea, dyspnea on exertion, and fatigue are indicators of left ventricular failure, resulting in pulmonary edema and right sided heart failure.

Complications

HF, life-threatening dysrhythmias, or endocarditis can occur.

Diagnostic Tests

ECG usually shows enlargement of the left ventricle and left atrium. A chest x-ray examination confirms hypertrophy of the left ventricle and calcification of the aortic valve. Left atrial enlargement may be seen but occurs primarily when mitral stenosis is also present. Two-dimensional and Doppler echocardiography show thickening of the left ventricular wall, impaired movement of the aortic valve, and the severity of the disease. Cardiac catheterization will show elevated left ventricular pressure and decreased cardiac output.

Therapeutic Measures

Generally, the treatment of choice is valve replacement because of the risk of sudden death when severe symptoms are present (see Box 23-2). If mechanical valves are used, they require lifelong anticoagulation. For older adults, biological valves are usually used because they do not require anticoagulation therapy and last about 12 years. For those considered too high risk for traditional open-heart surgery, an aortic valve implantation can be done with a catheter via the femoral artery (visit www.medtronic.com to view this procedure—Medtronic CoreValve® system). Valvotomy (expansion of a balloon to open the mitral valve) is used only for those who are unable to have valve replacement.

Symptoms of HF are treated. Medications that reduce the contractility of the heart and subsequently cardiac output are avoided to prevent further HF.

CRITICAL THINKING

Mrs. Pryor

■ Mrs. Pryor, age 48, has aortic stenosis and is admitted to the hospital with angina. She had an episode of syncope 2 days ago. She reports that she tires easily.

1. Mrs. Pryor asks what aortic stenosis is. What should the nurse tell her, and how should it be documented?
2. Why might Mrs. Pryor be experiencing angina?
3. What nursing care related to safety needs is important to include in Mrs. Pryor's plan of care? Think of how you would feel knowing you will continue to have episodes of syncope and fatigue. What concerns would you have regarding completing your activities of daily living?
4. What nursing diagnoses and care are relevant for Mrs. Pryor's report of being tired?
5. Digoxin (Lanoxin) 0.25 mg is prescribed for Mrs. Pryor. Digoxin is available in 0.125-mg tablets. How many tablets will the nurse give?

Suggested answers are at the end of the chapter.

Aortic Regurgitation

Pathophysiology

The aortic valve cusps may be scarred, thickened, or shortened in chronic aortic regurgitation. A backflow of blood from the aorta into the left ventricle occurs if the aortic valve cusps do not close completely. The left ventricle's blood volume increases with this backflow of blood that is in addition to the normal flow of blood from the left atrium. To handle the increased volume, the left ventricle compensates with dilation and hypertrophy to deliver a stronger contraction. This stronger contraction ejects more blood volume with each beat to maintain cardiac output. Over time, the heart's contraction is not effective, and the left ventricle fails, causing a cardiac output drop and pulmonary edema.

Etiology

Congenital defects, aging, rheumatic heart disease, syphilis, severe hypertension, and ankylosing spondylitis can cause aortic regurgitation. An acute cause of aortic regurgitation may be endocarditis or aortic dissection.

Signs and Symptoms

Symptoms may not become apparent for many years with chronic aortic regurgitation (see Table 23.1). Initially, the patient may report feeling a forceful heartbeat that is more pronounced when lying down. Also, palpitations and pounding in the head may be experienced. Then exertional dyspnea, fatigue, and worsening levels of dyspnea (orthopnea, paroxysmal nocturnal dyspnea) occur after years of progressive valvular dysfunction. A murmur is heard during diastolic after the second heart sound. The palpated pulse is forceful and then quickly collapses (Corrigan's pulse). The diastolic blood pressure decreases to widen the pulse pressure. This compensates for an increase in systolic blood pressure. Angina pectoris may occur late. The angina is atypical, often happening at rest or at night along with diaphoresis, when a lower pulse rate results in delivery of less oxygen to the myocardium. Eventually symptoms of HF develop if the left ventricle fails. In acute dysfunction, profound symptoms of pulmonary distress, chest pain, and shock symptoms occur.

Complications

Endocarditis is a risk due to the damaged valve. HF may occur.

Diagnostic Tests

The ECG shows left ventricle hypertrophy, ST-segment depression (see Fig. 25.10), and T-wave inversion (see Fig. 25.7) in some leads. A chest x-ray confirms hypertrophy of the left ventricle and aorta. With severe regurgitation, left atrial enlargement may also be seen. An echocardiogram, Doppler echocardiography, or transesophageal echocardiography show an enlarged left ventricle and severity of the aortic regurgitation. Cardiac catheterization reveals elevated left ventricular diastolic pressure and, with contrast injection, shows the regurgitation of blood into the left ventricle.

Therapeutic Measures

Treatment with vasodilator therapy may be useful for some patients to reduce systolic blood pressure and subsequently cardiac workload until surgery is needed. Occasionally, surgical valve repair can be done, but valve replacement is typically needed when symptoms develop (see Box 23-2).

Nursing Process for the Patient With a Cardiac Valvular Disorder

Data Collection

A history is obtained that includes information presented in Table 23.2. Vital signs are measured and recorded. Heart sounds are auscultated to detect murmurs. Any signs and symptoms of HF are noted and reported (see Chapter 26).

Nursing Diagnoses, Planning, Interventions, and Evaluation

The major nursing diagnoses for all valvular disorders are the same and include those for HF as well, if symptoms of HF are present. See "Nursing Care Plan for the Patient With a Cardiac Valvular Disorder."

Patient Education

Education, an important nursing intervention, promotes understanding of the valvular disorder, health maintenance, prevention of complications, and early recognition of symptoms so that medical care can be sought. For older adult patients, it is important to include caregivers or family members in teaching sessions to assist with understanding of the information being taught. Teaching is provided for medications the patient is taking. If the patient is on anticoagulants for atrial fibrillation or mechanical valve replacement, medical identification should be used, and monthly appointments to check international normalized ratio (INR)/prothrombin time (PT) values should be kept.

Information on endocarditis prevention is essential for patients with most valvular problems. Damaged cardiac valves are prone to developing infection from organisms such as *Streptococcus viridans* or *Staphylococcus epidermidis*. During invasive procedures in which bleeding is possible, these organisms can enter the circulation, attach to damaged valves, and multiply. Patients should discuss with their health care provider (HCP) the American Heart Association guidelines for prophylactic antibiotics to prevent endocarditis (see the prevention section for endocarditis later in this chapter).

Cardiac Valve Repairs

A balloon **valvotomy** opens a stenosed heart valve. A balloon catheter is inserted through the diseased valve and then inflated to open the stenosed valve leaflets. For mitral valve valvoplasty, the balloon catheter is inserted via the venous circulation into

TABLE 23.2 DATA COLLECTION FOR PATIENTS WITH CARDIAC VALVULAR DISORDERS

Data Collection	Subjective Data
Health History	Infections (rheumatic fever, endocarditis, streptococcal or staphylococcal, syphilis)? Congenital defects? Cardiac disease (myocardial infarction, cardiomyopathy)?
Respiratory	Dyspnea at rest, on exertion, when lying, or that awakens patient? Cough or hemoptysis?
Cardiovascular	Chest pain—when does it occur? Palpitations, dizziness, fatigue, activity intolerance?
Medications	What medications are you taking?
Knowledge of Condition	What is the reason that you are here today? What does your diagnosis mean to you?
Coping Skills	How does patient normally cope with stressors? Support system? Adaptations in lifestyle and/or environment?
	Objective Data
Respiratory	Crackles, wheezes, tachypnea
Cardiovascular	Murmurs, extra heart sounds, dysrhythmias, edema, jugular venous distention, Corrigan's pulse, increased or decreased pulse pressure
Integumentary	Clubbing; cyanosis; diaphoresis; cold, clammy skin; pallor
Diagnostic Test Findings	**Review ordered test results.**

the right atrium. Then the catheter is threaded through a small hole pierced into the right atrial septum that emerges into the left atrium. The catheter is passed through the mitral valve, and the inflation of the balloon within the mitral valve opens the stenosed valve flaps. Complications may include dysrhythmias, emboli, hemorrhage, and cardiac tamponade. A balloon valvuloplasty results in fewer complications than traditional open-heart surgery.

A **commissurotomy** repairs a stenosed valve. The valve flaps that have adhered to each other and thus closed the opening between them, known as the commissure, are separated to enlarge the valve opening. The patient is placed on cardiopulmonary bypass (CPB; see Chapter 21), and an

• WORD • BUILDING •
commissurotomy: commissura—joining together + tome—incision

NURSING CARE PLAN for the Patient with a Cardiac Valvular Disorder

Nursing Diagnosis: *Decreased Cardiac Output* related to valvular stenosis or insufficiency or heart failure

Expected Outcome: The patient will have adequate cardiac output as evidenced by vital signs within normal limits (WNL), no dyspnea, and minimal fatigue.

Evaluation of Outcome: Are patient's vital signs WNL with no dyspnea or fatigue?

Intervention Assess vital signs, oxygen saturation, chest pain, and fatigue. **Rationale** Vital signs, chest pain, and fatigue are indicators of cardiac output decline. **Evaluation** Are vital signs WNL with no chest pain?

Intervention Give oxygen as ordered. **Rationale** Supplemental oxygen provides more oxygen to the heart by increasing the oxygen saturation in the blood. **Evaluation** Is oxygen saturation WNL?

Intervention Provide bedrest or rest periods as ordered. **Rationale** Cardiac workload and oxygen needs are reduced with rest. **Evaluation** Are vital signs WNL and no fatigue reported?

Intervention Elevate head of bed 45 degrees. **Rationale** Venous return to heart is reduced and chest expansion improved, which increases the amount of oxygen coming into the lungs. **Evaluation** Are vital signs WNL without use of accessory muscles of respiration?

GERIATRIC
Intervention Note cardiac medication side effects and teach patient side effects to report. **Rationale** Toxic side effects are more common owing to altered metabolism and excretion of medications in the older adult. **Evaluation** Are side effects present for medications patient is taking? Does patient understand side effects to report?

Nursing Diagnosis: *Activity Intolerance* related to decreased oxygen delivery from decreased cardiac output

Expected Outcome: The patient will show normal changes in vital signs with less fatigue in response to activity.

Evaluation of Outcome: Does patient have normal changes in vital signs with activity? Does patient report decreased fatigue with activity?

Intervention Assist as needed with activities of daily living (ADLs). **Rationale** Conserve energy with ADL assistance. **Evaluation** Are all ADLs completed? Are vital signs WNL with activity?

Intervention Provide rest between activities. **Rationale** Cardiac workload and oxygen needs are reduced with rest. **Evaluation** Is patient able to perform activities when allowed extra time?

GERIATRIC
Intervention Slow pace of care and allow patient extra time to perform activities. **Rationale** Patients can often perform activities if allowed time to slowly perform them and rest at intervals. **Evaluation** Does blood pressure remain WNL when changing position?

Intervention Ensure safety when mobilizing older patient. **Rationale** Orthostatic hypertension is common in the older adult. **Evaluation** Does patient ambulate without injury?

atriotomy (incision into the atrium) is made to expose the valve. The valve cusps are either incised with a knife or broken apart with a dilator. The atrium is sewn closed, CPB is discontinued, and surgery continues as described in Chapter 21. Commissurotomy is most commonly performed on the mitral valve.

Annuloplasty is the repair or reconstruction of the valve flaps or annulus. It may involve the use of prosthetic rings. The mitral valve is the most common valve repaired in this way. Sutures or a ring may be placed in the valve annulus to improve closure of the leaflets. Similar procedures are used on the tricuspid valve; however, the aortic valve is not readily repaired in this manner.

Heart Valve Replacement

Valves used for cardiac valve replacement may be either mechanical or biological. Research is ongoing to develop tissue engineered heart valves. Biological (tissue) valves come from xenograft (porcine [pig] and bovine [cow]) or allograft (human donor) (see "Cultural Considerations"). Allografts are available in limited numbers because they rely on donors. An autograft (Ross procedure) uses the patient's own pulmonary valve to replace the removed aortic valve; an allograft (human donor) pulmonary valve then replaces the patient's pulmonary valve. Visit www.lifenet.org for more information on allografts.

For mitral valve replacement, a left atriotomy is made after the patient is on CPB. For an aortic valve replacement, an incision is made above the right coronary artery in the aorta. Then in either valvular procedure, the diseased valve is excised and the new valve sutured in place. The incision is closed, and surgery then continues as described in Chapter 21.

Complications of Valve Replacement

Tissue valves have a low incidence of thrombus formation and do not require lifelong anticoagulant therapy, but they do not last as long as mechanical valves because of degenerative changes and calcification. Mechanical valves are durable (lasting 20–30 years) but create turbulent blood flow, requiring lifelong anticoagulant therapy to prevent blood clots (Fig. 23.4). Anemia from hemolysis of red blood cells (RBCs) as they come in contact with mechanical valve structures can occur. Also endocarditis can occur due to micro-organisms growing on the valve leaflets or the sewing ring of mechanical valves. These

FIGURE 23.4 Mechanical valve prosthesis. An SJM Masters Series valve. *Courtesy of St. Jude Medical, Inc., St. Paul, MN.*

growths can make valves incompetent or break off to become emboli.

Nursing Process for the Preoperative Cardiac Surgery Patient

DATA COLLECTION. Baseline data collection is important for postoperative comparison and to begin discharge planning. Pain control needs and circulatory status are essential items. Results of diagnostic laboratory tests, x-ray examinations, and other studies are also significant. Typing and crossmatching for ordered units of blood is done.

NURSING DIAGNOSES, PLANNING, INTERVENTIONS, AND EVALUATION. See the "Nursing Process for Preoperative Patients" in Chapter 12.

Nursing Process for the Postoperative Cardiac Surgery Patient

After cardiac surgery, the patient goes to an intensive care unit (ICU) or cardiac universal bed unit (CUB). In the ICU,

• WORD • BUILDING •
annuloplasty: annulus—ring + plasty—formed

Cultural Considerations

Cardiac Valves

Because the pig is considered a forbidden animal to religious Jews and Muslims, only bovine, synthetic, or human valves should be used for these patients. Because the cow is sacred among Hindus, only porcine, synthetic, or human valves should be used for Hindu patients.

the patient is monitored for 1 to 2 days. As recovery progresses, the patient is transferred to a step-down or general surgical unit for continued cardiac monitoring. In the CUB unit, the patient recovers in the same room until discharge, which avoids transfers to other units and increases continuity of care.

DATA COLLECTION. The patient is accompanied to ICU/CUB by the anesthesiologist, who gives the nurse a report of the procedure, complications, and hemodynamic and ventilatory management of the patient. The patient is connected to a cardiac monitor and mechanical ventilator for up to 24 hours. The patient is placed under a warming device, such as a forced air blanket, as needed.

A head-to-toe assessment of the patient, including dressings, tubes (chest and, nasogastric tube, urinary catheter) and intravenous (IV) lines, is performed. Of importance are signs of awakening, shivering, pain, lung and heart sounds, and palpation of the entire chest and neck to detect crepitus (air in the subcutaneous tissue from opening the chest). Trends in cardiac output are monitored. Body temperature is continuously monitored if warming measures are used. Warming is discontinued when the core body temperature nears 98.6°F (37°C). Warming should occur slowly to avoid peripheral vasodilation, which can result in shock. While being rewarmed, patients are assessed for shivering, which may be felt as a fine vibration at the mandibular angle of the jaw. Shivering greatly increases cardiac oxygen needs. Paralyzing agents given with narcotics eliminate shivering. Complete blood count (CBC), electrolytes, coagulation studies, and arterial blood gases (ABGs) are monitored.

After the initial transfer assessment, vital signs, oxygen saturation, and cardiac pressures are monitored and recorded every 15 to 30 minutes, with decreasing frequency as the patient stabilizes. Input and output (I&O) is measured. A 12-lead ECG is done to detect perioperative MI. A chest x-ray examination is done to check central line and endotracheal tube placement and to detect a pneumothorax or hemothorax, diaphragm elevation, or mediastinal widening from bleeding. At this point, the family can see the patient.

Awakening with many questions, strange auditory and tactile sensations, and the inability to speak are frightening and frustrating to the patient. Give explanations regarding procedures in simple terms. Keeping eye contact with the patient and using touch appropriately can be soothing to the patient. If lip reading is unsuccessful, use simple closed-ended questions, nonverbal gestures, communication boards, or magic slates.

After cardiac surgery, pain is monitored in relation to the patient's preoperative anginal or infarction-associated pain. Chest pain after surgery can be frightening. Knowing that chest pain can occur from the surgical incision rather than from anginal or MI pain is comforting to the patient.

NURSING DIAGNOSES, PLANNING, INTERVENTIONS, AND EVALUATION. Nursing diagnoses for postoperative cardiac surgery are discussed in the "Nursing Care Plan for the Postoperative Patient Undergoing Cardiac Surgery." Additional general postoperative nursing care is discussed in Chapter 12.

NURSING CARE PLAN for the Postoperative Patient Undergoing Cardiac Surgery

Nursing Diagnosis: *Pain* related to sternotomy or pericarditis

Expected Outcomes: The patient will state that pain is relieved or tolerable. Patient will be able to rest and perform respiratory treatments.

Evaluation of Outcomes: Does patient state pain is within acceptable levels? Is patient able to rest and perform respiratory therapies?

Intervention Ask about characteristics of pain with each episode. **Rationale** A thorough description is needed to determine cause and plan actions. **Evaluation** Does patient describe pain on scale of 0 to 10?

Intervention Splint chest incision with all movement, including coughing and deep breathing. **Rationale** Stabilizes sternum and incision to increase comfort. **Evaluation** Can patient splint chest incision independently?

Intervention Encourage patient to report pain even when it is mild. **Rationale** It is easier to keep pain under control when mild. **Evaluation** Does patient report pain when mild?

Intervention Turn, reposition every 2 hours. **Rationale** Changes muscle position, relieving stiffness. **Evaluation** Is patient comfortable without stiffness?

NURSING CARE PLAN for the Postoperative Patient Undergoing Cardiac Surgery

Intervention Offer back rubs frequently. **Rationale** Relaxes tense muscles retracted during operation. **Evaluation** Is patient able to rest comfortably?

Intervention Instruct patient to take a deep breath before movement and exhale slowly during movement. **Rationale** Keeps muscles relaxed, minimizing tension with guarding and pain. **Evaluation** Can patient perform coughing and deep-breathing techniques as instructed?

Nursing Diagnosis: *Decreased Cardiac Output* related to myocardial depression, hypothermia, bleeding, unstable dysrhythmias, or hypoxemia

Expected Outcomes: The patient will remain free of major side effects of pharmacological support. The patient will maintain vital signs WNL, palpable peripheral pulses, urine output greater than 30 mL/hr, and normal sinus rhythm.

Evaluation of Outcomes: Is patient free of major side effects? Are vital signs WNL?

Intervention Monitor vital signs. **Rationale** Trends reflect problems. **Evaluation** Are vital signs WNL?

Intervention Monitor peripheral circulation. **Rationale** Mottling or weak pulses may indicate poor cardiac output (CO). **Evaluation** Do peripheral pulses remain strong with normal skin color, temperature, capillary refill?

Intervention Monitor intake and output. **Rationale** Fluid deficit or excess can alter CO. **Evaluation** Does total intake equal output?

Intervention Listen to lung sounds and note character of sputum. **Rationale** Wet lung sounds may indicate HF or pulmonary edema. **Evaluation** Are lungs clear?

Intervention Monitor temperature closely while rewarming the patient. **Rationale** Febrile state increases heart rate and myocardial oxygen consumption. **Evaluation** Does temperature remain less than or equal to 98.6°F (37°C)?

Intervention Monitor for shivering. **Rationale** Shivering increases the blood pressure, decreasing CO and increasing risk for bleeding. **Evaluation** Is patient's shivering controlled?

Intervention Monitor chest tube drainage for increase or sudden decrease. **Rationale** Drainage greater than 200 mL/hr may lead to hypovolemia and decreased CO. **Evaluation** Is patient free from cardiac tamponade and hypovolemia?

Intervention Monitor ECG. **Rationale** Premature ventricular contractions and atrial fibrillation decrease CO. **Evaluation** Does patient remain in normal sinus rhythm or controlled dysrhythmia?

Intervention Monitor electrolytes. **Rationale** Low calcium and magnesium and high potassium decrease contractility and CO. **Evaluation** Are electrolytes WNL?

Intervention Monitor arterial blood gases (ABGs). **Rationale** Acidosis decreases heart function, and a low CO may lead to further acidosis. **Evaluation** Are ABGs WNL?

Nursing Diagnosis: *Risk for Infection* related to inadequate primary defenses from surgical wound

Expected Outcome: The patient will remain free from infection.

Evaluation of Outcome: Does patient remain free from infection?

Continued

NURSING CARE PLAN for the Postoperative Patient Undergoing Cardiac Surgery—cont'd

Intervention Practice excellent hand hygiene, and always cleanse stethoscope with ethanol-based cleanser or alcohol between patients. **Rationale** Hands and stethoscopes carry infectious agents. **Evaluation** Are infectious preventive techniques used? Does patient remain free from infection?

Intervention Observe incision for signs and symptoms of infection, which are redness, warmth, fever, and/or edema. **Rationale** Redness, warmth, fever, and swelling indicate the body's response to an invading pathogen. **Evaluation** Are signs and symptoms of infection present?

Intervention Monitor drainage and maintain drains. **Rationale** Drains remove fluid from the surgical site to prevent infection development. **Evaluation** Are drainage amount and color normal for procedure? Are drains functioning?

Intervention Maintain sterile technique for dressing changes. **Rationale** Sterile technique reduces infection development. **Evaluation** Is incision free of signs and symptoms of infection?

Intervention Monitor and report abnormal findings for temperature, lung sounds, sputum, and urine consistency. **Rationale** Low-grade (immunosuppressed) or high-grade fever, crackles, yellow-green sputum color, or cloudy urine can indicate infection. **Evaluation** Is the patient's temperature WNL, and are lung sounds, sputum, and urine clear?

INFLAMMATORY AND INFECTIOUS CARDIAC DISORDERS

The layers of the heart—the endocardium, pericardium, and myocardium (Fig. 23.5)—can become inflamed or infected, leading to endocarditis, pericarditis, and myocarditis, respectively.

Infective Endocarditis

Infective endocarditis (IE) is an infection of the endocardium that mostly occurs in hearts with artificial or damaged valves. Men develop IE more often than women, as do older adults compared with younger.

Pathophysiology

Cardiac defects result in turbulent blood flow that erodes the normally infection-resistant endocardium. IE begins when the invading organism (most commonly a bacteria but possibly a fungi or other organism) attaches to eroded endocardium where platelets and fibrin deposits have formed a vegetative lesion. Then more platelets and fibrin cover the multiplying organism. This covering protects the microbes, reducing the ability to destroy them. Damage to valve leaflets occurs as the vegetations grow. As blood flows through the heart, these vegetations may break off and become **emboli**.

Damaged valves from conditions such as MVP with regurgitation, rheumatic heart disease, congenital defects, and valve replacements are especially prone to bacterial invasion. The mitral valve is the valve most commonly infected, with the aortic valve being second. HF may result from valve damage, especially of the aortic valve.

Etiology

Risk factors include the following:

- Compromised immune system
- Artificial heart valve

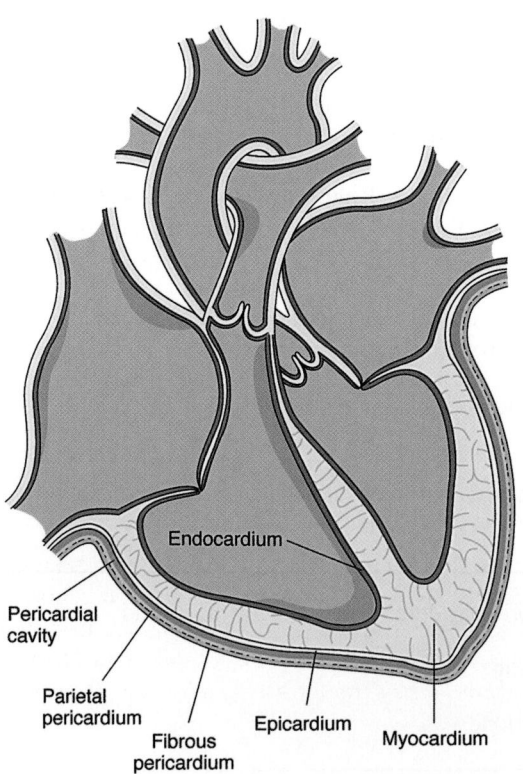

FIGURE 23.5 Layers of the heart.

Endocardium

Pericardial cavity

Parietal pericardium

Fibrous pericardium

Epicardium

Myocardium

• Congenital or valvular heart disease
• History of endocarditis
• IV drug use
• Gingival gum disease.

Prevention

Dental disease may be a contributing factor to IE, so daily oral care and regular dental care is an important preventive measure. Antibiotic prophylaxis guidelines have been updated. Before a dental procedure, the American Heart Association (2014) now recommends that only individuals with an artificial heart valve or a valve repaired with artificial material, a history of endocarditis, a heart transplant with abnormal valve function, or specific congenital heart defects receive antibiotics. Prophylaxis for procedures on the genitourinary or gastrointestinal (GI) tract or for most people who have orthopedic implants is no longer recommended.

Signs and Symptoms

The onset of symptoms can be rapid or slow. Fever (99°–103°F [37.2°–39.4°C]) is a common sign, although the older adult may be afebrile (Table 23.3). Chills, aching muscles and joints, fatigue, dyspnea, cough, edema, and hematuria may occur. A new or different murmur is heard with valvular damage. Splinter hemorrhages may be seen in the distal nailbed (black or red-brown longitudinal short lines). **Petechiae** (tiny red or purple flat spots) resulting from microembolization of the vegetation may occur on mucous membranes, conjunctivae, or skin (Fig. 23.6). Janeway lesions (small, painless red-blue lesions on palms and soles) are an acute finding. Osler's nodes (small, painful nodes on fingers and toes) from cardiac emboli are a late finding (Fig. 23.7). Have you ever seen petechiae or palpated an Osler's node? Look for the opportunity in clinical to see petechiae, Janeway lesions, or an Osler's node.

Complications

Vegetative emboli can be a major complication of IE. If organ embolization occurs, signs and symptoms that reflect the organ that was affected by the emboli are seen. Brain emboli may produce changes in level of consciousness or stroke. Kidney emboli cause pain in the flank area, hematuria, or renal failure. Emboli in the spleen cause abdominal pain. Emboli in the small blood vessels can impair circulation in the extremities. Pulmonary emboli result in sudden dyspnea, cough, and chest pain.

Heart structures can be damaged or destroyed by IE. Stenosis (narrowing) or regurgitation (leakage) of a heart valve may also result. As the infection progresses and causes more damage to heart structures, HF may occur. Abscesses may also develop in the heart or other parts of the body.

Diagnostic Tests

Table 23.3 lists diagnostic tests for IE. Positive blood cultures identify the causative organism, and echocardiography shows cardiac effects.

TABLE 23.3 INFECTIVE ENDOCARDITIS SUMMARY

Signs and Symptoms	Fever Chills Heart murmur Night sweats Fatigue Weight loss Weakness Aching in abdomen, joints, muscles, back Nailbed splinter hemorrhages Petechiae
Diagnostic Tests and Findings	Blood cultures Transesophageal echocardiography CBC Chest x-ray ECG
Therapeutic Measures	*Acute therapy:* IV antimicrobial medications such as penicillin, vancomycin, amphotericin B Antipyretics Rest Valve replacement Prophylactic antibiotic therapy per high-risk infective endocarditis criteria
Complications	Emboli Heart failure Abscesses
Priority Nursing Diagnoses	*Activity Intolerance* related to reduced oxygen delivery from decreased cardiac output *Decreased Cardiac Output* related to impaired valvular function or heart failure *Ineffective Tissue Perfusion* related to emboli

Note. CBC = complete blood count; ECG = electrocardiogram.

Therapeutic Measures

Initial treatment begins with hospitalization. An antimicrobial drug is selected that will destroy the organism identified by the blood culture. For bacterial infections, penicillin (or vancomycin for those allergic to penicillin) is commonly used. These medications are given IV over a period

• WORD • BUILDING •
petechiae: petecchia—skin spot

FIGURE 23.6 Petechiae. From Goldsmith, L. (1997). *Adult & pediatric dermatology* (p. 61). Philadelphia: F.A. Davis.

FIGURE 23.7 Osler's nodes. From Goldsmith, L. (1997). *Adult & pediatric dermatology* (p. 188). Philadelphia: F.A. Davis.

of 4 to 6 weeks, often once a day. A lengthy course of high-dose antibiotics is needed to penetrate the vegetations to reach all of the microbes inside to kill them. Rest and supportive symptom care are also used. If afebrile and without complications, the patient is discharged to continue IV antibiotic therapy at home. Response to the drug is monitored by the home care nurse and laboratory testing.

Surgical replacement or repair of valves is done for severely damaged heart valves, prosthetic valve infection, recurrent infection, multiple emboli from damaged valves, or HF. Antimicrobial therapy continues after surgery.

Nursing Process for the Patient With Infectious Endocarditis

DATA COLLECTION. A patient history is obtained that includes risk factors for IE and recent infections or invasive procedures (Table 23.4). Vital signs are recorded, and heart sounds are auscultated for murmurs. Signs of HF and emboli are noted. Notify the HCP immediately if circulatory impairment, such as cold skin, decreased capillary refill, cyanosis, or absent peripheral pulses in an extremity, or symptoms of organ-related emboli are detected.

NURSING DIAGNOSES, PLANNING, IMPLEMENTATION, AND EVALUATION. See "Nursing Care Plan for the Patient With Infective Endocarditis." Teaching provides patients and families with the ability to provide IV antibiotics at home and promotes health maintenance to prevent future IE. Good hygiene including dental care is essential. Skin care includes bathing, using proper hand-washing technique with soap, avoiding nail biting, not popping pimples or lancing boils, and washing and applying antibiotic ointment to cuts.

Brushing with a soft-bristle toothbrush (to prevent gum trauma) twice a day reduces the formation of plaque (which traps bacteria). Biannual dental cleaning (with prophylactic antibiotics as specified) is important. Recognition of symptoms (e.g., fever, chills, sweats), seeking prompt medical care, and having blood cultures drawn before antibiotics are started, along with the patient's statement of understanding and a willingness to follow lifestyle changes, support goal achievement.

CRITICAL THINKING

Mrs. Jones

■ Mrs. Jones, age 28, is admitted to the hospital with a fever of 100°F (37°C), chills, fatigue, anorexia, and pain in her joints. A physical assessment reveals splinter hemorrhages in the left index finger nailbed and petechiae on her chest. She is diagnosed with a heart murmur and infective endocarditis.

1. Why is a heart murmur heard with endocarditis?
2. What do splinter hemorrhages look like?
3. What do petechiae indicate?
4. How would Mrs. Jones's data collection findings be documented?
5. What type of medication would the nurse expect to be ordered to treat the infection?
6. Why does Mrs. Jones have chills if her temperature is elevated?
7. What signs and symptoms might occur if the complications of heart failure develop?
8. Tylenol 650 mg every 6 hours for pain is ordered. It comes as 325-mg tablets. How many tablets would be given per dose?

Suggested answers are at the end of the chapter.

TABLE 23.4 DATA COLLECTION FOR PATIENTS WITH INFECTIVE ENDOCARDITIS

	Subjective Data
Health History	Infections (rheumatic fever, scarlet fever, previous endocarditis, streptococcal or staphylococcal, syphilis)? Cardiac disease (valvular surgery, congenital)? Childbirth? Invasive procedures (surgery, dental, catheterization, IV therapy, cystoscopy, gynecological)? Malaise? Anorexia?
Medications	Steroids, immunosuppressants, prolonged antibiotic therapy, IV drug use, alcohol use?
Respiratory	Dyspnea on exertion or orthopnea (when lying down)? Cough?
Cardiovascular	Palpitations, chest pain, fatigue, or activity intolerance?
Musculoskeletal	Weakness, arthralgia, myalgia?
Knowledge of Condition	Patient's understanding
	Objective Data
Body Temperature	Fever, diaphoresis
Respiratory	Crackles, tachypnea
Cardiovascular	Murmurs, tachycardia, dysrhythmias, edema
Integumentary	Nailbed splinter hemorrhages; petechiae on lips, mouth, conjunctivae, feet, or antecubital area; paleness
Renal	Hematuria
Diagnostic Test Findings	Positive blood cultures, anemia, elevated WBC count, elevated ESR, ECG showing conduction problems, echocardiogram showing valvular dysfunction and vegetations, chest x-ray exam showing heart enlargement (cardiomegaly) and lung congestion

Note. ECG = electrocardiogram; ESR = erythrocyte sedimentation rate; IV = intravenous; WBC = white blood cell.

NURSING CARE PLAN for the Patient With Infective Endocarditis

Nursing Diagnosis: *Decreased Cardiac Output* related to impaired valvular function or heart failure as manifested by activity intolerance

Expected Outcome: The patient will have adequate cardiac output as evidenced by vital signs WNL, no dyspnea, and minimal fatigue in response to activity.

Evaluation of Outcome: Are patient's vital signs WNL with no dyspnea and minimal fatigue? Can patient participate in desired activities?

Intervention Assess vital signs, murmurs, dyspnea, and fatigue. **Rationale** Abnormal vital signs, dyspnea, and fatigue are indicators of cardiac output decline. **Evaluation** Are vital signs WNL with no dyspnea or fatigue?

Intervention Give oxygen as ordered. Measure oxygen saturation. **Rationale** Supplemental oxygen will increase oxygen level in the blood. **Evaluation** Is oxygen saturation WNL?

NURSING CARE PLAN for the Patient With Infective Endocarditis

Intervention Provide bedrest or rest periods as ordered. **Rationale** Cardiac workload and oxygen needs are reduced with rest. **Evaluation** Are vital signs WNL and no fatigue reported?

Intervention Elevate head of bed 45 degrees. **Rationale** Venous return to heart is reduced and chest expansion improved. **Evaluation** Are vital signs WNL and respirations easy with no reported dyspnea or use of accessory respiratory muscles?

Intervention Assist with activities of daily living (ADLs) as needed, providing rest periods. **Rationale** Assistance conserves energy. Cardiac workload and oxygen needs are reduced with rest. **Evaluation** Are ADLs completed? Does patient report less fatigue?

Nursing Diagnosis: *Deficient Diversional Activity* related to restricted mobility from prolonged IV therapy

Expected Outcome: The patient will state diversional activities are satisfying.

Evaluation of Outcome: Does patient participate in diversional activities? Does patient state satisfaction with activities?

Intervention Assess patient's preferred activities and hobbies. **Rationale** Activity preference should be known to plan satisfactory diversional activities. **Evaluation** Are patient's preferred activities known?

Intervention Plan patient's schedule around relaxing and fun activities, using the patient's input. **Rationale** Self-esteem is fostered with increased patient control. **Evaluation** Does patient offer input into scheduled care? Is input followed?

Intervention Use pet therapy. **Rationale** Individuals who interact with pets live longer and are healthier. **Evaluation** Does patient state enjoyment of pet therapy?

Intervention Provide a mix of physical, mental, and social activities on a rotating schedule. **Rationale** Rotating stimulating activities and visitors will keep patient interested and avoid fatigue. **Evaluation** Does patient state satisfaction in activities with no fatigue?

Pericarditis

Pathophysiology and Etiology

Pericarditis is an acute or chronic inflammation of the pericardium (the sac surrounding the heart). The inflammation creates a problem for the heart as it tries to expand and fill. As a result, ventricular filling is reduced, which then decreases cardiac output and blood pressure. Acute pericarditis usually resolves in less than 6 weeks. Recurrence is possible. Acute pericarditis can be caused by a variety of factors, including the following:

• Infections: viruses, bacteria, fungi, or Lyme disease
• Drug reactions
• Connective tissue disorders: systemic lupus erythematosus, rheumatic fever, or rheumatoid arthritis
• Neoplastic disease
• Postpericardiotomy (e.g., after cardiac surgery)
• Postmyocardial infarction
• **Dressler syndrome** (autoimmune response)
• Renal disease or uremia
• Trauma from chest injury or invasive thoracic procedures

There are several forms of chronic pericarditis. Chronic constrictive pericarditis is the result of fibrous scarring of the pericardium. The heart becomes surrounded by a thickened, stiff sac that limits the stretching ability of the heart's chambers for filling, which may result in HF. Chronic constrictive pericarditis results from neoplastic disease and metastasis, radiation, or tuberculosis.

Signs and Symptoms

Chest pain is the most common symptom of acute pericarditis (Table 23.5). The pain is located substernally and over the heart and may radiate to the clavicle, neck, left scapula, or epigastric area. Typically there is an intense, sharp, creaky, grating pain that increases with deep inspiration, coughing, moving of the trunk, or lying flat. For some the pain is not as intense and is instead a dull ache. The pain may be relieved by sitting up and leaning forward. Other symptoms depend on the cause of the pericarditis and may include orthopnea, low-grade fever, fatigue, cough, and edema.

TABLE 23.5 PERICARDITIS SUMMARY

Signs and Symptoms	Chest pain Dyspnea Low-grade fever Cough Pericardial friction rub
Diagnostic Tests	CBC ECG Echocardiogram MRI CT
Therapeutic Measures	Anti-inflammatory medication Corticosteroids Pericardiocentesis Pericardial window
Complications	Pericardial effusion Cardiac tamponade
Priority Nursing Diagnoses	*Acute Pain* related to inflammation of pericardium *Anxiety* related to disease process *Decreased Cardiac Output* related to cardiac constriction

Note. CBC = complete blood count; CT = computed tomography; ECG = electrocardiogram; MRI = magnetic resonance imaging.

A **pericardial friction rub**—a grating, scratchy, high-pitched sound—may be heard. The rub is a result of friction from the inflamed pericardial and epicardial layers rubbing together as the heart fills and contracts. Depending on the severity of the pericarditis, the rub may be faint when auscultated or loud enough to be audible without auscultation. The rub may be heard intermittently or continuously. It is usually heard over the lower left sternal border of the chest during each heartbeat. It is present in about 50% of those with pericarditis.

Chronic constrictive pericarditis produces dyspnea and signs and symptoms of right-sided HF and may also cause atrial fibrillation.

LEARNING TIP

To simulate the sound of a pericardial friction rub, hold the diaphragm of a stethoscope against the palm of one hand; listen through the stethoscope as you rub the index finger of the opposite hand over the knuckles of the hand holding the diaphragm. The sound you hear is similar to that of a pericardial friction rub.

Diagnostic Tests

Table 23.5 lists diagnostic tests for pericarditis. The ECG reveals ST-T wave elevation in all leads (see Fig. 25.11), which indicates cardiac injury. Echocardiogram results show **pericardial effusions** (buildup of fluid in pericardial space). Serum laboratory tests focus on causes of the pericarditis, such as an elevated white blood cell (WBC) count, indicating a bacterial or viral infection, or elevated blood urea nitrogen or creatinine levels, indicating uremia. Fluid obtained during **pericardiocentesis** (aspiration of fluid from pericardial sac) is examined to diagnose the cause. In chronic constrictive pericarditis, a CT scan or MRI may show a thickened pericardium.

Therapeutic Measures

Mild acute cases may resolve without treatment. The cause is determined so that appropriate treatment can be administered, such as antibiotics for bacterial infections. Bed rest is used to reduce the heart's workload during acute symptoms. Nonsteroidal anti-inflammatory drugs (NSAIDs) or aspirin are given along with colchicine (Colsalide) to resolve inflammation and reduce pain. Corticosteroids are used if initial treatment is not effective. Hemodialysis is used to treat uremic pericarditis. If the patient is unstable, prompt intervention is required, such as an emergency pericardiocentesis.

Chronic effusive pericarditis can be treated with a pericardial window to allow continuous drainage of pericardial fluid into the pleural space. A pericardial window is created surgically by removing a portion of the outer pericardial layer.

Chronic constrictive pericarditis is treated with **pericardiectomy**, which is the surgical removal of the entire tough, calcified pericardium. Pericardiectomy relieves constriction of the heart and allows normal filling of the ventricles.

Complications

A pericardial effusion is the most common complication of pericarditis. A rapidly developing effusion, such as one occurring from trauma, can produce symptoms with smaller amounts of fluid than slowly developing effusions, such as pericarditis from tuberculosis, with larger amounts of fluid. The increasing fluid presses on nearby tissue. Pressure on lung tissue can produce dyspnea, cough, and tachypnea. The heartbeat sounds distant. The body's compensatory mechanisms attempt to maintain blood pressure.

As the fluid accumulation grows, **cardiac tamponade**, another complication of pericarditis, can occur. Cardiac tamponade is a life-threatening compression of the heart

• WORD • BUILDING •

pericardiocentesis: peri—around + kardia—heart + centesis—puncture
cardiac tamponade: kardia—heart + tamponade—plug

by fluid accumulated in the pericardial sac. Cardiac output drops and, to compensate, the heart rate increases. Then blood pressure falls as compensatory mechanisms fail. The patient shows symptoms of decreased cardiac output, such as restlessness, confusion, tachycardia, and tachypnea. Jugular venous distention is present from increased venous pressure, and heart sounds are distant.

Cardiac tamponade requires immediate treatment with pericardiocentesis. The pericardium is punctured with a 16-gauge needle, and excess fluid in the pericardial sac is removed (Fig. 23.8). After the procedure, the patient is monitored for complications, such as dysrhythmias, laceration of a coronary artery, or laceration of the myocardium or pneumothorax.

Nursing Care

A patient history is obtained that includes any cardiac disease, recent infections, and current medications. Vital signs are documented, noting fever, tachycardia, as well as chest pain, pericardial friction rub, and signs of HF.

Nursing care focuses on relieving the patient's pain and anxiety and maintaining normal cardiac function. Pain is rated and treated as ordered. Allowing the patient to assume a position of comfort by sitting up and leaning forward also relieves pain. Teaching the patient about pericarditis and its treatment relieves anxiety and allows a feeling of control by allowing the patient to make knowledgeable health care decisions.

Myocarditis
Pathophysiology and Etiology

In **myocarditis**, inflammation of the myocardium occurs. The amount of muscle destruction and necrosis that occurs as a result of myocarditis determines the extent of damage to the heart. The heart may enlarge in response to the damaged muscle fibers, although most cases of myocarditis are benign, with few signs or symptoms.

Myocarditis is a rare condition that most commonly develops after a viral infection. Other causes are bacteria, parasites, fungi, rickettsiae, spirochetes, medications, lead toxicity, autoimmune factors, human immunodeficiency virus (HIV), rheumatic fever, systemic lupus erythematosus (SLE), pericarditis or IE, or cardiac transplant rejection.

Signs and Symptoms

Signs and symptoms of myocarditis vary from none to severe cardiac manifestations. Fatigue, fever, pharyngitis, malaise, dyspnea, palpitations, muscle aches, GI discomfort, and enlarged lymph nodes may occur early from a viral infection. Cardiac manifestations such as chest pain or tachycardia may occur about 2 weeks after a viral infection. Occasionally, sudden death may occur.

Diagnostic Tests

A myocardial biopsy during the first 6 weeks of inflammation is the preferred diagnostic test for myocarditis, although it is positive only about 30% of the time. Echocardiogram and MRI are helpful. An ECG shows dysrhythmias, commonly sinus tachycardia. Blood tests are done, including CBC, viral antibodies, and enzyme levels that look for heart damage.

Therapeutic Measures

Treatment is aimed at the cause, if known, such as antibiotics for bacterial infections. Interventions to reduce the heart's workload during recovery are essential and include bed rest and limited activity. Exercise increases myocardial inflammation and mortality and should be avoided until symptoms improve and inflammation is gone. The use of alcohol and tobacco should be avoided. Symptoms of HF are treated with medications such as beta blockers, ACE inhibitors, diuretics, or digoxin to reduce the heart's workload and oxygen needs. With myocarditis, the heart is sensitive to digoxin. The patient should be monitored closely for signs of digoxin toxicity, which may include anorexia, nausea, vomiting, bradycardia, dysrhythmias, or malaise.

Heart monitor

Attached to pressure monitor

Pericardium

Xyphoid

Heart

Excessive fluid-filled pericardial sac

Three-way stopcock

Syringe

Heart after pericardiocentesis

Heart

Pericardium

Pericardial sac

FIGURE 23.8 Pericardiocentesis.

• **WORD** • **BUILDING** •
myocarditis: myo—muscle + kardia—heart + itis—inflammation

Nursing Care

Recent illnesses, toxin exposure, cardiac diseases, activity tolerance, and current medications are documented. Vital signs and signs of heart failure, such as jugular venous distention, peripheral edema, crackles, and dyspnea are noted.

Nursing care is aimed at maintaining normal cardiac function by monitoring vital signs, symptoms, and administering medications as ordered. Interventions to reduce fatigue include providing assistance as needed, having frequent rest periods, and teaching energy conservation methods. Reducing the patient's anxiety and increasing his or her knowledge can be achieved by teaching about the disease. Determining diversional activities with the patient for times when activity is restricted further reduces patient anxiety.

Cardiac Trauma

Two types of cardiac trauma can occur: nonpenetrating and penetrating. Nonpenetrating injuries, or contusions, occur from blunt trauma such as motor vehicle accidents or contact sports in which direct compression or force is applied to the upper torso. Contusions may vary from small bruises to hemorrhage.

There may be few or no external injuries indicating traumatic cardiac injury. The patient may be asymptomatic or exhibit signs and symptoms identical to a MI. In severe contusions, laboratory results may show elevated creatine kinase MB (CK-MB, an enzyme) or troponin I (a protein) levels.

If bleeding into the pericardial sac occurs, cardiac tamponade can occur. If signs of shock are present, a pericardiocentesis must be performed. With its own pressure, the tamponade may seal the area of bleeding, so no cardiac decompensation occurs. In this case, only bed rest and observation are required. There are no long-term effects with most contusions. With severe contusions, however, scarring and necrosis of the myocardium may decrease cardiac output and increase the risk for cardiac rupture.

Penetrating traumas include an external injury to the chest, such as a stab or gunshot wound, or an internal injury, such as invasive lines that penetrate the cardiac muscle. Complications vary depending on the size, location, and cause of injury. Tamponade occurs from bleeding into the pericardial sac if the pericardium is sealed off by clot formation. A hemothorax develops if blood drains into the pleural space in the chest. A pneumothorax occurs if air collects in the pleural space. Signs and symptoms of hemorrhage and myocardial ischemia can be noted. Surgical repair may be indicated.

Cardiomyopathy

Cardiomyopathy is an enlargement of the heart muscle. There are three types of cardiac structure and function abnormalities in cardiomyopathy: dilated, hypertrophic, and restrictive (Fig. 23.9). A consequence of each type of cardiomyopathy can be HF (Fig. 23.10), myocardial ischemia, or MI due to reduced cardiac output. There is currently no cure. The greatest advancement for the cardiomyopathies has been in genetic research, which has identified genetic

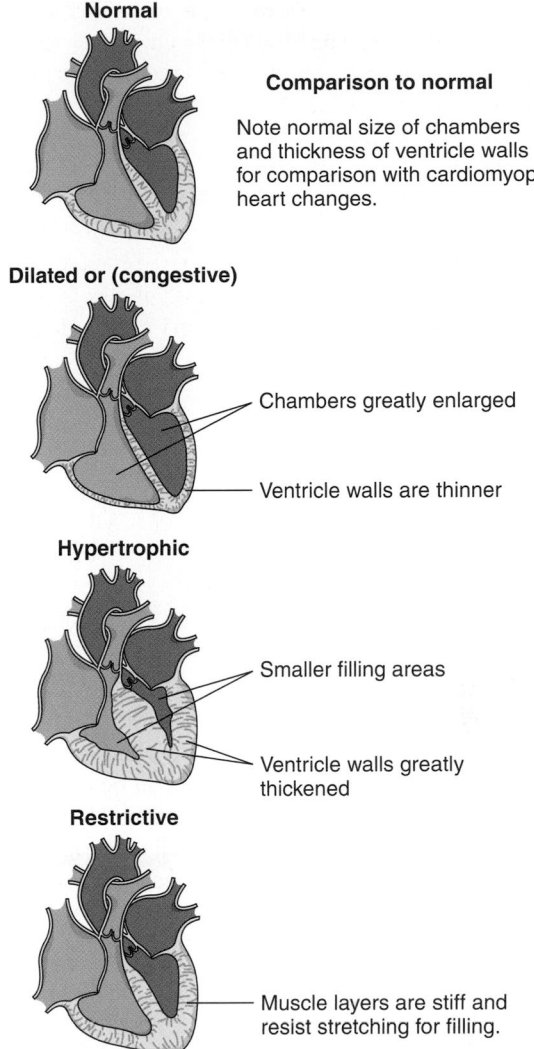

Normal

Comparison to normal

Note normal size of chambers and thickness of ventricle walls for comparison with cardiomyopic heart changes.

Dilated or (congestive)

Chambers greatly enlarged

Ventricle walls are thinner

Hypertrophic

Smaller filling areas

Ventricle walls greatly thickened

Restrictive

Muscle layers are stiff and resist stretching for filling.

FIGURE 23.9 Comparison of the normal heart structure with each type of cardiomyopic heart structure.

mutations that cause these diseases and are leading to better diagnosis and treatment.

Dilated Cardiomyopathy

In dilated cardiomyopathy, the size of the ventricular cavity enlarges with reduced cardiac output. Contractile function decreases as the myocardial tissue is destroyed. Blood moves more slowly from the left ventricle, which often results in blood clot formation. Dilated cardiomyopathy is the most frequent type of cardiomyopathy and one of the most frequent causes of HF. Dilated cardiomyopathy may be caused by genetics, infectious myocarditis, hypertension, heart valve disorders, myocardial infarction, chronic alcohol or cocaine use, metals such as lead, elevated iron levels, HIV, thiamine or zinc deficiencies, cardiac infections, chemotherapy, neuromuscular disorders, or other causes.

• WORD • BUILDING •

cardiomyopathy: kardia—heart + myo—muscle + pathy—disease

FIGURE 23.10 Each type of cardiomyopathy can lead to heart failure.

Hypertrophic Cardiomyopathy

Hypertrophic cardiomyopathy is enlargement of the cardiac muscle wall, often of the septum and left ventricle. The hypertrophy may occur asymmetrically. It can be a hereditary disorder that is transmitted as a dominant trait. Hypertrophic cardiomyopathy causes the ventricular wall to be rigid, which decreases ventricular filling. If an enlarged septum obstructs the outflow of blood through the aortic valve, it is known as obstructive hypertrophic cardiomyopathy. Death can occur suddenly and is likely due to an abnormal heart rhythm.

Restrictive Cardiomyopathy

Restrictive cardiomyopathy impairs ventricular stretch and limits ventricular filling. Cardiac muscle stiffness is present with no ventricular dilation, although systolic emptying of the ventricle remains normal. Restrictive cardiomyopathy is the rarest form of cardiomyopathy. It may be caused by infiltrative diseases such as amyloidosis that deposit the protein amyloid within the myocardial cells, making the muscle stiff and resistant to stretching for easy ventricular filling. Treating the underlying cause may help reduce heart damage.

Signs and Symptoms

Manifestations of cardiomyopathy depend on the type of abnormality. Most patients show varying degrees of signs and symptoms of heart failure (Table 23.6). With dilated cardiomyopathy, left ventricular and then right-sided heart failure with a poor prognosis are seen. Dyspnea on exertion, orthopnea, fatigue, and sometimes atrial fibrillation occur. In hypertrophic cardiomyopathy, exertional dyspnea related to the obstruction of cardiac output is the most common symptom. Angina is not common, but atypical chest pain that occurs at rest and is not relieved with nitrates may occur. With restrictive cardiomyopathy, heart failure symptoms result from the ventricles' inability to fill during diastole. Syncope, arrhythmias, and thrombi may occur.

TABLE 23.6 CARDIOMYOPATHY SUMMARY

Signs and Symptoms	Angina Arrhythmias Dyspnea Fatigue Syncope
Diagnostic Tests	Electrocardiogram Chest x-ray Cardiac catheterization Cardiac magnetic resonance imaging Echocardiography
Therapeutic Measures	Anticoagulants Antidysrhythmics *Dilated cardiomyopathy:* vasodilators, cardiac glycosides, biventricular pacing, ventricular assist device, heart transplant *Hypertrophic cardiomyopathy:* beta blockers, calcium channel blockers, myectomy, septal ablation *Restrictive cardiomyopathy:* vasodilators, heart transplant
Complications	Heart failure
Priority Nursing Diagnoses	*Decreased Cardiac Output* related to impaired myocardial function *Activity Intolerance* related to cardiac insufficiency *Anxiety* related to disease process

Diagnostic Tests

Cardiomegaly is visible on a chest x-ray examination. Echocardiography shows muscle thickness and chamber size to differentiate between the types of cardiomyopathy. Changes related to enlarged chamber size, tachycardia, and dysrhythmias can be seen on the ECG. Cardiac catheterization and biopsy may be useful as well as cardiovascular magnetic resonance. Blood tests may be done to identify infections or elevated metal or iron levels.

Therapeutic Measures

Treatment for both dilated and restrictive cardiomyopathies is palliative, aimed at managing HF and the underlying cause, if known (see Chapter 26). For dilated cardiomyopathy, treatment focuses on the symptoms of HF. ACE inhibitors, angiotensin II receptor blockers, beta blockers,

• WORD • BUILDING •
cardiomegaly: kardia—heart + mega—large

diuretics, aldosterone antagonists, and digoxin may be given. Biventricular pacing and implantable defibrillators may be used. Therapy is not very useful for restrictive cardiomyopathy. Diuretics or nitrates may be used to relieve venous congestion that occurs because of HF. However, a fine balance is needed when using these drugs so that preload is not reduced too greatly, which would worsen symptoms. Anticoagulants are given to prevent emboli formation in patients with atrial fibrillation. Antidysrhythmics or cardioversion is used for dysrhythmias.

For obstructive hypertrophic cardiomyopathy, beta blockers and calcium channel blockers are given to slow the heart rate to allow more filling time and lessen the strength of the heart's contraction. An antiarrhythmic agent might be used. Patients must remain hydrated at all times to maintain cardiac output.

In obstructive hypertrophic cardiomyopathy, digoxin and vasodilators are avoided because they can increase the obstruction. Strenuous exercise and athletic sports are restricted to prevent sudden death. Lower levels of exercise may be allowed. For patients in whom medical therapy is not effective, atrioventricular (AV) sequential pacemakers, implantable automatic defibrillators, or invasive procedures are considered. For those without obstruction, fewer treatment options exist. Diuretics are used to reduce elevated pressures along with beta blockers and calcium channel blockers.

If medical therapy is not successful, surgery is considered. For hypertrophied muscle, surgery to remove part of the ventricular septum (**myectomy**) is done to allow greater outflow of blood. Another option especially for those who are not candidates for surgery is septal ablation. In septal ablation, alcohol is delivered via a catheter to necrose and reduce septal heart wall thickness.

For severe HF, primarily in those with dilated cardiomyopathy, a heart transplant may be the only hope for survival. A ventricular assist device may be used until a donor is found. Many patients die while waiting for a donor heart because donated organs are limited.

Nursing Care

A patient history is obtained that includes signs and symptoms and data collection related to family support systems because of the chronic nature of the disease. A physical assessment is done, noting vital signs and any signs or symptoms of HF.

Nursing care focuses on maintaining normal cardiac function, increasing activity tolerance, relieving anxiety, and educating the patient about the disease and its treatment. Patients with cardiomyopathy can be very ill. Careful monitoring is done to detect complications, such as HF, emboli, or dysrhythmias. The HCP is immediately notified of problems. Home health care is often used for these patients to maintain their functional ability and reduce hospitalizations.

Maintenance of normal cardiac function includes increasing activity tolerance, planning rest periods, scheduling activities in small amounts, avoiding tiring activities, and providing small meals that require less energy to digest than large meals. Patients are encouraged to avoid alcohol because it decreases cardiac function.

Reducing anxiety is important and can be accomplished by providing education regarding procedures, as well as educating the patient about the disease and its treatment. This should provide patients with a greater sense of control and help them to make informed decisions. These patients and their families have a great need for emotional support because of the chronic nature of the disease (see Box 23-3).

VENOUS DISORDERS

Thrombophlebitis

Thrombophlebitis is the formation of a clot, followed by inflammation within a vein. Thrombophlebitis is the most common disorder of veins, with the legs being most often affected. Any superficial or deep vein in the body can be involved. Deep venous thrombosis (DVT) is the most serious form of thrombophlebitis because pulmonary emboli can result if the thrombus detaches (see Chapter 28).

Pathophysiology

A venous thrombus is made up of platelets, RBCs, WBCs, and fibrin. Platelets attach to a vein wall, and then a tail forms as more blood cells and fibrin collect. As the tail grows, it drifts in the blood flowing past it. The turbulence of the blood flow can cause parts of the drifting thrombus to break off and become emboli that travel to the lungs.

Etiology

Three factors, referred to collectively as Virchow's triangle, are involved in the formation of a thrombus: stasis of blood flow, damage to the lining of the vein wall, and increased blood coagulation (Table 23.7). Venous stasis occurs when blood flow is reduced, veins are dilated, muscle contractions are decreased, or vein valves are faulty. When the wall

• WORD • BUILDING •
myectomy: myo—muscle + ectomy—cutting out
thrombophlebitis: thromb—lump (clot) + phleb—vein + itis—inflammation

Box 23-3 Patient Education

Cardiomyopathy

Patients and families should understand the importance of the following:

• Adherence to medication regimen to prevent heart failure
• Having emergency telephone numbers readily available
• Cardiopulmonary resuscitation (CPR) training for family members
• The availability of hospice care and emotional support for families during the grieving process

TABLE 23.7 PREDISPOSING CONDITIONS FOR THROMBOPHLEBITIS (VIRCHOW'S TRIANGLE)

Condition	Type	Example
Venous stasis	Reduction of blood flow	Shock, heart failure, myocardial infarction, atrial fibrillation
	Dilated veins	Vasodilators
	Decreased muscle contractions	Immobility, sitting for long periods as in traveling, fractured hip, paralysis, anesthesia, surgery, obesity, advanced age
	Faulty valves	Varicose veins, venous insufficiency
Venous wall injury		Venipuncture, venous cannulation at same site for >48 hours, venous catheterization, surgery, trauma, burns, fractures, dislocation, intravenous (IV) medications (potassium, chemotherapy drugs, antibiotics, IV hypertonic solutions), contrast agents, diabetes, cerebrovascular disease
Increased coagulation of blood		Anemia, malignancy, antithrombin III deficiency, oral contraceptives, estrogen therapy, smoking, discontinuance of anticoagulant therapy, dehydration, malnutrition, polycythemia, leukocytosis, thrombocytosis, sepsis, pregnancy

of a vein is damaged, it provides a site for a thrombus to form. IV therapy and venipuncture cause trauma to the vein, and IV catheters in place longer than 48 to 72 hours increase the risk of inflammation and thrombus. Increased coagulation of the blood promotes thrombus formation. Patients on oral anticoagulants that are abruptly stopped experience increased clotting of the blood. Smoking, oral contraceptive use, and estrogen therapy also increase blood coagulation. Hematologic disorders can also lead to altered blood coagulation and increased risk of thrombus formation.

Prevention

Identification of risk factors for thrombosis (see Table 23.7) and patient education promote the use of interventions (discussed later) to prevent thrombosis (see "Evidence-Based Practice"). Because older adults are at increased risk for thrombus formation, a family member should also be instructed in techniques that may be difficult for the older person to perform. Dehydration should be avoided to reduce thrombus risk.

IMMOBILITY. People with sedentary jobs that require long periods of sitting, standing, or traveling long distances should change positions, perform knee and ankle flexion exercises, or walk at regular intervals to prevent stasis of blood. Patients on bed rest should have legs elevated above the level of the heart, if possible, and turn every 2 hours to prevent pooling of blood. Postoperatively or in times of bed rest, active or passive range-of-motion (ROM) exercises should be done to increase blood flow. Postoperatively, early ambulation is a major preventive technique for thrombosis. Patients' pain should be controlled to facilitate their ability to participate in early ambulation. Deep

breathing aids in improving blood flow in the large thoracic veins. Smoking should be avoided because nicotine causes vasoconstriction.

EVIDENCE-BASED PRACTICE

Clinical Question
Are statins effective in preventing venous thromboembolism?

Evidence
A large randomized controlled trial involving 17,802 participants aged 50 years or older for men and 60 years or older for women, without a history of cardiovascular disease, a low-density lipoprotein (LDL) cholesterol level of less than 3.4 mmol/L and a high-sensitivity C-reactive protein level of 2.0 mg/L or more found that rosuvastatin (Crestor), a statin, did reduce the incidence of venous thrombosis, especially in the presence of cancer, recent trauma, hospitalization, or surgery. However, the drug did not reduce complications that occurred after diagnosis of venous thrombosis.

Implications for Nursing Practice
It has been shown that statins are effective in reducing venous thromboembolism.

REFERENCE
Li, L., Sun, T., Zhang, P., Tian, J., Tian, J., & Yang, K. (2011). Statins for primary prevention of venous thromboembolism. *Cochrane Database of Systematic Reviews, 12,* CD008203.

BE SAFE!

For prevention of thrombophlebitis:

- Teach and encourage leg exercises if patient is immobilized in bed.
- Ambulate as early as possible.
- Change IV sites every 48 to 72 hours.

PROPHYLACTIC ANTIEMBOLISM DEVICES. Patients with peripheral vascular disease, those on bed rest, and those who have had surgery or trauma may use antiembolism devices to improve blood flow. Knee- or thigh-length elastic compression stockings apply pressure to the leg. They must be applied correctly to avoid a tourniquet effect. Older patients with decreased manual dexterity may need assistance. The skin should be inspected, cleansed, and moisturized daily for irritation under the stockings as ordered. Intermittent pneumatic compression (IPC) devices fill intermittently with air to move venous blood in the legs by simulating contraction of the leg muscles. They may be used in combination with elastic compression stockings. Research that compares the various preventive measures for DVT and rates of DVT in surgical patients has shown that the lowest incidence of DVT occurs with elastic compression stockings and IPC devices used together.

PROPHYLACTIC MEDICATION. Low molecular weight heparin (LMWH) is given postoperatively to prevent thrombosis (Table 23.8). Anticoagulation tests are not monitored with LMWH because of the predictability of its dose-related response. Subcutaneous heparin may also be used postoperatively to prevent thrombosis. Platelet counts must be monitored with either LMWH or heparin to detect heparin-induced thrombocytopenia.

Oral anticoagulants such as warfarin (Coumadin) can be used in the high-risk patient to decrease thrombosis. The

TABLE 23.8   ANTICOAGULANT MEDICATIONS

Medication Class/Action	Examples	Nursing Implications
Coumarin Inhibits liver synthesis of vitamin K dependent clotting factors: II, XII, IX, X.	warfarin (Coumadin)	Monitor INR/PT regularly. Monitor for bleeding, and teach patient to report bleeding. Acetaminophen (Tylenol) used instead of aspirin during therapy. Antidote: Vitamin K.
Heparins Bind to antithrombin III, which then inhibits fibrin formation.	heparin sodium	Do not give intramuscularly because of pain and hematoma. Monitor heparin antifactor Xa or PTT: 1.5–2 times control. Monitor platelet count for decrease. Monitor for bleeding, and teach patient to report bleeding. Antidote: Protamine sulfate.
Low Molecular Weight Heparins (LMWHs) Bind with antithrombin III, inhibiting making of factor Xa and the formation of thrombin.	dalteparin sodium (Fragmin) enoxaparin (Lovenox) fondaparinux (Arixtra)	Bleeding rare. Contraindicated with renal failure due to increased bleeding risk. Teach patient to give injection subcutaneously (with prefilled syringes, do not remove air bubble).
Thrombolytics Promote fibrinolysis to break down fibrin in blood clot.	rPA (Retavase, reteplase) TNK (TNKase, tenecteplase) tissue plasminogen activator (t-PA, alteplase)	Minimize blood draws for 24 hours. Monitor for bleeding. Avoid acetylsalicylic acid, nonsteroidal anti-inflammatory drugs.

Note. INR = international normalized ratio; PT = prothrombin time; PTT = partial thromboplastin time.

international normalized ratio (INR) measures the effectiveness of warfarin therapy using a standardized testing reagent. This means that INR can be used around the world with no variation in results as occurs with prothrombin time (PT) from lab to lab. INR is reported along with the PT. INR should be used; however, a discussion of how to interpret the PT is presented in the following "Learning Tip" for your understanding.

IV THERAPY. Monitoring of IV sites should be performed according to institutional policy time frames to detect signs of thrombophlebitis. Venous cannula sites should be changed regularly according to institutional guidelines (e.g., every 48–72 hours) to prevent thrombus formation.

LEARNING TIP

Before administering anticoagulants, laboratory values must be assessed to ensure patient safety.

- Normal and desired therapeutic INR values for the patient's disorder are provided on the laboratory report. These INR values do not require calculation of a therapeutic range because the values are given on the report.
- Compare the patient's INR value with the desired INR value to determine if it is safe to give the warfarin.
- Although INR is the preferred test for warfarin effectiveness, you might still want to know how to calculate a therapeutic range for PT. PT is measured in seconds. The normal value range gives the seconds required for a fibrin clot to form during the test. If a patient is on warfarin, the purpose is to increase the time (seconds) it takes the blood to clot.
- Because a therapy, warfarin, is being given, a PT range that safely considers the expected effects of the warfarin is needed. This is called the therapeutic range (i.e., a low and a high value). Warfarin's therapeutic range is 1.5 to 2 times the normal PT range. To monitor the patient's therapeutic PT, compare the patient's result with the therapeutic range that you calculate. For example: patient's value on warfarin: 16 seconds (sec)
- Normal PT range: 9 to 12 seconds

To calculate therapeutic range, multiply:

	1.5	2
	× 9 sec	× 12 sec

Therapeutic range: 13.5 sec to 24 sec
Compare the patient's value of 16 seconds with the therapeutic range of 13.5 to 24 seconds to determine that the patient's PT value is safely within the therapeutic range.

Signs and Symptoms

There are two locations for thrombophlebitis: superficial veins and deep veins. Up to 50% of patients have no symptoms with thrombophlebitis in the legs. For others, the symptoms vary according to the size and location of the thrombus, and for some the thrombus becomes an embolus (Table 23.9). If adequate collateral circulation is present near the involved area, symptoms are reduced.

SUPERFICIAL VEINS. Thrombophlebitis in a superficial vein may produce redness, warmth, swelling, and tenderness in the area around the site of the thrombus. The vein feels like a firm cord, which is referred to as induration. The saphenous vein is the most commonly affected vein in the leg. Varicosity of the vein is usually the cause. In the arm, IV therapy is the most common cause.

DEEP VEINS. In a DVT in the leg (femoral vein), swelling, edema, pain, warmth, venous distention, and tenderness with palpation of the calf may be present in the affected leg. Obstruction of blood flow from the leg causes edema and varies with the location of the thrombus. An elevated temperature

TABLE 23.9 THROMBOPHLEBITIS SUMMARY

Signs and Symptoms	*Superficial veins:* redness, warmth, swelling, and tenderness *Deep veins:* swelling, edema, pain, warmth, venous distention, and tenderness
Diagnostic Tests	Venous duplex ultrasound Magnetic resonance venography
Therapeutic Measures	*Superficial veins:* warm, moist heat; analgesics; NSAIDs; compression stockings *Deep veins:* low molecular weight heparin; heparin; warfarin; bedrest with extremity elevation above the level of the heart for 5–7 days; warm, moist heat; compression stocking therapy; thrombolytic therapy; thrombectomy; vena cava filter
Complications	Pulmonary embolism Chronic venous insufficiency Varicose veins Recurrent deep venous thrombosis
Priority Nursing Diagnoses	*Acute Pain* related to inflammation of vein *Impaired Skin Integrity* related to venous stasis *Anxiety* related to uncertain prognosis of disease

NSAID = nonsteroidal anti-inflammatory drugs.

may also be present. Pain in the calf with sharp dorsiflexion of the foot, a classic indication known as a positive Homans' sign, is present in less than 50% of those with thrombophlebitis and is not specific to DVT. Once a DVT is positively diagnosed, it is important to avoid performing Homans' sign because it may cause the clot to become dislodged. Cyanosis and edema may occur if the large veins such as the vena cava are involved.

Complications

The most serious complication of DVT is pulmonary embolism, which is a life-threatening emergency (see Chapter 28). Another complication, chronic venous insufficiency, results from damage to the valves in the vein and causes venous stasis. Signs and symptoms from venous insufficiency that may appear years after a thrombus include edema, pain, brownish discoloration and ulceration of the medial ankle, venous distention, and dependent cyanosis of the leg. This condition can be difficult to treat.

Diagnostic Tests

Diagnostic tests are done to guide treatment, with venous duplex ultrasound being the primary test used (see Table 23.9).

Therapeutic Measures

The goals of treatment are to relieve pain and to prevent pulmonary emboli, thrombus enlargement, and further thrombus development. Superficial thrombophlebitis is treated with warm, moist heat; analgesics; NSAIDs; and elastic compression stockings.

Patients with a proximal DVT may be treated at home if they do not have pulmonary embolism, cardiovascular or pulmonary disease, obesity, or renal failure and are able to adhere to follow-up care. LMWH is given subcutaneously daily or twice a day, and oral warfarin is started (see Table 23.8). Both are taken until the INR is within therapeutic range (about 5 days), then the LMWH is stopped.

Traditional medical care for some DVTs involves a hospital stay with bed rest, elevating the leg above heart level for 5 to 7 days; warm, moist heat; elastic compression stocking (initially on unaffected leg only until acute symptoms are gone on affected leg); and anticoagulants. An initial IV bolus of heparin and then a continuous heparin IV infusion is usually started and continued for up to 10 days to prevent further enlargement of the thrombus and development of new thrombi; it has no effect on the existing clot, which the body dissolves over time. Daily heparin antifactor Xa or partial thromboplastin times (PTTs) are monitored to maintain therapeutic heparin levels. Warfarin is begun 4 to 5 days before the heparin is stopped because it requires 3 to 5 days to reach a therapeutic level. To monitor warfarin's effects, INRs and PTs are done daily, and adjustments in warfarin doses are made based on the results. When the therapeutic INR goal is reached, the heparin is stopped. Warfarin is continued for several months, which necessitates regular monitoring of INR levels to ensure the drug's level is within therapeutic range. For second DVT episodes, lifelong warfarin therapy is used.

An endovascular procedure using the Trellis™ peripheral infusion system is used to remove new-onset proximal (high in leg) blood clots within 2 weeks of symptom onset. A catheter with two balloons is inserted into the vein and through the clot. The balloons are inflated. Then a thrombolytic medication is instilled into the clot through holes along the catheter between the two balloons. The balloons prevent the medication from being systemically absorbed and keep the clot material contained as it dissolves. A motor oscillates (moves) the catheter to disperse the medication along the clot to help dissolve it. Any clot material that remains is aspirated out of the vein through the catheter. Patients usually go home in 24 hours and return to normal activity as ordered. To see this procedure, visit www.bacchusvascular.com/products/trellis/animation.html. Early removal of the clot with this combined mechanical and pharmacological approach improves quality of life and reduces postphlebitic syndrome (PPS), which occurs in up to 50% of DVT patients within 1 year. PPS occurs after a DVT from damage to the vein valves and results in pain, swelling, and leg ulcers, which reduce quality of life. Little can be done for PPS, and treatment aims to prevent leg ulcers.

Other approaches are surgical treatment to prevent pulmonary emboli or chronic venous insufficiency when anticoagulant therapy cannot be used or the risk of pulmonary emboli is great. Venous thrombectomy removes the clot through a venous incision. In some cases, a vena cava filter is placed into the vena cava through the femoral or right internal jugular vein (Fig. 23.11). Once in place, it is opened and attaches to the vein wall. The filter traps clots traveling toward the lungs without hindering blood flow.

Nursing Process for the Patient With Thrombophlebitis

DATA COLLECTION. A patient history is obtained that includes questions regarding recent IV therapy or use of contrast

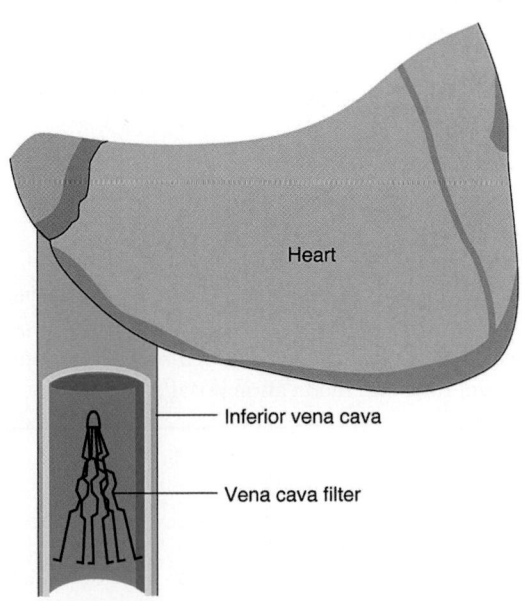

FIGURE 23.11 Vena cava filter placed in the inferior vena cava to prevent emboli from reaching the lungs.

media, surgery, extremity trauma, childbirth, bed rest, recent long trips, cardiac disease, recent infections, and current medications that can put the patient at high risk of thrombus. Physical assessment is done noting pain, fever, tenderness, positive Homans' sign, redness, warmth, swelling, edema, and a firm, cordlike vein in the affected extremity. Daily measurements are taken of bilateral thighs and calves and recorded to monitor swelling. Coagulation tests are monitored. Signs of a pulmonary embolism, such as dyspnea, tachycardia, tachypnea, blood-tinged sputum, chest pain, or changes in level of consciousness are immediately reported to the HCP.

NURSING DIAGNOSES, PLANNING, INTERVENTIONS, AND EVALUATION. See "Nursing Care Plan for the Patient With Thrombophlebitis" for specific nursing interventions. Teaching the patient about the disease and treatment is important to reduce anxiety about complications and to enhance adherence to treatment to prevent complications (see Box 23-4).

Box 23-4 **Patient Education**

Anticoagulant Therapy

Anticoagulants prolong the time it takes blood to clot, so it is important to prevent injury and to recognize and report signs of bleeding to the HCP.

To Prevent Injury
- Wear shoes or slippers; avoid going barefoot.
- Use an electric razor to shave.
- Use a soft toothbrush.

Signs of Bleeding to Report to Physician
- Easy bruising
- Nosebleeds
- Bleeding that does not stop
- Blood in urine
- Blood in sputum
- Blood in stools or black stools

Additional Instructions
- Avoid use of aspirin/NSAIDs because they further prolong the time it takes for a clot to form.
- Have lab work done as prescribed by HCP to monitor clotting time and medication dosage.

Home Health Hints

- On admission, measure the patient's midcalf area so you have a baseline size. Reassess measurements during each visit. Subtle changes in measurement can indicate a potential problem.
- Note whether pressure is being applied on the popliteal area or calf muscle when a patient with venous circulation problems is sitting in a recliner with the leg rest up. The angle of the recliner and the patient's height affect the position of the pressure. A small, flat pillow is placed underneath the knees and lower legs to open the angle and relieve the pressure.
- Report any abnormal findings following cardiovascular surgeries because patients are at a high risk for thrombophlebitis. They also are at risk for incisional infection, pneumonia, and pulmonary emboli.
- Encourage the patient to move often because immobility can contribute to thrombophlebitis.
- If the patient is bed bound, instruct both the patient and caregiver on simple active and passive ROM exercises. If necessary, consider involving occupational and physical therapists. Working collaboratively with therapy, an appropriate activity program can be planned.
- Assist patients to develop energy-conserving techniques by being observant of their lifestyles. For instance, notice the room and chair in which the patient spends most of the day. Trays and baskets can be used to hold items the patient may need or want, such as water, cup, medicines, tissues, a phone book, telephone, snacks, TV remote, reading material, paper, and pen. Other techniques to conserve energy are putting a carrying pouch on the front bar of a walker to carry items such as a portable phone or tissues and, if the house has stairs, putting a chair at the top and bottom of the stairs so the patient can rest.
- The caregiver should be the one to answer the door. When the patient is alone, a note can be placed on the door with instructions; however, the instructions should not convey that the patient is alone.
- Patients on oral anticoagulants should be instructed on dietary guidelines, adherence to follow-up labs, and potential complications. Many times, these patients are discharged with a booklet outlining his or her new medication. Spend time to review this information with the patient and family.

NURSING CARE PLAN for the Patient With Thrombophlebitis

Nursing Diagnosis: *Acute Pain* related to inflammation of vein

Expected Outcome: The patient will report satisfactory pain relief within 30 minutes of pain report.

Evaluation of Outcome: Does patient report satisfactory pain relief?

Intervention Assess pain using rating scale such as 0 to 10. **Rationale** Self-report is the most reliable indicator of pain. **Evaluation** Does patient report pain using scale?

Intervention Provide analgesics and NSAIDs as ordered. **Rationale** Pain is reduced when inflammation is decreased. **Evaluation** Is patient's rating of pain lower after medication?

Intervention Apply warm, moist soaks. **Rationale** Heat relieves pain and vasodilates, which increases circulation to aid comfort. Moist heat penetrates more deeply. **Evaluation** Does patient report increased comfort with warm, moist soaks?

Intervention Maintain bedrest with leg elevation above heart level. **Rationale** Elevation above heart level decreases swelling by aiding venous blood flow back to the heart. **Evaluation** Is swelling reduced, documented by measuring extremities?

Nursing Diagnosis: *Impaired Skin Integrity* related to venous stasis

Expected Outcome: The patient's skin will remain intact.

Evaluation of Outcome: Does patient's skin remain intact?

Intervention Observe skin for edema, skin color changes, and ulcers. Measure extremities, bilaterally at same location in each extremity. **Rationale** Monitoring will detect signs of skin integrity impairment and extremity swelling. Edematous skin breaks down more easily. **Evaluation** Are skin changes seen? Do daily measurements show a change in swelling?

Intervention Elevate feet above heart level. **Rationale** Elevation decreases swelling by increasing blood flow to heart. **Evaluation** Is swelling reduced?

Intervention Fit and apply elastic compression stockings after edema is reduced, as ordered. **Rationale** Elastic compression stockings are fitted after edema is reduced to avoid constriction. The compression of elastic stockings increases blood flow to reduce swelling. **Evaluation** Is swelling reduced?

Intervention Teach patient to avoid crossing legs or wearing constricting clothes. **Rationale** Crossing legs and constrictive clothes impair venous return. **Evaluation** Does patient state understanding of teaching?

SUGGESTED ANSWERS TO

CRITICAL THINKING

■ *Mrs. Tepley*

1. You might hear a murmur.
2. Stress and caffeine increase the occurrence of palpitations.
3. To help manage her condition, Mrs. Tepley needs a definition of MVP, stress management techniques, to know

she should reduce caffeine intake (e.g., drink decaffeinated coffee), and to understand symptoms of endocarditis to report to her HCP.

■ *Mrs. Pryor*

1. In aortic stenosis, the valve is narrowed, which makes it more difficult for blood to leave the left ventricle and go into the aorta. This means there can be less

SUGGESTED ANSWERS TO

blood flow to the body, which is most likely why Mrs. Pryor is feeling tired.

   Documentation using the SOAP method: S: "What is aortic stenosis?" O: Listened attentively during explanation that in aortic stenosis the valve is narrowed making it more difficult for blood to leave left ventricle to go to aorta. This means there can be less blood flow to the body. A: Interested in learning more about diagnosis. P: Provide more information written and verbal.

2. Angina results if the heart is not getting enough oxygen-rich blood.

3. Nursing care should include fall precautions due to syncope and fatigue. Teaching should be based on Mrs. Pryor's need for safety at home, assistance with ADLs, and her questions and concerns.

4. Diagnoses and care include the following: *Self-Care Deficits* related to fatigue, so plan for meeting ADL needs. *Activity Intolerance* related to fatigue, so plan rest periods between activity and monitor vital signs with activity.

5. You should give two tablets. Here is an example of how to solve this problem using the unit analysis method:

$$\frac{0.25 \text{ mg}}{} \left| \frac{1 \text{ tablet}}{0.125 \text{ mg}} \right. = 2 \text{ tablets}$$

■ *Mrs. Jones*

1. A heart murmur is heard from damaged heart valves.

2. Splinter hemorrhages appear as black or red lines in the nails.

3. Petechiae indicate that tiny pieces of a lesion on the endocardium or valves have broken off and become microemboli.

4. Subjective data collection findings might include patient statements such as, "I have pain in my joints and am chilled" or "I am fatigued and have no appetite." Objective findings are as follows: temperature 100°F (37°C), red splinter hemorrhages in left index finger nailbed, many petechiae on chest.

5. Expected medications include IV antibiotics.

6. Chilling is muscular work that raises the body's temperature. Raising the body's temperature is part of the inflammatory process and is the body's attempt at developing an unfavorable environment for the pathogen. Removing blankets to decrease fever results in chills and shivering, which further increases body temperature from the heat generated by muscular activity during shivering. Therefore, Mrs. Jones should be kept covered to prevent chills.

7. For left-sided HF, crackles, wheezes, cough, or dyspnea might be present. In right-sided HF, peripheral edema or jugular venous distention may be present.

8. Two tablets.

REVIEW QUESTIONS

1. The nurse is caring for a team of patients. After completing morning rounds, which of the following patients require priority care?
   1. A patient who is 2 days postsurgery reporting severe constipation.
   2. A patient with a DVT has peripheral edema.
   3. A patient with aortic stenosis who is reporting chest pain.
   4. A patient with mitral valve prolapsed has lost 2 pounds of weight this morning.

2. The nurse is evaluating patient teaching for mitral valve prolapse. The patient shows understanding of the prognosis of MVP by stating which of the following?
   1. "The prognosis is poor."
   2. "There are often no symptoms."
   3. "Heart failure often occurs."
   4. "Symptoms quickly progress."

3. The nurse is evaluating a patient's preoperative teaching for a commissurotomy. The patient shows understanding of the purpose of this procedure by stating which of the following?
   1. "Fused valve flaps are separated to enlarge the valve opening."
   2. "A mechanical valve is inserted to replace a valve."
   3. "The valve flaps are repaired or reconstructed."
   4. "A biological valve is inserted to replace a valve."

4. The nurse is evaluating understanding after a teaching session for mechanical cardiac valve replacement surgery. Which statement by the patient indicates understanding of teaching?
   1. "You will need anticoagulants for the first month after surgery."
   2. "You will not need to be on anticoagulant therapy."
   3. "You will need anticoagulant therapy for the first year after valve replacement."
   4. "You will need anticoagulant therapy for life."

5. The nurse evaluates the patient as understanding how to prevent rheumatic fever if the patient states that rheumatic fever can be prevented by treating streptococcal infections with which of the following?
   1. Penicillin
   2. Prednisone
   3. Cortisone
   4. Cyclosporine

6. The nurse is caring for a patient with cardiomyopathy. Which of the following symptoms, if reported by the patient, require priority action by the nurse?
   1. Left great toe pain
   2. Dyspnea
   3. Headache
   4. Decreased appetite

7. The nurse is collecting data on a patient who had surgery. Which of the following signs and symptoms indicate to the nurse the possible presence of a deep venous thrombus in the patient's leg? **Select all that apply.**
   1. Calf swelling
   2. Crackles
   3. Jugular venous distention
   4. Positive Homans' sign
   5. Warmth
   6. Redness

8. The nurse reviews medication orders and is to give warfarin (Coumadin). Which of the following actions should the nurse take first?
   1. Obtain a glass of water.
   2. Prepare the medication for administration.
   3. Review international normalized ratio result.
   4. Document the medication administration.

Answers can be found in Appendix C.

Reference

American Heart Association. (2014). Infective endocarditis. Retrieved February 16, 2014, from www.heart.org/HEARTORG /Conditions/CongenitalHeartDefects/TheImpactofCongenital HeartDefects/Infective-Endocarditis_UCM_307108_Article.jsp

 Davis*Plus* | For additional resources and information visit **davispl.us/medsurg5**

24

Nursing Care of Patients With Occlusive Cardiovascular Disorders

MAUREEN McDONALD

KEY TERMS

acute coronary syndrome (ah-KYOOT KOR-uh-nare-ee sin-dr-OME)

anastomosed (an-AST-tah-most)

aneurysm (AN-yur-izm)

angina pectoris (an-JYE-nah PEK-tuh-riss)

arteriosclerosis (ar-TEER-ee-oh-skleh-ROH-siss)

atherosclerosis (ATH-er-oh-skleh-ROH-siss)

collateral circulation (kuh-LAH-tur-al SIR-kew-LAY-shun)

coronary artery disease (KOR-uh-nare-ee AR-tuh-ree dih-ZEEZ)

endarterectomy (en-DART-tur-eck-toe-me)

embolism (EM-buh-lizm)

high-density lipoprotein (HY DEN-sih-tee LIH-poh-PROH-teen)

hyperlipidemia (HY-pur-LIH-pih-DEE-mee-ah)

intermittent claudication (IN-tur-MIT-tent KLAW-dih-KAY-shun)

low-density lipoproteins (LOH DEN-sih-tee LIH-poh-PROH-teen)

lymphangitis (lim-FAN-jee-EYE-tiss)

myocardial infarction (MY-oh-KAR-dee-yuhl in-FARK-shun)

peripheral arterial disease (puh-RIFF-uh-ruhl ar-TEER-ee-uhl dih-ZEEZ)

plaque (PLAK)

Raynaud's disease (rah-NOHZ dih-ZEEZ)

thrombosis (throm-BOH-siss)

varicose veins (VAR-ih-kohz VAINS)

venous stasis ulcers (VEE-nus STAY-siss UL-sers)

LEARNING OUTCOMES

1. Explain the etiologies, signs, symptoms, and therapeutic measures of coronary artery disease, angina pectoris, and myocardial infarction.

2. List data to collect for patients with coronary artery disease, angina pectoris, or myocardial infarction.

3. Describe what therapeutic measures are used to treat coronary artery disease, angina pectoris, and myocardial infarction.

4. Explain the etiologies, signs, and symptoms for each of the peripheral vascular disorders.

5. Identify therapeutic measures used to treat peripheral vascular disorders.

6. Plan nursing care for patients with a peripheral vascular disorder.

Cardiovascular diseases (CVDs) are the leading cause of disability and death in the United States. Diseases of the heart and peripheral vessels can affect quality of life and alter the ability of the individual to perform tasks of everyday living. Many factors leading to cardiovascular diseases can be controlled or modified. Education is important in preventing and treating occlusive CVDs.

An estimated 83.6 million American adults have one or more types of CVDs. In 2012, an estimated 785,000 Americans will have had a new **myocardial infarction** (MI) and 470,000 a recurrent MI. About every 25 seconds, a person in the United States will have a coronary event, and every minute someone will die from one (Roger et al, 2012).

More than one in three women have some form of CVD, which occurs on average about 6 years later than in men, often after menopause. In 2010, incidence of coronary heart disease (CHD) was greatest in people over age 65. The prevalence among men was 7.8% and in women, 4.6%. The average age for a person having a first heart attack is 64.5 for men and 70.3 for women. Smoking lowers this age for both genders but more so for women. Because women typically have heart attacks at older ages than men, they are more likely to die from heart attacks within a few weeks. It is interesting to note that the prevalence of CHD decreases with higher education. People with less than a high school education had rates of 9.2%, whereas those with a college degree had rates of 4.6 % (Centers for Disease Control and Prevention, 2011).

ARTERIOSCLEROSIS

Arteriosclerosis is a disorder characterized by thickening, loss of elasticity, and calcification of arterial walls. This condition is part of the aging process in which the intimal lining of the artery wall loses elasticity and weakens. This weakening is due to the high pressure that carries blood within arteries.

ATHEROSCLEROSIS

Atherosclerosis is the formation of plaque within the arterial wall. Arteriosclerosis and atherosclerosis are conditions that may begin in early childhood and progress without symptoms through adult life. It causes coronary artery disease (CAD), leads to CHD (Table 24.1).

Pathophysiology

Atherosclerosis is a multistep process that affects the inner lining of the artery (Fig. 24.1). First injury to the endothelial cells that line the walls of the arteries occurs, causing inflammation and immune reactions. Damage to the endothelium stimulates the growth of smooth muscle cells. These cells secrete collagen and fibrous proteins. Lipids, platelets, and other clotting factors accumulate. Scar tissue replaces some of the arterial wall.

• WORD • BUILDING •
arteriosclerosis: arterio—artery + sklerosis—hardness

TABLE 24.1 ATHEROSCLEROSIS SUMMARY

Diagnostic Tests	Cholesterol Triglycerides Arteriogram
Therapeutic Measures	Low-fat, low-cholesterol diet Smoking cessation Increased exercise—walk 30 minutes daily
Priority Nursing Diagnoses	*Deficient Knowledge* related to self-care and health promotion *Pain* related to reduced vascular or coronary artery blood flow

Normal artery

Atherosclerotic artery

FIGURE 24.1 (Top) Cross-section of normal coronary artery. (Bottom) Coronary artery with atherosclerosis narrowing the lumen.

An early indication of injury is a fatty streak on the lining of the artery. This buildup of fatty deposits is known as **plaque**. It is composed of smooth muscle cells, fibrous proteins, and cholesterol-laden foam cells. Plaque has irregular, jagged edges that allow blood cells and other material to adhere to the wall of the artery. The portion of the plaque that faces the bloodstream develops a fibrous cap, a firm shell that often contains calcium. Over time this buildup becomes calcified and hardened, causing turbulence that damages cells and increases the buildup within the vessel. Sometimes the plaque's fibrous cap tears or ruptures, and a blood clot forms. This blood clot can completely block the coronary artery, or it may break loose and lodge within a smaller artery leading to the heart. The vessel may also become stenosed (narrowed) by plaque buildup. This buildup of plaque may cause partial or total occlusion of the artery, resulting in reduced blood flow. The area distal to the occlusion may become ischemic as a result.

Etiology

Risk factors for atherosclerosis can be divided into two categories: those that can be modified and those that cannot (Table 24.2).

Diagnostic Tests

Total cholesterol levels above 200 mg/dL increase risk of MI (see Table 21.3). **Low-density lipoproteins** (LDLs) increase CAD risk, but **high-density lipoproteins** (HDL) are protective against CAD. A risk factor for premature CAD is a high Lp(a) cholesterol (a genetic variation of plasma LDL) level. Apolipoprotein B particles in LDL-type cholesterol are able to infiltrate the arterial wall, rapidly causing damage. People with a higher proportion of apolipoprotein B to apolipoprotein A are at a much higher risk for CVD. C-reactive protein (CRP) can indicate low-grade inflammation in coronary vessels and long-term heart disease risk. Elevated blood glucose levels can increase the risk for atherosclerosis. Radiological studies of the arteries can be performed to show narrowed or occluded vessels (see Chapter 21).

Therapeutic Measures

A healthy lifestyle, controlling risk factors, medications, and medical exams are helpful in controlling arteriosclerosis and atherosclerosis.

Diet

Because the formation of plaque within arteries is primarily caused by fatty deposits, an adherence to a healthy diet is recommended by the AHA. Heart-healthy foods include a variety of those colorful fruits and vegetables that have no trans fat; are low in saturated fat, cholesterol, sodium, and added sugars; and those that are high in whole-grain fiber and lean protein ("Nutrition Notes"). The AHA has guidelines and diets for decreasing fat and cholesterol intake at http://mylifecheck.heart.org.

Smoking

The risk of developing CAD is two to six times higher in cigarette smokers than in nonsmokers. Risk is proportionate to the number of cigarettes smoked. Smoking contributes to a

TABLE 24.2   RISK FACTORS FOR ATHEROSCLEROSIS/CORONARY ARTERY DISEASE

Risk Factors That Cannot Be Changed	
Age	Men have increased incidence after age 50. Women have increased incidence after menopause.
Ethnicity	African Americans have a higher incidence of atherosclerosis.
Gender	Men have more risk factors and higher incidence of coronary artery disease (CAD).
Genetics	CAD risk factors such as hyperlipidemia can run in families.
Risk Factors That Can Be Changed or Controlled	
Diabetes	Increases the risk of hypertension, obesity, and elevated blood lipids.
Hypertension	Vasoconstriction increases myocardial oxygen demand.
Elevated serum cholesterol	Level above 240 mg/dL increases the risk of developing CAD.
Elevated apolipoprotein B	Infiltrate arterial wall, rapidly causing damage
Elevated serum homocysteine	Increases CAD risk. Foods that contain folic acid (fruits, green leafy vegetables) reduce homocysteine level.
Excessive alcohol use	Raises blood pressure, increases triglycerides, causes irregular heartbeats.
Obesity	Increases heart workload and risk of hypertension, diabetes, glucose intolerance, hyperlipidemia.
Sedentary lifestyle	Increases obesity, hypertension, hyperlipidemia.
Stress	Increases heart workload and risk for hypertension.
Tobacco use including passive smoking (secondhand)	Causes vasoconstriction and increases myocardial oxygen demand. Decreases high-density lipoproteins.

Nutrition Notes

Controlling Blood Cholesterol With Diet

Two-thirds of the body's cholesterol is produced by the liver and intestines. Most people produce less cholesterol or increase its excretion in response to high levels of dietary cholesterol, but others respond weakly. In particular, obese individuals respond less to reductions in dietary saturated fat and cholesterol than do lean persons (Flock, Green, Kris-Etherton, 2011). Although only foods of animal origin contain cholesterol, some vegetable oil products contain trans fats, potent risk factors for cardiovascular disease.

The basis for the cholesterol-lowering diet is:
- Reducing saturated fat to less than 7% of total kilocalorie intake
- Reducing dietary cholesterol to less than 200 milligrams per day.

In dietary studies of about 1 month duration where all foods were provided, LDL cholesterol is reduced by 22 to 30%, whereas in community-based studies of more than 6 months' duration, where dietary advice is the basis of the intervention, reduction in LDL cholesterol is about 15%. This amount is possibly sufficient to reduce the need for pharmaceutical interventions (Harland, 2012).

Specific strategies to lower blood cholesterol include the following:
- Reducing saturated fat intake by choosing
- 2 to 3 servings per day of nonfat or low-fat dairy products
- 5 ounces of lean meat per day, trimming fat from meat, rinsing browned ground beef, and skimming fat from meat juices for soup or gravy
- 2 egg yolks per week; egg whites, egg substitutes as desired

Adding foods for which the U.S. Food and Drug Administration has approved health claims such as:
- Foods rich in marine omega-3 fatty acids (herring, mackerel, rainbow trout, salmon, sardines, swordfish, and tuna)
- Foods containing soluble fiber (Kellogg's Bran Buds, barley, oatmeal)
- Soy-containing foods
- Foods containing plant sterols (butter and margarine spreads, juices, salad dressings, soy milk) that interfere with intestinal absorption of cholesterol. Note, however, that they are contraindicated in a rare autosomal recessive disorder called sitosterolemia.

loss of HDL. These proteins are the best cholesterol to have in the body to decrease the risk of CVDs. Smoking also causes vasoconstriction, which leads to angina pectoris and cardiac dysrhythmias. The benefits of smoking cessation are dramatic and almost immediate. Education about the risks of smoking and effects of exposure to secondhand and third-hand (residual nicotine and other chemicals left on indoor surfaces—from skin, clothing, and hair to bedding, carpets, floors, furniture, and walls—by tobacco smoke) smoke should be presented to patients. The American Cancer Society has many programs to help patients quit smoking. Visit its website at www.cancer.org.

Exercise

Increased activity raises HDL levels. Increasing physical activity may also lower insulin resistance and facilitate weight loss. Over time, exercise also leads to the development of **collateral circulation**, which allows blood to flow around occluded sites. Before beginning an exercise program, consult a health care provider (HCP).

Medications

Lowering lipid levels is the primary therapy for atherosclerosis. When dietary control is not effective, medication is also used (Table 24.3). It may take 4 to 6 weeks before lipid levels respond to drug therapy. If one drug does not control lipids, another drug can be added.

CORONARY ARTERY DISEASE

Coronary artery disease is the obstruction of blood flow through the coronary arteries to the heart muscle cells, typically from atherosclerosis. Blood flow reduction resulting from CAD can cause angina, MI, or sudden death if blood flow is not restored.

Prevention

Risk factors for CAD are listed in Table 24.2. The risk factors that can be changed should be modified following the AHA's guidelines (see therapeutic measures for atherosclerosis). Low-dose aspirin as recommended by an HCP can be used to prevent the formation of a thrombus.

Angina Pectoris
Pathophysiology

When an increased workload is placed on the heart, as in exercise or strenuous activity, there is an increased demand for oxygen. Normally, when the heart muscle needs more oxygen, the coronary arteries dilate to carry more blood and oxygen. However, with CAD, the narrowed vessels are unable to dilate and supply the heart muscle with this extra blood and oxygen. This inability to supply more blood and oxygen causes myocardial ischemia and can produce its symptom, **angina pectoris** (chest pain). Angina may also result from other conditions that cause myocardial ischemia such as vasospasm, valvular heart disease, hypertension, or heart failure (HF).

• **WORD** • **BUILDING** •
angina pectoris: angina—to choke + pectora—chest

TABLE 24.3 MEDICATIONS USED TO LOWER LIPID LEVELS

Medication Class/Action	Examples	Nursing Implications
Statins First-line drugs to reduce low-density lipoprotein by reducing cholesterol synthesis.	atorvastatin (Lipitor) fluvastatin (Lescol XL) lovastatin (Mevacor) pravastatin (Pravachol) simvastatin (Zocor) rosuvastatin (Crestor)	Monitor liver function studies. Monitor for rhabdomyolysis (lethal breakdown of skeletal muscle). *Teaching:* Explain to take in the evening when cholesterol synthesis is highest. Teach patient to report any muscle pain.
Fibrates Reduce triglycerides.	fenofibrate (TriCor) clofibrate (Atromid-S) gemfibrozil (Lopid)	Tell patient to take 30 minutes before morning and evening meal. May increase the effects of anticoagulants and hypoglycemia.
Bile Acid Sequestrants Lower cholesterol by binding bile acids, so stored cholesterol is used to make more bile acids.	colestipol (Colestid) colesevelam HCl (Welchol, Sankyo) cholestyramine (Questran)	Fruits and vegetables high in fiber should be added to diet to reduce constipation and other gastrointestinal effects noted with bile acid sequestrants. May interfere with absorption of digoxin, thiazides, and beta blockers.
Niacin Prevents conversion of fats into very low-density lipoproteins. Rarely used because of flushing.	niacin (Nicotinic acid) extended-release niacin (Niaspan)	Take aspirin 30 minutes before taking drug to reduce flushing.
Cholesterol Absorption Inhibitor Inhibits the absorption of cholesterol. Decreases LDLs and increases HDLs.	ezetimibe (Zetia)	Tell patient to take with liquids and meals and to take other drugs 1 hour before or 4 hours after.
Combination Agent See each agent.	Vytorin (Zetia + Zocor)	See each agent.

LEARNING TIP

Angina pectoris is not a disease. It is the symptom of ischemia that results from a lack of oxygen and blood flow to the heart muscle.

Types of Angina

Angina can be classified as stable (less serious) or unstable.

STABLE ANGINA. Stable angina is chest pain that occurs with moderate exertion in a pattern that is familiar to the patient. The pain is predictable and can usually be managed with nitroglycerin (NTG) and rest. The pain of stable angina usually subsides when the activity is stopped.

VARIANT OR VASOSPASTIC ANGINA (PRINZMETAL'S ANGINA). This type of angina is caused by coronary artery spasms and is serious. The pattern of occurrence is often cyclical, with the pain presenting about the same time each day. The pain has a longer duration than stable angina, can occur with exercise or at rest, and often occurs at night.

Signs and Symptoms

Anginal pain manifests in several ways. Patients (especially men) often describe the pain as heaviness, tightness, squeezing, viselike, or crushing in the center of the chest or adjacent to the chest (Fig. 24.2). The pain can radiate down one or both arms, with pain in the left arm being more common, into the shoulder, neck, jaw, or back. Patients may also describe heaviness in their arms or a feeling of impending doom. During the episode of pain, the patient may be pale, diaphoretic, or dyspneic.

The pain is usually brought on by exertion and subsides with rest. It can be relieved with a vasodilator such as NTG. Episodes of chest pain may increase in frequency and severity over time. If patients do not heed the warning to stop their activity and rest, they may be at risk for MI or sudden death.

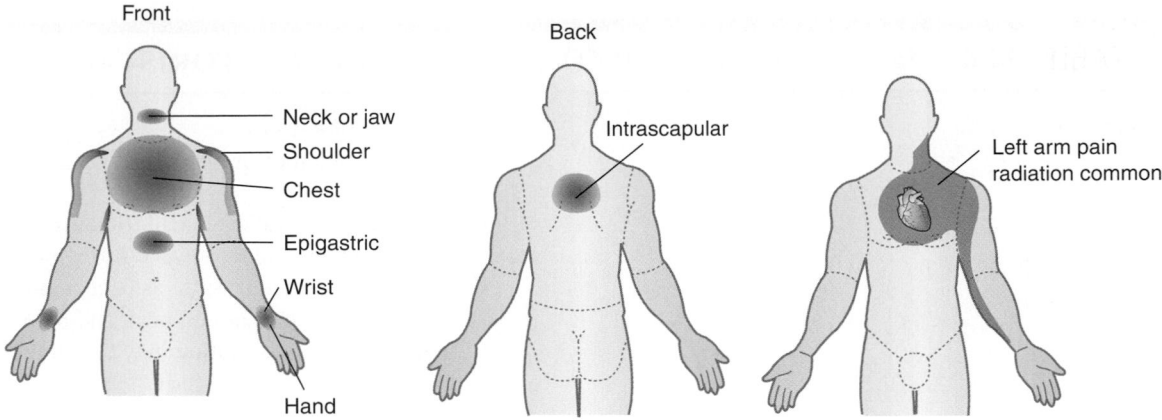

FIGURE 24.2 Common locations of anginal pain, which may vary in combination and intensity.

Any event that increases oxygen demand can cause an anginal attack. Most often, precipitating events include large meals, exercise, cold, stimulant drugs such as cocaine or amphetamines, stress, and emotional tension. Angina commonly occurs in the morning between 0600 and 1200 when the patient arises and the workload of the heart increases.

Women often experience angina symptoms atypically. They can experience chest pain, jaw pain, or heartburn but often have atypical symptoms of shortness of breath, fatigue, nausea, or less severe pain. Atypical symptoms should be recognized as possibly being cardiac related so that they are not ignored and treatment is sought. (See the "Women and Heart Health" section.)

Diagnostic Tests

Common tests for diagnosing CAD or angina causes include electrocardiogram (ECG), exercise stress test, echocardiography,

chemical stress testing, cardiac computed tomography (CT) scan, cardiac magnetic resonance imaging (MRI)/magnetic resonance angiogram (MRA), radioisotope imaging, and coronary angiography (see Table 21.3).

Therapeutic Measures

Treatment for CAD and angina is directed at relieving and preventing anginal episodes that could lead to a MI. The risk factors identified for the patient determine the course of treatment. Weight reduction following a heart healthy diet and stress reduction may help slow disease progression. The three major groups of medication used for reliving angina are vasodilators (nitrates), calcium channel blockers, and beta blockers (Table 24.4).

VASODILATORS. NTG, a nitrate, is the drug of choice for acute anginal attacks. Nitrates dilate coronary arteries to increase oxygen to the myocardium and dilate peripheral

TABLE 24.4 MEDICATIONS USED TO TREAT ANGINA PECTORIS

Medication Class/Action	Examples	Nursing Implications
Antiplatelets Inhibit platelet activation, adhesion, or procoagulant activity.	aspirin	Enteric coated may be given for daily dosing. Monitor for bleeding.
Statins *(See Table 24.2.)*		
Nitrates Vasodilate to reduce preload and afterload. Reduce oxygen consumption of myocardium.	nitroglycerin (Nitrostat, NitroQuick); nitroglycerin lingual spray (Nitrolingual Pumpspray) isosorbide dinitrate (Isordil) isosorbide mononitrate (Imdur, ISMO)	Document onset, type, radiation, location, and duration of chest pain. Take apical pulse and BP pre- and postadministration. Place sublingual (SL) tablet in buccal pouch to lessen burning sensation under tongue. Do not shake aerosol canister before administration of lingual spray.

Continued

TABLE 24.4   MEDICATIONS USED TO TREAT ANGINA PECTORIS—cont'd

Medication Class/Action	Examples	Nursing Implications
		Teaching: Explain to rise slowly, especially with SL spray. If chest pain is not relieved, call 911. Tablets should be replaced every 3 to 6 months. Keep tablets in original bottle as become inactive when exposed to light, air, heat, and moisture. Burning or tingling sensation may be felt under the tongue with SL nitroglycerin. Use of erectile dysfunction medications is contraindicated because they can cause a drop in blood pressure. Explain to avoid alcohol.
	nitroglycerin (Transderm Nitro, Nitro-Bid) nitroglycerin patch (Nitro-Dur, Nitrek)	Remove patch before MRI or defibrillation. *Teaching:* Remove old transdermal patch before applying new patch. Rotate application sites. Apply patch to clean, dry, hairless area. Remove at bedtime so tolerance does not develop.
Angiotensin-Converting Enzyme Inhibitors Block production of angiotensin II, a potent vasoconstrictor. Vasodilate and improve cardiac output and exercise tolerance.	captopril (Capoten) lisinopril (Prinivil, Zestril) ramipril (Altace) enalapril (Vasotec)	If pulse is less than 60 beats per minute or systolic blood pressure (BP) less than 90 mm Hg, notify HCP. Give 1 hour before meals. Give captopril on empty stomach. *Teaching:* Take first doses at night to adjust to lower BP. Rise slowly. Check BP weekly. Report development of dry cough or other side effects.
Calcium Channel Blockers Dilate peripheral arteries, decrease myocardial contractility, depress conduction system, and decrease workload of the heart. In variant angina, reduce coronary artery spasm.	diltiazem (Cardizem, Dilacor XR) amlodipine (Norvasc) nicardipine (Cardene) felodipine (Plendil)	If pulse less than 60 beats per minute or systolic BP less than 90 mm Hg, notify HCP. Administer before meals and at bedtime.
Beta Blockers Decrease pulse, BP, and cardiac output and suppress renin activity. Decrease the risk of sudden death.	metoprolol (Lopressor, Toprol XL) atenolol (Tenormin)	Beta blockers are contraindicated in asthma, heart block, bronchoconstriction. If pulse less than 60 beats per minute or systolic BP less than 90 mm Hg, notify HCP. *Teaching:* Explain to rise slowly. Abrupt withdrawal may result in diaphoresis, palpitations, headache, and tremors.
Anti-Ischemic Agent Antianginal agent used as combination therapy for those not responding to other antianginal.	ranolazine (Ranexa)	May not be as effective in women. Prolongs QT interval on ECG.

vessels so the heart does not have to work so hard to pump blood into them. NTG can be administered sublingually, orally, transdermally, intravenously (IV), or as a lingual spray. When administered sublingually, NTG may relieve chest pain within 1 to 2 minutes (Box 24-1).

BE SAFE!

Sublingual NTG:
AHA guidelines instruct people to immediately call 911 after one tablet and 5 minutes if pain remains unrelieved and symptoms of a MI are occurring.

Transdermal NTG:
Wear gloves to protect yourself from hypotension from touching the ointment or patch medication. Always remove the previous ointment or patch before applying a new one to prevent overdose.

Long-acting nitrates are used to prevent chest pain rather than to treat acute pain. They can be given orally, in ointment, or by transdermal patches. A problem with long-acting nitrates is the development of a tolerance to the drug. To prevent tolerance, the patch or ointment is usually removed at bedtime and reapplied in the morning, giving the patient an 8- to 12-hour nitrate-free period. Headaches may be experienced when nitrates are first begun. This side effect usually subsides after a week or two and can be relieved with aspirin.

CALCIUM CHANNEL BLOCKERS. Calcium is required for electrical excitability of cardiac cells and contraction of the myocardium and vascular smooth muscle. Calcium channel blockers relax vascular smooth muscle, which leads to decreased peripheral vascular resistance (afterload) and decreased myocardial oxygen demand. These drugs dilate main coronary arteries, increasing the myocardial oxygen supply. Calcium channel blockers are also used to decrease systolic and diastolic blood pressures and to slow the heart rate. Because these drugs are slow acting, they are ineffective in relieving acute anginal attacks. Side effects of calcium channel blockers are usually mild and include constipation, fluid retention, headache, and dizziness.

BE SAFE!

Those who take nitrates should not use drugs such as sildenafil (Viagra), tadalafil (Cialis), or vardenafil (Levitra) for erectile dysfunction because these types of drugs dilate blood vessels and may cause a significant drop in blood pressure if used together.

Box 24-1 Key Points for Using Sublingual Nitroglycerin

- Carry nitroglycerin (NTG) tablets at all times.
- Keep NTG tablets tightly sealed in the original container and protected from heat, light, and moisture.
- Replace NTG prescription at least every 6 months for maximum effect or every 3 to 4 months if carried in a pocket next to body heat.
- Take NTG tablet before an activity known to cause chest pain.
- Sit or lie down when taking NTG tablets, if possible.
- Take one NTG tablet. If the symptoms are not worsening but not completely relieved, your HCP may tell you to repeat a tablet every 5 minutes up to a total of three tablets. If pain is not relieved after three tablets, call 911.
- If pain is unrelieved after one NTG tablet and other symptoms of myocardial infarction are present, call 911 for emergency medical care.
- Tingling should be felt under the tongue when NTG tablets are used.
- NTG may cause a headache initially. Aspirin may relieve it.
- NTG may cause lightheadedness. Rise slowly to prevent falls.

BETA BLOCKERS. Beta blockers decrease heart rate, lower blood pressure, and prevent release of renin. This results in decreased workload on the heart to help prevent anginal attacks. Because of these decreased effects, beta blockers should be used with caution in patients with any degree of HF because it may make HF worse. There are nonselective and selective types of beta-adrenergic blockers. People with asthma or chronic obstructive pulmonary disease (COPD, including emphysema, bronchitis, and bronchiectasis) should avoid nonselective beta-adrenergic blockers because they cause bronchoconstriction. Metoprolol (Lopressor) and atenolol (Tenormin) are cardioselective and can be used in patients with asthma and COPD. Beta blockers are not effective for coronary artery spasms and should not be used for variant (Prinzmetal's) angina.

LEARNING TIP

To help you identify beta blockers, remember that their generic names end with -olol.

ANGIOTENSIN-CONVERTING ENZYME INHIBITORS. Angiotensin-converting enzyme (ACE) inhibitors block production of angiotensin II, which is a potent vasoconstrictor. This action reduces peripheral arterial resistance (vasodilation), which lowers blood pressure. ACE inhibitors may cause retention of potassium in some patients. If a patient taking an ACE inhibitor develops a dry cough, inform the HCP so the medication can be changed.

STATINS.   Cholesterol and inflammation in artery walls are involved in atherosclerosis development. Statins lower cholesterol levels by reducing cholesterol production in the liver (see Table 24.3). They also reduce inflammation and CRP levels, which improves patient outcomes in CAD. Statins are used to prevent and treat atherosclerosis and the disorders caused by it.

ANTIPLATELETS.   Aspirin and clopidogrel (Plavix) are commonly used antiplatelets that help prevent cardiovascular events.

Nursing Process for the Patient With Atherosclerosis, Coronary Artery Disease, and Angina

Data Collection

A health history is obtained regarding the patient's nonmodifiable and modifiable risk for atherosclerosis and CAD. A history of chest pain, fatigue, or activity intolerance is noted. Allergies and current medications, including over-the-counter and prescription drugs are documented. Height, weight, and diet history are recorded.

Assess anginal pain by patient's description of pain: type, location, and pain radiation to other areas of the body. Note skin color and temperature. Note any factors that may make the pain worse or better. This will provide information to determine improvement or lack of improvement in pain. Ask how long the patient has had angina, triggering activities, and how the pain has been relieved in the past. Note the presence of dyspnea, labored respirations, diaphoresis, or nausea. Obtain vital signs, blood pressure, apical pulse, respiration, and oxygen saturation to provide a baseline of the patient status.

Nursing Diagnoses, Planning, and Implementation

Acute Pain *related to reduced coronary artery blood flow and increased myocardial oxygen needs causing an imbalance between oxygen supply and demand*

EXPECTED OUTCOME: The patient will report an absence of pain.

- Ensure vascular access is established. *IV access may be necessary to use to administer drugs for pain relief.*
- Administer oxygen as ordered via nasal cannula *to increase oxygen availability to myocardium.*
- Obtain a 12-lead ECG as ordered *to determine ischemia or injury of the myocardium with evaluation of the ST segment.*
- Administer aspirin as prescribed *to decrease platelet aggregation.*
- Administer morphine as prescribed *to provide pain relief.*
- Administer nitroglycerin (sublingual, spray) as ordered. Notify HCP if pain is unrelieved after three doses of NTG or as prescribed, or if vital signs change. *Chest pain unrelieved by nitrates may represent unstable angina or MI.*
- Remain with patient and reassess pain in 5 minutes after administration of medication. *A patient who has chest pain should never be left alone.*

- Notify HCP of ECG changes. *ST-segment elevation may indicate a MI* (see Chapter 25).
- Offer the patient assurance and emotional support *to decrease anxiety. Emotional support is important because patients and their families are often afraid that the patient may die.*
- Promote rest and decrease anxiety for the patient with chest pain *to help relieve stress and chest pain.*
- Document patient data in the medical record *to communicate patient's problem and outcome.*

Deficient Knowledge *related to ineffective management of regimen for atherosclerosis or coronary artery disease*

EXPECTED OUTCOME: The patient will report understanding and management of atherosclerosis and CAD.

- Identify cognitive or physical impairments *that would interfere with the patient's ability to learn desired information.*
- Include significant other as appropriate *to support patient during learning.*
- Collect data on patient's present understanding of atherosclerosis and CAD *to determine baseline knowledge.*
- Collect data on patient's readiness to learn and desired learning needs and feelings about incorporating lifestyle changes into daily routine *to prioritize teaching topics.*
- Determine cultural beliefs *because they may influence learning.*
- Provide for patient's physical comfort during teaching *to increase learning.*
- Use appropriate teaching tools *to meet individual learning needs, such as pamphlets, diagrams, or other written materials in simple language.*
- Use an interpreter as needed and provide written materials in patient's native language *to facilitate understanding.*
- Explain pathophysiology of atherosclerosis and CAD, control of risk factors, and management of CAD symptoms *to promote understanding.*
- Explain action, side effects, and importance of taking medications as prescribed *to relieve pain and prevent complications.*
- Provide information about community resources *that can assist in making lifestyle changes, such as weight loss, smoking cessation, stress management, and exercise.*
- Teach patient to monitor blood pressure and heart rate as appropriate and to report chest pain or dyspnea, *which may point to the presence of complications from CAD.*
- Help patient plan how to incorporate information into daily life *to increase likelihood that change will occur.*
- Encourage questions and allow patient opportunity to verbalize new information and skills *to enhance learning.*
- Document teaching and evaluation of patient knowledge *to validate understanding.*

Evaluation

Interventions are successful if the patient is pain free and has an increased understanding of atherosclerosis and CAD and their management and states that he or she will modify risk factors of CAD.

ACUTE CORONARY SYNDROME

The term **acute coronary syndrome** (ACS) is used to encompass the continuum of CAD such as unstable angina pectoris and MI. Acute coronary syndrome is caused by a sequence of inflammatory processes mediated by activated macrophages, plaque rupture, tissue factor expressions and platelet activation leading to thrombus formation and coronary vessel occlusion.

Unstable Angina

Unstable angina occurs in patients with worsening CAD and is noted by its changing or unpredictable pattern. Rest does not decrease the chest pain of unstable angina. This pain may even occur when the patient is at rest. The episodes of chest pain with unstable angina increase in frequency and severity, placing the patient at risk for myocardial damage or sudden death. Symptoms of angina usually occur when an artery is narrowed by at least 60% to 70%.

Myocardial Infarction

An MI (heart attack), results in the death of heart muscle. The affected myocardial cells in the heart are permanently destroyed. An MI occurs from a partial or complete blockage of a coronary artery, which decreases the blood supply to the cells of the heart supplied by the blocked coronary artery. The extent of the cardiac damage varies depending on the location and amount of blockage in the coronary artery. This is a potentially devastating condition. The ability of the heart to contract, relax, and propel blood throughout the body requires healthy cardiac muscle. Results depends on the speed and effectiveness of treatment.

MI is identified by type. Non–ST-segment elevation MI (NSTEMI) is also known as a non–Q-wave MI. An ST-segment elevation MI (STEMI) is also known as a Q-wave MI and is the deadliest type because it is usually caused by a complete blockage of the artery. (See Chapter 25 for ST-segment definition.) With timely reperfusion, cell death may not occur, which reduces the amount of permanent damage.

Those experiencing an MI are typically men over age 40 with atherosclerosis. Although MIs can occur at any age in men or women, women who smoke and use oral contraceptives have a higher risk.

Silent Ischemia

Silent ischemia occurs without pain and can carry great risk. The older adult and those with hypertension or diabetes most often have silent ischemia.

Sudden Cardiac Death

Sudden cardiac death is cardiac arrest triggered by lethal ventricular dysrhythmias or asystole from an abrupt occlusion of a coronary artery (see Chapter 25). Prompt treatment is required in an attempt to prevent death.

Pathophysiology

MI does not happen immediately. Ischemic injury evolves over several hours before complete necrosis and infarction

take place. The ischemic process affects the subendocardial layer, which is most sensitive to hypoxia. This process leads to depressed myocardial contractility. The body's attempt to compensate for decreased cardiac function triggers the sympathetic nervous system to increase the heart rate. The change in heart rate increases myocardial oxygen demand, further depressing the myocardium.

Prolonged ischemia can produce severe cellular damage and necrosis of cardiac muscle. Once necrosis takes place, the contractile function of the muscle is permanently lost. The heart has a zone of ischemia and injury around the necrotic area (Fig. 24.3). The zone of injury is next to the necrotic area and is susceptible to becoming necrosed. If treatment is initiated within the first hour of symptoms of the MI, the area of damage can be minimized. Around the injury zone is an area of ischemia and viable tissue. If the heart responds to treatment, this area can rebuild and maintain collateral circulation. If prolonged ischemia takes place, the size of the infarction can be quite large. The size of the infarction depends on how quickly the blood supply from the blocked artery can be restored.

The area affected by an MI depends on the coronary artery involved and the extent of occlusive coronary disease (Fig. 24.4). Being familiar with the anatomy of the heart and the area of the MI helps the nurse anticipate dysrhythmias, conduction disturbances, and HF, which are the major complications of MIs (Table 24.5).

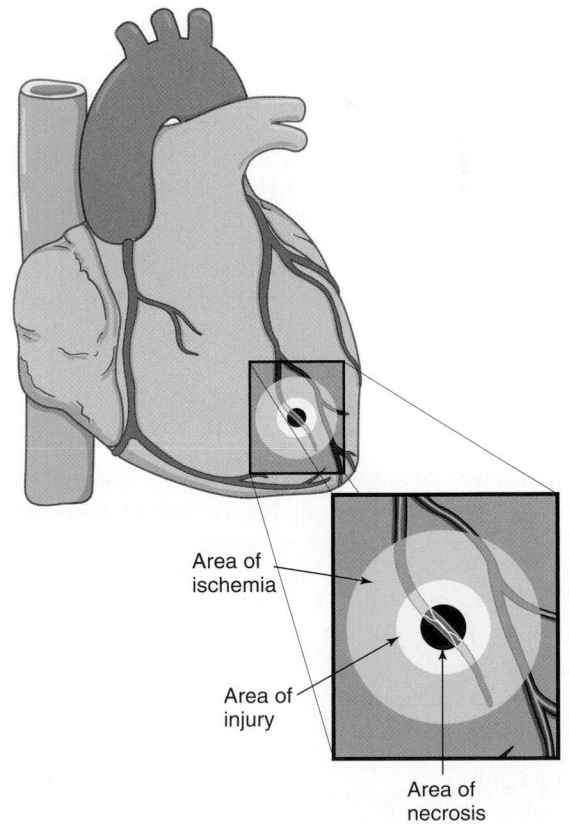

Area of ischemia

Area of injury

Area of necrosis

FIGURE 24.3 Myocardial infarction. Areas of ischemia, injury, and necrosis caused by a blockage in the left anterior coronary artery.

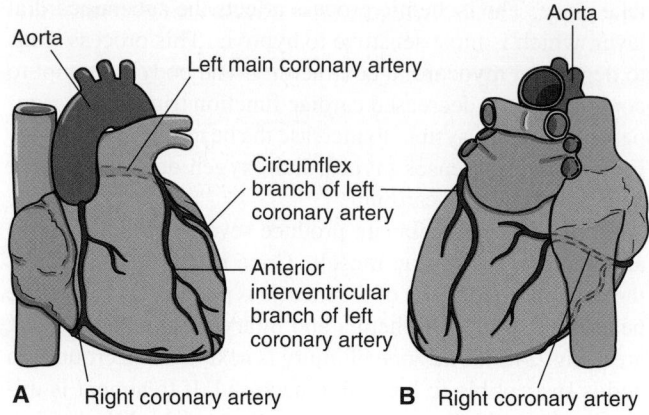

Aorta
Left main coronary artery

Aorta

Circumflex branch of left coronary artery

Anterior interventricular branch of left coronary artery

A Right coronary artery

B Right coronary artery

FIGURE 24.4 Coronary arteries. (A) Anterior view. (B) Posterior view.

The left coronary artery feeds the anterior wall of the heart, which also includes most of the left ventricle. An occlusion in this area causes an anterior wall MI. When the left ventricle is affected, there can be severe loss of left ventricular function, leading to severe changes in the hemodynamic status of the patient.

The right coronary artery (RCA) feeds the inferior wall and parts of the atrioventricular node and the sinoatrial node.

An occlusion of the RCA leads to an inferior MI and abnormalities in impulse formation and conduction. Serious dysrhythmias can occur early in an inferior MI that may be life threatening.

The left circumflex coronary artery feeds the lateral wall of the heart and part of the posterior wall of the heart. A lesion in the circumflex leads to a lateral wall infarction of the left ventricle.

LEARNING TIP

To remember which coronary artery occlusion results in a specific MI location, use coast-to-coast U.S. location initials such as those given below. You can personalize the locations with initials of landmarks familiar to you:

LOCATION	CORONARY ARTERY	RESULTING MI LOCATION
Los Angeles	Left anterior descending	Anterior
Cedar Point	Circumflex	Posterior
Rhode Island	Right	Inferior

TABLE 24.5 COMPLICATIONS OF MYOCARDIAL INFARCTION

Complication	Types or Symptoms	Interventions
Dysrhythmias	Premature ventricular contractions, ventricular tachycardia, ventricular fibrillation, heart block	Continuous cardiac monitoring Protocols for treatment of dysrhythmias (see Chapter 25)
Cardiogenic shock	Decreased blood pressure; increased heart rate; diaphoresis; cold, clammy, gray skin	Immediate initiation of treatment to decrease infarct size, control pain and dysrhythmias Intra-aortic balloon pump Thrombolytic therapy Dopamine and dobutamine
Heart failure/ pulmonary edema	Dizziness, orthopnea, weight gain, edema, enlarged liver, jugular venous distention, crackles	Correct underlying cause Relieve symptoms Increase cardiac contractility Administer furosemide (Lasix) and digoxin (Lanoxin)
Emboli	Dependent on location of emboli	Anticoagulants to prevent Supportive symptom treatment
Rupture of muscles or valves of the heart, septal rupture	Signs of cardiogenic shock, death	Mortality rate high Immediate treatment of MI to limit extent of damage
Pericarditis (inflammation of the heart muscle)	Chest pain, increased with movement, deep inspiration, or cough; pericardial friction rub (fine grating sound)	Relieved when sits up and leans forward Anti-inflammatory drugs (aspirin, indomethacin [Indocin])

Signs and Symptoms

Chest pain is a classic symptom of an MI. The pain begins suddenly and continues without relief with rest or administration of NTG. The pain in the center of the chest is usually described as crushing, viselike, or as if an elephant is standing on the chest. The pain may radiate to the back, one or both arms and shoulders, neck, or jaw. The pain can imitate indigestion or a gallbladder attack with abdominal pain and vomiting. Other classic MI symptoms include shortness of breath, dizziness, nausea, and sweating (Table 24.6). When listening to lung sounds, crackles or wheezing may be heard. The pulse may be rapid or irregular, and an extra heart sound (referred to as S_3 or S_4) may be present. The presence of an extra heart sound can mean ventricular failure is imminent.

TIMELY SYMPTOM TREATMENT. Individuals often deny or fail to recognize that an MI is occurring because they experience atypical MI symptoms or their symptoms are similar to other mild conditions such as indigestion ("Gerontological Issues"). Patients have reported that the symptoms of an MI that they experienced were not what they expected. If people expect to have the dramatic heart attack symptoms seen on television (which are usually not the same as those in real life) and they do not, they are likely to wait to seek treatment. Waiting 2 to 24 hours before seeking medical care is common, yet the first hour after symptom onset is crucial for administering the newer reperfusion treatments that restore blood flow, minimize tissue damage, and save lives. Individuals should not drive themselves or let someone else drive them to the hospital if they are having chest pain. Call emergency medical care (911 or local emergency services number) so lifesaving treatment can begin.

Because so few people arrive at the emergency room quickly enough to benefit from reperfusion treatment, several agencies have educational programs to address this issue. Individuals need to be educated that "time is muscle." As time passes during an MI, more muscle is lost. The National Heart, Lung, and Blood Institute and the AHA promote a campaign called "Act in Time to Heart Attack Signs." The purpose of the campaign is to educate people on the importance of recognizing heart attack symptoms, working with a HCP to create a heart attack survival plan, and calling 911 as soon as symptoms begin. For more information, visit:

> www.nhlbi.nih.gov/health/health-topics/topics /heartattack
> www.womenshealth.gov/heart-health-stroke/heart -disease-stroke-prevention/index.html
> www.heart.org/HEARTORG.

Women and Heart Health

Heart disease remains the leading cause of death in women in the United States. American women are six times more likely to die of heart disease than breast cancer. Heart disease kills more women than all cancers combined in the over-age-65 group. Ethnicity is also a factor among women. African American women are more likely than Caucasian women to develop heart disease. Women tend to have an acute MI at an older age than men. Women also have a higher mortality rate

Gerontological Issues

With age, the heart has decreased elasticity and decreased ability to respond to changes in pressure. This increases resistance to its pumping action and increases the workload of the myocardium.

Symptoms:

- Older patients should be taught never to neglect symptoms of shortness of breath, fatigue, fast or slow heartbeats, or chest discomfort.
- MIs that can occur without the presence of pain, a silent MI, most often occur in the older adult or those with diabetes regardless of age.
- When pain is not present, the only symptom may be a sudden onset of shortness of breath or fainting, restlessness, or a fall.
- Atypical presentation of MI symptoms is normal in older people, especially those older than age 85. Because the older adult has had more time to develop collateral circulation than younger people, they often do not have as many complications with an MI.

Therapies:

- In the older adult, reperfusion therapies such as angioplasty and bypass surgery seem to be superior in improving quality of life without increasing mortality risk. Statin therapy has also been shown to reduce mortality in those over age 80.

TABLE 24.6 MYOCARDIAL INFARCTION SUMMARY

Signs and Symptoms	Classic
	Crushing, viselike chest pain with radiation to arm, shoulder, neck, jaw, or back
	Shortness of breath
	Dizziness
	Nausea
	Sweating
	Atypical
	Absence of chest pain
	Fatigue
	Cramping in chest
	Anxiety
	Feeling of impending doom
	Falling
	More Common in Women
	Epigastric or abdominal pain
	Chest discomfort, pressure, burning

Continued

TABLE 24.6 MYOCARDIAL INFARCTION SUMMARY—cont'd

	Arm, shoulder, neck, jaw, or back pain Discomfort/pain between shoulder blades Shortness of breath Fatigue Indigestion or gas pain Nausea or vomiting
Diagnostic Tests	ECG Serum cardiac troponin I or T Serum myoglobin Serum CK-MB CBC Serum magnesium and potassium Vital signs, oxygen saturation, intake and output
Therapeutic Measures	Medications Oxygen Morphine sulfate Nitrates Fab Four cardiac medications: aspirin, statin, ACEI, beta blocker Platelet aggregation inhibitors Thrombolytics Anticoagulants Antidysrhythmics Vasodilators Percutaneous coronary interventions and stents Myocardial revascularization–CABG Fluid restriction Daily weights Bedrest with bedside commode/ bathroom privileges Low-sodium diet advanced to diet as tolerated; no caffeine Cardiac rehabilitation
Complications	Dysrhythmias Heart failure Cardiogenic shock Valvular insufficiency
Priority Nursing Diagnoses	*Acute Pain* *Anxiety* *Decreased Cardiac Output* *Deficient Knowledge*

and are more likely to have complications such as ventricular fibrillation and HF than men.

Women may have classic chest pain, but they are also likely to have other symptoms as well that men do not typically have. Research is focusing on understanding women and cardiac disease. Atypical symptoms reported by women may include extreme fatigue, epigastric pain, jaw pain, indigestion, nausea and vomiting, dyspnea, shortness of breath, or cramping in the chest. A high percentage of women (more than 50%) noted prodromal symptoms a month before an acute MI. These symptoms included unusual fatigue, sleep disturbances, and shortness of breath. Fewer than 30% reported chest discomfort.

Delay in seeking care has also been identified in women. Women also often do not associate their symptoms with a heart attack because they believe it is a male condition. Women with atypical symptoms usually delay treatment, and when treated have less aggressive management, which leads to increased mortality.

Diagnostic Tests

Patients with a strong familial history of MI should be considered at risk until an MI is ruled out. Indicators of an MI are patient history, ECG, and serum cardiac troponin I or T, myoglobin, and CK-MB levels (see Chapter 21). C-reactive protein levels are elevated in the presence of inflammation. Magnesium levels are also checked, especially for those on diuretic therapy. Before thrombolytic or heparin therapy, international normalized ratio (INR) and partial thromboplastin time (PTT) are determined. The ECG usually shows the area that has infarcted, as well as the ischemic areas of the heart. Myocardial damage can be seen as ST-segment elevation, the presence of a Q-wave, or T-wave abnormalities (Fig. 24.5). Serial ECGs are done to monitor changes indicating damage or ischemia.

FIGURE 24.5 Electrocardiogram changes during myocardial infarction. (A) Injury: ST-segment elevation. (B) Ischemia: ST-segment inversion. (C) Necrosis: large Q-wave and ST-segment elevation.

Therapeutic Measures

Treatment should be sought within 5 minutes for any unre-lieved chest pain. The AHA recommends chewing one un-coated adult aspirin at the onset of chest pain as directed by an HCP. Delays in seeking care can limit treatment options and result in more cardiac damage (Box 24-2).

Time until intervention is directly related to mortality. Guide-lines now consider first medical contact to intervention rather than "door-to-needle" time. The goal is to restore blood flow to the heart muscle within 90 minutes or less of the patient's arrival at the emergency department door. Percutaneous coronary in-tervention should be initiated within 90 minutes. A reperfusion drug, when used, should be given within 30 minutes of the patient arriving at the emergency department (Barto, 2013).

The presence of chest pain indicates a lack of oxygen to the myocardium. Patients reporting chest pain are treated as if they have an MI until proven otherwise through testing.

OXYGEN. Oxygen is administered immediately, usually at 2 L/min via nasal cannula. Oxygen therapy may be limited to the first 6 hours in stable patients. Too much oxygen can lead to systemic vasoconstriction, which may increase myocardial workload. Arterial blood gases (ABGs) are drawn to determine the patient's oxygen needs. Oxygen saturation should be mon-itored and kept above 94%. Oxygen can be administered via mask if higher concentrations are needed. Mechanical ventila-tion can be provided when indicated by ABGs.

PERCUTANEOUS CORONARY INTERVENTION. Percutaneous coronary intervention (PCI) is a mechanical procedure to in-crease blood flow and oxygen to the myocardium. Emer-gency PCI is being used frequently in the management of acute MI, with improved outcomes for patients.

BALLOON ANGIOPLASTY. In a cardiac catheterization labora-tory, a catheter with a balloon tip is inserted, usually via the femoral artery, and advanced into the heart to open the blocked coronary artery (Fig. 24.6). Once the blocked artery is entered, the balloon on the catheter is inflated and the atherosclerotic

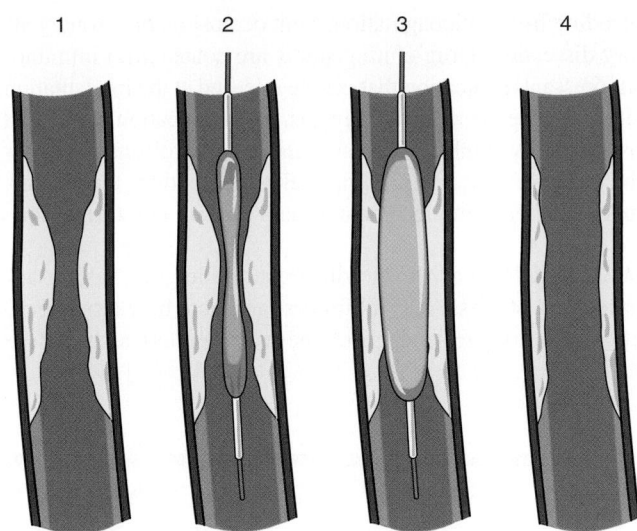

FIGURE 24.6 Percutaneous coronary intervention: Balloon an-gioplasty opens narrowed coronary arteries.

plaque is compressed. The dilated vessel is able to deliver more oxygen-rich blood to the myocardium. Angioplasty can be done with or without the placement of stents.

Coronary Artery Stent. A coronary artery stent, placed during angioplasty, is used to prevent closure of a coronary artery from an atherosclerotic lesion. A stent is an expandable metal mesh tube that is implanted at the site of blockage in the coronary artery (Fig. 24.7). A stent provides support to a coronary artery wall at the area of stenosis to keep blood flowing through the artery. Complications associated with stent placement include **thrombosis** (formation of a blood clot inside a blood vessel),

FIGURE 24.7 Insertion of a coronary artery stent: (A) A balloon catheter with a collapsed stent is advanced to the location of a coronary artery lesion. (B) The balloon is inflated, which expands the stent and compresses the lesion to increase the artery opening. (C) The balloon is then deflated and removed, leaving the expanded stent in place to prevent the artery from closing.

Box 24-2 Preventing Delays in Myocardial Infarction Treatment

- Understand symptoms and the "time is muscle" principle.
- Develop an action plan and rehearse it.
- Understand normal emotional responses of anxiety, denial, or embarrassment.
- Educate family to follow action plan.
- Establish protocols in workplaces for employees experiencing myocardial infarction.
- Establish emergency room policies that reduce delays, such as having equipment and medication readily available.

bleeding from anticoagulation, stent occlusion, or coronary artery dissection. Drug-eluting stents are coated with immunosuppressant medication that can be released at the implantation site to reduce the risk of restenosis. The medication is released over months to inhibit smooth muscle cell proliferation to reduce risk of restenosis. Antiplatelet medications are recommended after stent placement to help prevent clot formation.

MEDICATION. For those with unstable angina, taking antiplatelets, statins, ACE inhibitors, and beta blockers is beneficial. A drug from each of these drug classes should be considered. When taken together, these drugs have a synergistic effect in fighting plaque, which means they have a greater positive result for the patient. Research has shown that not all eligible patients are prescribed each of these medications. Patient teaching can include the need to ask the HCP about these drug classes to ensure they receive the ones for which they are eligible.

Table 24.7 summarizes pharmacological treatment of MI. MONA is a mnemonic in the Advance Cardiac Life Support guidelines for remembering the medications to give in treating a suspected MI: morphine, oxygen, nitroglycerin, and aspirin.

TABLE **24.7**   MEDICATIONS USED TO TREAT MYOCARDIAL INFARCTION

Medication Class/Action	Examples	Nursing Implications
Analgesics Opioid relieves pain. Reduces preload and afterload. Decreases anxiety.	morphine sulfate	Monitor vital signs before and after administration.
Angiotensin-Converting Enzyme Inhibitors *(See Table 24.4.)*		
Anticoagulants **Heparin** Inhibits conversion of prothrombin to thrombin to prevent thrombus formation.	Heparin sodium	Do not give if bleeding risk. Dose regulated by heparin anti-factor Xa or activated partial thromboplastin time (aPTT). PTT Goal: 1.5–2.5 times control. Monitor for bleeding.
Low Molecular Weight Heparin Antithrombotic. Prophylaxis of ischemic complications in unstable angina or NSTEMI with aspirin therapy.	dalteparin (Fragmin) enoxaparin (Lovenox)	Do not remove prefilled syringe air bubble. Give deep subcutaneously: hold fold of skin while giving injection. Rotate sites. *Teaching:* Monitor for bleeding.
Antidysrhythmics Inhibit ventricular arrhythmias.	amiodarone (Cordarone, Pacerone)	Contraindicated in AV block or pregnancy. Obtain baseline vital signs and ECG. Monitor for lung toxicity. *Teaching:* Avoid grapefruit juice with oral form.
Antiplatelets Inhibit platelet activation, adhesion, or procoagulant activity.	Aspirin Clopidogrel (Plavix)	Chewable aspirin as ordered should be taken as soon as ACS or MI is suspected. Enteric coated may be given daily. *Teaching:* Take with food. Report bleeding or bruising.
Glycoprotein 11b/111a inhibitors. Inhibit platelet aggregation. Given IV only during PCI.	bivalirudin (Angiomax) eptifibatide (Integrilin) tirofiban (Aggrastat) abciximab (ReoPro)	Prevent injury for bleeding risk. Monitor vital signs and ECG.

TABLE 24.7   MEDICATIONS USED TO TREAT MYOCARDIAL INFARCTION—cont'd

Medication Class/Action	Examples	Nursing Implications
Beta Blockers *(See Table 24.4.)*		
Nitrates Vasodilate to reduce preload and afterload. Reduce myocardial oxygen consumption. *(See Table 24.3 for other forms.)*	Nitroglycerin	Document onset, type, radiation, location, and duration of chest pain. Monitor apical pulse and BP. *Teaching:* Headache may occur but will resolve over time. Change position slowly to avoid orthostatic hypotension and fall risk.
Statins *(See Table 24.2.)*		
Thrombolytics Dissolve blood clots in blood vessels or catheters, such as dialysis catheters.	alteplase (Activase, tissue plasminogen activator [t-PA]) reteplase (Retavase) tenecteplase (TNKase)	Most effective when given within 6 hours of coronary event. Goal is 90 minutes from arrival. Baseline INR, aPTT, platelet count, and fibrinogen levels checked. Avoid venipunctures for 24 hours after administration.
Additional Medications as Needed Antiemetics Anxiolytics Antacids Stool softeners	Specific for drugs given.	Control nausea, vomiting, anxiety, gastric upset, or constipation.

ANALGESICS. Analgesics are given for relief of chest pain. Morphine sulfate is the most commonly used narcotic. It is usually given in increments of 2 to 8 mg IV every 5 to 15 minutes until pain is relieved. The patients should be monitored for hypotension, respiratory depression, oversedation, and morphine sensitivity. In addition to pain relief, morphine helps decrease anxiety, opens bronchioles, and increases peripheral blood pooling to decrease preload (blood returning to heart) and afterload (pressure within the aorta), which can help increase blood supply and oxygen to the myocardium.

VASODILATORS. NTG sublingually, topically, or by IV drip can be administered for vasodilation to supply more blood to the myocardium to reduce pain and the workload of the heart. In the acute phase, the IV route is usually used. Nitrates should not be given if the patient has a systolic blood pressure of less than 90 mm Hg or 30 mm Hg or more below baseline, severe bradycardia less than 50 beats per minute, or if the patient has taken a phosphodiesterase inhibitor for erectile dysfunction. Catastrophic hypotension may result.

THROMBOLYTICS. Thrombolytic therapy is used to dissolve a blood clot that is occluding a coronary artery. (Note, however, that PCI has greatly reduced the use of thrombolytics.)

Thrombolytic therapy must be started within a specified time range from the onset of symptoms, usually within 1 to 6 hours, before necrosis results. The goal is to give thrombolytics within 30 minutes of arrival at the emergency department door.

Glycoprotein 11b/111a inhibitors (Eptifibatide [Integrilin], abciximab [ReoPro], tirofiban [Aggrastat]) are examples of IV medication that can be used as an adjunct to thrombolysis or PCI in patients with unstable angina or non–ST-segment-elevation MI. These drugs work by inhibiting platelet aggregation and are used along with aspirin or Plavix, and heparin.

ACTIVITY. Initially, patients are kept on bed rest to decrease myocardial oxygen demand. A bedside commode for bowel movements is usually ordered to reduce straining. Then activity is advanced gradually as tolerated.

INTRA-AORTIC BALLOON PUMP. To support the ischemic heart, an intra-aortic balloon pump (IABP) may be used to increase circulation to the coronary arteries and reduce the work of the heart (see Chapter 26). While the heart is relaxed (diastole), the balloon is inflated, sending more blood into the coronary arteries. Just before the heart contracts (systole), the balloon deflates, creating a suction effect that allows blood to flow past it with less resistance (decreased afterload) into the aorta.

GLUCOSE CONTROL. Guidelines for managing hyperglycemia in critically ill patients are to maintain blood glucose levels at 140 to 180 mg/dL and avoid hypoglycemia. Strict glycemic control has been shown to increase the risk of death at 90 days (Dechant, 2012).

DIET AND WEIGHT LOSS. During the acute phase of an MI, small, easily digested meals are served. Caffeine is restricted because it increases heart rate and causes vasoconstriction. Fluids may be restricted if the patient is in heart failure as well. Initially a low-sodium clear liquid diet may be ordered. Then a heart-healthy diet may be ordered. If the patient is obese, weight loss can reduce cardiac workload. A dietitian can work with the patient and family to devise a weight-loss diet for the patient.

TOBACCO USE. Patients are instructed on the hazards of smoking or exposure to secondhand smoke. Referral to a tobacco cessation program can be made. The nurse can help patients understand and accept lifestyle changes.

Coronary Artery Bypass Graft

AHA guidelines help determine which type of procedure would benefit the patient, PCI or coronary artery bypass graft (CABG). During bypass surgery, the saphenous vein from the leg or an internal mammary artery from the chest wall is used to reroute blood around a segment of a coronary artery that is narrowed by atherosclerosis (Fig. 24.8). One or more vessels can be bypassed (see "Patient Perspective"). There are two types of bypass procedures: arrested heart surgery and beating heart surgery.

ARRESTED HEART SURGERY. Most bypasses are done while the heart is stopped with a cardiopulmonary bypass machine (on pump) in use (see Chapter 21). While the median sternotomy is made, the vein graft is being removed from the body. The graft is flushed with a heparinized solution to check for leaks and then set aside for use during the surgery. After the patient is placed on cardiopulmonary bypass and the heart is stopped, one end of the graft is **anastomosed** (joined) to the coronary artery distal to the occlusion, while the proximal end of the graft is anastomosed, often to the ascending aorta.

FIGURE 24.8 Myocardial reperfusion by coronary artery bypass graft surgery.

Patient Perspective

Keith: Coronary Artery Bypass Graft

I was 72 when I had coronary artery bypass surgery. I had some very minor symptoms, and a heart catheterization showed significant coronary artery blockage. I ended up having five bypass grafts performed. It was a long surgery. I felt disoriented for several days afterward—mostly while I was in the intensive care unit (ICU).

I have had a strange sensation in my legs at the incision sites ever since surgery, but not really pain! I also have experienced no depression, although postop depression is common, and have assumed an attitude that I am in better condition than before surgery, so why should I worry?

I was provided with excellent care at home after discharge from the hospital. The nursing and rehab personnel were outstanding. I had a capable visiting nurse, physical therapist, or occupational therapist practically every day. Physical therapy was difficult at first but shortly became routine and easy.

My experience during cardiac rehab was outstanding. I had three sessions per week for 12 weeks. I have always exercised a lot, so I had no problems attaining the exercise levels suggested. It was a very positive experience, and I enjoyed the association with others in the same situation. We even staged a graduation when we finished. I wore a tuxedo jacket with my gym shorts! Since completing my rehab, I have religiously maintained a minimum 40-minute exercise schedule three times per week. I do this because I want to stay healthy for a long time.

The only negative aspect I experienced was a minor stroke during surgery. As a result, my balance is not as good as I would like. I need to be more careful, particularly when running or bike riding. Perhaps this is just older age, but it started just after surgery, so that is the reason I assume it is due to the minor stroke.

The impact on my life and family has been minimal. The primary change is being more conscious of my diet and an emphasis on exercise. Otherwise, I live pretty much the same as before.

BEATING HEART SURGERY. This surgery is done with the heart beating and does not use the heart-lung machine (off pump). A device is used to stabilize a vessel while the surgeon works on it. Either traditional median sternotomy or minimally invasive surgery can be used.

MINIMALLY INVASIVE SURGERY. Less invasive approaches include the minimally invasive coronary artery bypass grafting (MICS CABG), which is done off pump, and totally endoscopic coronary artery bypass surgery (TECAB), which can be done on or off pump. MICS CABG is done through a small fifth intercostal incision. TECAB uses three or four chest holes for insertion of robotic arms and a camera that a surgeon then views to control the robotic arms.

CRITICAL THINKING

Mr. Jones

■ Mr. Jones is transferred to the critical care unit after a quadruple CABG. Preoperative vital signs were blood pressure 164/88 mm Hg, apical pulse 62 beats per minute and regular, respiratory rate 18 per minute, temperature 98.4°F (36.9°C). Data collection findings are blood pressure 100/56 mm Hg, apical pulse 105 beats per minute, and respiratory rate 28 per minute, irregular and shallow, temperature 99.8°F (37.7°C), lung sounds diminished with crackles in bilateral bases, pedal pulses weak bilaterally, chest and leg dressings dry and intact, and no urinary catheter. Mr. Jones is being monitored for first postoperative voiding.

1. Which findings may indicate pulmonary problems?
2. List four nursing interventions for the altered pulmonary status.
3. List three reasons why the apical pulse could be elevated.
4. Name two reasons why the blood pressure could be low.
5. With which health care team members will the nurse collaborate?

Suggested answers are at the end of the chapter.

Nursing Process for the Patient Experiencing Acute Coronary Syndrome or Acute Myocardial Infarction

DATA COLLECTION. A thorough history is obtained to identify risk factors that may contribute to an MI. All patients admitted with chest pain are treated as having a possible MI until it has been ruled out. Continuous cardiac monitoring, serial ECGs, and laboratory values help identify life-threatening dysrhythmias and determine the degree of cardiac damage. Controlling chest pain immediately helps diminish anxiety and the negative physiological effects pain has on the body. Assessment for depression for those experiencing an MI is important to ensure appropriate referrals are made for treatment (see "Evidence-Based Practice").

NURSING DIAGNOSES, PLANNING, IMPLEMENTATION, AND EVALUATION. See the "Nursing Care Plan for the Patient With Myocardial Infarction." Also see the "Nursing Care Plan for the Patient Undergoing Cardiac Surgery" for additional nursing care.

 EVIDENCE-BASED PRACTICE

Clinical Question
Do depression, stress, or other psychological stressors have an effect on patients with CVD?

Evidence
Depression is a risk factor for the development of CVD in healthy people and is predictive of adverse outcomes. Depression is more prevalent in populations with CVD. Poor health behaviors contribute to this association (Whooley & Wong, 2013). A study of 176 subjects showed a relationship between left ventricular ejection fraction (LVEF) and depression 3 months after an MI (Bagherian-Sararoudi, Gilani, & Bahrami Ehsan, 2013).

Implications for Nursing Practice
Depression affects a patient's adherence to post-MI lifestyle changes and medication adherence. After an MI, patients should be screened for depression, anxiety, sleep disorders, and social isolation at regular intervals during hospitalization and cardiovascular rehabilitation.

REFERENCES
Bagherian-Sararoudi, R., Gilani, B., & Bahrami Ehsan, H. (2013). Relationship between left ventricular ejection fraction and depression following myocardial infarction: An original article. ARYA Atherosclerosis, 9, 16–21.

Whooley, M. A., & Wong, J. M. (2013). Depression and cardiovascular disorders. Annual Review of Clinical Psychology, 9, 327–354.

 NURSING CARE TIP

When caring for a patient after a CABG, be sure to use infection-control procedures at all times to prevent surgical site infection. Surgical site infection following CABG (mediastinitis) is a "Never Event," which means that Medicare will not pay the hospital for care required for this condition.

Patient Education

Teaching about the therapeutic regimen includes information about the disease, medications, diet, activity, and rehabilitation needs that may require lifestyle changes. Diet, stress reduction, a regular exercise program, smoking cessation (if necessary), and following a medication schedule require extensive patient and family teaching. This disease can affect all aspects of a patient's lifestyle. Issues about family and job roles and sexual activities need to be addressed. Patients need time to understand information that has been presented and should be encouraged to express any questions, needs, or fears.

Cardiac Rehabilitation and Exercise

Cardiac rehabilitation begins when the patient's acute symptoms are relieved to improve cardiac function and quality of life. Phase 1 of rehabilitation occurs in the hospital. Activities for each hospital day, such as types and amounts of self-care and activity, are specified in protocols. Phase 2 occurs 4 to 6 weeks after discharge in an outpatient program and focuses on returning the patient to previous levels of activity and function. Phase 3 follows in which patients are encouraged to maintain optimal physical fitness and to continue healthy lifestyles that include exercising and losing weight to maintain an ideal body weight.

CRITICAL THINKING

Mrs. Sims

■ Mrs. Sims, age 43, is admitted to the ICU with a diagnosis of atypical chest pain that radiates to her left shoulder and down her left arm. She has a history of midsternal chest cramping. Her pain increases with activity and decreases with rest. She smokes one and a half packs of cigarettes per day and is 50 pounds overweight. The cardiac monitor shows normal sinus rhythm without dysrhythmias. She has NTG sublingual ordered prn (as needed) for chest pain.

One hour after admission, Mrs. Sims reports acute midsternal chest pain radiating to her left neck and jaw. The cardiac monitor shows sinus tachycardia with occasional premature ventricular contractions (PVCs). Her blood pressure is 100/70 mm Hg, respirations are 20 per minute and unlabored, and skin is warm and dry.

1. What actions should be taken?
2. What is happening to Mrs. Sims?
3. How is angina differentiated from an MI?
4. What are four indicators of an MI?
5. What medical interventions can be used for an MI?
6. What patient-centered education is indicated for Mrs. Sims?

Suggested answers are at the end of the chapter.

NURSING CARE PLAN for the Patient With Myocardial Infarction

Nursing Diagnosis: *Acute Pain* related to decreased coronary blood flow causing myocardial ischemia

Expected Outcomes: The patient will exhibit signs of decreased pain. Patient will exhibit signs of relaxation.

Evaluation of Outcomes: Does patient state that pain is reduced?

Intervention Monitor location, duration, intensity, and radiation of pain; use a scale of 0 to 10. **Rationale** Identifies type and severity of pain. **Evaluation** What is pain level, location, duration, intensity, and radiation?

Intervention Monitor blood pressure, pulse, and respiration. **Rationale** Vital signs may elevate with episodes of pain. **Evaluation** Are vital signs within normal limits?

Intervention Obtain ECG as ordered. **Rationale** Identifies location of infarction or ischemia. **Evaluation** Is ECG normal?

Intervention Administer oxygen as ordered. **Rationale** Helps prevent hypoxia. **Evaluation** Are ABGs within normal limits? Is oxygen saturation greater than 90%?

Intervention Instruct patient to report pain at first onset. **Rationale** Helps control pain quickly to prevent further ischemia. **Evaluation** Does patient report pain?

Intervention Instruct patient to rest during pain. **Rationale** Activity increases oxygen demand and can increase chest pain. **Evaluation** Does patient remain quiet and relaxed?

Intervention Remain with patient during chest pain until it is relieved. **Rationale** Provides comfort and reassurance to decrease anxiety and fear. **Evaluation** Are anxiety and fear decreased?

Intervention Assist with alternative pain relief measures; related to positioning, diversional activities, relaxation techniques. **Rationale** These measures help decrease painful stimuli, allowing the patient to focus on other things. **Evaluation** Does patient express relief and decreased stress?

Intervention Medicate as ordered. **Rationale** Helps eliminate pain. **Evaluation** Is pain relieved?

NURSING CARE PLAN for the Patient With Myocardial Infarction—cont'd

GERIATRIC

Intervention Monitor and ensure that older patient's pain is relieved. **Rationale** Pain is not an expected part of the aging process as many believe. **Evaluation** Does patient report pain is relieved?

Nursing Diagnosis: *Decreased Cardiac Output* related to ischemia or infarction, changes in heart rate and rhythm, and decreased contractility

Expected Outcomes: The patient will maintain adequate cardiac output and tissue perfusion. Patient will exhibit signs of improved cardiac output and tissue perfusion.

Evaluation of Outcomes: Does patient have heart rate greater than 60 and less than 100 beats per minute, blood pressure greater than 90/60 and less than 140/90 mm Hg, and urine output greater than 30 mL/hr?

Intervention Monitor blood pressure, heart rate, and urine output. **Rationale** Indirect indicators of cardiac output. **Evaluation** Are indicators within normal limits?

Intervention Listen to lung sounds. **Rationale** Crackles indicate heart failure. **Evaluation** Are lungs clear?

Intervention Monitor peripheral circulation, pulses, capillary refill, edema, color, and temperature. **Rationale** Indicators of adequate tissue perfusion. **Evaluation** Does patient have strong peripheral pulses, capillary refill less than 3 seconds, no edema, warm skin, pink nailbeds?

Intervention Monitor ECG. **Rationale** Identifies dysrhythmias. **Evaluation** Is patient's ECG within normal limits?

Intervention Administer medications, such as vasodilators, beta blockers, calcium channel blockers, and cardiac glycosides, as ordered by HCP. **Rationale** Helps improve contractility, cardiac output, and tissue perfusion. **Evaluation** Does patient show signs of improved contractility, increased cardiac output, and tissue perfusion?

Intervention Promote and provide for adequate rest, quiet environment, bedrest; place in semi-Fowler's position. **Rationale** Decreases cardiac workload and stress and allows for improved breathing. **Evaluation** Is patient relaxed?

GERIATRIC

Intervention Observe for atypical pain such as jaw pain or no pain with dyspnea or fatigue. **Rationale** In acute MI, older adults may not have had typical chest pain or have had a silent MI. **Evaluation** Does patient have atypical symptoms of MI?

Intervention Observe patient carefully for side effects of medications. **Rationale** Older patients are more likely to have medication toxicity owing to reduced renal and hepatic function. **Evaluation** Does patient exhibit toxic side effects of medications?

Nursing Diagnosis: *Fear* related to threat of death, changes in lifestyle, chest pain, and procedures

Expected Outcomes: The patient will verbalize reduced fear. Patient will demonstrate effective coping mechanisms.

Evaluation of Outcomes: Does patient verbalize reduced fear?

Intervention Assess level of fear and note nonverbal communication. **Rationale** Controlling anxiety will reduce sympathetic activity that may intensify condition. **Evaluation** Does patient report fear or have signs of being fearful?

Intervention Ask the patient's usual coping pattern. **Rationale** This allows building on patient's strengths. **Evaluation** What are patient's coping techniques?

Continued

NURSING CARE PLAN for the Patient With Myocardial Infarction—cont'd

Intervention Orient the patient and family to surroundings and equipment, oxygen, cardiac monitoring, IVs, and explain procedures. **Rationale** Information may promote trust and reduce emotional stress. **Evaluation** Does patient state understanding of environment and equipment?

Intervention Assure patient he/she will be closely monitored. **Rationale** Assurance of detection for prompt treatment of any complications will reduce fear. **Evaluation** Does patient state less fear due to continuous monitoring?

Intervention Allow patient to verbalize fear of dying. **Rationale** Ventilation helps identify and reduce fear. **Evaluation** Is patient able to verbalize fears?

Intervention Provide diversional materials such as newspapers, music, and television. **Rationale** Diversion can be relaxing and prevent feelings of isolation. **Evaluation** Does patient report that use of diversional activities reduces fear?

Intervention Offer family support. **Rationale** Significant others often ignore their own needs, experience anxiety, and need support, including ongoing information and explanations, being allowed to stay with patient, and being involved in patient's care. Nurses need to help spouses or significant others meet their own needs, so they can better support the patient. **Evaluation** Does family verbalize ability to offer support to patient without anxiety?

GERIATRIC

Intervention Provide protective, safe environment with consistent caregivers. **Rationale** Older adults adapt to change with more difficulty during illness than younger adults. **Evaluation** Is continuity of care provided? Does patient report less fear?

Nursing Diagnosis: *Activity Intolerance* related to imbalance between oxygen supply and demand, weakness, and fatigue

Expected Outcome: The patient will tolerate progressive activity as evidenced by heart rate, blood pressure, pulse oximetry, and respiratory rate within normal limits (WNL).

Evaluation of Outcome: Is patient's heart rate, blood pressure, pulse oximetry, and respiratory rate WNL with progressive activity?

Intervention Obtain patient's vital signs before activity. **Rationale** Identifies baseline data comparison with activity. **Evaluation** What are vital signs?

Intervention Observe patient during and after activity and document abnormal responses to activity, including heart rate over 120 beats per minute or 20 beats over resting rate, systolic BP increased over 20 mm Hg during activity, chest pain, dizziness, skin color changes, diaphoresis, dyspnea, dysrhythmias, excessive fatigue, and ST-segment changes on ECG. **Rationale** Observation allows detection of abnormal responses to stop activity. **Evaluation** Are vital signs WNL? Is activity tolerated without symptoms?

Intervention Position patient for comfort and ease in breathing. **Rationale** Semi-Fowler's position is usually preferred by patients in respiratory distress. When patient is sitting upright in bed, supporting arms on pillows reduces cardiac workload by eliminating force of gravity on unsupported arms. **Evaluation** Is patient able to breathe easily?

Intervention Maintain progression of activities as ordered by HCP or cardiac rehabilitation program. *Initial activities:* ADLs, dangle at bedside for 15 minutes, use commode with assistance. *Progressive activities:* Out of bed to chair for 30 to 60 minutes, partial bath, range-of-motion exercises. **Rationale** The patient should have increasing activity to condition the myocardium. **Evaluation** Is patient able to progress activity?

NURSING CARE PLAN for the Patient With Myocardial Infarction—cont'd

GERIATRIC

Intervention Slow the pace of care. **Rationale** Allow patient extra time to complete activity to reduce cardiac demand and fatigue. **Evaluation** Is patient able to complete care without symptoms or fatigue?

Intervention Refer patient to cardiac rehabilitation as able. **Rationale** Older adults benefit comparably to younger persons from exercise programs. **Evaluation** Does patient participate in cardiac rehab?

Intervention Encourage families to let patient be independent in activities. **Rationale** Families may believe being sedentary is helpful to the patient. **Evaluation** Do family members encourage patient to be as active as able?

NURSING CARE PLAN for the Patient Undergoing Cardiac Surgery

Nursing Diagnosis: *Acute Pain* related to sternotomy, leg incisions, internal mammary artery resection, or pericarditis

Expected Outcomes: The patient will state pain is relieved or tolerable. Patient will be able to rest and perform respiratory treatments.

Evaluation of Outcomes: Does patient state pain is within acceptable levels? Is patient able to rest and perform respiratory therapies?

Intervention Assess characteristics of pain with each episode. **Rationale** A thorough description is needed to determine cause and plan actions. **Evaluation** Does patient describe pain on scale of 0 to 10?

Intervention Encourage patient to report pain even when it is mild. **Rationale** It is easier to keep pain under control when mild. **Evaluation** Does patient report pain when mild?

Intervention Turn, reposition every 2 hours. **Rationale** Changes muscle position, relieving stiffness. **Evaluation** Is patient comfortable without stiffness?

Intervention Offer back rubs frequently. **Rationale** Relaxes tense muscles retracted during operation. **Evaluation** Is patient able to rest comfortably?

Intervention Teach patient "sternal precautions": • No pushing or pulling with arms. • Hug pillow for all movement, coughing, and deep breathing. • Do not use arms to raise yourself out of a chair. • No lifting over 5 to 10 lb. • Do not raise elbows higher than shoulders. • Bend elbows and lower head for grooming. **Rationale** Stabilizes sternum and incision to increase comfort. **Evaluation** Does patient understand sternal precautions and use them?

Intervention Instruct patient to take a deep breath before movement and exhale slowly during movement. **Rationale** Keeps muscles relaxed, minimizing tension with guarding and pain. **Evaluation** Can patient perform coughing and deep-breathing techniques as instructed?

Nursing Diagnosis: *Decreased Cardiac Output* related to myocardial depression, hypothermia, bleeding, unstable dysrhythmias, or hypoxemia

Expected Outcomes: The patient will remain free of major side effects of pharmacological support. Patient will maintain vital signs within normal limits (WNL), palpable peripheral pulses, urine output greater than 30 mL/hr, and normal sinus rhythm.

Continued

NURSING CARE PLAN for the Patient Undergoing Cardiac Surgery—cont'd

Evaluation of Outcomes: Is patient free of major side effects? Are vital signs WNL?

Intervention Monitor vital signs. **Rationale** Trends reflect problems. **Evaluation** Are vital signs WNL?

Intervention Check peripheral circulation. **Rationale** Mottling or weak pulses may indicate poor cardiac output (CO). **Evaluation** Do peripheral pulses remain strong with normal skin color, temperature, capillary refill?

Intervention Monitor intake and output. **Rationale** Fluid deficit or excess can alter CO. **Evaluation** Does total intake equal output?

Intervention Listen to lung sounds and note character of sputum. **Rationale** Wet lung sounds may indicate heart failure or pulmonary edema. **Evaluation** Are lungs clear?

Intervention Note shivering. **Rationale** Shivering increases the blood pressure, decreasing CO and increasing risk for bleeding. **Evaluation** Is patient's shivering controlled?

Intervention Monitor chest tube drainage for increase or sudden decrease. **Rationale** Drainage more than 200 mL/hr may lead to hypovolemia and a decrease in CO. **Evaluation** Is patient free from cardiac tamponade and hypovolemia?

Intervention Monitor ECG. **Rationale** Premature ventricular contractions and atrial fibrillation decrease CO. **Evaluation** Does patient remain in normal sinus rhythm or controlled dysrhythmia? (See Chapter 25.)

Intervention Monitor electrolytes. **Rationale** Low calcium and magnesium and high potassium decrease contractility and CO. **Evaluation** Are electrolytes WNL?

Intervention Monitor ABGs. **Rationale** Acidosis decreases heart function, and a low CO may lead to further acidosis. **Evaluation** Are ABGs WNL?

Nursing Diagnosis: *Risk for Infection* related to inadequate primary defenses from surgical wound

Expected Outcome: The patient will remain free from infection.

Evaluation of Outcome: Does patient remain free from infection?

Intervention Observe incision for signs and symptoms of infection. **Rationale** Redness, warmth, fever, and swelling indicate infection. **Evaluation** Are signs and symptoms of infection present?

Intervention Monitor drainage and maintain drains. **Rationale** Drains remove fluid from the surgical site to prevent infection development. **Evaluation** Are drainage amount and color normal for procedure? Are drains functioning?

Intervention Maintain sterile technique for dressing changes. **Rationale** Sterile technique reduces infection development. **Evaluation** Is incision free of signs and symptoms of infection?

Intervention Monitor and report abnormal findings for temperature, lung sounds, sputum, and urine consistency. **Rationale** Low-grade or high-grade fever, crackles, yellow-green sputum color, or cloudy urine can indicate infection. **Evaluation** Is the patient's temperature WNL and are lung sounds, sputum, and urine clear?

Intervention Encourage coughing and deep breathing and incentive spirometer use. **Rationale** Lung infections can be prevented with lung expansion and secretion removal. **Evaluation** Does patient perform coughing and deep breathing and use incentive spirometer?

PERIPHERAL VASCULAR SYSTEM

Peripheral vascular disease (PVD) may be either arterial or venous in origin. PVD is common in older people and people with diabetes. It is important for the nurse to understand whether the origin of the problem is arterial or venous to prevent serious complications from occurring.

Arterial Thrombosis and Embolism
Pathophysiology

Acute arterial occlusions are often sudden and dramatic. Occlusions are most common in the lower extremity but may occur in the upper extremity as well. A thrombus (blood clot) adheres to the vessel wall. Acute arterial thrombi occur where there is injury to an arterial wall, sluggish flow, or plaque formation secondary to atherosclerotic changes. Other causes of arterial thrombosis are polycythemia, dehydration, and repeated arterial needlesticks. If a thrombus breaks off and travels, it becomes an **embolism** that occludes an arterial vessel that is too small to allow it to pass. Some of the causes of an arterial embolism are dysrhythmias, prosthetic heart valves, MI, and rheumatic heart disease.

Signs and Symptoms

Usually there is an abrupt onset of symptoms with acute arterial occlusion. If a patient also has chronic arterial insufficiency, the symptoms may not occur as rapidly because collateral circulation has developed and can supply some blood to the occluded area. Symptoms depend on the artery occluded, the tissue supplied by that artery, and whether collateral circulation is present.

The six clinical signs of acute arterial occlusion are known as the "six Ps": *p*ain, *p*allor, *p*ulselessness, *p*aresthesia (numbness), *p*aralysis, and *p*oikilothermia (temperature). The patient experiences pain, numbness, and decreased movement in the extremity, which is pale, mottled and without pulses distal to the occlusion. The extremity feels cold because blood normally provides warmth. If treatment is not initiated immediately, ischemia occurs and can progress to tissue necrosis and gangrene development within hours.

Therapeutic Measures

Early treatment is necessary to protect and save the affected limb. Anticoagulant therapy is started immediately. IV heparin is the treatment of choice to prevent further clotting. Heparin has no effect on existing clots. An initial IV bolus of heparin, usually 5000 international units, is given. An IV infusion is then started as ordered. The patient remains on heparin therapy for several days. Daily heparin Xa or PTTs are monitored to maintain therapeutic heparin levels. After 3 to 7 days, typically, warfarin (Coumadin) is added. Warfarin, an oral anticoagulant, takes 3 to 5 days to reach therapeutic levels. The heparin is continued until a therapeutic warfarin level is reached. To monitor warfarin's effects, international normalized ratios (INRs) and prothrombin times (PTs) are done daily, and adjustments in warfarin doses are made based on the results.

For patients with severe occlusions, especially if the risk of limb loss is imminent, surgery or thrombolytic agents are used to save the extremity. During an emergency embolectomy or thrombectomy, the artery is cut open, the emboli or thrombus is removed, and the vessel is sutured closed. Thrombolytic agents dissolve the thrombus or embolus.

Peripheral Arterial Disease

Peripheral arterial disease (PAD) is a disorder of the arterial circulation usually caused by chronic, progressive narrowing of arterial vessels that leads to obstruction or occlusion. PAD usually affects the lower extremities. PAD is sometimes referred to as lower extremity arterial disease (LEAD). Atherosclerosis is the leading cause of occlusive disease. PAD can be described as organic or functional. Organic disease is caused by structural changes from plaque or inflammation in the blood vessels. Functional disease is a short-term localized spasm in the blood vessel as noted in Raynaud's disease.

Pathophysiology

The purpose of the arterial system is to deliver oxygen-rich blood to the vascular beds. Anything that impedes this flow causes an imbalance in supply and demand for oxygen. Decreased nutrition, cellular waste accumulation, and the development of ischemia occur at the area distal to the obstruction. With the increased debris and sluggish flow, thrombosis and embolism can become major problems.

CRITICAL THINKING

Mrs. May

■ Mrs. May is admitted with severe rheumatoid arthritis, which has left her relatively immobile for 7 months. She is returning to her room following a whirlpool treatment when she suddenly reports severe pain in her left groin.

1. What is your first action?
2. After assessing Mrs. May, what action should be taken next?
3. What are the possible causes of these sudden symptoms?
4. How would you document Mrs. May's symptoms?
5. What immediate interventions are necessary?
6. What medical interventions would you anticipate?
7. What surgical procedure may need to be done if the risk of losing the limb is imminent?

Suggested answers are at the end of the chapter.

The body has several mechanisms that attempt to compensate for reduced blood flow, including peripheral vasodilation, anaerobic metabolism, and development of collateral circulation. However, these mechanisms are not intended to meet the ongoing blood supply needs of the body. It takes time for collateral circulation to develop, blood vessels eventually reach their limit of dilation, and anaerobic metabolism is only a very short-term compensatory mechanism. Eventually this lack of blood supply produces signs of ischemia that, if not corrected, result in ulceration, gangrene, and necrosis of the extremity; amputation of the limb may then become necessary.

Signs and Symptoms

Many people with PAD, especially women, have no symptoms. Symptoms often occur late in the course of PAD when diminished blood flow begins to produce changes in the extremities. Pain in the calves associated with activity or exercise, called **intermittent claudication**, is a common symptom of arterial occlusive disease. When blood supply to the muscles is decreased, the muscles are unable to receive adequate oxygen, and ischemia develops. As ischemia increases, the muscle develops a cramping-type pain that usually subsides when the activity is stopped. As PAD progresses, the pain is present even at rest, thus indicating severe arterial occlusion.

Skin color changes are associated with decreased blood supply. The extremity is pale when the leg is elevated. If the leg is in a dependent position, it becomes reddish purple or cyanotic. The extremity is cool to touch even in warm environments. There may be hair loss on the lower calf, ankle, and foot. Other findings include dry, flaky, scaly, pale, or mottled skin. The toenails may be thickened. As occlusion of the arteries progresses, arterial pulses become diminished or absent. Pulses should be palpated in both legs. The loss of circulation leads to tissue death and gangrene.

Diagnostic Tests

Noninvasive studies can be used to diagnose occlusive disorders. The ABPI is used to determine pressures in the upper and lower extremities. Normally, blood pressure readings in the thigh and calf are higher than those in the upper extremities. With the presence of arterial disease, these pressures are lower than the brachial pressure. Normally the ankle pressure is equal to or greater than the brachial pressure. When an occlusion occurs in the lower extremities, the pressures between the upper and lower extremities become unequal. After treadmill exercise, the ABPI decreases in arterial insufficiency. A duplex ultrasound measures the velocity of the blood flow. MRI and CT scan can give definitive images of blood vessels and degrees of arterial closure. Plethysmography and angiography can also be used to evaluate arterial flow in lower extremities (see Chapter 21).

Therapeutic Measures

Conservative treatment is initiated with mild to moderate occlusive disease. This includes patients who experience pain on activity that ceases with rest. This type of patient usually receives medication for vasodilation and diet management if necessary. Surgical intervention is used for the patient who experiences pain at rest or who has leg ulcers that do not heal. Surgical treatment includes endarterectomy to remove atherosclerotic lesions, balloon angioplasty with stents, or grafting to bypass the occluded area. (See the discussion of vascular surgery later in this chapter.)

DIET. The diet should aim to control atherosclerosis development. Teaching the patient to eat a healthy diet is important.

MEDICATIONS. Drug therapy is geared toward the symptoms and causes of the occlusive disease. The same drugs used to decrease cholesterol and lipid levels in atherosclerosis are used with occlusive disease. Pentoxifylline (Trental) or cilostazol (Pletal) is used for patients with occlusive disorders who experience intermittent claudication. Trental makes red blood cells more flexible to improve perfusion. Pletal is an antiplatelet medication. The major side effect is gastrointestinal upset, so it should be taken with meals. Thrombolytic therapy is used when an occlusion is caused by a thrombus or an embolus.

INVASIVE THERAPIES. Percutaneous transluminal angioplasty (PTA) can be used to dilate a narrowed peripheral vessel, although it does not provide long-term results. It is similar to PCI, which was discussed earlier. Peripheral atherectomy is another invasive procedure used to remove plaque from atherosclerotic arteries. Intravascular stents can also be used to maintain patency of the artery. After stent placement, patients are given platelet aggregation inhibitors.

Raynaud's Disease

A vasoconstrictive response causing ischemia from exposure to cold and stress is known as **Raynaud's disease** or syndrome. It occurs more often in women who live in cold climates. Raynaud's disease primarily affects the hands but also can occur in the feet, ears, or nose. To be diagnosed with Raynaud's disease, the patient must experience intermittent attacks of ischemia for at least 2 years.

Pathophysiology

Raynaud's disease is characterized by spasms of small arteries in the digits. These spasms prevent arterial blood from perfusing the fingertips and sometimes the toes. The spasms can occur unilaterally and in one or two digits, but most often they occur bilaterally and in all digits. Raynaud's disease may be seen with collagen diseases such as rheumatoid arthritis, scleroderma, and systemic lupus erythematosus. This disease can progress over time; the vessels remain constricted and the severe decrease in blood flow can lead to fingers becoming gangrenous and necrotic.

Signs and Symptoms

The hands, when exposed to cold, exhibit vascular spasms and a marked decrease in blood flow to the tissues. The resulting effect in the tissues is ischemic pain. After several minutes of ischemia, hyperemia occurs. Hyperemia is intense reddening of the hands from dilation of all the vessels of the hands. Pain becomes more intense at this time. Patients with Raynaud's disease go through various phases, which include blanching of the skin, pain, and reddening of the skin.

Therapeutic Measures

Conservative treatment is attempted first. The patient is instructed to keep the hands warm. Gloves should be worn when going outside, cleaning a refrigerator, or preparing cold foods. Patients are instructed in the importance of protecting the hands from injury and avoiding things that contribute to vasoconstriction, such as smoking, alcohol, and caffeine. Reducing stress levels can also help prevent vasoconstriction. Immersing the hands in warm water may decrease the vasospasm. Vasodilators are sometimes prescribed to help the patient avoid peripheral vasoconstriction. Raynaud's disease is treated surgically with a sympathectomy. This blocks the sympathetic reflex.

Nursing Care

Education is essential for patients with Raynaud's disease. Teaching the patient to protect the hands is important. Stressing the use of gloves in cold climates, reducing vasoconstrictive activity, and decreasing stress levels helps reduce the number and severity of attacks.

Thromboangiitis Obliterans (Buerger's Disease)

Buerger's disease is a recurring inflammation and thrombosis of small and medium arteries and veins of the hands and feet. It is associated with tobacco use, both cigarettes and smokeless tobacco. The cause is unknown, but it is thought to be an autoimmune disorder. It is most prevalent in young men between ages 25 and 40. It is increasing in women likely due to increased tobacco use by women.

Intermittent claudication and other symptoms of occlusive disease are common in patients with Buerger's disease. Other symptoms include numbness or decreased sensation and cool extremities. Lower extremities can be red or cyanotic when in a dependent position, and pulses may be diminished. Depending on the degree of ischemia, ulceration or gangrene may be present.

Because the primary contributing factor is smoking, there is urgency in helping the patient to cease smoking and avoid secondhand smoke. The patient must be made aware of the effect smoking has on the body and that the disease will progress and further damage other vessels. There is no cure or effective treatment. The use of calcium channel blockers such as diltiazem (Cardizem) promotes vasodilation and may help with intermittent claudication. Surgery is not effective. Supportive therapy and nursing care for Buerger's disease is used with the goal of reducing complications of ulceration, gangrene, and amputation. Careful inspection of the lower extremities for signs of breakdown is important, so early treatment can begin.

Nursing Process for the Patient With a Peripheral Arterial Disorder

DATA COLLECTION. Monitoring peripheral circulation is most important for patients with arterial occlusive disorders. Careful assessment of pulses, capillary refill, temperature, color, and presence of edema helps identify patients at risk for complications. Absent pulses are reported immediately to prevent limb loss. Skin that is shiny and hairless points to chronic diminished blood flow to the extremity. Laboratory blood testing is not necessary to test for peripheral arterial disease, but a lipid panel and serum glucose can identify diabetes, which is a significant risk factor for PAD. The presence of skin lesions and ulcerations is noted.

NURSING DIAGNOSES, PLANNING, IMPLEMENTATION, AND EVALUATION. See the "Nursing Care Plan for the Patient With a Peripheral Arterial Occlusive Disorder."

NURSING CARE PLAN for the Patient With a Peripheral Arterial Occlusive Disorder

Nursing Diagnosis: *Acute Pain* related to impaired circulation to extremities causing intermittent or continuous pain

Expected Outcome: The patient will report that pain is controlled at an acceptable level.

Evaluation of Outcome: Does patient report relief from pain by nonpharmacological or pharmacological methods?

Intervention Note peripheral circulation, pulses, color, temperature, presence of edema, and skin breakdown. **Rationale** Determines the degree of tissue perfusion and complications. **Evaluation** Does patient have pulses, warm skin, capillary refill less than 3 seconds, no evidence of skin breakdown?

Intervention Monitor for intermittent claudication or pain at rest. **Rationale** Helps determine degree of occlusive disease. Pain at rest is an indicator that the arterial occlusion is becoming worse. **Evaluation** Does patient have pain during activity or at rest?

Intervention Administer medication as ordered: • Analgesics • Vasodilators • Calcium channel blockers **Rationale** Relieves chronic or acute pain. Increases blood flow to extremities. Decrease vasospastic episodes. **Evaluation** Does patient show signs of increased circulation and relief of pain following administration of medications?

Continued

NURSING CARE PLAN for the Patient With a Peripheral Arterial Occlusive Disorder—cont'd

Intervention Encourage rest if pain is present. **Rationale** Rest decreases muscle contraction and prevents further ischemia in extremities. **Evaluation** Is patient able to rest?

Intervention Position lower extremities below heart level. **Rationale** Increases arterial flow to lower extremities. **Evaluation** Are pulses strong, capillary refill less than 3 seconds, extremities pink and warm?

Intervention Protect extremities from cold or trauma. **Rationale** Extremities with decreased circulation have decreased sensation, which increases risk of injury. **Evaluation** Are extremities injury-free?

Intervention Teach the patient importance and use of relaxation techniques. **Rationale** Relaxation will decrease the stress response and vasoconstriction related to catecholamine release. **Evaluation** Does patient demonstrate use of relaxation techniques?

Nursing Diagnosis: *Ineffective Tissue Perfusion* related to interruption of arterial flow in arms and legs

Expected Outcome: The patient will show signs of increased arterial blood flow and tissue perfusion.

Evaluation of Outcome: Does patient have strong peripheral pulses, capillary refill less than 3 seconds, warm skin, absence of edema?

Intervention Check peripheral pulses, capillary refill, color, temperature, and presence of edema every 4 hours. **Rationale** Indication of adequate tissue perfusion. **Evaluation** Are peripheral pulses strong, nail beds pink, capillary refill less than 3 seconds with no edema noted?

Intervention Report absent or diminished pulses immediately. **Rationale** Indication of inadequate tissue perfusion requiring immediate treatment. **Evaluation** Are peripheral pulses present and strong?

Intervention Check skin for intactness, healed areas, signs of ulceration or infection. **Rationale** Chronic arterial occlusion leads to decreased blood flow, resulting in tissue damage and poor wound healing. **Evaluation** Is skin intact?

Intervention Place extremities lower than heart, feet on floor in sitting position, head of bed elevated on blocks. **Rationale** Dependent position increases blood flow to the legs and feet. **Evaluation** Does patient have adequate tissue perfusion signs?

Intervention Avoid bending knees, pillows under knees, prolonged sitting, or crossing legs. **Rationale** These activities impede blood flow to extremities. **Evaluation** Does patient exhibit understanding of improving blood flow?

Intervention Inspect lower extremities frequently. Clean feet with mild soap; dry carefully. Protect from injury. **Rationale** Cleaning prevents trauma to feet, protecting feet from things that can lead to ulcerations. **Evaluation** Is patient free from trauma or breaks in skin of the lower extremities?

Intervention Encourage use of shoes that fit well. **Rationale** Prevents irritation and tissue breakdown leading to ulcer. **Evaluation** Does patient verbalize that shoes fit well?

Intervention Refer to progressive activity program. **Rationale** Gradual progressive exercise promotes collateral circulation. **Evaluation** Does patient participate in exercise program?

Intervention Keep extremity warm with socks and blankets. **Rationale** Prevents vasoconstriction and promotes comfort. **Evaluation** Are extremities warm?

Nursing Diagnosis: *Activity Intolerance* related to activity pain and diminished blood flow

Expected Outcome: The patient will report that pain is relieved during desired activities.

NURSING CARE PLAN for the Patient With a Peripheral Arterial Occlusive Disorder—cont'd

Evaluation of Outcome: Does patient participate in activities without pain?

Intervention Begin walking program: Start on flat surface. Walk 30 minutes per day. **Rationale** Promotes collateral circulation without greatly increasing oxygen demand. **Evaluation** Does patient participate in walking program?

Intervention Walk every day, increasing the distance in small increments until experiencing claudication. Walk one-half city block after pain begins per HCP order. Stop and rest until pain subsides. **Rationale** Walking through the pain will promote collateral circulation. Pain should subside with rest. **Evaluation** Does patient increase distance with claudication? Does pain stop with rest?

Nursing Diagnosis: *Deficient Knowledge:* peripheral arterial disease related to complications, medications, or postoperative care

Expected Outcome: The patient and family will verbalize self-care measures to control disease and prevent complications.

Evaluation of Outcome: Do patient and family verbalize understanding of teaching?

Intervention Ask patient's and family's knowledge of the physiology of the disease, and treatment and preventive techniques. **Rationale** This will determine educational topics. **Evaluation** What is patient's and family's baseline knowledge of peripheral artery disease (PAD)?

Intervention Describe peripheral arterial disease, symptoms, diagnosis, treatment, and complications to patient and family. **Rationale** The patient should understand PAD to help control disorder. **Evaluation** Do patient and family verbalize understanding of PAD?

Intervention Teach healthy lifestyle and risk factor control: smoking cessation, healthy diet, walking programs, **hyperlipidemia**, and diabetes and hypertension control. **Rationale** Healthy lifestyle promotes circulation and decreases functional impairment and pain. **Evaluation** Is patient willing and able to incorporated healthy lifestyle into daily routine?

Intervention Explain daily foot care: • Inspect feet for ingrown toenails, redness, sores, or blisters, wash feet with warm soap and water, dry with gentle patting, lubricate skin to prevent cracking, wear clean socks. **Rationale** Daily foot care and reporting problems promptly can help prevent complications of PAD. **Evaluation** Does patient state that he or she will perform daily foot care and verbalize understanding?

Intervention • Do not walk barefoot, and inspect inside of footwear for foreign objects before inserting foot. **Rationale** Ulceration of the toes may follow trauma if foreign object is walked on, which can result in infection. **Evaluation** Does patient verbalize understanding of need to protect feet?

Intervention Explain prescribed drug treatment protocols. **Rationale** Medication explanation can help patient comply with therapy. **Evaluation** Does patient verbalize understanding of medications?

Aneurysms

An **aneurysm** is a bulging, ballooning, or dilation at a weakened point of an artery. The artery diameter is often increased by 50%. The cause is unknown, but anything that weakens the artery wall or causes loss of elasticity in the artery can cause an aneurysm. Atherosclerosis, hypertension, smoking, trauma, and congenital abnormalities are risk factors for an aneurysm. Heredity may also play a role.

Smoking is such a risk factor that Medicare allows a one-time screening for those over 65 with a smoking history. Aneurysms can occur in any artery in the body but are common in the abdominal aorta, which is the focus of the rest of this discussion.

• WORD • BUILDING •

hyperlipidemia: hyper—above + lipos—fat + emia—blood

An abdominal aortic aneurysm (AAA) is often silent if it is less than 4 cm. Men older than age 50 are at the highest risk of death from an AAA. The incidence of AAA increases with age. Survival improves with elective repair rather than having emergency surgery after the aneurysm ruptures.

Types of Aneurysms

The various types of aneurysms are shown in Figure 24.9. A fusiform aneurysm is the dilation of the entire circumference of the artery. A saccular aneurysm is one that bulges on only one side of the artery wall. A dissecting aneurysm occurs when a cavity is formed from a tear in the artery wall, usually the intimal (inner) layer. The layers of the artery are then separated as blood is pumped into the tear with each heartbeat, expanding the cavity, which is then prone to rupturing.

Signs and Symptoms

Aneurysms usually exhibit few if any symptoms (Table 24.8). As the AAA grows, symptoms may develop. Back or flank pain is the classic symptom; the pain is caused by the aneurysm pressing against nerves of the vertebrae. Depending on the location and size of the aneurysm, there may be reports of abdominal pain, a feeling of fullness, or nausea caused by pressure on the intestines. The pain may mimic pain associated with any abdominal or back disorder. Changing positions may temporarily relieve the symptoms. Because the symptoms are vague, they are often not associated with an AAA. There may be a pulsating mass in the abdomen caused by an AAA that is discovered during routine physical or x-ray examination.

Severe, sudden back, flank, or abdominal pain and a pulsating abdominal mass can indicate that the aneurysm may be about to rupture. With rupture, the patient's blood pressure may drop and signs of shock may be present. Immediate surgery is needed for a ruptured AAA. The mortality rate is high with a ruptured aneurysm.

Diagnostic Tests

Abdominal ultrasound, CT scan, MRA, or aortography can be done to diagnose an AAA. Small aneurysms are watched, usually with ultrasound every 6 to 12 months, for enlargement.

FIGURE 24.9 Types of aneurysms. (A) Fusiform: The entire circumference of the artery is dilated. (B) Saccular: One side of the artery is dilated. (C) Dissecting: A tear in the inner layer causes a cavity to form between the layers of the artery and fill with blood. The cavity expands with each heartbeat.

TABLE 24.8 ANEURYSM SUMMARY

Signs and Symptoms	Back pain Flank pain Abdominal fullness Nausea Pulsating mass in abdomen Severe sudden back pain with rupture Shock from blood loss
Diagnostic Tests	Ultrasound CT scan Aortography
Therapeutic Measures	Observe for growth of aneurysm Maintain blood pressure Surgical repair and graft
Complications	Rupture Shock Hemorrhage
Priority Nursing Diagnoses	*Acute Pain* *Risk for Deficient Fluid Volume* *Risk for Ineffective Tissue Perfusion*

Therapeutic Measures

Medical treatment consists of medication to maintain lower blood pressures to prevent arterial wall to rupture. Surgical treatment—a bypass graft—is performed when the patient is experiencing pain, showing signs of circulatory compromise, or has an aneurysm that is larger than 5 cm, which increases the risk of rupture.

An endovascular stent graft or a conventional open surgical repair may be done for an AAA. Endovascular grafting involves the placement (through the femoral artery) of a stent graft at the site of the AAA. A balloon catheter positions and opens the graft. Blood flows through the stent graft to reduce pressure on the aneurysm, which will shrink over time. A fenestrated (perforated) endograft is used when the AAA is near other arteries such as the renal arteries to maintain their blood flow. Endovascular surgery requires less hospitalization time (2–3 days) and a quicker recovery.

Nursing Process for the Patient With an Abdominal Aortic Aneurysm

DATA COLLECTION. Careful monitoring of a patient with a AAA is necessary. Patient understanding must be assessed so patients know their medications and the importance of taking antihypertensives as prescribed. Stress may be a risk factor that should be addressed. Lifting heavy objects can increase pressure within the artery and may be restricted even in the individual being treated with more conservative measures. Postoperatively, the patient should avoid lifting heavy objects (see "Home Health Hints").

Home Health Hints

Cardiac

Both patients and caregivers can experience stress and frustration related to cardiovascular disease. Patients who have undergone open-heart surgery may experience feelings of powerlessness, depression, and anger. The home health nurse can be instrumental in helping the family deal with these life-changing illnesses.

• Have a home health social worker visit a postsurgical cardiac patient. This can be useful to help the patient and family plan for lifestyle changes to reduce anxiety and environmental stress.

• Assess the ability of the patient's caregiver to provide necessary care. The support and resources available to the caregiver should be explored to prevent caregiver role strain.

• Assist the caregiver to identify a plan to distribute the care workload among family members, if possible.

• Determine the need for caregiver respite care, especially over time. If respite care is needed, assist the caregiver in identifying respite care resources in the family or community.

• Teach the caregiver stress management techniques to use. This can include deep-breathing exercises, reading a book, meditation, massage therapy, guided imagery, exercise, socializing with friends, and/or working on a favorite hobby.

• After open-heart surgery, many patients suffer from depression. If you encounter patients who appear withdrawn, offer limited eye contact during interaction, and seem uninterested with following through on postoperative instructions, discuss with them how they feel they have changed since having surgery. Report concerns to the patient's HCP; antidepressants might be helpful during this time. Also identify community resources that are available such as a support group and offer that information to your patient.

• Chest pain from esophageal reflux can mimic cardiovascular symptoms. Ask if the pain is related to consuming large meals, lying down, or bending over, or if it is relieved with antacids or food. Inform the HCP of these findings.

Vascular

• Instruct the patient to stop and rest if pain develops in the lower extremities during exercise.

• Monitor peripheral pulses and capillary refill to ensure adequate tissue perfusion. Report absent pulses or sluggish capillary refill to the patient's HCP.

• Instruct the patient to report changes in skin color, insect bites, and/or rashes to the HCP. Patients with peripheral vascular disorders are at a high risk for developing lower extremity wounds that are often slow to heal.

NURSING DIAGNOSES, PLANNING, IMPLEMENTATION, AND EVALUATION. See the "Nursing Care Plan for the Patient After Vascular Surgery."

Varicose Veins

Varicose veins are elongated, tortuous, dilated veins. The exact cause is unknown. The condition tends to be familial. Varicose veins are divided into primary and secondary varicosities.

Pathophysiology

Primary varicosities are believed to be caused by a structural defect in the vessel wall. Along with the defect, the dilation of the vessel can lead to incompetent venous valves. The valves help prevent blood from refluxing. If reflux occurs, it can cause further dilation of the vessel and blood pooling in the lower extremities. The superficial veins are the vessels most often involved in primary varicosities.

Secondary varicosities are caused by an acquired or congenital pathological condition of the deep venous system. This produces dilation of collateral and superficial veins. As a result, there is an interference of blood return to the heart, which leads to stasis, or pooling, of the blood in the deep venous system. This increases the pressure within the system, pushing blood into the collateral vessels and producing varicosities in the superficial veins.

Etiology

Wall defects have been identified as a familial tendency and may be inherited. Any factor that contributes to increasing hydrostatic pressure within the leg, such as prolonged standing, pregnancy, and obesity, can promote venous dilation. Incompetent valves within the veins can cause blockage of blood flow and lead to dilated veins.

Signs and Symptoms

The appearance of telangiectasias, or spider veins, indicates minor chronic venous disease. With more advanced disease there can be dull pain, cramping, edema, and feelings of heaviness in the lower extremities, especially after prolonged standing. This can usually be relieved by walking or elevating the extremity. With secondary varicosities, the pain and disfigurement can be more severe. Edema or ulceration can develop if circulation is severely compromised.

Therapeutic Measures

The primary goals are to improve circulation, relieve pain, and avoid complications. Conservative treatment is exercise, elevation, and elastic compression hose as ordered. Injection sclerotherapy or lasers treat superficial varicosities. Minimally invasive ablation procedures include radiofrequency ablation (closure procedure) or endovenous laser treatment.

Venous Insufficiency

Venous insufficiency is a chronic condition. Damaged or aging valves within the veins interfere with blood return to the heart, causing pooling of blood in the lower extremities. Chronic venous insufficiency can lead to venous stasis ulcers.

Venous Stasis Ulcers

PATHOPHYSIOLOGY. **Venous stasis ulcers** are the end result of chronic venous insufficiency. Dysfunctional valves in the venous system prevent or reduce venous blood return. As venous pressure increases, venous stasis occurs. Over time the congestion and decreased venous circulation lead to changes in the lower extremities. There may be edema and a brownish discoloration of the leg and foot, with the surrounding skin hardened and leathery in appearance. The brown color occurs

---

NURSING CARE PLAN for the Patient After Vascular Surgery

Nursing Diagnosis: *Acute Pain* related to surgical incision and reperfusion of tissue

Expected Outcomes: The patient will state that the pain is relieved or is tolerable within 30 minutes of pain report. The patient will rest comfortably, perform respiratory treatments as necessary, and perform activities of daily living (ADLs).

Evaluation of Outcomes: Does patient state that pain is relieved or acceptable? Is patient able to rest and participate in respiratory treatments and ADLs?

Intervention Ask about severity, as well as all other qualities, of pain. **Rationale** Peripheral vascular surgery pain is usually mild; severe pain may indicate reocclusion. Major vascular surgery pain is severe. **Evaluation** Does patient state that pain is at a tolerable level with a patent vessel?

GERIATRIC
Intervention Ask patient to rate pain after analgesic is given. **Rationale** Pain relief is individualized. **Evaluation** Does patient state that pain is controlled at a tolerable level?

Intervention Notify HCP if pain is unrelieved. **Rationale** Different analgesic may be needed to give relief. **Evaluation** Are patient's pain relief needs met?

Intervention Ensure that older patient's pain is relieved. **Rationale** Pain is not a normal part of aging, and older patients need and are entitled to adequate pain relief. **Evaluation** Does patient rate pain as none or at a tolerable level using a scale of 0 to 10?

Intervention Use opioid pain medications cautiously. Consider reducing frail older patients' first opioid dose by 25% to 50%, and increase as safe and needed and as ordered. **Rationale** Older patients are more susceptible to peak effects and duration of analgesia of opioids. **Evaluation** Are patient's vital signs and sedation levels within normal limits?

Nursing Diagnosis: *Ineffective Tissue Perfusion* related to hypotension, hypothermia, emboli, vascular spasm, or reocclusion

Expected Outcomes: The patient will have palpable peripheral pulses: adequate capillary refill, and normal color, temperature, motor, and sensory function of extremities. The patient will have reactive pupils and baseline cognitive function.

Evaluation of Outcomes: Is patient's circulatory status within normal limits? Does patient have reactive pupils and baseline cognitive function intact?

Intervention Monitor circulation, movement, and sensation to extremities every 1 to 4 hours. **Rationale** Early detection of spasm or reocclusion minimizes risk of ischemia and necrosis. **Evaluation** Does graft or vessel remain patent?

Intervention Mark location of pulses on affected extremity. **Rationale** Allows for quick location of pulses. **Evaluation** Are pulses located easily?

Intervention Perform neurologic checks every 2 to 4 hours (carotid). **Rationale** Allows early detection of complications. **Evaluation** Are major neurologic or circulatory problems detected?

NURSING CARE PLAN for the Patient After Vascular Surgery—cont'd

Intervention Perform circulation or neurologic check between nurses when changing caregiver. **Rationale** Subtle changes can be detected, and new caregiver has baseline for comparison. **Evaluation** Is baseline assessment done?

Intervention Measure abdominal girth every shift (abdominal aortic surgery). **Rationale** Increasing girth may indicate bleeding into abdomen. **Evaluation** Does abdominal girth remain unchanged?

Intervention Take temperature every 4 hours. **Rationale** May indicate infection or hypothermia with need for further warming. **Evaluation** Does patient remain normothermic?

Intervention Monitor complete blood cell count (CBC) as ordered. **Rationale** Red blood cell (RBC) count, hemoglobin, and hematocrit decrease with insidious bleeding into abdomen or significant hematoma formations. **Evaluation** Is CBC WNL?

Intervention Avoid constricting measures on affected extremity: knee gatch of bed, adhesive tape, tight dressings. **Rationale** Prevent further decrease in blood flow to compromised extremity. **Evaluation** Is blood flow to affected extremity maintained?

---

when veins rupture, releasing RBCs into the tissues; the RBCs then break down and stain the tissue brown.

Stasis ulcers develop from the increased pressure and rupture of small veins. Signs of skin breakdown are most commonly seen at the medial malleolus of the ankle. Stasis ulcers are a serious complication of venous insufficiency that are difficult to cure and can affect the patient's quality of life.

THERAPEUTIC MEASURES. The focus of treatment is to decrease edema and heal skin ulcerations. Compression wraps such as elastic stockings or bandage wraps are necessary to decrease edema. Bed rest and elevation of legs and feet above the heart are important to assist with drainage of lower extremities. Patients are advised not to keep legs dependent and to avoid long periods of standing or sitting to prevent increased pressure and pain. The foot of the bed should be elevated 5 to 6 inches. Additionally, patients should be encouraged to exercise and walk often during nonacute episodes. Patients should be taught not to cross their legs or wear constrictive clothing that would decrease venous blood return to the heart.

Skin ulcers are usually cultured and treated with topical antibiotics if needed. Wound care can be chronic and challenging (see Chapter 54). An Unna boot, which is a gauze dressing coated with zinc oxide, calamine, and glycerin, may be used to promote healing in severe ulcers. Zinc promotes wound healing and can be soothing. The Unna boot is applied snugly and provides compression therapy as well. It is changed every 2 to 7 days. Skin grafting may be necessary if ulcerations are severe or do not heal.

NURSING PROCESS FOR THE PATIENT WITH A VENOUS DISORDER.
Data Collection. Risk factors for varicose veins are identified. Symptoms and concerns about body image are noted. Leg appearance, presence of edema, and ulcerations are noted.

Patient-coping skills are assessed to determine patient's ability to cope with chronic ulcers that may affect quality of life. Baseline knowledge of contributing factors for venous disorders is determined for teaching plans.

Nursing Diagnoses, Planning, and Implementation.
Acute Pain related to edema and increased pressure
EXPECTED OUTCOME: The patient will report pain is at a tolerable level within 30 minutes of report of pain.

- Use rating scale such as 0 to 10 to identify pain level *to provide consistency in pain reporting.*
- Elevate legs above heart level (such as in a reclining chair) and avoid long periods of standing *to reduce pooling of fluid.*
- Apply compression therapy as ordered *to promote drainage and reduce edema.*
- Administer analgesics as prescribed *to provide pain relief.*

Impaired Tissue Integrity related to chronic venous congestion
EXPECTED OUTCOME: The patient will have intact tissue integrity.

- Assess and document size, shape, and depth of wound *to evaluate healing of wound over time.*
- Provide a comprehensive plan for wound care including methods of pressure relief from edema, treatments, and nutrition as ordered *to ensure that quality wound care is provided.*
- Provide wound care as ordered *to aid in wound healing.*

Ineffective Health Maintenance related to deficient knowledge of venous disease
EXPECTED OUTCOME: The patient will report understanding and management of his or her venous disorder.

- Assess the patient's present understanding of the disease *to determine baseline knowledge.*

- Explain to patient how to control risk factors and prevention of varicose veins: weight reduction, elevation of the extremities, walking, and exercise *help increase muscle strength and contraction.*
- Explain that tight-fitting clothes at tops of legs or waist should not be worn *to prevent venous occlusion.*
- Encourage patient with varicose veins to wear support hose *to assist blood flow return to the heart.*
- Explain need to avoid heating devices *because of decreased sensitivity and risk of burns.*
- Encourage questions and allow the patient the opportunity to verbalize new information and skills *to enhance learning.*
- Document teaching and evaluation of patient knowledge *to communicate patient progress toward goal attainment.*

See also the "Nursing Care Plan for the Patient After Vascular Surgery."

Evaluation. Interventions are successful if the patient reports understanding of venous disease and prevention and that pain is at an acceptable level.

Vascular Surgery

Vascular impairments requiring surgery may be acute or chronic and involve arteries, veins, or lymphatic vessels. When intermittent claudication becomes severe or disabling or when the limb is at risk for amputation, then surgical vascular grafting may be done.

Nursing Process for the Patient Undergoing Preoperative Vascular Surgery

DATA COLLECTION. A baseline assessment is important for postoperative comparison and discharge planning. Pain control needs and circulatory status are assessed. Diagnostic test results (CBC, electrolytes, PT, PTT, and bleeding time) are reviewed and typing and crossmatching of blood to be placed on hold is performed.

NURSING DIAGNOSES. The nursing diagnoses for preoperative vascular surgery may include the following:

- *Acute* or *Chronic Pain* related to ischemia of tissue distal to occlusion or aneurysm
- *Anxiety* related to unknown outcome, pain, powerlessness, or threat of death
- *Deficient Knowledge,* preoperative and postoperative procedures, related to unfamiliar process

See Chapter 12 for further preoperative nursing process information.

Embolectomy and Thrombectomy

When an artery becomes completely occluded by an embolus or thrombus, it is considered a surgical emergency. Emergency embolectomy is the procedure of choice only if the affected extremity is viable. Surgical removal to restore blood flow and oxygenation to the tissue distal to the occlusion is imperative to decrease ischemia and necrosis.

Vascular Bypasses and Grafts

Vascular bypass surgery involves the use of either autografts, such as the patient's own saphenous vein, or a synthetic graft material. The graft is anastomosed to the artery proximal to the occlusion and tunneled past the occlusion, where the distal end of the graft is anastomosed to the artery (Fig. 24.10). The graft is assessed for hemostasis and function, and then the wound is sutured closed.

Endarterectomy

Arteriosclerotic plaques are dissected from the lining of the arterial wall and removed in a procedure called an **endarterectomy**. This is most commonly performed on the carotid artery but may be done on peripheral arterial vessels as well. To control blood flow, the artery is clamped on both sides of the occlusion, and an incision is made into the artery. The plaque within the artery is removed with forceps. The artery is irrigated to remove any further debris and then closed with sutures. The clamps are removed, and the skin incision is closed. A drain may be placed to help prevent hematoma formation.

• WORD • BUILDING •

endarterectomy: end—inside + arter—artery + ectomy—excision

FIGURE 24.10 Aortofemoral bypass.

Angioplasty

Minimally invasive techniques can also be used to open plaque-blocked arteries. These techniques include balloon or laser angioplasty. A flexible laser-tipped catheter is inserted into an artery and advanced to the site of the blockage. The laser sends out pulsating beams of light, which vaporize the plaque. This procedure is used for patients with smaller occlusions in the distal superficial femoral, proximal popliteal, and common iliac arteries.

Stents

Stents are placed inside an artery to provide support to the artery walls and keep them open. Stents are placed in a procedure similar to PCI discussed earlier. Stents may also be used in combination with other procedures such as angioplasty.

Complications of Vascular Surgery

Bleeding and hemorrhage can occur with all vascular surgeries. Drainage can be expected with most surgeries. Drainage is usually small when peripheral vessels are involved. But with involvement of the great vessels, drainage is usually heavier and drains are often placed to prevent swelling and hematoma formation. If hemorrhage occurs, manual pressure is applied to the site of bleeding, and the HCP is notified immediately. Extensive surgeries may also result in significant blood loss, leading to fluid volume deficit or shock.

Reocclusion is possible with any vascular surgery. If thrombi or emboli develop and block blood flow, a surgical emergency results. Loss of a pedal pulse may signify reocclusion and must be immediately reported to the HCP. Blood flow needs to be reestablished within 4 to 6 hours to prevent risk of amputation of that extremity.

Nursing Process for the Patient After Vascular Surgery

DATA COLLECTION. Upon transfer postoperatively to either the ICU or surgical unit, the patient is positioned comfortably and a head-to-toe assessment is performed and documented. Abnormal findings are reported to the HCP. A patent airway is ensured and vital signs are monitored. The patient's pain level is rated on a scale of 0 to 10. All IVs and drains are monitored. Measurement of input and output (I&O) is done hourly, then every 4 to 8 hours. CBC, INR, PTT, and electrolytes are monitored. Increasing abdominal girth measurements (for AAA repair) can indicate hemorrhage. Any abnormal change is reported immediately to the HCP.

Initially, neurovascular checks are ordered every 15 minutes for the first 2 hours, then every 30 minutes for 1 to 3 hours, then hourly for aortic or extremity vascular surgery. Neurovascular checks include extremity movement and sensation, presence of numbness or tingling, pulses, temperature, color, and capillary refill (less than 3 seconds normally). Peripheral pulses are palpated, or assessed with Doppler ultrasound if not palpable, marked, and compared with the unaffected extremity to detect deficits. If a pulse is absent or weak or the extremity is cool or dusky, the HCP is notified immediately. A return to surgery for an embolectomy or other procedure is anticipated.

NURSING CARE TIP

Neurovascular checks refer to the assessment of an extremity. (Neurologic checks refer to assessment of the central nervous system.) The following are areas to examine on an extremity when doing neurovascular checks. They are identified under the category for which they provide information:

NEUROLOGIC	VASCULAR
Movement	Pulses
Sensation	Capillary refill
Numbness	Color (nailbed or skin)
Tingling	Temperature

CRITICAL THINKING

Mr. Janeway

■ The nurse is caring for Mr. Janeway, age 63, who has just returned from surgery after an embolectomy of the right lower leg. He has a history of insulin-dependent diabetes mellitus, hypertension, renal insufficiency, and an MI 2 weeks ago. He is 6 feet tall and weighs 316 pounds.

1. What four priority areas of data collection should the nurse focus on for Mr. Janeway?
2. What other information might the nurse want to know regarding Mr. Janeway's medical history?
3. List three priority nursing diagnoses for Mr. Janeway.
4. State one outcome for each nursing diagnosis.
5. What nursing interventions are appropriate for each nursing diagnosis identified?

Suggested answers are at the end of the chapter.

NURSING DIAGNOSES, PLANNING, IMPLEMENTATION, AND EVALUATION. See the "Nursing Care Plan for the Patient After Vascular Surgery."

LYMPHATIC SYSTEM

The lymphatic system returns fluid from other tissues in the body to the bloodstream. It is a pumpless system with one-way valves that return the fluid to the heart. Any interruption in the flow of lymph results in edema.

Lymphangitis

Lymphangitis is a bacterial infection of the lymphatic channels. The infection can occur in the arms or legs and is commonly caused by *Staphylococcus* or *Streptococcus* bacteria. It is a serious infection that can cause sepsis and be fatal. Symptoms include painful red streaks in the extremity. Fever and chills may be present. Lymph nodes in the area of infection can be enlarged and painful. Therapy is initiated with a broad-spectrum antibiotic as the drug of choice. The use of heat on the extremity, as well as elevating it, can help improve circulation. The use of a pneumatic pressure device can be ordered to help alleviate congestion.

Nursing Process for the Patient With Lymphangitis

DATA COLLECTION.   Frequent monitoring of the affected area for edema and skin breakdown is needed to prevent complications from edema. The nurse monitors the size of the extremity and notifies the HCP of any increase in size or possible spread of infection. Pain level and fever are monitored.

NURSING DIAGNOSES, PLANNING, AND IMPLEMENTATION.
Acute Pain related to tissue damage and edema from infection
EXPECTED OUTCOME: The patient will report an absence or acceptable level of pain within 30 minutes of reporting pain.

• Explain and have patient use pain rating *to report pain level for consistency.*
• Administer analgesics as prescribed *to provide pain relief.*
• Recheck pain level 30 to 60 minutes after analgesic given *to determine if pain relief has been obtained.*
• Position extremity *for comfort* and elevate *to reduce edema, which can cause pressure and pain.*

Risk for Excess Fluid Volume related to congested lymph nodes from infection
EXPECTED OUTCOME: The patient will exhibit no evidence of edema.

• Apply heat on the extremity as ordered *to increase circulation and reduce edema.*
• Elevate extremity *to help improve circulation and prevent edema.*

EVALUATION.   Interventions are successful if the patient reports pain is at an acceptable level and no edema is present.

SUGGESTED ANSWERS TO

CRITICAL THINKING

■ *Mr. Jones*

1. Irregular, respiratory rate 28 per minute and shallow, lung sounds diminished with crackles in bilateral bases.
2. Pain control, coughing and deep breathing, and incentive spirometer.
3. Pain, compensation for respiratory status, elevated temperature.
4. Hemorrhage, reduced cardiac output.
5. HCP for orders, pharmacist for medication orders, respiratory therapist for pulmonary concerns.

■ *Mrs. Sims*

1. Place on bedrest, administer oxygen via nasal cannula at 2 L/min, assess blood pressure and pulse, administer NTG sublingual as ordered, obtain ECG, and notify HCP.
2. She may be having an anginal attack versus acute MI.
3. NTG usually stops chest pain associated with angina. Rest may also alleviate chest pain. Neither NTG nor rest will relieve the pain of an acute MI.
4. Indicators of an MI include patient history, ECG changes with ST-segment elevation, elevated troponin I, and CK-MB elevation.

5. Medical interventions may include NTG drip, morphine, or anticoagulant therapy (heparin), as well as thrombolytic agents to dissolve the clot. A cardiac catheterization can determine which coronary artery is blocked. PCI or a coronary artery bypass graft may be done to reroute blood.
6. Educate Mrs. Sims about the risks of smoking and being overweight.

■ *Mrs. May*

1. Monitor the patient's left leg for color, temperature, capillary refill, and pulses: femoral, popliteal, dorsalis pedis, and posterior tibial. Compare findings with findings in the right leg.
2. If unable to palpate pulses, use a Doppler ultrasound that enhances sound to locate pulses.
3. The patient's symptoms could be caused by an embolism above left femoral artery.
4. To document finding, you would obtain more assessment data. A sample of SOAP charting for your additional findings is given:

   S: "I have a severe pain in my left groin that just started. It is at 9 on a scale of 0 to 10."

   O: Grimacing, moaning, and holding left upper leg. Left leg cool, color pale, nailbeds pale, capillary refill 10 seconds, unable to palpate pulses. Faint femoral and popliteal pulse, no dorsalis pedis or posterior tibial pulse heard with Doppler. Right leg warm, pink, capillary refill 3 seconds, with all pulses palpable.

A: Ineffective tissue perfusion.

P: Notify HCP stat.

5. Immediate interventions include complete bedrest, protecting the leg, and notifying the HCP.

6. Medical interventions could include medication for pain and use of an anticoagulant, such as heparin. If no pulses are present, a thrombolytic agent may be ordered. Surgery is possible.

7. Thrombectomy or embolectomy may be necessary to save the limb.

■ *Mr. Janeway*

1. Priority areas for data collection include respiratory status, circulatory status of right leg and foot, vital signs, and pain level.

2. A medical history should include Mr. Janeway's usual blood sugar values, insulin dose, ambulation aids, gait, knowledge base regarding his various disease processes, and what led to this hospitalization.

3. Priority nursing diagnoses include (1) *Pain* related to surgery of right lower leg; (2) *Ineffective Tissue*

Perfusion related to embolectomy of right lower leg, renal insufficiency; and (3) *Risk for Injury* related to leg surgery, diabetes, obesity.

4. Outcomes include (1) verbalizes relief of pain; (2) maintains adequate tissue perfusion as evidenced by palpable peripheral (pedal) pulses, warm and dry skin; and (3) remains free from injury.

5. Nursing interventions include the following: (1) position (especially right leg) for comfort; keep the right leg slightly elevated; educate the patient regarding the need to ask for pain medication before pain is too severe; educate the patient regarding the need to take pain medication to minimize the negative physiological effects of pain; monitor pain on a pain scale; evaluate the effectiveness of medication using the same pain scale; report ineffective pain measures. (2) Check pedal pulses, surgical dressing, pedal sensation and movement, and color, initially and every hour; report changes; check capillary refill; monitor for pain in extremities; monitor for edema in extremities; keep leg elevated slightly. (3) Make sure the nursing call light is within reach; provide assistance with ambulation; use walking aids.

REVIEW QUESTIONS

1. The nurse would evaluate the patient as understanding teaching on prevention of coronary artery disease if the patient stated that which of the following is a risk factor for coronary artery disease that can be controlled?
   1. Family history of cardiovascular disease
   2. Hypertension
   3. Ethnicity
   4. Family history of diabetes mellitus

2. The nurse is assisting with collecting data on a female patient in the emergency department. Which of these findings during data collection does the nurse report to the registered nurse as a possible atypical symptom of a myocardial infarction in the absence of chest pain?
   1. Fatigue
   2. Dizziness
   3. Sweating
   4. Nausea

3. The nurse would evaluate the patient as understanding teaching on the purpose of coronary artery bypass graft surgery if the patient made which of the following statements?
   1. "It cures coronary artery disease."
   2. "It is done to increase blood flow to the myocardium."
   3. "It prevents spasms of the coronary arteries."
   4. "It will decrease blood flow to the coronary arteries."

4. The nurse is reinforcing teaching for a patient prescribed sublingual nitroglycerin tablets. The nurse should instruct the patient to use this medication in which of the following ways?
   1. Take one tablet and lie down for 1 hour and repeat if pain unrelieved.
   2. Place two tablets under the tongue daily to prevent angina.
   3. Swallow one tablet, wait 10 minutes, swallow two tablets if pain persists, swallow 3 tablets if pain remains after 15 minutes.
   4. With symptoms of MI, place one tablet under the tongue and if after 5 minutes the pain is not relieved, call 911.

5. The nurse would evaluate the patient as understanding teaching on peripheral arterial occlusive disease if the patient stated that which of the following is the classic symptom?
   1. Angina
   2. Edema
   3. Intermittent claudication
   4. Stasis ulcers

6. Which of the following medications is used to treat intermittent claudication?
   1. Cholestyramine (Questran)
   2. Enoxaparin (Lovenox)
   3. Pentoxifylline (Trental)
   4. Ranolazine (Ranexa)

7. The nurse is caring for a patient who has peripheral arterial disease. Which of the following statements by the patient indicates understanding of how to manage the pain of peripheral arterial disease?
   1. "I will lie down frequently."
   2. "I will use a reclining chair."
   3. "I will sit with my legs down."
   4. "I will do knee flexion exercises."

Answers can be found in Appendix C.

References

American Heart Association. (2013). Statistical Fact Sheets 2013 updates.

Barto, D. (2013). Managing ST segment elevation myocardial infarction. *Nursing 2013 Critical Care, 8,* 22–25.

Centers for Disease Control. (2011). Prevalence of coronary heart disease—United States 2006–2010. *Morbidity and Mortality Weekly Report, 60,* 1377–1378.

Dechant, L. (2012). UA/NSTEMI: Are you following the latest guidelines? *Nursing 2012, 42,* 26–34.

Flock, M. R., Green, M. H., & Kris-Etherton, P. M. (2011). Effects of adiposity on plasma lipid response to reductions in dietary saturated fatty acids and cholesterol. *Advance Nutrition, 2,* 261–274.

Harland, J. I. (2012). Food combinations for cholesterol lowering. *Nutrition Research Review, 25,* 249.

Roger, V., Gol, A., Lloyd-Jones, D., Benjamin, E., Berry, J. D., Borden, W. B., . . . Turner, M. B.; American Heart Association Statistics Committee and Stroke Statistics Subcommittee. (2012). Heart disease and stroke statistics—2012 Update: A report from the American Heart Association. *Circulation, 125,* e2–e220.

 Davis*Plus* | For additional resources and information visit **davispl.us/medsurg5**

25

Nursing Care of Patients With Cardiac Dysrhythmias

LINDA S. WILLIAMS

LEARNING OUTCOMES

1. Describe how electrical activity flows through the heart.
2. List the six steps used for dysrhythmia interpretation.
3. Explain current medical treatments for each type of cardiac dysrhythmias.
4. Identify types of cardiac pacemakers and implantable cardioverter defibrillators and their uses.
5. Plan nursing care for patients with a dysrhythmia.
6. Plan nursing care for patients with an implanted device.

KEY TERMS

ablation (uh-BLAY-shun)
atrial depolarization (AE-tree-uhl DEE-poh-lur-ih-ZAY-shun)
atrial systole (AE-tree-uhl SISS-tuh-lee)
atrioventricular node (AE-tree-oh-ven-TRICK-yoo-lur NOHD)
bigeminy (bye-JEM-ih-nee)
bradycardia (BRAY-dih-KAR-dee-yah)
bundle of His (BUN-duhl of HISS)
cardioversion (KAR-dee-oh-VER-zhun)
defibrillation (dee-FIB-ri-lay-shun)
dysrhythmia (dis-RITH-mee-yah)
electrocardiogram (ee-LECK-troh-KAR-dee-oh-GRAM)
fluoroscopy (fluh-RAHS-kuh-pee)
hyperkalemia (HIGH-per-kuh-LEE-mee-ah)
hypomagnesemia (HIGH-poh-MAG-nuh-ZEE-mee-ah)
isoelectric line (EYE-so-e-LECK-trick LINE)
multifocal (MUHL-tee-FOH-kuhl)
sinoatrial node (SIGH-noh-AY-tree-al NOHD)
trigeminy (try-JEM-i-nee)
unifocal (YOO-ni-FOH-cull)
ventricular diastole (ven-TRICK-yoo-lar dye-AS-tuh-lee)
ventricular repolarization (ven-TRICK-yoo-lar RE-pol-lahr-i-ZAY-shun)
ventricular systole (ven-TRICK-yoo-lar SIS-tuh-lee)
ventricular tachycardia (ven-TRICK-yoo-lar TACK-ee-KAR-dee-yah)

CARDIAC CONDUCTION SYSTEM

The heart's electrical conduction system initiates an impulse whose purpose is to stimulate the mechanical cells of the heart to contract (Fig. 25.1). Electrical activity can be viewed on a cardiac monitor or recorded on an **electrocardiogram** (ECG) tracing. The activity seen on an ECG does not necessarily mean that the mechanical cells of the heart have contracted in response to the electrical impulse. So how can you verify heart muscle contraction and subsequent pumping of blood? By assessing the patient's blood pressure and apical and peripheral pulses, you will have evidence to determine if cardiac contraction occurred.

Do you recall what area of the conduction system is referred to as the normal pacemaker of the heart? Located in the upper posterior wall of the right atrium is the **sinoatrial** (SA) **node**. The SA node is the primary pacemaker of the heart because its inherent (built-in) rate is faster than those of the other conduction sites in the **atrioventricular** (AV) **node** or ventricles. It normally fires at a rate of 60 to 100 beats per minute (bpm). As a protective mechanism if the SA node slows or fails, other areas of the heart can initiate impulses to keep the heart beating. This mechanism is referred to as escape. The AV node has an inherent rate of 40 to 60 bpm. The body can usually function adequately with this rate. If the AV node is unable to initiate an impulse, then the ventricles can take over at 20 to 40 bpm. However, the ventricular rate of 20 to 40 bpm is not adequate to meet the body's oxygen needs, so the patient begins to show signs of inadequate cardiac output such as dyspnea, abnormal vital signs, and changes in level of consciousness. Treatment is usually needed to reestablish a normal heart rate as soon as possible.

After the SA node fires, the impulse spreads through the atria conduction system to the AV node, stimulating the atria to contract. This is known as **atrial systole**. The atrial contraction propels blood out of the atria and into the relaxed ventricles during **ventricular diastole**. At the AV node, the impulse is briefly delayed. Next the impulse travels down the **bundle of His**, which divides into right and left bundle branches through the Purkinje fibers. This stimulates both ventricles to contract upward from the apex of the heart, pushing blood toward the arteries. This contraction is known as **ventricular systole**.

Cardiac Cycle

A cardiac cycle is the period from the beginning of one heartbeat to the beginning of the next. The cardiac cycle is the electrical representation of the impulse that stimulates contraction and relaxation of the atria and ventricles. Within the normal cardiac cycle, there is a P wave, a QRS complex, and a T wave (Fig. 25.2).

ELECTROCARDIOGRAM

The electrical activity of the heart is seen either with an ECG that shows the activity for that moment when the ECG is obtained or with continuous cardiac monitoring. Electrodes placed on the patient's skin allow various views of the heart's electrical activity to be seen. Each view of the heart is referred to as a *lead*. A 12-lead ECG provides 12 different views of the heart's electrical activity, whereas an 18-lead ECG shows 18 views. For continuous monitoring of cardiac electrical activity, one lead providing a good view may be used, although

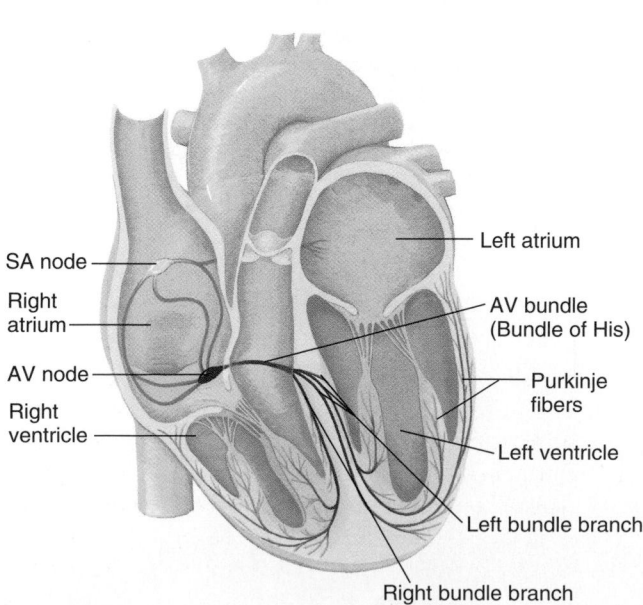

FIGURE 25.1 Conduction pathway of the heart. *From Scanlon, V., & Sanders, T. (2015). Essentials of anatomy and physiology (7th ed.). Philadelphia: F.A. Davis, with permission.*

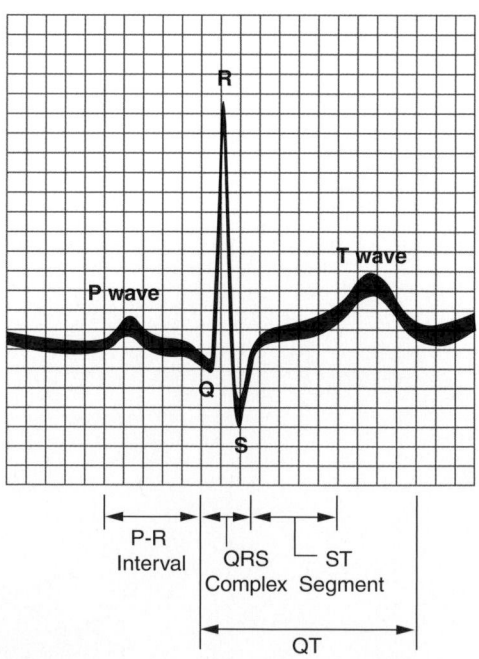

FIGURE 25.2 Components of the cardiac cycle. *From Scanlon, V., & Sanders, T. (2015). Essentials of anatomy and physiology (7th ed.). Philadelphia: F.A. Davis, with permission.*

with a five-electrode system, two views can be displayed at the same time. Continuous 12-lead monitoring can also be done.

Specialized training, usually obtained by physicians, is required to interpret ECGs for normal and abnormal heart rhythms. By learning the characteristics of a normal heart rhythm and rules for common **dysrhythmias**, you will be able to report rhythm changes to your supervisor or the health care provider (HCP).

 LEARNING TIP

Think of a 12- or 18-lead ECG as if you had a camera that you were using to take pictures (views) of an object such as an apple. To obtain views that showed you all of the areas of the apple—front, side, back, side—you would take a picture and then move the camera a little to get the view next to the one you had just taken. You would continue moving the camera until you had worked your way around the entire apple. This would then give you a view of the entire apple. This is what a 12- or 18-lead ECG does to allow viewing of the entire conduction system of the heart.

Electrocardiogram Graph Paper

The intervals of each of the components of a cardiac cycle can be measured in seconds of time on the ECG graph paper on which the heart rhythm is recorded. The graph paper is calibrated in a grid with small squares divided into heavy lined blocks of 25, five squares wide and five squares high (Fig. 25.3). Each small square is 0.04 seconds wide. There are five small squares, which equal 0.20 seconds of time, horizontally between two heavy vertical black lines (see Fig. 25.3). You will measure the waveforms horizontally from left to right on the graph paper. The height of waveforms (amplitude) is measured vertically.

You have probably seen a heart monitor, perhaps on television, with a straight line displayed on it. This straight line, called the **isoelectric line** (baseline), occurs when there is no electrical current, or the positive and negative electrical activity is equal. The isoelectric line is seen when there are no positive or negative electrical wave deflections. When cardiac cycle electrical impulses (seen as waveforms) occur, they are either upward (positive) or downward (negative) from the isoelectric line.

■ COMPONENTS OF A CARDIAC CYCLE

P Wave

The P wave is the first wave of the cardiac cycle and represents **atrial depolarization**. When the SA node fires, the electrical impulse spreads from the right to left atrium. The normal P wave appears rounded. When compared with other waveforms, it looks like a small hill. Disorders that change atrial size cause alterations in P-wave shape and size.

 LEARNING TIP

To make measuring waves easier:

- Identify the isoelectric line as you measure waveform tracings to help you determine the presence and type of wave. Place a straight edge along the isoelectric line so that it lays below this line, to then see any positive waves above the line; then lay the straight edge above the line to see any waves that fall below the line.
- If possible, find a wave that begins on a line to make it visually easier to see the interval being measured (Fig. 25.4).
- If the wave starts or ends in the middle of a small square, count it as one-half of a square, which is 0.02 seconds. Do not go smaller than one-half of a square.

PR Interval

The PR interval (PRI) represents the time it takes the electrical impulse to travel from the SA node to the AV node. The PRI starts at the beginning of the P wave and ends at the beginning of the QRS complex. Counting the number of small squares horizontally that the interval covers and then multiplying by 0.04 determines the length of the PRI (see Fig. 25.4). The normal PRI is 0.12 to 0.20 seconds (three to five small squares).

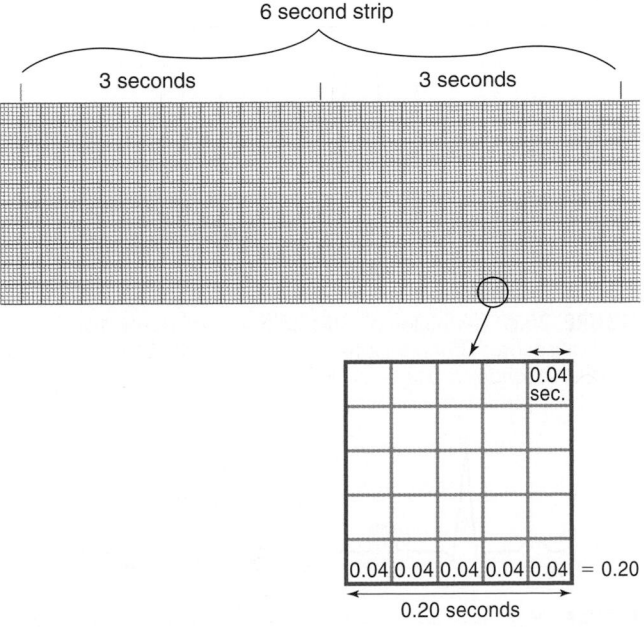

FIGURE 25.3 Electrocardiogram recording paper time intervals.

• **WORD** • **BUILDING** •

dysrhythmia: dys—difficult or abnormal + rhythm—rhythm

PR interval

FIGURE 25.4 PR interval. This PR interval covers four squares. Each square is 0.04 seconds; 4 × 0.04 = 0.16 seconds.

LEARNING TIP

To remember a normal PRI, you can use the "R" to think of normal respiratory rate and then add a decimal in front. A normal respiratory rate is 12 to 20 per minute, and a normal PRI is 0.12 to 0.20 seconds.

QRS Complex

The QRS complex represents ventricular depolarization and is composed of three waves: Q, R, and S. The Q wave is the first downward deflection after the P wave. The R wave is the first upward deflection after the P wave. The S wave is the first negative deflection after the R wave (see Fig. 25.2). The S wave ends when it returns to the isoelectric line (this is why locating the isoelectric line is helpful when first learning to identify waves). It is important to note that all three waves are not always present in every QRS complex. Even with absent waves, the QRS is still referred to as the QRS complex and can be considered normal (Fig. 25.5). The QRS complex is larger than the P wave because the ventricles have more muscle mass, so it looks like a mountain compared with the size of other waveforms.

FIGURE 25.5 (A) QRS complex with a Q wave. (B) QRS complex without a Q wave. (C) QRS complex without a Q or an S wave. (D) QRS complex with no R wave. The wave present is called a QS because it is not known if it is a Q or an S.

QRS Interval

The QRS interval represents the time it takes for the electrical impulse to travel from the AV node rapidly through the ventricles. To measure the QRS interval, count the number of squares from the wave that starts the QRS complex to the end of the wave that completes the QRS complex. For example, when a Q, R, and S are present, measure from the beginning of the Q wave to the end of the S wave (Fig. 25.6). If there is an R and an S present, measure from the beginning of the R to the end of the S. But if there is only an R present, measure from the beginning of the R to the end of the R. The normal QRS interval is 0.06 to 0.10 seconds (1.5–2.5 boxes).

T Wave

The T wave represents **ventricular repolarization**, the resting state of the heart, when the ventricles are filling with blood and preparing to receive the next impulse. It is a nicely rounded wave, and, in our size comparisons of other waves, it is a medium-size hill. In most leads, the T wave is an upward (positive) deflection, after the QRS complex, and ends with a return to the isoelectric line. An inverted (downward) T wave can indicate coronary ischemia (Fig. 25.7).

QT Interval

The QT interval measures the time from the start of the Q wave to the end of the T wave (see Fig. 25.2). This represents the time for ventricular depolarization and

QRS

FIGURE 25.6 QRS interval. This QRS interval covers two and one-half squares. Each square is 0.04 seconds. One-half square is 0.02 seconds; 2.5 × 0.04 = 0.10 seconds.

FIGURE 25.7 (A) T wave with positive deflection. (B) T wave with inverted, negative deflection, indicating ischemia.

repolarization. Normal ranges, 0.34 to 0.43 seconds, vary based on gender, heart rate, and age (a QT chart for identifying normal values is used). Prolonged or shortened QT intervals can lead to ventricular dysrhythmias. Abnormal intervals may be due to genetic causes, heart conditions, electrolyte imbalances, or medications that can prolong the QT interval.

U Wave

The U wave is small and often not seen. It occurs shortly after the T wave. It is most prominent in patients with hypokalemia (low serum potassium level; Fig. 25.8).

ST Segment

The ST segment reflects the time from completion of a contraction (depolarization) to recovery (repolarization) of myocardial muscle for the next impulse. The ST segment starts at the end of the QRS and ends at the beginning of the T wave (Fig. 25.9A). The ST segment is examined when patients experience chest pain. If a patient has nontransmural ischemia, the ST segment can become inverted or depressed (Fig. 25.9B). With transmural ischemia, the ST segment can elevate from the isoelectric line (Fig. 25.9C).

INTERPRETATION OF CARDIAC RHYTHMS

Six-Step Process for Dysrhythmia Interpretation

An orderly, systematic method for interpreting ECG rhythms should be used to increase understanding of items to examine and ensure nothing is overlooked. Six steps are examined in this process (Table 25.1). Use the findings of the first five steps to identify the ECG rhythm according to the five rules for each dysrhythmia. Then measure the QT

FIGURE 25.8 Various locations where U waves may appear.

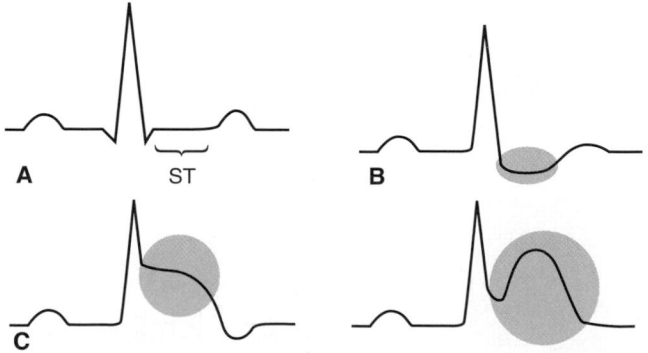

FIGURE 25.9 (A) ST segment. (B) ST segment inverted or depressed. (C) ST segment elevated.

TABLE 25.1   SIX-STEP PROCESS FOR DYSRHYTHMIA INTERPRETATION

After answering the questions listed here, you should be able to name the patient's dysrhythmia.		
Step	**Topic**	**Questions**
1	Regularity of rhythm	Is the rhythm regular? Irregular? Is there a pattern to the irregularity?
2	Heart rate	What is the heart rate?
3	P waves	Is there one P wave in front of every QRS complex? Is the atrial rate the same as the ventricular rate? Are the P waves smooth, rounded, and upright?
4	PR interval	Is the PR interval normal and constant? Does the PR interval vary?
5	QRS interval	Is the QRS interval normal and constant? Do the QRS complexes all look alike?
6	QT interval	Is the QT interval normal?

interval so that abnormalities can be reported to the HCP. A 6-second ECG tracing is used when interpreting rhythms (see Fig. 25.3).

Step 1. Regularity of the Rhythm

The regularity of the rhythm can be determined by looking at the R-to-R spacing on the ECG (Fig. 25.10). The same spacing between each R to R, with a rare variation of no greater than two small squares, is seen in a normal rhythm. To determine the regularity of a rhythm, count the number of small squares between each R wave, which normally should remain the same, or use a caliper (two-sided, movable metal instrument with sharp points) to measure the R-to-R spacing.

To use a caliper for measuring R waves, one point is placed on an R wave, and the other point is placed in the same spot on the next R wave. Then, without changing the distance between the caliper points, move the caliper from R wave to R wave across the ECG tracing (also known as an ECG strip) to see if R waves are regularly spaced. If the distance is the same, the rhythm is regular. If the distance varies, the rhythm is irregular. This can be further described by these fun terms: an irregular rhythm can be regularly irregular, which means it has a predictable pattern of irregularity, or irregularly irregular, without any pattern of irregularity.

A

B

FIGURE 25.10 Normal cardiac waves are equal distances apart. (A) R to R waves. (B) P to P waves.

LEARNING TIP

If a caliper is not available, a piece of paper can be placed on the ECG tracing. A mark can be made on the paper at the top of one R wave and another mark made on the paper at the top of the next R wave. The marks on the paper can then be moved across the R-to-R intervals on the tracing (just as caliper points would be) to determine the rhythm regularity.

Step 2. Heart Rate

After rhythm regularity is determined, a 1-minute heart rate is calculated. One of the two following methods is used:

1. Count the number of small (0.04-second) squares between two R waves and divide that number into 1500. This gives the beats per minute, because 1500 small squares equals 1 minute (Fig. 25.11). This method is used only for regular rhythms and is very accurate. A *rate meter* is a visual paper copy of this mathematical calculation for an entire 6-second ECG tracing that the nurse can view to

calculate the 1-minute heart rate. It is readily available in locations where these calculations are routinely done.

2. Six-second method: the 6-second method is used for irregular rhythms. It may also be used when a rapid estimate of a regular rhythm is needed, although it is not the most accurate method for regular rhythms. At the top of ECG graph paper are vertical marks at 3-second intervals (see Fig. 25.3). Count the number of R waves in a 6-second strip (three vertical marks) and multiply the total by 10 (the number of 6-second time periods in a minute) to obtain the beats per minute (6 seconds × 10 = 60 seconds or 1 minute; Fig. 25.12).

Step 3. P Waves

The P waves on the ECG tracing are examined to see if (1) there is one P wave in front of every QRS, (2) the P waves are regularly occurring, and (3) the P waves all look alike (see Fig. 25.10). If all of the P waves meet these criteria, they are considered normal. If they do not, further examination of the tracing is necessary to determine the dysrhythmia.

Step 4. PR Interval

All PR intervals are measured to determine whether they are normal (0.12–0.20 seconds) and constant. If the PRI is found

FIGURE 25.11 Rhythm regular: Count the small squares between two of the R waves and divide into 1500: 1500/25 = 60 beats per minute. Alternatively, count the large squares between two of the R waves and divide into 300: 300/5 = 60 beats per minute. Modified from Jones, S. A. (2008). *ECG success: Exercises in ECG interpretation*. Philadelphia: F.A. Davis, with permission.

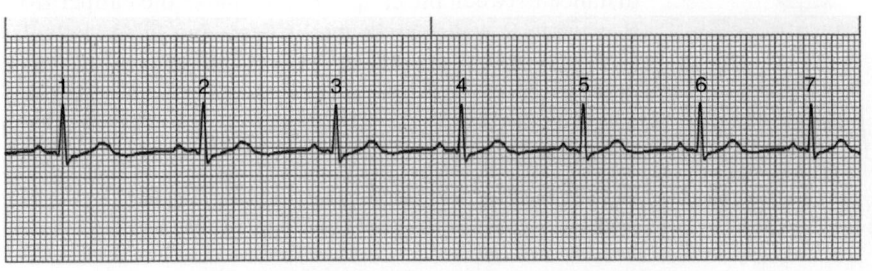

FIGURE 25.12 Rhythm irregular: Counting R waves in a 6-second strip. There are six R waves in this 6-second strip, and 6 × 10 = 60 beats per minute. Modified from Jones, S. A. (2008). *ECG success: Exercises in ECG interpretation*. Philadelphia: F.A. Davis, with permission.

to vary, it is important to note whether there is a pattern to the variation.

Step 5. QRS Interval

The QRS intervals are measured to determine whether they are all within normal range (0.06–0.10 seconds). Abnormal QRS complexes require further examination.

Step 6. QT Interval

Finally, the QT interval is measured to ensure that it is not shortened or prolonged, which can lead to dysrhythmias. Abnormal QT intervals should be reported to the HCP.

 ## NORMAL SINUS RHYTHM

Description

Normal sinus rhythm (NSR) is the heart's normal rhythm (Fig. 25.13). It originates in the SA node and has complete, regular cardiac cycles at 60 to 100 bpm.

NORMAL SINUS RHYTHM RULES
1. Rhythm: regular
2. Heart rate: 60 to 100 bpm
3. P waves: rounded, upright, precede each QRS complex, alike
4. PR interval: 0.12 to 0.20 seconds
5. QRS interval: less than or equal to 0.10 seconds.

 ## DYSRHYTHMIAS

Two terms are used for rhythm disturbances: *arrhythmia* (irregularity or loss of rhythm of the heartbeat) and *dysrhythmia* (abnormal, disordered, or disturbed rhythm). These two terms are used interchangeably, but *dysrhythmia* is the most accurate term for the discussion of most abnormal rhythms.

Several mechanisms can cause a dysrhythmia. Examples of these mechanisms are a disturbance in the formation of an impulse and a disturbance in the conduction of the impulse. When impulse formation is disturbed, the impulse may arise from the atria, the AV node, or the ventricles rather than the SA node. This disturbance can be seen as an increased or decreased heart rate, early or late beats, or atrial or ventricular fibrillation. With a disturbance in conduction, there may be normal formation of the impulse, but it becomes blocked within the electrical conduction system, resulting in abnormal conduction (as in heart block or bundle branch blocks). See www.heart.org for American Heart Association Guidelines for Cardiopulmonary Resuscitation and Emergency Cardiovascular Care Science.

Dysrhythmias Originating in the Sinoatrial Node

Rhythms arising from the SA node are referred to as *sinus rhythms*. Disturbances in conduction from the SA node can cause irregular rhythms or abnormal heart rates. Dysrhythmias arising from the SA node are rarely dangerous. Patients, especially those with heart, lung, or kidney disease, who cannot tolerate a rapid or slow heart rate, can require treatment.

 ### LEARNING TIP

The origin and the type of a problem are used to name a dysrhythmia. Let's name a slow dysrhythmia that originates in the sinoatrial node. The origin is sinus and the type of problem (slow rate) is bradycardia = sinus bradycardia. The term *normal* is not used because there is a problem. So what would a fast dysrhythmia originating in the SA node be called? Yes! Sinus tachycardia.

Sinus Bradycardia

Bradycardia is a rate slower than 60 bpm that can be asymptomatic or symptomatic (usually below 50 bpm). Sinus bradycardia has the same cardiac cycle components as NSR. The only difference between the two is a slower rate caused by fewer impulses originating from the SA node (Fig. 25.14). Do you see that the term *sinus bradycardia* tells you this difference? The name says the impulse is coming from the sinus node (sinus) but at a slower rate than normal (bradycardia). See, it is easy to understand what is happening in the dysrhythmia when you look at what the name is telling you.

• **WORD** • **BUILDING** •
bradycardia: bradys—slow + kardia—heart

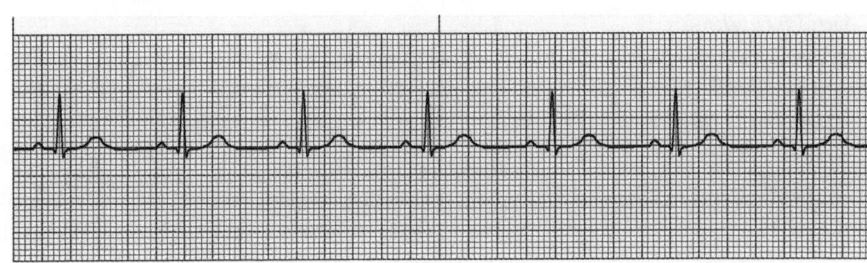

FIGURE 25.13 Normal sinus rhythm. Modified from Jones, S. A. (2008). *ECG success: Exercises in ECG interpretation.* Philadelphia: F.A. Davis, with permission.

FIGURE 25.14 Sinus bradycardia. Heart rate is 56. Modified from Jones, S. A. (2008). *ECG success: Exercises in ECG interpretation.* Philadelphia: F.A. Davis, with permission.

ETIOLOGY. Medications such as digoxin (Lanoxin) as well as myocardial infarction (MI) and electrolyte imbalances can cause bradycardia. Well-conditioned athletes can also have slower heart rates because their hearts work efficiently.

SINUS BRADYCARDIA RULES.
1. Rhythm: regular
2. Heart rate: less than 60 bpm
3. P waves: smoothly rounded, precede each QRS complex, alike
4. PR interval: 0.12 to 0.20 seconds
5. QRS interval: less than or equal to 0.10 seconds.

SIGNS AND SYMPTOMS. With symptomatic bradycardia decreased BP, respiratory distress, diminished or absent peripheral pulses, fatigue, or syncope can occur.

THERAPEUTIC MEASURES. Asymptomatic bradycardia does not require treatment. Observe the patient for symptom development, while the underlying cause is identified for correction. For the symptomatic patient, treatment is begun as the cause is corrected. Treatment can include intravenous (IV) atropine, or infusions of dopamine or epinephrine or transcutaneous pacing if atropine is ineffective (Table 25.2). Transvenous pacing can be considered, if needed.

Sinus Tachycardia

Tachycardia is defined as a heart rate greater than 100 bpm that originates from the SA node. Sinus tachycardia has the same components as NSR except the rate is faster (Fig. 25.15).

ETIOLOGY. Sinus tachycardia causes include physical activity; hemorrhage; shock; medications such as epinephrine, atropine, or nitrates; dehydration; fever; MI; electrolyte imbalance; fear; and anxiety. Tachycardia occurs as a compensatory mechanism for hypoxia when additional cardiac output is needed to deliver oxygen to tissues.

SINUS TACHYCARDIA RULES.
1. Rhythm: regular
2. Heart rate: 101 to 180 bpm
3. P waves: rounded, precede each QRS complex, alike
4. PR interval: 0.12 to 0.20 seconds
5. QRS interval: less than or equal to 0.10 seconds.

TABLE 25.2 MEDICATIONS USED TO TREAT DYSRHYTHMIAS

Medication Class/Action	Examples	Nursing Implications
Anticoagulant Increases clotting time. Reduces risk of blood clots in AF.	warfarin (Coumadin)	Monitor INR regularly. Monitor for bruising and bleeding. Acetaminophen (Tylenol) used instead of aspirin during therapy. Antidote: vitamin K.
	apixaban (Eliquis), dabigatran (Pradaxa), rivaroxaban (Xaletro)	No regular monitoring.
Antidysrhythmics Inhibit ventricular dysrhythmias, atrial fibrillation, atrial flutter.	amiodarone (Cordarone, Pacerone)	Contraindicated in AV block or pregnancy. Obtain baseline vital signs and ECG. Monitor for toxicity. Avoid grapefruit juice with oral form.
Inhibits atrial fibrillation, atrial flutter.	dronedarone (Multaq)	Less toxicity than amiodarone. Contraindicated in heart failure.

TABLE 25.2 MEDICATIONS USED TO TREAT DYSRHYTHMIAS—cont'd

Medication Class/Action	Examples	Nursing Implications
Anticholinergic Increases heart rate. Treats symptomatic bradycardia, asystole.	atropine	Contraindicated in angle closure glaucoma.
Beta Blockers Decrease myocardial contractility. Controls rate in sinus tachycardia, PAC, atrial flutter, atrial fibrillation, PVC.	atenolol (Tenormin), metoprolol succinate (Lopressor, Toprol XL)	Check apical pulse and BP before giving. If pulse <60 bpm, BP less than 100 mm Hg systolic, notify HCP. Instruct patient to rise slowly and not stop drug abruptly.
Calcium Channel Blocker Decreases myocardial contractility and depresses conduction system. Controls rate in sinus tachycardia, atrial flutter, and atrial fibrillation.	amlodipine (Norvasc)	Assess apical pulse and blood pressure. If BP <90 mm Hg systolic or apical rate less than 60 bpm, notify HCP. Administer before meals and at bedtime.
Inotrope—Cardiac Glycoside (Positive Inotrope and Negative Chronotrope)		
Slows heart rate. Maintains sinus rhythm for sinus tachycardia, atrial flutter, atrial fibrillation.	Digoxin (Lanoxicaps, Lanoxin)	Take apical pulse for 1 minute; if less than 60 bpm, notify HCP. Therapeutic digoxin levels: 0.5–2 mg/mL. Monitor drug level and electrolytes (hypokalemia, hypomagnesemia, hypercalcemia increase toxicity).
Vasopressors Cardiac stimulation, vasoconstriction, bronchodilation. Treats asystole, ventricular tachycardia, ventricular fibrillation, symptomatic bradycardia.	epinephrine (Adrenalin)	Contraindicated with nonselective beta blockers.
Vasoconstricts. Reduces urine volume. Single dose may replace dose of epinephrine. Treats pulseless ventricular tachycardia, ventricular fibrillation, asystole.	vasopressin (Pitressin)	Avoid IV site extravasation because of risk of necrosis and gangrene.
Increases cardiac output and blood pressure. Treats bradycardia.	dopamine	Monitor blood pressure.

Note. INR = international normalized ratio; PAC = premature atrial contraction; PVC = premature ventricular contractions.

SIGNS AND SYMPTOMS. Sinus tachycardia can be asymptomatic. But if the rate is very rapid (usually >150 bpm) and sustained for long periods, the patient may experience angina, dyspnea, syncope, or tachypnea. Older patients can become symptomatic more rapidly than younger patients ("Gerontological Issues—Dysrhythmia Risk"). Patients with MI might not tolerate a rapid heart rate and have more severe symptoms because cardiac workload is increased.

FIGURE 25.15 Sinus tachycardia. Heart rate is 115. Modified from Jones, S. A. (2008). *ECG success: Exercises in ECG interpretation.* Philadelphia: F.A. Davis, with permission.

THERAPEUTIC MEASURES. If stable, obtain an ECG and treat the cause. Medications such as adenosine, calcium channel blockers, or beta blockers can be used to slow the heart rate (when ≥150 bpm; see Table 25.2). The treatment goal is to decrease the heart's workload and resolve the cause, which then usually corrects the tachycardia. For example, if the patient is hemorrhaging, immediate intervention is needed to stop the bleeding and restore normal blood volume. Once normal blood volume is restored, the heart rate should return to normal.

Gerontological Issues

Dysrhythmia Risk

Factors that increase the risk of dysrhythmias in older adults include the following:
- Digitalis toxicity (most common)
- Hypokalemia
- Acute infection
- Hemorrhage
- Angina
- Coronary insufficiency or cardiomyopathy (exercise, stress)
- Thickness of the heart tissue
- Sleep apnea
- Hypothyroidism or hyperthyroidism.

Dysrhythmias that occur most often in older adults include the following:
- Atrial fibrillation (atria beating 400–700 times per minute)
- Sick sinus syndrome (alternating episodes of bradycardia, NSR, tachycardia, and periods of long sinus pause)
- Heart block (delayed or blocked impulses to the atria or ventricles)

Age-related effects of dysrhythmias include the following:
- Weakness
- Fatigue
- Forgetfulness
- Palpitations
- Dizziness
- Hypotension
- Bradycardia
- Syncope

- Dyspnea or shortness of breath
- Delayed capillary refill
- Diaphoresis
- Anxiety and fear
- Nausea and vomiting
- Stroke

Older adults are especially sensitive to changes in heart rate that increase the heart's workload. Whenever the heart works harder, as in tachycardia, the cardiac cells require more oxygen to function properly. Older adults have less ability to adapt to sudden changes or stressors, and they may not be able to tolerate tachycardia for very long. Any new-onset tachycardia in an older patient should be reported promptly.

LEARNING TIP

Tachycardia is often the first sign of hemorrhage. It is a compensatory mechanism to maintain cardiac output. If a patient develops sudden tachycardia, consider whether hemorrhage could be the cause, such as in postoperative patients, patients with gastrointestinal bleeding or cancer, or trauma patients. The bleeding may be external, or it may be internal and therefore not visible. Apply pressure to the site if the bleeding is obvious. Monitor the patient and report the tachycardia and any obvious bleeding promptly.

Dysrhythmias Originating in the Atria

As previously discussed, all areas of the heart can initiate an impulse. The SA node is the primary pacemaker, but if the atria initiate impulses faster than the SA node, they become the primary pacemaker. Atrial rhythms are usually faster than 100 bpm and can exceed 200 bpm. When an impulse originates outside the SA node, the P waves produced look different (flatter, notched, or peaked) from the rounded P waves from the SA node. This indicates that the SA node is not controlling the heart rate. These atrial impulses travel to the ventricles to initiate a normal QRS complex after each P wave.

LEARNING TIP

- If a QRS complex measures less than or equal to 0.10 seconds and a dysrhythmia is present, the problem originated above the ventricles. This is known as a supraventricular (above the ventricle) dysrhythmia.
- Ventricular originating dysrhythmias produce wide QRS complexes that are greater than 0.10 seconds.

Premature Atrial Contractions

The term *premature* refers to an "early" beat. When the atria fire an impulse before the SA node fires, a premature beat results. If the underlying rhythm is NSR, the distance between R waves is the same except where the early beat occurs. When looking at the ECG strip, a shortened R-to-R interval is seen where the premature beat occurs. The R wave preceding the premature atrial contraction (PAC) and the PAC's R wave are close together, followed by a pause, with the next beat being regular (Fig. 25.16).

ETIOLOGY. Causes of PACs include hypoxia, cigarette smoking, stress, myocardial ischemia, enlarged atria in valvular disorders, medications (such as digoxin), electrolyte imbalances, atrial fibrillation onset, and heart failure.

PREMATURE ATRIAL CONTRACTIONS RULES.
1. Rhythm: premature beat interrupts underlying rhythm where it occurs
2. Heart rate: depends on the underlying rhythm; if NSR, 60 to 100 bpm
3. P waves: early beat is abnormally shaped
4. PR interval: usually appears normal, but premature beat could have shortened or prolonged PR interval
5. QRS interval: less than or equal to 0.10 seconds (indicates normal conduction to ventricles).

SIGNS AND SYMPTOMS. Premature atrial contractions can occur in healthy individuals, as well as in the patient with a diseased heart. No symptoms are usually present. If many PACs occur in succession, the patient may report the sensation of palpitations.

THERAPEUTIC MEASURES. PACs are usually not dangerous, and often no treatment is required other than correcting the cause. Frequent PACs indicate atrial irritability, which may worsen into other atrial dysrhythmias. Beta blockers can be given to a patient having frequent PACs to slow the heart rate (see Table 25.2).

Atrial Flutter

In atrial flutter, the atria contract, or flutter, at a rate of 250 to 350 bpm. The very rapid P waves appear as flutter, or F waves, on ECG and appear in a sawtoothed pattern. Some of the impulses get through the AV node and reach the ventricles, resulting in normal QRS complexes. There can be from two to four F waves between QRS complexes. If impulses pass through the AV node at a consistent rate, the rhythm is regular (Fig. 25.17). The classic characteristics of atrial flutter are more than one P wave before a QRS complex, a sawtoothed pattern of P waves, and an atrial rate of 250 to 350 bpm.

ETIOLOGY. Causes of atrial flutter include rheumatic or ischemic heart diseases, congestive heart failure (CHF), hypertension, pericarditis, pulmonary embolism, and postoperative coronary artery bypass surgery. Many medications can also cause this dysrhythmia.

ATRIAL FLUTTER RULES.
1. Rhythm: atrial rhythm regular; ventricular rhythm regular or irregular depending on consistency of AV conduction of impulses
2. Heart rate: ventricular rate varies
3. P waves: flutter or F waves with sawtoothed pattern
4. PR interval: none measurable
5. QRS interval: less than or equal to 0.10 seconds.

FIGURE 25.16 Premature atrial contractions (PACs).

FIGURE 25.17 Atrial flutter. Modified from Jones, S. A. (2008). *ECG success: Exercises in ECG interpretation.* Philadelphia: F.A. Davis, with permission.

SIGNS AND SYMPTOMS. The presence of symptoms in atrial flutter depends on the ventricular rate. If the ventricular rate is normal, usually no symptoms are present. If the rate is rapid, the patient may experience palpitations, angina, or dyspnea.

THERAPEUTIC MEASURES. The ventricular rate and cardiac output guide treatment. The goal is to control the ventricular rate with conversion to NSR. For an unstable patient with a rapid ventricular rate, synchronized **cardioversion** (electrical shock) is used. Rapid atrial pacing may also stop the atrial flutter. Medications can be used to control the ventricular rate such as calcium channel blockers (see Table 25.2). Antiarrhythmic medications are used to convert atrial flutter. To terminate the atrial flutter in symptomatic patients, a radiofrequency catheter ablation (usually in the right atrium) may be done.

Atrial Fibrillation

In atrial fibrillation (AF), the atrial rate is extremely rapid and chaotic. An atrial rate of 350 to 600 bpm can occur. However, the AV node blocks most of the impulses, so the ventricular rate is much lower than the atrial rate. There are no definable P waves because the atria are fibrillating, or quivering, rather than beating effectively. No P waves can be seen or measured. A wavy pattern is produced on the ECG. Because the atrial rate is so irregular and only a few of the atrial impulses are allowed to pass through the AV node, the R waves are irregular. The ventricular rate varies from normal to rapid.

AF can be self-limiting, persistent, or permanent, which doubles the risk of death. Stroke risk is increased due to thrombus formation in the atria from blood stasis caused by poor emptying of blood from the quivering atria (Fig. 25.18).

ETIOLOGY. Causes of AF include aging (increases after age 60 and is the most common sustained dysrhythmia), history of cigarette smoking, rheumatic or ischemic heart diseases, heart failure, hypertension, pericarditis, pulmonary embolism, and postoperative coronary artery bypass surgery and some medications.

ATRIAL FIBRILLATION RULES.
1. Rhythm: irregularly irregular
2. Heart rate: atrial rate not measurable; ventricular rate under 100 is controlled response; greater than 100 is rapid ventricular response
3. P waves: no identifiable P waves
4. PR interval: none can be measured because no P waves are seen
5. QRS interval: less than or equal to 0.10 seconds.

LEARNING TIP

AF is easy to identify based on its two classic characteristics: a lack of identifiable P waves and an irregularly irregular rhythm (R waves).

SIGNS AND SYMPTOMS. With AF, most patients feel the irregular rhythm. Many describe it as palpitations or a skipping heartbeat. A patient's radial pulse may be faint because of a decreased stroke volume (volume of blood ejected with each contraction). If the ventricular rhythm is rapid and sustained, the patient can go into left-sided heart failure.

THERAPEUTIC MEASURES. The focus of AF treatment is to control rate, prevent thromboembolism, and restore normal rhythm. If the patient is unstable, synchronized cardioversion is done immediately to try to return the heart to NSR. For the patient who is stable, medications to control the ventricular rate such as beta blockers, calcium channel blockers, or digoxin are used (see Table 25.2). Anticoagulant therapy is given to reduce thrombi, which can cause a stroke. Pharmacological or electrical cardioversion may be performed to convert the rhythm after sufficient anticoagulation (about 3 weeks). Rhythm control medications such as sodium or potassium channel blockers are used to restore and maintain NSR. If known, the underlying cause of AF is treated.

For patients with AF who do not respond to medications or electrical cardioversion other therapies can be used.

Catheter Ablation. To isolate impulses coming from the pulmonary veins (most AF impulses arise from pulmonary veins) or AV node, catheter **ablation** may be used to cure AF. Intracardiac echocardiography maps the area of the heart requiring treatment. Then released energy such as radiofrequency waves create lesions either on all four pulmonary veins or near the AV node that heal and scar to block pathways for future impulses. Postprocedural care is similar to postangioplasty or postcardiac catheterization care (see Chapter 21).

Surgery. The MAZE procedure is often done as minimally invasive robotic-guided surgery. Incisions are made in the

• WORD • BUILDING •
ablation: ab—away from + lat—carry

FIGURE 25.18 Atrial fibrillation. Modified from Jones, S. A. (2008). *ECG success: Exercises in ECG interpretation.* Philadelphia: F.A. Davis, with permission.

atria that create a "maze," or route, for electrical impulses to travel to the AV node. These impulses cannot go off course because scar tissue surrounds the incision sites.

Ventricular Dysrhythmias

Premature ventricular contractions (PVCs) originate in the ventricles from an ectopic focus (a site other than the SA node). The ventricles are irritable and fire prematurely, before the SA node does. When the ventricles fire first, the impulses are not conducted normally through the electrical pathway. This results in a wide (>0.10 seconds), bizarre QRS complex on an ECG (Fig. 25.19).

PVCs can occur in different shapes. The shape of the PVC is referred to as **unifocal** (one focus) if all the PVCs look the same because they come from the same irritable ventricular area. **Multifocal** PVCs do not all look the same because they are originating from several irritable areas in the ventricle. There can be several repetitive cycles or patterns of PVCs:

- **Bigeminy** is a PVC that occurs every other beat (a normal beat and then a PVC; Fig. 25.20).
- **Trigeminy** is a PVC that occurs every third beat (two normal beats and then a PVC).
- Quadrigeminy is a PVC that occurs every fourth beat (three normal beats and then a PVC).
- When two PVCs occur together, they are referred to as a couplet (pair).

- If three or more PVCs occur in a row, it is referred to as a run of PVCs or ventricular tachycardia.

ETIOLOGY. Use of caffeine or alcohol, anxiety, hypokalemia, cardiomyopathy, ischemia, and MI are common causes of PVCs.

PREMATURE VENTRICULAR CONTRACTION RULES.
1. Rhythm: depends on the underlying rhythm; PVC usually interrupts rhythm
2. Heart rate: depends on underlying rhythm
3. P waves: absent before PVC QRS complex
4. PR interval: none for PVC
5. QRS interval: if PVC, is greater than 0.10 seconds; T wave is in the opposite direction of QRS complex (i.e., QRS upright, T downward; or QRS downward, T upright).

SIGNS AND SYMPTOMS. PVCs may be felt by the patient and are described as a skipped beat or palpitations. With frequent PVCs, cardiac output can be decreased, leading to fatigue, dizziness, or more severe dysrhythmias.

THERAPEUTIC MEASURES. Treatment depends on the type and number of PVCs and whether symptoms are produced. Occasional PVCs do not usually require treatment. However, if the PVCs are more than six per minute, regularly occurring, multifocal, falling on the T wave (known as "R-on-T phenomenon," which can trigger life-threatening dysrhythmias), or caused by an acute MI, they can be dangerous. Antidysrhythmic

FIGURE 25.19 Premature ventricular contractions. (A) Unifocal PVCs arise from one area and look the same. (B) Multifocal PVCs arise from different foci and may look different. Modified from Jones, S. A. (2008). *ECG success: Exercises in ECG interpretation.* Philadelphia: F.A. Davis, with permission.

FIGURE 25.20 Bigeminal premature ventricular contractions.

drugs that depress myocardial activity are used to treat PVCs such as amiodarone and beta blockers (see Table 25.2).

Ventricular Tachycardia

The occurrence of three or more PVCs in a row is referred to as **ventricular tachycardia** (VT) (Fig. 25.21). VT results from the continuous firing of an ectopic ventricular focus. During VT, the ventricles rather than the SA node become the pacemaker of the heart. The pathway of the ventricular impulses is different from normal conduction, producing a wide (>0.10 seconds), bizarre QRS complex.

ETIOLOGY. Myocardial irritability, MI, and cardiomyopathy are common causes of VT. Respiratory acidosis, hypokalemia, digoxin toxicity, cardiac catheters, and pacing wires can also produce VT.

VENTRICULAR TACHYCARDIA RULES.
1. Rhythm: usually regular, may have some irregularity
2. Heart rate: 150 to 250 ventricular bpm; slow VT is below 150 bpm
3. P waves: absent
4. PR interval: none
5. QRS interval: greater than 0.10 seconds.

SIGNS AND SYMPTOMS. The seriousness of VI is determined by the duration of the dysrhythmia. Sustained VT compromises cardiac output. Patients are aware of a sudden onset of rapid heart rate and can experience dyspnea, palpitations, and lightheadedness. Angina commonly occurs. The severity of symptoms can increase rapidly if the left ventricle fails and complete cardiac arrest results.

THERAPEUTIC MEASURES. If the patient is pulseless or not breathing, cardiopulmonary resuscitation (CPR) and immediate defibrillation are required. Advanced cardiac life support (ACLS) protocols for pulseless VT treatment should be followed. Medications may include epinephrine, vasopressin, and amiodarone (see Table 25.2).

If the patient is stable, medications are tried first, such as amiodarone. Magnesium can be used to help stabilize ventricular muscle excitability if the patient's magnesium level is low.

Ventricular Fibrillation

Ventricular fibrillation (VF) occurs when many ectopic ventricular foci fire at the same time. Ventricular activity is chaotic with no discernible waves (Fig. 25.22). The ventricle

CRITICAL THINKING

Mrs. Mae

■ Mrs. Mae, age 70, is 5 days post-MI without complications. You assist her back to bed at 1400 hours after she ambulates. Her oxygen is on at 2 L/min via nasal cannula. Her vital signs are BP 126/78 mm Hg, apical pulse 82 bpm, R 18 per minute. She has no pain and says she feels good after walking. The cardiac monitor shows normal sinus rhythm. Five minutes later, you see that the monitor shows sinus rhythm with PVCs of less than six per minute. Her vital signs are now BP 132/84 mm Hg, apical pulse 92 bpm, irregular, and R 22 per minute. She reports no pain but says, "I can feel my heart skipping. It takes my breath away." You call the registered nurse (RN) while staying with the patient to provide reassurance.

1. What should you do first?
2. What should you do regarding the dysrhythmia?
3. What might be some of the causes for this dysrhythmia?
4. What symptoms, if any, would you expect to be present?
5. What would you do if symptoms were present?
6. With which health care team members might you collaborate?
7. What type of orders would you anticipate from the HCP?
8. How would you document your findings?

Suggested answers are at the end of the chapter.

quivers and is unable to initiate a contraction. There is a complete loss of cardiac output. If this rhythm is not terminated immediately, death ensues.

ETIOLOGY. **Hyperkalemia** (elevated serum potassium), **hypomagnesemia** (low serum magnesium), electrocution, coronary

• WORD • BUILDING •
hyperkalemia: hyper—above + kalium—potassium + emia—blood
hypomagnesemia: hypo—below + magnes—magnesium +

FIGURE 25.21 Ventricular tachycardia.

CRITICAL THINKING

Mrs. Parker

■ You are caring for Mrs. Parker, age 66, on the cardiac medical unit. She had an MI and several episodes of VT while she was in the intensive care unit before transferring to your unit. At 1600 hours, you find her unresponsive, with no palpable pulses and shallow respirations and in VT on the ECG. Vital signs are BP 80/40 mm Hg, P 150 bpm, R 6 per minute.

1. Why are there no palpable pulses?
2. What is happening to the heart when VT is occurring?
3. What action should you take?
4. How will you document your findings?

Suggested answers are at the end of the chapter.

artery disease, and MI are all possible causes of VF. Placement of intracardiac catheters and cardiac pacing wires can also lead to ventricular irritability and then VF.

VENTRICULAR FIBRILLATION RULES.
1. Rhythm: chaotic and extremely irregular
2. Heart rate: not measurable
3. P waves: none
4. PR interval: none
5. QRS complex: none.

SIGNS AND SYMPTOMS. Patients experiencing VF lose consciousness immediately. There are no heart sounds, peripheral pulses, or blood pressure readings. These are all indicative of circulatory collapse. Additionally, respiratory arrest, cyanosis, and pupil dilation occur.

THERAPEUTIC MEASURES. Immediate defibrillation is the best treatment for terminating VF. Each minute that passes without defibrillation reduces survival. CPR is started until the defibrillator is available. Automatic external defibrillators (AEDs) provide quick access to easily used technology for defibrillation (see the later "Defibrillation" section). Endotracheal intubation and ventilation support respiratory function. Medications are given according to ACLS protocols and may include epinephrine, vasopressin, amiodarone, and magnesium (see Table 25.2).

Asystole

Asystole (the silent heart) is the absence of electrical activity in the cardiac muscle. It is referred to as cardiac arrest. A straight line appears on an ECG strip (Fig. 25.23).

ETIOLOGY. VF and a loss of a majority of functional cardiac muscle due to an MI are common causes of asystole. VF usually precedes this rhythm and must be reversed immediately to help prevent asystole. Hyperkalemia is another cause of asystole.

ASYSTOLE RULES.
1. Rhythm: none
2. Heart rate: none
3. P waves: none
4. PR interval: none
5. QRS interval: none.

SIGNS AND SYMPTOMS. Patients in asystole are unconscious and unresponsive. There are no heart sounds, peripheral pulses, blood pressure readings, or respirations.

THERAPEUTIC MEASURES. CPR is started immediately. Endotracheal intubation to support respirations is performed. Epinephrine or vasopressin can be administered per ACLS protocols (see Table 25.2).

FIGURE 25.22 Ventricular fibrillation.

FIGURE 25.23 Asystole.

CARDIAC PACEMAKERS

Pacemakers can be temporary (epicardial, transcutaneous, transvenous) or permanent (Fig. 25.24). They are used to generate an electrical impulse when there is a problem with the heart's conduction system.

Temporary pacemakers are used for bradycardia or tachycardia (overdrive pacing) that does not respond to medications or synchronized cardioversion. They may also be used after an MI to allow the heart time to heal when the diseased myocardium is unable to respond to or is not receiving electrical impulses because of damage within the conduction system. The temporary pacemaker becomes the electrical conduction system and stimulates the atria and ventricles to contract to maintain cardiac output. Temporary pacemakers can be inserted during valve or open heart surgery (epicardial), or in the cardiac catheterization lab or critical care unit (transvenous) as emergency treatment until surgery can be scheduled to implant a permanent pacemaker. Transcutaneous pacemakers are used in emergency situations because they are quick and easy to apply. Impulses are delivered to the heart through the skin from the external generator via electrodes that are attached to the chest and back.

FIGURE 25.24 Dual-chamber permanent pacemaker.

CRITICAL THINKING

Mr. Peet

■ You are making rounds. When you enter Mr. Peet's room, you note that he is having difficulty breathing and is unresponsive.

1. What are your initial actions?
2. What should you do after assessing and finding no pulse or respirations?
3. What is your responsibility during a cardiac/respiratory arrest code?

Suggested answers are at the end of the chapter.

Permanent Pacemaker Implantation

Permanent pacemaker implantation is a procedure in which **fluoroscopy**, a screen that shows an image similar to a radiograph, is used. The pacemaker generator is implanted subcutaneously and attached to leads (insulated conducting wires) that are inserted via a vein into the heart. The lead then delivers the impulse directly to the heart wall. A single-lead pacemaker paces either the right atrium or right ventricle depending on its chamber placement. Dual-chamber pacemakers have two leads, with one in the right atrium and the other in the right ventricle. This allows pacing of both chambers. Activity-responsive pacemakers provide a rate range (e.g., 60–115 bpm) in response to a person's activity level. This provides the patient with greater flexibility

for increasing cardiac output when needed, such as during exercise.

When a patient is in a paced rhythm, a small spike (vertical line) is seen on the ECG at the start of the paced beat. This spike is the electrical stimulus. It can precede the P wave, QRS complex, or both depending on what is being paced (Fig. 25.25). Patients may have 100% paced beats, a mixture of their own beats and paced beats, or all of their own beats. Pacemakers should not fire on patients' own beats.

Problems that can occur with pacemakers include the following:

• Failure to sense a patient's own beat
• Failure to pace because of a malfunction of the pulse generator
• Failure to capture, which is the heart's lack of depolarization

Nursing Care for Patients With Pacemakers

Patients' heart rhythm, apical pulse, and incision are monitored after implantation of a pacemaker. Irregular heart rhythms or a rate slower than the pacemaker's set rate can indicate pacemaker malfunction. Any change in heart rhythm, reports of chest pain, or changes in vital signs are reported immediately. The patient may remain in the hospital overnight.

Pacemaker care teaching before discharge includes the following:

• Report signs of incision infection (redness, swelling, warmth, pain, fever, or discharge) to the HCP.
• Care for incision as instructed (dressing removal, keep clean and dry, resuming showers).
• Report chest pain, dizziness, fainting, irregular heartbeats, palpitations, muscle twitching, or hiccups.
• Maintain ordered activity restrictions (limiting raising arm on pacemaker side, driving, return to work).

FIGURE 25.25 ECG tracings. (A) Atrial-only pacemaker (yellow spike before P wave). (B) Ventricular-only pacemaker (green spike before QRS). (C) AV sequential pacemaker that paces both atrial and ventricular chambers (yellow spike before P and green spike before QRS).

• Carry your pacemaker ID card to show to HCPs, airport security, or other security staff. Pacemaker metal may set off alarms but is not harmed if one walks normally through the security device. Avoid having a hand wand passed over the pacemaker.
• Understand electromagnetic restrictions to follow. Information is available on pacemaker manufacturer websites regarding various devices. Avoid strong electromagnetic fields (such as magnetic resonance imaging [MRI] unless it is the complete Revo MRI SureScan pacing system designed for use with MRI, welders above 130 amps, radio towers, or touching running car engines).
  • Microwaves and most common household devices may be used.
  • Keep cell phone of 3 watts or less 6 inches from your generator and on opposite side.
• If become lightheaded or dizzy near an electromagnetic device, move away from it.
• Keep scheduled appointments with the HCP. Periodic pacemaker checks will be done either by the HCP or remotely from home. The HCP can reprogram the pacemaker if needed.

CRITICAL THINKING

Mr. Treacher

■ Mr. Treacher, age 58, underwent pacemaker placement 6 days ago and is being transferred to the medical floor. After transfer, his vital signs are BP 138/72 mm Hg, apical pulse 72 bpm, and 100% paced rhythm.

Thirty minutes later, he says that he feels weak and tired. His vital signs are now BP 100/60 mm Hg, apical pulse 60 bpm, and irregular.

1. What is your first action?
2. What actions should be taken next?
3. What might be happening to Mr. Treacher?
4. What interventions should you anticipate next?

Suggested answers are at the end of the chapter.

DEFIBRILLATION

Defibrillation is a lifesaving procedure used for pulseless VT or VF. It delivers an electrical shock to reset the heart's rhythm. Self-adhesive pads, conductive jelly, or saline pads are placed on the patient's chest to prevent electrical burns and promote conduction of the electrical charge. After the defibrillator is charged, the paddles are pressed firmly and evenly against the chest wall to prevent burns or electrical arcing (Fig. 25.26).

For safety, the person who is defibrillating must announce "Clear." The phrase "One. I'm clear. Two. You're clear. Three. All clear" is suggested. No one, including the person defibrillating, should touch the bed or patient during this time to avoid also being shocked. ACLS protocols specify the guidelines for resuscitation.

• WORD • BUILDING •
defibrillation: de—from + fibrillation—quivering fibers

FIGURE 25.26 Placement of defibrillator paddles on chest.

After successful defibrillation, the patient is assessed for a pulse and adequate tissue perfusion. The patient is treated in the critical care unit (CCU) after successful resuscitation.

Emotional support for an alert patient having experienced cardiac arrest and defibrillation is an important aspect of nursing care. This can be an extremely frightening event for the patient. It is important to explain to the patient what happened and to listen and allow him or her to express concerns. The patient is reassured that continuous cardiac monitoring is done in the CCU. Families also require emotional support during resuscitation of a loved one and might be present during it per agency policy.

CARDIOVERSION

Cardioversion is performed with a defibrillator set in the synchronized mode. When the defibrillator is in the synchronized mode, it marks a highlighted area on the patient's R waves, which must be recognized to deliver a shock. When the discharge trigger is pressed, the shock is released when the machine senses it is safe to do so. The number of joules delivered with each shock usually ranges from 25 to 50. The procedure for delivering the shock is the same as for defibrillation.

Synchronized cardioversion is used for ventricular tachycardia with a pulse. Elective synchronized cardioversion is used for dysrhythmias such as AF, atrial flutter, and supraventricular tachycardia that are not responsive to drug therapy. The patient is given a sedative and monitored by anesthesia personnel during the procedure.

If cardioversion is successful, there should be a return to NSR. If the rhythm does not immediately convert, more cardioversion attempts can be made as determined by the HCP.

After the procedure, the patient is monitored for skin burns, rhythm disturbances, vital sign changes, respiratory problems, hypotension, and changes in the ST segment.

OTHER METHODS TO CORRECT DYSRHYTHMIAS

Automatic External Defibrillators

An AED is an external device that automatically analyzes rhythms and either automatically delivers or prompts operators to deliver an electrical shock if a shockable rhythm (VF or VT) is detected (Fig. 25.27). Minimally trained laypersons or hospital and rescue personnel can use these devices with little risk of injury to the patient because the AED analyzes the rhythm rather than the operator. The patient is connected to the AED with adhesive sternal-apex pads attached to cables coming from the device. This connection allows hands-free defibrillation.

AEDs are found in public places such as shopping malls, airports, stadiums, casinos, golf courses, and airplanes for immediate access because defibrillation attempts must occur within minutes of cardiac arrest to increase chance of survival. AEDs are available for home use. They are recommended for people at high risk of sudden cardiac arrest and for those at risk with rescue access that will take longer than 4 minutes, such as people living in rural areas, gated communities, or secured-access buildings.

Implantable Cardioverter Defibrillator

An implantable cardioverter defibrillator (ICD) or a combination pacemaker/ICD is placed into the chest of a patient who experiences life-threatening dysrhythmias or is at risk for sudden cardiac death (Fig. 25.28). ICDs have decreased the number of deaths from these dysrhythmias by analyzing and treating these heart rhythms. When an abnormal rhythm is detected that could cause death (VF), it automatically delivers an electrical shock. If the dysrhythmia does not convert on the initial shock, more shocks are delivered sequentially.

Automatic external defibrillator

FIGURE 25.27 Automatic external defibrillator.

Implanted cardioverter defibrillator

FIGURE 25.28 An implanted cardioverter defibrillator in place.

If the device detects VT, it cardioverts the rhythm using lower energy. ICDs also have antitachycardia pacing ability if a tachycardic rhythm is detected. Battery life depends on usage. When the battery is getting low, the entire unit needs to be changed within a few months.

Patients with ICDs can be extremely anxious about receiving shocks from the ICD. Defibrillator or cardioversion shocks may feel like a kick in the chest. Reinforcement of patient and family education is important. To prevent problems, those with ICDs should take the same precautions as discussed earlier with pacemakers. Provide emotional support, answer questions, and ensure that any misunderstood information is corrected before discharge.

NURSING PROCESS FOR THE PATIENT WITH DYSRHYTHMIAS

Data Collection

Patients at risk for dysrhythmias require careful monitoring so that any dysrhythmia is detected and treated. Obtaining apical and radial pulses at frequent intervals helps detect dysrhythmias. Most dysrhythmias are not life threatening. A patient's report of dizziness, chest pain, or palpitations should be reported to the HCP.

Nursing Diagnoses, Planning, Implementation, and Evaluation

See the "Nursing Care Plan for the Patient With Dysrhythmias."

Assist the patient and family in understanding the plan of care and the reasons for the prescribed interventions. Allow them to express their needs and fears. Family members should be taught CPR or given information on local CPR classes. This training gives the patient and family a sense of control and hope. In the event the patient requires CPR, the family can take action instead of simply standing by and feeling helpless. The patient will feel more secure in knowing that immediate help from family members is available at home until medical help arrives.

Home Health Hints

- A cell phone affords a home health nurse safety, convenience, and efficiency, especially if emergency help is needed, because some patients do not have phones.
- The nurse should have a pocket mask for CPR available at all times.
- Patients prone to dysrhythmias should avoid straining with bowel movements. If the patient reports straining, request a laxative or stool softener order from the HCP.
- Patients on beta blockers and inotropic agents (digoxin) need to know how to take their radial pulse, because bradycardia is a major side effect. For a pulse below 50 bpm, call the HCP.
- Visual disturbances can occur from digitalis toxicity. If the patient sees halos around lights or red-green tinting on everything, report this to the HCP.
- Blood drawn for digoxin (Lanoxin) levels, frequently prescribed for dysrhythmia, should be taken to the lab within 2 to 3 hours.
- Advise patients who are leaving home for the weekend or holidays to refill medicines ahead of time. Also, the HCP may write a prescription for patients to keep in their wallet for emergencies.
- Patients who come home with a pacemaker should be instructed to wear loose tops. Women should not wear tight bras.
- Follow patient teaching guidelines discussed earlier in the chapter.
- If the patient is discharged with a prescription for an anticoagulant, educate the patient and family regarding follow-up appointments, dietary needs, complication (signs and symptoms of active bleeding: hematuria, bleeding gums, frequent bruising, or dark stools).

NURSING CARE PLAN for the Patient With Dysrhythmias

Nursing Diagnosis: *Decreased Cardiac Output* related to dysrhythmias

Expected Outcomes: The patient's cardiac status will be stabilized. Patient will be able to tolerate activities of daily living (ADLs).

Evaluation of Outcomes: There is an absence of dysrhythmias. Patient is able to perform ADLs without tachycardia, chest pain, or weakness.

Intervention Take apical and radial pulses every 2 to 4 hours. Monitor blood pressure and urinary output. **Rationale** Monitors for dysrhythmias, impending cardiac arrest, or shock. Blood pressure, pulse, and urinary output are indicators of cardiac output. **Evaluation** Is the patient free of dysrhythmias with vital signs within normal limits?

Intervention Monitor mental status every 2 to 4 hours. **Rationale** Dizziness, confusion, and restlessness may indicate decreased cerebral blood flow. **Evaluation** Does patient show signs of decreased cerebral perfusion, such as confusion?

Intervention Listen to lung sounds every 2 to 4 hours. **Rationale** Dysrhythmias can cause heart failure. **Evaluation** Are lungs clear with no report of dyspnea?

Intervention Administer O_2 as ordered. **Rationale** Increases oxygenation to the heart and brain. **Evaluation** Is patient free of chest pain, confusion, and light-headedness?

Intervention Ensure that patient gets adequate rest and does not exceed activity tolerance. **Rationale** Reduces dyspnea and decreases O_2 demand on the myocardium. **Evaluation** Does patient rest and tolerate activity without dyspnea or chest pain?

GERIATRIC
Intervention Administer medications as ordered and observe for adverse reactions. **Rationale** Older patients may have decreased renal and liver function that may lead to rapid development of toxicity. **Evaluation** Does patient have signs of toxicity?

Nursing Diagnosis: *Anxiety* related to situational crisis

Expected Outcomes: The patient will be able to effectively manage anxiety. Patient will report decreased anxiety.

Evaluation of Outcomes: Patient uses effective coping mechanisms to manage anxiety. Patient expresses decreased anxiety.

Intervention Ask about level of anxiety. **Rationale** Establishes a baseline. **Evaluation** What is patient's level of anxiety?

Intervention Encourage patient and family to verbalize fears. **Rationale** Helps correct and clarify their concerns. **Evaluation** What are patient's feelings or fears?

Intervention Explain procedures to patient and family. **Rationale** Lack of knowledge increases anxiety. This knowledge will help with compliance of therapy. **Evaluation** Does patient express understanding of therapy with decreased anxiety?

Intervention Identify and reduce as many environmental stressors as possible. **Rationale** Anxiety often results from lack of trust in the environment. **Evaluation** Can patient describe two situations that increase tension?

Intervention Teach patient relaxation techniques to be performed every 4 to 6 hours, such as guided imagery, muscle relaxation, and meditation. **Rationale** These measures can restore psychological and physical equilibrium and help decrease anxiety. **Evaluation** Is patient successful in demonstrating relaxation methods?

Intervention Medicate with antianxiety agents as ordered. **Rationale** Aids the patient in decreasing anxiety. **Evaluation** Does patient show decreased anxiety?

SUGGESTED ANSWERS TO
CRITICAL THINKING

■ Mrs. Mae

1. Assess the patient's vital signs and heart sounds, note symptoms, obtain an ECG per agency protocol.
2. Report the patient findings to the RN or HCP.
3. Possible causes include hypokalemia or ischemia leading to irritability of the heart.
4. Symptoms might include lightheadedness, feeling of heart skipping, chest pain, or fatigue.
5. To alleviate symptoms, elevate head of bed to comfort, monitor vital signs, and maintain oxygen at 2 L/min via nasal cannula per agency protocol. Remain with the patient to help alleviate anxiety. Notify the RN.
6. RN, respiratory therapist, HCP
7. Orders might include ECG, oxygen, potassium, or electrolytes.
8. Documentation should include the following:
   - 1400: Ambulated 20 feet with one assist. Vital signs stable. Stated: "Feel good. Pain zero."
   - Tolerated well. Assisted to bed. Oxygen at 2 L/min via nasal cannula.
   - 1405: see ECG strip with intermittent PVCs. Vital signs: BP 132/84 mm Hg; apical 92 bpm, irregular; R 22 per minute.
   - "Pain zero. I can feel my heart skipping, it takes my breath away." RN notified.

■ Mrs. Parker

1. A heart in VT has an ectopic focus that is initiating impulses. The heart is unable to maintain adequate cardiac output with such a rapid heart rate. The rapid and irregular heart rhythm does not allow the heart chambers time to adequately fill and empty, thereby reducing the blood volume with each beat. This in turn affects the peripheral circulation, causing the absence of palpable pulses.
2. In VT, one or more sites in the ventricle may be initiating impulses. The rapid rate of VT overrides the normal pacemaker of the heart. The rhythm can be regular or irregular. The inability of the heart to conduct impulses along normal pathways prevents the chambers from emptying and filling properly. This leads to a decreased

cardiac output and can lead to cardiac arrest if the rhythm is not converted.
3. Call a code and begin CPR. Report findings to code team upon their arrival.
4. Documentation should include the following: 1600: Patient found in bed unresponsive to verbal and tactile stimuli. Respirations shallow. No palpable pulses. BP 80/40 mm Hg, P 150 bpm, R 6 per minute. Monitor shows VT (see strip). Code called from room. CPR started. Code team arrived at 1602. Report given to code team leader.

■ Mr. Peet

1. Initially you should assess responsiveness and the presence of a carotid pulse. Check for breathing.
2. Open the airway. Call for assistance or use the patient's phone to report a cardiac arrest. Initiate CPR until help arrives.
3. Once help or the code team arrives, the licensed practical nurse/licensed vocational nurse (LPN/LVN) reports the patient's status. The code team leader delegates responsibilities. Many facilities have protocols for each team member in a code. The LPN/LVN assists in the code as delegated by the RN in charge.

■ Mr. Treacher

1. Your first actions should be to obtain an ECG per agency protocol and to notify the RN or HCP.
2. You should keep the head of the bed elevated and administer oxygen at 2 L/min via nasal cannula per protocol. Turn the patient onto his side because this may help float the pacemaker wire to the chamber wall for better contact. Monitor the patient's ECG, vital signs, and symptoms, and remain with patient to provide emotional support.
3. Mr. Treacher could be experiencing pacemaker malfunction.
4. Interventions could include transfer to a step-down unit or CCU for reprogramming of the pacemaker, or a return to surgery for manipulation or replacement of the pacemaker wires.

REVIEW QUESTIONS

1. Place the following in the correct sequence for normal electrical impulse movement through the cardiac conduction system.
   1. AV node
   2. SA node
   3. bundle of His
   4. Purkinje fibers
   5. Internodal tracts
   Sequence: _____

2. The nurse prepares to document an ECG rhythm. The nurse uses a systematic method for analyzing the ECG tracing for which of the following reasons?
   1. So abnormalities are not missed.
   2. To save time.
   3. To develop a routine for examining tracings.
   4. To increase memory of the analysis steps.

3. The nurse responds to a call for assistance for a patient in pulseless ventricular tachycardia. The nurse should prepare for which of the following as the first choice of treatment for this rhythm?
   1. Synchronized cardioversion
   2. Pacemaker
   3. Defibrillation
   4. Antiarrhythmic medication

4. The nurse is to provide teaching to a patient after insertion of a pacemaker. Which of the following instructions should the nurse give the patient regarding pacemaker care?
   1. "Avoid microwaves."
   2. "All pacemaker types are compatible with MRI."
   3. "Avoid strong electromagnetic devices."
   4. "You will need to be on bedrest for 48 hours."

5. The nurse is ambulating a patient who is recovering from an MI when the patient develops chest pain with an irregular pulse. Which of these is safest way for the nurse to return the patient to bed?
   1. Ambulation to room with one assistant.
   2. With assistance by gurney.
   3. With assistance by a wheelchair.
   4. After completion of ambulation.

6. A patient has a radial pulse of 58 bpm. Which of the following should the nurse use to document this finding?
   1. Normal
   2. Asystole
   3. Tachycardia
   4. Bradycardia

7. The nurse is to give a patient amiodarone 800 mg/day PO in two divided doses. The nurse has available 200-mg tablets. How many tablets should the nurse give for each dose? **Fill in the blank.**
   Answer: _____ tablets

Answers can be found in Appendix C.

 DavisPlus | For additional resources and information visit **davispl.us/medsurg5**

Nursing Care of Patients With Heart Failure

KATHY BERCHEM

LEARNING OUTCOMES

1. Describe the pathophysiology of left- and right-sided heart failure.
2. Define acute heart failure.
3. List causes of acute and chronic heart failure.
4. Identify signs and symptoms of acute and chronic heart failure.
5. Plan nursing care for patients undergoing diagnostic tests for heart failure.
6. Explain medical treatments used for acute and chronic heart failure.
7. Plan nursing care for acute and chronic heart failure.
8. Plan teaching for patients with heart failure and their families.

KEY TERMS

afterload (AFF-ter-lohd)
cor pulmonale (KOR PUL-mah-NAH-lee)
cyanosis (SYE-an-NOH-siss)
hepatomegaly (HEP-aa-toh-MEH-gah-lee)
orthopnea (or-THOP-knee-ah)
paroxysmal nocturnal dyspnea (PEAR-ox-IS-mul knock-TURN-al DISP-knee-ah)
peripheral vascular resistance (puh-RIFF-uh-ruhl VAS-kyoo-lar ree-ZIS-tense)
preload (PREE-lohd)
pulmonary edema (PULL-muh-NARE-ee eh-DEE-muh)
splenomegaly (SPLEE-noh-MEG-ah-lee)

OVERVIEW OF HEART FAILURE

Heart failure (HF) is a clinical syndrome that occurs as a result of the inability of the ventricle(s) to fill or pump enough blood to meet the body's oxygen and nutrient needs. It may cause dyspnea, fatigue, and fluid volume overload in the intravascular and interstitial spaces, resulting in reduced quality and length of life. Causes of HF are varied and may include coronary artery disease (most often), myocardial infarction (MI), cardiomyopathy, heart valve problems, and hypertension. Any heart problem can potentially lead to HF. In the older adult, the most common cause of HF is cardiac ischemia. It may develop rapidly (acute), as with cardiogenic shock and pulmonary edema, or over time (chronic) as a result of another disorder, such as hypertension or pulmonary disease.

The incidence of HF is growing as the older adult population and patient survival rates increase. According to the American Heart Association (AHA; Go et al, 2014), 5.1 million people have HF with more than 670,000 new cases each year. HF is the most common reason for hospital admission in the older adult. The patient may experience many functional limitations and symptoms, and according to the Centers for Disease Control and Prevention (2013), the mortality rate is as high as 597,000 deaths per year. Quality of life is often impaired. Readmission rates to hospitals soon after discharge for HF treatment are high and pose a challenge for health care providers (HCPs). For more information, visit www.americanheart.org.

Congestive Heart Failure

Congestive HF is an older term for HF. It is still used interchangeably by some to indicate *HF,* the preferred term. This is because volume overload or "congestion" either in the lungs or periphery is not present in everyone with HF or at all times.

Pathophysiology

The heart is divided into two separate pumping systems, the right side of the heart and the left side of the heart. Proper cardiac functioning requires each ventricle to pump out equal amounts of blood over time. If the amount of blood returned to the heart becomes more than either ventricle can handle, the heart can no longer function effectively as a pump.

> **LEARNING TIP**
>
> To understand HF, compare it to a dam in a river:
>
> - In a river without a dam, the water flows freely; in the normal circulatory system, blood flows freely.
> - In a river with a dam, the water is blocked by the dam and builds up behind it; in HF, the failing ventricle acts like a dam in the river, causing blood to back up behind it.

> - When too much water builds up behind the dam, the riverbanks are flooded; in HF, if too much blood builds up behind the failing ventricle, the lungs (pulmonary edema) or peripheral tissues are flooded (peripheral edema).
> - HF can be the result of systolic (contractile) dysfunction, diastolic (relaxation) dysfunction, or a mixed systolic and diastolic dysfunction. Systolic dysfunction is a contractile problem in which the ventricle is unable to generate enough force to pump blood from the ventricle. Diastolic dysfunction is a problem with the ventricle's ability to relax and fill. Mixed systolic and diastolic dysfunction is a combination of the two defects.

Conditions that cause HF can affect one or both of the heart's pumping systems. Therefore, HF can be classified as right-sided HF, left-sided HF, or biventricular HF. The left ventricle typically weakens first because it has the greatest workload to eject blood against the resistance in the aorta. Because the right and left sides of the heart's pumping system work together in a closed system, failure of one side eventually leads to failure of the other side.

> **LEARNING TIP**
>
> To visualize and understand the effects of HF, trace the flow of blood backward from each ventricle. Along the backward path from the failing ventricle, congestion develops and produces the signs and symptoms seen in HF. If you understand the backward path of congestion, you can identify the signs and symptoms specifically associated with right- or left-sided HF.

Left-Sided Heart Failure

The left ventricle must generate a certain amount of force during a contraction to eject blood into the aorta through the aortic valve. This force is referred to as **afterload**. The pressure within the aorta and arteries acts as resistance and influences the force required to open the aortic valve to pump blood into the aorta. This pressure is called **peripheral vascular resistance** (PVR).

Hypertension is one of the major causes of left-sided HF because it increases the pressure within arteries. Increased pressure in the aorta makes the left ventricle work harder to pump blood into the aorta. Over time the strain caused by the increased workload causes the left ventricle to weaken and fail. Other conditions that can lead to left-sided HF are described in Table 26.1.

TABLE 26.1 CAUSES OF LEFT-SIDED HEART FAILURE

Cause	Primary Effect on Left Ventricular Workload
Aortic stenosis	Increased volume to pump from restricted blood outflow
Cardiomyopathy	Increased workload from impaired contractility
Coarctation of the aorta	Restricted outflow and increased resistance from narrowing of aorta
Hypertension	Resistance increased from elevated pressure
Heart muscle infection	Increased workload from damaged myocardium
Myocardial infarction	Increased workload from impaired contractility
Mitral regurgitation	Increased volume to pump from backward blood flow

With left-sided HF, blood backs up from the left ventricle into the left atrium and then into the four pulmonary veins and lungs (Fig. 26.1). This increases pulmonary pressure, causing movement of fluid first into the interstitium and then into the alveoli. Alveolar edema is more serious because it reduces gas exchange across the alveolar capillary membrane. Shortness of breath and cyanosis may result from the decreased

oxygenation of the blood leaving the lungs. If the fluid buildup is severe, acute pulmonary edema occurs, which requires immediate medical treatment.

Right-Sided Heart Failure

Conditions causing right-sided HF increase the work of the right ventricle. They increase the amount of contractile force needed or require pumping of excess blood volume (**preload**). Causes of right-sided HF are described in Table 26.2. The major cause of right-sided HF is left-sided HF. When the left side fails, fluid backs up into the lungs and pulmonary pressure is increased. The right ventricle must continually pump blood against this increased fluid and pressure in the pulmonary artery and lungs. Over time this additional strain eventually causes it to fail. When the right ventricle hypertrophies or fails because of increased pulmonary pressures, it is referred to as **cor pulmonale**.

When the right ventricle fails, it does not empty normally, and there is a backward buildup of blood in the systemic blood vessels. As the blood backs up from the right ventricle, right atrial and systemic venous blood volume increases. The jugular neck veins, which are not normally visible, become distended and can be seen when the person is in a 45-degree upright position. Edema may occur in the peripheral tissues, and the abdominal organs can become engorged (Fig. 26.2). Fluid congestion in the gastrointestinal (GI) tract causes anorexia, nausea, and abdominal pain. As the failure progresses, blood pools in the hepatic veins, and the liver becomes congested (**hepatomegaly**). This liver congestion also

• WORD • BUILDING •
cor pulmonale: cor—heart + pulm—lung
hepatomegaly: hep—liver + mega—large

FIGURE 26.1 Left-sided HF. Shaded areas indicate areas of congestion from blood backup caused by the failing left side of the heart.

TABLE 26.2 CAUSES OF RIGHT-SIDED HEART FAILURE

Cause	Primary Effect on Right Ventricular Workload
Atrial septal defect	Left atrial blood flow into right atrium increases right ventricular volume to pump
Cor pulmonale	Resistance increased from elevated pressure
Left-sided HF	Resistance increased from backup of fluid and elevated pressures
Pulmonary hypertension	Resistance increased from elevated pressure
Pulmonary valve stenosis	Increased volume to pump from restricted right ventricular blood outflow

FIGURE 26.2 Right-sided HF. Shaded areas indicate areas of congestion from blood backup due to the failing right side of the heart.

causes pain in the right upper quadrant of the abdomen and impairs liver function. Systemic venous congestion also leads to engorgement of the spleen (**splenomegaly**).

LEARNING TIP

To understand the signs and symptoms of left-sided versus right-sided HF, remember that left-sided signs and symptoms are found in the lungs. Left begins with L, as does Lung:

Left = Lungs = L.

Any signs and symptoms not related to the lungs (L) are caused by right-sided failure.

COMPENSATORY MECHANISMS TO MAINTAIN CARDIAC OUTPUT

Compensatory mechanisms help ensure that an adequate amount of blood is being pumped out of the heart. Although these mechanisms are designed to maintain cardiac output, they contribute to a cycle that, instead of being helpful, leads to further HF.

When the sympathetic nervous system detects low cardiac output, it speeds up the heart rate by releasing epinephrine and norepinephrine. Although this raises cardiac output (cardiac output = heart rate × stroke volume), the increased heart rate also increases the oxygen needs of the heart. In response to the resulting low renal blood flow, the kidneys activate the renin-angiotensin-aldosterone system, and antidiuretic hormone is

released from the pituitary gland to conserve water, causing decreased urine output. This adds to the fluid retention problem already found in HF.

Over time the heart responds to the increased workload by enlarging its chambers (dilation) and increasing its muscle mass (hypertrophy), referred to as remodeling. In dilation, the heart muscle fibers stretch to increase the force of myocardial contractions, which is known as the Frank-Starling phenomenon. In hypertrophy, the muscle mass of the heart increases, creating more contractile force. Both of these compensatory mechanisms temporarily improve patient symptoms but also increase the heart's oxygen needs, which further contributes to HF. Additionally, the heart walls stiffen, which further reduces pumping ability.

PULMONARY EDEMA (ACUTE HEART FAILURE)

Pulmonary edema, also known as acute HF, is sudden severe fluid congestion in the alveoli of the lungs and is life threatening. Pulmonary edema occurs with an acute event such as a MI or when the heart is severely stressed, causing the left ventricle to fail. Complications of pulmonary edema include dysrhythmias and cardiac arrest.

Pathophysiology

First, pressure rises in the lung's venous blood vessels as blood builds up. As pressures continue to rise, fluid moves into the interstitial spaces. Then, with continued pressure increases, fluid containing red blood cells (RBCs) leaks into the alveoli. Finally, the alveoli and airways become filled with fluid, reducing gas exchange and oxygen levels.

Signs and Symptoms

Signs and symptoms of pulmonary edema are listed in Table 26.3. Pink, frothy sputum is a classic symptom of pulmonary edema caused by the increased lung congestion and pressures that allow leaking of fluid and RBCs into the alveoli. Compensatory mechanisms increase the heart rate and blood pressure; however, as pulmonary edema worsens, the blood pressure may fall.

Diagnostic Tests

Diagnostic studies are listed in Table 26.3. The congestion in the pulmonary system can be seen on x-ray examination. Arterial blood gases (ABGs) show a decrease in Pa_{O_2} that continues as the edema worsens and an increase in $PaCO_2$, causing respiratory acidosis. The pulmonary artery catheter shows elevated pulmonary pressures and a decreased cardiac output.

Therapeutic Measures

Immediate treatment is needed to prevent patients from drowning in their own secretions (see Table 26.3). The goal

• **WORD** • **BUILDING** •

splenomegaly: splen—spleen + mega—large

TABLE 26.3 ACUTE HEART FAILURE SUMMARY

Signs and Symptoms	Rapid respirations with accessory muscle use Severe dyspnea, orthopnea Crackles and wheezes Coughing Pink, frothy sputum Anxiety, restlessness Pale skin and mucous membranes Clammy, cold skin
Diagnostic Tests	Chest x-ray examination Arterial blood gases Electrocardiogram Hemodynamic monitoring
Therapeutic Measures	Oxygen via cannula, mask, or mechanical ventilation Positioning in high or semi-Fowler's position Bedrest Intravenous (IV) drugs: morphine, diuretics, inotropic agents, vasodilators Frequent vital signs, urinary output Pulmonary pressures Daily weights Treatment of underlying cause
Priority Nursing Diagnoses	*Impaired Gas Exchange* *Decreased Cardiac Output* *Excess Fluid Volume*

of therapy is to reduce the workload of the left ventricle in order to improve cardiac output and reduce the patient's anxiety. Placing the patient in Fowler's position allows the lungs to expand more easily. Ask the patient what position provides him or her the most comfort in breathing. Oxygen is given, usually by mask to provide higher amounts. In severe cases of pulmonary edema, endotracheal intubation and mechanical ventilation may be necessary.

Medications are given intravenously to reduce anxiety, relax airways, increase peripheral blood pooling to decrease preload, reduce fluid congestion, strengthen heart contractions, reduce arterial pressure (afterload) and sodium and water retention to relieve dyspnea.

Nursing Care

The patient is typically critically ill and in an intensive care unit (ICU). Psychosocial supportive care is important because the patient will be anxious if alert.

 CHRONIC HEART FAILURE

Signs and Symptoms

Chronic HF is a progressive disorder. Signs and symptoms worsen over time (Table 26.4).

Fatigue and Weakness

Fatigue and weakness are the earliest symptoms of HF. They occur from the decreased amount of oxygen reaching the tissues. During the day, the fatigue worsens, especially with activity.

Dyspnea

Dyspnea is a common symptom of left-sided HF. It is a result of the pulmonary congestion that impairs gas exchange

TABLE 26.4 CHRONIC HEART FAILURE SUMMARY

	Right-Sided Heart Failure	Left-Sided Heart Failure
Signs and Symptoms	Jugular venous distention Dependent peripheral edema Ascites Weight gain Splenomegaly Hepatomegaly Gastrointestinal pain, anorexia, nausea Fatigue, weakness Tachycardia Nocturia	Dyspnea on exertion Dry hacking cough, especially when supine Crackles, wheezing Orthopnea Paroxysmal nocturnal dyspnea Cheyne-Stokes respirations Cyanosis Tachypnea, tachycardia Nocturia
Diagnostic Tests	History and physical examination Electrocardiogram Chest x-ray Two-dimensional echocardiography with Doppler Exercise stress test Coronary angiography	

Continued

TABLE 26.4   CHRONIC HEART FAILURE SUMMARY—cont'd

	Cardiac magnetic resonance imaging Nuclear imaging studies Cardiac catheterization Serum laboratory tests: CBC, BNP, electrolytes, BUN, creatinine, liver function tests, thyroid-stimulating hormone, fasting blood glucose, lipid profile, ferritin Arterial blood gases Urinalysis Sleep studies Hemodynamic monitoring
Complications	Hepatomegaly Splenomegaly Pleural effusion Left ventricular thrombus and emboli Cardiogenic shock
Therapeutic Measures	*Noninvasive* Treat underlying cause Oxygen by cannula or mask Drug therapy (see Table 26.5) Individualized activity plan Dietary sodium restriction Fluid restriction Daily weights
	Invasive Pacemaker ICD Resynchronization therapy Mechanical assistive devices Intra-aortic balloon pump Left ventricular assist device Total artificial heart Surgery: CABG, valvuloplasty, heart valve replacement, cardiac transplant
Priority Nursing Diagnoses	*Impaired Gas Exchange* *Decreased Cardiac Output* *Excess Fluid Volume*

Note. BNP = brain natriuretic peptide; BUN = blood urea nitrogen; CABG = coronary artery bypass graft; CBC = complete blood count; ICD = implantable cardioverter defibrillator.

between the alveoli and capillaries. Dyspnea stimulates compensatory mechanisms that produce short, rapid respirations. Dyspnea is classified in several ways:

- Exertional dyspnea is shortness of breath that increases with activity.
- **Orthopnea** is dyspnea that increases when lying flat. In an upright position, gravity holds fluid in the lower extremities. In a supine position, gravitational forces are removed, allowing fluid to move from the legs to the heart, which overwhelms the already congested pulmonary system. When orthopnea is present, two or more pillows are often used for sleeping. Documentation should state the number of pillows used. For example, use of three pillows would be "three-pillow orthopnea."
- **Paroxysmal nocturnal dyspnea** (PND) is sudden shortness of breath that occurs after lying flat for a time. PND results from excess fluid accumulation in the lungs. The sleeping person awakens with feelings of

• WORD • BUILDING •

orthopnea: orth—straight + pnea—to breathe

suffocation and anxiety. Relief is obtained by sitting upright for a short time, which reduces the amount of fluid returning to the heart.

Cough

A chronic, dry cough is common in HF. The coughing increases when lying down from increased irritation of the lung mucosa. This irritation is due to the increase in pulmonary congestion that occurs when gravity no longer keeps fluid in the legs and more fluid returns to the heart and lungs.

Crackles and Wheezes

Pulmonary congestion causes abnormal breath sounds such as crackles and wheezes. Crackles are produced from fluid buildup in the alveoli resulting from increased pressure in the pulmonary capillaries. Wheezes occur from bronchiolar constriction caused by the increased fluid.

Tachycardia

The sympathetic nervous system compensates for the decreased cardiac output in HF by releasing epinephrine and norepinephrine to increase the heart rate. Normally, this is helpful because the increased heart rate increases the amount of blood ejected by the heart to maintain an adequate cardiac output. However, whenever the heart works faster, the heart itself also requires more oxygen, which the failing heart finds difficult to supply.

LEARNING TIP

To simulate the sound of crackles, open a piece of Velcro or rub hair together next to your ear. These sounds are similar to the sound of crackles heard with a stethoscope.

Chest Pain

Chest pain may occur from ischemia in the patient with HF. Decreased cardiac output results in decreased oxygen delivery to the heart itself via the coronary arteries. Compensatory mechanisms designed to maintain cardiac output increase the workload and oxygen needs of the heart and are counterproductive in HF. Tachycardia increases the oxygen needs of the heart. The kidneys compensate by retaining sodium and fluid, which increases the fluid volume returning to the heart (preload) and therefore the heart's workload and oxygen needs. Pain also increases oxygen requirements, adding further to the cycle of HF.

Cheyne-Stokes Respiration

A breathing pattern of shallow respirations building to deep breaths followed by a period of apnea characterizes Cheyne-Stokes breathing. The apneic period occurs because the deep breathing causes carbon dioxide levels to drop to a level that does not stimulate the respiratory center. This apnea may last

up to 30 seconds and is then followed by the shallow to deeper respiratory pattern of Cheyne-Stokes as carbon dioxide levels rise again.

Edema

Edema occurs in HF as a result of (1) systemic blood vessel congestion and (2) sympathetic compensatory mechanisms that cause the kidneys to activate the renin-angiotensin-aldosterone system, in which antidiuretic hormone is released from the pituitary gland, causing sodium and water to be retained.

Systemic edema or pulmonary edema can occur in HF. The effect of backward buildup of pressure in the systemic blood vessels is seen with distention of the jugular veins, swelling of the legs and feet, sacral edema in the individual on bed rest, and increased fluid within the abdominal cavity and organs (ascites). An acute buildup of fluid in the lungs produces pulmonary edema.

Anemia

Many patients with HF are anemic due to hemodilution from fluid overload, and decreased angiotensin-converting enzyme (ACE) action. The reduced ACE action decreases erythropoietin release, resulting in decreased production of RBCs.

Nocturia

Nocturia is an increase in urine output at night during sleep. After lying down, fluid in the lower legs returns to the circulatory system. Renal blood flow and filtration are increased, resulting in greater urine production and the need to urinate frequently during the night. Nocturia may occur up to six times per night, contributing to the patient's fatigue from lack of sleep.

NURSING CARE TIP

Patients will often void shortly after going to bed due to fluid in the legs returning to the heart and then the kidneys for filtering after they lie down. To help patients get as much undisturbed rest as possible, teach them to recline with their legs at or above heart level for at least 30 minutes before going to bed. Then they can void before going to bed, instead of soon after.

Cyanosis

The skin, nail beds, or mucous membranes may appear blue, or cyanotic, from decreased oxygenation of the blood. **Cyanosis** is a late sign of HF. It is associated primarily with left-sided HF.

Altered Mental Status

Reduced cardiac output decreases the amount of oxygen delivered to the brain. As a result, restlessness, insomnia, confusion, decreased level of consciousness, and impaired memory may occur.

Malnutrition

Several factors contribute to malnutrition in the person with chronic HF. Altered mental status, dyspnea, and fatigue interfere with the ability to eat. Anorexia and GI upset occur from pressure exerted by excess fluid surrounding the GI structures (ascites). This pressure may also impair absorption of food.

CRITICAL THINKING

Mr. Shepard—Part 1

■ Mr. Shepard, age 66, has a family history of cardiac disease. He has been hypertensive for 10 years and takes captopril (Capoten) daily. His baseline vital signs are BP 122/78 mm Hg, pulse 80 beats per minute (beats/min), respirations 18 per minute, height 66 inches, and weight 170 lb. During a visit to his HCP, he states that he has been short of breath during his daily 2-mile walk and has been using two pillows at night for sleep. As he talks, the HCP notes that he has an intermittent dry cough. His physical examination shows BP 140/86 mm Hg, pulse 106 beats/min, respiration 24 per minute, weight 178 lb, and bilateral crackles in the lung bases.

1. What signs and symptoms of HF does Mr. Shepard have?
2. Do the signs and symptoms reflect right- or left-sided HF?
3. Why are each of the signs and symptoms occurring?
4. Why is Mr. Shepard using two pillows for sleeping?
5. What health care team members might collaborate on Mr. Shepard's care during the course of his HF?

Suggested answers are at the end of the chapter.

Complications of Heart Failure

Complications of HF are listed in Table 26.4. The liver and spleen enlarge from the fluid congestion, which causes impaired function, cellular death, and scarring. The elevated pressures in the capillaries of the lung can cause a pleural effusion, which is a leakage of fluid from the capillaries of the lung into the pleural space. Thrombosis and emboli can occur as a result of poor emptying of the ventricles, which leads to stasis of blood. Aspirin or anticoagulants are often prescribed to prevent thrombus formation in patients with HF. Cardiogenic shock, often caused by an MI that damages the left ventricle, occurs when the left ventricle is unable to supply the tissues with enough oxygen and nutrients to meet their needs. Cardiogenic shock is a life-threatening condition that requires immediate treatment (see Chapter 9).

Diagnostic Tests

Diagnostic tests are done to identify the cause of HF and determine the degree of failure present (see Table 26.4):

• Serum laboratory tests can evaluate contributing factors for HF, such as elevated serum blood urea nitrogen (BUN)

and serum creatinine from renal failure, elevated liver enzymes from liver damage, elevated ferritin with hemochromatosis (iron overload), and thyroid function tests.
• A serum B-type natriuretic peptide (BNP) or N-terminal proBNP (NT-proBNP) level may be obtained. Elevated levels indicate HF and severity; higher levels of this cardiac biomarker correlate with a worse prognosis. BNP is made by the heart to regulate blood volume to reduce cardiac workload. When the heart has to work harder over time, it releases more BNP.
• Elevated serum cystatin C (a protein produced by all nucleated cells) is a risk factor for HF.
• A chest x-ray examination shows the size, shape, and any enlargement of the heart as well as congestion in the pulmonary vessels.
• Cardiac dysrhythmias that precipitate and contribute to HF are diagnosed with an electrocardiogram (ECG; see Chapters 21 and 25).
• Echocardiography may measure ventricular size, wall thickness, motion, and ejection fraction and assess valvular function.
• Exercise stress testing and nuclear imaging studies show activity tolerance, which is usually limited in HF.
• Cardiac magnetic resonance imaging (MRI) shows both moving and still pictures of the heart and major blood vessels. Cardiac structure and function are analyzed to determine treatment for cardiac disease.
• Cardiac catheterization and angiography are used to detect underlying heart disease that may be the cause of HF.
• Sleep studies may be done because sleep apnea or breathing disorders can contribute to HF.
• Measurement of the pressure in the heart and lungs is done with hemodynamic monitoring to guide medical therapy.

CRITICAL THINKING

Mr. Shepard—Part 2

■ Mr. Shepard's chest x-ray examination shows an enlarged heart (cardiomegaly).

1. Why is Mr. Shepard's heart enlarged?
2. What is the significance of an enlarged heart?

Suggested answers are at the end of the chapter.

Therapeutic Measures

The overall goal of medical treatment for chronic HF is to improve the heart's pumping ability and decrease the heart's oxygen demands. Treatment of HF focuses on (1) identifying and correcting the underlying cause, (2) increasing the strength of the heart's contraction, (3) maintaining optimum water and sodium balance, and (4) decreasing the heart's workload. HF management requires a team approach that may involve physicians, nurse practitioners, case managers, nurses, dietitians, physical therapists, occupational therapists, pharmacists, social workers, and clergy. HF critical pathways (treatment guidelines) as well as HF clinics are used to ensure quality-based outcomes while reducing treatment costs.

The severity of HF determines the individualized therapy selected. Noninvasive approaches are usually tried first. If noninvasive treatment is not effective, invasive approaches may be used. Often, multiple therapies are used in combination for optimum patient outcomes.

Oxygen Therapy

One of the major problems caused by HF is a reduction in oxygen delivered to the tissues. The signs and symptoms of this are fatigue, dyspnea, altered mental status, and cyanosis. Oxygen therapy may assist in supplying the oxygen needs of the tissues. In mild HF, oxygen may be delivered via nasal cannula. For more severe cases, ABG values guide oxygen delivery, either via masks that provide high concentrations of oxygen or with mechanical ventilation.

Activity

Activity tolerance depends on the severity of HF signs and symptoms. Severe symptoms may require bed rest with restricted activity until treatment reduces the symptoms. For stable HF, a regular exercise program, such as one set up with referral to a cardiac rehabilitation program, has shown to improve cardiac function and reduce HF effects (see "Evidence-Based Practice"). Patients should be encouraged to stay as active as possible within the parameters of the collaborative plan set up with the health care team. An individualized walking program that increases activity over time is often prescribed. Patients are educated on how to exercise safely and how to identify symptoms they may have to prevent overexertion and worsening of symptoms.

EVIDENCE-BASED PRACTICE

Clinical Question
Do cardiovascular rehabilitation programs improve quality of life for HF patients?

Evidence
In a randomized controlled study of 123 medically stable HF patients over 10 years, exercise training demonstrated improved functional capacity and quality of life over patients who did not exercise regularly (Belardinelli, Georgiou, Cianci, & Purcaro, 2012).

Cardiac rehabilitation has shown long-term benefits also in a randomized controlled trial (Porto et al, 2012). In the study, patients with chronic HF who participated in a supervised cardiac rehabilitation program, compared with nonparticipants, demonstrated improved cardiovascular fitness, functional capacity, quality of life, and an increase

in survival along with a reduction in need for emergency treatment.

Implications for Nursing Practice
Cardiac rehabilitation programs for chronic HF patients have been shown to improve quality of life. Nurses should initiate referrals to cardiac rehabilitation programs and educate patients on their value toward overall cardiac health.

REFERENCES
Belardinelli, R., Georgiou, D., Cianci, G., & Purcaro, A. (2012). 10-year exercise training in chronic heart failure: A randomized controlled trial. *Journal of the American College of Cardiology, 60,* 1521–1528.

Porto, E. F., Kumpel, C., Leite, J. R., Andrade, A. A., Oliveira, N. C., & Portes, L. A. (2012). Quality of Life after Cardiac Rehabilitation for Patients with Heart Failure: 18 months followup. *American Journal of Medicine and Medical Sciences, 2*(5): 89–95.

Sodium Restriction and Weight Control

Dietary sodium is restricted to decrease fluid retention. Salt substitutes often use potassium in place of sodium, so the patient and HCP should discuss their use. A healthy weight range should be maintained, and a dietitian consult can include a plan for a low-sodium diet and weight reduction if needed.

BE SAFE!

In severe HF with abdominal discomfort present, malnutrition is a concern. The patient can be anorexic, but the weight gain that occurs with fluid retention can mask the weight loss occurring from the anorexia. Monitor food intake to ensure that weight gain from fluid retention does not allow malnutrition to go undetected.

Drug Therapy

There is no cure for HF. Medications, however, can improve symptoms and quality of life. The American College of Cardiology Foundation/American Heart Association (ACC/AHA) 2013 guidelines recommend medication classes with qualifiers for the following stages of HF development (Yancy et al, 2013):

- Stage A refers to people at high risk of HF.
- Stage B is those who have no HF symptoms but do have structural heart disease.
- Stage C applies to people with current or past symptoms of HF with structural heart disease. This includes most patients with HF.
- Stage D includes those with refractory HF, which requires extraordinary support or hospice care.

In general, drug categories begin with angiotensin-converting enzyme (ACE) inhibitors or angiotensin receptor blockers (ARBs) to control hypertension if present in Stage A, then add beta blockers (bisoprolol, carvedilol, metoprolol succinate SR) along with the ACE inhibitors or ARBs for Stage B, then diuretics for fluid retention, and consideration of aldosterone antagonists, nitrates, digitalis, and hydralazine (Apresoline) for Stage C (Table 26.5). Anticoagulants are also used on an individual risk basis.

 LEARNING TIP

To help you identify ACE inhibitors, remember that their generic names end with -pril.

ANGIOTENSIN-CONVERTING ENZYME INHIBITORS. ACE inhibitors are considered the first-choice drug over angiotensin receptor blockers (ARBs). They are used for their vasodilation effect, which lowers blood pressure and reduces workload on the heart. They also offer additional benefit by preventing remodeling, which is an effect that leads to progressive cardiac deterioration.

ANGIOTENSIN RECEPTOR BLOCKERS. ARBs are an alternative to ACE inhibitors for inhibiting the renin-angiotensin-aldosterone system, thereby lowering blood pressure and workload on the heart. They should be used carefully if ACE inhibitors are also used because hypotension, hyperkalemia, and renal dysfunction risks increase.

BETA-ADRENERGIC BLOCKERS. Initially the sympathetic nervous system (SNS) acts to compensate for HF. Long-term

TABLE 26.5 MEDICATIONS USED FOR HEART FAILURE

Medication Class/Action	Examples	Nursing Implications
ACE Inhibitors First-line therapy to decrease afterload. Decrease cardiac hypertrophy.	captopril (Capoten) benazepril (Lotensin) enalapril (Vasotec) fosinopril (Monopril) lisinopril (Prinivil, Zestril) moexipril (Univasc) quinapril (Accupril) perindopril (Aceon) ramipril (Altace) trandolapril (Mavik)	Check apical pulse and blood pressure (BP). If pulse less than 60 beats/min or systolic BP less than 90 mm Hg, notify HCP. Give 1 hour before meals. Give captopril and moexipril on empty stomach. *Teaching:* Take first doses at night to adjust to lower BP. Rise slowly. Check BP weekly. Report if persistent cough or other side effects develop.
Angiotensin II Receptor Inhibitors (ARBs) Block angiotensin II receptor blockers to prevent hypertension. May be used if ACE inhibitor not tolerated.	candesartan (Atacand) irbesartan (Avapro) losartan (Cozaar) valsartan (Diovan)	Check apical pulse and BP. If pulse below 60 beats/min or systolic BP below 100 mm Hg, notify HCP. *Teaching:* Rise slowly. Report rash, sore throat/mouth, fever, swelling, difficulty breathing, chest pain, or irregular heartbeat.
Beta-Adrenergic Blockers Reduce sympathetic nervous system input, cardiac remodeling; improve cardiac output to reduce symptoms, reduce disease progression and sudden death.	bisoprolol (Zebeta) carvedilol (Coreg) metoprolol succinate (Toprol XL)	Check apical pulse and BP. If pulse below 60 beats/min or systolic or BP below 100 mm Hg, notify HCP. *Teaching:* Take pulse daily and notify HCP if below 60. Take BP biweekly. Rise slowly.
Loop Diuretics Decrease fluid overload. • Potassium wasting	bumetanide (Bumex) furosemide (Lasix) torsemide (Demadex)	Check BP and pulse before giving. Monitor electrolyte levels (especially potassium and in those on digitalis) and fluid status (daily weight, intake, output, thirst, dry mouth, weakness, oliguria) throughout therapy. Administer per patient lifestyle (usually in the morning) to avoid nocturia.
• Potassium sparing	spironolactone (Aldactone)	Do not give potassium-sparing diuretic if hyperkalemic. *Teaching:* Report signs of hyperkalemia: weakness, fatigue, confusion, dyspnea, arrhythmias, confusion.

TABLE 26.5   MEDICATIONS USED FOR HEART FAILURE—cont'd

Medication Class/Action	Examples	Nursing Implications
Thiazide Diuretics Decrease fluid overload. Potassium wasting	chlorothiazide (Diuril) hydrochlorothiazide (Hydro DIURIL, HCTZ, Microzide) metolazone (Zaroxolyn)	Monitor potassium. *Teaching:* Use of potassium supplements and, if on dig- italis, increased risk of toxicity with hypokalemia. Monitor weight daily, and report 2- to 3-lb change over 1–2 days. Use sunscreen.
Inotropes—Cardiac Glycoside (Positive Inotrope and Negative Chronotrope)		
Increase force and contraction of myocardium, which increases cardiac output. Slow heart rate to reduce workload of heart and control atrial fibrillation, if present.	digoxin (Lanoxin)	Take apical pulse for 1 minute; if below 60 beats/min, notify HCP. Older patients are more susceptible to toxicity. Periodically monitor drug level and electrolytes (hypokalemia, hypomagnesemia, and hypercalcemia make more susceptible to toxicity). *Teaching:* Take medication exactly as directed, at the same time each day. Take pulse before taking med- ication; if below 60 beats/min hold and contact HCP. Signs of digitalis toxicity: abdominal pain, anorexia, nausea, vomiting, visual changes (blurred, yellow- green halos, photophobia, diplopia), bradycardia, dysrhythmias
Vasodilators Decrease afterload, which increases cardiac output and reduces cardiac workload. Used for patients who cannot take ACE inhibitors.	isosorbide dinitrate (Isorbid, Isordil) hydralazine (Apresoline) nitroglycerin	Take blood pressure and pulse before giving. Notify HCP if not within normal limits. *Teaching:* Rise slowly. Headache common initially, treated with aspirin.

ACE = angiotensin-converting enzyme.

sympathetic effects, however, are not helpful in HF. Beta-blockers block the adverse effects of the SNS. Improved cardiac output, reduced symptoms, reduced disease progression, and reduced sudden death are benefits of this therapy.

DIURETICS. Diuretics reduce fluid volume and decrease pulmonary venous pressure, which in turn decreases cardiac workload. Because they are given to help prevent edema, edema does not need to be present for their use. Diuretics act on various areas of the kidneys to promote the excretion of edema fluid. A combination of diuretics may be used to achieve the desired effect. Electrolytes (especially potassium levels to prevent hypokalemia) and fluid balance (to prevent dehydration) should be carefully monitored during therapy. Potassium supplements are often given with potassium-wasting diuretics.

ALDOSTERONE ANTAGONISTS. Spironolactone (Aldactone) blocks the effects of aldosterone, which causes the retention of sodium and fluid. Potassium must be monitored carefully, because spironolactone is a potassium-sparing agent and the risk of hyperkalemia increases if ACE inhibitors or ARBs are also used.

BE SAFE!

Always check potassium levels before giving a potassium-wasting diuretic such as the loop diuretics furosemide (Lasix), bumetanide (Bumex), or torsemide (Demadex) or before giving a potassium supplement, which the patient may be taking due to diuretic therapy. Do not give a diuretic if the potassium level is low or a potassium supplement if the potassium level is high.

INOTROPIC AGENTS. Inotropic drugs strengthen ventricular contraction to increase cardiac output. Inotropic agents include digitalis (digoxin), sympathomimetics (dobutamine), and phosphodiesterase inhibitors (milrinone). The sympathomimetics and phosphodiesterase inhibitors are usually used short term.

Digitalis. In addition to improving contraction strength, digitalis preparations decrease conduction time within the heart, which slows the heart rate to allow more complete emptying of the ventricles. Obtaining an apical pulse rate before administration of digitalis is required. Digitalis may increase myocardial oxygen needs, so it is used cautiously. Monitoring of serum drug levels is necessary to detect toxic levels of the drug. If toxic levels are present, the drug is stopped to allow digitalis levels to decrease over time.

CRITICAL THINKING

Mr. Shepard—Part 3

■ During Mr. Shepard's visit, the HCP tells him to continue the ACE inhibitor, the diuretic, and a 2-g sodium diet.

1. Why is the ACE inhibitor continued?
2. Will the ACE inhibitor affect preload or afterload?
3. Why is the diuretic ordered?
4. What lab test result is checked before administering diuretics?
5. Why is a 2-g sodium diet ordered?
6. What is the overall goal of the ordered treatment?

Suggested answers are at the end of the chapter.

Pacemakers and Implantable Cardioverter Defibrillator

For patients at risk of sudden death, pacemakers and implantable cardioverter defibrillators (ICDs) are used along with medication therapy. They can pace the heart rate and rhythm or deliver an electric countershock if a life-threatening rhythm occurs.

Cardiac Resynchronization Therapy

With HF, the ventricles do not always beat in normal synchrony with each other. This dyssynchrony results in less effective pumping by the ventricles and reduced stroke volume. Cardiac resynchronization therapy (CRT) restores normal contraction timing of the ventricles. It reduces symptoms and improves quality of life. A biventricular cardiac pacing system is used. An atrial lead senses or paces the atria as needed. A right and left ventricular lead stimulates the ventricles to synchronize their contractions in response to the atrial event. Left ventricular filling and thus contraction is then improved. CRT therapy is also available with an implantable cardioverter defibrillator (CRT-D). For more information and pictures of CRT devices, visit www.medtronic.com.

Mechanical Assistive Devices

Mechanical assistive devices can provide temporary support to patients in cardiogenic shock and act as a bridge to transplantation, destination therapy (long-term solution when other options are not available for the failing heart), or heart replacement. These devices increase the cardiac output of the patient. They include the intra-aortic balloon pump, ventricular assist devices, total artificial heart, and implantable replacement heart. Technology in this area is continually changing. For current information and to see pictures of these devices, see DavisPlus.

INTRA-AORTIC BALLOON PUMP. For acute care, an intra-aortic balloon pump (IABP) increases circulation to the coronary arteries and reduces the work of the heart. The IABP catheter is inserted into the femoral artery and positioned in the descending aortic arch (Fig. 26.3). It is attached to a computer that senses ventricular contraction and controls the balloon. While the heart is relaxed (diastole), the balloon is inflated, sending more blood into the coronary arteries. Just before the heart contracts (systole), the balloon deflates to allow blood to flow past it. The deflation of the balloon creates a suction effect, which allows the blood to flow past it with less resistance (decreased afterload) into the aorta. The IABP is inserted in a cardiac catheterization laboratory, critical care unit, or surgical suite and is used short term for several days.

VENTRICULAR ASSIST DEVICES. Ventricular assist devices (VADs) are implanted mechanical devices that assist cardiac pumping (Fig. 26.4). These devices maintain cardiac output and allow the failing ventricle to rest. VADs are used temporarily as a bridge to transplantation (while awaiting a donor heart), bridge to recovery (for hearts that potentially can recover), or as destination therapy (long-term therapy) for those who are not candidates for heart transplant. They may also be referred to as left ventricular assist devices (LVADs) if used in the left ventricle only, right ventricular assist devices (RVADs) if used in the right ventricle only, or bi-VADs

Diastole   Systole

FIGURE 26.3 Intra-aortic balloon pump.

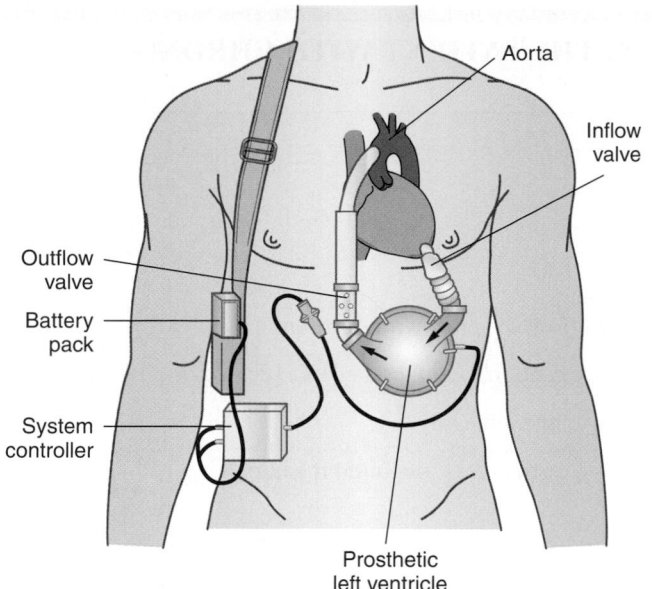

FIGURE 26.4 Schematic of a left ventricular assist device.

(biventricular assist devices) if used in both ventricles. VADs can pump blood directly from either the right atrium to the pulmonary artery (right ventricular failure) or the left atrium to the aorta (left ventricular failure). Two devices are used for biventricular failure.

Surgical Management

HF causes may be treated surgically with coronary artery bypass for coronary artery disease or valve replacement for valvular disease (see Chapters 23 and 24). Once these conditions are treated, HF symptoms should resolve.

Surgical ventricular reconstruction (SVR) reduces left ventricular volume in HF patients. It is often done along with coronary artery bypass surgery. The STICH trial data on further analysis showed that coronary artery bypass graft (CABG) with SVR increased survival when certain parameters occurred (end systolic volume index 70 mL/m² or less; Michler et al, 2013).

Nursing Process for the Patient With Chronic Heart Failure

Data Collection

While obtaining data for the patient with HF, focus on areas that might indicate the presence of HF (Table 26.6).

Nursing Diagnoses, Planning, Interventions, and Evaluation

See the "Nursing Care Plan for the Patient With Chronic HF" for common nursing diagnoses. The major focus of nursing care for chronic HF patients is to improve oxygenation and decrease the body's need for oxygen with rest, positioning, medications, fluid balance, and oxygen consumption control.

TABLE 26.6 NURSING DATA COLLECTION FOR THE PATIENT WITH CHRONIC HEART FAILURE

	Subjective Data
History Respiratory	Lung disease? How many flights of stairs can be climbed without dyspnea? How many pillows used for sleeping? Dyspnea at rest or that awakens from sleeping?
Cardiovascular	Any cardiac disease history: hypertension, myocardial infarction, valvular problem, anemia, dysrhythmias, palpitations? Chest pain: precipitating factors, severity, relieving factors? Can activities of daily living be performed? Can activities performed 6 months, 4 months, 2 months, 2 weeks ago still be done? Any dizziness (vertigo) or fainting (syncope)?
Fluid retention	Daily sodium intake? Weight gain? Are shoes tight? Do ankles swell?
Gastrointestinal	Is appetite good? Any nausea, vomiting, or abdominal pain?
Urinary	Decrease in daytime urine output? How often does patient go to the bathroom at night (nocturia)?
Neurologic	Any change in behavior?

Continued

TABLE 26.6 NURSING DATA COLLECTION FOR THE PATIENT WITH CHRONIC HEART FAILURE—cont'd

Medications *Knowledge* *of Condition* *Coping Skills*	
	Objective Data
Respiratory	Tachypnea, crackles, wheezing, respiratory effort, dyspnea with exertion
Cardiovascular	Tachycardia, dysrhythmias, jugular venous distention, peripheral edema (degree of pitting)
Gastrointestinal	Abdominal distention, ascites, hepatomegaly, splenomegaly
Neurologic	Confusion, decreased level of consciousness, restlessness, impaired memory
Integumentary	Cold, clammy skin; pallor; cyanosis
General	Weight
Diagnostic Test Findings	

OXYGEN. Oxygen therapy is ordered by the HCP and guided by blood gas analysis and patient symptoms. Before starting oxygen therapy, explain the therapy to the patient. For chronic HF, oxygen is administered at 2 to 6 L/min via nasal cannula. The effects of the oxygen should be monitored carefully.

REST AND ACTIVITY. Reduction of the body's oxygen demands decreases the workload of the heart. A balance of rest and activity that does not produce signs or symptoms of oxygen deprivation is essential. The activity level of the patient is determined by the severity of the HF. During times of exertion, monitor the patient's vital signs and respiratory effort for oxygen deprivation. If activity intolerance develops, the activity should be stopped.

POSITIONING. Semi-Fowler's or high-Fowler's position makes breathing easier. In upright positions, the lungs are able to expand more fully and gravity decreases the amount of fluid returned to the heart, thereby reducing the heart's workload.

FLUID RETENTION. Monitoring daily weights for weight gain is important in detecting fluid retention. Edema is usually not observed until 5 to 10 pounds of extra fluid are present. A baseline weight should be obtained when HF is diagnosed. Daily weights should be measured on the same scale, at the same time of day, and with the same type of clothing worn to ensure accuracy. A good time to obtain a daily weight is in the morning after the bladder is emptied. Documentation of daily weights should include the date and time of the weight, the scale used, the clothing worn, and the weight measurement. The patient can keep a weight journal. Tell patients to report weight gains of 2 to 3 pounds over 1 to 2 days.

NURSING CARE PLAN for the Patient With Chronic Heart Failure

Nursing Diagnosis: *Activity Intolerance* related to fatigue caused by oxygen imbalance

Expected Outcome: The patient will show increased activity tolerance with vital signs within normal limits (WNL) in response to activity.

Evaluation of Outcome: Does the patient participate in activities and maintain vital signs WNL?

Intervention Provide rest, space activities, and conserve energy. **Rationale** Myocardial oxygen need is decreased with rest and energy conservation. **Evaluation** Does patient participate in activity with minimal pulse rate or ECG changes?

Intervention Assist as needed with activities of daily living (ADLs). **Rationale** Conserve energy by assisting with ADLs. **Evaluation** Are patient's ADLs met?

NURSING CARE PLAN for the Patient With Chronic Heart Failure—cont'd

Intervention Teach use of assistive devices and lifestyle changes. **Rationale** Assistive devices can overcome limitations to increase activity. **Evaluation** Does patient incorporate assistive devices into lifestyle changes?

GERIATRIC
Intervention Increase time allowed to complete activities. **Rationale** Independence and participation are increased if extra time is allowed for tasks. **Evaluation** Does patient report greater ability to complete activities with fewer symptoms?

Nursing Diagnosis: *Excess Fluid Volume* related to HF and the secondary reduction in renal blood flow for filtration

Expected Outcomes: The patient will remain free from edema and dyspnea, have clear lung sounds, and maintain baseline weight at all times.

Evaluation of Outcomes: Does patient have clear lung sounds with baseline weight maintained?

Intervention Monitor for edema, weight gain, jugular venous distention (JVD), lung crackles. **Rationale** Excess fluid is indicated by edema, sudden weight gain, JVD, and crackles in the lungs. **Evaluation** Are edema, weight gain, JVD, or crackles present? Are they worsening or improving?

Intervention Monitor intake and output (I&O). **Rationale** I&O will show imbalances. **Evaluation** Are I&O balanced for 24 hours?

Intervention Administer diuretics. **Rationale** Diuretics promote fluid excretion. **Evaluation** Is output increased and edema or dyspnea reduced?

Intervention Decrease sodium intake as ordered. **Rationale** Sodium retains fluid. **Evaluation** Does patient restrict sodium intake?

Intervention Maintain fluid restriction as ordered. **Rationale** Excess fluid intake contributes to edema. **Evaluation** Does patient restrict fluid intake?

Nursing Diagnosis: *Disturbed Sleep Pattern* related to nocturia and inability to lie down and sleep comfortably

Expected Outcome: The patient will awaken refreshed and be less fatigued during the day at all times.

Evaluation of Outcome: Does patient wake up less frequently during the night and feel more refreshed with less fatigue during the day?

Intervention Identify barriers to sleep. **Rationale** Anxiety, nocturia, diuretics, orthopnea, or paroxysmal nocturnal dyspnea can make sleep difficult. **Evaluation** Does patient identify sleep barriers?

Intervention Assist patient in identifying positions of comfort for sleeping. **Rationale** Use of pillows or a recliner can decrease orthopnea. **Evaluation** Can patient identify a position of comfort?

Intervention Teach patient cause of dyspnea at night. **Rationale** Anxiety about falling asleep and waking up short of breath is reduced. **Evaluation** Can patient explain cause of dyspnea?

Intervention Encourage patient to recline for 30 to 60 minutes before bedtime. **Rationale** Reclining before bedtime redistributes fluid to the kidneys so that the patient can void before going to sleep instead of soon afterward. **Evaluation** Is patient awakened to void after going to bed less often?

GERIATRIC
Intervention Encourage patient to take diuretics according to sleep patterns. If sleeps during nighttime hours, then take diuretic early in the day. If sleeps during daytime hours, then take medications after rising. **Rationale** Nocturia is reduced if diuretics are taken earlier in the day. **Evaluation** Does patient take diuretics early and report less nocturia?

OXYGEN CONSUMPTION. Increased oxygen consumption by the heart should be avoided. Sustained tachycardia increases the oxygen needs of the heart and should be reported promptly to the HCP for treatment. Older patients are especially vulnerable to the effects of tachycardia because of their decreased reserves. Constipation should be prevented because straining during defecation, known as the Valsalva maneuver, increases the heart's workload by increasing venous return to the heart. Stool softeners should be administered, as ordered, to prevent straining.

Patients should be taught methods of saving energy while performing ADLs. Fatigue should be avoided by alternating activity with periods of rest. A referral to occupational therapy and physical therapy can be helpful for developing techniques that allow the patient to conserve energy during self-care. Some suggestions for conserving energy include placing frequently used objects at waist level to avoid reaching overhead, planning bathing activities to include rest periods, and using Velcro fasteners to make dressing easier.

MEDICATIONS. HF is a progressive, chronic condition, and patients may require lifetime medication. Combination drug therapy is often needed, and taking multiple pills daily can be challenging. Financial resources, adherence to therapy regimen, and ongoing monitoring are issues that must be considered.

Diuretics. Diuretics require monitoring of the patient's potassium levels and blood pressure. To prevent hypokalemia, potassium supplements may be prescribed during diuretic therapy, and a diet with high-potassium foods is encouraged. If too much fluid is removed, the patient may become hypotensive, and orthostatic hypotension can develop. The patient may then be dizzy and at risk of falling. Caution the patient to change positions and rise slowly to prevent falls during diuretic therapy.

Digitalis. Before administration of a digitalis drug, which slows the heart rate, the patient's apical pulse should be counted for 1 minute. If the pulse is below 60 beats/min, notify the HCP to determine if the drug should be given. Some patients are given digitalis even if their heart rates are between 50 and 60 beats/min, as long as their heart's conduction system is normal or if the rate is due to other medications such as a beta blocker. When giving digitalis, be aware that hypokalemia increases the heart's sensitivity to digitalis. A patient can become toxic on a normal dose of digitalis when hypokalemia is present. This is important to note because many people on digitalis also take diuretics, which may lower potassium levels. Monitoring for signs and symptoms of digitalis toxicity should be done routinely during patient assessment. Early signs and symptoms of digitalis toxicity are anorexia, nausea, and vomiting; bradycardia or other dysrhythmias; visual problems; and mental changes. Older adults are especially prone to the toxic effects of this drug and may exhibit confusion when levels are toxic.

Vasodilators. Medications with vasodilating effects reduce the heart's workload by decreasing vascular pressure. Blood pressure is monitored when administering vasodilators.

Medication Teaching. Patients and their families are taught the purpose, side effects, and precautions for prescribed medications. Patients should understand the importance of taking their medication as prescribed, even if they do not have symptoms. A schedule should be developed so patients remember to take their medications. Teach them to report side effects to the HCP. If dizziness occurs from drugs that reduce blood pressure, the drugs can be staggered so that they are not all taken at the same time. Patients taking digitalis or a beta blocker should be taught to take their pulse and to notify their HCP if it is below 60 beats/min or below the lower limit heart rate set by their HCP. Patients on diuretics should be taught the following:

- Take drug during the day before 1600 to decrease being awakened at night to void (if desired).
- Have a readily available and obstacle-free bathroom or commode to prevent incontinence and falls.
- Eat high-potassium foods if taking a potassium-wasting diuretic.
- Weigh oneself daily, and report weight gains of 2 to 3 pounds over 1 to 2 days.

LOW-SODIUM DIET AND WEIGHT CONTROL. A dietitian consult helps the patient and family understand the need for adherence to a special diet and ways to provide menus that are appealing and easy to use. Eating should remain pleasurable for the patient to avoid malnutrition. Discuss foods the patient likes and can still have rather than talking about only foods they cannot have. Patients are taught to read food labels to determine which foods are high and low in sodium content. They are also taught that salt substitutes may contain potassium. With this knowledge, patients can help design a daily meal plan using low-sodium foods that are appealing to them. Food preparers are taught not to salt food during cooking, and table salt should be eliminated. Spices, herbs, and lemon juice may be suggested to flavor unsalted foods.

For overweight patients, weight reduction may help eliminate the underlying cause of HF. Diet counseling and support should be given to the obese patient to encourage weight loss. The body mass index (BMI) and waist-to-hip ratio should guide weight loss.

If anorexia occurs in the later stages of HF, the patient's intake should be evaluated. Several small meals rather than three large meals will decrease the heart's workload. If the patient's nutritional needs are not being met, the HCP should be informed for a referral to a dietitian.

EDUCATION. Chronic management of HF requires patient and family understanding of the disease process, management of home oxygen therapy, diet and weight control, need for immunizations such as the annual flu shot, and medications (see "Home Health Hints"). The patient and family must recognize the importance of each of these factors to foster quality of life for the patient with chronic HF. A discussion of HF and signs and symptoms to report to the HCP using simple terms should be included in the teaching plan (Box 26-1, "Patient and Family Education").

Box 26-1 Patient and Family Education

HF Signs and Symptoms to Report to the Health Care Practitioner

- Shortness of breath
- Fatigue
- Dry cough
- Shortness of breath when lying down (orthopnea)
- Episodes of sudden awakening with shortness of breath (paroxysmal nocturnal dyspnea)
- Weight gain of 2 to 3 pounds over 1 to 2 days
- Ankle or foot edema
- Nocturia
- Anorexia

Home Health Hints

- Some patients may not have a scale in their home. It may be necessary to assist them in obtaining one or to leave an agency scale in the home for daily weights.
- The most objective way to document edema is to use a tape measure (marked in centimeters) on the abdominal girth, thigh, calf, and ankle. Measure at the same place each visit, such as measuring the girth of the calf at a specified distance above the medial malleolus. Edema may be present if the patient's waistband is getting tighter or shoes and socks feel tighter.
- The sacrum, back, and sides of a bedridden patient should be checked to note edema. These are dependent areas in the bedridden patient, so fluid accumulates in these areas instead of the ankles.
- Blood drawn for potassium levels needs to be transported to the laboratory within 1 hour. Ice should not be put directly on the blood-draw tube because this can cause destruction of the cells and a false elevation in the potassium level.
- Blood drawn for digoxin (Lanoxin) levels should be taken to the lab within 2 to 3 hours.
- Patients who are on sodium-restricted diets should use no-salt-added canned vegetables. If canned vegetables are not low-sodium, patients should be instructed to pour off the liquid and rinse the vegetables before heating them for serving. The use of herbs and spices can help make them more flavorful.
- For the patient on a low-sodium diet, an effective diet teaching technique is to have the patient name the foods highest in sodium. Asking the patient to rename the list on each visit helps knowledge retention and adherence to the diet.
- If patients have a poor appetite, ask their caregiver if they eat well when eating with others. Anorexia could be a sign of loneliness and depression if they eat well with others instead of an effect of HF.
- Assist patients in taking medications at times that fit their lifestyle. A morning dose of a diuretic may limit what they can do for the next few hours. An afternoon dose might encourage adherence to the medication regimen. Lack of adherence is a major factor in the rehospitalization of patients with HF. A dose of diuretic too late in the day may cause frequent awakenings during the night to void.
- The home health nurse should periodically check the contents of medicine bottles. If pills have been cut in half, question the patient because this is often an attempt by the patient to "stretch" the medicine to decrease expenses. Find out about community or drug company programs that help purchase medicines for patients with financial need. Eligible Medicaid patients can apply for medication cards. The new Medicare Part D prescription program, as well as retail drug discount programs, may be helpful as well.
- Visual disturbances can occur from digitalis toxicity. If the patient sees halos around lights or red-green tinting on everything, report this to the HCP.
- Troublesome side effects of an ACE inhibitor such as captopril (Capoten) are an intractable cough and hypotension. Note if the patient is coughing. Teach the patient to report the cough.
- Oxygen concentrators are widely used in home care. Instructions must be given on the proper use of the oxygen and safety precautions for oxygen use. Long tubing allows the patient ease in moving about the home. Patients need to be cautioned about keeping the tubing out of their way and not kinking it. Patients and caregivers should also be cautioned as to the explosive nature of oxygen and the danger of smoking in its presence.
- As the home health nurse becomes acquainted with the patient, it is easier to pick up on signs of oxygen deprivation and hypoxia, such as confusion, combativeness, or unusual expressions of anger.
- For patients with orthopnea, a foam wedge can be obtained from a medical equipment company to use under their head when sleeping instead of pillows.
- As patients with HF feel better, they may go back to the old habits that cause an increase in fluid. The home health nurse can help by providing information about the disease and help patients foster their own independence and ways of coping with the condition. Each home health visit is a teaching opportunity that empowers patients with a knowledge base to help them take control of their health.

COPING. Living with a chronic illness can be frustrating for both patients and their families. An assessment of coping skills used by patients and their families can be used to develop a plan for coping with this current illness. Available support systems are explained to patients. Referrals to social workers, sexual counselors, and nurse-managed clinics can be helpful in providing resources that may make living with HF easier. Providing patients options for traveling can help maintain quality of life.

Understanding the chronic nature of HF is important for patients, families, and caregivers so they can positively deal with the emotions and feelings that can result. Nurse-managed HF clinics have been shown to decrease hospitalization rates and increase effective management of the therapeutic regimen.

Should the patient's condition worsen irreversibly, a discussion regarding the possibility of organ donation could be considered. Such a discussion would require a team approach involving other members of the health care team (physician, social worker, clergy). As of 2013, 18 people will die each day waiting for an organ, yet one donation can save up to eight lives. For more information, visit www.organdonor.gov.

NURSING CARE TIP

Provide written discharge instructions for all patients with HF and their caregivers. Instructions should focus on medications (stressing adherence to following the medication regimen), diet, activity level, follow-up appointments, daily weights, and to report or seek care for symptoms that worsen.

CRITICAL THINKING

Mr. Shepard—Part 4

■ The nurse meets with Mr. Shepard after the HCP orders a continued ACE inhibitor, a diuretic, and a 2-g sodium diet.

1. What patient-centered information should the nurse teach Mr. Shepard based on the prescribed treatment?
2. What types of foods should be included in Mr. Shepard's diet?
3. Why does the nurse instruct Mr. Shepard to weigh himself daily?
4. Why does the nurse tell Mr. Shepard to weigh himself at the same time of day, on the same scale, and wearing the same type of clothing?
5. What guidelines does the nurse teach Mr. Shepard to follow with reporting of weight gain?

Suggested answers are at the end of the chapter.

■ CARDIAC TRANSPLANTATION

Cardiac transplantation is reserved for patients with end-stage cardiac disease. Guidelines for the selection of recipients and donors are applied to optimize survival (Box 26-2). Preoperative teaching is done once the recipient is accepted into the transplant program. For more information on heart transplantation, visit www.nhlbi.nih.gov/health/dci/Diseases/ht/ht_whatis.html.

To increase the availability of organs for transplant, a device has been developed that keeps the heart beating and nourished with the donor's blood during transport for up to 12 hours. The device, Organ Care Systems (Heart in a Box) is in use in Europe and in trials in the United States.

Surgical Procedure

Once a donor heart is found, the recipient is notified, admitted to the hospital, and prepared for surgery. The general procedures for this surgery are similar to those described in Chapter 21. Two types of cardiac transplant procedures are performed: orthotopic and heterotopic. In the orthotopic procedure, once the patient is on cardiopulmonary bypass (CPB), the recipient's diseased heart is removed, leaving the posterior wall of the atria, superior and inferior vena cava, and pulmonary vein (Fig. 26.5). The aorta and pulmonary artery are cut. The donor's atria, aorta, and pulmonary artery are then anastomosed to the recipient's atria, aorta, and pulmonary artery. The heterotopic procedure joins the donor heart and vessels to the recipient's heart and vessels without removing the recipient's heart. The donor heart rests in the right side of the chest.

Immunosuppressive therapy is required to prevent rejection of the transplanted heart. Medications such as cyclosporine

Box 26-2 Cardiac Transplant Guidelines

Donor Criteria

• Younger than age 45
• No significant cardiac or malignant disease
• No active infections
• No severe hypertension or diabetes mellitus
• Donor body weight no greater than 30% below recipients

Recipient Criteria

• Consideration of physiological age
• Class IV cardiac disease (not treatable with other medical or surgical treatment, less than 6 to 12 months survival)
• No irreversible pulmonary hypertension
• No unresolved pulmonary infarcts
• No systemic disease limiting survival
• No drug addiction or peptic ulcer disease

Aorta

Superior
vena cava
cannula

Pulmonary artery

Right atrium

Inferior
vena cava
cannula

To suction

Cardioplegia
catheter

Stapled donor aorta

Sinoatrial node

Donor right atrium
slit for attachment

Donor heart

Suture

Pericardial
pacing wire

FIGURE 26.5 Heart transplantation.

(Neoral, Sandimmune), mycophenolate mofetil (CellCept), tacrolimus (Prograf), sirolimus (Rapamune), and Prednisone are used ("Nutrition Notes"). It begins preoperatively with high loading doses of these medications. The risk for rejection is highest immediately after surgery and decreases with time but never goes away, so doses of immunosuppressive medication are also highest initially after surgery and decrease with time. Lifelong antirejection therapy is required and often involves the combination of three drugs to allow lower doses to help reduce side effects.

 NUTRITION NOTES

Cyclosporine, an immunosuppressant used to prevent transplant rejection, is metabolized by intestinal CYP3A4. Taking cyclosporine with grapefruit juice may cause elevated blood levels of the drug. In addition, St. John's wort, sold as a dietary supplement, has interacted with cyclosporine (through both CYP3A4 and P-glycoprotein mechanisms) sufficiently to cause organ rejection.

Complications

Heart transplantation complications may include those associated with cardiac surgery, as well as heart rejection, which is the major cause of death within the first year. To detect rejection, frequent biopsies of cardiac muscle or a newer blood test to detect activation of rejection genesis is done during the first year. If a biopsy shows damaged cells, indicating rejection, antirejection drug therapy may be changed.

In addition, as a result of immunosuppressive therapy, infection and cancer may occur. The medications used for immunosuppressive therapy also may cause adverse reactions such as increased cholesterol, diabetes, kidney disease, cataracts, or osteoporosis.

Therapeutic Measures

After CPB is stopped, the patient receives a diuretic to aid in excretion of excessive circulating fluid. Intake and output are monitored hourly, and the patient is observed for fluid overload. Lung sounds are monitored frequently for crackles, and weight and electrolyte levels are checked daily.

Postcardiotomy syndrome may occur from days 2 to 5 after surgery and last a few weeks. Patients may arouse normally and be oriented but exhibit mild confusion or psychosis. Pupillary reaction and motor response are assessed. The safety of the patient is maintained with side rails up, bed in low position, and nursing call light within reach. The patient is given as much rest and as little sensory stimulation as possible. The family is kept informed and involved in the patient's recovery.

Sleeping is difficult because of postoperative pain and the continuous level of activity in the ICU. Sleep is promoted in 90-minute intervals by dimming lights and decreasing all sensory stimulation near the patient. Additionally, listening to a favorite soothing type of music with earphones or the use of ordered narcotics for pain may also help sedate and relax the patient to allow for healing.

Temperature is monitored every 4 hours and complete blood cell count (CBC) and white blood cell (WBC) results are monitored for indications of infection. If oral thrush (white patches) develops, an antifungal agent is ordered. A urine culture to diagnose a urinary tract infection is ordered if cloudy urine or urinary tract burning occurs.

Nursing Process for the Preoperative Cardiac Transplant Patient

General preoperative and postoperative surgical care is discussed in Chapter 12. Postoperative needs for the patient undergoing cardiac surgery are discussed next.

Nursing Process for the Postoperative Cardiac Transplant Patient

Data Collection

The patient is accompanied to the ICU by the anesthesiologist, who gives the nurse a report of the procedure, complications, and hemodynamic and ventilatory management of the patient. The patient is connected to a cardiac monitor and a mechanical ventilator for 4 to 24 hours. A temporary pacemaker is connected to the epicardial pacing wires if they were placed during surgery as a precaution to treat bradycardia and other dysrhythmias. The patient is placed under a forced-air warming device, such as a blanket. The chest tubes are monitored, the nasogastric tube is placed to suction, and the urinary catheter is placed for gravity drainage.

A head-to-toe assessment of the patient, including dressings, tubes, and IV lines, is performed. Of importance are signs of awakening, shivering, pain, lung and heart sounds, and palpation of the entire chest and neck to detect crepitus (air in the subcutaneous tissue from opening the chest). CBC, electrolytes, coagulation studies, and ABGs are monitored. Cardiac transplant patients may be in isolation for their own protection, depending on the agency's policy.

After the initial transfer assessment, vital signs, oxygen saturation, and cardiac pressures are monitored and recorded every 15 to 30 minutes, with decreasing frequency as the patient stabilizes. Input and output (I&O) is measured and vital signs are monitored. An ECG is done to detect perioperative MI. A chest x-ray examination is done to check central line and endotracheal tube placement and to detect a pneumothorax or hemothorax, diaphragm elevation, or mediastinal widening from bleeding. At this point, the family may see the patient, and patient care is explained.

Nursing Diagnoses, Planning, Implementation, and Evaluation

Nursing diagnoses for postoperative cardiac surgery or transplant are discussed in the "Nursing Care Plan for the Postoperative Patient Undergoing Cardiac or Transplant Surgery."

Coping With Cardiac Transplant

Cardiac transplant patients may have feelings of sadness and grief for the donor and his family while also experiencing great elation, relief, and hope after a long wait for the transplant. Patients should be told that these feelings are normal and should be allowed to express their feelings when they are ready. Emotional support may be needed.

Transplant rejection is a possible complication of this surgery. Patients need to understand the importance of following instructions regarding medications and testing that are related to preventing or detecting rejection.

Cardiac transplant patients are followed in an exercise rehabilitation program that closely monitors their activity progression in relation to myocardial oxygen consumption and signs of activity intolerance. Most patients reach an activity level allowing them to participate in many recreational sports.

NURSING CARE PLAN for the Postoperative Patient Undergoing Cardiac or Transplant Surgery

Nursing Diagnosis: *Acute Pain* related to sternotomy, leg incisions, internal mammary artery resection, or pericarditis

Expected Outcomes: The patient will state pain is relieved or tolerable within 30 minutes of report of pain. Patient will be able to rest and perform respiratory treatments.

Evaluation of Outcomes: Does patient state pain is within acceptable levels? Is patient able to rest and perform respiratory treatments?

NURSING CARE PLAN for the Postoperative Patient Undergoing Cardiac or Transplant Surgery—cont'd

Intervention Obtain characteristics of pain with each episode. **Rationale** A thorough description is needed to determine cause and plan actions. **Evaluation** Does patient describe pain on scale of 0 to 10?

Intervention Splint chest incision with all movement and coughing and deep breathing. **Rationale** Stabilizes sternum and incision to increase comfort. **Evaluation** Can patient splint chest incision independently?

Intervention Encourage patient to report pain even when pain is mild. **Rationale** It is easier to keep pain under control when mild. **Evaluation** Does patient report pain when mild?

Intervention Turn, reposition every 2 hours. **Rationale** Changes muscle position, relieving stiffness. **Evaluation** Is patient comfortable without stiffness?

Intervention Offer back rubs frequently. **Rationale** Relaxes tense muscles retracted during operation. **Evaluation** Is patient able to rest in comfort?

Intervention Instruct patient to take a deep breath before movement and exhale slowly during movement. **Rationale** Keeps muscles relaxed, minimizing tension with guarding and pain. **Evaluation** Can patient perform coughing and deep-breathing techniques as instructed?

Intervention Explain that chest pain can occur from the surgical incision rather than the heart. **Rationale** Chest pain after surgery can be frightening for patients because they may not associate surgical chest pain with the incision and instead think the pain is anginal or infarction pain. **Evaluation** Does patient state understanding of pain sources?

Nursing Diagnosis: *Decreased Cardiac Output* related to myocardial depression, hypothermia, bleeding, unstable dysrhythmias, or hypoxemia

Expected Outcomes: The patient will remain free of major side effects of pharmacological support. The patient will maintain vital signs within normal limits (WNL), palpable peripheral pulses, urine output greater than 0.5 to 1 mL/kg/hr, and normal sinus rhythm posttransplant.

Evaluation of Outcomes: Is patient free of major side effects? Are vital signs WNL?

Intervention Monitor vital signs. **Rationale** Trends reflect problems. **Evaluation** Are vital signs WNL?

Intervention Monitor peripheral circulation. **Rationale** Mottling or weak pulses may indicate poor cardiac output (CO). **Evaluation** Do peripheral pulses remain strong with normal skin color, temperature, capillary refill?

Intervention Monitor I&O. **Rationale** Fluid deficit or excess can alter CO. **Evaluation** Does total intake equal output?

Intervention Listen to lung sounds and note character of sputum. **Rationale** Crackles may indicate HF or pulmonary edema. **Evaluation** Are lungs clear?

Intervention Monitor temperature closely while rewarming the patient. **Rationale** Febrile state increases heart rate and myocardial oxygen consumption. **Evaluation** Does temperature remain less than or equal to 98.6°F (37°C)?

Intervention Monitor chest tube drainage for increase or sudden decrease. **Rationale** Drainage = 200 mL/hr may lead to hypovolemia and a decrease in CO. **Evaluation** Is patient free from cardiac tamponade and hypovolemia?

Intervention Monitor ECG. **Rationale** Premature ventricular contractions and atrial fibrillation decrease CO. **Evaluation** Does patient remain in normal sinus rhythm or controlled dysrhythmia?

Intervention Monitor electrolytes. **Rationale** Low calcium and magnesium and high potassium decrease contractility and CO. **Evaluation** Are electrolytes WNL?

Continued

NURSING CARE PLAN for the Postoperative Patient Undergoing Cardiac or Transplant Surgery—cont'd

Intervention Monitor arterial blood gases (ABGs). **Rationale** Acidosis decreases heart function, and a low CO may lead to further acidosis. **Evaluation** Are ABGs WNL?

Nursing Diagnosis: *Risk for Infection* related to inadequate primary defenses from surgical wound or immuno-suppression (transplants)

Expected Outcome: The patient will remain free from infection posttransplant.

Evaluation of Outcome: Does patient remain free from infection?

Intervention Monitor and report abnormal findings for temperature, lung sounds, sputum, and urine consistency. **Rationale** Low-grade (immunosuppressed) or high-grade fever, crackles, yellow-green sputum color, or cloudy urine can indicate infection. **Evaluation** Is the patient's temperature WNL and are lung sounds, sputum, and urine clear?

Intervention Encourage coughing and deep breathing and incentive spirometer use. **Rationale** Lung infections can be prevented with lung expansion and secretion removal. **Evaluation** Does patient perform coughing and deep breathing and use incentive spirometer?

Intervention Observe incision for signs and symptoms of infection. **Rationale** Redness, warmth, fever, and swelling indicate infection. **Evaluation** Are signs and symptoms of infection present?

Intervention Monitor drainage and maintain drains. **Rationale** Drains remove fluid from the surgical site to prevent infection development. **Evaluation** Are drainage amount and color normal for procedure? Are drains functioning?

Intervention Maintain sterile technique for dressing changes. **Rationale** Sterile technique reduces infection development. **Evaluation** Is incision free of signs and symptoms of infection?

Nursing Diagnosis: *Deficient Knowledge* related to lack of prior experience with transplant

Expected Outcome: The patient will demonstrate understanding of posttransplant care before discharge.

Evaluation of Outcome: Does patient state understanding and ability to carry out posttransplant care?

Intervention Give information in small increments and use written and video materials. **Rationale** Cardiac transplant patients commonly have memory deficits, cognitive dysfunction, and short attention spans resulting from long-term decreased cerebral perfusion. **Evaluation** Does patient state understanding of information?

Intervention Include families in teaching sessions and encourage them to promote self-care by the patient. **Rationale** Family involvement in teaching sessions is important to promote understanding and retention. **Evaluation** Does family participate and state understanding of teaching sessions?

Intervention Address or refer sexual functioning questions with patients and their partners. **Rationale** Patients usually have questions regarding sexual functioning. Referrals can be made to sexual counselors. **Evaluation** Does patient state that questions have been addressed?

Intervention Discharge teaching includes treatment, complications, activity, medications, and enhancing quality of life. **Rationale** Patients need comprehensive information to comply with posttransplant care. **Evaluation** Does patient state understanding of discharge care?

CRITICAL THINKING

Mrs. Eden

■ Mrs. Eden, age 45, a single mother of two, is transferred to a surgical unit 5 days after a cardiac transplant. She is withdrawn and has a poor appetite. Her vital signs are stable. On ambulating to the bathroom, she is very weak, requiring two nurses to help her. Her respiratory rate increases from 20 to 32 per minute and is slightly labored, and her apical pulse increases from 88 to 103 mm Hg.

1. Is Mrs. Eden tolerating this activity? Why or why not?
2. List four reasons why Mrs. Eden has a poor appetite.
3. Give four patient-centered nursing interventions for Mrs. Eden's poor appetite.
4. Give three reasons why Mrs. Eden is withdrawn.
5. What health care team members might collaborate in Mrs. Eden's care?

Suggested answers are at the end of the chapter.

SUGGESTED ANSWERS TO

CRITICAL THINKING

■ Mr. Shepard—Part 1

1. Signs and symptoms of HF include shortness of breath, two-pillow orthopnea, dry cough, tachycardia (pulse 106 beats/min), tachypnea (respiration 24 per minute), and bilateral crackles.

2. Left-sided HF is indicated by the findings.

3. *Shortness of breath:* fluid in the lungs impairs gas exchange; *orthopnea:* lying flat increases fluid accumulation in the lungs, causing dyspnea; *dry cough:* fluid in the lungs irritates the mucosal lining of the lungs; *tachycardia:* sympathetic compensation to increase cardiac output; *tachypnea:* sympathetic compensation to increase blood oxygenation; *bilateral crackles:* fluid trapped in the lungs.

4. The two pillows help prevent orthopnea by using a more upright position, which allows gravity to decrease fluid accumulation in the lungs.

5. HCP (physician, physician's assistant, nurse practitioner), case manager, nurses, dietitian, physical therapist, occupational therapist, pharmacist, social worker, and clergy.

■ Mr. Shepard—Part 2

1. Mr. Shepard's heart is enlarged to compensate for the strain caused by increased peripheral vascular resistance from hypertension to maintain an adequate cardiac output.

2. An enlarged heart requires more oxygen, which often cannot be supplied in HF.

■ Mr. Shepard—Part 3

1. The ACE inhibitor is needed for vasodilation to reduce peripheral vascular resistance and decrease the heart's workload, which in turn prevents cardiac remodeling and improves functioning.

2. The ACE inhibitor will affect afterload.

3. The diuretic is ordered to decrease fluid volume, which reduces preload and decreases the heart's workload.

4. Potassium needs to be monitored because diuretics can be either potassium wasting or potassium sparing.

5. The low-sodium diet is ordered to reduce water retention, which decreases preload and decreases the heart's workload.

6. The goal is to decrease the heart's workload and increase its efficiency by reducing preload and peripheral vascular resistance and to decrease progression of chronic HF and improve survival.

■ Mr. Shepard—Part 4

1. After assessment of Mr. Shepard's knowledge base, medication teaching should be given on the ACE inhibitor and diuretic that includes their purpose, side effects, and precautions. A schedule for taking the medications can be planned. An explanation of the purpose of a low-sodium diet and menu planning based on Mr. Shepard's likes and dislikes should be done.

2. Low-sodium foods should be selected to prevent fluid retention, and high-potassium foods should be included to prevent hypokalemia from the diuretic if appropriate. Read food labels. Low-sodium foods include puffed rice, wheat cereals, fruits, chicken, beef, eggs, and potatoes. High-sodium foods include tomato juice, sauerkraut, softened water, buttermilk, cheese, smoked meats, canned tuna, canned soup, pickles, instant rice, and instant potatoes. High-potassium foods include salt substitutes, bran products, avocado, bananas, prunes, oranges, baked potato, sweet potato, spinach (cooked), chocolate, nuts, and molasses.

Continued

SUGGESTED ANSWERS TO—cont'd

3. Daily weighing is necessary to detect a rapid weight gain that indicates fluid retention (2 pounds in 24 hours) and to measure weight loss resulting from the diuretic.

4. These instructions ensure accuracy of the weight so that comparison to the baseline weight detects a weight gain or loss.

5. Weight increase reporting guidelines are as follows: increase of 2 to 3 pounds in 1 to 2 days.

■ *Mrs. Eden*

1. No, Mrs. Eden is not tolerating this activity, as evidenced by her increased respiratory rate and apical rate.

2. Steroids, immunosuppressive therapy, depression, and fatigue could be causing her poor appetite.

3. Nursing interventions related to Mrs. Eden's poor appetite could include the following: offering small, frequent meals; having family bring favorite foods from home; allowing the patient to rest before meals; providing oral hygiene before meals; administering antiemetics before meals; giving a high-calorie meal at peak appetite.

4. Mrs. Eden could be withdrawn because of changes in her lifestyle as a result of her transplant, extreme fatigue, concerns regarding how she will raise her children, grieving for the donor, and fear that she will reject her new heart.

5. HCP (surgeon, physician's assistant, nurse practitioner), case manager, nurses, dietitian, physical therapist, occupational therapist, pharmacist, social worker, and clergy.

REVIEW QUESTIONS

1. The nurse is providing patient education. The patient asks the nurse what HF is. Which of the following is the nurse's best response?
   1. "The heart pumps too much blood into the pulmonary veins."
   2. "The heart is unable to pump enough blood for the body's oxygen needs."
   3. "HF is a buildup of blood in the aorta from the heart's left ventricle."
   4. "With a failing heart, the heart stops beating, so blood is not pumped out."

2. The nurse is to give bumetanide (Bumex) to a patient and reviews laboratory results. Which of these results requires action by the nurse?
   1. potassium 3.0 meq/dL
   2. sodium 135 meq/dL
   3. International normalized ratio 0.8
   4. Partial thromboplastin time 36 seconds

3. A patient who has been treated for HF is being discharged from the hospital on 20 mg furosemide (Lasix) daily. Which of the following statements by the patient would indicate understanding to the nurse for instructions on taking this medication?
   1. "I will take the Lasix in the morning."
   2. "I will take the Lasix at bedtime."
   3. "I will drink lots of fluids with the Lasix."
   4. "I will take it with meals."

4. The nurse is caring for a patient receiving bumetanide (Bumex) to reduce preload for HF. While collecting data, the nurse sees the patient has less ankle edema and jugular venous distention than earlier. The next dose of bumetanide is scheduled in 1 hour. Which of the following actions should the nurse take?
   1. Notify the physician.
   2. Hold the bumetanide.
   3. Give the bumetanide as scheduled.
   4. Give the bumetanide early.

5. The nurse is reinforcing teaching for a patient with chronic HF. Which of the following assessments should the nurse teach the patient to perform to monitor fluid status at home?
   1. Weigh daily.
   2. Weigh weekly.
   3. Weigh biweekly.
   4. Weigh monthly.

6. A 160-pound patient is to receive cyclosporine (Neoral) 12.5 mg/kg daily in two divided doses. How many milligrams will the patient receive with each dose? **Fill in the blank.**
   Answer: _____ mg

Answers can be found in Appendix C.

References

Go, A. S., Mozaffarian, D., Roger, V. L., Benjamin, E. J., Berry, J. D., Blaha, M. J., Dai, S., . . . Turner, M. (2014). Heart disease and stroke statistics—2014 update: A report from the American Heart Association. *Circulation, 129,* e28–e292.

Michler, R., Rouleau, J., Al-Khalidi, H., Bonow, R. O., Pellikka, P. A., Pohost, G. M., . . . Donato, M. D. (2013). Insights from the STICH trial: Change in left ventricular size after coronary artery bypass grafting with and without surgical ventricular reconstruction. *The Journal of Thoracic and Cardiovascular Surgery, 146,* 1139–1145.e6.

Yancy, C. W., Jessup, M., Bozkurt, B., Butler, J., Casey, D. E., Drazner, M. H., . . . Wilkoff, B. L. (2013). 2013 ACCF/AHA Guideline for the Management of HF: A Report of the American College of Cardiology Foundation/American Heart Association Task Force on Practice Guidelines PDF. *Journal of American College of Cardiologists, 62,* e147–e239.

 DavisPlus | For additional resources and information visit **davispl.us/medsurg5**

unit SIX

Understanding the Hematologic and Lymphatic Systems

27

Hematologic and Lymphatic System Function, Assessment, and Therapeutic Measures

JANICE L. BRADFORD AND
LUCY L. COLO

LEARNING OUTCOMES

1. List the components of blood.

2. List the components of the lymphatic system.

3. Describe how changes in the blood or lymph systems can manifest as disease processes.

4. Describe the sequence of events in the process of blood clotting.

5. Identify data to collect when caring for a patient with a disorder of the hematologic or lymphatic system.

6. Identify laboratory and diagnostic studies that are used when evaluating the hematologic and lymphatic systems.

7. Plan nursing care for patients undergoing diagnostic tests of the hematologic or lymphatic systems.

8. List common therapeutic measures used for patients with hematologic and lymphatic disorders.

9. Discuss the role of the licensed practical nurse/licensed vocational nurse (LPN/LVN) in administering blood products.

NORMAL HEMATOLOGIC AND LYMPHATIC SYSTEM ANATOMY AND PHYSIOLOGY

The hematologic system includes the bone marrow, blood, and blood components. The lymphatic system includes lymph nodes and nodules, which filter pathogens for destruction, and lymph vessels, which return lymph to the blood.

Blood

The general functions of blood are transportation of substances; regulation of body temperature, pH, and fluid balance; and transport of cells that offer the body protection.

The human body contains 4 to 6 L of blood; approximately 45% is formed elements, and the remainder is plasma (Figure 27.1). All formed elements are produced from stem cells in the red bone marrow (hematopoietic tissue), found in flat bones, irregular bones, and the epiphyses of long bones (Figure 27.2). T-lymphocyte maturation and differentiation occurs in the thymus. Table 27.1 shows normal blood cell counts.

Plasma

Plasma, the transporting medium, is about 91% water. Plasma proteins are synthesized by the liver and include clotting factors, albumin, and globulins. Clotting factors such as prothrombin and fibrinogen circulate until activated for coagulation. Albumin helps maintain blood volume and pressure by pulling tissue fluid into the venous ends of the capillary networks. Alpha and beta globulins are carrier molecules for substances such as fats, and gamma globulins are antibodies produced by lymphocytes.

Plasma is also important in maintaining body temperature. The water of plasma is warmed by passage through active organs, such as the liver or skeletal muscles; then blood distributes this heat throughout the body. This process may be visible in people with fair skin. The flush of fever or vigorous exercise is caused by vasodilation in the dermis, allowing blood to circulate near the body surface resulting in heat loss. A person in a cold environment may appear pale, because vasoconstriction in the dermis shunts blood toward the core of the body for heat retention.

The normal pH range of blood is 7.35 to 7.45. Buffer systems in the blood moderate acid–base changes to maintain homeostasis.

Red Blood Cells

Mature red blood cells (RBCs) are biconcave disks without nuclei; they carry oxygen bonded to the iron in hemoglobin (Hgb). *Oxyhemoglobin* is formed in the pulmonary capillaries when oxygen bonds to the iron of hemoglobin (Hgb). Once hemoglobin gives up its oxygen to the cells of the body, it becomes *reduced hemoglobin*. The amount of hemoglobin in RBCs, the amount of iron in that hemoglobin, and the number of RBCs determine the amount of oxygen the blood can carry. Reduced oxygen-carrying capacity causes anemia, which results in symptoms such as shortness of breath and fatigue.

Hypoxia stimulates the kidneys to secrete erythropoietin, which increases the rate of RBC production and thus the oxygen-carrying capacity of the blood. A reticulocyte (immature RBC) becomes a mature RBC when it ejects its nucleus. This causes the characteristic biconcave disk shape. The presence of large numbers of reticulocytes in peripheral blood indicates an insufficient number of mature RBCs to meet the oxygen demands of the body.

Sufficient dietary intake of protein and iron to synthesize hemoglobin is required for normal production of RBCs. The vitamins folic acid and vitamin B_{12} are needed for DNA synthesis in the stem cells of the red bone marrow; mitosis is dependent on the ability to produce new sets of chromosomes. Vitamin B_{12} is called *extrinsic factor* because it comes from an

The main component of plasma is water; however, plasma also contains proteins (the main one being **albumin**), nutrients, electrolytes, hormones, and gases. Plasma proteins play roles in blood clotting, the immune system, and the regulation of fluid volume. Plasma without the clotting proteins (which occurs when blood is allowed to clot and the solid portion is removed) is called **serum**.

Plasma is the clear, extracellular matrix of this liquid connective tissue. It accounts for 55% of blood.

WBCs and platelets form a narrow buff-colored band just underneath the plasma. Called the *buffy coat*, these cells constitute 1% or less of the blood volume.

Formed elements—which include cells and cell fragments—make up 45% of blood. Specific blood cells include **erythrocytes** (red blood cells, or RBCs), **leukocytes** (white blood cells, or WBCs), and **platelets**.

RBCs are the heaviest of the formed elements and sink to the bottom of the sample. They account for most of the formed elements. This value—the percentage of cells in a sample of blood—is called the **hematocrit**.

FIGURE 27.1 Components of blood. From Thompson, G. S. (2013). *Understanding anatomy and physiology*. Philadelphia: F.A. Davis, p. 245.

FIGURE 27.2 Blood cell formation. From Thompson, G. S. (2013). *Understanding anatomy and physiology.* Philadelphia: F.A. Davis, p. 246.

TABLE 27.1 REVIEW OF BLOOD CELL VALUES AND DISORDERS

Test	Normal Value	Significance of Abnormal Findings
Red Blood Cells		
Red blood cells (RBCs)	*Male:* 4.71–5.14 million/mm³	Increased in chronic hypoxia
	Female: 4.2–4.87 million/mm³	Decreased in anemia or blood loss
Hematocrit (cellular portion of blood)	*Male:* 43%–49%	Increased in dehydration or chronic hypoxia
	Female: 38%–44%	Decreased in anemia or blood loss
Hemoglobin (reflects oxygen-carrying capacity of blood)	*Male:* 13.2–17.3 g/100 mL	Increased in chronic hypoxia
	Female: 11.7–15.5 g/100 mL	Decreased in blood loss or anemia
Reticulocytes (number of circulating immature RBCs)	1.5%–2.5%	Increased in hypoxia or anemia
		Decreased in RBC maturation defect
White Blood Cells		
White blood cells (WBCs)	4500–11,000/mm³	Increased in infection

TABLE 27.1   REVIEW OF BLOOD CELL VALUES AND DISORDERS—cont'd

Test	Normal Value	Significance of Abnormal Findings
Neutrophils	59%	Increased in infection
(Bands)	(3%)	
(Segments)	(56%)	
Eosinophils	2.7%	Increased in allergic response, some leukemias
Basophils	0.5%	Increased in hyperthyroidism, some bone marrow disorders, ulcerative colitis
Lymphocytes	34%	Increased in viral infections, chronic bacterial infection, some leukemias
Monocytes	4%	Increased in chronic inflammatory disorders, some leukemias
Platelets		
Thrombocytes/platelets	150,000–450,000/mm³	Increased from trauma Decreased with blood disorders Increased risk of bleeding with low platelet count

extrinsic source: food. The parietal cells of the stomach lining produce *intrinsic factor,* which is a chemical that combines with vitamin B_{12} to promote its absorption in the small intestine.

RBCs live for about 120 days and then become fragile and are phagocytized by fixed macrophages in the liver, spleen, and red bone marrow (Fig. 27.3). Diseases such as malaria and sickle cell anemia cause an accelerated destruction of RBCs **(hemolysis).** The resulting release of excess hemoglobin can cause the blood level of bilirubin to rise. Elevated bilirubin levels discolor the sclerae, skin, and mucous membranes to a yellowish orange hue; this condition is known as jaundice.

Each person has an inherited blood type, which is determined by the antigens present on the RBCs. The two most important type categories are the ABO group and the Rh factor. The ABO type (A, B, O, or AB) indicates the antigens present (or not present, as in type O) on the RBCs. The plasma contains antibodies for antigens that are not present in the blood. These antibodies can interact with antigens in transfused blood if the donor's blood does not match the recipient's blood (Table 27.2). To be Rh-positive means that the D antigen is present on the RBCs; Rh-negative means that the antigen is not present. Rh-negative people do not have natural antibodies to the D antigen but will produce them if given Rh-positive blood.

White Blood Cells

WBCs are larger than RBCs and have nuclei when mature. The granular WBCs (neutrophils, eosinophils, and basophils) and the agranular WBCs (lymphocytes and monocytes) are produced in the red bone marrow; the T lymphocytes complete their development in the thymus. The T lymphocytes and B lymphocytes become activated, proliferate, and differentiate in the lymph nodes, spleen, and lymphatic nodules. Table 27.1 shows normal values and percentages for each

type of WBC in a differential count. WBCs function within tissue fluid, as well as the blood; all are involved in the immune or inflammatory response to injury.

Monocytes become macrophages in tissues, which phagocytize pathogens and viral-infected cells; neutrophils are more numerous and phagocytize foreign materials. Eosinophils combat the effects of histamine, detoxify foreign proteins during allergic reactions, and respond to parasitic infections. Basophils release heparin and histamine as part of inflammatory reactions. There are two groups of lymphocytes: T cells and B cells. T cells may be helper, suppressor, killer, or memory T cells. B cells become memory cells and plasma cells; plasma cells produce antibodies to foreign antigens.

Platelets

Platelets are formed in the red bone marrow; they are fragments of large cells called megakaryocytes. Platelets are involved in all mechanisms of hemostasis: vascular spasm, platelet plugs, and chemical clotting.

After a platelet plug is formed, one of two pathways initiates a cascade of events to bring about coagulation. When a blood vessel or surrounding tissues *outside* the blood are damaged, the extrinsic pathway begins. Conversely, when platelets adhere to damaged endothelium and release clotting factors, this initiates the *intrinsic* pathway. Either way, the end result is a fibrin clot (Figure 27.4).

Excessive clotting in the vascular system is prevented in several ways. The smooth endothelial lining of blood vessels repels platelets so that they do not stick to intact vessel walls. Heparin produced by mast cells inhibits the clotting mechanism, and

• WORD • BUILDING •

hemolysis: heme—blood + lysis—dissolution

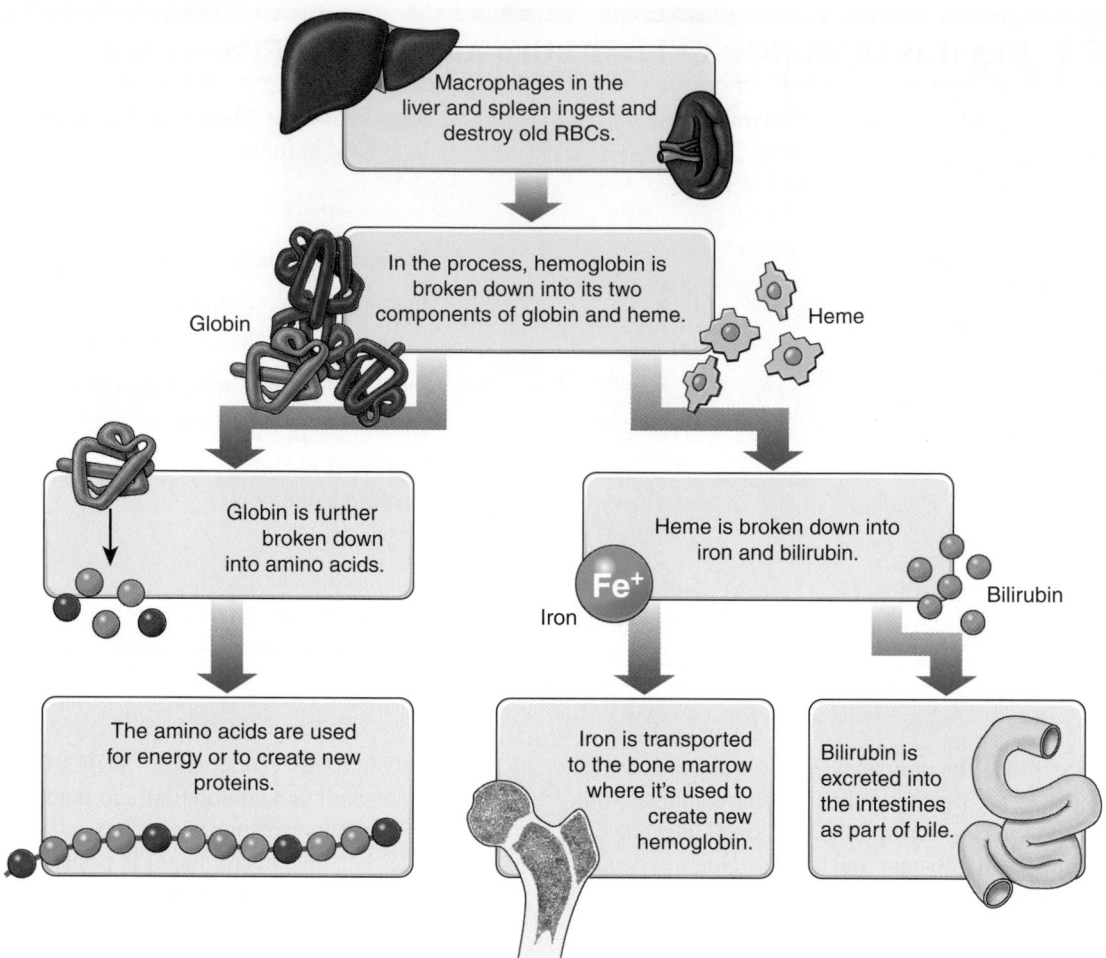

FIGURE 27.3 Breakdown of red blood cells. From Thompson, G. S. (2013). *Understanding anatomy and physiology*. Philadelphia: F.A. Davis, p. 250.

TABLE 27.2   ABO BLOOD TYPES

Type	Antigens Present on Red Blood Cells	Antibodies Present in Plasma
A	A	Anti-B
B	B	Anti-A
AB	Both A and B	Neither anti-A nor anti-B
O	Neither A nor B	Both anti-A and anti-B

antithrombin inactivates excess thrombin to prevent the clotting mechanism from becoming a vicious cycle.

Lymphatic System

The lymphatic system consists of lymph, lymph vessels, lymph nodes and nodules, the spleen, and the thymus (Fig. 27.5). Functions of the lymph system include the return of tissue fluid to maintain blood volume and protecting the body against pathogens and other foreign material. (Immunity is covered in Unit 4.)

Lymphatic Vessels

Lymph is tissue fluid that has entered lymph capillaries. Lymph must be returned to the blood to maintain blood volume and blood pressure. Lymph capillaries are found in most tissue spaces; they anastomose, forming larger and larger lymph vessels, which have valves to prevent backflow. Lymph from areas below the diaphragm and the upper left half of the body enters the thoracic duct and is returned to the blood in the left subclavian vein. Lymph from the upper right body enters the right lymphatic duct and is returned to the blood in the right subclavian vein.

Lymph Nodes and Nodules

Lymph *nodes* are masses of lymphatic tissue along the pathways of the lymph vessels. They house activated lymphocytes and macrophages. Nodes are scattered throughout the body and are concentrated in the cervical, axillary, and inguinal regions, where they are well situated to remove pathogens before the lymph is returned to the blood. Foreign materials are phagocytized by fixed macrophages; lymphocytes form immune responses.

Lymph *nodules* (or mucosa-associated lymphatic tissue) are small masses of lymphatic tissue found just beneath the

Both the extrinsic and intrinsic pathways result in the formation of factor X. (This occurs in a single reaction in the extrinsic pathway, while, in the intrinsic pathway, four different reactions are required to activate factor X.) Either way, once factor X is activated, the formation of a blood clot follows a common pathway, as shown here.

The end result of both the extrinsic and intrinsic pathways is the production of an enzyme called **prothrombin activator**.

Prothrombin activator acts on a globulin called **prothrombin** (factor II)...

...converting it to the enzyme **thrombin**. Thrombin transforms the soluble plasma protein fibrinogen into fine threads of insoluble **fibrin**.

The sticky fibrin threads form a web at the site of the injury. Red blood cells and platelets flowing through the web become ensnared, creating a clot of fibrin, blood cells, and platelets. A blood clot can effectively seal breaks in a smaller vessel; however, blood clotting alone may not stop a hemorrhage from a large blood vessel.

FIGURE 27.4 Formation of a blood clot. From Thompson, G. S. (2013). *Understanding anatomy and physiology*. Philadelphia: F.A. Davis, p. 256.

epithelium of all mucous membranes. Mucosal-lined tracts (respiratory, digestive, urinary, and reproductive) have openings to the external environment. Any natural body opening is a potential portal of entry for pathogens; microbes that penetrate the epithelium are usually destroyed by the macrophages in the lymph nodules. The tonsils, which protect the oral and nasal portions of the pharynx, are familiar examples of lymph nodules.

Spleen

The spleen is located in the upper left quadrant of the abdominal cavity, just below the diaphragm, behind the stomach. The lower rib cage protects the spleen from mechanical injury. In the fetus, the spleen produces RBCs, a function assumed by the bone marrow after birth.

The spleen has several functions after birth. It contains B cells and T cells, which conduct immune responses. It also contains fixed macrophages that phagocytize pathogens and worn or defective blood cells and platelets. The heme unit

from RBC destruction forms bilirubin. Bilirubin is sent to the liver by way of portal circulation for excretion in the bile. The spleen stores up to one-third of the body's platelets.

The spleen is not considered a vital organ because other organs compensate for its functions if the spleen must be removed. The liver and red bone marrow also remove worn RBCs from circulation, and the many lymph nodes and nodules produce lymphocytes and macrophages for protection. However, a person without a spleen is somewhat more susceptible to certain bacterial infections, such as pneumonia and meningitis.

Thymus

The thymus is located in the mediastinum, anterior to the trachea. With increasing age, the thymus atrophies; relatively little thymic tissue is found in adults. The thymus contains T lymphocytes, or T cells, that mature and proliferate. Thymic hormones contribute to the maturation of the T cells. (Immunity is covered in Unit 4.)

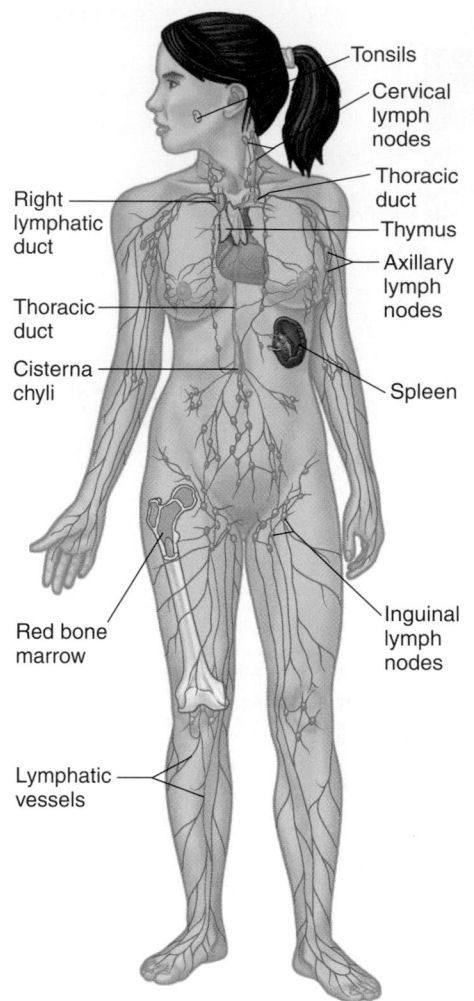

Tonsils
Cervical lymph nodes
Thoracic duct
Thymus
Axillary lymph nodes
Right lymphatic duct
Thoracic duct
Cisterna chyli
Spleen
Red bone marrow
Inguinal lymph nodes
Lymphatic vessels

FIGURE 27.5 The lymphatic system. From Thompson, G. S. (2013). *Understanding anatomy and physiology.* Philadelphia: F.A. Davis, p. 307.

Aging and the Hematologic and Lymphatic Systems

Older adults undergo a number of changes in the hematologic and lymphatic systems (Fig. 27.6).

NURSING ASSESSMENT OF HEMATOLOGIC AND LYMPHATIC SYSTEMS

Health History

A thorough nursing assessment starts with an in-depth patient history (Table 27.3). Specific problems that might be seen in

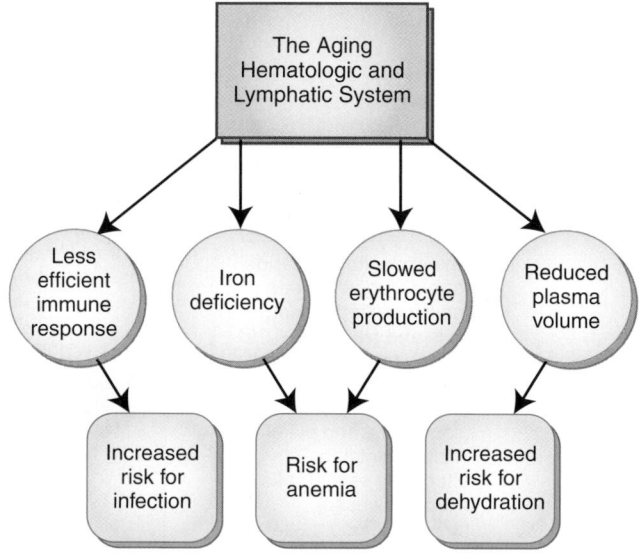

FIGURE 27.6 Effects of aging on the hematologic and lymphatic systems.

TABLE 27.3   SUBJECTIVE DATA COLLECTION FOR THE HEMATOLOGIC AND LYMPHATIC SYSTEMS

Category	Questions to Ask During the Health History	Rationale/Significance
Reason for Seeking Health Care	Why are you seeking health care?	Signs and symptoms of hematologic/lymphatic disorders may be nonspecific. Any body system can be involved.
Family History	How is the health of your blood relatives? Does anyone in your family have any blood-related diseases?	Some blood and immune disorders are hereditary.
Diet History	Describe your usual diet.	Dietary deficiencies can lead to anemia or altered immune responses.
Medications/Supplements	What medications do you take?	Herbs and drugs can cause adverse reactions in the blood and immune systems.

TABLE 27.3   SUBJECTIVE DATA COLLECTION FOR THE HEMATOLOGIC AND LYMPHATIC SYSTEMS—cont'd

Category	Questions to Ask During the Health History	Rationale/Significance
	What herbs or alternative therapies do you use? How much alcohol do you drink each day?	Excess alcohol intake can lead to folic acid–deficiency anemia.
Occupational/Exposure History	What is your occupational history? What is your military history?	Exposure to certain hazardous substances can lead to anemias, leukemias, or other cancers.
Fatigue	Have you noticed any change in your energy level?	Anemia and many cancers are associated with fatigue.
Bleeding Tendency	Have you experienced nosebleeds or any other unusual bleeding? Have you had bloody or black bowel movements?	Bleeding may indicate low platelet levels or a clotting factor deficiency.
Respiratory	Do you experience shortness of breath or faintness?	Red blood cells (RBCs) carry oxygen, so a reduced RBC count can cause dyspnea.
Integumentary	Have you noticed any changes in your skin?	Bleeding into the skin or mucous membranes can indicate a bleeding disorder.
Lymphadenopathy	Have you noticed swelling in your neck, armpits, or groin?	Swollen lymph nodes may indicate inflammation, infection, or some cancers.

patients with hematologic disorders include abnormal bleeding, **petechiae** (small purplish hemorrhagic spots under the skin), **ecchymoses** (larger areas of discoloration from hemorrhage under the skin), and **purpura** (hemorrhage into the skin, mucous membranes, and organs), as well as fatigue, weakness, shortness of breath, and fever. Fatigue, malaise, and weight loss can accompany cancers of the lymphatic system.

Begin by obtaining the patient's biographical data, marital status, occupation, religion, age, sex, and ethnic background. This information can give you valuable clues to risk factors. For example, even though hemophilia almost always occurs in males, females can carry the gene. Sickle cell anemia occurs mostly in African Americans but also affects people of Mediterranean or Asian ancestry. Pernicious anemia occurs most often in people of northern European ancestry. By carefully collecting this information, you can obtain important clues that will help pinpoint a patient's problem. Finally, focus on collecting data about symptoms by using the **WHAT'S UP?** format presented in Chapter 1.

A complete review of past illnesses and family history is always indicated and can provide some valuable information. A social history is also useful. After developing good rapport with the patient, explore dietary and alcohol intake habits, any drug use or abuse, and sexual habits, all of which can cause changes in the hematologic system.

An occupational review can reveal exposure to some hazardous substances that can cause bone marrow dysfunction. Certain occupations, such as working in a paint factory, tool and dye processing, and even dry cleaning can be related to the formation of some hematologic cancers. Military history can also reveal sources of exposure that can help during the diagnostic phase for hematologic and lymphatic disorders.

Physical Examination

Hematologic and lymphatic disorders can involve almost every body system, so each system must be assessed. Signs and symptoms of hematologic and lymphatic disorders can be vague, such as shortness of breath or fatigue. A careful assessment will guide nursing care but may also uncover important data that should be reported to the primary care provider. Table 27.4 reviews objective data that should be collected and possible interpretations of findings.

 NURSING CARE TIP

If abdominal girth must be monitored for changes, use a marker to identify the site where you measure so it can be measured at the same place each time.

TABLE 27.4 OBJECTIVE DATA COLLECTION FOR THE HEMATOLOGIC AND LYMPHATIC SYSTEMS

Category	Abnormal Findings	Possible Hematologic/Lymphatic Causes
Vital Signs	Fever	Poor immune function, infection
	Subnormal temperature	Possible overwhelming Gram-negative infection
	Elevated heart rate	Blood loss
	Elevated respiratory rate	Anemia, decreased oxygen supply
Level of Consciousness	Decreased level	Hypoxia, fever, intracranial bleeding
Skin, Mucous Membranes	Pallor	Anemia
	Cyanosis	Poor oxygenation of red blood cells
	Jaundice (yellow color)	Hemolysis, liver involvement
	Inflammation, redness, swelling, drainage	Poor immune function, infection
	Purpura, ecchymoses, petechiae	Bleeding disorder
	Dry or coarse skin	Some anemias
	Itching	Blood or lymph disorders, jaundice, liver involvement
Fingernails	Striations	Anemia
	Spoon-shaped nails	Anemia
	Clubbed fingers	Long-term hypoxia, anemia
Abdomen	High-pitched, tinkling bowel sounds	Intestinal obstruction
	Increasing abdominal girth	Ascites, bleeding
Neck, Axillae	Lymph nodes >1 cm in size or tender nodes	**Lymphedema**, inflammation, some cancers
Sternum	Tenderness	Bone marrow packed with abnormal cells

DIAGNOSTIC TESTS FOR THE HEMATOLOGIC AND LYMPHATIC SYSTEMS

Blood Tests

Examples of laboratory studies routinely done for patients with hematologic disorders include complete blood count (CBC), total hemoglobin concentration (Hgb), hematocrit level (Hct), and platelet level. See normal values in Table 27.1.

CRITICAL THINKING

Mrs. Brown

■ Mrs. Brown is on warfarin (Coumadin) therapy because of a blood clot in her leg. She has a prothrombin time (PT) drawn at the lab, and the result is 12 seconds. Will the health care provider (HCP) most likely increase Mrs. Brown's daily dose of warfarin, decrease it, or leave it the same? (Use Table 27.5 to figure out the answer.)

Suggested answers are at the end of the chapter.

Coagulation Tests

Coagulation tests are shown in Table 27.5. Agglutination tests include ABO blood typing, Rh typing, crossmatching of blood samples, and direct antiglobulin tests (also known as Coombs' test).

Bone Marrow Biopsy

Biopsy information can be obtained through removal of a small amount of bone marrow with a needle. Aspiration of marrow is done to obtain a specimen that can be viewed under the microscope. Purposes of this test include the diagnosis of hematologic disorders; monitoring the course of treatment; discovery of other disorders, such as primary and metastatic tumors, infectious diseases, and certain granulomas; and isolation of bacteria and other pathogens by culture.

An accurate bone marrow specimen in an adult can be obtained from the sternum, the spinous processes of the

• WORD • BUILDING •

lymphedema: lymph—fluid found in lymphatic vessels + edema—swelling

LEARNING TIP

When a patient has a bacterial infection, the neutrophils, which are the most numerous of the WBCs, rise in number to help fight it. There are two forms of neutrophils: segmented (mature) and bands (immature). Initially, the number of segmented neutrophils rises. Then, as the infection becomes more severe, the number of immature bands begins to rise.

An easy way to remember this is that the WBCs are part of the body's defenses, just like the military is part of a country's defenses. When needed, sergeants who are fully trained or mature are called to assess the battle first. If they are unable to fight off the invading enemy, new recruits being trained in boot camp are called in to help.

So segmented neutrophils (called **S**egs) are like the **S**ergeants, fully mature and ready to fight. The **B**ands are like **B**oot camp recruits, immature and not fully trained. However, in an acute infection, bands are needed to keep the body from being overwhelmed by the infection and losing the battle.

As you look at the differential WBC count, if the segs are elevated but the bands are normal, the infection is probably new. If the bands are also elevated, the infection is worsening. The more elevated they are, the more severe the infection.

Lymphocytes fight viral infections and are elevated during a virus. A common pattern in the WBCs is produced for either a bacterial or viral infection. If the infection is acute bacterial:

Segs ↑ Bands ↑ Lymphocytes ↓

If the infection is viral:

Segs ↓ Bands ↓ Lymphocytes ↑

This can be remembered as the bone marrow producing the cells most needed during the time of viral infection and reducing production of those cells least needed. When the infection is resolved, all of the cells should return to their normal production levels.

vertebrae, or the anterior or posterior iliac crest. Bone marrow biopsy is considered a minor surgical procedure and is carried out under aseptic conditions. For iliac crest aspiration, the patient is placed comfortably on the side with the back slightly flexed. The posterior iliac crest is cleansed and covered with antiseptic solution. The skin, subcutaneous tissue, and periosteum are anesthetized using 1% or

TABLE 27.5 COAGULATION STUDIES

Test	Normal Value	Significance of Abnormal Findings
Prothrombin time (PT) (affected by activity of clotting factors V, VII, X, prothrombin, and fibrinogen)	*Male:* 9.6–11.8 seconds *Female:* 9.5–11.3 seconds *Therapeutic range:* 1.5–2.0 times normal for patient on warfarin (Coumadin) therapy	Abnormalities in these values when the patient is not receiving anticoagulant therapy can indicate liver malfunction and bleeding tendency.
International normalized ratio (standardized test adopted by World Health Organization)	Less than 1.3 *Therapeutic range:* 2.0–3.0 for patient on warfarin (Coumadin) (3.0–4.5 for recurrent problems)	
Activated Partial thromboplastin time (aPTT; evaluates factors I, II, V, VIII, IX, X, XI, XII)	25–39 seconds *Therapeutic range:* 1.5–2.0 times normal for patient on heparin therapy	
Bleeding time (measures time for small puncture wound to stop bleeding)	2.5–9.5 minutes	Prolonged bleeding time indicates a platelet disorder.
Capillary fragility test	Fewer than 10 petechiae appearing in a 2-inch circle after application of a blood pressure cuff at 100 mm Hg for 5 minutes	Tests ability of capillaries to resist rupture under pressure. More than 10 petechiae could be related to fragile capillaries or thrombocytopenia.

2% lidocaine (Xylocaine). A 2- to 3-mm incision is made to facilitate penetration with a 14-gauge, 2- to 4-cm-long bone marrow needle. The incision is made to avoid introducing a skin plug into the marrow cavity, which can cause infection.

The nurse's role in bone marrow biopsy is multifaceted. You may need to help coordinate between the laboratory and the HCP, establishing a time to do the procedure and determining who obtains the supplies, such as the disposable bone marrow aspiration tray and specialized needles, from the central supply department. Be sure to obtain an order for an analgesic and administer it before the procedure. Assist with positioning the patient before and during the procedure, help the patient maintain the needed position, and observe the aspiration site for bleeding and infection. You can also provide emotional support to the patient before, during, and after the procedure.

BE SAFE!

For all surgical and nonsurgical invasive procedures, the intended procedure site should be marked. Before the start of any invasive procedure, a final verification process is conducted to confirm the correct procedure, for the correct patient, at the correct site. The patient is involved in the verification process when possible (Joint Commission's 2014 National Patient Safety Goals, © The Joint Commission, 2013. Reprinted with permission.).

Lymphangiography

Problems in the lymph system, such as lymphoma or metastatic cancers, can be evaluated using lymphangiography. This procedure involves injection of a dye into the lymphatic vessels of the hand or foot. X-ray views are then taken to determine lymph flow or blockages. X-ray examinations are repeated in 24 hours to assess lymph node involvement.

Following the procedure, the HCP may order a pressure dressing and immobilization of the injected limb to prevent bleeding at the site. Continue to monitor the limb for swelling, circulatory status, and changes in sensation. Warn the patient that the skin, urine, or feces may be tinged blue from the dye for about 2 days.

Lymph Node Biopsy

If a lymph node is enlarged, it may be biopsied to determine whether the cause is infection or malignancy. A biopsy is done with a needle aspiration or surgical incision. A small dressing or bandage is applied to the site. Following the procedure, review signs of bleeding and infection with the patient that should be reported to the HCP.

THERAPEUTIC MEASURES FOR THE HEMATOLOGIC AND LYMPHATIC SYSTEMS

Blood Administration

Blood may be administered by a registered nurse (RN) or licensed practical nurse/licensed vocational nurse (LPN/LVN), depending on the state in which you practice. Some states require that only RNs administer blood. As an LPN/LVN, you may be called on to assist with proper identification procedures and monitoring of vital signs during the transfusion.

Table 27.6 lists blood components that may be ordered. The main goals are to administer them safely and to avoid mistakes. Make sure to use proper identifying information to ensure that the right patient is receiving the right blood products (Fig. 27.7). In addition, it is important to note that some institutions require a special transfusion consent form to be completed and present in the patient's chart. A careful system most often used in health care institutions is found on DavisPlus.

TABLE 27.6   BLOOD PRODUCTS

Product	Use
Packed RBCs	Severe anemia or blood loss
Frozen RBCs	Autotransfusion (blood taken from patient and saved for future surgery), prevention of febrile reactions
Platelets	Bleeding caused by thrombocytopenia
Albumin	Hypovolemia caused by hypoalbuminemia
Fresh frozen plasma	Provides clotting factors for bleeding disorders; occasionally used for volume replacement
Cryoprecipitates	Bleeding caused by specific missing clotting factors

FIGURE 27.7 Two nurses check a patient's identification before administering a unit of blood.

BE SAFE!

BE VIGILANT! Eliminate transfusion errors related to patient misidentification. Before initiating a blood or blood component transfusion:

- Match the blood or blood component to the order.
- Match the patient to the blood or blood component.
- Use a two-person verification process or a one-person verification process accompanied by automated identification technology, such as bar coding.
  - When using a two-person verification process, one individual conducting the identification verification is the qualified transfusionist who will administer the blood or blood component to the patient.
  - When using a two-person verification process, the second individual conducting the identification verification is qualified to participate in the process, as determined by the hospital.

Source: Joint Commission's 2014 National Patient Safety Goals, © The Joint Commission, 2013. Reprinted with permission.

Special Precautions

FLUID COMPATIBILITY. Make sure to use only normal saline solution to help dilute the blood and to flush the intravenous (IV) lines before and after the transfusions. Solutions that contain dextrose can cause red cells to lyse (i.e., their cell membranes are destroyed), and solutions with calcium can cause the blood product to clump, clot, or not infuse at all.

TIMING. Transfuse each unit of packed cells over 2 hours. If it must transfuse more slowly because of the patient's condition, make sure the unit does not hang longer than 4 hours to prevent deterioration and bacterial proliferation.

FILTERING. Filters are used with blood administration tubing to prevent potentially harmful particles from entering the patient. Most often, the filter that comes with the transfusion tubing is sufficient for each unit of packed RBCs. In some situations, special filters may be needed to remove leukocytes or microaggregates. The blood bank can advise in these situations.

WASHED OR LEUKOCYTE-DEPLETED BLOOD. In some instances packed RBCs (PRBCs) are ordered as "washed" and often arrive from the blood bank in a special round bag. The washing process removes almost all of the plasma and can decrease the risk or severity of a febrile reaction. In addition, leukocyte filters may be used to completely remove all WBCs. This removal process is used in cases in which many transfusions are anticipated, because it decreases the chance of antigen sensitization. It can also reduce transmission of certain viruses, such as cytomegalovirus.

WARMED BLOOD. If the patient has had a severe bleeding episode and the nurses are helping to give replacement therapy through rapid, multiple transfusions, the HCP may consider ordering a blood warmer. It works just as the name implies, warming the cold blood from the blood bank to the standard body temperature of 98.6°F (37.0°C). This warming helps prevent hypothermia, which can cause heart dysrhythmias, and shivering, which can destroy blood cells and platelets.

Monitoring

Whether or not you actually administer the blood, you will likely participate in monitoring to prevent complications or to detect and treat them quickly if they occur. Stay with the patient for the first 15 minutes of the blood transfusion to assess for any immediate reactions. The 15 minutes begins when the blood enters the vein. If saline solution is in the tubing, it may take several minutes before the blood reaches the patient. Check and document vital signs before starting the transfusion, after the blood has begun to infuse, and after the infusion is complete. Some institutions require vital sign monitoring every 15 to 30 minutes during the earliest part of the transfusion and then slightly less often for the duration of the infusion. Always follow institution guidelines. During the transfusion, assess the patient for signs and symptoms of complications.

Complications

Quick detection of complications can be lifesaving. It is easy to think of transfusing blood components as a routine procedure because it is a common activity. Do not be fooled. *It is a serious procedure that can be life threatening if errors occur.* Complications include febrile reactions, hypersensitivities, hemolytic reactions, anaphylaxis, circulatory overload, and even death. Regular monitoring according to institution policy can help detect complications early when treatment can be most effective.

FEBRILE REACTION. By far the most common reaction is fever (febrile reaction). It occurs up to 2% of the time. Make sure that blood never transfuses for more than 4 hours. The risk of a febrile reaction goes up with each unit of blood product given to the patient. Many times, febrile reactions occur after the transfusion is completed, but they can occur at any time. This is the reason for obtaining a set of baseline vital signs, including the patient's temperature. Once a febrile reaction begins, the most common signs are an increasing fever and shaking chills, which can be severe. Other symptoms can include headache and back pain. If febrile symptoms occur, stop the transfusion and notify the HCP. Acetaminophen may be ordered. If a hemolytic reaction is not suspected, the HCP may order the transfusion to continue once the patient is more comfortable. Administering leukocyte-depleted blood can usually prevent future febrile reactions.

URTICARIAL REACTION. Urticarial (hive) reactions are considered to be minor allergic reactions and are usually associated with antigens in the plasma accompanying the transfusion.

There may be a fever, but the cardinal sign is the appearance of urticaria, a hive-like rash. On discovery of this reaction, stop the transfusion and notify the HCP immediately. Expect that the patient will be given a dose of an antihistamine, such as diphenhydramine (Benadryl). If the transfusion is restarted, continue to monitor the patient closely. Again, make sure the 4-hour administration rule is not violated.

HEMOLYTIC REACTION. The most deadly and, fortunately, the rarest of the possible reactions is an acute hemolytic reaction. The cause of this reaction is transfusion of incompatible blood. The result is hemolysis (destruction) of RBCs. This type of serious reaction is usually noticed within minutes of starting the transfusion. The patient may report back pain, chest pain, chills, fever, shortness of breath, nausea, vomiting, or a feeling of impending doom. As the reaction progresses, the patient begins to show signs of shock, hypotension, oliguria, and decreased consciousness. Late signs and symptoms include those associated with disseminated intravascular coagulation: uncontrollable bleeding from many different sites at the same time, usually ending in death.

At the first sign of this type of reaction, immediately stop the transfusion and stay with the patient. Institute emergency procedures to notify the charge nurse, the HCP, and the blood bank. Keep the vein open with normal saline using a new tubing set (ensuring that no more incompatible blood is administered) so that emergency drugs can be administered. High volumes of fluids are administered to decrease shock and hypotension, and high doses of diuretics are given to promote urine flow because the kidneys are the most likely organs to be damaged. Dialysis may be necessary.

ANAPHYLACTIC REACTION. Anaphylactic reactions are not common but may be seen more often in patients who have received many transfusions or have had many pregnancies. Usually, the source of the anaphylaxis is sensitization to immune globulins passed from the donor blood product. In this type of reaction, the very first milliliters of blood containing the allergens to pass into the patient's system may be enough to cause the patient to develop respiratory or cardiovascular collapse. Other more common symptoms include severe gastrointestinal cramping, instant vomiting, and uncontrollable diarrhea.

If the patient exhibits these signs and symptoms, stop the transfusion at once and stay with the patient. Have someone else notify the RN and the HCP, using institutional emergency procedures. Emergency resuscitation measures, including cardiopulmonary resuscitation if necessary, must be instituted until the Rapid Response or code team arrives. Expect the patient to be intubated and receive oxygen, steroids, and other drugs as needed for life support. After the emergency has passed, this patient will likely need to receive transfusions from frozen, deglycerolized blood cells.

CIRCULATORY OVERLOAD. Circulatory overload is caused by rapid transfusion in a short period, particularly in older and debilitated patients. Usual signs and symptoms include chest pain, cough, frothy sputum, distended neck veins, crackles and wheezes in the lung fields, and increased heart rate. If symptoms occur, stop the transfusion and notify the HCP. Anticipate administration of diuretics, which help get rid of the excess fluid. The transfusion may be restarted later at a slower rate (see "Gerontological Issues").

Gerontological Issues

Older patients have less cardiac and renal ability to adapt to changes in blood volume, so they have a much higher risk of fluid overload when receiving IV infusions or blood transfusions. Carefully monitor lung sounds and vital signs both before and during a blood transfusion. New onset of dyspnea, crackles, hypertension, or bounding pulse during any infusion should be reported to the registered nurse or HCP immediately.

SUGGESTED ANSWERS TO
CRITICAL THINKING

■ *Mrs. Brown*
The HCP will most likely increase Mrs. Brown's warfarin dose. Note in Table 27.5 that the PT for a patient on warfarin should be 1.5 to 2.0 times normal. That is the reason the warfarin is ordered—to prolong the time it takes for blood to clot. If a normal PT is 9.5 to 11.3 seconds, a therapeutic PT for Mrs. Brown would be 14.25 seconds (9.5×1.5) to 22.6 (11.3×2.0). Her result of 12 seconds is not therapeutic.

REVIEW QUESTIONS

1. Which of the following actions should the nurse prioritize when taking care of a patient with a platelet count of 23,000/mm^3?
   1. Request an order for an anticoagulant.
   2. Protect the patient from injury.
   3. Encourage the patient to drink plenty of fluids.
   4. No action is necessary. This is a normal level.

2. A nurse is assessing a patient and finds small red-purple dots over most of his skin surfaces. The patient denies noticing them before. Which action should the nurse take first?
   1. Report the findings immediately to the RN or HCP.
   2. Document the findings objectively in the medical record.
   3. Assist the patient to apply lotion.
   4. Administer an antihistamine as needed.

3. A nurse is preparing a patient for lymphangiography. Which statement by the patient shows that more teaching is needed?
   1. "My skin might turn a bluish color."
   2. "I will need a sandbag on my groin to prevent bleeding."
   3. "My nurse will be checking my circulation routinely after the procedure."
   4. "I will need more X-rays tomorrow."

4. Which of the following activities should be carried out to keep the patient safe before starting a blood transfusion? **Select all that apply.**
   1. Match the blood to the order.
   2. Match the patient to the blood.
   3. Match the room number to the order.
   4. Check the patient's vital signs.
   5. Check the temperature of the blood.
   6. Check the patient's weight.

5. A nurse is monitoring a patient during a blood transfusion. After the blood has been hanging for 30 minutes, the patient's temperature rises from 98.6°F (37.0°C) at baseline to 101.0°F (38.3°C). The patient also experiences severe chills. Which action should the nurse take first?
   1. Document the vital signs in the medical record.
   2. Administer acetaminophen for the fever.
   3. Notify the HCP of the change.
   4. Stop the transfusion and hang normal saline solution.

Answers can be found in Appendix C.

Reference

Joint Commission. (2013). *2014 National Patient Safety Goals.* Retrieved June 1, 2013, from www.jointcommission.org /patientsafety/nationalpatientsafetygoals

 Davis*Plus* | For additional resources and information visit **davispl.us/medsurg5**

28

Nursing Care of Patients With Hematologic and Lymphatic Disorders

LUCY L. COLO

KEY TERMS

anemia (uh-NEE-mee-yah)
aplastic (ay-PLAS-tik)
disseminated intravascular coagulation (dis-SEM-ih-NAY-ted IN-trah-VAS-kyoo-lar koh-AG-yoo-LAY-shun)
glossitis (gloss-SY-tiss)
hemarthrosis (HEEM-ar-THROH-sis)
hemolysis (hee-MAHL-eh-sis)
hemolytic (HEE-moh-LIT-ik)
hemophilia (HEE-moh-FILL-ee-ah)
idiopathic thrombocytopenic purpura (ID-ee-oh-PATH-ik THROMB-boh-SY-toh-PEE-nik PURR-purr-rah)
leukemia (loo-KEE-mee-ah)
lymphoma (lim-FOH-mah)
pancytopenia (PAN-sy-toh-PEE-nee-ah)
panmyelosis (PAN-my-eh-LOH-sis)
pathological fracture (PATH-uh-LAW-jik-uhl FRAK-chur)
phlebotomy (fleh-BAW-tuh-mee)
polycythemia (PAW-lee-sy-THEE-mee-ah)
splenectomy (spleh-NEK-tuh-mee)
splenomegaly (SPLEE-noh-MEG-ah-lee)
thrombocytopenia (THROM-boh-SY-toh-PEE-nee-ah)

LEARNING OUTCOMES

1. Explain the pathophysiology of each of the hematologic and lymphatic disorders discussed in this chapter.
2. Describe the etiologies, signs, and symptoms of each disorder.
3. Identify tests used to diagnose each of the disorders.
4. Describe current therapeutic measures for each disorder.
5. List data you should collect when caring for patients with disorders of the hematologic or lymphatic systems.
6. Plan nursing care for patients with hematologic disorders.
7. Plan nursing care for patients with lymphatic disorders.
8. Explain how you will know if your nursing interventions have been effective.
9. Describe precautions you should institute to prevent bleeding in patients with clotting disorders.
10. Identify nursing care and teaching you will provide for patients undergoing a splenectomy.

HEMATOLOGIC DISORDERS

Patients with hematologic disorders have problems related to their blood. What do you suppose happens when there are too many blood cells, or too few, or the cells are defective?

- When red blood cells (RBCs) are affected, oxygen transport is also affected, causing symptoms related to poor oxygenation.
- When white blood cells (WBCs) are affected, the patient is unable to effectively fight infections.
- If platelets or clotting factors are affected, bleeding disorders occur.

DISORDERS OF RED BLOOD CELLS

Anemias

The term **anemia** describes a condition in which there is a deficiency of RBCs, hemoglobin, or both, in the circulating blood. Because hemoglobin carries oxygen, this results in a reduced capacity to deliver oxygen to the tissues, producing symptoms such as weakness and shortness of breath, which lead the patient to seek medical help.

Pathophysiology

A decrease in the number of RBCs can be traced to three conditions: (1) impaired production of RBCs, as in **aplastic** anemia and nutrition deficiencies; (2) increased destruction of RBCs, as in **hemolytic** or sickle cell anemia; or (3) massive or chronic blood loss. Some anemias are related to genetic problems in certain cultures ("Cultural Considerations"). It is important to remember that the general term *anemia* refers to a symptom or a condition secondary to another problem and is not a diagnosis in itself. Different types of anemia are discussed later in this chapter.

Etiology

DIETARY DEFICIENCIES. Iron, folic acid, and vitamin B_{12} are all essential to the production of healthy RBCs. A deficiency of any of these nutrients can cause anemia. Pernicious anemia is associated with a lack of intrinsic factor in stomach secretions, which is necessary for absorption of vitamin B_{12}. See "Nutrition Notes" for more information.

HEMOLYSIS. **Hemolysis** is the destruction, or lysis, of RBCs. Destruction of RBCs leads to a type of anemia called hemolytic anemia. This may be a congenital disorder, or it may be caused by exposure to certain toxins.

OTHER CAUSES. Thalassemia anemia is a hereditary anemia found in persons from Southeast Asia, Africa, Italy, and the Mediterranean islands. People with thalassemia do not synthesize hemoglobin normally. People with chronic disease also develop anemia ("Gerontological Issues"). Additional causes of anemia are discussed under the separate headings of aplastic and sickle cell anemias.

Signs and Symptoms

Symptoms of anemia include pallor, tachycardia, tachypnea, irritability, fatigue, and shortness of breath (Table 28.1). These symptoms occur because of the reduced number of functioning RBCs, with reduced ability to carry oxygen to tissues. In addition to these symptoms, the patient with pernicious (vitamin B_{12}) anemia may experience numbness of the hands or feet and weakness because vitamin B_{12} is needed for normal neurologic function. Pernicious anemia is also associated with a sore, beefy red tongue. Patients with iron deficiency may have fissures at the corners of the mouth, an inflamed tongue (**glossitis**), and spoon-shaped fingernails.

Diagnostic Tests

A complete blood cell count (CBC) is done to determine the number of RBCs and WBCs per cubic millimeter. The size,

- WORD • BUILDING •
anemia: a—not + emia—blood
aplastic: a—not + plastic—develop
hemolytic: heme—blood + lytic—break down
hemolysis: heme—blood + lysis—dissolution
glossitis: glos—tongue + itis—inflammation

Cultural Considerations

In the past, Iranian cross-cousin marriages have resulted in an increased incidence of several forms of anemia and hemophilia. These marriages are now being addressed through genetic counseling and premarital screening for carriers.

A sex-linked genetic disease common in the Chinese is glucose-6-phosphate dehydrogenase (G6PD) deficiency, an enzyme deficiency affecting the person's RBCs and resulting in anemia. Mediterranean G6PD deficiency is common, causing a hemolytic crisis when fava beans are eaten, when aspirin or certain other drugs are taken, or in acidotic or hypoxemic states. Mediterranean-type G6PD deficiency is an inherited disorder most fully expressed in males, with a carrier state in females.

Among Asian Indians, sickle cell disease (SCD) is highly prevalent; the gene is detected in 16.5% of selected populations. Sickle cell anemia is the most common genetic disorder among African American populations. Sickle cell anemia is also found in individuals who live in areas where malaria is endemic, such as the Caribbean, the Middle East, the Mediterranean region, and Asia.

Nutrition Notes

Understanding Common Nutritional Anemias

Nutritional deficiencies can produce some forms of anemia. Nutrients vital to the synthesis of RBCs include iron, folic acid, and vitamin B_{12}. Even if the cause of the anemia is dietary, other therapies may be used in addition to nutritional interventions.

Microcytic Anemia

Iron-deficiency anemia, the most common nutrient deficiency in the world, is characterized by smaller-than-normal RBCs. Insufficient intake of iron, excessive blood loss, or lack of stomach acid can lead to iron-deficiency anemia. Those at greatest risk of iron deficiency are women of childbearing age and young children. Even before obvious anemia is seen, cognitive abilities can be impaired.

   Good sources of iron include the following:

- Meat, fish, and poultry contain 50 to 60% heme iron that is absorbed intact.
- Plant sources and the other 40% of iron in meat, fish, and poultry must be reduced by stomach acids to an absorbable form. Vitamin C assists in this conversion of iron in:
  - Cooked dark green leafy vegetables
  - Lima and navy beans
  - Dried fruits
  - Enriched, fortified, or whole-grain products

Techniques to enhance absorption of iron from nonheme sources include the following:

- Consuming foods rich in vitamin C with iron-rich foods
- Adding small amounts of meat, fish, or poultry to plant sources of iron
- Stewing acidic foods such as tomatoes in iron cookware that leeches iron from the pot

If iron supplements are given to treat iron deficiency, they should be continued for several months after hemoglobin and hematocrit levels return to normal to enable the body to rebuild iron stores.

Macrocytic Anemia

Folic acid or vitamin B_{12} deficiencies produce anemias characterized by larger-than-normal RBCs.

   Folic acid aids in the formation of DNA and heme, the iron-containing portion of hemoglobin and is particularly necessary for rapidly growing cells, including those in the gastrointestinal (GI) tract, blood, and fetal tissue. Many drugs including alcohol, anticonvulsants, and aspirin interfere with the use of folic acid and can lead to anemia.

   Good food sources of folic acid include the following:

- Fortified flours, grains, cereals, wheat germ
- Liver
- Green leafy vegetables: asparagus, endive, lettuce
- Legumes: peanuts, dried peas, beans, and lentils

Because folic acid markedly decreases the occurrence of fetal neural tube defects such as spina bifida, women capable of becoming pregnant are advised to consume 400 mcg of synthetic folic acid daily from fortified foods or supplements in addition to the food folate furnished by a varied, balanced diet.

   Vitamin B_{12} is essential for the manufacture of DNA, RBCs, and for synthesis and maintenance of myelin, the fatty covering of nerves that facilitates rapid transmission of impulses. Vitamin B_{12} requires a highly specific protein-binding factor called intrinsic factor, secreted by glands in the stomach, to protect vitamin B_{12} from digestive enzymes and intestinal bacteria until the complex reaches the ileum where the vitamin is absorbed.

   Vitamin B_{12} is found in foods such as these:

- Meat, fish, shellfish, poultry
- Milk, cheese
- Eggs
- Vitamin B_{12} fortified soymilk or tofu

A healthy person eating these foods regularly is not at risk of vitamin B_{12} deficiency, but strict vegetarians may be at risk and have passed that risk to their breastfed infants. Pregnant and lactating vegan women's diets should be evaluated carefully for deficiency of vitamin B_{12}.

   Because the deficiency in this case is dietary, a dietary supplement is the treatment. Continued lack of vitamin B_{12} can cause irreparable nerve damage.

   Vitamin B_{12} deficiency should be considered in a person being evaluated for dementia.

Gerontological Issues

Hemoglobin and hematocrit levels should remain unchanged in healthy older adults; anemia is usually brought on by an underlying medical condition that causes altered iron metabolism, deficiency of erythropoietin, or shortened life span of RBCs. Unfortunately, anemia of chronic disease is often mistaken for iron-deficiency anemia; however, nutritional deficiencies and blood loss are common causes of iron-deficiency anemia.

color, and shape of the blood cells are determined by microscopic examination. Hemoglobin and hematocrit levels are below normal in anemia. Serum iron, ferritin, and total iron-binding capacity measurements are done to diagnose iron-deficiency anemia. Serum folate is measured if folic acid deficiency is suspected. A bone marrow biopsy and analysis may also be done.

   Patients with pernicious anemia have low gastric acid levels, and many have antibodies to intrinsic factor. Both abnormalities are associated with poor absorption of vitamin B_{12}. If blood loss is suspected, additional tests are done to determine the source of bleeding.

TABLE 28.1   CLINICAL MANIFESTATIONS OF ANEMIA

Body System	Mild (Hgb 10–14 g/dL)	Moderate (Hgb 6–10 g/dL)	Severe (Hgb <6 g/dL)
Skin	None	None	Pallor, jaundice, pruritus
Eyes	None	None	Jaundiced conjunctivae and sclerae, retinal hemorrhages, blurred vision
Mouth	None	None	Glossitis, smooth tongue
Cardiovascular	Palpitations	Increased palpitations	Tachycardia, increased pulse pressure, systolic murmurs, angina, congestive heart failure, myocardial infarction
Lungs	Exertional dyspnea	Significant dyspnea	Tachypnea, orthopnea, dyspnea at rest
Neurologic	None	None	Headache, vertigo, irritability, depression, impaired thought processes
Gastrointestinal	None	None	Anorexia, hepatomegaly, splenomegaly
Musculoskeletal	None	None	Bone pain
General	None	Fatigue	Sensitivity to cold, weight loss, lethargy

Therapeutic Measures

Treatment begins with elimination of contributing causes. Intake of the deficient nutrient can sometimes be increased in the diet or administered as a supplement (see "Nutrition Notes"). Changing cooking habits, taking dietary supplements, decreasing alcohol intake, and controlling chronic diarrhea can help correct folic acid deficiency. If symptoms of anemia are acute, a blood transfusion may be needed.

Nursing Process for the Patient With Anemia

DATA COLLECTION. Monitor hemoglobin and hematocrit levels and other laboratory studies as ordered and report any downward trend. Monitor responses to therapy, the patient's fatigue level, and the patient's ability to ambulate safely and perform activities of daily living (ADLs). Monitor degree of dyspnea and oxygen saturation, but be aware that at lower hemoglobin levels, oxygen saturation values may not be accurate. Assess for pallor in the skin and conjunctivae.

NURSING DIAGNOSES, PLANNING, AND IMPLEMENTATION. Possible nursing diagnoses are listed next along with outcomes and interventions.

Activity Intolerance related to tissue hypoxia and dyspnea
EXPECTED OUTCOME: The patient will be able to tolerate activity as evidenced by the ability to complete ADLs with minimal assistance. The patient will have knowledge about conserving energy as evidenced by a verbal statement.

• Monitor vital signs to evaluate tolerance to activity. *The patient experiencing activity intolerance may have tachycardia, increased respiratory rate, and decreased blood pressure with activity.*

• If the pulse or respiratory rate increases more than 20% from baseline during activity, reduce the activity level. *This is evidence that the activity is too strenuous and can result in increased hypoxia and dyspnea.*

• Plan care to conserve energy after periods of activity. *Balancing activities and rest periods assists the patient in conserving energy.*

• Assist the patient with self-care activities as needed. *Assisting with ADLs helps to decrease the amount of energy expended by the patient.*

• Place articles within easy reach of the patient *to reduce physiological demands on the body.*

• Encourage the patient to limit visitors, telephone calls, and unnecessary interruptions *to conserve energy.*

• Administer oxygen as ordered to relieve dyspnea. *The patient with anemia does not have enough hemoglobin to carry oxygen to vital organs.*

• Assist with blood transfusion as ordered if hemoglobin levels are very low or symptoms are severe. *A blood transfusion is a quick way to raise hemoglobin levels and to correct severe symptoms.*

Imbalanced Nutrition: Less Than Body Requirements related to disease, treatment, or lack of knowledge about adequate nutrition
EXPECTED OUTCOME: The patient will (1) have improved nutrition as evidenced by stable weight and stable hemoglobin and hematocrit and (2) will be able to appropriately select foods that will meet nutritional requirements.

• Consult a dietitian *to provide diet instruction if the anemia is caused by a dietary deficiency.*

• Teach the patient with folic acid deficiency that daily requirements can be met by including foods from each food group at every meal. *A balanced diet includes adequate amounts of folic acid.*

- Instruct the patient to take the supplements as ordered by the health care provider (HCP). *The patient should not stop taking the medication until the HCP advises him or her to do so.*
- Instruct the patient that vitamin B$_{12}$ injections are given for lifetime with pernicious anemia *because it is a chronic disease.*
- Instruct the patient with iron deficiency about high-iron foods and the correct use of an iron supplement. *An iron supplement should be taken with vitamin C to enhance absorption.*
- Instruct the patient to notify the primary care provider of any side effects related to iron supplements *such as nausea, diarrhea, constipation, and dark stools.*
- Administer intramuscular iron injections by the Z-track method *to avoid staining the injection site.*
- Administer oral iron 1 hour before or 2 hours after meals *to enhance absorption.*
- Administer liquid supplements with a drinking straw *to avoid staining the teeth.*

Risk for Falls related to weakness and dizziness

EXPECTED OUTCOME: The patient will remain safe from injuries related to a fall.

- Assess the patient at risk for falls using a fall risk assessment tool *to determine risk.*
- Assist the patient in changing positions slowly *to decrease dizziness and risk of falls.*
- Assist the patient with ambulation *to prevent a fall.*
- Protect the patient with pernicious anemia from injuries resulting from decreased sensation (e.g., take special care with heating pads and turning and positioning) *because the ability to sense pain may be impaired.*

Impaired Oral Mucous Membranes related to altered dietary status

EXPECTED OUTCOME: The patient will have intact oral mucous membranes.

- Monitor condition of oral mucous membranes *to detect changes.*
- Provide good oral hygiene *to keep the oral cavity clean and prevent infection.*
- Encourage soft, bland foods, *which are more tolerable until healing can occur.*
- Instruct the patient to use a soft toothbrush for oral care *because it is gentler until healing can occur.*

EVALUATION. When successfully treated, the patient should be able to tolerate a normal level of activity without shortness of breath or excess fatigue. The patient should be able to explain the correct treatment plan and therapeutic measures for long-term prevention of problems, including dietary choices and supplements as well as self-care measures. The patient will remain free from injury, and the oral mucosa will be intact.

Aplastic Anemia

PATHOPHYSIOLOGY. Aplastic anemia differs from other types of anemia in that the bone marrow becomes fatty and incapable of producing the needed numbers of RBCs. Also known as hypoplastic anemia, the cells that are produced are normal in size and shape, but there are not enough of them to sustain life. The resulting **pancytopenia** (reduced numbers of all formed elements from the bone marrow—RBCs, platelets, and WBCs) is the indicator that something is wrong with the bone marrow. Left untreated, aplastic anemia is almost always fatal.

ETIOLOGY. Aplastic anemia may be congenital—that is, the person is born with bone marrow incapable of producing the correct number of cells. Or it may be due to exposure to toxic substances such as industrial chemicals (e.g., benzenes and insecticides), chemotherapy medications, or use of cardiopulmonary bypass during surgery. Other causes include certain bacterial and viral infections, such as tuberculosis and hepatitis, or autoimmune disease.

SIGNS AND SYMPTOMS. The clinical features of aplastic anemia vary with the severity of the bone marrow failure. As with other anemias, early symptoms include progressive weakness, fatigue, pallor, shortness of breath, and headaches. As the disease progresses and the pancytopenia worsens, other symptoms, such as tachycardia and heart failure, may appear. Ecchymoses and petechiae appear on the skin surface because of the reduced platelet count (Fig. 28.1; also see Fig. 28.5). Blood may ooze from mucous membranes. Injection sites may progress from oozing to frank bleeding. There is often overt bleeding into vital organs. Infection occurs because of reduced WBCs. When aplastic anemia is left untreated, most patients die from infection or bleeding.

DIAGNOSTIC TESTS. The diagnosis of aplastic anemia begins with a CBC. Usually all values are very low, with the occasional exception of the RBC count, in part because of the

---

• WORD • BUILDING •
pancytopenia: pan—all + cyto—cell + penia—poverty

FIGURE 28.1 Petechiae on the skin from thrombocytopenia. From Goldsmith, L. A., et al (1997). *Adult and pediatric dermatology* (p. 61). Philadelphia: F.A. Davis, with permission.

longer life span of RBCs. Eventually the RBCs are also depleted. If the patient is having gross bleeding internally or externally, the RBC level can drop rapidly and dramatically. The most definitive test is a bone marrow biopsy. Because the bone marrow is essentially dead, the result is often described as a "dry tap" in which pale, fatty, yellow, fibrous bone marrow is extracted instead of the red, gelatinous bone marrow normally seen. Not surprising, the more fatty and pale the marrow is, the more dysfunctional it is. Other diagnostic tests include total iron-binding capacity (TIBC) and serum iron level. It is common to find both of these levels elevated because the RBCs are not being produced and are using up the stores of iron in the production of hemoglobin.

THERAPEUTIC MEASURES. Early identification of the cause of the anemia and correction of the underlying problem are important to survival. Unfortunately, it is often difficult to determine the cause, and there is no way to reverse the damage already done. Aggressive supportive measures may be the only treatment. Most of these measures are aimed at prevention of infection and bleeding. Transfusions may be administered to replace deficient cells.

Today the most effective treatment for aplastic anemia is bone marrow transplantation (see "Patient Perspective"). Another common therapy is the administration of steroids to stimulate production of cells in the weakened bone marrow. Immunosuppressant agents may be given if an autoimmune disorder is the underlying cause. Occasionally the administration of hormones may work to increase the viability of the marrow. Steroid or other treatments may be tried before attempting a bone marrow transplant.

Patient Perspective

Bone Marrow Transplant

In June 2002, I took my daughter to the doctor for her sports physical. Later that day, I received a call telling me to take her to the university hospital immediately because she had a serious life-threatening illness. I kept telling myself and my husband that our small-town hospital must have made some sort of error. As it turned out, they had not. My daughter was diagnosed with aplastic anemia and needed a bone marrow transplant. I became obsessed with the illness, poring over every tidbit of medical information I could find. Sometimes I found myself out in the car unable to remember where I was going; sometimes I had to pull over because my eyes were filled with tears and I could no longer see.

My daughter was 16 at the time of her illness, yet it is the parents who sign consent forms and make the choices in care. When the chemotherapy was started and running through the IV tubing, I felt like grabbing the tubing and pinching it off, yelling, "I need more time to think about this decision," but time was running out. Without a bone marrow transplant, she had about 8 months to live.

After transplantation, my daughter was in an isolation room for a month. I stayed with her every day, and at night I stayed at the inn that was attached to the hospital. If I was needed, I wanted to be no more than a minute away. I was one of the luckier parents because I had the financial means to manage this process. I thought about how horrible it would be if I had other children at home. Sometimes I would have such an urge to run away and escape from it all. I attended support groups that were held on the hospital unit. I got to know a lot of other parents with sick kids, and it became very upsetting to me at times. One day parents told me how well their child was doing; the next day I saw the child's room empty and thought he must have gone home, only to find out later that he had died during the night. I wondered if my daughter would be next.

I look at my daughter now, 4 years later, alive and perfectly healthy, and I tell myself that I made the right choices for her. But she tells me that if it happens again, she will not go through chemotherapy. I wonder, is chemo worse than death?

In many treatment institutions, limited success is being obtained with the use of colony-stimulating factors, natural elements that can now be produced synthetically. (You can read more about these medications in Chapter 11.) For example, erythropoietin (Epogen) stimulates production of RBCs, and filgrastim (granulocyte colony stimulator [Neupogen]) stimulates production of WBCs. The major drawback to this type of therapy is the high cost. Many of the pharmaceutical manufacturers have patient access programs that help reduce the costs of these medications.

NURSING MANAGEMENT. Nursing care of patients with symptoms related to reduced RBCs was presented earlier in the "Nursing Process for the Patient With Anemia" section. If the patient's platelet count is low (usually less than 20,000), the patient is placed on bleeding precautions (Box 28-1). If the WBC count is low, the patient must be protected from infection (Box 28-2).

BE SAFE!

BE VIGILANT! Watch carefully for even subtle signs of bleeding, such as early skin changes, or pink-tinged urine. Report findings before bleeding worsens.

Sickle Cell Anemia

PATHOPHYSIOLOGY. Sickle cell anemia is an inherited anemia in which the RBCs have a specific mutation that makes the hemoglobin in the red cells very sensitive to oxygen

Box 28-1 Interventions to Prevent Bleeding in the Patient With Thrombocytopenia

- Use an electric razor instead of a safety razor for shaving.
- Use a soft toothbrush or gauze to clean the teeth. Avoid flossing.
- Avoid invasive procedures as much as possible, including enemas, douches, suppositories, and rectal temperatures.
- Avoid intramuscular injections.
- To avoid injury when checking blood pressure, pump cuff up only until pulse is obliterated.
- Avoid blood draws whenever possible. Use established access sites or group specimen collections into once-daily draws.
- Maintain pressure on intravenous (IV), blood draw, and other puncture sites for 5 minutes.
- Encourage use of shoes or slippers when out of bed.
- Keep area clutter-free to prevent bumps and bruises.
- Avoid use of drugs that interfere with platelet function, such as aspirin products and nonsteroidal anti-inflammatory drugs (aspirin, ibuprofen, naproxen, and others).
- Administer stool softeners as ordered to prevent straining to have a bowel movement.
- Move and turn patient gently to avoid bruising.
- Instruct patient to blow nose very gently and only when necessary.
- Advise patient to consult with health care provider about whether sexual intercourse is safe.

Box 28-2 Interventions for the Patient at Risk for Infection

- Place the patient in a private room.
- Ensure that all staff and visitors wash hands before entering the room.
- Teach the patient to wash hands before and after using the toilet and before and after eating.
- Teach the patient and family to wash hands before touching each other.
- Prevent staff or visitors with known infections from entering the patient's room.
- Teach the patient to not handle flowers or plants brought into the room.
- Teach the patient to avoid raw fruits, vegetables, and milk products.
- Avoid use of indwelling urinary catheters and other invasive devices.
- Use strict aseptic technique if invasive procedures are needed.
- Use acetaminophen if an antipyretic is needed; aspirin can induce bleeding.

changes. Any time a decrease in the oxygen tension is sensed, the cells begin an observable physical change from their usual spherical shape to a sickle or crescent shape (Fig. 28.2). Sickled cells are very rigid and easily cracked and broken. The abnormal shape also causes the cells to become tangled in the blood vessels and organs. The result is congestion, clumping, and clotting.

As RBCs are broken, the cellular contents spill out into the general circulation. The resulting increase in the bilirubin level causes jaundice. Gallstones (cholelithiasis) may develop because of the increased amounts of bile pigments. The spleen and liver may enlarge because of the increase in retained cells and cellular materials.

Because the cells are fragile, the life span of the RBCs in patients with sickle cell anemia is significantly decreased. Normal red cells live about 120 days. Sickled cells survive only about 10 to 20 days, an 80% to 90% decrease in cell survival.

ETIOLOGY. Sickle cell disease (SCD) is an autosomal recessive hereditary disorder. This means that if both parents pass

FIGURE 28.2 (A) Normal red blood cells (RBCs) flowing freely in a blood vessel. The inset image shows a cross-section of a normal RBC with normal hemoglobin. (B) Abnormal, sickled RBCs blocking blood flow in a blood vessel. The inset image shows a cross-section of a sickle cell with abnormal (sickle) hemoglobin forming abnormal strands.

on the abnormal hemoglobin, the child will have the disease. If only one parent passes on the abnormal hemoglobin, the child will have the sickle cell trait and will be able to pass the trait (or the disease if the other parent is also affected) on to his or her child.

In the United States, sickle cell anemia is most often found in those of African or Eastern Mediterranean heritage. Worldwide, many persons residing in Asia, the Caribbean, the Middle East, and Central America are affected. Nearly 10% of African Americans have the sickle cell trait; 1 of every 500 African American infants born has inherited the two sets of abnormal genes needed to have the disease. Symptoms do not appear in infants until after the age of 6 months because up to that age, the infant is using hemoglobin manufactured during fetal life, which is not affected by the sickling process.

SIGNS AND SYMPTOMS. The sickling changes just described are a daily occurrence. The rapid return of the oxygen level to normal usually returns the cells to their normal shape.

Occasionally, the sickling process cannot be reversed, and the problem continues unabated. This sudden and severe sickling is called a sickle cell crisis. As more and more sickling occurs, the blood becomes sluggish and does not flow easily. It tends to collect in the capillaries and veins of chest and abdominal organs, as well as joints and bones, and can cause infarction (tissue necrosis resulting from lack of blood supply). Tissue necrosis causes pain, fever, and swelling.

Any condition that leads to decreased oxygenation can contribute to the development of a sickle cell crisis. Some examples include pneumonia with hypoxia, exposure to cold, diabetic acidosis, and severe infection. Sickle cell anemia presents problems for the patient who needs surgery. Anesthesia and blood loss during surgery and postoperative dehydration can trigger a crisis.

Common symptoms produced during sickle cell crises include severe pain and swelling in the joints, especially of the elbows and knees, as the sickled cells impede circulation. Abdominal pain is common with swelling of the spleen and engorgement of the vital organs. Hypoxia occurs as fever and pain increase, causing the patient to breathe rapidly. A male patient may have a continuous, painful erection (priapism) from impaired blood flow through the penis. Symptoms of renal failure are common as circulation is slowed and the kidneys become clogged with cellular debris.

Repeated crises and infarctions lead to chronic manifestations such as hand-foot syndrome, an unequal growth of fingers and toes from infarction of the small bones in the hands and feet (Fig. 28.3). Additional manifestations of SCD are shown in Figure 28.4.

The patient with sickle cell anemia has impaired quality of life. Often, strenuous exercise or more exotic activities, such as scuba diving, are impossible because of the risk of crisis. Crises may occur without any apparent cause. In general, crises last from 4 to 6 days. They may occur in cycles close together for a time and then become dormant for months to years. The cause of death in patients with sickle cell anemia is usually infection, stroke, or organ involvement.

DIAGNOSTIC TESTS. The most telling feature of SCD is a blood smear that shows sickle-shaped RBCs in circulation. The Sickledex test is a screening test that shows sickling of RBCs when oxygen tension is low. Hemoglobin electrophoresis is a test used to determine the presence of hemoglobin (Hgb) S, the abnormal form of hemoglobin. Also, there is a decreased amount of hemoglobin, a lowered RBC count, an elevated WBC count, and a decreased erythrocyte sedimentation rate.

THERAPEUTIC MEASURES. Treatment depends on the severity of the disease. All patients should receive patient education to prevent crises and supportive care when crises occur. Some patients may be placed on low-dose oral penicillin to help prevent infections, decreasing the risk of crises.

During acute crises, the patient is admitted to the hospital. The nurse can anticipate that the patient will require sedation and analgesia for severe pain and blood transfusions to replace the sickled red cells lost by their being caught, crushed, and destroyed. Oxygen therapy decreases dyspnea caused by the anemia, and large amounts of oral and intravenous (IV) fluids are given to flush the kidneys of the byproducts of the many broken cells' debris. Antibiotics are used to treat infection that may have triggered the crisis.

New treatments are being developed to treat SCD. Frequent blood transfusions, often monthly, are one of the newest treatment recommendations. However, frequent transfusions can cause high levels of iron to build up in the body.

FIGURE 28.3 Hand-foot syndrome. Note different lengths of fingers and toes. *Courtesy of Sandoz Pharmaceutical Corp., East Hanover, NJ.*

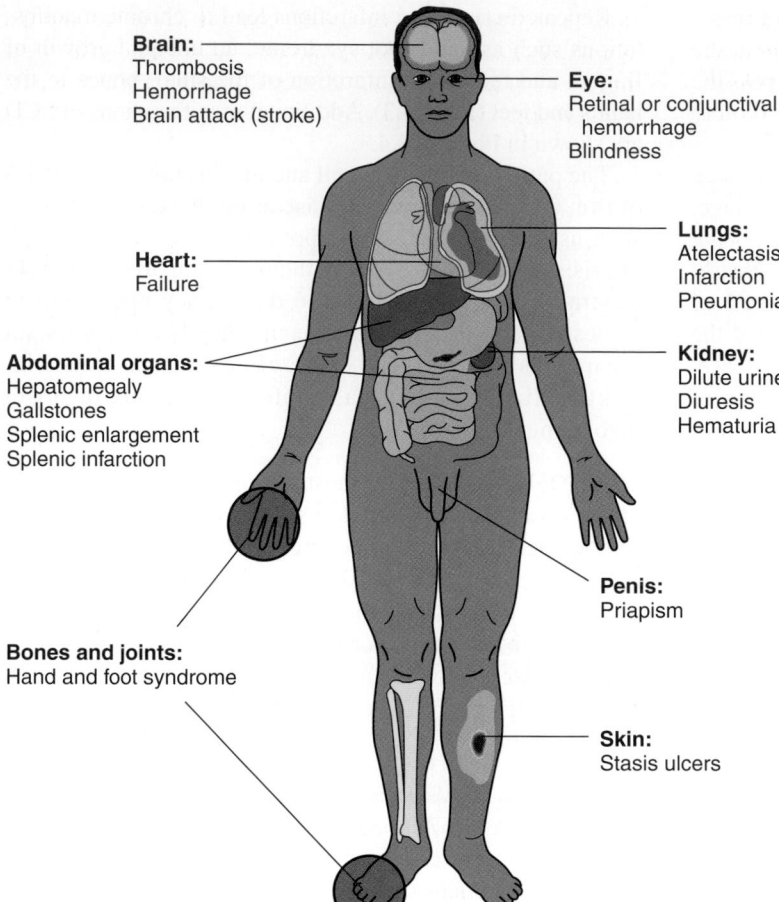

Brain:
Thrombosis
Hemorrhage
Brain attack (stroke)

Eye:
Retinal or conjunctival
    hemorrhage
Blindness

Heart:
Failure

Lungs:
Atelectasis
Infarction
Pneumonia

Abdominal organs:
Hepatomegaly
Gallstones
Splenic enlargement
Splenic infarction

Kidney:
Dilute urine
Diuresis
Hematuria

Penis:
Priapism

Bones and joints:
Hand and foot syndrome

Skin:
Stasis ulcers

FIGURE 28.4 Clinical manifestations of sickle cell anemia.

Deferasirox (Exjade) is a medication that may be given to decrease the excess iron levels. Corticosteroids may reduce the need for analgesics and oxygen. Hydroxyurea (Droxia) is a drug that has been shown to decrease crises, but it can cause life-threatening side effects; it should also be used with caution in women of childbearing years because of the risk of birth defects. Patients may not adhere to hydroxyurea therapy because they don't feel different; it may take months to years to make a difference in outcomes.

Bone marrow transplantation has shown promise in the treatment of SCD, although it is not without risk. In 2012, Johns Hopkins released data from a study of 17 patients with SCD who received bone marrow transplant. Eleven of the 17 patients had successful outcomes at the 2-year follow-up. Eight of the 11 transplants were half-matched transplants, meaning donor marrow came from parents, children, and siblings that were half-identical to the patient's tissue. The transplant process is similar to the regimen for bone marrow transplant for cancer diagnoses. Because of the numerous blood transfusions throughout the life of a patient with SCD, antibodies have been acquired that make it difficult to administer donor marrow. Researchers continue to look for methods to improve the engraftment for transplants in the sickle cell population (Johns Hopkins, 2012).

NURSING PROCESS FOR THE PATIENT WITH SICKLE CELL ANEMIA.

Data Collection. In the patient in crisis, assess circulation in the extremities every 2 hours, including pulse oximetry, capillary refill, peripheral pulses, and temperature. Frequent pain assessment is also essential.

Nursing Diagnoses, Planning, and Implementation
Risk for Ineffective Tissue Perfusion related to sickled cells and infarction

EXPECTED OUTCOME: *The patient will have adequate tissue perfusion as evidenced by the presence of peripheral pulses, warm extremities, urine output within normal limits, and a capillary refill time of less than 3 seconds.*

• Encourage oral fluids, and assist the registered nurse (RN) to monitor IV fluids *to dilute and aid in elimination of cell debris.*

• Apply warm compresses as ordered to the painful areas, cover the patient with a blanket, and keep the room temperature above 72°F (22°C) *to reduce the vasoconstricting effects of cold.*

• Avoid cold compresses *because they decrease circulation and increase the number of sickled cells caught in a painful area.*

- Avoid restrictive clothing and raising the knee gatch (the adjustable joint in the hospital bed, which allows for the patient's knee to be flexed and the legs supported). *These can restrict circulation.*

Acute Pain related to tissue infarction

EXPECTED OUTCOME: The patient will state pain is controlled at an acceptable level at all times.

- Administer opioid analgesics such as morphine as ordered *for acute pain.* (Analgesics may be given intravenously or by use of patient-controlled analgesia.)
- Administer acetaminophen (Tylenol) *to control fever.*
- Avoid giving aspirin *because it may increase acidosis, which can worsen the crisis.*
- Encourage bedrest during the acute phase of the crisis *to reduce oxygen demand.*

Evaluation. If nursing care has been effective, the patient will state that he or she is comfortable, and will not have signs of poor circulation.

Risk for Nonadherence to Treatment

EXPECTED OUTCOME: The patient will state reasons why treatment is important, and follow therapeutic regimen as prescribed.

- Assess patient and family's understanding of rationale for treatment and expected effects. *Assessment of knowledge base should guide teaching.*
- Assess patient's ability to obtain medication, including ability to make trips to laboratory and pharmacy. *One study looked at the patients enrolled in the North Carolina Medicaid program who were prescribed hydroxyurea between 1999 and 2008. Only 35% of the patients were adherent to the therapy. Reasons for nonadherence included difficulty in getting to the pharmacy monthly to fill the prescription and to the clinic for lab tests (Brandow & O'Brien, 2010).*
- Refer the patient and family for in-depth education as needed about treatment regimen. *Patients must understand therapy in order to adhere to it.*
- Refer the patient and family to a support group with others who have sickle cell anemia. *Support groups are a venue for sharing stories about personal experiences with the disease and to encourage each other to stay adherent to the medication.*

Evaluation. If interventions have been effective, the patient will state that he is comfortable, will have evidence of adequate circulation, will state understanding of importance of adhering to treatment plan, and will have fewer crises.

PATIENT EDUCATION. During remission, teach the patient how to prevent acute episodes. Advise the patient to avoid tight-fitting clothing that restricts circulation. Also urge the patient to avoid strenuous exercise, which increases oxygen demand, as well as cold temperatures and smoking, which cause vasoconstriction. Alcoholic beverages can also trigger a crisis and should be avoided. Patients should never fly in unpressurized aircraft or undertake mountain climbing or other sports that can cause hypoxia. Encourage patients to get a pneumococcal

vaccine and yearly flu vaccine. Encourage fluids to maintain hydration and reduce blood viscosity. Genetic counseling is important to prevent passing on the trait or disease to offspring. For more information, visit www.sicklecelldisease.org.

Polycythemia
Pathophysiology and Etiology

Polycythemia is really two separate disorders that are easily recognizable by similar characteristic changes in the RBC count. In both forms of polycythemia, the blood becomes so thick with an overabundance of RBCs that it closely resembles sludge. This thickness does not allow the blood to circulate easily. Laboratory tests show a hemoglobin level greater than 18 mg/dL, an RBC mass greater than 6 million, and a hematocrit of more than 55%.

Polycythemia vera (PV) is known as primary polycythemia. Most people with PV have a specific genetic mutation. In PV, the RBCs, platelets, and WBCs are all overproduced, and the bone marrow becomes packed with too many cells. As this overabundance of cells spills out into the general circulation, the organs become congested with cells and the tissues become packed with blood. The skin takes on a plethoric (dark, flushed) appearance from the buildup of red cells. The thick blood and excess platelets can cause thrombosis and occlusion of vessels. PV is usually found in patients over age 50.

In contrast, secondary polycythemia is the result of long-term hypoxia. Common coexisting conditions that may predispose a patient to secondary polycythemia include pulmonary diseases such as chronic obstructive pulmonary disease (COPD), cardiovascular problems such as chronic heart failure, living in high altitudes, and smoking. The body makes more RBCs in response to the low oxygenation associated with these conditions. Secondary polycythemia is a compensatory mechanism rather than an actual disorder.

Signs and Symptoms

A patient with PV commonly presents with hypertension, vision changes, headache, vertigo, dizziness, and ringing in the ears (tinnitus). Laboratory results show an increased level of all bone marrow components (RBCs, WBCs, platelets), which is called **panmyelosis**. Patients with extreme thrombocytopenia are also at risk for developing a bleeding disorder called acquired von Willebrand syndrome. The patient may have nosebleeds and bleeding gums, retinal hemorrhages, exertional dyspnea, and chest pain because of the increased pressure exerted by the excess cells. The patient usually has a dark, flushed complexion. Intense itching is related to excess mast cells (and, therefore, histamine) in the skin. Abdominal pain with an early feeling of fullness with meals occurs because of the enlarged liver and spleen. Nearly all of the symptoms in PV are due to the major problems of hypervolemia, hyperviscosity, and engorgement of capillary beds. Without treatment, patients with PV die of thrombosis or hemorrhage.

• WORD • BUILDING •

polycythemia: poly—many + cyt—cells + emia—in the blood

Diagnostic Tests

Diagnosis of PV is made based on a CBC and bone marrow aspiration. A low level of erythropoietin is present, caused by negative feedback to the kidneys, where erythropoietin is made. The bone marrow or blood will also show the genetic mutation if it is present.

Therapeutic Measures

Treatment of PV takes place in two stages. The first stage is to decrease the hyperviscosity problem. The most common first-line treatment is therapeutic **phlebotomy**. Phlebotomy involves withdrawal of blood, which is then discarded. From 350 to 500 mL of blood are removed each time on an every-other-day basis, with the goal being a hematocrit of about 45%. This reduces the RBC level, and the patient usually feels more comfortable quickly. Repeated phlebotomies eventually cause iron-deficiency anemia, which in turn stabilizes RBC production; phlebotomies can then be reduced to every 2 to 3 months. Low-dose aspirin reduces the risk of blood clots.

The problem that remains is the increased WBC and platelet counts because phlebotomy does little to correct these overloads. Chemotherapeutic agents or radiation therapy, including radioactive phosphorus, may be used to suppress production of blood cells in some patients. Leukemia is a side effect of this therapy, so it is used only if the benefits outweigh the risks.

Nursing Management

Explain the phlebotomy procedure and reassure the patient that the treatment will relieve the most distressing symptoms. The procedure is the same as that used for donating blood. The patient should be active and ambulatory to help prevent thrombus formation. When bedrest is needed, passive and active range-of-motion exercises should be implemented. Monitor the patient for complications such as hypovolemia and bleeding.

If the patient has more advanced manifestations, such as an enlarged liver or spleen, offer several small meals each day so the patient will be more comfortable while still receiving adequate nutrition. A dietitian can be consulted to discuss ways to maintain good nutrition. If the patient is on drug therapy, monitor CBC and platelet counts.

Patient Education

Instruct the patient to drink at least 3 L of water daily to reduce blood viscosity. Encourage smoking cessation, avoidance of tight or restrictive clothing, and elevation of feet when resting to prevent impairment of circulation. Use of support hose when active also promotes circulation. If anticoagulants or antiplatelet agents are ordered, instruct the patient about side effects to watch for and the importance of routine laboratory tests. Routine bleeding precautions are implemented (see Box 28-1). Warn the patient to stop activities at the first sign of chest pain. Instruct the patient to report chest pain, increased joint pain, decreased activity tolerance, or fever, as well as signs of iron-deficiency anemia, such as pallor, weight loss, and dyspnea. Advise the patient to report any signs or symptoms of bleeding or thrombosis immediately.

 HEMORRHAGIC DISORDERS

Disseminated Intravascular Coagulation

Pathophysiology

Disseminated intravascular coagulation (DIC) involves a series of events that result in severe hemorrhage.

As its name implies, this syndrome is a catastrophic, overwhelming state of accelerated clotting throughout the peripheral blood vessels. In a short period, all of the clotting factors and platelet supplies are exhausted, and clots can no longer be formed. This results in bleeding from nearly every bodily route possible. DIC is not a disease; it is a syndrome that develops secondary to some other severe physical problem. Once this deadly syndrome develops, the progression of symptoms is rapid.

Massive clotting in blood vessels leads to organ and limb necrosis. Organs most often affected include the kidneys and the brain, but other blood-engorged organs, such as the lungs, the pituitary and adrenal glands, and the GI mucosa, are commonly involved. DIC is usually acute in onset, although in some patients it becomes a chronic condition. The prognosis depends on early diagnosis and intervention and the severity of the hemorrhaging. DIC has a very high mortality rate.

Etiology

DIC can develop after any condition in which the body has sustained major trauma. The sources of trauma are varied and can include an overwhelming infection; obstetric complications such as abruptio placentae, amniotic fluid embolism, or a retained dead fetus; or cancer-related causes such as acute leukemia or lung cancer. Massive tissue necrosis found in severe crush or burn injuries may increase the risk of DIC. Tissue necrosis secondary to extensive abdominal surgery with leakage of the intestinal contents can also be related to DIC onset. Rarer causes of this condition have included heatstroke, shock, and poisonous snakebites, as well as fat embolism secondary to broken long bones.

Signs and Symptoms

Abnormal bleeding without a history of a serious hemorrhagic disorder is a cardinal sign of DIC. Early signs of bleeding include petechiae, ecchymoses (Fig. 28.5), and bleeding from venipuncture sites. Bleeding may progress to IV sites, skin tears, surgical sites, incisions, and the GI tract and oral mucosa. Joints become painful and enlarged if bleeding into the joints occurs. All of these signs and symptoms may occur at the same time. Massive bleeding may also be accompanied by nausea, vomiting, dyspnea, oliguria, convulsions, coma, shock, major organ system failure, and severe muscle, back, and abdominal pain.

Diagnostic Tests

Initial laboratory findings in DIC include a prolonged prothrombin time (PT) and partial thromboplastin time (PTT), decreased platelet count, and increased evidence of fibrin degradation products (Table 28.2). A decrease in hemoglobin is the result of spilled hemoglobin from the increased numbers of broken red cells. Blood urea nitrogen (BUN) and serum creatinine levels may also be increased.

FIGURE 28.5 Extensive hemorrhage into the skin in disseminated intravascular coagulation. Note how the area is outlined in pen so the nurse can assess if the area is spreading. From Harmening, D. M. (1997). *Clinical hematology and fundamentals of hemostasis* (3rd ed., p. 520). Philadelphia: F.A. Davis, with permission.

TABLE 28.2 LABORATORY ABNORMALITIES IN DISSEMINATED INTRAVASCULAR COAGULATION

Screening Test	Finding
Prothrombin time (PT)	Prolonged
Partial thromboplastin time (PTT)	Prolonged
Activated partial thromboplastin time (APTT)	Prolonged
Thrombin time (TT)	Prolonged
Fibrinogen	Reduced
Platelets	Reduced
Fibrin split products (FSP; also known as fibrin degradation products [FDP])	Elevated
Protamine sulfate	Strongly positive
Dimers (cross-linked fibrin fragments)	Elevated
Antithrombin III	Reduced
Factor assays (for factors V, VII, VIII, X, and XIII)	Reduced

Therapeutic Measures

Effective treatment of DIC depends on early recognition of the condition. Treatment is first aimed at correcting the underlying cause. Additional treatment consists of supportive interventions, including administration of blood, fresh frozen plasma, platelets, vitamin K, and the infusion of cryoprecipitate (containing clotting factors) to support hemostasis. IV heparin may be used to help prevent the

initial microembolization and may also be used for chronic DIC cases. Additional therapies are being investigated.

Nursing Management

Care of the patient with DIC is a nursing challenge. Early intervention requires vigilance in recognizing and reporting signs of bleeding. In addition to supportive care, focus on the prevention of further bleeding episodes. Care should be taken to avoid any trauma that might cause bleeding. Be careful not to dislodge clots from any site because another clot may not form, and the patient will hemorrhage. See Box 28-1 for bleeding precautions.

Patient Education

Because a patient with DIC is often cared for in the intensive care unit, there are many opportunities for patient and family teaching. Explain all diagnostic tests to the patient if he or she is alert. If not, keep the family informed. A large part of family education is preparing the family for what the patient may look like in terms of bleeding and bruising, as well as specific equipment that may be in place, such as IV lines, a nasogastric (NG) tube, and an indwelling urinary catheter. It may be helpful to enlist the aid of social workers, chaplains, and other members of the health care team to help support the family.

CRITICAL THINKING

Mrs. Johns

■ Mrs. Johns is admitted to your unit with DIC following the difficult delivery of her new baby.

1. What data will you collect as you care for Mrs. Johns?
2. What treatment do you anticipate?
3. What concerns is Mrs. Johns likely to have?
4. Mrs. Johns is to receive IV fresh frozen plasma 300 mL over 30 minutes. How many milliliters per hour should be set on the IV controller?
5. What members of the health team should you anticipate collaborating with?

Suggested answers are at the end of the chapter.

Idiopathic Thrombocytopenic Purpura
Pathophysiology and Etiology

Acute **idiopathic thrombocytopenic purpura** (ITP) results from increased platelet destruction by the immune system. Any time platelet numbers are reduced, the risk for bleeding increases. Acute ITP usually affects children between ages 2 and 6, whereas chronic ITP mainly affects adults over age 60.

• WORD • BUILDING •

idiopathic thrombocytopenic purpura: idio—unknown + pathic—disease + thrombo—clot + cyto—cell + penic—lack + purpura—hemorrhage in the skin

Acute ITP usually occurs after an acute viral illness such as rubella or chickenpox. Hepatitis C virus and human immunodeficiency virus (HIV) can also be triggers. It may be drug-induced or associated with pregnancy. ITP is believed to be related to an immune system dysfunction. Antibodies responsible for platelet destruction have been found in nearly all diagnosed patients.

Signs and Symptoms

ITP produces clinical changes that are common to all forms of **thrombocytopenia**: petechiae, ecchymoses, and bleeding from the mouth, nose, or GI tract. Bleeding may occur in vital organs, such as the brain, which may prove fatal. In the acute type, onset may be sudden and without warning, causing easy bruising, nosebleeds, and bleeding gums. Onset of chronic ITP is usually insidious.

Diagnostic Tests

A platelet count of less than $20,000/mm^3$ and a prolonged bleeding time suggest ITP. The greatly decreased platelet level places the patient at serious risk for hemorrhage. Examination of platelets under the microscope shows them to be small and immature. Anemia may be present if there has been a bleeding episode. If a bone marrow aspiration is performed, the results show an adequate amount of the precursor cells for platelets, the megakaryocytes. However, instead of the 7- to 10-day life span that platelets usually have, these immature platelets have a life span of just a few hours.

Therapeutic Measures

The goal of treatment is to have an adequate (if not normal) platelet count and no bleeding. Most cases of acute ITP resolve spontaneously without treatment. Initial treatment, if needed, often involves the administration of steroids. The purpose of the steroids is to prolong the life of the platelets by decreasing immune activity. In acute situations, immune globulin may be given to quickly increase the blood count. Some patients receive chemotherapeutic drugs. The spleen may be removed because it is the primary site of platelet destruction. Often the patient undergoing splenectomy has tried all other courses of treatment unsuccessfully and may be having bleeding episodes. Acute bleeding episodes are treated with transfusions of blood, platelets, and vitamin K.

Nursing Care

Care for the patient with ITP is the same as any patient with a bleeding disorder. See Box 28-1 for bleeding precautions. Teach the patient to watch for and report signs and symptoms of bruising and bleeding (Box 28-3, "Patient Education"). The patient should avoid trauma and restrict activity during severe episodes.

Hemophilia

Hemophilia is a group of hereditary bleeding disorders that result from a severe lack of specific clotting factors. The two most common are hemophilia A (classic hemophilia) and hemophilia B (Christmas disease). Von Willebrand's disease is

---

Box 28-3 **Patient Education**

Signs and Symptoms of Bleeding

Notify your health care provider if the following occur:

- Easy bruising of skin
- Petechiae (small red spots on skin)
- Blood in urine
- Black tarry stools
- Bleeding from nose or gums
- Increase in vaginal bleeding
- New onset of painful joints

---

another related bleeding disorder, but it represents a minority of cases and is not discussed in this chapter.

Pathophysiology

Recall that many different clotting factors make up the clotting mechanism. Hemophilia A accounts for 80% of all types of hemophilia and results from a deficiency of factor VIII. Hemophilia B is a factor IX deficiency; about 15% of people with hemophilia have this type. The severity and prognosis of hemophilia depend on the degree of deficiency of the specific clotting factors. Mild hemophilia has the best prognosis because it does not cause spontaneous bleeding and joint deformities like severe hemophilia can.

After an injury, the person with hemophilia forms a platelet plug (which differs from a clot) at the site of an injury as would normally be expected, but the clotting factor deficiency keeps the patient from forming a stable fibrin clot. Continued bleeding washes away the platelet plug that initially formed. Contrary to popular myths, people with hemophilia do not bleed faster and are not at risk from small scratches.

Etiology

Hemophilia A and B are inherited as X-linked recessive traits. This means that the female carrier (daughter of an affected father) has a 50% chance of transmitting the gene to each son or daughter. Daughters who receive the gene are carriers, and sons who receive the gene are born with hemophilia. It is technically possible for daughters to be affected with hemophilia, although it is rare.

Signs and Symptoms

Bleeding occurs as a result of injury or, in severe cases, spontaneously (unprovoked by injury). Bleeding into the muscles and joints (**hemarthrosis**) is common and can cause acute pain. Severe and repeated episodes of joint hemorrhage cause joint deformities, especially in the elbows, knees, and ankles, which decrease the patient's range of motion and ability to walk.

• WORD • BUILDING •
thrombocytopenia: thrombocyte—platelet + penia—lack
hemophilia: hemo—blood + philia—to love
hemarthrosis: hem—bleeding + arthr—joint + osis—condition

In mild hemophilia, excessive bleeding is usually associated only with surgery or significant trauma. However, once a person with mild hemophilia begins to bleed, the bleeding can be just as serious as that of the patient with a more severe form.

The patient with moderate hemophilia has an occasional bout of spontaneous bleeding. In severe hemophilia, spontaneous bleeding occurs more frequently. It would be possible for the patient to develop hemarthrosis or bleeding into the brain without any precipitating trauma. Severe episodes can produce large subcutaneous and deep intramuscular hematomas. Major trauma can cause bleeding so severe that it becomes life threatening.

Another unfortunate problem related to hemophilia treatment is the frequent need to replace clotting factors and other blood products. Before 1986, blood banks and other centers did not routinely test for human immunodeficiency virus (HIV) antibodies. Depending on the patient's age and frequency of treatment, many patients may have been exposed to HIV or hepatitis. Blood banks and pharmacies have checked their blood supplies for the presence of HIV since 1986. Today, the plasma proteins are artificially created or thoroughly cleansed to prevent transmission of disease.

Diagnostic Tests

Laboratory data reveal a prolonged PTT. The various clotting factor levels are measured to determine which is missing. Once the missing factor is identified, the type of hemophilia is determined and necessary treatments can be implemented. In some cases of mild hemophilia, a surgical procedure or trauma is the first time a bleeding problem is noticed.

Therapeutic Measures

Hemophilia is not curable. However, treatment advances have improved outcomes, and many patients can now live a normal life span. Treatment is aimed at preventing crippling deformities and increasing life expectancy and involves stopping bleeding episodes by administering the missing clotting factors. Mild hemophilia A may be treated with injection or nasal inhalation of desmopressin (DDAVP, antidiuretic hormone), which can stimulate the body to release more clotting factors. More severe hemophilia A is treated with factor VIII; hemophilia B is treated with factor IX. Each is available in a freeze-dried powder that is reconstituted with water and administered intravenously. The newest treatment employs factors made using recombinant DNA technology without the use of any human blood products. Blood transfusions are uncommon but may be necessary after severe trauma or surgery.

Complications occur when therapy is started too late. Minor trauma typically needs to be treated with at least 72 hours of added clotting factors; major traumas and surgeries may require up to 14 days of added factors to prevent sudden bleeding. Health care workers should pay careful attention to the patient who says that bleeding is starting even when no outward signs are evident. The patient usually knows from experience if bleeding is starting. If treatment is delayed at this time, the results can be disastrous. Some patients with severe disease are treated prophylactically to prevent bleeding.

Nursing Process for the Patient With Hemophilia

DATA COLLECTION. Because a major goal is prevention of bleeding episodes, assess the patient and family for knowledge of the disease and its treatment and understanding of preventive measures. Most patients care for themselves at home, starting their own IVs and administering treatment independently. Hospitalization is needed only for surgery or major trauma. During an acute episode of bleeding, monitor hemoglobin and hematocrit carefully. Monitor factor VIII or IX levels to determine if factor replacement has reached adequate levels. Monitor vital signs for falling blood pressure and rising pulse rate, which are signs of hypovolemic shock. All body systems are assessed for signs of bleeding (Box 28-3). Perform a pain assessment using the **WHAT'S UP?** format.

NURSING DIAGNOSES, PLANNING, AND IMPLEMENTATION.
Acute Pain related to bleeding into tissues
EXPECTED OUTCOME: The patient's pain will be controlled as evidenced by verbalization that pain is relieved to a satisfactory level within a specified time frame depending on medication and route of intervention.

• Have the patient report the location, intensity, and quality of the pain. *Assessment provides the caregiver with data that can be used to develop a treatment plan.*
• Administer opioids as prescribed, including patient-controlled analgesia. *Analgesics are the primary way to manage moderate to severe pain.*
• Avoid the administration of intramuscular injections *because of the risk of bleeding into the muscle.*
• Reassess the level of pain after administration of analgesia *to determine the effectiveness of the treatment ordered. IV medications will work almost immediately; oral medications may take 30 to 60 minutes.*
• Monitor sedation and respiratory status of the patient receiving opioids for pain. *Opioids depress the respiratory center of the brain.*

Risk for Bleeding related to factor deficiencies
EXPECTED OUTCOME: The patient will experience no signs or symptoms of bleeding. The patient will verbalize understanding of bleeding precautions.

• Instruct the patient on bleeding precautions (see Box 28-1). *Identification of signs of bleeding will promote early intervention to prevent injury.*
• Assist with administration of factor concentrates, fresh frozen plasma, cryoprecipitate, blood, or a combination of these as ordered *to treat acute episodes of bleeding.* See Chapter 27 for transfusion of blood products.
• Apply ice or pressure on bleeding sites *to help slow bleeding.*
• Avoid intramuscular, subcutaneous, or rectal medications. *These routes can cause bleeding into tissues.*
• Instruct the patient that preventive care will be needed if surgery or dental procedures are needed. *These invasive procedures can be life-threatening events for the patient with hemophilia.*

Risk for Ineffective Self Health Management related to deficient knowledge

EXPECTED OUTCOME: The patient will be able to manage self-care requirements as evidenced by verbalization of understanding/demonstration of the treatment regimen.

• Assess knowledge base and determine readiness to learn and incorporate new information. *Each patient is unique in the way he or she learns new information.*
• Instruct the patient on ways to prevent bleeding and recognition of signs and symptoms of bleeding (see Boxes 28-1 and 28-3). *Identification of signs of bleeding will promote early intervention to prevent injury.*
• Instruct the patient to obtain emergency care in the event that bleeding occurs. *Intervention is critical for survival of an acute bleeding episode.*
• Instruct the patient to administer factor treatments at home. *Treatment can often be administered at home and can be given more promptly if a trip to the emergency department is not needed.*
• Instruct patients and families on the community services and hemophilia treatment centers available to the patient. *These centers are nationwide and coordinate care for patients with hemophilia.*
• Instruct the patient that the approach to care is multidisciplinary in nature and includes social services, dental, rehabilitation, nursing, financial, and medical needs. *These are all areas that have an impact on the care of the patient with hemophilia.*

EVALUATION. If interventions have been effective, the patient will be comfortable, and bleeding will be prevented or complications minimized. The patient and family will be able to state appropriate measures to prevent and treat bleeding episodes. The patient will be knowledgeable about the resources available to cope with the diagnosis of hemophilia.

 DISORDERS OF WHITE BLOOD CELLS

Leukemia

The term *leukemia* literally means "white blood." It was first identified in 1845 when the blood of victims was examined and found to have an excess of "colorless" cells.

Pathophysiology

Leukemia is a malignant disease of the WBCs that affects all age groups. The immature WBCs (blast cells) generate in an explosive fashion in the bone marrow, lymph tissue, and spleen. The cells are abnormal and unable to effectively fight infection. So many abnormal cells develop and are dumped into the peripheral circulation that they tend to collect in the body tissues and organs, especially where circulation is sluggish. Areas especially prone to infiltration with immature WBCs are the oral mucosa, anus, sinuses, and lungs. At the time of diagnosis, these areas are often inflamed, painful, and infected. It is common for patients to be diagnosed only after experiencing an infection that does not clear up easily with treatment.

As the disease progresses, the bone marrow continues to produce large numbers of the useless cells; the peripheral circulation is filled with them, and the bone marrow is packed with blast cells. Because so many of the blood stem cells are being used to make defective white cells, production of most other normal cells is impossible. The patient becomes anemic because of the lack of RBC production, and bleeding becomes a problem as fewer and fewer platelets are manufactured. But most importantly, even though the WBC count is very high, there are few normal, mature, and active white cells with which to fight infection. Thus, the patient often begins to have raging infections that do not respond to antibiotics. Without treatment, leukemia leaves the patient unable to fight infection, unable to control bleeding, and in a downward spiral of fatigue and anorexia. Untreated leukemia is almost always fatal.

Classifications

• Leukemias are classified as either acute or chronic and either lymphoid or myeloid. Symptoms of the acute leukemias begin suddenly, and the patient is very sick, whereas chronic leukemias develop slowly and patients can be surprised by the diagnosis because they feel well. Lymphoid leukemias affect the lymphocytes. Myeloid leukemias originate in the stem cells of the bone marrow that develop into monocytes, granulocytes, erythrocytes, and platelets. The most common leukemias are discussed next.

ACUTE LEUKEMIAS. Acute lymphocytic leukemia (ALL) is the most common cancer in children and involves abnormal growth of the lymphocyte precursors (lymphoblasts). Acute myelogenous (myeloblastic) leukemia (AML) usually affects people over age 60 and has a poor prognosis. The patient with acute leukemia may present with sudden onset of high fever, abnormal bleeding from the mucous membranes, petechiae, ecchymoses, and easy bruising after minor trauma. Death usually results from infection.

CHRONIC LEUKEMIAS. Chronic lymphocytic leukemia (CLL) predominantly affects the B and T lymphocytes and usually occurs in adults. Chronic myelogenous leukemia (CML) is characterized by the Philadelphia chromosome and occurs most often in older adults.

Chronic leukemia usually develops in a three-phase process. The first, insidious phase is characterized by anemia and mild bleeding abnormalities. During this phase, the patient often feels well and is not even aware of being sick. After a time, generally years, the disease progresses to the accelerated and acute phases, in which the scenarios are similar to the events seen in acute leukemias. Chronic leukemia is almost always fatal; the average survival time is 3 to 5 years after onset of the chronic phase and 3 to 6 months after onset of the acute phase. With advances in treatments, however, it is not uncommon to encounter patients who have been living with chronic leukemia for 10 years or more.

Etiology

The cause of leukemia is unknown. Risk factors are thought to include certain viruses because remnants of viruses have been found in leukemic cells. Genetic and immunological factors are often involved. For example, persons with Down syndrome are more likely to develop leukemia. Exposure to radiation is believed to be a factor, in part because radiologists have been found to have a higher than average development of leukemia. Some patients have developed leukemia after being treated for another unrelated malignancy using radiation or chemotherapy. Researchers have noted the higher occurrence rate of leukemia in persons who lived through the Hiroshima and Nagasaki atomic bombings during World War II. Water polluted with benzenes and other chemicals may be a factor. There is no single clear-cut cause for the development of leukemia.

Signs and Symptoms

Symptoms are similar for all types of leukemia and include low-grade fever caused by infection and pallor, weakness, lethargy, shortness of breath, and malaise caused by anemia. These symptoms may be present weeks or months before the appearance of other symptoms. The patient also may have fatigue, tachycardia, palpitations, and abdominal pain. Sternal pain and rib tenderness may result from crowding of bone marrow. If the leukemia has invaded the central nervous system, the patient may experience confusion, headaches, and personality changes. During the acute phase the patient may have high fevers from infection. Ecchymosis or petechiae may result from thrombocytopenia.

Diagnostic Tests

Although a simple CBC often points toward the diagnosis, only bone marrow aspiration can show the degree of proliferation of the malignant WBCs and confirm the diagnosis of leukemia. The CBC may also show a decrease in the numbers of platelets, RBCs, and mature WBCs. A lumbar puncture helps determine if the central nervous system is involved. Genetic analysis of the peripheral blood and bone marrow components may show the presence of the Philadelphia chromosome in patients with CML.

Therapeutic Measures

CHEMOTHERAPY. Systemic chemotherapy aims to eradicate the leukemic cells and induce a remission. Remission means that the bone marrow is free to produce normally occurring cells in normal proportions without production of the immature WBCs. The type of chemotherapy used varies with the type of leukemia and the level of involvement.

The overall goal of the initial treatments is to get the patient to a state of remission. Occasionally, partial remission is achieved when everything looks good except for an occasional leukemic cell seen in the bone marrow. Remission is not the same as cure.

There are four phases to the treatment of leukemia: induction, intensification, consolidation, and maintenance. Induction is the period in which an attempt is made to get the patient into remission. This first phase is difficult because chemotherapy is given in very high doses and on an aggressive timetable. Often the patient becomes quite ill from

complications of the treatment. The patient may become depressed because the treatment seems worse than the disease at this stage. The nurse must help the patient deal with anemia, thrombocytopenia, and leukopenia, as well as other side effects (Table 28.3; also see Box 28-2 and Chapter 11).

If the first remission is accomplished, the other phases of treatment are begun. Intensification is similar to the initial induction phase, using the same drugs at even higher doses. The next phase, consolidation, is used to ensure that all leukemic cells have been eradicated from the body. Finally, the patient graduates to maintenance therapy in which the patient is kept free of leukemic cells and in remission for a period of years (and hopefully a lifetime). This requires years of continued chemotherapy treatments, often on a monthly basis.

RADIATION THERAPY. Radiation therapy is sometimes used in addition to chemotherapy for initial treatment of leukemia. It may be directed at the entire body or at specific areas where leukemic cells are collecting.

BONE MARROW TRANSPLANT. Bone marrow transplant (BMT) is sometimes used to treat leukemia. Preparation for BMT includes high-dose chemotherapy and/or total body irradiation. The goal is to destroy all of the patient's malignant bone marrow and then, at the last possible moment, replace it with a donor's clean and healthy bone marrow (allogenic transplant). Another type of bone marrow transplant, known as an autologous transplant, uses the patient's own diseased bone marrow, which is harvested, chemically treated and cleaned, stored, and later reinfused. Transplanted bone marrow is given to the patient like a blood transfusion; typically through a central line placed in the chest. Once infused into the bloodstream, the new marrow travels to the bones, where, ideally, it will begin to grow and function normally. Bone

TABLE 28.3 LEUKEMIA SUMMARY

Signs and Symptoms	Fever (related to infection) Pallor Weakness, malaise Tachycardia Dyspnea Bone pain Headaches, confusion
Diagnostic Tests	CBC Bone marrow aspiration Lumbar puncture
Therapeutic Measures	Chemotherapy Radiation therapy Bone marrow transplant
Priority Nursing Diagnoses	*Risk for Injury* (infection, bleeding) related to pancytopenia *Fatigue* related to decreased tissue oxygenation

marrow transplants are being performed at more and more centers across the United States.

A new and promising treatment for leukemia is peripheral blood stem cell transplantation. Hematopoietic stem cells can be collected from the patient during remission and then reinfused at a later time. Donor stem cells are also sometimes used if a good match can be found.

OTHER THERAPIES. Biological therapies may be used to boost the patient's immune system. They may be used to help the body attack cancer cells, or to control side effects by boosting red cell or white cell production. Kinase inhibitors (the most common is mesylate [Gleevec]) may be used to inhibit abnormal proteins in leukemic cells in CML. By targeting just the cancer cells, the incidence of side effects is reduced.

Nursing Process for the Patient With Leukemia

The patient with leukemia is at risk for many problems, including fatigue, bleeding, infection, and other complications of the disease and its treatment. The patient must understand the disease process and treatment regimen to participate in self-care. See the "Nursing Care Plan for the Patient With Leukemia" for interventions to deal with these problems. Additional diagnoses include *Deficient Knowledge* and *Anxiety*. The following websites provide resources for patients and families with leukemia:

> American Cancer Society, www.cancer.org
> Leukemia and Lymphoma Society, www.lls.org
> National Cancer Institute, www.cancer.gov
> Also see Chapter 11 for general care of the patient with cancer.

NURSING CARE PLAN for the Patient With Leukemia

Nursing Diagnosis: *Risk for Injury* (infection, bleeding) related to pancytopenia

Expected Outcomes: The patient will be free from injury and infection as evidenced by temperature within normal limits and no signs or symptoms of bleeding. Signs and symptoms of infection or bleeding will be reported promptly.

Evaluation of Outcomes: Is the patient free from infection and bleeding, or are problems reported so that quick intervention can prevent further complications?

Intervention Monitor vital signs every 4 hours and as needed. **Rationale** Elevated temperature is a sign of infection. Falling blood pressure and elevated pulse rate may indicate sepsis or blood loss. **Evaluation** Are vital signs stable?

Intervention Monitor patient for swelling, redness, purulent drainage. **Rationale** These are signs of infection and should be reported promptly. **Evaluation** Are signs of infection present?

Intervention Protect patient from sources of infection (see the "Evidence-Based Practice" box; also see Box 28-2). **Rationale** Patient is at risk for infection because of ineffective WBCs. **Evaluation** Are precautions being observed to prevent infection?

Intervention Observe for tarry stools, petechiae, ecchymosis (Box 28-3). **Rationale** These are signs of bleeding and should be reported promptly. **Evaluation** Are signs of bleeding present?

Intervention Protect patient from injury that could cause bleeding (see Box 28-1). **Rationale** Patient is at risk for bleeding because of reduced platelet count. **Evaluation** Are precautions being observed to prevent injury and bleeding?

Nursing Diagnosis: *Fatigue* related to decreased red cell count and oxygenation and effects of treatments as evidenced by patient statement of lack of energy, inability to participate in desired activities

Expected Outcome: The patient's fatigue will be controlled at a level that is acceptable to the patient as evidenced by patient ability to participate in activities that are important to him or her.

Evaluation of Outcome: Is patient able to identify and participate in activities as desired?

Intervention Assess fatigue using the **WHAT'S UP?** format. **Rationale** A good assessment establishes a baseline and aids in planning. **Evaluation** Is fatigue present? To what degree?

NURSING CARE PLAN for the Patient With Leukemia—cont'd

Intervention Assist patient to identify activities that are important to him or her (e.g., ADLs, attending a child's wedding, taking a trip). Assist in setting goals to work toward the desired activity. **Rationale** If the patient cannot do everything he or she wishes, it may help to focus on the most important things. **Evaluation** Can patient identify important activities? What are they? How can the nurse assist the patient to reach activity goals?

Intervention Encourage a balanced diet. Contact dietitian as needed. **Rationale** Poor nutrition contributes to fatigue. **Evaluation** Is patient eating a balanced diet? Is weight stable?

Intervention Allow periods of rest between activities. **Rationale** Any activity (ADL, x-rays, even talking) can increase fatigue. **Evaluation** Is patient able to rest?

Intervention Ensure adequate sleep. Obtain order for sleeping aid if indicated. **Rationale** Lack of sleep worsens fatigue. **Evaluation** Does patient state feeling rested on awakening? Is medication needed?

Intervention Provide for ADLs when patient is unable to do so independently. **Rationale** Extreme fatigue may prevent the patient from participating in self-care. **Evaluation** Does patient need total assistance?

Nursing Diagnosis: *Impaired Oral Mucous Membranes* related to chemotherapy and pancytopenia as evidenced by bleeding, ulcerations, statement of pain, difficulty eating

Expected Outcomes: The patient's oral mucous membranes will remain intact as evidenced by pink, moist, smooth tissue without ulceration. The patient will be able to eat a balanced diet.

Evaluation of Outcomes: Are oral mucous membranes intact, without lesions? Is patient eating a balanced diet?

Intervention Assess mouth daily for redness, edema, and lesions. **Rationale** Routine assessment helps identify problems early so treatment can be implemented. **Evaluation** Are mucous membranes intact?

Intervention Encourage adequate nutrition and fluids. **Rationale** Poor nutrition and dehydration increase the risk of oral lesions. **Evaluation** Is patient eating and drinking?

Intervention Encourage patient to brush teeth after meals with a soft toothbrush. If irritation is severe or if the patient is at risk for bleeding, use swabs or sponge Toothettes instead of a toothbrush. **Rationale** Brushing the teeth controls tooth and gum disease; a toothbrush may be too harsh if the patient is at risk for bleeding. **Evaluation** Is mouth care being provided after meals? Is mouth care irritating? Are alternative methods needed?

Intervention Avoid use of lemon-glycerin swabs for mouth care. **Rationale** Lemon-glycerin swabs are drying to oral mucosa. **Evaluation** Are products used appropriate?

Intervention Obtain an order for a mouthwash containing diphenhydramine (Benadryl). Obtain an order for a topical anesthetic if mouth is very inflamed and painful. **Rationale** Diphenhydramine reduces inflammation; anesthetics reduce pain. **Evaluation** Does mouthwash soothe pain?

Intervention Encourage the patient to avoid smoking, alcohol, acidic food or drinks, extremely hot or cold foods and drinks, and commercial mouthwash. **Rationale** These things can be irritating to the mucosa. **Evaluation** Does patient state understanding of things to avoid?

GERIATRIC
Intervention Advise patient to remove dentures for cleaning and at bedtime. **Rationale** Dentures left in for long periods can impair circulation and increase risk of lesions. **Evaluation** Are oral mucous membranes intact?

BE SAFE!

BE VIGILANT! Monitor the patient carefully for subtle signs of infection. With inadequate or immature white cells, symptoms may not be obvious. Any redness, swelling, or even slight increase in temperature should be reported.

EVIDENCE-BASED PRACTICE

Clinical Question
Is the use of protective isolation required for all patients with neutropenia after chemotherapy?

Evidence
The most current information related to protective or reverse isolation suggests that this type of isolation be considered for a limited group of patients being treated in specialty areas such as bone marrow transplant. Rooms with special airflow systems and filters are an important part of protecting patients at high risk for infection. Patients who develop neutropenia after chemotherapy treatment show some benefit from being in a private room but do not necessarily require protective isolation (Pieszak, 2011).

Implications for Nursing Practice
Isolation is unpleasant and lonely for patients. Question the use of protective isolation in rooms without special airflow systems and filters and in patients with postchemotherapy neutropenia.

REFERENCE

Pieszak, S. (2011). Putting evidence into practice: Prevention of infection in patients receiving cancer treatments. *American Nurse Today, 6*(12). Retrieved July 10, 2013, from www.americannursetoday.com/article.aspx?id=8574

CRITICAL THINKING

Mr. Washington

■ Mr. Washington is on your unit undergoing initial treatment for leukemia. You enter his room and find it full of visitors.

1. What concerns do you have?
2. What do you do?
3. How can you promote patient-centered care during Mr. Washington's treatment?

Suggested answers are at the end of the chapter.

MULTIPLE MYELOMA

Multiple myeloma is a deadly cancer of the plasma cells in the bone marrow. When the disease is caught in its early stages, treatment can prolong life by 3 to 5 years. More important, early detection can decrease the amount of pain and disability due to bony destruction and **pathological fractures**. Unfortunately, almost half of patients die within the first 3 months after diagnosis because of the silent and deadly nature of the disease; another 40% of patients die within 2 years after diagnosis. Multiple myeloma currently has a 45% survival rate at 5 years (www.cancer.net/cancer-types/multiple-myeloma/statistics, 2012). Multiple myeloma most often affects men aged 50 to 70.

Pathophysiology

In this disorder, cancerous plasma cells in the bone marrow begin reproducing uncontrollably. These cells infiltrate bone tissue all over the body and produce hundreds of tumors that begin to devour the bone tissue. X-ray examination may show holes in the bones forming a Swiss cheese pattern (Fig. 28.6). As more and more of these holes are formed, the integrity of the bone is compromised and weakened. Multiple myeloma usually affects the bones of the skull, pelvis, ribs, and vertebrae.

As the disease progresses, plasma cells infiltrate the major organs, including the liver, spleen, lymph nodes, lungs, adrenal glands, kidneys, skin, and GI tract. Because the diagnosis is usually made only after widespread invasion of the bones is well under way, the prognosis for patients with this disease is poor. Although the overall result of the disease is the devastating destruction of the bone and widespread osteoporosis, death is often from sepsis.

FIGURE 28.6 X-ray of bone destruction in multiple myeloma. From Huether, S. E., & McCance, K. L. (1996). *Understanding pathophysiology* (p. 548). St. Louis, MO: Mosby, with permission.

Etiology

The cause of multiple myeloma is unknown. Research suggests genetics may be one factor. People who work in rubber, leather, farming, and petroleum industries are more likely to develop multiple myeloma. Obesity, exposure to radiation, and long-term exposure to hair dyes also increase risk.

Signs and Symptoms

Skeletal pain is the most common complaint. The patient may describe the pain as constant severe back pain that increases with exercise or movement or as pain in the ribs. Other signs and symptoms include achiness of the long bones, joint swelling and tenderness, low-grade fever, and general malaise. Sometimes there is evidence of early peripheral neuropathy secondary to vertebral collapse and spinal cord compression. The patient may be unable to feel the true temperature of bath water and be burned or may be unable to feel wounds and infections on the feet. In more severe cases of cord compression, the patient may lose control of bladder and bowels. This is a true oncological emergency. Prompt emergency treatment is needed to keep the patient from becoming paralyzed.

Occasionally, patients have pathological fractures of the long bones. These are fractures that occur with no trauma, such as the person who breaks a leg just turning over in bed or breaks a rib while sneezing. In advanced disease there is anemia, weight loss, thoracic spinal deformities from multiple rib destruction, and a loss of height because of pathological fractures and compacting of the vertebrae.

Because calcium is mobilized from the bones and into the blood, the patient is at risk for hypercalcemia. Signs and symptoms of hypercalcemia include anorexia, nausea, vomiting, mental changes (especially confusion), seizures, weakness, and fatigue. Kidney stones may result as the excess calcium passes through the kidneys.

Patients are susceptible to infection because of compromised immune function. Pneumonia is a common finding in patients with multiple myeloma. They may develop anemia because of bone marrow dysfunction and reduced erythropoietin formation by diseased kidneys. Risk for bruising and bleeding occurs due to thrombocytopenia.

Patients often develop kidney failure because the filtering capacity of the kidney becomes blocked by calcium. Other factors include recurrent infections and deposits of myeloma cells in the kidneys.

Diagnostic Tests

A CBC shows moderate to severe anemia. The WBC count may show an increase in the number of white cells secondary to infection. Blood and urine studies are positive for M-type globulins (called Bence-Jones proteins when found in the urine) in 40% of patients. X-ray examinations or magnetic resonance imaging (MRI) may show changes in the lungs and diffuse osteoporosis in bones not already riddled with holes. Bone marrow biopsy is done to confirm the diagnosis and determine the stage of the disease.

Blood chemistries often show an increased amount of calcium in the blood. Hypercalciuria results when the calcium released out of the bones is flushed out in the urine. An IV pyelogram may be done to see how much calcium is collecting in the kidneys. A 24-hour urine collection is done to evaluate protein excretion.

C-reactive protein (CRP) is elevated in multiple myeloma; it is believed that the CRP actually promotes the cancer cells' proliferation and protects them from the effects of chemotherapy agents. Measurement of CRP helps determine prognosis. Elevated CRP levels are also associated with increased fatigue.

Therapeutic Measures

Long-term treatment of multiple myeloma consists of a two-pronged approach: (1) managing the disease and (2) managing the symptoms. To manage the disease, corticosteroids (prednisone or dexamethasone) and oral or IV chemotherapy agents are given. Thalidomide may be given to slow the progression of the disease. Lenalidomide (Revlimid) is chemically similar to thalidomide but has fewer side effects. The goal of drug therapy is to suppress plasma cell proliferation, which then helps decrease the amount and speed of bone destruction.

Another medication for multiple myeloma is bortezomib (Velcade). Bortezomib is a proteasome inhibitor that inhibits enzymes to disrupt cancer cell growth and survival.

Another option is high-dose chemotherapy combined with stem cell transplantation. Donor stem cells can be used, or a patient's own peripheral stem cells can be removed and reinfused. These stem cells can then differentiate into new, healthy cells. Methods of cleaning the cells to prevent contamination with malignant cells are being researched.

The second approach is control of symptoms. The patient is monitored for signs and symptoms of hypercalcemia, hyperuricemia, dehydration, respiratory infection, renal problems, and pain. The HCP may order the administration of IV bisphosphonate agents such as pamidronate (Aredia). This class of drugs inhibits bone resorption and is used to help keep serum calcium levels controlled. Oral compounds are also available to help keep the calcium within normal limits. The goal is to get the serum calcium level below 10 mg/dL. If hypercalcemia occurs, the HCP will order an IV infusion of normal saline solution at a high rate, followed by regular administration of diuretics.

External beam irradiation may be given to especially painful areas of bone involvement. Fortunately, this treatment is quite effective, usually decreasing pain intensity in just a few days. The patient can expect to have a daily (or perhaps a twice-daily) treatment over a course of 10 to 14 days that is delivered directly to the painful bony areas. Vigorous attention to administering pain medications during the early course of treatment greatly reduces the patient's pain levels.

The patient may need a laminectomy if vertebral collapse occurs. Because of demineralization of the bone, with resulting large amounts of calcium in the blood and urine, surgery for kidney stones and eventual dialysis for acute or chronic kidney failure may be needed.

Nursing Process for the Patient With Multiple Myeloma

The patient with multiple myeloma is at risk for many problems. In addition to those below, the diagnoses in the "Nursing Care Plan for the Patient With Leukemia" are appropriate.

Data Collection

Assess for fever or malaise, which can signal the onset of infection. Other conditions to be alert for include anemia, hypercalcemia, fractures, and renal complications. Monitor intake and output, and strain urine for stones. Elevated BUN and creatinine levels will alert you to possible renal failure. Report back pain, leg weakness, sensory loss, or loss of bowel or bladder function because these can indicate spinal cord compression. Monitor the patient for elevated CRP and low hemoglobin, which are associated with increased fatigue.

Nursing Diagnoses, Planning, and Implementation

Risk for Infection related to compromised immune function
EXPECTED OUTCOME: Patient will remain free from infection as evidenced by temperature within normal limits and no signs or symptoms of infection.

- Intervene as appropriate *to reduce the risk of infection* (see Box 28-2).
- Encourage deep breathing, and keep patient active *to decrease the risk of respiratory complications.*

Risk for Injury: Fracture related to weakened bones; complications of immobility; complications due to hypercalcemia
EXPECTED OUTCOME: Patient will remain free from injury as evidenced by no fracture and no complications related to immobility or hypercalcemia.

- Keep the patient mobile. Consult physical and occupational therapy as needed. Bones in use are strongest, so the patient should remain up and moving as much as possible *to help stimulate calcium resorption and decrease demineralization.*
- Assist the patient with walking *to reduce the risk of pathological fractures of the long bones.*
- If the patient is unsteady, use a walker or a support belt *to reduce the risk of falls.*
- If the patient is bedridden, reposition every 2 hours *to prevent complications related to immobility.*
- Use a lift sheet to move the patient gently in bed *to decrease the risk of skin damage and pathological fractures.*
- Provide passive range-of-motion exercises *to maintain mobility if the patient is unable to be independently mobile.*
- Administer fluids so that daily output is never less than 1500 mL *to flush kidneys and reduce the risk of kidney stones.*
- Teach the patient the importance of good hydration at all times *to minimize complications of hypercalcemia.* Depending on time of year and the type and level of patient activities, the patient may need to have an intake of more than 4 L daily.

Evaluation

If nursing care has been effective, the patient will be free of infection or infection will be recognized and treated promptly. The patient will avoid injury, with no fracture, skin breakdown, or complications related to hypercalcemia. See "Home Health Hints" at the end of this chapter for additional suggestions for patients being cared for at home.

LYMPHATIC DISORDERS

Lymphatic disorders include Hodgkin's disease and the non-Hodgkin's **lymphomas**. Because the spleen is part of the lymph system, this section also discusses splenectomy.

Hodgkin's Disease

Despite its name, Hodgkin's disease is a lymphoma, which is a cancer of the lymph system. Its distinguishing feature is the presence of Reed-Sternberg cells, which make it different from all the other forms of lymphoma. Hodgkin's disease is more prevalent in men than in women and occurs most often in young adults ages 15 to 40. After a decrease in incidence in persons aged 40 to 55, the incidence peaks again in adults older than age 55. Of all the lymphomas, Hodgkin's disease is the most curable type even when the disease is widespread at the time of diagnosis.

Pathophysiology

Lymph nodes are made of tightly bound fibers and cells that serve as filtering devices for the body's immune system. Most often, Hodgkin's disease begins as a single changed lymph node, usually in the cervical lymph nodes of the neck. As the disease progresses, the cancer invades the lymph node chains node by node. The path of cancer infiltration is usually the same as the path of lymph fluid flow. Left untreated, other lymphoid tissues such as the spleen become infiltrated with Hodgkin's disease. The major organs eventually become involved. Common reports of patients with organ involvement include shortness of breath, feelings of fullness, weakness, and malaise. These organ-related symptoms usually motivate the patient to seek medical help.

A tentative diagnosis of Hodgkin's disease is based on one or more painlessly enlarged nodes in the cervical, axillary, or inguinal areas. A biopsy of several of the enlarged nodes is performed to search for the presence of Reed-Sternberg cells, which confirms the diagnosis.

Etiology

The exact cause of Hodgkin's disease is unknown. A possible viral origin has been proposed; it is more common in people who have had mononucleosis. Sometimes it occurs in families, suggesting a genetic link. Patients with

• WORD • BUILDING •
lymphoma: lymph—fluid found in lymphatic vessels + oma—tumor

impaired immune function, such as those with acquired immunodeficiency syndrome (AIDS) or those taking immunosuppressant drugs after organ transplant, are also at higher risk.

Signs and Symptoms

Painless swelling in one or more of the common lymph node chains is a usual presentation (Fig. 28.7). Swelling can range from barely perceptible to the size of a softball, occasionally even larger. The patient may report generalized pruritus. One other curious event, alcohol-induced pain, is occasionally present. With just a few sips of any type of alcohol-containing beverage (beer, wine, or liquor), the patient may describe intense pain at the site of disease. Because the lymph nodes in the upper chest and neck are often involved, the patient may have symptoms of obstruction, such as cough, dysphagia, or stridor.

Other common symptoms include persistent low-grade fever, night sweats, fatigue, weight loss, and malaise. When these additional symptoms are present, the prognosis is worse. In older adults, enlarged lymph nodes might not be

FIGURE 28.7 Cervical Hodgkin's disease. (A) Young boy with extensive cervical Hodgkin's disease. (B) Appearance several years later, when axillary manifestation developed. (C) Appearance 23 years after initial treatment with radiation. From del Regato, J. A., Spjut, H. J., & Cox, J. D. (1985). *Cancer: Diagnosis, treatment, and prognosis* (6th ed.). St. Louis, MO: Mosby, with permission.

visible, so these secondary symptoms may be the only presenting symptoms. Other symptoms associated with late-stage disease include edema of the neck and face, possible jaundice, nerve pain, enlargement of the retroperitoneal nodes, and infiltration of the spleen; liver and bones may also be involved.

Diagnostic Tests and Staging

Diagnosis usually begins with a lymph node biopsy of the easiest lymph node to access. Lymph node biopsies are done to check for abnormal histiocyte proliferation, nodular fibrosis, and necrosis. Other tests include bone marrow biopsy and aspiration, liver and spleen biopsies, routine chest x-ray examination, abdominal computed tomography (CT) scan to check for disease in the liver and spleen, lung scan, and bone scan. Lymphangiography may be performed to view the flow of lymph in the lymph network. A gallium scan can also be done to view lymph tissue.

Hematologic tests (e.g., CBC) may show wide variability of RBCs, indicating mild to severe anemia. The WBC count is often abnormal and extreme (either very high or very low) because of bone marrow infiltration by disease. These same tests are used for staging the disease into one of four stages:

- Stage I disease is limited to a single lymph node or site or a single organ.
- Stage II disease occurs when two or more nodes are involved on the same side of the diaphragm.
- Stage III disease affects nodes on both sides of the diaphragm.
- Stage IV, the most serious form of the disease and the least curable, includes widely disseminated disease in both lymph nodes and other organs such as bone marrow or liver.

Therapeutic Measures

Appropriate therapy includes the use of radiation and chemotherapy and depends on the stage of the disease. Radiation therapy, administered on an outpatient basis over a 4- to 6-week period, can cure most patients with stage I or stage II disease. Combinations of chemotherapy and radiation therapy are used for patients with stage III and stage IV disease. Results vary depending on the location and the stage of disease. If the disease recurs after initial treatment, bone marrow or stem cell transplant may be considered.

Nursing Management

Most nursing interventions are aimed at symptom management. If the patient is experiencing pruritus or night sweats, nursing interventions are aimed at alleviation of discomfort. These may include changing the gown and bed linens several times a night and helping the patient remain clean and dry. Keeping the patient and family involved in the plan of care may relieve anxiety.

Later, nursing interventions are tailored to alleviate problems that arise secondary to chemotherapy and radiation therapy. See Chapter 11 for nursing interventions for these problems. Also see the "Nursing Care Plan for the Patient With Lymphoma."

Patient Education

In addition to the teaching needs outlined above, make sure that the patient and the family know about local chapters of the American Cancer Society and the Leukemia and Lymphoma Society. Both of these organizations provide information, financial assistance, and counseling referral sources, which most patients find valuable. For more information visit the www.lls.org or www.cancer.org.

CRITICAL THINKING

Jeanie

■ Jeanie is a 60-year-old nurse diagnosed with stage II Hodgkin's disease. She wishes to continue working at her job on a respiratory unit at the local hospital while she undergoes treatment. What concerns do you have about this?

Suggested answers are at the end of the chapter.

NURSING CARE PLAN for the Patient With Lymphoma

Nursing Diagnosis: *Activity Intolerance* related to fatigue and anemia as evidenced by inability to carry out ADLs without excessive fatigue or dyspnea

Expected Outcome: The patient will have ADL needs met by self or caregiver as evidenced by patient statement of met needs.

Evaluation of Outcome: Is patient able to carry out ADLs or are ADL needs met by a caregiver?

Intervention Assess amount of activity that causes fatigue or dyspnea. **Rationale** Assessment helps guide plan of care. **Evaluation** How much can patient do before becoming fatigued or dyspneic?

Intervention Assist patient with activities as needed. **Rationale** The patient may need assistance with ADLs if fatigue is extreme. **Evaluation** Does the patient need assistance? Can family members assist?

Intervention Provide oxygen therapy as ordered. **Rationale** Oxygen therapy can increase oxygen levels and activity tolerance. **Evaluation** Does patient tolerate activity better with oxygen therapy?

Intervention Instruct patient to space rest with activities. **Rationale** Rest periods decrease oxygen needs and allow patient to conserve energy for next activity. **Evaluation** Is patient able to tolerate activity better after a rest period?

Nursing Diagnosis: *Risk for Infection* related to bone marrow involvement and side effects of treatment as evidenced by elevated temperature, redness, swelling, or other signs and symptoms based on infection site

Expected Outcome: The patient will remain infection free as evidenced by temperature within normal limits and no signs or symptoms of infection.

Evaluation of Outcome: Are signs and symptoms of infection absent? Is temperature within normal limits?

Intervention Assess patient for risk factors for infection. **Rationale** The WBC count may be very high or very low, placing the patient at risk for infection. **Evaluation** Is the patient at risk? Are additional interventions indicated?

Intervention Monitor patient for signs and symptoms of infection, such as cough, fever, malaise, erythema, pain, or drainage and report immediately. **Rationale** Early detection and treatment of infection provide the best results. **Evaluation** Are signs and symptoms of infection present?

Intervention Teach patient and significant others signs and symptoms of infection to watch for and report. **Rationale** The patient must be involved in monitoring for infection when at home. **Evaluation** Does patient verbalize understanding of signs and symptoms of infection and importance of reporting?

NURSING CARE PLAN for the Patient With Lymphoma—cont'd

Intervention Teach the patient to avoid exposure to others with influenza or other infections. **Rationale** Exposure increases risk for infection, especially with compromised immune function. **Evaluation** Does patient verbalize understanding of sources of infection to avoid?

Intervention Teach patient proper hand washing and good oral and personal hygiene. **Rationale** These activities reduce risk of infection. **Evaluation** Does patient demonstrate proper hand washing and hygiene?

Intervention Teach hand hygiene and infection risk reduction to family members. **Rationale** Family caregivers can be sources of infection. **Evaluation** Do family members demonstrate appropriate hand hygiene and infection control measures?

Nursing Diagnosis: *Ineffective Coping* related to new diagnosis and potential lifestyle changes to accommodate treatments as evidenced by poor problem solving, lack of goal-directed behavior, statement of poor coping

Expected Outcome: The patient will be able to cope effectively as evidenced by statement of ability to manage lifestyle changes and medical management of condition.

Evaluation of Outcome: Does patient carry out self-care necessary to manage treatment?

Intervention Assess patient's level of distress related to uncertainty about the future, bothersome symptoms, changes in self-concept, and past coping mechanisms. **Rationale** Obtaining information regarding past experiences helps the nurse identify and correct misconceptions. The nurse can support effective coping mechanisms that worked in the past. **Evaluation** Is patient able to identify sources of anxiety? Are past coping mechanisms effective?

Intervention Assess for signs of maladaptive behaviors that interfere with responsible health practices, such as missed appointments or failure to attend to symptoms. **Rationale** Long-term survival depends on keeping the scheduled therapy appointments. The ability to manage and report symptoms early keeps the patient out of the hospital and in control of his or her own life. **Evaluation** Does the patient keep appointments? Does the patient participate in self-care activities and report symptoms promptly?

Intervention Assist the patient to identify support systems and resources. Refer to social worker or other community resources as needed. **Rationale** Resources can assist with participation in treatment plan, home care, or financial assistance. **Evaluation** Are resources identified and helpful?

Intervention Refer patient and family to a cancer survivors' support group. **Rationale** Others who have been through treatment can be a good support for patients with cancer. **Evaluation** Does the patient state that the support group is helpful?

Non-Hodgkin's Lymphomas

All of the other types of lymphomas are clumped into a diverse classification known as the non-Hodgkin's lymphomas (NHLs). It is possible to sort these other types of lymphomas into different categories based on the degree of malignancy. Non-Hodgkin's lymphomas arise in the lymphoid tissues of the body, just as Hodgkin's disease does, but they differ in several ways (Table 28.4).

Pathophysiology

The most distinguishing difference is the absence of the Reed-Sternberg cells in NHL. Instead, many of these lymphomas arise from the B cells and T cells. The B cells are involved in recognizing and destroying specific antigens. Cells specifically involved include the memory B cells and the plasma cells. The T cells also are involved in registering antigens, but there are many more kinds of T cells. These include the amplifier T cells, helper T cells, suppressor T cells, memory T cells, cytotoxic T cells, and delayed hypersensitivity T cells. An abnormality in any of these cells can result in a type of NHL. Most cases of NHL are of B-cell origin. Cancerous cells are found most commonly in the lymph nodes, but they can also be found in other lymph tissues such as the tonsils, thymus, or bone marrow.

TABLE 28.4 HODGKIN'S DISEASE VERSUS NON-HODGKIN'S LYMPHOMA

	Hodgkin's Disease	Non-Hodgkin's Lymphomas
Age	15–40 and over 55 years	Usually over 50 years
Incidence	Less common	More common
Prognosis	Good	Poorer
Reed-Sternberg cells	Present	Absent
Alcohol-induced pain	May be present	Absent

Etiology

The cause of NHL is unclear, but some viruses, such as the Epstein-Barr and herpes viruses, are thought to play a role in their development. *Helicobacter pylori,* the bacterium that causes ulcers, has been associated with NHL. Genetics plays a role, as do immune problems such as AIDS. People working in farming, printing, medicine, electronics, and leather also have a higher risk for developing NHL.

Signs and Symptoms

Clinical features of malignant lymphomas include enlarged, painless, rubbery nodes in the cervical and supraclavicular areas, axillae, and groin; enlarged tonsils and adenoids; and occasional symptoms of dyspnea and cough. As the disease progresses, the patient may report fatigue, malaise, weight loss, and night sweats similar to Hodgkin's disease. NHL usually progresses more rapidly than Hodgkin's disease.

Diagnostic Tests

Diagnosis is confirmed by histological evaluation of biopsied lymph nodes, tonsils, bone marrow, liver, bowel, skin, or other affected tissues. Other relevant tests include bone scans, chest x-rays, lymphangiography, liver and spleen scans, CT of the abdomen, MRI, positron emission tomography (PET) scan, and IV pyelogram to determine the extent of the disease. Laboratory tests include a CBC (which often indicates anemia), serum uric acid level, and liver function studies. Serum calcium level may be elevated if bone lesions are present.

Therapeutic Measures

Treatment usually involves multimodal therapy, including the use of chemotherapy and radiation therapy in combination. Radiation therapy is given to affected areas in advanced stages of NHL. Stem cell transplant may be tried in patients with advanced disease. Newer therapies include the use of monoclonal antibodies to target and destroy cancer cells and interferon therapy to help boost the immune system to fight the cancer.

Nursing Management

You can provide emotional support by keeping the patient and family informed during the testing phase. Symptoms such as night sweats can be managed with frequent linen and gown changes. Help the patient maintain nutrition with attractively prepared meals. Spend time listening to the patient's concerns; involve the hospital chaplain in the patient's care if the patient desires. See Table 28.5 and the "Nursing Care Plan for the Patient with Lymphoma" for more information.

■ SPLENIC DISORDERS

The spleen is involved in a number of disorders, including cancers of the blood, lymph, and bone marrow; hereditary conditions such as SCD; and acquired problems such as idiopathic thrombocytopenia. Under normal circumstances, the spleen is not paid much attention; it generally performs its functions without much fanfare.

If the spleen enlarges markedly, the condition is referred to as **splenomegaly**. Other times, the spleen may or may not be enlarged, but the function is out of control so that too many RBCs and platelets are removed from the peripheral circulation. Sometimes the spleen is not able to perform its job because of bleeding into the pulp of the organ, which renders it useless. Bleeding into the spleen can occur from various illnesses or from trauma. Regardless of the nature of the malfunction, one treatment option may be splenectomy.

Splenectomy

Splenectomy is the surgical removal of the spleen. This is sometimes used to treat selective hematologic disorders and

---

• WORD • BUILDING •
splenomegaly: splen—spleen + megaly—large
splenectomy: splen—spleen + ectomy—excision

TABLE 28.5 LYMPHOMA SUMMARY

Signs and Symptoms	Swollen lymph nodes Fatigue Low-grade fever Night sweats
Diagnostic Tests	CBC Lymph node biopsy Lymphangiography CT scan
Therapeutic Measures	Chemotherapy Radiation Bone marrow or stem cell transplant
Priority Nursing Diagnoses	*Activity Intolerance* *Risk for Infection* *Risk for Ineffective Coping*

is also used, under different circumstances, to determine the stage of lymphomas. It may be done with traditional, open surgery or laparoscopically. Splenectomy is performed fairly often in the United States, but, like any surgery, it is not without risk. Some patients have splenic autotransplantation, which involves implantation of some of the removed tissue, usually in the peritoneal cavity. This allows for return of some splenic function.

Patient Education

Explain to patients that this surgery removes the spleen, usually under general anesthesia. Inform patients that they can live a normal life after the surgery but that they may be more prone to infection and that they should receive the influenza vaccine each year, preferably in the early autumn.

Preoperative Care

Before the surgery, ensure that the CBC and coagulation profile are completed and reported to the HCP. Blood transfusion may be ordered to correct underlying anemia and to prepare for the loss of a great deal of blood stored in the spleen. Vitamin K is often ordered to correct clotting factor deficiencies.

Check the patient's vital signs, and perform a baseline respiratory assessment. Note especially any signs of respiratory infections such as fever, chills, crackles, wheezes, or cough. If any of these are noted, make sure that the surgeon is aware of them because surgery may need to be delayed. Teach the patient routine coughing and deep-breathing techniques to help prevent postoperative respiratory complications.

Postoperative Care

During the early postoperative period, watch carefully for bleeding, either external or internal. Be prepared to administer opioids for pain, usually on an around-the-clock schedule so the patient is comfortable enough to deep breathe, cough, and ambulate. After opioid administration, be sure to observe for side effects, which may include incomplete pain relief or hypoventilation. Monitor for fever every 4 hours, and expect a mild, low-grade, transient fever postoperatively. A persistent fever may indicate abscess or hematoma formation.

If the surgery was performed to decrease the numbers of cells being removed from the peripheral circulation, monitor the platelet count. Often the count begins to rise in just a few days, but it may take up to 2 weeks for the platelets to normalize.

Complications

A splenectomy can lead to complications such as bleeding, pneumonia, and atelectasis (collapsed alveoli). Respiratory problems occur because of the spleen's position close to the diaphragm. This placement requires the need for a high surgical incision that is very painful. Often the patient tries to restrict lung expansion after surgery to keep from hurting, but this splinting behavior may leave the patient at risk for pneumonia and respiratory problems. In addition, splenectomy

patients are usually more vulnerable to infection, especially influenza, because the spleen's role in the immune response is no longer filled.

Another possible complication of splenectomy includes the development of pancreatitis. This is because the tail of the pancreas is close to the spleen, and irritation may have occurred.

Another serious complication is overwhelming postsplenectomy infection (OPSI). The causative agents in OPSI include streptococci, *Neisseria* spp., and influenza bacteria (as opposed to a flu virus). OPSI can occur at any time from 1 week to 20 years after the splenectomy. Patients most at risk are those with poor immune function.

Early symptoms of OPSI include fever and malaise that seem unremarkable. However, the infection may progress within a few hours to sepsis and death. Unfortunately, OPSI has a mortality rate as high as 70%. Be sure to include the signs and symptoms of OPSI in presplenectomy patient education. Also, stress the need to promptly obtain medical attention for the patient at the first signs and symptoms of OPSI. The patient should be directed to continue to receive lifetime vaccinations against these bacteria.

Home Health Hints

- Patients who are at risk for infection can place a sign on the front door of their homes to limit visitors or ask persons with colds to come back when they are well. The patient may appreciate the home nurse giving permission to be assertive in such circumstances.
- Teach patients with infection risk to avoid working with dirt or soil, to avoid manicures and pedicures, to avoid hot tubs or Jacuzzis, and to wash hands after contact with pets, fresh flowers, or plants.
- To prevent bruising, have the patient cut the feet off of long, white sport socks and wear them on the arms. They can be hidden under long-sleeve shirts and blouses and provide a cushion when doing housework.
- Teach patients with thrombocytopenia to avoid contact sports and to consult with their HCP about whether sexual intercourse is safe.
- Teach patients with thrombocytopenia to avoid over-the-counter medications unless approved by the HCP. Many such agents contain aspirin or nonsteroidal anti-inflammatory drugs (NSAIDs).
- Patients with sickle cell anemia usually have lower blood pressures. It is important to report even mild hypertension in these patients.
- If fatigue or nausea causes poor appetite, discuss eating smaller, more frequent meals. Ask the HCP for an antiemetic order if needed.

SUGGESTED ANSWERS TO

CRITICAL THINKING

■ *Mrs. Johns*

1. Monitor Mrs. Johns's vital signs and report falling blood pressure and rising pulse immediately. Inspect her skin for petechiae and ecchymoses. Outline ecchymotic areas with a marker to see if the area is increasing in size. Monitor urine for signs of blood. Test stools for occult blood. Monitor vaginal discharge for increasing bleeding. Report any changes promptly.

2. Anticipate assisting the RN with administration of blood or blood products. Instruct Mrs. Johns in the importance of preventing injury that could cause further bleeding. Other care will be supportive.

3. Mrs. Johns will be concerned for her new baby, who is most likely on another unit or already discharged home. Allow Mrs. Johns to talk about her concerns. Arrange visits with her family and baby if permitted by her condition and her HCP.

4.

$$\frac{300 \text{ mL}}{30 \text{ min}} \left| \frac{60 \text{ min}}{1 \text{ hour}} \right. = 600 \text{ mL per hour}$$

5. Collaborate with the RN, internist, obstetrician, hematologist, neonatal nurse, husband, family, and social worker to provide holistic, patient-centered care for this new mother.

■ *Mr. Washington*

1. Because of his leukemia and his treatment, Mr. Washington is at risk for infection. If he develops an infection, he will have great difficulty getting over it. With so many visitors in the room, it is likely that one or more has a cold or virus. They may not be aware of the risk this poses to Mr. Washington. Mr. Washington is probably also fatigued because of his disease and treatment, and visiting requires energy.

2. You should kindly explain that although family visits are important, Mr. Washington is very susceptible to catching colds or other illnesses and that it would be best to limit visitors to one or two at a time. Point out that persons with symptoms of colds or flu should not enter the room at all. Visits should also be brief to prevent overtiring the patient.

   Ask Mr. Washington about his preferences, and attempt to honor them if possible. He may choose one or two (healthy!) visitors to come regularly, or choose a time of day when he is less fatigued to have visitors. As his nurse, you can help enforce visiting limitations so Mr. Washington does not have to feel ungracious toward his visitors.

■ *Jeanie*

Jeanie will probably be fatigued from her disease, and fatigue may increase further as a side effect of treatment. Staff nursing jobs can be tiring even for healthy nurses. In addition, she will be around patients with respiratory diseases, many of whom are contagious. Because of the risk of infection secondary to the disease process and the treatment regimen, Jeanie might want to take a leave of absence during treatment or ask to be reassigned to an area that is less demanding and away from direct patient care until her treatments have been completed.

REVIEW QUESTIONS

1. The nurse is caring for a patient admitted with pancytopenia with complaints of dyspnea upon exertion. This symptom would be most directly related to which condition?
   1. Pain
   2. Thrombocytopenia
   3. Anemia
   4. Neutropenia

2. A nurse is teaching a patient with sickle cell anemia about activities to avoid. Which of the following activities the patient plans to do shows that more teaching is needed?
   1. Going to the beach
   2. Taking a long car trip
   3. Running in a marathon
   4. Listening to a concert

3. The family of a patient with DIC has questions about the bleeding that is occurring. Which statement by the nurse is the best response to explain why the patient is bleeding?
   1. "He is bleeding because he does not have enough RBCs."
   2. "He is bleeding because his white cells are depleted."
   3. "He is bleeding because his blood pressure is so high that it forces blood from mucous membranes."
   4. "He is bleeding because his body's clotting factors have all been used up."

4. The nurse is teaching the parent of a child with hemophilia. Which of the following statement by the parent demonstrates understanding about preventing bleeding episodes?
   1. "My son will have to avoid contact sports."
   2. "My son will have to avoid irritating foods in his diet."
   3. "My son will have to grow a beard."
   4. "My son will always have to live near a major hospital."

5. Which family member should be restricted from visiting a patient with newly diagnosed leukemia?
   1. The one who has a new baby at home
   2. The one who has a history of asthma
   3. The one who has received recent radiation treatment for cancer
   4. The one who has a runny nose

6. Which of the following nursing interventions is a priority for the patient with multiple myeloma found in the ribs and femur?
   1. Implement safety measures to prevent falls.
   2. Assist with all ADLs.
   3. Provide a high-protein, low-sodium diet.
   4. Institute neutropenic precautions.

7. Which of the following nursing interventions are appropriate for a patient with thrombocytopenia? **Select all that apply.**
   1. Avoid intramuscular injections.
   2. Keep visitors who are ill away from the patient.
   3. Encourage 4 L of fluid daily.
   4. Avoid use of aspirin and NSAIDs.
   5. Allow rest between activities.
   6. Encourage use of shoes or slippers.

8. A patient with hypercalcemia needs to drink at least 3 L of fluid per day. Today, he has had 1 measuring cup of coffee, 1 L of water, a can of soda that says it has 355 mL, and a half cup of juice. How many milliliters has he had so far today? **Fill in the blank.**
   Answer: _____ mL

9. What assessment data will best help the nurse determine if interventions for neutropenia have been effective?
   1. Temperature
   2. Fatigue level
   3. Oxygen saturation
   4. Hemoglobin level

10. Which circumstance places the patient at most risk for postoperative pneumonia following a splenectomy?
    1. Disturbance of clotting factors
    2. Nothing by mouth (NPO) status
    3. Need for frequent dressing changes
    4. Location of surgical incision

Answers can be found in Appendix C.

References

Brandow, A., & O'Brien, S. (2010). Is patient compliance a significant barrier to hydroxyurea treatment of children with sickle cell disease? *HemOnc Today.* Retrieved July 12, 2013, from www.healio.com/hematology-oncology/news/print/hematology-oncology/%7B07ce7dc3-c132-40f2-aab3-885e1dffef5d%7D/is-patient-compliance-a-significant-barrier-to-hydroxyurea-treatment-ofchildren-with-sickle-cell-disease

Johns Hopkins. (2012). Half-match bone marrow transplants wipe out SCD in selected patients. Retrieved June 20, 2013, from www.hopkinsmedicine.org/news/media/releases/half_match_bone_marrow_transplants_wipe_out_sickle_cell_disease_in_selected_patients

Cancer.net. (2012). Multiple myeloma. Retrieved July 10, 2013, from www.cancer.net/cancer-types/multiple-myeloma/statistics

 For additional resources and information visit **davispl.us/medsurg5**

unit SEVEN

Understanding the Respiratory System

29

Respiratory System Function, Assessment, and Therapeutic Measures

KEY TERMS

adventitious (add-ven-TISH-uss)
apnea (AP-nee-ah)
crepitus (KREP-ih-tuss)
cyanosis (SY-uh-NOH-siss)
dyspnea (DISP-nee-ah)
respiratory excursion (RESS-prah-TOR-ee eks-KUR-zhun)
retraction (rih-TRAK-shun)
thoracentesis (THOR-uh-sen-TEE-siss)
tidaling (TY-dah-ling)
tracheostomy (TRAY-key-AW-stuh-mee)
tracheotomy (TRAY-key-AW-tuh-mee)

PAULA D. HOPPER AND
JANICE L. BRADFORD

LEARNING OUTCOMES

1. Describe the normal structures and functions of the respiratory system.
2. Identify how aging affects the respiratory system.
3. List data to collect when caring for a patient with a respiratory disorder.
4. Recognize expected findings when inspecting, palpating, percussing, and auscultating the chest.
5. Identify common diagnostic tests performed to diagnose disorders of the respiratory system.
6. Plan nursing care for patients undergoing each of the diagnostic tests.
7. Discuss therapeutic measures used to help patients with respiratory disorders.

592

NORMAL RESPIRATORY SYSTEM ANATOMY AND PHYSIOLOGY

The respiratory system is basically a tract, divided into upper and lower respiratory portions. The upper tract is above the thoracic cavity, and the lower portion is within the thoracic cavity. The alveoli of the lungs are the site of gas exchange between the air and the blood of pulmonary circulation; the rest of the system moves air into and out of the lungs. Together with the cardiovascular system, the respiratory system supplies the body with oxygen and eliminates carbon dioxide.

Nose and Nasal Cavities

The nose is made mostly of bone and cartilage covered with muscle and epithelium. Hairs inside the nostrils block the entry of dust and other particles. The nasal cavities are separated at midline by the nasal septum, which is made of bone and cartilage. The nasal mucosa is highly vascular, ciliated epithelium that warms and moistens inhaled air. Dust and microorganisms become trapped on mucus produced by goblet cells and are swept back into the pharynx by the cilia. See Table 29.1 for a summary of protective mechanisms in the respiratory system.

The paranasal sinuses are air cavities in the maxillary, frontal, sphenoid, and ethmoid bones that open into the nasal cavities, releasing mucus. The sinuses lessen the weight of the skull and provide resonance for the voice.

Pharynx

The pharynx is posterior to the nasal and oral cavities. It has three regions (Figure 29.1). The soft palate and uvula rise to block the nasopharynx during swallowing. The lingual tonsils, the adenoid (pharyngeal tonsil), and the palatine tonsils form a ring of lymphatic tissue around the pharynx and destroy pathogens that penetrate the mucosa.

Larynx

The larynx is the airway between the pharynx and trachea. It houses the vocal cords and produces sound that can be formed

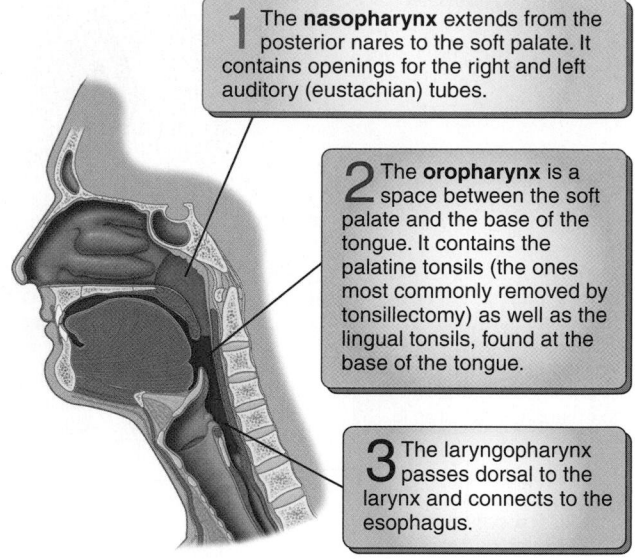

1. The **nasopharynx** extends from the posterior nares to the soft palate. It contains openings for the right and left auditory (eustachian) tubes.

2. The **oropharynx** is a space between the soft palate and the base of the tongue. It contains the palatine tonsils (the ones most commonly removed by tonsillectomy) as well as the lingual tonsils, found at the base of the tongue.

3. The laryngopharynx passes dorsal to the larynx and connects to the esophagus.

FIGURE 29.1 Pharynx. From Thompson, G. S. (2013). *Understanding anatomy and physiology.* Philadelphia: F.A. Davis, p. 328.

into speech. The epiglottis at the top of the larynx prevents ingested materials from entering the trachea (Figure 29.2). The cartilaginous walls are lined with ciliated epithelium. The vagus and accessory cranial nerves innervate the larynx.

Trachea and Bronchial Tree

The trachea descends from the larynx to the primary bronchi (Figure 29.3). The mucosa is ciliated epithelium; mucus with trapped dust and microorganisms is swept upward toward the pharynx and is swallowed.

Deeper into the bronchial tree, cartilage diminishes, and smooth muscle in the walls increases. The bronchioles have no cartilage in the walls to maintain patency, therefore they can be closed completely by bronchoconstriction.

Lungs and Pleural Membranes

The lungs occupy the thoracic cavity on each side of the heart, extending from the clavicles to the diaphragm, and are protected by the ribs (costae). On the medial (mediastinal) surface of each lung is an indentation called the hilus, where the primary bronchus and the pulmonary vessels enter the lung (Figure 29.4). A thin layer of fluid between the visceral and parietal pleural membranes provides lubrication to reduce friction during lung expansion.

The functional units of the lungs are the millions of alveoli, the air sacs where gas exchange occurs. Both the alveoli and the surrounding alveolar capillaries are made of simple squamous epithelium; that is, their walls are only one cell in thickness to permit diffusion of gases (see Fig. 29.5).

Each alveolus is lined with a thin layer of tissue fluid that is essential for the diffusion of gases, but the surface tension of the fluid tends to make the walls of an alveolus stick together internally. Alveolar cells secrete *surfactant,* a lipoprotein that mixes with the tissue fluid and decreases surface tension to permit inflation.

TABLE 29.1 PROTECTIVE MECHANISMS IN THE RESPIRATORY SYSTEM

Nasal hairs and turbinates	Trap dust and microorganisms.
Mucous membranes	Warm and moisten inhaled air; trap inhaled particles.
Cilia	Move particles toward pharynx to be swallowed or coughed out.
Irritant receptors in nose and airways	Trigger sneeze and cough to remove foreign debris.
Alveolar macrophages	Phagocytize foreign particles and bacteria.

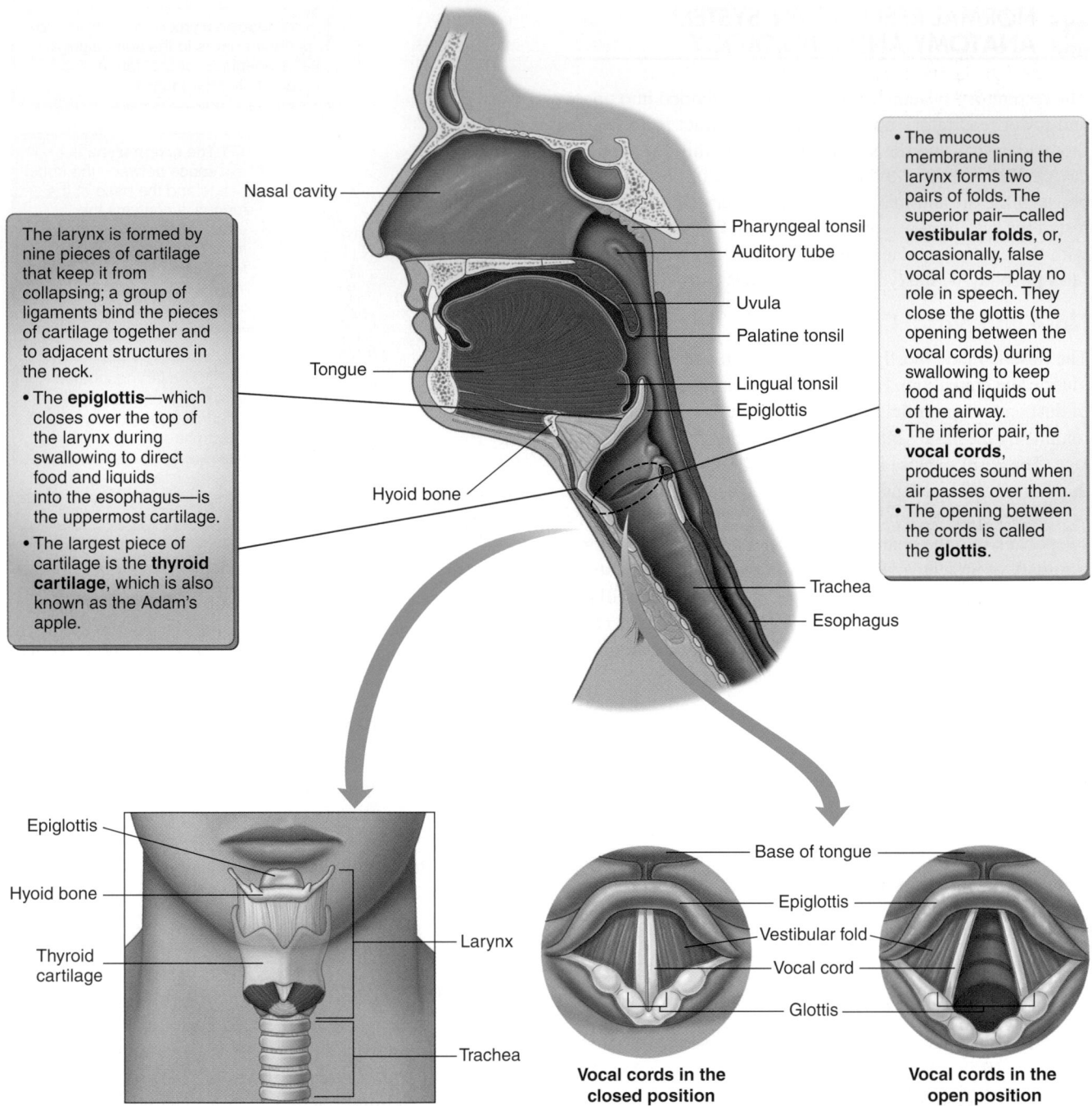

The larynx is formed by nine pieces of cartilage that keep it from collapsing; a group of ligaments bind the pieces of cartilage together and to adjacent structures in the neck.
- The **epiglottis**—which closes over the top of the larynx during swallowing to direct food and liquids into the esophagus—is the uppermost cartilage.
- The largest piece of cartilage is the **thyroid cartilage**, which is also known as the Adam's apple.

- The mucous membrane lining the larynx forms two pairs of folds. The superior pair—called **vestibular folds**, or, occasionally, false vocal cords—play no role in speech. They close the glottis (the opening between the vocal cords) during swallowing to keep food and liquids out of the airway.
- The inferior pair, the **vocal cords**, produces sound when air passes over them.
- The opening between the cords is called the **glottis**.

Nasal cavity

Pharyngeal tonsil
Auditory tube

Uvula
Palatine tonsil

Tongue

Lingual tonsil
Epiglottis

Hyoid bone

Trachea
Esophagus

Epiglottis
Hyoid bone
Thyroid cartilage

Larynx

Trachea

Base of tongue
Epiglottis
Vestibular fold
Vocal cord
Glottis

Vocal cords in the closed position

Vocal cords in the open position

FIGURE 29.2 Larynx. From Thompson, G. S. (2013). *Understanding anatomy and physiology.* Philadelphia: F.A. Davis, p. 329.

Between clusters of alveoli is elastic connective tissue that can stretch during inhalation and recoil during exhalation. The recoil of this tissue allows passive exhalation without the expenditure of energy.

Mechanism of Breathing

Ventilation is the term for the movement of air into and out of the alveoli. The primary respiratory muscles are the diaphragm, inferior to the lungs, and the external intercostal muscles, between the ribs. Accessory muscles of respiration are used during exercise and times of respiratory distress. These include muscles for deep inspiration (sternocleidomastoid, scalene, pectoralis minor) and for forced expiration (internal intercostal muscles and abdominal musculature; Figure 29.6). Respiratory centers of the brain, located in the medulla oblongata and pons, innervate muscles of respiration via the intercostal and phrenic nerves. A normal respiratory rate is 12 to 20 breaths/minute.

Ventilation is accomplished by respiratory muscle contractions, causing changes in lung volumes. Movement of air follows Boyle's Law, which states that in a closed container of gases, volume and pressure are inversely related. Air moves from high-pressure to low-pressure areas.

Trachea

Lying just in front of the esophagus, the trachea is a rigid tube about 4.5 inches (11 cm) long and 1 inch (2.5 cm) wide. C-shaped rings of cartilage encircle the trachea to reinforce it and keep it from collapsing during inhalation. The open part of the "C" faces posteriorly, giving the esophagus room to expand during swallowing.

The trachea extends from the larynx to a cartilaginous ridge called the **carina**.

Bronchial Tree

At the carina, the trachea branches into two primary bronchi. Like the trachea, the primary bronchi are supported by C-shaped rings of cartilage. (All of the divisions of the bronchial tree also consist of elastic connective tissue.)

The right bronchus is slightly wider and more vertical than the left, making this the most likely location for aspirated (inhaled) food particles and small objects to lodge.

Immediately after entering the lungs, the primary bronchi branch into **secondary bronchi**: one for each of the lung's lobes. Since the left lung consists of two lobes, it has two secondary bronchi; the right lung has three lobes, so it has three bronchi.

Secondary bronchi branch into smaller **tertiary bronchi**. The cartilaginous rings become irregular and disappear entirely in the smaller bronchioles.

Tertiary bronchi continue to branch, resulting in very small airways called **bronchioles**. Less than 1 mm wide and lacking any supportive cartilage, bronchioles divide further to form thin-walled passages called **alveolar ducts**.

Alveolar ducts throughout the lungs terminate in clusters of alveoli called **alveolar sacs**, the primary structures for gas exchange.

Larynx

Left primary bronchus

Left secondary bronchus

Left tertiary bronchus

Bronchioles

FIGURE 29.3 Trachea and bronchial tree. From Thompson, G. S. (2013). *Understanding anatomy and physiology*. Philadelphia: F.A. Davis, p. 330.

Inhalation

Inhalation, also called inspiration, occurs when motor impulses from the medulla cause contraction of the respiratory muscles. Impulses travel along the phrenic nerves and cause the dome-shaped diaphragm to contract and flatten inferiorly. Intercostal nerves cause the external intercostal muscles to expand the thoracic cavity in the anteroposterior dimension. These movements then expand the pleural membranes and therefore the lungs due to adhesion from serous fluid. As the lungs expand, alveolar pressure falls below atmospheric pressure, and air enters the nose and respiratory passages. A deeper inhalation requires a more forceful contraction of the respiratory muscles (including accessory inspiratory muscles) to expand the thoracic cavity and lungs even further. Ease of thoracic and lung expansion is called compliance.

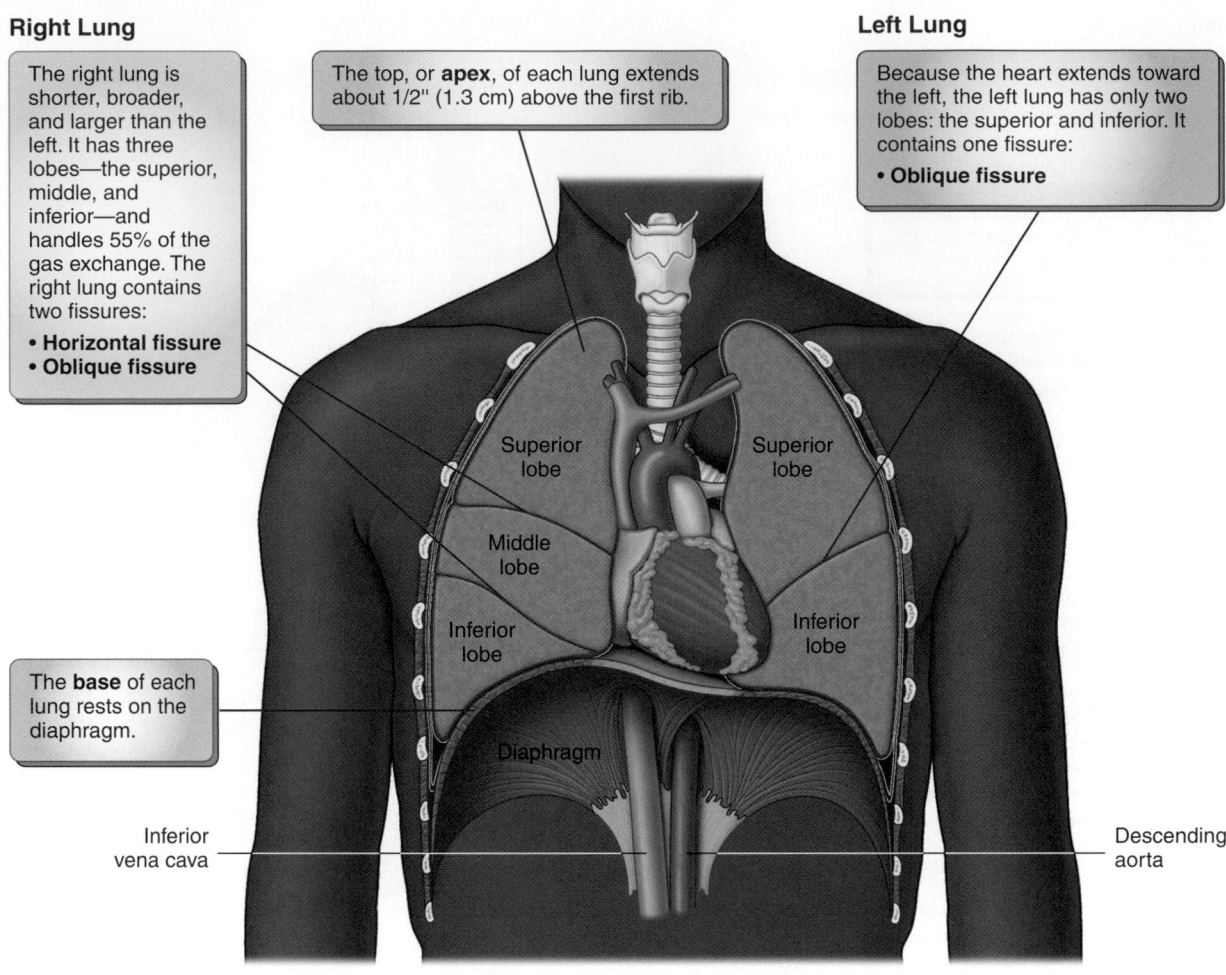

Right Lung

The right lung is shorter, broader, and larger than the left. It has three lobes—the superior, middle, and inferior—and handles 55% of the gas exchange. The right lung contains two fissures:
• **Horizontal fissure**
• **Oblique fissure**

The top, or **apex**, of each lung extends about 1/2" (1.3 cm) above the first rib.

Left Lung

Because the heart extends toward the left, the left lung has only two lobes: the superior and inferior. It contains one fissure:
• **Oblique fissure**

Superior lobe

Superior lobe

Middle lobe

Inferior lobe

Inferior lobe

The **base** of each lung rests on the diaphragm.

Diaphragm

Inferior vena cava

Descending aorta

FIGURE 29.4 Lungs. From Thompson, G. S. (2013). *Understanding anatomy and physiology.* Philadelphia: F.A. Davis, p. 332.

Exhalation

Normal exhalation is a passive process. The lungs are compressed as the thoracic cavity reduces volume and the recoil of the elastic lung tissue compresses the alveoli. Alveolar pressure rises above atmospheric pressure, and air is forced out of the lungs. At rest, energy is not used in exhalation because no muscle contraction is required. Forced exhalation is an active process, requiring contraction of the internal intercostal muscles compressing the thorax, and abdominal muscles that force the diaphragm superiorly, increasing compression of the lungs.

Transport of Gases in the Blood

Ninety-eight-and-a-half percent of oxygen is carried in the blood, bound to iron of hemoglobin (Hgb) in red blood cells (RBCs). Oxyhemoglobin is formed in the lungs, where the partial pressure of oxygen (PO_2) is high. In tissues where the PO_2 is low, hemoglobin releases much of its oxygen. The remaining oxygen is dissolved in the plasma.

Most carbon dioxide (70%) is carried as bicarbonate ion in the blood plasma. These ions form when carbon dioxide enters RBCs and is converted to carbonic acid (H_2CO_3), which ionizes into bicarbonate ions (HCO_3^-) and hydrogen ions (H+). The bicarbonate ions leave the RBCs for the plasma, and the remaining hydrogen ions are buffered by the hemoglobin in the RBCs. When the blood reaches the lungs, an area of lower partial pressure of carbon dioxide (PCO_2), these reactions are reversed—carbon dioxide is reformed and diffuses into the alveoli to be exhaled. Carbon dioxide is also transported as carbaminohemoglobin (23%) and dissolved in plasma (7%).

Chemical Regulation and Respiration

Chemoreceptors (in the carotid and aortic bodies), monitor blood levels of oxygen, carbon dioxide, and pH. The medulla responds by increasing respiration during hypoxemia, hypercapnia, and/or acidemia.

Respiration and Acid–Base Balance

Because of its role in regulating the amount of carbon dioxide in body fluids, the respiratory system is important in the maintenance of acid–base balance, measured by blood pH. Any decrease in the rate or efficiency of respiration permits excess carbon dioxide to accumulate in the blood. The

Pulmonary venule
Terminal bronchiole
Pulmonary arteriole
Alveolar duct

The alveoli are wrapped in a fine mesh of capillaries. The extremely thin walls of the alveoli, and the closeness of the capillaries, allow for efficient gas exchange.

The exchange of air occurs through what's called the **respiratory membrane**, which consists of the alveolar epithelium, the capillary endothelium, and their joined basement membranes.

Alveolar sac

Alveoli

Alveoli

O_2

CO_2

Capillary

FIGURE 29.5 Alveoli. From Thompson, G. S. (2013). *Understanding anatomy and physiology.* Philadelphia: F.A. Davis, p. 331.

resulting accumulation of excess hydrogen ions lowers pH. This is called respiratory acidosis and can occur as a consequence of pulmonary disease or any impairment of gas exchange in the lungs.

Respiratory alkalosis occurs when the rate of respiration increases, eliminating exhaled carbon dioxide rapidly. Less carbon dioxide in the blood means fewer hydrogen ions are formed and the pH rises. Although it is not a common condition, respiratory alkalosis may occur during states of anxiety and hyperventilation, or when acclimating to a high altitude, before RBC production increases to provide sufficient oxygenation of tissues.

The respiratory system also helps compensate for pH changes that are metabolic—that is, due to any cause other than respiratory. Metabolic acidosis occurs when the concentration of hydrogen ions in body fluids is above normal due to lowered HCO_3^- buffer. Common causes include kidney disease, uncontrolled diabetes mellitus, and severe

diarrhea. Respiratory compensation involves an increase in the rate and depth of respiration to exhale more carbon dioxide, which decreases hydrogen ion formation and raises the pH toward normal. Metabolic alkalosis can be caused by overingestion of antacid medications or by vomiting acidic gastric contents. Respiratory compensation involves a decrease in the breathing rate to retain carbon dioxide in the body, increasing the formation of hydrogen ions, which lowers the pH toward normal.

Respiratory compensation for an ongoing metabolic pH imbalance (such as kidney failure) cannot be complete because the amount of carbon dioxide that may be exhaled or retained is limited. At most, respiratory compensation is only about 75% effective.

Acid–base balance is discussed further in Chapter 6.

Effects of Aging on the Respiratory System
See Figure 29.7 for the effects of aging on respiration.

Inspiration

- The **external intercostal** muscles pull the ribs upward and outward, widening the thoracic cavity.

- The **internal intercostals** help elevate the ribs.

- The **diaphragm** contracts, flattens, and drops, pressing the abdominal organs downward and enlarging the thoracic cavity.

- Air rushes in to equalize pressure.

Expiration

- The **internal intercostal** muscles pull the ribs downward as the external intercostals relax.

- The **diaphragm** relaxes, bulging upward and pressing against the base of the lungs, reducing the size of the thoracic cavity.

- Air is pushed out of the lungs.

Sternocleidomastoid
Scalenes
Pectoralis minor
External abdominal oblique
Rectus abdominis

FIGURE 29.6 Respiratory muscles. From Thompson, G. S. (2013). *Understanding anatomy and physiology*. Philadelphia: F.A. Davis, p. 334.

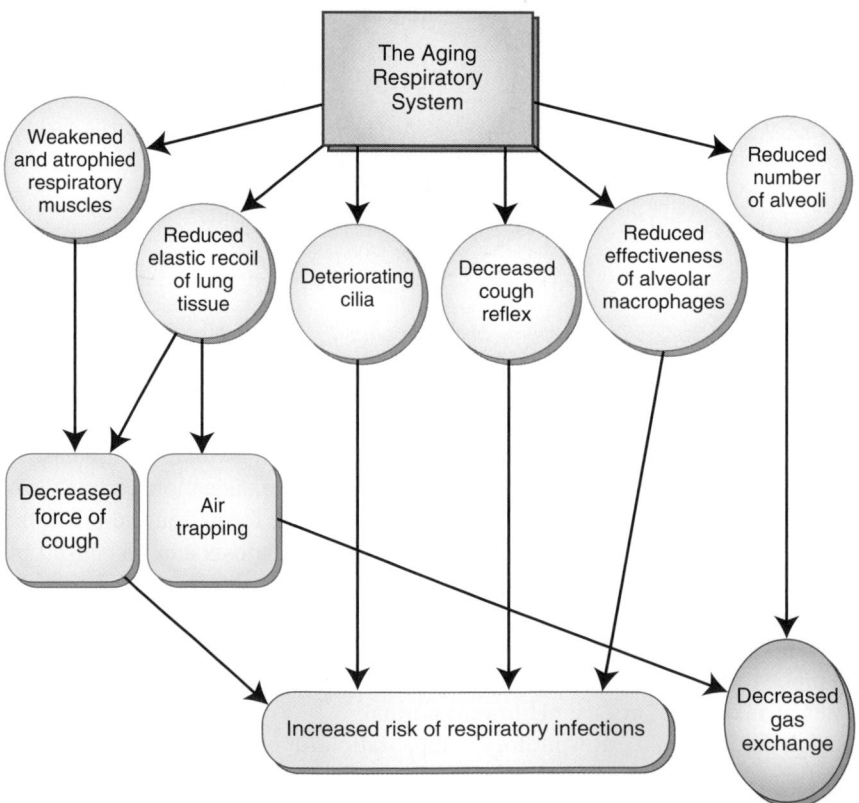

The Aging Respiratory System

Weakened and atrophied respiratory muscles

Reduced elastic recoil of lung tissue

Deteriorating cilia

Decreased cough reflex

Reduced effectiveness of alveolar macrophages

Reduced number of alveoli

Decreased force of cough

Air trapping

Increased risk of respiratory infections

Decreased gas exchange

FIGURE 29.7 Effects of aging on respiration.

NURSING ASSESSMENT OF THE RESPIRATORY SYSTEM

Health History

Many factors in a patient's personal and family history affect respiratory function. Questions to ask while assessing the patient with a history of respiratory dysfunction are presented in Table 29.2. If at any time while you are taking the history the patient relates a specific symptom, redirect the line of questioning to further assess that symptom. One such line of questioning, as presented in Chapter 1, is the **WHAT'S UP?** format. For example, if the patient reports shortness of breath, respond with the following questions:

- *Where is it?* (Doesn't apply to shortness of breath, so it may be skipped.)
- **H**ow does it feel? Does your breathing feel tight, gasping, painful, suffocating?
- **A**ggravating and alleviating factors? How much activity causes your shortness of breath? Does anything else aggravate it? What do you do to lessen your shortness of breath?

TABLE 29.2 SUBJECTIVE DATA COLLECTION FOR THE RESPIRATORY SYSTEM

Category	Questions to Ask During the Health History	Rationale/Significance
Upper Respiratory Tract	Do you often have headaches or sinus tenderness? Do you often experience nosebleeds? Has your voice changed?	These may indicate sinusitis. A history of nosebleeds may indicate an abnormality that can predispose to future nosebleeds. A voice change may indicate a variety of disorders of the nose or throat, including cancer.
Lower Respiratory Tract	Do you ever feel short of breath, like you can't get enough air? Do you have a cough? Is it productive? What does the sputum look like? Have you recently experienced night sweats, chills, or fever? Do you ever feel confused, light-headed, or restless? Have you had any chest surgeries?	Many respiratory and cardiac problems result in shortness of breath. A cough indicates respiratory irritation or excessive secretions. Yellow, tan, or green sputum may accompany an infection. Blood in the sputum is usually serious; it can occur with pneumonia, tuberculosis, pulmonary embolism, or cancer. These are symptoms of tuberculosis. These symptoms might indicate a low PO_2, reducing oxygen to the brain. This may reveal problem areas the patient has not yet mentioned.
Exposures	Do you have any allergies that cause respiratory symptoms? How do you treat them? Do you smoke? How many packs per day? For how many years? Are you exposed to environmental smoke? Have you been exposed to airborne pollutants at home or work?	The patient may take over-the-counter medications for allergies that affect respiratory function or interact with prescribed medications. Many respiratory disorders are caused or aggravated by exposure to tobacco smoke. Pollutants such as asbestos, radon, coal dust, or chemicals can cause lung disease.
Treatments	Do you take any medications or use inhalers (prescribed or over-the-counter) for your respiratory problems? Do you use home oxygen or other home respiratory treatments?	Information about medications gives further information about disorders, severity, and treatment. You should also consider drug interactions and side effects. This helps determine the severity of disease and the treatment.
Family History	Do any of your blood relatives have respiratory problems such as emphysema, asthma, or tuberculosis?	Some respiratory disorders have a hereditary tendency. Tuberculosis is contagious.

- **T**iming? When did you first experience shortness of breath? Does it happen more at any particular time of day or year?
- **S**everity? Rate your shortness of breath on a scale of 0 to 10, with 0 being easy breathing and 10 being the worst shortness of breath you can imagine.
- **U**seful other data? Do you have any other symptoms that occur along with the shortness of breath?
- **P**atient's perception? What do you think is causing your shortness of breath?

Because smoking is such a major risk factor for many types of lung disease, it is essential to ask about smoking history and encourage the patient to quit (see the discussion of smoking cessation later in this chapter). Document the patient's smoking history in terms of pack-years. For example, if a patient has smoked two packs of cigarettes per day for 20 years, he has a 40 pack-year smoking history ($2 \times 20 = 40$ pack-years). It is also important to be aware of cultural influences on the patient's respiratory health (see "Cultural Considerations").

Physical Examination

Inspection

Inspection begins during the nursing history and continues during the physical assessment. Start with the nose, observing for symmetry, swelling, or other abnormalities. Note whether the patient is short of breath while speaking or moving. If the patient feels very breathless, he or she may speak in short sentences.

Observe the patient for use of accessory muscles of breathing (Fig. 29.8). Use of the sternocleidomastoid muscles causes the shoulders to rise during labored inspiration. During forced expiration, the abdominal and intercostal muscles contract. The use of accessory muscles for breathing indicates respiratory distress. **Retraction** of the chest wall between the ribs occurs when airways are obstructed and can indicate serious distress. When the patient inhales and air can't easily

FIGURE 29.8 Accessory muscles of breathing. Note the prominent sternocleidomastoid muscles.

flow into the lungs, negative pressure in the chest pulls the soft tissue between the ribs inward.

Note the color of the skin, lips, mucous membranes, and nailbeds. A bluish color is called **cyanosis** and is a late sign of oxygen deprivation. Observe the trachea and chest for symmetry. Count the number of respirations per minute, noting depth and rhythm. Irregular respirations, or periods of **apnea** (absence of respirations), can indicate a pathological condition and are described in Figure 29.9. Observe the

- • WORD • BUILDING •
cyanosis: cyan—dark blue + osis—condition
apnea: a—not + pnea—breath

Cultural Considerations

Pulmonary diseases associated with Japanese people include asthma related to dust mites in the straw mats that cover floors in Japanese homes and air pollution from living in urban areas. Encourage patients who have straw mats and who wish to keep them to have them sterilized.

Patients from Poland, Ireland, or other countries where mining is a primary occupation may have an increased incidence of respiratory disease. It is essential for health care providers (HCPs) to carefully screen Polish and Irish immigrants for respiratory conditions.

HCPs also should be aware of variations among ethnic peoples of color when assessing for cyanosis. Cyanosis and decreased blood hemoglobin levels in darker-skinned individuals give the skin an ashen color instead of the bluish color seen in light-skinned people. Thus, the nurse must examine the sclerae, conjunctivae, buccal mucosa, tongue, lips, nailbeds, and palms and soles of the feet to assess for cyanosis.

Smoking is deeply ingrained in the Arab-American culture. Offering cigarettes is a rite of Arab hospitality. Arab individuals may have difficulty stopping smoking because of these cultural rituals.

Strategies to increase the effectiveness of smoking cessation in African Americans include working with community and church groups in African American communities. Populations living in inner cities are at increased risk for respiratory diseases related to pollution.

Respiratory patterns

When assessing a patient's respirations, the nurse should determine their rate, rhythm, and depth. These schematic diagrams show different respiratory patterns.

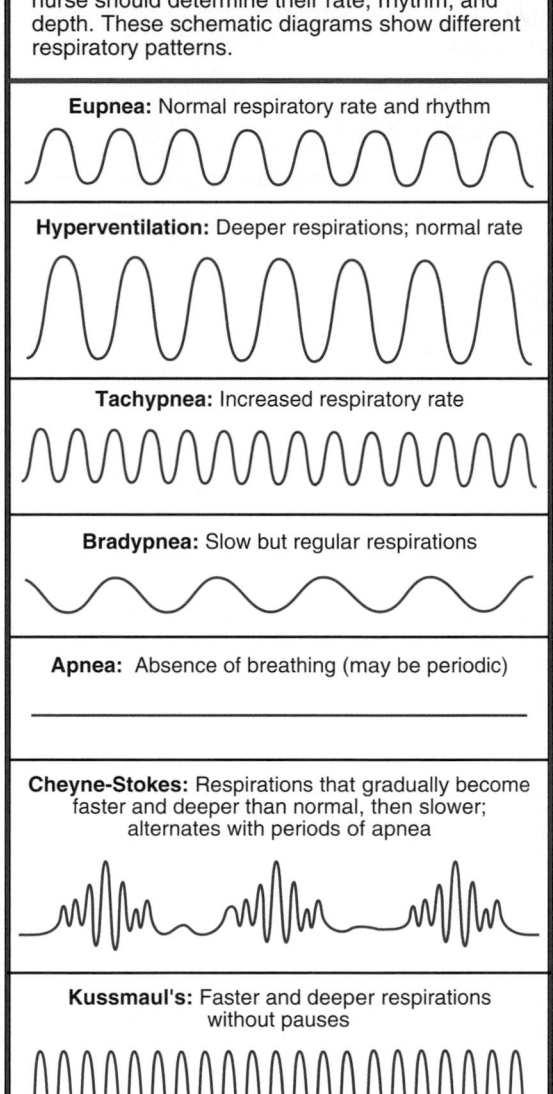

Eupnea: Normal respiratory rate and rhythm

Hyperventilation: Deeper respirations; normal rate

Tachypnea: Increased respiratory rate

Bradypnea: Slow but regular respirations

Apnea: Absence of breathing (may be periodic)

Cheyne-Stokes: Respirations that gradually become faster and deeper than normal, then slower; alternates with periods of apnea

Kussmaul's: Faster and deeper respirations without pauses

FIGURE 29.9 Abnormal respiratory patterns.

shape of the chest. Normally the chest is about twice as wide (side to side) as it is deep (front to back). If it is more rounded, it is called a barrel chest, which is associated with trapped air in the lungs. See Table 29.3 for a summary of objective data.

Palpation

Palpate the frontal and maxillary sinuses if sinus inflammation is suspected (Fig. 29.10). Use your thumbs to palpate gently below the eyebrows and below each cheekbone. Tenderness may indicate sinus inflammation or infection.

Respiratory excursion can also be palpated. This is a rough measurement of chest expansion on inspiration. It is not necessary to palpate expansion on every patient, but it may be helpful if hypoventilation or asymmetry is suspected. Figure 29.11 illustrates how to palpate for respiratory excursion. You can palpate for **crepitus** (also called subcutaneous emphysema) if indicated. Crepitus feels like Rice Krispies under the skin when felt with the fingers. It occurs when air leaks into subcutaneous tissues because of pneumothorax or a leaking chest tube site. Palpation for crepitus is not done routinely but rather when the possibility of an air leak exists.

Percussion

Percussion is typically done by the experienced nurse. It involves tapping on the anterior and posterior chest, in each intercostal space, and comparing sounds from side to side. A normal chest sounds resonant and is the same bilaterally except over the heart. If other percussion notes are heard, they can indicate a pathological condition and should be reported.

Auscultation

Auscultation provides valuable information about respiratory status. Use the diaphragm of your stethoscope to listen to the anterior, lateral, and posterior chest during an entire inspiration and expiration at each interspace (Fig. 29.12). Auscultation of the posterior chest is easiest if the patient is sitting, but if necessary, it may be done with the patient in a side-lying position. Asking the patient to breathe deeply through the mouth can help enhance the sounds. Allow the patient to

TABLE 29.3 OBJECTIVE DATA COLLECTION FOR THE RESPIRATORY SYSTEM

Category	Abnormal Findings	Possible Causes
Respiratory	Respiratory rate <12 or >20 per minute	Respiratory depression may be from opioid or sedative use; elevated respiratory rate indicates respiratory distress
	Use of accessory muscles	
	Barrel chest	Restrictive or obstructive disorders
	Adventitious sounds	Air trapping from obstructive disorder (chronic obstructive pulmonary disorder)
	Cough	*See Table 29.4.*
	Sputum	Airway irritation or secretions
		Yellow, tan, or green sputum may indicate infection; blood in sputum can indicate pneumonia, tuberculosis, cancer, or pulmonary embolism

Continued

TABLE 29.3   OBJECTIVE DATA COLLECTION FOR THE RESPIRATORY SYSTEM—cont'd

Category	Abnormal Findings	Possible Causes
Integumentary	Cyanosis	Tissue hypoxia
	Nail clubbing	Chronic tissue hypoxia
Neurologic	Confusion	Lack of oxygen to the brain
Gastrointestinal	Weight loss	Dyspnea interfering with eating; use of calories for breathing

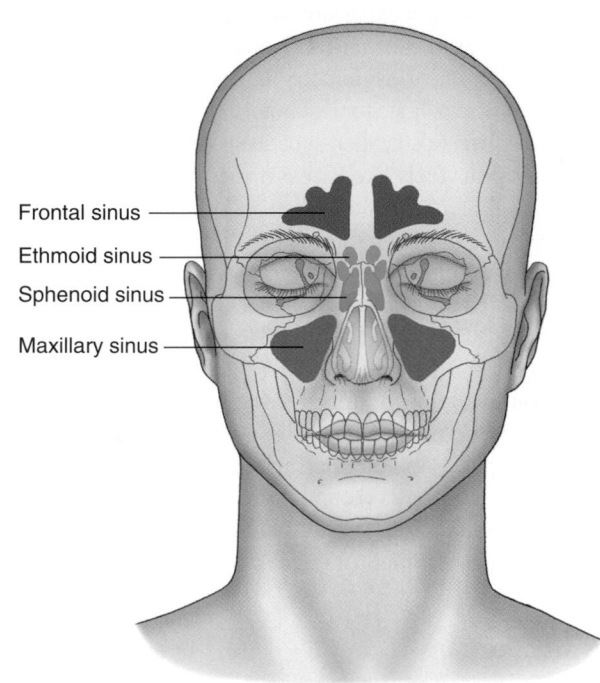

Frontal sinus
Ethmoid sinus
Sphenoid sinus
Maxillary sinus

FIGURE 29.10 Paranasal sinuses.

FIGURE 29.11 Palpation of respiratory excursion. Left: during exhalation. Right: after inhalation.

rest at intervals to prevent hyperventilation. Regular and frequent practice helps you learn to distinguish normal from abnormal breath sounds. Abnormal extra sounds (another term is **adventitious**) indicate a pathological condition and are described in Table 29.4.

LEARNING TIP

Listen to breath sounds on all your friends and family members. Assuming they are normal, this will give you a good baseline so when you hear an abnormal or adventitious sound on a patient, you will recognize it as "not normal."

CRITICAL THINKING

Timothy

■ Timothy is a 16-year-old whose mother brought him to the emergency room because of an asthma attack. He says he feels short of breath, but when you listen to his lungs, you hear no wheezing.

1. Does Timothy really need to be in the emergency room?
2. What should you do?
3. What do you think could be happening?
4. What other team members can you collaborate with as you care for Timothy?

Suggested answers are at the end of the chapter.

DIAGNOSTIC TESTS FOR THE RESPIRATORY SYSTEM

Laboratory Tests

For normal values for the following laboratory tests, see Appendix B.

Blood Tests

COMPLETE BLOOD COUNT. Measurement of RBCs and hemoglobin can give information about the oxygen-carrying capacity of the blood. **Dyspnea** (shortness of breath) can be caused by a reduction in RBCs or hemoglobin. Elevated white blood cells (WBCs) indicate infection. See Table 29.5 for normal blood count values.

• WORD • BUILDING •
dyspnea: dys—bad + pnea—breathing

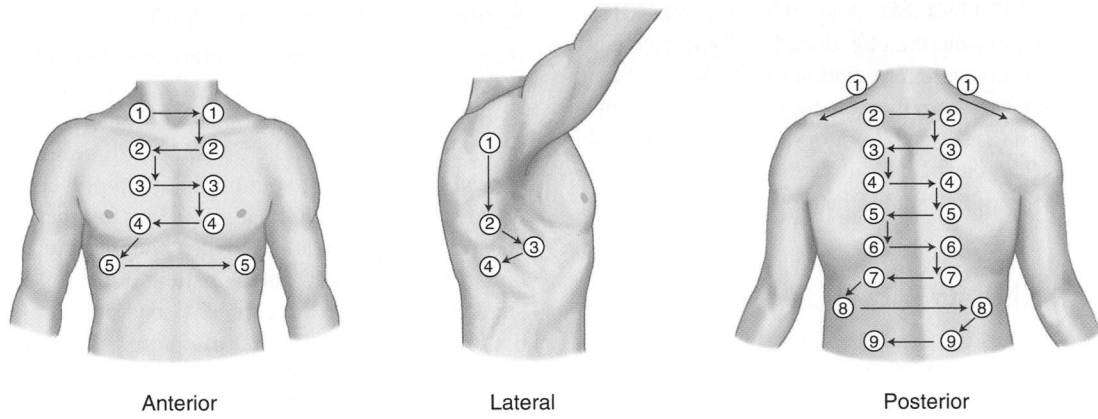

Anterior   Lateral   Posterior

FIGURE 29.12 Auscultation of the chest. Use a systematic approach to auscultate the chest, comparing sounds from side to side.

TABLE 29.4   ABNORMAL LUNG SOUNDS

Abnormal (Adventitious) Sound	Cause of Sound	Description	Associated Disorders
Coarse crackles (sometimes called rales)	Fluid in airways	Moist bubbling sound, heard on inspiration or expiration	Pulmonary edema, bronchitis, pneumonia
Fine crackles (rales)	Alveoli popping open on inspiration	Velcro being torn apart, heard at end of inspiration	Heart failure, atelectasis
Wheezes	Narrowed airways	Fine high-pitched violins mostly on expiration	Asthma
Stridor	Airway obstruction	Loud crowing noise heard without stethoscope	Obstruction from tumor or foreign body
Pleural friction rub	Inflamed pleura rubbing together	Sound of leather rubbing together; grating sound	Pleurisy, lung cancer, pneumonia, pleural irritation
Diminished	Decreased air movement	Faint lung sounds	Emphysema, hypoventilation, obesity, muscular chest wall
Absent	No air movement	No sounds heard	Pneumothorax, pneumectomy

TABLE 29.5   DIAGNOSTIC LABORATORY TESTS FOR THE RESPIRATORY SYSTEM

Test	Normal Values	Associated Conditions
Red Blood Cell Count	*Male:* 4.5–6.2 million cells/mm^3 venous blood *Female:* 4.2–5.4 million cells/mm^3 venous blood	↑ in chronic lung disease, dehydration ↓ in anemia, hemorrhage, overhydration with intravenous (IV) fluids
Hemoglobin	*Male:* 13.5–18 g/dL *Female:* 12–16 g/dL	Same as red blood cell count
White Blood Cell Count	5000–10,000 cells/mm^3 venous blood	↑in infection

ARTERIAL BLOOD GAS ANALYSIS. Arterial blood gases (ABGs) are measured to determine the effectiveness of gas exchange. See Table 29.6 for a basic interpretation of ABGs. The blood sample is usually taken from the radial artery in the wrist by a respiratory therapist (RT) or laboratory technician specially trained to do this. This can be painful for the patient. Place pressure on the site for 5 minutes after the test to prevent bleeding.

LEARNING TIP

If you remember that a normal blood pH is 7.35 to 7.45, then it is easy to remember that a normal $PaCO_2$ is 35 to 45 mm Hg.

LEARNING TIP

Remember 50! If the Pao_2 falls below 50 and the $PaCO_2$ is above 50, the patient is in trouble and the health care provider should be notified. This is a crude analysis, but it is helpful when a quick assessment is needed.

D-DIMER. This blood test measures fibrin degradation products, which are present if there is a blood clot in the body. It helps diagnose the presence of a pulmonary embolism.

TABLE 29.6 ARTERIAL BLOOD GAS ANALYSIS

	Normal Values	Interpretation
Pao_2	75–100 mm Hg	↑ in hyperventilation ↓ in impaired respiratory function
$PaCO_2$	35–45 mm Hg	↑ in impaired gas exchange ↓ in hyperventilation
pH	7.35–7.45	↑ in respiratory alkalosis with low $PaCO_2$ ↓ in respiratory acidosis with high $PaCO_2$
HCO_3^-	22–26 mEq/L	↑ to buffer $PaCO_2$ in acidosis ↓ to buffer $PaCO_2$ in alkalosis
Oxygen saturation	95%–100%	↓ in impaired respiratory function

Sputum Culture and Sensitivity

A sputum culture identifies pathogens present in the sputum. The sensitivity test determines which antibiotics will be effective against those pathogens. To obtain a sputum specimen, first obtain a sterile container. Some institutions have special containers for sputum that help prevent transmission of infection to the HCP (Fig. 29.13). Instruct the patient to take several deep breaths and then cough sputum into the container. It is important that the patient not simply spit saliva or sinus drainage into the cup. The specimen must come from the lungs. It may be easiest to obtain a specimen first thing in the morning (after mouth care) because secretions build up during the night. Send the specimen to the laboratory immediately. If the patient is unable to cough up sputum, extra fluids or a bedside humidifier may help. An RT may be able to help obtain a specimen with a nebulized mist treatment or with a special suction catheter with a sputum trap. A HCP's order may be needed for these procedures.

BE SAFE!

If the HCP orders a "sputum for AFB," tuberculosis is suspected, which is caused by an acid-fast bacillus (AFB). Ask whether the patient should be placed in isolation while waiting for test results.

Throat Culture

A throat culture is done to determine the presence of viral or bacterial pathogens in the pharynx. Use a swab to reach into the posterior pharynx behind the uvula (without touching the patient's mouth) and swab the red area or lesions. Use a tongue blade to help hold the tongue down while

FIGURE 29.13 A special container that helps prevent transmission of infection is often used to collect sputum for culture.

obtaining the culture. Warn the patient that a gag reflex may be triggered. Once the culture has been obtained, place it in a sterile tube with culture medium, according to package instructions. Send it to the laboratory immediately for analysis.

Nasal Samples

A nasopharyngeal swab or a nasal wash can be used to identify flu or other respiratory viruses. To be accurate, it must be done in the first few days a person has symptoms. The sample may be obtained by swabbing the nasal passages or pharynx or by using a small amount of saline to wash out the nose, depending on the type of test ordered.

Oxygen Saturation

The oxygen saturation test (also called pulse oximetry, O_2 sat, or SpO_2) is a simple and noninvasive way to measure arterial oxygenation. A sensor is placed on the patient's finger or ear. The sensor measures the percentage of hemoglobin that is saturated with oxygen. Oxygen saturation can be measured at rest or while the patient is walking to determine the patient's exercise tolerance. It is also often done with and without supplemental oxygen to determine the patient's need for oxygen supplementation at home. See Table 29.6 for normal values. Collaborate with the HCP for an appropriate SpO_2 level for your patient. Although 95% or greater is considered normal, some patients with chronic lung disease may be maintained at 90% to 92%. If the SpO_2 is less than 75%, prepare for emergency intervention.

Oxygen saturations may be inaccurate in patients with low blood flow or decreased perfusion, patients who are moving, and patients who have smoke inhalation injury or carbon monoxide poisoning. Dark-skinned patients may have falsely high readings. Acrylic nails may need to be removed for accurate readings. Always correlate SpO_2 results with patient assessment findings.

Capnography

The process of measuring a person's exhaled carbon dioxide level is called capnography. It provides a continuous measurement of the patient's ventilation status. In the past, capnography was done primarily during surgery by an anesthetist. Now it is becoming more common in emergency departments and intensive care units; even emergency medical technicians are using it. It is most often used when patients are intubated. A special sensor is placed between the endotracheal tube and the ventilator to measure the exhaled carbon dioxide. Special nasal cannulas with sensors are also now available. Results are displayed on a special monitor.

Other Tests

For explanations of the following diagnostic tests, see Appendix A.

Chest X-Ray Examination

A chest x-ray examination may be ordered to help diagnose a variety of pulmonary disorders. Usually, posterior–anterior (PA) and side views (lateral) are taken. If a hospitalized patient is too ill to go to the radiology department, a portable chest x-ray machine can be used at the bedside to obtain a PA view.

Computed Tomography

A computed tomography (CT) scan can show cancers, pneumonia, emphysema, and more. It may be used to obtain more information after an abnormal chest x-ray. A spiral CT scan can be useful for evaluating trauma or blood vessel abnormalities in the chest.

Ventilation-Perfusion Scan

During a ventilation-perfusion scan (also called a lung scan or VQ scan), a radioactive substance is injected intravenously, and a scan is done to view blood flow to the lungs (perfusion). Another radioactive substance is inhaled, and scanning shows how well oxygen is distributed in the lungs (ventilation). If an area of the lungs is well ventilated but has no blood supply, a pulmonary embolism is suspected. Chronic lung disease may cause poor ventilation and perfusion.

Pulmonary Function Studies

Pulmonary function studies are a series of tests done to determine lung volume, capacity, and flow rates. These are commonly used to help diagnose and monitor restrictive or obstructive lung disease. The patient is asked to use a special mouthpiece to blow into a cylinder that is connected to a computer. A computer printout is generated to show the results. See Table 29.7 for normal values. Some patients use handheld peak expiratory flow rate (PEFR) meters at home to monitor asthma symptoms. They might notice changes in PEFR before symptoms occur, allowing them to begin treatment before the problem becomes more serious.

Pulmonary Angiography

Pulmonary angiography involves an x-ray examination of the pulmonary vessels after intravenous (IV) administration of a radiopaque dye. Pulmonary angiography is used to help diagnose pulmonary embolism or other pulmonary vessel disorders.

Bronchoscopy

Bronchoscopy involves the use of a flexible endoscope to examine the larynx, trachea, and bronchial tree. Bronchoscopy can be used diagnostically for visualization or to obtain a biopsy specimen for examination. It can also be used therapeutically to remove an obstruction, foreign body, or thick secretions.

TABLE 29.7 MEDICATION REGIMEN OPTIONS FOR H. PYLORI INFECTION

Test	Definition	Normal Values*
Tidal volume (TV)	Air inspired and expired in one breath	400–600 mL at rest
Residual volume (RV)	Air remaining in lungs after maximum exhalation	1000–1500 mL
Functional residual capacity (FRC)	Air remaining in lungs after normal expiration	2300 mL
Inspiratory reserve	Amount of air beyond tidal volume that can be taken in with the deepest possible inhalation	2000–3000 mL
Expiratory reserve	Amount of air beyond tidal volume in the most forceful exhalation	1000–1500 mL
Forced vital capacity (FVC)	Maximum amount of air expired forcefully after maximum inspiration	3000–5000 mL
Forced expiratory volume in 1 second (FEV_1)	Amount of air expired in first second of forced exhalation, expressed as percent of FVC	65%–85% of the FVC
Peak expiratory flow rate (PEFR)	Maximum flow of air expired during FVC (this is a rate rather than a volume)	450 L/min

*Normal values are approximate. They are individualized based on patient's sex, height, and age.

THERAPEUTIC MEASURES FOR THE RESPIRATORY SYSTEM

Smoking Cessation

Probably the most important intervention for preventing and treating respiratory disease is smoking cessation. Many respiratory disorders are caused or aggravated by smoking, and stopping can prevent disease from occurring or slow its progression significantly. Table 29.8 lists interventions to help patients stop smoking. Remind patients that if they have tried quitting before and failed, that does not mean that they will never be able to quit (see "Evidence-Based Practice"). Many patients try several times before quitting

TABLE 29.8 INTERVENTIONS TO STOP SMOKING

Intervention	Rationale
Behavior modification	If the patient can identify situations associated with smoking, such as eating a meal or experiencing stress, then other healthier behaviors can be substituted, such as going for a walk.
Counseling	Counseling by a health care worker alone or in combination with other methods can greatly increase success.
Setting a quit date	The "cold turkey" (all-at-once) method is more effective than slow tapering, although the patient may choose to taper before the quit date.
Nicotine replacement therapy	Nicotine gum, patches, nasal sprays, lozenges, and inhalers can reduce withdrawal symptoms.
Drug therapy (bupropion [Zyban], varenicline [Chantix])	Bupropion may help reduce cravings. Varenicline attaches to nicotine receptors in the brain to block nicotine and reduce its pleasurable effects.
Acupuncture	Acupuncture may help curb the desire to smoke, but studies are not yet conclusive.
Hypnosis	Hypnosis is believed to help the person be open to the suggestion that smoking is undesirable.
Physical activity	Physical activity reduces cravings and post-cessation weight gain.

successfully. Formal smoking cessation programs and support groups can be helpful.

EVIDENCE-BASED PRACTICE

Clinical Question
Can nurses make a difference in helping patients stop smoking?

Evidence
Thirty-one randomized trials comparing targeted nursing interventions to controls (usual care interventions) found that nursing intervention significantly increased the likelihood of patients quitting smoking (Rice & Stead, 2008). Nursing interventions were more effective in hospital settings but less effective in outpatient settings.

Implications for Nursing Practice
Advice and support from nursing staff can increase people's success in quitting smoking, especially in a hospital setting.

REFERENCE
Rice, V. H., & Stead, L. F. (2008). Nursing interventions for smoking cessation. *Cochrane Database of Systematic Reviews 2008*, 1 (Art. No. CD001188; DOI 10.1002/14651858 .CD001188.pub3).

Many Internet sites have information to help people stop smoking. Among these are the American Lung Association site at www.lungusa.org and the National Lung Health Education Program at www.nlhep.org. Or simply type "smoking cessation" into any search engine. The American Lung Association has a "Freedom From Smoking" online smoking cessation program that can be accessed at www.ffsonline.org. Alternatively, individuals can call 1-800-QUIT NOW to speak with a representative who will assist with cessation strategies.

Deep Breathing and Coughing

Effective coughing can keep the airways clear of secretions. An ineffective cough is exhausting and fails to bring up secretions. Instruct the patient to take two or three deep breaths, using the diaphragm. This helps get the air behind the secretions. After the third deep inhalation, tell the patient to hold the breath for a few seconds and then cough forcefully. This is repeated as necessary, usually every 1 to 2 hours. Good hydration can facilitate mucous removal.

Huff Coughing

Patients with chronic obstructive pulmonary disease (COPD) typically have a weak cough and airways that collapse easily. *Huff* coughing may work better for them. Instruct the patient to deep breath and cough, as above. Instead of closing the glottis to generate a forceful cough, the patient should keep the glottis and mouth open, and use the abdominal muscles to create a series of forced expirations, moving air and mucus up the bronchial tree. This creates "huff" or "who" sounds. A short "huff" helps clear larger airways, and a longer "huff" held out for several seconds helps open and clear smaller airways. Finally, the patient should take one more controlled inhalation and a final huff cough to expel the mucus.

Autogenic Drainage

Autogenic drainage is a variation on deep breathing and coughing that may be more effective for patients with thick secretions that are difficult to raise, such as those with cystic fibrosis or severe COPD. It is also gentler and less likely to cause declines in oxygen saturation or uncontrolled coughing than other methods. The patient is taught to sit upright and breathe in more deeply than usual, slowly through the nose, and then hold the breath for 2 to 4 seconds. When holding the breath, the patient should keep the glottis open, to prevent airway collapse. Exhaling is done as a quiet sigh, as if trying to steam up a mirror.

Using these breathing techniques, the patient is taught three phases:

1. *Unstick.* The patient breathes out completely and then takes a slow breath and exhales fully several times, suppressing the urge to cough. This loosens mucus in the lower airways.
2. *Collect.* The patient takes 10 to 20 slightly deeper breaths, exhaling normally, still suppressing the urge to cough. This helps move mucus up to the middle airways.
3. *Evacuate.* The patient takes 10 to 20 breaths and huff coughs to move the mucus up and out.

During the *unstick* and *collect* phases, airflow should be high enough to produce a rattle if secretions are present. This is a complex process that is typically taught by an RT.

Breathing Exercises

Breathing exercises are essential for patients with chronic lung disease. Diaphragmatic and pursed-lip breathing increase the effectiveness of breathing and help reduce panic when dyspnea occurs.

Diaphragmatic Breathing

The diaphragm is the major muscle of breathing, but patients often use less efficient accessory muscles when they are short of breath. Conscious use of the diaphragm during breathing can be relaxing and conserve energy. With practice, the patient should be able to use diaphragmatic breathing all the time without thinking about it. Teach the patient to do the following:

1. Place one hand on the abdomen and the other on the chest.
2. Concentrate on pushing out the abdomen during inspiration and relaxing the abdomen on expiration. The chest should move very little.

Pursed-Lip Breathing

This technique can be used any time the patient feels short of breath. It helps keep airways open during exhalation, which promotes carbon dioxide excretion. It should be done with diaphragmatic breathing. Counting during breathing also distracts the patient, reducing panic. Teach the patient to do the following:

1. Inhale slowly through the nose to the count of two (using diaphragmatic breathing).
2. Exhale slowly through pursed lips to the count of four.

NURSING CARE TIP

When teaching a patient to do pursed-lip breathing, try teaching them to "smell the roses" while inhaling slowly through the nose, and "blow out the candle" while exhaling. If you remind them not to let the wax splatter, then they'll blow slowly and gently!

Positioning

The patient who is short of breath should be positioned to conserve energy while allowing for maximum lung expansion. Most respiratory patients do not tolerate lying flat. The patient in bed can use Fowler's or semi-Fowler's position to keep abdominal contents from crowding the lungs. Some patients prefer to sit in a chair while leaning forward and placing their elbows on their knees or an overbed table (tripod position, Fig. 29.14).

FIGURE 29.14 The tripod position may help reduce dyspnea.

Patients with unilateral (one-sided) lung disease can benefit from the "good lung down" lateral position. This is a side-lying position with the good lung in the dependent position. Gravity causes greater blood flow to the dependent, "good" lung, thereby increasing oxygen saturation. Some patients may also benefit from prone positioning.

NURSING CARE TIP

Patients at home may choose to sleep in a recliner or La-Z-Boy–type chair to keep their head elevated. Others may use a wedge under their mattress, or a hospital bed.

Oxygen Therapy

Oxygen therapy is ordered by the HCP when the patient is unable to maintain oxygenation. Patients are typically placed on supplemental oxygen when their oxygen saturation is less than 90% on room air. The HCP's order should include the method of administration and the flow rate. A variety of delivery methods are described in the following sections. The role of the nurse in oxygen therapy includes monitoring the flow rate, ensuring that the cannula and tubing or other device remain properly placed, and monitoring the patient's response to treatment. If the patient becomes short of breath while on oxygen therapy, an RT, registered nurse (RN), or HCP should be notified. Instruct the patient to avoid smoking, using electrical equipment, and performing other activities that can cause fire in the presence of oxygen. The RT is knowledgeable about oxygen therapy and is an excellent resource when questions arise.

NURSING CARE TIP

If a patient suddenly becomes confused, check the SpO_2 and oxygen delivery system. The patient may have taken off the cannula, or the tubing may be kinked or disconnected, resulting in hypoxia and confusion.

Low-Flow Devices

NASAL CANNULA. The nasal cannula is the most common method of oxygen administration. Oxygen is delivered through a flexible catheter that has two short nasal prongs (Fig. 29.15). For the nasal cannula to be most effective, the patient must breathe through his or her nose. The cannula allows the patient to eat and talk, and it is generally more comfortable than other methods of administration. If the nasal mucous membranes become dry, a water source can be placed on the system to humidify the oxygen. Oxygen can

FIGURE 29.15 Nasal cannula for oxygen delivery.

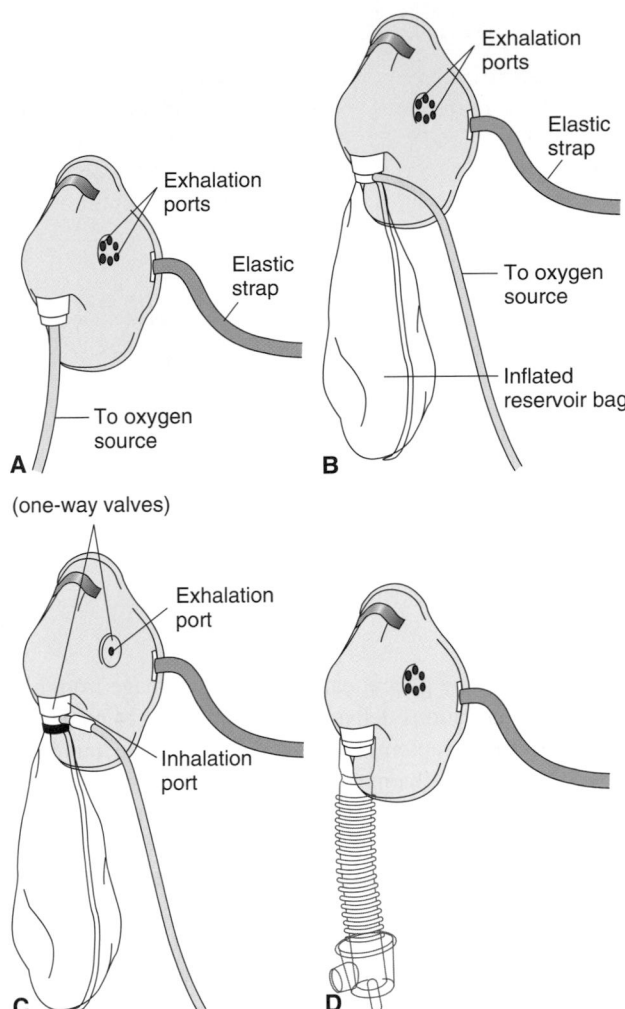

FIGURE 29.16 Oxygen masks. (A) Simple mask. (B) Partial rebreather mask. (C) Nonrebreathing mask. (D) Venturi mask.

be delivered at 1 to 6 L/min via a nasal cannula; special high-flow cannulas can deliver much higher rates.

Masks. Masks are used when a higher oxygen concentration is needed (Fig. 29.16). A disadvantage of masks is that they make some patients feel claustrophobic. Also, a mask must be replaced by a cannula while the patient eats.

• *Simple face mask.* A rate of 5 to 10 L/min can deliver oxygen concentrations from 40% to 60% with a simple face mask.
• *Partial rebreather mask.* A partial rebreather mask uses a reservoir to capture some exhaled gas for rebreathing. Vents on the sides of the mask allow room air to mix with oxygen. It can deliver oxygen concentrations of 50% or greater.
• *Nonrebreather mask.* A nonrebreather mask has one or both side vents closed to limit the mixing of room air with oxygen. The vents open to allow exhalation but remain closed on inhalation. The reservoir bag has a valve to store oxygen for inhalation but does not allow entry of exhaled air. It is used to deliver oxygen concentrations of 70% to 100%.

NURSING CARE TIP

When a patient is using a partial rebreather or nonrebreather mask, ensure that the reservoir bag is never allowed to collapse to less than half full.

High-Flow Devices

VENTURI MASK. A Venturi mask is used for the patient who requires precise percentages of oxygen, such as the patient with chronic lung disease with CO_2 retention. A combination of valves and specified flow rates determines oxygen concentration.

Transtracheal Catheter

A transtracheal catheter is a small tube that is surgically placed through the base of the neck directly into the trachea to deliver oxygen (Fig. 29.17). This is an attractive alternative for some patients who are on long-term oxygen therapy at home because it does not obstruct the nose or mouth and can be easily covered with a loose scarf or collar. The patient is taught to remove and clean the catheter two or three times a day to prevent mucus obstruction. Check institution policy and procedure for specific care instructions.

Risks of Oxygen Therapy

Patients with COPD usually have chronically high $PaCO_2$ levels. Therefore, they depend on low Pao_2 levels to stimulate breathing, and high supplemental oxygen flow rates can depress respirations. Patients with COPD who retain CO_2 should be maintained on no more than 1 to 2 L of oxygen per minute. Occasionally, hospitalized patients require higher flow rates, but they must be carefully monitored and may require mechanical ventilation.

FIGURE 29.17 Transtracheal oxygen catheter

In addition, any patient can suffer lung damage from high oxygen concentrations delivered for more than 24 hours. If a patient exhibits symptoms of dry cough, chest pain, numbness in the extremities, lethargy, or nausea, the HCP should be contacted. A Pao_2 greater than 100 mm Hg should also be reported.

Nebulized Mist Treatments

Nebulized mist treatments (NMTs) use a nebulizer to deliver medication directly into the lungs (Fig. 29.18). Such topical use of medication reduces systemic side effects. Bronchodilators such as albuterol, mixed with normal saline solution and sometimes with supplemental oxygen, are most commonly administered. Other medications, including corticosteroids, mucolytics, and antibiotics, may also be given. An RT or a specially trained nurse administers the NMT. The patient uses a handheld reservoir with tubing and a mouthpiece to breathe in the medication. NMTs are commonly ordered every 4 to 6 hours and as needed. You may call for an NMT as needed (prn) when a patient with chronic pulmonary disease becomes acutely dyspneic. Some patients are taught to administer their own NMTs at home.

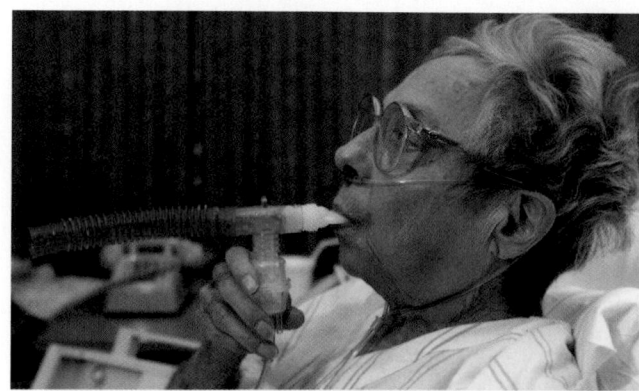

FIGURE 29.18 Patient receiving nebulized mist treatment.

Metered-Dose Inhalers

Inhalers are another way to administer topical medication directly into the lungs, minimizing systemic side effects. Medications that can be inhaled include corticosteroids, bronchodilators, and mast cell inhibitors. Metered-dose inhalers (MDIs) use propellants to deliver medication. Figure 29.19 shows use of a

1. Gently twist the canister into the inhaler unit. Shake the inhaler and remove the cap.

2. Exhale.

3. Place the inhaler mouthpiece in your mouth.

4. Press the canister down to actuate a dose of medication. As you do so, breathe in slowly and deeply. Time the dose and breath so the medication goes into the lungs and not onto the tongue.

5. Hold your breath for 5 – 10 seconds. Repeat steps 2 – 4 if two puffs are ordered.

FIGURE 29.19 Instructions for use of a metered-dose inhaler. See package inserts for specific instructions because many types of inhalers are available.

traditional MDI. Use of a spacer can increase the amount of medication that gets to the lungs (Fig. 29.20).

Before December 31, 2008, many MDIs used a chlorofluorocarbon (CFC) as a propellant, but CFC damages the ozone, so new ways to deliver inhaled medications have been developed. Many new models of inhalers such as dry powder inhalers do not use any propellants, and some use an HFA (hydrofluoroalkane) propellant. With so many different types of inhalers, it is important to carefully read the instructions for use before assisting a patient.

The RT or nurse must carefully instruct the patient because improper use can reduce the effectiveness of the medication. It is also important to teach the patient to avoid overuse of adrenergic bronchodilator inhalers. Patients with chronic lung disease may tend to use extra puffs when they feel short of breath. Adrenergic bronchodilators, however, can cause severe rebound bronchoconstriction and even death when used too often.

Incentive Spirometry

Incentive spirometers (Fig. 29.21) are used to encourage deep breathing in patients at risk for collapse of lung tissue, a condition called *atelectasis*. These devices are commonly ordered for postoperative patients. Patients are instructed to use the spirometer 10 times each hour they are awake. Because a variety of spirometers are available, consult with an RT and read package inserts for specific directions for use.

Chest Physiotherapy

Chest physiotherapy (CPT), which includes postural drainage, percussion, and vibration, helps move secretions from deep inside the lungs (Fig. 29.22). It is indicated for the patient who has a weak or ineffective cough and is at risk for retaining secretions. Patients with retained secretions due to conditions such as COPD, cystic fibrosis, or bronchiectasis and patients on ventilators benefit from CPT.

CPT is performed by an RT or specially trained nurse. For postural drainage, the patient is placed in various positions (head down to help drain secretions) and turned periodically

FIGURE 29.21 Incentive spirometers. (A) Voldyne volumetric deep-breathing exerciser. (B) Triflow II incentive breathing exerciser. Modified from Barnes, T. A. (1991). *Respiratory care principles.* Philadelphia: F.A. Davis, p. 434.

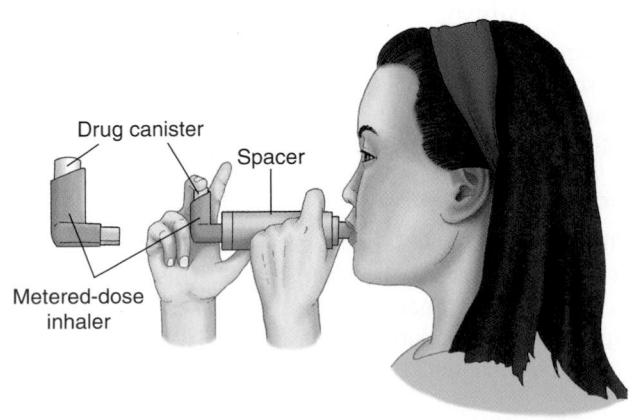

FIGURE 29.20 Use of a spacer increases the amount of medication that gets to the lungs.

FIGURE 29.22 Patient receiving chest physiotherapy.

during the treatment so all lobes of the lungs are drained. The therapist uses cupped hands to strike the chest repeatedly (percussion), producing sound waves that are transmitted through the chest, loosening secretions. The therapist may also apply vibration to the patient's chest, using the hands or a vibrator, to loosen secretions. An NMT should be given before CPT to humidify secretions. The patient is instructed to cough and deep breathe at intervals during and after the treatment.

High-Frequency Chest Wall Oscillation Vest

The high-frequency chest wall oscillation vest (sometimes called vest therapy) is an alternative to CPT. Because it does not require the presence of a RT, it is less expensive over time. An inflatable vest is placed on the patient, and a compressor generates pulses of air into the vest to vibrate the patient's chest. Like CPT, this helps loosen secretions so that they can be expectorated. The patient must cough during and after the therapy for it to be effective. It can easily be used at home.

Vibratory Positive Expiratory Pressure Device

Another alternative to chest physiotherapy is a small hand-held device called a vibratory positive expiratory pressure (PEP) device. (One brand is the Flutter mucus clearance device shown in Fig. 29.23.) When the patient blows into the mouthpiece, it makes a heavy steel ball inside bounce around in its chamber, which then sends vibrations back into the airways to help loosen mucus. Blowing into the device also creates positive pressure, which opens airways.

Thoracentesis

Thoracentesis involves the insertion of a needle into the pleural space. It is commonly done to aspirate fluid in patients with pleural effusion (fluid trapped in the pleural space, see Chapter 31). The procedure may be diagnostic to determine the source of fluid or therapeutic to remove fluid and reduce respiratory distress. It may also be performed to aspirate blood or air or to inject medication.

Perforated cover

Stainless steel ball

Mouthpiece

FIGURE 29.23 Flutter® mucus clearance device. When the patient blows into the mouthpiece, the stainless steel ball bounces up and down, causing airways to vibrate. This helps open airways and loosens mucus. Consult package instructions before use. *Courtesy of Axcan Scandipharm, Birmingham, AL.*

When assisting an HCP with a thoracentesis, first verify that the patient understands the procedure and that written consent has been obtained if required by institution policy. Have the patient void before the procedure. The patient should be aware that a sensation of pressure may be felt, but that severe pain is rare. Administer an analgesic, if ordered, before the procedure. Obtain a special procedure tray that has the equipment needed by the HCP. Place the patient in a sitting position, bending over a bedside table, or in a side-lying position if unable to sit. You can position yourself in front of the patient and encourage relaxation during the procedure. If you are asked to hand equipment to the HCP, be sure to keep everything sterile.

The HCP uses a local anesthetic before inserting a needle into the patient's back through the desired interspace. Specimens are withdrawn through the needle, labeled, and sent to the laboratory. If the thoracentesis is being done for therapeutic reasons, a sterile container is used to collect the remaining fluid. As much as 2 L can be removed, sometimes more, and the patient will usually report immediate reduction of dyspnea.

    BE SAFE!

BE VIGILANT! Label all medications, medication containers, and other solutions on and off the sterile field in perioperative and other procedural settings (Joint Commission 2014 National Patient Safety Goals, © The Joint Commission, 2013. Reprinted with permission.).

After the procedure, the HCP may apply a petroleum jelly dressing to prevent air leakage into the wound. Assess vital signs, breath sounds, and the puncture site according to the HCP's orders (e.g., every 15 minutes times two, every 30 minutes times two, then every 4 hours for 24 hours). The patient is usually maintained on bedrest for 1 hour after the procedure. Label and send specimens to the laboratory as ordered. The HCP may order a postprocedure x-ray examination to ensure that the lung was not punctured, causing a pneumothorax.

Chest Drainage

Continuous chest drainage involves insertion of one or two chest tubes by the HCP into the pleural space to drain fluid or air. The tubes are connected to a chest drainage system that collects the fluid or allows escape of the air.

Indications

Chest tubes and a chest drainage system are used when fluid or air has collected in the pleural space. This can occur with a collapsed lung (pneumothorax), pleural effusion, penetrating chest injury, or during chest surgery. These conditions are covered in Chapter 31.

• **WORD** • **BUILDING** •
thoracentesis: thoraco—chest + centesis—puncture

Chest Tube Insertion

The HCP inserts drainage tubes through the chest wall into the pleural space either in surgery or at the bedside. If removal of air from around a collapsed lung is the goal, the tube is inserted into the upper anterior chest, in the second to fourth intercostal space. If removal of fluid is the goal, such as after an injury, the tube is inserted in the lower lateral chest, in the eighth or ninth intercostal space. If a patient has both air and fluid to drain, two tubes are inserted and may be joined with a Y connector before connecting to the tubing that leads to a drainage system.

You can assist the HCP by obtaining a chest tube insertion tray and chest drainage system and preparing it according to the manufacturer's directions. Ensure that the patient understands the procedure and that written consent has been obtained according to institutional policy. Administer an analgesic as ordered, and help position the patient as directed by the HCP. Chest tube insertion is often an emergency intervention, which necessitates preparing the patient quickly.

Once the tube has been inserted and the system is in place, ensure that each connection is securely taped to prevent a break in the system. Petroleum jelly gauze and a sterile occlusive dressing are applied over the insertion site to prevent air leakage. If the dressing becomes soiled, do not change it; reinforce it with additional dressings, and notify the RN or HCP. Some nurses may change chest tube dressings with special training.

Obtain two padded clamps to keep at the bedside. These are used for clamping the chest tube if the chest drainage system becomes accidentally disconnected from the tubing, for changing the drainage system, or for a trial period before chest tube removal. The tubes are never clamped for more than a few seconds, however, because this prevents air escape and can cause a buildup of air in the pleural space. This can create a tension pneumothorax, which is a life-threatening emergency (see Chapter 31).

Chest Drainage System

The drainage system has evolved from a set of glass bottles to a one-piece molded plastic system with chambers that correspond to the bottles. Studying the bottle system will help you understand the one-piece system (Fig. 29.24). One, two, or three bottles can be used. Study the picture as you read the following sections.

WATER SEAL BOTTLE OR CHAMBER. Each time the patient exhales, trapped air also escapes the pleural space and travels through the chest tube to the water seal bottle or chamber, under the water, and then bubbles up and out of the bottle. The water acts as a seal, allowing air to escape from the pleural space but preventing air from getting back in during the negative pressure of inspiration. When the system is initiated, bubbling will occur on each exhalation until the lung is re-expanded. Once most of the pneumothorax is resolved, water in the tube fluctuates up with each inspiration and down with each expiration, as much as 5 to 10 cm. This is called **tidaling**. When the lung is fully reinflated, tidaling stops. If

FIGURE 29.24 Pleur-evac® chest drainage system. *Courtesy of Deknatel Snowden Pencer, Inc., Tucker, GA.*

tidaling stops before the lung is reinflated, the tubing should be checked for a kink or occlusion. If constant bubbling occurs in the water seal chamber, the system should be checked immediately for leaks.

 LEARNING TIP

Think of blowing bubbles through a straw into a glass of water as a child; the air could escape through the water, but you could not suck the air back through the water after it escaped. This is the same principle as a water seal chamber.

SUCTION BOTTLE OR CHAMBER. Sometimes a suction source is used to speed lung reinflation. A separate bottle with tubing attached to suction is used. The amount of suction depends on the level of water in the bottle, not the amount of suction set on the machine. (Look at the picture—some air is being suctioned from the atmosphere from the center straw, and some is being suctioned from the patient. The farther the straw is immersed in the water, the harder it will be for the suction to draw air from the atmosphere, and more will be suctioned from the patient.) The suction level is ordered by the HCP and is almost always negative 20 cm of water. The suction source should be turned on far enough to cause gentle bubbling in the suction bottle or chamber. Vigorous bubbling causes water evaporation, which alters the amount of suction. If water evaporates, more must be added to maintain the correct amount of suction. Some newer one-piece systems use special valves to eliminate the need for water.

DRAINAGE BOTTLE OR CHAMBER. Sometimes a third bottle is needed to catch fluid drained from the pleural space. Drainage may be from pleural effusion, chest trauma, or surgery. Sometimes a small amount of drainage occurs because of the insertion of the chest tube. The drainage chamber is not emptied to measure drainage. Rather the drainage level in the bottle or chamber is marked and timed each shift to monitor the amount. It is documented as output on the intake and output record. If drainage suddenly increases or becomes very bloody, notify the HCP. If the drainage chamber fills up, either the chamber or the entire unit will need to be changed, depending on the type of system used.

Nursing Care of the Patient With a Chest Tube

Nursing care of a patient with a chest tube involves regular assessment of the patient and the drainage system. See Box 29-1 for specific assessment and care. If permitted by the HCP, patients can be free to move around with the chest tube and drainage system. The drainage system must always be kept upright and below the level of the chest. If the patient must be transported, the drainage system is transported with the patient. Ask the HCP if the patient can be safely transported without suction. If the answer is yes, the suction control chamber is then left open to allow air to escape. Do not clamp tubing for transport.

If a chest tube is accidentally pulled out before the pneumothorax is resolved, air can reenter the pleural space. Some HCPs want an occlusive dressing placed over the site to prevent air from reentering. However, an occlusive dressing increases the risk of trapped air building up and placing pressure on the heart. Contact the RN or HCP immediately if this occurs.

Stripping and Milking

In the past, it was routine to strip or milk the tubing from the patient toward the drainage system to dislodge clots and maintain patency. Stripping is done by holding the proximal end of the tubing and using the other hand to squeeze the tubing between two fingers while sliding the fingers toward the drainage system. This is repeated on small sections of tubing until all have been stripped. It is now known, however, that this process can create negative pressure at the openings in the tubing that are within the pleural space, which can suck lung tissue in and cause damage. Stripping should be done only if it is ordered by the HCP, and even then only with specific instructions.

Milking is done by gently squeezing portions of tubing from the patient to the system without any sliding motion. This is somewhat safer for the patient but is still not done routinely. If tubing appears to be occluded, consult with the HCP for specific orders.

Box 29-1 Care of the Patient With a Chest Drainage System

Assess the patient according to institution policy. Start with the patient and move toward the drainage system.

PATIENT

1. Observe respiratory rate, effort, and symmetry.
2. Assess shortness of breath, pain, anxiety, or other discomforts.
3. Auscultate lung sounds (lung sounds may initially be muffled or absent on the side of a collapsed lung but should gradually return to normal as the lung reinflates).
4. Confirm that dressing is intact; observe for drainage. If necessary, reinforce the dressing and notify the HCP. Do not change the dressing unless specifically ordered to and trained to do so.
5. Palpate around insertion sites for crepitus.

TUBING

6. Check all tubing for kinks, breaks, or broken connections. Verify that all connections are securely taped.
7. Ensure that there are no dependent loops of tubing. Excess tubing should be coiled on the bed.

DRAINAGE SYSTEM

8. Verify that drainage system is below level of patient's chest at all times.
9. Check drainage system for cracks or leaks.
10. Check water seal chamber for correct water level and for tidaling (unless lung is reinflated). Add water if evaporation has decreased level. If continuous bubbling is present, check entire system for leaks and notify HCP.
11. Check suction control chamber for gentle bubbling (or open to air). Confirm correct amount of water as ordered. Add water if needed.
12. Check and mark amount of drainage in collection chamber every 8 hours and prn or as ordered. Report any marked increase in bloody drainage. Record drainage as output.
13. Document findings.
    Notify RN or HCP if any of the following occur:
- *The patient suddenly reports increasing dyspnea.*
- *There is a change in the patient's assessment findings.*
- *The drainage chamber is full and needs to be changed.*

CRITICAL THINKING

Miss Israel

■ Miss Israel has a chest tube in place for a spontaneous pneumothorax.

1. You note that the water seal chamber is bubbling vigorously. What could cause this? What should you do?
2. You are totaling intake and output for your 8-hour shift. There is 240 mL of serous fluid in the drainage chamber of the drainage system at 2200. At 1400, there was 190 mL. How much output should you record?

Suggested answers are at the end of the chapter.

Removal of Chest Tube

When the reason for the chest tube is resolved, the HCP removes it and places petroleum jelly gauze and a sterile occlusive dressing over the site. Continue to watch for development of crepitus and monitor the patient's respiratory status and dressing site.

Tracheostomy

A **tracheotomy** is a surgical opening through the base of the neck into the trachea. It is called a **tracheostomy** when it is more permanent and has a tube inserted into the opening to maintain patency (Fig. 29.25). The patient breathes through this opening, bypassing the upper airways. A tracheostomy is performed for a variety of reasons, such as in patients who have had a cancerous larynx removed, patients with airway obstruction caused by trauma or a tumor, patients who have

difficulty clearing secretions from the airway, or patients who need prolonged mechanical ventilation.

The tracheostomy tube consists of three parts: an outer cannula, an inner cannula, and an obturator (Fig. 29.26A and B). The obturator is a guide that is used only during insertion of the tube. After insertion, the obturator is immediately removed

• WORD • BUILDING •
tracheotomy: trach—trachea + otomy—incision
tracheostomy: trache—trachea + ostomy—opening or mouth

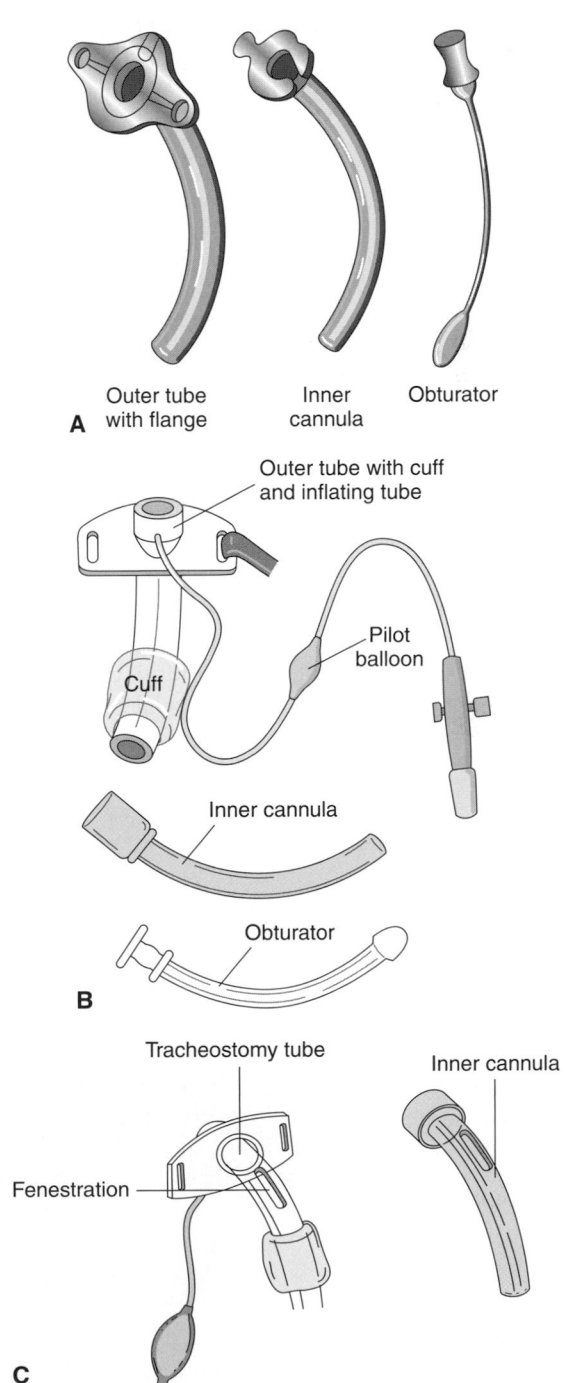

A Outer tube with flange   Inner cannula   Obturator

Outer tube with cuff and inflating tube

Pilot balloon

Cuff

Inner cannula

Obturator

B

Tracheostomy tube

Inner cannula

Fenestration

C

FIGURE 29.26 Tracheostomy tube. (A) Metal tube. (B) Cuffed plastic tube. (C) Fenestrated tube.

FIGURE 29.25 Patient with tracheostomy.

and kept at the bedside (commonly in a plastic bag taped to the wall above the bed) for emergency use if the tracheostomy tube is accidentally removed. The outer cannula remains in place at all times and is secured by ties to prevent dislodging. The inner cannula is removed at intervals, usually every 8 hours and as needed for cleaning. Some newer tracheostomy tubes eliminate the need for an inner cannula.

The tube may be metal or plastic. Plastic tubes typically have disposable inner cannulas, which can be replaced rather than cleaned. Plastic tubes also may have balloon-like cuffs that are inflated to prevent air escape during mechanical ventilation. You know that the cuff is inflated if the small pilot balloon on the tubing used to inject air is inflated (Fig. 29.26B and C). Cuffs are deflated routinely to prevent tissue damage. See the "Tracheostomy Care Procedure" on DavisPlus for steps required for a routine tracheostomy cleaning.

Communication is problematic for the patient with a tracheostomy tube because air is diverted out the tube rather than past the vocal cords and out the mouth. Fenestrated tubes are tubes with openings (fenestra) in the cannula to allow air to flow up into the larynx for speaking (see Fig. 29.26C). The patient can be taught to plug the opening of the tube while speaking to divert air through the fenestra. Another option is a valve such as the Passy-Muir® tracheostomy speaking valve (Fig. 29.27). This is a special valve that allows air into the tracheostomy during inspiration but closes and redirects air up around the tracheostomy tube, through the vocal cords, and out the nose and mouth on expiration, allowing the patient to speak. Use of the valve eliminates the need for the patient to use a finger over the opening to speak. For the valve to be used safely and effectively, the tracheostomy tube must be small enough for air to flow around it or it must be fenestrated to allow air to flow up through the vocal cords. If cuffed, the cuff must be completely deflated. A patient with a tracheostomy tube in place due to laryngectomy surgery will not have vocal cords, and the trachea will no longer connect to the nose and mouth. The patient will not be able to plug the tube or use a valve to talk; plugging a laryngectomy tube would cause suffocation. Laryngectomy is covered in Chapter 30.

Some tracheostomies are permanent. However, some patients can be weaned from the tracheostomy tube when their condition has improved enough to allow breathing without it. The HCP may replace the tube with a smaller tube to prepare the patient for its removal. This allows a plug to be inserted into the tracheostomy tube at intervals to force the patient to breathe around the tube through the nose and mouth. When the tracheostomy tube has been removed, the opening may be taped shut and covered with gauze until it is healed. The gauze often becomes saturated with secretions and is changed as needed.

FIGURE 29.27 The Passy-Muir® tracheostomy speaking valve allows air into the tracheostomy during inspiration but closes and redirects air up through the vocal cords and out the nose and mouth on expiration, allowing the patient to speak. *Courtesy of Passy-Muir, Inc., Irvine, CA.*

Exhaled air

Larynx and vocal folds
Esophagus (food pipe)
Trachea (windpipe)
Passy-Muir
Speaking valve

Inhaled air

CRITICAL THINKING

Mr. Smith

■ Mr. Smith had a plastic, cuffed tracheostomy tube that was small enough to allow airflow around it for talking when the cuff was deflated. A friend stopped by for a chat and assisted Mr. Smith to plug his tracheostomy so he could talk. Mr. Smith's face turned dark red, and his expression showed extreme anxiety.

1. What happened?
2. How could you help prevent this in the future?
3. How would you document this occurrence?

Suggested answers are at the end of the chapter.

Nursing Process for the Patient With a Tracheostomy

See the "Nursing Care Plan for the Patient With a Tracheostomy."

Suctioning

Suctioning involves the use of a flexible catheter to remove secretions from the respiratory tract of a patient who is unable to cough effectively. This may be a patient with overwhelming secretions or a patient with a tracheostomy or endotracheal tube who is unable to clear the tube with coughing.

The procedures for suctioning are found on DavisPlus. A procedure manual should be consulted for more detailed instruction. Remember that suctioning is both frightening and uncomfortable for a patient. Patients sometimes feel as though oxygen is being "vacuumed" from their lungs. Suctioning can cause hypoxia, vagal stimulation with resulting bradycardia, and even cardiac arrest. It is done only when necessary rather than on a routine basis. Coughing is the most effective way to clear secretions and should be encouraged if the patient is capable. Signs that suctioning is needed include crackles or wheezes heard with or without a stethoscope or a dropping oxygen saturation value. Each step should be explained to the patient during suctioning even if he or she is unresponsive.

NURSING CARE PLAN for the Patient With a Tracheostomy

Nursing Diagnosis: *Risk for Ineffective Airway Clearance* related to excessive secretions

Expected Outcome: The patient's airway will be free of secretions as evidenced by no audible crackles or wheezes in airway and a clear cannula.

Evaluation of Outcome: Is airway free of secretions?

Intervention Assess lung sounds every 4 hours and as needed (prn). **Rationale** Coarse crackles or wheezes may indicate secretions in airways. **Evaluation** Are coarse crackles or wheezes present?

Intervention Monitor oxygen saturation every 4 hours and prn. **Rationale** Secretions may reduce gas exchange. **Evaluation** Is oxygen saturation less than 90%, indicating a problem?

Intervention Encourage patient to deep breathe and cough as able. **Rationale** Patients may be able to clear own secretions without suctioning. **Evaluation** Is patient able to cough up secretions effectively?

Intervention Encourage fluids if not contraindicated. **Rationale** Fluids help hydrate secretions, making them easier to cough up. **Evaluation** Is patient taking adequate fluids? Are secretions thin?

Intervention Provide humidified oxygen or a room humidifier. **Rationale** Humidification helps prevent drying of mucosa and secretions. **Evaluation** Are mucosa moist and secretions easily removed?

Intervention Encourage ambulation as able, or turn every 2 hours. **Rationale** Movement helps mobilize secretions. **Evaluation** Is patient mobilized as much as possible?

Intervention Clean tracheostomy according to agency policy. **Rationale** Cleaning helps remove excess mucus and keeps airway clear. **Evaluation** Does cleaning help maintain an open airway?

Intervention Suction patient using sterile technique, only when needed. **Rationale** Suctioning clears secretions from airways. Unnecessary suctioning irritates airways. **Evaluation** Is suction necessary? Is airway free of secretions after suctioning?

Intervention Monitor and document amount, color, and character of secretions. Report change in secretions accompanied by fever. **Rationale** Purulent sputum accompanied by fever can indicate pneumonia. **Evaluation** Is sputum clear or white and scant in amount? Is purulent sputum reported?

Nursing Diagnosis: *Risk for Infection* related to bypass of normal respiratory defense mechanisms and increased aspiration risk

Expected Outcome: The patient will be free of infection, as evidenced by vital signs within normal limits and clear secretions.

Evaluation of Outcome: Is patient free from symptoms of infection?

Intervention Monitor and report signs and symptoms of infection: fever, increased respiratory rate, purulent sputum, elevated white blood cell (WBC) count. **Rationale** Early recognition and treatment of infection enhances outcome. **Evaluation** Are signs of infection present?

Intervention Use good hand hygiene practice. **Rationale** Hand hygiene is important in preventing infection. **Evaluation** Do all caregivers use good hand hygiene technique?

Intervention Protect tracheostomy opening from foreign material: food, sprays, powders. **Rationale** Foreign materials in the tracheostomy can cause pneumonia. **Evaluation** Is tracheostomy adequately protected?

Continued

NURSING CARE PLAN for the Patient With a Tracheostomy—cont'd

Intervention Use meticulous sterile technique for all tracheostomy care and suctioning. **Rationale** Use of non-sterile technique may introduce microorganisms into the respiratory tract. **Evaluation** Is sterile technique used by all caregivers?

Intervention Encourage a well-balanced diet. Consult dietitian prn. **Rationale** A well-balanced diet enhances immune function. **Evaluation** Is patient eating a balanced diet or receiving adequate supplementation?

Intervention Keep head of bed elevated 30 to 45 degrees. **Rationale** Elevation helps reduce aspiration of gastric contents, which can lead to pneumonia. **Evaluation** Is head of bed elevated?

Intervention Consult with speech therapist and HCP about whether to have cuff inflated or deflated on cuffed tube. **Rationale** An inflated cuff can impair swallowing in some patients, and help prevent aspiration in others. **Evaluation** Is cuff properly inflated or deflated according to specific orders?

Nursing Diagnosis: *Impaired Verbal Communication* related to presence of tracheostomy tube

Expected Outcomes: The patient will use alternate methods of communication effectively. The patient will express satisfaction with ability to communicate needs.

Evaluation of Outcomes: Is patient able to use alternative methods to express needs? Does patient express satisfaction with ability to do so?

Intervention Take time to allow patient to communicate needs. **Rationale** Patient may become frustrated if hurried. **Evaluation** Does patient feel he or she is given adequate time for communication of needs?

Intervention Watch for patient's nonverbal cues. **Rationale** Gestures and facial expression can provide valuable cues. **Evaluation** Is the patient attempting to communicate with nonverbal cues?

Intervention Offer pen and paper or magic slate (if patient is literate). **Rationale** The patient may be able to write out his or her needs/concerns. **Evaluation** Is patient able to write out needs?

Intervention Use picture board (available from speech therapy department). **Rationale** The patient can point to a picture (water, toileting) that indicates his or her need. **Evaluation** Is patient able to point appropriately to needs?

Intervention Teach patient with fenestrated or small tracheostomy tube how to cover opening with a plug or clean finger to talk, or to use Passy-Muir valve, according to HCP or speech therapy recommendations. **Rationale** Covering opening or using valve diverts air into larynx and allows speech. **Evaluation** Is patient able to communicate in this manner?

Intervention Consult with speech therapist. **Rationale** Speech therapist may have additional methods for communicating with patient. **Evaluation** Are alternative methods effective?

Nursing Diagnosis: *Disturbed Body Image* related to presence of tracheostomy

Expected Outcomes: The patient will verbalize acceptance of tracheostomy. Patient will be willing to participate in tracheostomy care.

Evaluation of Outcomes: Does patient verbalize acceptance of tracheostomy? Does patient participate in learning to care for tracheostomy?

Intervention Assess patient's and family members' feelings about tracheostomy. **Rationale** Assessment provides basis for care. **Evaluation** Are the patient's feelings within an expected range for such a change in body image? Are family members accepting?

NURSING CARE PLAN for the Patient With a Tracheostomy—cont'd

Intervention Approach patient with an accepting attitude. **Rationale** The patient will be aware of the nurse's nonverbal body language. **Evaluation** Does the patient indicate a feeling of acceptance from the nurse?

Intervention Allow patient opportunity to share concerns about tracheostomy. **Rationale** Sharing concerns helps the patient to sort out feelings and problem solve. **Evaluation** Does the patient share feelings as needed? (*Note:* Some patients do not wish to share feelings and should not be forced to do so.)

Intervention Refer patient to support group if available. **Rationale** The patient may benefit from communicating with others with tracheostomies. **Evaluation** Is patient receptive to a support group referral?

Intervention Assist patient in finding attractive ways to conceal tracheostomy if desired. **Rationale** Loose scarves or collars can help conceal and protect the tracheostomy. **Evaluation** Is patient satisfied with appearance of tracheostomy?

Nursing Diagnosis: *Deficient Knowledge* related to care of new tracheostomy

Expected Outcomes: The patient and significant other will verbalize understanding of self-care, demonstrate tracheostomy self-care procedures, and state resources for help after discharge.

Evaluation of Outcomes: Are patient and significant other able to verbalize self-care actions and rationale? Are patient and significant other able to correctly demonstrate care procedures? Is patient able to state how to obtain help after discharge?

Intervention Assess patient's and significant other's baseline knowledge of self-care. **Rationale** Teaching should only be initiated if a knowledge deficit exists. **Evaluation** Does patient exhibit knowledge of self-care?

Intervention Instruct patient and significant other in the following: • Tracheostomy cleaning • Deep breathing and coughing • Suctioning • Prevention of infection and symptoms to report to health care provider • Protection of tracheostomy from pollutants, water (no swimming, careful showering) **Rationale** The patient will need to care for self after discharge. **Evaluation** Does patient verbalize understanding of self-care and demonstrate all procedures correctly?

Intervention Provide follow-up with home health nurse after discharge. **Rationale** A home health nurse can provide reinforcement of instruction at home. **Evaluation** Is patient receptive to having a home health nurse assist?

Intubation

Some patients are unable to breathe effectively and maintain adequate oxygenation because of airway obstruction or respiratory failure. These patients are intubated with a special endotracheal (ET) tube through the nose or mouth and into the trachea (Fig. 29.28). Patients in cardiopulmonary arrest are intubated during advanced cardiac life support, and patients undergoing general anesthesia during surgery are intubated. Most intubated patients are also mechanically ventilated. Some patients have advance directives that indicate they do not wish to be intubated. You should be familiar with the patient's wishes and bring them to the attention of the HCP if necessary.

Because intubation can damage the vocal cords and surrounding tissues, it is usually a short-term intervention. Patients who need long-term ventilatory support have a tracheostomy tube placed.

Nursing Care for the Intubated Patient

Nursing care of the intubated patient includes regular assessment of the patient's respiratory status and tube placement. Lung sounds are auscultated bilaterally to ensure that the tube has not been displaced into one bronchus. The tube is carefully secured with tape or a Velcro holder to avoid dislodging. Oral tubes are repositioned and resecured to the opposite side of the mouth every 24 hours or according to institution policy to prevent tissue damage. An adhesive skin barrier should be applied under the tape to protect the skin. If the patient is alert, he or she is instructed to be careful not to pull on the tube. You may need to obtain an order for soft wrist restraints if absolutely necessary for the confused patient. Restraints can be avoided if a family member is available to sit with the patient. Many nursing interventions for the patient with a tracheostomy are also appropriate for

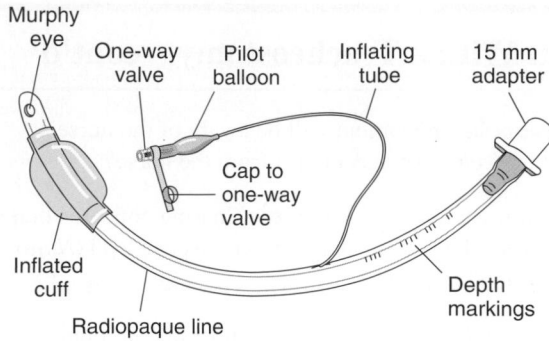

Murphy eye
One-way valve
Pilot balloon
Inflating tube
15 mm adapter
Cap to one-way valve
Inflated cuff
Radiopaque line
Depth markings

Placement of tube in airway

FIGURE 29.28 Endotracheal tube. Modified from Barnes, T. A. (1991). *Respiratory care principles.* Philadelphia: F.A. Davis, p. 425.

the intubated patient. (See the "Nursing Care Plan for the Patient With a Tracheostomy.")

Endotracheal tubes have a cuff (a balloon-like area around the tube) to help maintain proper placement and to prevent leakage of air around the tube. An RT usually inflates the cuff and maintains a specific cuff pressure and should be consulted for assistance with this activity.

Patients with ET tubes may need suctioning if they are unable to cough effectively. Visible secretions in the tube, crackles or wheezes heard with or without the stethoscope, or a drop in Sao$_2$ without another obvious cause are signs that suctioning is necessary. The ET tube suctioning procedure is sterile and is the same as suctioning a tracheostomy tube. Some institutions have in-line suctioning devices, which are connected to the ET tube within a sterile sleeve. This maintains sterility, protects the nurse, and simplifies the suctioning procedure. Oral suction may also be necessary to keep the mouth free of secretions.

The intubated patient is often extremely anxious, especially if she or he is alert. Explain the purpose of all care activities. Suctioning is a particularly anxiety-producing activity and should be explained carefully even if the patient is unresponsive.

Intubated patients are at risk of developing ventilator-associated pneumonia (VAP) because normal respiratory

defense mechanisms are bypassed. Good hand hygiene and frequent mouth care to reduce risk of aspirating oral microorganisms can help prevent VAP. The head of the bed should also be kept elevated 30 to 45 degrees at all times.

Because the ET tube passes between the vocal cords, the patient is unable to speak. Provide paper and pencil or a picture board for communication. Yes/no questions can be answered by a nod or shake of the head.

Monitor arterial blood gas and oxygen saturation values and notify the HCP of changes. If oxygen values drop or the patient becomes confused or agitated, the patient should be immediately assessed for a disconnected oxygen source or excessive secretions.

If the HCP determines that the patient can breathe effectively without the tube, the tube will be removed. The patient will be slowly weaned from the ventilator first. Before tube removal, the patient's mouth and tube are suctioned, and the cuff is deflated. After removal, the patient is observed closely for laryngeal edema or respiratory distress. The patient is maintained in high Fowler's position to maximize chest expansion.

Mechanical Ventilation

Ventilators are devices that provide ventilation (respirations) for patients who are unable to breathe effectively on their own (Fig. 29.29). Ventilators use positive pressure to push oxygenated air via a cuffed ET or tracheostomy tube into the lungs at preset intervals. Patients may need mechanical ventilation after some surgeries, after cardiac or respiratory arrest, for declining arterial blood gases related to worsening respiratory disease, or for neuromuscular disease or injury that affects the muscles of respiration.

Ventilator Modes

Ventilators can control ventilation or assist the patient's own respirations. See Table 29.9 for terms related to ventilator

FIGURE 29.29 Patient on ventilator.

TABLE 29.9 VENTILATOR TERMINOLOGY

FIO_2	Fraction of inspired oxygen.
Tidal volume	Amount of air delivered with each breath.
Rate	Frequency of breaths delivered.
Assist control mode (AC; also called continuous mechanical ventilation, or CMV)	Ventilator delivers a breath each time patient begins to inspire. If patient does not breathe, the machine continues to deliver a preset number of breaths per minute.
Synchronized intermittent mandatory ventilation (SIMV)	Allows patient to breathe independently but delivers a minimum number of ventilations per minute as necessary. Synchronized to patient's own respiratory pattern.
Pressure support (PS)	Provides positive pressure on inspiration to decrease the work of breathing.
Continuous positive airway pressure (CPAP)	Provides positive pressure on inspiration and expiration to keep alveoli open in a spontaneously breathing patient.
Positive end-expiratory pressure (PEEP)	Provides positive pressure on expiration to help keep small airways open.

function. There are many types and models of ventilators. Consult with the respiratory care department for an explanation of a patient's ventilator and how to troubleshoot alarms.

Ventilator Alarms

Several types of alarms are found on ventilators. Low-pressure alarms sound if the ventilator senses reduced pressure in the system. This can be caused by disconnected tubing, leaks in tubing or around the ET tube, or an underinflated cuff. A low-pressure alarm may also sound if the patient has attempted to remove the tube.

High-pressure alarms sound for higher-than-normal resistance to airflow. This might occur if the patient needs to be suctioned; if the patient is biting on the tube, coughing, or trying to talk; if tubing is kinked or otherwise obstructed; or if worsening respiratory disease causes decreased lung compliance. In addition, the high-pressure alarm may be triggered if the patient is anxious and unable to time his or her breaths with those of the ventilator. Water in the tubing might also cause a high-pressure alarm. Consult with the respiratory care department for guidance in draining the tubing.

A loss-of-power alarm may signal a power failure or a disconnected plug. Be aware of emergency power sources and be prepared to ventilate the patient manually if necessary. Volume and frequency alarms sound when tidal volume or number of breaths per minute fall outside preset parameters.

When an alarm sounds, always check the patient first. If the patient is stable, the machine may be checked. Determine why the alarm is sounding and correct the problem quickly. If no cause can be found, disconnect the patient from the ventilator and call for help. Use a manual resuscitation bag until help arrives.

NURSING CARE. Before initiating mechanical ventilation, it is important for the health care team to be aware of any advance directives and consult with the patient and family, because many patients do not wish to be intubated and mechanically ventilated. Some patients accept mechanical ventilation if it is a temporary measure but not if it might be a permanent intervention.

Until recently, ventilators were used only in intensive care units. Now ventilators are seen on medical-surgical units, in nursing homes, and even in patients' homes. It is important that a team approach be used when caring for a patient who is mechanically ventilated. The social worker; RT; physical, occupational, and speech therapist(s); dietitian; nurse; and HCP all work together to provide the comprehensive care needed by the patient. RTs usually take responsibility for routine monitoring and equipment maintenance.

The nurse is responsible for monitoring the patient, ensuring that ventilator settings are maintained as prescribed, providing initial response to alarms, keeping tubing free from water accumulation, and keeping the patient's airway free from secretions. In addition, the nurse keeps a manual resuscitation bag at the bedside for emergencies. Good nursing care is essential for preventing ventilator-associated complications, especially pneumonia. Keep the head of the bed at a 45-degree angle to reduce the risk of aspiration. Oral care with 0.12% chlorhexidine solution can significantly reduce the incidence of VAP (Zurmehly, 2013). Regular suctioning helps keep the airway clear. Good nutrition is also essential and has been shown to be related to eventual successful weaning.

Patients who are mechanically ventilated are unable to talk and can become very uncomfortable and anxious if there is no easy way to communicate. See Box 29-2 for one nurse's tips for making ventilated patients feel more secure. These tips were developed after the author interviewed 12 patients who had been intubated. They shared their fears, anxieties, and physical discomforts.

Box 29-2 Tips for Caring for Patients Who Are Mechanically Ventilated

- Mechanically ventilated patients report feeling panicky but less so if relatives or nursing staff are present.
  - Speak to the patient each time you enter the room and explain everything you do.
  - Encourage family to visit.
  - Answer the patient's call light and attend to ventilator alarms promptly.
  - Use restraints only as a last resort.
- Patients may have difficulty relaxing and sleeping while on a ventilator.
  - Administer sedatives or antianxiety drugs as ordered. Request an order if necessary.
  - Allow uninterrupted blocks of time for sleep.
- Patients with endotracheal tubes report pain and discomfort.
  - Assess for comfort and reposition at regular intervals.
  - Be careful not to pull on the ventilator tubing.
  - Administer analgesics as ordered.
  - Provide good oral care, moistening the lips with a cool washcloth and water-based lubricant.
- Suctioning is painful and frightening for patients.
  - Suction quickly and smoothly, and avoid inserting the catheter too deeply.
  - Avoid the use of saline with suctioning, which can reduce SpO_2.
  - Allow the patient to suction him or herself if possible (with HCP order and appropriate instruction).
- Communication is very difficult for the patient.
  - Be patient when trying to understand communication efforts.
  - Provide a pencil and paper, but be aware that even writing can be exhausting.
  - Ask yes or no questions when possible. Establish a response system with the patient such as blinking (once for no, twice for yes), hand squeezes, or nodding.
  - Validate patient expressions and body language; don't assume that a patient is sad or wants to be left alone based on facial expression.
  - Make sure the call light is within reach at all times.

Noninvasive Positive-Pressure Ventilation

Noninvasive positive-pressure ventilation (NIPPV) is an alternative to intubation and mechanical ventilation for patients who are able to breathe on their own but are unable to maintain normal blood gases. Patients with severe respiratory disease, sleep apnea, or neuromuscular diseases such as amyotrophic lateral sclerosis (ALS) that weaken respiratory muscles can benefit from this treatment. Instead of the invasive endotracheal or tracheostomy tube, NIPPV uses an external masklike device that fits over the nose or mouth and nose (Fig. 29.30). It can be successful in patients who are alert, able to cooperate, do not have excessive secretions, and are able to breathe on their own for periods of time. It can be used with or without supplemental oxygen. In an acutely ill patient, oxygen saturations are monitored.

Two basic types of NIPPV are available: continuous positive airway pressure (CPAP) and bilevel positive airway pressure (BiPAP). With CPAP, the same amount of positive pressure is maintained throughout inspiration and expiration to prevent airway collapse. In BiPAP, a lower level of positive pressure is used on expiration.

Problems to be alert for in patients receiving NIPPV include skin irritation from the mask and gastric distention from swallowing air. Apply an adhesive skin barrier to the areas that come in contact with the mask to prevent irritation. To prevent gastric distention, place the patient in semi-Fowler's position and consult with the RT to adjust air delivery pressure if necessary. Topical saline or a special humidifier on the machine can reduce nose and mouth dryness. An air leak around the mask can cause air to blow in the patient's eyes, which can be irritating. If this happens, remove the mask and reposition it. Another problem is patient acceptance of NIPPV. Many patients do not like the tight mask covering their nose or mouth. Be patient in explaining the reason for this treatment and check the patient frequently to help control anxiety. Be sure to assess the patient's goals for therapy. Some patients may choose not to use NIPPV, but they must be fully aware of possible consequences.

Patients can use NIPPV nearly continuously, removing it to eat or use the bathroom. Other patients who are able to breathe effectively on their own during the day use it only when they are sleeping. Some use it for a few days until an acute exacerbation of disease is resolved, and others continue its use indefinitely at home.

FIGURE 29.30 Noninvasive positive-pressure ventilation. Note round face from steroid use.

SUGGESTED ANSWERS TO

CRITICAL THINKING

■ *Timothy*

1. There is no way to know whether Timothy needs to be in the emergency room without further assessment. Remember that shortness of breath is very subjective and must be evaluated before discharge.

2. Collect further data. Have Timothy rate his shortness of breath. Look at his color and use of accessory muscles. Check his vital signs, peak expiratory flow rate, and oxygen saturation.

3. If Timothy is having an asthma attack, one explanation for the absence of wheezing on auscultation is that he is not moving enough air to generate the wheezing sound. If his airways are extremely tight, breath sounds may be so diminished that wheezing is not heard. This is a bad sign rather than a good one.

4. If Timothy's assessment findings are abnormal, call for help. The HCP may want to begin treatment quickly before further evaluation is done. A RT can be helpful with both further assessment and treatment. Collaborate with the RN to determine the cause of Timothy's problems and provide appropriate education to prevent repeat episodes.

■ *Miss Israel*

1. Bubbling in the water seal chamber indicates a leak in the system. Vigorous bubbling may indicate a large leak, and the HCP should be contacted immediately. After you check the patient, check the entire system for cracks or leaks and correct any problems discovered.

2. 50 mL.

■ *Mr. Smith*

1. Mr. Smith plugged his tracheostomy while the cuff was still inflated, so no air could get to his lungs. If the plug is not removed immediately, he will be totally unable to breathe. Whenever the plug is in place, air must be able to travel around the tracheostomy tube or through the opening of a fenestrated tube so the patient can breathe.

2. To prevent this from happening in the future, Mr. Smith should be taught how his tracheostomy tube works and how to care for it. He can be taught to check the pilot balloon if he is unsure.

3. "Answered call for help at 12:30, found patient dark red in color, unable to breathe, trach plugged. Trach unplugged, respirations restored, vital signs stable. Patient stated he plugged trach so he could talk to his friend. Function of trach cuff explained to patient and friend. Both verbalize understanding to only plug trach when cuff is deflated or to call for nurse if unsure."

REVIEW QUESTIONS

1. How should the nurse record smoking history on a patient who has smoked 2.5 packs of cigarettes per day for 10 years?
   1. Patient has smoked cigarettes for 10 years.
   2. Patient smokes 2.5 packs of cigarettes per day.
   3. Patient has a 12.5 pack-year smoking history.
   4. Patient has a 25 pack-year smoking history.

2. Which term should be used to document the musical sounds generated by airflow through narrowed airways?
   1. Crackles
   2. Wheezes
   3. Friction rub
   4. Stridor

3. Which laboratory result should alert the nurse to perform further assessment on a patient admitted with respiratory distress?
   1. $PaCO_2$ <50 mm Hg
   2. HCO_3^- <27 mEq/L
   3. Pao_2 <90 mm Hg
   4. Spo_2 <90%

4. Place the following steps in the correct sequential order for obtaining a sputum specimen for culture.
   1. Have the patient cough deeply from the lungs.
   2. Teach the patient to inhale deeply several times.
   3. Check the order for the test.
   4. Send the specimen immediately to the laboratory.
   5. Obtain the appropriate container.

5. Which instruction is correct when teaching a patient how to use a traditional metered-dose inhaler?
    1. "Inhale deeply, place canister in mouth, depress top of canister, exhale."
    2. "Exhale, place canister in mouth, depress canister and inhale at the same time."
    3. "Cough, place canister in mouth, inhale deeply, cough again."
    4. "Exhale, depress canister, place in mouth, inhale deeply."

6. A patient with a continuous positive airway pressure (CPAP) mask develops dry irritated eyes from the blowing air. What nursing intervention will help prevent eye irritation while maintaining the positive pressure ventilation?
    1. Offer moisturizing eyedrops.
    2. Discontinue the CPAP.
    3. Reposition the mask.
    4. Tape the patient's eyes closed.

Answers can be found in Appendix C.

References

Joint Commission. (2013). *2014 National Patient Safety Goals.* Retrieved July 3, 2013, from www.jointcommission.org /assets/1/18/NPSG_Chapter_Jan2013_HAP.pdf

Karlsson, V., Lindahl, B., & Bergbom, I. (2012). Patients' statements and experiences concerning receiving mechanical ventilation: A prospective video-recorded study. *Nursing Inquiry, 19,* 247–258. doi:10.1111/j.1440-1800.2011.00576.x

Laakso, K., Markström, A., & Hartelius, L. (2009). Communication and quality of life in individuals receiving home mechanical ventilation [including commentary by Happ, M. B.,

Salahuddin, N., Carone, M., & Antoniu, S. A.]. *International Journal of Therapy & Rehabilitation, 16,* 648–658.

Zurmehly, J. (2013). Oral care education in the prevention of ventilator-associated pneumonia: Quality patient outcomes in the intensive care unit. *The Journal of Continuing Education in Nursing, 44,* 67–75.

 DavisPlus | For additional resources and information visit **davispl.us/medsurg5**

Nursing Care of Patients With Upper Respiratory Tract Disorders

30

PAULA D. HOPPER

LEARNING OUTCOMES

1. Explain the pathophysiologies of disorders of the upper respiratory tract.
2. Describe etiologies, signs, and symptoms of disorders of the upper respiratory tract.
3. Describe current therapeutic measures for disorders of the upper respiratory tract.
4. Plan nursing care for the patient with an upper respiratory disorder.
5. Discuss how you will know if your care has been effective.
6. Identify the special needs of the patient who has undergone a laryngectomy.

KEY TERMS

dysphagia (dis-FAY-jee-ah)
epistaxis (EP-iss-TAX-iss)
exudate (EKS-yoo-dayt)
laryngectomee (lare-in-JEK-tuh-mee)
laryngitis (lare-in-JY-tiss)
myalgia (my-AL-jyah)
nasoseptoplasty (NAY-zoh-SEP-toh-plass-tee)
pharyngitis (fair-in-JY-tiss)
rhinitis (rye-NYE-tiss)
rhinoplasty (RY-noh-plass-tee)
sinusitis (SY-nuss-EYE-tuss)

Disorders of the upper respiratory tract include problems occurring in the nose, sinuses, pharynx, larynx, and trachea. Many of these problems are minor illnesses that can be cared for at home. Others can become serious if they are not recognized and treated in a timely manner.

 DISORDERS OF THE NOSE AND SINUSES

Epistaxis

Pathophysiology

Epistaxis is more commonly known as a nosebleed. The nose can bleed either from the anterior or posterior region. Anterior bleeds are much more common and originate from a group of vessels called the Kiesselbach plexus. Anterior bleeds are easier to locate and treat than posterior bleeds. The blood vessels of the posterior nose are larger, and bleeding can be severe and difficult to control.

Etiology

The most common cause of epistaxis is dry, cracked mucous membranes. Trauma, forceful nose blowing, nose picking, and tumors are also factors. Anything that reduces the blood's ability to clot, such as hemophilia or leukemia, regular aspirin use, anticoagulant therapy, or chemotherapy can predispose a patient to nosebleeds. Cocaine use can also cause epistaxis. High blood pressure can prolong a nosebleed but is not usually the cause.

Therapeutic Measures

Instruct a patient with a nosebleed to sit in a chair and lean forward slightly to avoid aspirating or swallowing blood. If the patient swallows blood, it will be difficult to assess the extent of bleeding, and it might cause nausea and vomiting. Be sure to wear gloves and follow standard precautions. Place pressure on the nares for 5 to 10 minutes to stop bleeding. However, avoid placing pressure on the nose if a fracture is suspected to avoid further trauma. Ice packs to the nose and eye area may be used to constrict the bleeding vessels.

If first aid measures are ineffective in stopping bleeding, a physician may attempt more invasive treatment. Local application of a vasoconstrictive agent such as oxymetazoline (Afrin) or phenylephrine might be used to constrict the bleeding vessels. If the bleeding vessel can be located, the physician may cauterize it by use of an electrical cauterizing device or by application of silver nitrate.

Gauze may be used to pack the anterior nasal cavity. The cavity is packed firmly but gently, usually with half-inch petroleum or iodoform gauze. Placement and removal of packing can be uncomfortable for the patient. If there is time, administration of an analgesic before the procedure is helpful. Petroleum jelly on the packing helps prevent gauze from adhering to the nasal mucosa. If the packing is to remain in place for several days, it is coated with an antibiotic ointment to reduce the risk of infection, or oral antibiotics may be ordered.

Commercial products such as compressed sponges and nasal tampons are available to pack the nose. For anterior and posterior bleeds, balloon catheters such as the Rapid Rhino® device can be inserted and inflated near the bleeding vessels in the nasal cavity (Fig. 30.1). The inflated balloon places pressure on the bleeding vessels to stop the bleeding. A small Foley catheter can also be used for this procedure. If these measures are not effective, materials such as a gelatin sponge or a tiny coil can be inserted into the bleeding artery. Patients who are treated for posterior bleeding are typically hospitalized until they are stable.

If the patient has lost a significant amount of blood, intravenous (IV) fluid replacement or a transfusion may be needed. Nosebleeds rarely cause death because blood loss lowers blood pressure, which in turn slows the bleeding. Ultimately the cause of the epistaxis is determined and corrected if possible. Rarely, surgical correction may be necessary for repeat episodes of epistaxis.

Nursing Care for the Patient With Epistaxis

Monitor bleeding, noting the amount and color of drainage. Monitor vital signs and hemoglobin level for signs of excessive blood loss. If the patient swallows repeatedly, inspect the back of the throat for bleeding. If bleeding does not stop within 10 to 15 minutes, or if it worsens, notify a registered nurse (RN) or health care provider (HCP) immediately.

If posterior packing has been used, monitor the patient for airway obstruction from a slipped device. Know how to remove

FIGURE 30.1 Rapid Rhino®. *Courtesy of ArthroCare, Inc.*

the device in case of emergency. Institute comfort measures, and maintain the placement of the external portion of the device. The HCP will remove the packing or catheter. Once bleeding is controlled, caution the patient not to blow the nose for up to 48 hours and to avoid nose picking. The patient should also avoid bending over, which can increase pressure in the nose. If the cause of the bleeding is dryness, teach the patient to use nasal saline spray or a room humidifier.

CRITICAL THINKING

Mr. Jondahl

■ Mr. Jondahl is brought to the emergency room with a nosebleed. His vital signs are blood pressure 140/90 mm Hg, pulse 92 beats per minute, respirations 20 per minute. He states that he has never had a nosebleed before. He denies any history of coagulation disorders. His current medications include captopril (Capoten), furosemide (Lasix), and ibuprofen (Motrin). What are two areas you should assess further in trying to determine a cause? (*Hint:* If you are not familiar with Mr. Jondahl's medications, look them up.)

Suggested answers are at the end of the chapter.

Nasal Polyps
Pathophysiology and Etiology

Polyps are grapelike clusters of mucosa in the nasal passages. They are usually benign, but they can obstruct the nasal passages and are sometimes complicated by sinus infections. Although the exact cause is unknown, they are related to chronic inflammation, and people with allergies are prone to developing them. They are also associated with cystic fibrosis. Some patients with nasal polyps also have asthma and are allergic to aspirin. This is called *aspirin triad asthma* because the three components often occur together.

Therapeutic Measures

Control of allergy symptoms may help control polyp development. Oral antihistamines or nasal corticosteroid sprays can help control inflammation. Antibiotics are used if there is a related sinus infection. If polyps obstruct breathing, they can be removed. This is done as an outpatient procedure under local anesthesia, using laser or endoscopic surgery. Patients are taught to avoid aspirin products after surgery because they increase the risk of postoperative bleeding and recurrence of the polyps.

Deviated Septum
Pathophysiology and Etiology

The septum dividing the nasal passages is slightly deviated in most adults. This may result from nasal trauma but often has no cause. Some septa may be so deviated that they block sinus drainage or interfere with breathing.

Signs and Symptoms

The patient may report a chronically stuffy nose or discomfort from blocked sinus drainage. Some patients have headaches, sinus infections, or nosebleeds.

Therapeutic Measures

Symptoms may be treated with decongestants, antihistamines, or intranasal cortisone sprays to reduce inflammation. However, if the deviated septum is causing chronic problems, a **nasoseptoplasty** can be done. This surgery involves revising or removing the deviated portion of the septum. Nasal packing is then placed to reduce bleeding. This is typically done as an outpatient surgical procedure under local anesthesia.

Nursing Care for the Patient After Nasoseptoplasty

After surgery, monitor vital signs and bleeding until the patient is stable. Excessive swallowing should alert you to check for blood running down the back of the throat. The patient will have nasal packing and a "mustache dressing" of folded gauze under the nose to catch drainage.

Most patients are discharged home once they are stable, so teaching is important. The patient should maintain a semi-Fowler's position as much as possible and avoid anything that might increase pressure and cause bleeding, such as sneezing, coughing, or straining to move the bowels.

Stool softeners and cough suppressants may be ordered by the HCP if needed. Aspirin and related medications are avoided because they increase the risk of bleeding. Antibiotics may be ordered if packing is in place because of the risk of infection from nasal bacteria. The HCP should be contacted for specific orders if the patient is on anticoagulant therapy at home.

Ice can be used to reduce swelling and bruising. Instruct the patient to contact the HCP if fever, excessive pain, swelling, or bleeding occurs and to return in 24 to 48 hours for removal of nasal packing (Box 30-1, "Patient Education").

Rhinoplasty

Rhinoplasty is the surgical reconstruction of the nose, usually for cosmetic purposes. It may also be done to correct deformity caused by trauma. Nursing care is similar to that for the patient after nasoseptoplasty.

Sinusitis
Pathophysiology and Etiology

Sinusitis is inflammation of the mucosa of one or more sinuses. It can be either acute or chronic. Chronic sinusitis is diagnosed if symptoms have existed for more than 3 months and are unresponsive to treatment. The maxillary and ethmoid sinuses are the most commonly affected. The inflammation is often the

---

• WORD • BUILDING •

nasoseptoplasty: naso—nose + septo—septum + plasty—to mold, as in plastic surgery

rhinoplasty: rhin—nose + plasty—to mold, as in plastic surgery

sinusitis: sinu—sinus + itis—inflammation

Box 30-1 Patient Education

Nasal Surgery

1. Your nose will feel stuffy and may drain. Change the moustache dressing as often as needed. Do *not* blow your nose. If you must sneeze, do so with your mouth open.
2. Avoid strenuous exercise, including swimming, for several weeks.
3. Drink plenty of fluids unless your HCP advises otherwise.
4. Use a cool mist vaporizer to humidify air and prevent nasal drying.
5. Keep your head elevated on two pillows or sleep in a recliner chair.
6. Expect some bruising around your eyes.
7. Use an ice pack on your face to help reduce swelling.
8. Take pain medication as prescribed.
9. Call your HCP if you have a fever higher than 101°F (38.3°C).
10. Return to see your HCP as directed. Check hospital or surgeon policy for specific instructions.

result of a bacterial infection and may follow a cold or other viral upper respiratory illness. Because the mucous lining of the nose and sinuses is continuous, nasal organisms easily travel to the sinuses. When the infected mucous lining of the sinuses swells, drainage is blocked. Bacteria that normally reside in the sinuses multiply in the retained secretions. The most common infecting organisms are *Streptococcus pneumoniae* and *Haemophilus influenzae*. Other causes of sinusitis include swelling caused by allergies, nasal polyps, fungal infection, or intubation with a nasotracheal or nasogastric tube.

Signs and Symptoms

The patient usually has pain over the region of the affected sinuses and purulent nasal discharge. If a maxillary sinus is affected, the patient will have pain over the cheek and upper teeth. In ethmoid sinusitis, pain occurs between and behind the eyes. Pain in the forehead typically indicates frontal sinusitis. Fever may be present in acute infection, with or without generalized fatigue and foul breath.

Complications

The patient who has received inadequate treatment or who has not complied with treatment is at risk for complications. Uncontrolled sinusitis may spread to surrounding areas, causing osteomyelitis, cellulitis of the orbit (infection of the soft tissues around the eye), abscess, or meningitis. Sinusitis can also trigger asthma symptoms.

Diagnostic Tests

Uncomplicated sinusitis may be diagnosed based on symptoms alone. If repeated episodes occur, x-ray examination,

nasal endoscopy, computed tomography (CT) scan, or magnetic resonance imaging (MRI) may be done to confirm the diagnosis and determine the cause. Nasal discharge may be cultured to determine appropriate antibiotic therapy.

Therapeutic Measures

Treatment is aimed at relieving pain and promoting sinus drainage. Nasal irrigation with normal saline solution helps some sufferers of chronic sinusitis. Corticosteroids, usually via a nasal spray (such as fluticasone [Flonase]) reduce inflammation. Adrenergic nasal sprays such as oxymetazoline (Afrin) constrict blood vessels and therefore reduce swelling, but they should be used cautiously by patients with heart disease or hypertension because vasoconstriction increases blood pressure. Adrenergic sprays may be used for up to 3 days; longer use may cause rebound congestion. Warm moist packs over the affected sinus for 1 to 2 hours twice a day may help decrease inflammation. Acetaminophen or ibuprofen is given for pain and fever. Opioids may be used if pain is severe. Expectorants such as guaifenesin (Robitussin, Mucinex), fluids, and a room humidifier can help loosen secretions. Antihistamines dry and thicken secretions and usually are avoided. Antibiotics are not recommended for most sinus infections. If conservative treatment does not relieve symptoms, the physician may surgically drain the affected sinus and irrigate it with normal saline or an antibiotic solution.

One such drainage procedure is the Caldwell-Luc procedure. The surgeon enters the maxillary sinus above the upper teeth, under the upper lip. The infected mucosa and bone are removed, and a new, larger opening is made to drain the sinus. Newer procedures, now more common, use nasal endoscopy to open and drain a chronically infected sinus.

Nursing Care for the Patient With Sinusitis

Patients with uncomplicated sinusitis are cared for at home. Instruct the patient to increase water intake to 8 to 10 glasses per day unless contraindicated. Excess water might be contraindicated in patients with fluid overload, such as those with cardiovascular or kidney disease. Pressure may be relieved if the patient maintains a semi-Fowler's position, as in a reclining chair. Explain the use of warm moist packs, analgesics, and prescribed medications. Instruct the patient to finish the antibiotic prescription even if he or she is feeling better before it is completed and to call the primary care provider if pain becomes severe or if signs of complications such as a change in level of consciousness occur.

Sleep Apnea
Pathophysiology and Etiology

The patient with obstructive sleep apnea (OSA) has periods of apnea during sleep. This most often occurs when sleeping supine. The muscles of the throat relax, and the tongue and soft tissues fall back to obstruct the airway (Fig. 30.2). Transient hypoxemia results, and a signal to take a breath causes a sudden, loud inhalation. This can occur up to 100 times an hour throughout the night. Men are affected more often than women, as are people who are overweight, smokers, and

FIGURE 30.2 Obstructive sleep apnea. (A) Normal open airway. (B) Obstructed airway in OSA. *Courtesy of Philips Respironics, Murraysville, PA.*

those with high arched palates or receding jawlines. OSA is associated with increased risk for heart disease, high blood pressure, stroke, and diabetes.

Signs and Symptoms

Ask the sleeping partner of someone with sleep apnea, and he or she will tell you that sleep apnea is noisy. When the tongue falls back and obstructs the airway, the result is total silence. When breathing resumes, it is like a very loud snore. Spouses often find themselves lying awake waiting for the next breath. Because the quality of sleep is impaired, the sufferer may awaken with a headache, often is not rested on awakening, is sleepy throughout the day, and may have difficulty with memory and attention. Sudden sleepiness can make driving dangerous.

Diagnostic Tests

A sleep study involves an overnight stay at a sleep center. (The proper name for this test is nocturnal polysomnography.) The patient is hooked up to electroencephalogram (EEG), electrocardiogram (EKG), electromyography (EMG), oxygen saturation, and eye movement monitors and then observed while sleeping. Many people find it somewhat difficult to fall asleep hooked up to so many wires, but a sedative would alter the results of the test. A less sophisticated form of the test can sometimes be performed at home.

Therapeutic Measures

Teach patients self-care measures such as avoiding alcohol or sedatives at bedtime; these can worsen apnea by increasing relaxation of the muscles in the pharynx. Advise against sleeping on the back, and encourage smoking cessation. Weight loss may help reduce sleep apnea and is also a good idea for reducing cardiovascular and diabetes risks. A newer treatment involves nasal patches (such as Provent®) that have valves that impede airflow on exhalation, causing increased pressure in the airway. This holds the airway open during exhalation.

New evidence-based guidelines from the American College of Physicians provide three treatment recommendations: (1) weight loss, (2) noninvasive positive pressure ventilation (NIPPV, see Chapter 29), and (3) use of a mandibular advancement devices (a mouthpiece to advance the mandible (Qaseem et al, 2013). If all other measures have failed, surgery may be necessary to remove excess tissue.

NURSING CARE TIP

If your patient has trouble avoiding sleeping on his back, have him sew a pocket onto the back of an old tee shirt and put a tennis ball in it. As soon as he rolls over onto the ball, he'll quickly be back on his side!

 INFECTIOUS DISORDERS

Viral Rhinitis/Common Cold
Pathophysiology and Etiology

Rhinitis (also called coryza) is inflammation of the nasal mucous membranes. The release of histamine and other substances causes vasodilation and edema. It may occur as a

• WORD • BUILDING •

rhinitis: rhin—nose + itis—inflammation

reaction to allergens (sometimes called hay fever) such as pollen, dust, molds, or some foods, or it may be caused by viral or bacterial infection. Viral rhinitis is another name for the common cold. The most common cold virus is the rhinovirus, which is contagious.

Signs and Symptoms

Common symptoms include nasal congestion, localized itching, sneezing, sore throat, and nasal discharge. Viral or bacterial rhinitis may also be accompanied by fever and malaise. Sometimes it is difficult to differentiate between a cold and influenza (flu). See Table 30.1 for signs and symptoms of each.

Diagnostic Tests

A throat culture or rapid flu test can help identify whether symptoms are caused by the flu virus.

Therapeutic Measures

Treatment of viral rhinitis is symptomatic. Because colds are caused by viruses, antibiotics are not effective. Inappropriate use of antibiotics can lead to antibiotic-resistant infections. Explain to the patient that taking antibiotics for a viral infection is not only ineffective but also potentially dangerous.

Acetaminophen can be used for generalized discomfort. Decongestants cause vasoconstriction, which reduces swelling and congestion. Any drugs that cause vasoconstriction should be used cautiously in patients with heart disease or hypertension. Cough syrups and cold medicines should be used with caution, because they do not treat the underlying cause of the cold and often contain several drugs, many of which are not really needed. Teach the patient that rest and fluids are the most effective treatment (see the "Nursing Care Plan for the Patient With an Upper Respiratory Infection"). Echinacea, vitamin C, and zinc are alternative remedies that might help reduce the severity or length of symptoms by supporting the immune system, but there is not enough evidence to be sure at this time.

 EVIDENCE-BASED PRACTICE

Clinical Question
Are antibiotics useful for the common cold or purulent rhinitis?

Evidence
Eleven research studies were reviewed. Researchers found that patients receiving antibiotics did not do better than those receiving placebos and had higher risk for adverse effects.

Implications for Nursing Practice
Routine use of antibiotics for the common cold or purulent rhinitis is not recommended.

REFERENCE
Kenealy T, Arroll B. Antibiotics for the common cold and acute purulent rhinitis. Cochrane Database of Systematic Reviews 2013, Issue 6. Art. No.: CD000247. DOI: 10.1002 /14651858.CD000247.pub3

TABLE 30.1 DIFFERENTIATING RESPIRATORY TRACT INFECTIONS

Signs and Symptoms	Cold	Influenza	Bacterial Infection
Onset	Slow	Sudden	Usually slow
Fever	None or low grade	Common, may exceed 101°F (38.3°C)	Common, may exceed 101°F (38.3°C)
Headache	Rare	Common	Less common
Muscle aches	Less common	Common, may be severe	Less common
Cough	Present	Present, usually dry	Present, may be dry or productive
Chest pain	Absent	Common	Common
Fatigue	Slight	Common, prolonged, may be severe	Common
Runny nose	Common	Less common	Less common
Sore throat	Common	Less common	Less common
Complications	Rare	Pneumonia	Pneumonia
Treatment	Rest and fluids	Rest and fluids, antiviral agents in some cases	Antibiotics

Pharyngitis
Pathophysiology and Etiology

Pharyngitis, or inflammation of the pharynx, is usually related to bacterial or viral infection. It may also occur as a result of trauma to the tissues. Five percent to 15% of pharyngitis cases are caused by beta-hemolytic streptococci, commonly referred to as strep throat. If strep throat is not treated with antibiotics, it can lead to rheumatic fever, glomerulonephritis, or other serious complications.

Signs and Symptoms

The most common symptom of pharyngitis is a sore throat. Some patients may also experience **dysphagia** (difficulty swallowing). The throat appears red and swollen, and **exudate** (drainage or pus) may be present. Exudate usually signifies bacterial infection and may be accompanied by fever, chills, headache, and generalized malaise.

Diagnostic Tests

The HCP may order a rapid streptococcal antigen test or a throat culture and sensitivity test (explained in Chapter 29) to identify the causative organism and determine which antibiotic will be effective.

Therapeutic Measures

If the pharyngitis is bacterial, antibiotics are ordered. Penicillin is commonly used for streptococcal infection. Acetaminophen or throat lozenges may be used to relieve discomfort. Saltwater gargles (a teaspoon salt in a glass of warm water) or honey and lemon mixed with warm water help soothe inflamed tissues. Encourage fluids (if not contraindicated) and rest. (See the "Nursing Care Plan for the Patient With an Upper Respiratory Infection.")

Laryngitis
Pathophysiology and Etiology

Laryngitis is an inflammation of the mucous membrane lining the larynx (voice box). It can be caused by irritation from smoking, alcohol, chemical exposure, gastroesophageal reflux disease (GERD), or a viral, fungal, or bacterial infection.

- WORD • BUILDING •
pharyngitis: pharyng—pharynx + itis—inflammation
dysphagia: dys—bad + phagia—to swallow
exudate: to sweat out
laryngitis: laryng—larynx + itis—inflammation

NURSING CARE PLAN for the Patient With an Upper Respiratory Infection

Nursing Diagnosis: *Impaired Comfort* related to infectious process

Expected Outcomes: The patient will be comfortable as evidenced by statement of increased comfort and ability to swallow and sleep at night.

Evaluation of Outcomes: Does the patient express comfort? Is the patient able to sleep?

Intervention Assess for cause of discomfort: malaise, muscle aches, fever, sore throat. **Rationale** Knowing cause of discomfort helps guide intervention. **Evaluation** Can interventions be directed toward specific symptoms?

Intervention Offer acetaminophen or nonsteroidal anti-inflammatory drugs (NSAIDs) as ordered. **Rationale** Analgesics relieve pain. Antipyretics relieve fever, which may contribute to discomfort. **Evaluation** Do analgesics/antipyretics relieve discomfort?

Intervention Offer throat lozenges, saltwater, or honey and lemon gargles as ordered for irritated throat. **Rationale** Lozenges or gargles soothe irritated mucous membranes. **Evaluation** Do measures relieve throat irritation?

Intervention Encourage rest. **Rationale** Physical stress increases need for sleep. Rest boosts immune function. **Evaluation** Is patient resting comfortably?

Nursing Diagnosis: *Hyperthermia* related to infectious process

Expected Outcomes: The patient will have a temperature lower than 103°F (39.4°C) and show no signs/symptoms of dehydration.

Evaluation of Outcomes: Is the patient's fever controlled at safe level? Is the patient well hydrated?

Continued

NURSING CARE PLAN for the Patient With an Upper Respiratory Infection—cont'd

Intervention Monitor temperature daily; every 4 hours if fever present. **Rationale** Screening helps detect temperature changes early. **Evaluation** Is patient febrile?

Intervention If patient begins chilling, recheck temperature when chilling subsides. **Rationale** Chilling indicates rising temperature. **Evaluation** Is chilling present? Should temperature be checked more often?

Intervention Monitor for signs of dehydration: dry skin and mucous membranes, thirst, weakness, hypotension. **Rationale** Fever causes loss of body fluids. **Evaluation** Are signs of dehydration present?

Intervention Encourage oral fluids if not contraindicated. **Rationale** Fluids prevent or treat dehydration. **Evaluation** Is patient taking fluids well?

Intervention Administer antipyretic such as acetaminophen if fever is higher than 102°F (39°C) or for discomfort. **Rationale** Antipyretics reduce fever. Fever enhances immune function and so should be treated only if very high, patient has a history of febrile seizures, or patient is uncomfortable. **Evaluation** Is fever higher than 102°F (39°C)? Are antipyretics indicated? Are they effective?

Intervention If fever rises above 103°F (39.4°C), contact health care provider. **Rationale** A fever above 103°F (39.4°C) can indicate more serious infection and may require treatment. **Evaluation** Is fever above 103°F? Has provider been contacted?

Nursing Diagnosis: *Risk for Infection:* transmission to others related to presence of infectious disease

Expected Outcomes: Risk for infection of others will be reduced, as evidenced by the patient stating measures to prevent transmission and the patient taking precautions against spread.

Evaluation of Outcomes: Is transmission to others prevented?

Intervention Assess patient's understanding of infection transmission. **Rationale** Understanding of mode of transmission is essential to prevention. **Evaluation** Does patient understand how infection is transmitted?

Intervention Based on patient's previous knowledge, teach patient and all caregivers: • the importance of good hand hygiene after contact with patient or patient's belongings • to cover nose and mouth when coughing or sneezing • not to share eating or drinking utensils. See cough etiquette guidelines in Chapter 8. **Rationale** The nurse should build on patient's previous understanding and not repeat information. Hand hygiene prevents spread of infection. Covering nose and mouth prevents spread of infectious droplets. Many infections are transmitted via contaminated objects. **Evaluation** Does patient take precautions to prevent spread of infection?

It often follows an upper respiratory infection. Laryngeal cancer can also cause symptoms of laryngitis.

Signs and Symptoms

The most common symptom is hoarseness. Cough, dysphagia, or fever may also be present.

Diagnostic Tests

The HCP may use a tiny mirror to view the larynx. If hoarseness persists for more than 2 weeks, a laryngoscopy and biopsy may be done to rule out cancer of the larynx.

Therapeutic Measures

Treatment includes rest, fluids, humidified air, and aspirin (in adults) or acetaminophen. Antibiotics are used if bacterial infection is present. Medication to control acid reflux is used if GERD is the cause. Encourage the patient to avoid speaking, which will help rest the voice. Also advise the patient that whispering strains the voice even more than normal speech. Obtain a "magic slate" (from the speech therapy department) or paper and pen to help the patient communicate. Throat lozenges may help increase comfort. Help the patient to identify and avoid causative factors. (See the

"Nursing Care Plan for the Patient With an Upper Respiratory Infection.")

Tonsillitis/Adenoiditis

Pathophysiology and Etiology

The tonsils are masses of lymphoid tissue that lie on each side of the oropharynx. They filter microorganisms to protect the lungs from infection. Tonsillitis occurs when the filtering function becomes overwhelmed with a virus or bacteria and infection results. The adenoids, a mass of lymphoid tissue located at the back of the nasopharynx, can also become involved. Tonsillitis is more common in children but is more serious when it occurs in adults. Tonsillitis is usually viral, but bacteria that are commonly associated with tonsillitis include *Streptococcus* species, *Staphylococcus aureus, Haemophilus influenzae,* and *Pneumococcus* species.

Signs and Symptoms

Tonsillitis usually begins suddenly with a sore throat, fever, chills, and pain on swallowing. Generalized symptoms include headache, malaise, and **myalgia**. On examination, the tonsils appear red and swollen and may have yellow or white exudate on them. If the adenoids are involved, the patient may mention snoring, a nasal obstruction, and a nasal tone to the voice.

Diagnostic Tests

A throat culture is done to discover the causative organism and determine effective treatment. A white blood cell count and differential can also help identify whether the infection is viral or bacterial. A chest x-ray may be done if respiratory symptoms are present.

Therapeutic Measures

Antibiotics are prescribed for bacterial infection. Acetaminophen, lozenges, and saline gargles help promote comfort. For care of the patient who is not having a tonsillectomy, see the "Nursing Care Plan for the Patient With an Upper Respiratory Infection."

If tonsillitis becomes chronic or if breathing or swallowing is affected, a tonsillectomy may be considered, although this is not a common procedure in an adult. An adenoidectomy may be performed at the same time. After the tonsillectomy, the patient is maintained in a semi-Fowler's position to reduce swelling and promote drainage. Monitor the patient for bleeding and airway patency, and provide comfort measures. Encourage fluids for hydration; cold fluids may help reduce pain and bleeding. Red-colored drinks are avoided because they interfere with observation for bleeding. A room humidifier helps prevent drying. Keep suction equipment available for emergencies.

Influenza

Pathophysiology and Etiology

Influenza, commonly called the *flu,* is a viral infection of the respiratory tract. Many different flu viruses have been identified, and new strains appear each year. Influenza is the cause of millions of lost workdays each year. Young children,

---

CRITICAL THINKING

Mrs. Hiler

■ You are caring for Mrs. Hiler after a tonsillectomy. She is sleeping, but you notice that she swallows every few seconds. She has an IV line of normal saline solution running at 100 mL per hour.

1. How do you respond?
2. What should you be vigilant for?
3. How many drops per minute do you set on her IV if the tubing has a drop factor of 15?

Suggested answers are at the end of the chapter.

---

chronically ill patients, and older adults are at particular risk for complications and even death from influenza because of compromised immune function.

Influenza is easily transmitted via droplets from coughs and sneezes of infected people, or it may be transmitted by physical contact with a person or object that harbors the virus. The incubation period from time of exposure to onset of symptoms is 1 to 3 days.

Prevention

The Centers for Disease Control and Prevention (CDC) recommends a yearly flu vaccine for anyone over 6 months of age (2013). Although Medicare covers the cost of a flu shot, many older adults do not get one. Emphasize to older people that they will not get the flu from the shot because it does not contain any live virus. Once the shot has been administered, it takes about 2 weeks for antibodies to develop; it is then effective for about 4 months. Other important preventive measures include hand hygiene and avoidance of people with influenza.

 BE SAFE!

Reduce the risk of health care–associated infections. Comply with either the current CDC hand hygiene guidelines or the current World Health Organization hand hygiene guidelines (Joint Commission's 2014 National Patient Safety Goals, © The Joint Commission, 2013. Reprinted with permission.).

Signs and Symptoms

Symptoms of flu include abrupt onset of fever, chills, myalgia, sore throat, cough, general malaise, and headache. Flu can last for 2 to 5 days, with malaise lasting up to several weeks.

• WORD • BUILDING •
myalgia: myo—muscle + algia—pain

Complications

The most common complication of influenza is pneumonia, which may be caused by the same virus as the flu or by a secondary bacterial infection. This should be suspected if the patient has persistent fever and shortness of breath or if the lungs develop crackles or wheezes.

Diagnostic Tests

Viral cultures of throat or nasal swabbing can be done to identify influenza, but results may take 3 to 10 days. Rapid tests can identify the presence of flu virus in less than 15 minutes in an office setting but are less reliable than cultures. Cultures may also be done to rule out bacterial infection. Once influenza has been identified in a geographical area, HCPs will test less often and treat based on symptoms.

Therapeutic Measures

Treatment is primarily symptomatic. Acetaminophen is given for fever, headache, and myalgia. Aspirin is avoided in children because it increases the risk of Reye's syndrome. Rest and fluids are essential. Antibiotics are used only if a secondary bacterial infection is present.

Antiviral medications such as zanamivir (Relenza, an inhaled agent) and oseltamivir (Tamiflu, an oral medication) may reduce the severity and duration of symptoms if given within 48 hours of becoming ill. Antiviral agents may also be given prophylactically to high-risk people who have not been immunized or to control outbreaks in high-risk situations, such as in long-term care facilities.

Nursing Care for the Patient With Influenza

Older adults or other high-risk patients may be hospitalized for treatment of influenza. These patients are closely monitored for complications. Assess lung sounds and vital signs every 4 hours and monitor for dehydration. Report changes to an RN or HCP. Encourage rest and fluids (if not contraindicated), and provide comfort measures. Teach patients and families not to give aspirin to treat influenza symptoms in children aged under 18 years because of the risk of Reye's syndrome. (See the "Nursing Care Plan for the Patient With an Upper Respiratory Infection.")

For an excellent tutorial for you or your patients, visit www.nlm.nih.gov/medlineplus/tutorials/influenza/htm/index.htm.

CRITICAL THINKING

Mrs. Murdock

■ Mrs. Murdock is a 97-year-old resident of a long-term care facility who develops flu symptoms. She is lethargic, confused, and feverish. Because of her mental status changes, you want to send her to the hospital, but her son asks you to please keep her where she is. She has a history of chronic obstructive pulmonary disease (COPD) and diabetes.

1. How could Mrs. Murdock have caught the flu?
2. How could it have been prevented?
3. What can be done now to prevent her from developing complications that could lead to pneumonia or even death?
4. What other concerns do you have?
5. What other team members should you involve in her care?

Suggested answers are at the end of the chapter.

Other Viral Infections

In recent years, new viruses have become a worldwide concern. Several of these are described in this section. Continuous research is being conducted to learn more about the spread, prevention, and treatment of new viral infections.

Bird Flu

Avian influenza, more commonly known as bird flu, is an influenza virus that infects wild and domestic birds (often poultry), just as people get infected by the flu. Humans can contract it from contact with infected birds or their secretions or excrement. Transmission does not occur from eating infected poultry and eggs as long as they have been properly prepared and cooked. Eggs from infected poultry typically do not make it to stores. Transmission from human to human is rare, but is a potential concern.

Symptoms of bird flu are similar to the influenza symptoms described earlier, but complications can be more severe and deadly. Conventional vaccines are not effective in preventing bird flu. Oseltamivir (Tamiflu) may be useful in treatment, along with supportive measures.

SARS

Severe acute respiratory syndrome (SARS) is another newer viral disease that has influenza-like symptoms. High fever, body aches, and respiratory symptoms often progress to pneumonia. SARS first appeared in Asia in 2003. Transmission is believed to occur from close contact with a contaminated person or object or through respiratory droplets when an ill person coughs or sneezes. SARS is treated with antiviral medications, steroids, and oxygen.

Swine Flu

The H1N1 and H3N2 viruses cause what is commonly known as the swine flu. It was first recognized in humans in 2009. It is called swine flu because the virus usually affects pigs, but it is also transmitted to humans and from human to human. It cannot be contracted by eating cooked pork. Symptoms and prevention are similar to those for other types of flu. Seasonal flu vaccines protect against H1N1. Antiviral agents may be used, but no agent is specific to swine flu.

West Nile Virus

West Nile virus is less deadly than some other flu viruses but can still cause serious complications. West Nile virus is transmitted from birds to humans by mosquitoes and causes either no symptoms or flulike symptoms. However, in a few people, especially older adults, it can progress to encephalitis (inflammation of the brain) and meningitis (inflammation of the covering of the brain and spinal cord). Teach patients to prevent exposure by using mosquito repellant and to eliminate standing water where mosquitoes lay eggs. There is no specific treatment for West Nile virus. Patients who develop complications are hospitalized for supportive care.

 MALIGNANT DISORDERS

Cancer of the Larynx
Pathophysiology

Cancer of the larynx (the voice box) usually develops in the squamous cells of the mucosal epithelium. It is evaluated based on the tumor-node-metastasis (TNM) staging system described in Chapter 11. It is most often a primary cancer and can spread to the lungs, liver, or lymph nodes. The prognosis for a patient with laryngeal cancer is good with early diagnosis but is often poor because many patients delay seeking help.

Etiology

Risk factors for cancer of the larynx include a history of alcohol and tobacco use. Exposure to industrial chemicals or hardwood dust, chronic overuse of the voice, and a diet low in fruits and vegetables are also factors. Men are more likely to be affected than women.

Prevention

Prevention begins with education. You can help educate patients about the relationship between cancer of the larynx and use of alcohol and tobacco. It is also important to teach patients to seek help when symptoms first occur because a delayed diagnosis may mean metastasis of the cancer and a poor prognosis. Teach that any hoarseness that lasts longer than 2 weeks should be investigated by a HCP.

Signs and Symptoms

The most common symptom is persistent hoarseness because the vocal cords are located in the larynx (Table 30.2). The patient may also have throat or ear pain, shortness of breath, a chronic cough, and difficulty swallowing. Stridor may indicate a tumor obstructing the airway. Late signs include weight loss and halitosis (foul breath).

Diagnostic Tests

The larynx can be examined with a laryngeal mirror. Laryngoscopic examination and biopsy are used to diagnose and determine the stage of laryngeal cancer. A CT scan, MRI, or other diagnostic tests may be done to determine the presence or extent of metastasis.

Therapeutic Measures

If laryngeal cancer is diagnosed early in the disease, it may be treatable with radiation therapy; this treatment can preserve the patient's voice. Chemotherapy may be used with radiation or surgery, but it is not usually used alone. New targeted chemotherapy attacks only certain cells in the body. Surgery may be done

TABLE 30.2 LARYNGEAL CANCER SUMMARY

Signs and Symptoms	Hoarse voice Pain Cough Shortness of breath Difficulty swallowing Weight loss Foul breath
Diagnostic Tests	Examination with laryngeal mirror Laryngoscopy with biopsy Additional blood and radiographic studies to detect metastasis
Therapeutic Measures	Radiation therapy Chemotherapy (adjunct to radiation or surgery) Endoscopic laser surgery to destroy tumor Partial laryngectomy (preserves some voice) Radical neck dissection with total laryngectomy (loss of voice)
Nursing Diagnoses	*Risk for Ineffective Airway Clearance* *Acute Pain* *Impaired Verbal Communication* *Risk for Imbalanced Nutrition: Less Than Body Requirements* *Impaired Swallowing* *Grieving* *Disturbed Body Image*

at any stage of the disease. The larynx will be either partially or completely removed (Fig. 30.3). If cancer has spread beyond the larynx, a radical neck dissection, which removes adjacent muscle, lymph nodes, and tissue, may be done. Surgery can be done using laser technology, endoscopy, or traditional methods.

After a partial laryngectomy, the patient may have a permanently hoarse voice. If a total laryngectomy is done, the patient will have a permanent tracheostomy (in this case called a laryngectomy) tube in place and no voice. The patient will need to learn alternative methods of communication. A person who has had a total laryngectomy is sometimes referred to as a **laryngectomee**.

Several alternatives for long-term speech exist:

- Esophageal speech involves swallowing air and forming words as the air is regurgitated back up the esophagus.
- Electronic devices are available, which the patient places next to the neck or mouth. These devices use sound vibrations to help the patient form words. UltraVoice®

• WORD • BUILDING •

laryngectomee: laryng—larynx + ectome—excision (person who has undergone laryngectomy)

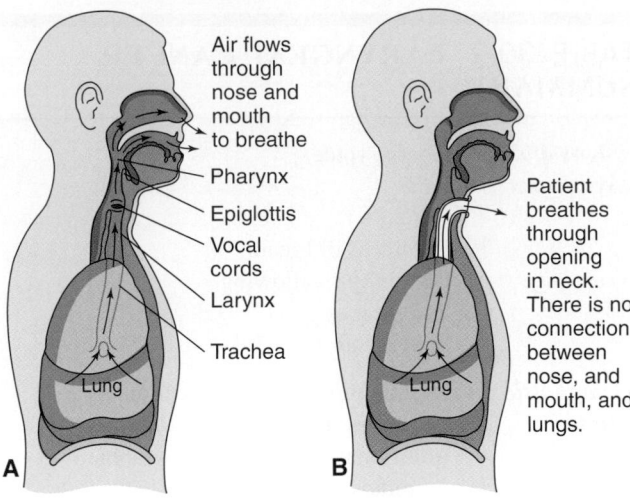

Air flows
through
nose and
mouth
to breathe

Pharynx

Epiglottis

Vocal
cords

Larynx

Trachea

Lung

A

Patient
breathes
through
opening
in neck.
There is no
connection
between
nose, and
mouth, and
lungs.

Lung

B

FIGURE 30.3 (A) Before laryngectomy. (B) After laryngectomy.

(UltraVoice Ltd.) is an electronic device that is placed inside an upper denture or retainer, and the patient speaks into a small microphone (Fig. 30.4A).
- Another alternative is a tracheoesophageal puncture (TEP), such as the Blom-Singer voice prosthesis (In-Health Technologies), which uses a surgically implanted voice prosthesis that creates a valve between the trachea and esophagus. If the patient holds a finger over the laryngectomy, air is diverted into the esophagus and the patient forms words as the air exits the mouth (Fig. 30.4B).

All of these devices take time to adjust to, and the patient will need support after discharge to continue to develop communication skills.

 LEARNING TIP

Did you ever "burp the ABCs" as a child? If not, ask most any child to demonstrate! This uses the same idea as esophageal speech.

Nursing Process for the Patient Undergoing Total Laryngectomy

PREOPERATIVE CARE. In addition to routine preoperative teaching, the patient undergoing a total laryngectomy surgery must be prepared for the loss of ability to breathe through the mouth and nose and loss of ability to speak. Initial instruction in communication techniques should take place before surgery to prevent the patient from feeling panicky after surgery when he or she cannot communicate needs. A variety of techniques and devices are available. Consult a speech therapist before surgery to provide a picture board, magic slate, or paper and pencil (see Chapter 49). The patient is instructed to point to the picture that corresponds with the need or to write out his or her concern. A dietary consult is also important before surgery if the patient has been undernourished.

POSTOPERATIVE CARE.
Data Collection. Collecting data about the patient's physical and psychosocial status, comfort, nutritional status, and ability to swallow is important both before and after surgery. After surgery, assessment of airway patency and respiratory function takes priority. Monitor lung sounds, oxygen saturation, and arterial blood gases. In addition, be sure to assess the patient's understanding of the disease process and self-care needs after surgery. It is important to evaluate the patient's support systems and ability to cope with the partial or total loss of voice after surgery.

Nursing Diagnoses, Planning, and Implementation

Risk for Ineffective Airway Clearance related to excessive secretions and new tracheostomy/laryngectomy
EXPECTED OUTCOME: The patient will maintain a clear airway as evidenced by clear lung sounds and ability to cough up secretions.

- Monitor and record amount, color, and consistency of secretions; vital signs; oxygen saturation; lung sounds; and signs of respiratory distress. *Visible secretions, a drop in oxygen saturation (Spo$_2$), or an increase in crackles may indicate airway compromise and a need for suctioning. A change in amount or color of secretions, an increased temperature, or presence of adventitious sounds can indicate infection and should be reported to the HCP immediately.*
- Provide tracheostomy care and suctioning according to agency policy (see Chapter 29). *This keeps the airway clear.*
- Maintain strict sterile technique with tracheostomy care and suctioning. *Prevention of infection is essential, because the airway no longer has the protection of normal upper airway defense mechanisms.*
- Place the patient in semi-Fowler's position *to allow for lung expansion and more effective coughing.*
- Encourage the patient to deep breathe and cough every hour *to keep airway free of secretions.*
- Administer oxygen as ordered. A special tracheostomy collar should be used. *Supplemental oxygen helps maintain oxygenation. The oxygen must be applied to the stoma because there is no connection between the nose and lungs.*
- Provide room or oxygen humidification. *Humidification can help keep secretions mobile.*
- Avoid use of powders, sprays, or other airborne materials near the patient. *These can cause irritation or infection if they enter the laryngectomy.*

Acute Pain related to surgical procedure
EXPECTED OUTCOME: The patient will state his or her pain level is acceptable.

- Assess pain level every 4 hours and as needed (prn). *A good assessment must guide treatment.*
- Assess sedation and respiratory status often. Opioids are given carefully *because they may reduce respiratory rate and cough reflex, which is vital to clearing the airway.*

Tracheoesophageal Voice Prosthesis

Location of tissue vibration for voice

Tracheoesophageal Puncture and Blom-Singer® Voice Prosthesis

Esophagus

Trachea and air from lungs

Speech

Stoma closure with thumb (low pressure prosthesis pictured.)

ATSV II with HumidiFilter cap and indwelling voice prosthesis.

INHEALTH® TECHNOLOGIES

Blom-Singer® voice restoration systems

FIGURE 30.4 Devices to aid speech in the laryngectomy patient. (A) UltraVoice is an electronic device placed inside a denture or retainer; the patient speaks into a small microphone. *Courtesy of UltraVoice Ltd.* (B) The Blom-Singer voice prosthesis diverts air into the esophagus and out the mouth to form tracheoesophageal speech. *Courtesy of InHealth Technologies, Carpinteria, CA.*

- Include nonpharmacological pain control interventions (see Chapter 10). *Interventions such as distraction and relaxation may help with pain control and reduce (not eliminate) the need for opioids.*
- Administer analgesics as ordered, on an around-the-clock basis or via patient-controlled pump, for the first few days after surgery. If the liver has been damaged from previous alcohol use, dosages are adjusted by the HCP. *The patient who is comfortable will be better able to participate in care and take measures to prevent complications, such as coughing and ambulating.*

Impaired Verbal Communication related to loss of vocal cords

EXPECTED OUTCOME: The patient will be able to communicate his or her needs.

- Use a picture board or paper and pencil *so the patient can communicate without speaking.*
- Make sure the patient has a call light or bell nearby at all times. *Patients can become panicky if they have a need and no way to summon a nurse.*
- Work with the speech therapist and HCP to provide the patient with a method of communication that best fits his

or her needs (see Fig. 30.4). *Different patients prefer different long-term communication methods.*

Risk for Imbalanced Nutrition: Less Than Body Requirements related to absence of oral feeding immediately following surgery and possible previous alcohol use or abuse
EXPECTED OUTCOME: The patient's weight will be within normal limits for height and age.

- Monitor weight. *Underweight or weight loss reflects inadequate nutrition.*
- Monitor parenteral nutrition or tube feedings after surgery until the neck has begun to heal and swallowing can be evaluated. *Nutrition must be maintained to support healing.*
- Consult a dietitian for nutrition guidance. If the patient has a history of alcohol abuse, he or she may have been undernourished before surgery. *You may need to advocate for the patient and ensure that he or she is receiving adequate calories for healing. A dietitian can assist with specific recommendations.*

Impaired Swallowing related to edema or presence of laryngectomy tube
EXPECTED OUTCOME: The patient will be able to swallow safely.

- Consult a speech therapist to assist with a swallowing assessment and recommendations. *Speech therapists are trained to assess and treat swallowing disorders.*
- Assure the patient that aspiration will not occur *because there is no longer a connection between the mouth and the lungs.*
- Place the patient in high-Fowler's position *to make swallowing easier.*
- Stay with the patient during the first attempts *to eat to help alleviate anxiety.*

Grieving related to loss of voice
EXPECTED OUTCOME: Patient will express feelings of loss and begin to plan for the future.

- Assess patient's feelings of loss. *Inability to speak is a loss that cannot be overemphasized. The patient may also be facing a career change if job-related exposure contributed to the disease or if loss of voice prevents return to a previously held job.*
- Actively attend to the patient's communication of feelings *to show your support and validate feelings.*
- Assess and involve support systems. *Family support is important to the patient's long-term adjustment to a laryngectomy.*
- Contact the patient's clergy if patient wishes. *A religious counselor can help with grief and spiritual distress.*

Disturbed Body Image related to change in body structure and function
EXPECTED OUTCOME: The patient will verbalize acceptance of new laryngectomy and participate in self-care.

- Portray an accepting attitude. *Patients are very aware of nurses' nonverbal behavior, and looks of distaste can be disturbing.*
- Allow the patient to share feelings if he or she indicates a need to do so. *This may help the patient to work through feelings about the changes to his or her body image.*
- With the patient's permission, contact a local support group that may have names of people who have had similar experiences who are willing to visit with the patient. *Such visitors can provide firsthand information and support.*
- Assist the patient to find ways to camouflage the change, such as scarves or necklines that conceal but do not obstruct the airway. *Camouflage can help the patient feel less conspicuous and also protect the airway.*

EVALUATION. When evaluating the patient's progress toward goals, ask the following questions:

- Is the airway clear, without signs of infection or obstruction?
- Does the patient verbalize an acceptable level of comfort?
- Do the patient and significant others demonstrate understanding of self-care at home or have referrals to continue learning self-care at home?
- Does the patient indicate satisfaction with the level and quality of communication?
- Is the patient's weight stable?
- Is the patient able to swallow if taking oral nutrition?
- Is the patient able to grieve appropriately?
- Does the patient have someone to talk to if he or she wishes?
- Does the patient show acceptance of the laryngectomy by learning to care for it?

Note that many of these evaluative criteria are long term and may not be seen while the patient is hospitalized, so follow-up by a home care nurse is essential.

PATIENT EDUCATION. After assessing the patient's readiness to learn, teach the patient self-care measures for the laryngectomy, including how to perform cleaning and suctioning (see Chapter 29). Involve the significant other or family whenever possible.

The patient must also be instructed to perform gentle range-of-motion exercises of the neck. Some patients may avoid extending the neck because of the location of the incision, causing muscle contracture.

Referral to home nursing after discharge will provide assessment of the home environment, as well as follow-up instruction. A social service referral may be made for financial or psychosocial concerns if needed. Consult with the health care provider or check the local phone directory for laryngectomee support groups, and refer the patient to them if appropriate. The local branch of the American Cancer Society may also be able to provide information. Assist the patient in finding resources to support alcohol and smoking cessation. Continued alcohol and tobacco use will increase the patient's risk of cancer recurrence.

To find additional information for laryngectomees, visit the National Cancer Institute's website at www.cancer.gov.

SUGGESTED ANSWERS TO

CRITICAL THINKING

■ *Mr. Jondahl*

Explore the amount of ibuprofen being taken daily because NSAIDs can interfere with platelet aggregation. In addition, high blood pressure can aggravate the bleeding.

■ *Mrs. Hiler*

1. Mrs. Hiler may be swallowing blood. Examine the back of her throat with a flashlight. Check vital signs for evidence of impending shock. Notify an HCP if bleeding is confirmed.

2. Continue to be vigilant for signs of bleeding: frequent swallowing, or bright red blood from the mouth. Monitor for changes in vital signs and report even small changes to the RN or HCP.

3. Use this formula to determine drops per minute:

$$\frac{100 \text{ mL}}{1 \text{ hour}} \mid \frac{1 \text{ hour}}{60 \text{ minutes}} \mid \frac{15 \text{ gtt}}{1 \text{ mL}} = 25 \text{ gtt per minute}$$

■ *Mrs. Murdock*

1. Mrs. Murdock may have contracted the flu from a visitor or a staff person at the long-term care facility. She is susceptible because of her age and comorbid conditions (COPD, diabetes).

2. Mrs. Murdock's flu could probably have been prevented with a flu vaccination, but her son refused it because he believed it could cause her to get the flu. Good hand hygiene by staff and urging visitors not to visit when ill will also help.

3. If it is within 48 hours of symptom onset, an HCP may prescribe an antiviral agent to help reduce her symptoms and shorten the course of her illness. In addition, you can provide fluids, acetaminophen, and comfort measures. You should also monitor her closely for evidence of bacterial infection or pneumonia and report signs or symptoms immediately to the HCP.

4. A major concern is that Mrs. Murdock could transmit the flu to other residents or staff. Hopefully, they have all been vaccinated. In addition, you must decide whether to send Mrs. Murdock to the hospital. Check her advance directives, and talk to her son about goals for her care. If needed, educate him about differences in long-term care and hospital care.

5. Involve the RN, supervisor or director, and infection control nurse. Collaborate to determine how to manage Mrs. Murdock but also to protect other residents.

REVIEW QUESTIONS

1. Which is the best explanation to a patient by a nurse for why a health care provider does not prescribe antibiotics for influenza?
   1. "Most cases of influenza are caused by antibiotic-resistant bacteria."
   2. "Influenza is caused by viruses."
   3. "Antibiotics have too many serious side effects."
   4. "Antibiotics can interact with other medications used for influenza."

2. After a laryngectomy, which of the following assessments takes priority?
   1. Airway patency
   2. Nutritional status
   3. Lung sounds
   4. Patient acceptance of surgery

3. Which of the following responses is correct when a patient asks why the health care provider did not order a new antiviral drug for flu symptoms that started 3 days ago?
   1. "Antiviral drugs are for AIDS, not the flu."
   2. "The side effects of the antiviral drugs are worse than having the flu."
   3. "Antiviral drugs are only prescribed for children."
   4. "Antivirals work only if you start them within 48 hours after flu symptoms begin."

4. Which of the following positions is recommended for a patient experiencing a nosebleed?
   1. Lying down with feet elevated
   2. Sitting up with neck fully extended
   3. Lying down with a small pillow under the head
   4. Sitting up leaning slightly forward

5. The nurse knows that the patient understands teaching related to prevention of influenza transmission when the patient demonstrates which behaviors? **Select all that apply.**
   1. Washing hands frequently
   2. Covering the nose and mouth during coughing or sneezing
   3. Taking acetaminophen as ordered
   4. Drinking extra fluids
   5. Avoiding sharing eating utensils with others
   6. Taking antibiotics until the entire prescription is finished

6. Which of the following communication methods is inappropriate for the patient with a total laryngectomy?
   1. Placing a finger over the stoma
   2. Providing a special valve that diverts air into the esophagus
   3. Obtaining a picture board
   4. Teaching the patient esophageal speech

Answers can be found in Appendix C.

References

Joint Commission. (2014). *2014 National Patient Safety Goals.* Retrieved June 20, 2013, from www.jointcommission.org/assets/1/18/NPSG_Chapter_Jan2013_HAP.pdf

Centers for Disease Control and Prevention. (2013). *Seasonal influenza (flu).* Retrieved October 30, 2013, from www.cdc.gov/flu/protect/whoshouldvax.htm

Qaseem, A., Holty, J., Owens, D., Dallas, P., Starkey, M., & Shekelle, P. (2013). Management of obstructive sleep apnea in adults: a clinical practice guideline from the American College of Physicians. *Ann Intern Med, 159,* 471–483. Published online September 24, 2013. Retrieved October 20, 2013 from http://annals.org/article.aspx?articleID=1740756

 For additional resources and information visit **davispl.us/medsurg5**

31

Nursing Care of Patients With Lower Respiratory Tract Disorders

PAULA D. HOPPER

LEARNING OUTCOMES

1. Explain the pathophysiology of each of the disorders of the lower respiratory tract.
2. Describe the etiologies, signs, and symptoms of each of the disorders.
3. Identify tests that are used to diagnose lower respiratory disorders.
4. Describe therapeutic measures used for disorders of the lower respiratory tract.
5. List data to collect when caring for patients with disorders of the lower respiratory tract.
6. Plan nursing care for patients with disorders of the lower respiratory tract.
7. Identify interventions for patients experiencing impaired gas exchange, ineffective airway clearance, or ineffective breathing pattern.
8. Explain how you will know if your nursing interventions have been effective.

KEY TERMS

anergy (AN-ur-jee)
antitussive (AN-tee-TUSS-iv)
atelectasis (AT-eh-LEK-tah-siss)
atypical (ay-TIP-ih-kuhl)
bleb (BLEB)
bronchiectasis (BRONG-key-EK-tah-siss)
bronchitis (brong-KY-tiss)
bronchodilator (BRONG-koh-DY-lay-ter)
bronchospasm (BRONG-koh-spazm)
bulla (BULL-ah)
ectopic (ek-TOP-ik)
emphysema (EM-fih-SEE-mah)
empyema (EM-pye-EE-mah)
exacerbation (egg-ZASS-ur-BAY-shun)
expectorant (eks-PEK-ta-rant)
exudate (EKS-yoo-dayt)
hemoptysis (hee-MOP-tih-siss)
hemothorax (HEE-moh-THOR-aks)
hypostatic (HYE-poh-STAH-tik)
induration (IN-dyoo-RAY-shun)
lobectomy (loh-BEK-tuh-mee)
mucolytic (MYOO-koh-LIT-ik)
paradoxical respiration (PEAR-uh-DOK-sih-kuhl RESS-per-AY-shun)
pleurodesis (PLOO-roh-DEE-siss)
pneumonectomy (NOO-moh-NEK-tuh-mee)
pneumothorax (NOO-moh-THOR-aks)
polycythemia (PAW-lee-sye-THEE-mee-ah)
status asthmaticus (STAT-us az-MAT-ih-kus)
tachypnea (TAK-ip-NEE-uh)
thoracotomy (THOR-ah-KOT-ah-mee)

Disorders of the lower respiratory tract include problems of the lower portion of the trachea, bronchi, bronchioles, and alveoli. These disorders may be related to infection, noninfectious alterations in function, neoplasm (cancer), or trauma. Any pathological condition of the lower respiratory tract can seriously impair carbon dioxide and oxygen exchange.

 INFECTIOUS DISORDERS

Acute Bronchitis

Bronchitis is an inflammation of the bronchial tree, which includes the right and left bronchi, secondary bronchi, and bronchioles. When the mucous membranes lining the bronchial tree become irritated and inflamed, excessive mucus is produced. The result is congested airways. Acute bronchitis is usually an isolated episode. If it occurs more than 3 months out of the year for 2 consecutive years, chronic bronchitis is diagnosed. See the discussion of chronic bronchitis later in this chapter for more information that applies to both the acute and chronic forms.

Bronchiectasis

Pathophysiology

Bronchiectasis is a dilation of the bronchial airways (Fig. 31.1). The dilated areas become flabby and scarred. Bronchiectasis can remain localized or spread throughout the lungs. Secretions pool in these areas and are difficult to cough up. This creates an environment where bacteria can flourish, and infection is common.

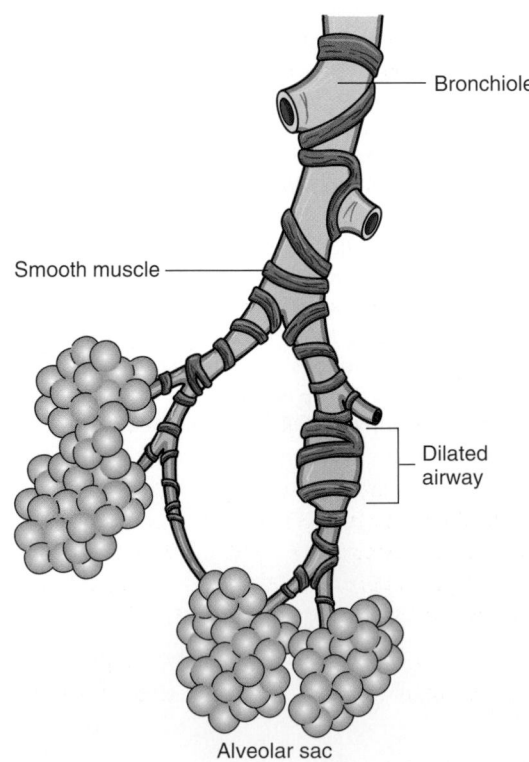

FIGURE 31.1 Bronchiectasis. Note dilated airway.

Labels: Bronchiole, Smooth muscle, Dilated airway, Alveolar sac

Etiology

Bronchiectasis usually occurs secondary to another chronic respiratory disorder, such as cystic fibrosis, asthma, tuberculosis, bronchitis, or exposure to a toxin. Airway obstruction from a tumor or foreign body can also be a predisposing factor. Infection and inflammation of the airways in these underlying disorders weaken the bronchial walls and reduce ciliary function. Airway obstruction from excessive secretions then predisposes the patient to development of bronchiectasis. Vitamin D deficiency may be related to risk of infection in bronchiectasis, but the mechanism for this link is not clear (Chalmers, 2013).

Signs and Symptoms

The patient with bronchiectasis has recurrent lower respiratory infections. Sputum is copious and purulent. The accompanying cough can produce as much as 200 mL of thick, foul-smelling sputum in a single episode of coughing. Interestingly, if the sputum is allowed to sit for a couple of hours, it will separate into a purulent bottom layer, a clear center layer, and a cloudy top layer. Extreme airway inflammation may cause sputum to be bloody. If bronchiectasis is widespread throughout the lungs, the patient may experience dyspnea even with minimal exertion. Wheezes and crackles may be auscultated. Fever is present during active infection. Cor pulmonale (right-sided heart failure; covered in Chapter 26) and clubbing of the fingers may develop with chronic disease.

Diagnostic Tests

A chest x-ray examination may be done, but it may not show early disease. A computed tomography (CT) scan provides a better view of the dilated airways. Bronchoscopy may be done if needed. Sputum cultures determine infecting organisms and guide antibiotic therapy. Additional testing may be done to determine the cause of bronchiectasis.

Therapeutic Measures

Treatment is aimed at keeping the airways clear of secretions, controlling infection, and correcting the underlying problem. Antibiotics may be used intermittently or for prolonged periods. Azithromycin may reduce exacerbations (Wong et al, 2012). Measures to prevent infection, including vaccinations for flu and pneumonia, should be implemented. **Bronchodilators** improve airway obstruction. **Mucolytic** agents and expectorants help loosen and mobilize secretions so they can be coughed up. Bronchitol, a form of mannitol, is an inhaled drug that is still being studied to promote mucus clearance. It is a sugar that draws fluid into the airways to help liquefy mucus. Inhaled beta-agonist bronchodilators help

• WORD • BUILDING •

bronchitis: bronch—airway + itis—inflammation
bronchiectasis: bronch—airway + ectasis—dilation or expansion
bronchodilator: broncho—airway + dilator—to expand
mucolytic: muco—mucus + lytic—break up

keep airways open. Chest physiotherapy (CPT) or a high-frequency chest wall oscillation vest can help mobilize secretions. Oxygen is used if hypoxemia is present. Oral fluids are encouraged. If the affected area of the lung is localized and symptoms are severe, surgery may be considered to remove the diseased area. Lung transplant may be considered in severe cases. Nursing care is found in "Nursing Care Plan for the Patient With a Lower Respiratory Tract Disorder."

NURSING CARE TIP

If your patient is coughing up a lot of sputum, line an emesis basin with a white tissue. This makes it easier to assess the color of the sputum and also simplifies cleaning out the basin!

Pneumonia

Pneumonia is the cause of many hospital admissions each year and is a common cause of death from infection. Persons at risk for pneumonia are the very young, adults over age 65, and people who are immunocompromised, such as those with acquired immunodeficiency syndrome (AIDS), alcoholism, or another underlying illness. Pneumonia is categorized according to where it is acquired. For example, hospital-acquired pneumonia (HAP) is defined as pneumonia that develops at least 48 hours after a hospital admission. One type of HAP is ventilator-associated pneumonia, or VAP. Health care–associated pneumonia (HCAP) is pneumonia that develops in outpatient settings or nursing homes. Community-acquired pneumonia (CAP) develops in the community and is usually less serious than other forms. Each type of pneumonia may be caused by different organisms.

Pathophysiology

Pneumonia is an acute inflammation and/or infection of the lungs that occurs when an infectious agent enters and multiplies in the lungs of a susceptible person. Infectious particles can be transmitted by the cough of an infected individual, from contaminated respiratory therapy equipment, infections in other parts of the body, or aspiration of bacteria from the mouth, pharynx, or stomach. Organisms from the mouth and pharynx may be related to poor oral hygiene or may be present because of a cold or influenza virus. When pathogens enter the body of a healthy person, normal respiratory defense mechanisms and the immune system prevent the development of infection. In a person who is immunocompromised, however, even microorganisms that are normally present in the oropharynx can cause an infection.

When the microorganisms multiply, they release toxins that induce inflammation in the lung tissue, causing damage to mucous and alveolar membranes. This leads to the development of edema and **exudate**, which fills the alveoli and reduces the surface area available for exchange of carbon dioxide and oxygen. Some bacteria also cause necrosis of lung tissue.

Pneumonia may be confined to one lobe (lobar pneumonia), or it may be scattered throughout the lungs (bronchopneumonia). Bronchopneumonia occurs more often as a nosocomial infection in hospitalized patients, the very young, or the very old, and can be quite serious. Patients may use terms such as walking pneumonia or double pneumonia. These are not medical terms, but it is helpful to understand them. *Walking pneumonia* refers to a mild infection that may not even keep the patient from working (or walking); *double* is a lay term for bilateral.

Etiology

Pneumonia has a variety of causes, as discussed next.

BACTERIAL PNEUMONIA. The most common cause of community-acquired bacterial pneumonias is *Streptococcus pneumoniae,* also called pneumococcal pneumonia. Other community-acquired infections are caused by *Staphylococcus aureus, Chlamydia trachomatis,* and *Mycoplasma pneumoniae.* HAPs are often antibiotic-resistant, and tend to be much more serious than CAP. They can be caused by *Escherichia coli, Haemophilus influenzae,* and *Klebsiella pneumoniae,* among others. Methicillin-resistant *Staphylococcus aureus* (MRSA), *Pseudomonas aeruginosa,* and other antibiotic-resistant pneumonias are especially difficult to treat.

VIRAL PNEUMONIA. Influenza viruses are the most common cause of viral pneumonia. The presence of viral pneumonia increases the patient's susceptibility to a secondary bacterial pneumonia. Generally, patients are less ill with viral pneumonia than with bacterial pneumonia, but they may be ill for a longer period because antibiotics are ineffective against viruses.

FUNGAL PNEUMONIA. *Candida* and *Aspergillus* are two types of fungi that can cause pneumonia. *Pneumocystis carinii* pneumonia (PCP) is caused by a fungus and typically causes pneumonia in patients with AIDS.

ASPIRATION PNEUMONIA. Some pneumonias are caused by aspiration of foreign substances. This most often occurs in patients with decreased levels of consciousness or an impaired cough or gag reflex. These conditions can occur with alcohol ingestion, stroke, general anesthesia, seizures, gastrointestinal reflux disease (GERD), or other serious illness. Aspiration pneumonia increases the risk for subsequent bacterial pneumonia.

VENTILATOR-ASSOCIATED PNEUMONIA. A type of aspiration pneumonia, ventilator-associated pneumonia (VAP), develops in patients who are intubated and mechanically ventilated. The endotracheal tube keeps the glottis open, so secretions can be easily aspirated into the lungs. A cuff on the tube is kept inflated to attempt to protect the lower airway, and suction can keep secretions under control, but risk of aspiration is still significant.

HYPOSTATIC PNEUMONIA. Patients who hypoventilate because of bedrest, immobility, or shallow respirations are at risk

• WORD • BUILDING •
exudate: to sweat out

for **hypostatic** pneumonia. Secretions pool in dependent areas of the lungs and can lead to inflammation and infection.

CHEMICAL PNEUMONIA. Inhalation of toxic chemicals can cause inflammation and tissue damage, which can lead to chemical pneumonia. This increases the risk for subsequent bacterial infection.

Prevention

Both flu and pneumonia vaccination are essential to preventing pneumonia. See Box 31-1 for current Center for Disease Control and Prevention (CDC) vaccine recommendations.

Box 31-1 2013 CDC Guidelines for Flu and Pneumonia Vaccination

Flu Vaccine

Everyone who is at least 6 months of age should get a flu vaccine this season. It's especially important for some people to get vaccinated. Those people include the following:

- People who are at high risk of developing serious complications like pneumonia if they get sick with the flu. This includes:
  - People who have certain medical conditions including asthma, diabetes, and chronic lung disease.
  - Pregnant women.
  - People 65 years and older.
- People who live with or care for others who are high risk of developing serious complications. This includes household contacts and caregivers of people with certain medical conditions including asthma, diabetes, and chronic lung disease.

Pneumococcal Vaccine

The CDC now recommends two kinds of pneumococcal vaccines for adults.

- One dose of pneumococcal conjugate vaccine (PCV13) is recommended for adults aged 19 years and older with asplenia, sickle cell disease, cerebrospinal fluid leaks, cochlear implants, or conditions that cause weakening of the immune system.
- Adults 19 through 64 years old with certain medical conditions (for example, certain kidney diseases, cigarette smoking, chronic heart or lung disease, asplenia, and conditions that cause weakening of the immune system) should receive one or two doses of pneumococcal polysaccharide vaccine (PPSV23).
- All adults 65 years and older should still get one dose of pneumococcal polysaccharide vaccine (PPSV23).

  If you are recommended to get both PPSV23 and PCV13 vaccines, you should get the PCV13 vaccine first, followed by PPSV23 eight weeks later.

Note. From CDC (2013a).

Gerontological Issues

Advanced age is a significant risk factor for serious complications from respiratory infections such as influenza, pneumococcal pneumonia, and aspiration pneumonia. Therefore, it is recommended that people over age 65 and people with chronic disease have yearly influenza vaccines and pneumococcal vaccine with repeat dose as needed. Consistent oral care is also a significant nursing intervention to help prevent morbidity and mortality from aspiration pneumonia.

Nursing care plays an important role in the prevention of HAP. Regular coughing, deep breathing, and position changes for patients on bedrest or after surgery, prevention of aspiration for patients at risk, and good hand hygiene practices by both patients and health care personnel can help prevent many cases (see "Gerontological Issues").

The risk of VAP can be reduced with frequent mouth care, including toothbrushing, and use of a special endotracheal tube that allows continuous suctioning of secretions above the inflated cuff. All patients should be positioned with the head of the bed elevated 30 to 45 degrees to help prevent aspiration. Medication to reduce gastric acid secretion and stress ulcers may help reduce aspiration but may also increase bacterial growth.

CRITICAL THINKING

Mr. Smith

■ Mr. Smith is an 86-year-old man who was watching television when he couldn't sleep one night. After seeing a commercial for toilet cleaner, he decided his own toilet could use some attention. He used bleach and ammonia "to get it really clean." The combination created toxic fumes, which caused a severe chemical pneumonia. He was brought to the emergency room in acute respiratory distress.

1. As his nurse, what questions might you ask as you further assess the cause of his pneumonia?
2. What can you teach Mr. Smith related to prevention of similar episodes in the future?
3. How can you be vigilant in preventing complications in Mr. Smith?

Suggested answers are at the end of the chapter.

Signs and Symptoms

Patients with pneumonia present with fever, shaking, chills, chest pain, dyspnea, fatigue, and a productive cough. Sputum is purulent or may be rust-colored or blood-tinged. Crackles and wheezes may be heard on lung auscultation because of the exudate in the alveoli and airways.

• WORD • BUILDING •
hypostatic: hypo—below + static—standing

BE SAFE!

Reduce the risk of health care–associated infections. Adhere to either the current Centers for Disease Control and Prevention (CDC) hand hygiene guidelines or the current World Health Organization (WHO) hand hygiene guidelines (Joint Commission's 2014 National Patient Safety Goals, © The Joint Commission, 2013. Reprinted with permission.).

Some bacterial and many viral pneumonias cause **atypical** symptoms. The patient may experience fatigue, sore throat, dry cough, or nausea and vomiting.

Older adult patients may not exhibit expected symptoms of pneumonia. New-onset confusion or lethargy in an older patient can indicate reduced oxygenation and should alert you to look for other symptoms or request evaluation by the health care provider (HCP). New onset of fever or dyspnea should also cause suspicion of pneumonia in older adults.

Complications

Complications from pneumonia most commonly occur in patients with other underlying chronic diseases. Pleurisy and pleural effusion (discussed later in this chapter) are two of the most common complications and generally resolve within 1 to 2 weeks. **Atelectasis** (collapsed alveoli) can occur as a result of trapped secretions and may be resolved by efforts to keep the airways clear, especially use of an incentive spirometer. Other complications result from spread of infection to other parts of the body, causing septicemia, meningitis, septic arthritis, pericarditis, or endocarditis. Treatment for each of these is antibiotics. Although antibiotics can greatly reduce the incidence of death related to pneumonia, it is still a common cause of death in older people.

Diagnostic Tests

A chest x-ray examination is done to identify the presence of pulmonary infiltrate, which is fluid leakage into the alveoli from inflammation (Fig. 31.2). In addition, sputum and blood cultures are obtained to identify the organism causing the pneumonia and determine appropriate treatment. If the patient is unable to produce a sputum specimen, a nebulized mist treatment may be ordered to promote sputum expectoration. If this is unsuccessful, nasotracheal suctioning or a bronchoscopy can be done to obtain a specimen from a very ill patient.

NURSING CARE TIP

Obtain culture specimens before antibiotics are started to avoid altering culture results. The best time to obtain a specimen is first thing in the morning, before breakfast. If the patient has eaten, be sure he has rinsed his mouth to keep food particles out of the specimen.

FIGURE 31.2 Chest x-ray examination showing infiltrates in pneumonia.

Therapeutic Measures

Broad-spectrum antibiotics are initiated as soon as cultures are sent to the lab, even if results are not completed. Once the culture and sensitivity report is available, antibiotic orders may change to more narrow-spectrum agents. Many patients can be treated with oral antibiotics as outpatients, but hospitalization and intravenous (IV) therapy may be necessary in older adults or in individuals who are chronically or acutely ill. If the pneumonia is caused by a virus, rest and fluids are recommended. Occasionally, antiviral medications are used.

Expectorants, bronchodilators, and analgesics may be given for comfort and symptom relief. Nebulized mist treatments or metered-dose inhalers may be used to deliver bronchodilators. Supplemental oxygen via nasal cannula or mask is used as needed. Nursing care is found in "Nursing Care Plan for the Patient With a Lower Respiratory Tract Disorder." (See "Evidence-Based Practice" and Table 31.1 for a pneumonia summary.)

• WORD • BUILDING •

atypical: a—not + typical—usual
atelectasis: atel—imperfect + ectasis—expansion
expectorant: ex—out of + pec—chest

EVIDENCE-BASED PRACTICE

Clinical Question
Is noninvasive ventilation with oxygen an effective treatment for adult patients with pneumonia?

Evidence
Three randomized controlled trials found that noninvasive ventilation with oxygen in patients with pneumonia reduces risk of death in the intensive care unit (ICU) and may be more beneficial than oxygen alone.

Tuberculosis

Pathophysiology and Etiology

Tuberculosis (TB) is an infectious disease caused by the bacterium *Mycobacterium tuberculosis.* TB primarily affects the lungs, although other areas, such as the kidneys, liver, brain, and bone, may be affected as well. *M. tuberculosis* is an acid-fast bacillus (AFB), which means that when it is stained in the laboratory and then washed with an acid, the stain remains, or stays "fast." *M. tuberculosis* can live in dark places in dried sputum for months but is killed in a few hours of direct sunlight. It is spread by inhalation of the tuberculosis bacilli from respiratory droplets (droplet nuclei) of an infected person.

Once the bacilli enter the lungs, they multiply and begin to disseminate to the lymph nodes and then to other parts of the body. The patient is then infected but may or may not go on to develop clinical (active) disease. TB infection without disease is called latent TB infection (LTBI). During this time the body develops immunity, which keeps the infection under control. If the lungs are involved, the immune system surrounds the infected area in the lung with neutrophils and alveolar macrophages. This process creates a lesion called a tubercle, which seals off the bacteria and prevents spread. Similar processes take place in other affected areas of the body. The bacteria within the tubercle die or become dormant, and the patient is no longer infectious. If the patient's immune system becomes compromised, however, some of the dormant bacteria can become active, causing active disease. Only 5% to 10% of infected people in the United States actually develop the disease, and even then it may not occur for many years (see "Gerontological Issues").

Risk Factors

Crowded or poorly ventilated living conditions place people at risk for becoming infected with tuberculosis. Although tuberculosis can infect any age group, older people are especially at risk. They may have contracted the disease many years before, but it can reactivate as the aging process diminishes immune function. AIDS, chronic alcohol abuse, and cancer chemotherapy can also compromise immune function and increase risk of activation. In the United States, tuberculosis is also prevalent among the urban poor and minority groups.

Before 1985, the incidence of TB in the United States was steadily decreasing. Since that time, it has increased in incidence, in part because of the prevalence of AIDS, the development of antibiotic-resistant strains of the TB bacillus, and ineffective treatment programs. One-third of the world's population is currently infected with TB (WHO, 2013).

Prevention

Clean, well-ventilated living areas are essential to the health of all people. If a hospitalized patient is known or suspected to have tuberculosis, he or she is placed in respiratory isolation to prevent spread to staff or other patients. Special negative-pressure isolation rooms are ventilated to the outside. Staff should wear special high-efficiency filtration masks when in the patient's room; a regular surgical mask is not effective against TB. Verify with the institution's infection control department that the masks provided are effective for use with TB patients. If the patient must travel through the hallway for tests or other activities, he or she must wear

TABLE 31.1 PNEUMONIA SUMMARY

Signs and Symptoms	Fever, chills Chest pain Dyspnea Productive cough Crackles and wheezes
Diagnostic Tests	Chest x-ray Sputum cultures
Therapeutic Measures	Antibiotics Supplemental oxygen Bronchodilators, expectorants Rest, fluids
Complications	Pleurisy, pleural effusion Atelectasis
Priority Nursing Diagnoses	*Impaired Gas Exchange* *Ineffective Airway Clearance* *Activity Intolerance*

Gerontological Issues

The age-related decline in immune system function can decrease the effectiveness of the tuberculosis antibodies in someone who previously had latent infection. The tuberculosis bacilli can be activated, causing active disease. Because of the risk of false-negative tuberculin test results, a two-step test is recommended, with the second test done 1 to 3 weeks after the first. Decline in immune system function can also have an impact on clinical manifestations of tuberculosis. Patients may exhibit fewer symptoms, making recognition difficult.

a mask. Additional protective barriers, such as gowns, gloves, or goggles, are used when contact with sputum is likely.

A vaccine against tuberculosis, the Bacillus Calmette–Guérin (BCG) vaccine, is available and is used in areas where TB is prevalent. It is not used routinely in the United States because of the low risk for infection. Individuals who have had the vaccine will have a positive skin test for TB, so alternative methods for screening must be used.

Ultimately, prevention will come from adequate treatment of patients with TB. A current concern is the development of antibiotic-resistant strains of the tuberculosis bacillus, which can develop when patients are noncompliant with drug therapy. When antibiotics are taken intermittently or discontinued early, the more virulent (stronger) bacteria survive and multiply and become resistant to the drugs being used. This multi-drug-resistant TB (MDR-TB) can then be passed on to someone else. Some strains are resistant to nearly all antibiotics. They are called extensively drug resistant, or XDR-TB. It is therefore vital to teach all patients the importance of strict adherence to drug therapy. Patients who are at risk for nonadherence to drug therapy must have a visiting nurse or other health professional observe each dose of antibiotic taken. This is called directly observed therapy (DOT) or directly observed therapy—short course (DOTS). DOT transfers responsibility for making sure the drugs are taken from the patient to the health care worker. The WHO reports the highest treatment success rates with DOT/DOTS.

In 2006, the WHO launched a global plan to stop TB, with a goal of eliminating it by 2050. The six components of the plan include the following:

1. Pursuing high-quality DOTS expansion
2. Addressing TB in HIV infection, MDR-TB, and other challenges
3. Contributing to health system strengthening
4. Engaging all care providers
5. Empowering people with TB, and communities
6. Enabling and promoting research (WHO, 2013)

Signs and Symptoms

Active pulmonary tuberculosis is characterized by a chronic productive cough, blood-tinged sputum, and drenching night sweats. Chest pain, fatigue, poor appetite, weight loss, and a low-grade fever are common. If effective treatment is not initiated, a downhill course occurs, with pulmonary fibrosis, **hemoptysis**, and progressive weight loss.

Complications

Spread of the tuberculosis bacilli throughout the body can result in pleurisy, pericarditis, peritonitis, meningitis, bone and joint infections, genitourinary or gastrointestinal (GI) infection, or infection of many other organs.

Diagnostic Tests

Routine screening for tuberculosis infection is usually done with a purified protein derivative (PPD) skin test. The PPD is injected intradermally; the test is considered positive if a raised area of **induration** occurs within 48 to 72 hours. If a red area appears around the induration, this is not measured. The size of induration that indicates a positive test varies based on the individual's history (Table 31.2). A red area without induration is considered a negative result. A positive

• WORD • BUILDING •
hemoptysis: hem—blood + ptysis—to spit
induration: in—in + durus—hard

TABLE 31.2 CLASSIFYING A TUBERCULIN SKIN TEST REACTION

Size of Induration	Considered Positive for
5 mm or more	People infected with human immunodeficiency virus (HIV)
	Recent contacts of infectious TB cases
	Persons with fibrotic changes on chest radiograph consistent with prior TB
	Organ transplant recipients
	Those who are immunosuppressed for other reasons (taking equivalent of 15 mg/day or more of prednisone for 1 month or more), or those taking TNF-α antagonists
10 mm or more	Recent immigrants (within last 5 years) from high-prevalence countries
	Injection drug users
	Residents or employees of high-risk congregate settings
	Mycobacteriology laboratory personnel
	Persons with clinical conditions that place them at high risk
	Children younger than age 4
	Infants, children, or adolescents exposed to adults in high-risk categories
15 mm or more	People with no risk factors for TB

Source: Centers for Disease Control and Prevention. (2012). *Tuberculosis skin testing.* Retrieved June 22, 2013, from www.cdc.gov/tb/publications/factsheets/testing/skintesting.htm

result indicates that a person has been exposed to TB; it does not mean that active TB disease is present.

Some health care institutions use a two-step process for baseline testing of employees and residents. If an individual has a negative PPD test, he or she is retested in 1 to 3 weeks. This is because someone who was exposed many years ago may not react to the first test. The first test acts as a reminder to the immune system to react. The second test will then be positive in the person with a past TB infection.

NURSING CARE TIP

You have probably had a PPD skin test so you can do your clinical practice for school. When you have it checked, the clinician should touch your arm. Just looking at it is not adequate to judge whether there is a raised area of induration.

The QuantiFERON-TB Gold (QFT-G) test is a newer blood test that detects the cell-mediated immune response to TB bacteria in blood. Unlike the PPD skin test, the QFT-G is a simple blood test and is valid in individuals who have been vaccinated against TB.

A chest x-ray examination is used as a screening tool in someone with a known positive test. Final diagnosis is made based on sputum culture results.

BE SAFE!

While awaiting culture results on a hospitalized patient, ask the HCP if the patient should be isolated to protect staff and other patients.

NURSING CARE TIP

A *Candida* or mumps skin test may be ordered along with a PPD skin test. This does not mean the patient is being tested for *Candida* or mumps because everyone generally reacts to these. Rather the patient is being tested for **anergy,** or the inability of the immune system to react to an antigen. A positive *Candida* or mumps test means the immune system is intact, and the TB results are considered to be reliable.

The *Candida* or mumps test is administered in the same way as the PPD test. If more than one test is administered, use a permanent marker to identify which test is which, and clearly document (draw a picture) on the chart where each

test was placed. Check institution policy; it may direct where the tests are administered—PPD in the right arm and *Candida* in the left, for example.

Therapeutic Measures

Treatment consists of specific antibiotic therapy. First-line drugs have the fewest adverse effects (Box 31-2), but they can still be toxic to the liver and nervous system and have other side effects. Second-line drugs are more toxic and are reserved for cases that do not respond to first-line drug therapy. Generally, two or three antibiotics are given simultaneously to allow lower doses of each individual drug, reducing the incidence of serious side effects, and reducing the risk of developing resistant bacteria. Drugs must be taken for 6 to 9 months or up to 2 years for MDR-TB. Because of the length of therapy and the incidence of side effects, adherence to therapy is often a problem.

Additional treatment is supportive. Rest and good nutrition are important for helping the patient's own immune system to work. Patients must be isolated until their sputum no longer contains TB bacteria.

Patients with latent TB infection do not need to be treated, but some health departments recommend treatment to reduce the risk of progression to active disease and subsequent spread to others. Latent TB is easier to treat than active TB.

The CDC has an excellent website with lots of information about TB at www.cdc.gov. Simply type "tuberculosis" into the search window.

Nursing Process for the Patient With Tuberculosis

DATA COLLECTION. Perform a thorough history and head-to-toe physical examination, because TB can affect many systems. Focus on respiratory and psychosocial assessments.

Box 31-2 Antibiotics Used to Treat Tuberculosis

First-Line Drugs

Isoniazid
Rifampin
Ethambutol
Pyrazinamide

Second-Line Drugs

Linezolid
Rifabutin
Rifapentine
Para-aminosalicylic acid
Streptomycin
Levofloxacin
Ethionamide
Amikacin
and others

The severity of the disease determines the impact on the patient's lifestyle. It is also important to determine the patient's knowledge of the disease and treatment and his or her adherence to drug treatment.

NURSING DIAGNOSES, PLANNING, AND IMPLEMENTATION. Nursing interventions for impaired gas exchange, ineffective airway clearance, and activity intolerance are found in the "Nursing Care Plan for the Patient With a Lower Respiratory Tract Disorder." Additional nursing diagnoses for the patient with TB follow.

Risk for Ineffective Self Health Management related to deficient knowledge and length of treatment

EXPECTED OUTCOME: The patient will follow treatment regimen and infection will be resolved, as evidenced by negative cultures.

• Assess patient's and family's ability and intent to follow treatment regimen. *It is essential for patients to be diligent about taking their drugs to eradicate the infection and to prevent spread to others.*
• Teach patient and family that drugs must be taken as scheduled for the entire course (6 months or longer) or a drug-resistant form of disease may develop. *Patients may be more willing to adhere to treatment if they understand the rationale for taking their medications.*
• Forewarn the patient that rifampin turns urine and other body fluids red. *This might frighten the patient and prevent adherence to treatment.*
• Teach patient to report side effects of medications. *If side effects can be managed, the patient is more likely to adhere to therapy.*
• Request an order for a visiting nurse. *A visiting nurse can monitor adherence to therapy. Directly observed therapy (DOT) has been found to increase adherence to medication therapy.*

Risk for Infection: Transmission to Others related to deficient knowledge about how infection is spread, or nonadherence to control measures

EXPECTED OUTCOME: The patient will verbalize understanding of and employ measures to prevent spreading infection.

• Assess patient's understanding of how TB is spread. *Teaching should build on patient's current knowledge.*
• Teach the patient how TB is spread and the importance of following measures to avoid spread. *The patient will be more likely to adhere to prevention measures if he understands the rationale for his actions.*
• Teach the patient to use a tissue to cover the mouth and nose when coughing or sneezing. *TB is spread by droplet nuclei that can be contained with a tissue.*
• Teach patient to flush tissues down the toilet or dispose of carefully in the trash. *TB bacteria can live in dried sputum for months, so careful disposal is essential.*
• Teach all family members the importance of careful hand hygiene. *Hand hygiene is an important measure in preventing all kinds of infections.*
• Instruct the patient in the importance of adherence to having follow-up sputum cultures. *Once sputum cultures are negative, the patient is no longer contagious.*

EVALUATION. If nursing care has been effective, the patient will understand his or her disease and the importance of taking care of himself or herself. The patient will take medications and receive follow-up care as ordered. He or she will take measures to protect others from catching TB. Additional evaluation is found in the "Nursing Care Plan for the Patient With a Lower Respiratory Tract Disorder."

NURSING CARE PLAN for the Patient With a Lower Respiratory Tract Disorder

Note: The most commonly used nursing diagnoses related to respiratory disorders are presented in the following care plan. This is not a care plan for any one respiratory disorder. Rather, use it as a reference when one of the nursing diagnoses applies to the patient, based on a thorough respiratory assessment.

Nursing Diagnosis: *Impaired Gas Exchange* related to decreased ventilation or perfusion as evidenced by Pao_2 less than 80 mm Hg, $PaCO_2$ greater than 45 mm Hg, or Spo_2 less than 90%, statement of dyspnea

Expected Outcomes: The patient will experience improved gas exchange, as evidenced by improving arterial blood gases (ABGs) or pulse oximetry and statement of acceptable level of dyspnea.

Evaluation of Outcomes: Are the patient's blood gases or Spo_2 improving? Does the patient state that dyspnea is resolved or controlled at an acceptable level?

Intervention Monitor arterial blood gas values and pulse oximetry as ordered. **Rationale** Pao_2 less than 80 mm Hg, $PaCO_2$ greater than 45 mm Hg, or Spo_2 less than 90% indicate impaired gas exchange. **Evaluation** Are values within patient's baseline values?

Continued

NURSING CARE PLAN for the Patient With a Lower Respiratory Tract Disorder—cont'd

Intervention Assess degree of dyspnea on a scale of 0 to 10, with 0 = no dyspnea and 10 = worst dyspnea. **Rationale** The patient's subjective report is the best measure of dyspnea; dyspnea indicates impaired gas exchange. **Evaluation** Is patient's degree of dyspnea within parameters that are acceptable to patient?

Intervention Assess lung sounds, respiratory rate and effort, use of accessory muscles. **Rationale** Respiratory rate less than 12 per minute or more than 24 per minute or use of accessory muscles indicates distress. Diminished or adventitious lung sounds can indicate risk factors for impaired gas exchange. **Evaluation** Are lung sounds clear and audible? Is respiratory rate 12 to 20 per minute and unlabored?

Intervention Observe skin and mucous membranes for cyanosis. **Rationale** Cyanosis indicates poor oxygenation. Oral mucous membrane cyanosis indicates serious hypoxia. **Evaluation** Are skin and mucous membranes pink?

Intervention Monitor for confusion or changes in mental status. **Rationale** Changes in mental status can signal impaired gas exchange. **Evaluation** Is patient alert and oriented? If not, could poor gas exchange be the reason?

Intervention Elevate head of bed or help patient to lean on over-bed table. **Rationale** Upright positioning promotes lung expansion. **Evaluation** Did change of position relieve some distress?

Intervention Position with good lung dependent ("good lung down"). **Rationale** This position allows the healthier lung to be better perfused and increases gas exchange. **Evaluation** Is SpO_2 improved in this position?

Intervention Administer supplemental oxygen at ≤2 L/min unless ordered otherwise. **Rationale** Supplemental oxygen decreases hypoxia. Rates more than 2 L/min may depress hypoxic drive. **Evaluation** Is oxygen placed properly on patient? Does it provide relief from dyspnea?

Intervention Place a fan in the patient's room, or provide a hand-held fan. **Rationale** The hand-held fan directed toward the face reduces feelings of breathlessness (Galbraith et al, 2010). **Evaluation** Is a fan available to the patient, and does it help?

Intervention Teach patient relaxation exercises. **Rationale** Relaxation exercises decrease perceived dyspnea. **Evaluation** Does patient use relaxation effectively?

Intervention For chronic disease, teach patient diaphragmatic and pursed-lip breathing. (See Chapter 29.) **Rationale** Breathing exercises promote relaxation and increase CO_2 excretion. **Evaluation** Does patient use breathing exercises correctly? Do they help?

Intervention Encourage patient to stop smoking if patient is a current smoker. **Rationale** Smoking is damaging to lungs and respiratory function. **Evaluation** Is patient receptive to smoking cessation? Are resources available?

Intervention For severe dyspnea, ask HCP about an order for IV morphine sulfate. **Rationale** Low doses of IV morphine reduce anxiety and cause peripheral vasodilation, which helps relieve pulmonary edema. **Evaluation** Does morphine provide relief from dyspnea?

Nursing Diagnosis: *Ineffective Airway Clearance* related to excessive secretions as evidenced by crackles or wheezes, ineffective cough

Expected Outcome: The patient will have improved airway clearance as evidenced by clear breath sounds and ability to cough up secretions.

Evaluation of Outcome: Are the patient's breath sounds clear? Is the patient able to effectively cough up and expectorate secretions?

NURSING CARE PLAN for the Patient With a Lower Respiratory Tract Disorder—cont'd

Intervention Assess lung sounds every (q) 4h and as needed (prn). **Rationale** Crackles and wheezes may indicate excess secretions in airways. **Evaluation** Do lung sounds indicate retained secretions?

Intervention Monitor amount, color, and consistency of sputum. **Rationale** Thick, purulent sputum indicates infection and should be reported to the HCP. **Evaluation** Does sputum indicate infection?

Intervention Turn patient q2h or encourage ambulating if able. **Rationale** Movement mobilizes secretions. **Evaluation** Is patient mobile?

Intervention Encourage oral fluids; use cool steam room humidifier. **Rationale** Hydration decreases viscosity of secretions and aids expectoration. **Evaluation** Is patient able to take oral fluids? Are secretions thin and easily expectorated?

Intervention Encourage patient to cough and deep breathe every hour and prn. **Rationale** Controlled coughing following deep breaths is more effective in clearing airway. **Evaluation** Does patient cough and deep breathe effectively?

Intervention Administer expectorants or mucolytics as ordered. **Rationale** Expectorants help liquefy secretions and trigger the cough reflex. **Evaluation** Are expectorants effective?

Intervention If patient is unable to cough up secretions, suction per institution policy. **Rationale** Suctioning is necessary to remove secretions when the patient is unable to cough effectively. **Evaluation** Is suctioning necessary? Does it help remove secretions?

Intervention Obtain order for CPT or vibratory positive expiratory pressure (PEP) device if indicated. **Rationale** CPT helps mobilize secretions. **Evaluation** Is CPT effective and well tolerated by the patient?

Nursing Diagnosis: *Ineffective Breathing Pattern* related to anxiety or pain as evidenced by respiratory rate less than 12 per minute or greater than 24 per minute, labored or shallow respirations, abnormal ABGs and Spo_2 values.

Expected Outcomes: The patient will maintain an effective breathing pattern as evidenced by respiratory rate between 12 and 20 per minute, even, and unlabored; and arterial blood gas and oxygen saturation results within patient's normal range.

Evaluation of Outcomes: Is the patient's respiratory rate within normal limits and unlabored? Does the patient's breathing pattern support normal blood gas and Spo_2 values?

Intervention Assess respiratory rate, depth, and effort every q4h and prn. **Rationale** Respirations less than 12 per minute or more than 20 per minute may indicate an ineffective pattern. **Evaluation** Is respiratory pattern ineffective?

Intervention Monitor blood gas and oxygen saturation values. **Rationale** An ineffective breathing pattern will not maintain oxygenation. **Evaluation** Is breathing pattern adversely affecting oxygenation?

Intervention Determine and treat the cause of ineffective breathing pattern. **Rationale** Pain or anxiety can cause a patient to change the breathing pattern. **Evaluation** Is a contributing factor identifiable and correctable?

Intervention Place patient in Fowler's or semi-Fowler's position. **Rationale** This allows for maximum chest expansion. **Evaluation** Is the patient in a comfortable position that enables adequate expansion?

Continued

NURSING CARE PLAN for the Patient With a Lower Respiratory Tract Disorder—cont'd

Intervention Teach patient to use diaphragmatic breathing, with a regular 2 second in, 4 second out pattern. **Rationale** Breathing exercises promote relaxation and increase CO_2 excretion. **Evaluation** Is the patient able to demonstrate an effective breathing pattern?

Nursing Diagnosis: *Activity Intolerance* related to imbalance between oxygen supply and demand as evidenced by dyspnea or drop in SpO_2 with routine activity

Expected Outcomes: The patient will tolerate increasing activity level as appropriate based on prognosis, as evidenced by stable respiratory rate and SpO_2 with activity. The patient will receive assistance with self-care until he or she is able to carry out own activities of daily living (ADLs) and will space rest and activity to provide as much self-care as possible.

Evaluation of Outcomes: Are the patient's care needs met by self or caregiver?

Intervention Assess amount of activity the patient can tolerate without becoming short of breath. **Rationale** Patients should be encouraged to do as much as they can for themselves to avoid becoming deconditioned. **Evaluation** What is patient able to do?

Intervention Monitor vital signs and oxygen saturation with activities. **Rationale** Respiratory rate will rise and SpO_2 will drop if activity is not tolerated. **Evaluation** Are vital signs and SpO_2 stable?

Intervention Allow patient to rest between activities. Bedrest may be needed during acute dyspnea. **Rationale** Even talking or eating can be exhausting to a patient who is dyspneic. **Evaluation** Is patient able to catch his or her breath between activities?

Intervention Obtain bedside commode, shower chair, handheld showerhead, if needed. **Rationale** Assistive devices can help the patient conserve energy. **Evaluation** Do assistive devices allow patient more independence?

Intervention Obtain portable oxygen if patient is able to ambulate. **Rationale** Portable oxygen may enable the patient to ambulate and prevent deconditioning. **Evaluation** Is patient able to ambulate and maintain SpO_2 within normal limits with portable oxygen?

Intervention Allow uninterrupted rest at night as much as possible. **Rationale** Lack of sleep can contribute to activity intolerance. **Evaluation** Is patient able to sleep uninterrupted? Can interferences be delayed until morning?

Intervention Slowly increase activity as able. **Rationale** Increasing activity helps maintain muscle tone and endurance. **Evaluation** Is patient able to increase a little each day? Is this a realistic goal for patient?

Intervention Refer patient with chronic lung disease to a pulmonary rehabilitation program. **Rationale** Pulmonary rehabilitation programs can help patient increase exercise tolerance. **Evaluation** Is patient willing to participate in a rehabilitation program?

CRITICAL THINKING

Mr. Woo

■ Mr. Woo is being tested for tuberculosis. You check his skin tests and find that the PPD test in his left forearm is negative, with no redness or induration. You also find that the *Candida* test in his right forearm is negative, with no redness or induration.

1. How do you document these results?
2. How do you interpret them?

Suggested answers are at the end of the chapter.

NURSING PROCESS FOR THE PATIENT WITH A LOWER RESPIRATORY TRACT INFECTION

Priority nursing diagnoses and interventions for patients with lower respiratory infections are presented in the "Nursing Care Plan for the Patient With a Lower Respiratory Tract Disorder."

RESTRICTIVE DISORDERS

Restrictive disorders are those problems that limit the ability of the patient to expand his or her lungs and, therefore, inhale air. Restrictive disorders can be intrinsic, involving lung tissue (such as pulmonary fibrosis), or extrinsic, involving structures outside the lungs (such as pleural effusion). Restrictive disorders covered below include pleurisy, pleural effusion, empyema, pulmonary fibrosis, and atelectasis.

Pleurisy (Pleuritis)
Pathophysiology

Recall that the visceral and parietal pleurae are the membranes that surround the lungs. Between these membranes is a small amount of serous fluid that prevents friction as the pleurae slide over each other during inhalation and exhalation. If the membranes become inflamed for any reason, they do not slide as easily. Instead of sliding, one membrane may "catch" on the other, causing it to stretch as the patient attempts to take a breath. This causes the characteristic sharp pain on inspiration. The irritation causes an increase in the formation of pleural fluid, which in turn reduces friction and decreases pain.

Etiology

Pleurisy is usually related to another underlying respiratory disorder, such as pneumonia, tuberculosis, a tumor, or trauma. Nonrespiratory disorders such as pancreatitis or certain autoimmune disorders can also result in pleurisy.

Signs and Symptoms

Pleurisy causes a sharp pain in the chest on inspiration. Pain also occurs during coughing or sneezing. Breathing may be shallow and rapid because deep breathing increases pain. The patient may also exhibit fever, chills, and an elevated white blood cell (WBC) count if the cause is infectious. A pleural friction rub is heard on auscultation.

Complications

As pleural membranes become more inflamed, serous fluid production increases, which may result in pleural effusion (see next section). If pleuritic pain is not controlled, patients have difficulty breathing deeply and coughing, which may lead to atelectasis. If infection goes untreated, empyema can result.

Diagnostic Tests

Diagnosis is based on signs and symptoms, including auscultation of a pleural friction rub. A chest x-ray examination or ultrasound and complete blood cell count (CBC) may be done. FVC (forced vital capacity) is reduced more than FEV_1 (forced expiratory volume in 1 second) because expansion is limited by the restrictive disorder; airways and FEV_1 may be normal. Additional testing is done to determine the underlying cause.

Therapeutic Measures

Treatment is aimed at correcting the underlying cause. Nonsteroidal anti-inflammatory drugs (NSAIDs) or opioids are given to control pain and facilitate deep breathing and coughing. The physician may perform a nerve block by injecting anesthetic near the intercostal nerves to block pain transmission. Patients may also experience some pain relief when lying on their affected side.

Pleural Effusion
Pathophysiology

When excess fluid collects in the pleural space, it is called a pleural effusion. Fluid normally enters the pleural space from surrounding capillaries and is reabsorbed by the lymphatic system. When a pathological condition causes an increase in fluid production or inadequate reabsorption of fluid, excess fluid collects. A normal amount of pleural fluid around each lung is 1 to 15 mL. More than 25 mL of fluid is considered abnormal; in pleural effusion, as much as several liters of fluid can collect at one time. The effusion can be either transudative, forming a watery fluid from the capillaries, or exudative, with fluid containing WBCs and protein from an inflammatory or infectious process.

Etiology

Like pleurisy, pleural effusion is generally caused by another lung disorder. It is a symptom rather than a disease. Transudative effusions may result from heart failure, liver disorders, or kidney disorders. Exudative effusions more commonly occur with lung cancer, infection, or inflammation.

Signs and Symptoms

Symptoms depend on the amount of fluid in the pleural space. The patient may or may not experience pleuritic pain. Increasing shortness of breath occurs because of the decreasing space for lung expansion. Cough and **tachypnea** may be present. A dull sound is heard when the affected area is percussed. Lung sounds are decreased or absent over the effusion, and a friction rub may be auscultated.

Diagnostic Tests

A chest x-ray examination is done to determine whether pleural effusion is present. If a thoracentesis is done, fluid samples are sent to the laboratory for culture and sensitivity and cytological examination. Further tests are done to determine the cause of the effusion.

• **WORD • BUILDING •**

tachypnea: tachy—rapid + pnea—breathing

Therapeutic Measures

Bedrest is recommended to enhance spontaneous resolution of the effusion. If symptoms are severe, a therapeutic thoracentesis is done to remove the excess fluid from the pleural space and relieve the patient of dyspnea. (Chapter 29 discusses how to assist with a thoracentesis.) Patients usually experience immediate improvement in dyspnea following thoracentesis. The physician will use x-ray examinations and percussion, or sometimes ultrasound, to determine where to insert the needle to obtain the fluid. If the fluid accumulation is large or recurring, a chest tube might be placed to continuously drain the pleural space. Occasionally talc or another irritating agent will be instilled via the chest tube to cause the pleural membranes to adhere to each other, eliminating the pleural space and preventing future episodes of pleural effusion. Treatment of the underlying cause of the effusion is necessary to prevent recurrence.

Empyema

Empyema is the collection of pus in the pleural space. It is a pleural effusion that is infected. Empyema is usually a complication of pneumonia, tuberculosis, or lung abscess. Symptoms, diagnosis, therapeutic measures, and nursing care are the same as the care of the patient with a pleural effusion, with an added emphasis on identifying and resolving the infection. A chest tube or surgery may be necessary to drain the area.

Pulmonary Fibrosis

Pathophysiology

Pulmonary fibrosis (PF), sometimes called interstitial lung disease, is a group of disorders that cause scarring and fibrosis of lung tissue. PF may evolve from injury to the alveoli, causing chronic inflammation; inflamed tissues are gradually replaced by fibrous connective tissue. Alveoli become thick and scarred, and gas exchange becomes difficult.

Etiology

Various factors are linked with pulmonary fibrosis, including heredity, exposure to certain viral illnesses, wood and metal dust exposure, medications, radiation therapy, and smoking. It may also be associated with some autoimmune disorders such as lupus erythematosus or rheumatoid arthritis. Chronic GERD may play a role. Often PF is called idiopathic PF because no specific cause can be found.

Signs and Symptoms

Patients with PF experience progressive shortness of breath. Inspiratory crackles and chronic cough are present. Some experience flulike symptoms. Fatigue is common, and clubbing of fingers may be present. Patients usually follow a downhill course.

Diagnostic Tests

A chest x-ray may show lung infiltrates. A CT scan may be done. Spirometry is done to verify that the condition is restrictive. ABGs may show reduced Pao_2. A bronchoscopy and lung biopsy can help rule out other causes of the patient's symptoms and can show inflammation and fibrosis. A blood test (ANA titer) may show whether an autoimmune process is involved.

Therapeutic Measures

Glucocorticoids (steroids) are used to reduce inflammation. Drugs to suppress the immune system may reduce autoimmune activity. Patients should be encouraged to stop smoking and to avoid secondhand smoke. Oxygen is used if needed to maintain oxygenation. Patients should receive flu and pneumococcal vaccines. Younger patients may be considered for a lung transplant. Pulmonary rehabilitation helps patients maintain optimum activity tolerance.

Atelectasis

Atelectasis is the collapse of alveoli. It most commonly occurs in postsurgical patients who do not cough and deep breathe effectively, although it can be caused by anything that causes hypoventilation. Areas of the lungs that are not well aerated become plugged with mucus, which prevents inflation of alveoli. As a result, alveoli collapse. Compression of lung tissue from effusion or a tumor can also cause atelectasis. The focus of nursing care is on prevention. Patients should be taught the importance of coughing and deep breathing, or use of an incentive spirometer whenever the risk for hypoventilation is present. Frequent position changes and ambulation are also helpful.

NURSING PROCESS FOR THE PATIENT WITH A RESTRICTIVE DISORDER

Data Collection

Perform a routine respiratory assessment. Monitor lung sounds for friction rub or decreasing breath sounds in any of the lobes. Assess pain level and vital signs. Be vigilant for an increase in dyspnea, tachypnea, changes in vital signs or pulse oximetry, or an increased white blood cell count or temperature.

Nursing Diagnoses, Planning, and Implementation

Priority nursing diagnoses are similar to those for other respiratory disorders and are addressed in the "Nursing Care Plan for the Patient With a Lower Respiratory Tract Disorder." In addition, it is essential to address pain (see below), because pain can prevent the patient from breathing effectively.

Risk for Ineffective Breathing Pattern related to acute pain
EXPECTED OUTCOME: The patient will be comfortable enough to breathe deeply and cough effectively and will have a respiratory rate of 12 to 20 per minute.

- Monitor respiratory rate and depth and pain location and level. *Some types of pain can cause shallow respirations, especially pleuritic pain.*
- Position patient for comfort. *Sometimes laying on the affected side for short periods will help reduce chest wall movement and pain.*

- Administer pain medication as ordered, preferably around the clock, to prevent pain from becoming severe. *Pain must be controlled so the patient can breathe deeply and prevent further complications. NSAIDs or acetaminophen are usually tried first because they will not suppress cough and respirations.*
- If opioids are required to control pain, carefully monitor respirations and cough. *Opioids can suppress respirations and cough, which can further complicate the underlying disorder.*
- Teach patient the importance of effective deep breathing and coughing (see Chapter 29). *This can help prevent further complications. If opioids have suppressed cough reflex, patient will need to purposefully deep breath and cough.*
- Request an order for an incentive spirometer. *Incentive spirometry can help encourage the patient to breathe deeply.*

Evaluation

If interventions have been effective, the patient should report a decrease in dyspnea and anxiety. Pain will be controlled so that the patient is able to take deep breaths and cough effectively. Breath sounds will be clear and equal bilaterally, and the patient will be free of signs and symptoms of infection.

■ OBSTRUCTIVE DISORDERS

Obstructive disorders are characterized by air trapping and difficulty getting air out of the lungs. Obstructive disorders covered in this chapter include COPD, emphysema, chronic bronchitis, asthma, and cystic fibrosis.

Chronic Obstructive Pulmonary Disease/Chronic Airflow Limitation

According to the National Heart, Lung, and Blood Institute (NHLBI), chronic obstructive pulmonary disease (COPD) is the third leading cause of death in the United States. More than 12 million adults have been diagnosed with COPD, and another 12 million likely have it but have not yet been diagnosed. COPD kills more than 120,000 Americans each year (NHLBI, n.d.). In the past, it was more common in men, but the incidence in women is rising because more women now smoke.

Pathophysiology

COPD is a group of pulmonary disorders characterized by difficulty exhaling because of airways that are narrowed or blocked by inflammation and mucus and because the loss of elastic fibers causes an increase in compliance. More effort is required for the weakened alveoli to push air out through obstructed airways (Fig. 31.3). Emphysema, chronic bronchitis, and asthma are disorders that limit airflow. A patient with COPD may have some degree of both emphysema and chronic bronchitis, although usually bronchitis is the dominant disorder. Asthma may also be present, but it differs somewhat because the airway limitation in asthma is usually reversible. A patient with unremitting asthma is treated as

having COPD. Airflow limitation in emphysema and bronchitis is progressive and minimally reversible (Fig. 31.4).

AIR TRAPPING IN CHRONIC AIRFLOW LIMITATION

Air trapping from excess mucus

Air trapping from decreased elastic recoil and narrowed airways

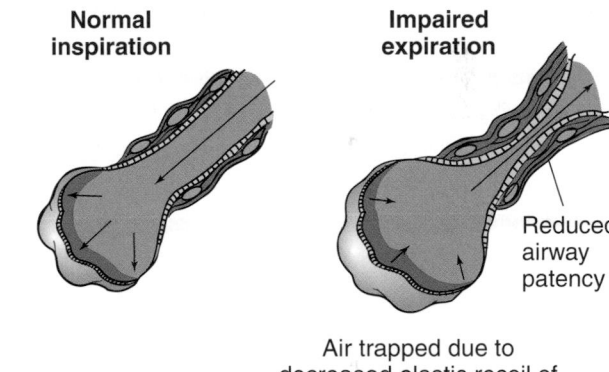

FIGURE 31.3 Air trapping in COPD.

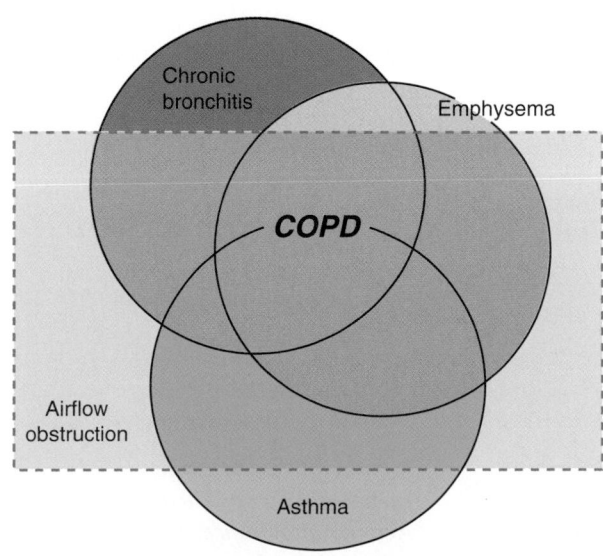

FIGURE 31.4 Chronic bronchitis and emphysema are the primary underlying disorders in COPD. Asthma also may play a role.

COPD may also be referred to as chronic airflow limitation (CAL) or chronic obstructive lung disease (COLD). COPD develops slowly and may be present for many years before symptoms become evident, and it may be advanced by the time the patient seeks treatment. It is characterized by periods of relative stability and **exacerbations** (acute worsening of symptoms), which may be triggered by respiratory infection or other stressors. (See Table 31.3 for a COPD summary.)

LEARNING TIP

*Restrictive disorders cause difficulty with inhala-tion or air ente**R**ing the lungs. **O**bstructive disor-ders are associated with difficulty exhaling or getting air **O**ut.*

TABLE **31.3** COPD SUMMARY

Signs and Symptoms	Cough
	Chronic sputum production
	Dyspnea that occurs every day, worsens with exercise
	Activity intolerance
	Crackles, wheezes, diminished breath sounds
	Barrel chest
	Use of accessory muscles
Diagnostic Tests	Chest x-ray examination, CT scan
	ABG analysis
	CBC
	Sputum analysis
	Spirometry
	α_1AT level if hereditary deficiency suspected
Therapeutic Measures	Smoking cessation
	Bronchodilators (PO, NMT, MDI)
	Corticosteroids, expectorants
	Flu and pneumonia vaccinations
	Supplemental oxygen
	Breathing exercises
	Chest physiotherapy
	Pulmonary rehabilitation
Priority Nursing Diagnoses	*Impaired Gas Exchange*
	Ineffective Airway Clearance
	Activity Intolerance

ABG = Arterial blood gases; CBC = complete blood count; CT = computed tomography; MDI = metered-dose inhaler; NMT = nebulized mist treatment; PO = *per os,* by mouth.

CHRONIC BRONCHITIS PATHOPHYSIOLOGY. Chronic bronchitis is similar to acute bronchitis, with symptoms occurring for at least 3 months of the year for 2 consecutive years. Patients may have multiple exacerbations, each lasting 2 weeks or more. The bronchial tree becomes inflamed from inhaled irritants, and impaired ciliary function reduces the ability to remove the irritants. The mucus-producing glands in the airways become hypertrophied, producing excessive thick, tenacious mucus, which obstructs airways and traps air (Fig. 31.5A). These changes lead to chronic low-grade infection.

EMPHYSEMA PATHOPHYSIOLOGY. **Emphysema** affects the respiratory bronchioles and alveoli distal to the terminal bronchioles, causing destruction of the alveolar walls and loss of elastic recoil (see Fig. 31.5C). This also causes damage to adjacent pulmonary capillaries. Because of the loss of elastic recoil, passive exhalation is impaired and air is trapped in the alveoli. The combination of damaged alveoli and capillaries causes reduced surface area for gas exchange. Emphysema can occur primarily in the respiratory bronchioles (centrilobular emphysema), with delayed alveolar damage, or in the respiratory bronchioles and alveoli (panlobular emphysema; Fig. 31.6).

Etiology

Smoking is the single most important risk factor for COPD. Other factors include passive (secondhand and possibly third-hand) smoking, indoor and outdoor air pollution, and exposure to industrial chemicals. Some familial predisposition to chronic bronchitis has been demonstrated. A small number of individuals have an inherited deficiency of the enzyme alpha-antitrypsin (α_1AT), which causes a predisposition to the development of emphysema. Patients with this inherited tendency who also smoke have a very high risk of developing the disease. Children of smoking parents are at higher risk because of smoke exposure.

Prevention

Prevention is important because no cure for COPD is currently available. Avoidance of smoking and other inhaled irritants is vital, especially in those individuals with parents or siblings with COPD. According to the Global Initiative for Chronic Obstructive Lung Disease (GOLD; 2013) guidelines, "Smoking cessation is the intervention with the greatest capacity to influence the natural history of COPD."

• WORD • BUILDING •
emphysema: to inflate

NURSING CARE TIP

This is a self-care tip. If you are a smoker, now is a good time to quit. COPD is deadly. Check Chapter 29 for ways to quit smoking. Or visit www.tobaccofreenurses.org. You CAN do it! Good luck!

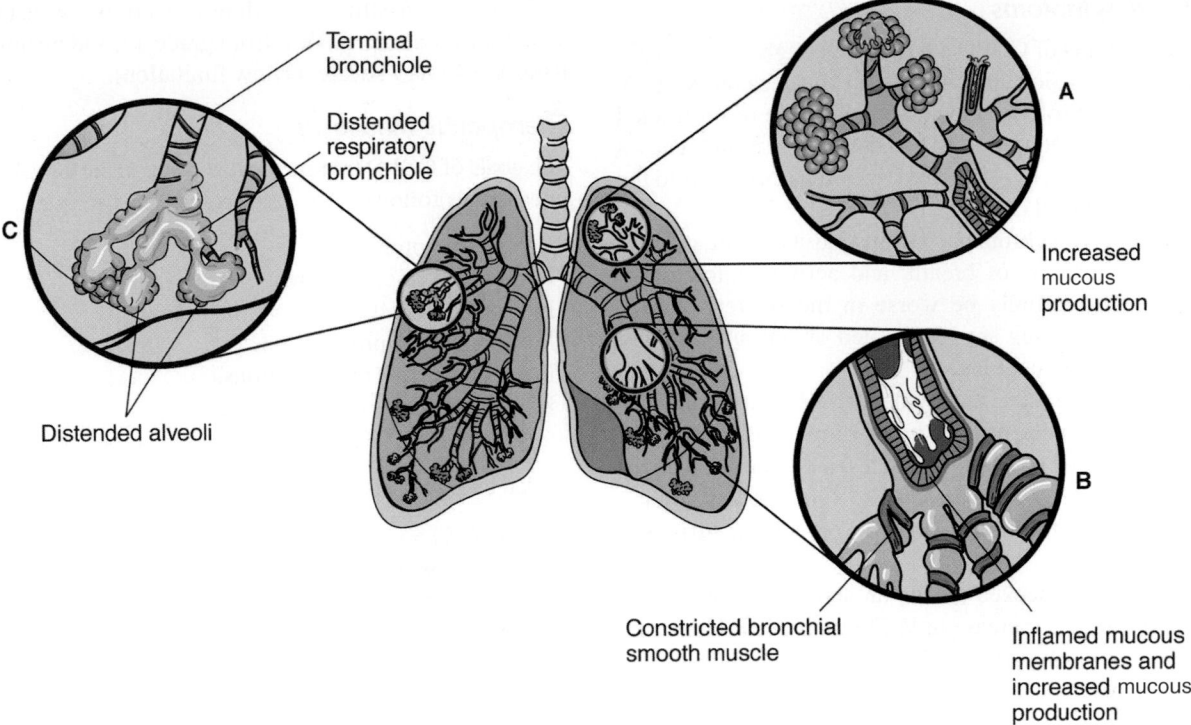

FIGURE 31.5 (A) Chronic bronchitis. Note inflamed airways and excessive mucus. (B) Asthma. Note narrowed bronchial tubes and swollen mucous membranes. (C) Emphysema. Note distended respiratory bronchioles and alveoli.

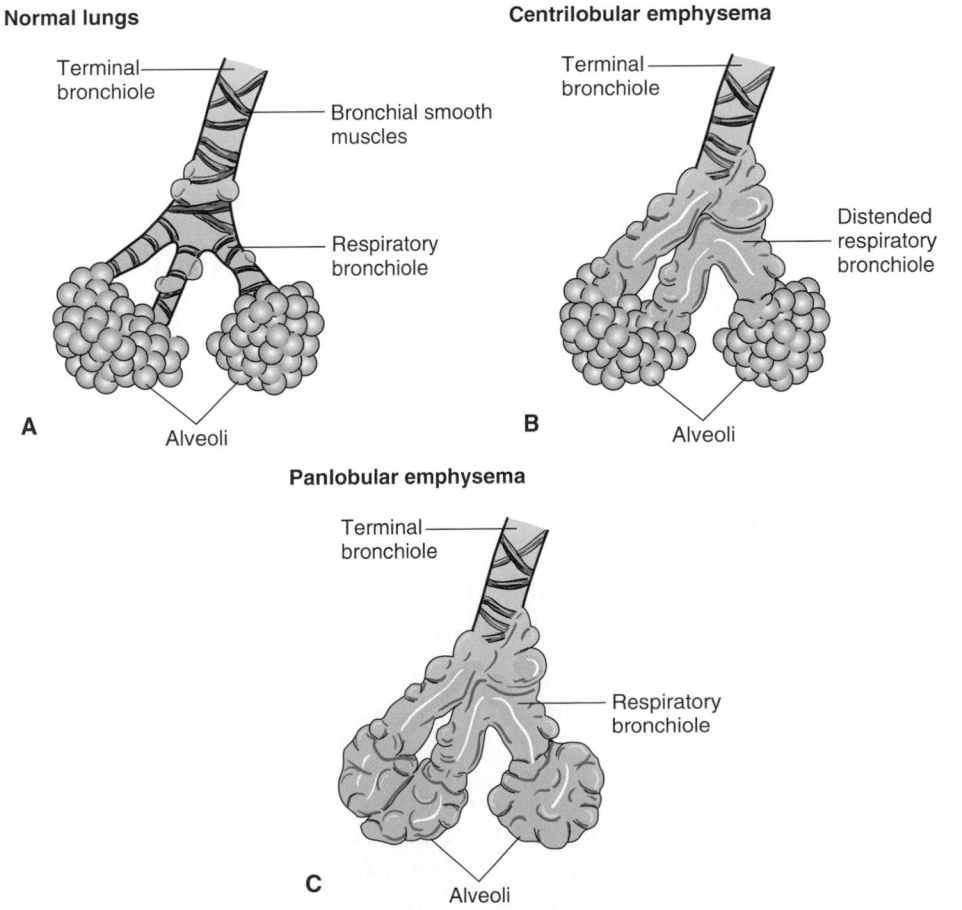

FIGURE 31.6 Types of emphysema. (A) Normal lungs. (B) Centrilobular emphysema. (C) Panlobular emphysema.

Signs and Symptoms

Classic symptoms of COPD are chronic cough with or without sputum production, and progressive dyspnea on exertion. Patients exhibit prolonged exhalation because of obstructed air passages and reduced elastic recoil. Air trapping causes the lungs to become hyperinflated, which in turn leads to the classic barrel-shaped chest.

The patient with chronic bronchitis has a chronic productive cough, shortness of breath, and activity intolerance. Symptoms may initially be worse in the winter months. Crackles and wheezing are often noted on auscultation and may improve after coughing.

The most characteristic symptom of emphysema is progressive shortness of breath, accompanied by activity intolerance. Use of accessory muscles is evident. Auscultation reveals diminished breath sounds. Remember that many patients have symptoms of both chronic bronchitis and emphysema.

ABGs may be checked during an acute exacerbation of COPD and show an increase in $PaCO_2$ and a low PaO_2. The patient develops **polycythemia** in response to chronic hypoxemia, which results in a ruddy skin color. Cyanosis may also be present.

In late stages of COPD, patients may lose weight and become malnourished. They have difficulty eating because of severe dyspnea, and the increased work of breathing expends more calories. Chronic hypoxemia causes release of certain chemicals that may also lead to weight loss. Patients use accessory muscles to breathe and tend to assume the classic tripod position to aid breathing.

Complications

Some patients with emphysema develop large air spaces within the lung tissue (**bullae**) or adjacent to the pleurae (**blebs**). These are like blisters that can rupture and cause the lung to collapse. Right-sided heart failure may develop because the heart has to work harder to pump blood to the diseased lungs. (See the section on cor pulmonale in Chapter 26.) Death usually results from respiratory infection or respiratory failure.

Diagnostic Tests

Information from spirometry, chest x-ray examination, and blood gas analysis is correlated with the history and physical examination to diagnose COPD. Spirometry is essential for diagnosis. Normally, the forced expiratory volume in 1 second (FEV_1) is about 70% to 80% of the forced vital capacity (FVC). In COPD, the FEV_1 following bronchodilator use is less than 70%. This is because the patient with airflow limitation is unable to forcefully exhale as much air in the first second as would normally be expected.

If lung function improves after administration of a bronchodilator, asthma is suspected rather than COPD. A α_1AT level is checked if deficiency is suspected, especially in patients with a family history of COPD. CBC, electrolytes, and sputum culture may also be assessed during exacerbations.

COPD is classified according to spirometry results and symptoms into four grades, from grade 1 (mild airflow limitation) to 4 (very severe airflow limitation).

Therapeutic Measures

The goals of COPD treatment, according to the GOLD guidelines, are as follows:

- Relieve symptoms.
- Improve exercise tolerance.
- Improve health status.
- Prevent disease progression.
- Prevent and treat exacerbations.
- Reduce mortality (GOLD, 2013).

In addition, cessation of cigarette smoking should be included as a goal throughout any management program.

SMOKING CESSATION. Even late in the disease process, stopping smoking can slow disease progression and prolong life. Exposure to other respiratory contaminants should also be minimized. Hair spray, other household aerosols, and body powder should be avoided. Figure 31.7 shows the benefit of smoking cessation and impact on the length of time to disability and death. "Patient Perspective" is a personal account from one woman who understood too late the importance of smoking cessation.

OXYGEN. Oxygen therapy is usually delayed until grade 4 disease, and then is used to keep SpO_2 at or above 90%. It

---

• WORD • BUILDING •

polycythemia: poly—many + cyt—cells + emia—in the blood

Patient Perspective

Sarah

At age 17, I started the habit that would change my life. I started to smoke.

At first it was just a few cigarettes, but as time passed I smoked more and more until I reached two packs a day. This habit continued for 42 years. I disregarded all the warnings about what could happen. I was sure this would never happen to me.

Now at age 75, I must do three breathing treatments a day and carry an inhaler with me at all times. I have a cough that cannot be controlled. I can no longer ride a bike with my grandchildren, play badminton, or even bowl. My lungs won't let me. Going shopping is no longer fun—it's a chore. I have to walk slowly or I can't breathe.

All the things I enjoyed most I've given up because for 42 years I was a slave to cigarettes. If any of you smoke, stop now. Smell the coffee and roses without coughing.

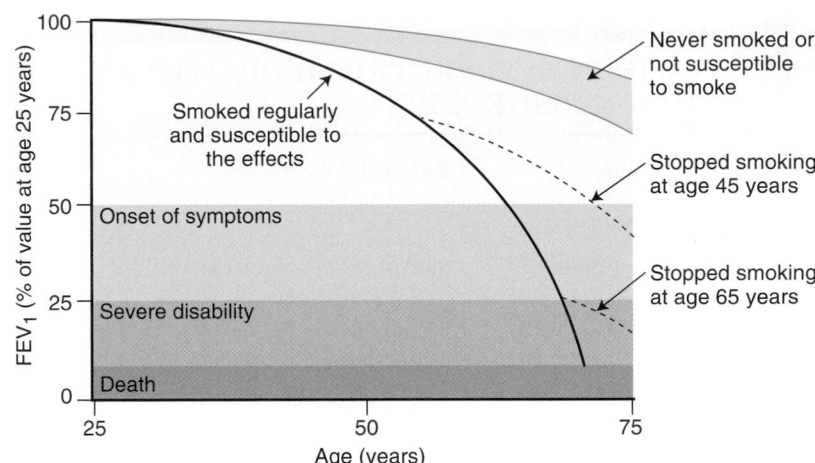

FIGURE 31.7 Fletcher and Peto chart. From Fletcher, C., & Peto, R. (1977). The natural history of chronic airflow obstruction. *British Medical Journal, 1,* 1645–1648.

usually is ordered at a flow rate of 1 to 2 L/min. Higher flow rates may suppress the hypoxic drive in patients who are chronic CO_2 retainers, although this is uncommon. Higher flow rates may be used during acute exacerbations in a monitored setting. Patients with chronic oxygen saturation levels of 88% or less should be placed on oxygen at home.

MEDICATIONS. Medications commonly used include adrenergic and anticholinergic metered-dose inhalers or nebulized mist treatments to open airways, corticosteroid inhalers to control inflammation, and intermittently when needed, antibiotics. Much focus is now placed on a combination of long-acting adrenergic agents and corticosteroids (Advair, Symbicort) and a new long-acting anticholinergic agent (tiotropium [Spiriva]), all of which may reduce exacerbations

and prolong survival. **Antitussive** agents should be avoided in patients with COPD because they need to be able to cough up secretions.

Oral theophylline bronchodilators are sometimes used but have significant side effects so are avoided if possible. Oral or IV corticosteroids are used for acute exacerbations. Replacement of $\alpha 1 AT$ may be used in emphysema patients who are deficient. See Table 31.4 for a more detailed list of medications used in the treatment of COPD.

Patients with COPD should also be assessed for depression. Depression is common with chronic illness and often

• WORD • BUILDING •

antitussive: anti—against + tussive—cough

TABLE 31.4   SELECTED MEDICATIONS USED FOR LOWER RESPIRATORY TRACT DISORDERS

Drug Class/Action	Examples	Nursing Implications
Adrenergic Bronchodilators Stimulate beta receptors to dilate bronchioles	albuterol (Ventolin-HFA, Proventil-HFA, ProAir-HFA) metaproterenol (Alupent, Metaprel) pirbuterol (Maxair)	Use with care in patients with cardiac disease. Overuse can cause rebound bronchospasm. Short acting; used as rescue inhalers.
Anticholinergic Agents Block parasympathetic response, causing bronchodilation	ipratropium (Atrovent) tiotropium (Spiriva)	Anticholinergics should be avoided with narrow-angle glaucoma and prostatic hypertrophy. Tiotropium is a capsule that is placed in a device and activated before inhalation. Instruct patient not to swallow capsules.
Methylxanthines Relax bronchial smooth muscle to dilate airways	theophylline (Theo-24, Uniphyl) aminophylline	Narrow therapeutic index; can become toxic. Therapeutic theophylline level 10–20 mcg/mL.

Continued

TABLE 31.4 SELECTED MEDICATIONS USED FOR LOWER RESPIRATORY TRACT DISORDERS—cont'd

Drug Class/Action	Examples	Nursing Implications
Corticosteroids Reduce inflammation in airways	methylprednisolone (Medrol, Solu-Medrol) prednisone triamcinolone acetonide (Azmacort) beclomethasone (Beclovent, QVAR) fluticasone (Flovent) budesonide (Pulmicort)	Must be used regularly to prevent symptoms. Never discontinue abruptly; must be tapered. Monitor blood glucose while on high doses. Rinse mouth after inhaler use to prevent local infection (candidiasis). If using glucocorticoid and adrenergic MDIs together, use adrenergic inhaler first to open airways.
Combination agents	albuterol and ipratropium (Combivent) fluticasone and salmeterol (Advair) budesonide and formoterol (Symbicort)	See individual agents. Salmeterol and formoterol are long-acting beta agonists that are unsafe for use alone but appear to be safer when used with inhaled corticosteroids. Use only as directed. Not for use as rescue inhalers.
Phosphodiesterase-4 inhibitors Reduces COPD exacerbations	roflumilast (Daliresp)	NOT effective for acute symptoms. Used prophylactically to reduce exacerbations.
Mast Cell Stabilizers Stabilize mast cells to reduce histamine release	cromolyn sodium (Intal) nedocromil (Tilade)	Effective for allergic asthma. May be used prophylactically before exercise or allergen exposure.
Expectorants Liquefy secretions and stimulate cough	guaifenesin (Robitussin, Mucinex)	Encourage fluids.
Antileukotrienes Inhibit leukotriene synthesis or activity, a mediator of inflammation in asthma	zafirlukast (Accolate) montelukast (Singulair) zileuton (Zyflo)	Must be taken regularly to prevent symptoms. Monitor for elevation of liver enzymes.
Antitussives Suppress cough reflex	codeine dextromethorphan (DM suffix in cough preparations)	Avoid giving to patient who has secretions that need to be expectorated.

Note. This table is an overview. A drug guide should be consulted for complete administration guidelines. MDI = metered-dose inhaler.

goes undiagnosed. Patients may not report feeling depressed but may experience more physical symptoms. Antidepressant medications, if indicated, can increase quality of life for COPD patients.

Morphine or other opioids may be effective in reducing acute dyspnea and anxiety. They are reserved for end-stage disease.

SUPPORTIVE CARE. A pneumococcal vaccination and yearly influenza vaccinations are recommended to reduce the risk of respiratory infection. Avoidance of crowds and exposure to people with respiratory infections is advised.

Good hydration and a cool mist humidifier help keep secretions loose. Chest physiotherapy may be used to help the patient remove excessive secretions. A dietitian consultation is helpful for the patient who is unable to maintain a desirable weight. Typically a high-protein, high-fat, low-carbohydrate diet is prescribed. Breathing exercises help improve oxygenation and reduce anxiety (see Chapter 29).

REHABILITATION. Pulmonary rehabilitation programs can help patients increase exercise tolerance and maintain a sense of well-being (Fig. 31.8). Patients exercise in a monitored environment and benefit from the support of other patients with similar problems. Some groups of pulmonary rehabilitation patients have even formed harmonica clubs! Playing their harmonicas mimics pursed-lip breathing and may strengthen the diaphragm, the major muscle of breathing.

SURGERY. Surgical removal of emphysematous lung tissue (called lung volume reduction surgery, or LVRS) increases the space available for good lung tissue to expand, reducing dyspnea and increasing exercise tolerance. This is a high-risk procedure, but it has allowed some patients to return to a more normal activity level and improved quality of life. Surgery may also be performed to remove blebs in an attempt to prevent pneumothorax. Lung transplant may be an option in select patients.

ENDOBRONCHIAL VALVE. A newer treatment is similar to lung reduction surgery, but without the surgery. It is placement of a tiny one-way valve via bronchoscopy into an area of emphysematous lung, which causes the diseased area to collapse. This then allows the healthy lung tissue more space to expand. It has been shown to increase FEV_1 and exercise tolerance. Research is ongoing on this intervention.

MECHANICAL VENTILATION. If arterial blood gases worsen despite treatment, intubation and mechanical ventilation may be considered, depending on the patient's advance directive.

Unfortunately, mechanical ventilation will not make a patient's disease better, and weaning may be difficult or impossible once it is initiated. Use of noninvasive positive-pressure ventilation (NIPPV; see Chapter 29) may be a good alternative for many patients.

END-OF-LIFE PLANNING. It is important to assess whether the patient has a living will or durable power of attorney for health care (DPOA; see Chapter 17). COPD is a progressive disease, and patients can increase the quality of their life and death by making decisions in advance. Patients should make decisions about whether they would want to be intubated and mechanically ventilated, or have cardiopulmonary resuscitation (CPR) in event of a cardiac arrest. CPR is rarely successful in a patient with end-stage disease. Patients should be made aware of palliative care options and assured that they will be kept as comfortable as possible.

Research is ongoing to determine which treatments will alter long-term outcomes of the disease. Check the American Lung Association website for more information at www.lungusa.org.

Nursing Process for the Patient With COPD

See "Nursing Process for the Patient With an Obstructive Disorder" and the "Nursing Care Plan for the Patient With a Lower Respiratory Tract Disorder." Priority nursing diagnoses for the patient with COPD include *Impaired Gas Exchange, Ineffective Airway Clearance,* and *Activity Intolerance.*

Asthma

The incidence of asthma is on the rise. Nearly 19 million adults and 7.1 million children in the United States have asthma (CDC, 2013b). It accounts for 3.1 million urgent care and emergency department visits each year. Asthma is more prevalent in African Americans than in whites. Asthma deaths are more common in lower socioeconomic groups, possibly because of poor access to treatment or less compliance with treatment. With careful monitoring and treatment, however, patients with asthma can manage their symptoms and lead normal lives.

Pathophysiology

Asthma is characterized by chronic inflammation and edema of the mucosal lining of the airways and hyperresponsiveness of the bronchial smooth muscles (**bronchospasm**). This causes narrowed airways and air trapping, which is why it is considered an obstructive disorder (see Fig. 31.5B). Inflammation occurs in part because things that trigger asthma (asthma triggers) cause release of inflammatory substances such as histamine and leukotrienes. Symptoms are intermittent and generally reversible, with periods of normal airway function. Some people develop permanent changes in their airways, called remodeling; this leads to a progressive loss of lung function.

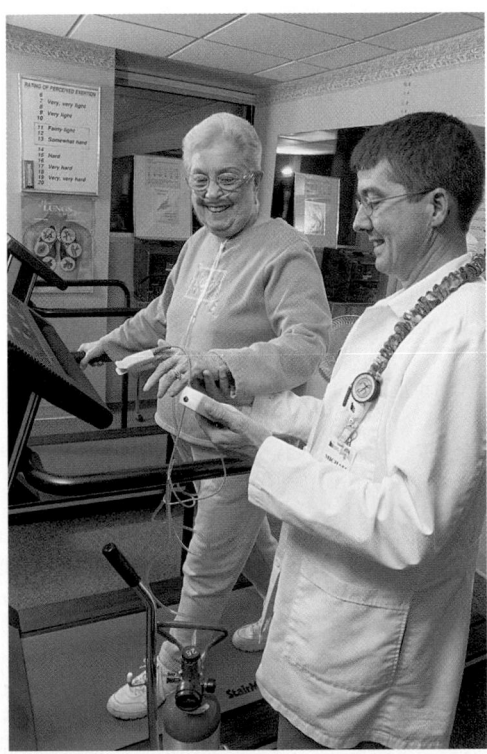

FIGURE 31.8 Patients build exercise tolerance in pulmonary rehabilitation programs. Note therapist monitoring oxygen saturation.

• **WORD • BUILDING •**

bronchospasm: broncho—airway + spasm—convulsion, involuntary narrowing

About 50% of patients develop the disorder in childhood, and some outgrow it. However, a significant number develop symptoms again later in life. Children with asthma should be counseled that smoking can increase the risk of recurrence in adulthood. Asthma may also complicate chronic bronchitis or emphysema.

Etiology

The tendency to develop asthma is inherited. The most common predisposing factor is the genetic tendency to be allergic to airborne allergens such as pollen or molds. Viral respiratory infections are also a contributing factor to asthma diagnosis and exacerbation. Tobacco smoke, air pollution, early use of antibiotics, and sensitization to house-dust mites and cockroaches have also been linked to asthma development.

Asthma Triggers

Once asthma develops, a number of triggers can cause an acute attack. Exposure to allergens such as dust mites, cockroaches, cat and dog dander, or pollen can trigger an attack. Other possible triggers include emotional upset, exercise, medications (aspirin, beta blockers), and GERD. GERD can trigger an attack because stomach acid can reflux into the esophagus and then be aspirated, causing an exacerbation of symptoms. This occurs especially at night. GERD and its treatment are discussed in Chapter 33.

Prevention

Although asthma cannot be prevented at this time, research is ongoing to determine factors associated with its development. Some studies have suggested that the presence of older siblings in the home, early exposure to day care, certain infections, or a rural environment may be protective against asthma development in childhood. Appropriate control of childhood asthma may prevent more serious asthma in later years. Avoidance of smoking may reduce the risk of recurrence of asthma that started in childhood. To prevent acute attacks, it is important that the patient identify triggers of asthma symptoms and avoid them whenever possible. Monitoring of symptoms and compliance with prophylactic and maintenance therapy is also important.

Signs and Symptoms

Asthma symptoms are intermittent and are often referred to as attacks, which may last from minutes to days. Patients report chest tightness, dyspnea, coughing, and difficulty moving air in and out of the lungs. Symptoms are often worse at night. Some patients experience coughing but no wheezing. Once initial symptoms are controlled, airways may remain hypersensitive and prone to asthma symptoms for many weeks.

On examination, you will note an increased respiratory rate as the patient attempts to compensate for narrowed airways. Inspiratory and expiratory wheezing is heard because of turbulent airflow through swollen airways with thick secretions; wheezing may sometimes be audible even without a stethoscope. Air is trapped in the lungs, and expiration is prolonged. A cough is common and may produce thick, clear sputum. Use of accessory muscles to breathe is a sign that the attack is severe and warrants immediate attention.

Be aware that an absence of audible wheezing may not signal improvement but rather may be an ominous sign that the patient is not moving enough air to make any sound. If wheezing is not heard, use of accessory muscles and peak expiratory flow rate values must be carefully evaluated. Once treatment begins to open the airways, wheezing may become audible.

Asthma is classified according to frequency of symptoms (Table 31.5).

TABLE 31.5   CLASSIFICATION OF ASTHMA FOR PATIENTS NOT CURRENTLY TAKING LONG-TERM CONTROL MEDICATIONS

	Symptoms	SABA Use	Activity	Lung Function
Intermittent	Asthma symptoms 2 days per week or less; nighttime awakenings twice a month or less.	SABA for symptom control 2 days a week or less.	No interference with normal activity.	Normal FEV_1 between exacerbations.
Mild persistent	Asthma symptoms more than twice a week, but not daily; nighttime awakenings 3 to 4 times per month.	SABA more than 2 days a week but not more than once daily.	Minor limitation of normal activity.	FEV_1 greater than 80% predicted. FEV_1/FVC normal.
Moderate persistent	Asthma symptoms every day; nighttime awakenings more	SABA use daily.	Some activity limitation.	FEV_1 greater than 60% but less than 80% predicted.

TABLE 31.5   CLASSIFICATION OF ASTHMA FOR PATIENTS NOT CURRENTLY TAKING LONG-TERM CONTROL MEDICATIONS—cont'd

	Symptoms	SABA Use	Activity	Lung Function
	than once a week but not every night.			FEV$_1$/FVC reduced 5%.
Severe persistent	Symptoms throughout the day; nighttime symptoms often 7 times per week.	SABA several times daily.	Activity extremely limited.	FEV$_1$ less than 60% predicted. FEV$_1$/FVC reduced more than 5%.

Note. FVC = forced vital capacity; FEV$_1$ = forced expiratory volume in 1 second; SABA = short-acting beta agonist (such as albuterol).
Adapted from the National Heart, Blood, and Lung Institute, Expert Panel Report 3. (2007). *Guidelines for the diagnosis and management of asthma.* Bethesda, MD: Author. Retrieved June 25, 2013, from www.nhlbi.nih.gov/guidelines/asthma/asthgdln.htm

Complications

Status asthmaticus occurs if bronchospasm is not controlled and symptoms are prolonged. As the patient increases the respiratory rate to compensate for narrowed airways, a lot of carbon dioxide is blown off and respiratory alkalosis occurs. If the attack is not resolved and the patient begins to tire, the patient will no longer be able to compensate, and PaCO$_2$ will rise, resulting in respiratory acidosis. This can lead to respiratory failure and death if untreated.

Diagnostic Tests

Diagnosis is based on the patient's report of symptoms, physical examination, and spirometry results. Peak expiratory flow rate and FEV$_1$ are reduced, especially during symptomatic periods. Asthma can be differentiated from COPD during spirometry testing by administering an adrenergic agonist (such as an albuterol inhaler) and then retesting. Asthma symptoms can generally be reversed with the medication, but COPD cannot. Allergy skin testing and increased serum immunoglobulin E and eosinophil levels indicate allergic involvement and may help determine appropriate treatment. ABGs may be evaluated during an acute severe attack.

On a long-term basis, asthma control can be evaluated using FEV$_1$ or peak flow measurements, frequency and severity of exacerbations and nighttime awakenings, and frequency of short-acting beta-agonist use.

Therapeutic Measures

Patients must learn to manage asthma at home. If they can monitor and manage their symptoms, acute episodes and hospitalizations can be avoided.

SELF-MONITORING. All patients benefit from learning to monitor their asthma symptoms and make treatment decisions accordingly. This can be done by carefully monitoring symptoms or by monitoring peak expiratory flow rate (PEFR; Fig. 31.9). PEFR is a measurement, in liters per minute, of the amount of air a patient can blow into a peak flow meter from fully inflated lungs. The patient determines his or her baseline PEFR during symptom-free times. Readings can be

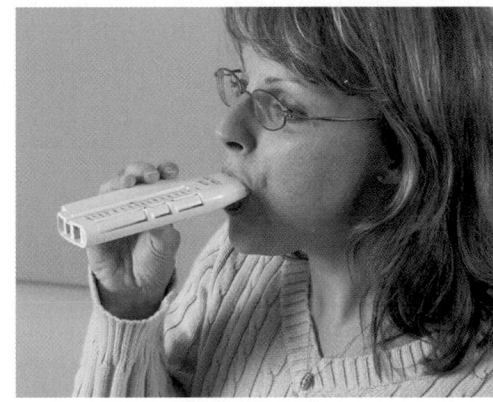

FIGURE 31.9 Patient with asthma using a peak flowmeter to monitor peak expiratory flow rate.

charted to keep track of progress (Fig. 31.10). If symptoms worsen or PEFR begins to fall below the patient's baseline, treatment that has been predetermined with the HCP should be initiated (Fig. 31.11). If treatment does not improve PEFR to the expected degree, the patient is advised to go to the emergency room. PEFR results may indicate the onset of asthma before the patient experiences any obvious symptoms.

AVOIDANCE OF TRIGGERS. The patient is instructed to identify and avoid asthma triggers. If triggers cannot be avoided, the patient can use bronchodilator or mast cell stabilizer inhalers as prescribed before exposure. Inhalers can be especially useful before exercise. Recent studies have shown that a high-salt diet may worsen exercise-induced airway inflammation. Animal dander and foods that cause symptoms are best avoided when possible. Eliminating carpets and curtains in bedrooms, using vinyl mattress and pillow covers, and installing a portable or central air filter can reduce dust mite exposure. Maintenance of indoor humidity between 40% and 50% can reduce mold growth. If cold air triggers symptoms, the patient should keep the nose and mouth covered when outside in cold weather. Smoking and exposure to secondhand smoke are strongly discouraged.

Name															
Green zone _____ Yellow zone _____ Red zone _____															
Date															
	AM	PM	AM	PM	AM	PM	AM	PM	AM	PM	AM	PM	AM	PM
800														
750														
700														
650														
600														
550														
500														
450														
400														
350														
300														
250														
200														
150														
100														
Notes														

FIGURE 31.10 Peak flow chart. The green zone is 80% to 100% of the patient's normal peak flow rate. The yellow zone is 50% to 80% of normal. The red zone is less than 50% of normal. The patient works with the HCP to determine which actions to take when readings fall in the yellow or red zones.

Aspirin and NSAIDs can cause asthma symptoms in some individuals. Beta-blocking medications (propranolol, metoprolol), used commonly for hypertension, block beta receptors in the lungs, preventing the sympathetic nervous system from promoting bronchodilation. These drugs should be avoided if they make symptoms worse.

MEDICATIONS. Medications for asthma treatment may be used intermittently or continuously, depending on the persistence of symptoms. Inhaled medications are preferred because they cause fewer adverse effects than oral or injected medications. See Table 31.4 for a summary of medications used in the treatment of lower respiratory disorders.

For patients with intermittent symptoms, short-acting beta agonists (SABAs) such as albuterol are used to dilate bronchioles. They are administered via metered-dose inhaler when symptoms occur and are often called rescue inhalers. They can also be administered preventively before exercise or other events that trigger asthma.

If the patient needs to use a rescue inhaler more than two times a week for symptoms, maintenance medications to prevent symptoms will likely be started. Inhaled corticosteroids such as fluticasone or budesonide are generally added first to control inflammation. Instruct the patient that corticosteroids must be used regularly to prevent symptoms and that they do not provide immediate symptom relief during an acute attack.

Long-acting beta-agonist bronchodilators (LABAs) such as salmeterol (Serevent) or formoterol (Foradil) can also help prevent symptoms by keeping airways dilated for up to 12 hours or more. Research in recent years, however, has questioned their safety, and they are no longer recommended to be used alone. If they are used, they should be used in combination with inhaled corticosteroids (Advair, Symbicort).

Mast cell stabilizers (cromolyn sodium, nedocromil) may help prevent symptoms but are often not useful. Some patients use mast cell stabilizers 10 to 15 minutes before exposure to allergens or exercise to reduce symptoms.

If inhaled medications do not control symptoms or if the patient has nocturnal symptoms, oral antileukotrienes may be added; theophylline bronchodilators are generally used as a last resort because of their many side effects. Immunotherapy (allergy shots) may be used for some patients with allergic asthma.

An acute asthma attack may be treated with an inhaled (metered dose inhaler or nebulized mist treatment) or subcutaneous short-acting beta agonist (bronchodilator) or, rarely, IV aminophylline. IV or oral corticosteroids (methylprednisolone, prednisone) are potent anti-inflammatory agents that are useful in an acute episode but are avoided for long-term therapy if possible because of their cushingoid side effects. (See the section on Cushing's syndrome in Chapter 39.) Corticosteroids must be tapered before discontinuing to prevent withdrawal symptoms. (See the section on addisonian crisis in Chapter 39.)

NURSING CARE TIP

If separate short-acting bronchodilator and corticosteroid inhalers are used at the same time, instruct the patient to use the bronchodilator first. This opens the airways and allows for better distribution of the corticosteroid in the lungs.

Asthma Action Plan for _____ Doctor's Name _____ Date _____

Doctor's Phone Number _____ Hospital/ Emergency Room Phone Number _____

GREEN ZONE: Doing Well

- No cough, wheeze, chest tightness, or shortness of breath during the day or night
- Can do usual activities

And, if a peak flow meter is used,

Peak flow: more than _____
(80% or more of my best peak flow)

My best peak flow is: _____

Take These Long-Term-Control Medicines Each Day (include an anti-inflammatory)

Medicine	How much to take	When to take it

Before exercise   ☐ _____   ☐ 2 or ☐ 4 puffs   5 to 60 minutes before exercise

YELLOW ZONE: Asthma Is Getting Worse

- Cough, wheeze, chest tightness, or shortness of breath, or
- Waking at night due to asthma, or
- Can do some, but not all, usual activities

-Or-

Peak flow: _____ to _____
(50% – 80% of my best peak flow)

First ▷ **Add: Quick-Relief Medicine – and keep taking your GREEN ZONE medicine**

_____   ☐ 2 or ☐ 4 puffs, every 20 minutes up to 1 hour
(short-acting beta$_2$-antagonist)   ☐ Nebulizer, once

Second ▷ **If your symptoms (and peak flow, if used) return to GREEN ZONE after 1 hour of above treatment**

☐ Take the quick-relief medicine every 4 hours for 1 to 2 days

☐ Double the dose of your inhaled steroid for _____ (7–10) days

-Or-

If your symptoms (and peak flow, if used) do not return to GREEN ZONE after 1 hour of above treatment

☐ Take:_____   ☐ 2 or ☐ 4 puffs or ☐ Nebulizer
(short-acting beta$_2$-antagonist)

☐ Add: _____ mg/day For _____ (3–10) days
(oral steroid)

☐ Call the doctor before/ ☐ within _____ hours after taking the oral steroid.

RED ZONE: Medical Alert!

- Very short of breath, or
- Quick-relief medicines have not helped, or
- Cannot do usual activities, or
- Symptoms are same or get worse after 24 hours in Yellow Zone

-Or-

Peak flow: less than _____
(50% of my best peak flow)

Take this Medicine

☐ _____   ☐ 4 or ☐ 6 puffs or ☐ Nebulizer
(short-acting beta$_2$-antagonist)

☐ _____ mg
(oral steroid)

Then call your doctor NOW. Go to the hospital or call for an ambulance if:

✔ You are still in the red zone after 15 minutes AND
✔ You have not reached your doctor

DANGER SIGNS

- **Trouble walking and talking due to shortness of breath**
- **Lips or fingernails are blue**

▷ ✔ Take ☐ 4 or ☐ 6 puffs of your quick-relief medicine AND
✔ Go to the hospital or call for an ambulance (_____) NOW!

WHITE – PATIENT COPY   YELLOW – WORK/SCHOOL COPY   PINK – PROVIDER COPY

FIGURE 31.11 Asthma action plan.

It is important for patients to understand the difference between long-acting maintenance medications and rescue medications and to use them appropriately. Oxygen is generally not necessary because many patients hyperventilate during an acute attack. If the attack is prolonged and the patient becomes cyanotic or Pao$_2$ levels begin to fall, oxygen therapy will be used.

 NURSING CARE TIP

Instruct the patient to contact the HCP if using more than two adrenergic metered dose inhaler canisters per month. This has been associated with an increased risk of death.

Nursing Process for the Patient With Asthma

See the "Nursing Process for the Patient With an Obstructive Disorder" section, following the section on cystic fibrosis in

this chapter. Primary nursing diagnoses include *Impaired Gas Exchange, Ineffective Airway Clearance,* and *Anxiety.* See Table 31.6 for an asthma summary.

Cystic Fibrosis

In the past, cystic fibrosis (CF) was thought to be just a childhood disease because most affected children did not survive past puberty. However, with new treatments, patients with CF are living longer and more productive lives. Some CF patients now marry, have careers, and live well into their 30s.

Pathophysiology

CF is a disorder of the exocrine glands that affects primarily the lungs, GI tract, and sweat glands. The disease varies in severity; some patients have no GI involvement. Abnormal sodium and chloride transport across cell membranes, causing thick, tenacious secretions, is responsible for many of the characteristic symptoms. Thick, sticky respiratory secretions that are difficult to remove cause airway obstruction, resulting in air trapping and frequent respiratory infections.

TABLE 31.6 ASTHMA SUMMARY

Signs and Symptoms	Chest tightness, dyspnea, cough Wheezing
Diagnostic Tests	Spirometry, before and after bronchodilator ABGs in acute attack

Therapeutic Measures	Identification and avoidance of
	    triggers
	Inhaled corticosteroids
	Inhaled bronchodilators
	Oral bronchodilators and steroids if
	    inhaled ineffective

Complications	Status asthmaticus
Priority Nursing Diagnoses	*Impaired Gas Exchange* *Ineffective Airway Clearance* *Anxiety*

Similar abnormalities in the pancreas cause blocked ducts and retained digestive enzymes. These retained enzymes digest and destroy the exocrine pancreas. The absence of digestive enzymes in the intestines causes malabsorption of essential nutrients; frequent foul-smelling, fatty stools; and excess flatus.

Patients with CF secrete sweat that is high in sodium and chloride because these electrolytes are not reabsorbed as they pass through the sweat ducts.

Etiology

CF is a genetic disorder. Both parents must be carriers of the defective gene for CF to be present in a child. Patients with CF who marry are counseled on the risk of potential offspring having the disease.

Signs and Symptoms

Symptoms usually first appear in infancy or childhood, although a few individuals are not diagnosed until adulthood. Respiratory symptoms are often the first visible manifestation of the disease and range from chronic sinusitis to production of thick, tenacious sputum. Patients with CF are at risk for frequent respiratory infections, with coughing and purulent sputum. Finger clubbing is common. Late in the disease, hemoptysis may occur related to damaged blood vessels within the lungs. Over time, bouts of infection become more frequent, with eventual loss of lung function and respiratory failure. Antibiotic-resistant infections are a threat to life in these individuals.

Frequent foul-smelling stools result from the lack of enzymes in the small intestine. Inability to absorb fat-soluble vitamins and poor appetite due to respiratory disease result in malnutrition. Bowel obstruction, cirrhosis, cholecystitis, and cholelithiasis are associated findings. Chronic disease causes delayed sexual maturation in both males and females, and infertility is common.

Complications

Patients with CF are at risk for a variety of complications, including bronchiectasis, pneumothorax, cor pulmonale, and respiratory failure. Bowel obstructions can occur as a result of thick mucus binding with poorly digested fecal matter. Diabetes from pancreatic islet cell involvement may be present late in the disease. Death is usually the result of pulmonary complications, especially antibiotic-resistant infection.

Diagnostic Tests

Because so many different gene mutations can occur in CF, genetic testing may be used to confirm a suspicion of CF but not for screening. Testing can also help prospective parents determine if they are carriers. The standard diagnostic test is the sweat chloride test. If respiratory symptoms are accompanied by excessive amounts of sodium chloride in sweat, CF is diagnosed. You may recall public health campaigns that advise parents to kiss their babies and report any salty taste to their HCPs. Genetic testing can be done on blood samples of newborns who have respiratory symptoms. Chest x-ray and spirometry also may be done.

Therapeutic Measures

Because there is no cure for CF, treatment is aimed at controlling infection and relieving symptoms. Removal of thick sputum is promoted with hydration, use of a vibratory PEP device, chest physiotherapy, or high-frequency chest wall oscillation vest (see Chapter 29) up to four times a day. Regular exercise also helps mobilize secretions; pulmonary rehabilitation may be beneficial. All forms of smoke should be avoided. A hot shower may be an easy occasional alternative to loosen secretions. Nebulized mist treatments using normal or hypertonic saline or mucolytic medications may be used before chest physiotherapy. An inhaled medication called dornase alpha (Pulmozyme) is an enzyme that breaks up and loosens mucous; it has been shown to reduce lung infections and improve lung function. Bronchitol, mentioned earlier in the section on bronchiectasis, is also being studied for CF. Inhaled beta-agonist bronchodilators help keep airways open. Ivacaftor (Kalydeco) is a new oral medication that is being studied to improve the function of a protein that is defective in patients with CF. It is the first drug that will target the underlying cause of CF rather than treat symptoms. High doses of ibuprofen (Motrin) may slow lung deterioration. Breathing exercises, incentive spirometry, and effective coughing techniques such as autogenic drainage (see Chapter 29) are also helpful. Lung transplant is a potentially promising treatment.

Prevention of infection is vital to slowing progression of lung damage. Patients should receive a yearly flu vaccination. Antibiotics must be administered as soon as signs of infection occur. Prophylactic antibiotic therapy may be used. Some patients use inhaled antibiotics for chronic infection; others are on home IV antibiotic therapy. Antibiotic-resistant infections are a deadly threat to the patient with CF. Patients must be vigilant in avoiding others with infections.

Pancreatic enzyme replacement (Pancrease, Viokase) helps reduce symptoms related to malabsorption and improve nutritional status. An increase in calorie requirements necessitates a high-calorie, nutrient-dense diet. For more information, visit the Cystic Fibrosis Foundation at www.cff.org.

Nursing Process for the Patient With Cystic Fibrosis

See the "Nursing Process for the Patient With an Obstructive Disorder" section next. Also, be sure to remember the special needs of the adolescent patient with this chronic, debilitating disease. Not only are normal physical growth and development delayed, but psychosocial development is also affected by repeated hospitalizations and the necessity of routine daily medication and treatments.

CRITICAL THINKING

Mr. Jenkins

■ Mr. Jenkins is a 36-year-old accountant with bronchiectasis secondary to cystic fibrosis. You enter his room during an episode of uncontrollable coughing and offer him support. You observe his sputum as you dispose of it—a whole Styrofoam coffee cup full of thick, bright yellow sputum; the smell makes you nauseated. Even after coughing, his lungs sound congested from retained secretions. You offer him mouth care before you leave his room.

1. What questions can you ask Mr. Jenkins to assess his cough?
2. What nursing diagnosis is most appropriate for Mr. Jenkins?
3. What nursing care can you provide to enhance secretion removal?
4. How would you document this episode of coughing?
5. What other team members can you collaborate with to provide the best care for Mr. Jenkins?

Suggested answers are at the end of the chapter.

 ## NURSING PROCESS FOR THE PATIENT WITH AN OBSTRUCTIVE DISORDER

Data Collection

Perform a complete respiratory assessment as presented in Chapter 29. Frequency of assessment is dictated by the severity of the patient's condition. Note orientation and level of consciousness; poor gas exchange can cause confusion and lethargy. Assess respiratory rate and effort. Observe skin and mucous membranes for cyanosis. Auscultate lungs for adventitious sounds. Monitor cough and the color, viscosity, odor, and amount of sputum. Note exercise tolerance, and have patient report degree of dyspnea on a scale of 0 to 10. Monitor vital signs, oxygen saturation, and arterial blood gases if ordered. Careful documentation of findings allows you to be vigilant for trends in the patient's progress.

Nursing Diagnoses, Planning, and Implementation

A number of nursing diagnoses are appropriate for the patient with an obstructive disorder. As always, choose diagnoses based on defining characteristics and the patient's individual assessment findings.

Priority nursing diagnoses for most chronic respiratory patients include *Impaired Gas Exchange, Ineffective Airway Clearance, Ineffective Breathing Pattern,* and *Activity Intolerance.* Interventions for these diagnoses are presented in the "Nursing Care Plan for the Patient With a Lower Respiratory Tract Disorder." Related diagnoses are discussed next.

Imbalanced Nutrition: Less Than Body Requirements related to poor appetite and increased calorie expenditure as evidenced by weight loss or low weight for height
EXPECTED OUTCOME: *The patient's weight will be stable at desired weight for height.*

• Monitor food intake and weekly weight. *Regular monitoring can help identify nutrition problems before they are severe.*
• If the patient is too dyspneic to eat, schedule rest periods and bronchodilator treatments before meals. *Eating takes a lot of energy, and resting can help conserve energy before a meal. Bronchodilators can reduce dyspnea while eating.*
• Create a pleasant eating environment. *Unpleasant views or odors can spoil an appetite.*
• Provide smaller, more frequent meals of the patient's favorite foods. *Eating a lot at one time can fill up the stomach and reduce room for lung expansion.*
• Encourage family members to bring favorite foods from home for the hospitalized patient. *A large tray of unappetizing food may be more than a patient can handle and may spoil the appetite. Be sure to note sodium or other restrictions; although the patient with end-stage disease may be allowed a more lenient diet, excess sodium can cause fluid retention and increase dyspnea.*
• Consult a dietitian for liquid supplement recommendations. *A specialized supplement such as Pulmocare provides less carbon dioxide than other supplements when metabolized and may be used for patients with chronic respiratory disease.*
• See also "Nutrition Notes—Optimizing Nutrition in Patients With Respiratory Disease."

Nutrition Notes

Optimizing Nutrition in Patients With Respiratory Disease

Malnutrition affects up to 60% of COPD patients and is associated with poor outcomes. Calorie requirements commonly are increased in patients with pulmonary disease. When caloric intake is inadequate, the body begins to break down muscle stores, including the respiratory and GI muscles, which only worsens the problem.

Causes of inadequate food intake can include the following:
- Anorexia
- Shortness of breath
- Fatigue (too tired to eat)
- Pressure from the GI tract impinging on the chest
- Medication side effects

Many patients with COPD have carbon dioxide retention and oxygen depletion. Because fat calories produce less carbon dioxide when metabolized than carbohydrate calories, diets with increased fat and decreased carbohydrate have been suggested, and special supplements for pulmonary patients have been designed and marketed. Energy needs may be 140% of normal and protein needs 150% of normal for maintenance. Nevertheless, it is important not to overfeed the patient. Excess intake can raise the demand for oxygen and the production of carbon dioxide beyond the patient's capacity to manage them.

For the patient with inadequate intake, useful dietary strategies include the following:
- Offer small, frequent feedings of nutrient-dense foods by adding butter, peanut butter, margarine, mayonnaise, sauces, and gravies.
- Select foods that require little or no chewing: eggs, custards, puddings, soups with additional whole milk or powdered milk.
- Include sources of the following vitamins:
  - A (fortified milk, carrots) for healthy epithelial tissue
  - C (citrus fruit, peppers) to prevent infections.
- Discourage gas-producing foods to lessen abdominal pressure on the diaphragm.
- Offer oral nutritional supplements that have shown improved total intake, anthropometric measures, and grip strength in COPD clients (Collins, Stratton, & Elia, 2012).

Nutrition support also improves the likelihood of successful weaning in patients receiving mechanical ventilation.

From Collins, P. F., Stratton, R. J., & Elia, M. (2012). Nutritional support in chronic obstructive pulmonary disease: A systematic review and meta-analysis. *American Journal of Clinical Nutrition, 95*, 1385.

Anxiety related to acute dyspnea as evidenced by statement of anxiety, tense appearance, tremors

EXPECTED OUTCOME: The patient will state that anxiety is controlled; appearance of tension and tremors will be absent. The patient will use techniques to control dyspnea and anxiety when they occur.

- Stay with a patient who is acutely dyspneic and anxious. *Feeling alone during episodes of dyspnea can increase anxiety.*
- Calmly remind the patient to breathe slowly in through the nose and out through pursed lips. *During acute episodes of dyspnea, the patient may forget that breathing exercises can help.*
- Teach relaxation exercises during times when anxiety is minimal, and remind the patient to use them during acute anxiety. *Relaxation exercises can help reduce muscle tension and distract the patient.*
- Administer antianxiety medications as ordered. *Medications can reduce anxiety but can also depress respirations, so should be used with caution.*
- Administer IV morphine (or contact RN to do so). *Morphine helps acute dyspnea and anxiety in patients with end-stage disease.*

Evaluation

If interventions have been effective, the patient will learn techniques to make breathing as comfortable as possible and will be able to cough up secretions and maintain a clear airway. He or she will be able to manage anxiety symptoms and complete ADLs or other desired activity without dyspnea. The patient's intake should be adequate to maintain a stable weight. If any of the patient's goals have not been met, the plan of care should be revised.

Patient Education

The patient must be aware of the contributing factors to the disease and eliminate them if at all possible. The patient who is a smoker should not simply be told to quit smoking; he or she should be referred to a smoking cessation program and be provided with medication, nicotine patches, or other resources and support as necessary to quit (see Chapter 29). Techniques for effective breathing and anxiety control should also be taught. A formal pulmonary rehabilitation program is an excellent resource for patient education.

CRITICAL THINKING

Mr. Franklin

■ Mr. Franklin is admitted to the respiratory unit with exacerbated COPD. He has a history of emphysema and now has an acute infection complicating his disease. His lung sounds are very diminished, and he is short of breath at rest, even on 2 L of oxygen per nasal cannula. You walk into his room when he puts on his call light and find him sitting on the bedside commode with a look of panic in his eyes. He is gasping for breath, his color is gray, and his respiratory rate is 36 per minute.

1. What do you do first? What assessment is appropriate? Whom can you call for assistance?
2. What can you teach Mr. Franklin to prevent an acute dyspneic episode in the future?
3. How will you document this episode?

Suggested answers are at the end of the chapter.

PULMONARY VASCULAR DISORDERS

Pulmonary Embolism

Pathophysiology

An embolism is a foreign object that travels through the bloodstream. It may be a blood clot, air, or fat. A pulmonary embolism (PE), sometimes called a pulmonary thromboembolism (PTE), is usually a blood clot that has traveled into a pulmonary artery (Fig. 31.12). Resulting obstruction of blood flow causes a ventilation-perfusion mismatch, which in this case means that an area of the lung is well ventilated with air but has no blood flow, or perfusion. Because reduced or no blood supply is available to pick up the oxygen in the affected

Pulmonary embolism

FIGURE 31.12 Pulmonary embolism.

portion of the lung, it becomes pulmonary "dead space," causing seriously impaired gas exchange.

Occasionally, damage occurs to a portion of the lung because of lack of oxygen. This is called lung infarction, and it is not common because oxygen is delivered to lung tissue not only from the pulmonary arteries but also via the bronchial arteries and the airways.

Etiology

Most pulmonary emboli originate in the deep veins of the lower extremities (deep venous thrombosis [DVT]). Some risk factors for DVT, and therefore PE, include surgical procedures done under general anesthesia, heart failure, fractures of the lower extremities, immobility, obesity, oral contraceptive use, smoking, and a previous history of DVT or PE. Prolonged immobility on airline flights is also a risk factor. Less common causes of PE include fat emboli from compound fractures, amniotic fluid embolism during labor and delivery, and air embolism from entry of air into the bloodstream.

Prevention

Prevention of thrombi in the deep veins of the legs is the most important factor in the prevention of a PE. Regular ambulation is advised if the patient is able. If a patient is at risk for DVT or PE, such as following surgery or during times of immobility, low-dose subcutaneous heparin or enoxaparin, or oral warfarin (Coumadin) may be used for anticoagulation. Intermittent compression stockings may also be used. If a DVT is diagnosed, prompt treatment is essential to prevent PE.

Signs and Symptoms

The most common symptom of PE is a sudden onset of dyspnea for no apparent reason. The patient may be gasping for breath and appear anxious. Tachycardia, tachypnea, cough, and pleuritic chest pain may be present. Auscultation may reveal crackles or a friction rub. If lung infarction has occurred, hemoptysis may also be present. Some patients have no symptoms at all. Be vigilant for the presence of risk factors and obtain immediate assistance if the cause of dyspnea might be PE. Death can occur if treatment is not fast and effective.

Complications

High blood pressure within the pulmonary circulation (pulmonary hypertension) may result from arterial occlusion and lead to right ventricular failure. This occurs because the right ventricle is unable to push blood into the occluded artery. As a result, the contraction becomes weak, cardiac output falls, and the patient becomes hypotensive.

Diagnostic Tests

A spiral CT scan with contrast dye is noninvasive and can diagnose PE quickly. If this is not available, a lung scan (ventilation-perfusion scan) is done to assess the degree of ventilation of lung tissue and the areas of blood perfusion. If an area is well ventilated but poorly perfused (i.e., a mismatch), PE is suspected.

A pulmonary angiogram is an invasive test that can outline the pulmonary vessels with a radiopaque dye injected via a cardiac catheter. It can show where blood flow is diminished or absent, suggesting an embolism.

Chest x-ray examination, electrocardiogram (ECG), arterial blood gas analysis, or magnetic resonance imaging (MRI) may also be done. However, many of these show changes only in the presence of a very large embolism or infarction.

A D-dimer blood test can be helpful to rule out PE. Results can be obtained in less than an hour. D-dimer is a fibrin fragment that is found in the blood after any thrombus formation. It can be present in a number of disorders, but if it is negative, PE can be eliminated as a possible cause of the patient's symptoms.

Therapeutic Measures

Thrombolytic agents such as alteplase (Activase) or reteplase (Retavase) may be used in life-threatening emergencies to dissolve the clot; heparin is used to prevent new clots from forming. Thrombolytics must be administered within 4 to 6 hours of the clot's occurrence and are associated with risk for hemorrhage.

In patients who cannot tolerate a thrombolytic agent, the clot may be removed with a cardiac catheter, or a surgical embolectomy can be performed. This is a rare procedure that is reserved for emergency situations.

Oxygen is administered even if SpO_2 is normal, because it may help dilate pulmonary vessels. Intubation and mechanical ventilation may be required in some cases.

Long-term use of anticoagulants follows initial treatment to prevent formation of additional clots. Initially, heparin, a potent anticoagulant medication, is administered via continuous IV infusion. Sometimes an intermittent IV or subcutaneous route is used. Clotting studies are monitored and maintained at 1.5 to 2 times the control value. Sometimes heparin therapy is initiated even before a diagnosis of PE is made. It is believed that it is safer to begin therapy and then stop if PE is ruled out than to wait until all test results are available.

An oral anticoagulant is used for at least 3 to 6 months after PE to prevent recurrence. It can also be used for long-term prevention of repeated clots in patients who have risk factors that cannot be resolved. Oral therapy can begin 2 to 3 days after the heparin therapy begins. Because it has a slow onset of action, it may take several days for the full anticoagulant effect to occur. See Chapter 23 for nursing care of patients on anticoagulant therapy.

If clots are a recurring problem, a filter may be placed into the inferior vena cava via the jugular or femoral vein to filter out clots traveling from the lower extremities toward the heart and lungs.

Nursing Process for the Patient With a Pulmonary Embolism

DATA COLLECTION. Assess the patient for respiratory distress, including respiratory rate and effort, cyanosis, confusion, chest pain, and subjective feelings of dyspnea and anxiety.

Auscultate lung sounds. Note sputum color and amount, watching especially for hemoptysis. Monitor ABGs and oxygen saturation. Monitor heart sounds and peripheral edema for signs of heart failure. Contributing factors, such as calf pain, should be noted. Remember, any sudden onset of dyspnea should be taken seriously and reported quickly.

NURSING DIAGNOSES, PLANNING, AND IMPLEMENTATION. The priority nursing diagnosis for a patient with a pulmonary embolism is *Impaired Gas Exchange* (see the "Nursing Care Plan for the Patient With a Lower Respiratory Tract Disorder" for interventions). Because of the impaired perfusion of the affected area of the lung, oxygen and carbon dioxide exchange are limited. Anxiety occurs related to dyspnea. Risk for injury related to anticoagulant therapy is a concern once treatment is initiated (also see Chapter 23).

Risk for Injury (Bleeding) related to anticoagulant therapy
EXPECTED OUTCOME: The patient will remain safe as evidenced by absence of bleeding. The patient will verbalize understanding of self-care measures.

- Monitor coagulation studies and report results to the HCP. *Anticoagulant therapy may be adjusted as often as every 6 hours on the basis of laboratory results.*
- Protect the patient from injury *so that excessive bleeding does not occur.*
- Encourage the patient to wear shoes or slippers when ambulating *to protect from injury.*
- Teach patient to use a soft toothbrush and an electric razor *to prevent injury.*
- Avoid use of intramuscular (IM) injections. *An IM injection can result in hematoma in an anticoagulated patient.*
- Instruct the patient to report any signs of bleeding, such as hematuria or easy bruising. *Bleeding may be associated with excessively prolonged clotting and may require a change in anticoagulant dosing or administration of an antidote.*

EVALUATION. The patient should state that dyspnea and anxiety are resolved and verbalize understanding of anticoagulant therapy and precautions. (See Table 31.7 for a pulmonary embolism summary.)

 CHEST TRAUMA

Pneumothorax

The term **pneumothorax** literally means "air in the chest" and is used to describe conditions in which air has entered the space between the visceral and parietal pleurae. If the pneumothorax occurs without an associated injury, it is called a spontaneous pneumothorax. A secondary spontaneous pneumothorax may occur due to underlying lung disease. Traumatic pneumothorax results from a penetrating chest injury. Iatrogenic (caused by medical treatment) pneumothorax results from complications

---

• WORD • BUILDING •
pneumothorax: pneumo—air + thorax—chest

TABLE **31.7** PULMONARY EMBOLISM SUMMARY

Signs and Symptoms	Sudden-onset dyspnea, tachypnea Chest pain Tachycardia Hemoptysis Crackles History of blood clot
Diagnostic Tests	D-dimer CT scan Ventilation-perfusion lung scan Angiogram
Therapeutic Measures	Thrombolytic therapy Anticoagulants Oxygen
Complications	Pulmonary hypertension
Priority Nursing Diagnoses	*Impaired Gas Exchange* *Anxiety* *Risk for Injury* from anticoagulant therapy

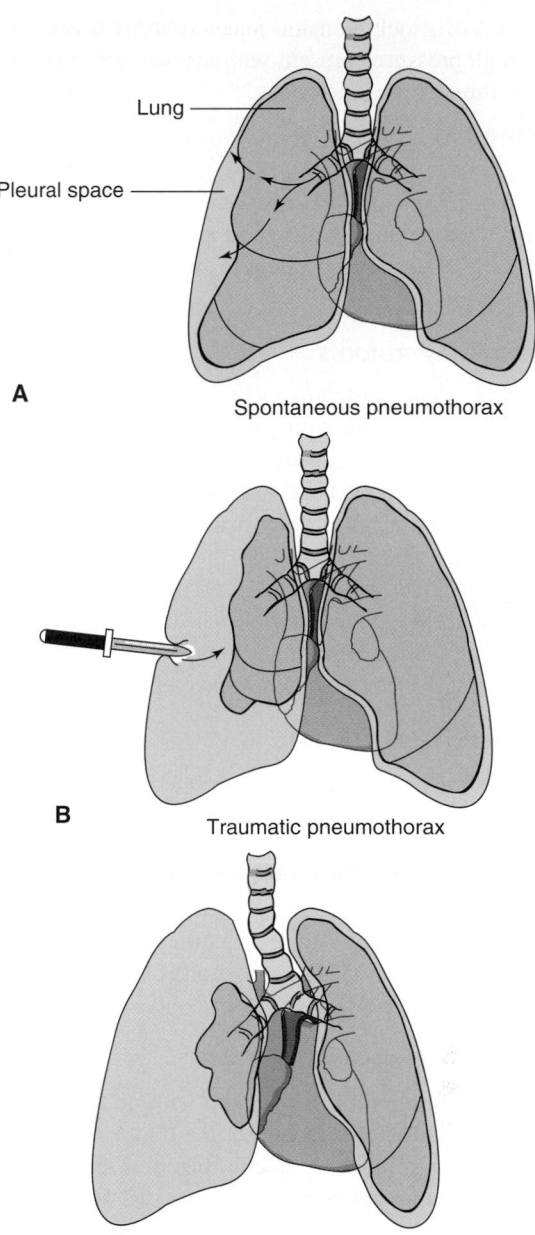

FIGURE 31.13 Types of pneumothorax. (A) Spontaneous pneumothorax. (B) Traumatic pneumothorax. (C) Tension pneumothorax with mediastinal shift.

of hospital procedures such as central line insertion, pleural biopsy, or positive pressure ventilation.

Pathophysiology and Etiology

Recall that the lungs are surrounded by the visceral and parietal pleurae. These membranes are normally separated only by a thin layer of pleural fluid. Each time a breath is taken in, the diaphragm descends, creating negative pressure in the thorax. This negative pressure pulls air into the lungs via the nose and mouth. If either the visceral pleura or the chest wall and parietal pleura are perforated, air will enter the pleural space, negative pressure will be lost, and the lung on the affected side will collapse (Fig. 31.13). Each time the patient takes a breath, the temporary increase in negative pressure will draw more air into the pleural space via the perforation. During exhalation, air may or may not be able to escape through the perforation.

SPONTANEOUS PNEUMOTHORAX. If no injury is present, the pneumothorax is considered spontaneous. This occurs mostly in tall, thin individuals and in smokers. Patients who have had one spontaneous pneumothorax are at greater risk for a recurrence. Patients with underlying lung disease (especially emphysema) may have blister-like defects in lung tissue (called bullae or blebs) that can rupture, allowing air into the pleural space. Weakened lung tissue from lung cancer can also lead to pneumothorax.

TRAUMATIC PNEUMOTHORAX. Penetrating trauma to the chest wall and parietal pleura allows air to enter the pleural space. This can occur as a result of a knife or gunshot wound or from protruding broken ribs.

OPEN PNEUMOTHORAX. If air can enter and escape through the opening in the pleural space, it is considered an open pneumothorax.

CLOSED PNEUMOTHORAX. If air collects in the space and is unable to escape, a closed pneumothorax exists.

TENSION PNEUMOTHORAX. If a pneumothorax is closed, air, and therefore tension, builds up in the pleural space and is unable to escape. As tension increases, pressure is placed on the heart and great vessels, pushing them away from the affected side of the chest. This is called a mediastinal shift. When the heart and vessels are compressed, venous return to the heart is impaired, resulting in reduced cardiac output and symptoms of shock. Tension pneumothorax is often related to the high pressures present with mechanical ventilation. It is a life-threatening emergency.

HEMOTHORAX. The term **hemothorax** refers to the presence of blood in the pleural space. This can occur with or without accompanying pneumothorax (when they occur together it is called a hemopneumothorax) and is often the result of traumatic injury. Other causes include lung cancer, PE, and anticoagulant use.

Signs and Symptoms

Sudden dyspnea, chest pain, tachypnea, tachycardia, restlessness, and anxiety occur with pneumothorax. On examination, asymmetrical chest expansion on inhalation may be noted. Breath sounds may be absent or diminished on the affected side. In a "sucking" chest wound, air can be heard as it enters and leaves the wound.

If tension pneumothorax develops, the patient becomes hypoxemic and hypotensive as well. The trachea may deviate to the unaffected side. Heart sounds may be muffled. Bradycardia and shock occur if emergency intervention is not provided.

Diagnostic Tests

History, physical examination, ultrasound, chest x-ray examination, and CT scan can be used to diagnose pneumothorax. In the emergency department, bedside ultrasound can shorten the time required for diagnosis and intervention and avoid the wait for a chest x-ray to be completed. Chest x-ray examination may be done to monitor the resolution of the pneumothorax after treatment. Arterial blood gases and oxygen saturation are monitored as needed throughout the course of treatment.

Therapeutic Measures

A small pneumothorax may absorb with no treatment other than rest or high-flow oxygen, or the trapped air can be removed with a small-bore needle inserted into the pleural space. Chest tubes connected to a water seal drainage system are used to remove larger amounts of air or blood from the pleural space. See Chapter 29 for complete information about chest drainage. Smaller devices that have special one-way valves to allow air to escape but not reenter the chest may be used for some patients who are treated at home. Some injuries require surgical repair before the pneumothorax can be resolved. Oxygen and positioning help maintain oxygenation.

If the pneumothorax is recurrent, other treatments can be used to prevent additional episodes. Sterile talc or certain antibiotics (such as doxycycline) can be injected into the pleural space via thoracentesis, irritating the pleural membranes and making them stick together. This is called **pleurodesis**, or sclerosis, and prevents recurrent pneumothorax. Pleurodesis is painful; prepare the patient with an analgesic before the procedure.

Nursing Care of the Patient With a Pneumothorax

Nursing care of the hospitalized patient with a pneumothorax involves close monitoring of the condition. Frequent and thorough assessments should be done, including level of consciousness, skin and mucous membrane color, vital signs, oxygen saturation, respiratory rate and depth, and presence of dyspnea, chest pain, restlessness, or anxiety. Regular auscultation of lung sounds provides information about reinflation of the affected lung. Be especially vigilant for signs of increasing or tension pneumothorax, and report them to the HCP immediately. Nursing diagnoses to consider include *Impaired Gas Exchange, Acute Pain,* and *Anxiety.* See Chapter 29 for care of patient with a chest tube and water seal drainage system. See Table 31.8 for a pneumothorax summary.

Rib Fractures
Etiology and Signs and Symptoms

Chest trauma is often accompanied by fractured ribs. Uncontrolled coughing, especially in the presence of osteoporosis or cancer, can also fracture ribs. Falls are a common cause of broken ribs in older people. The fourth through ninth ribs are the most commonly affected. Broken ribs can be painful and often prevent the patient from breathing deeply or coughing effectively, which can result in atelectasis or pneumonia. Displaced ribs can also damage abdominal organs or lung tissue, causing pneumothorax.

Therapeutic Measures

In the past, elastic rib belts were used to stabilize the ribs while healing took place. These are no longer used because it restricts deep breathing. Pain control is the most important treatment.

• WORD • BUILDING •

hemothorax: hem—blood + thorax—chest
pleurodesis: pleur—pleural membrane + desis—binding

TABLE 31.8 PNEUMOTHORAX SUMMARY

Signs and Symptoms	Sudden-onset dyspnea, chest pain, tachypnea Asymmetrical chest expansion Diminished or absent breath sounds on affected side
Diagnostic Tests	Ultrasound Chest x-ray, computed tomography (CT) scan Arterial blood gases (ABGs)
Therapeutic Measures	Chest tube and water seal drainage Pleurodesis for recurrent pneumothorax
Complications	Tension pneumothorax Shock
Priority Nursing Diagnoses	*Impaired Gas Exchange* *Acute Pain* *Anxiety*

Keeping the patient comfortable allows coughing and deep breathing, which in turn prevents complications such as pneumonia and atelectasis. If traditional pain control measures such as NSAIDs or opioids are ineffective, intercostal nerve blocks may be used. Ribs generally heal in about 6 weeks.

Flail Chest

Pathophysiology and Etiology

When multiple ribs are fractured, the structural support of the chest is impaired. As a result, the affected part of the chest collapses with the negative pressure of inhalation and bulges with exhalation. This is called **paradoxical respiration**, which may be ineffective in ventilating the lungs and result in hypoxia.

Signs and Symptoms

The patient with a flail chest exhibits chest movement that is opposite to that usually seen with respiration. The patient is dyspneic and anxious and may also be tachypneic and tachycardic.

Therapeutic Measures

Treatment includes supplemental oxygen and analgesics. Intubation and mechanical ventilation may be necessary but are avoided if possible because of related risk for infection. If lung damage has occurred, treatment for pneumothorax may be needed. Surgical stabilization of the ribs may be done in some cases.

 NURSING PROCESS FOR THE PATIENT WITH CHEST TRAUMA

The following nursing process is based on the stabilized patient. For emergency care of the trauma patient, see Chapter 13.

Data Collection

When caring for the patient following chest trauma, it is important to monitor respiratory status continuously. Be vigilant for any sign of worsening status, such as a change in vital signs, oxygen saturation, or lung sounds; change in respiratory rate; increase in dyspnea, chest pain, pallor, or cyanosis; development of tracheal deviation; or new onset of anxiety or restlessness. Report changes to the HCP immediately. Monitor pain and condition of the chest wound, if present. Additional assessment may be necessary depending on the type of injury sustained.

Nursing Diagnoses, Planning, and Implementation

Priority nursing diagnoses for the patient with chest trauma include *Impaired Gas Exchange, Ineffective Breathing Pattern,* and *Acute Pain.* Additional diagnoses may be appropriate depending on the individual patient's assessment. See the "Nursing Care Plan for the Patient With a Lower Respiratory Tract Disorder" for interventions for *Impaired Gas Exchange* and *Ineffective Breathing Pattern;* see next for *Acute Pain.*

Acute Pain related to chest trauma as evidenced by pain rating

EXPECTED OUTCOME: The patient will state pain is controlled and will be able to cough and deep breathe effectively.

- Administer NSAIDs or opioids as ordered. *Pain must be controlled so the patient is able to breathe deeply and prevent atelectasis and pneumonia.*
- If opioids are used, monitor for depressed respirations and reduced cough reflex. *Depressed respirations and cough increase the risk of atelectasis and pneumonia.*
- Teach the patient to splint the chest with a pillow for coughing. *This may help reduce chest movement and pain during coughing.*

Evaluation

Are pain, anxiety, and dyspnea controlled? Are respiratory rate and SpO$_2$ within normal limits? Are vital signs stable? Frequent evaluation is essential, so that failure to progress can be quickly reported.

 RESPIRATORY FAILURE

Acute Respiratory Failure

Pathophysiology

Acute respiratory failure is diagnosed when the patient is unable to maintain adequate blood gas values. Hypoxemia may result from inadequate ventilation (air movement in and out of lungs) or poor oxygenation (adequate ventilation but inability to get the oxygen into the blood and therefore the cells) or both. Hypercapnia and respiratory acidosis occur when the diseased lungs are unable to effectively eliminate carbon dioxide.

Etiology

An acute respiratory infection in a patient with chronic obstructive disease is often the precipitating factor in acute respiratory failure. Other causes include central nervous system (CNS) disorders that affect the muscles of breathing, such as a stroke, spinal cord injury, or myasthenia gravis; inhalation of toxic substances; opioid overdose; and aspiration.

Prevention

Avoidance of respiratory infections in patients with chronic respiratory disease is important. Instruct patients to notify their HCP immediately if sputum becomes purulent so treatment can be initiated.

Sedatives and narcotics should be used carefully or avoided in patients with chronic respiratory disease because these are respiratory depressants and can precipitate failure. Careful monitoring and early intervention are essential in patients at risk for respiratory failure.

Signs and Symptoms

The patient with impending respiratory failure may become restless, confused, agitated, or sleepy. Arterial blood gases show decreasing PaO_2 and pH and increasing $PaCO_2$, which lead to respiratory acidosis. The patient is cyanotic and dyspneic, and respirations becomes rapid and deep in an effort to blow off excess CO_2.

Diagnostic Tests

Respiratory failure is diagnosed when PaO_2 falls below 60 mm Hg or $PaCO_2$ is elevated above 50 mm Hg. Some patients with chronic respiratory disease have adapted to impaired gas exchange. In these patients a drop in PaO_2 of 10 to 15 mm Hg is considered acute failure. Sputum cultures or chest x-ray examinations may be used to identify underlying respiratory problems. Additional tests may be done to determine nonpulmonary causes and guide treatment. Pulse oximetry is used to continuously monitor oxygen saturation. Patients cared for in ICUs may have additional monitoring, including capnography (Chapter 29).

Therapeutic Measures

Carefully observe the patient and report significant findings to the HCP immediately. It is easy to mistakenly treat symptoms of agitation or confusion with sedatives, which will speed the onset of respiratory failure. Oxygen therapy via nasal cannula or mask is provided. High-flow oxygen may be necessary to oxygenate the patient, but if the patient has a chronically high $PaCO_2$, the high flow can interfere with the hypoxic drive. (Remember the rule "Never give a chronic CO_2 retainer more than 2 liters of oxygen"? This is an exception to the rule.) If a flow rate greater than 1 to 2 L/min is necessary, mechanical ventilation via an endotracheal tube or NIPPV may be required. Before invasive ventilation is undertaken, it is important to check the patient's advance directives.

Antibiotics or other treatments are ordered to correct the underlying cause of the failure. Bronchodilators promote ventilation and secretion removal. Interventions for ineffective airway clearance and impaired gas exchange are initiated. Suctioning is indicated if the patient is unable to cough effectively.

Acute Respiratory Distress Syndrome/ Acute Lung Injury

Acute respiratory distress syndrome (ARDS) is a group of disorders that has diverse causes but similar pathophysiology, symptoms, and treatment.

Pathophysiology and Etiology

ARDS occurs because of acute lung injury (ALI). The most common cause of injury is widespread sepsis. Other causes include pneumonia, trauma, shock, narcotic overdose, inhalation of irritants, burns, pancreatitis, and aspiration. Each of these causes begins a chain of events leading to alveolocapillary damage and noncardiogenic pulmonary edema (pulmonary edema that is not caused by heart failure). ARDS usually affects patients without a previous history of lung disease.

Tired respiratory muscles, in combination with edema and atelectasis, reduce gas exchange and result in hypoxia. As the condition progresses, atelectasis and edema worsen and the lungs may hemorrhage. A chest x-ray examination appears white because of the excessive fluid in the lungs. These changes explain some of the older names for what is now known as ARDS: wet lung, white lung, shock lung, and stiff lung.

Prevention

Early recognition and treatment of underlying disorders is important in prevention of ARDS. Good nursing care can help reduce aspiration and some types of pneumonia.

Signs and Symptoms

The patient presents with dyspnea, tachypnea, and cyanosis. Initial respiratory alkalosis (from tachypnea) develops into acidosis as the patient tires. Fine inspiratory crackles are auscultated. The patient is often confused and lethargic. If ARDS is not reversed, eventually hypoxemia leads to decreased cardiac output, shock, and death.

Complications

Complications that can result from ARDS include heart failure, pneumothorax related to mechanical ventilation, infection, and disseminated intravascular coagulation (DIC). The death rate for ARDS in the past was 100%. With newer treatments, it is now closer to 40%. Most patients who survive ARDS recover completely.

Diagnostic Tests

Diagnosis is made based on history of a causative injury, physical examination, chest x-ray examination, CT scan, and blood gas analysis. An ECG is done to rule out a cardiac-related cause.

Therapeutic Measures

The patient with ARDS is cared for in an ICU. Treatment is supportive and also aimed at the underlying cause. Oxygen therapy is adjusted on the basis of repeated ABG results. Noninvasive positive pressure ventilation or intubation and mechanical ventilation are necessary in most cases, with the use of positive end-expiratory pressure (PEEP) to keep the airways open. Diuretics may be used to reduce pulmonary edema, but care must be taken to prevent fluid depletion. IV fluids are administered if blood pressure or urine output is low. A pulmonary artery catheter may be used to monitor hemodynamic status. If infection or sepsis is the underlying cause, antibiotics are administered. Tube feeding or total parenteral nutrition (TPN) maintain nutritional status while the patient is acutely ill. Positioning the patient with the less involved lung in the dependent position ("good lung down") allows the better lung to be well perfused with blood and may increase PaO_2. Prone positioning has also been shown to increase oxygenation and reduce death rate in patients with ARDS.

Nursing Process for the Patient Experiencing Respiratory Failure
Data Collection

Assess the patient's degree of dyspnea on a scale of 0 to 10 if the patient is able to participate. Monitor respiratory rate and effort, use of accessory muscles, arterial blood gases, and oxygen saturation values. Note the presence of cyanosis.

Monitor mental status, including restlessness, confusion, and level of consciousness, because reduced oxygenation can produce CNS symptoms. Monitor symptoms of the underlying cause of respiratory failure. If the cause is infectious, monitor temperature and WBC counts; if the infection is respiratory in origin, monitor cough and sputum.

All assessment findings should be compared with earlier data. Even subtle changes in the assessment findings can be significant and should be reported.

Nursing Diagnoses, Planning, and Implementation

Priority nursing diagnoses include *Impaired Gas Exchange, Ineffective Airway Clearance,* and *Ineffective Breathing Pattern* (see the "Nursing Care Plan for the Patient With a Lower Respiratory Tract Disorder"). Related diagnoses include *Activity Intolerance, Anxiety, Disturbed Thought Processes,* and *Self-Care Deficit.*

 NURSING CARE TIP

The "good lung down" position can help increase oxygenation in patients with lung disease. Gravity results in more blood in the dependent lung, where it can receive oxygen from the healthier lung tissue. If both lungs are diseased, the right lung down position may be beneficial because the right lung has a larger surface area (Yeaw, 1992).

Evaluation

If interventions have been effective, the patient will state that dyspnea is controlled. Mental status will be at baseline for the patient. Airways will be kept clear at all times, and Spo_2 and respiratory rate will be within normal limits.

 LUNG CANCER

Lung cancer is the leading cause of cancer death in the United States for both men and women. In 2009, the most recent year for which statistics are available, 110,190 men and 95,784 women were diagnosed with lung cancer, an increase from 2005; 87,694 men and 70,387 women died from lung cancer (CDC, 2013c).

Pathophysiology

Lung cancers originate in the respiratory tract epithelium; most originate in the lining of the bronchi (Fig. 31.14). The four major types of lung cancer are identified by the type of cells that are affected: small cell lung cancer (SCLC), large cell carcinoma, adenocarcinoma, and squamous cell carcinoma. The latter three types are classified as non–small cell lung cancer (NSCLC).

About 20% of lung cancers are SCLC (sometimes called oat cell carcinoma). SCLC grows rapidly and often has

FIGURE 31.14 Cross-section of a human lung. The white area in the upper lobe is cancer, the black areas indicate the patient was a smoker. *From the National Cancer Institute, June, 1998.*

metastasized by the time of diagnosis. It is usually caused by smoking and is most often found centrally, near the bronchi. The patient with SCLC has a poor prognosis, with survival time averaging less than 1 year.

The remaining 80% of lung cancers are NSCLC. Large cell carcinoma is a rapidly growing cancer that can occur anywhere in the lungs. It metastasizes early in the disease, so these patients also have a poor prognosis.

Adenocarcinoma occurs more often in women, and most often in the peripheral lung fields. It is slow growing but often is not diagnosed until metastasis has occurred. It is less closely linked with smoking.

Squamous cell carcinoma is the most common form of NSCLC and usually originates in the lining of the bronchi; it metastasizes late in the disease. It is associated with a history of smoking. The prognosis for individuals with squamous cell carcinoma may be better than for some other lung cancers.

Etiology

Tobacco smoke causes 80% to 90% of lung cancers. Cigarettes contain chemicals that cause DNA to mutate, creating changes in cells and development of tumors. If a patient stops smoking, the risk of lung cancer decreases significantly. Unfortunately, even with all this information, 19% of adults in the United States continue to smoke (CDC, 2013d).

Environmental tobacco smoke has also been shown to cause lung cancer. It is estimated that about 3,400 lung cancer deaths, 46,000 heart disease deaths, and 430 sudden infant death syndrome deaths occur each year due to environmental tobacco smoke (National Cancer Institute, 2007). Other factors that contribute to increased lung cancer risk are exposure to asbestos, radon, arsenic, air pollution, diesel exhaust, and radiation. Genetic predisposition and a diet poor in fruits and vegetables may also be factors.

NURSING CARE TIP

Exposure to radon gas, which can be found in homes, is a significant risk factor for lung cancer. Check out www.epa.gov/radon/pubs/citguide.html for more information and to find out if radon is a concern in your area. Many local health departments and hardware stores have inexpensive radon test kits available for purchase.

Prevention

The single most important way to prevent lung cancer is to reduce smoking. Many programs educate school children about the dangers of smoking. Smoking cessation programs are available for people who desire to quit. Contact your local American Cancer Society chapter for smoking cessation programs that can be recommended to patients. See Chapter 29 for more information on smoking cessation.

Signs and Symptoms

Manifestations of lung cancer depend on the location of the tumor. Commonly, patients exhibit a persistent cough with sputum production. The patient may ignore these symptoms because they are also associated with smoking and other chronic respiratory disorders. Repeated respiratory infections may occur, producing thick, purulent sputum. Sputum may become bloody (hemoptysis). The patient may experience dyspnea. If the airway becomes obstructed by the tumor, wheezing or stridor may be heard. Late signs include chest pain, weight loss, anemia, and anorexia.

Complications
Pleural Effusion

Fifty percent of patients with lung cancer develop pleural effusion. Pleural fluid collects in the pleural space as a result of irritation or obstruction of lymphatic or venous drainage by the tumor (see earlier "Pleural Effusion" section).

Superior Vena Cava Syndrome

If the tumor obstructs the superior vena cava, blood flow is interrupted, causing distention of the jugular veins and swelling of the chest, face, and neck. Diuretics may help relieve the fluid buildup. Radiation may be used to shrink the obstruction.

Ectopic Hormone Production

Some lung cancers produce **ectopic** hormones that mimic the body's own hormones. Ectopic production of antidiuretic hormone (ADH) can produce syndrome of inappropriate ADH production (SIADH), which is associated with fluid retention. Ectopic production of adrenocorticotropic hormone (ACTH) can cause Cushing's syndrome. High calcium levels can be caused by ectopic secretion of a parathyroid-like hormone. These disorders are discussed in Chapter 39.

Atelectasis and Pneumonia

Atelectasis occurs when tumor growth prevents ventilation of areas of the lung. Patients with lung cancer also have a greater risk for pneumonia. (See earlier sections on both of these disorders.)

Metastasis

Common sites of lung cancer metastasis include the brain, bones, opposite lung, liver, adrenal gland, and lymph nodes.

Diagnostic Tests

A complete medical history and physical examination are done to look for symptoms and risk factors for lung cancer. A chest x-ray examination is done to identify a mass. However, all tumors may not show up on a radiograph. A CT or positron emission tomography (PET) scan or MRI may be done to provide more specific information about the size and location of a tumor. Sputum is analyzed for abnormal cells. Brain and bone scans are done to find metastatic lesions.

Diagnosis is confirmed with a biopsy of the lesion. A biopsy specimen may be obtained via bronchoscopy, percutaneous biopsy (a needle through the skin guided by radiograph), or mediastinoscopy (placement of an endoscope into the mediastinum to look for changes in mediastinal lymph nodes).

Therapeutic Measures

Tumors are staged based on the tumor-node-metastasis (TNM) staging system. Staging helps determine appropriate treatment (Table 31.9). If NSCLC is localized and in an early stage, it may be cured with surgical removal of the tumor. This can be accomplished with a segmental or wedge resection, which removes only the affected lung segment. A **lobectomy** (removal of a lobe) or removal of an entire lung may be done in more advanced cases (Fig. 31.15). Chemotherapy or radiation may be done alone or in addition to surgery. Patients with Stage IV cancer may opt for using experimental drugs in clinical research trials. Palliative surgery may be done to make a patient more comfortable.

Chemotherapy is the treatment of choice in SCLC, because usually it has metastasized by the time of diagnosis. Radiation may be used in combination with chemotherapy.

• WORD • BUILDING •
ectopic: displaced
lobectomy: lobe—lobe (of lung) + ectomy—excision

TABLE 31.9 STAGES OF LUNG CANCER

Cancer Type	Stage	Characteristics
Non–small cell lung cancer	I	No metastasis to lymph nodes; tumor smaller than 5 cm
	II	Cancer has spread to local lymph nodes or chest wall, or tumor larger than 5 cm
	III	Cancer has invaded chest wall and mediastinum and usually has spread to lymph nodes
	IV	Tumor has metastasized to distant organs and lymph nodes
Small cell lung cancer	Limited	Cancer is limited to one side of the chest
	Extensive	Cancer cells are found outside one side of the chest or in distant sites

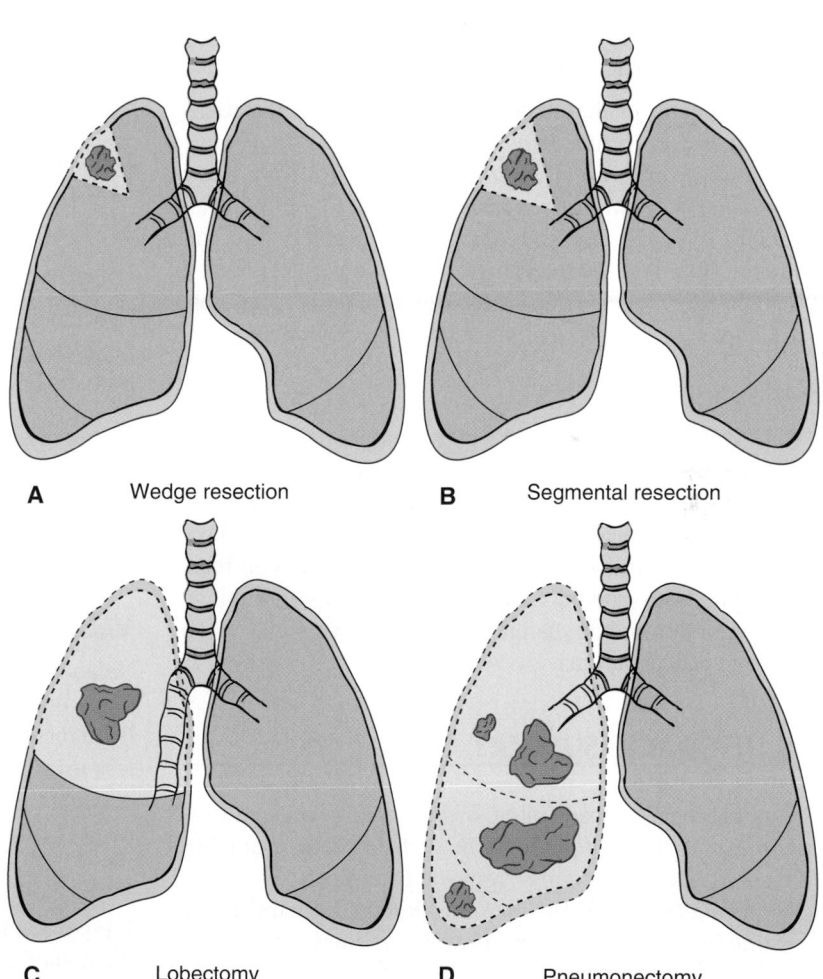

A   Wedge resection

B   Segmental resection

C   Lobectomy

D   Pneumonectomy

FIGURE 31.15 Types of surgeries for lung cancer. (A) Wedge resection. (B) Segmental resection. (C) Lobectomy. (D) Pneumonectomy.

Surgery is not usually indicated in SCLC; the goal of treatment may be palliation of symptoms rather than cure.

Newer therapies for lung cancer include targeted therapies, such as monoclonal antibodies, antiangiogenesis agents, and growth factor inhibitors. Targeted therapies attack the cancer cells and spare normal cells from damage. Vaccines and gene therapy are also being studied to treat lung cancer.

For more information about cancer treatment and nursing care, see Chapter 11. For more on lung cancer, visit the American Cancer Society at www.cancer.org.

NURSING PROCESS FOR THE PATIENT WITH LUNG CANCER

Data Collection

Perform a complete biopsychosocial assessment of the patient with lung cancer. Assess and document respiratory rate and depth, skin and mucous membrane color, lung sounds, oxygen saturation, cough, and sputum amount and character. Ask the patient to rate the degree of pain and dyspnea on appropriate scales. Ask about appetite and weight loss, as well as symptoms of other complications. Note activity tolerance and fatigue.

The patient will likely be grieving about his or her illness and prognosis. Assessment of the patient's coping strategies and support systems will help you plan care for psychosocial needs. The presence of a living will or durable power of attorney and the desire for assistance with end-of-life planning should be noted (see Chapter 17).

Nursing Diagnoses, Planning, and Implementation

Possible diagnoses that may be experienced by the patient with lung cancer include *Impaired Gas Exchange, Ineffective Airway Clearance, Imbalanced Nutrition: Less Than Body Requirements, Pain, Constipation* related to opioid use, *Anticipatory Grieving,* and *Activity Intolerance.* See the "Nursing Care Plan for the Patient With a Lower Respiratory Tract Disorder" for care of patients with respiratory diagnoses. See Chapter 11 for interventions related to cancer diagnoses.

Evaluation

Carefully consider the patient's individual goals when evaluating care. Is the patient comfortable and free from unnecessary dyspnea? Is the airway clear, and is nutrition being maintained? Are medication side effects manageable? Have patients with terminal conditions come to terms with their impending death, and have they been able to do those things most important to them before their death? See Table 31.10 for a lung cancer summary.

THORACIC SURGERY

A surgical incision made into the chest wall is called a **thoracotomy**. A thoracotomy may be performed for a number of reasons, including biopsy; removal of tumors, lesions, or foreign objects; to repair trauma following penetrating or crushing injuries; or to repair or revise structural problems.

Pneumonectomy

A **pneumonectomy** is the surgical removal of a lung. This is usually done to treat lung cancer. It may also be used to treat severe cases of tuberculosis, bronchiectasis, or lung abscesses. Chest drainage is not usually used following a pneumonectomy because once the lung is removed, the air in the thoracic cavity is absorbed, and the cavity fills with serosanguineous fluid. At about 6 months after surgery, the fluid is coagulated, and the thoracic cavity is stabilized.

TABLE 31.10   LUNG CANCER SUMMARY

Signs and Symptoms	Cough, hemoptysis Dyspnea, wheezing Repeat respiratory infections
Diagnostic Tests	Chest x-ray Computed tomography scan Biopsy
Therapeutic Measures	Surgery Chemotherapy Radiation Targeted therapies
Complications	Pleural effusion Superior vena cava syndrome Ectopic hormone production Atelectasis Metastasis
Priority Nursing Diagnoses	*Impaired Gas Exchange* *Ineffective Airway Clearance* *Activity Intolerance*

Lobectomy

Lobectomy is the surgical removal of one lobe. This also may be done for lung cancer, tuberculosis, or another localized problem.

Resection

Resection refers to removal of a smaller amount of lung tissue—that is, less than one lobe. A segmental resection is the removal of one segment of a lobe; a wedge resection is removal of a small wedge of lung tissue (see Fig. 31.15).

Video-Assisted Thorascopic Surgery

Video-assisted thorascopic surgery (VATS) is a newer technique that uses a specialized endoscope to perform surgery. It can be done with two or three small incisions, so is much less invasive than a traditional thoracotomy, which requires opening the chest. It can be used for biopsy, staging, or treatment of tumors.

Lung Transplantation

Lung transplant can benefit patients with a variety of serious pulmonary disorders, including pulmonary hypertension, emphysema, cystic fibrosis, and bronchiectasis. Either a single lung, both lungs, or heart and lungs have been successfully transplanted. Better criteria for selecting patients and donors, as well as advancements in surgical techniques, have improved outcomes for transplant patients.

• WORD • BUILDING •
thoracotomy: thora—chest + otomy—incision
pneumonectomy: pneum—lung + ectomy—excision

NURSING PROCESS FOR THE PATIENT UNDERGOING THORACIC SURGERY

Preoperative Nursing Care

Work with the RN to perform a thorough assessment before surgery, with a focus on the respiratory system. This gives a baseline against which to judge changes postoperatively. Routine preoperative teaching is done by the nurse in collaboration with the health team. The patient should understand that he or she will wake up in an intensive care environment. If at all possible, it is helpful to have the patient and family tour the ICU before the surgery to decrease anxiety postoperatively. Prepare the patient for waking up after surgery with an endotracheal tube connected to a ventilator, oxygen, chest tubes, IV fluids, cardiac monitor, Foley catheter, and possibly an epidural catheter for pain control. Let the patient know he or she will not be able to talk while the ET tube is in, and explain the use of the call light, picture board, or alternate communication techniques. Consult the surgeon for specific plans.

Advise the patient that position changes and early ambulation help prevent complications following surgery. Also instruct the patient in the use of an incentive spirometer and coughing and deep-breathing techniques for after the endotracheal (ET) tube is removed.

Postoperative Nursing Care
Data Collection

Following thoracic surgery, patients initially are in an ICU. Larger hospitals have special ICUs specifically for surgical or thoracic patients, where patients can be closely monitored for complications. Frequent assessment of vital signs and hemodynamic stability; respiratory rate, depth, and effort; and lung sounds is performed. Remember that lung sounds are absent on the side of a pneumonectomy. An increase in pulse rate or a falling blood pressure may indicate internal bleeding and should be reported immediately. Oxygen saturation is monitored continuously. Often patients report an immediate improvement in breathing because the pulmonary blood supply is no longer being routed to diseased lung tissue.

Assessment for tracheal deviation alerts you to the possible complication of mediastinal shift. The trachea is normally positioned straight above the sternal notch. If the trachea deviates from the midline position, the surgeon should be notified immediately. Secretions are monitored and reported to the HCP if they become thick, yellow or green, or foul smelling. ABGs are monitored closely. Chest tubes are usually present (except following pneumonectomy) and are monitored as explained in Chapter 29. Pain is assessed using a pain rating scale, and incision sites are monitored for redness, edema, or drainage. If the patient is mechanically ventilated, additional assessment of the endotracheal tube and ventilator settings will be needed.

Nursing Diagnoses, Planning, and Implementation

See the "Nursing Care Plan for the Patient With a Lower Respiratory Tract Disorder" for basic interventions. Following are some additional interventions specific to the patient following thoracic surgery.

Ineffective Airway Clearance related to presence of ventilator, inability to cough, and sedation, as evidenced by presence of crackles and wheezes, and high-pressure ventilator alarm

EXPECTED OUTCOME: The patient will have a clear airway as evidenced by clear lung sounds and by absence of airway noise and high-pressure ventilator alarms.

- Suction according to agency policy. *The airway must remain free of secretions to prevent ventilator-associated pneumonia and dyspnea.*
- Once extubated, remind the patient to cough and deep breathe regularly. *This helps clear the airway.*
- Administer analgesics as ordered. *Postoperative pain must be controlled for the patient to be able to cough effectively.*

Impaired Gas Exchange related to surgical intervention, opioid use, and removal of lung tissue, as evidenced by ABGs and by SpO$_2$ not within normal limits

EXPECTED OUTCOME: The patient's gas exchange will be within acceptable limits as evidenced by SpO$_2$ of 90% or above.

- Monitor SpO$_2$. *Interventions should maintain SpO$_2$ at 90% or above.*
- Reposition patient every 1 to 2 hours. Consult surgeon for specific positioning orders. *Some surgeons want patients positioned with the operative side up, others with the operative side down. Fowler's position allows room for lung expansion and helps prevent aspiration.*
- Encourage use of an incentive spirometer as ordered following extubation *to encourage the patient to deep breathe and maximize oxygenation.*
- Monitor chest tube and water seal drainage system, if used. *This helps reexpand the lung and must remain intact at all times.*
- Administer oxygen and bronchodilators as ordered *to maintain oxygenation.*

Acute Pain related to surgical procedure as evidenced by pain rating

EXPECTED OUTCOME: The patient will be comfortable as evidenced by statement or indication that pain is controlled. If unable to communicate, objective signs of acute pain (increase in vital signs, restlessness) will be absent.

- Administer analgesics as ordered, around the clock. *Pain control is important for the patient to be able to ambulate and deep breathe and cough effectively.*
- Monitor respiratory rate and effort if not mechanically ventilated. *Opioids depress respirations.*
- Teach the patient to splint the incision while coughing. *This can stabilize the site and reduce pain, increasing the likelihood of effective coughing.*

Impaired Physical Mobility related to discomfort at surgical site as evidenced by inability or unwillingness to move

EXPECTED OUTCOME: The patient will maintain mobility as evidenced by ability to move arm and shoulder through range-of-motion exercises.

• Perform range-of-motion exercises, passively at first, then actively when the patient is able. *This helps prevent contracture of the arm and shoulder on the affected side.*

• Assist the patient to ambulate as tolerated on first or second postoperative day as ordered. *Ambulation helps maintain mobility and prevent postoperative complications.*

Risk for Infection related to intubation, Foley catheterization, surgical incision, and major surgery

EXPECTED OUTCOME: The patient will be free of signs of infection as evidenced by clean and dry incision, temperature and WBC count within normal limits, clear sputum, and clear urine.

• Monitor temperature, WBC count, incision, sputum, and urine for signs of infection *so infection can be identified and treated quickly.*

• Use standard infection control precautions, including careful hand hygiene, *because the patient is at increased risk for infection.*

• Use meticulous sterile technique for all invasive procedures: suctioning, dressing changes, catheter insertion. *This prevents introduction of pathogens.*

• Monitor nutritional intake. Consult dietitian for recommendations. *Adequate nutrients are essential for wound healing and immune function.*

• Maintain head of bed at minimum 30 degrees elevation *to help prevent aspiration of gastric contents.*

• Provide frequent oral care *to reduce risk of aspiration of oral bacteria.*

• Assist with ventilator weaning and extubation as soon as possible. *Mechanical ventilation is associated with increased risk of pneumonia.*

• Request order to remove Foley catheter as soon as possible. *Foley catheter insertion is associated with risk of urinary tract infection (UTI).*

Evaluation

The patient's airway should remain clear, and secretions should be easily coughed up. The patient should report an acceptable comfort level and be able to cough, deep breathe, and ambulate without excessive discomfort. The patient's breathing should be unlabored, with a respiratory rate of 12 to 20 per minute. The patient's affected arm and shoulder should maintain full range of motion. Urine should be clear. Signs of infection should be absent.

Home Health Hints

• When a patient is using oxygen by nasal cannula, the area around the ears can become irritated or excoriated. A small sponge-type hair roller can be placed around the tubing to protect the ears. Avoid using gauze for this purpose. It can be abrasive and worsen the problem.

• When a home health patient has a metered-dose inhaler, the nurse should not assume he or she is using it correctly. The patient should be observed using it.

• When a patient requires more than one metered-dose inhaler, number the canisters in the order they are to be used.

• Read inhaler package inserts to find how many puffs are in an inhaler, and help the patient devise a system for keeping track of how many puffs are used so he does not run out. Manufacturers no longer recommend seeing if canisters float or sink in water to determine if they are empty because this method can be unreliable.

• To help the COPD patient conserve energy, he or she can be encouraged to sit on a stool when cooking at the stove or doing dishes. A shower stool can be obtained from a medical supply store. Personal care activities should be spaced throughout the day.

• Support bars, also obtained from a medical supply store, can be strategically placed in the shower area, on the walls along hallways, and in a passageway to the restroom. This can help the patient ambulate when fatigued and also help prevent falls.

• If the COPD patient is tempted to adjust his or her own oxygen flow rate, equipment suppliers can put on a locking flowmeter. Increasing the flow rate can reduce hypoxic drive and cause hypoventilation.

• Nebulizer parts should be cleaned at least three times a week, using warm water and a common home disinfectant solution for 30 minutes.

• When in the home, it is important not only to assess your patient but also the primary caregiver. Many times he or she is experiencing caregiver role strain. Discuss options available and consider having a social worker consulted to assist with counseling and community resources. Contact the HCP to discuss your concerns and ideas.

SUGGESTED ANSWERS TO

CRITICAL THINKING

■ *Mr. Smith*

1. A complete respiratory history is taken as described in Chapter 29. An open-ended question such as, "What happened to bring you to the hospital?" elicits information about the incident. In addition, questions to determine mental status and ability to make decisions and function safely on his own are appropriate. If any concerns arise, a social service consultation will be helpful for discharge planning.

2. Mr. Smith should be instructed to always read label warnings before using any cleaning products in the future and to never mix bleach and ammonia!

3. Monitor Mr. Smith closely for signs or symptoms of bacterial pneumonia. Assist with good mouth care, and maintain careful hand-washing and infection-control practices. Discourage ill visitors.

■ *Mr. Woo*

1. Document exactly what you see: "No redness or induration at either the PPD or *Candida* test sites." Date and time your entry, and sign.

2. Everyone has been exposed to, and should react to, *Candida* with some degree of redness and induration. The fact that Mr. Woo has no reaction at all may mean that his immune system is not working well—he is "anergic." Therefore, the fact that his PPD test shows no redness and swelling could just be because of his anergy even though he may be infected with TB. So this is an unreliable test for him. Mr. Woo will need a chest x-ray and a sputum culture to be sure he is not infected.

■ *Mr. Jenkins*

1. Ask questions based on the **WHAT'S UP?** format:

   Where (not applicable)

   How does it feel? Does the coughing cause chest pain? Are you short of breath?

   Aggravating and alleviating factors. What makes the cough worse? What seems to help? Do you use any techniques at home that are helpful?

   Timing. How often do you cough during a day? Is it interfering with sleep and rest?

   Severity. How bad is it on a scale of 0 to 10? How much sputum are you coughing up? Is it usually this color?

   Useful other data. Are you experiencing any other symptoms with your cough (such as shortness of breath, nausea, loss of appetite)?

   Patient's perception. Is it better or worse than usual today? How can I help? (The patient with long-standing disease often knows what will help but is hesitant to ask.)

2. The most appropriate nursing diagnosis is *Ineffective Airway Clearance* related to excessive secretions and ineffective cough.

   Provide hydration with oral liquids and a room humidifier to liquefy secretions. Administer expectorants as ordered. Instruct the patient in coughing and deep-breathing exercises such as autogenic drainage to increase the effectiveness of his cough. Provide good oral care following expectoration of sputum to freshen the patient's mouth. Obtain an order for chest physiotherapy or a vibratory PEP device (Chapter 29) to help loosen and drain secretions.

3. "Patient expectorated 200 mL of bright yellow, foul-smelling sputum. Lungs have scattered crackles and wheezes throughout after coughing episode. Expectorant given; fluids encouraged. Mouth care provided."

4. Respiratory therapy should be involved with nebulized mist treatments and assistance with airway clearance interventions. Occupational or physical therapy can help with mobilization and increasing exercise tolerance. Discharge planning may be needed to help set up home therapies. Social work or pastoral care can help with emotional distress related to having a chronic disease.

■ *Mr. Franklin*

1. You need to do several things at once. You will begin by speaking in a calm voice and trying to help Mr. Franklin to calm himself by doing pursed-lip breathing. Assure him that you will help him and won't leave. At the same time, check his oxygen to make sure it is on the ordered number of liters and that his tubing is not kinked or disconnected. Grab the bedside table for him to lean on. Call for someone to page a respiratory therapist to do a nebulized mist treatment if ordered. Have someone bring a pulse oximeter to check his oxygen saturation. Also call for the RN to administer IV morphine if ordered. All this should take about 1 minute! Once Mr. Franklin is a bit calmer, you can find out what happened. Did the exertion of moving to the bedside commode cause his dyspnea? Check his vital signs and lung sounds, and work with the RN to determine if this represents a change in Mr. Franklin's condition that should be reported to the HCP.

2. Teach Mr. Franklin that he should probably stay on bedrest until his acute exacerbation is resolved. Once he is able to start moving around, he should call for help to get up. Review his controlled breathing exercises, which he can use during movement, and encourage rest between activities.

Continued

SUGGESTED ANSWERS TO—cont'd

3. "3:00: Patient up on bedside commode (BSC), respiratory rate (RR0 36 per minute and labored, color gray, appeared very apprehensive. O_2 on at 2 L per min per nasal cannula (NC), assisted to lean on over-bed table. Encouraged pursed-lip breathing. Vital signs (VS) 146/64 mm Hg, 102 beats per minute, 36 per minute, SpO_2 82%. RT paged; administered as needed (prn) NMT. Breath sounds diminished, no cough. At 3:15, patient appears much calmer, RR 24 per minute and less labored, SpO_2 90%."

REVIEW QUESTIONS

1. A patient asks the nurse why he doesn't feel sick even though his TB test is positive. The nurse knows the patient has been diagnosed with LTBI. Which explanation is best to provide the patient?
   1. "TB often does not make people feel sick, but it is contagious nevertheless."
   2. "You have latent disease, which just stays in your system but won't ever make you sick."
   3. "You have TB infection, but not active disease. As long as your immune system stays strong, it can keep the infection from making you sick."
   4. "Even though you do not feel sick, the positive test shows that you have the disease and must be treated."

2. Which of the following assessment findings does the nurse expect in the patient with emphysema?
   1. Purulent sputum
   2. Diminished breath sounds
   3. Generalized edema
   4. Dull chest pain

3. A patient with shortness of breath is being tested for lung cancer. Which diagnostic test will be most conclusive?
   1. Chest x-ray
   2. MRI
   3. Sputum culture
   4. Biopsy

4. A patient with recurrent pneumothorax is scheduled to have pleurodesis done in 1 hour. Which nursing intervention should take priority at this time?
   1. Encourage fluids.
   2. Encourage coughing and deep breathing.
   3. Administer a prn analgesic as ordered.
   4. Administer a prn bronchodilator as ordered.

5. Which of the following assessment findings in the patient with pneumonia most indicates a need to remind the patient to cough and deep breathe?
   1. The patient reports chest pain.
   2. The patient has removed her oxygen.
   3. The patient develops coarse wheezes and crackles.
   4. The patient has a fever of 101°F (38.3°C).

6. A patient is admitted to the hospital with shortness of breath. The nurse notes increasing confusion and combativeness during the past hour. Which of the following actions is appropriate first?
   1. Assess SpO_2 and apply oxygen per protocol if indicated.
   2. Page the physician stat.
   3. Put up the patient's side rails and apply soft restraints.
   4. Administer a prn dose of intramuscular sedative.

7. Which of the following interventions is most appropriate for the patient with an ineffective breathing pattern?
   1. Encourage the patient to cough and deep breathe.
   2. Teach the patient controlled diaphragmatic breathing.
   3. Encourage oral fluids.
   4. Allow the patient to rest between activities.

8. A patient with end-stage COPD has a nursing diagnosis of *Impaired Gas Exchange.* Which assessment finding shows that interventions have been effective?
   1. The patient's SpO_2 is 92% on 2 L of oxygen.
   2. The patient appears comfortable.
   3. The patient is coughing up copious white sputum.
   4. The patient is able to move in bed without difficulty.

Answers can be found in Appendix C.

References

Centers for Disease Control and Prevention. (2013a). *2013 vaccine recommendations.* Retrieved June 25, 2013, from www.cdc.gov/features/adultvaccines

Centers for Disease Control and Prevention. (2013b). Asthma. Updated May 30, 2013. Retrieved June 25, 2013, from www.cdc.gov/nchs/fastats/asthma.htm

Centers for Disease Control and Prevention. (2013c). *Lung cancer statistics.* Retrieved June 26, 2013, from www.cdc.gov/cancer/lung/statistics

Centers for Disease Control and Prevention. (2013d). *Current cigarette smoking among adults—United States, 2011.* Retrieved June 26, 2013, from www.cdc.gov/mmwr/preview/mmwrhtml/mm6144a2.htm

Chalmers, J. D., McHugh, B. J., Docherty, C., Govan, J. R. W., & Hill, A. T. (2013). Vitamin-D deficiency is associated with chronic bacterial colonisation and disease severity in bronchiectasis. *Thorax, 68,* 39–47.

Galbraith, S., Fagan, P., Perkins, P., Lynch, A., & Booth, S. (2010). Does the use of a handheld fan improve chronic dyspnea? A randomized, controlled, crossover trial. *Journal of Pain Symptom Management, 39,* 831–838.

Global Initiative for Chronic Obstructive Lung Disease. (2013). Global strategy for the diagnosis, management, and prevention of chronic obstructive pulmonary disease. Retrieved June 22, 2013, from www.goldcopd.org/guidelines-global-strategy-for-diagnosis-management.html

Joint Commission. (2013). *2014 National Patient Safety Goals.* Retrieved June 20, 2013, from www.jointcommission.org/assets/1/18/NPSG_Chapter_Jan2013_HAP.pdf

National Cancer Institute. (2007). Cancer trends progress report—2007 update. Retrieved June 26, 2013, from http://progressreport.cancer.gov/2007/index.asp

National Heart, Lung, and Blood Institute. (n.d.). *Take the first step to breathing better. Learn more about COPD.* Retrieved June 22, 2013, from www.nhlbi.nih.gov/health/public/lung/copd/index.htm

Wong, C., Jayaram, L., Karalus, N., Eaton, T., Tong, C., Hockey, H., . . . Ashton, T. (2012). Azithromycin for prevention of exacerbations in non-cystic fibrosis bronchiectasis (EMBRACE): A randomised, double-blind, placebo-controlled trial. *The Lancet, 380,* 660–667.

World Health Organization. (2013). *Tuberculosis.* Retrieved June 22, 2013, from www.who.int/mediacentre/factsheets/fs104/en

Yeaw, E. (1992). How position affects oxygenation: Good lung down? *American Journal of Nursing, 92,* 26.

 DavisPlus | For additional resources and information visit **davispl.us/medsurg5**

unit EIGHT

Understanding the Gastrointestinal, Hepatic, and Pancreatic Systems

32

Gastrointestinal, Hepatobiliary, and Pancreatic Systems Function, Assessment, and Therapeutic Measures

KEY TERMS

basal cell secretion test (BAY-zuhl SELL seh-KREE-shun TEST)
bowel sounds (bough-UL SOWNDS)
caput medusa (KAP-ut meh-DOO-see)
carcinoembryonic antigen (KAR-sin-oh-EM-bree-aw-nick AN-tih-jen)
colonoscopy (KOH-lun-AW-skuh-pee)
endoscopy (EN-daw-skuh-pee)
esophagogastroduodenoscopy (ee-SOFF-ah-go-GAS-troh-doo-AW-den-AW-skuh-pee)
esophagoscopy (ee-SOFF-ah-GAW-skuh-pee)
fluoroscope (FLOOR-oh-skohp)
gastric acid stimulation test (GAS-trick AS-id STIM-yoo-LAY-shun TEST)
gastric analysis (GAS-trick ah-NAL-ih-siss)
gastroscopy (gas-STRAW-skuh-pee)
gastrostomy (gas-STRAW-stoh-mee)
gavage (gah-VAZH)
icterus (ICK-tur-us)
impaction (im-PACK-shun)
jaundice (JAWN-diss)
lavage (lah-VAZH)
lower gastrointestinal series (LOH-er GAS-troh-in-TESS-tih-null SEER-ees)
occult blood (uh-KULT BLUHD)
peripheral parenteral nutrition (puh-RIFF-uh-ruhl par-EN-teh-ruhl new-TRISH-un)
peristalsis (pear-ih-STALL-sis)
proctosigmoidoscopy (PROCK-toh-SIG-moy-DAWS-kuh-pee)
retrograde cholangiopancreatography (RET-roh-grayd koh-LAN-jee-oh-PAN-kree-ah-TOG-rah-fee)
spider angioma (SPY-der AN-jee-OH-mah)
steatorrhea (STEE-ah-toh-REE-ah)
striae (STREYE-ee)
upper gastrointestinal series (UH-pur GAS-troh-in-TES-tih-nuhl SEER-ees)

LAZETTE V. NOWICKI, LINDA S. WILLIAMS, AND JANICE L. BRADFORD

LEARNING OUTCOMES

1. List the structures of the gastrointestinal tract and of the accessory glands: liver, gallbladder, and pancreas.
2. Describe the functions of each organ of the gastrointestinal tract and of the accessory glands: liver, gallbladder, and pancreas.
3. Discuss how age affects the gastrointestinal tract and accessory glands.
4. List data to collect when caring for a patient with a disorder of the gastrointestinal system, liver, gallbladder, or pancreas.
5. Differentiate normal and abnormal data collection findings.
6. Explain techniques used to conduct a physical examination of the abdomen.
7. Plan nursing care for patients having diagnostic tests of the gastrointestinal tract.
8. Explain types of nasogastric tubes and their uses.
9. Plan nursing care for insertion and maintenance of nasogastric tubes.
10. Describe therapeutic measures used for patients with gastrointestinal diseases.

NORMAL GASTROINTESTINAL, HEPATOBILIARY, AND PANCREATIC SYSTEMS ANATOMY AND PHYSIOLOGY

The gastrointestinal (GI) tract (or alimentary tract) is part of the digestive system (Fig. 32.1). Digestion begins in the oral cavity and continues in the stomach and small intestine. Most absorption of nutrients takes place in the small intestine. The large intestine is where the majority of water is reabsorbed. Indigestible material, mainly cellulose, is then eliminated from the large intestine. Accessory organs include teeth, tongue, salivary glands, liver, gall bladder, and pancreas.

Oral Cavity and Pharynx

The boundaries of the oral cavity are the hard and soft palates superiorly, the cheeks laterally, and the floor of the mouth inferiorly. Within the oral cavity are the teeth, tongue, and the openings of the ducts of the salivary glands.

The teeth begin mechanical digestion to create more surface area for the chemical digestion regulated by enzymes. The roots of the teeth are in sockets in the mandible and maxillae. The tongue is made of skeletal muscle innervated by the hypoglossal nerve. Taste buds surround the base of each papilla. Innervation for tasting is by the facial, glossopharyngeal, and vagus nerves. Elevation of the tongue is the first step in swallowing.

The three pairs of salivary glands are the parotid, submandibular, and sublingual glands. Their ducts secrete saliva to the oral cavity. Salivation is a parasympathetic response mediated by the facial and glossopharyngeal nerves. Saliva is mostly water, which is used to dissolve food for gustation and moisten the food for swallowing. The only digestive enzyme in saliva that functions in the mouth is amylase, which digests starch to maltose. However, food does not remain in the mouth long enough for significant starch digestion. There is also lingual lipase, however, which when activated by acidic pH begins its action in the stomach.

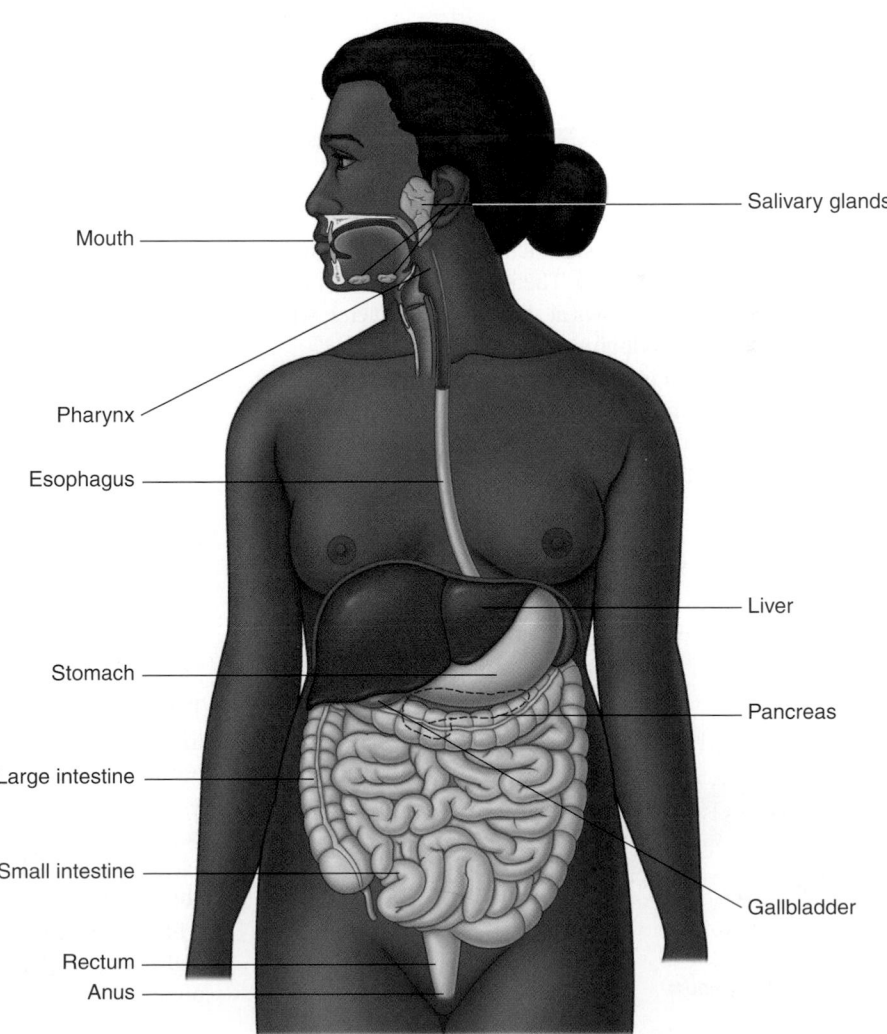

FIGURE 32.1 Digestive system. From Thompson, G. S. (2013). *Understanding anatomy and physiology.* Philadelphia: F.A. Davis, p. 377.

Mouth

Salivary glands

Pharynx

Esophagus

Liver

Stomach

Pancreas

Large intestine

Small intestine

Gallbladder

Rectum

Anus

The pharynx is a muscular tube connecting the oral cavity to the esophagus. When a mass of food is pushed posteriorly by the tongue, the smooth muscles of the pharynx contract as part of the swallowing reflex. This reflex is regulated by the medulla and pons. The uvula closes off the nasopharynx while the epiglottis closes the opening to the larynx.

Esophagus

The esophagus is about 10 inches long and carries ingested items from the pharynx to the stomach. No digestion takes place in the esophagus. **Peristalsis** of the muscle layer in the wall of the esophagus propels food inferiorly to the stomach. At the junction with the stomach, the lumen of the esophagus is surrounded by the lower esophageal sphincter (LES; also cardiac sphincter, gastroesophageal sphincter, or esophageal sphincter), a circular smooth muscle. The LES relaxes to permit food to enter the stomach and then contracts to prevent the backflow of stomach contents. The esophagus penetrates the diaphragm at the esophageal hiatus. The remainder of the digestive system is within the abdominopelvic cavity.

Stomach

The stomach is in the upper left abdominal quadrant, to the left of the liver and in front of the spleen. It is a J-shaped, saclike organ that extends from the esophagus to the duodenum of the small intestine. Some digestion takes place in the stomach; it mainly serves as a reservoir for food so that digestion may take place gradually.

The four regions of the stomach are the cardia, fundus, body, and pylorus (Fig. 32. 2). The pylorus is divided into an antrum and canal and narrows at the pyloric sphincter, which guards entry to the duodenum.

When the stomach is empty, the mucosa (inner lining) has folds called rugae that permit expansion of the lining. The mucosa contains gastric pits with glands of the stomach that produce gastric juice.

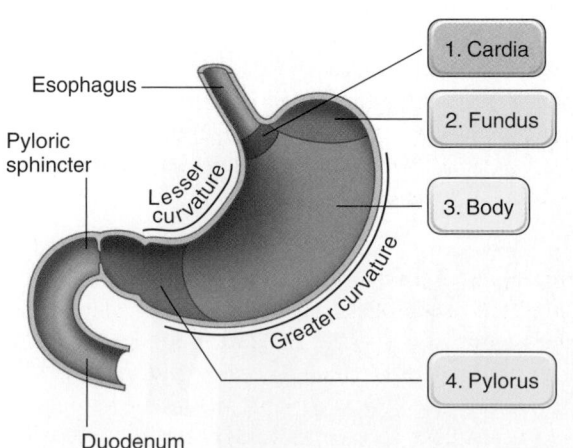

FIGURE 32.2 Parts of the stomach. From Thompson, G. S. (2013). *Understanding anatomy and physiology*. Philadelphia: F.A. Davis, p. 383.

Gastric juice begins secretion at the sight or smell of food; this is a parasympathetic response. The presence of food in the stomach stimulates the secretion of the hormone gastrin by the gastric mucosa. Gastrin increases the secretion of gastric juice.

The three layers of smooth muscle in the stomach wall achieve efficient mechanical digestion, changing ingested food to a thick liquid called chyme. The pyloric sphincter contracts when the stomach is churning food and relaxes at intervals to allow small amounts of chyme to pass into the duodenum. Carbohydrates are most readily digested by the stomach, followed by proteins and fats.

Small Intestine

The small intestine is about 1 inch in diameter and approximately 20 feet long. Within the peritoneal cavity, the coils of the small intestine are encircled by the colon. The small intestine extends from the stomach to the cecum of the colon. The duodenum is the first 10 inches and contains the hepatopancreatic ampulla (ampulla of Vater), the entrance of the common bile duct and the pancreatic duct. The jejunum is about 8 feet long; the ileum is about 11 feet in length.

Digestion is completed in the small intestine, and the end products of digestion are absorbed into the blood and lymph. Bile from the liver and enzymes from the pancreas function in the small intestine (Table 32.1). When chyme enters the duodenum, the intestinal mucosa produces the enzymes sucrase, maltase, and lactase, which complete the digestion of disaccharides to monosaccharides; the peptidases, which complete the digestion of proteins to amino acids; and the nucleosidases and phosphatases, completing nucleotide digestion.

The absorption of nutrients requires a large surface area; the small intestine has extensive folds for this purpose. Macroscopic circular folds and microscopic villi with apical border microvilli greatly expand the absorptive surface. Water-soluble nutrients (monosaccharides, amino acids, minerals, water-soluble vitamins) are absorbed into the blood in the capillary networks. Fat-soluble vitamins and fatty acids and glycerol are absorbed into the chyle of the lacteals.

Large Intestine

The large intestine extends from the ileum of the small intestine to the anus. It is about 5 feet long and 2.5 inches in diameter. No further digestion takes place in the colon; it temporarily stores and then eliminates indigestible material. The mucosa absorbs significant amounts of water and minerals, as well as the vitamins produced by the normal bacterial flora.

Elimination of feces is accomplished by involuntary and voluntary actions. Parasympathetic control initiates the defecation reflex, from centers in the sacral region of the spinal cord. Baroreceptor input produces returning motor impulses, which cause contraction of the smooth muscle of the rectum and relaxation of the internal anal sphincter. Voiding is voluntarily controlled via actions of the external anal sphincter.

• **WORD** • **BUILDING** •
peristalsis: peri—around + stellein—to place

TABLE 32.1 **DIGESTIVE SECRETIONS**

Organ	Enzyme or Other Secretion	Function	Site of Action
Salivary glands	Amylase	Converts starch to maltose	Oral cavity
Stomach	Pepsin Hydrochloric acid	Converts proteins to polypeptides Changes pepsinogen to pepsin Maintains pH of 1–2 Destroys pathogens	Stomach
Liver	Bile salts	Emulsify fats	Small intestine
Pancreas	Amylase Lipase Trypsin	Converts starch to maltose Converts emulsified fats to fatty acids and glycerol Converts polypeptides to peptides	Small intestine
Small intestine	Peptidases Sucrase, maltase, lactase	Convert peptides to amino acids Convert disaccharides to monosaccharides	Small intestine

Liver

The liver occupies the right side and center of the upper abdominal cavity just below the diaphragm. Its right lobe is larger than the left lobe.

The blood supply of the liver differs from that of other organs. The liver receives oxygenated blood by way of the hepatic artery. By way of the hepatic portal vein, blood from the abdominal digestive organs and the spleen is brought to the liver before being returned to the heart. This special pathway is called hepatic portal circulation and permits the liver to regulate blood levels of nutrients or to remove potentially toxic substances such as alcohol from the blood before the blood circulates to the rest of the body. All blood leaving the liver exits via the hepatic vein.

The only digestive function of the liver is the production of bile by the hepatocytes. Bile flows to the duodenum via ducts from either the liver or gall bladder (Fig. 32.3).

Bile is mostly water and bile salts. Its excretory function is to carry bilirubin and excess cholesterol to the intestines for elimination in feces. The digestive function of bile is accomplished via bile salts, which emulsify fats in the small intestine. Emulsification is a type of mechanical digestion in which large fat globules are broken into smaller globules producing greater surface area for chemical catabolism. Secretion of bile is stimulated by the hormone secretin and ejection of bile from the gallbladder is stimulated by cholecystokinin.

Functions of the Liver

The liver is involved in a great variety of functions, most of which involve organic molecule metabolism. These functions can be grouped into categories.

CARBOHYDRATE METABOLISM. The liver regulates the blood glucose level by storing excess glucose as glycogen and performing glycogenolysis when the blood glucose level is low. The liver also changes other monosaccharides to glucose, which is more readily used by cells for energy production.

AMINO ACID METABOLISM. The liver regulates the blood levels of amino acids based on tissue needs for protein synthesis. Of the 20 amino acids needed for the production of human proteins, the liver is able to synthesize 12, called the nonessential amino acids, by the process of transamination. The other 8 amino acids, which the liver cannot synthesize, are called the essential amino acids. Essential amino acids are required in the diet.

Excess amino acids (those not needed for protein synthesis) undergo the process of deamination in the liver; the amino group is removed, and the remaining carbon chain is converted to a simple carbohydrate that is used for energy production or converted to fat for energy storage. The amino groups are converted to urea, a nitrogenous waste product that is removed from the blood by the kidneys and excreted in urine.

LIPID METABOLISM. The liver forms lipoproteins for the transport of lipids in the blood to other tissues. The liver also synthesizes cholesterol and excretes excess cholesterol into bile to be eliminated in feces.

Beta oxidation is another task of the liver, in which fatty acid molecules are split into two-carbon acetyl groups. These acetyl groups may be used by the liver to produce energy, or they may be combined to form ketones to be transported to other cells for energy production.

SYNTHESIS OF PLASMA PROTEINS. The liver synthesizes albumin, clotting factors, and globulins. Albumin, the most abundant plasma protein, maintains osmotic balance. Clotting factors produced by the liver include prothrombin and fibrinogen, which circulate in the blood until needed for coagulation. Globulin functions include becoming part of lipoproteins, acting as carriers, and acting as antibodies.

PHAGOCYTOSIS BY KUPFFER CELLS. The fixed macrophages of the liver (named Kupffer cells or stellate reticuloendothelial cells), phagocytize worn formed elements and pathogens.

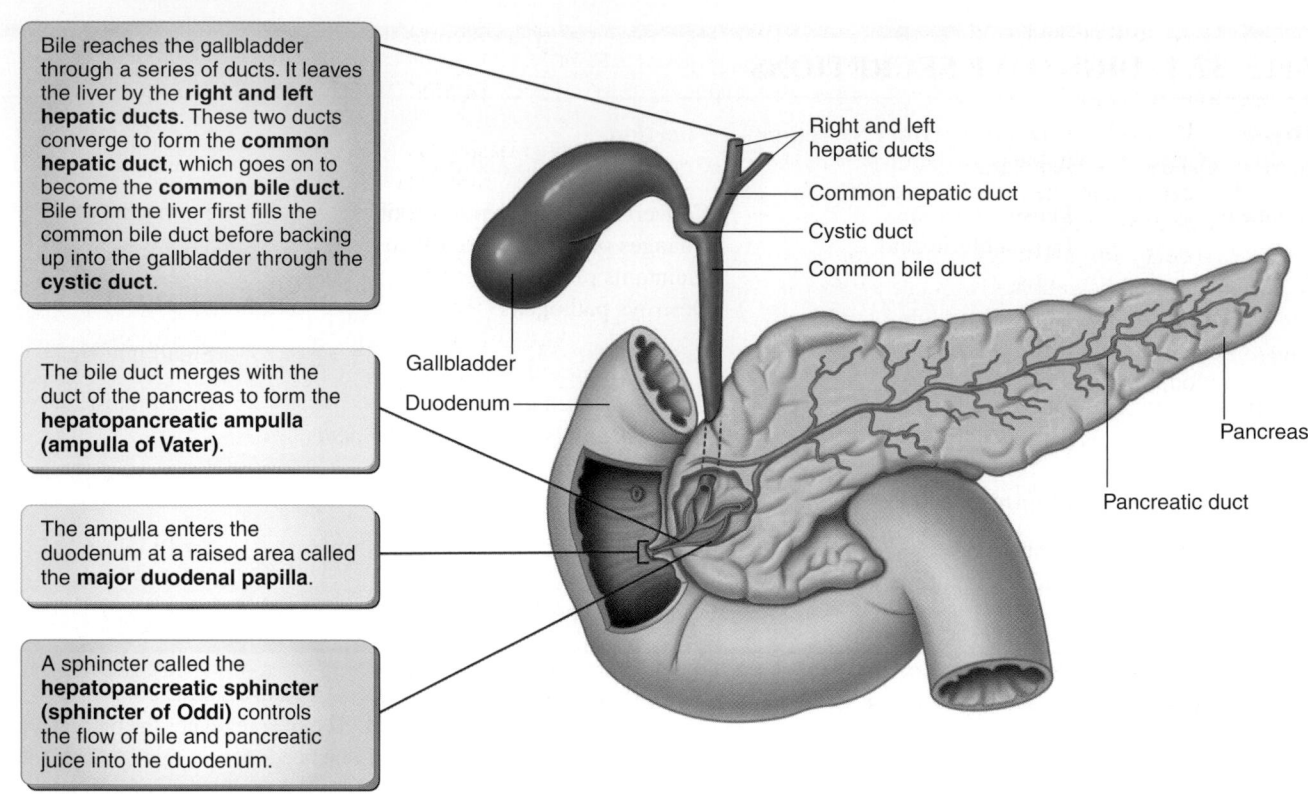

Bile reaches the gallbladder through a series of ducts. It leaves the liver by the **right and left hepatic ducts**. These two ducts converge to form the **common hepatic duct**, which goes on to become the **common bile duct**. Bile from the liver first fills the common bile duct before backing up into the gallbladder through the **cystic duct**.

The bile duct merges with the duct of the pancreas to form the **hepatopancreatic ampulla (ampulla of Vater)**.

The ampulla enters the duodenum at a raised area called the **major duodenal papilla**.

A sphincter called the **hepatopancreatic sphincter (sphincter of Oddi)** controls the flow of bile and pancreatic juice into the duodenum.

Right and left hepatic ducts
Common hepatic duct
Cystic duct
Common bile duct
Gallbladder
Duodenum
Pancreas
Pancreatic duct

FIGURE 32.3 Gall bladder and pancreas. From Thompson, G. S. (2013). *Understanding anatomy and physiology*. Philadelphia: F.A. Davis, p. 388.

FORMATION OF BILIRUBIN. Hepatocytes form bilirubin from the *heme* portion of hemoglobin removed from worn erythrocytes and collect bilirubin from the spleen. Bilirubin is excreted as a part of bile to be eliminated in feces.

STORAGE. The liver stores the minerals iron and copper; the fat-soluble vitamins A, D, E, and K; and the water-soluble vitamin B_{12}.

DETOXIFICATION. The liver synthesizes enzymes that convert harmful substances to less harmful ones. Alcohol and medications are examples of potentially toxic chemicals. The liver also converts ammonia from protein metabolism to urea, a less toxic substance.

ACTIVATION OF VITAMIN D. The skin, kidneys, and liver each perform a role in providing the body with activated vitamin D.

Gallbladder

The gallbladder is a muscular sac approximately 4 inches long located on the undersurface of the liver. Bile in the common hepatic duct from the liver flows through the cystic duct into the gallbladder, which stores bile until it is needed in the small intestine (see Fig. 32.3). The gallbladder concentrates bile by absorbing water.

When fatty foods or partially digested proteins enter the duodenum, the duodenal mucosa secretes the hormone cholecystokinin. One function of cholecystokinin is to stimulate contraction of the smooth muscle of the wall of the gallbladder. Contraction of the gallbladder forces bile into the cystic duct, then into the common bile duct, which empties into the duodenum.

Pancreas

The pancreas is about 6 inches long and is located posterior to the greater curvature of the stomach. Digestive secretions enter the duodenum either via the pancreatic duct or the alternate accessory duct (see Fig. 32.3).

The pancreatic digestive enzymes are involved in the digestion of all four of the organic molecule categories. The enzyme pancreatic amylase digests starch to maltose. Pancreatic lipase converts emulsified fats to fatty acids and monoglycerides. Trypsinogen is an inactive enzyme that is changed to active trypsin in the duodenum. Trypsin digests polypeptides to shorter chains of amino acids. Pancreatic juice also contains proteolytic enzymes: chymotrypsin, carboxypeptidase, and elastase. Ribonuclease and deoxyribonuclease, for the digestion of RNA and DNA, respectively, are contributed by the pancreas as well.

Secretion of pancreatic juice is stimulated by the hormones of the duodenal mucosa. Secretin stimulates the production of bicarbonate pancreatic juice, and cholecystokinin stimulates secretion of the pancreatic enzyme juice.

Aging and the Gastrointestinal, Hepatobiliary, and Pancreatic Systems

Many changes occur in the aging gastrointestinal (GI) system (Fig. 32.4). The sense of taste becomes less acute, and the likelihood of developing periodontal disease or oral cancer increases. If teeth have been lost, an older person may experience difficulties with chewing. Secretions throughout the GI tract are reduced, and the effectiveness of peristalsis diminishes because of loss of muscle elasticity and slowed motility. Indigestion may become more common, especially if the LES loses its tone, and peptic ulcers are more common. In the colon, diverticula may form. Constipation may be a problem, as may hemorrhoids. The risk of colon cancer also increases with age.

The liver usually continues to function well into old age, unless damaged by pathogens such as the hepatitis viruses or by toxins such as alcohol ("Gerontological Issues"). There is a greater tendency for gallstones to form, sometimes necessitating removal of the gallbladder. In the absence of specific pathological conditions, the pancreas usually functions well, although acute pancreatitis of unknown cause is somewhat more common in older adults.

Gerontological Issues

With increasing age, the liver decreases in volume, mass, and blood flow. These changes are significant because the liver acts to metabolize many drugs. If a patient has impaired liver function, toxic levels of a drug may be present in the blood. It is important to assess liver function tests and perform a medication review to determine those that are metabolized by the liver. Older adults may require reduced doses of many drugs.

NURSING ASSESSMENT OF THE GASTROINTESTINAL, HEPATOBILIARY, AND PANCREATIC SYSTEMS

Health History

Assessment of current signs and symptoms includes asking the **WHAT'S UP?** questions as presented in Chapter 1 (Tables 32.2 and 32.3). Demographic data are obtained, including travel

history, which may help in diagnosing the cause of GI symptoms such as diarrhea.

Ask the patient about any nausea, vomiting, or abdominal distention. Information about the timing or other common triggers of episodes of nausea or vomiting may help the practitioner identify their cause. Such information may also help determine appropriate treatment for any future nausea or vomiting. Abdominal distention in the presence of nausea

FIGURE 32.4 The effects of aging on the gastrointestinal, hepatic, and pancreatic systems is shown on this concept map.

TABLE 32.2 SUBJECTIVE DATA COLLECTION FOR THE GASTROINTESTINAL SYSTEM

Category	Questions to Ask During the Health History	Rationale/Significance
Health History	Identify current symptoms using the **WHAT'S UP** format.	This will help you adequately assess the patient's current problem.
	What are your bowel patterns? How often do you usually have a bowel movement?	Changes in bowel habits could indicate new disease process.
	What is the color? Consistency?	
	Diarrhea or constipation?	
	Have you had any blood in your stool or on the toilet tissue?	Blood in stool may indicate hemorrhoids, early sign of cancer, or inflammatory diseases such as ulcerative colitis.
	Have you had any change in appetite?	Appetite changes can be common with gastrointestinal disorders.
	Nausea and/or vomiting?	
	Bloating? Excess gas?	Can be associated with GI disorders.
	Do you have any history of gastrointestinal illnesses or surgeries?	Patient may have a recurring problem.
	Do you smoke?	Nicotine can irritate the GI mucosa. Smoking is related to esophagitis, ulcers, and GI cancers such as esophagus and mouth cancer.
Medications	What medications are you currently taking?	Provides baseline information about patient.
	How do the drugs relate to the GI system?	
	Are they working? How do you know?	
	Have you recently taken any NSAIDs, aspirin, anticoagulants, or steroids?	These medications can cause gastric upset and/or bleeding.
	Do you routinely take laxatives? Fiber?	Patient may have dependency on laxatives.
	Are you taking or have you recently taken antibiotics?	Diarrhea due to *Clostridium difficile* can be caused by recent antibiotic use.
Nutrition	Describe your usual diet. Tell me what you ate yesterday for the entire day.	Provides information about your patient's nutritional status. Older adults may be on a fixed income and unable to afford adequate nutrition.
	Do you have any food allergies?	These may interfere with proper nutrition.
	Do you have indigestion, dysphagia, heartburn, nausea, vomiting, diarrhea, constipation, flatulence, or bowel incontinence?	If patient has any of these symptoms, use the **WHAT'S UP** format to gather more specific information.
	Have you had a change in appetite?	
	Have you had a change in weight—gain or loss?	
	Are there any foods that you cannot eat?	
Family History	Do you have a family history of any GI disorders such as cancer?	Some diseases are thought to be hereditary.
Cultural Influences	Are there any cultural considerations I should be aware of regarding your food intake or care?	Many societies use herbs, vitamins, or home remedies to care for disorders.

Note. GI = gastrointestinal; NSAID = nonsteroidal anti-inflammatory drug.

and vomiting may indicate intestinal obstruction. Patients with liver, gallbladder, or pancreatic disease may also report feeling bloated, having gas or belching frequently, or right upper quadrant (RUQ) tenderness.

Question the patient about any observed changes in bowel elimination. Diarrhea may be caused by irritation of the bowel. Constipation may indicate decreased water intake or excessive water loss. Observe the patient's stool for evidence of bacteria (a foul smell), fat (stool floats on the water surface and appears greasy), pus, blood, or mucus. Patients with liver or gallbladder disease may have pale or clay-colored stools.

TABLE 32.3 SUBJECTIVE DATA COLLECTION FOR THE HEPATOBILIARY AND PANCREATIC SYSTEMS

Category	Questions to Ask During the Health History	Rationale/Significance
Health History	Do you have abdominal pain? (Use **WHAT'S UP?** format to further identify.) Do any foods cause pain?	Pain can be associated with disease of the liver, gallbladder, or pancreas. Fatty foods can cause pain related to gallbladder disease.
	What do your stools look like?	Clay-colored stools indicate liver or gallbladder disease. Black stools may indicate bleeding, which can be related to liver disease. Fatty stools occur with pancreatic disease.
	Does your abdomen feel distended or full?	Fluid in the abdomen, or ascites, occurs with liver disease.
	How much alcohol do you drink each day?	Excess alcohol intake is associated with liver disease and pancreatitis.
	Do you bruise or bleed easily?	Bleeding is associated with liver disease, because clotting factors are made in the liver.
	Have you had any recent blood transfusions or blood products, dental procedures, body piercing or tattooing, or IV injection with a potentially contaminated needle?	Breaks in skin may be the route of entry for hepatitis (type B or C) or other pathogens.
Nutrition	Have you experienced nausea and vomiting?	These are generalized symptoms that may be associated with disease of the liver, gallbladder, or pancreas.
	Has your appetite or weight changed?	Anorexia and weight loss accompany many liver, gallbladder, and pancreatic disorders.
Family History	Does anyone in your family have liver, gallbladder, or pancreatic disease or alcoholism?	These disorders tend to run in families.
Medications	Do you use any over-the-counter drugs or herbal remedies?	Many drugs and herbs are toxic to the liver.

Determine if the patient has had any recent blood transfusions or blood products, dental procedures, body piercing or tattooing, or intravenous (IV) injection with a potentially contaminated needle. These procedures cause a break in the skin that can become an entry point for hepatitis virus (type B or C) as well as other pathogens.

Ask about the patient's usual work activities and work setting. Document exposure to chemicals such as paint fumes, industrial dyes, acids, farm pesticides, or other liver-toxic substances.

Investigate the patient's activities other than work. Document reports of fatigue along with information about when the fatigue occurs. Ask the patient about stressors such as financial concerns, problems dealing with the health care environment, and any family or personal problems. Attempt to determine what coping mechanisms the patient usually employs to deal with stressors.

Medications

The patient is asked about medication use such as nonsteroidal anti-inflammatory drugs (NSAIDs), aspirin, vitamins, laxatives, enemas, or antacids. Heavy use of medications that can cause irritation and bleeding in the GI tract, such as NSAIDs or aspirin, should be carefully noted. Older patients with arthritis often use these types of medications for pain control. The patient's knowledge of the side effects of these medications should be assessed to identify important teaching needs. Older patients may use laxatives regularly and develop a dependence on them. Teaching may be needed on normal bowel patterns and laxative use. Also ask the patient what medications are being taken with or without a health care provider's (HCP's) prescription, such as acetaminophen, which can be hepatotoxic. Many people do not consider it necessary to report over-the-counter preparations and herbal, natural, or other nonprescription products and must be asked specifically about them.

CLOSTRIDIUM DIFFICILE. Question the patient about uncontrolled diarrhea, recent hospitalizations, or antibiotic use. Hospitalization or recent antibiotic use is a risk factor for *Clostridium difficile* (see Chapter 8). With antibiotic use, a decrease in normal flora can result, allowing an overgrowth of *C. difficile*. The toxins produced by *C. difficile* can cause diarrhea, colitis, toxic megacolon, dehydration, or colonic perforation. Monitor patients closely for signs of *C. difficile* infection such as diarrhea, nausea, anorexia, and abdominal tenderness or pain. Report these symptoms to the HCP because this infection can be fatal.

CRITICAL THINKING

Mrs. Todd

■ Mrs. Todd, age 74, has arthritis and takes eight aspirin daily for pain control. She is scheduled for an esophagogastroduodenoscopy (EGD) for suspected GI bleeding causing unexplained anemia.

1. What is a likely cause of the GI bleeding?
2. What could you do to help prevent future bleeding episodes for Mrs. Todd?
3. What nursing care will need to be completed before the test and after the test?

Suggested answers are at the end of the chapter.

Nutritional Assessment

A diet history should include usual foods and fluids, allergies, appetite patterns, swallowing difficulty, and use of nutritional and herbal supplements. A food diary can be used to provide more detailed information. Older patients may be on fixed incomes, which may limit their food budget and result in meal skipping or purchasing of inexpensive foods. The older patient's daily food intake should be explored, especially if malnutrition, financial limitations, or living alone is noted.

Also explored during a nutritional assessment are patterns of gastric acid reflux, indigestion, heartburn, nausea, vomiting, diarrhea, constipation, flatulence, and bowel incontinence, all of which may interfere with proper nutrition ("Gerontological Issues"). Acid reflux can be assessed by asking patients if they experience reflux with a bile taste or awaken with an unpleasant taste in their mouth.

Family History

Family history of close relatives with conditions that may influence the patient's GI status is noted. Some GI problems such as colon cancer are thought to be hereditary. The patient's history should note whether there is a family history of liver, pancreas, or gallbladder diseases, such as diabetes mellitus, alcoholism, cancer, heart disease, or bleeding tendencies. These diseases tend to run in families.

Cultural Influences

Many cultures have special dietary practices and restrictions ("Cultural Considerations"). See Box 32-1, "Cultural Assessment Questions," for assessment questions. Understanding these cultural influences, respecting them, and assisting the patient to maintain desired cultural practices are important for nutritional maintenance.

Gerontological Issues

A complete bowel history should be obtained for older adults before beginning a bowel program. A bowel history includes the following:
- Normal bowel evacuation pattern
- Characteristics of stool
- Presence of any bleeding or mucus with the stool
- Use of products and medications to stimulate or slow bowel function
- Report of usual diet
- Amount of fluids—number and size of beverages, glasses per day (beverages containing caffeine, such as coffee, tea, and sodas, do not count as fluids because of the diuretic effect of caffeine)
- Exercise and physical activity

Patients with disease of the liver, pancreas, or gallbladder commonly have changes in appetite such as anorexia or alterations in eating preferences. Ask the patient about any abnormal weight loss or unexpected weight gain and changes in food tolerance, including the type or amount of offending foods. For example, patients with gallbladder disease may report that they feel nauseated or bloated after eating fried or greasy foods. Ask if the patient smokes, ingests alcohol, or uses other recreational drugs. If the patient acknowledges alcohol or other drug use, record the type, frequency, and amount used.

Box 32-1 Cultural Nutritional Assessment

Questions to ask when performing a cultural nutritional assessment:
- What types of your cultural foods are available in your community?
- What are your preferred foods over foods available and eaten?
- Which foods do you most commonly consume?
- How and where are your foods chosen and purchased?
- Who prepares the food in your household?
- Who purchases the food in your household?
- How is your food stored for future use?
- How is your food prepared before being eaten?
- How is any uneaten food discarded?
- What foods do you eat to maintain your health?
- What foods do you avoid to maintain your health?
- What foods do you eat when you are ill?
- What foods do you avoid when you are ill?

Cultural Considerations

African Americans

Obesity is seen as positive among many African Americans. They often view individuals who are thin as "not having enough meat on their bones." One needs to have adequate meat on his or her bones so that when an illness occurs, one can afford to lose weight. Many African American diets are high in animal fat and fried foods and low in fiber, fruits, and vegetables.

Appalachians

The diet of some Appalachians is deficient in vitamin A, iron, and calcium. The nurse working with this population needs to do a dietary assessment and teach patients food selections that include adequate vitamin A, iron, and calcium.

Arabs

Many Arabs eat food only with their right hand because it is regarded as the clean hand. The left hand, commonly used for toileting, is considered unclean. Thus, the nurse should feed the Arab patient with the right hand regardless of the nurse's dominant handedness. Additionally, some may not drink beverages with their meals because some consider it unhealthy to eat and drink at the same meal. Likewise, mixing hot and cold foods may be seen as unhealthy.

Muslim Arabs may refuse to eat meat that is not *halal* (slaughtered and prepared in a ritual manner). Because Muslim Arabs are prohibited from ingesting alcohol or eating pork, they may refuse medication that includes alcohol, such as mouthwashes, toothpaste, alcohol-based syrups and elixirs, and products derived from pigs, such as insulin, gelatin-coated capsules, and skin grafts. However, if no substitute is available, Muslims are permitted to use these preparations.

The condition of the alimentary tract has priority over all other body parts in the Arab's perception of health. GI problems are the most common reasons for which Arab Americans seek care.

Asian Indians

Among Asian Indians, nutritional deficiencies are patterned from the region of emigration. For example, *beriberi* (thiamine deficiency) is found in people emigrating from rice-growing areas. Pellagra (niacin deficiency), causing skin and mental disorders and diarrhea, is found in people emigrating from maize-millet areas. Thorough milling of rice, washing rice before cooking, and allowing the cooked rice to remain overnight before consumption the following day result in the loss of thiamine.

Asian Indians use chili, which may make it difficult for them to eat food that is tasteless, or the use of chili may cause problems with upper GI conditions.

The commitment to the sacred cow concept encourages dairy and milk use by Hindus. However, lactose intolerance affects more than 10% of adults. The adequacy or inadequacy of the ability to digest lactose may be due to genetic differences among Asian Indians.

Goiter is prevalent among some Asian Indian immigrants as a result of an iodine deficiency in food and water from their homeland. Fluorosis occurs in other parts of India from drinking water high in fluoride. Osteomalacia is prevalent where diets are deficient in calcium and vitamin D. Endemic dropsy is prevalent among Asian Indians emigrating from West Bengal, resulting from the use of mustard oil for cooking. The nurse needs to be aware of these conditions and their causes when working with Hindus and Asian Indians and teach patients prevention.

Brazilians

Brazilians experience an increase in GI distress when they first come to the United States, partially because many have a lactose intolerance and partially because of different methods of milk pasteurization. The nurse can assist with identifying alternative food sources for Brazilian patients to obtain needed calcium in their diet.

Jews

Among Jews, the laws regarding food are commonly referred to as the laws of Kashrut, or the laws of what foods are permissible in accordance with the religious law. The term *kosher* means "fit for eating"; it is not a brand or form of cooking.

Continued

Cultural Considerations—cont'd

Foods are divided into those that are permitted (clean) and forbidden (unclean). The kosher slaughter of animals prevents undue cruelty to the animal and ensures the animal's health for its consumer. Care must be taken that all blood is drained from the animal before eating it.

Among the more conservative and Orthodox Jews, dairy products and meat may not be mixed together, whether in cooking, serving, or eating. This involves separating the utensils used to prepare foods and the plates used to serve them. To avoid mixing foods, religious Jews have two sets of dishes, pots, and utensils: one set for dairy products and one for meat.

Cheeseburgers, meat lasagna, and grated cheese on meatballs and spaghetti are not acceptable. Milk cannot be used in coffee if served with a meat meal. Nondairy creamers can be used as long as they do not contain sodium caseinate, which is derived from milk.

Fish, eggs, vegetables, and fruits are considered neutral and may be used with either dairy or meat dishes. A "U" with a circle around it or a "K" is used on food products to indicate that a food is kosher.

When working in a Jewish person's home, the nurse should not bring food into the house without knowing whether the patient is kosher. If the patient is kosher, do not use any cooking items, dishes, or silverware without knowing which are used for meat and which are used for dairy. It is important for the nurse to understand the dietary laws so as not to offend the patient. The nurse should advocate for kosher meals if they are requested and plan medication times accordingly.

Although nonreligious Jews decide for themselves which dietary laws, if any, they follow, many still avoid pork and pork products out of a sense of tradition and symbolism. It would be insensitive to serve pork products to Jewish patients unless they specifically request them.

Kosher meals are available in hospitals and long-term care facilities. Even though the organization may not have a kosher kitchen, frozen kosher meals can be obtained from several organizations, most of which are located in large cities with large Jewish populations. The address and telephone number of the kosher kitchen closest to your organization can be obtained by calling the nearest Jewish synagogue. Kosher meals arrive on paper plates with plastic utensils sealed in plastic. The nurse should not unwrap the utensils if the patient is able to do so or change the foodstuffs to another serving dish. Determining a patient's dietary preferences and practices regarding dietary laws should be done during the admission assessment.

Mexican Americans

Good health to Mexican Americans, which is largely a part of "God's will," can be maintained by dietary practices that keep the body in balance. To provide culturally competent care, the nurse must be aware of the hot-and-cold theory of disease when offering health teaching. Many diseases are thought to be caused by a disruption in the hot-and-cold balance theory of the body. Thus, by eating foods of the opposite variety, one may either cure or prevent specific hot-and-cold illnesses and conditions.

Examples of hot disease conditions include infection, diarrhea, sore throats, stomach ulcers, liver conditions, kidney problems, GI upset, and febrile conditions. Foods that are considered "cold" are therefore viewed as remedies for hot illness conditions. Cold foods include fresh fruits and vegetables, dairy products, barley water, fish, chicken, goat meat, and dried fruits. However, significant differences are seen in terms of what are considered hot and cold foods and illnesses among Mexican American families depending on their native region in Mexico.

Examples of cold illness conditions include cancer, malaria, earaches, arthritis and related conditions, pneumonia and other pulmonary conditions, headaches, menstrual cramping, and musculoskeletal conditions. Hot substances used to treat these conditions typically include cheeses, liquor, beef, pork, spicy foods, eggs, grains other than barley, vitamins, tobacco, and onions.

Physical Examination

Table 32.4 summarizes findings from the objective assessment of the GI, hepatobiliary, and pancreatic systems discussed next.

Height, Weight, and Body Mass Index

The patient's height and weight are obtained for planning care. It is compared with the patient's ideal body weight obtained using current reference charts. Body mass index (BMI) is calculated to measure body fat and used with waist-to-hip ratio measurements to determine patient's health risk factors (Table 32.5). Excess waist circumferences (for women, more than 35 inches; for men, more than 40 inches) place people at greater risk for diabetes and cardiovascular disease. Also the location of excess fat, mainly around the waist, increases the risk of health problems even with a normal BMI.

TABLE **32.4 OBJECTIVE DATA COLLECTION FOR THE GASTROINTESTINAL, HEPATOBILIARY, AND PANCREATIC SYSTEMS**

Category	Physical Examination Findings	Possible Abnormal Findings/Causes
Height, Weight, and Body Mass Index (BMI)	Normal height, weight and BMI	Decreases in height, weight, and BMI could indicate inadequate nutrition or malabsorption problems. Current weight loss could indicate new onset of a disease such as cancer.
Oral Cavity	Moist, pink oral mucosa, without lesions, inflammation, tenderness, or discolorations. Pink, rough tongue. Teeth should be intact. Dentures should fit properly.	Foul odor may indicate infection or poor oral hygiene. Dry tongue with cracked furrows could indicate dehydration possibly due to vomiting or diarrhea. Broken teeth or ill-fitting dentures can contribute to inadequate nutrition.
Abdomen Inspection	Abdomen contour should be flat, rounded, or convex. Shape should be symmetrical. Skin color should be consistent with overall skin tone. No visible scars or discolorations.	Irregularities in contour such as bulging or masses may be due to distention, tumors, hernia, or previous surgeries. Any scars, dressings, appliances such as an ostomy should be noted. Indicate what the stoma looks like. Scars may be present if the patient has had previous surgeries or injuries. Striae are present if the skin has been stretched (i.e., with pregnancy or weight gain). Bruising could be related to injury or altered liver function. Note any caput medusae or spider angiomas. Jaundice color may indicate liver or gallbladder disease.
Auscultation	Soft bowel sounds should be heard in all quadrants every 5–15 seconds. Circulatory sounds should be absent.	Hyperactive sounds are heard with increased motility such as diarrhea. Hypoactive sounds are associated with decreased motility such as abdominal surgery, paralytic ileus, or bowel obstruction. A humming sound may be heard over the liver in patients with chronic liver failure.
Percussion	Completed by health care provider.	
Palpation	No pain, muscle tension, rigidity, or masses should be felt on light palpation. The abdomen should feel soft. Abdominal girth should be appropriate for patient without increasing. Deep palpation is done by the advanced practitioner.	Muscle tension, rigidity, or pain may occur in many abdominal disorders. Patients with ascites from liver disease may have an increased girth that increases as the disease worsens.
Anus	No lumps, rashes, scars, erythema, bleeding, fissures, or hemorrhoids.	Hemorrhoids may be present. Patients with diarrhea may have skin breakdown or rash.

TABLE 32.5 CALCULATING BODY MASS INDEX AND WAIST-TO-HIP RATIO MEASUREMENT

To calculate body mass index:	*Formulas:* *Pounds and inches:* weight (lb) / [height (in.)]^2 × 703 Step 1. Multiply height (in inches) by height. Step 2. Divide weight (in pounds) by Step 1 answer. Step 3. Multiply Step 2 answer by 703. *Kilograms and meters:* weight (kg) / [height (m)]^2 Step 1. Multiply height (in meters) by height. Step 2. Divide weight (in kilograms) by Step 1 answer.
Findings	Below 18.5: underweight 18.5–24.9: normal 25–29.9: overweight 30 and over: obese
To obtain waist measurement:	Step 1. Place measuring tape around bare waist at top of the iliac crest. Step 2. Pull snugly around the waist. Step 3. Read measurement at end expiration.
To obtain waist-to-hip ratio measurement*	Step 1. Place measuring tape at the level of the top of the iliac crest. Step 2. Pull snugly around the waist. Step 3. Read measurement at end expiration. Step 4. Place measuring tape around hip at widest part and read measurement. Step 5. Waist measurement is divided by hip measurement.
Findings/risk for health complications:	Female: ≤ 0.8—low risk; > 0.85—high risk Male: ≤ 0.95—low risk; > 1.0—high risk

*Method for patients who are overweight or obese.

Oral Cavity

GI assessment begins with the oral cavity. The lips are examined for lesions, abnormal color, and symmetry. With a penlight and tongue blade, the oral cavity is inspected for inflammation, tenderness, ulcers, swelling, bleeding, and discolorations. Any odor of the patient's breath is noted. A foul odor may indicate infection or poor oral care. The tongue should be pink with a rough texture and assessed for signs of dehydration such as dryness, cracks, or furrows. The patient's gums should be pink without swelling, redness, or irregularities. The teeth or dentures are examined for loose, broken, or absent teeth and the fit of the dentures or dental work. Ill-fitting dentures can affect the patient's nutritional intake and obstruct the airway. Loose teeth can become dislodged and aspirated into the airway. Broken teeth can be a source of pain and contribute to poor nutritional intake.

The patient's knowledge of dental and oral care is assessed. The ability of the patient to perform oral care is noted and included in the plan of care if there are deficits. Oral health is very important to a person's overall health and well-being.

Abdomen

Be prepared to assist with a thorough physical assessment of the patient. Instead of following the usual inspect-palpate-percuss-auscultate (IPPA) format, assess the abdomen starting with inspection, then auscultation, percussion, and palpation. This is to prevent palpation from altering other assessment findings.

INSPECTION. To inspect the abdomen, patients are placed in a supine position with their arms at their sides. The abdomen is visually inspected to note the condition of the skin and the contour. The contour may be rounded, flat, concave, or distended, depending on the patient's body type. Abdominal pulsatile masses are noted. Such masses may be visible in thin persons or they may indicate an abdominal aortic aneurysm. Irregularities in contour may be due to distention, tumors, hernia, or previous surgeries. Also note any wounds, tubes, or ostomy devices including type and location.

Inspect the patient's skin for scars, **striae** (commonly called stretch marks; light silver-colored or thin red lines on the abdomen), bruising, **caput medusae** (bluish purple swollen vein pattern extending out from the navel), and **spider angiomas** (thin reddish purple vein lines close to the skin surface). Note any petechiae. The patient's abdomen

• WORD • BUILDING •
caput medusae: caput—head + medusae—Medusa's snaky locks

is observed for any visible masses, visible movement or peristalsis, or **jaundice** (also called **icterus**; a yellowing of the skin and the sclerae of the eyes).

Jaundice is a cardinal symptom of liver or gallbladder disease and red blood cell disorders. Old red blood cells are cleared from the circulatory system by phagocytes in the spleen, liver, lymph nodes, and bone marrow. In the process, the compound heme (part of hemoglobin) is split into iron and another substance that is metabolized to bilirubin. The liver is then responsible for converting bilirubin to a water-soluble compound that can be excreted in bile. If the liver is unable to convert or conjugate bilirubin to a water-soluble compound or if bile drainage is obstructed, serum bilirubin is elevated and pigments are deposited in body tissues.

When serum bilirubin levels elevate, the patient's skin color changes to yellow. The yellow color varies from pale yellow to a striking golden orange. The color intensity is directly related to the amount of elevation of the serum bilirubin. Jaundice can be seen in nearly every body tissue and fluid where there is any amount of albumin ("Cultural Considerations"). Pigment may occasionally be seen in cerebrospinal fluid or joint fluid. Pigment is not seen in saliva or tears. Urine becomes dark, and if bile flow to the bowel is obstructed, stools will be a light clay color. Describe any abnormal finding completely in the patient's record, and report your findings promptly.

The perianal and anal areas are inspected. Inspect the area for color, rashes, scars, fissures, external hemorrhoids, or skin breakdown. Describe any abnormal findings.

AUSCULTATION. When auscultating the patient's abdomen, the upper right quadrant is auscultated first (Fig. 32.5). Then a clockwise direction is followed to listen to the other quadrants. The stethoscope is pressed lightly on the abdomen to listen for **bowel sounds**, which are soft clicks and gurgles that may be heard every 5 to 15 seconds, occurring irregularly 5 to 30 times per minute. Bowel sounds at this rate are considered normal.

Bowel sounds are produced when peristalsis moves air and fluid through the GI tract, and they are categorized as normal, hyperactive, hypoactive, or absent. Hyperactive bowel sounds are usually rapid, high pitched, and loud and may occur with hunger or gastroenteritis. Hypoactive bowel sounds are bowel sounds that are infrequent and can occur in patients with a paralytic ileus or following abdominal surgery (see "Evidence-Based Practice"). Bowel sounds are considered absent if no sounds are auscultated after listening to all four quadrants for 2 to 5 minutes in each quadrant. However, this timing is an area for further research because, in practice, auscultation for this amount of time is rarely done. With a bowel obstruction, a high-pitched tinkling sound that is proximal to the obstruction and absent distal to the obstruction may be heard. Abnormal or absent bowel sounds are important findings and should be documented and reported to the HCP.

Note the presence of any vascular sounds or bruits (swooshing sounds), which are normally not present, are heard with the stethoscope over the aorta. Patients with chronic liver failure may have a humming sound over their liver. This finding usually indicates overloaded venous circulation in the liver.

PERCUSSION. Percussion produces a sound that identifies the density of the organs beneath the area being percussed and is performed by the HCP. Percussion is used to detect fluid, air, and masses in the abdomen and to identify size and location of abdominal organs (especially the liver and spleen). Tympanic high-pitched sounds indicate the presence of air, and dull thuds indicate fluid or solid organs.

 LEARNING TIP

In a complete bowel obstruction, air and fluid are propelled forward by peristalsis proximal to the obstruction. This produces proximal high-pitched bowel sounds when the air and fluid create turbulence as they hit the obstruction and are unable to pass. Absent bowel sounds are heard distal to the obstruction. If a patient has a nasogastric (NG) tube for suction, turn off the suction before listening for bowel sounds.

PALPATION. Light palpation of the abdomen concludes the physical assessment. If the patient is having pain, that area should be palpated last. Using the same quadrant approach as previously mentioned (see Fig. 32.5), lightly depress the abdomen not more than 0.5 to 1.0 inch during the palpation using the finger pads. Note any muscle tension, rigidity, masses, or expressions of pain.

Deep palpation of the abdomen is done only by the HCP. Rebound tenderness is determined by pressing down on the abdomen a few inches and quickly releasing the pressure. If the patient feels a sharp pain during this procedure, appendicitis may be indicated.

• **WORD • BUILDING •**
jaundice: jaune—yellow

 ## Cultural Considerations

The nurse should be aware of the variations among people of color when assessing for jaundice. To assess for jaundice in a patient with dark skin, look at the sclerae, conjunctivae, palms of hands, soles of feet, and in the buccal mucosa for patches of bilirubin pigment.

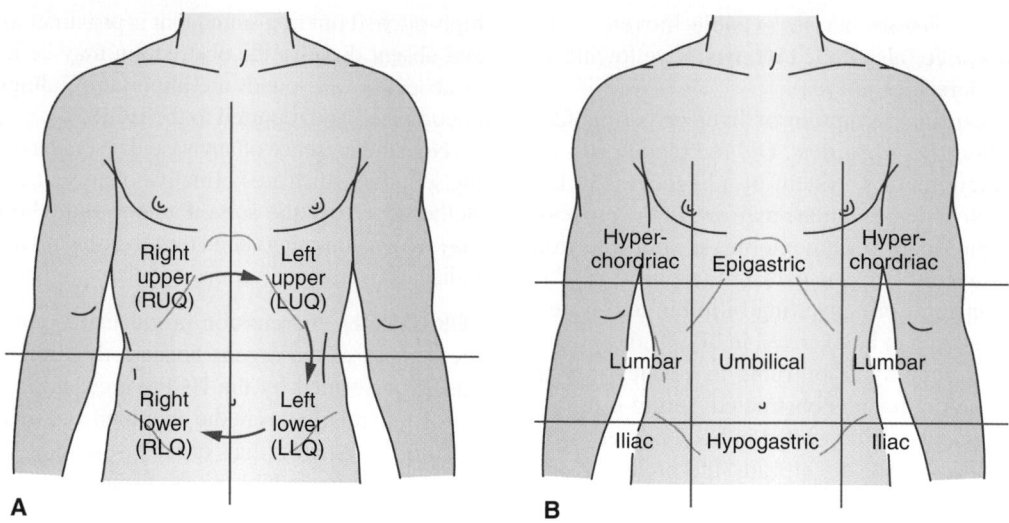

FIGURE 32.5 (A) Abdominal quadrants are auscultated from the right upper quadrant in a clockwise manner. (B) Nine abdominal regions.

Abdominal girth is measured by placing a tape measure around the patient's abdomen at the iliac crest. A mark is made at the measurement site so measurements are made at the same location for comparison. Abdominal girth is increased in patients with distention or conditions such as ascites (accumulation of fluid in the peritoneal cavity). When abdominal girth is abnormal, daily measurements should be obtained and recorded to monitor changes.

EVIDENCE-BASED PRACTICE

Clinical Question
Can gum chewing reduce the incidence of post-operative ileus?

Evidence
A meta-analysis of four studies of early gum chewing after surgery demonstrated that there can be a reduction time in the first flatus after surgery by 12 hours, reduction of time in the first bowel movement by 1 day, and a decreased length of hospital stay by 1 day.

Implications for Nursing Practice
Early gum chewing after surgery can reduce time of flatus after surgery, decrease time of first bowel movement, and length of hospital stay by 1 day. Patients should chew sugarless gum three or four times a day for 5 to 30 minutes, unless not tolerated.

REFERENCE
Lafon, C., & Lawson, L. (2012). Gum chewing as a strategy to reduce the duration of postoperative ileus. *Gastrointestinal Nursing, 10,* 17–22.

DIAGNOSTIC TESTS FOR THE GASTROINTESTINAL, HEPATOBILIARY, AND PANCREATIC SYSTEMS

See Appendix B for general information on common diagnostic tests.

Laboratory Tests

The complete blood cell count (CBC) reveals if anemia or infection is present. Anemia may occur with GI bleeding or cancer. Electrolyte imbalances often occur with GI illness as a result of vomiting, diarrhea, malabsorption, or use of GI suction. **Carcinoembryonic antigen** and carbohydrate antigen 19-9 are markers used to monitor GI cancer treatment effectiveness and detect recurrence (Tables 32.6 and 32.7). These markers are also found in patients with cirrhosis, hepatic disease, and alcoholic pancreatitis and in heavy smokers. Genetic testing can be done to identify family members at risk of developing serious conditions such as the polyps associated with colon cancer.

Bilirubin level is an excellent measure of liver and gallbladder functioning. In addition, certain enzymes such as alanine aminotransferase, aspartate aminotransferase, and lactic dehydrogenase are released by damaged liver cells. Elevations in these blood values in the absence of known trauma or heart muscle damage such as a heart attack are excellent indicators of liver damage.

Stool Tests

Stool samples can be tested for **occult blood** (blood not seen by the naked eye). A series of three tests is usually done to increase the chances of detecting blood. False-positive occult blood results can occur with bleeding gums following a dental procedure; ingestion of red meat within 3 days before testing; ingestion of fish, turnips, or horseradish; and use of drugs, including anticoagulants, aspirin, colchicine, iron preparations in large doses, NSAIDs, and steroids.

TABLE 32.6   LABORATORY TESTS USED TO ASSESS GASTROINTESTINAL FUNCTION

Test	Definition	Normal Range	Significance of Abnormal Findings
Carcinoembryonic Antigen	Blood test to detect protein that is usually found in fetal gut tissue.	Less than 5 nanograms/mL (nonsmokers)	Increased values indicate possible colorectal cancer, other cancers, or inflammatory bowel disease.
Fecal Analysis Stool for occult blood	Normally minimal quantities of blood are passed into the GI tract. Stool sample is taken to determine if blood is present in the stool.	Negative	Presence indicates possible peptic ulcer, cancer of the colon, ulcerative colitis.
Stool for ova and parasites	Stool sample to determine if pathogenic bacteria or parasites are present in the stool.	Negative	Presence indicates infection.
Stool cultures	Same as above.	No unusual growth	Presence of pathogens may indicate *Shigella, Salmonella, Staphylococcus aureus,* or *Bacillus cereus* infections.
Stool for lipids (fecal fat)	Test that measures the fat content in the stool. Used to confirm diagnosis of steatorrhea.	2–5 g per 24 hours (normal diet)	Increased values indicate possible malabsorption syndrome or Crohn's disease; increased in pancreatic disease.

TABLE 32.7   COMMON LABORATORY TESTS FOR HEPATOBILIARY AND PANCREATIC SYSTEMS DISORDERS

Test	Definition	Normal Range	Significance of Abnormal Findings
Blood Alanine aminotransferase (ALT)	Determines serum ALT levels. ALT is found mainly in the liver. With liver injury or disease, ALT is released into bloodstream.	5–35 international unit/dL	↑ in chronic liver failure and hepatitis
Albumin	Measures serum protein level.	3.1–4.3 g/dL	↓ in liver disease
Amylase	Detects and monitors status of pancreatitis.	53–123 unit/L	↑ in pancreatitis, gallstones

Continued

TABLE 32.7 COMMON LABORATORY TESTS FOR HEPATOBILIARY AND PANCREATIC SYSTEMS DISORDERS—cont'd

Test	Definition	Normal Range	Significance of Abnormal Findings
Ammonia	Determines serum levels. Ammonia is a by-product of protein catabolism.	12–55 mol/L	↑ in chronic liver failure, hepatitis
Aspartate aminotransferase (AST)	Enzyme found in highly metabolic tissues such as the liver. AST is released into bloodstream when cells lyse.	8–20 unit/L	↑ in chronic liver failure, viral hepatitis, acute pancreatitis
Bilirubin	Evaluates liver function.		
• Total serum bilirubin	Sum of the conjugated and unconjugated bilirubin.	0.1–1.0 mg/dL	↑ in liver and gallbladder disease with red blood cell destruction
• Conjugated (direct) bilirubin	Bilirubin that is conjugated in the liver (joined with glucuronide).	0.0–0.4 mg/dL	↑ with gallstones, gallbladder obstruction, extensive liver metastasis
• Unconjugated (indirect) bilirubin	Bilirubin in the bloodstream that has not yet passed through the liver.	0.1–1.0 mg/dL	↑ with red blood cell destruction or liver disease such as hepatitis or cirrhosis
Calcium	Identifies serum calcium level.	9–10.5 mg/dL	↓ with acute pancreatitis, liver disease, or malabsorption
Cholesterol	Identifies serum cholesterol level. Patient should fast 12–14 hours before test.	150–200 mg/dL	↑ in pancreatitis, gallbladder disease ↓ may indicate severe liver disease
Lactic dehydrogenase (LDH)	Determines level of this intracellular enzyme, which is released with injury or disease.	110–250 IU/L	↑ in liver disease
Lipase	Determines serum levels to detect and monitor pancreatitis.	0–110 unit/L	↑ in acute pancreatitis. ↑ in acute cholecystitis.
Potassium	Determine serum levels. Major cation in the cell.	3.5–5.0 mEq/L	↓ with diarrhea, intestinal fistulas, vomiting, suctioning
Prothrombin time	Determines adequacy of clotting mechanism.	11–13.5 seconds	↑ in liver disease, vitamin K deficiency

TABLE 32.7   COMMON LABORATORY TESTS FOR HEPATOBILIARY AND PANCREATIC SYSTEMS DISORDERS—cont'd

Test	Definition	Normal Range	Significance of Abnormal Findings
	Used to monitor anti-coagulation therapy with warfarin (Coumadin).		
Urine			
Urine amylase	Assists in making diagnosis of pancreatitis.	Depends on test	↑ in acute pancreatitis
Urine bilirubin	Measures predominantly conjugated bilirubin.	Negative	↑ in chronic liver failure, hepatitis, biliary obstruction Used primarily for screening purposes
Urobilinogen	Included in a routine urinalysis to support the diagnosis of hemolysis.	0.3–1.0 Ehrlich unit in 2 hr	↑ with destruction of red blood cells, hepatitis, chronic liver failure, obstructive jaundice

Stool is collected to detect intestinal infections caused by parasites and their ova (eggs). The test usually requires a series of three stool specimens collected every second or third day. The stool specimen is collected using a tongue blade, placed in a container with a preservative, and sent immediately to the laboratory. The stool must be examined within 30 minutes of collection. False-negative results can occur as a result of urine in the specimen or if the specimen is not fresh.

Stool cultures (sterile collection technique) are done to determine the presence of pathogenic organisms in the GI tract. Stool can also be examined for lipids (fat). Excessive secretion of fecal fats (**steatorrhea**) may occur in various digestive and absorptive disorders. The stools are collected for 72 hours and stored on ice if necessary before being sent to the laboratory.

Radiographic Tests

Upper Gastrointestinal Series (Barium Swallow)

An **upper gastrointestinal (GI) series** is an x-ray examination of the esophagus, stomach, duodenum, and jejunum using an oral liquid radiopaque contrast medium (barium) and a **fluoroscope** (an x-ray source and fluorescent screen between which the patient is placed) to outline the contours of the organs. An upper GI series is used to detect such things as strictures, ulcers, tumors, polyps, hiatal hernias, and motility problems.

The patient receives nothing by mouth (NPO) for 6 to 8 hours before the procedure. Usually the patient has a clear liquid supper the night before the procedure and is then NPO until the procedure is done. Because smoking can stimulate gastric motility, the patient is discouraged from smoking the morning of the procedure. Patient teaching includes information about the patient's diet before and after

the procedure, the barium ingestion, and the appearance of stools afterward. During the procedure, the patient drinks thick, chalky barium while standing in front of a fluoroscopic tube. X-ray films are taken in various positions and at specific intervals to visualize the outline of the organs and to note the passage of the barium through the GI tract. The patient should understand that the procedure may take several hours depending on the rate at which the barium moves through the patient's GI tract.

A laxative is usually ordered after the procedure to expel the barium and prevent constipation or a barium **impaction** (impassable mass of stonelike feces). The patient is instructed to drink 12 eight-ounce glasses of water per day for several days to prevent dehydration, which can lead to constipation. The abdomen is assessed for distention and bowel sounds. The stool is monitored to determine whether the barium has been completely eliminated. Initially, the barium causes the patient's stool to be white, but it should return to its normal color within 3 days. Constipation with distention indicates a barium impaction.

Lower Gastrointestinal Series

The **lower GI series** (barium enema) is performed to visualize the position, movements, and filling of the colon. Tumors, diverticula, stenosis, obstructions, inflammation, ulcerative colitis, and polyps can be detected. The patient is placed on a low-residue or clear liquid diet for 2 to 5 days before the test to empty the bowel. Laxatives, bowel-cleansing solutions and enemas may be administered the

• WORD • BUILDING •

steatorrhea: steato—fat + rrhea—flow
fluoroscope: fluor—a flowing + skopein—to look at

evening before the test or split between the evening before and very early on the morning of the examination. GoLYTELY is chilled and drunk full strength with no ice, 8 ounces every 10 minutes for a total of 4 L. Drinking this solution can be unpleasant for the patient. Inform the patient that a watery diarrhea will begin in about 1 hour and continue for up to 5 hours as the bowel is cleared. Other bowel preparations are available such as sodium picosulfate/magnesium oxide/anhydrous citric acid or polyethylene glycol (Miralax). Bowel preparation is necessary for adequate visualization during the procedure. Inadequate bowel preparation may result in poor test results or test cancellation (Fig. 32.6). The patient either receives a clear liquid diet the morning of the test up to 2 to 4 hours before the test or is NPO after midnight the night before. The area around the rectum should be clean before the patient is sent for the procedure. If the patient has active inflammatory disease of the colon or suspected perforation or obstruction, a barium enema is contraindicated. Active GI bleeding may also prohibit the use of laxatives and enemas.

During the procedure, barium is instilled rectally and x-ray films are taken with or without fluoroscopy. The patient may experience some abdominal cramping and an urge to have a bowel movement during the procedure. The patient is told to take slow, deep breaths and to tighten the anal sphincter. The rate of flow of the barium is slowed until the cramping diminishes. The procedure takes about 15 minutes, and the patient is allowed to use the bathroom immediately after the procedure.

The patient's stools are monitored after the procedure to note if all the barium is passed, as with the UGI series. Constipation development is monitored. The patient is encouraged to drink at least one 8-ounce glass of liquid per hour for the next 24 waking hours to help remove the barium. Laxatives may be ordered to help clear the barium from the colon. The patient is told to report any abdominal pain, bloating, or absence of stool, all of which could indicate constipation or bowel obstruction, as well as any rectal bleeding.

FIGURE 32.6 (A) An image of a patient who was poorly prepared for a barium enema. (B) An image of a patient who was adequately prepared for a barium enema. *Courtesy Dr. Russell Tobe.*

CRITICAL THINKING

Mrs. Pearl

■ Mrs. Pearl is a 95-year-old woman undergoing a lower GI series for abdominal pain. As her nurse, what concerns might you have for Mrs. Pearl as she undergoes this test? How can you address them?

Nuclear Scanning

Nuclear scanning of the gallbladder involves injecting a patient with a small amount of radioactive isotope. The scan is called a cholescintigraphy, DISIDA, HIDA, or PIPIDA scan, depending on the radioactive isotope and exact procedure that is used. A patient may be given a fatty meal or cholecystokinin to stimulate emptying of the gallbladder. Any biliary disease, ejection problem, or obstruction can be confirmed with this examination.

Liver Scan

A liver scan involves injecting a slightly radioactive medium that is taken up by the liver. An instrument is passed over the liver that records the amount of material taken up by the liver and forms a composite picture of the liver. The HCP may be able to determine tumors, masses, and abnormal size and patterns of blood vessels. The procedure takes a short time.

Endoscopy

Esophagogastroduodenoscopy

Esophagogastroduodenoscopy (EGD) visualizes the esophagus (**esophagoscopy**), the stomach (**gastroscopy**), and the duodenum (Fig. 32.7). Conscious sedation, for example, midazolam (Versed), is used to relax and ease pain during the procedure. Sometimes a local anesthetic in spray or gargle form is given to inhibit the gag reflex. Abnormalities such as inflammation, cancer, bleeding, injury, and infection can be seen. Biopsy or cytology specimens can be obtained.

After the procedure, vital signs are monitored. If the patient had a local anesthetic for the throat, keep patient NPO and check for gag reflex return before allowing fluids or food (usually within 4 hours). Patients are assessed for signs of perforation, which include bleeding, fever, and dysphagia. Midesophageal perforation can cause referred substernal or epigastric pain. Blood loss secondary to perforation can lead to hematoma formation, which in turn can result in cyanosis and referred back pain. Distal esophageal perforation may result in shoulder pain, dyspnea, or symptoms similar to those of a perforated ulcer. The patient may have a sore throat for a few days.

Capsule **endoscopy** makes use of a capsule with a microchip in it that is swallowed. As the capsule moves through the GI tract, pictures are taken of the stomach and small intestine to diagnose conditions such as bleeding, tumors, or Crohn's disease. It is most helpful in the small intestine, which is difficult to scope because of its length and twists. Advances in this technology are focusing on the power supply and performing treatments as with an endoscope.

Endoscopic Retrograde Cholangiopancreatography

Endoscopic **retrograde cholangiopancreatography** (ERCP) permits the HCP to visualize the liver, gallbladder, and pancreas (Fig. 32.8). The procedure allows both direct viewing and use of contrast medium and intervention if needed such

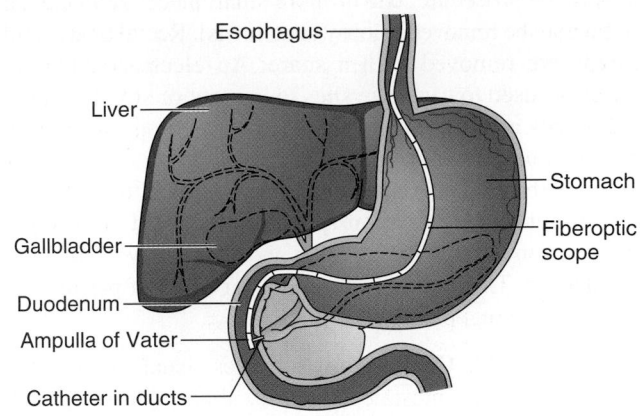

FIGURE 32.8 Endoscopic retrograde cholangiopancreatography. Modified from Watson, J., & Jaffe, S. (1995). *Nurse's manual of laboratory and diagnostic tests* (2nd ed.). Philadelphia: F.A. Davis, p. 525, with permission.

as biopsy, stone or tumor removal, stricture balloon dilation, or bile duct stent placement. An endoscope is passed through the esophagus to the duodenum, where dye is injected that outlines the pancreatic and bile ducts.

The patient is prepared for an ERCP in the same manner as for an EGD. NPO times can vary (8–12 hours) before the procedure. In addition, the patient is asked about allergies to contrast agents. Ensure that any ordered laboratory studies have been done before the procedure and that the patient has removed dentures. Postprocedure pancreatitis can develop. A pancreatic stent may be placed to help prevent this in certain patients. Follow-up care is similar to that for an EGD. In addition, the nurse is alert to patient reports of increased right upper quadrant pain, fever, or chills, which may indicate infection. Hypotension, tachycardia or rapid heart rate, increasing RUQ pain, nausea, or vomiting may indicate perforation or the onset of pancreatitis. Report such findings immediately.

Lower Gastrointestinal Endoscopy

PROCTOSIGMOIDOSCOPY. **Proctosigmoidoscopy** is the examination of the distal sigmoid colon, the rectum, and the anal canal using a flexible endoscope (sigmoidoscope). Ulcerations, punctures, lacerations, tumors, hemorrhoids, polyps, fissures, fistulas, and abscesses can be detected. Malignancies at an early stage can be detected, so an examination for patients age 50 and older is recommended every 5 years.

Proctosigmoidoscopy requires the lower bowel to be cleaned out. The patient usually receives a clear liquid diet 24 hours before the test and a laxative the night before the test. The morning of the procedure a warm tap-water enema, or sodium biphosphate (Fleet) enema may be given. Bowel preparation may not be ordered for patients with bleeding or severe diarrhea.

The patient is positioned in a left lateral knee-to-chest position, which allows the sigmoid colon to straighten by gravity. A rigid proctoscope is used to visualize the rectum. A flexible scope is then used to permit visualization above the rectosigmoid junction. Patients are told they may feel pressure as though they are going to have a bowel movement.

FIGURE 32.7 Gastroscopy.

During the procedure, one or more small pieces of intestinal tissue may be removed (biopsy specimens). Rectal or sigmoid polyps are removed with a snare. An electrocoagulating current is used to cauterize sites to prevent or stop bleeding. Specimens are labeled and sent to the pathology laboratory immediately for examination.

After the procedure, the patient is allowed to rest for a few minutes in the supine position to avoid orthostatic hypotension when standing. Pain and flatus may occur from instilled air. The patient is observed for signs of perforation such as bleeding, pain, and fever.

COLONOSCOPY. **Colonoscopy** provides visualization of the lining of the large intestine to identify abnormalities through a flexible endoscope, which is inserted rectally. A biopsy specimen may be obtained or polyps removed during the colonoscopy.

The patient receives a clear liquid diet 24 hours before the test and is NPO after midnight before the procedure. A bowel preparation solution is given the night before the procedure such as a laxative, suppository (bisacodyl [Dulcolax]), or enema. Bowel preparations similar to lower GI series can be used.

BE SAFE!

Older patients may experience fatigue and weakness during bowel preparation and may be unable to complete it. Monitor the patient for distress. Consult the HCP if you note any patient distress during bowel preparation. Observe the patient often because defecation urgency, especially in unfamiliar surroundings, may create a fall risk.

Conscious sedation is used. The patient is positioned on the left side with the knees bent. A small amount of air is instilled into the colon to help the HCP visualize the bowel. The air causes pressure and may be uncomfortable for the patient. The patient is encouraged to relax and take slow deep breaths through the nose and out the mouth. Vital signs are monitored throughout the procedure to watch for a vasovagal response, which can lead to hypotension and bradycardia.

After the procedure, the patient is monitored until stable. Complications such as hemorrhage or severe pain are reported. When giving the patient discharge instructions, explain that flatus and cramping will occur for several hours after the test, that blood may be present in the stool if a biopsy specimen was taken, and to report problems to the HCP.

Gastric Analysis

Gastric analysis measures the secretions in the stomach. Diagnoses of duodenal ulcer, gastric carcinoma, pyloric or duodenal obstruction, and pernicious anemia are made with

this test. A diagnosis of pernicious anemia is ruled out by the finding of acid. A diagnosis of gastric carcinoma may be made by the presence of cancer cells in the gastric secretions. The two gastric analysis tests performed are the **basal cell secretion test** and the **gastric acid stimulation test**.

Before the basal cell secretion test, the patient should avoid taking any drugs that could interfere with gastric acid secretion, such as cholinergics and antacids. The patient is NPO after midnight the night before the test. For the procedure, a NG tube is inserted and the contents of the stomach are suctioned out through the tube using a syringe. The NG tube is connected to wall suction, and stomach contents are collected every 15 minutes for 1 hour. The specimens are labeled according to the time they were collected and the order in which they were obtained. The gastric acid is tested for pH using indicator paper or a pH meter. The amount of gastric acid is also measured. Too much hydrochloric acid may indicate a peptic ulcer; too little could be a sign of cancer or pernicious anemia.

The gastric acid stimulation test measures the amount of gastric acid for 1 hour after subcutaneous injection of a histamine drug. If abnormal results occur, radiographic tests or endoscopy can be done to determine the cause.

Percutaneous Liver Biopsy

If less invasive tests do not aid in diagnosis of liver disease, a liver biopsy can be done. This type of biopsy can identify cancer, cirrhosis, hepatitis, or other causes of liver disease. The HCP generally inserts a needle through the skin and into the liver to withdraw a small sample for examination. This procedure places the patient at risk for bleeding because the liver is highly vascular and because many patients with liver disease have reduced clotting ability.

During the procedure the nurse assists the HCP to position the patient on his or her back or left side and assists the patient to hold very still while the needle is being introduced. The HCP may also ask the patient to exhale and hold his or her breath during the needle insertion.

After the biopsy, the patient should remain on bed rest for 24 hours. The patient lies on the right side for the first 2 hours with a small pillow or rolled towel under the biopsy site to provide pressure and prevent bleeding. Vital signs and the site are monitored for signs of bleeding. The patient is advised to avoid coughing or straining. Analgesics are offered for comfort if ordered.

See Table 32.8 for a summary of diagnostic procedures for the GI system.

CRITICAL THINKING

Mr. Wozynski

■ Mr. Wozynski is admitted with chronic liver failure and jaundice. What specific laboratory value can you expect to be elevated related to his jaundice? Mr. Wozynski's HCP orders a liver biopsy. Why is it important for you to check Mr. Wozynski's laboratory reports before the procedure?
Suggested answers are at the end of the chapter.

TABLE 32.8   DIAGNOSTIC PROCEDURES FOR THE GASTROINTESTINAL SYSTEM

Procedure	Definition/Normal Finding	Significance of Abnormal Findings	Nursing Management
Noninvasive Upper GI series	X-ray examination of esophagus, stomach, duodenum, and jejunum using oral liquid radiopaque contrast medium. Fluoroscope outlines contours of the organs. Normal finding should show normal anatomical structures.	Used to detect strictures, ulcers, tumors, polyps, hiatal hernias, and motility problems.	Clear liquid diet night before procedure. NPO for 6–8 hours before test. No smoking the morning of procedure. Provide increased fluids and laxative after procedure.
Lower GI series (barium enema)	Colon is filled with barium and x-rays taken to visualize position, movements, and filling of colon. Normal finding would be no polyps, inflammation, diverticula, stenosis, or tumors.	Tumors, diverticula, stenosis, obstructions, inflammation, ulcerative colitis, and polyps can be detected.	Patient is placed on low-residue or clear liquid diet for 2 days before test. Laxatives, bowel cleansing solutions, and enemas may be given the evening before the test. Bowel needs to be adequately cleaned for adequate visualization during the test. Encourage fluids and possibly laxatives to clear barium from colon.
Invasive Nuclear scanning (cholescintigraphy, di-isopropyl iminodiacetic acid scintigraphy [DISIDA], hepatobiliary iminodiacetic acid [HIDA] scan, or iminodiacetic acid [IDA])	Involves injecting patient with a small amount of IV radioactive isotope. Serial images of gallbladder, bile duct, and duodenum are recorded. Normal finding is no evidence of biliary disease, obstruction, or ejection problems.	Confirms any biliary disease, ejection problem, or obstruction.	Fast for 2–6 hours before procedure. May be given cholecystokinin.
Esophagogastroduodenoscopy (EGD)	Endoscopy that visualizes esophagus, stomach, and duodenum. Biopsy or cytology specimens can be obtained. Normal findings indicate all normal structures without inflammation, bleeding, or cancer.	Abnormalities such as inflammation, cancer, bleeding, injury, and infection can be detected.	May use a preoperative checklist. NPO for 8–12 hours. May need to premedicate to relax patient. Monitor vital signs and prevent aspiration after procedure. Monitor for pain, bleeding, fever, and dysphagia after procedure.
Endoscopic retrograde cholangiopancreatography (ERCP)	Endoscopy that permits HCP to visualize liver, gallbladder, and pancreas.	Liver, gallbladder, or pancreas disease.	See EGD. NPO after 20:00 the night before exam. Check prothrombin time before procedure.

Continued

TABLE 32.8   **DIAGNOSTIC PROCEDURES FOR THE GASTROINTESTINAL SYSTEM—cont'd**

Procedure	Definition/Normal Finding	Significance of Abnormal Findings	Nursing Management
	May use contrast medium. Endoscope passed through esophagus to duodenum, where dye is injected that outlines pancreatic and bile ducts. Normal findings indicate all normal structures without inflammation, bleeding, or cancer.		Monitor for pain, fever, chills, which could indicate infection. Monitor for onset of pancreatitis.
Proctosigmoidoscopy	Examination of distal sigmoid colon, rectum, and anal canal using a rigid or flexible endoscope (sigmoidoscope). Normal finding would be no ulcerations, punctures, laceration, tumors, hemorrhoids, polyps, fissures, or fistulas.	Ulcerations, punctures, lacerations, tumors, hemorrhoids, polyps, fissures, fistulas, early malignancies, and abscesses can be detected.	Clear liquid diet for 24 hours before exam. Laxative the night before exam. Enemas the morning of exam.
Colonoscopy	Visualization of lining of the large intestine to identify abnormalities through a flexible endoscope, inserted rectally. Biopsy specimen may be obtained or polyps removed. Normal finding would show a normal colon without signs of inflammation, ulcers, polyps, or cancer.	Colon cancer, polyps, inflammation.	Clear liquid diet for 24 hours before exam. Bowel preparation the night before exam. Possibly enemas the evening before exam and morning of exam. Patient will receive conscious sedation during exam. Monitor for complications, such as hemorrhage and severe pain. Explain that cramping may last several hours after test, and blood may be present in stool if specimen was taken.
Analysis • Basal cell secretion test	Measures secretions in the stomach. For basal cell secretion test, nasogastric tube is inserted and contents of stomach suctioned out through tube using a syringe. Stomach contents are collected at intervals.	Diagnosis of duodenal ulcer, gastric carcinoma, pyloric or duodenal obstruction, and pernicious anemia are made.	Patient should avoid drugs that could interfere with gastric acid secretion, such as cholinergics and antacids. Patient is NPO after midnight the night before test.
• Gastric acid stimulation test	Measures amount of gastric acid for 1 hour after subcutaneous injection of a histamine.		

TABLE 32.8   DIAGNOSTIC PROCEDURES FOR THE GASTROINTESTINAL SYSTEM—cont'd

Procedure	Definition/Normal Finding	Significance of Abnormal Findings	Nursing Management
• Percutaneous liver biopsy	Usually a needle inserted through skin and into liver to withdraw a small sample for examination. Normal finding would be negative for cancer, cirrhosis, hepatitis, or other liver diseases.	May identify cancer, cirrhosis, hepatitis, or other causes of liver disease.	Signed consent needed. Ensure laboratory tests such as complete blood count and coagulation studies have been ordered and reviewed. NPO for 6–8 hours before procedure. Rest for several hours after procedure; restricted activity 1 day. Monitor biopsy site pressure dressing for bleeding. Monitor vital signs after procedure. Coughing and straining avoided after the procedure. Medicate for pain.

THERAPEUTIC MEASURES FOR THE GASTROINTESTINAL, HEPATOBILIARY, AND PANCREATIC SYSTEMS

Gastrointestinal Intubation

GI intubation is the placement of a tube within the GI tract for therapeutic or diagnostic purposes (Fig. 32.9). When the GI tube is inserted orally into the stomach it is an orogastric tube. When it goes from the nares into the stomach, it is referred to as a nasogastric tube. A variety of tubes are available, each designed for specific purposes (Table 32.9). Orogastric tubes reduce sinus infection risk because they do not block normal drainage of the sinuses, as can nasal tubes. GI intubation is done for a variety of reasons:

• To remove gas and fluids from the stomach (decompression)
• To diagnose GI motility and to obtain gastric secretions for analysis
• To relieve and treat obstructions or bleeding within the GI tract
• To provide a means for nutrition (**gavage** feeding), hydration, and medication when the oral route is not possible or is contraindicated
• To promote healing after esophageal, gastric, or intestinal surgery by preventing distention of the GI tract and strain on the suture lines
• To remove toxic substances (**lavage**) that have been ingested either accidentally or intentionally and to provide for irrigation.

Feeding tubes include nasogastric, esophagostomy, **gastrostomy**, or jejunostomy tubes (see Fig. 32.9). NG tubes are usually temporary and short term. Esophagostomy, gastrostomy, or jejunostomy tubes are generally used for longer-term nutrition delivery.

Provide emotional support and explanations to the patient and significant others to facilitate the process of tube insertion and maintenance. Assessing tube placement is essential to prevent complications or death from incorrect tube placement. NG tube placement must be assessed after insertion and then intermittently to ensure that it is in the correct position and not in the lungs (most common), esophagus, pleural space, or brain. (See DavisPlus for procedures on the insertion and maintenance of nasogastric tubes.)

Gastrostomy or jejunostomy tube placement is verified by comparing current exposed length with documented exposed length at insertion. The tube may not be in the desired position if the current and insertion exposed tube lengths are different, so the HCP should be consulted before using the tube.

Enteral Nutrition

Enteral nutrition supplies patients with nutrition when oral intake is not possible. Feedings can be given to the patient as a supplement or to provide the patient's total nutritional needs. The esophagus and stomach might need to be bypassed due to inability to swallow, severe burns or trauma to the face or jaw, debilitation, and oropharyngeal or esophageal paralysis. Enteral feedings are delivered directly into the duodenum or proximal jejunum. Patients may benefit

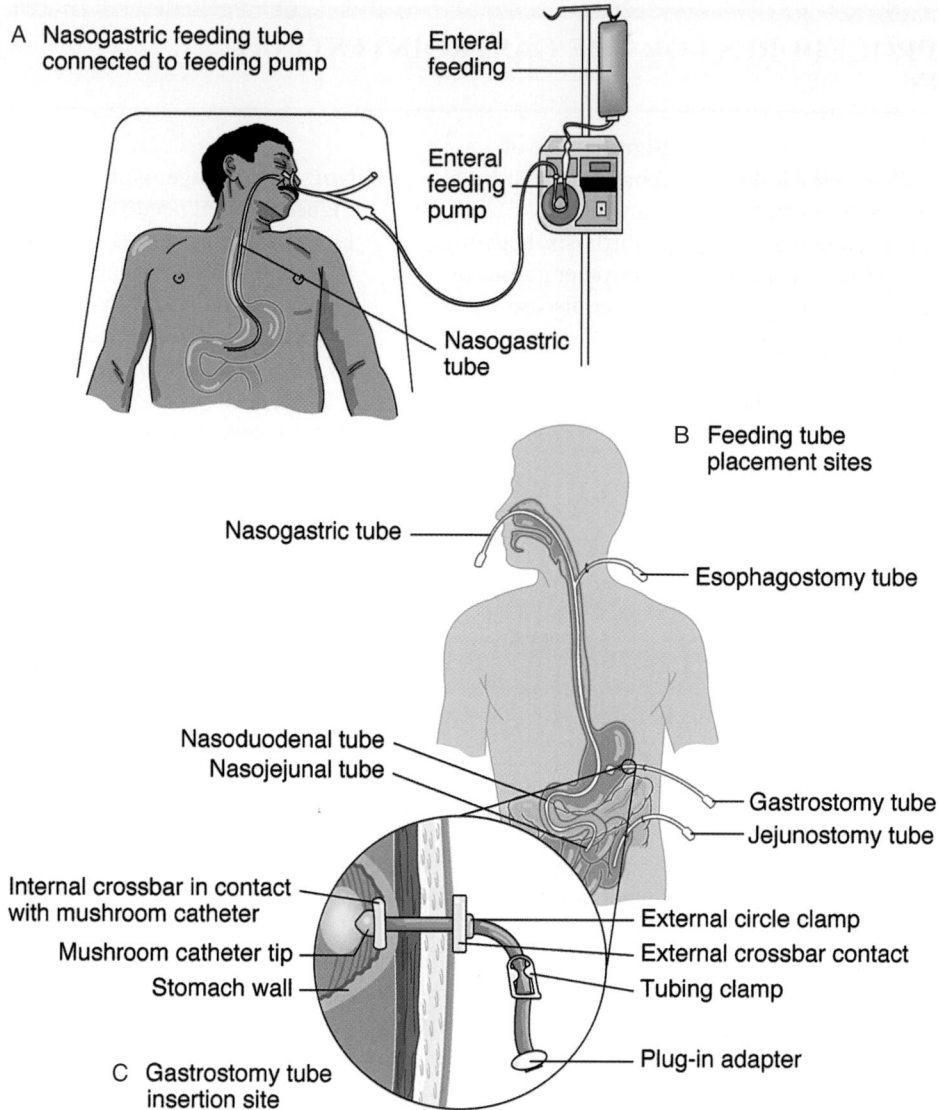

A Nasogastric feeding tube connected to feeding pump

Enteral feeding

Enteral feeding pump

Nasogastric tube

B Feeding tube placement sites

Nasogastric tube

Esophagostomy tube

Nasoduodenal tube
Nasojejunal tube

Gastrostomy tube
Jejunostomy tube

Internal crossbar in contact with mushroom catheter

Mushroom catheter tip

Stomach wall

External circle clamp

External crossbar contact

Tubing clamp

Plug-in adapter

C Gastrostomy tube insertion site

FIGURE 32.9 Feeding tubes. (A) Nasogastric tube connected to feeding tube pump. (B) Feeding tube placement sites (esophagostomy, nasointestinal, gastrostomy, and jejunostomy). (C) Gastrostomy tube insertion site.

from either oral or enteral nutrition within 24 hours postoperatively from GI surgery. Complications associated with enteral nutrition are presented in Table 32.10.

Enteral Nutrition Formulas

Enteral nutrition formulas are prescribed by the HCP based on the patient's nutritional needs, the consistency of the formula, the size and location of the tube, the method of delivery, and the convenience for the patient at home. Commercially prepared formulas are composed of protein, carbohydrates, and fats. When patients receive enteral nutrition, their daily water needs in addition to any water supplied by the feeding should be considered. Dietitians can help calculate the patient's free water needs. The water used to flush the tube or administer medications can be considered as meeting part of the patient's daily total water needs. Dehydration can occur if the patient's water needs are not met.

Method of Enteral Feeding Delivery

Feedings are administered either by gravity or by a controlled pump that delivers continuous volume through the feeding tube. Gravity feedings are placed above the level of the stomach and dripped in by gravity slowly or given as a bolus feeding over a few minutes. Intermittent feedings are defined as either being delivered by a pump that runs continuously throughout the day and is discontinued each night or as a 4- to 6-hour volume of feeding given over 20 to 30 minutes. Intermittent feedings via a pump allow the stomach to rest at night and more closely simulate normal eating and nutrient absorption patterns. A continuous feeding administered 24 hours a day through a pump allows for small amounts to be given over a long period. Pumps are set at the specified rate to control the speed of the feeding being delivered to the patient.

When feedings are administered, patients must be positioned in a sitting or high-Fowler's position to reduce the risk

TABLE 32.9 GASTRIC TUBES

Tube	Uses and Description	Nursing Considerations
Levin tube	Single lumen. May be used for gastric decompression, irrigation, lavage, and feeding.	Tube is not vented. Avoid use with continuous suction to prevent injury to stomach lining.
Salem sump tube	Double lumen, "pigtail" acts as an air vent and prevents excess suction, which could damage stomach lining. Air vent must not be plugged off. Used for decompression, irrigations, and lavage.	May be used with continuous suction because of air vent.
Weighted, flexible feeding tubes with stylets	Small-bore tube for enteral feeding only. Less injury. Remains in place for extended periods.	Suction collapses tube. Use 10-mL syringe or greater because smaller syringe creates too much pressure, possible rupture of tube. Inject 30 mL of air with a 60-mL syringe immediately before withdrawing fluid to make it easier to withdraw.

Note. NPO = nothing by mouth.

TABLE 32.10 COMMON MECHANICAL, GASTROINTESTINAL, AND METABOLIC COMPLICATIONS OF TUBE-FED PATIENTS AND PREVENTION STRATEGIES

Complication	Prevention Strategies
Mechanical Tube irritation	Consider oral tubes and avoid nasal tubes due to sinus infection risk. Oral tubes also help prevent ventilator-associated pneumonia. Consider using a smaller or softer tube. Lubricate tube before insertion. Make sure tube is secured in place.
Tube obstruction	Flush tube with water after each use and before and after medication administration. Do not mix medications with tube-feeding formula. Use liquid medications if available. Crush other medications thoroughly (if not contraindicated). Use infusion pump to maintain constant flow (see Fig. 32.9).
Aspiration and regurgitation	Feeding should not be started until tube placement is radiographically confirmed. Avoid use of blue dye to detect aspiration because it has not been shown predictive, and dye can be absorbed in critically ill patients, who then turn blue and can die. Elevate head of patient's bed 30 degrees or more at all times. Discontinue feeding at least 30–60 minutes before treatments requiring head to be lowered (e.g., chest percussion). If patient has an endotracheal tube in place, keep cuff inflated during feeding.
Tube displacement	Place a black mark at the point where tube, when properly placed, exits the nostril. Measure exposed length for future placement verification. Replace tube and obtain HCP's order to confirm with x-ray imaging.

Continued

TABLE 32.10 COMMON MECHANICAL, GASTROINTESTINAL, AND METABOLIC COMPLICATIONS OF TUBE-FED PATIENTS AND PREVENTION STRATEGIES—cont'd

Complication	Prevention Strategies
Gastrointestinal	
Cramping, distention, bloating, gas pains, nausea, vomiting, diarrhea*	Practice good personal hygiene when handling any feeding product. Bring formula to room temperature before feeding. Initiate and increase amount of formula gradually. Change to a lactose-free formula. Decrease fat content of formula. Administer drug therapy as ordered (e.g., Lactinex, kaolin-pectin, Lomotil). Change to formula with a lower osmolality. Change to formula with a different fiber content. Evaluate diarrhea-causing medications patient may be receiving (e.g., antibiotics, digitalis preparations).
Metabolic	
Dehydration	Note patient's fluid requirements before treatment. Monitor hydration status. Provide adequate daily water.
Overhydration	Note patient's fluid requirements before treatment. Monitor hydration status.
Hyperglycemia	Initiate feeding at a slow rate. Monitor blood glucose. Use hyperglycemic medication if needed. Select a low-carbohydrate formula.
Hypernatremia	Note patient's fluid and electrolyte status before treatment. Provide adequate fluids.
Hyponatremia	Note patient's fluid and electrolyte status before treatment. Restrict fluids. Supplement feeding with rehydration solution and saline. Diuretic therapy may be beneficial.
Hypophosphatemia	Monitor serum level. Replenish phosphorus before refeeding.
Hypercapnia	Select a low-carbohydrate, high-fat formula.
Hypokalemia	Monitor potassium level. Supplement feeding with potassium if needed.
Hyperkalemia	Reduce potassium intake. Monitor potassium level.

Note. Modified from Lutz, C. A., & Przytulski, K. R. (2014). *Nutrition & diet therapy* (6th ed.). Philadelphia: F.A. Davis.
  *The most commonly cited complication of enteral feeding is diarrhea.

of aspiration. Monitor the rate carefully to avoid administering feedings too rapidly, and watch for signs that the feeding is not being absorbed. Abdominal distention, patient report of a feeling of fullness, and nausea or vomiting are indicators that the feeding is not being absorbed and should be stopped to prevent aspiration. A residual check to see how much feeding, if any, has not been absorbed is done hourly when the feeding is initiated, then every 4 hours or before giving any medications or adding more feeding for infusion. If there is more than 100 mL or the amount specified by the agency or HCP, the feeding should be stopped to prevent vomiting or aspiration and the HCP notified. Continuous or intermittent feedings reduce the risk of aspiration, distention, nausea, vomiting, and diarrhea.

If medications are administered during enteral feeding, understand possible drug–nutrient interactions. Some medications cannot be given with certain substances. Other medications, such as enteric-coated or sustained-release medications, should not be crushed. Liquid medications should be used when possible to reduce clogging of the tube. Pharmacists and dietitians should be consulted for special considerations.

Gastrointestinal Decompression

GI decompression may be necessary when the stomach or small intestine becomes filled with air or fluid. Swallowed air and GI secretions enter the stomach and intestines and collect there if they are not propelled through the GI tract by peristalsis. Accumulating air or fluid causes distention, a feeling of fullness, and possibly pain in the abdomen. Gastric distention may occur after major abdominal surgery. Ambulating or turning the patient frequently can help prevent this. However, when GI decompression is necessary, a NG tube or occasionally a nasointestinal tube may be inserted and suction applied. Nasointestinal tubes are more difficult and slower to place and may be uncomfortable, so they are not used often. The tube remains in place until full peristaltic activity (active bowel sounds and passage of flatus) has returned. The diet is then progressed as ordered and tolerated by the patient.

BE SAFE!

Incorrect connection of enteral feeding equipment is a hazard to patient safety. An enteral feeding incorrectly connected and administered through a nonenteral system (such as an IV line, peritoneal dialysis catheter, oxygen tubing, or tracheostomy tube cuff) can result in patient injury or death. Luer connections require extra caution. Equipment redesigns have been undertaken to make these types of faulty connections less possible. Nurses must be vigilant to ensure that they understand the appropriate use of the equipment and all tubing connections being made to prevent harmful errors:

- Avoid rigging connections that may impair designed safety features.
- Package together all parts needed for enteral feeding within the agency to avoid improper equipment being selected and connected.
- Label or color-code feeding tubes and connectors within the institution.
- Verify the solution's label (a 3-in-1 parenteral nutrition solution looks similar to enteral nutrition).

- Label enteral bags with large words such as "ALERT! For Enteral Use Only."
- Use adequate room lighting when working with equipment.
- Route tubes/catheters with different purposes in standardized directions (IV lines routed toward the patient's head; enteric lines routed toward the feet).
- If disconnection occurs, only staff familiar with the equipment should make a reconnection.
- During a reconnection, always trace the lines back to their origins and then ensure that they are secure.
- During the handoff process, trace all tubes to their origin and check connections.

CRITICAL THINKING

Mrs. Wood

■ Mrs. Wood is receiving enteral nutrition because of dysphagia, the cause of which is being investigated. Mrs. Wood is not receiving any medications. You note that Mrs. Wood's tongue is bright red with deep furrows. She states her mouth is very dry. Her skin remains tented when skin turgor is checked.

1. What do Mrs. Wood's data collection findings indicate?
2. How would you document your findings?
3. What other data should you gather?
4. Why might Mrs. Wood be exhibiting this condition?
5. What actions could you take for this condition?
6. How would you record the total of Mrs. Wood's 8-hour intake, which is an enteral feeding at 50 mL per hour?

Suggested answers are at the end of the chapter.

Parenteral Nutrition

Parenteral nutrition (PN) is a method of supplying nutrients to the patient by a **central or peripheral IV** route. PN solutions usually contain dextrose (sugar), amino acids (protein), vitamins, minerals, and fat (intralipid) emulsions. PN solutions are designed to improve the patient's nutritional status, achieve weight gain, and enhance the healing process. Patients with conditions such as burns, trauma, cancer, acquired immunodeficiency syndrome (AIDS), malnutrition, anorexia nervosa, or fever and those undergoing major surgery may need PN.

NURSING CARE TIP

Patients with any of the following may need to be considered for PN:

- Any significant weight loss (10% or more of healthy weight)
- A decrease of oral food intake for more than 3 days
- Any significant sign of protein loss: serum albumin levels below 3.2 g/dL
- Muscle wasting
- Decreased tissue healing
- Persistent vomiting and diarrhea.

Usually, RNs are responsible for administering PN. A filter might be required with PN solutions and possibly lipid solutions. It is important to monitor glucose levels as ordered and to look for signs of hyperglycemia in the patient receiving PN. Refer to agency policy for obtaining glucose levels when a hyperglycemic reaction is suspected in the patient receiving PN.

During PN administration, the following laboratory values, as ordered, are usually monitored:

- CBC
- Albumin
- Glucose
- Electrolytes
- Platelet count
- PT

PN can be irritating to the peripheral veins because it is five or six times more concentrated than blood. Therefore, PN dextrose more than 12% is administered through a central venous catheter into a large vein such as the subclavian or internal jugular (see Fig. 7.7). The volume in the large vein dilutes the PN solution, so it is less irritating.

LEARNING TIP

- Patients may respond to PN with an elevated serum glucose level, even though they do not have diabetes. This is due to the high concentration of glucose used in PN. These elevated serum glucose levels do not usually indicate that the patient who does not have diabetes has acquired the disease. After the PN is discontinued, the serum glucose levels should return to baseline or normal levels.
- Regular insulin is given, as ordered, to control hyperglycemia during PN therapy. The insulin is ordered on a sliding scale (regular insulin given based on blood glucose levels measured at ordered intervals over 24 hours) or as an additive to the PN solution, or both.
- Administration of insulin according to a sliding scale requires a current blood glucose level. Based on the obtained glucose level, if it is elevated, specified regular insulin units may be ordered. Usually blood glucose is measured before meals, but for a patient who is not eating, as with most patients receiving PN, there is no mealtime. Instead, specified time intervals are ordered (typically every 6 hours).
- Insulin given on a sliding scale is always regular insulin. Can you figure out why? Regular insulin is rapid acting, which is what is needed to treat the current blood glucose level that was obtained to determine what insulin coverage was needed, if any.

Home Health Hints

- Be familiar with community nutritional support services: the Women, Infants, and Children (WIC) program, nutrition sites for older adults, Meals on Wheels, school food programs, and government surplus food programs.
- Observe patient's food preparation facilities to ensure the patient's nutritional needs can be met. Some older patients may have outdated or spoiled food in their refrigerators or cupboards because they are unable to see dates or mold growing on foods.
- Ensure that patients are able to use appliances to heat food safely. Patients with limited vision may not see gas flames and can ignite their clothing. Confused patients might try to heat foods in

Peripheral Parenteral Nutrition

Peripheral parenteral nutrition (PPN) is a method of supplying nutrients to the patient by an IV route that is not a central vein. PPN is used for less than 10 days when the patient does not need more than 2000 calories daily. PPN solutions can contain a mixture of dextrose (of less than 12%), amino acids, and lipids, in addition to electrolytes or water, which can be found in routine IV solutions. The all-in-one PPN system mixes dextrose, amino acids, and lipids all in one container, which causes less vein irritation.

cardboard containers. If the patient is able to obtain and learn to use a microwave, it may be a safer cooking appliance than a stove.
- A feeding tube can be prevented from kinking by slipping a split straw lengthwise around the area

that tends to kink and lightly taping over the split in the straw.
- Wire coat hangers make good hooks for enteral feeding solution bags. They can be bent and hung over doorways or closet bars.

SUGGESTED ANSWERS TO

CRITICAL THINKING

■ *Mrs. Todd*

1. Daily aspirin use is the most likely cause of her bleeding.

2. Medication teaching including side effects can help Mrs. Todd prevent future bleeding episodes. Mrs. Todd should be instructed to take aspirin with food to minimize GI upset and help prevent formation of ulcers. Assessment of pain relief needs and consultation with the HCP will also help.

3. See Table 32.8.

■ *Mrs. Pearl*

Mrs. Pearl is at risk for dehydration and electrolyte loss as a result of the laxative and enema preparation and NPO status. This risk is increased because of her age. Her fluid and electrolyte status should be monitored closely.

Mrs. Pearl will likely have a concern about "making it" to the bathroom during the preparation and should have a bedside commode placed within easy reach. Her call light should be answered promptly. If enemas are ordered "until clear," Mrs. Pearl will be at greater risk for fluid and electrolyte loss. If more than two or three enemas are required, the HCP should be notified.

Older patients can become very fatigued during testing and test preparation. Mrs. Pearl should be allowed plenty of rest before and after the test. She may also have a concern about being able to hold the barium in her bowel during the test without having an "accident." She should be assured that the barium is held in with a balloon that is on the end of the enema catheter and that bathrooms are nearby.

■ *Mr. Wozynski*

You can expect to find that Mr. Wozynski's serum bilirubin is elevated because his liver is unable to convert

or conjugate bilirubin into a water-soluble compound that can be eliminated in feces. Mr. Wozynski is at risk for bleeding because the liver is highly vascular and prone to bleed when a biopsy specimen is taken. In addition, he may not be manufacturing the necessary amount of prothrombin needed for blood clotting and is less likely to stop bleeding once the biopsy has been performed. It will be especially important to check his coagulation studies and report any elevations to the HCP before the biopsy.

■ *Mrs. Wood*

1. Assessment of Mrs. Wood indicates dehydration.

2. Document as follows: "0800 'Mouth very dry.' Tongue bright red with deep furrows, tented turgor. Enteral feeding infusing (include solution and rate). Physician notified. K. Ohno, LVN."

3. You would assess Mrs. Wood's vital sign to look for changes such as increased heart rate, decreased blood pressure, and possibly mildly elevated temperature. The nurse would review current lab work if available for indications of dehydration such as elevated blood urea nitrogen (BUN) and elevated hematocrit (see Chapter 6).

4. Mrs. Wood's daily water needs are not being met. She is not receiving medications that would incidentally provide water during their administration.

5. Consult a dietitian and/or HCP to review Mrs. Wood's daily water needs. Divide the water needs over 24 hours and ensure that water is administered. Ensure tubing is flushed per agency policy, and calculate water used toward daily water needs. Monitor intake and output. Continue assessing Mrs. Wood's signs and symptoms, and report abnormal findings.

6. 50 mL × 8 hours = 400 mL.

REVIEW QUESTIONS

1. The nurse is collecting data on a patient with a ruptured appendix that is painful. Where would the nurse expect the patient's pain to be located?
   1. Right upper quadrant
   2. Right lower quadrant
   3. Left upper quadrant
   4. Left lower quadrant

2. The nurse is contributing to the plan of care for a 78-year-old patient's elimination needs. Which of the following interventions should the nurse recommend to reduce complications from the aging change of slowed motility?
   1. Decrease ambulation.
   2. Decrease fluid intake.
   3. Increase dairy products.
   4. Increase dietary fiber.

3. The nurse is listening to a patient's bowel sounds and hears them at an irregular rate every 5 to 15 seconds. How should the nurse document the findings?
   1. Normal bowel sounds heard every 5 to 15 seconds
   2. Hyperactive bowel sounds heard every 5 to 15 seconds
   3. Hypoactive bowel sounds heard every 5 to 15 seconds
   4. Abnormal bowel sounds heard every 5 to 15 seconds

4. Which of the following best describes the technique of palpation?
   1. Firmly place hands on abdomen, depressing tissues 1 to 2 inches.
   2. Randomly feel the patient's abdomen with fingertips.
   3. Lightly depress the abdomen 0.5 to 1 inch.
   4. Light palpation is completed by an experienced practitioner.

5. The nurse is contributing to the plan of care for a patient who is to have a lower GI series. Which of the following measures should the nurse recommend be included in the plan of care?
   1. Have the patient cough and deep breathe hourly while awake.
   2. Encourage fluids.
   3. Check for return of a gag reflex.
   4. Keep the patient in semi-Fowler's position.

6. A patient is admitted with an order for a sump tube (Salem sump). The nurse knows this tube is used for which of the following purposes? **Select all that apply.**
   1. Supplemental feeding
   2. Decompression
   3. Irrigation
   4. Lavage
   5. Gavage
   6. Parenteral nutrition

7. The nurse assisted with the insertion of a flexible feeding tube into a patient. Which of the following actions should the nurse take to confirm tube placement?
   1. Aspirate gastric contents for green-colored fluid.
   2. Measure the pH of secretions from tube.
   3. Obtain x-ray to check placement.
   4. Look in the back of the mouth for a coiled tube.

8. The nurse is caring for a patient who is receiving a PN infusion. The nurse would perform blood glucose monitoring every 6 hours to detect which complication?
   1. Hyponatremia
   2. Hyperkalemia
   3. Hypocalcemia
   4. Hyperglycemia

Answers can be found in Appendix C.

 DavisPlus | For additional resources and information visit **davispl.us/medsurg5**

Nursing Care of Patients With Upper Gastrointestinal Disorders

LAZETTE V. NOWICKI

LEARNING OUTCOMES

1. Explain nausea, vomiting, anorexia, anorexia nervosa, and bulimia nervosa.
2. Describe therapeutic measures and nursing care for nausea, vomiting, anorexia, anorexia nervosa, and bulimia nervosa.
3. Describe medical, surgical, and nursing management for obesity.
4. Plan nursing care for a patient with stomatitis.
5. Plan nursing care for patients with acute or chronic gastritis.
6. Explain the pathophysiology, signs and symptoms, and diagnostic testing for hiatal hernia, peptic ulcer disease, gastric bleeding, and gastric cancer.
7. List current pharmacological treatments used for peptic ulcer disease.
8. Plan nursing care for patients with hiatal hernia, peptic ulcer disease, gastric bleeding, and gastric cancer.

KEY TERMS

anorexia (AN-uh-REK-see-ah)
anorexia nervosa (AN-uh-REK-see-ah nur-VOH-sah)
aphthous stomatitis (AF-thus STOH-mah-TY-tiss)
bariatric (BEAR-ry-AT-trick)
bulimia nervosa (buh-LEE-mee-ah ner-VOH-sah)
gastrectomy (gast-TREK-tuh-mee)
gastritis (gas-TRY-tiss)
gastroduodenostomy (GAS-troh-DOO-oh-den-AW-stuh-mee)
gastrojejunostomy (GAS-troh-JAY-joo-NAW-stuh-mee)
Helicobacter pylori (HEH-lih-koh-back-tur PIE-lore-ee)
hiatal hernia (hy-YAY-tuhl HER-nee-ah)
obesity (oh-BEE-sih-tee)
peptic ulcer disease (PEP-tick UL-sir dih-ZEEZ)
Roux-en-Y (roo-ehn-WHY)
steatorrhea (STEE-ah-toh-REE-ah)
stomatitis (STOH-mah-TY-tiss)

NAUSEA AND VOMITING

Nausea is the subjective feeling of the urge to vomit. Vomiting is the act of expelling stomach contents from the body through the esophagus and mouth. It is a protective function to rid the body of harmful substances from the gastrointestinal (GI) tract. This reflex is controlled by the vomiting center of the brain. Stimuli and conditions that are directly related to the GI tract or independent of it can trigger nausea and vomiting. Viral GI infection and other infections, motion sickness, stress, pregnancy, medications (narcotics), myocardial infarction, uremia, and other conditions may cause nausea and vomiting.

Therapeutic Measures

Nausea and vomiting may be self-limited and require no intervention. If it is prolonged, however, dehydration and electrolyte imbalances can occur. The loss of hydrochloric acid from the stomach can result in metabolic alkalosis. Emesis that looks like coffee grounds (dark brown) occurs from bleeding in the stomach and requires further assessment.

 BE SAFE!

Protection of the airway during vomiting is a priority to prevent aspiration. Those at risk of aspiration are persons who are unconscious, older, and experiencing gag reflex impairments. Place these types of persons on their side when they begin to vomit. This allows the gastric contents to be expelled from the mouth rather than pooling at the back of the throat and being aspirated.

If the cause of vomiting is known, it is treated. Antiemetics can be given to control nausea and vomiting. Ginger used with antiemetic medications may help ease nausea (see "Evidence-Based Practice"). For severe or prolonged vomiting, intravenous (IV) fluids and possibly nutrition need to be provided. Occasionally, an orogastric or nasogastric (NG) tube with suction may be ordered to decompress the stomach. After the vomiting is resolved, clear liquids are started, with water preferred. If liquids are tolerated, crackers or dry toast may be tolerated as well.

 EVIDENCE-BASED PRACTICE

Clinical Question
Does ginger help alleviate chemotherapy-induced nausea and vomiting (CINV)?

Evidence
Ginger has been used as a nonpharmacologic intervention to prevent and treat CINV as well as postoperative and pregnancy induced nausea and vomiting. Studies have been conducted to evaluate the effectiveness of ginger at relieving CINV in many patients. A systematic review was conducted of five randomized, controlled trials involving 872 patients with cancer. Ginger was compared with placebo or metoclopramide. The incidence and severity of acute and delayed CINV were subject to meta-analysis. The incidence of acute nausea ($p = .67$), incidence of acute vomiting ($p = .37$), and severity of acute nausea ($p = .12$) did not differ significantly between the ginger and control groups (Lee & Ho, 2013). In another meta-analysis, Marx et al (2013) found mixed results in that some patients experienced relief from CINV, but others had mixed results and some patients had no relief.

Implications for Nursing Practice
Research has not established that ginger is an effective means to control CINV. More research and controlled studies are needed before clinical use can be recommended.

REFERENCE
Lee, J., & Oh, H. (2013). Ginger as an antiemetic modality for chemotherapy-induced nausea and vomiting: A systematic review and meta-analysis. *Oncology Nursing Forum, 40,* 163–170.

Marx, W., Teleni, L., McCarthy, A., Vitetta, L., McKavanagh, D., Thomson, D., & Isenring, E. (2013). Ginger (*Zingiber officinale*) and chemotherapy-induced nausea and vomiting: A systematic literature review. *Nutrition Reviews, 71,* 245–254.

Nursing Process for the Patient With Nausea and Vomiting
Data Collection

The characteristics of the episodes of the nausea and vomiting are noted. Medical conditions, medications, and treatments are documented to aid in diagnosing the cause. Signs of early fluid deficit, such as weakness, headache, muscle cramps, restlessness, inability to concentrate, and postural hypotension, are reported for treatment. Later signs include confusion, oliguria, cold clammy skin, and chest or abdominal pain.

Nursing Diagnoses, Planning, and Implementation
Nausea related to various causes
EXPECTED OUTCOME: Patient will report no nausea or relief from nausea within 30 minutes of reporting nausea.

• Provide quiet, odor-free, visually clean environment *to avoid triggering stimuli.*
• Give antiemetics as ordered *to relieve nausea.*
• Provide frequent oral care *to remove emesis taste and enhance patient comfort.*

• Teach patient to avoid triggering fluids or foods *to prevent nausea and vomiting.*

Risk for Aspiration related to decreased gag reflex or unconsciousness

EXPECTED OUTCOME: Patient's airway and lung sounds will remain clear at all times.

• Identify patients who are nauseated and at risk of aspiration *to plan preventive care.*
• Turn patient onto side if nauseated and vomiting *to protect airway and prevent aspiration.*

Deficient Fluid Volume

EXPECTED OUTCOME: Patient's vital signs will remain within normal limits. Monitor for early signs of hypovolemia in patients with vomiting *to allow treatment and prevent complications.*

• Obtain daily weight on same scale, at same time of day, with same type of clothing *to detect fluid losses.* (A 1-pound weight loss reflects a fluid loss of 500 mL.)
• Monitor intake and output and vital signs including orthostatic blood pressure per shift or daily or more frequently as patient's condition indicates *to report changes for prompt treatment.*
• Provide fluids as ordered to hydrate patient. *IV fluids allow the GI tract to rest. Slightly chilled sports replacement drinks or ginger ale may be given in small amounts at frequent intervals.*
• Monitor older adults for excess fluid volume during treatment of deficient fluid volume *to prevent and detect fluid overload, which may occur quickly in the older adult.*

Evaluation

The patient's goals are met if nausea is not present, lung sounds remain clear, and vital signs remain within normal limits.

EATING DISORDERS

Anorexia

Anorexia, which is a lack of appetite, is a common symptom of many diseases and can be caused by noxious food odors, certain drugs (as an intended or side effect), emotional stress, fear, psychological problems, and infections. Prolonged anorexia with an inadequate nutritional intake can lead to serious electrolyte imbalances, which in turn can lead to cardiac dysrhythmias. Although eating is the preferred method of weight gain, other measures such as tube feedings and IV infusion can be used. Ask patients what causes them to lose their appetite and what improves it to plan their care. Nursing actions for the patient with anorexia include documenting accurate intake and output; monitoring vital signs, electrolytes, and electrocardiograms (ECGs); and monitoring the rate of the IV infusion and tube feeding.

Anorexia Nervosa

Anorexia nervosa is an eating disorder recognized by the American Psychiatric Association. This disease most commonly occurs in females between ages 12 and 18 who are from the middle and upper classes of Western culture. Males account for less than 10% of those with anorexia nervosa. Young women with low self-esteem seem to be at highest risk. Anorexia nervosa is thought to be psychological in origin. Patients may have a phobia about weight gain, be afraid of a loss of control, and be mistrusting.

Signs and Symptoms

Early signs and symptoms of anorexia nervosa include severe weight loss, low self-esteem, compulsive dieting, and an altered body image (patients imagine themselves as fat, although they are within or below normal weight range). As the disease progresses, additional symptoms appear, including electrolyte imbalance, cardiac dysrhythmias, constipation, dry skin, lanugo (downy hair covering body), bradycardia, hypothermia, hypotension, muscle wasting, and facial puffiness. Often patients with anorexia nervosa deny the existence of any problem. They may develop bizarre food rituals and sometimes weigh themselves several times a day.

Complications

Chronic poor nutritional health takes its toll on the body. Complications from starvation occur as the body tries to conserve energy. Pulse and blood pressure fall. Heart and kidney failure are a risk. Osteoporosis and muscle loss occur. Vitamin and electrolyte imbalances result. Diabetes may develop with a high morbidity.

Therapeutic Measures

Treating this disorder is complex and requires a multidisciplinary approach. Patients often do not see the need for medical intervention. They do not usually seek help on their own and are often resistant to treatment. When treatment is sought, often through a concerned person's urgings, a medical and psychological workup is necessary. Nutritional status is also evaluated to determine the urgency of intervention. Establishing a trusting relationship, which can be difficult, is a key element in initiating treatment. Early treatment results in a better prognosis.

What do you think would be the most important initial intervention for anorexia nervosa? The answer is the restoration of nutritional health. Up to 18% of anorexia patients eventually die as a result of starvation and complications. For those who are underweight with severe weight loss, life-threatening electrolyte imbalances and dysrhythmias or other symptoms, nutrition is supplied by IV infusions containing electrolytes. Oral food supplements may also need to be given. Restoring normal weight is a long, slow process. Gains may be small with setbacks along the way. Praise and rewards for small achievements in weight gains (not food intake) are positive reinforcements that aid recovery. Programs that treat eating disorders are often set up on a reward system, with privileges being increased as progress occurs.

The patient's damaged self-image and self-esteem are underlying causes of the disorder that must be addressed in conjunction with the nutritional aspect. Psychotherapy and behavior modification that include participation of the patient's significant others are used in treatment of anorexia nervosa. The altered body image is the main focus of therapy. Educating the patient on normal body weight can be helpful. Individual or group therapy is used. Family counseling may be used because childhood events often create the negative self-image. During treatment, a support system is vital to success. Visit www.nationaleatingdisorders.org for resources for patients and families.

Bulimia Nervosa

Bulimia nervosa is compulsive eating with self-induced vomiting, which is commonly known as binge–purge. A high percentage of patients with bulimia are young women.

The patient with bulimia typically eats massive amounts of food at one sitting and then purges the food by intentionally inducing vomiting so weight is not gained. Laxatives are also sometimes used by the bulimic patient to purge the body of food to avoid weight gain. Excessive exercise may also be used to control weight.

Signs and Symptoms

Patients with bulimia nervosa exhibit many of the same signs and symptoms as patients with anorexia nervosa, with a few exceptions. Bulimic patients often have enamel erosion of the front teeth and staining caused by the acid content of the emesis. They also spend a great deal of time locked in the bathroom vomiting, especially after meals. Electrolyte imbalances occur from dehydration. The loss of potassium and sodium may result in dysrhythmias, heart failure, and death. As the electrolyte imbalance worsens, metabolic alkalosis develops as a result of the loss of gastric acid in the stomach contents. Signs and symptoms of metabolic alkalosis include hypokalemia and hypocalcemia. Laxative use results in irregular bowel movements.

Therapeutic Measures

The treatment for bulimia nervosa is essentially the same as for the patient with anorexia nervosa.

Nursing Process for the Patient With an Eating Disorder

Why do you think caring for patients with eating disorders is challenging? Gaining the patient's genuine cooperation by using therapeutic communication and setting realistic, mutual goals is important for establishing trust and preventing relapse. To work with patients with an eating disorder, a therapeutic relationship must be developed to facilitate effective interactions. Empathy, acceptance of the patient, trust, warmth, and being nonjudgmental are important.

Data Collection

Data are collected related to inadequate nutrition. Note changes in weight (15% or more below expected weight), poor skin turgor, poor muscle tone, lanugo, amenorrhea, electrolyte imbalances, and hypothermia. Data collection findings may also include a normal weight, enamel erosion of front teeth, and metabolic alkalosis for the patient with bulimia. Note abnormal diagnostic studies such as anemia, electrolyte imbalances, altered endocrine studies, and ECG changes.

Nursing Diagnoses, Planning, and Implementation

Imbalanced Nutrition: Less Than Body Requirements related to inadequate food intake, self-induced vomiting, and/or chronic/excessive laxative use

EXPECTED OUTCOME: The patient will establish dietary pattern and gain weight toward desired individual weight range.

- Monitor patient's weight *to determine baseline and monitor patient's progress toward goal.*
- Monitor vital signs and laboratory studies *to detect changes in cardiac function related to electrolyte imbalances.*
- Promote consistent approach *to enhance acceptance by patient and to build trust.*
- Promote pleasant eating environment and record intake *to enhance patient intake.*
- Provide six small meals and snacks *to prevent gastric dilation.*

Disturbed Body Image related to psychosocial or cognitive/perceptual changes

EXPECTED OUTCOME: The patient will verbalize satisfaction with body appearance.

- Assess and document patient's verbal and nonverbal responses to own body *to provide baseline understanding of patient's perceptions of body image.*
- Listen to patient and acknowledge reality of concerns regarding treatment and progress *to establish therapeutic relationship.*
- Monitor frequency of negative statements about self *to determine if interventions are helping patient.*
- Assist with referrals to social services or counseling *to help patient overcome psychosocial issues.*
- Provide care in a nonjudgmental manner *to maintain the patient's dignity.*
- Use positive praise when patient verbalizes positive comments about own body.
- Encourage patient to verbalize consequences of eating disorder that have influenced self-concept *to help patient realize the negative impact of the eating disorder.*

Evaluation

The patient's goals are met if the patient gains weight toward expected weight goal and if the patient verbalizes satisfaction with body appearance and increases the number of positive statements about own appearance.

 OBESITY

Several methods can be used to diagnose a patient as overweight or obese, although there is no single, definitive measure of either. Factors such as age, body frame size, and gender can influence these measurements:

- *Height-weight chart:* Weight 10% to 20% above ideal body weight is overweight; 20% or more above ideal body weight is obese.
- *Waist-to-hip ratio:* Waist-to-hip ratio is waist measurement divided by hip measurement.
- *Body mass index (BMI):* BMI, calculated using height-to-weight ratios, is one of the best methods for defining **obesity** (see Fig. 33.1).

People who are overweight or obese are at increased risk for developing other diseases. Diseases associated with being overweight or obesity are called comorbidities and can include atherosclerosis, gallbladder disease, heart disease, hypertension, osteoarthritis, sleep apnea, type 2 diabetes mellitus, decreased mobility, lack of self-esteem, and depression. When combined with a high-fat diet, there is also an increased risk of breast, colon, rectum, and prostate cancer. For more information, visit the Centers for Disease Control and Prevention (CDC) at www.cdc.gov/nccdphp/dnpa/obesity/defining.htm.

Obesity is caused by a caloric intake that exceeds energy expenditure. Only a small percentage of obesity is associated with a metabolic or endocrine abnormality. Obesity that interferes with activities of daily living, such as breathing or walking, is known as morbid obesity. Morbid obesity refers to people whose BMI is above 40, which is about 100 lb overweight for men and about 80 lb overweight for women. Surgery can be an option for people whose BMI is above 40 or for people whose BMI is between 35 and 40 and who have life-threatening obesity-related diseases such as severe sleep apnea or heart disease. For more information, visit the CDC (www.cdc.gov/obesity/adult/defining.html) or American Obesity Association (www.obesity.org).

Therapeutic Measures

Initial treatment for obesity is weight loss through education regarding a healthy and balanced diet, exercise, and calorie restriction. For weight loss to occur, the patient must cooperate and have sustained motivation. Support groups such as Take Off Pounds Sensibly (TOPS.org) and Weight Watchers can help patients be successful. Behavior modification methods that provide rewards for successful weight loss are often included in a weight loss plan. Short-term use of medications that suppress appetite or block fat absorption may also be used.

Bariatric Surgery

Patients who do not respond to medical methods of weight loss, who weigh 100 pounds over ideal body weight, have a BMI over 40, or have a BMI over 35 with severe health effects as a result might be candidates for surgical weight loss ("Patient Perspective"). Additional screening for psychiatric and social stability is required.

Weight loss surgery is called bariatric surgery. The word **bariatric** comes from the Greek word *baros,* which means "weight." Surgical techniques produce weight loss by limiting how much the stomach can hold and/or decreased calorie and nutrient absorption ("Nutrition Notes"). One benefit of the gastric surgeries is that type 2 diabetes can improve by varying degrees with each type of surgery. For a list of surgical weight loss centers and surgical procedures, visit the American Society for Bariatric Surgeons at www.asbs.org.

Adjustable Gastric Banding

Laparoscopic adjustable gastric banding is done with an inflatable silicone band placed around the upper portion of the

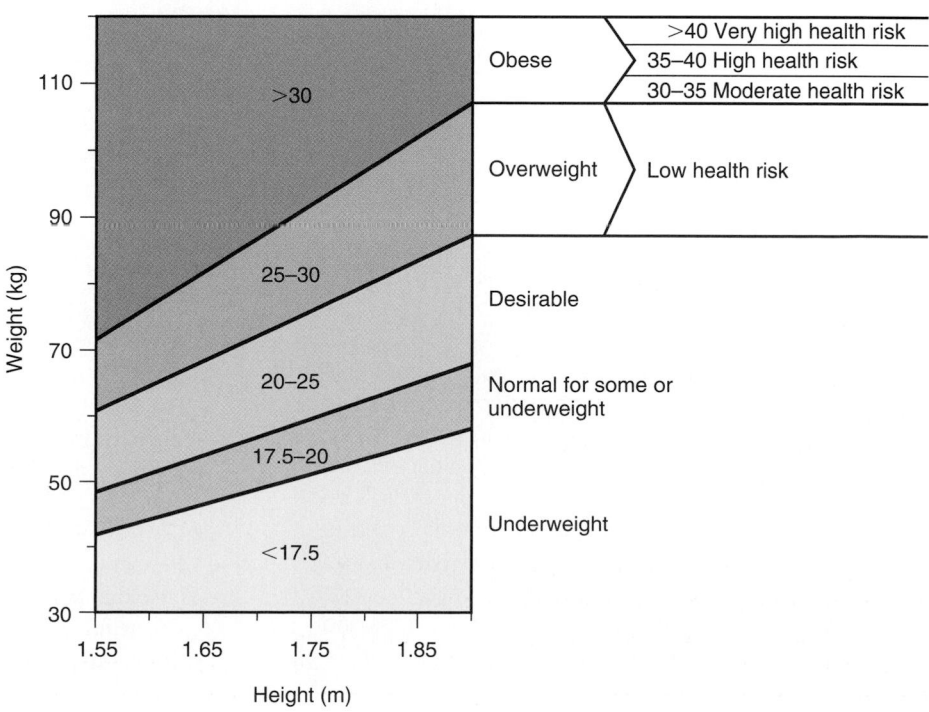

FIGURE 33.1 Body mass index ranges and associated level of health risk with obesity.

Patient Perspective

Curtis

I am 47, with eight children. For many years, I experienced weight control problems. By the time I was in high school, I weighed 250 pounds, and the weight just kept building from there. I had tried many weight control programs, including some medications that now have been removed from the market.

When I was about 38, I began to look into weight loss surgeries such as the Roux-en-Y. Many of the older techniques were dangerous and risky. Even the newer procedures are major procedures with many risks.

I had spoken to many people who had bariatric surgery. Many pointed out the psychological aspect, talking about how differently people treated you after weight loss, and how some couples ended up divorcing. This was a very scary aspect to me.

However, after much research and after reaching a weight of about 380 pounds, I arranged to have the surgery. I had my surgery at a facility that did only bariatric surgery. I felt very comfortable through the whole process. This included all the presurgical testing, including psychological evaluation and counseling.

One of the nice features was that the facility itself was patient-friendly, with large chairs and other amenities for larger people. When I had the surgery I had a rough first 24 hours, spent in the critical care unit. The nursing staff was very professional and understanding. The care was personal and responsive to my needs. The staff was courteous and made me comfortable.

I think that understanding the medical field you are working in is important to this feeling of patient comfort. Several of my nurses had gone through the procedure themselves. This really helped them to know what I was experiencing. Nurses should be well informed about the procedures.

It has been 6+ years now, and I have continued to keep my weight down around 230 to 250 pounds, which is a loss of approximately 120 pounds. My health has improved a good deal. I would do it again, even though at about day 21, I would have said "never again."

As nursing professionals, it is very important to treat all patients as human beings and with much respect regardless of their socioeconomic status or medical needs. If patients are treated with respect and caring, it is a step for them in the right direction. I believe it is not only kind but helps in the healing and recovery processes as well. I was treated with a great deal of kindness and respect during my procedure and I greatly appreciated this. Thanks to all the professional nurses out there who do a great job.

Nutrition Notes

Supplying Nutrition in Upper Gastrointestinal Conditions

Bariatric Surgery

Candidates for bariatric surgery should be carefully selected and instructed that the procedure is a tool to assist with weight control, along with behavioral changes, diet and exercise. If the patient overeats, the small pouch can be stretched and the weight regained.

Intake is rigidly controlled in type and amount immediately after the surgery and during approximately 12 weeks of rehabilitation. Long-term dietary strategies include the following:
- Eating three to six small balanced meals daily
- Choosing high protein, low fat, low sugar foods
- Chewing thoroughly and eating slowly
- Drinking sufficient fluids, mostly between meals
- Taking vitamin and mineral supplements as prescribed.

Nutritional ramifications following bariatric surgery are legion. The most common clinically relevant micronutrient deficiencies after gastric bypass include those of thiamin, vitamin B_{12}, vitamin D, iron, and copper. Also, intakes of less than recommended amounts of calcium, magnesium, and phosphorus have been reported. As many as 30% of postoperative patients reported intolerance to certain foods. One case of severe scurvy was diagnosed 3 months postoperatively in a patient who rejected dietary advice.

Potential complications of these surgeries include nausea, vomiting, bloating, heartburn, staple disruption, obstruction, dumping syndrome (rapid entry of food into the jejunum without proper mixing of the food with digestive juices), gout, gallstones, kidney stones, and osteoporosis.

Gastroesophageal Reflux and Hiatal Hernia

Thorough chewing and correct timing of intake is helpful in controlling symptoms:
- Eat six small meals
- Limit liquids with meals if they cause distention or satiety
- No food within 3 hours of bedtime
    Avoiding certain substances can alleviate symptoms.
- Those that relax the sphincter:
    - Fat and chocolate
    - Peppermint and spearmint
    - Caffeine and alcohol
- Those that stimulate gastric secretions:
    - Coffee and tea, regular or decaffeinated
    - Pepper
- Those that may be irritating:
    - Citrus juices
    - Tomatoes, tomato juice and sauces

Postprandial Hypotension

This refers to a drop in systolic blood pressure of 20 mm Hg or more within 2 hours of beginning a meal. Symptoms are dizziness, weakness, lightheadedness, falls, disturbed speech, and vision changes. Complications are angina pectoris and stroke.

Normally, the body compensates for the increased blood flow to the digestive tract after meals, but in older adults, the mechanisms maintaining adequate circulation to the rest of the body become less effective. Most at risk are people with hypertension or impaired control of the autonomic nervous system. Greater effects are seen when the stomach empties rapidly.

To prevent postprandial hypotension, a person should:

- Drink 12 to 18 ounces of water 15 minutes before meals to enhance fluid balance.
- Limit carbohydrate intake.
- Eat frequent small meals.
- Lie in a semirecumbent position for 90 minutes after eating.
- Schedule antihypertensive medications between rather than just before meals.

Special dietary additives or medications to delay gastric emptying are sometimes prescribed.

Dumping Syndrome

The recommended meal pattern for patients with dumping syndrome includes six small meals per day that are high in protein and fat but low in simple sugars; fluids between rather than with meals; and reclining for 30 to 60 minutes after meals. Supplementation with the vitamins B_{12} and D, folic acid, and the minerals calcium and iron may be necessary to prevent deficiencies.

Gastric Cancer

If a patient has a poor prognosis after a total **gastrectomy** for cancer, dietary interventions should focus on symptoms the patient wishes to control. An overly restricted diet that causes the patient discomfort or distress is inappropriate.

stomach (Fig. 33.2). This creates a small pouch to limit the amount of food the patient eats. The band is adjustable with a saline solution injected into the band through a port in the skin, making a larger or smaller pouch. The procedure is reversible.

Gastric Plication

Laparoscopic gastric plication folds the stomach inwardly, and then sutures hold the folds in place. This reduces the stomach's volume and limits the food that can be ingested at one time. It can be reversed. Research is ongoing relevant to its success.

Sleeve Gastrectomy

Laparoscopic sleeve gastrectomy removes about 75% of the stomach to leave a slim gastric "sleeve." This reduces the stomach's

volume and limits food intake at one time. It also may decrease the hormone produced by the stomach that causes hunger.

Gastric Bypass

The **Roux-en-Y** gastric bypass is a commonly done surgery that reduces stomach size and bypasses some of the small intestine (see Fig. 33.2). It can be done as an open or laparoscopic surgery. First, a small stomach pouch the size of a thumb is created. This small pouch causes a quick satisfactory feeling of fullness during a meal, which is the key to the success of this procedure. Next, the small intestine is divided and the pouch is connected to the lower part of the cut small intestine to allow food to bypass the lower stomach, duodenum, and part of the jejunum. Digestive juice flow is maintained, and food enters the jejunum within 10 minutes of eating. There is little malabsorption of food.

Biliopancreatic Diversion With Duodenal Switch

Like the sleeve gastrectomy, a small tubular pouch is created. Then most of the small intestine is bypassed, so that with the connection of a piece of the distal small intestine to the pouch, the food goes directly to the end portion of the small intestine. The end of the bypassed small intestine is reconnected to this end portion of the small intestine so that digestive juices are not lost and can mix with the food.

Complications of Gastric Surgeries

A common side effect of stomach size reducing gastric surgery is vomiting caused by overeating or by not chewing food well. Protein, vitamin, and mineral deficiencies can result. Lifelong supplements are required. Band slippage or intestinal leakage can occur.

 NURSING CARE TIP

When caring for a patient after bariatric surgery, use infection control procedures at all times to prevent surgical site infection. Surgical site infection following bariatric surgery is a Medicare-designated "never event"—hospitals will not be paid by Medicare for the care required for this condition.

Postoperative Care

Patients who have had bariatric surgery require care similar to that for most types of gastric surgeries. (See the "Nursing Process for the Patient Having Gastric Surgery" section later in this chapter.) The bariatric diet, however, is very different and requires individualized dietary education. Some patients will have an NG tube placed in surgery. It is important to

• WORD • BUILDING •
gastrectomy: gastr—stomach + ectomy—to remove

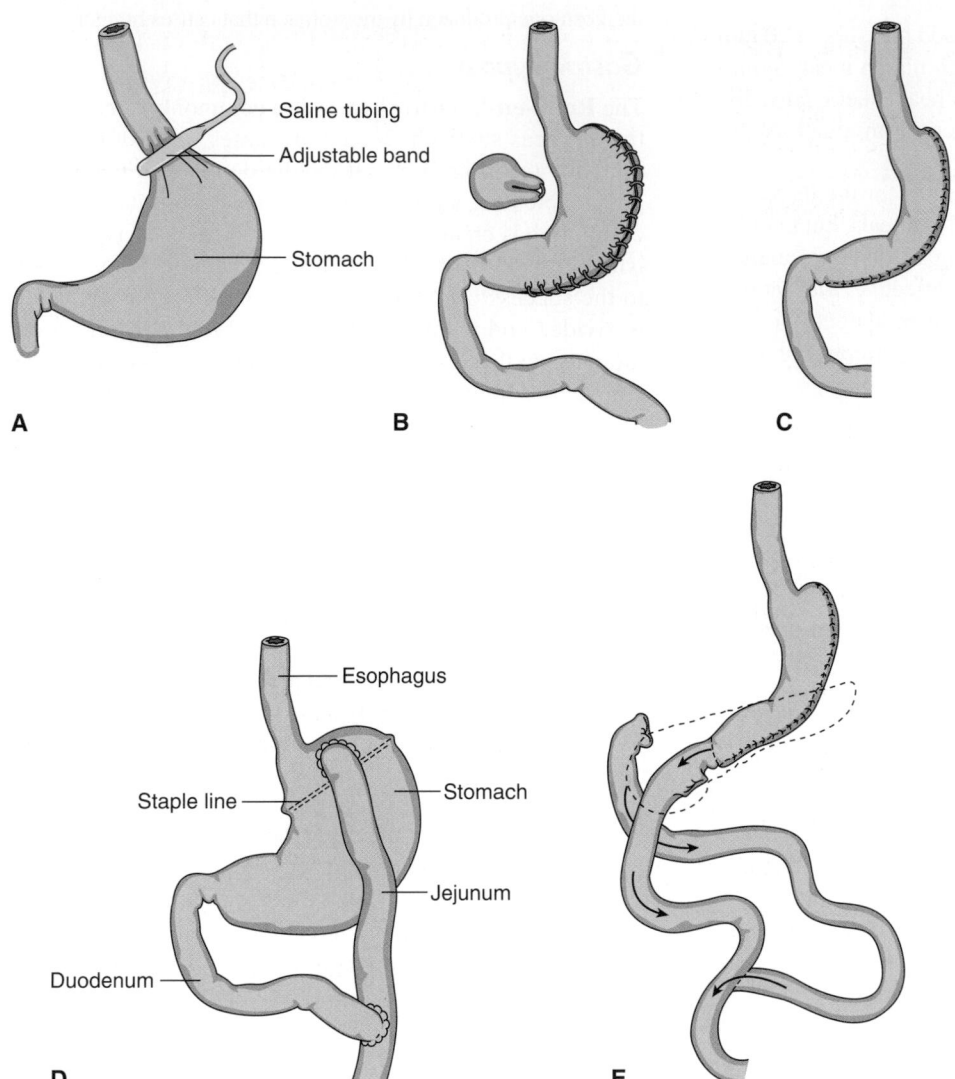

FIGURE 33.2 (A) Adjustable gastric band. (B) Gastric plication. (C) Sleeve gastrectomy. (D) Roux-en-Y gastric bypass. (E) Biliopancreatic diversion with duodenal switch.

keep the head of the bed elevated to ensure adequate lung expansion. Patients are started on a clear liquid diet because of the small stomach pouch that has been created. Only a small amount of fluid, 30 mL, is allowed at a time. Then the diet progresses to full liquids, pureed foods, and, finally, at about 6 weeks after surgery, regular foods as tolerated. Patients will need to be taught to restrict the amount of food ingested at one time.

Bariatric patients will need long-term follow-up. Many patients experience significant weight loss by 6 to 8 months after surgery. This can lead to a large amount of flabby skin. It is recommended that they wait at least 1 full year before having reconstructive surgery to remove the excess skin.

Nursing Process for the Patient Who Is Obese
Data Collection

Data collection for the patient with obesity should include measurements of height, weight, and BMI. Information about eating patterns and exercise patterns should be obtained. The nurse should determine if any problems exist for the patient related to excess weight such as physical limitations, social interaction issues, and personal issues (e.g., changes in sexuality or financial status). The nurse should complete a complete physical assessment noting any abnormalities. Assessment should include any areas in which the patient has expressed concerns or problems. Persons who are overweight have an increased risk for other diseases. The nurse should assess for signs and symptoms of disease.

Nursing Diagnoses, Planning, and Implementation
Imbalanced Nutrition: More Than Body Requirements related to caloric intake greater than metabolic needs and/or decreased activity level

EXPECTED OUTCOME: The patient will achieve and maintain weight loss to specified weight.

• Establish desired weight goal and monitor weight *to track progress toward goal.*

• Modify eating habits and patterns *to lose weight and then maintain weight loss.*

• Establish and maintain increased activity pattern *to lose weight and then maintain weight loss.*

• In collaboration with a dietician, implement eating plan for patient *to safely reduce weight and maintain adequate protein intake.*

• Discuss realistic weight loss goals of 1 to 2 lb/week *to achieve lasting weight loss effects.*

• Discuss emotions, events, and patterns of eating *to help patient identify when she or he is eating to satisfy an emotional need versus a physiological hunger.*

• In collaboration with physician, establish increased activity pattern *to promote weight loss.*

• Provide preoperative instructions if surgical interventions are planned *to help patient understand the procedure.*

Evaluation

The patient's goals are met if the patient maintains progressive weight loss to specified weight goal and safely progresses through the perioperative period if a surgical intervention is completed.

NURSING CARE TIP

For the patient who is obese, it is often necessary to have on hand special bariatric equipment for patient care. Some items you may need include:

• Larger hospital bed, wheelchair, or walker
• Patient lifting devices
• Extra pillows to ease breathing
• Larger hospital gowns
• Larger blood pressure cuff

ORAL HEALTH AND DENTAL CARE

Good oral health care is important to overall health. Nutrition can be affected if oral problems interfere with eating and drinking. Respiratory illness and cardiac disease are associated with pathogens in the mouth. Regular mechanical oral hygiene is needed to remove plaque and prevent infections. Functional limitations may interfere with self-care for oral hygiene especially for older adults ("Gerontological Issues"). Regular dental care is also important in the prevention of infections (Box 33-1). Providing oral hygiene using oral chlorhexidine gluconate (germicidal) mouthwash has been shown to be effective in preventing pneumonia in long-term care residents as well as reducing ventilator-associated pneumonia in cardiac surgery patients. Suction toothbrushes are available for those patients who are unable to control secretions (see Fig. 2.2).

Aging changes as well as disease and treatment can result in oral inflammation and infection. Those who are

Box 33-1 Common Concerns in Oral Health and Dental Care

Oral care is important throughout life and has been found to have a link to cardiac health. The importance of daily and ongoing oral care should be considered for all patients, especially older adults.

Patients who have artificial joints or some heart conditions who must undergo a dental procedure need to take prophylactic antibiotics before some dental procedures to prevent bacteria entry and bacterial endocarditis. The dentist should be informed of the patient's history so that appropriate antibiotics can be prescribed.

Xerostomia (Dry Mouth)

As people age, it is not unusual for them to experience a condition known as xerostomia (dry mouth). Also, some medications and radiation treatment of the head and neck areas can cause it. Xerostomia can lead to rampant tooth decay in older adults, putting their dentition at risk. Before any radiation therapy of the head or neck area, a thorough oral examination and any needed restorative dental procedures should be completed.

Although water is used as a common substitute for saliva, it does not contain the necessary compounds, such as lubricants, to protect the teeth. There are many products available for dry mouth, such as Biotene gel, Act rinse, and sprays to help with the discomfort of dry mouth. Brushing with a high fluoride toothpaste that is available by prescription is also recommended.

Dentures

It is helpful to have a person's name implanted into his or her dentures to avoid lost or mixed up dentures, especially when the person lives in an extended care facility. This service can be requested when the dentures are made, and the dentist will place a small identity tag in the acrylic of the denture with the person's name on it.

Those with complete dentures still need to be routinely screened by a dentist or dental hygienist for proper denture fit, sore areas, oral cancer detection, and oral fungal infections.

Gingival Recession

As people age, it is not unusual for their gingivae (gums) to recede or shrink, exposing the root surfaces of the teeth. This can lead to root sensitivity, tooth decay, or both.

To protect the teeth from tooth decay as a result of dry mouth or gingival recession, a fluoride gel (Gel-Kam), rinse (Act), or a prescription toothpaste with high fluoride is strongly recommended.

Continued

Gingivitis

As people get older, the gingivae have a greater tendency to bleed, a condition known as gingivitis. If the supporting tissues in the sockets of the teeth become inflamed, bone loss occurs, resulting in a condition known as periodontitis (pyorrhea). Periodontitis can lead to tooth mobility or loss.

Good oral hygiene habits cannot be overemphasized in the prevention of gum disease. Flossing every day is very important. If the patient is unable to floss due to arthritis or other conditions, an electric toothbrush or a Waterpik device is helpful in providing oral hygiene.

Candida Albicans Infection (Yeast Infection)

Older adults are susceptible to oral yeast infections (caused by *Candida albicans*) due to certain medications, systemic conditions, or chemotherapy. Nystatin (Mycostatin, Nadostine) as an oral rinse treats this infection.

Angular Cheilosis

A condition known as angular cheilosis (red, raw corners of the mouth) develops more often in older adults. It may be from infection, deficiency of riboflavin (vitamin B_2), or loss of facial profile due to worn-down or damaged dentures or the patient not wearing his or her dentures. Depending on the cause, it is treated with anti-infective medications, vitamins, or new dentures.

Dental Implants

Dental implants are gaining in popularity. An implant is an artificial root placed in the jawbone. The implant is usually tubular and made of titanium. Implants can be used to replace one tooth, multiple teeth, or an entire arch. They can also be used to stabilize a complete denture.

Source: *Dr. Ralph Kluk and Dr. Cheryl Kluk. Jackson, Michigan.*

immunosuppressed (i.e., with acquired immunodeficiency syndrome; AIDS) or undergoing chemotherapy or who have vitamin deficiencies are more at risk. Candidiasis is a common oral infection that is treated with nystatin oral swish and swallow. During data collection, especially in these higher risk patients, the nurse should note any oral signs of inflammation or infection requiring prompt treatment.

Gerontological Issues

Nurses can have a positive impact on older patients' outcomes by providing mechanical oral hygiene. Studies have shown that because mechanical oral care removes plaque, it helped to prevent pneumonia and pneumonia-related death in older patients who were either hospitalized or in an extended care facility.

 ORAL INFLAMMATORY DISORDERS

Stomatitis

Stomatitis is inflammation of the oral cavity. There are many causes of stomatitis, such as an infection or a systemic disease.

Aphthous Stomatitis (Canker Sores)

Aphthous stomatitis appears as small, white, painful ulcers on the inner cheeks, lips, tongue, gums, palate, or pharynx and typically lasts for several days to 2 weeks. Self-induced trauma such as biting the lips and cheeks can cause these ulcers to develop, as can stress or exposure to irritating foods. Application of topical tetracycline several times a day usually shortens the healing time. A topical anesthetic such as benzocaine or lidocaine provides pain relief and makes it possible to eat with minimal pain.

Herpes Simplex Virus Type 1 Infection

Herpes simplex virus type 1 (HSV-1) infection may appear as painful cold sores or fever blisters on the face, lips, perioral area, cheeks, nose, or conjunctivae. These lesions recur over time but last only for a few days each time. The onset can be provoked by fever or stress, among other things. Acyclovir ointment can be used to ease the pain, but it does not cure the lesions. Oral acyclovir may reduce recurrences. These lesions are infectious, and standard precautions should be used when ointment is applied or oral care is given.

 ORAL CANCER

Pathophysiology and Etiology

Oral cancer can occur anywhere in the mouth or throat. If detected early enough, it is curable. Oral cancer is found most commonly in patients who use alcohol or any form of tobacco. The highest incidence of oral cancer is found in the pharynx (throat), with the lowest incidence being on the lips.

Signs and Symptoms

Any oral sore that does not heal in 2 weeks should be assessed by the patient's physician. Cancerous ulcers are often painless but may become tender as the cancer progresses. In the later stages, the patient may report difficulty chewing, swallowing, or speaking or may have swollen cervical lymph glands.

Diagnostic Tests

Biopsy specimens are taken to determine the presence of cancer.

Therapeutic Measures

Oral cancer treatment varies depending on the individualized diagnosis. Radiation, chemotherapy, and surgery are used alone or in combination to treat oral cancer. Radical or modified neck dissection is often performed because this type of

• WORD • BUILDING •
stomatitis: stoma—mouth + itis—inflammation

cancer frequently has metastasized to cervical lymph nodes by the time it is diagnosed (Fig. 33.3). The tumor is removed along with lymph nodes, muscles, blood vessels, glands, and part of the thyroid, depending on the extent of the cancer. Drains are inserted into the incision to prevent fluid accumulation. A tracheostomy is usually performed to protect the airway and prevent obstruction.

Nursing Care

Preoperative and postoperative nursing care is discussed in Chapter 12. Preoperatively, the use of alcohol or tobacco is addressed and referrals to cessation programs and support groups offered. Preoperative teaching includes how the patient will communicate if a tracheostomy is placed. Postoperatively, major concerns are airway patency, communication, and nutritional needs. Nursing care for the patient with a tracheostomy is discussed in Chapter 29. The airway must be monitored and secretions controlled to prevent aspiration. Determining that the methods the patient is using for communication are satisfactory is evaluated. Tube feedings (see Chapter 32) are usually given to meet the patient's nutritional needs because swallowing is difficult.

ESOPHAGEAL CANCER

Pathophysiology and Etiology

As with oral cancer, esophageal cancer is associated with the use of tobacco or alcohol. Barrett's esophagus, a precancerous condition, is a risk factor. Esophageal cancer is usually

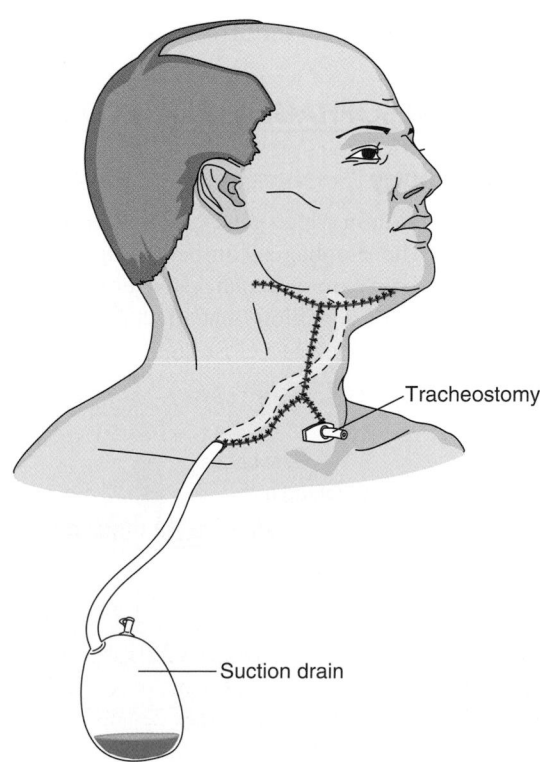

FIGURE 33.3 Radical neck dissection with tracheostomy tube and drains inserted.

detected in advanced stages because of its location near many lymph nodes that allow it to metastasize. As the cancer progresses, obstruction of the esophagus can occur, with possible perforation or fistula development that may cause aspiration.

Signs and Symptoms

Signs and symptoms may include progressive dysphasia (difficulty swallowing), a feeling of fullness, pain in the chest after eating, foul breath, or regurgitation of foods if there is an obstruction.

Diagnostic Tests

Diagnosis of esophageal cancer can be made by barium swallow studies, biopsy, or endoscopy procedures such as esophagogastroduodenoscopy (EGD) or mediastinoscopy (endoscopic examination of mediastinum). Mediastinoscopy is used to determine whether the cancer has spread to the lymph nodes and surrounding structures.

Therapeutic Measures

Treatment for esophageal cancer includes surgery (most common), radiation, chemotherapy, laser therapy, and electrocoagulation. These therapies may be used alone or in combination. Surgical procedures include esophageal resection (esophagectomy), resection of the esophagus and anastomosis to the remaining part of the stomach (esophagogastrostomy), Dacron esophageal replacement, or use of a section of colon to replace the esophagus (esophagoenterostomy). If the tumor is inoperable, esophageal dilation or stent placement can be done to relieve dysphagia and allow food to pass through the esophagus.

Nursing Process for the Patient With Esophageal Cancer

The patient with esophageal cancer may undergo various forms of treatment: chemotherapy, radiation, or surgery. Nursing care is provided based on the effects of the therapies (see Chapters 11 and 12).

Data Collection

Patient data are collected for risk factors of esophageal cancer, pain, dysphagia, and nutritional status.

Nursing Diagnoses, Planning, and Implementation

Pain related to tumor and pressure exerted on surrounding tissues

EXPECTED OUTCOME: Patient will state a reduction of pain to acceptable level or total relief of pain within 30 minutes of report of pain.

• Assess pain level using pain rating scale *to identify pain level.*
• Provide pain medications as ordered *to provide pain relief.*

Risk for Deficient Fluid Volume related to decreased intake

EXPECTED OUTCOME: Patient's vital signs will remain within normal limits and intake and output will be balanced for 24 hours at all times.

• Assess fluid intake and swallowing ability with fluids *to plan care.*

- Obtain daily weights *to detect changes in fluid volume.*
- Provide fluids as able to swallow *to ensure adequate intake.*
- Monitor IV infusion as ordered *to prevent hypovolemia.*
- Monitor vital signs and report abnormal findings *for prompt treatment.*

Imbalanced Nutrition: Less Than Body Requirements related to dysphagia

EXPECTED OUTCOME: Patient will maintain weight within normal limits for body frame, and laboratory values such as albumin, electrolytes, and lymphocytes will be within normal limits.

- Obtain patient height and weight, and weigh weekly *to monitor changes during care.*
- Identify patient's ability to swallow and eat food *to determine plan of care.*
- Provide oral care frequently *to refresh mouth and encourage desire to eat.*
- Provide nutrition as ordered in form patient is able to tolerate (liquid supplements, tube feedings, parenteral nutrition, etc.) *to maintain adequate nutrition.*

Evaluation

The goals are met if the patient reports pain is relieved and fluid volume and nutritional needs are met.

 HIATAL HERNIA

Pathophysiology

The esophagus passes through an opening in the diaphragm called the hiatus. A **hiatal hernia** is a condition in which the stomach slides up through the hiatus of the diaphragm into the thorax (Fig. 33.4). A sliding hiatal hernia is the most common type in which the junction of the stomach and esophagus slides up into the thoracic cavity when a patient is supine and then usually goes back into the abdominal cavity when the patient stands upright. A paraesophageal hernia is rarer but serious as part of the stomach squeezes through the hiatus and is at risk for strangulation (blood supply is cut off). Hiatal hernia occurs most commonly in smokers, those who are older than age 50, obese, or pregnant. People with hiatal hernia often have gastroesophageal reflux disease (GERD) as well (discussed later).

Signs and Symptoms

A small hernia may not produce any discomfort or require treatment. However, a large hernia can cause pain, heartburn, a feeling of fullness, or reflux, which can injure the esophagus with possible ulceration and bleeding.

Diagnostic Tests

Hiatal hernias are diagnosed by x-ray studies and fluoroscopy.

Therapeutic Measures

Lifestyle changes for symptomatic hiatal hernia include losing weight, taking antacids, eating small meals that pass easily through the esophagus, not reclining for 3 to 4 hours after eating, elevating the head of the bed 6 to 12 inches to prevent reflux, and avoiding bedtime snacks, spicy foods, alcohol, caffeine, and smoking (see "Nutrition Notes").

Surgical Management

Surgery is done for symptomatic hiatal hernia when GERD, strangulation, or obstruction is present. Fundoplication, in which the stomach fundus is wrapped around the lower part of the esophagus, is the most common surgical procedure performed (Fig. 33.5).

Nursing Care

The patient is taught lifestyle interventions to reduce the symptoms of hiatal hernia. If the patient undergoes surgery, general postoperative nursing care is provided. In addition, following fundoplication, patients are assessed for dysphagia during their first postoperative meal. If dysphagia occurs, the physician should be notified because the repair may be too tight, causing obstruction of the passage of food.

 GASTROESOPHAGEAL REFLUX DISEASE

Pathophysiology

GERD is a condition in which gastric secretions reflux into the esophagus. The esophagus can be damaged by acidic gastric secretions and exposure to digestive enzymes. GERD is caused primarily by conditions that affect the ability of the lower esophageal sphincter to close tightly, such as hiatal hernia.

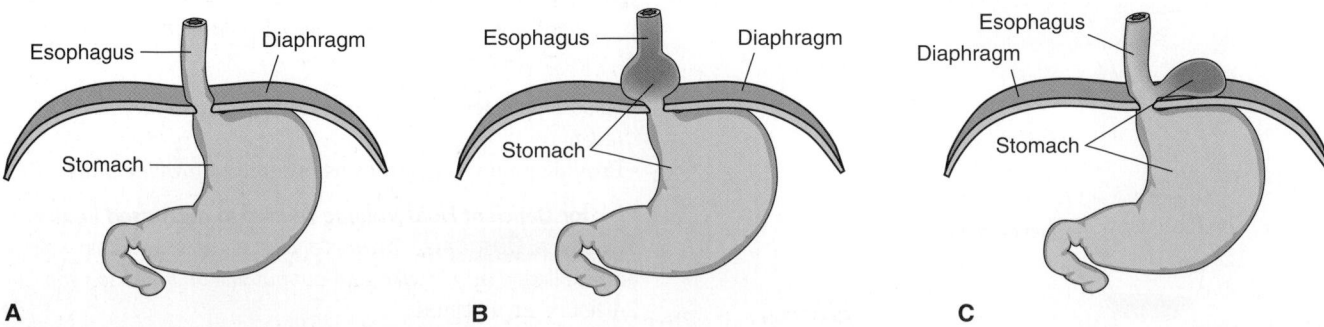

FIGURE 33.4 Hiatal hernia. (A) Normal esophagus and stomach. (B) Sliding hiatal hernia. (C) Rolling hiatal hernia.

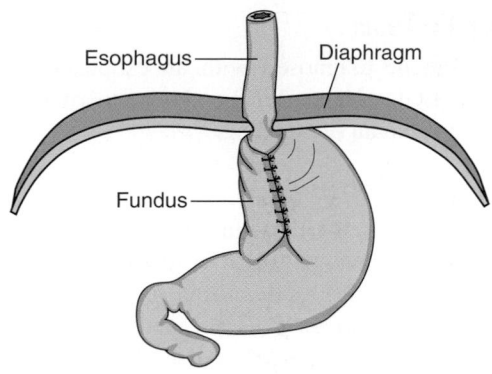

FIGURE 33.5 Hiatal hernia repair. Nissen fundoplication wraps the stomach fundus around the esophagus and then sutures it onto itself to hold it in place.

Signs and Symptoms

Signs and symptoms of GERD include heartburn, regurgitation, dysphagia, and bleeding (Table 33.1). Aspiration is a concern. Scar tissue can develop from the inflammation.

Diagnostic Tests

Diagnostic tests include a barium swallow, esophagoscopy (an endoscopic procedure), or pH monitoring of the normally alkaline esophagus.

Complications

Complications of GERD can result in esophagitis (inflammation of the esophagus) due to acid reflux. Over time this can lead to changes in the epithelium of the esophagus and lead to Barrett's esophagus. This is a precancerous lesion that puts the patient at risk of developing esophageal cancer. Barrett's tissue can be removed during a 30-minute outpatient endoscopic procedure using radiofrequency ablation (the BARRx system). Normal tissue returns, and the risk of cancer is reduced. Respiratory complications such as bronchospasm, laryngospasm, and aspiration pneumonia can also occur owing to aspiration of gastric contents. There is the potential for asthma, chronic bronchitis, or pneumonia due to the aspiration of gastric contents.

Therapeutic Measures

Lifestyle changes are recommended along with medications. Obese patients are encouraged to lose weight. A low-fat, high-protein diet is recommended because fat causes decreased functioning of the lower esophageal sphincter. See "Nutritional Notes" for additional things to avoid. Patient teaching includes eating small meals often during the day, drinking fluids between meals instead of with meals, avoiding late evening meals, snacking, and fluids 2 to 3 hours before bedtime. Medications may include nonprescription antacids for mild symptoms. Histamine (H_2) receptor antagonists (acid reducers) that are available in nonprescription and prescription strengths are used for mild to moderate symptoms. Proton pump inhibitors (PPIs) reduce acid in the stomach and are used for frequent, severe symptoms and Barrett's esophagus. (Table 33.4 later

TABLE 33.1 GERD SUMMARY

Signs and Symptoms	***Heartburn*** Regurgitation Dysphagia Bleeding
Diagnostic Tests	X-ray studies Endoscopy Fluoroscopy
Therapeutic Measures	Medications to decrease acid, improve gastric emptying, and function of lower esophageal sphincter: antacids, histamine (H_2) receptor antagonists, proton pump inhibitors, cytoprotective agents (sucralfate), and cholinergic drugs Controlling symptoms Low-fat, high-protein diet Avoiding triggers Raising head of bed on 4- to 6-inch blocks Instructing patient to drink fluids between meals rather than with meals Avoid eating and drinking before bedtime
Complications	Esophagitis Barrett's syndrome Respiratory symptoms
Priority Nursing Diagnoses	*Acute Pain* *Deficient Knowledge*

in this chapter provides information on PPIs.) There are suspected risks associated with PPI use that includes a possible increased risk of osteoporosis and *Clostridium difficile* infection. If diarrhea occurs that does not stop, patients should contact a health care provider (HCP; Janarthanan, Ditah, Adler, & Ehrinpreis, 2012).

Surgery can be done if necessary to alleviate symptoms. A fundoplication or endoscopic procedures can be done. As you read, what do you think the benefit of the following procedure is over fundoplication surgery? A minimally invasive procedure, transoral incisionless fundoplication (TIF) is performed through the mouth without incisions. It employs the EsophyX device to create an esophagogastric fundoplication that is up to 270° and 2 to 3 cm in length. EsophyX, uses an endoscope to tighten the lower esophageal sphincter, which aids in improving or eliminating gastroesophageal reflux with good success (www.endogastricsolutions.com/TIF.aspx). If you thought that the benefit of TIF is that it's minimally invasive and, therefore, has a speedier recovery, you would be correct. Other endoscopic procedures that use radiofrequency waves, such as the Stretta, can be done. The radiofrequency waves are injected into the lower esophageal sphincter muscle to form collagen contraction, which leads to a barrier against reflux.

Nursing Process for the Patient With GERD
Data Collection

Assessment of the patient with GERD includes evaluation of reports of heartburn. The onset, duration, characteristics, and precipitating or relieving factors are noted.

Nursing Diagnoses, Planning, and Implementation

Acute Pain related to inflammation of esophageal tissues
EXPECTED OUTCOME: The patient will state a reduction of pain to an acceptable level or total relief of pain within 30 minutes of report of pain.

- Identify factors that increase pain *to develop teaching plan.*
- Monitor pain level using pain rating scale *to identify pain level.*
- Instruct patient regarding factors that aggravate pain *to enhance management of condition.*
- Instruct patient to sleep with head of bed elevated 4 to 6 inches, eat small meals, and avoid lying down for 2 hours after eating *to prevent reflux of gastric contents into esophagus.*
- Instruct patient to avoid smoking and alcohol *because they decrease functioning of the lower esophageal sphincter.*
- Instruct patient to avoid foods that cause discomfort *to avoid pain.*
- Review medication schedule and teach patient to take medications even if symptoms are relieved *because the underlying pathology still exists.*
- Provide pain medications on routine schedule, especially postoperatively, *to provide optimum pain relief and control.*

Evaluation

The goals are met if the patient is able to manage medications, pain is controlled, and symptoms are relieved.

 ## MALLORY-WEISS TEAR

Pathophysiology

A Mallory-Weiss tear (MWT) is a longitudinal tear in the mucous membrane of the esophagus at the stomach junction (gastric cardia). These tears occur from a sudden powerful or prolonged force due to coughing, vomiting, seizures, prolapse of the stomach into the esophagus, or cardiopulmonary resuscitation (CPR). Hiatal hernia is present in most patients with MWTs.

Signs and Symptoms

Bleeding may result from the tear. Up to 15% of GI bleeding is caused by MWTs. Symptoms include bright red, bloody emesis or bloody or tarry stools.

Diagnostic Tests

The tear can be diagnosed with an esophagogastroduodenoscopy (EGD). Hemoglobin and hematocrit are checked to determine amount of bleeding.

Therapeutic Measures

The tears usually self-heal without intervention in several days, and bleeding stops within a few hours. It is rare to have it happen again. Medications such as a PPI and an antiemetic may be given. Alcohol use should be avoided. Up to 75% of those with MWT use alcohol excessively. Rarely, excessive bleeding may occur, resulting in shock and/or the need for a blood transfusion. Bleeding is treated with injection of epinephrine to constrict the blood vessel, and during endoscopy, endoclips can be placed to stop the bleeding. The prognosis for MWTs is good. The condition is seen in men more often than in women.

Nursing Care

Monitoring the patient for signs of bleeding and reporting them to prevent complications from hemorrhage are the focus of nursing care. If excessive bleeding occurs, shock symptoms may occur and require prompt intervention. Teaching about medications and the avoidance of alcohol use is also done. See the section on gastric bleeding later in the chapter for more information.

 ## ESOPHAGEAL VARICES

Esophageal varices are dilated blood vessels in the esophagus (see Chapter 35). Their rupture can precipitate a life-threatening event. Varices develop from portal hypertension. This occurs when pressure rises in the portal vein from blocked blood flow in the liver. This is often due to cirrhosis of the liver.

 ## GASTRITIS

Gastritis is inflammation of the stomach mucosa and can be acute or chronic. Causes are listed in Box 33-2.

Acute Gastritis
Pathophysiology

Gastritis results when the protective mucosal barrier is broken down and allows autodigestion from hydrochloric acid and pepsin to occur. This results in edema of the tissue and possible hemorrhage. With severe gastritis, the gastric mucosa can become gangrenous and perforate, which can lead to peritonitis (infection of the peritoneum). Scarring may also occur, resulting in pyloric obstruction.

• **WORD** • **BUILDING** •
gastritis: gastr—stomach + itis—inflammation

Box 33-2 **Causes of Gastritis**

Diet
- Alcohol
- Spicy foods

Microorganisms
- *Helicobacter pylori*
- *Salmonella*

Medications
- Aspirin
- Nonsteroidal anti-inflammatory drugs
- Corticosteroids
- Digitalis
- Chemotherapy drugs

Stress
- Physiological
- Psychological

Trauma

Other Factors
- Reflux of bile
- Smoking
- Radiation
- Nasogastric suctioning

Endoscopic procedures

Signs and Symptoms

The major symptom of gastritis is abdominal pain, which is often accompanied by nausea and anorexia. The patient may also experience abdominal tenderness, a feeling of fullness, reflux, belching, and hematemesis. If the cause of the gastritis is contaminated food, symptoms including diarrhea usually start within 5 to 6 hours.

Therapeutic Measures

Treatment of gastritis is removal of the irritating substance and provision of a bland diet of liquids and soft foods along with antacids. Medication therapy may include antiemetics to control vomiting and antacids and/or histamine receptor antagonists to control pain. With a bland diet, the patient usually recovers in a short period of time.

Chronic Gastritis

Chronic gastritis occurs over time and is classified as type A or type B.

Type A

Type A chronic gastritis is often referred to as autoimmune gastritis and occurs in the fundus (body of stomach). Chronic gastritis type A is diagnosed by endoscopy, upper GI x-ray examination, and gastric aspirate analysis (see Chapter 32). Type A gastritis is often asymptomatic. Patients with type A gastritis usually do not secrete enough intrinsic factor from their stomach cells and as a result have difficulty absorbing vitamin B_{12}, which leads to pernicious anemia (discussed later).

Type B

Type B chronic gastritis affects the antrum and pylorus (lower end of the stomach near the duodenum) and is associated with *Helicobacter pylori* bacterial infection. Type B is the most common type of chronic gastritis. Signs and symptoms include poor appetite, heartburn after eating, belching, a sour taste in the mouth, and nausea and vomiting. Type B gastritis can also be diagnosed by endoscopy, upper GI x-ray examination, and gastric aspirate analysis. *H. pylori* infection is treated with antibiotics.

Stress-Induced Gastritis

A small number of patients who are critically ill may develop GI mucosal damage from ischemia. The stress response to the illness causes reduced blood flow to the stomach and small intestine, resulting in ischemia and damage to the mucosa. The damaged mucous barrier then allows acid secretions to create ulcerations. Preventive treatment has dramatically reduced stress ulceration, which can have a high mortality rate because of the multiple bleeding ulcer sites. This treatment includes trauma care that quickly restores oxygen to the stomach, as well as early feeding within 24 hours of the trauma and prophylactic sucralfate (forms a gel that binds to the base of an ulcer), antacids, or histamine blockers.

PEPTIC ULCER DISEASE

Pathophysiology

Peptic ulcer disease (PUD) is a condition in which the lining of the stomach, pylorus, duodenum, or the esophagus is eroded, usually from infection with *H. pylori*. The erosion may extend into the muscular layers or the peritoneum. Peptic ulcers occur in the portions of the GI tract that are exposed to hydrochloric acid and pepsin. The erosion is due to an increase in the concentration or activity of hydrochloric acid and pepsin. The damaged mucosa is unable to secrete enough mucus to act as a barrier against the hydrochloric acid. Some individuals have more rapid gastric emptying, which, combined with hypersecretion of acid, creates a large amount of acid moving into the duodenum. As a result, peptic ulcers occur more often in the duodenum. Ulcers are named by their location: esophageal, gastric, or duodenal. Duodenal ulcers are more common than gastric ulcers.

Etiology

Until 1982, the cause of peptic ulcers was poorly understood and thought to be related to stress, diet, and alcohol or caffeine ingestion. However, research results have found that PUD is primarily caused by infection with the Gram-negative bacterium *H. pylori*. This bacterium is responsible for 80% of gastric ulcers and more than 90% of duodenal ulcers. Two-thirds of all people are infected with *H. pylori*, and it is most common in those who are older adult Hispanics, African Americans, or in lower socioeconomic groups in the United States. The discovery of *H. pylori* has led to changes in treating and curing peptic ulcers. It is not known how *H. pylori* is transmitted, although the oral-oral or fecal-oral route is likely. Contaminated water may also play a role. Vaccines to prevent peptic ulcers are being developed.

> ## LEARNING TIP
>
> Most peptic ulcers are caused by an infection (H. pylori) that can be cured with antibiotics. Risk factors that contribute to peptic ulcer disease include smoking, chewing tobacco, stress, caffeine use, and medications such as steroids, aspirin, and nonsteroidal anti-inflammatory drugs (NSAIDs). Peptic ulcer development is influenced by smoking because it increases the harmful effects of H. pylori, alters protective mechanisms, and decreases gastric blood flow. For more information on H. pylori, visit www.cdc.gov.

Signs and Symptoms

Symptoms vary with the location of the ulcer (Table 33.2). Symptoms, including pain, may not be experienced with gastric or duodenal ulcers until complications such as hemorrhage, obstruction, or perforation develop. If pain does occur, patients with gastric ulcers commonly experience a burning and gnawing pain in the high left epigastric region, and may increase with food ingestion or 1 to 2 hours after a meal. Duodenal ulcers produce cramping or burning pain in the midepigastric or upper abdominal area, which occurs 2 to 4 hours after meals or in the middle of the night. This intermittent pain may be relieved by the ingestion of food or antacids. Anorexia and nausea and vomiting may also occur with either ulcer location. Bleeding may occur with massive hemorrhaging or slow oozing. Patients often have low hematocrit and hemoglobin levels, and gastric or fecal occult blood may be found, depending on where the ulcers are located.

TABLE 33.2 PEPTIC ULCER DISEASE SUMMARY

Signs and Symptoms	Gastric ulcer	Intermittent high left epigastric or upper abdominal burning or gnawing pain, increased 1–2 hours after meals or with food
		Variable pain pattern possibly made worse by food
		Antacids ineffective
		Can lead to gastric cancer
		Patient may be malnourished
		Hematemesis more common than melena
	Duodenal ulcer	Intermittent midepigastric or upper abdominal burning or cramping pain, increased 2–4 hours after meals or in the middle of the night
		Relieved by food or antacids
		Patient usually well nourished
		Melena more common than hematemesis
		Anorexia
		Nausea and vomiting
		Bleeding (stomach secretions or stool positive for occult blood)
Diagnostic Tests	H. pylori	Urea breath test
		Immunoglobulin G antibody detection test for H. pylori
		Biopsy
		Culture
	Peptic ulcer	Upper GI series (barium swallow)
		Esophagogastroduodenoscopy
Therapeutic Measures	Antibiotics	
	Proton pump inhibitors	
	H₂ antagonists	
	Bismuth subsalicylate	
	Sucralfate (Carafate)	
	Antacids	
	Bland diet	

TABLE 33.2 PEPTIC ULCER DISEASE SUMMARY—cont'd

	Avoiding irritants, such as smoking, caffeine, alcohol, trigger foods
Complications	Bleeding Perforation Obstruction
Priority Nursing Diagnoses	*Acute Pain* *Risk for Injury* *Deficient Knowledge*

Complications

Major complications can result from PUD. These include bleeding, perforation, and obstruction. Bleeding can occur in varying degrees from occult blood in stool and emesis to massive bright red bleeding. Hemorrhage tends to occur more often with gastric ulcers in older adults. The patient may experience signs and symptoms of shock. Treatment includes stopping the bleeding, replacing fluid and electrolytes, and possibly administering vasopressin to stop the bleeding.

Diagnostic Tests

H. pylori can be diagnosed with several tests. The urea breath test is performed by having the patient drink carbon-labeled urea. The urea is metabolized rapidly if *H. pylori* is present, allowing the carbon to be absorbed and measured in exhaled carbon dioxide. An immunoglobulin G antibody detection test for *H. pylori* identifies whether the patient is infected with *H. pylori*. These are both noninvasive detection tests. Biopsy specimens for the *Campylobacter*-like organism (CLO) biopsy urease test and a histological examination can be obtained during EGD. Biopsy is the most conclusive test for *H. pylori*. Cultures of the biopsy specimen may also be done to determine antimicrobial susceptibility.

Peptic ulcers are diagnosed on the basis of symptoms, upper GI series (barium swallow), and EGD. Endoscopy allows direct visualization of the ulcer and mucosal tissues.

Therapeutic Measures

Several treatment options are used to cure *H. pylori* without recurrence (Table 33.3). For better effectiveness, triple therapy

TABLE 33.3 MEDICATION REGIMEN OPTIONS FOR *H. PYLORI* INFECTION

Type of Therapy	Included in Therapy	Examples of Therapy Options
Triple therapy*	Two antibiotics + proton pump inhibitor	Amoxicillin (Amoxil) + clarithromycin (Biaxin) + omeprazole (Prilosec) Amoxicillin (Amoxil) + clarithromycin (Biaxin) + lansoprazole (Prevacid) (available as Prevpac, combined for convenience)
Dual therapy	Antibiotic + proton pump inhibitor Antibiotic + H$_2$ antagonist	Clarithromycin (Biaxin) + omeprazole (Prilosec) Amoxicillin (Amoxil) + lansoprazole (Prevacid) Clarithromycin (Biaxin) + H$_2$ antagonist
Other therapy	Two antibiotics + bismuth subsalicylate + H$_2$ antagonist	Metronidazole (Flagyl) + tetracycline + bismuth subsalicylate (Pepto-Bismol) + H$_2$ antagonist

*Triple therapy has the best eradication rate.

with two antibiotics to decrease resistance of the bacteria and a PPI or H_2 antagonist is used. Treatment lasting 14 days has better eradication rates than 10-day treatments. Bismuth subsalicylate (e.g., in Pepto-Bismol™) may also be used for its antibacterial effects.

PPIs are powerful agents that stop the final step of gastric acid secretion to reduce mucosa erosion and aid in healing ulcers (Table 33.4). H_2 antagonists block H_2 receptors to decrease acid secretion, although they are not as powerful as gastric acid pump inhibitors. A bland diet may also be recommended, and foods known to cause discomfort to the patient, such as spicy foods, carbonated drinks, and caffeine, should be avoided until the ulcer heals. Alcohol should also be avoided during the healing period.

TABLE 33.4 MEDICATIONS USED TO PROMOTE HEALING OF PEPTIC ULCERS

Drug Class/Action	Examples	Nursing Implications
Hyposecretory Agents		
H_2 *receptor blocking agents:* Inhibit gastric acid secretion by blocking H_2 receptors on gastric parietal cells.	cimetidine (Tagamet)	Monitor mental status of older adults. Do not give antacids within 1 hour of Tagamet. Give with meals and at bedtime. Interacts with theophylline, phenytoin, warfarin, and beta blockers.
	ranitidine (Zantac)	Give antacids at least 1 hour before or 2 hours after Zantac. Can be given in single bedtime dose.
	famotidine (Pepcid)	May be given with antacids. Can be given in single bedtime dose.
	nizatidine (Axid)	Give antacids at least 1 hour before or 2 hours after Axid. Can be given in single bedtime dose or, if given twice a day, one dose at bedtime. Monitor for excessive drowsiness and monitor and record stools.
Proton pump inhibitors: Bind to an enzyme in the presence of acidic gastric pH, preventing final transport of hydrogen ions into the gastric lumen.	dexlansoprazole (Dexilant)	Delayed release. Capsule swallowed whole.
	omeprazole (Prilosec)	Give before meal in morning. Capsule swallowed whole. Assess for abdominal pain and bleeding. Monitor CBC and liver enzymes. Notify physician of bleeding, diarrhea, headache, or abdominal pain.
	lansoprazole (Prevacid)	Give before meals. Capsule not to be crushed or chewed. May be sprinkled on applesauce and taken immediately. Packet mixed as liquid, but not for nasogastric (NG) tube because it sticks to tube. Sublingual tablet may be dissolved and given through NG tube. Notify physician of bleeding, diarrhea, headache, or abdominal pain.
	rabeprazole (Aciphex)	Tablets to be swallowed whole.
Antacids Increase gastric pH to reduce pepsin activity; strengthen gastric mucosal barrier and esophageal sphincter tone.	aluminum-magnesium combinations (Riopan, Maalox, Mylanta, Gelusil)	Do not give to patients with renal disease. Monitor bowel movements and signs of hypermagnesemia. Riopan low in sodium.

TABLE 33.4 MEDICATIONS USED TO PROMOTE HEALING OF PEPTIC ULCERS—cont'd

Drug Class/Action	Examples	Nursing Implications
	calcium carbonate (Tums, Titralac)	Do not give within 1 to 2 hours of H₂ receptor antagonists, tetracycline, or enteric-coated tablets. Do not give with milk. Do not give within 1 to 2 hours of H₂ receptor antagonists, tetracycline, or enteric-coated tablets. Monitor for hypercalcemia and constipation.
Mucosal Barrier Fortifiers In presence of mild acid condition, forms viscid and sticky gel and adheres to ulcer surface, forming a protective barrier.	sucralfate (Carafate)	Take on an empty stomach, 1 hour before meals and at bedtime. Monitor for constipation.

Do not give within 1 to 2 hours of H_2 receptor antagonists, tetracycline, or enteric-coated tablets. Do not give with milk. Do not give within 1 to 2 hours of H_2 receptor antagonists, tetracycline, or enteric-coated tablets. Monitor for hypercalcemia and constipation.

CRITICAL THINKING

Mr. Smith

■ Mr. Smith, a patient on your medical unit, has a duodenal ulcer. His wife runs to the nursing station and says that you need to help her husband, he is in terrible pain. As you enter the room, you see Mr. Smith curled up in a knee-to-chest position on the bed. He is crying and says he has excruciating abdominal pain.

1. What additional data would you gather?
2. What nursing actions would you complete?
3. What emotional support would you offer to Mrs. Smith?
4. What complication do you suspect Mr. Smith is experiencing?
5. What member(s) of the health team should you anticipate collaborating with?
6. After orders are obtained, what nursing actions will you anticipate implementing?

Suggested answers are at the end of the chapter.

A perforated ulcer is a medical emergency and usually requires surgical intervention. Gastroduodenal contents escape through the perforation into the peritoneal cavity. This can result in peritonitis, septicemia, and hypovolemic shock. Perforation most often occurs with duodenal ulcers and presents with an acute onset of sharp, severe pain. Surgical treatment includes cleaning the peritoneal cavity, closing the perforation, and possibly a vagotomy and hemigastrectomy or pyloroplasty.

Obstruction may be due to scar tissue because of repeated ulcerations and healing in a patient with long-standing PUD. Obstruction frequently occurs at the pylorus, causing pain at night and vomiting. A pyloroplasty is completed to correct the problem.

Nursing Process for the Patient With Peptic Ulcer Disease

Data Collection

The primary focus of nursing care for peptic ulcer disease is educating patients regarding the importance of this diagnosis because ulcers may be caused by an infection that can be cured with antibiotics. Patients may still believe that all ulcers are caused by stress, lifestyle, or diet. Assessing the patient's knowledge aids in providing accurate information to assist the patient in managing peptic ulcer disease. Data are also collected about the patient's disease history. Identifying factors that trigger or relieve symptoms is important.

The nurse assesses and monitors for complications of bleeding, such as occult blood in stool or emesis, perforation, including acute onset of severe pain, obstruction, changes in vital signs, and signs of shock.

Nursing Diagnoses, Planning, Implementation, and Evaluation

See the "Nursing Care Plan for the Patient With Peptic Ulcer Disease." The care plan should focus on the patient's understanding of the importance of taking all medication as directed, even if symptoms are gone.

GASTRIC BLEEDING

Gastric bleeding may be caused by ulcer perforation, tumors, gastric surgery, or other conditions. Bleeding peptic ulcers are the most common cause of blood loss into the stomach or intestine. Blood loss can be hidden (occult) blood in the stool, observable vomited blood (hematemesis), or black tarry stools (melena). When blood mixes with hydrochloric acid and enzymes in the stomach, a dark, granular material resembling coffee grounds is produced. This material can be vomited or passed through the GI system and mixed with stools. Melena occurs from slow bleeding in an upper GI area.

NURSING CARE PLAN for the Patient With Peptic Ulcer Disease

Nursing Diagnosis: *Acute Pain* related to gastric mucosal erosion

Expected Outcome: The patient's pain will be relieved as evidenced by no report of pain and the absence of nonverbal pain cues within 30 minutes of report of pain.

Evaluation of Outcome: Is pain relieved to patient's satisfaction?

Intervention Ask patient to rate pain level on scale of 0 to 10 every 3 hours and as needed. Note location, onset, intensity, characteristics of pain, and nonverbal pain cues. **Rationale** Prompt assessment can lead to timely intervention and relief of pain. **Evaluation** Does patient rate pain using scale and describe pain?

Intervention Ask about factors precipitating and relieving pain. **Rationale** Peptic ulcer pain may be relieved by food, antacids, or other interventions. **Evaluation** Is patient able to state precipitating and relieving pain factors?

Intervention Ask patient to help identify techniques for pain relief. **Rationale** Gaining the patient's cooperation increases compliance. **Evaluation** Is patient willing to participate in planning how to relieve pain?

Intervention Administer antiulcer medications as ordered. **Rationale** H_2 receptor antagonists reduce amount of gastric acid produced, and antacids neutralize gastric acid to help relieve pain. **Evaluation** Do medications reduce patient's symptoms?

Intervention Provide small, frequent meals four to six times a day. **Rationale** Small, frequent meals dilute and neutralize gastric acid. **Evaluation** Does patient report relief of gastric pain between meals?

Intervention Encourage nonacidic fluids between meals. **Rationale** Nonacidic fluids decrease irritation to gastric mucosa. **Evaluation** Does patient identify and drink nonacidic fluids?

Nursing Diagnosis: *Risk for Injury* related to complications of peptic ulcer activity such as hemorrhage and perforation

Expected Outcomes: The patient's vital signs will be maintained within normal limits and bleeding or hemorrhage will be promptly detected.

Evaluation of Outcomes: Are patient's vital signs within normal limits?

Intervention Monitor for signs and symptoms of hemorrhage such as hematemesis (vomiting blood) and melena (blood in the stool). **Rationale** Rapid assessment can lead to prompt intervention. **Evaluation** Does patient have any bleeding?

Intervention Monitor vital signs: blood pressure, pulse, respirations, and temperature. **Rationale** Severe blood loss of more than 1 L per 24 hours may cause evidence of shock, such as hypotension; weak, thready pulse; chills; palpitations; and diaphoresis. **Evaluation** Are vital signs normal?

Intervention Maintain IV infusion as ordered. **Rationale** Normal fluid balance prevents hypovolemia and shock due to hemorrhage. **Evaluation** Are intake and output balanced?

Intervention Monitor hematocrit and hemoglobin levels as ordered. **Rationale** Decreased hematocrit and hemoglobin levels indicate a decrease in circulating blood volume and reduced oxygen-carrying capacity to the tissues. **Evaluation** Are hematocrit and hemoglobin levels normal?

Signs and Symptoms

With mild bleeding, the patient may experience only slight weakness or diaphoresis (Table 33.5). Severe blood loss (more than 1 L in 24 hours) may result in hypovolemic shock, with signs and symptoms such as hypotension; a weak, thready pulse; chills; palpitations; and diaphoresis.

Therapeutic Measures

What do you think are important interventions to promote patient safety when patients experience blood loss? The goal of treatment for a massive GI bleed is to prevent or treat hypovolemic shock and prevent dehydration, electrolyte imbalance, and further bleeding. The following steps are taken:

- The patient is kept on nothing by mouth (NPO) status.
- An IV line is started to replace lost fluids and administer blood if necessary.
- A complete blood cell count is obtained to determine the amount of blood lost.
- A urinary catheter might be inserted to monitor output.
- An NG tube is inserted to assess the rate of bleeding, decompress the stomach, monitor the pH of gastric secretions, and administer saline lavage if ordered.
- Oxygen therapy may be required if the patient has lost a large amount of blood.
- To prevent aspiration with vomiting, the head of the bed is elevated.
- The physician may perform endoscopy to help control the bleeding.
- Drugs may also be instilled into the GI tract by use of an endoscope.
- For severe cases, surgery may be needed to remove the bleeding area or ligate bleeding vessels.

TABLE 33.5   GASTRIC BLEEDING SUMMARY

Signs and Symptoms	Occult blood in stool Hematemesis Melena Hypovolemic shock
Diagnostic Tests	Endoscopy Low hemoglobin and hematocrit
Therapeutic Measures	Treat hypovolemic shock: NPO (nothing by mouth), IV fluids, oxygen therapy, nasogastric tube Removal or ligation of bleeding area Medications to decrease gastric acid
Complications	Hypovolemic shock
Priority Nursing Diagnoses	*Deficient Fluid Volume* *Risk for Deficient Fluid Volume*

- Histamine (H_2) receptor antagonists are given to decrease the secretion of gastric acid.

Nursing Process for the Patient With Gastric Bleeding

Data Collection

The nurse should assess patients at risk for bleeding for signs and symptoms of bleeding. Assess any emesis and stool for occult or obvious bleeding. Assess for signs of hypovolemic shock such as hypotension, tachycardia, tachypnea, chills, palpitations, and diaphoresis. The nurse should also assess for changes in level of consciousness, confusion, dry mucous membranes, reports of thirst, and fatigue, which could indicate a decrease in circulating blood volume.

Nursing Diagnoses, Planning, and Implementation

Deficient Fluid Volume or Risk for Deficient Fluid Volume related to vomiting and diarrhea
EXPECTED OUTCOME: The patient's vital signs will remain within normal limits and intake and output will be balanced over 24 hours.

- Monitor color, amount, and frequency of fluid loss *to determine fluid balance changes.*
- Monitor vital signs and report abnormal findings *for prompt treatment.*
- Monitor level of consciousness, mucous membranes, and skin turgor *to assess for changes in fluid volume.*
- Obtain daily weights *to detect changes in fluid volume.*
- Offer oral fluids *to ensure adequate intake.*
- Monitor IV infusion as ordered *to prevent hypovolemia.*
- Monitor hematocrit and hemoglobin levels as ordered *to detect a decrease in circulating blood volume.*

Evaluation

If interventions have been effective, vital signs are within the normal range and the patient has a balanced intake and output over 24 hours.

GASTRIC CANCER

Gastric cancer refers to malignant lesions found in the stomach. It is more common in men than in women. *H. pylori* infection plays a role in gastric cancer development. Other factors that may be associated with gastric cancer development include pernicious anemia; exposure to occupational substances such as lead dust, grain dust, glycol ethers, or leaded gasoline; and a diet high in smoked fish or meats. A poor prognosis is often associated with gastric cancer because most patients have metastasis at the time of diagnosis (see "Nutrition Notes").

Signs and Symptoms

Gastric cancer is rarely diagnosed in its early stages because symptoms do not appear until late in the disease (Table 33.6). In the early stages, there may not be any symptoms at all, and metastasis to another organ, such as the liver, may have already occurred. The symptoms of gastric cancer are often

TABLE 33.6 GASTRIC CANCER SUMMARY

Signs and Symptoms	Rarely detected during early stages Symptoms often mistaken for PUD: indigestion, anorexia, pain, weight loss, nausea, vomiting, anemia Late symptoms include involvement of other organs such as the liver
Diagnostic Tests	X-ray studies Gastroscopy Gastric fluid analysis Serum gastrin levels
Therapeutic Measures	Medical treatment not very effective Surgical treatment: subtotal or total gastrectomy
Complications	Related to disease and surgery: hemorrhage, acute gastric distention, nutritional problems
Priority Nursing Diagnoses	*Acute Pain* *Fear*

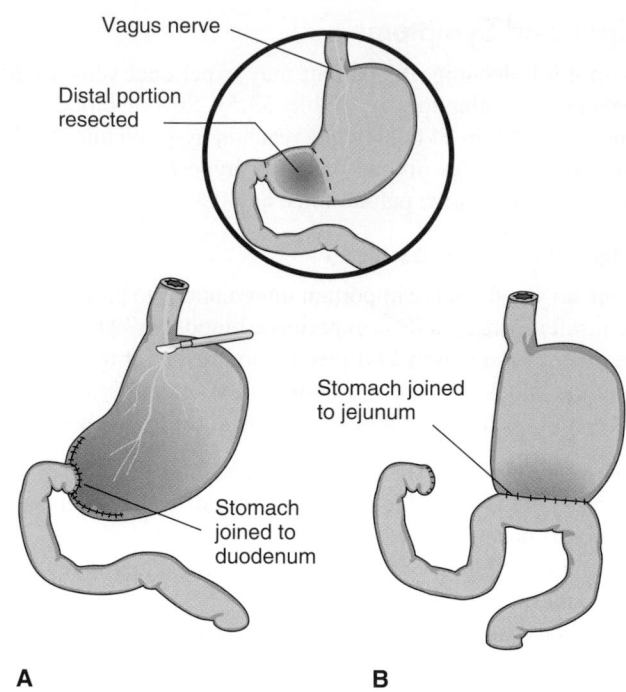

FIGURE 33.6 Subtotal gastrectomy involves removing the distal portion of the stomach. The remaining portion of the stomach is then sutured (A) to the duodenum (Billroth I procedure) or (B) to the proximal jejunum (Billroth II procedure).

mistaken for peptic ulcer disease: indigestion, anorexia, pain relieved by antacids, weight loss, and nausea and vomiting. Anemia from blood loss commonly occurs, and occult blood may be present in the stool.

Diagnostic Tests

Diagnosis of gastric cancer is made by upper GI x-ray examination, gastroscopy, gastric fluid analysis, and measurement of serum gastrin levels.

Therapeutic Measures

There is little effective medical treatment available for gastric cancer. Surgical removal of the cancer is the most effective treatment. Most often the cancer has already metastasized, and surgery is performed only to relieve the symptoms. Chemotherapy and radiation are sometimes used in conjunction with surgery. Biological therapies with natural substance to boost the immune system might also be tried.

■ GASTRIC SURGERY

Two types of surgical interventions are typically used to treat upper GI diseases: subtotal gastrectomy and total gastrectomy. There are two types of subtotal gastrectomy, which is partial removal of the stomach. It is used to treat cancer or rarely peptic ulcer disease that does not respond to therapy. For a **gastroduodenostomy** (Billroth I), the distal portion of the stomach is removed, and the remainder of the stomach is anastomosed (surgically attached) to the duodenum (Fig. 33.6). A

gastrojejunostomy (Billroth II) involves removal of a larger amount of the distal stomach and reanastomosis of the proximal remnant of the stomach to the proximal jejunum (see Fig. 33.6). Because it results in bypassing of the duodenum, the Billroth II procedure is used to treat duodenal ulcers. Pancreatic secretions and bile are necessary for digestion and continue to be secreted from the common bile duct even after partial gastrectomy. Total gastrectomy, the total removal of the stomach, is the treatment for extensive gastric cancer. This surgery involves total removal of the stomach, with anastomosis of the esophagus to the jejunum (Fig. 33.7). Rarely, a vagotomy may also be performed.

Nursing Process for the Patient Having Gastric Surgery

Data Collection

Identify the patient's fears or concerns and provide knowledge about postoperative care and discharge instructions to teach them how to assist in their recovery. This teaching includes incisional care, activity or dietary restrictions, and information about prescribed medications.

Postoperatively, the patient's vital signs are monitored as ordered. Respiratory status is carefully monitored because

• WORD • BUILDING •

gastroduodenostomy: gastro—stomach + duoden—duodenum + ostomy—mouth or opening

gastrojejunostomy: gastro—stomach + jejeun—jejunum + ostomy—mouth or opening

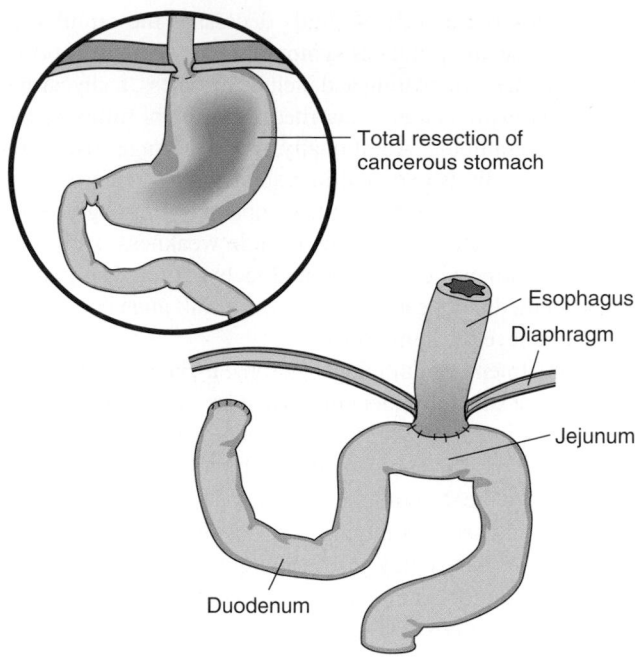

FIGURE 33.7 Total gastrectomy.

the high location of the surgical incision may cause pain, which interferes with deep breathing and coughing. Atelectasis or pneumonia can develop as a result of guarding and shallow breathing. The patient's pain is assessed and relieved, which also helps the patient's ability to deep breathe or cough without pain. The patient's IV site and infusion are monitored, and intake and output are recorded. The incisional site and dressings are observed for drainage and bleeding. Early ambulation is encouraged to promote a quicker recovery by improving respiratory and gastrointestinal function.

Patients may have an NG tube inserted during surgery. The drainage from the NG tube is monitored for color and amount. If bleeding or excessive amounts of drainage or abdominal distention are noted, they are reported to the physician.

 BE SAFE!

After gastric surgery, do not irrigate or reposition an NG tube to prevent damaging the suture line.

Nursing Diagnoses, Planning, and Implementation

Acute Pain related to postoperative status

EXPECTED OUTCOME: The patient's pain will be controlled or reduced to a tolerable level of 2 to 3 on a pain scale of 0 to 10 within 30 minutes of report of pain.

• Evaluate pain regularly, noting characteristics, location, and intensity on pain scale of 0 to 10 *to provide information regarding patient's pain level and effectiveness of interventions.*

• Assess religion, culture, beliefs, and circumstances *to determine impact on patient's pain and response to interventions.*
• Monitor incision noting any drainage, redness, swelling, or increased pain *to assess for postoperative infection, which can increase pain level.*
• Take vital signs (note if tachycardia, hypertension, or tachypnea is present), *which may indicate acute pain is present.*
• Provide comfort measures such as positioning every 2 hours and back rub *to improve circulation and reduce tension associated with pain.*
• Use relaxation techniques such as deep breathing, guided imagery, music, and distraction therapy *to enhance relaxation and improve pain relief.*
• Medicate as ordered on routine schedule for 24 to 48 hours *to control postoperative pain and prevent pain from becoming unbearable for patient.*
• Ensure functioning of NG tube (usually low intermittent suction) *to prevent distention and increased pain.*
• Notify physician if pain control measures are unsuccessful *to allow revision of treatment plan.*

Fear related to body image changes, treatment, and life-threatening illness

EXPECTED OUTCOME: The patient will understand and discuss disease process and treatment options and possible outcomes of treatment before surgical procedure.

• Use open communication and convey acceptance of patient's fears *to help patient cope with fears.*
• Explain disease process and treatment options, reinforce as needed *to decrease patient's fear of the unknown.*
• Explain all postoperative procedures and interventions (such as medications, NG tube, drains) *to help decrease the patient's fear.*

Evaluation

If interventions have been effective, the patient will report a reduction of pain to a tolerable level or the total absence of pain and will also verbalize understanding of the disease process, treatment options, and possible outcomes of treatment.

Complications of Gastric Surgery

Complications that can occur after gastric surgery include hemorrhage, acute gastric distention, dumping syndrome, nutritional problems, **steatorrhea** (fat in stools), and pyloric obstruction.

Hemorrhage

The incidence of hemorrhage after gastric surgery is very low and most often caused by a dislodged clot at the surgical site or slippage of a suture. The patient experiencing hemorrhage exhibits restlessness, cold skin, increased pulse and respirations, and decreased temperature and blood pressure. The patient may have a change in level of consciousness and become confused. In addition, the patient may vomit bright red blood. To prevent aspiration during vomiting, the patient is turned to one side and the head of the bed is elevated.

Following gastric surgery, patients usually have an NG tube that has been inserted in the operating room. The drainage from the tube should be assessed for color and amount. A small amount of pink or light red drainage may be expected for the first 12 hours, but moderate or excessive bleeding should be immediately reported to the physician. The abdominal dressing should also be assessed for any drainage or bleeding.

Gastric Distention

In the immediate postoperative period, distention of the stomach can occur if an inserted NG tube is clogged or if an NG tube has not been inserted. Symptoms of gastric distention include an enlarged abdomen, epigastric pain, tachycardia, and hypotension. The patient may say she is feeling full and may hiccup or gag repeatedly. These symptoms must be reported to the physician.

CRITICAL THINKING

Mr. Wong

■ You are working the evening shift on a surgical unit. A patient, Mr. Wong, has had gastric surgery earlier that morning. He has an IV infusion of 1000 mL dextrose 5% in 0.45 normal saline over 8 hours and a NG tube set to low intermittent suction. Mr. Wong is restless and reporting pain. His abdomen is distended. The suction canister contains no gastric output.

1. What nursing interventions in order of priority are needed to help Mr. Wong?
2. What equipment do you need to care for Mr. Wong?
3. As you monitor the IV, you know it is set for how many drops per minute with a 10-drop factor IV set?

Suggested answers are at the end of the chapter.

The physician usually inserts the NG tube during surgery so that the suture line is not damaged. If suction is desired, a physician's order is required. Irrigating or repositioning the NG tube is not performed by the nurse to prevent harm to the suture line. Any problems with distention or an improperly functioning NG tube are reported to the physician. The physician may need to reposition the NG tube to correct the problem. The patient's vital signs should be monitored until the patient's distention is relieved and the patient is stable.

Dumping Syndrome

Dumping syndrome is one of the most common complications of gastric surgery. It occurs with the rapid entry of food into the jejunum without proper mixing of the food with digestive juices. On entering the jejunum, the hyperosmolar food draws extracellular fluid into the bowel from the circulating blood volume to dilute the high concentration of electrolytes and

sugars. This rapid shift of fluids decreases the circulating blood volume and produces symptoms. The symptoms occur 5 to 30 minutes after eating and include dizziness, tachycardia, fainting, sweating, nausea, diarrhea, a feeling of fullness, and abdominal cramping. Additionally, the blood sugar rises, and excessive insulin is excreted in response. This release of insulin causes the patient to have symptoms of hypoglycemia about 2 hours later. Symptoms include weakness, sweating, anxiety, shakiness, confusion, and tachycardia. The patient should immediately eat some candy or drink juice containing sugar to relieve the symptoms.

The treatment for dumping syndrome includes teaching the patient to eat small, frequent meals that are high in protein and fat and low in carbohydrates, especially refined sugars (see "Nutrition Notes"). The patient is also taught to avoid fluids 1 hour before meals, with meals, or for 2 hours after meals to prevent rapid gastric emptying. It is best for the patient to lie down after meals to delay gastric emptying. The patient is told that these symptoms may last for up to 6 months after gastric surgery but usually slowly subside over time.

CRITICAL THINKING

Mrs. Lindsay

■ Mrs. Lindsay has had gastric surgery. You have taught her about dumping syndrome, and she is concerned about what she will eat. Create a 1-day meal plan for Mrs. Lindsay.

Suggested answers are at the end of the chapter.

Nutritional Problems

Nutritional problems that commonly occur after removal of part or all of the stomach include vitamin B_{12} and folic acid deficiency and reduced absorption of calcium and vitamin D. Also, rapid entry of food into the bowel often results in inadequate absorption of food.

Following gastric surgery, patients may be NPO until the physician resumes a diet. IV fluid provides hydration. However, if patients are to be NPO for any length of time, they will need an alternate form of nutrition such as parenteral nutrition with an IV solution to meet their caloric and nutritional needs.

After removal of the nasogastric tube, clear fluids may be ordered with progression to full liquids, then soft foods as the patient tolerates. Foods and fluids should be introduced into the diet gradually following gastric surgery. If the patient eats too much or too fast, regurgitation may result.

PERNICIOUS ANEMIA. Vitamin B_{12} deficiency may occur after some or all of the stomach is removed because intrinsic factor secretion is reduced or absent. Normally vitamin B_{12} combines with intrinsic factor to prevent its digestion in the stomach and promote its absorption in the intestines. Lifelong replacement of vitamin B_{12} is required to prevent the development of pernicious anemia, and patients must be taught the importance of complying with this treatment. Traditionally after gastric surgery, it is given by the parenteral route. However, other routes such as oral tablets or nasal gel may be effectively used. Vitamin B$_{12}$ injections are given daily initially, then weekly, and then monthly for life. Symptoms of pernicious anemia include anemia, weakness, sore tongue, numbness and tingling, and GI upset.

Steatorrhea

Steatorrhea is the presence of excessive fat in the stools and is the result of rapid gastric emptying, which prevents adequate mixing of fat with pancreatic and biliary secretions. In most cases, steatorrhea can be controlled by reducing the intake of fat in the diet.

Pyloric Obstruction

Pyloric obstruction can occur after gastric surgery as a result of scarring, edema, inflammation, or a combination of these. The signs and symptoms are vomiting, a feeling of fullness, gastric distention, nausea after eating, loss of appetite, and weight loss. As the obstruction increases, it gradually becomes more difficult for the stomach to empty, and symptoms worsen. Conservative methods are used first, such as replacing fluids and electrolytes through IV fluids and decompressing the distended stomach using a NG tube. Surgery may be necessary if conservative measures do not relieve the signs and symptoms. Pyloroplasty widens the exit of the pylorus to improve emptying of the stomach.

SUGGESTED ANSWERS TO

CRITICAL THINKING

■ *Mr. Smith*

1. Additional data would include vital signs (looking for signs of shock), assessment of Mr. Smith's abdomen (looking for location of pain, tenderness, rigidity), assessment for any vomiting and characteristics of emesis including any blood, and assessment for IV site access.

2. Assist Mr. Smith to a comfortable position and stay with him. Call for help. Inform the RN so the physician can be notified immediately and provide data regarding Mr. Smith's change in condition. Administer oxygen, monitor IV fluids, and continue to monitor vital signs. Medicate for pain as ordered.

3. Explain that you will stay with Mr. Smith as you gather data and take vital signs. State that you have informed the RN, who will assess Mr. Smith and report findings to the physician. Explain that the treatments as ordered by the physician will be started: oxygen, IV fluids, pain medication. State that explanation will be provided related to Mr. Smith's care. Invite questions and have a nursing assistant provide Mrs. Smith with comfort needs: beverage, tissues, chair.

4. You suspect a perforated duodenal ulcer, which is a medical-surgical emergency.

5. RN, HCP

6. Prepare Mr. Smith for surgery. Interventions would include maintaining NPO status, starting an IV, ensure that the consent is signed, obtain labs (may include complete blood count (CBC), chemistry panel, type and crossmatch for blood), and administer antibiotics as ordered.

■ *Mr. Wong*

1. Prioritize your interventions:

   a. Take Mr. Wong's vital signs to determine whether he is stable. Pain can sometimes increase the blood pressure and pulse rate.

However, gastric distention can cause pain, and once the distention is relieved, the pain caused by distention subsides.

b. Check placement of Mr. Wong's NG tube by aspirating gastric contents and verifying the pH of the contents as ordered. It is important to check for abdominal placement of Mr. Wong's NG tube to make sure it is not misplaced in the lungs. After abdominal placement is determined, if there is a physician's order, the NG tube can be connected to suction equipment, usually set on low intermittent suction. Do not reposition an NG tube in a patient who has had gastric surgery. Repositioning the NG tube could damage the surgical suture line.

c. Next check the suction equipment for ordered settings and to ensure that it is turned on. The suction setting normally is ordered to be on low. A whistling sound is heard when the tube is disconnected from the suction setup. The seals should be tight on the suction canister. When the tubing is hooked to suction, gastric contents should start moving into the suction canister. It is important to make sure equipment is functioning properly to ensure patient safety.

d. Check the NG tube for clogs only if the physician orders aspiration or irrigation to be done. The tube is gently aspirated with a 60-mL catheter-tipped syringe. If the tube remains clogged, it is gently flushed as ordered with 10 to 20 mL of sterile normal saline.

e. After the gastric distention has been relieved, Mr. Wong's pain level is reassessed to determine if he needs pain medication. Considering that he is less than 1 day postoperative, he probably needs it.

2. Necessary equipment includes stethoscope, 60-mL catheter-tipped syringe, gloves, goggles, and normal saline for irrigation.

Continued

SUGGESTED ANSWERS TO—cont'd

3.

$$\frac{1000 \text{ mL}}{480 \text{ min}} \times \frac{10 \text{ gtt}}{\text{mL}}$$

$$= \frac{10,000 \text{ drops}}{480\text{min}} = 21 \text{ drops/min}$$

■ *Mrs. Lindsay*

Although there are many variations, the following is an example of a 1-day meal plan for Mrs. Lindsay:

Breakfast: one egg, any style; 1/2 orange; one glass milk

Snack: one slice toast with apple butter, jelly, or jam

Lunch: 2 oz ham, 1/2 cup cottage cheese, four asparagus spears

Snack: 1/2 serving chicken salad on bed of lettuce

Dinner: 2 oz broiled fish, 1/2 serving corn, 1/2 serving broccoli

Snack: 1/2 cup yogurt or sherbet

REVIEW QUESTIONS

1. The nurse is planning care for a patient with an eating disorder. The patient is 40 kg and 68 inches tall. Serum laboratory data: potassium 2.6 mEq/dL, sodium 126 mEq/dL, chloride 95 mEq/dL, calcium 10.8 mg/dL. Which of these is the priority intervention for this patient?
   1. Weigh the patient daily at the same time.
   2. Maintain IV of dextrose and electrolytes.
   3. Praise intake of any type of food.
   4. Document intake and output.

2. The nurse is planning care for a team of patients. To provide care safely, for which patient should the nurse use specialized mobility equipment designed for the patient who is obese?
   1. A 25-year-old woman with body weight 5% above ideal body weight
   2. A 45-year-old man with waist-to-hip ratio measurement of 0.5
   3. A 50-year-old man with body mass index of 31
   4. A 21-year-old woman with anorexia nervosa weighing 98 pounds

3. A patient is diagnosed with aphthous stomatitis (canker sore). Which of the following actions would be appropriate?
   1. Tell patient to avoid brushing teeth until the sore has healed.
   2. Encourage patient to use a mouthwash four times a day.
   3. Apply acyclovir ointment to ease the pain of the lesion.
   4. Teach patient to apply topical tetracycline several times a day to sore.

4. The nurse is caring for a patient with gastritis. Which of the following interventions would be appropriate for a patient with acute gastritis?
   1. Monitor patient for bloody diarrhea.
   2. Explain that aspirin rarely causes gastritis.
   3. Administer phenothiazine to control vomiting.
   4. Encourage a regular diet during the acute phase of gastritis.

5. The nurse is planning a teaching session for a patient with a peptic ulcer. Which of the following would the nurse include in the teaching plan as the primary cause of peptic ulcers?
   1. Eating spicy foods
   2. A stressful life
   3. A bacterial infection
   4. Excessive caffeine intake

6. The nurse provides teaching for a patient with a peptic ulcer. Which patient statement indicates patient understanding of the purpose of H_2 antagonists?
   1. Neutralize gastric acid
   2. Form a protective paste
   3. Determine gastric pH levels
   4. Inhibit secretion of gastric acid

7. A patient who has just returned from surgery after a total gastrectomy begins to vomit bright red blood. Which of the following is the priority action for the nurse to take?
   1. Increase the IV rate.
   2. Take blood pressure.
   3. Place patient onto side.
   4. Administer oxygen.

8. The nurse is teaching a patient with dumping syndrome about food choices. Which of these foods would the nurse instruct the patient to avoid?
   1. Spinach and avocado salad
   2. Coffee and glazed doughnut
   3. Sausage and liver
   4. Creamed chipped beef

9. To deliver 1000 mL of 5% dextrose in 0.45 normal saline (at 150 mL per hour using 10 drop tubings), the nurse would monitor the IV infusion at how many drops per minute? **Fill in the blank.**
   Answer: _____ drops per minute

   Answers can be found in Appendix C.

Reference

Janarthanan, S., Ditah, I., Adler, D. G., & Ehrinpreis, M. N. (2012). *Clostridium difficile*–associated diarrhea and proton pump inhibitor therapy: A meta-analysis. *American Journal of Gastroenterology, 107,* 1001–1010.

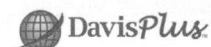 Davis*Plus* | For additional resources and information visit **davispl.us/medsurg5**

34

Nursing Care of Patients With Lower Gastrointestinal Disorders

KEY TERMS

appendicitis (uh-PEN-dih-SYE-tiss)
colectomy (koh-LEK-tuh-me)
colitis (koh-LYE-tiss)
colostomy (kuh-LAW-stuh-mee)
constipation (KON-stih-PAY-shun)
diarrhea (DYE-uh-REE-ah)
diverticulitis (DYE-ver-tik-yoo-LYE-tiss)
diverticulosis (DYE-ver-tik-yoo-LOH-siss)
enteritis (en-tur-EYE-tiss)
fissures (FISH-ers)
fistulas (FIST-yoo-lahs)
hematochezia (HEM-uh-toh-KEE-zee-uh)
hemorrhoids (HEM-uh-royds)
hernia (HER-nee-uh)
ileostomy (ILL-ee-AW-stuh-mee)
impaction (im-PAK-shun)
intussusception (IN-tuh-suh-SEP-shun)
megacolon (MEG-ah-KOH-lun)
melena (muh-LEE-nah)
obstipation (OB-stih-PAY-shun)
peristomal (PEAR-ih-STOH-muhl)
peritonitis (pear-ih-toh-NYE-tiss)
stoma (STOH-mah)
volvulus (VOL-view-luss)

LEARNING OUTCOMES

1. List data to collect when caring for patients with lower gastrointestinal disorders.
2. Identify the causes, signs and symptoms, and therapeutic measures of constipation and diarrhea.
3. Plan nursing care and teaching for patients with constipation or diarrhea.
4. Describe pathophysiology, therapeutic measures, nursing care, and teaching for patients with inflammatory and infectious disorders of the lower gastrointestinal tract.
5. Describe pathophysiology, therapeutic measures, nursing care, and teaching for inflammatory bowel disease.
6. Plan nursing care for an abdominal hernia.
7. Plan nursing care and teaching for patients with absorption disorders.
8. Describe causes, signs and symptoms, therapeutic measures, and nursing care for intestinal obstruction.
9. Plan nursing care for anorectal problems.
10. Describe causes, signs and symptoms, therapeutic measures, and nursing care for lower gastrointestinal bleeding.
11. Describe the causes, signs and symptoms, therapeutic measures, and nursing care for colon cancer.
12. Plan nursing care and teaching for a patient with an ostomy.
13. Discuss how to know if nursing care for various lower gastrointestinal disorders is effective.

The lower gastrointestinal (GI) system includes the small and large intestines, rectum, and anus.

 PROBLEMS OF ELIMINATION

Constipation
Pathophysiology

Constipation occurs when the fecal mass is held in the rectal cavity for a period of time that is not usual for the patient. While the feces are held for a prolonged time in the rectum, more water is absorbed. This makes the feces drier, harder, and more difficult and sometimes painful to pass.

If a patient repeatedly ignores the urge to have a bowel movement (laxation), the musculature and rectal mucous membrane become insensitive to the presence of feces. Eventually a stronger stimulus is needed to produce the peristaltic rush required for defecation. Prolonged constipation is called **obstipation**.

Etiology

There are many causes of constipation. Medications such as narcotics, tranquilizers, and antacids with aluminum decrease motility of the large intestine and may contribute to constipation. Rectal or anal conditions such as hemorrhoids or fissures may lead to a delay in defecation because of the associated pain. Metabolic or neurologic conditions such as diabetes mellitus, multiple sclerosis, lupus erythematosus, or scleroderma may interfere with normal bowel innervation and function. Colon cancer may cause an obstruction that prevents normal bowel function and leads to constipation. Low intake of dietary fiber and fluids decreases the bulk of the feces and causes constipation. Decreased mobility, weakness, and fatigue, especially in the older adult, reduce the strength of the muscles used for defecation, increasing the likelihood of constipation.

Prevention

Regular exercise and a diet high in fiber and fluids are the best preventive measures for constipation. Laxatives should be used only occasionally to prevent complications.

Signs and Symptoms

Abdominal pain and distention, indigestion, rectal pressure, a sensation of incomplete emptying, and intestinal rumbling are indications of constipation (Table 34.1). The patient may also report headache, fatigue, decreased appetite, straining at stool, and elimination of hard, dry stool.

Complications

A variety of problems can result from constipation. Fecal **impaction** may result when the fecal mass is so dry it cannot be passed. Pressure on the colon mucosa from a mass of stool may cause ulcers to develop. Often, small amounts of liquid stool ooze around the fecal mass and cause incontinence of liquid stools. The incontinence may be treated with an antidiarrheal medication, which will worsen the constipation

TABLE 34.1	CONSTIPATION SUMMARY
Signs and Symptoms	Abdominal distention Indigestion Rectal pressure Feeling of incomplete emptying Straining at stool Hard, dry stool Intestinal rumbling
Diagnostic Tests	History Physical examination
Therapeutic Measures	High-fiber diet 2–3 L fluid daily Strengthening of abdominal muscles Exercise Bulk-forming agents Stool softeners
Priority Nursing Diagnoses	*Constipation* *Deficient Knowledge*

if a thorough assessment is not performed to rule out impaction. Straining to have a bowel movement (Valsalva's maneuver) can result in cardiac, neurologic, and respiratory complications. If the patient has a history of heart failure, hypertension, or recent myocardial infarction, straining can lead to cardiac rupture and death. Grossly dilated loops of the colon, known as **megacolon**, can occur proximal to the dry fecal mass and obstruct the colon. Abdominal distention occurs, and in severe cases, loops of bowel can be palpated through the abdominal wall.

Chronic laxative abuse can lead to colonic mucosal atrophy, muscle thickening, and fibrosis. These conditions can result in perforation of the colon and necessitate an emergency **colectomy**.

Diagnostic Tests

Constipation is usually self-diagnosed or diagnosed by history and physical examination. If complications are suspected, a radiographic examination, sigmoidoscopy, and stool testing for occult blood may be needed.

Therapeutic Measures

Treatment of constipation depends on the cause. Fiber should be added to the diet, and exercises to strengthen abdominal muscles should be done. Behavior changes, such as setting a daily defecation time, appropriately responding to the urge to defecate, and drinking 8 oz of warm water

• **WORD** • **BUILDING** •
megacolon: mega—large + colon—colon
colectomy: col—pertaining to colon + ectomy—surgical excision

every morning and 2 to 3 L of water every day, if not contraindicated for other reasons, can help establish a more normal bowel pattern. Chronic laxative use should be discontinued. Bulk-forming agents such as psyllium (Metamucil) or stool softeners such as docusate sodium (Colace) should be used instead of laxatives. Enemas and rectal suppositories are used only in extreme cases and are discontinued when an acute episode is resolved. Methylnaltrexone (Relistor) given subcutaneously treats opioid-induced constipation for patients receiving palliative care when other laxatives have not been effective. It does not treat other forms of constipation.

Nursing Process for the Patient With Constipation

DATA COLLECTION. The patient may feel self-conscious or embarrassed when interviewed about bowel habits and history. Consideration should be given to the patient's feelings by postponing the discussion until rapport has been established. Data gathered in privacy should include the onset and duration of constipation, past elimination pattern, current elimination pattern, occupation, lifestyle (stress, exercise, nutrition), history of laxative or enema use, medical-surgical history, and current medications being taken. Color, consistency, and any odor of the stool, as well as any intestinal symptoms, are also important.

After the interview, the patient's abdomen is inspected and palpated for distention and symmetry. Inspection of the perianal area may reveal fissures, external hemorrhoids, or irritation.

NURSING DIAGNOSES, PLANNING, AND IMPLEMENTATION.
Constipation related to irregular defecation habits
EXPECTED OUTCOME: The patient will maintain passage of soft, formed stool every 1 to 3 days without straining.

- Assess normal pattern of defecation, diet and fluid intake, medications, surgeries, and use of laxatives *to help identify factors contributing to constipation.*
- Determine patient's access to the bathroom and ability to use the toilet *to ensure barriers to safe toileting, such as unsafe obstructing furniture arrangements or clutter, are removed.*
- Set a specific time for defecation, such as after a meal, *to facilitate the urge reflex.*
- Place feet on a footstool *to promote flexion of the hips, which aids defecation.*
- Provide a high-fiber, high-residue diet including fresh fruits, vegetables, and whole grains with 2 g of bran added to cereal daily for constipation caused by decreased motility and muscle tone or a low-fiber diet *to significantly increase bowel movements and decrease the number of laxatives, enemas, or stool softeners required* ("Nutrition Notes").
- Increase fluid if not contraindicated to 2 to 3 L per day *to aid in ability to discontinue laxative use.*
- Increase activity through a daily walking program and abdominal exercises designed to improve the muscle tone *to improve peristalsis and promote more spontaneous defecation.*

Nutrition Notes

Treating Constipation With Food Formula

Constipation may be successfully treated with 1 to 2 oz of the following mixture taken with the evening meal:
   1 cup applesauce,
   1 cup All-Bran cereal, and
   1/2 cup 100% prune juice.
   Mixture may be stored in the refrigerator for 5 days and then should be discarded. In all cases of constipation, especially when increased fiber is given, adequate fluid intake is essential.

Treating Constipation With Food Choices

Achieving the recommended fiber intake of 21 to 38 grams per day is a matter of prudent choices at every meal. Listed below are examples of high fiber foods on the left and foods in the same category on the right with less fiber.

Higher Fiber Foods	Grams of Fiber	Lower Fiber Foods	Grams of Fiber
Breakfast			
All-bran buds, 1/3 cup	13	Corn flakes, 1 cup	1
Orange sections, 1 cup	4	Orange juice from frozen concentrate, 1 cup	0
Lunch			
Wendy's chili, small	5	Campbell's microwavable chicken noodle soup, 1 cup	2
Raw apple with skin, 2 3/4" diameter	4	Raw apple peeled, 2 3/4" diameter	2
Dinner			
Whole wheat spaghetti, 1 cup cooked	6	White spaghetti, 1 cup cooked	3
Banana, 1 cup sliced	4	Watermelon 1 cup diced	1
Totals	**36**		**9**

Many other foods also contribute to fiber intake and can be evaluated via nutrition labels or at http://ndb.nal.usda .gov or http://nutritiondata.self.com. Individuals who wish to correct constipation without medications should determine their present fiber intake and increase it gradually to the U.S. Department of Agriculture Recommended Dietary Allowance while also drinking sufficient water.

╔══════════════════════════════════════╗
║ **CRITICAL THINKING**   ║
║   ║
║ *Mrs. Burns*   ║
║   ║
║ ■ Mrs. Burns is a 93-year-old resident in an assisted liv-║
║ ing facility. The nurse notes that she has not had a bowel║
║ movement in 5 days. What action should the nurse take║
║ to provide patient centered care?   ║
║ *Suggested answers are at the end of the chapter.*║
╚══════════════════════════════════════╝

Deficient Knowledge related to practices to prevent constipation
EXPECTED OUTCOME: The patient will state understanding and ability to carry out preventive measures for constipation.

• Teach factors leading to constipation, such as a low-fiber diet, and preventive interventions such as increasing fiber or fluid intake. *Prevention of constipation may be as simple as correcting the contributing factors.*

• Explain the physiology of defecation and the importance of responding to the urge to defecate when it occurs *to help prevent constipation.*

• Explain that regular laxative use may increase motility and pressure in the bowel and cause further complications *to promote understanding and use of other preventive measures.*

EVALUATION. The plan has been effective if the patient has established a regular bowel function pattern (Table 34.2), verbalizes understanding of self-care measures, and expresses satisfaction with the outcomes.

Diarrhea

Diarrhea occurs when fecal matter passes through the intestine rapidly, resulting in decreased absorption of water, electrolytes, and nutrients and causing frequent, watery stools. Classification and severity of diarrhea are based on the number of unformed stools in 24 hours.

Pathophysiology and Etiology

The most common cause of acute diarrhea is a bacterial or viral infection. Bacteria (normal flora) are normally found in

---

TABLE 34.2   CRITERIA FOR REGULAR BOWEL FUNCTION

1. A regular time for defecation is routine.
2. A regular exercise program is followed.
3. Laxative use is avoided.
4. Water consumption is 2–3 L per day.
5. High-fiber and high-residue foods are added to the diet.
6. Consistency of stools reported is soft and formed.
7. Frequency of stools is every 1 to 3 days.

---

the intestines. If these bacteria grow out of control or if bacteria or viruses are ingested in contaminated food or water, infection results. Some bacteria release toxins that irritate the intestinal mucosa, causing an inflammatory response and an increase in mucus production. Hyperperistalsis occurs, which lasts until the irritants have been excreted. The most common infectious agents are *Escherichia coli, Campylobacter jejuni, Shigella* spp., *Clostridium difficile, Giardia* spp., and *Salmonella* spp.

Poor tolerance or allergies to certain foods may cause diarrhea. Foods that most commonly cause diarrhea are additives (such as nutmeg or sorbitol), caffeine, milk products, meats, wheat, and potatoes. Acute diarrhea usually resolves in 7 to 14 days.

Chronic diarrhea may result from inflammatory disease, osmotic agents, excessive secretion of electrolytes, or increased intestinal motility. Inflammatory diseases such as Crohn's disease or ulcerative colitis (discussed later) may impair absorption, resulting in frequent, watery stools. Osmotic diarrhea results from ingestion of laxatives or other agents that prevent absorption of water or nutrients in the intestine. Additional causes of malabsorption include surgical resection or disease of certain areas of the intestinal tract, such as the terminal ileum or pylorus. Radiation therapy for cancer also may induce a malabsorption syndrome. Enteral feedings can result in diarrhea, especially when malnutrition has caused edema in the gut wall, which decreases absorption.

Increased secretion of water and electrolytes by the intestinal mucosa associated with certain hormonal disorders results in high-volume fecal output. An irritable bowel or a neurologic disorder may cause increased motility problems.

Prevention

To prevent diarrhea, proper handling, storage, and refrigeration of all fresh foods helps to minimize contact with infectious agents. Milk and milk products must be kept refrigerated and protected. Hand hygiene and cleaning of the kitchen and the food preparation and serving items are extremely important. Also enteral feedings should be given using full-strength formula rather than diluting the formula. This reduces the risk of contaminating the formula.

Signs and Symptoms

Initial diarrhea stools may be foul smelling and have undigested food particles and mucus (Table 34.3). The stools may also contain blood or pus. Diarrhea resulting from food poisoning usually has an explosive onset and may be accompanied by nausea and vomiting. Abdominal cramping, distention, anorexia, intestinal rumbling, and thirst are common. Fever indicates infection. Weakness and dehydration from fluid loss may occur ("Gerontological Issues").

• WORD • BUILDING •
diarrhea: dia—through + rhea—to flow

TABLE 34.3 DIARRHEA SUMMARY

Signs and Symptoms	Frequent, watery stools Abdominal cramping Distention Anorexia Intestinal rumbling
Causes	Inflammatory diseases such as Crohn's disease and ulcerative colitis Infectious organisms Recent antibiotic use Surgical procedures such as bowel resection Laxatives Enteral tube feedings Radiation therapy
Diagnostic Tests	History Laboratory examinations of stool
Therapeutic Measures	Replacement of fluids and electrolytes Antidiarrheal medications Antimicrobials Lactinex
Priority Nursing Diagnoses	*Diarrhea* *Deficient Fluid Volume* *Deficient Knowledge*

Gerontological Issues

Dehydration and Hypokalemia

Diarrhea can cause older people to quickly become dehydrated and hypokalemic because both fluid and potassium are lost in stools. The signs and symptoms of hypokalemia include muscle weakness, hypotension, anorexia, paresthesia, and drowsiness. It can also cause cardiac dysrhythmias, such as atrial and ventricular tachycardia, premature ventricular contraction, and ventricular fibrillation, which can be fatal.

If the older person has decreased mobility, quick access to the bathroom is important. Because of poor muscle control, older patients may be incontinent. This might embarrass patients or cause them to hurry, which increases chances of patients falling and causing other problems such as fracture, dislocation, or hematoma. Also, because older patients' skin is more sensitive resulting from poor turgor and a reduction in subcutaneous fat layers, perirectal skin excoriation can occur secondary to the acidity and digestive enzyme content of diarrheal stools.

Diagnostic Tests

The diagnosis of diarrhea is determined by the onset and progression of the condition, presence of fever, laboratory examinations, and visual inspection of the stool for bacteria, pus, or blood. Diarrhea mixed with red blood cells (RBCs) and mucus is associated with cholera, typhoid, typhus, large-bowel cancer, or amebiasis. Diarrhea mixed with white blood cells (WBCs) and mucus is associated with shigellosis, intestinal tuberculosis, salmonellosis, regional **enteritis**, or ulcerative colitis. Bulky, frothy stool is seen in celiac disease. Pasty stools usually have a high fat content and may be associated with common bile duct obstruction and celiac disease.

Therapeutic Measures

Replacing fluids and electrolytes is the first priority. This can be done by increasing oral fluid intake and using solutions with glucose and electrolytes if ordered by the health care provider (HCP). Intravenous (IV) fluid replacement may be necessary for rapid hydration, especially in the very young or very old. An elimination diet can be tried to identify foods that may contribute to diarrhea. Foods known to cause diarrhea are eliminated to see if a change in bowel function occurs. Each food item is then added back into the diet, one at a time, to see which ones cause diarrhea.

If the patient has three or more watery stools per day, motility of the intestines can be decreased with the use of drugs, such as diphenoxylate (Lomotil), difenoxin HCl (Motofen), and loperamide (Imodium). If diarrhea is thought to be caused by antibiotics that change the normal flora of the bowel, a *Lactobacillus* granule probiotic supplement (Lactinex) may be used to help restore the normal flora. Fecal transplant can restore the normal intestinal flora in those who are ill (Chapter 32). Antimicrobial agents are prescribed if infectious agents have been identified.

Nursing Process for the Patient With Diarrhea

DATA COLLECTION. Observation of the patient's behaviors and symptoms assists in identifying the cause of diarrhea. Ask the patient to describe any symptoms, when they started, and how long they have been present. Questions should include "Is there any abdominal pain, urgency, or cramping?" and "What time of the day does it happen?" Stool consistency, color, odor, and frequency are documented.

Observe for symptoms of dehydration, such as tachycardia, hypotension, decreased skin turgor, weakness, thready pulse, dry mucous membranes, and oliguria. Obtain the patient's height and weight to establish a baseline. Abnormal laboratory studies that may indicate dehydration include increased serum osmolality, increased specific gravity of urine, and increased hematocrit. Decreased serum potassium may result from intestinal loss of potassium.

Inspect the abdomen for distention. The patient's usual dietary habits and any changes or recent exposure to contaminated

• WORD • BUILDING •
enteritis: entero—intestine + itis—inflammation

food or water are noted. Determine if medications such as antibiotics or laxatives could have contributed to the diarrhea. If the patient has traveled recently, determine the geographic location and whether exposure to an infected person or someone with similar symptoms occurred.

Data are collected on the patient's coping mechanisms for use if the patient needs to express concerns or anxiety regarding incontinence of liquid stools and embarrassment.

NURSING DIAGNOSES, PLANNING, AND IMPLEMENTATION.
Diarrhea related to infection or possible ingestion of irritating foods

EXPECTED OUTCOME: The patient will maintain formed, soft stool every 1 to 3 days.

- Obtain history including medications regarding diarrhea episode *to help identify cause.*
- Monitor and record stool characteristics, amount, and frequency *to plan care.*
- Ensure hand hygiene by patient, family, and health care staff *to prevent the spread of infection.*
- Identify potentially infected persons or contaminated foods *to prevent the spread of infection.*
- Consider private patient room *to prevent infection transmission.*
- Maintain nothing by mouth (NPO) as ordered *to promote bowel rest.*
- Give antidiarrheal medications as ordered. *Controlling diarrhea controls comfort and fluid balance.*
- Keep skin clean, dry, and protected with a moisture barrier, such as petrolatum or medicated ointment, after each bowel movement or use a fecal incontinence appliance to protect perianal skin from contact with liquid stools and their enzymes (see "Evidence-Based Practice").
- Provide clear liquids, such as water, juices, bouillon, and gelatin, with progression to a low-residue diet when the acute diarrhea phase is over ("Nutrition Notes").
- Limit caffeine intake *because it stimulates intestinal motility.*

Risk for Deficient Fluid Volume related to frequent passage of stools and insufficient fluid intake

EXPECTED OUTCOME: The patient will maintain a stable weight and vital signs, and urine output will remain within normal limits at all times.

- Record intake and output (including diarrheal stools) *to determine fluid balance.*
- Weigh patient daily *to determine fluid loss.*
- Maintain IV fluid replacement as ordered *to maintain fluid balance if output is greater than intake.*
- Encourage fluids when acute diarrhea subsides *to maintain fluid balance.*
- Teach patient signs and symptoms of dehydration to report *to allow prompt treatment.*

EVALUATION. Goals have been met if frequency of diarrheal stools is decreased and balance of fluid and electrolytes is achieved.

Nutrition Notes

Deciding When to Refer an Adult With Diarrhea for Medical Care

Most instances of diarrhea in healthy adults are self-limiting and resolve without treatment. Indications for medical consultation include the following:

- Lasts for more than 3 days
- Causes severe pain in the abdomen or rectum
- Provokes a fever of 102°F or higher
- Produces blood in the stool or black, tarry stools
- Is accompanied by signs of dehydration
- Occurs in a person with medical conditions for which fasting, dehydration, or infectious disease is a hazard

Healthy adults at minimal risk of electrolyte imbalance may institute self-treatment as follows:

- *For the first 12 hours:* Water or oral rehydration solutions at room temperature. Easily absorbed fluids maintain hydration. Hot or cold liquids are more likely to stimulate peristalsis.
- *For the second 12 hours:* Clear liquids, no caffeine or extremes of temperature. If more than 5% of body weight is lost, seek medical attention.
- *For the third 12 hours:* Full liquids. Experiment with milk in case temporary lactose intolerance has developed as a result of intestinal inflammation.
- *For the fourth 12 hours:* Soft diet. Include applesauce or banana for pectin and also rice, pasta, and bread without fat (digested by enzymes usually unaffected in gastroenteritis).
- *By the 48th hour:* Regular diet. If diarrhea has not resolved and regular diet is not tolerated, seek medical treatment.

INFLAMMATORY AND INFECTIOUS DISORDERS

Many diseases of the lower GI tract are a result of inflammation in the bowel. Sometimes the inflamed areas become infected, resulting in a worsening of symptoms.

Appendicitis

Pathophysiology

Appendicitis is the inflammation of the appendix, the small, finger-like appendage attached to the cecum of the large intestine (see Fig. 32.1). Because of the small size of the appendix, obstruction may occur, causing inflammation and making it susceptible to infection.

Signs and Symptoms

Signs and symptoms of appendicitis include fever, increased WBCs, and generalized pain in the upper abdomen. Within

EVIDENCE-BASED PRACTICE

Clinical Question

Can a traditional indwelling fecal incontinence device (mushroom catheter with soft flared tip or urinary catheter with balloon) be safely used for patients with diarrhea or fecal incontinence?

Evidence

A literature review conducted on the use of indwelling rectal tubes and practices that nurses might use to improve patient care revealed safer options to use before using a traditional indwelling rectal tube. First, the cause of diarrhea should be evaluated and treated. If the diarrhea continues, other methods of external fecal containment should be tried such as anal bags or pouches. External fecal containment devices protect the perigenital skin, save money and prevent damage to the rectal sphincter or internal mucosa. A nasopharyngeal airway can be safely used to contain fecal incontinence and protect the skin. Bowel management systems, such as the FlexiSeal® Fecal Management System, consist of soft flexible catheters and containment drainage systems that contain liquid stools, keep skin intact and rectal mucosa healthy, provide accurate input and output (I&O), and limit exposure to feces.

Implications for Nursing Practice

Identifying the cause of diarrhea is essential. When diarrhea persists, external devices and bowel management systems are preferred over the use of traditional rectal tubes.

REFERENCE

Makic, M. B., Vonrueden, K. T., Rauen, C. A., & Chadwick, J. (2011). Evidence-based practice habits: Putting more sacred cows out to pasture. *Critical Care Nurse, 31,* 38–62.

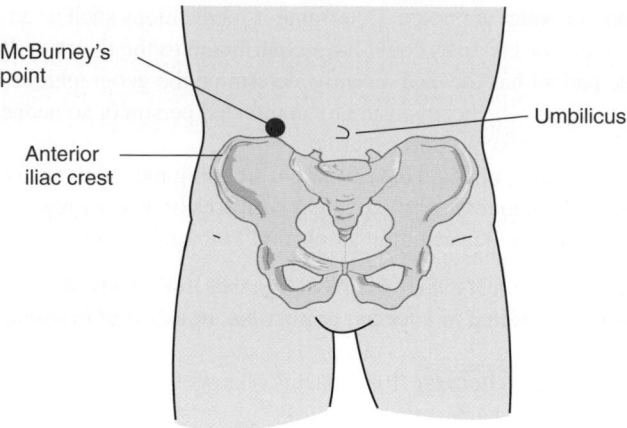

FIGURE 34.1 Pain at McBurney's point is a symptom of appendicitis.

Diagnostic Tests

A complete blood cell count (CBC) reveals elevated leukocyte (WBC) and neutrophil counts. An ultrasound or computed tomography (CT) scan reveals an enlargement in the area of the cecum.

Therapeutic Measures

The patient is kept NPO, and surgery is done immediately unless there is evidence of perforation or peritonitis. Applying ice to the site of pain and keeping the patient in a semi-Fowler's position may help reduce pain while the diagnosis is being made.

Laxatives and enemas are avoided because they may cause or complicate a rupture. The use of a heating pad on the abdomen is avoided because the warmth may increase inflammation and risk of rupture. If the appendix has ruptured, IV fluids and antibiotic therapy are started to treat infection and peritonitis. Surgery may or may not be done right away. If infection is present, a drain may be inserted into the abdomen by a radiologist. Surgery may then be delayed for up to several weeks while the infection is resolved.

After surgery, the diet is advanced as ordered and tolerated. If the appendix has ruptured, the patient may have an orogastric or nasogastric (NG) tube to decompress the stomach. Vital signs and abdominal data are collected to monitor for signs and symptoms of peritonitis. Pain control to promote early ambulation, coughing, deep breathing, and movement help prevent respiratory complications.

Complications

Perforation, abscess of the appendix, and peritonitis are major complications of appendicitis. With perforation, the pain is severe, and temperature is elevated to at least 100°F (37.7°C). An abscess is a localized collection of pus separated from the peritoneal cavity by the omentum or small bowel. This is usually treated with IV antibiotics and surgical drainage. An appendectomy is done about 6 weeks later.

hours of onset, the pain usually becomes localized to the right lower quadrant at McBurney's point, midway between the umbilicus and the right iliac crest (Fig. 34.1). This is one of the classic symptoms of appendicitis. Nausea, vomiting, and anorexia are also usually present.

Physical examination reveals slight abdominal muscular rigidity (guarding), normal bowel sounds, and local rebound tenderness (intensification of pain when pressure is released after palpation) in the right lower quadrant of the abdomen. Sometimes there is pain in the right lower quadrant when the left lower quadrant is palpated (Rovsing's sign). The patient may keep the right leg flexed for comfort and experience increased pain if the leg is straightened.

Peritonitis

Peritonitis is inflammation of the peritoneum that occurs from a variety of causes. It is a serious condition that can be life threatening.

Pathophysiology and Etiology

Trauma, ischemia, or tumor perforation in any abdominal organ causes leakage of the organ's contents into the peritoneal cavity. The most common cause of peritonitis is a ruptured appendix, but it can also occur after perforation of a peptic ulcer, gangrenous gallbladder, intestinal diverticula, incarcerated hernia, or gangrenous small bowel. It may also be a complication of peritoneal dialysis. Peritonitis results from the inflammation or infection that is caused by the leakage. The tissues become edematous and begin leaking fluid containing increasing amounts of blood, protein, cellular debris, and WBCs. Initially, the intestinal tract responds with hypermotility, but this is soon followed by paralysis (paralytic ileus).

Signs and Symptoms

Generalized abdominal pain evolves into localized pain at the site of the perforation or leakage. The area of the abdomen that is affected is extremely tender and aggravated by movement. Rebound tenderness and abdominal rigidity are present. Decreased peristalsis results in nausea and vomiting. Infection causes fever, increased WBCs, and an elevated pulse.

Diagnostic Tests

Rapid diagnosis is essential in preventing complications. Tests include an abdominal x-ray or computed tomography (CT) scan to show distention or perforation, WBCs significantly elevated, paracentesis and laboratory studies to identify a causative organism, or exploratory surgery to identify the cause.

Therapeutic Measures

The patient is NPO because of impaired peristalsis. Fluid and electrolyte replacement is crucial to correct hypovolemia and prevent or treat shock. Abdominal distention is relieved through insertion of an orogastric (or NG) tube with low intermittent suction. Antibiotics are used to treat or prevent sepsis. Depending on the cause of the peritonitis, surgery may be performed to excise, drain, or repair the cause. An ostomy may be formed to divert stool, allowing resolution of the infection. After surgery, the patient usually has a wound drain, a NG tube, and a urinary catheter. Pain control is essential to overall recovery. Severely compromised patients may receive parenteral nutrition (PN) to meet nutritional needs.

Complications

Wound dehiscence (separation of layers of a surgical wound) or evisceration (protrusion of abdominal viscera) can occur if the patient has had abdominal surgery. Complications of peritonitis are intestinal obstruction (discussed later), hypovolemia caused by the shift of fluid into the abdomen, and septicemia from bacteria entering the bloodstream. Shock and ultimately death may result.

Diverticulosis and Diverticulitis

Pathophysiology

A diverticulum is a herniation or outpouching of the bowel mucous membrane caused by increased pressure within the colon and weakness in the bowel wall. **Diverticulosis** is a condition in which multiple diverticula are present without evidence of inflammation (Fig. 34.2). Many people have diverticulosis without knowing it because it develops gradually. When food and bacteria are trapped in a diverticulum, inflammation and infection develop. This is called **diverticulitis**.

Etiology

Chronic constipation usually precedes the development of diverticulosis by many years. When the patient is chronically constipated, pressure within the bowel is increased, leading to development of diverticula. A major cause of the disease is a decreased intake of dietary fiber. Diverticulosis is most common in the sigmoid colon. A small percentage of patients with diverticulosis develop diverticulitis. People older than age 60 are the most common group to experience diverticulitis.

• **WORD • BUILDING •**
peritonitis: periton—pertaining to peritoneum + itis—inflammation
diverticulosis: diverticul—blind pouch + osis—condition
diverticulitis: diverticul—blind pouch + itis—inflammation

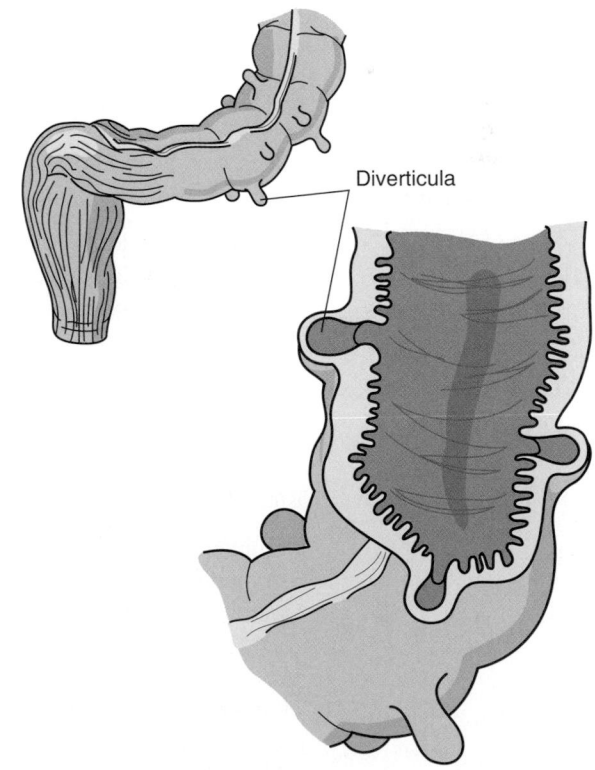

Diverticula

FIGURE 34.2 A diverticulum is a herniation or outpouching of the bowel mucous membrane. Having multiple diverticula is a condition called diverticulosis. If they become inflamed or infected, the condition is called diverticulitis.

Prevention

Diverticulitis can be prevented by increasing dietary fiber to prevent constipation and onset of diverticulosis.

Signs and Symptoms

The patient with diverticulosis is generally asymptomatic. When diverticulitis is present, the patient exhibits bowel changes, possibly alternating between constipation and diarrhea (Table 34.4). Steady or crampy pain in the left lower quadrant of the abdomen is the most common symptom. As the condition worsens, bleeding may occur, along with weakness, fever, fatigue, and anemia. Guarding and rebound tenderness may be present. If an abscess develops, the diverticulum may rupture, leading to peritonitis ("Gerontological Issues").

Diagnostic Tests

Diverticulosis is confirmed with sigmoidoscopy, colonoscopy, or barium enema. The diverticula and specific areas of inflammation can be seen during a colonoscopy or sigmoidoscopy. If an abscess is suspected, a CT scan may be done. Barium enema may show irregular narrowing of the colon and thickened muscle walls. A stool specimen may show occult blood. An abdominal x-ray examination may be done to identify a perforated diverticulum.

TABLE 34.4 SYMPTOMS ASSOCIATED WITH DIVERTICULITIS

W—Where is the pain?	Usually in the left lower quadrant
H—How does it feel? (Describe quality)	Tender, crampy
A—Aggravating and alleviating factors	Constipation and low-fiber diet may aggravate; treatment of constipation may alleviate
T—Timing (onset, duration, frequency)	Gradual onset, intermittent, gradual increase in frequency of pain events
S—Severity (0–10)	Usually 5–7
U—Useful other data/associated symptoms	Intermittent rectal bleeding; straining at stool; constipation alternating with diarrhea; elevated white blood cells and sedimentation rate; elevated temperature and pulse rate; and pus, mucus, and blood in stool
P—Patient's perception	Fear of cancer diagnosis

Gerontological Issues

With aging, the incidence of diverticular disease increases. Clinical manifestation of this condition may include abdominal pain, rectal bleeding, nausea, and vomiting. Patients may not notice the abdominal pain until infection is present. Many times the symptoms are not reported early because patients fear it may be cancer. Blood in the stool, which can be an indication of diverticulitis, may not be seen by the older adult due to impaired vision.

Therapeutic Measures

Diverticulosis is managed by preventing constipation. With acute diverticulitis, the patient may be hospitalized for administration of IV antibiotics and pain control. An NG tube, IV fluids, and NPO status may be ordered until pain, nausea or vomiting, fever, and inflammation decrease. When the acute period is over, a progressive diet is started. Whether or not perforation occurs, surgical resection with anastomosis or a temporary colostomy (discussed later) may be done to allow the inflammation to subside and the diseased portion of the colon to rest.

Dietary considerations for a patient with diverticulosis (without evidence of inflammation) include foods that are soft but high in fiber, such as prunes, raisins, and peas. Unprocessed bran can be added to soups, cereals, and salads to give added bulk to the diet. Fiber should be increased in the diet slowly to prevent excess gas and cramping. Some health care providers recommend avoiding nuts or foods with small seeds that can get caught in diverticula, such as tomatoes and raspberries, but this has not been shown to prevent diverticulitis. If the patient is overweight, he or she is encouraged to lose weight.

Surgery may be needed for ruptured diverticula. Laparoscopic surgery can be used to decrease the morbidity and mortality associated with this emergency surgery.

Nursing Process for the Patient With an Inflammatory or Infectious Disorder

Data Collection

Assessment of pain is essential for patients with inflammation or infection. Monitor the patient closely and notify the HCP immediately if pain increases, especially if associated with abdominal rigidity. Increased pain may indicate that the bowel has ruptured and peritonitis is developing. Abdominal distention is monitored and recorded. With diverticulitis, a firm mass may be palpated in the sigmoid area.

Vital signs are monitored for fever or signs of septic shock. Intake and output are monitored and recorded accurately so that appropriate fluid replacement therapy is ordered. Monitoring for reduced urinary output, dropping blood pressure, and rising pulse rate can show fluid volume imbalance. If a fever is noted, the patient may be developing sepsis. All symptoms are reported to the HCP promptly.

Nursing Diagnoses, Planning, and Implementation

Acute Pain related to inflammatory process

EXPECTED OUTCOME: The patient will report pain is at an acceptable level within 30 minutes of report of pain.

- Have patient rate pain on objective scale such as 0 to 10 *to determine pain level.*
- Give analgesics or antispasmodic drugs as ordered *to relieve pain.*
- Use position changes, diversion, and relaxation exercises to help relieve pain. *Semi-Fowler's position may reduce tension on the abdomen.*
- Provide frequent mouth care if an NG tube is in place *to increase comfort.*

Risk for Deficient Fluid Volume related to diarrhea or fluid shifting from the circulation to the peritoneal cavity

EXPECTED OUTCOME: The patient will maintain vital signs and urine output within normal limits at all times.

- Record intake and output *to determine fluid balance.*
- Weigh patient daily *to determine fluid loss.*
- Monitor vital signs and urine output and report changes *to detect changes from within normal limits.*
- Maintain IV fluid replacement as ordered *to maintain fluid balance if output is greater than intake.*

For constipation related to a low-fiber diet, see the earlier section on constipation.

Evaluation

The goals are met if the patient reports that pain is controlled, vital signs and urinary output are stable, and patient has regular, comfortable bowel elimination.

 INFLAMMATORY BOWEL DISEASE

Crohn's Disease

Pathophysiology

Crohn's disease is an inflammatory bowel disease (IBD) that can involve any part of the GI tract but most commonly affects the terminal portion of the ileum, or first part of the large intestine. The inflammation extends through the intestinal mucosa, which leads to the formation of abscesses, **fistulas** (abnormal connections between structures), and fissures (unnatural tracts or ulcers). The inflamed areas from Crohn's disease can alternate with areas of healthy tissue, so the inflamed areas are referred to as "skip lesions" (because they are not continuous lesions along the intestine). As the disease

progresses, obstruction occurs because the intestinal lumen narrows with inflamed mucosa and scar tissue.

Etiology

Although the exact cause of Crohn's disease has not been identified, it tends to occur within families. Other possible influences are autoimmune processes and infectious agents. Crohn's disease is most often diagnosed between the ages of 15 and 30 and occurs more often in women than men. Smoking increases the risk for Crohn's disease. The patient experiences periods of remissions and exacerbations. Physical or psychological stress may trigger exacerbations ("Cultural Considerations").

Signs and Symptoms

Crampy abdominal pains (unrelieved by defecation), weight loss, fever, and diarrhea occur. Because the crampy pains occur after eating, the patient often does not eat to avoid the pain. A lack of eating and poor absorption of nutrients results in weight loss and malnutrition. Chronic diarrhea contributes to fluid deficit and electrolyte imbalance. The inflamed intestine may perforate, leading to the formation of intra-abdominal or anal fissures, abscesses, or fistulas. Symptoms outside the GI tract, such as arthritis, skin lesions, and inflammatory disorders of the eyes, and abnormalities of liver function may also occur.

Complications

In addition to malnutrition, the development of fissures, abscesses, strictures, or fistulas is the most common complication of Crohn's disease. Fistulas may include enterovaginal (small bowel to vagina), enterovesical (small bowel to bladder), enterocutaneous (small bowel to skin), enteroentero (small bowel to small bowel), or enterocolonic (small bowel to colon) (Fig. 34.3). Fistulas communicating with organs that then drain externally can cause tremendous skin irritation, as well as increased risk of developing infections. Fistulas are corrected surgically and antibiotics may be used.

Diagnostic Tests

Laboratory testing looks for anemia, infection, liver function, low albumin due to poor absorption of protein, and stool infections or occult blood. Endoscopy (colonoscopy and sigmoidoscopy), with multiple biopsies of the diseased colon and terminal ileum, is used to diagnose Crohn's disease. Other endoscopic tests include capsule endoscopy (swallowed camera the size of a pill), ultrasound to identify fistulas and areas of bleeding, and double balloon enteroscopy, which

Cultural Considerations

Ulcerative colitis and Crohn's disease are more common in Caucasians, persons of Jewish descent, and upper-middle-class urban populations. The incidence of Crohn's disease is increasing rapidly in western Europe and North America. These findings support possible hereditary or environmental risk factors for inflammatory bowel disease.

FIGURE 34.3 Fistulas are a common complication of Crohn's disease.

provides views of the inside of tissue folds. Crohn's disease is confirmed by granulomas in the biopsy specimen. Imaging tests include multiphase CT enterography and magnetic resonance enterography (MRE), which provide detailed images of the intestines.

Therapeutic Measures

Management of Crohn's disease is aimed at achieving remission and maintaining it because there is no cure. Symptoms are controlled by reducing the intestinal inflammation that is the underlying cause of the symptoms. The classes of medications used to achieve these goals are aminosalicylates, biologics, corticosteroids, and immunomodulators (Table 34.5). Treatment is individualized. Aminosalicylates reduce inflammation and have various formulations to be delivered to specific sites in the intestines. They do not prevent acute episodes. Biologics selectively target agents in the inflammatory process to block their action and effects. Corticosteroids are used during an acute inflammation, then tapered and discontinued. Budesonide (Entocort EC), an anti-inflammatory synthetic corticosteroid, acts locally rather than affecting the whole body. Immunomodulators modify the immune system to decrease inflammation. They may be used with steroids to treat acute episodes because they have a longer onset of action. Traditionally, corticosteroids, then azathioprine, then infliximab, which inhibits tumor necrosis factor, a primary cause of the inflammation, are given.

TABLE 34.5 MEDICATIONS FOR CROHN'S DISEASE AND/OR ULCERATIVE COLITIS

Medication/Action	Examples	Nursing Implications
Aminosalicylates Decrease intestinal inflammation.	sulfasalazine (Azulfidine)	Contraindicated in sulfa allergy. Some patients do not tolerate sulfasalazine but can tolerate other drugs in this class.
	mesalamine (Asacol, Canasa, Pentasa, Rowasa)	Monitor for signs of reduced kidney function.
	olsalazine (Dipentum) balsalazide (Colazal)	Take with food. Continue drugs even if feeling better to maintain remission.
Biologics Selectively target inflammatory agents to interfere with inflammatory response.	adalimumab (Humira) certolizumab pegol (Cimzia) infliximab (Remicade) Natalizumab (Tysabri)	Tuberculosis test must be done before therapy begins and annually. Monitor for infections, bone marrow suppression, central nervous system disorder.

TABLE 34.5 MEDICATIONS FOR CROHN'S DISEASE AND/OR ULCERATIVE COLITIS—cont'd

Medication/Action	Examples	Nursing Implications
Corticosteroids Decrease inflammation and suppress immune system. May be used with aminosalicylates.	prednisone (Deltasone) methylprednisolone (Medrol, Solu-Medrol) hydrocortisone (Cortenema)	Teach patient not to stop taking medication abruptly. Patient should lie on left side for 30 minutes and retain enema for 1 hour if not retaining all night.
Anti-Inflammatory Synthetic Corticosteroid Reduce inflammation locally for Crohn's disease.	budesonide (Entocort EC)	Grapefruit and grapefruit juice should be avoided. Take in morning. Swallow whole.
Immunomodulators Immunosuppression to reduce inflammation.	azathioprine (Imuran) 6-mercaptopurine (6-MP, Purinethol) cyclosporine (Sandimmune, Neoral) tacrolimus (Prograf) methotrexate (MTX, Mexate, Rheumatrex)	Report symptoms of infection when taking any immunomodulators. Monitor for infection. Blood pressure and renal function are monitored. Blood pressure and renal function are monitored. Monitor for infections.

Antidiarrheal medications such as diphenoxylate with atropine (Lomotil) or loperamide (Imodium) are used. Bulk-forming laxatives may help reduce loose stools and subsequently skin irritation.

As complications develop, surgery may be indicated for obstruction, stricture, fistula, abscess, excessive bleeding, perforation, toxic megacolon (loss of muscle tone and dilation in colon), or symptoms that do not respond to treatment. Surgery does not cure Crohn's disease because it can recur elsewhere in the GI tract. Surgical procedures include strictureplasty to widen areas of stricture, resection of the affected area with anastomosis, colectomy with ileorectal anastomosis, or proctocolectomy (rectum and colon) with ileostomy. See details regarding intestinal ostomies later in this chapter. A Kock pouch is not recommended for those with Crohn's disease because the disease may affect the pouch.

A healthy diet is important in overall health, but there is no special diet for Crohn's disease. A dietitian referral is important for nutritional support. Malnutrition is a concern if the small intestine is affected and nutrients are not absorbed properly. Folic acid and vitamin B$_{12}$ supplements may be needed. Calcium intake may be decreased and osteoporosis is a concern. Calcium 1500 mg daily and vitamin D supplements are considered. Foods that increase symptoms should be avoided. Enteral feedings may be required and can be done at night through a gastrostomy tube (G tube) or nasogastric feeding tube. For acute flare-ups, PN may be used to rest the GI tract. Adequate fluid intake is essential to prevent dehydration if diarrhea is present.

Nursing Process for the Patient With Crohn's Disease

Because of the similarities between Crohn's disease and ulcerative colitis, the nursing processes for both are discussed together in the "Nursing Process for the Patient with Inflammatory Bowel Disease" section that follows.

Ulcerative Colitis
Pathophysiology

Ulcerative **colitis** is similar to Crohn's disease. Crohn's disease, however, can occur anywhere in the GI system, whereas ulcerative colitis occurs in the large colon and rectum. Multiple ulcerations and diffuse inflammation occur in the superficial mucosa and submucosa of the colon. The lesions spread in a continuous pattern throughout the large intestine and usually involve the rectum.

Etiology

Infection, allergy, and autoimmune response are possible causes of ulcerative colitis. Environmental agents such as

• WORD • BUILDING •
colitis: col—pertaining to colon + itis—inflammation

pesticides, tobacco, radiation, and food additives may precipitate an exacerbation. Diet or psychological stress may trigger or worsen an attack of symptoms. Ulcerative colitis usually begins between ages 15 and 40.

Signs and Symptoms

Abdominal pain, diarrhea, rectal bleeding, and fecal urgency are common symptoms of ulcerative colitis (Table 34.6). Anorexia, weight loss, cramping, vomiting, fever, and dehydration associated with passing 5 to 20 liquid stools a day may also occur. Along with the potential for fluid and electrolyte imbalance, calcium is lost. Anemia often develops as a result of rectal bleeding. Serum albumin level may be low because of malabsorption. Like Crohn's disease, arthritis, skin lesions, inflammatory disorders of the eyes, and abnormalities of liver function may also occur. Symptoms are usually intermittent, with remissions lasting from weeks to years.

Complications

Malnutrition occurs less often with ulcerative colitis than with Crohn's disease. Other complications include the potential for hemorrhage during an acute phase, bowel obstruction, perforation, and peritonitis. The risk for colorectal cancer is also increased in patients with ulcerative colitis.

TABLE 34.6 INFLAMMATORY BOWEL DISEASE SUMMARY

Signs and Symptoms	Abdominal pain or cramping Weight loss Diarrhea Fluid and electrolyte imbalance Fissures, fistulas, abscesses Arthritis and skin lesions Inflammatory eye disorders Abnormal liver function
Diagnostic Tests	Endoscopy with biopsy Barium enema Laboratory examination Stool examination Absent bowel sounds
Therapeutic Measures	Medications: anti-inflammatories, antidiarrheal, antibiotics, immunosuppressants, corticosteroids Surgery if necessary Avoidance of offending foods Elemental formula or total parenteral nutrition (TPN) if required
Priority Nursing Diagnoses	*Constipation* *Diarrhea* *Deficient Fluid Volume* *Deficient Knowledge*

Diagnostic Tests

Anemia and infection are checked with blood tests. Anemia is often present because of blood loss. Examination of stool specimens is done to rule out the presence of any bacterial or amebic organisms. The stool is positive for blood in the presence of ulcerative colitis. Electrolytes may be depleted from chronic diarrhea. There is protein loss because of liver dysfunction and malabsorption. Barium enema is an x-ray with contrast that looks at the lower GI tract. A flexible sigmoidoscopy to view the lower colon or a colonoscopy to see the whole colon is done. Biopsy specimens show inflamed cells. Leukocyte scintigraphy, a noninvasive imaging test, uses the patient's white blood cells tagged with a radioactive material to detect infection and inflammation in the colon.

Therapeutic Measures

Diet and lifestyle changes and then medications are used for treatment. Foods that cause gas or diarrhea should be avoided. Because the offending foods may be different for each patient, foods are tried in small amounts if they are thought to cause symptoms. In general, high-fiber foods, caffeine, spicy foods, and milk products are avoided. Parenteral nutrition may be needed to meet nutritional needs during acute exacerbations. Diarrhea may increase the need for fluids to prevent dehydration.

Many of the medication classes used with Crohn's disease are used for ulcerative colitis (see Table 34.5).

Surgery is considered for excessive bleeding, severe symptoms, perforation, or toxic megacolon. Because ulcerative colitis usually involves the entire large intestine, surgery removes the entire colon and rectum. An ileoanal pouch (restorative proctocolectomy) or proctocolectomy with ileostomy (discussed later) are the procedures done. Surgery cures ulcerative colitis if the colon is removed.

An ileoanal pouch does not require an ostomy pouch to be worn and is the more common surgery performed. Because the anus and sphincter are saved, stool still passes through the anus. The rectum and colon are removed and the end of the ileum, which is made into a J-shaped pouch, is attached to the anus. A temporary ileostomy is created to allow the pouch to heal. After about 12 weeks, the ileostomy is closed. Several bowel movements per day occur. The stool is of soft consistency. Surgical complications can include a bowel obstruction, or an inflammation of the pouch (pouchitis), which is treated with antibiotics.

Nursing Process for the Patient With Inflammatory Bowel Disease
Data Collection

A history obtained from the patient includes symptoms, including the onset, duration, frequency, and severity. Ask if there has been any correlation between exacerbations of symptoms related to dietary changes or stress. Determine the presence of any food allergies or intolerances that may increase diarrhea. Also, note the daily and weekly intake of caffeine, nicotine, and alcohol because all these stimulate the bowel and can cause cramping and diarrhea.

Assess the patient for nutritional status and signs of dehydration. Ten to 20 pounds can be lost in a 2-month period. Perianal skin should be assessed for irritation and excoriation.

Assessment of emotional status, coping skills, and verbal and nonverbal behaviors is essential. The patient may withdraw from family and friends because of frequent bowel movements. Anxiety, sleep disturbances, depression, and denial can be problems. If surgery involving an ileostomy is planned, the patient is at risk for altered body image.

Nursing Diagnoses, Planning, and Implementation

Acute Pain related to increased peristalsis and cramping
EXPECTED OUTCOME: The patient will state pain is relieved or at an acceptable level within 30 minutes of report of pain.

- Have patient rate pain on objective scale such as 0 to 10 *to determine pain level.*
- Document the character of the pain (dull, cramping, burning) and ask whether the pain is associated with meals or other activities *to plan care.*
- Give analgesics and medications *to relieve cramping, as prescribed.*

Diarrhea related to the inflammatory process
EXPECTED OUTCOME: The patient will maintain formed, soft stool every 1 to 3 days.

- Document characteristics of stools, including color, consistency, amount, frequency, and odor *to plan care.*
- Ensure patient has quick access to the bathroom or provide a bedside commode *to prevent incontinence.*
- Administer antidiarrheal medication as prescribed. *Controlling diarrhea controls comfort and fluid balance.*
- Encourage bed rest *to decrease peristalsis.*
- Keep the environment clean and odor free *to help alleviate anxiety.*
- Teach the patient to avoid high-fiber foods such as whole grains and raw fruits and vegetables, as well as caffeine, alcohol, and nicotine *because they stimulate intestinal motility.*

Risk for Deficient Fluid Volume related to diarrhea and insufficient fluid intake
EXPECTED OUTCOME: The patient will maintain vital signs and urine output within normal limits at all times.

- Weigh patient daily *to determine fluid loss.*
- Record intake and output (including diarrhea stools) *to determine fluid balance.*
- Document and report signs of deficient fluid volume to the HCP *to allow treatment.*
- Maintain IV fluids as ordered *to maintain fluid balance.*
- Encourage fluids when acute diarrhea subsides *to maintain fluid balance.*
- Teach patient signs and symptoms of dehydration to report *to allow prompt treatment.*

Anxiety related to symptoms and frequency of stools and treatment
EXPECTED OUTCOME: The patient will report that anxiety is reduced.

- Answer questions; talk in a calm, confident manner; and actively listen to the patient *to reduce anxiety, which aggravates symptoms of inflammatory bowel disease.*

Impaired Skin Integrity related to frequent loose stools
EXPECTED OUTCOME: The patient's skin will remain intact at all times.

- Keep perianal skin clean, dry, and protected with a moisture barrier, such as petrolatum or medicated ointment, after each bowel movement *to protect perianal skin from contact with liquid stools and their enzymes.*
- Provide sitz baths, which may be comforting and helpful in keeping skin clean *to prevent excoriation.*

Imbalanced Nutrition: Less Than Body Requirements related to malabsorption
EXPECTED OUTCOME: The patient will maintain weight within normal range for height and age.

- Weigh weekly *to detect weight loss.*
- Give special liquid (elemental) formula that is absorbed in the upper bowel as ordered *to allow the colon to rest.*
- Maintain PN as ordered to provide nourishment *if the patient is unable to tolerate oral intake.*

See the "Nursing Care Plan for the Patient With Inflammatory Bowel Disease."

Evaluation

Goals have been met if pain is relieved, frequency of diarrhea stools is decreased, fluid and electrolyte balance is achieved, anxiety is reduced, skin is intact, and weight is within normal range for height and age.

IRRITABLE BOWEL SYNDROME

Pathophysiology

Irritable bowel syndrome (IBS) is not a disease but rather a functional problem. The colon mucosa is not damaged by the condition, and there is no increased risk of colorectal cancer. IBS is a disorder of altered intestinal motility in which the colon muscle contracts more easily. It contracts in a disorderly way that can be violent and last for long times or, at times, it may not contract at all. The abnormal contractions lead to changes in bowel patterns. Thus, the disorder may be classified as IBS with diarrhea, IBS with constipation, or IBS with mixed diarrhea and constipation. Additionally, patients experience increased abdominal discomfort or pain. Localized prolonged contractions may cause stool to be retained for a long time, causing it to become hardened as water is absorbed from it. Bloating may also occur because air is unable to be expelled. Mucus may be seen in the stool, although this

NURSING CARE PLAN for the Patient With Inflammatory Bowel Disease

Nursing Diagnosis: *Ineffective Coping* related to inflammatory bowel disease

Expected Outcome: The patient will identify strategies that promote effective coping.

Evaluation of Outcome: Is the patient able to state strategies for effective coping?

Intervention Identify patient's knowledge of Crohn's disease or ulcerative colitis. **Rationale** Many people have little knowledge of a disease unless they know someone who has it. Inaccurate information must be corrected. **Evaluation** Does the patient verbalize information about ulcerative colitis and its effects on the body?

Intervention Encourage the patient to express feelings about the disease and how it may affect his or her life. **Rationale** Expressing feelings about the disease and its perceived effect enables the patient to identify and talk about concerns. Once identified, the health care team can then address these concerns. **Evaluation** Does the patient talk about feelings regarding the potential impact of the disease on his or her life?

Intervention Determine whether the patient would like to speak with a person of similar age from the Crohn's and Colitis Foundation of America. **Rationale** Speaking with someone close in age with the same disease lets the patient know that he or she is not the only person having to cope with this disorder. It can also help him or her learn some strategies for effectively coping with the disease. **Evaluation** Does the patient show an interest in speaking with someone with the same disease?

Intervention Identify strategies for effective coping that are acceptable to the patient. **Rationale** Talking about concerns and possible solutions is a positive step. Coping strategies identified with the patient are more likely to be implemented. **Evaluation** Is the patient able to identify strategies for effective coping that he or she believes will work?

CRITICAL THINKING

Judy Moore

■ Judy Moore is an 18-year-old college student who has just been diagnosed with Crohn's disease.

1. What questions should the nurse ask Judy to identify her symptoms?
2. What nursing diagnoses would be relevant for Judy's condition?
3. What patient-centered care can help Judy adapt to this disease?
4. If Judy's condition were to worsen, what manifestations would be exhibited?
5. What members of the health team might the nurse collaborate with?

Suggested answers are at the end of the chapter.

is not abnormal and does not typically cause a problem. Symptoms may be exacerbated by psychological stress or food intolerances. The nerves in the bowel are overly sensitive in people with IBS. At times of stress in daily living, abnormal contractions may result.

Etiology

There is a hereditary tendency for IBS. IBS is more common in women than men and in those who are young to middle-aged. Flare-ups can be caused by other illnesses, infections, or the menstrual cycle.

Signs and Symptoms

IBS is characterized by reports of gas, bloating, constipation, diarrhea, or alternating constipation and diarrhea. The patient also has feelings of abdominal bloating, with or without visible abdominal distention. Other symptoms include the rectal passage of mucus, a feeling of incomplete evacuation, abdominal pain, depression, anxiety, and palpitations.

Diagnostic Tests

Diagnosis of IBS is made based on history and physical examination along with stool examination, colonoscopy, and sigmoidoscopy to rule out other disorders. Avoiding milk products for a time may be advised to rule out lactose intolerance.

Therapeutic Measures

IBS is a chronic condition, but symptoms can generally be controlled through lifestyle, diet, stress management, and medication. See "Nutrition Notes" for diet. A high-fiber and high-bran diet (psyllium [Metamucil] or methylcellulose [Citrucel]) may help to form softer, larger stools but may increase other symptoms in some people. Eating smaller, frequent meals can be helpful in reducing bowel contractions. Patients can keep a diary of foods eaten, stressors, and symptoms. This can help the HCPs identify flare-up triggers. Stress management, behavioral therapy (biofeedback, hypnosis, psychotherapy), and exercise are helpful in relaxing the bowel as well as contributing to overall health.

Various medications are used depending on the type of IBS. Antidepressants are given to block the brain's perception of abdominal pain. For IBS with constipation, selective serotonin reuptake inhibitors (SSRIs) such as paroxetine HCl (Paxil) are given. Tricyclic antidepressants (such as amitriptyline HCl [Elavil]) are used for IBS with diarrhea because they tend to cause constipation. Antispasmodics such as hyoscyamine (Levbid) or dicyclomine (Bentyl) are used in IBS for diarrhea to relieve the painful colon spasms.

For women in whom treatment for IBS with constipation has not been successful, lubiprostone (Amitiza) may be used. It is a chloride channel activator that increases fluid secretion in the small intestine to help pass stool.

Nursing Process for the Patient With IBS
Data Collection

Height, weight, and data on the symptoms, including pain that the patient experiences, are collected. Timing of the

- Mannitol—mushrooms, cauliflower, sugar-free mints/gums (Barrett & Gibson, 2012; Thomas, Nanda, & Shu, 2012).

Not all FODMAPs will trigger symptoms for all patients. Only those that are malabsorbed are likely to be clinically significant. Fructans and GOSs are always malabsorbed and fermented by intestinal bacteria, resulting in gas production and associated flatulence even in healthy people.

The remaining FODMAP carbohydrates will only induce symptoms in the patients with IBS that malabsorb them. Identification of susceptible patients can be achieved by breath tests after ingestion of lactose or fructose or by eliminating all FODMAP foods and relating their reintroduction to returning symptoms.

Individualizing the diet is important, particularly for vegetarians who may depend on legumes for protein intake, as it may show patients that they can cope with garlic as a minor ingredient, or wheat products occasionally which would expand the nutritional composition of their diet. The key issue is the total FODMAPS ingested at a meal, not the individual items. The low-FODMAP diet requires a registered dietitian's expertise both to maximize compliance with instigating the complete list of FODMAP sources and to avoid an overly restrictive approach unnecessarily. The latter is of great import in the event the diet is successful and likely to be followed long term. Considerable evidence supports the efficacy of the low-FODMAP diet for IBS suggesting that this should be the first dietary strategy tried (Barrett & Gibson, 2012).

Nutrition Notes

Low FODMAP Diet

The Low FODMAP diet restricts certain carbohydrates that are known to cause symptoms in patients with IBS because of their poor absorption, osmotic activity, and rapid fermentation. FODMAP stands for Fermentable Oligosaccharides, Disaccharides, Monosaccharides, And Polyols. Up to 86% of patients with IBS have achieved relief of overall GI symptoms from the Low FODMAP Diet (Barrett, 2013).

The richest sources of the FODMAPs are:

- Fructooligosaccharides (fructans)—wheat, rye, onions, garlic, artichokes
- Galacto-oligosaccharides (GOSs)—legumes (soy, beans, chickpeas, lentils), cabbage, Brussels sprouts
- Lactose—milk, dairy products, beer, prepared soups and sauces
- Fructose—honey, apples, dates, mangoes, papaya, pears, prunes, watermelon, high fructose corn syrup
- Sorbitol—apples, pears, stone fruits, sugar-free mints/gums

---

symptoms, food and fluid intake, elimination patterns, effects on self-esteem, socialization, and personal and family roles are explored because IBS is a significant cause of missed work and school and also causes social withdrawal and embarrassment for people with it. Knowledge of the syndrome and its treatment are determined. Readiness for managing the syndrome is determined to plan care.

Nursing Diagnoses, Planning, and Implementation
Constipation related to irregular motility of GI tract

EXPECTED OUTCOME: The patient will maintain passage of soft, formed stool every 1 to 3 days without straining.

- Assess normal pattern of defecation, diet and fluid intake, and medications *to help identify factors contributing to constipation for planning care.*
- Increase fluid intake, if not contraindicated, to 2 to 3 L per day *to prevent hard stools.*
- Teach patient about the benefits of increasing fiber and bran in the diet *to promote soft, larger stools that are easier to pass.*
- Give medication as ordered *to control symptoms.*

Diarrhea related to irregular motility of GI tract

EXPECTED OUTCOME: The patient will maintain formed, soft stool every 1 to 3 days.

- Obtain history including medications regarding diarrhea episodes *to help identify cause.*
- Monitor and record stool characteristics, amount, and frequency *to plan care.*
- Give antidiarrheal medications as ordered. *Controlling diarrhea controls comfort and fluid balance.*
- Limit caffeine intake *because it stimulates intestinal motility.*
- Keep skin clean, dry, and protected with a moisture barrier, such as petrolatum or medicated ointment, after each bowel movement *to protect perianal skin from contact with liquid stools and their enzymes.*

Readiness for Enhanced Self Health Management related to desire to manage symptoms of IBS

EXPECTED OUTCOME: The patient will state understanding and ability to carry out preventive measures to control symptoms before discharge.

- Explain IBS including symptoms, aggravating factors, and treatments *to promote understanding, which will aid ability to follow therapeutic regimen.*
- Encourage use of food diary documenting foods eaten and timing of symptom occurrence *to identify food triggers for symptoms including lactose intolerance.*
- Consult registered dietitian and share food diary *to allow identification of food connection with symptoms and meal planning to prevent symptoms.*
- If lactose intolerant, teach patient to avoid dairy products and substitute yogurt *to reduce symptoms.*

Evaluation

The plan has been effective if the patient has regular bowel function pattern, verbalizes understanding of self-care measures, and expresses satisfaction with the outcomes.

 ABDOMINAL HERNIAS

Pathophysiology and Etiology

A **hernia** is an abnormal protrusion of an organ or structure through a weakness or tear in the wall of the cavity normally containing it, which in this case is the abdominal wall. Hernias are caused by a weakness in the abdominal wall along with increased intra-abdominal pressure, such as the pressure from coughing, straining, and heavy lifting. Obesity, pregnancy, and poor wound healing are also risk factors. The hernial sac is formed by the peritoneum protruding through the weakened muscle wall. Contents of the hernia can be small or large intestine or the omentum. Indirect hernias are caused by a defect of structural closure. Direct hernias are acquired and arise from a weakness in the abdominal wall, usually at old incisional sites.

Figure 34.4 illustrates the various types of hernias. Inguinal hernias are located in the groin where the spermatic cord in males or the round ligament in females emerges from the abdominal wall. This common hernia is an example of an indirect hernia and is usually seen in males.

Umbilical hernias are seen most often in obese women and in children. They are caused by a failure of the umbilical orifice to close. Ventral (incisional) hernias usually result from a weakness in the abdominal wall after abdominal surgery, especially in the obese patient, if a drainage system was used, the patient experienced poor wound healing, or the patient received inadequate nutrition.

Prevention

Congenital defects cannot be prevented. However, reducing strain on abdominal muscles is helpful. Those who do heavy lifting, tugging, or pushing should wear a support binder or avoid the lifting. A healthy lifestyle of maintaining normal weight, not smoking, and eating high-fiber foods is recommended.

Signs and Symptoms

Unless complications occur, few symptoms are associated with hernias. An abnormal bulging can be seen in the affected area of the abdomen, especially when straining or coughing. The patient may have some discomfort due to tension on tissues around the hernia. The herniation may disappear when the patient lies down. If the intestinal mass easily returns to the abdominal cavity or can be manually placed back in the abdominal cavity, it is called a reducible hernia. When adhesions or edema occur between the sac and its contents, the hernia becomes irreducible or incarcerated.

Umbilical hernia   Direct inguinal hernia   Indirect inguinal hernia   Femoral hernia

FIGURE 34.4 Types of hernias.

Complications

An incarcerated hernia may become strangulated if the blood and intestinal flow are completely cut off in the trapped loop of bowel. Strangulated hernias do not develop in adults very often. Incarceration leads to an intestinal obstruction and possibly gangrene and bowel perforation. Symptoms are pain at the site of the strangulation, nausea and vomiting, and colicky abdominal pain.

Therapeutic Measures

Hernias are diagnosed by physical examination. Treatment options include no treatment, observing the hernia, using short-term support devices, or surgery to cure the hernia. A supportive truss or brief applies pressure to keep the reduced hernia in place. Emergency surgery is needed for strangulation or the threat of bowel obstruction. Surgical repair is recommended for inguinal hernias. Surgical procedures are most often done laparoscopically and include hernioplasty (open or laparoscopically) or herniorrhaphy (open hernia repair). Herniorrhaphy involves making an incision in the abdominal wall, replacing the contents of the hernial sac, sewing the weakened tissue, and closing the opening. Hernioplasty involves replacing the hernia into the abdomen and reinforcing the weakened muscle wall with wire, fascia, or mesh. Bowel resection or a temporary colostomy may be necessary if the hernia is strangulated.

Nursing Care

The patient is instructed to avoid activities that increase intra-abdominal pressure, such as lifting heavy objects. The patient is taught to recognize signs of incarceration or strangulation and the importance of notifying the HCP immediately. If a support truss or brief has been ordered, the patient is taught to apply it before arising from bed each morning while the hernia is not protruding. Special attention should be paid to maintenance of skin integrity beneath the truss.

Postoperative Care

Care following inguinal hernia repair is generally similar to any abdominal postoperative care (see Chapter 12). Patients can perform deep breathing to keep lungs clear postoperatively but should avoid coughing. Coughing increases abdominal pressure and could affect the hernia repair. The male patient may experience swelling of the scrotum. Ice packs and elevation of the scrotum may be ordered to reduce the swelling. Because most patients are discharged the same day of surgery, they are taught to change the dressing and report difficulty urinating, bleeding, and signs and symptoms of infection, such as redness, incisional drainage, fever, or severe pain. The patient is also instructed to avoid lifting, driving, or sexual activities for 2 to 6 weeks as specified by the HCP. Most patients can return to nonstrenuous work within 2 weeks.

 ABSORPTION DISORDERS

The process of digestion reduces nutrients to a liquid form that can be absorbed through intestinal mucosa into the portal bloodstream. More than 8000 mL of liquid with nutrients and electrolytes is absorbed, mostly proximal to the ileocecal valve.

Pathophysiology and Etiology

Malabsorption occurs when the GI system is unable to absorb one or more of the major nutrients (carbohydrates, fats, or proteins). Some causes of malabsorption are ileal dysfunction, jejunal diverticula, parasitic disease, celiac disease, enzyme deficiency, and inflammatory bowel diseases such as Crohn's disease and ulcerative colitis. The primary malabsorption disorders are celiac disease and lactose intolerance.

In *celiac disease,* a sensitivity to gluten is thought to cause malabsorption of protein. Gluten is a protein found in wheat, barley, and rye. Oats may become contaminated with gluten in the milling process of these other grains ("Nutrition Notes").

 Nutrition Notes

Treating Celiac Disease

Celiac disease, or gluten-sensitive enteropathy, is classically diagnosed in infants after gluten-containing foods are introduced to the diet. Many adults have the disease for a decade or more before they are diagnosed, but this is changing with the advent of serologic testing. Adults with celiac disease may present with anemia or have the disease discovered through endoscopy for symptoms not suggestive of celiac disease. A previous diagnosis of IBS is common.

The etiology is considered to be multifactorial involving a combination of

- genetic predisposition (only a few genetically susceptible individuals develop the disease),
- ingestion of gluten, and
- an autoimmune response that produces chronic inflammation of the small intestine.

Definitive diagnosis is made with a biopsy of the small intestine. In all cases, the patient should continue consuming gluten until the diagnostic testing has been completed.

Treatment requires permanent elimination of wheat, rye, and barley from the diet. Although gluten free, oats can pick up gluten from other grains during milling and may have to be avoided also. Careful selection of prepared foods is mandatory because of the widespread use of these grains as thickeners. If a patient with celiac disease ingests gluten, damage to the intestine continues even in the absence of symptoms. Because dietary restriction is permanent, instruction from and follow-up by a registered dietitian are indicated to ensure adequate nutritional intake despite the many dietary limitations.

A deficiency in lactase, an enzyme that breaks down lactose (milk sugar), causes lactose intolerance. When lactose is not digested, a high concentration of it occurs in the intestines, causing an osmotic retention of water in the colon and watery stools.

Signs and Symptoms

Weight loss, weakness, and general malaise resulting from malnutrition are associated with malabsorption disorders. Lactose intolerance causes abdominal cramping, excessive gas, and loose stools after eating milk products. Signs and symptoms of celiac disease can range from none to many in various body systems (see www.csaceliacs.org). Frequent loose, bulky, foul stools that are gray in color with an increased fat content may occur in celiac disease. Increased fat in the stool is named steatorrhea. Nutritional issues with celiac disease include iron-deficiency anemia secondary to poor iron absorption.

Complications

Vitamin K deficiency and resulting hypoprothrombinemia can increase the risk of bleeding. Calcium deficiency can be severe enough to cause bone pain and neuromuscular hyperirritability, including tetany. Folic acid, vitamin B_{12}, and iron deficiencies can result in glossitis, stomatitis, anemia, and dry, rough skin.

Diagnostic Tests

See Table 34.7 for diagnostic studies used to identify malabsorption diseases.

Therapeutic Measures

CELIAC DISEASE. Patients with celiac disease are ordered a high-calorie, high-protein, gluten-free diet to relieve the symptoms, promote intestinal healing, and improve nutritional status. However, because gluten is used as a filler or binder in many products, even those labeled "wheat free," diligence in identifying potentially offending foods is essential.

LACTOSE INTOLERANCE. Lactose intolerance is treated by removing foods from the diet that contain lactose, such as milk and milk products. Some fermented milk products, such as cheese and yogurt, may be lower in lactose and better tolerated. Lactaid is an over-the-counter lactase substitute that can be taken when milk products cannot be avoided. It can be added to milk in liquid form or taken as a tablet before eating foods containing lactose. Lactaid digests about 70% of the lactose in foods, making them more tolerable.

Nursing Care

Nursing care involves monitoring fluid and electrolyte balance, nutritional status, and skin integrity. Recording daily weight and intake and output helps determine if fluid loss is occurring. Intake of electrolyte-rich fluids is encouraged to replace losses. Antidiarrheal agents are given if ordered. Electrolyte levels, especially potassium, are monitored as ordered. The patient is instructed in dietary limitations. Nutritional supplements may be ordered if needed. Perianal skin is kept clean and dry, and barrier ointments are used as needed to protect the skin from excoriation.

 INTESTINAL OBSTRUCTION

Intestinal obstructions occur when the flow of intestinal contents is blocked. The two types of intestinal obstruction are mechanical and nonmechanical, both of which can be either partial or complete.

Mechanical obstruction occurs when a blockage occurs within the intestine from conditions causing pressure on the intestinal walls such as adhesions, twisting of the bowel, or strangulated hernia. Nonmechanical obstruction occurs when peristalsis is impaired and the intestinal contents cannot be propelled through the bowel. Nonmechanical obstruction is seen following abdominal surgeries, trauma, mesenteric ischemia, or infection. The severity of the obstruction depends

TABLE 34.7   DIAGNOSTIC TESTS FOR DISORDERS OF MALABSORPTION

Diagnostic Test	Test Result and Associated Malabsorption Syndrome
Hemoglobin and hematocrit	Decreased if anemia is present.
Mean corpuscular volume	Decreased values are found with malabsorption of vitamin B_{12}.
Upper GI series	Thickening of the intestinal mucosa, narrowed mucosa of the terminal ileum, or a change in fecal transit time are indicative of malabsorption syndrome.
D-xylose absorption test	Decreased excretion of xylose after 5 hours is indicative of malabsorption.
Sudan stain for fecal fat	Malabsorption can be distinguished from maldigestion if this test shows abnormally large numbers of fat droplets.
72-hour stool collection for fat	Stool fat greater than 5 g per 24 hours after ingestion of 80 g of fat in 2 days implies a fat digestion disorder.
Biopsy	Shows flattened mucosa and loss of villi with celiac disease

Note. GI, gastrointestinal.

on the area of bowel affected, the amount of occlusion within the lumen, and the amount of disturbance in the blood flow to the bowel (Table 34.8).

Small-Bowel Obstruction

Pathophysiology

When obstruction occurs in the small bowel, a collection of intestinal contents, gas, and fluid occurs proximal to the obstruction. The distention that results stimulates gastric secretion but decreases the absorption of fluids. As distention worsens, the intraluminal pressure causes a decrease in venous and arterial capillary pressure, resulting in edema, necrosis, and eventually perforation of the intestinal wall.

Etiology

Following abdominal surgery, loops of intestine may adhere to areas in the abdomen that are not healed. This may cause a kink in the bowel that occludes the intestinal flow. These adhesions, or bands of scar tissue, are the most common cause of small-bowel obstruction and are usually acquired from previous abdominal surgery or inflammation. Hernias and neoplasms are the next most common causes, followed by inflammatory bowel disease, foreign bodies, strictures, volvulus, and intussusception. A **volvulus** occurs when the bowel twists, occluding the lumen of the intestine. **Intussusception**

occurs when peristalsis causes the intestine to telescope into itself (Fig. 34.5).

These conditions are mechanical obstructions. Paralytic, or adynamic, ileus is a nonmechanical obstruction that occurs when the intestinal peristalsis decreases or stops because of a vascular or neuromuscular pathological condition. Box 34-1 lists causes of nonmechanical obstructions.

Signs and Symptoms

The patient initially reports wavelike abdominal pain and vomiting. Initially, flatus and feces that are low in the bowel and blood and mucus may be passed, but this stops as the obstruction becomes worse. The symptoms progress as the obstruction worsens or becomes complete. As the obstruction becomes more extreme, peristaltic waves reverse, propelling the intestinal contents toward the mouth, eventually leading to fecal vomiting. Peristaltic waves may be visible in a thin person. Pain and abdominal distention are present. Pain that is sharp and sustained may indicate perforation. In mechanical obstructions, high-pitched, tinkling bowel sounds are heard proximal

• WORD • BUILDING •

intussusception: intus—within + suscept—to receive

TABLE 34.8   BOWEL OBSTRUCTION SUMMARY

Signs and Symptoms	Abdominal pain Blood and mucus from rectum Feces and flatus cease Visible peristaltic waves in thin person Possible fecal vomiting Bowel sounds high pitched, tinkling, or absent Abdominal distention Fluid and electrolyte imbalance
Diagnostic Tests	Abdominal x-ray examination Computed tomography scan Complete blood count and electrolytes
Therapeutic Measures	Nothing by mouth (NPO) status Frequent mouth care Nasogastric tube Fluid and electrolyte replacement Medications: antibiotics, antiemetics, analgesics Surgery
Priority Nursing Diagnoses	*Pain* *Deficient Fluid Volume* *Risk for Electrolyte Imbalance* *Risk for Dysfunctional Gastrointestinal Motility*

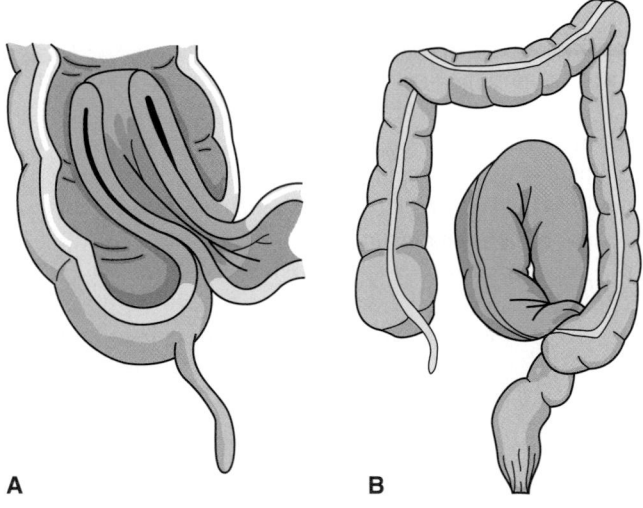

A   **B**

FIGURE 34.5 Mechanical bowel obstructions. (A) Intussusception. (B) Volvulus.

Box 34-1 Causes of Nonmechanical Obstruction

• Abdominal surgery and trauma
• Pneumonia
• Spinal injuries
• Hypokalemia
• Myocardial infarction
• Peritonitis
• Vascular insufficiency

to the obstruction and are absent distal to it. If the obstruction is nonmechanical, there is an absence of bowel sounds.

Loss of fluid and electrolytes leads to dehydration, with its associated symptoms of extreme thirst, drowsiness, aching, and general malaise. The lower in the GI tract the obstruction is, the greater the abdominal distention. An uncorrected obstruction can lead to shock and possibly death.

Diagnostic Tests

Dilated loops of bowel are evident in radiographic studies and CT scans. If strangulation or perforation occurs, leukocytosis is evident. Hemoglobin and hematocrit levels are elevated if the patient is dehydrated, and serum electrolyte levels are decreased.

Therapeutic Measures

In most cases, the patient is NPO and the bowel is decompressed using a NG (or, rarely, a tungsten-weighted intestinal) tube, which relieves symptoms and may resolve the obstruction. An IV solution with electrolytes is initiated to correct the fluid and electrolyte imbalance. Sometimes IV antibiotics are begun. Complete mechanical obstruction requires surgical intervention, such as removal of tumors, release of adhesions, or bowel resection with anastomosis.

Large-Bowel Obstruction

Pathophysiology

Obstruction in the large bowel is less common and not usually as dramatic as small-bowel obstruction. Dehydration occurs more slowly because of the colon's ability to absorb fluid and distend well beyond its normal full capacity. If the blood supply to the colon is cut off, the patient's life is in jeopardy because of bowel strangulation and necrosis.

Etiology

Most large-bowel obstructions occur in the sigmoid colon and are caused by carcinoma, inflammatory bowel disease, diverticulitis, or benign tumors. Impaction of stool may also cause obstruction.

Signs and Symptoms

Symptoms of large-bowel obstruction develop slowly and depend on the location of the obstruction. If the obstruction is in the rectum or sigmoid, the only symptom may be constipation. As the loops of bowel distend, the patient may report crampy lower abdominal pain and abdominal distention. Vomiting, if it occurs, is a late sign and may be fecal. High-pitched tinkling bowel sounds may be heard. A localized tender area and mass may be felt on palpation. Large-bowel obstructions, if not diagnosed and treated, can lead to gangrene, perforation, and peritonitis.

Therapeutic Measures

Radiological examination reveals a distended colon. If impaction is present, enemas and manual disimpaction may be effective. Other mechanical blockages may require surgical intervention.

Surgical resection of the obstructed colon may be necessary. A temporary colostomy may be indicated to allow the bowel to rest and heal. Sometimes an ileoanal anastomosis is done. A patient who is a poor surgical risk may have a cecostomy (an opening from the cecum to the abdominal wall) to allow diversion of stool.

Nursing Process for the Patient With a Bowel Obstruction

DATA COLLECTION. Each quadrant of the abdomen is auscultated for bowel sounds to identify the location of the obstruction. The abdomen is palpated for distention, firmness, and tenderness. The amount and character of stool, if any, are documented. Pain is assessed using the institution's pain scale and described according to location and character, such as crampy or wavelike. Vital signs are monitored for signs of infection or shock. Daily weight and intake and output are monitored. Skin turgor is assessed for fluid deficit. If a nasogastric or nasointestinal tube is in place, the amount, color, and character of drainage are documented.

NURSING DIAGNOSES, PLANNING, AND IMPLEMENTATION.
Acute Pain related to abdominal distention
EXPECTED OUTCOME: The patient will state pain is relieved or at an acceptable level within 30 minutes of report of pain.

• Assess pain level using rating scale *to consistently communicate patient level.*
• Give medications ordered for pain cautiously *because they may mask symptoms of perforation and decrease intestinal motility.*
• Position patient in semi-Fowler's position *to reduce tension on the abdomen.*

Risk for Deficient Fluid Volume related to vomiting
EXPECTED OUTCOME: The patient will maintain vital signs and urine output within normal limits at all times.

• Accurately monitor intake and output and note trends *to identify fluid deficit.*
• Maintain fluid replacement as ordered *to prevent dehydration.*

Risk for Electrolyte Imbalance related to suctioning
EXPECTED OUTCOME: The patient will maintain vital signs and urine output within normal limits at all times.

• Monitor electrolyte values *to identify imbalances.*
• Monitor vital signs, and watch for signs of electrolyte imbalances such as weakness accompanied by low potassium levels *to identify imbalances for prompt treatment.*
• Give ice chips sparingly if ordered by the HCP. *Melted ice increases electrolyte and hydrochloric acid removal when suctioned from the stomach, and electrolyte imbalance and metabolic alkalosis occur.*

Risk for Dysfunctional Gastrointestinal Motility
EXPECTED OUTCOME: The patient will maintain passage of flatus and stool.

• Monitor GI function for presence of flatus and bowel movements *to detect problems.*

- Maintain orogastric, NG, or nasointestinal tube on low intermittent suction as ordered *to relieve discomfort from distention.*
- Maintain NPO status *to rest the bowel and promote comfort.*

EVALUATION. Goals are met if the patient states that pain is controlled, fluid is balanced, electrolytes are within normal limits, and GI motility is normal.

CRITICAL THINKING

Mrs. Loos

■ Mrs. Loos is admitted for abdominal pain. She has a history of abdominal surgery. Her abdomen is distended, firm, and tender to touch. She states that she feels nauseated.

1. How would the nurse know if Mrs. Loos might be developing a small-bowel obstruction?
2. Is she at risk for developing an obstruction?
3. If she is at risk, what data should be collected?
4. What findings would be normal?
5. How would the nurse recognize that an obstruction is developing?
6. What should the nurse do if the patient's assessment has changed?
7. How will the nurse document the findings?
8. After treatment is started, how will the nurse know the patient is improving, getting worse, or developing complications as a result of a bowel obstruction?

Suggested answers are at the end of the chapter.

ANORECTAL PROBLEMS

Hemorrhoids

Hemorrhoids are enlarged veins within the anal tissue. They are caused by an increase in pressure in the veins, often from increased intra-abdominal pressure. Internal hemorrhoids occur above the internal sphincter, and external hemorrhoids occur below the external sphincter. Most hemorrhoids are caused by straining during bowel movements. They are common during pregnancy. Prolonged sitting or standing, obesity, and chronic constipation also contribute to hemorrhoids. Portal hypertension related to liver disease may also be a factor.

Internal hemorrhoids are usually not painful unless they prolapse. They may bleed during bowel movements. External hemorrhoids cause itching and pain when inflamed and filled with blood (thrombosed). Inflammation and edema occur with thrombosis, causing severe pain and possibly infarction of the skin and mucosa over the hemorrhoid.

Treatment is aimed at preventing constipation, avoiding straining during defecation, maintaining good personal hygiene, and making lifestyle changes to relieve hemorrhoid symptoms and discomfort. Increased fluid intake and stool softeners can be used to reduce the need for straining. Daily sitz baths increase circulation to the area and aid in comfort and healing. Prolonged standing and sitting are avoided. Astringents, such as witch hazel, can be used for symptom relief. Anti-inflammatory medications may be tried, such as steroid creams or suppositories. Alternating ice and heat helps relieve edema and pain for thrombosed hemorrhoids. The blood clot will be removed by a HCP.

If surgery is required for internal hemorrhoids methods include rubber-band ligation using a rubber band around the hemorrhoid that cuts off the blood supply, causing the hemorrhoid to slough off into the stool; infrared coagulation that burns off the hemorrhoid; sclerotherapy that shrinks the hemorrhoid with a chemical solution; hemorrhoidectomy to surgically remove the hemorrhoid.

Patient education includes prevention and self-care. The patient should be instructed to consume a high-fiber diet and 2 to 3 L of fluid a day to promote regular bowel movements. The effects and side effects, proper dosage, and frequency of local or topical medications should be explained.

If the patient has surgery, analgesics are given as needed because the many nerve endings in the anal canal can cause severe pain. Comfort measures such as a side-lying position and fresh ice packs can be used to relieve pain. After the first postoperative day, sitz baths may be ordered. Unfortunately, a side effect of opioid analgesics is constipation, which needs to be avoided, especially in the immediate postoperative period. Because the first bowel movement can be painful and anxiety provoking, stool softeners are given and analgesics administered before the first bowel movement.

Anal Fissures

Anal **fissures** are cracks or ulcers in the lining of the anal canal. They are most commonly associated with constipation and stretching of the anus with passage of hard stool, although Crohn's disease or other factors may also play a role. The patient may experience bright red bleeding. Pain may be so severe that the patient delays defecation, leading to further constipation and worsening symptoms. Treatment of anal fissures involves measures to ensure soft stools to allow fissures time to heal. Sitz baths may be used to promote circulation to the area to aid in healing. Anesthetic suppositories and nonopioid analgesics may be ordered for comfort. If conservative measures are not helpful, surgical excision of the fissure may be needed.

Anorectal Abscess

An anorectal abscess is a collection of pus in the rectal area. Common causative organisms include *Escherichia coli, Proteus* spp., staphylococci, or streptococci. Symptoms include pain, redness and swelling, fever, and sometimes drainage. Abscesses are treated with antibiotics and surgical incision and drainage of pus. The area may be left open to drain, with gauze packing placed to assist with drainage and healing.

Nursing Care

Nursing care includes dressing or packing changes as ordered. Sitz baths are used to keep the area clean and promote healing,

be contacted for follow-up. Most colorectal cancers are identified by biopsy done at the time of endoscopy (proctosigmoidoscopy, sigmoidoscopy, or colonoscopy). A CT scan can perform a virtual colonoscopy to view the inside of the colon. The carcinoembryonic antigen blood test is used to assess response to treatment of GI cancer. Carcinoembryonic antigen is present when epithelial cells rapidly divide and provides an early warning that the cancer has returned.

Therapeutic Measures

Small, localized tumors may be excised and treated during endoscopy or laparoscopy. These procedures can also be used as palliative care for patients with advanced tumors who cannot tolerate major surgery. If a tumor is causing obstruction, a stent can be placed to keep the colon open for bowel function until surgery.

Surgery is performed either to resect larger tumors and anastomose the remaining bowel or to create a fecal diversion by forming an ostomy. A variety of surgical procedures can be done depending on the location and extent of the cancer (Table 34.10 and Fig. 34.6). Medical management can include radiation therapy, chemotherapy, and monoclonal antibody therapy. When used, along with surgery, increased survival rates have been demonstrated.

Monoclonal antibody therapy uses antibodies that are made in a laboratory and work like normal antibodies do. They can enhance immune system function, interfere with the cancer cell's growth, or even carry treatment such as drugs

TABLE 34.10 INTESTINAL SURGERIES

Types of Intestinal Surgery	Definition	Effect on Stool Elimination
colectomy	Affected part of colon and nearby lymph nodes removed with laparoscope through smaller incisions.	Anastomosed ends. Stool is passed via rectum and anus.
Open colectomy	Affected part of colon and nearby lymph nodes removed through traditional incision.	Anastomosed ends. Stool is passed via rectum and anus.
Ileocolectomy	Right side of colon and diseased portion of ileum removed.	Anastomosed ends. Stool is passed via rectum and anus.
Hemicolectomy	Right or left side of colon removed.	Right: Colon attached to small intestine. Left: Anastomosed ends. Stool is passed via rectum and anus.
Total colectomy	Entire colon removed; rectum and anus remain.	Ileorectal anastomosis. Stool is passed via rectum and anus.
Total proctocolectomy	Entire colon, rectum, and sometimes anus removed.	Ileostomy. If anus left, ileal pouch-anal anastomosis and stool is passed via anus.
Rectal Cancer		
Local transanal resection: Cancer in lower area of rectum Transanal endoscopic microsurgery: Cancer higher in rectum	No incision. Rectal cancer removed through anus.	Anastomosed ends. Stool is passed via anus.
Lower anterior resection: cancer in upper two-thirds of rectum	Affected part of colon and nearby lymph nodes removed through traditional incision.	Anastomosed ends. Stool is passed via rectum and anus.
Abdominoperineal resection: cancer in lower one-third of rectum	Sigmoid colon, rectum, anus removed.	End colostomy. Stool passed via ostomy.
Proctectomy: cancer in lower two-thirds of rectum	Rectum removed.	Coloanal anastomosis. Stool passed via anus.

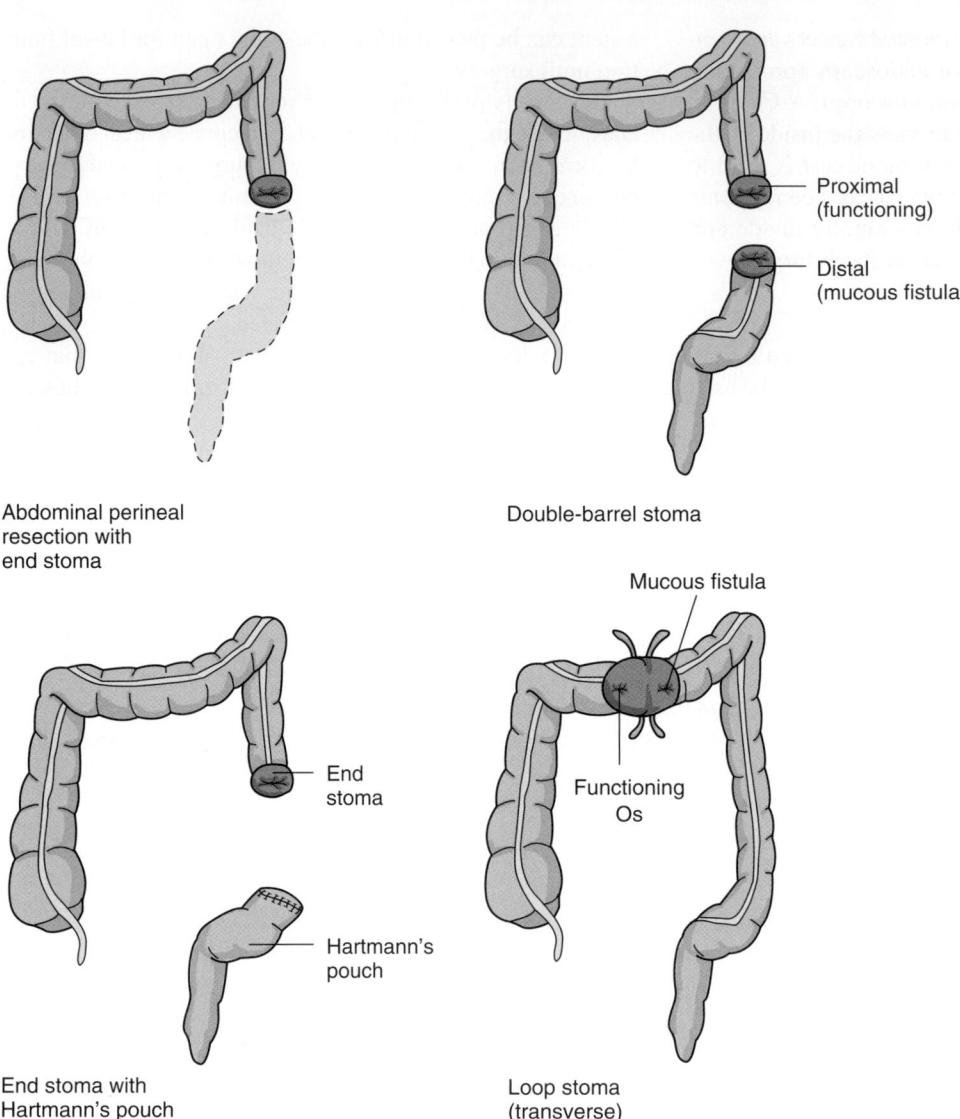

Abdominal perineal
resection with
end stoma

Double-barrel stoma

Proximal
(functioning)

Distal
(mucous fistula)

End
stoma

Hartmann's
pouch

Mucous fistula

Functioning
Os

End stoma with
Hartmann's pouch

Loop stoma
(transverse)

FIGURE 34.6 Types of stomas.

or radiation to cancer cells. The antibody is designed to attach to cancer cells to flag them for the immune system so they can be destroyed. Bevacizumab (Avastin) blocks the making of new blood vessels to deprive cancer cells of nourishment. Cetuximab (Erbitux) blocks the cell's growth signal to stop it from growing.

Complications

Complications include bleeding, complete obstruction of the colon, perforation, anastomosis leaking leading to peritonitis, and extension of the tumor to adjacent organs. Colorectal cancer can metastasize to the lymphatic system and liver.

If the patient has an anastomotic leak, the location of the leak determines the effects that are seen. The patient may need to be NPO for up to 4 weeks to rest the GI tract and prevent more leakage and also receive high-dose antibiotic therapy such as ciprofloxacin (Cipro) or metronidazole (Flagyl). Ongoing monitoring includes WBCs, sedimentation rate, and fever. The patient will likely go home with special home care needs. A peripherally inserted central catheter line is placed to continue the antibiotic therapy.

Nursing Process for the Patient With Colorectal Cancer

Data Collection

Risk factors for colorectal cancer are identified by asking questions about the patient's personal and family history: Is there a history of inflammatory bowel disease? What were the patient's dietary habits? What foods were usually eaten, and how much fluid was usually consumed? Prior to diagnosis, did the patient experience constipation or diarrhea? Has there been a change in bowel habits? Has mucus or blood been noted in the stools? What social habits does the patient have? Did the patient smoke, drink alcoholic beverages, exercise? Has there been a recent weight loss? If so, how much and over what period of time? Does the patient admit to unusual fatigue or insomnia? Stool should be checked for mucus or blood.

If the patient has surgery, postoperative assessment includes monitoring vital signs and the return of flatus and bowel movements. Lung sounds are monitored for response to coughing and deep breathing and early ambulation. Dressings are observed for drainage. Large amounts of drainage or bleeding are reported. If a drain is inserted in the perineal wound, moderate amounts of serosanguineous (light pink) drainage are expected. If the patient has an ostomy, it is monitored (see ostomy section later in the chapter).

Nursing Diagnoses, Planning, and Implementation

Acute Pain related to tissue compression from the tumor

EXPECTED OUTCOME: The patient will report pain relieved or at an acceptable level.

• Have patient identify pain using a rating scale *to identify pain level consistently.*
• Administer analgesics as prescribed postoperatively *to relieve pain.*

Fear related to serious threat to well-being

EXPECTED OUTCOME: The patient will state fear is reduced after information is given related to patient's condition.

• Assist patient in identifying fears *to develop plan for reducing fears.*
• Set aside time to allow the patient who so desires to talk, cry, or ask questions about the diagnosis and planned surgery *to help reduce fear.*
• Answer questions accurately *to provide a trusting relationship.*

Imbalanced Nutrition: Less Than Body Requirements related to nausea and anorexia

EXPECTED OUTCOME: The patient will maintain normal weight for height and age.

• Give antiemetics as ordered *to relieve nausea.*
• Identify foods patients like and provide them *to stimulate appetite.*
• Give parenteral nutrition as ordered *to provide depleted vitamins, minerals, and nutrients if the patient has been anorexic for any length of time or has had a significant weight loss.*
• Provide the patient with a high-protein, high-calorie diet, as ordered, that is low in residue *to decrease excessive peristalsis and minimize cramping.*

Evaluation

Expected outcomes are that the patient verbalizes control of pain and less fear and attains an optimum level of nutrition.

OSTOMY AND CONTINENT OSTOMY MANAGEMENT

An ostomy is a surgically created opening (traditional abdominal incision or laparoscopic) that diverts stool or urine to the outside of the body through an opening on the abdomen called a **stoma**. A stoma is the portion of bowel that is sutured onto the abdomen. A continent ostomy uses an internal reservoir to collect stool. The types of abdominal ostomies include ileostomy, colostomy, and urostomy. (Urinary ostomies are discussed in Chapter 37.) The stomas can be end, loop, or double barrel (see Fig. 34.6). How do you think a patient would feel when being told he or she needs an ostomy?

Ileostomy

An **ileostomy** is an end stoma formed by bringing the terminal ileum out to the abdominal wall following a total proctocolectomy. Two types of ileostomies can be formed: a conventional ileostomy and a continent ileostomy, such as a Kock pouch (sometimes called a Koch pouch) or Barnett's continent internal reservoir, which is a modification of a Kock pouch (Fig. 34.7). A conventional ileostomy has a small stoma in the right lower quadrant that requires a pouch at all times because of the continuous flow of liquid effluent.

Continent ileostomies are formed by taking a portion of the terminal ileum to construct an internal reservoir with a nipple valve. A stoma is created and the patient is taught to insert a catheter into the stoma three or four times a day to empty the reservoir. A continent ileostomy surgical procedure takes longer and requires additional instruction for the patient to be able to do self-care. It is important for the patient to empty the pouch routinely to prevent pouch rupture. Complications can occur, especially for the Kock pouch, such as valve slippage or leaking, pouch rupture, or pouchitis. Corrective surgery may be required.

• WORD • BUILDING •
ileostomy: ileo—pertaining to ileum + stoma—mouth or opening

FIGURE 34.7 Surgical formation of continent ileostomy (Kock pouch). (A) Loop of terminal ileum. (B) Both limbs of ileum are brought together and sutured into a U shape. (C) Pouch created with nipple valve. (D) Pouch sutured to abdominal wall.

LEARNING TIP

As stool travels through the colon, water is absorbed and the stool becomes firmer. Therefore, an ileostomy produces the most liquid effluent, followed by an ascending colostomy. A descending or sigmoid colostomy produces the firmest stool. Those with an ileostomy are at increased risk for dehydration due to greater water loss.

TABLE 34.11 LOCATION OF STOMA AND TYPE OF EFFLUENT

Location of Stoma	Type of Effluent
Ileostomy	Liquid to mushy
Cecostomy, ascending colostomy	Liquid to mushy, foul odor
Right transverse colostomy	Mushy to semiformed
Left transverse colostomy	Semiformed, soft
Descending or sigmoid colostomy	Soft to hard formed

An ileoanal anastomosis connects the ileum to the anus and avoids the need for a stoma (Fig. 34.8). This is usually a two-step procedure. During the first surgery, the diseased bowel is removed. A reservoir (named by its shape: J [most common], S, W, or H pouch) is then formed from part of the ileum and connected to the anus. A temporary ileostomy is also formed to divert stool while the reservoir heals. After about 3 months, the temporary ileostomy is reversed and the patient can have bowel movements from the anus. Problems with perianal skin irritation resulting from frequent liquid stools may occur. An ileorectal anastomosis can also be performed, but this may not be a curative procedure for a patient with ulcerative colitis because the rectum may still be diseased.

Colostomy

A **colostomy** is named according to where in the bowel it is formed: it may be an ascending, transverse, descending, or sigmoid colostomy. The type of effluent is dependent on the location of the bowel used (Table 34.11).

End Stoma

An end stoma is formed when the proximal end of the bowel is brought to the outside abdominal wall. If an abdominoperineal (AP) resection is done, the rectum is removed, and the proximal sigmoid or descending colon is brought out as a stoma. Another procedure that may be done involves removing the segment of diseased or injured bowel and using the proximal portion to form the stoma. The remaining limb of bowel is sutured closed and left in the peritoneal cavity so that the rectum is intact. This is called a Hartmann's pouch, or mucous fistula, and may be permanent or temporary depending on the diagnosis. Because the rectum is intact, the patient may feel the urge to defecate. This is normal because the colon continues to produce mucus. As the rectal stump fills with mucus, the sphincter is triggered and alerts the patient as if it were stool.

Loop Stoma

To create a loop stoma, a loop of bowel, usually the transverse colon, is pulled to the outside abdominal wall and a bridge is slipped under the loop to hold it in place. An incisional slit is made in the top of the exposed colon to allow stool to exit. The entire loop of bowel is not cut through.

Double-Barrel Stoma

With a double-barrel stoma, the bowel is completely dissected, and both ends of the colon are brought to the outside abdominal wall to form two separate stomas. The proximal stoma is the functioning stoma that expels stool. The distal stoma is called a mucous fistula because mucus produced by the bowel passes from it. A double-barrel stoma is often temporary, allowing the bowel to rest during healing after trauma or surgery.

Preoperative Care

A wound ostomy continence nurse (WOCN) should be consulted before surgery. The WOCN can help prepare the patient both emotionally and physically for the surgery. In addition, the WOCN has expertise in selecting the stoma site for the surgeon to ensure that it is easy to sit with it, care for

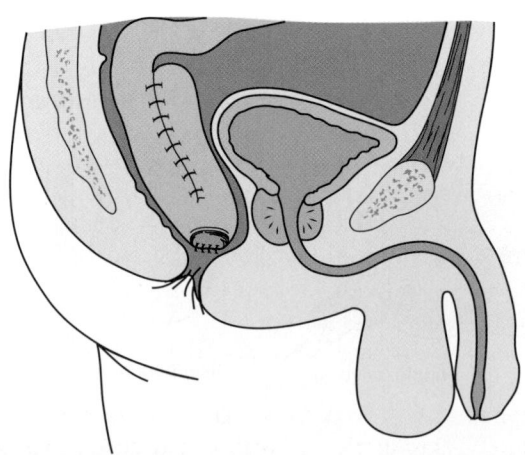

FIGURE 34.8 Ileal J pouch-anal anastomosis. The two-loop ileal pouch is simple to construct, provides adequate storage capacity, and is evacuated spontaneously and fully.

• WORD • BUILDING •

colostomy: colo—pertaining to colon + stoma—mouth or opening it, and wear clothing over it. This involves observing the abdomen as the patient assumes different positions and noting how clothing is worn, such as where the belt rides. The site for the stoma can then be chosen so it is visible to the patient for self-care, avoids skin or fat folds, and is where clothing will not interfere with the appliance. Properly planned stoma placement can prevent discomfort when sitting, inability to perform self-care, and uncomfortable, leaking, or poorly fitting appliances postoperatively.

Routine preoperative instruction, including the importance of coughing and deep breathing, splinting, and early ambulation, is provided. Orders for cleansing of the bowel are performed to reduce the risk for infection following surgery. Unless the patient has chronic diarrhea related to IBD, an oral agent to cleanse the bowel is given. Oral and IV antibiotics are given as ordered.

Nursing Process for the Patient With a New or Established Ostomy or Continent Ostomy

Data Collection

For a patient with a new ostomy, in addition to routine postoperative assessment, a stoma should be inspected at least every 8 hours. The stoma should be pink to red, moist (similar to the inside of the mouth), and well attached to the surrounding skin (Fig. 34.9). A bluish stoma indicates inadequate blood supply; a black stoma indicates necrosis. Either complication should be reported to the HCP immediately for treatment, which may require that the patient return to surgery. Note edema of stoma. The stoma size gradually decreases over the first few weeks following surgery.

For both new and established ostomies, skin is assessed for irritation around the pouch and under the pouch each time it is changed. Ostomy discharge (effluent) is monitored and documented. Unexpected changes, such as liquid stool from a descending ostomy, are reported. For the patient with a continent ostomy pouch, assessing that regular emptying of the pouch is done is important to prevent rupture and leakage. The characteristics of the stool are noted for any type of continent ostomy so that problems can be reported.

Nursing Diagnoses, Planning, and Implementation

See the "Nursing Care Plan for the Patient With an Intestinal Ostomy" and Table 34.12.

Deficient Knowledge related to ostomy

EXPECTED OUTCOME: Patient will demonstrate how to care for ostomy.

- Determine patient readiness and ability to learn and perform self-care. *The patient experiencing pain, nausea, or vomiting is not likely to be ready to look at the ostomy or learn about ostomy care.*
- Provide special instructions or a specific type of ostomy appliance for patients with special needs, such as blindness, deafness, language barrier, severe arthritis, or other physical conditions that limit ability to perform self-care, *so they will be able to perform self-care.*

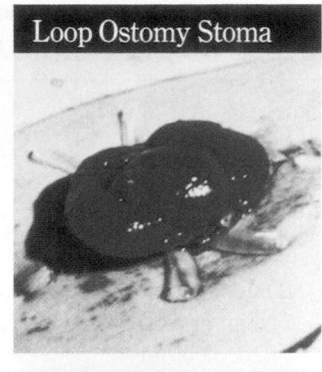

Man above has a descending or "dry" colostomy.

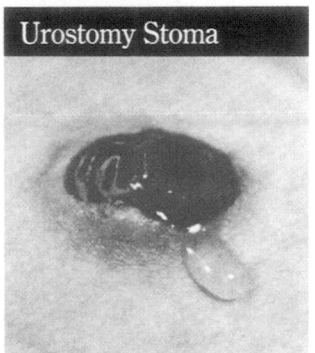

FIGURE 34.9 Types of stomas. Note moist, pink to red appearance of healthy stoma. *Reproduced with permission of Hollister Inc., Libertyville, IL.*

- Include caregiver in teaching if the patient is not ready or able to learn. *With short hospital stays, time for teaching is limited and must begin soon after surgery.*
- Ensure referral to home care nurse is made *to continue teaching in the patient's home.*
- Consult a WOCN or ostomy equipment supplier if needed *to identify appliances suited to individual patient's needs.* Figure 34.10 shows types of appliances.
- Explain how to change appliance (Fig. 34.11) *to promote self-care.*
- Demonstrate how to apply appliance using moldable or traditional skin barrier to promote self-care. *Moldable (able to change shape) skin barrier does not require measuring a pattern or cutting and does not leave a gap around the stoma.*

TABLE 34.12 SUMMARY OF RECOVERY FROM INTESTINAL SURGERY

Intestinal Surgery	Elimination Needs	Discharge Teaching Needs	Possible Psychological Needs
Total colectomy	Normal or continent anal passage	Continent ostomy care. Soft diet until first doctor visit. Monitor for constipation and report.	Chronic sorrow related to inflammatory bowel disease (IBD)
Hemicolectomy (right or left) or ileocolectomy	Normal, no appliance needed	Avoid stress to abdomen: heavy lifting, sit-ups. Soft diet until first doctor visit. Monitor for constipation and report.	Fear of cancer Chronic sorrow related to IBD
Partial colectomy	Normal, no appliance needed	Monitor for constipation.	Fear of cancer
Abdominoperineal resection	Pouch	Ostomy care.	Fear of cancer Body image changes
Proctosigmoidectomy	Normal, no appliance needed	Soft diet until first doctor visit. Monitor for constipation and report.	Fear of cancer
Total proctocolectomy	Continent anal passage or pouch	Continent ostomy care. Soft diet until first doctor visit. Monitor for constipation and report.	Chronic sorrow related to IBD

FIGURE 34.10 Appliances used for ostomies. The long sleeve at the lower left of the photograph is used to drain the bowel following irrigation. *Reproduced with permission of Hollister Inc., Libertyville, IL.*

- For the traditional skin barrier:
  - Measure stoma with a stoma-sizing guide initially with each appliance change *because the stoma will shrink for up to 6 months.*
  - Trace the stoma pattern on the cut to fit skin barrier and cut to fit, if using a nonmoldable barrier, *to teach the*

patient proper size and shape because most stomas are not round.
  - Apply a moldable barrier ring or strips to the skin barrier as needed to fill in gaps or fit convex shapes *to protect the skin and prevent leakage.*
  - Fit the traditional skin barrier over the stoma on the skin with no gaps around the base of the stoma *to prevent skin contact with stool.*
- Change appliance first thing in the morning every 3 days or every 10 to 14 days depending on the type of appliance *to reduce skin shearing from frequent removal.*
- Change appliance immediately if leakage occurs *to avoid* **peristomal** *skin irritation.*
- Use an open-ended or drainable pouch for all colostomies or ileostomies, especially during the first 8 weeks after surgery *to facilitate emptying and comfort.*
  - Explain to the patient who has a left-sided (descending or sigmoid) colostomy that the bowel can be regulated either by diet or regular irrigation of the stoma. After bowel regulation has been achieved, the patient may use a closed-end pouch or a stoma cap.
- Explain daily care and hygiene:
  - Empty pouch when it is one-third to one-half full. The amount of effluent and the frequency of emptying depend on the location of the stoma in the bowel. *If the pouch is allowed to get more than half full of stool, the weight of the effluent will pull on the pouch and weaken the seal of the skin barrier.*

- **WORD • BUILDING** •

peristomal: peri—surrounding + stoma—mouth or opening

Preparation of the Stomahesive Wafer with Sur-Fit Flange

1. Cleanse the peristomal area with water and pat thoroughly dry. Measure your stoma size with the measuring guide provided and trace the proper opening on the white paper backing of the Stomahesive® disc.

2. Leaving the white paper backing of the wafer in place, cut a hole in the wafer to the same shape and size as the base of the stoma. The best result is usually obtained by cutting from the reverse side of the wafer, using curved, short-bladed scissors.

3. Peel the white paper backing from the wafer just prior to application.

4. Gaps between the wafer and the base of the stoma may be further protected by applying Stomahesive® Paste to the wafer.

Application of the Stomahesive Wafer with Sur-Fit Flange

5. Center the enlarged hole over the stoma, place on abdomen, and apply light pressure.

FIGURE 34.11 Preparation to apply an ostomy appliance. *Courtesy ConvaTec, a Bristol-Myers Squibb Company, Princeton, NJ, with permission.*

- Empty pouch and then clean inside of the tail of the pouch before the self-seal or clamp is replaced *to help control odor.*
- Place deodorants in the pouch *to control odor.*
- Bathe or shower with the appliance in place but check seal and retape or change it if it is loosening. Water will not harm stoma or leak into stoma.
- Explain dietary considerations:
  - Identify foods that contribute to odor and gas. If foods that are known to cause odor or gas are eaten, the patient should know to empty the pouch of flatus more often and to be aware that more odor is probable.
  - Identify foods that contribute to and control diarrhea and what to do for constipation. A list of foods that may contribute to ileostomy blockage must be given to the ileostomy patient (Box 34-2 and "Nutrition Notes").

Readiness for Enhanced Self Health Management related to difficulty carrying out self-care measures
EXPECTED OUTCOME: Patient will demonstrate ability to perform self-care measures.

- Identify financial ability to obtain supplies. *The cost and availability of ostomy supplies is problematic for*

Nutrition Notes

Anticipating Dietary Management of Ostomies

Ostomy patients receive a soft diet initially, progressing to a general diet as the surgeon prescribes. Stringy, high-fiber foods are initially avoided until a definite tolerance has been demonstrated and then are best tried in small amounts, one at a time. Stringy, high-fiber foods include the following:
- Cabbage (including coleslaw, sauerkraut), corn, peas, spinach
- Coconut, dried fruit, pineapple, membranes on citrus fruits
- Popcorn, nuts, seeds, skins of fruits and vegetables.

Some patients avoid beans, cruciferous vegetables (broccoli, Brussels sprouts), eggs, fish, beer, and carbonated beverages because they produce excessive odor. Dietary restrictions are usually based on individual tolerance.

Certain foods may be therapeutic because they thicken the stool, including:
- Applesauce, banana
- Cheese
- Creamy peanut butter
- Pasta, white bread, white rice

Patients with ostomies should be encouraged to do the following:
- Eat at regular intervals.
- Chew food well to avoid blockage at the stoma site.
- Drink adequate amounts of fluid.
- Avoid foods that produce excessive gas, loose stools, offensive odors, and undesirable bulk.
- Avoid excessive weight gain.
- Explain colostomy irrigation if ordered for descending or sigmoid colostomies (more formed stool):
  - Explain that colostomy irrigation is done *to regulate bowel movements at a regular time.*
  - Show how to perform irrigation (similar to an enema), with special equipment used to instill fluid into the bowel via the stoma. *Because a stoma does not have a sphincter, specially designed tubing with a cone at the end is used to irrigate the ostomy. The cone prevents the fluid that is being instilled from flowing back out of the stoma.*

many patients. Most insurers, including Medicare, pay for ostomy supplies, although some limit the type of appliance and number allowed per month. Each state-funded Medicaid system is different. The type of appliance needed to eliminate leakage may not always be covered, requiring the patient either to pay the difference or wear what the insurance company will provide. If the patient has no insurance, costs can be high. Some patients find they have to choose whether to purchase ostomy appliances or prescriptions with their limited funds. Fortunately, the pouches in most two-piece systems can be washed out and reused to save money (see "Home Health Hints").

Box 34-2 Foods That Can Cause Ileostomy Blockage

Vegetables: celery, Chinese vegetables, coleslaw, corn, green leafy (collards, lettuce, mustards, spinach), mushrooms, popcorn, potato skins
Fruits: apple skins, coconut, dried fruits (apricots, dates, figs, raisins), grapes, orange membranes, pineapple, seedy fruits (raspberries, strawberries)
Nuts and seeds (e.g., coconut, poppy seeds)
Meats with casings: bologna, frankfurters, salami, other sausages

---

Home Health Hints

- Patients with ostomies may be able to have some of their supplies covered by insurance. The home health nurse can work with the medical supply store to assist the patient in receiving the needed equipment. Most companies will deliver supplies to the patient's home.
- Foods such as broccoli, cauliflower, Brussels sprouts, and cabbage can cause increased malodorous gas production. Encourage the patient with a colostomy to eat these in moderation. Offer alternative choices, such as green leafy vegetables, carrots, and cucumbers.
- If the patient requires a stool for occult blood test, deliver a collection device (hat) before you visit to assist with obtaining the specimen. Plan to deliver the specimen to the laboratory the day it is collected.
- Dietary instruction is important for home health patients with lower GI disorders. Give instructions both verbally and in writing. Written format allows the patient to have the information available for review and to assist with creating a shopping list.

Sexual Dysfunction related to body image change or erectile dysfunction
EXPECTED OUTCOME: Patient will discuss satisfying acceptable sexual practices for self and partner.

- Identify if male patient who had an AP resection is experiencing erectile dysfunction. *This impotence may be transient, depending on the severity of nerve damage or edema associated with the surgery.*
- Ensure consultation with urologist is made *to treat erectile dysfunction if present.*
- Encourage patients to discuss any concerns regarding sexuality with his or her sexual partner. *This may help them work through any fears or embarrassment.*
- Explain that attractive pouch covers can be purchased and worn *to help disguise the pouch and its contents.*
- Encourage personal hygiene and emptying ostomy pouch before sexual encounters *to decrease odors and enhance experience*
- Refer to sex counselor *who can suggest alternative sexual positions to increase satisfaction for partners.*

Risk for Injury related to skin and stomal complications
EXPECTED OUTCOME: The patient will remain free from injury with intact skin, red, moist stoma, and functioning ostomy.

- Identify allergies *to prevent complications because allergic dermatitis from sensitivity to the adhesive may develop.*
- Consult WOCN for complications associated with care of the ostomy. *A WOCN has had specialized instruction in caring for the stoma and peristomal skin and has a wealth of information to offer.*
- Use a protective skin paste *to prevent skin breakdown from leakage.*
- Apply a stoma powder to absorb moisture from broken skin around the stoma *to allow the skin to heal.*
- Remove tape and adhesive only when necessary *to prevent skin shearing from frequent removal.*
- Leave pouches on for several days unless leakage occurs *to prevent skin shearing from frequent removal.*
- Monitor for peristomal hernia *to detect hernias that may develop around the stoma as a result of weakened abdominal muscles and cause leakage by the change in body contours associated with the hernia.*
- Use a more flexible ostomy appliance if peristomal hernia is present *to fit body contours better.*
- Monitor for and report stomal prolapse, especially in older adults. *Weakened abdominal muscles contribute to the falling down (or out) of the intestinal mucosa, which can make pouching difficult.*
- Monitor stoma color and immediately report dusky or blue color, *which occurs when there is circulatory compromise. This may arise as a result of vascular collapse, blockage in the mesentery of the intestines, or edema in the intestine from obstruction proximal to the stoma. Usually, necrotic tissue occurs only at the very end of the stoma and will eventually slough off, revealing viable mucosa.*

• Explain signs and symptoms of an ileostomy blockage: absent stool, abdominal cramping, edematous stoma, and stoma color that is pale or dusky *to detect it for treatment.*

• Have patient consider what was eaten in the past 24 hours if blockage occurs *because certain foods are considered to cause stomal blockage (see Box 34-2).*

• Have the patient get into a tub of warm water (not too hot or cold), get into a knee-to-chest position, and sip on warm liquid, such as coffee, tea, bouillon, broth, or hot chocolate for an ileostomy blockage. *If the blockage is partial, relief will occur fairly soon after these measures are taken.*

• Explain to patient that if no relief is obtained, medical treatment should be sought. *For a complete blockage, an ileostomy lavage must be performed by a HCP or WOCN.*

Evaluation

The plan of care has been effective if the patient is able to accept the change in body image, competently care for the ostomy (or caregiver will), carry out self-care, is satisfied with sexual practices, and describes self-care measures to prevent or treat complications.

Rehabilitative Needs

Ensuring that the patient is becoming comfortable with self-care, is able to perform the ostomy appliance change, and is able to return to work or civic activities as before are the goals of care. The patient can generally perform any activity he or she was able to do before the ostomy including swimming. Several support resources are available (see DavisPlus).

NURSING CARE PLAN for the Patient With an Intestinal Ostomy

Nursing Diagnosis: *Disturbed Body Image* related to new ostomy

Expected Outcome: The patient will verbalize acceptance of intestinal ostomy before discharge.

Evaluation of Outcome: Is the patient able to verbalize acceptance of the ostomy?

Intervention Identify knowledge of self-care of ostomies. **Rationale** Many people have misconceptions regarding ostomies. Identification of misconceptions and "hearsay" knowledge is important to clarify or correct. **Evaluation** Does the patient verbalize appropriate knowledge of ostomy care?

Intervention Encourage patient to verbalize feelings about the stoma. **Rationale** Allowing the patient to express his or her feelings provides opportunity to identify and verbalize concerns, which then can be addressed by HCPs. **Evaluation** Does the patient discuss his or her feelings regarding the stoma with the nurse or significant other?

Intervention Explain the normal characteristics of the stoma before the patient's first look. **Rationale** Helping the patient understand what to expect will help relieve anxiety. Being available to answer questions immediately also relieves anxiety. **Evaluation** Does the patient look at the stoma without hesitation?

Intervention Demonstrate ostomy appliance change and daily care and encourage patient participation. **Rationale** When the patient observes and participates in self-care, his or her self-concept improves. **Evaluation** Is the patient participating in self-care? Has the patient performed return demonstration of appliance change and emptying of pouch?

SUGGESTED ANSWERS TO

CRITICAL THINKING

■ *Mrs. Burns*

You need to assess the situation before intervening. First, ask Mrs. Burns or her caregivers if she had a bowel movement that was inadvertently not charted. Next, ask Mrs. Burns if she feels constipated or if she has abdominal discomfort. Assess Mrs. Burns' abdomen for distention and presence or absence of bowel sounds. A digital examination may be necessary to determine if a fecal impaction is present. If simple constipation appears to be the problem, the medical record should be checked for as-needed laxative or enema orders. Once Mrs. Burns has had a bowel movement, laxatives should be discontinued and preventive measures such as regular fluids, fiber, and exercise should be instituted.

Continued

SUGGESTED ANSWERS TO—cont'd

■ *Judy Morrow*

1. Characteristics of pain: location, quality, intensity, precipitating factors, relieving factors.

   Characteristics of bowel elimination: frequency, characteristic of stool, amount, color, consistency.

   Nutritional status: Weight loss, appetite, daily food intake, food likes/dislikes, irritating foods, fluid intake.

   Anxiety and coping skills: Support systems, usual coping methods.

2. *Acute Pain* related to increased peristalsis and cramping

   Diarrhea related to inflammatory process

   Risk for Deficient Fluid Volume related to diarrhea and insufficient fluid intake

   Anxiety related to symptoms and frequency of stools and treatment

   Impaired Skin Integrity related to frequent loose stools

   Imbalanced Nutrition, Less Than Body Requirements related to malabsorption

   Ineffective Coping related to frequency of stools.

3. Further assess how Judy perceives that Crohn's disease will affect her lifestyle. What does she know about Crohn's disease? What is she concerned about? How has Crohn's disease affected her ability to sleep, what she eats, her participation in sports, and her relationships with other people?

   Convey a caring manner to Judy by being accepting of her, listening actively to her concerns, and helping her to find acceptable ways of resolving them. Provide her with information that she needs about Crohn's disease. Arrange to have a well-adapted person of approximately the same age from the Crohn's and Colitis Foundation of America meet with her to share coping strategies with her.

4. Increased frequency of stools leading to fluid volume deficit and possibly shock symptoms; bleeding leading to anemia and hypovolemia and possibly shock symptoms.

5. HCP, dietician, psychologist, registered nurse.

■ *Mrs. Loos*

1. The first consideration is to be aware of whether the patient is at risk for a small-bowel obstruction. After abdominal surgery, loops of intestine may adhere to areas in the abdomen that are not healed, causing a kink in the bowel that occludes the intestinal flow.

2. Yes, due to her history of abdominal surgery she is at risk of adhesion development that can cause obstruction. If assessment findings confirm this possibility, the HCP should be contacted. Because of the nausea and the potential obstruction, withhold food and oral fluids until the HCP can be contacted.

3. Begin by asking the **WHAT'S UP?** questions, including exactly where the pain is occurring, how it feels, if there is anything that aggravates or alleviates the pain, when it started, how bad it is on a scale of 0 to 10, whether there are associated symptoms, and if Mrs. Loos has some insight regarding the cause of her problem. Then, in this order, inspect, auscultate, and palpate (doing the exam in this order prevents palpation from changing other assessment findings). Inspect her abdomen to note distention. Listen for bowel sounds for 5 minutes in each quadrant. Lightly palpate her abdomen noting tenderness or rigidity. Ask when her last bowel movement was.

4. Bowel sounds normal in all quadrants, abdomen flat, soft with no tenderness, flatus present.

5. Abnormal bowel sounds; either absent for a nonmechanical obstruction or for a mechanical obstruction, high-pitched, tinkling bowel sounds proximal to the obstruction and absent distal to it; pain; abdominal distention.

6. Findings should be discussed with the registered nurse or HCP. New orders such as an NG tube, NPO status, and pain management should be anticipated.

7. When documenting, answer the questions what, why, when, where, how, who (either explicitly or implicitly by professional knowledge, in narrative or flow sheet format) for completeness.

   What = Patient is experiencing large, firm, tender to touch abdomen with nausea (additional assessment data should be included).

   Why = Unknown, HCP notified

   When = Current date and time

   Where = Abdomen

   How = Unknown

   Who = S. Mazur, LPN

8. If improving, symptoms will be resolving: no nausea, abdomen soft, bowel sounds present in all quadrants, flatus present, and bowel movements normal. If condition is worsening or complications are developing, symptoms will not improve, and fecal vomiting and shock may occur.

REVIEW QUESTIONS

1. The nurse is collecting data on a patient admitted with a history of severe diarrhea. Findings include cool, pale skin, red tongue with furrows, blood pressure 102/74 mm Hg, pulse 106 beats per minute, respirations 20 per minute, temperature 99.9°F (37.7°C). Which action should the nurse take now?
   1. Report findings to registered nurse.
   2. Give acetaminophen (Tylenol) as ordered.
   3. Obtain bedside commode.
   4. Apply warm blankets.

2. The nurse is reinforcing patient teaching about laxative use. The nurse would evaluate the patient as understanding the teaching if the patient stated which of the following?
   1. "Laxatives may be used as needed."
   2. "Regular laxative use can be harmful."
   3. "Daily use of laxatives prevents constipation."
   4. "Laxative use has no complications."

3. The nurse is caring for a patient after an appendectomy. Which of the following interventions should the nurse include in the patient's plan of care to prevent respiratory complications? **Select all that apply.**
   1. Pain control
   2. Early ambulation
   3. Bedrest
   4. Coughing, deep breathing
   5. Incentive spirometer

4. The nurse is reinforcing patient teaching. Which of the following foods would the nurse reinforce that the patient with ulcerative colitis is to avoid?
   1. Fresh fruits
   2. White bread
   3. Sweet dessert
   4. Meat

5. The nurse participated in a patient's teaching session for care to prevent respiratory complications after a hernia repair. Which statement by the patient would indicate to the nurse that the patient understood the teaching?
   1. "I will cough every hour while awake."
   2. "I will deep breathe four times daily."
   3. "I will cough and deep breathe every hour."
   4. "I will deep breathe every hour while awake."

6. The nurse would evaluate the patient as understanding diet teaching for celiac disease if the patient selected which of the following foods to eat?
   1. Fresh fruit and oatmeal with milk
   2. Tomato juice and waffles
   3. Hard-boiled egg, bacon, and blueberries
   4. Banana, cream of wheat cereal, and coffee

7. The nurse is caring for a patient with a small-bowel obstruction who is NPO with an orogastric tube on low intermittent suction. Which of the following ongoing data would be a priority for the nurse to monitor and collect? **Select all that apply.**
   1. Intake and output
   2. Pain level
   3. Bowel sounds
   4. Pulse rate
   5. Edema

8. The nurse is caring for a patient who has a sudden onset of diarrhea with black tarry stools. Which action should the nurse take?
   1. Obtain vital signs
   2. Monitor output
   3. Ask about a history of food allergies
   4. Place the patient on NPO status

9. Which of these patient's dietary habits does the nurse understand may increase the risk for development of colon cancer?
   1. High-fat, low-fiber intake
   2. High intake of milk and milk products
   3. Low-meat and protein intake
   4. Low-fat, high-carbohydrate intake

10. The nurse is caring for a 1-day postoperative patient who has a new end colostomy that is a dusky color. Which action is the priority for the nurse to take?
    1. Inform the HCP now.
    2. Monitor the stoma color in 4 hours.
    3. Check the stoma drainage in 1 hour.
    4. Place a new ostomy appliance over the stoma.

11. A patient with Crohn's disease is to receive sulfasalazine (Azulfidine), 500 mg oral suspension four times daily. The oral suspension is available as 250 mg/5 mL. How many milliliters should the nurse give for the 0800 dose?
    1. 5 mL
    2. 10 mL
    3. 20 mL
    4. 50 mL

Answers can be found in Appendix C.

References

Barrett, J. S. (2013).Extending our knowledge of fermentable, short-chain carbohydrates for managing gastrointestinal symptoms. *Nutrition in Clinical Practice, 28*(3), 300–306.

Barrett, J. S., & Gibson, P. R., (2012). Fermentable oligosaccharides, disaccharides, monosaccharides and polyols (FODMAPs) and nonallergic food intolerance: FODMAPs or food chemicals? *Therapeutic Advances in Gastroenterology, 5*(4), 261–268.

Thomas, J. R., Nanda, R., & Shu, L. H. (2012). A FODMAP diet update: Craze or credible? *Practical Gastroenterology, 36*(12), 37–46.

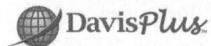 Davis*Plus* | For additional resources and information visit **davispl.us/medsurg5**

Nursing Care of Patients With Liver, Pancreatic, and Gallbladder Disorders

LAZETTE V. NOWICKI

LEARNING OUTCOMES

1. Explain the causes, risk factors, and pathophysiology of the various types of liver disease.
2. Describe therapeutic measures used for patients with liver disease.
3. Plan nursing care for the patient experiencing a liver disorder.
4. Explain the causes, risk factors, and pathophysiology of the various pancreatic disorders.
5. Describe therapeutic measures used for patients with pancreatic disorders.
6. Plan nursing care for a patient with a pancreatic disorder.
7. Explain the causes, risk factors, and pathophysiology of gallbladder disorders.
8. Describe therapeutic measures used for patients with gallbladder disorders.
9. Plan nursing care for the patient with a gallbladder disorder.

KEY TERMS

ascites (ah-SYE-teez)
asterixis (AS-tur-IK-siss)
cholecystitis (KOH-lee-siss-TYE-tiss)
choledocholithiasis (koh-LED-oh-koh-lih-THIGH-ah-siss)
cholelithiasis (KOH-lee-lih-THIGH-ah-siss)
cirrhosis (sih-ROH-siss)
colic (KAW-lick)
encephalopathy (en-SEF-uh-LAW-pah-thee)
extracorporeal shock-wave lithotripsy (EKS-trah-kor-POR-ee-uhl SHAWK-WAYV LITH-oh-TRIP-see)
fetor hepaticus (FEE-tur heh-PAT-tih-kuss)
hepatitis (HEP-uh-TYE-tiss)
hepatorenal syndrome (heh-PAT-oh-REE-nuhl SIN-drohm)
laparoscopy (LAP-uh-ROSS-kuh-pee)
pancreatectomy (PAN-kree-uh-TEK-tuh-mee)
pancreatitis (PAN-cree-uh-TYE-tiss)
portal hypertension (POR-tuhl HYE-per-TEN-shun)
T-tube (TEE-toob)
transjugular intrahepatic portosystemic shunt (TRANZ-jug-you-lur in-trah-heh-PAT-tik por-toe-siss-TEM-ik SHUNT)
varices (VAR-i-seez)

DISORDERS OF THE LIVER

Hepatitis

Hepatitis is an inflammation of the liver resulting from viral or bacterial infection, drugs, alcohol, or chemicals toxic to the liver, and metabolic or vascular disorders. Symptoms of hepatitis range from no symptoms to life-threatening symptoms due to death of liver tissue. Many people who are infected with hepatitis C, especially baby boomers (people born 1945–1965), are not aware of it and can live for 20 years without symptoms. Those infected can develop chronic infection, chronic liver disease, cirrhosis, or liver cancer. Risk factors for becoming infected with hepatitis C include sharing needles or other equipment to inject drugs. Also, health care providers (HCPs) who are exposed to the virus can become infected in the health care setting. Before 1992, when widespread screening of the blood supply began in the United States, hepatitis C was also commonly spread through blood transfusions and organ transplants. It is recommended by the Centers for Disease Control and Prevention (CDC; www.cdc.gov) that all baby boomers be tested for hepatitis C. Viral hepatitis is quite common and discussed below.

Pathophysiology and Etiology

Viral hepatitis is usually caused by one of five viruses:

- Hepatitis A virus (HAV)
- Hepatitis B virus (HBV)
- Hepatitis C virus (HCV)
- Hepatitis D virus (HDV)
- Hepatitis E virus (HEV)

The viral agents vary by mode of transmission, incubation period, symptoms, diagnostic tests, and preventive vaccines (Table 35.1). The infecting organism causes inflammation of the liver, with resulting damage to liver cells and loss of liver function. If damage involves the bile canaliculi (thin tubes that collect secreted bile), obstructive jaundice will occur. If complications do not occur, cells regenerate and normal liver function eventually resumes.

There are an estimated 72,000 new hepatitis A, B, and C infections in the United States each year (CDC, 2013). The incidence of all types of viral hepatitis is at a historic low. HAV is overall the most common cause of hepatitis and has a low mortality rate. However, HBV is more common among some groups, including health care workers and intravenous (IV) drug users.

Prevention

The hepatitis viruses are very resistant to a wide range of anti-infective measures, such as drying, heat, ultraviolet light exposure, freezing, and bleach and other disinfectants. At least 30 minutes in boiling water is required to destroy them. The best methods for preventing the transmission of the hepatitis viruses are careful attention to cleanliness and the use of vaccines to HAV and HBV or the use of immunoglobulin (Ig)

after exposure. Ig can be given up to 2 weeks after exposure to HAV; up to 1 week with a second dose of Ig in 1 month after HBV exposure. Infection control precautions used should reflect the usual mode of transmission of the particular hepatitis virus.

Ig provides temporary, passive, nonspecific immunity to hepatitis. A vaccine for HAV and HBV is available that provides permanent, active immunity. Health care workers are strongly encouraged (and often required by employers as a condition of employment) to be vaccinated for HBV. Permanent, active immunity is acquired from the body's own antibodies in response to an actual viral infection. The active immunity is to the specific virus to which the body has developed antibodies.

Public health measures such as health education programs, licensing and supervision of public facilities, screening of blood donors, and screening of food handlers are general measures to prevent the transmission of hepatitis viruses.

BE SAFE!

In the United States, 27 (93%) of the 29 HBV outbreaks involving adults in long-term-care facilities reported to the CDC since 1996 have been among residents with diabetes receiving assistance in blood glucose monitoring, and in recent years, the majority of these outbreaks have occurred in assisted living facilities (CDC, Morbidity and Mortality Weekly Report [MMWR], May 18, 2012).

Breaks in infection control procedures were identified in an assisted living facility in which all eight residents who contracted acute hepatitis B infection (six died) were assisted in blood glucose monitoring by staff whereas none of the residents performing their own glucose monitoring were infected (Centers for Disease Control, MMWR, February 18, 2011).

Follow infection control procedures whenever performing invasive procedures to keep your patients protected and safe!

Signs and Symptoms

Hepatitis usually shows a typical pattern of loss of liver function, which generally occurs in three stages:

1. The prodromal (preicteric [prejaundice]) stage occurs about 2 weeks after exposure to the hepatitis virus and lasts about 1 week. The patient reports flulike symptoms of malaise, headache, anorexia, low-grade fever, possibly dull right upper quadrant (RUQ) pain, nausea, vomiting, and diarrhea or constipation.

- WORD - BUILDING -

hepatitis: hepat—liver + itis—inflammation

TABLE 35.1 COMPARISON OF TYPES OF VIRAL HEPATITIS INFECTION

	Hepatitis A Virus	Hepatitis B Virus	Hepatitis C Virus	Hepatitis D Virus	Hepatitis E Virus
Mode of transmission	Oral-fecal contamination of water, shellfish, eating utensils, or equipment	Blood or body fluids such as saliva, semen, and breast milk; equipment contaminated by blood	Blood transfusions, IV drug use Rarer: unprotected sex	Blood or body fluids as with HBV Strongly linked as a co-infection with HBV	Usually contaminated water
Incubation period	3–7 weeks	2–5 months	1 week to months	Same as HBV	2–9 weeks
Symptoms	Early (prodromal): fatigue, anorexia, malaise, nausea, or vomiting Icteric: jaundice, pale stools, amber or dark urine, RUQ pain	Early (prodromal): 1–2 months of fatigue, malaise, anorexia, low-grade fever, nausea, headache, abdominal pain, muscle aches May have no early symptoms Icteric: jaundice, rashes	Same as HBV, usually less severe	Similar to HAV and to HBV but more severe	Similar to HAV
Diagnostic tests	**Anti-HAV IgM** Acute infection **Anti-HAV IgG** Recovery and immunity to virus	**HBsAg** Surface antigen of virus Disappears by month 5 Continued presence: chronic or carrier state **Anti-HBs IgM** Antibody to surface antigen Acute illness and infectiousness Protective, immunity **Anti-HBc IgM** Antibody to core antigen during acute illness and recovery **HBeAg** Active viral replication **Anti-HBe** Lower infectivity but still possible	**Anti-HCV** Antibody to virus several weeks after exposure Does not provide immunity **HCV EIA** If positive, RIBA to confirm **HCV RIBA** If positive with elevated ALT, diagnosis of HCV **HCV-RNA** Presence of replicating virus **Liver biopsy** Shows liver damage **HCV genotype (1-6)** Guides treatment type	**HDV-RNA** Presence of replicating virus **HDAg** Acute infection	**Anti-HEV** Acute infection
Preventive vaccine	Ig; hepatitis A vaccine	Hepatitis B Ig (HBIg); hepatitis B vaccine	None	None	None
Groups at risk	Individuals in military or day care Travelers to endemic areas	Correctional facility employees, health care workers, IV drug users, men who have sex with men, transplant or hemodialysis patients	Same as HBV	Same as HBV	Travelers to endemic areas

Note. Anti = antibody; ALT = alanine aminotransferase; EIA = enzyme-linked immunosorbent assay (ELISA-2); Ig = immunoglobulin; IV = intravenous; RUQ = right upper quadrant; RIBA = recombinant immunoblot assay.

2. With the appearance of jaundice (see Chapter 32), the icteric stage begins (Fig. 35.1). It occurs about 5 to 10 days after the prodromal stage and lasts 2 to 6 weeks. The patient continues to have prodromal symptoms. Dark urine can be present due to increased bilirubin. The liver is usually enlarged and tender on examination.

3. The convalescent stage (posticteric) begins when the patient starts feeling better. It can last from 2 to 6 weeks. Recovery varies and depends on the type of hepatitis. Full recovery is measured by the return to normal of all liver function tests and may take as long as 1 year. The effects of hepatitis can be considered reversible if the patient adheres to a medical regimen of adequate rest, proper nutrition, and abstinence from alcohol and other liver-toxic agents for at least 1 year after liver function laboratory values return to normal.

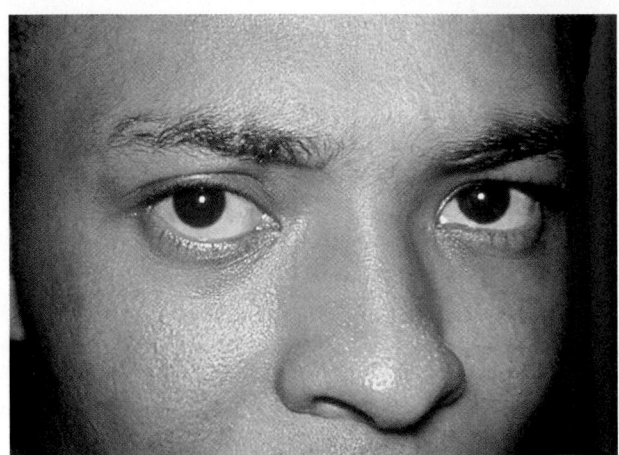

FIGURE 35.1 Jaundice of the conjunctivae and facial skin. *From the Centers for Disease Control and Prevention/ Dr. Thomas F. Sellers; Emory University, 1963.*

Complications

Hepatitis may lead to fulminant (sudden, severe), acute or chronic liver failure. Chronic infection can develop in those with HBV or HCV. Some people are asymptomatic carriers of HBV or HCV and never have an active illness. However, they can infect others and have a greater risk of developing cancer of the liver.

Diagnostic Tests

Serum liver enzymes are elevated (Table 35.2). Serum bilirubin may be elevated. In patients with severe hepatitis, prothrombin time may be prolonged. Serological tests can determine the specific virus causing the hepatitis via viral antigens and also identify the presence of antibodies to the virus (see Table 35.1). Abdominal x-ray examination may show an enlarged liver. Liver biopsy is done to assess liver damage and healing.

TABLE 35.2 LABORATORY TESTS FOR LIVER FUNCTION IN HEPATITIS AND CIRRHOSIS

Test	Normal Value	Significance of Abnormal Findings
Indicate Liver Damage		
Alanine aminotransferase (ALT)	*Male:* 10–40 units/L *Female:* 7–35 units/L	Most specific enzyme for liver damage. Released with death of liver cells.
Aspartate aminotransferase (AST)	*Male:* 15–40 units/L *Female:* 13–55 units/L	Enzyme found in liver and heart; released and elevates 10 times or greater than normal with death of liver cells.
Alkaline phosphatase (ALP)	*Male:* 35–142 units/L *Female:* 25–125 units/L	Enzyme found in liver and bone; released and elevates greatly with severe liver damage.
Measures Functioning of Liver		
Albumin	3.4–4.8 g/dL	Decreased because of impaired protein synthesis; edema and ascites may result.
Ammonia	15–45 mcg/dL	Increased because liver cannot metabolize protein end product; contributes to hepatic encephalopathy.
Bilirubin	0.3–1.2 mg/dL	Increased because the liver is unable to use it to produce bile.
Prothrombin time (PT)	11–13.5 seconds	Prolonged. Liver can no longer make prothrombin; patient bleeds easily.

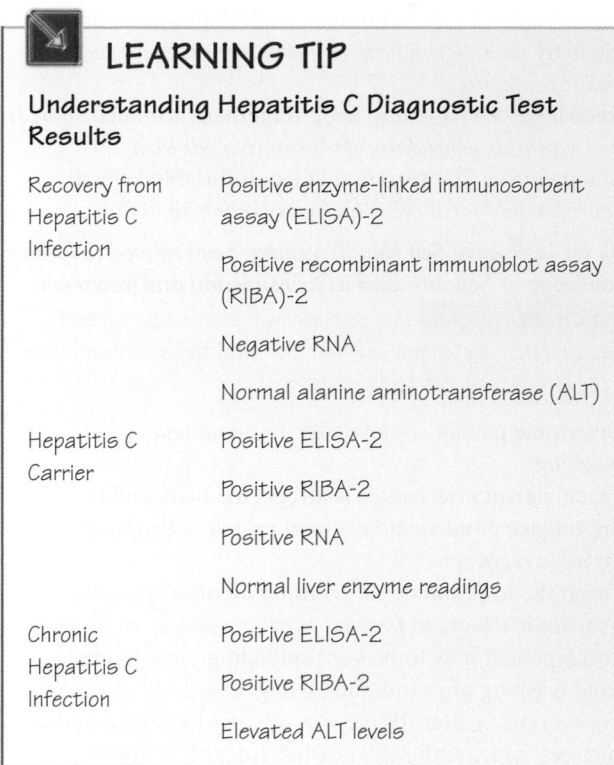

LEARNING TIP

Understanding Hepatitis C Diagnostic Test Results

Recovery from Hepatitis C Infection	Positive enzyme-linked immunosorbent assay (ELISA)-2
	Positive recombinant immunoblot assay (RIBA)-2
	Negative RNA
	Normal alanine aminotransferase (ALT)
Hepatitis C Carrier	Positive ELISA-2
	Positive RIBA-2
	Positive RNA
	Normal liver enzyme readings
Chronic Hepatitis C Infection	Positive ELISA-2
	Positive RIBA-2
	Elevated ALT levels

Therapeutic Measures

Treatment goals are to identify the cause of hepatitis, monitor liver status, and provide symptom relief and supportive care. To promote healing with acute infection, limited activity with bathroom privileges and adequate nutrition and fluids are ordered. As the patient improves, activity may be increased as tolerated. Patients should avoid using alcohol or drugs that are known to be toxic to the liver (Box 35-1).

To manage chronic hepatitis B infection, the antivirals adefovir (Hepsera) or lamivudine (Epivir) may be used. Interferon therapy (peginterferon alpha-2b [Peg-Intron] or interferon alpha-2a [Pegasys]) along with an antiviral medication (oral ribavirin [Rebetol]) is considered to prevent chronic hepatitis C infection. A new drug, sofosbuvir (Sovaldi; a nucleotide analog inhibitor) was approved for treating adults with chronic hepatitis C infection. For more information, visit the websites of the Hepatitis Foundation International (www.hepfi.org), the CDC (www.cdc.gov), or the American Liver Foundation (www.liverfoundation.org).

Nursing Process for the Patient With Hepatitis

DATA COLLECTION. Identify subjective data such as malaise, fatigue, pruritus (itching), nausea, anorexia, and RUQ abdominal pain. Objective data, such as baseline weight, vomiting, pale stools, dark-colored (tea-colored) urine, and jaundice, are recorded. The patient's vital signs are taken, and a low-grade fever or any abnormal bruising or bleeding is reported immediately. Ask the patient about his or her knowledge of disease process and how to prevent spread of the disease.

Box 35-1 Common Causes of Hepatic Inflammation

Medications

- Acetaminophen (Tylenol)
- Acetylsalicylic acid (aspirin)
- Allopurinol (Zyloprim)
- Captopril (Capoten)
- Carbamazepine (Tegretol)
- Diazepam (Valium)
- Erythromycin estolate (Ilosone)
- Estrogen
- Halothane (Fluothane)
- Isoniazid (INH)
- Methotrexate (Trexall)
- Methyldopa (Aldomet)
- Oral contraceptives
- Phenobarbital (Luminal)
- Phenytoin (Dilantin)
- Sulfonamides
- Tetracycline (Sumycin)

Metabolic Disorders

- Alpha-1 antitrypsin deficiency
- Hemochromatosis (iron buildup)
- Wilson's disease (copper buildup)

Toxins

- Ethyl alcohol
- Carbon tetrachloride
- Cholecystographic dyes
- Kava-containing products (herb)
- Poisonous wild mushrooms
- Trichloroethylene
- Toluene

Vascular Disorders

- Budd-Chiari syndrome (hepatic vein occlusion)
- Heart failure
- Shock

Viruses

- Cytomegalovirus
- Epstein-Barr
- Hepatitis A, B, C, D, E
- Herpes
- Yellow fever

NURSING DIAGNOSES, PLANNING, AND IMPLEMENTATION.
Pain related to inflammation and enlargement of the liver
EXPECTED OUTCOME: The patient will state that pain level is acceptable.

- Monitor pain level on 10-point scale, including **WHAT'S UP?** questions *to determine treatment needs.*

- For continuous pain, provide analgesics around the clock and as needed (prn) analgesics for intermittent breakthrough pain *to provide comprehensive pain relief.*
- Give analgesics as ordered, recognizing that lower doses might be needed with liver dysfunction, *to control pain.*
- Avoid use of acetaminophen (Tylenol) and combination drugs containing acetaminophen *due to risk of liver toxicity.*
- Encourage nondrug pain relief, such as distraction, imagery, and relaxation *to supplement and possibly decrease need for analgesics.*

Imbalanced Nutrition, Less Than Body Requirements related to anorexia, nausea, or vomiting

EXPECTED OUTCOME: The patient's weight will be stable and appropriate for height.

- Obtain baseline nutritional status with a nutritional screening tool *to identify malnutrition and plan nutritional needs.*
- Monitor weight and nutritional intake recording percentage of food eaten *to determine ongoing treatment needs.*
- Make dietary referral *to develop* nutritional plan.
- Administer antiemetic drugs as ordered *to reduce nausea and increase appetite.*
- Provide frequent, smaller meals *because these may be better tolerated than larger meals.*
- Place the patient in an upright or sitting position for meals *to decrease abdominal discomfort.*
- Serve meals in a quiet environment without unpleasant noise or odors *to increase intake by making eating as pleasant as possible.*
- Teach patient to avoid alcohol and vitamin supplements unless specifically prescribed by the physician *to prevent further damage to liver because alcohol and some vitamins are metabolized by the liver.*

Risk for Impaired Liver Function related to viral infection

- Monitor liver function tests *to detect liver infections.*
- Monitor for signs of liver dysfunction: ascites, mental changes (check ammonia levels), bleeding (check coagulation studies) *to report for implementation of supportive interventions.*
- Review medications for hepatotoxicity *to protect liver function.*
- Calculate acetaminophen daily dosage so daily limit of 3000 mg or less is not exceeded if applicable *to protect liver function.*
- Administer medication as ordered carefully in consideration of liver effects *to preserve liver function.*
- Refer to alcohol cessation program if applicable *to preserve liver function.*

Risk for Impaired Skin Integrity related to itching secondary to bilirubin pigment deposits in skin

EXPECTED OUTCOME: The patient's skin will remain intact and free from secondary infection.

- Administer antihistamines as ordered *to decrease itching.*

- Encourage the patient not to scratch but to press firmly on the itchy area. *Scratching can damage skin and increase risk for infection.*
- Encourage the patient to keep fingernails trimmed short *so that vigorous scratching does not tear the skin.*
- Maintain room temperature at a comfortable level *to decrease perspiration, which may increase itching.*

Risk for Ineffective Self Health Management related to lack of knowledge of hepatitis and its transmission and treatment

EXPECTED OUTCOME: The patient will state how to self-manage the treatment regimen for viral hepatitis and how to prevent spread of the disease.

- Determine patient's knowledge of hepatitis *to plan teaching.*
- Teach patient how hepatitis affects the body and the importance of adequate rest and proper nutrition *to promote recovery.*
- Teach the importance of avoiding alcohol and other liver-toxic drugs, *to prevent further damage to liver.*
- Teach patient how to prevent spreading virus to others: hand washing after toileting, using soap and hot water to clean eating utensils, cookware, and food preparation surfaces, practicing safer sex (abstinence, condoms, monogamy), and not sharing needles *because hepatitis is contagious.* (See "Home Health Hints.")

Home Health Hints

- For patients with hepatitis, home health nurses are concerned with proper treatment and patient education to prevent transmission in the community.
- If possible, the patient with hepatitis should have a separate bedroom and bathroom. The person cleaning the bathroom should wear disposable gloves or rubber gloves and then clean the gloves with a 10% bleach solution. The family is advised to use liquid soap instead of bar soap.
- Contaminated linens used by a patient with hepatitis should be washed separately from household laundry and in hot water. One cup of bleach should be added with the detergent to each load. Rubber gloves should be worn to wash the patient's laundry.
- A patient with abdominal ascites needs a hospital bed at home so the patient can be positioned to aid in breathing. A physician's order must be obtained for insurance coverage.
- Measure abdominal girth of the patient with ascites at each visit and record in the nurse's notes. The patient should weigh on the same scale, first thing in the morning, and record the weight so the nurse can document the findings.

EVALUATION. Management of the patient with hepatitis has been successful if the patient reports pain is satisfactorily relieved; body weight is maintained within 2 pounds of pre-illness weight; skin has no breaks, cuts, or tears, or secondary infections; patient can define disease; and patient follows transmission precautions and treatment.

CRITICAL THINKING

Carl Young

■ Carl Young, 23, has returned from a missionary trip in Africa. He reports that during his time there, he sustained a serious laceration that required sutures. Carl also mentions his fondness for seafood and that, since his return, he has had several "feasts" that have included raw oysters. Carl states that since his return, he has lost nearly 8 pounds, is nauseated, has frequent headaches, tires easily, and is very irritable.

1. What information might lead you to suspect hepatitis A infection? Hepatitis B infection?
2. What precautions should be instituted for Carl until a diagnosis is made?
3. What health care team members in addition to nursing will be beneficial to Carl's care?
4. What patient-centered care actions might you implement to help Carl improve his nutrition?
5. What medications should Carl avoid?
6. What information should be included in a teaching plan related to hepatitis for Carl?

Box 35-2 Patient Education

Liver Failure Prevention

To avoid causes of liver failure:

- Wash hands after using the bathroom and before handling food.
- Do not share personal grooming items (especially toothbrushes or razors).
- Obtain hepatitis A and B vaccine.
- Eat a balanced diet.
- Do not exceed 3000 mg of acetaminophen in 24-hour period or a prescribed drug with more than a 325-mg dose of acetaminophen in it.
- Review prescribed and over-the-counter medications to know which are combination drugs that contain acetaminophen to prevent excessive dosage. There are more than 600 drugs containing acetaminophen, such as Norco, NyQuil, Percocet, Vicodin, Tylenol with Codeine, or Tylox.
- Know how to read your medicine label and dosage found in the active ingredient list on the label. Visit www.knowyourdose.org to interactively read a drug label.
- Avoid alcohol or drink it only in moderation. Do not drink alcohol when taking acetaminophen.
- Avoid exposure to blood.
- Use condoms for safer sex.
- Ensure sanitary conditions and equipment when obtaining a body piercing or tattoo.
- Do not share IV needles.

Acute Liver Failure

Acute liver failure is a rare but serious condition that can develop rapidly, sometimes in just 2 days. When the liver is severely damaged, its many functions are impaired. The outcome of the disease may be decided within 48 to 72 hours of diagnosis. Possible outcomes are liver recovery, need for liver transplantation, or death. See Box 35-1 for causes. Box 35-2 ("Patient Education") teaches patients ways to prevent liver damage and possible liver failure.

Acetaminophen Toxicity

Acetaminophen (Tylenol) overdose is the most common cause of acute liver failure. Acetaminophen should not exceed 3000 mg in a 24-hour period. Prescription drugs containing more than 325 mg of acetaminophen should not be prescribed or taken per Food and Drug Administration (FDA) guidelines. Visit www.knowyourdose.org, an acetaminophen awareness program, for more information and a list of more than 600 medications containing acetaminophen.

Review prescribed and over-the-counter medications to know which are combination drugs that contain acetaminophen

to prevent excessive dosage. If overdose of acetaminophen is the cause, activated charcoal is given if it is within 4 hours of the overdose. N-acetylcysteine is then given to protect the liver. Aminoglycosides or nonsteroidal anti-inflammatory drugs (NSAIDS) are never given to patients with acetaminophen toxicity because nephrotoxicity can then be more severe.

 BE SAFE!

You should understand how to monitor the 24-hour dosage of acetaminophen taken by a patient. Look back at the previous 24-hour timeframe from the current time and add up the dosage of any acetaminophen taken alone and in combination drugs. This is a floating 24-hour period, not shift times or a calendar day. The acetaminophen dose should not exceed 3000 mg in a 24-hour period. Also teach the patient how to do this.

Signs and Symptoms

Initial symptoms of liver failure—fatigue, gastrointestinal (GI) upset, and diarrhea—are vague and make detection difficult. As the condition worsens, symptoms become more severe: jaundice, hepatic encephalopathy, bleeding, and abdominal distention. The patient may suddenly lapse into an extremely serious illness, starting with confusion and progressing to coma. In a matter of hours, on x-ray, the liver shows a rapid reduction in size, a typical sign of onset of acute liver failure. In addition, there is a sudden elevation of liver enzymes, ALT, aspartate aminotransferase (AST), and bilirubin. Prothrombin time is elevated, with marked elevation being an ominous sign. Potassium and blood glucose levels drop.

Therapeutic Measures

Treatment is directed toward stopping and reversing the damage to the liver. The patient needs intensive amounts of supportive care. Maintaining the airway (head elevated 30°, NPO [nothing by mouth], nasogastric [NG] tube, endotracheal intubation) is important as encephalopathy progresses. An attempt is made to put the liver completely at rest. The patient is on bed rest. Stimulation is avoided. Most medications are discontinued because they are metabolized by the liver. Dialysis may be ordered if the liver damage results from an overdose of a hepatotoxic substance to filter the substance from the blood. Nutrition may be provided via enteral or parenteral nutrition. Lactulose, neomycin, magnesium citrate, or sorbitol may be given to decrease ammonia levels (see later section on hepatic encephalopathy). If a liver transplant is needed, an otherwise healthy patient may be a priority organ recipient, depending on age and whether the patient is alcohol dependent.

Nursing Process for the Patient With Acute Liver Failure

Nursing care of the patient with acute liver failure is the same as for the patient with cirrhosis, which is discussed next.

Cirrhosis

Cirrhosis is the progressive, irreversible replacement of healthy liver tissue with scar tissue. It is caused by chronic liver disease. In 2010, chronic liver disease/cirrhosis was the 12th leading cause of death in the U.S. population (Murphy, Xu, & Kochanek, 2013). It occurs more commonly among men than women ("Cultural Considerations"). There are a variety of causes of cirrhosis (see Box 35-1). Chronic alcohol use is the most common cause of cirrhosis in the United States.

BE SAFE!

Many consequences of alcohol abuse such as cirrhosis can take years to develop but not acute alcohol toxicity. Ingesting a large quantity of ethanol (or a smaller quantity of alcohols not intended for beverages) in a short time can be fatal within a few hours. Alcohol poisoning is especially heartbreaking when it kills a young person whose companions let the victim "sleep it off" through ignorance or fear of retribution. Teaching young people about the hazards of alcohol and counseling adult patients about the responsible use of alcohol are appropriate health-teaching functions in all settings.

Pathophysiology

Healthy liver cells exposed to toxins become inflamed. Then the liver cells are infiltrated with fat and white blood cells (WBCs) and are replaced by fibrotic tissue. The liver makes some repairs. But if the damage continues over many years, and an increasing number of liver cells are replaced with fatty tissue and scar tissue, cirrhosis can develop. Liver regeneration continues abnormally, disrupting the lobes of the liver and creating nodules. The liver becomes hardened and lumpy. Early in the disease, the liver is enlarged, firm, and hard from the inflammatory process. Blood flow through the liver becomes impaired due to the nodules, resulting in portal venous hypertension. Later, the liver shrinks and is covered with gray connective tissue. As the disease progresses, liver function is impaired and after many years cirrhosis can lead to chronic liver failure.

Signs and Symptoms

Initially, symptoms are not usually seen with cirrhosis. As liver function becomes impaired, symptoms may begin to be seen. They include anorexia, nausea, vomiting, weight loss, and fatigue, which is due to decreased metabolic function of the liver. Jaundice may be present. The patient's skin may be dry from bile products deposited in the skin. The patient may report severe pruritus (itching). The liver may be

• **WORD** • **BUILDING** •
cirrhosis: cirrh—orange yellow + osis—condition

Cultural Considerations

The incidence of liver disease is more common among Mexican Americans. Risk factors include working in occupations such as mining, factories using chemicals, and farming while using pesticides.

Egyptian Americans may suffer from schistosomiasis (a parasitic disease), known as bilharziasis in Egypt. Schistosomiasis can lead to cirrhosis, liver failure, portal hypertension, esophageal varices, bladder cancer, and renal failure. Thus, the nurse may need to screen newer Egyptian American immigrants for this disease.

enlarged, firm, and tender. Laboratory values reflect progressive loss of liver function. As cirrhosis progresses, signs and symptoms of increasing loss of liver function and complications related to the increasing loss of function develop (Fig. 35.2, Table 35.3).

Complications

Complications of cirrhosis include blood clotting defects, portal hypertension, ascites, hepatic encephalopathy, and hepatorenal syndrome.

CLOTTING DEFECTS. Blood clotting defects may develop because of impaired prothrombin and fibrinogen production in the liver. Furthermore, the absence of bile salts prevents the absorption of fat-soluble vitamin K, which is essential for some blood clotting factors. Patients with cirrhosis have a tendency to bruise easily and can develop disseminated intravascular coagulation or hemorrhage.

PORTAL HYPERTENSION. **Portal hypertension** is persistent blood pressure elevation in the portal circulation of the abdomen. Liver damage causes a blockage of blood flow in the portal vein. Increased resistance from delayed drainage causes enlargement of the visible abdominal veins around the umbilicus (called *caput medusae*), rectal hemorrhoids, enlarged spleen (splenomegaly), and esophageal **varices** (dilated veins; Fig. 35.3).

The most serious result of portal hypertension is bleeding esophageal varices. The walls of the esophageal veins are thin and tear easily. Varices usually develop from the fundus of the stomach upward and may extend into the upper esophagus. The blood-filled, thin-walled varices may tear easily from sudden excessive pressure, such as the intra-abdominal pressure that results from coughing, lifting, or straining, causing severe bleeding.

TABLE 35.3   CIRRHOSIS SUMMARY

Signs and Symptoms	Anorexia, nausea Dull RUQ pain Bruising Jaundice Ascites
Diagnostic Tests	Elevated ALT, AST, ALP, ammonia, bilirubin, PT Decreased albumin Liver biopsy
Therapeutic Measures	Prevent disease progression and treat complications.
Complications	*C:* Clotting defects *H:* Hepatorenal syndrome *E:* Encephalopathy *A:* Ascites *P:* Portal hypertension
Priority Nursing Diagnoses	*Pain* *Excess or Deficient Fluid Volume* *Imbalanced Nutrition*

Note. ALT = alanine aminotransferase; ALP = alkaline phosphatase; AST = aspartate aminotransferase; IV = intravenous; PT = prothrombin time; RUQ = right upper quadrant.

Hepatic encephalopathy
Behavior changes
Flapping tremor
Confusion
Fetor hepaticus
Gradual progression
to coma

Portal hypertension
Hemorrhoids
Ascites
Caput medusae
Enlarged spleen
Esophageal varices
Spider angiomas

Hepatorenal syndrome
Oliguria
Sodium retention

Skin
Jaundice
Itching

Gastrointestinal
Diarrhea
Constipation
RUQ pain
Anorexia
Nausea
Clay-colored stools

Reproductive
Amenorrhea
Testicular atrophy
Gynecomastia (male)
Erectile dysfunction

Hematologic
Bruising
Abnormal bleeding
Anemia
Petechiae

FIGURE 35.2 Signs and symptoms of cirrhosis.

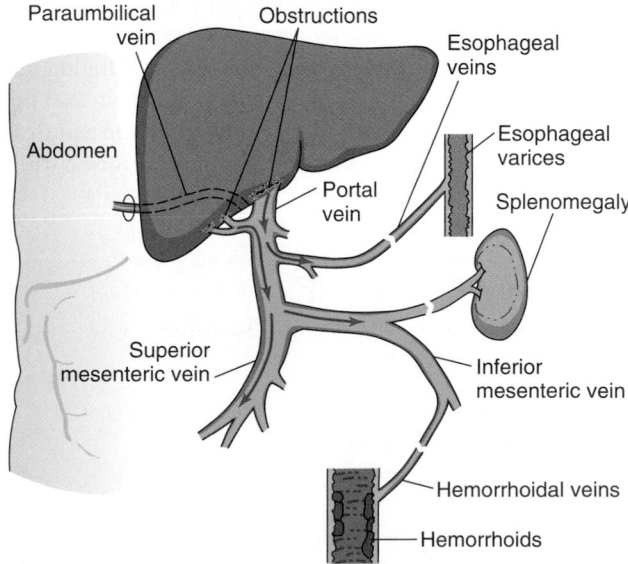

FIGURE 35.3 Portal hypertension. Obstruction of normal blood flow through the liver causes blood to back up into the venous system, leading to esophageal varices, splenomegaly, hemorrhoids, and caput medusae.

ASCITES. **Ascites** is an accumulation of serous fluid in the abdominal cavity. The fluid accumulates from portal hypertension and low production of albumin by the failing liver and aldosterone accumulation. An insufficient amount of albumin causes plasma to seep into the abdominal cavity. The kidneys respond to the decreased circulating blood volume by saving sodium and water. The accumulated fluid causes a markedly enlarged abdomen. The fluid may cause severe respiratory distress as a result of elevation of the diaphragm.

HEPATIC ENCEPHALOPATHY. Hepatic **encephalopathy** is caused by elevated ammonia, a byproduct of protein metabolism, which disrupts mental status. The damaged liver is unable to make the ammonia water soluble for excretion in the urine. Signs and symptoms of hepatic encephalopathy include progressive confusion; **asterixis**, or flapping tremors in the hands caused by toxins at peripheral nerves; and **fetor hepaticus**, or foul breath caused by metabolic end products related to sulfur.

Stages of hepatic encephalopathy and signs and symptoms of the stages are as follows:

- *Early:* The patient exhibits subtle changes in personality, fatigue, drowsiness, and changes in handwriting (the best assessment for the early stage).
- *Stupor and confusion:* The patient is often belligerent and irritable and develops asterixis, muscle twitching, hyperventilation, and marked confusion.
- *Comatose:* The patient gradually loses consciousness and becomes comatose.

With treatment, if ammonia levels decrease, the patient gradually regains consciousness. Hepatic encephalopathy represents end-stage liver failure and has a mortality rate as high as 90% once coma begins.

HEPATORENAL SYNDROME. **Hepatorenal syndrome** is a secondary failure of the kidneys in some patients with cirrhosis. Symptoms of hepatorenal syndrome include oliguria without detectable kidney damage, reduced glomerular filtration rate (GFR) with essentially no urine output or less than 200 mL per day, and nearly total sodium retention. Albumin and fresh frozen plasma to increase intravascular volume is given while avoiding diuretics.

LEARNING TIP

For complications of cirrhosis, remember the pneumonic "CHEAP":

C: Clotting defects
H: Hepatorenal syndrome
E: Encephalopathy
A: Ascites
P: Portal hypertension

Diagnostic Tests

Tests that show liver damage and functioning of the liver are shown in Table 35.2. Abdominal radiographs of patients

with cirrhosis may show ascites and enlargement of the liver. An abdominal ultrasound may show liver enlargement early in cirrhosis or a small liver later in the disease. An esophagogastroduodenoscopy (EGD) detects esophageal varices and bleeding (discussed later in the chapter). A liver biopsy may be done to determine the extent and nature of the liver damage (see Chapter 32).

NURSING CARE TIP

Patients with cirrhosis undergoing a liver biopsy need careful observation for bleeding after the procedure due to possible impaired clotting.

Therapeutic Measures

Interventions for cirrhosis are to prevent advancement of the disease and treat complications.

ASCITES. Ascites is treated with diuretics such as spironolactone (Aldactone) or furosemide (Lasix), sodium and fluid restriction (800–1000 mL/day), and albumin infusions for severe ascites. Paracentesis can be done to remove accumulated fluid from the peritoneal cavity when the fluid is compromising the patient's breathing, causing abdominal discomfort, or posing a threat of ruptured umbilical hernia. If large amounts of fluid are removed, albumin may be given to replace lost proteins to prevent fluid shifting.

Ascites can be treated by the placement of a shunt, called a **transjugular intrahepatic portosystemic shunt**, under fluoroscopy (Fig. 35.4). Access to place the shunt is gained through the jugular vein. A stent is placed to connect the portal vein to the hepatic vein, in the middle of the liver. This reduces portal pressure by allowing blood to bypass the liver and be carried to the heart. It reduces fluid accumulation and aids in reducing the risk of bleeding.

ESOPHAGEAL VARICES. The medical goals for managing bleeding from esophageal varices are to stop the bleeding immediately, maintain normal clotting, and treat infection. Bleeding varices can be treated with vasoconstrictors such as vasopressin, octreotide (Sandostatin), beta blockers or nitrates, and endoscopic variceal ligation (banding) or sclerotherapy to close the varices. Vitamin K, which is often deficient in liver

- WORD - BUILDING -
encephalopathy: encephalo—brain + pathy—disease
asterixis: a—not + sterixis—fixed position
fetor hepaticus: fetor—offensive odor + hepat—liver + icas—related to
hepatorenal syndrome: hepato—liver + renal—kidneys + syndrome—group of symptoms
transjugular intrahepatic portosystemic shunt: trans—across + jugular—jugular vein + intra—within + hepatic—liver + porto—portal (liver circulation) + systemic—systemic (circulation) + shunt—to divert

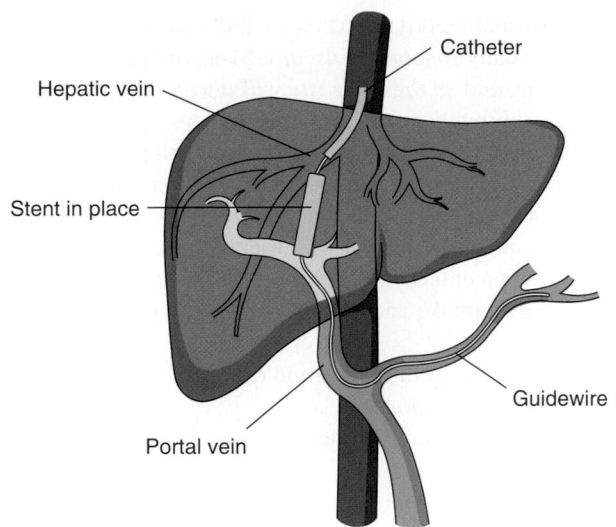

FIGURE 35.4 Transjugular intrahepatic portosystemic shunt (TIPS). A stent is placed to shunt blood from the portal vein to the hepatic vein and systemic circulation to divert blood flow around the diseased liver.

disease, is given to assist with the clotting process. Antibiotic prophylaxis is given with hemorrhage because severe bacterial infection is a risk and can be a precursor to rebleeding varices.

Banding of varices with rubber bands during endoscopy is done to stop the bleeding (Fig. 35.5). Sclerotherapy is another method of treatment during endoscopy. The varices are injected with a sclerosing agent that causes thickening and closing of the dilated vessels. Postprocedure the patient may report chest pain for up to 72 hours. Give prescribed analgesics, and monitor the patient for relief of pain. Report severe pain unrelieved by the prescribed analgesic immediately because the patient may have an esophageal perforation or ulceration, which is a complication of sclerotherapy.

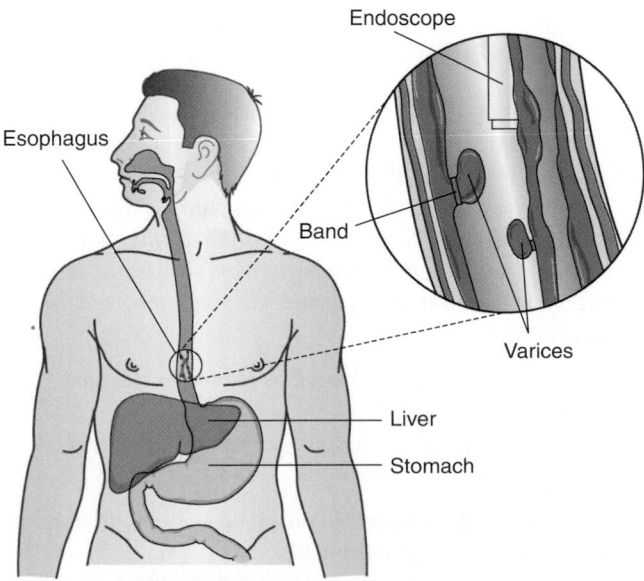

FIGURE 35.5 Variceal banding.

In emergency cases when other methods are not available, temporary tamponade (application of pressure) of the bleeding varices may be done with a multilumen esophagogastric tube that has a balloon on the end for inflation (Sengstaken-Blakemore tube or Minnesota tube). Complications of esophagogastric tamponade may include aspiration, erosion of the mucosa, perforation, and suffocation, so it is not often used.

HEPATIC ENCEPHALOPATHY. Lactulose may be given by mouth, NG tube, or enema (depending on how alert the patient is) to make the colon contents more acidic. This creates an insoluble form of ammonia that is then excreted in the stool. Neomycin, an intestinal antibiotic, occasionally may be given to reduce colonic bacteria that change ammonium to ammonia. See "Nutrition Notes."

Nutrition Notes

Supplying Nutrients to Patients With Liver Disease

A registered dietitian may modify the diet daily for patients with serious liver disease. Usually these patients suffer from severe anorexia, as well as nausea, often displaying their best appetites for breakfast.

Restriction of dietary protein was long considered a mainstay in the management of liver disease and hepatic encephalopathy until studies showed the strategy was not only ineffective but possibly harmful (Ambühl, 2011; Bémeur, Desjardin, & Butterworth, 2010).

Nutritional Care for Hepatitis Patients

A high-kilocalorie, high-protein, moderate-fat diet is frequently prescribed for hepatitis patients:

- Up to 400 grams of carbohydrate provides energy intake.
- Up to 100 grams of protein promotes healing.
- Up to 35% of kilocalories in fat to use a dense energy source. Emulsified fats in dairy products and eggs may be better tolerated than other fats.
- Up to 3 to 3.5 liters of fluid intake per day.
- Supplemental between-meal feedings may be prescribed.

Nutritional Care for Cirrhosis Patients

In general, dietary interventions for patients with stable cirrhosis features these key components:
- Avoidance of alcohol
- Ingestion of four to six meals per day
- Late evening snack to avoid fasting-associated catabolism
- Protein intake of 1.0 to 1.2 grams per kilogram of body weight
- Sufficient kilocalories to avoid muscle catabolism
- Monitored vitamin status and appropriate supplementation
- Sodium restriction based upon ascites level

Some evidence shows supplementation with branched-chain amino acids (isoleucine, leucine, and valine) may delay the progression of cirrhosis. Branched-chain amino acids do not require oxidation by the liver and are available for direct use by other tissues. A special formula for oral or enteral feeding is Hepatic-Aid II®.

Nutritional Care for Patients With Hepatic Encephalopathy

Hepatic encephalopathy is associated with increased serum levels of ammonia caused by the liver's inability to degrade ammonia to urea. Ammonia is toxic to all cells, including those of the liver and the brain. The goal of nutritional management of patients with hepatic encephalopathy is to promote protein synthesis by supplying ample amounts of amino acids. Only in cases of severe protein intolerance should protein be restricted and then for as short a time as possible with supplemental branched-chain amino acids administered until normal protein intake is resumed.

Complication of Alcoholic Liver Disease: Wernicke-Korsakoff Syndrome

This disorder of the central nervous system, caused by thiamin deficiency, is diagnosed mainly in alcoholics but also occasionally in malnourished patients with no history of alcohol abuse, including women with hyperemesis gravidarum.

Wernicke's encephalopathy is an acute neuropsychiatric condition caused by inadequate thiamin supplied to the brain. When caused by dietary deficiency, it can usually be successfully treated with oral or subcutaneous thiamin and rarely progresses to Korsakoff's psychosis, the result of damage to the brain tissue. Thiamin given at this stage will not reverse the effects. These patients display an abnormal mental state in which memory and learning are affected out of all proportion to other cognitive functions in an otherwise alert and responsive patient.

Nursing Process for the Patient With Acute Liver Failure and Cirrhosis

DATA COLLECTION. A complete history and physical assessment are done. Be alert to subjective symptoms of liver dysfunction, such as abdominal pain, anorexia, nausea, severe itching, and dull, aching RUQ pain. Note objective evidence of liver problems, such as jaundice, light-colored stools, ascites, ecchymosis (bruising) of the skin, GI bleeding, and any evidence of alterations in thought processes, such as confusion, disorientation, or inability to make decisions.

NURSING DIAGNOSES, PLANNING, AND IMPLEMENTATION. Common nursing diagnoses for patient with cirrhosis include the following.

Excess Fluid Volume related to portal hypertension (ascites)
EXPECTED OUTCOME: Fluid volume will be controlled as evidenced by stable weight and abdominal girth within normal limits for the patient.

• Weigh the patient on admission and daily *to measure fluid retention.*

• Measure and record the patient's abdominal girth (circumference) daily *to monitor ascites.* Mark the place where you measured *so the same site will always be measured during subsequent assessments.*
• Report any weight gain or increase in girth promptly *so treatment can be ordered and complications minimized.*
• Monitor the patient's vital signs and lung sounds; report changes and any evidence of difficulty breathing or changes in mental status promptly *to detect fluid overload.*
• Measure all intake and output *to accurately detect fluid overload.*
• Maintain a low-sodium diet and order fluid restrictions *to reduce fluid retention.*
• Administer ordered diuretics as scheduled *to reduce fluid volume.*
• If IV fluids or albumin have been ordered, assist in careful monitoring of the rate of infusion *to prevent or detect fluid overload.*

Imbalanced Nutrition: Less Than Body Requirements related to anorexia and impaired metabolism of needed nutrients
EXPECTED OUTCOME: The patient's (dry) weight will be within normal limits for height.

• Monitor weight; report unexpected (nonfluid) weight loss *so timely intervention can be implemented.*
• Monitor serum prealbumin, total protein, vitamin, and mineral levels *because these may be better indicators of nutrition if nutritional status is masked by fluid overload in weight measurement.*
• Offer frequent mouth care *to increase comfort and make food more palatable.*
• Make sure that odors and other unpleasant stimuli are eliminated *to prevent further worsening of appetite.*
• Offer the patient frequent, small, high-calorie meals *to reduce feeling of fullness that can occur with larger meals.*
• Administer vitamins or supplements as ordered *to correct deficiencies.*

Pain related to abdominal pressure
EXPECTED OUTCOME: The patient will state pain level is acceptable.

• Monitor pain level using a 10-point scale and **WHAT'S UP?** questions *to guide treatment.*
• Give analgesics as ordered to control pain. *Lower doses may be needed for the patient with liver dysfunction.*
• Encourage nondrug pain relief activities, such as distraction, imagery, and relaxation *to possibly decrease the need for analgesics.*

Risk for Disturbed Thought Processes related to elevated ammonia levels
EXPECTED OUTCOME: The patient will remain alert and oriented to person, place, and time.

• Assess the patient's level of consciousness and orientation often *to allow prompt treatment.*
• Assess neuromuscular function by asking the patient to hold his or her arms out straight in front and steady.

If asterixis, or liver flap, is present, the patient's hands will unwillingly dip and return to the horizontal position in a flapping motion due to elevated ammonia.

- Look for changes in the patient's handwriting *because changes can indicate altered neuromuscular function.*
- Give lactulose, neomycin, magnesium citrate, or sorbitol as scheduled *to decrease serum ammonia levels.*
- Be aware that lactulose causes loose stools, and do not withhold the medication when the patient develops diarrhea. *Loose stools are a sign that the medication is working, not a reason to withhold it when treating ammonia levels.*
- Question giving medications such as sedatives, opioids, and tranquilizers *because these can precipitate hepatic encephalopathy.*
- Reorient the patient to time and place as needed and helpful *to reinforce reality.*
- Give simple, clear explanations of care, and give the patient time to understand the explanation *because short, simple explanations are easier to process.*
- Provide a safe environment for the confused or unsteady patient *to prevent injury.*

Risk for Ineffective Breathing Pattern related to excess fluid in the abdomen

EXPECTED OUTCOME: The patient's respirations will be even and unlabored, 16 to 20 per minute.

- Assess the patient's respiratory rate, rhythm, chest movement, skin color, and oxygen saturation frequently *to determine if breathing pattern is effective.*
- Assist the patient to use an incentive spirometer and to cough gently every 2 to 4 hours *to encourage deep breathing and keep airways clear.*
- Elevate the head of the patient's bed *so that the patient's lungs have maximum room for expansion.*
- Administer analgesics carefully, as ordered, if pain is causing shallow respirations. *Reducing pain with breathing allows for a more effective breathing pattern.*
- Reposition the patient at least every 2 hours *to ventilate all areas of the lungs.*
- Assist with treatments to decrease ascites as ordered *to increase room for lung expansion.*

Risk for Deficient Fluid Volume related to bleeding esophageal varices or gastrointestinal bleeding secondary to clotting dysfunction

EXPECTED OUTCOME: Fluid volume will remain within normal limits without bleeding as evidenced by no signs and symptoms of bleeding, and vital signs within normal limits for the patient.

- Monitor gastric secretions, stool, and urine at least every 8 hours, and report any signs of bleeding. *Early identification of bleeding is essential to prompt treatment.*
- Monitor blood clotting laboratory studies such as prothrombin time and report any abnormal values *to identify risk for bleeding.*
- Caution the patient to use a soft-bristle toothbrush and an electric rather than straight razor *to avoid injury and bleeding.*

- Avoid suctioning the patient if possible *because suctioning can cause esophageal varices to bleed.*
- Use a small-gauge needle for injections and apply direct pressure to all puncture sites *to avoid bleeding.*
- Teach the patient to avoid hot, spicy, or irritating foods *because these may irritate the esophageal mucosa and increase risk of bleeding.*
- Instruct the patient to avoid forceful coughing or nose blowing, straining, vomiting, or gagging if at all possible. Administer medications as ordered to prevent their occurrence. *These can increase pressure and risk of bleeding varices.*

Risk for Infection related to impaired immune function

EXPECTED OUTCOME: The patient will be free from infection as evidenced by WBC count within normal limit, afebrile.

- Monitor for signs of infection and report promptly *so treatment can begin.*
- Be aware that the earliest warning signs of infection may be subtle changes in the patient's behavior, such as sudden restlessness, an increase in confusion, or irritability. *Early recognition is essential to prompt treatment.*
- Carefully evaluate laboratory studies such as the WBC count. *The WBC count may not elevate or may elevate slowly because the white cell activity is impaired.*
- Teach the patient careful hand hygiene and avoidance of people who are ill *to prevent exposure to infection.*

EVALUATION. Nursing care has been effective if the patient is alert and oriented and has no signs of fluid retention, a stable weight appropriate for height, no abdominal pain or pain reported as tolerable using a 10-point scale, a respiratory rate between 16 and 20 respirations per minute with no cyanosis or changes in level of consciousness, no bleeding, no infection, no injuries, and an accurate knowledge of cirrhosis and proper disease management requirements.

PATIENT EDUCATION. Teach patients how cirrhosis is affecting their bodies. In particular, patients need to know about portal system hypertension and hepatic encephalopathy. In addition, teach:

- How to observe for and report any confusion, tremors, or personality changes
- The importance of adequate rest and avoidance of strenuous activity
- See "Nutrition Notes"
- The need to use opioids, sedatives, and tranquilizers cautiously due to potential mental function impairment
- The need to promptly report any bleeding; any sign of low potassium, such as muscle cramps, nausea, or vomiting caused by diuretics; changes in mental status, such as confusion or personality changes; changes in weight; and any increase in current symptoms
- The importance of avoiding alcohol
- The importance of frequent follow-up care and laboratory studies

CRITICAL THINKING

Mrs. Conner

■ Mrs. Conner, a 76-year-old retired businesswoman, has lived alone for the past 20 years since the death of her husband. She has a long history of poor nutritional habits but does not consume alcohol. She is admitted with cirrhosis.

1. What risk factors does Mrs. Conner have for cirrhosis?
2. What symptoms would you expect Mrs. Conner to exhibit with early cirrhosis?
3. What values do you expect to see for serum albumin? Prothrombin time?
4. What are the two greatest concerns with portal hypertension?
5. What is the usual treatment for ascites?

Suggested answers are at the end of the chapter.

Liver Transplantation

The patient with end-stage liver failure from cirrhosis, hepatitis, biliary disease, metabolic disorders, or hepatic vein obstruction might be evaluated for a liver transplant. The patient will be evaluated for emotional and physical stability and must accept that he or she will be on daily medications for life ("Cultural Considerations").

After the surgical implantation of a donor liver, the patient must be closely observed for evidence of donor organ rejection. The patient will be on drugs to suppress immune system responses and prevent tissue rejection. Observe the patient for the following signs of impending rejection:

• Pulse greater than 100 beats per minute
• Temperature greater than 101°F (38°C)
• Reports of RUQ pain
• Increased jaundice
• Decrease in bile from the T-tube or change in bile color.

In addition, laboratory studies may show increased serum transaminases (ALT and AST), serum bilirubin, alkaline phosphatase, and prothrombin time. Symptoms of acute tissue rejection usually develop between the 4th and 10th postoperative days. The patient who has received an organ transplant needs extended medical follow-up. Teach the patient to promptly report to the physician any symptoms of infection, bleeding episodes, or RUQ pain.

As a short-term bridge to liver transplant, bioartificial livers with filtering membranes have been used. Under study, for longer term support is hepatocyte transplantation via a splenic artery catheter.

Cancer of the Liver

Cancer of the liver usually results from metastasis from a primary cancer at a distant location. The liver is a likely area of involvement if cancer originated in the esophagus, lungs, breast, stomach, colon, pancreas, kidney, bladder, or skin. For some patients, liver cancer is the primary tumor site. Patients with a history of chronic hepatitis B or C infection, nutritional deficiencies, heavy alcohol use or smoking, and exposure to hepatotoxins have an increased risk for cancer of the liver.

Symptoms of cancer of the liver include encephalopathy, abnormal bleeding, jaundice, and ascites. Laboratory tests show elevated serum alkaline phosphatase. Radiologic examinations may include abdominal radiographs or radioisotope scans, which show tumor growth. Liver cancer is definitively diagnosed with a positive needle biopsy combined with an ultrasound exam of the liver.

Liver cancer is staged upon diagnosis. If found early, surgery can be curative. Rarely, though, is it found early. Care of the postsurgical patient is similar to other abdominal surgery patients. If surgery is not an option, the patient may receive chemotherapeutic drugs by injection directly into the affected lobe of the liver or into the hepatic artery; sorafenib, which, slows the spread of cancer cells; or radiation therapy. The overall survival rate for liver cancer is low. (See Chapter 11 for care of patients with cancer.)

 DISORDERS OF THE PANCREAS

Pancreatitis

Pancreatitis, inflammation of the pancreas, may be either acute or chronic. The two forms of pancreatitis have different courses and are considered two different disorders.

 ## Cultural Considerations

Jewish law addresses organ transplantation from the perspectives of the recipient, the living donor, the cadaver donor, and the dying donor. If a recipient's life can be prolonged without considerable risk, transplant is ordained. For a living donor to be approved, the risk to the life of the donor must be considered. One is not obligated to donate a part of himself or herself unless the risk is small. The use of a cadaver for transplant is usually approved if it is saving a life. The nurse may need to help a patient who is Jewish contact a rabbi when making a decision regarding organ donation or transplantation.

Acute Pancreatitis

Pathophysiology

Inflammation of the pancreas appears to be caused by a process called autodigestion. Recall that the pancreas normally secretes digestive enzymes. For reasons not fully understood, pancreatic enzymes can be activated while they are still in the pancreas and begin to digest the pancreas. In addition, large amounts of enzymes are released by inflamed cells. As the pancreas digests itself, chemical cascades occur. Trypsin destroys pancreatic tissue and causes vasodilation. As capillary permeability increases, fluid is lost to the retroperitoneal space, causing shock. In addition, trypsin appears to set off another chain of events that causes the conversion of prothrombin to thrombin, so that clots form. The patient may develop disseminated intravascular coagulation (see Chapter 28).

Etiology

Acute pancreatitis is most commonly associated with heavy alcohol consumption or gallstones. Alcohol appears to act directly on the acinar cells of the pancreas and the pancreatic ducts to irritate and inflame the structures. Cholelithiasis (gallstones) or cholangitis (inflammation of the bile ducts) can also trigger pancreatitis. Gallstones may plug the pancreatic duct and cause inflammation from excessive fluid pressure on sensitive ducts. The irritant effect of bile itself may cause inflammation. Elevated triglycerides, pancreatic tumors, or, rarely, medications can cause pancreatitis.

Prevention

Caution patients who drink alcohol to stop. Patients with biliary disease need to seek medical treatment for these conditions so that pancreatitis does not develop as a complication.

Signs and Symptoms

Patients with acute pancreatitis are very ill, with dull abdominal pain, guarding, a rigid abdomen, hypotension or shock, and respiratory distress from accumulation of fluid in the retroperitoneal space. The abdominal pain usually is located in the midline just below the sternum, with radiation to the spine, back, and flank. The location and degree of pain indicate the area of the pancreas involved and to some extent the amount of involvement. Respirations are likely to be shallow as the patient attempts to splint painful areas. Eating makes the pain worse.

The patient may have a low-grade fever, dry mucous membranes, and tachycardia. If the primary cause is biliary, the patient may report nausea and vomiting, and jaundice may be evident. The islets of Langerhans in the terminal one-third of the pancreas are usually not impaired.

Complications

It may be useful to think of acute pancreatitis as a chemical burn to the organ. As with other severe burns, death is likely to occur from secondary causes. From the onset of symptoms, cardiovascular, pulmonary (including acute respiratory distress syndrome), and renal failure are the most likely causes of death. Hemorrhage, peripheral vascular collapse, and infection are also major concerns. A purplish discoloration of the flanks (Turner's sign) or a purplish discoloration around the umbilicus (Cullen's sign) may occur with extensive hemorrhagic destruction of the pancreas.

Diagnostic Tests

Diagnosis of acute pancreatitis is made when two of these are present: abdominal pain, serum amylase (normal: 80–180 units/dL) and/or serum lipase (normal: 0 to 160 units/L) more than 3 times normal, abdominal imaging is indicative of it. Serum amylase rises quickly and then returns to normal in 3 to 5 days. Serum lipase is thought to be more specific for acute pancreatitis and elevates and stays elevated for a longer period of time. Glucose, bilirubin, alkaline phosphatase, lactic dehydrogenase, ALT, AST, cholesterol, and potassium are all elevated. Decreases are seen in serum albumin, calcium, sodium, and magnesium. Ultrasonography may show pleural effusion from local inflammatory reaction to pancreatic enzymes or a change in the size of the pancreas.

Therapeutic Measures

Early aggressive IV hydration during the first 24 hours for hypovolemia treatment is recommended. In asymptomatic mild acute pancreatitis, oral nutrition is given ("Nutrition Notes"). In severe cases, enteral feeding is maintained (see "Evidence-Based Practice"). A histamine (H_2) antagonist can help decrease acid stimulation of pancreatic secretions (Table 35.4). Additional drug orders include electrolytes such as calcium and magnesium to replace losses, short-acting insulin to combat hyperglycemia, and antibiotics to treat sepsis (Table 35.5). Surgery may be needed for debriding necrotic tissue. Abscesses or pseudocysts may need to be drained.

Nutrition Notes

Nourishing the Patient With Pancreatitis

Nutritionally, mild acute pancreatitis can be treated with the following:
- Aggressive hydration with IV fluids
- Nothing by mouth for 48 hours to avoid stimulating the pancreas
- Clear liquids after pain has been controlled and nausea and vomiting end
- Low-fat, soft diet
- Soft to general diet over 3 or 4 days if satisfactory progress

If the disease progresses to severe pancreatitis, the goal of nutritional support is to meet the elevated metabolic demands as much as possible without stimulating pancreatic secretion and self-digestion. The more distally the feeding enters the gut, the less it stimulates pancreatic secretions. In general, feedings should:

- Begin as early as possible following admission to the hospital
- Consist of a high-protein, low-fat, semielemental (partially predigested) formula
- Start slowly, 20 to 25 mL/hour for 24 hours
- Increase in 25 mL increments to goal of 25 kcal/kg/ideal body weight/day

General dietary management principles for chronic pancreatitis depend on the stage of disease but progressively are likely to include the following:

- Total abstinence from alcohol (and, although not dietary, smoking)
- Small, frequent nutritionally balanced meals, avoiding fatty foods
- Vitamin-mineral supplements as appropriate
- If underweight
  - 35 calories per kilogram of body weight daily
  - to 1.5 grams of protein per kilogram of body weight per day
- Pancreatic enzyme supplements, which help but do not substitute for normal function
- Jejunal tube feeding
- Rarely, short-term parenteral nutrition to replace nutrient stores
- Monitoring and treating diabetes resulting from loss of endogenous insulin and glucagon secretions.

Pain relief is essential, and opioids such as morphine or hydromorphone (Dilaudid) are ordered for pain. The patient may be given antianxiety agents to decrease oxygen demand. Supplemental oxygen may be required if abdominal pressure, pleural effusion, or acidosis cause impaired gas exchange or an ineffective breathing pattern.

 EVIDENCE-BASED PRACTICE

Clinical Question
Does the use of enteral nutrition have outcomes similar to parenteral nutrition in patients with acute pancreatitis?

Evidence
A systematic review of literature from 1999 through 2011 to develop guidelines for pancreatitis and nutrition was conducted. Based on the evidence the following guideline was developed: Nutrition support therapy is generally not needed for mild to moderate disease; nutrition support therapy is needed for severe disease. Enteral nutrition is preferred over parenteral nutrition; parenteral nutrition is only used when enteral nutrition is contraindicated or not feasible.

Implications for Nursing Practice
Enteral nutrition is a cost-effective method with fewer complications (infection) for providing nutritional support to patients with acute pancreatitis. Being informed about options for nourishment allows nurses to advocate for patient nourishment to promote healing.

REFERENCE
Mirtallo, J., Forbes, A., McClave, S., Jensen, G., Waitzberg, D., & Davies, A. (2012). International consensus guidelines for nutrition therapy in pancreatitis. *Journal of Parenteral and Enteral Nutrition, 36*, 284–291.

CRITICAL THINKING

Mrs. Samuels

■ Mrs. Samuels, an 85-year-old retired librarian, is admitted to the nursing unit from the emergency department with severe midepigastric pain that radiates to her back. On admission, she is noted to have guarding of the abdomen, and her abdomen is full and tense. Her medical record documents that she had an endoscopic retrograde cholangiopancreatograph (ERCP) 2 days ago for recurrent episodes of RUQ abdominal pain. She has no history of excessive alcohol intake.

1. What is the most common cause of acute pancreatitis? Does Mrs. Samuels fit the description?
2. Why do patients such as Mrs. Samuels have difficulty breathing?
3. Why is Mrs. Samuels at risk for hemorrhage?
4. What laboratory test is most likely to be abnormal in early acute pancreatitis?
5. Why are opioids commonly ordered for acute pancreatitis?
6. Why does the HCP usually order a histamine antagonist?
7. What nutrition orders will likely be given for Mrs. Samuels?

Suggested answers are at the end of the chapter.

Chronic Pancreatitis

Chronic pancreatitis is ongoing pancreatic cellular damage and decreased pancreatic enzyme functioning often following repeated occasions of acute pancreatitis.

Pathophysiology

Chronic pancreatitis is a continuous, progressive disease that replaces functioning pancreatic tissue with fibrotic tissue as a result of inflammation. Pancreatic ducts become

TABLE 35.4 MEDICATIONS USED FOR LIVER, GALLBLADDER, OR PANCREATIC DISORDERS

Medication Class/Action	Examples	Nursing Implications
Antiemetics Reduce nausea	prochlorperazine (Compazine) metoclopramide (Reglan) promethazine (Phenergan) odansetron (Zofran)	Contraindicated in glaucoma or prostatic hypertrophy. Give antacids 2 hours before or after. Monitor for extrapyramidal symptoms. Administer 30 minutes before meals. May be additive when used with opioids. Monitor I&O, sedation, urine retention. Monitor for hypersensitivity.
Antihistamines Reduce itching	diphenhydramine (Benadryl)	If using topical preparation, do not apply to open skin. Can cause confusion in older adults.
Anticholinergics Decrease GI secretions	dicyclomine hydrochloride (Bentyl)	Contraindicated in glaucoma or prostatic hypertrophy.
Bile Acid Sequestrants Bind with circulating bile acids for excretion in the stool to relieve itching.	cholestyramine (Questran, LoCholest) colestipol (Colestid)	Give 4–6 hr before or 1 hr after other medications.
Bile Acid Agents Prevent or dissolve (noncalcified) cholesterol gallstones	ursodiol (Actigall) chenodiol (Chenix)	Give with a full glass of water. Aluminum antacids may reduce absorption.
Histamine (H₂) antagonists Lock histamine receptors in acid, producing cells to inhibit gastric acid secretion	famotidine (Pepcid) ranitidine (Zantac)	If ordered once a day, give at bedtime. Smoking may interfere with action.
Proton Pump Inhibitors Inhibit proton pump to reduce gastric acid production	rabeprazole (AcipHex) esomeprazole (Nexium) lansoprazole (Prevacid) omeprazole (Prilosec) pantoprazole (Protonix) dexlansoprazole (Dexilant, Kapidex)	Monitor bowel sounds, liver function (AST, ALT). Can result in serious infection with cirrhosis. Delayed release. Capsule swallowed whole.
Pancreatic Supplements Replace pancreatic digestive enzymes: lipase, protease, amylase	pancrelipase (Cotazym, Creon Pancrease, Ultrase, Viokase)	Give with meals. Teach not to hold medication in mouth because it may irritate inside of mouth.

Note. ALT = alanine aminotransferase; AST = aspartate aminotransferase; I&O = input and output.

TABLE 35.5 PANCREATITIS SUMMARY

Signs and Symptoms	Midline abdominal pain Low-grade fever Nausea and vomiting
Diagnostic Tests	Elevated serum amylase and lipase
Therapeutic Measures	Pain control NPO NG suction IV fluids, parenteral nutrition, enteral nutrition
Complications	Hemorrhage, shock, infection
Priority Nursing Diagnoses	*Pain* *Imbalanced Nutrition* *Risk for Ineffective Breathing Pattern*

Note. IV = intravenous; NG = nasogastric; NPO = nothing by mouth.

obstructed, dilated, and finally atrophied. The acinar, or enzyme-producing, cells of the pancreas ulcerate in response to inflammation. The ulceration causes further tissue damage and tissue death, and it may cause cystic sacs filled with pancreatic enzymes to form on the surface of the pancreas. The pancreas becomes smaller and hardened, and progressively smaller amounts of pancreatic enzymes are produced.

Etiology and Incidence

The major cause of chronic pancreatitis in men is excessive alcohol ingestion that causes repeated attacks of acute pancreatitis. The major cause in women is chronic obstructive biliary disease, which leads to persistent inflammation of the pancreatic ducts. Other conditions known to cause chronic pancreatitis are prolonged malnutrition, cancer of the pancreas or duodenum, and prolonged use of enteral feedings, which can cause atrophy of the pancreas. The usual age for chronic pancreatitis to develop is between ages 45 and 60. The patient's mean life span is 25 years after the diagnosis of chronic pancreatitis is made. Death is often not related to pancreatic failure.

Prevention

Advise patients with acute pancreatitis from heavy alcohol ingestion that abstinence could prevent recurrence of the pancreatitis and prevent the possibility of chronic pancreatitis. Advise all patients with obstructive biliary disease to seek medical treatment for their condition to prevent the progression from acute to chronic pancreatitis. Carefully monitor patients who are unable to feed themselves for nutritionally adequate diets. Monitor routine laboratory values. Report any trend toward reduced functioning of the pancreas.

Signs and Symptoms

The signs and symptoms of chronic pancreatitis are less severe than for acute pancreatitis but are long term. The patient's history will show a pattern of remissions and exacerbations over years. The patient will report epigastric or lower upper quadrant (LUQ) pain, weight loss, and anorexia.

Complications

A variety of complications can result from chronic pancreatitis. Abscesses and fistulas may develop when cysts filled with pancreatic enzymes burst into the abdominal cavity, causing severe inflammation and tissue necrosis. Pleural effusion may develop from inflammation just under the diaphragm. Pancreatic enzymes are essential for normal absorption of nutrients from the intestines. Fat intolerance and malabsorption syndrome with fatty stools and diarrhea may develop in response to the limited amount of pancreatic enzymes produced. In addition, biliary obstruction may further complicate fat absorption. As the terminal third of the pancreas becomes involved and the islets of Langerhans are destroyed, the patient exhibits symptoms of insulin-dependent diabetes mellitus (discussed in Chapter 40).

Diagnostic Tests

Serum amylase and serum lipase levels elevate only in acute disease. In chronic pancreatitis, enzymes will be normal or below normal. Fecal fat analysis shows higher than normal amounts of fat. Both computed tomography (CT) and ultrasonography show characteristic pancreatic structural changes such as masses, calcification of ducts, cysts, and change in pancreatic size. ERCP can locate specific obstructions and detect ductal leaks.

Therapeutic Measures

Treatment is aimed at promoting comfort and maintaining adequate nutrition (see "Nutrition Notes: Nourishing the Patient With Pancreatitis"). Pain is managed with analgesics. Surgery may be necessary to treat biliary disease, repair fistulas, drain cysts, or repair other damage.

Nursing Process for the Patient With Pancreatitis

See the "Nursing Care Plan for the Patient With Acute and Chronic Pancreatitis."

Cancer of the Pancreas

Pancreatic cancer is the fourth leading cause of cancer deaths in the United States, killing more than 38,000 people each year. The incidence of pancreatic cancer has slowly been rising over the past 10 years. Nearly 45,000 new cases of cancer of the pancreas are diagnosed yearly (American Cancer Society, 2013); it most often affects people between ages 65 and 79.

Pathophysiology

Most primary tumors of the pancreas are ductal adenocarcinomas and occur in the exocrine (digestive secretion) parts of the pancreas. The tumors in the head and body of the pancreas tend to be large. Cancer of the pancreas spreads rapidly by direct extension to the stomach, gallbladder, and duodenum. Cancer located in the body of the pancreas usually spreads farther and more rapidly than do masses in the head. Cancer of the pancreas may spread by the lymphatic and vascular systems to distant organs and lymph nodes.

Etiology

The cause of pancreatic cancer is associated most commonly with smoking, then dietary factors (obesity, especially during early adulthood; red meat; processed meat), diabetes mellitus, chronic pancreatitis, and heredity. African American males have the highest rate of pancreatic cancer. Protection may be provided with high folate and lycopene fruits and vegetables.

Signs and Symptoms

The patient with pancreatic cancer experiences vague symptoms early in the disease. Epigastric or back pain, anorexia, nausea, fatigue, and malaise are early symptoms. Detection is often difficult because of the nonspecific symptoms identified by the patient. Weight loss is the classic sign of pancreatic cancer. The patient may report abdominal pain that is worse at night. The pain is described as gnawing or boring, and it radiates to the back. The pain may be lessened by a side-lying position with the knees drawn up to the chest or by bending over when walking. The pain becomes increasingly severe and unrelenting as the cancer grows. Pruritus is annoying. Depression may be experienced. The patient may report a bloated feeling or fullness after eating. If the cancer obstructs the bile duct, the patient may have jaundice, dark urine, pruritus, and light-colored stools. The patient's health history may include a recent diagnosis of diabetes mellitus.

Complications

Complications may occur before or after surgical treatment. Preoperative complications include malnutrition, spread of the cancer, and gastric or duodenal obstruction. Postoperative complications include infection, breakdown of the surgical site, fistula formation, diabetes mellitus, and malabsorption syndrome. If the patient has had chemotherapy or radiation therapy, complications specific to those therapies can also occur.

Thrombophlebitis is a common complication of cancer of the pancreas. As the tumor grows, by-products of the tumor growth appear to increase the levels of thromboplastic (clotting) factors in the blood, making clotting easier. The potential for thrombophlebitis increases if the patient is confined to bed or has surgery.

Diagnostic Tests

Serum alkaline phosphatase, glucose, and bilirubin levels may be elevated. Amylase and lipase are elevated if the cancer has caused a secondary pancreatitis. Blood coagulation tests, such as clotting time, are done. Carcinoembryonic antigen is ordered to confirm the presence of cancer (normal: less than 5 ng/mL).

Abdominal x-rays determine the size of the pancreas and the presence of masses. CT scan, magnetic resonance imaging (MRI), or ultrasonography are done to precisely locate masses in the pancreas. ERCP can be used to visualize the common ducts and to take tissue samples for microscopic analysis. Pancreatic biopsy is necessary for definitive diagnosis of pancreatic cancer. A tissue sample may be obtained by needle aspiration during ultrasonography. This procedure may cause seeding of the tumor along the needle pathway.

Therapeutic Measures

The prognosis for pancreatic cancer is poor. Survival time is often 4 to 6 months. If diagnosed early, treatment may be aimed at cure. If the patient's cancer has progressed to distant involvement of other organ structures and lymph

---

NURSING CARE PLAN for the Patient With Acute and Chronic Pancreatitis

Nursing Diagnosis: *Pain* related to edema and inflammation

Expected Outcome: The patient will state pain level is less than 2 on a scale of 0 to 10 within 30 minutes of pain report.

Evaluation of Outcome: Does patient state pain level is less than 2 on a pain scale of 0 to 10?

Intervention Assess the patient every 2 hours for pain by: • Asking the patient to rate pain on a scale of 0 to 10. **Rationale** Intense pain is likely to occur with acute pancreatitis. A pain scale allows for a consistent and individual evaluation of pain. **Evaluation** Does patient state that pain is tolerable and less than 2 on a pain scale of 0 to 10, where 0 = no pain and 10 = worst possible pain?

Intervention • Observing the patient for pain behaviors such as grimacing, irritability, reluctance to move, or inability to lie quietly. **Rationale** Observation of pain behaviors, such as reluctance to move, shallow respirations, grimacing, or irritability, may be a reliable indicator of pain. However, the patient in pain may have no observable pain behaviors. **Evaluation** Does patient exhibit pain behaviors that differ from his or her report of pain?

Continued

NURSING CARE PLAN for the Patient With Acute and Chronic Pancreatitis—cont'd

Intervention Administer analgesics as ordered, before pain becomes severe. **Rationale** Analgesics are most effective if given before pain becomes too great. **Evaluation** Are analgesics effective?

Intervention Assist the patient to a position of comfort, usually high Fowler's or leaning forward slightly. **Rationale** An upright position keeps abdominal organs from pressing against the inflamed pancreas. **Evaluation** Does positioning promote comfort?

Intervention Keep the environment free from excessive stimuli. **Rationale** Quiet, restful, anxiety-free atmosphere permits the patient to relax and may decrease pain perception. **Evaluation** Does patient state atmosphere is relaxing?

Intervention Teach the patient alternative pain control strategies such as guided imagery and relaxation techniques. **Rationale** Successful use of pain control strategies may decrease the amount of analgesics needed and give the patient a greater sense of control. **Evaluation** Are alternative strategies effective?

Nursing Diagnosis: *Imbalanced Nutrition: Less Than Body Requirements* related to pain, anorexia, and treatment

Expected Outcome: The patient will experience improved nutrition as evidenced by stable weight and serum albumin level greater than 3.5 g/L.

Evaluation of Outcome: Is weight stable? Is serum albumin level greater than 3.5 g/L?

Intervention Assess the patient's nutritional status by: • Weighing the patient every other day. **Rationale** A loss of 1 lb of body weight occurs when the body uses 3500 calories more than is taken in. **Evaluation** Has patient lost less than 5% of total baseline body weight?

Intervention • Monitoring serum albumin levels as ordered. **Rationale** Serum albumin of 3.5–5.5 g/L indicates normal protein metabolism in the absence of liver or renal disease. **Evaluation** Is patient's albumin level above 3.5 g/dL?

Intervention • Observing for nausea or vomiting. **Rationale** Nausea, vomiting, and pain are risk factors for inadequate intake. **Evaluation** Does nausea need to be treated to prevent vomiting? Is intake adequate?

Intervention • Monitoring blood sugar at least every 6 hr if the patient is on parenteral nutrition. **Rationale** Patients on parenteral nutrition are more likely to have high blood glucose. **Evaluation** Is blood sugar normal?

Intervention • Observing for diarrhea, bloating, or steatorrhea (fatty stools). Report steatorrhea immediately. **Rationale** Diarrhea, bloating, or fatty stools may indicate malabsorption syndrome. Steatorrhea (fatty stools) may indicate that the enzyme replacement doses are not meeting the patient's needs. **Evaluation** Are stools normal?

Intervention Administer nutritional supplements, including pancreatic enzymes, as ordered. **Rationale** Provides adequate nutrition. **Evaluation** Does patient take any supplements?

Intervention Teach the patient to avoid alcohol. **Rationale** Alcohol may trigger another episode of pancreatitis. **Evaluation** Does patient verbalize understanding of importance of avoiding alcohol? Is follow-up support for alcohol avoidance provided?

Intervention Teach the patient and family the signs and symptoms of diabetes mellitus. **Rationale** Patients with pancreatitis are at great risk for developing diabetes mellitus. **Evaluation** Does patient verbalize signs and symptoms of diabetes to report?

NURSING CARE PLAN for the Patient With Acute and Chronic Pancreatitis—cont'd

Intervention Teach the patient and family to self-monitor for symptoms of malabsorption syndrome, such as fatty stools, weight loss, dry skin, or bleeding. **Rationale** Absence of pancreatic enzymes causes problems with digestion of fats, carbohydrates, and proteins. **Evaluation** Does patient verbalize understanding of symptoms of malabsorption to report?

Nursing Diagnosis: *Risk for Ineffective Breathing Pattern* related to abdominal pressure and pain

Expected Outcome: The patient will have an effective breathing pattern as evidenced by unlabored respirations, 16 to 20 per minute, Sao_2 95% or greater at all times.

Evaluation of Outcome: Are respirations unlabored, 16–20 per minute, Sao_2 95% or greater?

Intervention Assess the patient's breathing patterns: • Observe respirations for depth, regularity, and rate. • Observe respiratory effort. • Observe for evidence of respiratory distress, such as use of accessory muscles, use of intercostal muscles, Sao_2 less than 95%, and rapid or difficult breathing. **Rationale** Abdominal pressure from inflammation and tissue damage under the diaphragm may cause the patient to take shallow, rapid respirations, which can tire the patient. **Evaluation** Are patient's respirations 16–20 per minute, unlabored, and regular? Is patient alert and oriented? Has there been a change in the level of patient's arousal? Does patient exhibit signs of distress?

Intervention Administer oxygen as ordered. **Rationale** Oxygen can decrease the amount of effort the patient must expend to breathe. **Evaluation** Does oxygen help patient breathe easier?

Intervention Place the patient in an upright or slightly forward-leaning position. **Rationale** Relieves pressure on the diaphragm. **Evaluation** Is positioning effective?

Intervention Prepare the patient's food by opening cartons and lids and cut food into bite-size portions. **Rationale** Decreases the demand for oxygen. **Evaluation** Does patient accept assistance with food preparation?

Intervention Teach the patient to move slowly and to take frequent rests. **Rationale** Helps decrease the demand for oxygen. **Evaluation** Does patient tolerate activity?

Nursing Diagnosis: *Risk for Injury* related to hemorrhage or fluid and electrolyte imbalances

Expected Outcome: The patient will experience no injury during illness.

Evaluation of Outcome: Is there evidence of injury? Are signs and symptoms of impending injury recognized and reported early?

Intervention Monitor sodium, potassium, calcium, and magnesium levels daily. **Rationale** Electrolyte levels can become imbalanced in pancreatitis. **Evaluation** Do laboratory studies show that patient's electrolytes are within acceptable ranges?

Intervention Evaluate neuromuscular status by checking Chvostek's/Trousseau's signs. **Rationale** These are signs of calcium depletion (see Chapter 6). **Evaluation** Are signs of calcium depletion present?

Intervention Monitor the patient's hematocrit, hemoglobin, and blood clotting times frequently. **Rationale** Destruction of the pancreas can result in hemorrhage. **Evaluation** Does patient have any abnormal bruising, bleeding gums, or pink urine?

Intervention Observe abdomen and flanks for Cullen's and Turner's signs. **Rationale** These are signs of hemorrhage. **Evaluation** Are signs of hemorrhage present?

Continued

NURSING CARE PLAN for the Patient With Acute and Chronic Pancreatitis—cont'd

Intervention Weigh the patient daily. **Rationale** To monitor fluid balance. **Evaluation** Is weight stable?

Intervention Measure and record intake and output every shift. **Rationale** To monitor fluid balance. **Evaluation** Is urinary output greater than 30 mL/hr?

Intervention Observe for nausea and vomiting. **Rationale** Vomiting can contribute to fluid loss. **Evaluation** Does nausea need to be treated to prevent vomiting?

Intervention Report any drop in blood pressure greater than 5% of the patient's baseline. **Rationale** May indicate severe fluid loss. **Evaluation** Are vital signs stable? Is patient's blood pressure within 5% of baseline?

Intervention Teach the patient to report any weakness or muscle twitching. **Rationale** May indicate electrolyte imbalance. **Evaluation** Does patient verbalize understanding of signs and symptoms of electrolyte imbalance to report?

nodes, treatment is directed at easing symptoms and making the patient more comfortable.

Surgery is the primary treatment. A total pancreatectomy is one option. For tumors in the body and tail of the pancreas, a distal **pancreatectomy** is done. When the tumor is located at the head of the pancreas, the Whipple procedure is done to remove the head of the pancreas, the lower portion of the common bile duct, most of the duodenum, and possibly parts of the stomach nearby (Fig. 35.6). Potential postoperative problems after the Whipple procedure include failure of the suture lines to hold, causing leakage of pancreatic enzymes and bile into the abdomen; pneumonia or atelectasis from shallow breathing because the incision line is directly under the diaphragm;

paralytic ileus; gastric retention or ulceration; wound infection; fistula formation; unstable diabetes mellitus; and renal failure.

Relief of biliary obstruction can sometimes be accomplished by implanting a stent or plastic tube in the common bile duct during an endoscopic procedure. Pain can be reduced by surgical removal of a portion of the greater splanchnic nerve.

Chemotherapy and or radiation therapy can be used to shrink or destroy the tumor, treat or prevent metastasis, or provide relief of symptoms if the cancer has become too widespread for surgery. (See Chapter 11 for care of the patient undergoing radiation or chemotherapy.)

Nursing Process for the Patient With Pancreatic Cancer

DATA COLLECTION. Observe the patient with cancer of the pancreas for evidence of malnutrition and fluid imbalance, including weight loss, inelastic skin turgor, vomiting, fatty stools, and reports of anorexia or nausea. Review laboratory tests, especially blood glucose, liver function studies, and clotting studies. Evaluate the patient every 2 to 4 hours for pain. Observe the skin for bruising, scaling, and yellowing, and question the patient about itching. Evaluate the patient's mental status for evidence of depression.

NURSING DIAGNOSES, PLANNING, AND IMPLEMENTATION. The patient with cancer of the pancreas will have numerous problems. Interventions for *Imbalanced Nutrition: Less Than Body Requirements* related to inability to digest food, anorexia, nausea, and vomiting, and *Pain* related to pancreatic tumor or surgical incision are the same as for patients with pancreatitis and are found in the "Nursing Care Plan for the Patient With Acute and Chronic Pancreatitis." Other care is listed next. Additional interventions for patients with cancer, including psychosocial interventions, can be found in Chapter 11.

FIGURE 35.6 Pancreatoduodenectomy (Whipple procedure) for cancer of the head of the pancreas.

• **WORD** • **BUILDING** •
pancreatectomy: pancreat—pancreas + ectomy—excision

Risk for Deficient Fluid Volume

EXPECTED OUTCOME: The patient will have adequate fluid volume as evidenced by stable vital signs, elastic skin turgor, and moist mucous membranes.

- Monitor the patient's intake and output carefully. *Low intake increases risk of deficient fluid volume; low output is a sign of deficient fluid.*
- Monitor vital signs. *Tachycardia, tachypnea, and low blood pressure may indicate excessive fluid loss.*
- Monitor laboratory values, especially serum sodium, potassium, calcium, and chloride levels. Report abnormal values. *If electrolyte values are low, the physician may order IV replacement solutions.*
- Report low serum albumin level (normal is 3.4–4.8 g/dL) and assist with monitoring IV albumin therapy if ordered. *Low albumin places the patient at risk for fluid imbalances.*
- Carefully observe the patient for signs of blood loss *that may indicate abnormal bleeding:*
  - Bruising, bleeding gums, or pink-tinged urine
  - Cullen's sign (bluish discolorations around the umbilicus)
  - Turner's sign (bluish discolorations on the flanks)
  - Bleeding at incision and drain sites and in drainage tubing
- Teach the patient to use a soft-bristle toothbrush and electric razor rather than a straight razor *to reduce risk of injury and bleeding.*
- Administer vitamin K as ordered *to replace deficiency and to reduce risk for bleeding.*

Risk for Impaired Tissue Integrity related to itching and to leaking around drainage tubes

EXPECTED OUTCOME: The patient's skin will remain intact.

- Monitor the patient for reports of itching *because scratching can cause a break in the skin.*
- Help the patient keep fingernails short *to reduce damage to skin with scratching.*
- Provide frequent skin care with products free of soap or alcohol *to prevent further dryness and itching.*
- Protect skin around drains with skin-protective barrier products and ostomy bags *to prevent skin damage.*
- Apply products such as calamine lotion as ordered *to decrease itching.*
- Exercise special care of any drains *to prevent unnecessary tension that may cause sutures to give way.*
- Keep all drains patent, and keep drainage tubing and bags free from kinks *to prevent fluid leakage onto the skin.*
- Place the patient in semi-Fowler's position *to help with gravity drainage and reduce risk of fluid leakage.*

EVALUATION. The plan of care for the patient with pancreatic cancer is successful if the patient maintains body weight within 5% of normal body weight and experiences no nausea or vomiting; states that pain remains tolerable at 2 or less on a pain scale of 0 to 10; has urinary output greater than 30 mL/hr,

elastic skin turgor, moist mucous membranes, pulse and blood pressure within 10% of patient's baseline, no sudden, excessive abdominal pain or rigidity, and incisions heal at the expected rate; demonstrates the appropriate self-care procedures for tubes, drains, dressings, and medication administration; and states the signs and symptoms of complications that are to be reported immediately.

PATIENT EDUCATION. Teach the patient and family self-care measures such as blood glucose monitoring, insulin administration, signs and symptoms of hyperglycemia and hypoglycemia (see Chapter 40), and the regimen for pancreatic enzyme replacement. Instruct the patient on how to manage dressing changes if he or she is to be discharged with tubes or drains. Patient and family should know the signs and symptoms of hemorrhage, gastric ulceration, infection, and fistula formation. A patient being cared for at home should have a referral for hospice care or home nursing care.

For more information, visit the National Pancreas Foundation at www.pancreasfoundation.org.

▮ DISORDERS OF THE GALLBLADDER

Cholecystitis, Cholelithiasis, and Choledocholithiasis

Gallstones and inflammations of the gallbladder and common bile duct are the most common disorders of the biliary system.

Pathophysiology

Cholecystitis is an acute or chronic inflammation of the gallbladder. It is most often a response to obstruction of the common bile duct resulting in edema and inflammation. Bacteria can invade stagnant bile and add to the inflammation and irritation of the gallbladder. Chronic cholecystitis may be the result of repeated attacks of acute cholecystitis or chronic irritation from gallstones. The gallbladder then becomes fibrotic and thickened and does not empty easily or completely. This is a risk factor for gallbladder cancer.

Cholelithiasis is the formation of gallstones in the gallbladder that are most often composed of cholesterol in the United States. They can be asymptomatic for decades. **Choledocholithiasis** refers to gallstones within the common bile duct. Gallstones form when bile becomes supersaturated with a substance such as cholesterol, which then crystallizes, forming sludge with continued enlargement to form stones. Another type of gallstone is a pigment stone. Pigment stones are composed of calcium bilirubinate, which occurs when free bilirubin combines with calcium.

• WORD • BUILDING •

cholecystitis: chole—bile + cyst—bladder + itis—inflammation
cholelithiasis: chole—bile + lith—stone + iasis—condition
choledocholithiasis: chole—bile + docho—duct + lith—stone + iasis—condition

Etiology and Incidence

CHOLELITHIASIS. Gallstones occur most in women, from aging, obesity, pregnancy, stasis of bile, fasting, medications, and heredity. Stasis may be caused by a decreased gallbladder-emptying rate, a partial obstruction in the common duct, or pregnancy. Excessive cholesterol intake combined with a sedentary lifestyle is linked to an increased incidence of cholelithiasis, as are hemolytic blood disorders such as sickle cell disease and bowel disorders such as Crohn's disease. After age 50, the rate of gallstones is about the same for men and women ("Cultural Considerations").

CHOLECYSTITIS. Cholelithiasis is responsible for most cases of cholecystitis, or inflammation of the gallbladder.

Signs and Symptoms

Signs and symptoms of cholecystitis and cholelithiasis are similar. Subjective symptoms include epigastric pain, RUQ tenderness, nausea, and indigestion, especially after eating foods high in fat. Objective symptoms include evidence of inflammation, such as an elevated temperature, pulse, and respirations; vomiting; and jaundice. The patient may have a positive Murphy's sign, which is the inability to take a deep breath when an examiner's fingers are pressed below the liver margin. Family history of either cholecystitis or cholelithiasis, dietary habits such as high fat intake or a recent low-fat diet, and reports of flatulence (gas), eructation (belching), nausea, vomiting, or abdominal discomfort after a high-fat meal are common evidence of a gallbladder disorder.

CHOLELITHIASIS. The epigastric pain caused by cholelithiasis may also be called biliary **colic**. The pain is a steady, aching, severe pain in the epigastrium and RUQ that may radiate back to behind the right scapula or to the right shoulder. The pain usually begins suddenly after a fatty meal and lasts for 1 to 3 hours. If the pain is caused by a stone in the common bile duct (choledocholithiasis), the pain may last until the stone has passed into the duodenum. Jaundice is more commonly present with acute choledocholithiasis because the common bile duct is blocked or inflamed.

CHOLECYSTITIS. The biliary colic caused by cholecystitis typically lasts 4 to 6 hours. The pain is made worse with movement such as breathing. The patient usually has nausea, vomiting, and a low-grade fever with the pain. Heartburn, indigestion, and flatulence are more common with chronic cholecystitis. Patients often report repeated attacks of acute cholecystitis symptoms (Table 35.6).

CRITICAL THINKING

Donna Stewart

■ Donna Stewart, a 23-year-old woman, is diagnosed with possible acute cholecystitis. She is 5 feet, 6 inches tall and weighs 138 pounds. She is 4 months pregnant. Her HCP wishes to delay surgery until her inflammation has subsided.

1. What risk factors does Donna have for cholecystitis?
2. What diagnostic tests might be ordered to confirm Donna's diagnosis of cholecystitis?
3. What considerations should be weighed when scheduling diagnostic tests?
4. What medications can you anticipate that the physician will order for Donna?
5. What type of diet will Donna need to eat after discharge?
6. If the diagnosis of cholecystitis is confirmed, what type of surgical treatment might be ordered?

Suggested answers are at the end of the chapter.

Complications

Complications of cholecystitis include cholangitis (inflammation of the bile ducts), necrosis or perforation of the gallbladder, empyema (a collection of purulent drainage in the gallbladder), fistulas, and adenocarcinoma of the gallbladder. A major complication of choledocholithiasis is acute pancreatitis if the pancreatic duct is obstructed.

Diagnostic Tests

An ultrasound of the gallbladder is the classic test done to detect stones, inflamed walls of the gallbladder, and dilated

• WORD • BUILDING •
colic: colic—spasm

Cultural Considerations

Gallbladder disease is more common among Mexican Americans. Risk factors include working in occupations such as mining, factories using chemicals, and farming with pesticides. The disease has a lower incidence in blacks in Africa and in blacks living in the Western world. Native Americans have an increased incidence of pancreatic and gallbladder disease. It is unknown how much increased dietary risk factors may contribute to gallbladder disease. The nurse can positively affect the nutritional status of at-risk patients by teaching food preparation practices that use less fat.

TABLE 35.6 SYMPTOMS OF GALLBLADDER DISORDERS

	Acute Cholecystitis	Chronic Cholecystitis	Cholelithiasis and Choledocholithiasis
Biliary colic	Lasts 4–6 hr Worse with movement	Only during acute attack	Sudden onset
Jaundice	Present (if common bile duct is inflamed or blocked)	Present	Lasts 1–3 hr Radiates to right scapula or shoulder
Low-grade fever	Present	Present	Present
Nausea, vomiting	Present	Only during acute attack	Present
Repeated attacks		Present	
Heartburn, indigestion, and flatulence		Present	
Complications	Cholangitis Necrosis or perforation Fistulas	Empyema Fistulas Adenocarcinoma	Acute pancreatitis

ducts. An ERCP can be done to directly visualize the pancreatic ducts and bile ducts to determine the presence of stones in the common duct and allows the ability to remove stones from the common duct. Further examination may include a radionuclide scan, such as a hepatobiliary iminodiacetic acid scan. For this procedure, the patient will be given an IV injection of a radioactive isotope that is metabolized by the liver and excreted in the bile. The scanning camera then traces the path of the isotope as it travels through the bile ducts, gallbladder, and intestines to identify blockages.

The patient may have an elevated WBC count (normal: 5000–10,000 cells/mm^3). If direct bilirubin is elevated (normal: 0.3–1.2 mg/dL), its cause is likely obstruction in the biliary or liver areas. Liver enzymes can rise from hepatic inflammation. Serum amylase and lipase may be elevated if the pancreas is involved or if there is a stone in the common duct.

Therapeutic Measures

Treatment of an acute episode of cholecystitis centers on pain control, prevention of infection, and maintenance of fluid and electrolyte balance. Pain control is achieved with analgesics. For itching relief if the patient is jaundiced from bile acid deposits in the skin, colestipol (Colestid) or cholestyramine (Questran, LoCholest) is given. These drugs bind with the circulating bile acids for excretion in the stool. If the patient has nausea and vomiting, an antiemetic may be ordered (see Table 35.4). See "Nutrition Notes."

SURGERY. Treatment for cholelithiasis typically involves cholecystectomy (surgical removal of gallbladder) via

 Nutrition Notes

Modifying the Diet for Patients With Gallbladder Disease

During an acute attack of cholecystitis, a full liquid diet with minimal fat is usually allowed. For treatment of chronic cholecystitis, the patient is instructed to do the following:
- Correct obesity.
- Avoid troublesome and gas-forming foods (fried foods are worst offenders).
- Decrease dietary fat by (1) selecting skim-milk dairy products, (2) limiting fats or oils to 3 teaspoons, and (3) consuming no more than 6 ounces of very lean meat.

Cholelithiasis has been associated with a long overnight fast that permits concentrated bile to remain in the gallbladder for an extended period. Eating a light bedtime snack or drinking two glasses of water on arising if breakfast is delayed alter this risk factor.

After traditional cholecystectomy, the patient may initially receive nothing by mouth or clear liquids. Then the diet is progressed as tolerated. Following laparoscopic cholecystectomy, patients may receive a general diet immediately.

Later in convalescence, balanced meals should be well tolerated because bile enters the duodenum continuously. Patients who became nauseated and suffered pain after eating certain foods preoperatively, however, may continue to avoid them postoperatively because of the association.

laparoscopy. A laparoscopic cholecystectomy is done with a laparoscope through four small puncture wounds in the abdomen. Patients are usually discharged in 24 hours or less, and recovery time is reduced with laparoscopic surgery.

For large stones or an infected gallbladder, a traditional open cholecystectomy may be required. A **T-tube** may be inserted into the common duct to ensure that bile drainage is not obstructed (Fig. 35.7). T-tube drainage ranges from 500 to 1000 mL the first day and decreases to 200 mL by the third day. The patient with a traditional cholecystectomy has incisional pain that creates difficulty with coughing and deep breathing postoperatively because deep breathing causes the diaphragm to press on the operative site. Patients are hospitalized for 2 to 3 days with a traditional cholecystectomy.

EXTRACORPOREAL SHOCK-WAVE LITHOTRIPSY (ESWL). **Extracorporeal shock-wave lithotripsy** is done less frequently now due to the availability of laparoscopic cholecystectomy. It uses shock waves to destroy stones in the gallbladder or biliary ducts. Patients who have few cholesterol stones that are not calcified are the most likely candidates for ESWL. After ESWL, the patient is usually put on a course of oral dissolution drugs to ensure complete removal of all stones and stone fragments.

MEDICATION.   Dissolution of small noncalcified stones (less than 2 centimeters) with the bile acid drugs ursodiol (Actigall) is used for those who are not surgical candidates. Treatment with the dissolution drugs may take months and stones may return.

Nursing Process of the Patient With a Gallbladder Disorder

DATA COLLECTION.   Monitor the patient frequently for pain, using the **WHAT'S UP?** questions. Take the patient's vital signs, particularly the temperature and pulse, frequently to monitor for signs of infection. Weigh the patient and inspect mucous membranes, skin turgor, and urinary output for signs of dehydration. Measure intake and output, including any emesis or drainage from NG tubes or T-tubes.

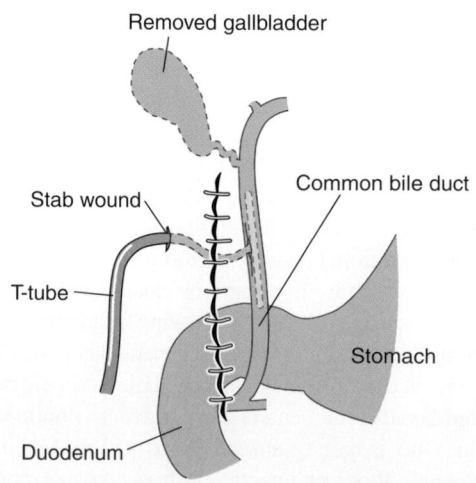

FIGURE 35.7 T-tube. A T-tube is used to drain bile after a cholecystectomy until swelling of the duct subsides.

Observe stools and urine for color and consistency. Obstruction of bile flow may result in stools that are clay colored or have a foul, greasy appearance or urine that is dark amber or tea colored. Report either new finding immediately. Evaluate laboratory studies for elevation in the WBC count or abnormalities in electrolytes or serum bilirubin levels.

NURSING DIAGNOSES, PLANNING, AND IMPLEMENTATION. Common nursing diagnoses for the patient with cholecystitis include pain and risk for deficient fluid volume. Additional nursing diagnoses for the patient with cholelithiasis who has a surgical procedure include risk for impaired skin integrity related to surgical incision and T-tube drainage and risk for ineffective breathing pattern related to abdominal incision.

Acute Pain related to biliary colic
EXPECTED OUTCOME: The patient will rate pain as 2 or less on a 10-point scale.

- Assess the patient frequently for pain *to guide treatment.*
- Administer analgesics as ordered *to reduce pain.*
- Administer antispasmodics or anticholinergics as ordered *for biliary colic.*
- Assist patient with positioning *to assume whatever position provides the most comfort.*

Risk for Deficient Fluid Volume related to anorexia, nausea, vomiting, or excessive tube drainage
EXPECTED OUTCOME: The patient will have adequate fluid volume as evidenced by stable vital signs, elastic skin turgor, and moist mucous membranes at all times.

- Monitor intake and output, daily weights, and skin turgor *to monitor fluid balance.*
- Monitor T-tube drainage. Carefully observe the T-tube drainage unit to prevent kinking of the tubing. *Pressure in the biliary drainage system from poor drainage may greatly increase the patient's pain and the risk for infection.*
- Give antiemetics as needed *to control nausea and vomiting.*
- Assist with administration of IV fluids and electrolytes as ordered while the patient is on restricted oral intake *to maintain hydration.*

Risk for Impaired Skin Integrity related to surgical incision and T-tube drainage
EXPECTED OUTCOME: The patient's skin will remain intact at all times.

- Inspect the patient's skin and the sclerae of the eyes for jaundice, and report jaundice or pruritus, *to provide treatment to reduce itching injury to skin.*
- Inspect the cholecystectomy incision for excessive drainage or evidence of infection such as redness, edema, or warmth, *which can irritate and break down skin.*

• WORD • BUILDING •
laparoscopy: laparo—pertaining to flank + scopy—to examine
extracorporeal shock-wave lithotripsy: extra—outside + tripsy—rub or crush

- Change dressings frequently *to protect the skin around the incision site from irritating drainage.*
- Protect the skin with a skin barrier product or bag such as those used with colostomies if bile is leaking around the T-tube site. An ostomy care nurse (if available) can be consulted for the best choice of dressing. *A skin barrier can protect skin from breakdown due to contact with bile.*

Risk for Ineffective Breathing Pattern related to abdominal incision

EXPECTED OUTCOME: The patient will have effective breathing pattern as evidenced by a respiratory rate of 16 to 20 per minute, even, unlabored, depth within normal limits at all times.

- Monitor respiratory rate, depth, and effort, and ability to cough effectively. *The high abdominal incision can cause pain with deep breathing and coughing.*
- After surgery, encourage the patient to cough and deep breathe at every encounter. Instruct the patient in the proper techniques before surgery and give the opportunity to practice. *Deep breathing and coughing after any surgical procedure helps prevent atelectasis and respiratory tract infections.*

- If the patient is reluctant to cough because of pain, evaluate the pain medication regimen *so that pain is controlled.*
- Assist the patient with splinting when coughing *to make coughing less painful.*
- Encourage the patient to walk as soon as able *to help mobilize secretions.*

EVALUATION. The plan of care for a patient with cholecystitis or cholelithiasis is successful if the patient reports tolerable pain not greater than 2 on a pain scale of 0 to 10, no weight loss, excessive thirst, urinary output greater than 50 mL/hour; has moist mucous membranes, elastic skin turgor, intact skin with no warmth, redness, swelling, or purulent drainage at the wound site; no jaundice or itching; clear breath sounds; and a normal white blood cell count (Table 35.7).

PATIENT EDUCATION. Discharge education focuses on diet. Patients are put on high-protein, low-fat diets. Encourage obese patients to lose weight. After a cholecystectomy, fat should be slowly reintroduced into the diet. Once the duodenum becomes accustomed to a constant infusion of bile, the patient's individual tolerance for fat becomes the only restriction for diet.

TABLE 35.7   CHOLECYSTITIS SUMMARY

Signs and Symptoms	Epigastric/RUQ pain, especially after a fatty meal Elevated temperature, pulse, respirations Jaundice if common bile duct blocked
Diagnostic Tests	Ultrasound ERCP Radionuclide scan (hepatobiliary iminodiacetic acid scan [HIDA]) WBC count elevated
Therapeutic Measures	Pain control Laparoscopic or open cholecystectomy Extracorporeal shock-wave lithotripsy Medications (see Table 35.4) Low-fat diet
Priority Nursing Diagnoses	*Pain* *Risk for Deficient Fluid Volume* *Risk for Ineffective Breathing Pattern* *Risk for Impaired Skin Integrity*

Note. RUQ = right upper quadrant; WBC = white blood cell.

SUGGESTED ANSWERS TO

CRITICAL THINKING

■ *Carl Young*

1. Foreign travel within the past 2 months, eating raw oysters, fatigue, nausea, and irritability suggest hepatitis A virus infection. Recent possible exposure to materials contaminated with blood or body fluids and fatigue, headache, and nausea suggest hepatitis B virus infection.

2. Careful hand hygiene and standard precautions when handling any body fluids or feces should be instituted.

3. Infectious disease HCP, dietician for nutritional needs, social worker for financial information during recovery period.

4. The nurse should plan to give an antiemetic if Carl is nauseated. Larger meals should be given early in the day, with Carl in an upright or sitting position. The nurse should also ensure that the environment is free of noxious stimulants such as unpleasant odors. The diet should be high calorie, high protein, high carbohydrate, and low fat.

5. Any medication that is known to be hepatotoxic, such as acetaminophen, aspirin, and diazepam (Valium), should be avoided.

6. Carl should be taught that cleanliness, especially with food preparation, is essential; that he should avoid eating raw oysters or raw or undercooked shellfish; that frequent hand washing is crucial; and that alcohol and other liver-toxic substances should be avoided.

■ *Mrs. Conner*

1. Mrs. Conner has a history of poor nutrition that puts her at risk, as does her age.

2. Mrs. Conner may report that she has malaise, nausea, weight loss, a change in bowel habits, and dull, aching RUQ pain.

3. Serum albumin level may be less than 3.2 g/dL. Her prothrombin time will probably be greater than 25 seconds.

4. Esophageal varices and ascites are the two greatest concerns for the patient with portal hypertension.

5. The physician will usually order diuretics, a sodium-restricted diet, and possibly IV albumin infusions.

■ *Mrs. Samuels*

1. The most common cause of acute pancreatitis is heavy alcohol intake. Mrs. Samuels reports no alcohol consumption, but she does have the risk factor of having had a recent ERCP, which may have dislodged a gallstone or irritated the pancreatic duct.

2. Respiratory distress may result from excess fluid accumulation in the retroperitoneal space and from shallow respirations that seek to decrease pressure from the diaphragm on the inflamed pancreas and surrounding tissues.

3. Pancreatitis is similar to a chemical burn and may cause erosion of major blood vessels in surrounding tissue.

4. Serum amylase rises quickly and then returns to normal in 3 to 5 days. Serum lipase is thought to be more specific for acute pancreatitis and elevates and stays elevated for a longer period of time.

5. Opioids are ordered because pain is intense, and pain with anxiety stimulates the autonomic nervous system, which may stimulate greater production of pancreatic enzymes.

6. Stomach acid stimulates the production of pancreatic enzymes. Histamine antagonists decrease stomach acidity.

7. Enteral nutrition until symptoms (pain) are resolved, then oral nutrition.

■ *Donna Stewart*

1. Some low-fat diets have been linked to the development of cholesterol gallstones, which then irritate the gallbladder and cause inflammation.

2. Donna's physician might order a white blood cell count, which will be elevated if she has cholecystitis. In addition, the physician may order an ultrasound or radionuclide scan to visualize the gallbladder and its contents and the common bile duct.

3. Donna is 4 months pregnant. Radionuclide scans should be cleared with her obstetrical care provider before being scheduled.

4. You can anticipate that the HCP will order an antibiotic and an analgesic.

5. Donna will need to eat a low-fat diet after discharge. Eventually she may be able to add more fats to her diet as her body adjusts.

6. If the diagnosis is confirmed, Donna will probably have a laparoscopic cholecystectomy unless her HCP decides that she needs a traditional cholecystectomy.

REVIEW QUESTIONS

1. The nurse is planning care for a patient with cirrhosis. For which condition would the nurse place the patient on bleeding precautions?
   1. Encephalopathy
   2. Low vitamin K
   3. Elevated liver enzymes
   4. Hepatorenal syndrome

2. The nurse is caring for a patient with cirrhosis. The nurse would cautiously use sedatives for the patient due to which of the following?
   1. The liver's ability to synthesize protein is altered.
   2. Sedatives may increase the risk of jaundice.
   3. Sedatives are potentially toxic to the cirrhosis patient.
   4. Sedatives promote the conversion of ammonia to ammonium ion.

3. The nurse is collecting data for a patient with suspected acute hepatitis A infection. Which clinical manifestations would the nurse expect the patient to report?
   1. Brown urine and anorexia
   2. Malaise, lighter colored stools, and pruritus
   3. Headache, nausea, and flulike symptoms
   4. Abdominal pain and jaundice

4. The nurse is caring for a patient with chronic pancreatitis. While reviewing laboratory data to contribute to the plan of care, the nurse would expect an elevation in which laboratory value?
   1. Serum bilirubin
   2. Serum calcium
   3. Serum albumin
   4. Serum amylase

5. A patient with acute pancreatitis is started on early aggressive IV hydration. Which laboratory result indicates the need to consult the dietitian for initial nutritional support?
   1. Potassium 4.2 mEq/L
   2. Sodium 130 mEq/L
   3. Fasting glucose 82 mg/dL
   4. Serum albumin 2.9 g/dL

6. The nurse is planning care for a newly admitted patient with acute pancreatitis. Which patient outcome should receive the *highest* priority in the plan of care?
   1. Patient expresses satisfaction with pain control.
   2. Patient verbalizes understanding of medications at discharge.
   3. Patient increases activity tolerance.
   4. Patient maintains normal bowel function.

7. The nurse is collecting data for a patient who develops jaundice and dark, amber-colored urine. The nurse recognizes that which of the following is most likely the cause of these manifestations?
   1. Encephalopathy
   2. Pancreatitis
   3. Bile duct obstruction
   4. Cholecystitis

8. The nurse reinforces teaching for a patient after a cholecystectomy who is on a low-fat diet. The nurse will know that the patient understands the diet if which menu items are selected?
   1. Roast chicken, rice, gelatin dessert
   2. Cream of chicken soup, milk, gelatin dessert
   3. Meat loaf, mashed potatoes with small amount of gravy, green beans
   4. Turkey and cheese sandwich on whole-grain bread, apple, milk

9. The nurse is caring for a patient who had an open cholecystectomy 24 hours ago. Which actions should the nurse take to assist the patient to maintain an effective breathing pattern? **Select all that apply.**
   1. Place in a supine position.
   2. Provide analgesics for pain relief.
   3. Encourage coughing and deep breathing.
   4. Monitor bowel sounds.
   5. Assist with splinting during coughing.
   6. Maintain bed rest for 48 hours after surgery.

10. The nurse is to administer promethazine 12.5 mg intramuscularly and has 50 mg/mL on hand. How many milliliters should be drawn up? **Fill in the blank.**
    Answer: _____ mL

Answers can be found in Appendix C.

References

Ambühl, P. M. (2011). Protein intake in renal and hepatic disease. *International Journal of Vitamin and Nutrition Research, 81,* 162–172.

American Cancer Society. (2013). *Estimated new cancer cases and deaths by sex, United States, 2013.* Retrieved June 28, 2013 from www.cancer.org/acs/groups/content /@epidemiologysurveilance/documents/document /acspc-031941.pdf

American Cancer Society. (2013). *Estimated new cancer cases and deaths by sex, United States, 2013.* Retrieved June 28, 2013 from www.cancer.org/cancer/pancreaticcancer /detailedguide/pancreatic-cancer-key-statistic

Bémeur, C., Desjardins, P., & Butterworth, R. F. (2010, December 22). Role of nutrition in the management of hepatic encephalopathy in end-stage liver failure. *Journal of Nutrition and Metabolism,* 489823. Retrieved May 12, 2013, from www.ncbi.nlm.nih.gov /pmc/articles/PMC3017957

Centers for Disease Control and Prevention. (2013). *Viral hepatitis.* Retrieved June 28, 2013, from www.cdc.gov /hepatitis/Statistics/index.htm

Murphy, S. L., Xu, J., & Kochanek, K. D. (2013). Deaths: Final data for 2010. *National Vital Statistics Reports, 57*(14). Hyattsville, MD: National Center for Health Statistics. Retrieved June 28, 2013, from www.cdc.gov/nchs/data/nvsr /nvsr61/nvsr61_04.pdf

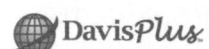 Davis*Plus* | For additional resources and information visit **davispl.us/medsurg5**

Understanding the Urinary System

36

Urinary System Function, Assessment, and Therapeutic Measures

MAUREEN McDONALD
AND JANICE L. BRADFORD

KEY TERMS

cystoscopy (sist-TAW-skuh-pee)
dysuria (diss-YOO-ree-ah)
hematuria (HEE-muh-TOOR-ee-ah)
incontinence (inn-CON-tin-ense)
nephrotoxic (NEF-row-TOCKS-sick)
nocturia (knock-TOO-ree-ah)
percutaneous (PURR-kyoo-TAY-nee-us)
pyelogram (PIE-eh-loh-gram)
uremia (yoo-REE-mee-ah)

LEARNING OUTCOMES

1. Identify the normal anatomy of the urinary system.
2. Describe the normal function of the urinary system.
3. Discuss the effects of aging on the urinary system.
4. List data to collect when caring for a patient with a disorder of the urinary system.
5. Plan preparation and postprocedure care for patients undergoing diagnostic tests of the urinary system.
6. Plan nursing care for patients with incontinence.
7. Discuss nursing actions to decrease the risk of infection in urinary catheterized patients.

NORMAL URINARY SYSTEM ANATOMY AND PHYSIOLOGY

The urinary system consists of two kidneys and two ureters, the urinary bladder, and the urethra. The kidneys form urine, and the rest of the system eliminates urine. The purpose of urine formation is the removal of potentially toxic waste products from the blood; however, the kidneys have other equally important functions as well:

- Regulation of blood pressure, volume, and composition by the excretion or conservation of water
- Regulation of the electrolyte balance of the blood by the excretion or conservation of minerals
- Regulation of the acid–base balance of the blood by the excretion or conservation of ions such as hydrogen or bicarbonate
- Regulation of all of the above in tissue fluid
- Production of erythropoietin, which then stimulates erythrocyte production in the bone marrow
- Activation of vitamin D, which maintains bone health

The process of urine formation thus helps maintain the normal composition, volume, and pH of blood and tissue fluid.

Kidneys

The bilateral kidneys are located against the posterior wall of the abdominal cavity and are retroperitoneal. The superior portions of both kidneys rest on the inferior surface of the diaphragm and are protected by the lower rib cage. The kidneys are cushioned by surrounding adipose tissue, which is in turn covered by a fibrous connective membrane called the renal fascia. On the medial surface of each kidney is an indentation called the hilus, where the renal artery enters and the renal vein and ureter emerge. The ureter carries urine from the kidney to the urinary bladder.

Internal Structure of the Kidney

A frontal section of the kidney shows three distinct areas: the cortex, medulla, and pelvis (Fig. 36.1).

Blood Vessels of the Kidney

The pathway of blood flow through the kidney is an essential part of the process of urine formation. Blood enters the kidney from the renal artery and exits through the renal vein. Extensive branching within the kidney eventually leads arterial blood to each afferent arteriole. This vessel begins the microcirculation at the nephron, the functional unit of the kidney. The exchanges that take place in the capillaries of the nephrons form urine from blood plasma.

Nephron

Urine is formed in the approximately 1 million nephrons per kidney. The two major parts of a nephron are the renal corpuscle with glomerulus, and the renal tubule with peritubular

The **renal cortex** forms the outer region of the kidney.

The **renal medulla** forms the inner region.

Extensions from the renal cortex, called **renal columns**, divide the interior region into cone-shaped sections.

The cone-shaped sections are called **renal pyramids**. Consisting of tubules for transporting urine away from the cortex, the base of each pyramid faces outward toward the cortex. The point of the pyramid, called the **renal papilla**, faces the hilum.

The renal papilla extends into a cup called a **minor calyx**. The calyx collects urine leaving the papilla.

Two or three minor calyces join together to form a **major calyx**.

The major calyces converge to form the **renal pelvis**, which receives urine from the major calyces. The renal pelvis continues as the **ureter**, a tube-like structure that channels urine to the urinary bladder.

Fibrous capsule

Hilum

Renal papilla

Ureter

FIGURE 36.1 Interior of the kidney. From Thompson, G. S. (2013). *Understanding anatomy and physiology*. Philadelphia: F.A. Davis, p. 348.

capillaries (Fig. 36.2). These are the two sites of exchange between blood plasma and urinary filtrate within the nephron. All parts of the renal tubule are surrounded by the peritubular capillaries, which arise from the efferent arteriole and receive the materials reabsorbed by the renal tubules.

Formation of Urine

The formation of urine involves three major processes: glomerular filtration, tubular reabsorption, and tubular secretion.

Glomerular Filtration

In glomerular filtration, blood pressure forces water and small solutes out of the glomeruli and into Bowman's capsules. This fluid is then called renal filtrate (Fig. 36.3).

Tubular Reabsorption and Secretion

Exiting the glomerular capsule, renal filtrate then enters the renal tubules. Tubular reabsorption is the recovery of useful materials from the renal filtrate and their return to the blood in the peritubular capillaries (Table 36.1). In tubular secretion, substances are actively secreted from the blood in the peritubular capillaries into the filtrate in the renal tubules.

The Kidneys and Acid–Base Balance

Other than exhalation of carbon dioxide by the respiratory system, the kidneys are the organs most responsible for maintaining the normal pH range of blood and tissue fluid. They compensate for the pH changes that are part of normal body metabolism or the result of disease. In acidosis, the kidneys secrete more hydrogen ions into the renal filtrate and return more bicarbonate ions back to the blood. When body fluids become too alkaline, the kidneys return hydrogen ions to the blood and excrete bicarbonate ions in urine.

Elimination of Urine

The ureters, urinary bladder, and urethra do not change the composition or volume of urine but are responsible for its elimination.

1 In the cortex, a series of **afferent arterioles** arise from the smaller arteries. Each afferent arteriole supplies blood to one nephron.

2 Each afferent arteriole branches into a cluster of capillaries called a **glomerulus**. The glomerulus is enclosed by Bowman's capsule, which will be discussed later in this chapter.

3 Blood leaves the glomerulus through an **efferent arteriole**.

4 The efferent arteriole leads to a network of capillaries around the renal tubules called **peritubular capillaries**. These capillaries pick up water and solutes reabsorbed by the renal tubules.

5 Blood flows from the peritubular capillaries into larger and larger veins that eventually feed into the renal vein.

Nephron
Proximal convoluted tubule
Distal convoluted tubule
Cortex
Collecting duct
Medulla
Loop of Henle

FIGURE 36.2 Nephron. From Thompson, G. S. (2013). *Understanding anatomy and physiology.* Philadelphia: F.A. Davis, p. 349.

1 Blood flows into the glomerulus through the afferent arteriole, which is much larger than the efferent arteriole. Consequently, blood flows in faster than it can leave, which contributes to higher pressure within the glomerular capillaries.

2 The walls of glomerular capillaries are dotted with pores, allowing water and small solutes (such as electrolytes, glucose, amino acids, vitamins, and nitrogenous wastes) to filter out of the blood and into Bowman's capsule. Blood cells and most plasma proteins, however, are too large to pass through the pores.

3 The fluid that has filtered into Bowman's capsule flows into the renal tubules. The amount of fluid filtered by both kidneys—called the **glomerular filtration rate (GFR)**—equals about 180 liters each day, which is 60 times more than the body's total blood volume. The body reabsorbs about 99% of this filtrate, leaving 1 to 2 liters to be excreted as urine.

Plasma protein

Afferent arteriole

Efferent arteriole

Filtrate

FIGURE 36.3 Glomerular filtration. From Thompson, G. S. (2013). *Understanding anatomy and physiology.* Philadelphia: F.A. Davis, p. 351.

TABLE 36.1   EFFECTS OF HORMONES ON THE KIDNEYS

Hormone (Gland)	Function
Aldosterone (adrenal cortex)	Promotes reabsorption of sodium ions from the filtrate to the blood and excretion of potassium ions into the filtrate. Water is reabsorbed after the reabsorption of sodium.
Antidiuretic hormone (posterior pituitary)	Promotes reabsorption of water from the filtrate to the blood.
Atrial natriuretic hormone (atria of heart)	Decreases reabsorption of sodium ions, which remain in the filtrate. More sodium and water are eliminated in urine.
Parathyroid hormone (parathyroid glands)	Promotes reabsorption of calcium ions from filtrate to blood and excretion of phosphate ions into filtrate.

Source: Scanlon, V., & Sanders, T. (2015). *Essentials of anatomy and physiology* (7th ed., p. 470). Philadelphia: F.A. Davis, with permission.

Ureters

The ureters are behind the peritoneum of the dorsal abdominal cavity. Each ureter extends from the hilus of a kidney to the lower, posterior side of the urinary bladder. The smooth muscle in the wall of the ureter contracts in peristaltic waves to propel urine toward the urinary bladder. As the bladder fills, it expands and compresses the lower ends of the ureters to prevent backflow of urine.

Urinary Bladder and Urethra

The urinary bladder is a muscular sac inside the peritoneum just posterior to the pubic symphysis. In women, the bladder is anterior and inferior to the uterus; in men, the bladder is superior to the prostate gland. The functions of the bladder are the temporary storage of urine and its elimination. Urethra anatomy is different in some ways between men and women.

Urination Reflex

Urination (micturition) is a spinal cord reflex over which voluntary control may be exerted. Muscles involved include the detrusor of the bladder wall and two urethral sphincters.

Characteristics of Urine
Amount

Normal urinary output is 1000 to 2000 mL per 24 hours. Any changes in fluid intake or other fluid output (such as sweating) change this volume.

Color

The color of urine is often referred to as straw or amber. Dilute urine is a lighter color than is concentrated urine. Freshly voided urine is clear. Cloudy urine may indicate an infection.

Specific Gravity

Specific gravity is a measure of the dissolved materials in urine. The specific gravity of urine is 1.002 to 1.035. (The specific gravity of distilled water is 1.000.) The higher the specific gravity, the more dissolved material is present. Specific gravity of urine is a measure of the concentrating ability of the kidneys. They must excrete the waste products that are constantly formed in as little water as possible.

pH

The pH range of urine is 4.6 to 8.0, with an average of 6.0. Diet has the greatest influence on urine pH. A vegetarian diet results in more alkaline urine; a high-protein diet results in more acidic urine.

Constituents

Urine is about 95% water, which is the solvent for waste products and salts. Nitrogenous wastes include urea, creatinine, and uric acid. Urea is formed by liver cells when excess amino acids are deaminated (metabolized) to be used for energy production. Creatinine is a product of metabolism of creatine phosphate, an energy source in muscles. Uric acid results from the metabolism of nucleic acids. Other solutes, such as enzymes and hormones, are present in small quantities.

Aging and the Urinary System

With age, the number of nephrons in the kidneys decreases, often to half the original number by age 70 or 80 (Fig. 36.4).

The glomerular filtration rate (GFR) also decreases. This results in part from arteriosclerosis and diminished renal blood flow. The urinary bladder decreases in size, and the tone of the detrusor muscle decreases. This may result in the need to urinate more often or in residual urine in the bladder after voiding. Older adults are also more subject to infections of the urinary tract, and the changes of aging may influence medication therapy for older adults (see "Gerontological Issues").

■ NURSING ASSESSMENT OF THE URINARY SYSTEM

If the patient has impaired kidney function, complete head-to-toe data collection is needed because kidney disease can affect every system of the body (see Chapter 37).

Health History

Table 36.2 describes questions to ask for a health history, along with the use of the **WHAT'S UP?** format (Chapter 1) for symptoms.

Physical Examination

Table 36.2 also lists objective data that should be collected.

Pain

Pain in the flank or abdominal areas can be an indicator of renal problems or disease.

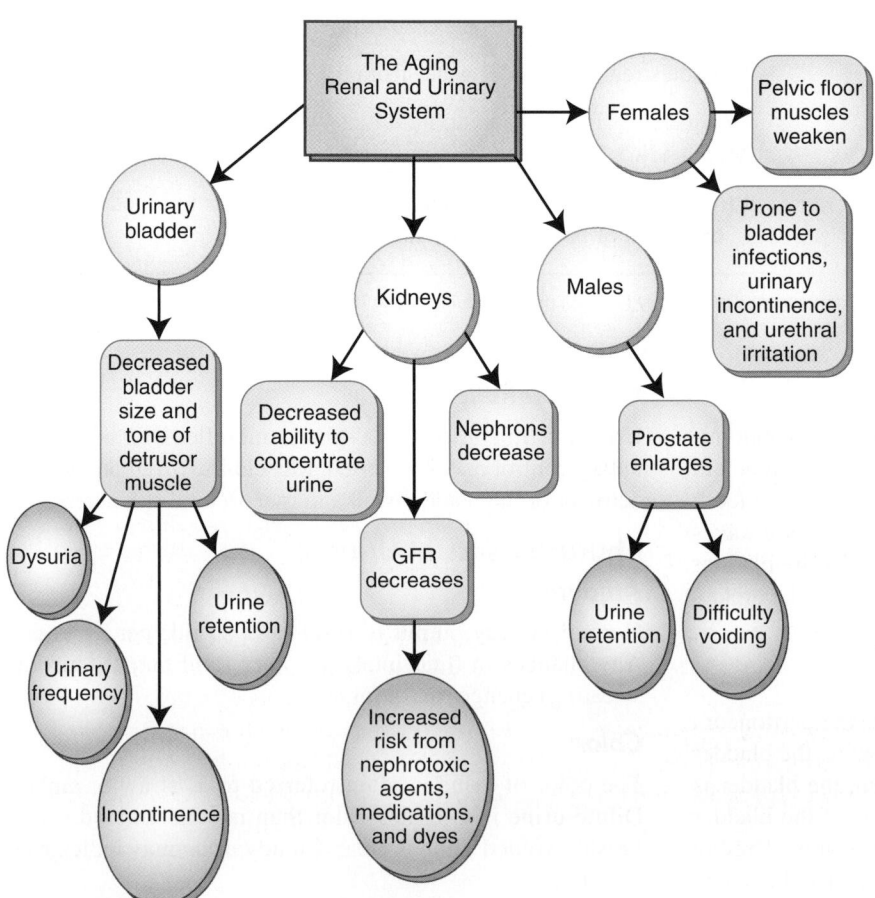

FIGURE 36.4 Aging and the urinary system. This concept map shows effects of the aging process on the urinary system.

Gerontological Issues

Age-Related Renal Changes

Certain changes typically occur in the renal system as people age. They include the following:
- The renal mass becomes smaller.
- Renal flow decreases by 50%, with subsequent decreased glomerular filtration rate.
- Tubular function and the exchange of substances decrease.
- Bladder muscles weaken and bladder capacity decreases, leading to increased frequency and **nocturia** (awakening from sleep at night to urinate).
- The voiding reflex is delayed.

Also, keep in mind that most drugs are excreted through the kidneys. Consequently, dehydration—which the older adult is prone to having—and changes in renal function become a serious consideration for older adults who need drug therapy. Decreased renal function could slow the excretion of some drugs, keeping them in the body longer. This can increase the risk of adverse drug reactions, such as toxicity and overdose. It is important to monitor kidney function (such as serum creatinine and blood urea nitrogen levels) in an older person receiving drug therapy.

Skin

The skin is inspected for color, texture, edema, or swelling. With chronic kidney disease there can be a yellow or gray cast to the skin. The presence of crystals on the skin is called uremic frost and is a late sign of waste products building up in the blood (**uremia**). When the waste products are not filtered by the kidneys or with treatment, they can come out through the skin and look like a coating of frost in the winter.

Vital Signs

If renal disease is suspected, blood pressure should be assessed and documented while the patient is lying, sitting, and standing. An increase in blood pressure is common with renal disease. A rapid respiratory rate may indicate fluid retention in the lungs.

Lung Sounds

If the patient retains more fluid than the heart can effectively pump, fluid may build up in the lungs. This is manifested as crackles (popping sounds heard on inspiration and sometimes on expiration). Wheezes may also be present. New-onset crackles and wheezes should be reported to a physician (see Chapter 29).

(Text continued on page 820)

• WORD • BUILDING •

nocturia: nox—night + uria—urine
uremia: ur—urine + emia—blood

TABLE 36.2 DATA COLLECTION FOR THE URINARY SYSTEM

Health History

Category	Questions to Ask	Rationale/Significance
Age	How old are you?	Aging is associated with a gradual loss of nephrons and decreased urine-concentrating ability and bladder capacity.
Gender	Male or female?	Men are at risk for prostate problems. Women have a high incidence of incontinence.
Ethnicity	What is your ethnic origin?	African American men over age 40 have a higher incidence of prostate and bladder cancer; those between ages 25 and 35 have an increased incidence of testicular cancer.
	Do you prefer to speak in a language other than English?	Language barriers may exist for gathering data.
Occupation	What type of work do you do?	Renal cancers may occur with occupational exposure to nephrotoxic chemicals, such as phenol and ethylene glycol.
	Have you had any exposure to chemicals in your present or past jobs or hobbies?	Some occupations and hobbies are related to a higher incidence of bladder tumors.
	Has your job affected your health, if so how?	Stress may predispose to hypertension and cardiovascular disease.

Continued

TABLE 36.2 DATA COLLECTION FOR THE URINARY SYSTEM—cont'd

Category	Questions to Ask	Rationale/Significance
Health habits	Do you use alcohol, caffeine, tobacco, or recreational drugs?	Alcohol can irritate the bladder and increase urinary output. Tobacco use increases risk of renal cancer.
Medical history	Have you been diagnosed with any of the following: • Beta-hemolytic streptococci • Cancer • Diabetes • Glomerulonephritis • Gout • Heart disease • Hyperlipidemia • Hypertension • Lupus erythematosus • Polycystic kidney disease • Renal stones • Sickle cell disease • Systemic infections • Urinary tract infection	Diabetes is the most common cause of chronic kidney disease worldwide, and hypertension is a significant risk factor. Systemic diseases such as gout, lupus, sickle cell disease, coronary artery disease, and atherosclerosis increase the risk of renal disease. Streptococcal infection may precede renal disease.
	Do you have any history of falls, motor vehicle accidents, or other trauma?	Risk of renal damage secondary to infection, abscess formation, and strictures.
	How many children do you have?	Increased parity may affect pelvic floor muscles, which can lead to stress incontinence.
Family history of urinary disorders	Is there a family history of hypertension, diabetes, kidney stones, polycystic kidney disease, or other kidney or urinary problems?	Hereditary tendency for some renal conditions.
Current medications, over-the-counter medications, or herb use	What prescription or over-the-counter medications are you taking?	Nephrotoxic drugs increase risk for kidney damage. Treatment with vasopressors, angiotensin-converting enzyme (ACE) inhibitors, or nonsteroidal anti-inflammatory drugs (NSAIDs) can impair renal perfusion and impair kidney function.
	What herbs or minerals are you taking?	Herbs with aristolochic acid may be renal toxic.
	Do you have any allergies to antibiotics, contrast media, or dyes?	Allergies and contrast media can lead to renal disease.
Renal/urinary problems	Have you experienced any of the following? • Pain, burning with urination • Blood in urine • Use of urinary catheter • Kidney or bladder surgery	Painful voiding may indicate an infection. **Hematuria** may indicate an infection or cancer.
	Have you noticed changes in your urination patterns? • Urgency, frequency • Difficulty starting stream of urine • Nocturia • Incontinence	Urgency with diminished amounts of urine suggests urinary retention. Difficulty starting urination may indicate a prostate obstruction. Nocturia occurs with nephrotic syndrome, diabetes, and heart failure.

• WORD • BUILDING •
hematuria: hemat—blood + uria—urine

TABLE 36.2   DATA COLLECTION FOR THE URINARY SYSTEM—cont'd

Category	Questions to Ask	Rationale/Significance
	Have you had changes in the color, odor, clarity, or amount of urine?	Cloudy urine or foul odor indicates possible infection; decreased amount may indicate renal disease; increased amount may indicate diabetes or inability to concentrate urine.
	Have you had any pain in the costovertebral angle (the area formed by the rib cage and the vertebral column)?	Renal calculus (stone) may produce dull ache in kidney area or colicky pain radiating to genital area or leg on affected side.
	Have you noticed any swelling of your lower legs or around your eyes in the morning?	Edema occurs with fluid retention; periorbital edema is noted around the eyes in the morning.
New onset of symptoms	Have you noticed any of the following symptoms? • Fatigue • Shortness of breath • Fever or chills • Nausea, vomiting, anorexia • Blurred vision • Headache • Lethargy • Confusion • Itchy skin • Metallic taste • Bone or joint problems	Fatigue and shortness of breath may be from anemia due to reduced erythropoietin, which is produced in the kidney. Fever occurs with urinary tract infections. Uremic toxins may produce many symptoms in multiple body systems. Metallic taste may be due to electrolyte imbalances. Bone and joint problems may be due to problems with calcium and vitamin D metabolism.
	Have you had pain in your back, lower abdomen, or perineum? Pain over the bladder? Leg pain?	May indicate infection, obstruction, or inflammation of the urinary system. Kidney pain: dull, aching, steady, flank area. Ureteral pain begins in the costovertebral angle radiating into lower abdomen and groin. Bladder pain felt over symphysis pubis. Back or leg pain may be due to prostrate or metastasis of cancer.
Diet and fluid intake	Describe your appetite, fluid intake, and nutritional status. Have you noticed any changes in weight over the last year? Are you able to shop and cook for yourself?	Anorexia occurs with renal disease. Large intake of protein or dairy products may lead to kidney stone formation. The person who is obese is at greater risk for renal ischemia from fluid losses and dehydration. Inability to take care of shopping and cooking can have a direct effect on diet.

Objective Assessment

Category	Possible Abnormal Findings	Possible Causes
Vital signs:	Hypertension	Hypertension is related to renal disease and fluid volume overload.
• Blood pressure • Pulse	Orthostatic hypotension	Orthostatic hypotension may be due to dehydration.
• Respiratory rate	Irregular heart rate	Hyperkalemia causes arrhythmias.
• Temperature	Fever	Infection elevates temperature.

Continued

TABLE 36.2 DATA COLLECTION FOR THE URINARY SYSTEM—cont'd

Category	Possible Abnormal Findings	Possible Causes
Cognitive function	Confusion Lethargy Insomnia	Changes in level of consciousness may be due to changes in electrolytes and fluid balance or a urinary tract infection.
Neurologic status	Diminished deep tendon reflexes Hyperesthesia Paresthesias Peripheral neuropathy	Increased levels of altered fluid balance, urea, creatinine, ammonia levels, and parathyroid hormone may interfere with nerve function and contribute to neuropathies.
Skin, hair, and nail assessment	Skin pallor, color, yellow gray cast Dry skin Excoriations Changes in turgor Bruising Distal portion of nailbeds white Capillary refill less than 3 seconds Impetigo—a streptococcal infection of the skin	Pallor may be due to anemia. Scratching from dry skin, pruritus may lead to excoriations. Dehydration is associated with oliguria. Thrombocytopenia. Distal portion of nailbeds turn white with kidney disease. Increased capillary refill may result from poor blood flow to the extremity or anemia. Streptococcal infections may precede glomerulonephritis.
Eyes	Conjunctival pallor Corneal calcification Retinal arteriosclerotic changes Blurred vision	Anemia Corneal calcification results from phosphate retention Retinal changes in blood vessels result from prolonged hypertension or diabetes. Retinitis pigmentosa may accompany hereditary nephropathies.
Ears, nose, and throat	Deafness Strep throat	High-frequency deafness may accompany hereditary nephritis. Acute glomerulonephritis may be accompanied by pharyngitis or group A beta-hemolytic streptococcal infections.
Cardiovascular	Hypertension Friction rub Cardiac enlargement of the left ventricle Angina or chest pain Distended neck veins, pericardial effusion, heart failure, pulmonary edema Dysrhythmias Edema	Causes renal disease; can result from alterations of sodium and renal secretion of vasoconstrictors. Friction rub may occur with uremia. Occurs from hypertension, increased fluid volume. Angina may occur from chronic anemia. Results from increased fluid volume. Dysrhythmias may occur as a result of imbalances of potassium, magnesium, and calcium. Edema occurs from decreased serum albumin.
Respiratory	Shortness of breath Tachypnea Rales Acid-base disturbances Kussmaul's respirations	Shortness of breath, tachypnea, and rales result from fluid volume overload. Metabolic acidosis occurs early in renal disease and causes Kussmaul's respirations.

TABLE 36.2   DATA COLLECTION FOR THE URINARY SYSTEM—cont'd

Category	Possible Abnormal Findings	Possible Causes
Hematologic	Anemia Bruising Bleeding tendencies	Result from decreased erythropoietin production in the kidneys. All blood cells are defective in renal disease.
Gastrointestinal	Weight changes Malnutrition Gastroparesis Gastritis Metallic taste Foul urine odor to breath Constipation Diarrhea	Nausea and changes in taste may lead to diminished appetite. Metabolic and hormonal changes in renal disease lead to gastrointestinal upset, malnutrition, and decreased nutrient intake. Urea buildup causes metallic taste in the mouth or foul breath odor. Alterations in elimination occur with renal disease.
Genitourinary	Nocturia Hematuria Dysuria Anuria Oliguria Polyuria Interrupted urine stream, dribbling, urine retention Incontinence Cloudy urine, foul odor Perineal pain	Kidneys lose concentrating ability. Blood in the urine may indicate urinary infection, irritation, obstruction, or cancer. Dysuria is a sign of urinary tract infection or interstitial cystitis. Less than 100 mL of urine in 24 hours seen in acute renal disease, end-stage renal disease, bilateral ureteral obstruction. Urine output of 100–400 mL in 24 hours with severe dehydration, shock, transfusion reactions, end-stage renal disease. Occurs with diabetes, diabetes insipidus, and chronic kidney disease. Urine flow difficulty may be due to prostate problems. Incontinence may be a sign of urological disorders or neurologic disease. Cloudy, foul-smelling urine may indicate a urinary tract infection. Occurs with infection, foreign body in urinary tract, urethritis, pyelonephritis, and renal colic or stone.
Musculoskeletal	Muscle weakness Bone and joint problems Gait disturbances Osteoporosis Fractures	Vitamin D synthesis decreases with the increase of parathyroid hormone causing changes in the calcium-phosphorus ratio and hyperparathyroidism. Bone and mineral disease occurs from low calcium level, high phosphorus level, and inability to activate vitamin D.
Endocrine system	Hypertension Hyperglycemia	Renin produced in the kidney activates angiotensin II, which is a potent vasoconstrictor that elevates blood pressure. Renal disease inhibits kidney's ability to break down insulin.

Edema

Fluid retention can be manifested as edema (excess fluid in tissues). The degree and location of edema is documented (see Chapter 21).

Daily Weights

Weight is the best indicator of fluid balance in the body. Patients with renal disease often have fluid imbalances. The patient should be weighed at the same time each day, in the same or similar clothing, and with the same scale. The nurse looks for trends in weight gain or loss. If the patient's weight is steadily increasing, fluid retention is suspected and should be reported.

Intake and Output

The patient with kidney disease is often on a fluid restriction. Intake and output (I&O) should be carefully measured. Intake includes oral, intravenous (IV), irrigation, tube feeding, and other fluids. Output includes urine, emesis, nasogastric effluent, wound drainage if it is copious, and any other drainage.

I&O totals are analyzed and recorded per agency policy, usually every 8 to 12 hours or more often for unstable patients. As with daily weights, the nurse notes trends in retention or loss of fluid to report to the physician. Accurate documentation is vital because the physician may base medication and IV fluid orders on intake and output results.

CRITICAL THINKING

Mr. Nolan

■ It is the end of the shift. As you empty Mr. Nolan's urinary collection bag, you find that it has only 50 mL of concentrated urine in it. What do you do?

Suggested answers are at the end of the chapter.

 ## DIAGNOSTIC TESTS FOR THE URINARY SYSTEM

Laboratory Tests

Urine Tests

URINALYSIS. A urinalysis (urine analysis) is a commonly performed diagnostic test for the urinary system, kidney disease, and systemic diseases that may affect the kidneys (Table 36.3).

A urine specimen for routine analysis may be collected at any time of day; however, the first morning specimen is best. First morning specimens are usually concentrated and more likely to contain abnormal constituents if they are present. The specimen should be examined within 1 hour of collection. Urine that cannot be examined promptly should be refrigerated. Urine standing at room temperature longer than 2 hours has more bacteria present, changes in pH, and hemolysis of red blood cells (RBCs). Urine collected for cytology should not be a first morning specimen due to changes in epithelial cells in urine held overnight. Random specimens are used for cytology. If a urinalysis is ordered for a patient with an indwelling urinary catheter, the nurse obtains the sterile urine specimen (see the DavisPlus site for this book).

Composite urine specimens (such as 24-hour urine) are collected over a period of time that may range from 2 to 24 hours. These specimens are usually used to examine the urine for specific components such as glucose, electrolytes, protein, 17-ketosteroids, catecholamines, creatinine, urea nitrogen, and minerals. These specimens may need refrigeration or may have preservatives added to the collection container.

For a composite urine collection, the patient is instructed to urinate and then discard this urine. The time is recorded and becomes the start time of the test. During the designated time period all urine voided is saved in the container and kept refrigerated or on ice. Exactly at the end of the time frame, the patient is asked to void, and this is the last amount added to the container. Reminding the patient to save all of the urine is critical for accurate results. Incomplete collections result in inaccurate results. Blood is often drawn from the patient at the end of the test for analysis as part of the test.

Renal Function Tests

A number of blood and urine tests reflect kidney function (Table 36.4). If the kidneys are not filtering adequately, the serum test values, such as the creatinine and blood urea nitrogen, will be elevated. These tests are useful because they provide information about the severity of a patient's kidney disease and also the patient's response to any treatments or medications being used. Renal function test values may still be within the normal range until the glomerular filtration rate is less than 50% of normal.

Diagnostic Procedures

Table 36.5 summarizes diagnostic procedures for the urinary system. For explanations of computed tomography (CT) scan, magnetic resonance imaging, and ultrasound testing and routine nursing care, see Appendix A.

Contrast-Induced Nephropathy

Contrast media used in diagnostic testing and procedures can be nephrotoxic and cause contrast-induced nephropathy resulting in acute kidney injury within 48 hours of contrast exposure. This condition is serious and can result in death. It is usually asymptomatic with a decline in renal function as shown by a rise in serum creatinine. Treatment is the same as for acute kidney injury (see Chapter 37).

Risk factors are having azotemia (increased creatinine and blood urea nitrogen) and diabetes mellitus–associated renal impairment. Creatinine levels are checked before the procedure and should be monitored afterward. A risk assessment should be done before testing regarding allergies/allergic reactions, diabetes, use of oral metformin (Glucophage), kidney disease, other medical conditions, medications: anti-inflammatories, antibiotics, antifungals, immunosuppressives. When contrast media are used, metformin hydrochloride (Glucophage) must not be given before and for 48 hours after administration of contrast media. Severe lactic acidosis as well as acute kidney injury can occur.

(Text continued on page 827)

TABLE 36.3 URINALYSIS RESULTS

Test	Normal Results	Significance of Abnormal Results
Color of urine	Pale yellow to amber	Dark-amber urine suggests dehydration. Yellow-brown to green urine indicates excessive bilirubin. Dark, smoky color suggests hematuria. Orange-red or orange-brown color caused by phenazopyridine (Pyridium). Cloudiness of freshly voided urine indicates infection. Nearly colorless urine is seen with a large fluid intake, renal disease, or diabetes insipidus.
Odor of urine	Aromatic	With infection, urine becomes foul smelling. In diabetic ketoacidosis, urine has a fruity odor. Urine that has been standing for a while develops a strong ammonia smell.
pH	4.6-8.0	pH is greatly affected by food eaten. pH below 4.6 is seen with metabolic and respiratory acidosis. pH above 8.0 is seen when urine has been standing or with infection because bacteria decompose urea to form ammonia.
Specific gravity	1.002-1.035	Low specific gravity indicates excessive fluid intake or diabetes insipidus. High specific gravity is seen with dehydration. Specific gravity fixed at 1.010 indicates kidney dysfunction. The specific gravity of glomerular filtrate is 1.010.
Protein	0-18 mg/dL 0-150 mg/24 hr	Persistent proteinuria, creating foamy urine, is seen with damage to the glomerulus. Proteinuria is a significant sign of renal disease. Intermittent protein in urine can result from strenuous exercise, dehydration, or fever. Vaginal secretions may contaminate urine and give a positive reading.
Glucose	None	Glucose in urine indicates diabetes mellitus, excessive glucose intake, or low renal threshold for glucose reabsorption.
Ketones	None	Ketones in urine indicate diabetes mellitus with ketonuria or starvation from breakdown of body fats into ketones. Can also be seen with carbohydrate-free diets, severe diarrhea, dehydration, and vomiting.
Bilirubin	None	Bilirubin in urine indicates liver disorders causing jaundice. Bilirubin may appear in the urine before jaundice is visible.
Nitrite	Negative	Nitrites in urine indicate infection. Bacteria in urine convert nitrate to nitrite, which gives a positive reading.
Leukocyte esterase	Negative	Positive leukocyte esterase in urine indicates infection in urine. It determines the presence of an enzyme released by WBCs in the urine.
Red blood cells	0-4/hpf	Blood in urine may be caused by kidney stones, infection, cancer, renal disease, or trauma.
White blood cells	0-5/hpf	WBCs in urine indicate infection or inflammation in the urinary tract.
Casts	None to occasional hyaline cast	Casts are formed when abnormal urine contents settle into molds of the renal tubules and may be made of protein, WBCs, RBCs, or bacteria. A few hyaline casts may be found in normal urine. The presence of casts usually indicates renal damage or infection.

Note. hpf = high-power field; RBC = red blood cells; WBC = white blood cells.

TABLE 36.4 DIAGNOSTIC LABORATORY TESTS FOR THE URINARY SYSTEM

Test	Definition/Normal Value	Significance of Abnormal Findings
Urine Studies		
Residual urine	Shows amount of urine left in the bladder after voiding. *Reference value:* Less than 50 mL (increases with age)	Bladder ultrasound equipment may be used to determine amount of urine remaining after voiding. Increased residual volume may occur in urethral strictures, sphincter impairment, or neurogenic bladder.
Urinalysis	Used to establish baseline information, confirm or establish a diagnosis, or determine if further testing needs to be done.	May be used to monitor progress of an existing condition or plan a program of care.
Urine culture	Determines number of bacteria in urine and identifies organism causing urinary tract infection. Sensitivity test also may be ordered to determine most effective antibiotic against offending bacteria. *Reference value:* Negative if less than 10,000/mL of urine Positive if 100,000 or more/mL of urine. An amount less than 100,000 may result from contamination during specimen collection.	Urine should be collected before antibiotic treatment starts to avoid altering results. Catheterized specimen may be ordered to avoid risk of contamination from vagina if female patient is menstruating or patient is incontinent.
Urine specific gravity	Evaluates the concentration of urine. Reference value: 1.002–1.035	Low specific gravity may occur in patients with diabetes insipidus, glomerulonephritis, or severe renal damage. High specific gravity may occur from diabetes mellitus, high urine glucose level, nephrosis, congestive heart failure, or dehydration.
Quantitative test for protein	A 12- or 24-hour urine collection is obtained to measure protein. *Reference values:* Less than 150 mg/24 hours (conventional units) Less than 0.15 g/24 hours (SI units)	Persistent proteinuria is usually seen with glomerular renal disease.
Creatinine clearance	Measures amount of creatinine cleared from blood in a specified time by comparing amount of creatinine in blood with creatinine in urine. An excellent indicator of renal function. *Reference value:* 85–135 mL/min	Creatinine clearance is computed in the laboratory and is expressed in volume of blood that is cleared of creatinine in 1 minute. Minimum creatinine clearance of 10 mL per minute is needed to live without dialysis. To carry out the test, urine is collected for a 24-hour period, and a sample for serum creatinine is collected sometime during the 24 hours.

TABLE 36.4   DIAGNOSTIC LABORATORY TESTS FOR THE URINARY SYSTEM—cont'd

Test	Definition/Normal Value	Significance of Abnormal Findings
		The following procedure should be followed: 1. At start of test, patient is directed to void and discard that urine. 2. Urine is collected for 24 hours in a large container provided by the laboratory. The container is kept refrigerated. 3. Twenty-four hours after test started, patient is instructed to void again. This urine is added to the collection container. 4. Laboratory collects serum creatinine during this 24-hour period.
Urine cytology	Microscopic examination of urine to detect atypical epithelial cells shed from the surface of the urinary tract.	Used to screen people at high risk for cancer in the urinary system. Atypical cells indicate need for further testing.
Bladder tumor antigen (a bladder cancer marker)	Measurement of a protein produced by bladder tumor cells. *Reference value:* Less than 14 units/mL	No special preparation needed. A single voided specimen collected before noon is taken directly to the laboratory.
NMP22 (a bladder cancer marker)	Measurement of a protein deposited into urine during nuclear disruption (apoptosis) of bladder cells. *Reference value:* Less than 10 units/mL	No special preparation needed. A single voided specimen collected before noon is taken directly to the laboratory.
Blood Chemistry Studies—Kidney Function		
Blood urea nitrogen (BUN)	Urea is a waste product of protein metabolism that is excreted by the kidneys. *Reference value:* 8–20 mg/dL	Not as sensitive an indicator of kidney function as creatinine level because BUN is affected by increased protein intake, dehydration, and other factors in the body. Elevated level: kidney disease, shock, severe heart failure, dehydration, high-protein diet, gastrointestinal bleeding, steroid use.
Serum creatinine	Creatinine is a waste product from muscle metabolism and is released into the bloodstream at a steady rate. *Reference value:* 0.6–1.5 mg/dL	Very good indicator of kidney function. The higher the creatinine level, the more impaired the kidney function. More than 1.5 mg/dL indicates kidney dysfunction.
BUN-to-creatinine ratio	Evaluates hydration status. *Reference value:* About 10:1	An elevated ratio occurs in hypovolemia. A normal ratio with an elevated BUN and creatinine occurs in intrinsic renal disease.
Cystatin C (Cys C)	Proteinase inhibitor produced by all cells with chromosomes and genetic material at their center at a constant rate, filtered out of blood by the glomerulus, and reabsorbed by tubular epithelial cells.	Cystatin C is a sensitive marker that reflects glomerular filtration rate independent of body weight and height. Cystatin C level increases with impaired renal function.

Continued

TABLE 36.4   DIAGNOSTIC LABORATORY TESTS FOR THE URINARY SYSTEM—cont'd

Test	Definition/Normal Value	Significance of Abnormal Findings
	Reference values: 0.53– 0.95 mg/dL In young adults, less than 0.70 mg/mL (0.9 micromol/mL) In older adults, less than 0.85 mg/mL (3.5 micromol/mL)	
Uric acid	Uric acid is an end product of purine metabolism and the breakdown of body proteins. Uric acid is not as diagnostic as creatinine because many factors can cause an elevated uric acid level. Reference value: 2–7 mg/dL	Elevated uric acid level can be caused by kidney disease, gout (patients with gout metabolize uric acid abnormally), malnutrition, leukemia, use of thiazide diuretics (because of impaired uric acid clearance by the kidney).
Blood Chemistry Studies Sodium (Na$^+$)	Extracellular electrolyte regulating blood volume. Reference value: 135–145 mEq/L	Remains within normal range until late stages of renal disease. Decreases with fluid retention (dilutional effect).
Potassium (K$^+$)	Intracellular electrolyte excreted by kidneys. Reference value: 3.5–5.5 mEq/L	In renal disease, K$^+$ is one of the first electrolytes to become abnormal. Level greater than 6 mEq/L can lead to muscle weakness and cardiac arrhythmias.
Calcium (Ca^{2+})	Main mineral in bone and aids in muscle contraction, neurotransmission, and blood clotting. Reference values: 4.5–5.5 mEq/L and 9–11 mg/dL	In renal disease decreased reabsorption of calcium leads to bone and mineral disease.
Phosphorus	Mineral found in bone, teeth, bloodstream, cells. Many functions. Reference values: 2.8–4.5 mg/dL and 0.95–1.45 mmol/L	Phosphorus balance is inversely related to calcium balance. Elevated in renal disease.
Bicarbonate (HCO$_3^-$)	An alkaline that indicates status of acid–base system. Reference value: 22–28 mEq/L	Most patients with renal disease have metabolic acidosis and low serum HCO$_3^-$ levels
Magnesium	Found in bone and intracellularly and excreted by the kidney. Reference value: 1.3–2.1 mEq/L	Elevated in chronic renal disease. Symptoms of elevated magnesium level include lethargy, nausea, vomiting, and slurred speech.
Serum albumin	Plasma protein maintaining oncotic pressure in vascular system. Reference value: 3.5–5.0 g/dL	Low level occurs in nephrotic syndrome and renal disease and leads to edema.

TABLE 36.5 DIAGNOSTIC PROCEDURES FOR THE URINARY SYSTEM

Procedure	Uses and Possible Abnormal Findings	Nursing Management
Noninvasive		
Renal ultrasound or ultrasonography	Congenital disorders of the kidney, abscesses, hydronephrosis, kidney stones or tumors, kidney enlargement, structural changes with chronic infection	No special preparation or aftercare. No known complications. No radiation exposure.
Bladder ultrasound	Portable ultrasound instrument computes residual urine volume, bladder wall thickness, bladder calculi, tumors, diverticula	Determines postresidual voiding accurately to reduce catheterizations for bladder distention.
Kidney-ureter-bladder x-ray	Renal calculi, kidney size, masses in the kidney	Usually, no special care is needed. If done as preliminary study, bowel prep may be done.
Computed tomographic scan (with/ without contrast)	Evaluation of kidneys, ureters, bladder, abdominal and pelvic organs for kidney size, tumors, cysts, abscesses, malignant masses, metastases, lymph node enlargement; nonfunctioning kidneys, renal stones, obstructions, infections	*Precare:* Check allergies, creatinine levels before patient receives contrast media. Withhold metformin before and for 48 hours after contrast is given. *Postcare:* Maintain hydration if contrast media given.
Magnetic resonance imaging (with/ without contrast media)	Staging of cancers of the kidney, bladder, and prostate	Know contraindications for metallic objects in body, surgical clips, or pacemakers not designed for magnetic resonance imaging. Metal objects, jewelry, and clothing with metal clips must be removed.
Invasive **Pyelogram:** X-ray examination of renal tissue, calyces, pelvises, ureters, and bladder (with/without contrast media)	Abnormal size or shape of kidneys, absent kidneys, polycystic kidney disease, tumors, hydronephrosis, renovascular hypertension (see Fig. 36.5).	*Precare:* Enemas may be given the evening before the test to empty the colon. Check allergies, creatinine levels before patient receives contrast media. Explain warm, flushing sensation up arm and sometimes all over the body when the dye is injected. Strange taste may occur as well. *Postcare:* Maintain hydration if contrast media given. Monitor urine output.
Renal angiography or arteriogram with contrast media.	Visualizes renal blood vessels. Hypervascular tumors, renal cysts, renal artery stenosis, renal artery aneurysms, pyelonephritis, obstructions, renal infarction, renal trauma evaluation. May be used during renal angioplasty.	*Precare:* Check allergies, creatinine levels before patient receives contrast media. Enemas may be given the evening before the test. *Postcare:* Bedrest up to 12 hours to prevent bleeding at injection site. Check distal pulses in leg every 30–60 minutes. Instruct patient not to bend leg or raise head of bed more than 45 degrees. Monitor vital signs, dressing, and pulses in leg frequently.

Continued

• WORD • BUILDING •
pyelogram: pyelo—pelvis of the kidney + gram—radiograph

TABLE 36.5 DIAGNOSTIC PROCEDURES FOR THE URINARY SYSTEM—cont'd

Procedure	Uses and Possible Abnormal Findings	Nursing Management
Nephrotomogram: Series of x-rays with contrast media creating three-dimensional image of the kidney	Renal cysts, tumors, areas of nonperfusion, renal fractures or lacerations following renal trauma	*Precare:* Prepare patient as for a pyelogram, Check allergies, creatinine levels before patient receives contrast media. Monitor fluid intake and output before and after test. *Postcare:* Maintain hydration.
Renal scan	Renovascular hypertension diagnosis; kidney function; renal blood flow; glomerular filtration rate; tubular function; excretion of urine; kidney size and shape; abscesses, cysts, and tumors, which may appear as cold spots because of nonfunctioning kidney tissue; determination of vascular supply to the kidneys in patients with renal trauma, dissecting aneurysm, and other disorders affecting blood flow to the kidneys	Assesses kidneys' ability to perfuse blood and secrete urine. Usually, no special preparation needed. Determine if any of patient's medications will interfere with test, such as nonsteroidal anti-inflammatory drugs or antihypertensives. Patient may be asked to drink two glasses of water before test. Level of radiation is very low and produces no side effects. Pregnant and nursing mothers are advised to be cautious. If captopril given monitor for hypotension.
Renal biopsy	Microscopic examination of kidney tissue for diagnosis or treatment of renal disorder, benign and malignant masses, causes of renal disease, renal transplant rejection, lupus	*Precare:* Before biopsy, patient is NPO for 6 to 8 hours. Mild sedative is given. No anticoagulants, CBC, coagulation studies. *During:* Prone position, with sandbag under the abdomen, for biopsy through flank area. Patient instructed to hold breath while needle is inserted to prevent kidney from moving. *Postcare:* Bandage is applied. Patient vital signs and output monitored. Grossly bloody urine, falling blood pressure, and rising pulse are signs of bleeding and are reported immediately. Encourage fluids. Teaching: No heavy lifting for 2 weeks.
Cystoscopy and pyelogram: Minor surgical procedure with lighted fiber-optic cystoscope	Diagnostic: Inspect inside of bladder, collect urine specimen from either kidney, take x-rays or biopsy growths. Therapeutic: Remove small bladder tumors, polyps, stones from bladder/ureters, dilation of ureters, treat enlarged prostate or congenital abnormalities	*Precare:* Surgical preparation. *Postcare:* Measure urine output to detect retention from swelling of urinary meatus. Encourage fluid intake. Expect dysuria for 24 hours and initial voidings to be blood tinged. *Complications:* UTI, urine retention, bladder perforation.
Cystogram or voiding cystourethrogram: X-ray of bladder/lower urinary tract with contrast media or radioisotope instilled into bladder via catheter or cystoscope	Evaluates bladder filling and emptying. Incomplete bladder emptying, distention, reflux, obstruction to urine outflow identified.	No special prep. After the scan, can have slight dysuria and pink urine for 1–2 days. Bright red urine, fever, or persistent discomfort should be reported to physician.

• WORD • BUILDING •
cystoscopy: cysto—bladder + scopy—to examine

FIGURE 36.5 IV pyelogram x-ray. Contrast media injected intravenously with x-ray images taken as the contrast is excreted by the kidneys.

Protective measures continue to be studied. IV hydration with normal saline or a sodium bicarbonate infusion is likely one of the main preventative measures in use. Acetylcysteine (Mucomyst) before and after the procedure is also used.

Renal Biopsy

A renal biopsy diagnoses or provides information about kidney disease. A CT scan or ultrasound is done first to locate the kidney for biopsy. A small section of the renal cortex is obtained for laboratory analysis either **percutaneously** (local anesthetic, needle through skin) or with a small flank incision. Patients with bleeding tendencies, uncontrolled hypertension, or a solitary kidney generally do not undergo renal biopsy.

Nursing Process for Diagnostic Tests of the Urinary System Assessment

The patient is assessed for baseline understanding testing procedures to plan teaching sessions. Identified contraindications to testing are reported to the health care provider (HCP).

Nursing Diagnoses, Planning, and Implementation

Anxiety related to unfamiliar environment, procedure, diagnostic test, health status, or severity of disease
EXPECTED OUTCOME: The patient will have reduced anxiety concerning health status or severity of disease before a procedure or test.

- Assess patient for signs and symptoms of anxiety: verbalization, tenseness, tachycardia, elevated blood pressure, facial pallor, and self-focused behaviors. *A high level of*

fear will interfere with teaching and learning and also diminish cooperation during testing.
- Examine patient's health beliefs *to provide insight into patient behaviors that may affect outcome.*
- Acknowledge patient's anxiety and the perceived threat of the situation *to facilitate communication and trust.*
- Maintain a calm, supportive, and confident environment and manner when interacting with patient *to reduce anxiety.*
- Encourage patient to verbalize feelings, concerns, or specific stressors *to provide a baseline of information to develop an individualized teaching plan.*
- Provide patient with access to timely information regarding outcome of diagnostic testing *to facilitate trust and promote comfort.*
- Engage support from patient's family throughout diagnostic testing *for patient's coping.*
- Instruct patient in relaxation techniques and facilitate their use *to reduce anxiety.*
- Respond to patient's request for assistance as soon as possible *to reduce anxiety.*
- Reinforce explanations and correct misconceptions the patient has about diagnostic tests or disease condition *to facilitate trust and promote comfort.*

Acute Pain related to infection, edema, obstruction, or bleeding along the urinary tract or to invasive diagnostic tests
EXPECTED OUTCOME: The patient will report a decrease in discomfort or pain within 30 minutes of report of discomfort or pain.

- Assess location and level of pain, **dysuria**, burning on urination, or abdominal or flank pain *to provide baseline data to evaluate progression of pain and effectiveness of treatment plan.*
- Provide comfort measures *to relieve pain.*
- Provide analgesics and antispasmodics as prescribed *for pain relief.*
- Report severe pain to HCP. *Severe pain may indicate complications are present or the need for a change in pain control medications.*

Impaired Urinary Elimination related to complications from diagnostic tests of the urinary system
EXPECTED OUTCOME: The patient will maintain urine output greater than 30 mL per hour in the postprocedure period.

- Maintain hydration with ordered IV infusion before and after diagnostic testing *to protect kidneys and facilitate contrast removal from the body.*
- Monitor fluid intake and output closely *to ensure adequate renal function.*
- Monitor serum creatinine level *to assess for complications from diagnostic testing.*
- Observe patient for hypersensitivity reactions to contrast media or injectable materials *to help prevent renal complications.*

• WORD • BUILDING •
percutaneous: per—through + cutaneous—skin

- Assess patient for pruritus, rashes, breathing difficulties, generalized edema, or urinary retention *to detect possible reaction symptoms.*

Deficient Knowledge related to unfamiliar environment, procedure, diagnostic test, and health status

EXPECTED OUTCOME: The patient will report understanding of the environment, procedure, or diagnostic test before the procedure.

- Collect data on patient's understanding of the procedure *to provide a baseline for teaching.*
- Introduce staff members who will be caring for the patient. *Familiarity with staff will decrease anxiety.*
- Include family members or significant others in orientation and teaching sessions *to encourage their support of the patient.*
- Orient patient to the environment, equipment, and routines *to increase understanding.*
- Explain all activities that will take place before, in the diagnostic area, and afterward *to reduce fear and promote cooperation during testing.*
- Provide information at the patient's level *to promote understanding.*
- Reinforce physician's explanations and correct misconceptions about the diagnostic test or procedure *to help alleviate anxiety.*
- Provide information about self-care following procedure or diagnostic test *to facilitate the patient in self-care.*

Evaluation

If interventions have been effective, the patient will report reduced anxiety, maintain urine output greater than 30 mL per hour, and a decrease in pain and increased understanding of the procedure.

 ## THERAPEUTIC MEASURES FOR THE URINARY SYSTEM

Management of Urinary Incontinence

Urinary incontinence is defined as the involuntary leakage of urine and is very common. There are several types of incontinence. The incidence is rising and affects both men and women. Urinary incontinence is often underdiagnosed and underreported because many patients are too embarrassed to talk about the problem. Most patients do not seek treatment until the problem profoundly affects quality of life. With any type of incontinence, the nurse or patient should keep a voiding diary for at least several days to determine when incontinence occurs and to look for any predisposing events. The patient should be referred to a urologist specializing in the area of incontinence or a continence clinic for a careful examination to determine the cause and identify potential medical or surgical treatment. Incontinence that cannot be treated is managed by the use of padding and absorptive products worn by the patient.

Stress Incontinence

Stress incontinence is the involuntary loss of less than 50 mL of urine associated with increasing abdominal pressure during coughing, sneezing, laughing, or other physical activities. Stress incontinence is commonly seen in women after childbirth and after menopause. In men, stress incontinence is associated with prostatectomy and radiation.

Urge Incontinence

Urge incontinence is the involuntary loss of urine associated with an abrupt and strong desire to void. The patient typically reports being "unable to make it to the bathroom in time." Urge incontinence is the most common type of urinary incontinence in older adults. Patients with stress incontinence or urge incontinence can be taught Kegel exercises to increase perineal muscle tone (Box 36-1, "Patient Education").

Functional Incontinence

Functional incontinence is the inability to reach the toilet because of environmental barriers, physical limitations, loss of memory, or disorientation. People with functional incontinence are often dependent on others and have no other urinary

---

Box 36-1 **Patient Education**

Kegel Exercises

Kegel exercises decrease incontinence by strengthening the pubococcygeal muscle, which supports the pelvic organs. By increasing the tone of this muscle, the patient has an increased ability to tighten the muscle that encircles the urinary meatus and stop the flow of urine. These exercises can also help prevent uterine prolapse, enhance sensation during sexual intercourse, and hasten postpartum healing. It may be used by the older male patient to control dribbling.

1. Establish awareness of pelvic muscle function by instructing the patient to "pull in" the muscles in the perineum as if to control urination or defecation. The muscles of the buttocks, inner thigh, and abdomen are not used to do Kegel exercises.
2. To help identify the correct muscles to tighten, ask the patient to tighten the muscles that control urination. It can be helpful to use an analogy of an elevator: start squeezing at the bottom floor and then squeeze upward to the top floor.
3. Instruct the patient to tighten the pelvic muscles for 10 seconds, followed by at least 10 seconds of relaxation.
4. Advise the patient to perform these exercises 30 to 80 times per day. Help devise cues to remind the patient to perform the exercises, such as stopping the stream of urine 10 times each time the patient urinates.

Source: Adapted from Agency for Healthcare Research and Quality. (2012). *Nonsurgical treatments for urinary incontinence in adult women: diagnosis and comparative effectiveness.* Executive Summary April 9, 2012. Retrieved from www.ahrq.gov/news /newsletters/research-activities/may12/0512RA3.html problems. This is a common cause of incontinence in those who are institutionalized.

Overflow Incontinence

Overflow incontinence is the involuntary loss of urine associated with overdistention of the bladder. It occurs with acute or chronic urinary distention with dribbling of urine. The bladder is unable to empty normally despite frequent urine loss. Spinal cord injuries or an enlarged prostate may cause this type of incontinence.

Total Incontinence

Total incontinence is a continuous and unpredictable loss of urine. It usually results from surgery, trauma, or a malformation of the ureter. Bladder training has been tried and proven ineffective. Often the patient with total incontinence is neurologically impaired. In these situations, the nurse's priority is to keep the patient clean and dry using absorptive products. For the male patient, an external condom catheter can be effective in some situations.

Nursing Process for the Patient With Stress or Urge Incontinence

The medical diagnoses of stress and urge incontinence are also nursing diagnoses. Many nursing interventions can help to improve these types of incontinence. See the "Nursing Care Plan for the Patient With Stress or Urge Incontinence and the Nursing Care Plan for the Patient with Functional Incontinence."

NURSING CARE PLAN for the Patient With Stress or Urge Incontinence

Nursing Diagnosis: *Stress Incontinence* or *Urge Incontinence* related to decreased tone of perineal muscles

Expected Outcomes: The patient will be continent of urine and will state three actions that can be taken to decrease incidence of stress or urge incontinence.

Evaluation of Outcomes: Is the patient continent? Is the patient able to state three actions that can be taken to decrease the incidence of stress or urge incontinence?

STRESS INCONTINENCE OR URGE INCONTINENCE

Intervention Ask about the history of incontinence. Have patient keep a voiding journal. **Rationale** A journal helps identify the severity and timing of incontinence. **Evaluation** Does patient complete the voiding journal?

Intervention Instruct patient on how to perform Kegel exercises (see Box 36-1). **Rationale** Kegel exercises increase perineal muscle tone and help prevent incontinence. **Evaluation** Does patient explain how to perform Kegel exercises?

Intervention Work with the patient to incorporate Kegel exercises into normal activities of daily living (e.g., do 10 pelvic muscle contractions during each voiding). **Rationale** An excellent time to perform Kegel exercises is when voiding because the correct muscles are used. **Evaluation** Does patient perform Kegel exercises when voiding or at other cued times during the day?

Intervention Encourage patient to drink at least 2000 mL of fluid per day, preferably 3000 mL per day unless medical reason for fluid restriction. **Rationale** Concentrated urine is irritating to the urinary tract and can increase the incidence of urge incontinence and dribbling. **Evaluation** Is urine dilute?

Intervention Encourage patient to avoid alcohol and caffeine. **Rationale** Alcohol serves as a diuretic. Caffeine is irritating to the urinary tract. **Evaluation** Does patient explain the need to avoid alcohol and fluids containing caffeine?

Intervention Discuss use of and provide small adhesive peripads to wear in underclothing. **Rationale** Peripads provide protection in case of incontinence. **Evaluation** Does patient have and use peripads if desired?

Intervention Refer patient to a continence clinic or to a physician specializing in incontinence. **Rationale** Specialists in the area of incontinence can use medical or surgical interventions to decrease incontinence. **Evaluation** Does patient understand what resources are available to further assist with treatment of incontinence?

Continued

NURSING CARE PLAN for the Patient With Stress or Urge Incontinence—cont'd

Intervention Refer patient to supportive and educational groups such as National Association for Continence (www.nafc.org). **Rationale** Support groups can help patients deal with the embarrassment of incontinence and learn methods and resources to prevent incontinence. **Evaluation** Does patient know the names and addresses of support groups to help with incontinence?

URGE INCONTINENCE

Intervention Teach patient to void at frequent intervals (every 2 hours), and then gradually increase the length of time between voidings. **Rationale** By emptying the bladder at frequent intervals, the incidence of urge incontinence can be decreased. **Evaluation** Does patient follow a frequent voiding schedule?

Intervention Teach urge inhibition techniques (distraction), such as counting back from 100 by sevens and relaxation breathing. **Rationale** These distraction techniques can help patients reach the bathroom in time to prevent incontinence. **Evaluation** Do distraction techniques help patient prevent incontinence?

NURSING CARE PLAN for the Patient With Functional Incontinence

Nursing Diagnosis: *Functional Urinary Incontinence* related to interference with rapid voiding

Expected Outcomes: The patient will be continent of urine and will state three measures to increase continence.

Evaluation of Outcomes: Is the patient continent of urine? Is the patient able to state three measures to increase continence?

Intervention Ask about the history of incontinence. Keep a voiding log of when patient is incontinent. **Rationale** A voiding log helps demonstrate when incontinence is most likely to occur and can help determine the cause of incontinence. **Evaluation** Does the patient cooperate so that a voiding log can be kept?

Intervention Determine any acute causes of incontinence, including new onset of urinary tract infection, constipation or impaction, medication effect, or poor fluid intake. **Rationale** These may be readily treatable causes of incontinence. **Evaluation** Does the patient have any easily treatable causes of incontinence?

Intervention Determine if clothing is inhibiting timely voiding. If needed, Velcro™ fasteners or sweatshirts and sweatpants might be appropriate. **Rationale** Clothing can be difficult to remove for older adults, resulting in voiding before the clothing can be removed. Clothing can be modified so that it comes off quickly. **Evaluation** Does the patient have easy-to-remove clothing?

Intervention Determine if there are any obstacles to reaching appropriate urine receptacle, such as poor lighting, busy bathroom, lack of assistive devices. **Rationale** Obstacles can make it impossible for the patient to reach the voiding receptacle in time to prevent incontinence. **Evaluation** Does the patient have ready access to a voiding receptacle?

Intervention Provide appropriate urinary receptacles, such as a three-in-one commode, female or male urinal, or no-spill urinal. **Rationale** Assistive devices can be helpful for the patient to increase continence. **Evaluation** Does the patient need and have access to an appropriate assistive device?

Intervention Initiate a voiding schedule of every 2 hours, or base schedule on voiding log. **Rationale** Frequent scheduled voiding using prompting techniques can increase continence. **Evaluation** Does the patient receive help to do bladder training with prompted voiding?

Intervention Always assist patient to the toilet when patient first awakens and before sleep. **Rationale** These are the main times when toileting is needed. **Evaluation** Are patient's toileting needs met?

NURSING CARE PLAN for the Patient With Functional Incontinence—cont'd

Intervention Use prompted voiding techniques, including checking patient regularly, providing positive reinforcement if dry, prompting patient to toilet, praising patient after toileting, and returning patient to toilet in a specified time. **Rationale** Maintaining a regular toileting schedule will help patient remain dry. **Evaluation** Does patient remain dry?

Intervention Teach patient to set up schedule of voiding using environmental cues such as meals, bedtime, and television shows. **Rationale** Environmental cues help the patient remember when it is time to void. **Evaluation** Can the patient indicate cues throughout the day that prompt voiding?

Management of Urine Retention

Urinary retention is the inability to empty the bladder completely during attempts to void. Many factors can be the cause. It can be acute, with a sudden onset of retention and no urine output, or chronic, with a slower onset of retention of urine and some urine being expelled. Acute retention often results from surgery and is caused by anesthesia, medications, or local trauma to the urinary structures. Acute retention can be a medical emergency causing extreme pain, a large bladder, and the possibility of bladder rupture or acute kidney injury. Chronic urine retention may be related to an enlarged prostate gland, diabetes, pregnancy, a medication effect, strictures, or other causes of obstruction of the urinary tract.

Gentle palpation and percussion of the bladder may be done by the licensed practical nurse/licensed vocational nurse (LPN/LVN) if urine retention is suspected. If the patient has a feeling of fullness but is unable to urinate, the nurse gently palpates the suprapubic area for a full bladder or performs a bedside bladder ultrasound. Normally, the bladder is not palpable. If the fluid-filled bladder is percussed, it sounds dull over the bladder and may extend up to and beyond the umbilicus.

A bladder scan assesses the volume of urine in the bladder (Fig. 36.6). Sound waves estimate the amount of urine in the bladder. It is painless, noninvasive, and requires no patient preparation. The nurse performs this scan at the bedside. It helps guide the need for urinary catheterization, thereby reducing unnecessary catheterizations and associated risks. The bladder scan may be used instead of catheterization (the gold standard for determining urine retention) after the patient urinates to determine the amount of urine remaining in the bladder. Normally the bladder contains less than 50 mL after urination. A residual volume of 150 to 200 mL of urine indicates a need for treatment for urine retention. Bladder scanning may also be used as a tool for incontinent patients to plan their care.

Urinary Catheters
Indwelling Catheters

Indwelling urinary catheters can be inserted into hospitalized patients for various justifiable reasons, such as shock, heart failure, or urinary tract obstruction. The Joint Commission (2014) recommends using indwelling urinary catheters short term and only when necessary because of the high risk of urinary tract infections (UTIs). Urinary incontinence is not a justification for insertion of an indwelling urinary catheter. Indwelling catheters result in UTI the longer they are in place. The incidence of infection is decreased when intermittent straight urinary catheterization is used instead of an indwelling urinary catheter.

With an indwelling urinary catheter, bacteria enter the bladder mainly in one of two ways: (1) through the outlet at the end of the collection bag contaminating the urine, which is then inadvertently drained back into the bladder, or (2) around the catheter up the urethra and into the bladder. Routine perineal care during the daily bath is sufficient to minimize infection from an indwelling urinary catheter (see "Evidence-Based Practice"). Box 36-2 outlines steps that should be followed to decrease infection in the patient with an indwelling catheter. (See also "Home Health Hints.")

FIGURE 36.6 A bladder scan can be used to determine the volume of urine in a patient's bladder.

BE SAFE!

Implement evidence-based practices to prevent indwelling catheter–associated UTIs (Joint Commission's 2014 National Patient Safety Goals; © The Joint Commission, 2013. Reprinted with permission.).

Box 36-2 Guidelines for Care of the Patient With an Indwelling Urinary Catheter

1. Maintain a closed system. Do not separate the catheter from the tubing of the bag. Instead, sterilely collect specimens and irrigate through the specimen port in the tubing.
2. Secure the catheter with tape or fastener as directed. This decreases traction on the catheter and the back-and-forth movements of the catheter that can help bacteria enter the bladder.
3. Encourage fluid consumption to naturally irrigate the catheter, if fluids are not contraindicated.
4. Use aseptic technique when emptying the collection bag by washing hands, wearing clean gloves, and using a clean container for single-patient use to collect the urine.
5. Wash the perineum with soap and water once a day and again if there is any bowel incontinence.
6. Keep the tubing coiled on the bed and positioned to allow free urine flow. Keep the catheter bag below the level of the bladder at all times.
7. Do not clamp catheters. Clamping a catheter results in obstruction and increases risk of infection. Periodic clamping has not been found to be effective in bladder retraining.
8. Replace the urine collection system as required.
9. Remove indwelling catheters as soon as possible.

After an uncircumcised male is catheterized, the foreskin must be properly repositioned over the glans penis and not left retracted to prevent injury. If left retracted, subsequent swelling may make it impossible to pull the foreskin over the glans penis later. This can then cause ischemia of the glans penis, which is an emergency. A physician must be notified immediately and may need to perform an emergency circumcision if the foreskin cannot be properly positioned. Always make sure that the foreskin is positioned properly after catheterization or perineal care.

EVIDENCE-BASED PRACTICE

Clinical Question
Does the practice of daily meatal cleansing decrease the incidence of UTIs in patients with indwelling urinary catheters?

Evidence
Catheter care and meatal cleansing with antimicrobials or antiseptic soap have not shown a reduction in catheter-related UTIs. Administration of prophylactic antibiotics can increase resistant microorganism and increase susceptibility to Clostridium difficile infection (Muzzi-Bjornson, 2011). Current guidelines recommend routine hygiene of cleansing the meatal surface during bathing or showering (Gould, 2009).

Implications for Nursing Practice
Normal daily genital hygiene with soap and water is sufficient to achieve meatal cleanliness. Avoid vigorous and specific regimens because they may lead to meatal trauma from catheter manipulation.

REFERENCES

Gould, C. et al (2009). Guideline for prevention of catheter-associated urinary tract infections. Healthcare Infection Control Practices Advisory Committee, Centers for Disease Control and Prevention.

Muzzi-Bjornson, L. (2011). Preventing infection in elders with long term indwelling urinary catheters. *Journal of American Academy of Nurse Practitioners*, 23, 127–134.

Intermittent Catheterization

For the patient who is unable to void, the best intervention is intermittent catheterization. A postoperative patient or a patient with a neurologic disorder or urine retention may benefit from intermittent catheterization. It reduces the risk of infection as long as the bladder is not allowed to overfill. A full bladder stretches the muscle fibers, which in turn reduces circulation to the bladder and increases the risk of infection.

Intermittent catheterization involves the use of a straight plastic or rubber catheter that is inserted into the urethra about every 3 hours to empty the bladder. Once the bladder is empty, the catheter is removed. Patients may be taught to do intermittent self-catheterization (ISC) at home. Patients doing ISC may be taught to wash and reuse the same catheter repeatedly when they are in their own environment. In the hospital, however, sterile technique is used.

Suprapubic Catheter

After some surgeries of the urinary tract and in some long-term situations, a suprapubic catheter may be used. This is an indwelling catheter that is inserted through a surgical incision in the lower abdomen directly into the bladder.

Nursing care of a suprapubic catheter involves keeping the area clean and dry, changing the dressing when the site is new, and keeping the catheter taped to prevent tension. A skin barrier such as Stomahesive may help protect the skin from urine leakage. All other care is the same as for any indwelling urinary catheter. See DavisPlus for resources related to the urinary system and its disorders.

Home Health Hints

- The home health nurse should always have a sterile specimen container available. This provides a quick way to get a specimen to the physician's office without the nurse having to obtain the container, saving time and money.
- When catheters become plugged and irrigation fails, families can be taught to take the catheter out. A syringe for removing water from the balloon should be left in the home for this purpose. The family is instructed to avoid cutting the valve stem.
- The family should contact the nurse to reinsert the catheter. For incontinence the patient's bed or chair can be padded with waterproof items such as adult briefs or plastic bags on the mattress. The family must be instructed to notify the nurse immediately if the catheter is plugged or has been removed.

- Not all homes have adequate lighting, which is a must for inserting a catheter. If lighting is inadequate, a caregiver can be asked to hold a flashlight while the nurse inserts the catheter, while respecting the patient's privacy. The nurse should always have a flashlight available. Having two catheters and catheter trays is also wise in case of a defect or contamination.
- Urine collection bags can be used safely for up to 4 weeks. Cleansing instructions might be provided.
- To encourage fluid intake, urge patient and family to keep a large container of water (1 to 2 quarts) next to the place the patient usually sits. The goal is to drink 2 quarts of water by the end of each day, unless contraindicated by other medical problems. This also simplifies measuring intake. A sports bottle helps to keep water at hand while moving about the home.

SUGGESTED ANSWERS TO

CRITICAL THINKING

■ Mr. Nolan

You should realize that 50 mL of concentrated urine for 8 to 12 hours is not adequate or normal. Further investigation is needed to determine the cause and seriousness of the problem. Some items to assess include the following:

1. Consider Mr. Nolan's diagnosis. Is he experiencing acute kidney injury? Is he severely dehydrated and retaining water?
2. Ask if anyone emptied Mr. Nolan's bag earlier in the shift.
3. Look at the trends in Mr. Nolan's intake and output record. Has his output been decreasing? Is this a change?
4. Has Mr. Nolan been taking in enough fluids?
5. Look at trends in daily weights. Is Mr. Nolan's weight increasing? Is this an expected finding?
6. Listen to Mr. Nolan's lung sounds. Check for edema. Do findings indicate fluid retention?
7. Palpate Mr. Nolan's bladder. Is it distended? Maybe the catheter is blocked.
8. If a problem is identified, the physician should be contacted.

REVIEW QUESTIONS

1. A home health nurse visits a patient who is 82 years old, uses a cane, and is not incontinent. Which of the following interventions should be included in the plan of care, based on an understanding of normal age-related changes of the urinary system, to promote patient safety?
   1. Encourage fluids after 18:00.
   2. Limit fluids to 1000 mL per day.
   3. Provide a nightlight in the bathroom.
   4. Provide adult briefs to absorb dribbling.

2. The nurse is caring for a patient with acute kidney injury. Which of the following actions should the nurse take to obtain the most accurate assessment of fluid balance for the patient?
   1. Document voiding pattern
   2. Obtain daily weight
   3. Review laboratory studies
   4. Observe skin turgor

3. The nurse is caring for a patient who is to have a urine culture and sensitivity done. Which of the following should be included in patient teaching for collecting a midstream clean-catch urine specimen for culture and sensitivity?
   1. A second voided specimen is preferred.
   2. A 24-hour urine specimen is needed.
   3. As soon as the urine starts to flow, it should be collected in a sterile container.
   4. Women should keep the labia separated while voiding.

4. The nurse is caring for a patient who has had a pyelogram with IV contrast. Which of the following care should the nurse provide? **Select all that apply.**
   1. Maintain nothing by mouth.
   2. Encourage fluids.
   3. Check gag reflex.
   4. Measure urine output.
   5. Position patient prone.
   6. Maintain bed rest for 24 hours.

5. A patient is experiencing stress incontinence with frequent involuntary loss of urine. Which of the following directions would be most appropriate when teaching the patient how to perform Kegel exercises?
   1. "Tighten your rectum at frequent intervals throughout the day."
   2. "Keep your abdominal muscles tightened; do this every time you stand up."
   3. "Do at least 20 sit-ups per day."
   4. "When urinating, stop and start the stream of urine by tightening the perineal muscles."

6. The nurse is caring for a patient with a urinary catheter. Which of the following is the most important nursing action for the nurse to take to prevent urinary tract infection in this patient?
   1. Force fluids to 4000 mL every 24 hours.
   2. Empty the Foley bag every 4 hours around the clock.
   3. Maintain a closed catheter system.
   4. Wash the perineum every 8 hours.

7. The nurse is documenting the patient's shift output. What is the patient's total output as recorded during the 0700 to 1500 shift?
   0800 voided 165 mL
   1130 voided 450 mL
   1300 emesis 42 mL
   1500 voided 255 mL
   Answer: _____ mL

8. The nurse is reviewing the urinalysis of a patient. Which of the following are abnormal findings to report to the HCP? **Select all that apply.**
   1. Blood 7/hpf
   2. Glucose none
   3. Protein 4 mg/dL
   4. White blood cells 11/hpf
   5. Nitrites positive

Answers can be found in Appendix C.

 DavisPlus | For additional resources and information visit **davispl.us/medsurg5**

Nursing Care of Patients With Disorders of the Urinary System

MAUREEN McDONALD

LEARNING OUTCOMES

1. Explain the predisposing causes, symptoms, laboratory abnormalities, and treatment of urinary tract infections (UTIs).
2. Explain the predisposing causes, symptoms, treatment, and teaching for kidney stones.
3. List risk factors and signs and symptoms of cancer of the bladder.
4. List risk factors and signs and symptoms of cancer of the kidneys.
5. Discuss nursing care for a patient with an ileal conduit or continent reservoir.
6. Explain the pathophysiology and nursing care for diabetic nephropathy, nephrosclerosis, hydronephrosis, and glomerulonephritis.
7. Describe the signs and symptoms for patients with acute kidney injury.
8. Describe the signs and symptoms for patients with chronic kidney disease.
9. Plan nursing care for patients with acute kidney injury.
10. Plan nursing care for patients with chronic kidney disease.
11. Discuss nursing care for a vascular blood access site.
12. Plan nursing care for patients on hemodialysis.
13. Plan nursing care for patients on peritoneal dialysis.

KEY TERMS

anuria (an-YOO-ree-ah)
azotemia (AH-zoh-TEE-mee-ah)
calculi (KAL-kyoo-lye)
cystitis (siss-TYE-tiss)
glomerulonephritis (gloh-MURR-yoo-loh-neh-FRY-tiss)
hemodialysis (HEE-moh-dye-AH-lih-siss)
hydronephrosis (HYE-droh-neh-FROH-siss)
nephrectomy (neh-FREK-tuh-mee)
nephrolithotomy (NEH-froh-lih-THAW-tuh-mee)
nephropathy (neh-FROP-uh-thee)
nephrosclerosis (NEH-froh-skleh-ROH-siss)
nephrostomy (neh-FRAW-stoh-mee)
nephrotoxin (NEH-froh-TOK-sin)
oliguria (AW-lih-GYOO-ree-ah)
peritoneal dialysis (PEAR-ih-toh-NEE-uhl dye-AL-ih-siss)
polyuria (PAW-lee-YOOR-ee-ah)
pyelonephritis (PYE-eh-loh-neh-FRY-tiss)
stent (STENT)
uremia (yoo-REE-mee-ah)
urethritis (YOO-reh-THRYE-tiss)
urethroplasty (yoo-REE-throw-PLAS-tee)
urosepsis (YOO-roh-SEP-siss)

Disorders of the urinary tract include a variety of problems involving the kidneys, ureters, bladder, and urethra. These problems may arise from infection, obstructions, cancer, hereditary disorders, and metabolic, traumatic, or chronic diseases. Some may lead to chronic kidney disease (CKD) if not treated or controlled. Infection may be found in three anatomic parts of the urinary tract: the urethra, resulting in urethritis; the bladder, with a diagnosis of cystitis; or the kidneys, with a diagnosis of pyelonephritis. When problems occur with the kidney, homeostasis of the body is affected.

 URINARY TRACT INFECTIONS

Urinary tract infection (UTI) refers to invasion of the urinary tract by bacteria. Normally, the urinary tract is sterile above the urethra. UTI is the second most common bacterial disease. In the hospital, UTIs are the most common hospital-acquired infection (HAI). Lower UTIs include urethritis, prostatitis, and cystitis. Upper UTIs include pyelonephritis and ureteritis. Infections may result in sepsis or CKD.

Risk Factors for Urinary Tract Infections

UTIs are caused most often by an ascending infection, starting at the external urinary meatus and progressing toward the bladder and kidneys. Most UTIs are caused by the bacterium *Escherichia coli,* which is commonly found in feces. Other less common pathogens include *Staphylococcus saprophyticus, Klebsiella* spp., and *Enterobacter.* Risk factors for UTI include (a) incomplete emptying of the bladder; (b) contamination in the perineal and urethral area; (c) instruments or tubes inserted into the urinary meatus; (d) reflux of urine because of faulty valves; previous UTIs; (e) anatomical and genetic aspects of females; (f) pregnancy and asymptomatic bacteriuria; and aging.

Incomplete Bladder Emptying

Stasis of urine in the bladder can result from obstruction or simply from not voiding frequently enough. Urine overdistends the bladder, decreasing the blood supply to the wall of the bladder, which keeps white blood cells (WBCs) from fighting contamination that may have entered the bladder. The standing urine then serves as a culture medium for bacterial growth. Incomplete emptying of the bladder prevents flushing out of the bacteria and allows bacteria to ascend to higher structures.

Contamination in Perineal and Urethral Areas

Contamination in the perineal and urethral areas can be from fecal soiling, from sexual intercourse in which bacteria are massaged into the urinary meatus, or from infection in the area, such as vaginitis, epididymitis, or prostatitis.

Instrumentation Infection

Having instruments or tubes inserted into the urinary meatus can cause infection. The most common cause of instrumentation infection is urinary catheterization. Bacteria ascend around or within the catheter, causing infection. Within 48 hours of catheter insertion, bacterial colonization begins.

Many patients develop a UTI within 2 weeks of placement of an indwelling urinary catheter.

Faulty Valves Causing Reflux of Urine

Faulty valves that do not maintain one-way flow can cause reflux of urine from the urethra to the bladder or the bladder to the ureter. Reflux can be congenital, or it may be acquired as a result of previous infections.

Previous Urinary Tract Infections

Previous UTIs are thought to provide a reservoir of persistent bacteria that cause reinfection. Incomplete bladder emptying can precipitate infections as well.

Female Anatomic and Genetic Differences

Women are more susceptible to UTIs than men because of the short length of the female urethra and its proximity to the anus and vagina. Some women with recurrent UTIs have a shorter mean distance from the urethra to anus. This can facilitate colonization of the urinary tract. Genetic factors have been found that may play a role in women who have a certain phenotype for developing UTIs.

Pregnancy

Pregnant women may have asymptomatic bacteriuria. Untreated, 40% to 50% will develop pyelonephritis. Pregnant women may be prone to infection with group B streptococci. Most commonly, infection occurs in the second and third trimesters.

Aging and the Urinary Tract

Older adults have an increased incidence of UTIs due to diminished immune function, diabetes, and neurogenic bladder which fails to completely empty. Aging increases the risk of lower UTIs and may also mask symptoms. UTI is the most common cause of acute bacterial sepsis in patients over age 65. Older men are predisposed to infection because an enlarged prostate obstructs urine flow. In older women, the decline in estrogen can also contribute to the risk of UTI.

 NURSING CARE TIP

When caring for a patient at risk for a catheter-related UTI, limit the use of a urinary catheter, use infection control procedures at all times, and discontinue the use of the catheter as soon as possible. Catheter-related UTI is a "never event"—that is, hospitals will not be paid by Medicare for the costs of care provided if this condition occurs during hospitalization.

• WORD • BUILDING •

urethritis: urethr—urethra (canal that discharges urine from bladder) + itis—inflammation
cystitis: cyst—closed sac containing fluid + itis—inflammation
pyelonephritis: pyelo—pelvis + nephr—kidney + itis—inflammation

Signs and Symptoms

UTIs are characterized by common symptoms of dysuria, urgency, frequency, incontinence, nocturia, hematuria, back pain, and cloudy, foul-smelling urine (Table 37.1). In the older adult, the most common presenting symptom of UTI is generalized fatigue. Atypical symptoms or a change in cognitive functioning, especially noted in patients without dementia, can be seen. A decline in mental status and fever in any patient with an indwelling catheter meets the diagnostic criteria for a UTI.

Types of Urinary Tract Infections

Urethritis

Urethritis is inflammation of the urethra that may result from a chemical irritant, bacterial infection, trauma, or exposure to a sexually transmitted infection (STI). Posttraumatic urethritis can occur with intermittent catheterization or instrumentation of the urethra. Bubble bath and bath salts are common urethral irritants and should not be used by anyone with a history of UTIs. Urethritis can also be caused by spermicidal agents. Gonorrhea and chlamydiosis are STIs that can cause urethritis in men. It is common to have some degree of urethritis in association with bladder or prostatic infections.

Symptoms of urethritis include urinary frequency, urgency, and dysuria. The male patient may have discharge from the penis. A urinalysis or urine culture is done to diagnose urethritis.

The treatment of urethritis is based on the cause. If it is a chemical irritant, it is avoided. If urethritis is caused by bacteria, an antibiotic is prescribed based on the results of a culture. Phenazopyridine (Pyridium), a urinary analgesic, is often used to treat dysuria. The patient should be forewarned that urine will turn orange while taking phenazopyridine. If urethritis was sexually transmitted, it is important that the sexual partner also be treated.

Cystitis

Cystitis is inflammation and infection of the bladder wall. It can be due to bacteria, viruses, fungi, or parasites. About 90% of UTIs are caused by *Escherichia coli*. In most cases, the causative organisms first grow in the perineal area and then ascend into the bladder.

Symptoms include dysuria, frequency, urgency, and cloudy urine. Cystitis acquired outside the hospital is diagnosed with a routine urinalysis collected as a midstream, clean-catch specimen. Changes seen in the urinalysis include cloudy urine and the presence of WBCs, bacteria, and sometimes red blood cells (RBCs) in the specimen. Nitrites are usually positive. Some laboratories also examine for leukocyte esterase, which is positive if infection is present in the urine. In complicated UTIs, such as one acquired in the hospital or a repeat infection, a urine culture and sensitivity should be done. Hospital-acquired UTIs are often caused by bacteria that are resistant to the usual antibiotics used for UTIs. A sensitivity test can identify which antibiotics will be effective against the offending organism.

Treatment of uncomplicated cystitis is most often a combination of sulfa medication, such as sulfamethoxazole and trimethoprim (Bactrim, Septra), or nitrofurantoin (Macrodantin).

Complicated cystitis is often treated with ciprofloxacin (Cipro). Other antibiotics may be prescribed depending on the results of the urine culture and sensitivity. Estrogen used as an intravaginal cream may prevent recurrent UTIs in postmenopausal women. The patient is told to finish all prescribed medications, force fluids unless contraindicated, and return for a follow-up urinalysis or culture after the antibiotic course is complete to ensure that the infection is gone.

Pyelonephritis

PATHOPHYSIOLOGY. **Pyelonephritis** is infection of the renal pelvis, tubules, and interstitial tissue of one or both kidneys. Pyelonephritis usually begins with colonization and infection of the lower urinary tract by means of the ascending urethral route. A preexisting condition is usually present, such as obstruction, strictures, stones, or vesicoureteral reflux. Risk factors include urological surgery, lymphatic infection, urinary stasis, and decreased immunity. Acute pyelonephritis begins in the renal medulla and spreads to the adjacent cortex.

Pathophysiology includes formation of small abscesses throughout the kidney and gross enlargement of the kidney. On occasion, kidney infection is caused by bacteria spreading

TABLE 37.1   URINARY TRACT INFECTION (URETHRITIS, CYSTITIS, PYELONEPHRITIS) SUMMARY

Signs and Symptoms	Urinary urgency, frequency, dysuria Flank pain, fever, chills, costovertebral tenderness Cloudy urine with casts, bacteria, and WBCs Urine positive for nitrites
Diagnostic Tests	Urinalysis culture greater than 100,000 bacteria Elevated WBCs Elevated sedimentation rate Increased neutrophils
Therapeutic Measures	Antibiotic therapy sensitive to organism cultured from urine Force fluids
Complications	Pyelonephritis Urosepsis CKD
Priority Nursing Diagnoses	*Pain* *Impaired Urinary Elimination: Frequency* *Ineffective Health Maintenance*

Note. CKD = chronic kidney disease; WBCs, white blood cells.

from a distant site through the bloodstream and entering the kidney through the glomerulus. **Urosepsis** is a severe infection of the urinary tract with systemic inflammatory response syndrome. Prompt diagnosis and treatment are essential to prevent septic shock and death.

SIGNS AND SYMPTOMS. Symptoms include fatigue, urgency, frequency, dysuria, flank pain, fever, and chills. Costovertebral tenderness on the right or left side (tenderness posteriorly at angle where rib and vertebrae join when struck gently with heel of examiner's closed fist), which is associated with renal disease, is noted. The urine is cloudy with increased WBCs, bacteria, casts, RBCs, and positive nitrites. In contrast to cystitis, the patient with pyelonephritis is much sicker and shows signs of systemic disease. In acutely ill patients, blood cultures may be obtained.

DIAGNOSTIC TESTS. Several tests are helpful to differentiate pyelonephritis from cystitis. With kidney infection, the urinalysis will show casts. Casts are microscopic particles formed in the kidney from abnormal constituents in the urine such as WBCs, RBCs, or pus. The urine specimen will have more than 100,000 colonies of bacteria per milliliter. The presence of casts always indicates a problem in the kidneys. The complete blood cell (CBC) count will show an elevated WBC count. There will also be an increase in sedimentation rate.

THERAPEUTIC MEASURES. Treatment of pyelonephritis includes administration of antibiotics based on the results of the culture and sensitivity (Table 37.2). With severe Gram-negative infections, the patient is hospitalized for intravenous (IV) antibiotics. The patient with acute pyelonephritis generally heals completely after treatment and has no lasting kidney damage.

COMPLICATIONS. Repeated kidney infections can result in scarring and loss of kidney function, leading to CKD.

Nursing Process for the Patient With a Urinary Tract Infection

Data Collection

Listen to the patient's concerns about the diagnosis. Ask about pain on urination, flank pain, or general symptoms of infection, such as fever, chills, and malaise. The patient's usual pattern of voiding and any urinary frequency, burning, or pain on urination is documented. Note presence of pain in the lower abdomen, flank, or costovertebral angle. Document the presence of a catheter, recent instrumentation, surgery, or other predisposing factors. Inspect the urine for volume, color, concentration, cloudiness, blood, or foul odor. Review urinalysis and culture results.

Nursing Diagnoses, Planning, and Implementation

Acute Pain *related to inflammation of the urethra, bladder, and other urinary structures*

EXPECTED OUTCOME: The patient will report relief from pain and discomfort.

- Administer antimicrobial therapy as ordered *to relieve pain and discomfort from inflammation and infection.*
- Administer antispasmodic agents as ordered *to relieve bladder irritability and pain.*

- Encourage fluids at 2 to 3 L per day *to flush bacteria from urinary tract and promote renal blood flow.*
- Apply heat to suprapubic area *to relieve discomfort.*
- Encourage voiding every 3 hours *to empty the bladder, lower bacterial counts, reduce stasis, and prevent reinfection.*
- Suggest consuming cranberry juice or capsules *to prevent bacteria from sticking on the walls of the bladder* (see "Evidence-Based Practice").
- Teach patient to finish all prescribed medications *to prevent recurrent infection.*
- Teach patient to avoid cola, coffee, tea, and alcohol *because they are urinary irritants.*
- Teach patient to empty bladder as soon as urge is felt and after sexual intercourse *to flush bacteria out of the body.*
- Teach patient to avoid substances such as bubble bath and scented toilet paper, *which can be irritants.*
- Teach patient to wear cotton underwear *to reduce perineal moisture.*

EVIDENCE-BASED PRACTICE

Clinical Question
Do cranberries or cranberry juice prevent UTI?

Evidence
In a systematic review of studies that compared the use of cranberries containing products to prevent UTI with placebo or nonplacebo controls, it was found that cranberry-containing products are associated with a protective effect against UTIs. Cranberries contain a substance that can prevent bacteria from sticking on the walls of the bladder. Other compounds found in cranberries inhibit the adherence of *E. coli* to the urogenital mucosa (Wang et al, 2012). It was also found that cranberries are effective in reducing the annual number of UTI episodes by 63.9% in clients after renal transplantation (Pagonas et al, 2012).

Implications for Nursing Practice
Teach patients that cranberry products might help prevent recurrent UTI.

REFERENCE
Pagonas, N., Hörstrup, J., Schmidt, D., Benz, P., Schindler, R., Reinke, P., . . . Westhoff, T. H. (2012). Prophylaxis of recurrent urinary tract infection after renal transplantation by cranberry juice and L-methionine. *Transplant Proceedings, 44,* 3017–3021.

Wang, C., Fang, C. C., Chen, N. C., Liu, S. S., Yu, P. H., Wu, T. Y., . . . Chen, W. T. (2012). Cranberry-containing products for prevention of urinary tract infections in susceptible populations. *Archives of Internal Medicine, 172,* 988–996.

• WORD • BUILDING •
urosepsis: uro—urine + sepsis—infection in the blood

TABLE 37.2   MEDICATIONS USED TO TREAT URINARY TRACT INFECTIONS

Medication Class/Action	Example	Nursing Considerations
Antibiotics Effective against *Escherichia coli*, *Klebsiella* spp., *Serratia*	aztreonam (Azactam)	Contraindicated in patients allergic to penicillins and cephalosporins or if creatinine clearance is less than 30 mL/min. Check blood urea nitrogen and creatinine before administration.
Effective against *E. coli* and *Enterococcus faecalis*	fosfomycin (Monurol)	Dissolve packet in 3–4 oz of cold water.
Effective against *E. coli*, enterococci, *Staphylococcus aureus*, *Klebsiella* spp., and *Enterobacter.*	nitrofurantoin (Macrobid, Macrodantin)	Give with food or milk and full glass of water. Avoid antacids.
Fluoroquinolones Effective against *E. coli*, *Klebsiella* spp., *Pseudomonas,* and other organisms.	ciprofloxacin (Cipro) levofloxacin (Levaquin)	Absorption may be decreased if given within 2 hr of aluminum antacids. Give with large amounts of water. Teach to avoid sunlight and report tendon aches promptly.
Sulfonamides Effective against *E. coli* and *Pseudomonas.* Used for uncomplicated UTIs.	trimethoprim-sulfamethoxazole (Bactrim, Septra)	Teach to avoid sunlight. Give with large amounts of water. Contraindicated in severe renal or liver disease.
Urinary Antiseptic Antibacterial action in the urine; not systemic. Effective against *E. coli*, *Klebsiella* spp., and other Gram-negative organisms.	cinoxacin (Cinobac)	Teach to avoid sunlight. Encourage fluids. May discolor urine. Absorption may be decreased if given within 2 hr of aluminum or magnesium antacids.
Urinary Analgesic Topical analgesic. Relieves pain urgency and frequency associated with UTI.	phenazopyridine (Pyridium)	Urine color changes to red-orange. Avoid in renal insufficiency. Changes urine glucose testing.

Impaired Urinary Elimination related to frequency, nocturia, dysuria, and incontinence

EXPECTED OUTCOME: The patient will return to previous voiding patterns.

- Monitor urinary elimination, including frequency, consistency, volume, and color, *to identify signs and symptoms of UTI.*
- Administer antimicrobial drugs as ordered *to eliminate symptoms produced by microbial growth.*
- Encourage adequate fluids *to prevent infection and dehydration.*
- Encourage women to void after sexual intercourse *to flush bacteria out of the urethra.*
- Teach patient to recognize signs and symptoms of UTI *to monitor effectiveness of treatment and detect recurrence.*

Risk for Injury related to sepsis, kidney disease, or kidney injury

EXPECTED OUTCOME: The patient will be free from injury due to sepsis or recurrent infection.

- Administer antimicrobial drugs as prescribed *to prevent recurrent infection or complications.*
- Monitor intake and output *to ensure adequate intake and normal output.*
- Monitor patient for signs and symptoms of bacteriuria and bacteremia such as fever, chills, recurrent pain.
- Explain need for follow-up urine culture and imaging studies *when indicated by recurrent symptoms.*
- Teach need for adequate fluid intake *to prevent dehydration and renal impairment.*
- Teach signs and symptoms of UTI *so patient can detect recurrence or complications.*

Evaluation

The outcomes have been met if the patient verbalizes relief of pain and discomfort, returns to previous voiding patterns, and is free from injury related to sepsis, CKD, or recurrent infection.

CRITICAL THINKING

Mrs. Milan

■ Mrs. Milan is a 25-year-old woman who recently had a 3-day weekend getaway with her husband. On Monday she notices that she has symptoms of dysuria, frequency, and urgency. She visits her health care provider (HCP) and is diagnosed with a UTI. She is placed on an antibiotic.

1. What do you think could have predisposed Mrs. Milan to developing a UTI?
2. What should Mrs. Milan be taught to prevent further occurrences of a UTI?
3. What urinalysis findings would you expect for Mrs. Milan?
4. What should you include in her teaching plan based on her therapeutic regimen?

Suggested answers are at the end of the chapter.

Patient Education

It is very important that patients be advised to take the entire prescribed antibiotic until it is gone. It is not uncommon for patients to take medication for several days until symptoms are gone, and then stop. Stopping the antibiotic too early allows the infection to continue. It may become chronic and resistant to antibiotics as a result. In addition to encouraging fluids, cranberry products may be helpful.

Patients who have one UTI commonly develop repeat infections. It is important that such patients receive education to prevent repeated infections of the urinary tract (Box 37-1 and "Nutrition Notes").

Nutrition Notes

Urinary Tract Infections

An effective intervention for UTI is increasing fluid intake, both for its flushing effect and to excrete urinary drugs. Instructions to increase fluid intake should specify amounts to consume or the amount of urine to be produced. Patients have developed electrolyte imbalances by overenthusiastically forcing fluids.

Box 37-1 **Patient Education**

Preventing Urinary Tract Infection

1. Void frequently—at least every 3 hours while awake.
2. Drink up to 3000 mL of fluid a day if there are no fluid restrictions from the HCP. Preferably drink water.
3. Drink one glass of cranberry juice (10 oz) per day.
4. Take showers; avoid tub baths.
5. Wipe perineum from the front to the back after toileting.
6. Urinate after sexual intercourse.
7. Avoid bubble bath and bath salts, perfumed feminine hygiene products, synthetic underwear, and constricting clothing such as tight jeans.
8. Take medication prescribed for urinary tract infection (UTI) until it is all gone.
9. If UTI is associated with another source of infection, such as vaginitis or prostatitis, ensure that both infections are treated.

UROLOGICAL OBSTRUCTIONS

Urinary tract obstruction is an interference with the flow of urine at any location along the urinary system. It is always a significant problem. The obstruction of urine flow causes dilation and thinning of the renal tubules with eventual atrophy of renal tissues. Renal blood flow is compromised. Eventually renal tissue is destroyed by the compression.

Urethral Strictures

A urethral stricture is a narrowing of the lumen of the urethra caused by scar tissue. Urethral strictures are becoming more prevalent due to the rising incidence of STIs in young adults. Most strictures are acquired from injury or infection. Some strictures are a result of trauma from insertion of catheters or surgical instruments, untreated gonorrhea, and congenital abnormalities.

The patient with a urethral stricture has a diminished urinary stream and is prone to developing UTIs because of obstruction of urine flow. Urethral strictures are often seen in older men. The problem becomes more apparent when attempts to insert a urinary catheter are unsuccessful because of the narrowed lumen.

Initially the treatment of a urethral stricture is mechanical dilation by the urologist, who inserts instruments to stretch open the urethra and then inserts a urinary catheter. If the stricture continues to be a problem after dilation, the area can be surgically repaired (**urethroplasty**) and a stent inserted.

• WORD • BUILDING •
urethroplasty: urethro—urethra + plasty—surgical repair

The dilation process can be done at the bedside. This is a painful experience for the patient, and it is helpful and caring to administer pain medication before the procedure. The nursing diagnosis of *Acute Pain* is very relevant. An indwelling catheter is typically inserted after the dilation, so the nursing diagnosis of *Risk for Infection* is also present. Patients are taught about UTI prevention (see Box 37-1).

Renal Calculi

Renal **calculi** (kidney stones; one stone is a *calculus*) are hard, usually small stones that form somewhere in the renal structures (Table 37.3). The stones are masses of crystals and protein that form when the urine becomes supersaturated with a salt capable of forming solid crystals. Diet and lifestyle can account for the prevalence of stones in some patients. Symptoms occur when the stones become impacted in the urinary tract. When stones are found in the kidneys, the condition is called nephrolithiasis (Fig. 37.1).

Pathophysiology

Normally, substances dissolved in urine, including urinary salts, are diluted and readily excreted from the body. Calculi are formed when urinary salts are concentrated enough to settle out; the salts often collect and deposit around a nucleus (see Table 37.3). Substances that can serve as a nucleus include pus, blood, dead tissue, a catheter, and crystals. Stones usually grow on the papillae or in the renal tubules, calyces, or renal pelvis. Stones may also form in the ureter or bladder. Stones less than 5 mm are readily passed in the urine.

Etiology

Causes of calculi formation include a family history of stones, chronic dehydration (causing more concentrated urinary salts), and infection, because the latter provides a nucleus for stone formation. Additional contributing causes of calcium stones include dietary factors ("Nutrition Notes") and medications (Table 37.4). Excessive amounts of calcium in the water in some geographic areas may also be a factor. Immobility causes stone formation because of the resulting urinary stasis; in addition, calcium leaves the unstressed bones during immobility, so more calcium is in the blood, which is then filtered through the kidneys. Stones are more common in men than women. A diet high in sodium and animal protein increases the amount of calcium in the urine (hypercalciuria)

TABLE 37.3   OVERVIEW OF RENAL CALCULI

Type of Stone	Features	Possible Causes	Interventions
Calcium oxalate, calcium phosphate, or mixture	Accounts for two-thirds of stones Small, rough, and hard Shaped like needles Colors vary from gray to white	Excessive calcium Excessive urea Hyperparathyroidism, Cushing's disease, immobility, osteolysis from tumors of the breast, lung	Force fluids. Restrict protein and sodium in the diet. Administer hydrochlorothiazide. Treat hyperparathyroidism. Cellulose sodium phosphate (Calcibind) may prevent calcium stones by binding calcium from food in the GI system.
Struvite—magnesium ammonium phosphate	Calculi crumble easily Stones have a yellow color	Infection by urea splitting microbes, usually *Proteus*. May cause abscess formation in the kidney.	Force fluids. Decrease urine pH. Administer antibiotics.
Uric acid stones	Dye enhancement needed for x-ray visualization Small Color varies from yellow to red Hard	Gout High uric acid levels Decreased fluid intake	Force fluids. Administer sodium citrate to alkalinize urine. Administer allopurinol to reduce urinary uric acid levels. Low-purine diet. Avoid shellfish, anchovies, asparagus, organ meats, and mushrooms.
Cystine stones	Small, smooth calculi Smooth, waxy stones	Cystine-containing crystals appear in the urine	Force fluids. Use low-protein diet; urine is alkalinized. Give penicillamine to decrease amount of cystine in urine.

FIGURE 37.1 Location of calculi in the urinary tract.

TABLE 37.4 MEDICATIONS AFFECTING STONE FORMATION

Acetazolamide (Diamox)	Decreases urinary citrates and increases uric acid concentration in urine.
Adrenocorticosteroids	Increases urinary calcium.
Allopurinol	Used to prevent uric acid calculi. May cause the rarer xanthine calculi.
Antacids such as magnesium trisilicate (Gaviscon)	May cause rare silicon-based calculi. Phosphate binding nonabsorbable antacids can increase urinary calcium.
Aspirin	Increases urinary uric acid levels in patients with hyperuricemia.
Chemotherapeutic agents and external radiation	May cause cellular breakdown and cause acute hyperuricemia.
Hydrochlorothiazide (used to prevent calcium calculi)	May cause uric acid calculi by increasing urinary uric acid levels.
Furosemide (Lasix)	May cause hyperuricemia.
Vitamin C in large doses	Increases oxalate excretion in urine.
Vitamin D	Increases calcium and oxalate excretion in urine.

and may contribute to the formation of stones. The risk peaks between ages 30 and 50.

Signs and Symptoms

Symptoms of renal calculi include excruciating flank pain and renal colic. When a stone is lodged in the ureter, it is common to have pain radiate down to the genitalia. The pain results when the stone prevents urine from draining. Additional symptoms include hematuria from irritation by the stone, dysuria, frequency, urgency, and enuresis. The patient also may have costovertebral tenderness. Some people develop nausea, vomiting, and diarrhea because of the proximity of the GI structures. Table 37.5 summarized the discussion of renal calculi.

Prevention

Consult with the HCP and dietitian to determine if any foods should be avoided, depending on the type of stone found. "Nutrition Notes: Renal Calculi" discusses foods that may contribute to calculi development (see also "Cultural Considerations"). Encourage fluid intake to prevent dehydration. Encourage the patient to walk, which promotes the excretion of stones and reduces bone calcium resorption (release). Urocit(r)-K (potassium citrate), which restores chemicals in the urine that prevent crystals from forming to decrease calcium oxalate and uric acid stones, might be prescribed.

Complications

The presence of renal calculi increases the risk for UTIs because of obstruction of the free flow of urine. Untreated obstruction of a stone in a ureter or the urethra can also result

Nutrition Notes

Renal Calculi

Concentrated urine enhances the formation of crystals, so sufficient fluid should be consumed to produce 2000 mL of urine per day. About 3000 mL or 13 cups of water per day are needed to produce this amount of urine.

About 80% of kidney stones are composed of calcium oxalate, which led to early prescriptions for low-calcium diets, but it was later found that a high-calcium intake binds dietary oxalate in the gastrointestinal (GI) tract and prevents its absorption, thereby reducing urinary oxalate formation. If a low-oxalate diet is prescribed, a long list of foods may be restricted beginning with spinach, rhubarb, beets, nuts, chocolate, tea, wheat bran, and strawberries.

Uric acid kidney stones can be a complication of gout, which is a disorder of purine metabolism. Purines are end products of digestion of certain proteins and are present in some medications. High-purine foods include organ meats, anchovies, herring, sardines, meat extracts, consommé, and gravies.

Cultural Considerations

Recurrent Calculus Development

Filipino immigrants are at high risk for developing renal stones, hyperuricemia, and gout. A shift from a traditional Filipino diet to an American diet increases the occurrence of hyperuricemia, with some older Filipinos developing gout. The nurse may need to assist Filipino patients to identify food choices that will help prevent these conditions.

    Caucasians have the highest incidence of kidney stones, followed by Mexican Americans. African Americans have the lowest risk. Prevalence of stones is increased in the southern United States and lowest in the western United States.

TABLE 37.5   RENAL CALCULI SUMMARY

Signs and Symptoms	Costovertebral angle pain Groin pain Renal colic Flank pain radiating to genitalia Hematuria Anuria Restlessness Pallor Temperature Diminished or absent bowel sounds with ileus
Diagnostic Tests	Urinalysis Crystals and urine pH 24-hour renal creatinine clearance BUN Creatinine KUB—reveals most calculi Retrograde pyelography Ultrasound
Therapeutic Measures	Treat pain Chemolysis—stone dissolution using infusions of chemicals to dissolve stone Lithotripsy Surgery—Nephrolithotomy Pyelolithotomy Percutaneous nephrostomy tube
Complications	Shock Sepsis Hydronephrosis Hydroureter CKD
Priority Nursing Diagnoses	*Acute Pain* *Risk for Infection* *Deficient Knowledge*

Note. BUN = blood urea nitrogen; CKD = chronic kidney disease; KUB = kidney, ureter, and bladder x-ray.

in retention of urine and damage to the kidney. This process is called **hydronephrosis** (discussed later).

Diagnostic Tests

Helical computed tomography (CT) without contrast is the preferred diagnostic test. It requires no contrast agent and has the ability to detect stones in the distal ureters as well as small stones less than 1 to 2 mm. Other tests include an abdominal x-ray or an IV pyelogram, which will identify the anatomic location of the stone. Renal ultrasound may be done to identify a stone in the renal pelvis, calyx, or ureter. This is the preferred test for pregnant women suspected of having a kidney stone. Urinalysis may indicate gross or microscopic hematuria and could indicate abrasion of the urinary tract. The presence of crystals or urinary pH may indicate calculus type. Two consecutive 24-hour urine collections should be done while the patient follows his or her usual diet. The 24-hour urine collection should measure total urine volume, calcium, oxalate, citrate, uric acid, sodium, potassium, phosphorus, pH, and creatinine as well as cystine and magnesium.

Therapeutic Measures

Renal calculi are treated medically if possible. Most small stones are flushed out of the body during urination. Patients can pass stones in the urine if they are 5 mm or smaller. Drinking 2 to 3 quarts of fluids, taking analgesics such as Tylenol or ibuprofen, and perhaps a prescribed alpha-blocker medication (such as tamsulosin [Flomax]) to relax ureter muscles will help pass a small stone.

    Patients who develop severe renal colic are usually admitted to the hospital. IV fluids are given to hydrate the patient and help flush the stone out of the body. All urine is strained to detect passage of stones, and pain medication is given. If the patient is unable to pass the stone and infection, impaired renal function, or severe pain continues, intervention is needed. The solubility of stone-forming substances can be changed by altering the pH of the urine. Calcium stones may be treated with thiazide diuretics and allopurinol (Aloprim,

• WORD • BUILDING •

hydronephrosis: hydro—pertaining to water + nephrosis—degenerative change in kidney

Zyloprim). Surgical removal may be required for large stones, obstructions, or intractable pain.

LITHOTRIPSY. Lithotripsy is the use of sound, laser, or dry shock-wave energies to break the stone into small fragments. Types of lithotripsy include extracorporeal shock-wave lithotripsy (ESWL), electrohydraulic lithotripsy, laser lithotripsy, and percutaneous ultrasonic lithotripsy.

With ESWL, a form of lithotripsy, sedated or anesthetized patients lie down on the lithotriptor with a water-filled device supporting their back. Ultrasonic shock waves are used to break up the stone into sand particles, which are then urinated out over a week with small discomfort or be small enough to be removed. Some lithotripsy procedures do not require submersion and use other means of initiating shock waves (Fig. 37.2). Occasionally, a stent is placed in the ureter to facilitate the passage of the stone fragments. After the procedure, the patient is usually discharged home after being told to increase fluid intake to help flush the sand particles out, strain the urine to catch stone fragments for analysis, and notify the urologist if there are any problems. Blood in the urine is common after lithotripsy. ESWL is most effective with stones that are in the kidney. ESWL may increase the risk of kidney disease or hypertension later in life.

SURGERY FOR RENAL CALCULI. Some patients may need surgery for stone removal. The particular procedure chosen—endoscopic or open surgery—depends on the location of the stone.

Endoscopic procedures for the bladder include cystoscopy for small stones and cystolitholapaxy for larger stones. For cystolitholapaxy, an instrument is inserted through the urethra to the bladder to crush the stone. The stone is then washed out with an irrigating solution. If the stone is lodged in a ureter, the urologist may insert an instrument into the ureter through a cystoscope to crush the stone or use an ultrasonic lithotripsy instrument to break the stone into fragments. Postoperative care following these procedures is similar to care following any cystoscopy (see Chapter 36). The open surgery procedure for stones in the bladder is a cystotomy and for the ureter an ureterolithotomy.

For kidney stones, a percutaneous **nephrolithotomy** is performed in which a scope is inserted through the skin into the kidney to aid in breaking up the stone and to irrigate the renal pelvis. A nephrostomy tube is often left in place at first to prevent stone fragments from passing through the urinary system. If the stone is very large, a nephrolithotomy may be needed, which involves a surgical incision into the kidney to remove the stone. A pyelolithotomy is done to remove stones lodged in the renal pelvis.

Nursing Process for the Patient With Renal Calculi

DATA COLLECTION. Patients with stones are often in extreme pain and should be monitored for pain. Patients over age 60 should have an abdominal aneurysm ruled out. A health history may identify a family or patient history of previous stone formation. People who have had stones usually have a recurrence. Why would renal colic usually begin suddenly, progress rapidly, and peak over a 30-minute period? Because it occurs as urine attempts to pass the stone. Flank pain may radiate to the genitals. Diminished or absent bowel sounds may progress to an ileus. The patient may also be restless, pale, and lightheaded.

Nursing care of a patient with a renal calculus involves careful measurement of intake and output and observation of urine for abnormalities such as hematuria, pyuria, or passage of a stone. Obstruction may occur at the bladder neck or urethra. With obstruction, **anuria** (less than 50 mL of urine output daily) or **oliguria** (less than 400 mL of urine output daily) is noted. This is an emergency situation and must be treated immediately to preserve kidney function. Temperature is monitored for onset of fever, which would indicate infection.

• WORD • BUILDING •

lithotripsy: litho-stones + tripso-breaking stones
nephrolithotomy: nephro—kidney + lith—stone + otomy—incision
anuria: an—without + uria—urine
oliguria: olig—small + uria—urine

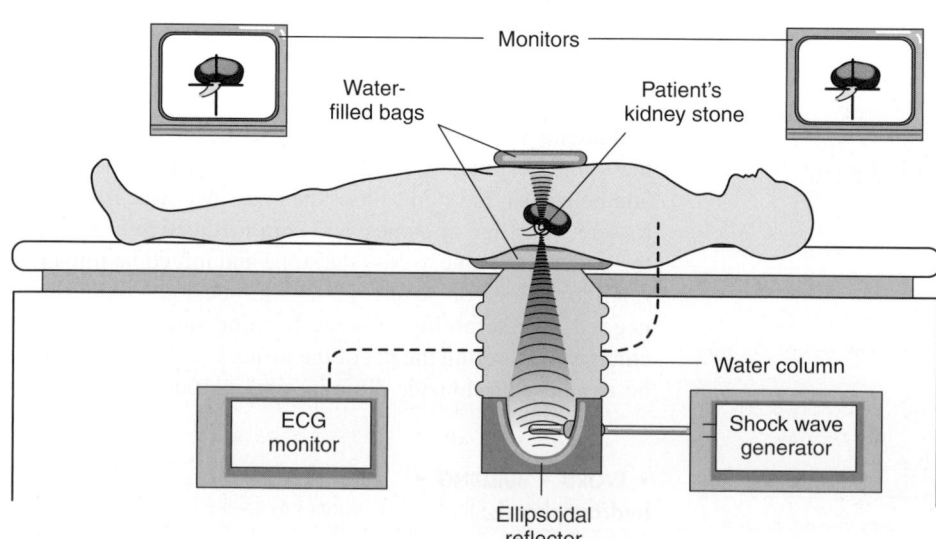

FIGURE 37.2 Extracorporeal shock-wave lithotripsy.

Blood pressure may decrease if severe pain causes shock. A special strainer is used to strain all urine for stones. If a stone is found, it is saved for analysis in the laboratory. The patient is also asked about a recent history of infection, diet or activity changes, or other risk factors for renal calculi. If the cause can be identified, teaching can be done to help prevent recurrent calculi.

NURSING DIAGNOSIS, PLANNING, AND IMPLEMENTATION.
Acute Pain related to the presence of, obstruction, or movement of a stone within the urinary system
EXPECTED OUTCOME: The patient will verbalize the relief of pain or ability to tolerate pain.

- Ask severity, location, and duration of pain using a pain scale. *Pain is typically in the flank or costovertebral angle and may radiate to the pelvic, groin, or abdominal area.*
- Monitor patency of drains, and catheters. *Obstruction of urine flow will increase pain.*
- Encourage fluid intake, unless contraindicated, *to promote the passage of stone, dilute the urine, and reduce the risk of further stone formation.*
- Administer pain medication as ordered *to promote comfort.*
- Apply heat to flank area *to reduce pain and promote comfort.*
- Ambulate if possible *to facilitate the passage of the stone through the urinary system.*
- Strain urine through gauze or strainer *to identify stones that may have been passed providing pain relief.*

Risk for Infection related to the introduction of bacteria from obstructed urinary flow and instrumentation
EXPECTED OUTCOME: The patient will remain infection free.

- Monitor vital signs, and observe for chills, cloudy, foul-smelling urine, or bleeding. *Abnormalities may indicate an infection.*
- Monitor urine amount, color, clarity, and odor *to ensure patency of urinary system or tubes. Foul-smelling or cloudy urine may indicate an infection.*
- Encourage fluid intake *to flush bacteria and stones and prevent further stone formation.*

Deficient Knowledge related to lack of knowledge about prevention of recurrence, diet, and symptoms of renal calculi
EXPECTED OUTCOME: The patient will verbalize an understanding of the factors related to the recurrence of renal calculi, infection, and treatment options.

- Note recurrence of renal stones. *Recurrence may indicate knowledge deficit.*
- Note family history of renal stones and explain relevance to patient. *Stones have a higher incidence in patients with a positive family history.*
- Determine the relationship between activity and stones. *Sedentary lifestyle or limited mobility may increase risk of stone formation.*
- Ask the patient's understanding of possible courses of therapy to treat renal stones *to establish baseline knowledge.*
- Teach the importance of maintaining a fluid intake of 2 to 3 quarts per day. *Low-solute (dilute) urine helps prevents stone formation.*

- Teach patient about medications used to prevent recurrence of renal stones:
  - *Diuretics (thiazide type) increase tubular reabsorption of calcium, making it less available for calculi formation in the urinary tract.*
  - *Allopurinol (Zyloprim) reduces uric acid production.*
  - *Antibiotics prevent chronic UTI, which may precede renal calculus formation.*
- As applicable, teach patient about management of stones. *Most stones pass spontaneously. There may be pain, nausea, and vomiting. Medical management consists of fluids, pain management, and antibiotics. Mechanical interventions with percutaneous catheters and nephroscopic procedures, lithotripsy, or surgery can be used to eliminate stones.*
- Teach patient to strain all urine. *Stone fragments may continue to pass for weeks after stone crushing or lithotripsy.*
- Teach patient to report signs of infection, pain not relieved by medication, nausea, chills, or the appearance of foul-smelling urine *for treatment.*

EVALUATION. Outcomes have been achieved if the patient remains comfortable, free from infection, and gains understanding about prevention of the reoccurrence of renal stones.

Hydronephrosis

Hydronephrosis is distention of the renal pelvis and calices. This condition results from untreated obstruction of urine flow in the urinary tract. The kidney enlarges as urine collects in the pelvis and kidney tissue. Hydronephrosis is usually treatable once the condition is detected.

Obstruction of urine flow can result from a stricture in a ureter or the urethra, kidney stones, a tumor, or an enlarged prostate. Because of the unrelieved obstruction, urine backs up and distends the ureters and then progresses to the kidney (Fig. 37.3). The capacity of the renal pelvis is normally 5 to 8 mL. Obstruction in the renal pelvis quickly distends it. Kidney pressure increases as the volume of urine increases. This enlargement of the kidney can be either unilateral or bilateral. Unrelieved pressure on the kidneys from urine causes the kidneys to become sacs filled with urine instead of functioning kidneys. Sometimes, in a matter of hours, the blood vessels and renal tubules can be damaged extensively.

If the onset of obstruction is gradual, the patient initially may be asymptomatic. Patients commonly develop UTIs because of the obstruction of urine flow and may have symptoms of frequency, urgency, and dysuria. As the disease progresses, flank and back pain may occur. Eventually the patient develops symptoms of CKD (discussed later).

Treatment of hydronephrosis always involves relieving the obstruction. Initial removal of the obstruction may be done by insertion of an indwelling urinary catheter. Long-term correction depends on the cause and includes treatments and surgeries to relieve obstruction from strictures, stones, tumor, or an enlarged prostate. At times, the obstruction cannot be relieved because a stone is too large or removal of tumor growth would result in the patient's death. In these situations, **stents**, which are tiny tubes, may be placed inside the ureters during

FIGURE 37.3 Hydronephrosis. Progressive thickening of bladder wall and dilation of ureters and kidneys results from obstruction of urine flow.

a cystoscopy and pyelogram (C&P) to hold the ureters open, or a **nephrostomy** tube may be inserted directly into the kidney pelvis to drain urine. A nephrostomy tube exits through an incision in the flank area and allows urine to drain into a collecting bag so that function of the kidney can be maintained. Figure 37.4 shows a stent in place in a ureter and a nephrostomy tube.

Complications associated with hydronephrosis include increased incidence of UTIs because of obstruction of urine flow and kidney failure from unrelieved pressure on the kidneys.

Intake and output are carefully measured. Urine retention can worsen the condition and must be recognized and reported promptly. If the patient has a nephrostomy tube, ensure that it is draining adequately and prevent kinking or clamping of the tube. Kinking of the tube results in continuation of the hydronephrosis, and the resulting pressure will destroy kidney function. If both a nephrostomy tube and urinary catheter are present, output from each should be measured and documented separately.

TUMORS OF THE RENAL SYSTEM

Cancer of the Bladder

Cancer of the bladder is the most common kind of cancer of the urinary tract. It is most common in men, with the average age being 73. It is more common in Caucasians than in African Americans. The incidence of bladder cancer has been rising in the United States, and the American Cancer Society (ACS) estimates that more than 72,570 new cases of bladder cancer occurred in 2013.

Pathophysiology

Cancer of the bladder often starts as a benign growth on the bladder wall that undergoes cancerous changes. Most bladder cancers begin in the inner lining of the bladder called the

urothelium. They are called transition cell cancers. They come in a variety of forms and can behave in different ways. Some occur as small wartlike growths on the inside of the bladder. Others form large tumors that grow into the muscle wall of the bladder and require surgical removal. If the cancer affects only the inner lining of the bladder, it is known as a superficial cancer. If it has spread to the muscle wall, it is called an invasive cancer. Common sites for metastasis include the liver, bones, and lungs.

Etiology

There is a strong correlation between cigarette smoking and bladder cancer. Those who smoke get bladder cancer twice as often as people who do not smoke. Specific chemicals that cause bladder cancer have been found in cigarette smoke. The more cigarettes smoked, the greater the risk. The lung absorbs the chemicals from tobacco. These chemicals are then passed via the bloodstream to the kidneys and collected in the urine. From there, they accumulate in the urine and damage the cells that line the bladder. Exposure to industrial pollution such as aniline dyes, benzidine and naphthylamine, leather finishings, metal machinery, and petroleum processing products also increases the incidence. It can take about 25 years after exposure to chemicals for bladder cancer to develop. Bladder cancer is often diagnosed at a later stage in women.

Signs and Symptoms

Cancer of the bladder usually causes painless hematuria. The patient may notice that the urine is darker or more reddish in color than usual. Blood in the urine is one of the ACS's seven warning signs of cancer. Initially the bleeding is intermittent,

---

• **WORD** • **BUILDING** •

nephrostomy: nephr—pertaining to the kidney + ostomy— surgically formed artificial opening to the outside

B   **Posterior view**

FIGURE 37.4 (A) Ureteral stents. (B) Nephrostomy tube inserted into renal pelvis; catheter exits through an incision on flank.

which often causes the patient to delay seeking treatment. As the disease progresses, the patient develops frank hematuria, bladder irritability, urine retention from clots obstructing the urethra, and fistula formation (an opening between the bladder and an adjoining structure such as the vagina or bowel). Other common signs and symptoms of bladder cancer include pelvic pain, pain in the lower back, painful urination, changes in bladder habits, and inability to void.

Diagnostic Tests

Routine urinalysis can detect evidence of bladder cancer. A urine test for the enzyme telomerase has been found to be 90% accurate in detecting bladder cancer in early and late stages. Urine for cytology can be obtained to determine if cancer cells are present in the urine. Urine culture should also be done. Symptoms of bladder infection may be similar to those of bladder cancer. Diagnosis of bladder cancer may also

be made with cystoscopy and transurethral biopsy. An IV pyelogram or CT scan also may be done.

Therapeutic Measures

Treatment depends on the type and staging (severity) of the bladder cancer. For small, confined tumors, chemotherapeutic agents are instilled into the bladder through a urinary catheter, allowed to dwell, and then removed along with the catheter. Systemic chemotherapy is also used and can be helpful to prolong life when other treatments are no longer indicated. The bacille Calmette-Guérin vaccine may be instilled into the bladder to prevent recurring tumors.

Photodynamic therapy, in which drugs are given that make tumors sensitive to light, may be used. When light is applied to the tumor area, cancer cells are killed.

Surgical treatment of bladder cancer includes a number of procedures. A cystoscopy and pyelogram with fulguration (destruction of tissue with electrical current) may be done to burn off cancerous tissue. An alternate method is use of a laser to destroy tumor tissue. Partial cystectomy can be done for cancer limited to one area. Advances in surgical techniques involve robotic and laparoscopic techniques. If the bladder requires removal, robotic laparoscopic radical cystectomy with urinary diversion is an option. In this procedure, robotic surgical equipment, which imitates surgical movements guided by the surgeon, allows more precision, steadiness, and maneuverability than manual surgery, as well as the use of small openings rather than larger incisions into the abdomen. Recovery time is reduced as a result.

INCONTINENT URINARY DIVERSION. If the patient has a potentially curable disease with significant bladder involvement, complete removal of the bladder and creation of a urinary diversion may be done. A urinary diversion means that urine leaves the body in a different manner. A common surgery for urinary diversion is called an ileal conduit, an involved surgery in which a 6- to 8-inch section of the ileum or colon is removed and used as a conduit for urine. The remaining portions of the bowel are stitched back together. The surgeon is careful to keep the blood and neurologic supply intact to the section of bowel that has been removed. The isolated section of bowel is closed off on one end, the ureters are stitched into it, and the other end is brought out as a stoma on the abdomen (urostomy) that almost continuously drains urine (Fig. 37.5). The urine from an ileal conduit contains mucus because it comes through the ileum, which normally secretes mucus. The patient must wear an ostomy appliance at all times over the stoma to collect urine. Box 37-2 explains how to apply an appliance to an ileal conduit stoma.

CONTINENT URINARY DIVERSION. Continent urinary diversion surgeries are being done for patient convenience. One version is the Kock pouch (continent internal ileal reservoir), which is created from a segment of ileum that has been made into a reservoir for urine (see Fig. 37.5B). The ureters are implanted into the side of the reservoir. A special nipple valve is constructed and is the passageway through which the patient inserts a catheter at 4- to 6-hour intervals

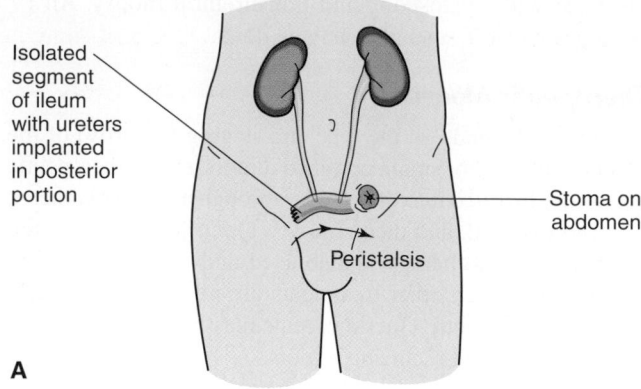

Isolated segment of ileum with ureters implanted in posterior portion

Stoma on abdomen

Peristalsis

A

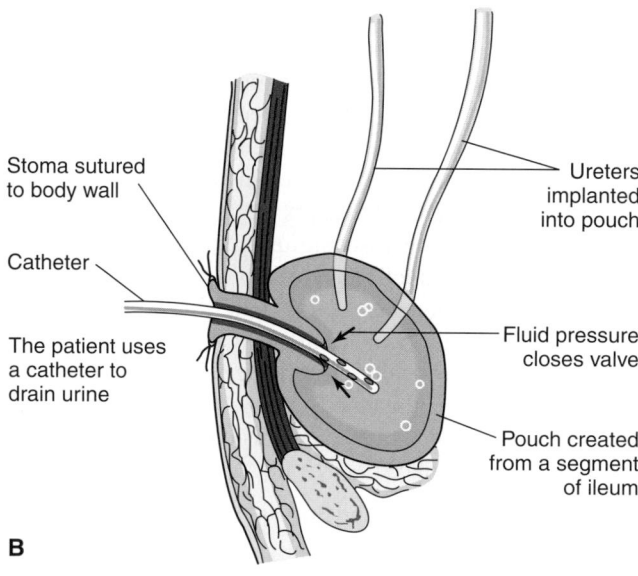

Stoma sutured to body wall

Catheter

The patient uses a catheter to drain urine

Ureters implanted into pouch

Fluid pressure closes valve

Pouch created from a segment of ileum

B

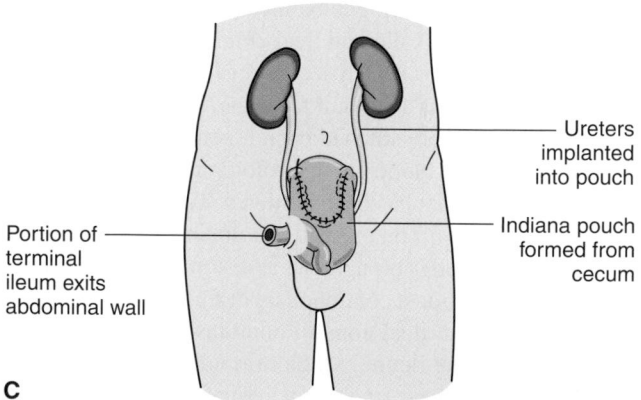

Ureters implanted into pouch

Portion of terminal ileum exits abdominal wall

Indiana pouch formed from cecum

C

FIGURE 37.5 Urinary diversion surgery. (A) Ileal conduit. (B) Kock pouch. (C) Indiana pouch.

to drain urine. Another version of this surgery is the Indiana pouch (see Fig. 37.5C). A reservoir is created using a portion of the ascending colon and terminal ileum, making a larger pouch than the Kock pouch. Additional versions of this type of surgery use other parts of the bowel and include the Mainz pouch or Florida pouch.

Box 37-2 Application of a Disposable Pouch to an Ileal Conduit

1. Gather all supplies: a washcloth, towels, and water; a pouch to apply with a Stomahesive flange; and wicks such as gauze to absorb continually flowing urine. Wear clean gloves.
2. Empty the old pouch.
3. Gently remove soiled pouch by pushing down on skin while lifting up on the flange. Discard soiled pouch and flange.
4. Place a towel around the stoma to catch urine.
5. Mold or cut an opening in the flange that is only 1/16 to 1/8 inch larger than the stoma. Once stomal shrinkage is complete, a presized pouch can be used that fits the stoma.
6. Remove paper backing from the Stomahesive and set the flange to one side.
7. Clean the skin around the stoma with water. Pat dry. Immediately wrap the stoma in wicks to absorb urine. Otherwise urine will leak onto the skin, and the flange will not adhere.
8. Center the flange over the stoma, remove the wick, and immediately apply the flange. Then snap the pouch onto the flange. *Note:* The flange and pouch may be snapped together before application to the stoma.
9. Use the heat of your hand to compress the flange to ensure a good seal.
10. Ensure that the bottom of the pouch is closed off, or connect to a urinary catheter bag at night or if patient is in bed most of the time.

ORTHOTOPIC BLADDER SUBSTITUTION. This surgery involves formation of an orthotopic bladder using a section of the intestine to make a neobladder (*neo* = new) and implanting both the ureters and the urethra into the neobladder. Various types of orthotopic bladder substitution surgery include the Studer pouch, hemi-Kock pouch, and ileal W-neobladder. After this surgery, the patient can void through the urethra, although incontinence may be a problem and intermittent catheterization may be needed.

Nursing Care

Nursing care of the postoperative patient is similar to care following any major surgical procedure (see Chapter 12). It is important to ensure adequate urinary output and to detect and report any obstruction of urine drainage early to prevent complications. The skin around the stoma will require special care to prevent skin breakdown. The patient is taught how to care for the urinary diversion after surgery, either by frequent draining with a catheter or by wearing an appliance. Be sensitive to the patient's anxiety about caring for the urinary diversion.

Body image disturbance may occur because of the change in body function. A consultation with a nurse who specializes in wound, ostomy, and continence care (WOC nurse) or an ostomy support group may be helpful both before and after surgery.

Cancer of the Kidney
Pathophysiology and Etiology

Cancer of the kidney is among the 10 most common cancers in both men and women. The ACS (2013) estimates about 65,150 new cases of kidney cancer will occur in 2013. The lifetime risk of kidney cancer is 1 in 63. Risk factors include genetics, smoking, obesity, hypertension, years of kidney dialysis, and exposure to radiation, asbestos, and industrial pollution. Most patients with kidney cancer are over age 55. It is rare under the age of 45. Men have twice the incidence of women. Often the cancer has metastasized before it is diagnosed because the kidney has such a large volume of circulating blood, which increases the risk of tumor spread. In addition, the disease has few early symptoms.

Signs and Symptoms

The three classic symptoms of kidney cancer are hematuria, dull pain in the flank area, and a mass in the area. Often, symptoms of kidney cancer do not occur until the tumor invades surrounding tissue. Less specific symptoms include fever, weight loss, night sweats, hypertension, anemia, polycythemia, swelling in the legs, fatigue, anorexia, and constipation. Symptoms of metastasis may be the first evidence of kidney cancer and include weight loss, cough, bone fractures, liver abnormalities, and increasing weakness.

Diagnostic Tests

A number of diagnostic tests will be done, including an IV pyelogram, cystoscopy and pyelogram, ultrasound examination of the kidneys, CT scans of the abdomen, and magnetic resonance imaging (MRI). A definitive diagnosis is made with a renal biopsy.

Therapeutic Measures

Surgery is the commonly used treatment for cancer of the kidney. A radical **nephrectomy** removes the entire kidney along with the adrenal gland and other surrounding structures, including fascia, fat, and lymph nodes, in the area. Radiation therapy, immunotherapy, or chemotherapy may be used after the surgery. In nephron-sparing surgery, only the tumor is removed, and the healthy part of the kidney is saved.

Nursing Care

After nephrectomy, provide postoperative nursing care for any major surgery (see Chapter 12). Because the kidney is highly vascular, it is essential that the nurse watch for onset of bleeding and any signs of hypovolemic shock. Urine output is monitored. Changes in urine amount or color, bleeding, and signs of infection are reported. The patient should be assessed for shortness of breath or diminished breath sounds on the affected side. Surgically induced or spontaneous pneumothorax may occasionally occur after a nephrectomy.

RENAL SYSTEM TRAUMA

Renal trauma is the most common injury to the urinary system. The kidneys are highly vascular and have a lot of mobility, so they are vulnerable to vascular and tissue damage. The many causes of trauma to the kidney, ureters, and bladder include motor vehicle accidents, sports injuries, falls, gunshot wounds, and stabbing.

Data collection includes a history of the injury and inspection of the abdomen and flank for asymmetry and bruising or swelling of the flank area. Flank pain and hematuria may be present. Diagnostic tests include urinalysis, IV pyelogram, ultrasound, CT, and MRI. Treatment depends on the extent of the injury and ranges from bedrest to surgical intervention. Nursing care includes measuring intake and output, monitoring vital signs, and providing IV fluids and pain relief.

Bladder trauma may occur with pelvic fractures and multiple trauma from a blow to the lower abdomen when the bladder is full. The weakest part of the bladder wall, which is the dome located at the top of the bladder, may rupture. Urine leaks out of the peritoneal cavity and around the bowel. The patient can have symptoms of hematuria, abdominal pain, inability to void, shock, and pelvic hematoma noted on rectal examination. IV pyelogram and x-ray of the abdomen may be done. A urinary or suprapubic catheter is placed until the bladder heals.

POLYCYSTIC KIDNEY DISEASE

Polycystic kidney disease is a hereditary disorder that can result in CKD. The disease affects men and women equally. Polycystic kidney disease is characterized by formation of multiple cysts in the kidney that can eventually replace normal kidney structures. The cysts are grapelike and contain serous fluid, blood, or urine. The patient typically first shows signs of the disease in adulthood. The initial symptoms include a dull heaviness in the flank or lumbar region and hematuria. Other symptoms include hypertension and UTIs. People with inherited polycystic kidney disease may also experience aneurysms in the brain and diverticulosis in the colon. As the disease progresses, the patient develops symptoms of CKD (discussed later). The renal cysts are usually diagnosed with ultrasound imaging. Ultrasound uses no dyes or radiation, so it is safe for all patients, including pregnant women. Often there is a strong family history of polycystic kidney disease.

There is no treatment to stop the progression of polycystic kidney disease. Complications such as UTIs are treated as needed. Headaches that are severe due to hypertension or seem to feel different might be caused by aneurysms in the brain. A patient with severe or recurring headache should see a HCP. As the disease progresses, treatment for hypertension

• **WORD** • **BUILDING** •
nephrectomy: nephr—kidney + ectomy—excision

and eventual CKD may be needed. Because polycystic disease is hereditary, patients should be counseled about the risks of children inheriting it.

 ## CHRONIC RENAL DISEASES

Diabetic Nephropathy

Diabetic **nephropathy** is the most common cause of CKD. It is a long-term complication of diabetes mellitus in which the effects of diabetes result in damage to the small blood vessels in the kidneys. Microalbuminuria may be detected within 5 years of the onset of type 1 diabetes and 10 to 15 years after the onset of type 2 diabetes. Renal damage appears about 15 to 20 years after onset of type 1 diabetes, but it may also be a complication of type 2 diabetes. Risk factors for development of diabetic nephropathy include hypertension, genetic predisposition, smoking, and chronic hyperglycemia. Careful control of blood glucose levels reduces the risk of nephropathy in patients with diabetes.

Pathophysiology

Multiple factors contribute to diabetic nephropathy. It begins with increased osmotic pressure from hyperglycemia, increased diuresis and compensatory cell growth and expansion, and increased glomerular filtration rate (GFR). Widespread atherosclerotic changes occur in the blood vessels of patients with diabetes, decreasing the blood supply to the kidney. Abnormal thickening of glomerular capillaries damages the glomerulus, allowing protein to leak into urine. Patients with diabetes also commonly develop pyelonephritis and renal scarring. Another complication of diabetes, neurogenic bladder, causes incomplete bladder emptying. This results in urine retention, which can cause infection or obstruction of urine, further damaging the kidneys.

Initially, patients lose only small amounts of protein in their urine (microalbuminuria); this disease can be detected only with careful watching by the HCP, using frequent examinations of the urine. As the disease progresses, high-output CKD (nonoliguria) can develop, in which a large amount of diluted urine is excreted without the usual amounts of waste products dissolved in the urine. The patient can lose large amounts of protein in the urine and develop nephrotic syndrome, which causes massive edema because of low levels of albumin in the blood. As renal function decreases, the patient needs smaller doses of insulin because the kidney normally degrades insulin. Because the kidney is no longer able to break down insulin and excrete it, small doses of insulin circulate in the body for long periods.

Symptoms

The progression of nephropathy is marked by microalbuminuria advancing to proteinuria. Hypertension accelerates the renal damage. As diabetic nephropathy progresses, urine output decreases, toxic wastes accumulate, and the patient develops CKD. For symptoms, see the discussion of CKD in a later section.

Complications

Patients with diabetic nephropathy often have a guarded prognosis because they are vulnerable to all the complications of long-term diabetes in addition to kidney disease. The risk of cardiovascular disease is significant with the progression of protein spilling in the urine.

Diagnostic Tests

Diabetic nephropathy is diagnosed by carefully watching the patient with diabetes for onset of protein spillage or microalbuminuria in the urine, which is an early sign of the disease. Serum creatinine levels and 24-hour creatinine clearance tests are then done to confirm the presence and extent of diabetic nephropathy.

Therapeutic Measures

In the early stages of diabetic nephropathy, strict control of blood glucose levels and blood pressure can help slow the progress of the disease and reduce symptoms. Angiotensin-converting enzyme (ACE) inhibitors or angiotensin II receptor blockers (ARBs) may be given to slow the decline of the GFR and microalbuminuria. As the disease progresses, the patient needs dialysis to maintain life. Unfortunately, other complications related to diabetes cause patients to tolerate dialysis less well than patients with CKD from other causes. Kidney or kidney-pancreas transplant, when available, is the treatment of choice for the patient with diabetic nephropathy and often improves the patient's chance for a healthier life.

Nephrotic Syndrome

Nephrotic syndrome is the excretion of 3.5 g or more of protein in the urine per day. Nephrotic syndrome may occur as a result of other disease processes. In nephrotic syndrome, large amounts of protein are lost in the urine from increased glomerular membrane permeability. As a result, serum albumin and total serum protein are decreased. Normally, albumin and other serum proteins maintain fluid within the vascular space. When levels of these proteins are low, fluid leaks from the blood vessels into tissues, resulting in edema. With very low levels of protein, ascites and massive widespread edema (anasarca) occur. In response to the low protein levels, the liver produces lipoproteins. As a result, serum cholesterol, low-density lipoproteins, and triglyceride levels are elevated. Urine may appear foamy from lipoproteinemia. Loss of immunoglobulins may lead to increased susceptibility to infection. Elevated blood pressure readings are noted.

Treatment is focused on the cause and symptoms of nephrotic syndrome. To control edema, sodium intake is restricted. Protein intake is based on the severity of urinary protein loss. Diuretics may be used. Lipid-lowering drugs may be tried. Anticoagulants are given for thrombosis prevention. In some cases, corticosteroids may be used to reduce inflammation.

Complications of nephrotic syndrome include impaired immune function, nutritional imbalances, and, most importantly,

• WORD • BUILDING •
nephropathy: nephro—pertaining to the kidney + pathy—disease

increased blood coagulation, which is due to urinary loss of clotting inhibitors such as antithrombin III and plasminogen.

Nursing care focuses on the edema and preventing infection. For edema, daily weights, careful measurements of intake and output, and abdominal girth measurements are performed and documented. Edematous tissue must be protected from injury. Preventing malnutrition is challenging but important in maintaining normal body functions.

Nephrosclerosis

Hypertension damages the kidneys by causing sclerotic changes in the small arteries and arterioles, such as arteriosclerosis with thickening and hardening of the renal blood vessels (**nephrosclerosis**). Arteriosclerotic changes in the kidney blood vessels result in a decreased blood supply to the kidney (ischemia of the kidney) and can eventually destroy the kidney. The remaining nephrons try to compensate with vasodilation to increase blood flow to the glomeruli. This results in increased glomerular pressure and filtration, which thickens the blood vessels. High pressure in the kidneys causes the vessels to weaken and hemorrhage. Large areas of the kidney become damaged. Symptoms of nephrosclerosis include proteinuria, hyaline casts in the urine, and, as it progresses, symptoms of CKD.

The treatment for nephrosclerosis is to reduce blood pressure and treat the hypertension. The patient is placed on antihypertensive medications or, if already on these, changed to stronger antihypertensive medications. The patient is placed on a low-sodium diet. Dialysis may be used to maintain life.

The prognosis is often poor because by the time the patient has developed nephrosclerosis, there is widespread arteriosclerosis throughout the body. Arteriosclerosis makes the patient prone to myocardial infarctions or cerebrovascular accidents.

The major nursing diagnosis that is relevant when the patient develops nephrosclerosis is *Ineffective Health Maintenance.* The priority is to help the patient learn as much about the control of hypertension as possible. The patient should also be taught the symptoms of CKD. Once the patient has lost renal function, the nursing care plan for CKD is appropriate.

> ## CRITICAL THINKING
>
> ### Mr. Stevens
>
> ■ Mr. Stevens is a 35-year-old African American man admitted to the intensive care unit with uncontrolled hypertension. His blood pressure is controlled by IV medication. His laboratory tests show protein and hyaline casts in the urine. He is diagnosed with nephrosclerosis.
>
> 1. What data should the nurse collect as part of the morning evaluation of the patient's condition?
> 2. What other renal function tests are appropriate for the nurse to check?
> 3. What teaching does Mr. Stevens need when his condition is more stable?
>
> *Suggested answers are at the end of the chapter.*

GLOMERULONEPHRITIS

Pathophysiology

Glomerulonephritis is an inflammatory disease of the glomerulus. It can be caused by a variety of factors including immunological abnormalities, toxins, vascular disorders, and systemic diseases. Inflammation occurs as a result of the deposition of antigen-antibody complexes in the basement membrane of the glomerulus or from antibodies that specifically attack the basement membrane. The resulting immune reaction in the glomerulus causes inflammation, which in turn causes the glomerulus to be more porous, allowing proteins, WBCs, and RBCs to leak into the urine.

Etiology
Acute Poststreptococcal Glomerulonephritis

Glomerulonephritis is most commonly associated with a group A beta-hemolytic streptococcal infection following a streptococcal infection of the throat or skin. This is the most common cause in children and young adults. Antibodies form complexes with the streptococcal antigen and are deposited in the basement membrane of the glomerulus, inducing damage from inflammation. Damaged glomeruli become unable to filter blood correctly, and protein leaks into the urine. Edema, oliguria, and hypertension result. Glomerulonephritis typically develops about 6 to 10 days after the preceding infection. The disease has an abrupt onset. Other kinds of bacteria and viruses can also be the offending infectious agent.

Goodpasture's Syndrome

Occasionally glomerulonephritis is caused by an autoimmune response, in which the person, for unknown reasons, forms antibodies against his or her own glomerular basement membrane. Glomerulonephritis caused by an autoimmune response usually progresses rapidly and often leads to CKD.

Chronic Glomerulonephritis

Chronic glomerulonephritis occurs over years as a result of glomerular inflammatory disease. There may be no history of renal disease before the diagnosis. Often, proteinuria and hematuria may have been noted previously before the diagnosis. Systemic lupus erythematosus and insulin-dependent diabetes mellitus may precede chronic glomerular injury. It is often discovered during an examination for another concern. Ultrasound, CT scan, or renal biopsy is used to diagnose the cause.

Symptoms

Symptoms of glomerulonephritis include fluid overload with oliguria, hypertension, electrolyte imbalances, and edema

• WORD • BUILDING •
nephrosclerosis: nephro—pertaining to the kidney + sclerosis—hardening
glomerulonephritis: glomerulo—glomerulus + nephr—kidney + itis—inflammation

(Table 37.6). Edema may begin around the eyes (periorbital edema) and face and progress to the abdomen (ascites), lungs (pleural effusion), and extremities. Flank pain may be present. Blood urea nitrogen (BUN) and creatinine levels may be elevated. Urinalysis shows RBCs, WBCs, albumin, and casts. The urine is dark or cola colored from old RBCs and may be foamy because of proteinuria.

Complications

The prognosis is good for acute glomerulonephritis acquired in childhood, and most children recover completely. Adults who develop glomerulonephritis may recover renal function or progress to chronic glomerulonephritis. Some patients develop rapidly progressive glomerulonephritis, which can quickly lead to acute renal injury. Chronic glomerulonephritis is a slow process characterized by hypertension, gradual loss of renal function, and eventual CKD.

Diagnostic Tests

Glomerulonephritis is diagnosed with urinalysis, which shows protein, casts, or RBCs and elevated serum levels of nitrogenous wastes (creatinine, urea). Hypertension may be present. Kidney ultrasound, x-ray, or biopsy may be done to determine abnormal kidney shape, size, blood flow, inflammation, or scarring of the glomeruli.

TABLE 37.6   GLOMERULONEPHRITIS SUMMARY

Signs and Symptoms	Fluid volume overload Hypertension Electrolyte imbalances Edema Periorbital edema Flank pain
Diagnostic Tests	Urinalysis shows red cells, WBCs, protein, and casts Urine dark or cola colored Foamy urine Creatinine, urea level elevated Renal biopsy
Therapeutic Measures	Treatment is symptomatic Nonsteroidal anti-inflammatory drugs Steroids Antibiotics prophylactically to prevent further kidney damage
Complications	CKD
Priority Nursing Diagnoses	*Fluid Volume Excess* *Decreased Tissue Perfusion*

Note. CKD = chronic kidney disease; WBCs = white blood cells.

Therapeutic Measures

Most cases of acute glomerulonephritis resolve spontaneously in about a week, but some progress to CKD. Treatment is primarily symptomatic. Sodium and fluid restrictions may be ordered, along with diuretics to treat fluid retention. Medications may be given to control hypertension. If associated with a streptococcal infection, antibiotics are given to treat any remaining infection. If fluid overload is severe, dialysis may be done.

Nursing Care

Nursing care for a patient with glomerulonephritis focuses on symptom relief. Vital signs are monitored because the patient may be critically ill. During the acute phase, rest is encouraged. Edema is controlled with fluid and sodium intake restrictions. Protein intake may be limited if the kidneys are not filtering protein waste products (as seen by increased serum BUN and creatinine levels). Other care is discussed in the next section on CKD. Teaching the patient about preventing glomerulonephritis is important. Antibiotics for diagnosed streptococcal throat infections should be taken for prevention.

ACUTE KIDNEY INJURY OR CHRONIC KIDNEY DISEASE

Kidney disease is diagnosed when the kidneys are no longer functioning adequately to maintain normal body processes. This results in dysfunction in almost all other parts of the body as a result of imbalances in fluid, electrolytes, and calcium levels, as well as impaired RBC formation and decreased elimination of waste products. It can be acute (acute kidney injury) with sudden onset of symptoms, or it can be chronic (CKD), occurring gradually over time. For more information on kidneys, visit the American Kidney Fund (www.kidneyfund.org), the National Kidney Foundation (www.kidney.org), and the American Association of Kidney Patients (www.aakp.org).

Acute Kidney Injury

Acute kidney injury (AKI) is the sudden (hours to days) loss of the kidneys' ability to clear waste products and regulate fluid and electrolyte balance. Rapid accumulation of toxic wastes from protein metabolism in the blood (**azotemia**) occurs. In azotemia, the serum urea level (measured by BUN) and creatinine level are elevated. Potassium imbalances may lead to tachycardia. Most types of AKI are reversible if diagnosed and treated early; however, AKI can lead to CKD. It is often associated with a urine output of less than 30 mL/hr or 400 mL/day. It may be caused by hypotension, dehydration, vascular obstruction, glomerular disease, or acute tubular necrosis, in which the tubules are damaged. This may occur after administration of diagnostic contrast agents (contrast-induced nephropathy).

• WORD • BUILDING •
azotemia: azo—nitrogenous waste products + temia—blood

NURSING CARE TIP

To protect patients' kidneys, be aware of the following:

- The patient's renal function status: GFR is the best indicator, serum creatinine, and BUN levels.
- Nephrotoxic substances:
  - Diagnostic contrast agents (dyes)
  - Medications—IV aminoglycosides (gentamicin [Garamycin], tobramycin [Tobrex]), amikacin (Amikin), cisplatin (Platinol), Vancomycin
  - Chemicals—arsenic, carbon tetrachloride, lead, mercuric chloride
- Preventive measures:
  - Before administering nephrotoxic contrast agents or medications, check serum BUN and creatinine levels.
  - With contrast agent (dye) tests, encourage fluids before and after to maintain renal blood flow throughout the renal capillaries and reduce hypoxia in the kidney (Jorgensen, 2013). Volume expansion with normal saline may reduce the incidence of contrast-induced nephropathy (Dirkes, 2012). Ensure peak and trough drug levels of nephrotoxic drugs are obtained on an ongoing basis per institutional policy.

Pathophysiology

There are three major mechanisms of injury in AKI. These mechanisms are hypoperfusion, direct tissue injury, and hypersensitivity reactions causing renal inflammation. In AKI, rapid damage to the kidney causes waste products to accumulate in the bloodstream, resulting in signs and symptoms. The patient becomes oliguric, with urine output decreasing to less than 20 mL/h. Treatment is directed toward correcting the cause, supporting the patient with dialysis, and preventing complications that may lead to permanent damage. Many patients with AKI recover completely. About 40% to 50% of patients hospitalized with intrarenal AKI die from complications, such as infection, pneumonia, or sepsis (Pannu et al, 2011).

AKI can progress through four stages, with an intrarenal cause taking a longer recovery time because there is actual renal damage. Once an event causes AKI in the initial phase, symptoms occur in hours to days.

OLIGURIC PHASE. In the oliguric phase, less than 400 mL of urine is produced in 24 hours. Fifty percent of those with AKI experience this phase, which occurs from 24 hours to 7 days after the initial phase. This phase can last up to 2 weeks to several months. Prognosis for renal recovery is decreased the longer this phase lasts.

In the oliguric phase, fluid is retained, electrolytes become imbalanced, and waste products are not excreted as urine output decreases. Signs of fluid overload arise. Serum potassium rises while sodium is lost in the urine, creating a normal or low serum sodium level. The longer this phase lasts, the more effects that are seen. These may include metabolic acidosis from reduced hydrogen ion excretion and sodium bicarbonate levels, increased phosphate and decreased calcium levels, abnormal blood cells (RBCs, WBCs, platelets), neurologic effects ranging from confusion to seizures to coma, and finally effects on all body systems as is seen in chronic renal failure (discussed later).

DIURETIC PHASE. As the kidneys begin to excrete waste products again, 1 to 3 L/day of urine is produced. Osmotic diuresis occurs from the elevated waste products (urea), which the body is attempting to eliminate. The kidneys are not yet able to concentrate urine, so dehydration and hypotension are a concern. It is important for the nurse to monitor for hypovolemia, hyponatremia, hypokalemia, and hypotension in this phase. Serum BUN and creatinine levels are high until the end of this phase, when they begin to return to normal. This phase may last 1 to 3 weeks.

RECOVERY PHASE. In this final phase, recovery begins as the glomerular filtration rate rises. Waste product levels (BUN, creatinine) decrease greatly within the first 2 weeks of this phase. However, recovery can take up to 1 year. Those who do recover usually do so without complications. Older adults are more at risk for reduced recovery of renal function. In those who do not recover renal function, CKD occurs.

Etiology

AKI is often classified as prerenal, intrarenal, or postrenal. These categories relate to the causes leading to the injury. Each category is associated with the location of the cause in the kidney. Understanding the cause can point to the direction of treatment plans helpful to the patient.

PRERENAL INJURY. Prerenal (before the kidney) injury, the most common cause of AKI, is associated with a decrease or interruption of blood supply to the kidneys. Causes may include decreased blood pressure from dehydration, blood loss, shock, or trauma to or blockage in the arteries that carry blood to the kidneys. When the nephrons receive an inadequate blood supply, they are unable to make urine, and waste products are not adequately removed. Use of nonsteroidal anti-inflammatory drugs (NSAIDs) and cyclooxygenase-2 (COX) inhibitors can also lead to prerenal injury. These drugs impair the autoregulatory responses of the kidney by blocking prostaglandin, which is needed for renal perfusion.

Prerenal injury can be diagnosed by evaluating possible causes. If dehydration is the cause, then an IV fluid challenge may be given. With increased IV fluid, more blood flows to the kidneys for filtering, which increases urine output and waste product filtering. An arteriogram of the renal arteries is helpful to determine if the blood supply to the kidneys is decreased or blocked; angioplasty may be used to open the blockage. Serum creatinine increases and creatinine clearance decreases. Urinalysis may be helpful in determining the cause as well.

Newer biomarkers such as interleukin 18, neutrophil gelatinase–associated lipocalin (NGAL), and kidney injury molecule-1 (KIM-1) might be able to provide more information on the type of kidney injury. These markers are under ongoing study.

INTRARENAL INJURY. Intrarenal (inside the kidney) injury occurs when there is damage to the nephrons inside the kidney. The most common causes are ischemia, reduced blood flow, and toxins. Other causes are infectious processes leading to glomerulonephritis, trauma to the kidney, exposure to **nephrotoxins**, allergic reactions to contrast agents, and severe muscle injury, which releases substances that are harmful to the kidneys.

A number of substances can be toxic to the kidneys (nephrotoxic) when they enter the body (Table 37.7). Kidney damage is most likely to occur when these substances enter

TABLE 37.7 COMMON NEPHROTOXINS

Antibiotics	Aminoglycosides Amphotericin B Cephalosporins Sulfonamides Tetracyclines
Analgesics	Acetaminophen Nonsteroidal anti-inflammatory drugs Salicylates
Other Drugs	ACE inhibitors Amphetamines Cisplatin Dextran Heroin Interleukin-2 Mannitol
Heavy Metals	Arsenic Copper Gold Lead Lithium Mercury
Contrast Media	Contrast agents used for diagnostic testing such as IV pyelograms, cardiac catheterizations
Organic Solvents	Gasoline Glycols Kerosene Tetrachloroethylene Turpentine

ACE = angiotensin-converting enzyme; IV = intravenous.

the body in high concentrations or when preexisting kidney damage is present for some other reason. Many commonly administered medications can be nephrotoxic. Aminoglycosides are nephrotoxic antibiotics; when they are administered, blood levels of the drugs are carefully monitored to avoid toxic levels.

CONTRAST-INDUCED NEPHROPATHY. Contrast agents used during tests such as IV pyelograms and CT scans can cause kidney damage, especially when the patient is dehydrated and has preexisting renal damage. The incidence increases with age greater than 60 years, decreased renal function, poor renal perfusion, or exposure to nephrotoxic drugs. Contrast media has the potential to cause renal vasoconstriction, hypoxia, and alteration of renal blood flow (Jorgensen, 2013). Loss of regulation of renal blood flow causes decreased oxygen transport with causes increasing renal medullary hypoxia, necrosis and renal cell tubular collapse (Isaac, 2012). Before administration of contrast media, patients should be assessed for risk factors: diabetes mellitus, hypertension, dyslipidemia, advanced age over 70, renal surgery. Anemia, proteinuria, hyperuricemia, and the use of diuretics and other nephrotoxic drugs increases the likely hood of contrast-induced nephropathy. Prevention strategies should focus on screening patients for dehydration and risk factors. IV hydration with normal saline is most effective. Hydration is inexpensive and usually without risks. Studies are being done on the use of sodium bicarbonate infusion as well as the use of N-acetylcysteine to prevent contrast-induced nephropathy. (Jorgensen, 2013).

POSTRENAL INJURY. Postrenal (after the kidney) injury is associated with an obstruction that blocks the flow of urine out of the body. Only 5% of acute kidney injuries are classified as postrenal. In this case, the blood supply to the kidneys and nephron function initially may be normal, but urine is unable to drain out of the kidney, resulting in the backup of urine and impaired nephron function. Common causes are kidney stones, tumors of the ureters or bladder, and an enlarged prostate that blocks the flow of urine.

Diagnosis of causes can be done with x-ray examination of the kidneys, ureters, and bladder. Cystoscopy will show tumors, stones, or prostate enlargement. Renal ultrasound can measure kidney size, detect tumors and blockages, and reveal cystic disease. Surgical intervention may be needed to correct the problem.

Measures

AKI is treated by relieving the cause. Prevention of permanent damage is the goal of treatment. Signs and symptoms are managed as they develop, and supportive care is given. Treatment may include restoring fluid and electrolyte balance, discontinuing nephrotoxic drugs that may have caused the problem, bypassing urinary tract obstructions with catheters, or using short-term continuous renal replacement

• WORD • BUILDING •
nephrotoxin: nephro—kidney + toxin—poison

therapy to filter blood and restore potassium and other electrolytes to normal. Some symptoms, such as anemia, may not have time to develop in the patient with AKI as they do in CKD. The care of the patient with AKI is similar to care of the patient with CKD.

CONTINUOUS RENAL REPLACEMENT THERAPY. Continuous renal replacement therapy (CRRT) is used to remove fluid and solutes in a controlled, continuous manner in unstable patients with AKI. Unstable patients may not be able to tolerate the rapid fluid shifts that occur in hemodialysis, so CRRT provides an alternative therapy that results in less dramatic fluid shifting. CRRT can be used with **hemodialysis**, which is needed if severe symptoms of **uremia** (hyperkalemia) are present. CRRT is not as complex as hemodialysis and can be done for more than a month, if needed, via temporary vascular access.

During CRRT, a permeable hemofilter is attached to the vascular access. Blood flows through the hemofilter and excess fluids and solutes move into a collection bag. The remaining blood returns to the patient via the venous access. If desired, replacement fluid and electrolytes can be given through the vascular access. Monitoring intake and output, fluid and electrolytes, daily weights, hourly vital signs, and vascular access is important.

Chronic Kidney Disease

Kidney disease is the eighth leading cause of death in the United States (U.S. Renal Data System, 2013), where CKD affects about 26 million people and the incidence is on the rise. This disease is a progressive, irreversible deterioration in renal function in which the body is unable to maintain metabolic, fluid, and electrolyte balance. It occurs with a gradual decrease in the function of the kidneys over time. The result is accumulation of nitrogenous waste products in the blood and uremia. CKD affects every body system (Table 37.8).

Pathophysiology

When a large proportion of the body's nephrons are damaged or destroyed, AKI or CKD occurs. As the nephrons die off, the undamaged ones increase their work capacity and take over the work previously done by the dead ones, so the patient may experience significant kidney damage without showing symptoms.

CKD is a progressive disease process. In the early, or silent, stage (decreased renal reserve), the patient is usually without symptoms, even though up to 50% of nephron function may have been lost (Table 37.9). This stage is often not diagnosed.

The renal insufficiency stage occurs when the patient has lost 75% of nephron function and some signs of mild kidney disease are present. Anemia and the inability to concentrate

TABLE 37.8 CHRONIC KIDNEY DISEASE SUMMARY

Signs and Symptoms	Decreased urine output Acute kidney injury symptoms appear rapidly Fatigue Nausea and vomiting Shortness of breath Platelet dysfunction
Diagnostic Tests	Urinalysis Elevated BUN, creatinine levels Urine sodium level less than 10 mEq/L Acidosis Anemia Electrolyte abnormalities Elevated potassium, magnesium levels Hypertension Pericarditis Platelet dysfunction Dialysis
Therapeutic Measures	Transplant Diet Dialysis
Complications	Accelerated atherosclerosis Anemia Anorexia, nausea, and vomiting Dry itchy skin, ecchymosis, and subcutaneous bruises Headache Heart failure Hypertension Impotence Osteomalacia Osteoporosis Pulmonary edema Uremic encephalopathy—lethargy, coma, seizures Uremic pericarditis
Priority Nursing Diagnoses	*Fluid Volume Excess* *Risk for Electrolyte Imbalance* *Imbalanced Nutrition: Less Than Body Requirements* *Sexual Dysfunction* *Urinary Retention* *Anxiety* *Infection* *Noncompliance* *Ineffective Coping*

• WORD • BUILDING •

hemodialysis: hemo—blood + dialysis—passage of a solute through a membrane

uremia: ur—urea + emia—in the blood

TABLE 37.9 STAGES OF CHRONIC KIDNEY DISEASE

Stage	Kidney Function Description	GFR mL/min
1	Slight decrease	≥90
2	Mild decrease	60–89
3	Moderate decrease	30–59
4	Severe decrease	15–29
5	Dialysis/Transplant	<15

Note. GFR = glomerular filtration rate.

urine may occur. BUN and creatinine levels are slightly elevated. These patients are at risk for further damage caused by infection, dehydration, drugs, heart failure, and use of diagnostic x-ray dyes. The goal of care is to prevent further damage, if possible, by control of blood glucose levels and blood pressure.

End-stage renal disease occurs when 90% of the nephrons are lost. Patients at this stage experience chronic and persistent abnormal kidney function. BUN and creatinine levels are always elevated. These patients may make urine but not filter out the waste products, or urine production may cease. Dialysis or a kidney transplant is required to survive.

Uremia (urea in the blood) is present in CKD. Patients eventually develop problems in all body systems (Table 37.10). If left untreated, the patient with uremia dies, often within weeks.

TABLE 37.10 EFFECTS OF CKD ON BODY SYSTEMS

Body System	Disease Process
Cardiovascular	Hypertension due to fluid overload and accelerated arteriosclerosis Congestive heart failure/pulmonary edema due to fluid overload, increased pulmonary permeability, left ventricular failure Angina due to coronary artery disease, anemia Dysrhythmias due to electrolyte imbalance, coronary artery disease Edema due to fluid overload and a decrease in osmotic pressure Pericarditis due to presence of waste products in the pericardial sac
Gastrointestinal	Stomatitis due to fluid restriction, presence of waste products in the mouth, secondary infections Anorexia, nausea, vomiting due to uremia Gastritis/gastrointestinal bleeding due to urea decomposition in gastrointestinal tract releasing ammonia that irritates and ulcerates the stomach or bowel; patient is also under stress, increasing ulcer formation, and may have platelet dysfunction Constipation due to electrolyte imbalances, decrease in fluid intake, decrease in activity, phosphate binders Diarrhea, hypermotility due to electrolyte imbalance
Hematopoietic	Anemia due to impaired synthesis of erythropoietin, a substance needed by the bone marrow to stimulate formation of RBCs; also due to decreased life span of RBCs from uremia and interference in folic acid action Bleeding tendency due to abnormal platelet function from effects of uremia Prone to infection due to a decrease in immune system function from uremia; renal patients can rapidly become septic and die from septic shock
Integumentary	Dry, itchy, inflamed skin due to calcium-phosphate deposits in the skin Pale yellow skin color due to urobilins, which give urine its yellow color. Skin will have an odor of urine because skin is an organ of excretion and the body attempts to remove toxins Decreased function of oil and sweat glands
Neurologic	Confusion due to uremic encephalopathy from an increase in urea and metabolic acids Peripheral neuropathy due to effects of waste products on neurologic system Cerebrovascular accidents due to accelerated atherosclerosis
Pulmonary	Pleurisy/pleural effusion due to waste products in the pleural space causing inflammation with pleurisy pain and collection of fluid resulting in effusion
Reproductive	Loss of libido, impotence, amenorrhea, infertility due to a decrease in hormone production
Skeletal	Bone and mineral disease due to hyperphosphatemia and hypocalcemia

Note. RBCs = red blood cells.

Etiology

The causes of CKD are numerous. The most common include diabetes mellitus resulting in diabetic nephropathy, chronic high blood pressure causing nephrosclerosis, glomerulonephritis, and autoimmune diseases. Diabetes and hypertension account for close to 70% of all CKD (U.S. Renal Data System, 2013).

Symptoms of Kidney Disease

Patients in either AKI or CKD have multiple symptoms. Figure 37.6 illustrates symptoms and some of the more common ones are explained next.

Disturbance in Water Balance

Disturbances in the removal and regulation of water balance in the body occur with signs of fluid accumulation. An early symptom is edema (swelling) of the extremities, sacral area, and abdomen. Patients may report shortness of breath. Crackles and wheezes (signs of fluid accumulation) may be present on auscultation of the lungs. Blood vessels in the neck may be distended, and the patient may be hypertensive. These patients may produce a large amount of dilute urine (**polyuria**), small amounts of urine (oliguria), or no urine (anuria).

Disturbance in Electrolyte Balance

As kidney function decreases, the kidneys lose their ability to absorb and excrete electrolytes. Important electrolytes are sodium, potassium, and magnesium. When the kidneys are unable to maintain normal amounts of electrolytes in the blood, these substances accumulate at high levels and may be life threatening.

When the kidneys are unable to regulate sodium levels adequately, the patient may show signs of hypernatremia (excessive sodium in the blood), which causes water retention, edema, and hypertension. Hyponatremia (too little sodium) may occur when too much sodium is lost. This can occur when the patient has experienced prolonged episodes of vomiting or diarrhea or is urinating large amounts of diluted urine. Patients with hyponatremia may show signs of confusion. The sodium may be normal or low due to being diluted from excess fluid.

Hyperkalemia (potassium level exceeding 5 mEq/L) can be life threatening if the level goes above 7 mEq/L. The patient may have dysrhythmias and cardiac arrest if the potassium level is too high. Patients with hyperkalemia report muscle weakness, abdominal cramping, and diarrhea. The nurse may identify that the patient is confused or disinterested in care. These patients should be placed on a cardiac monitor and observed for cardiac dysrhythmias.

A high potassium level in the patient with CKD may be caused by a diet high in potassium-rich foods, injuries, or blood transfusions. Monitoring daily laboratory values, restricting potassium intake, and reporting abnormalities are important. IV insulin with glucose, or calcium gluconate may be used as a temporary measure to drive excess potassium into the cells. Sodium polystyrene sulfonate (Kayexalate) may be given either orally or as a retention enema; it causes potassium to be eliminated through the stool. The definitive treatment for hyperkalemia is hemodialysis, which removes potassium from the body. Dietary education is extremely important. The patient is instructed to avoid foods that are high in potassium (Box 37-3).

Calcium levels decrease because the kidneys are unable to produce the hormone that activates vitamin D, the vitamin needed for calcium absorption. Hypocalcemia exists when the calcium level falls below 8.5 mg/dL. Also associated with a low calcium level is hyperphosphatemia, a phosphorus level above 5 mg/dL. These imbalances cause the bones to release

• WORD • BUILDING •
polyuria: poly—much + uria—urine

FIGURE 37.6 Symptoms of chronic kidney disease.

Box 37-3 Foods High in Potassium

- Beans: lima, lentils, kidney, navy, northern, pinto, refried, soy
- Chocolate
- Dairy products (cheese, ice cream, milk, yogurt)
- Dried fruit: apricots, dates, figs, prunes, raisins
- Fruit: avocado, banana, kiwi, mango, melons (cantaloupe, honeydew), nectarine, oranges, orange juice, papaya, pumpkin, tomato paste
- Juice: carrot, prune, tomato, vegetable
- Nuts
- Vegetables: beet greens, potatoes (chips, sweet, white, yams), spinach, squash
- Salt substitutes
- Seeds

calcium, increasing the risk of fractures. These patients should ambulate regularly to prevent further calcium loss from the bone. Many patients who are on dialysis develop hypercalcemia due to hyperparathyroidism (excess release of parathyroid hormone). Cinacalcet (Sensipar) reduces excess levels of parathyroid hormone, which then reduces calcium levels.

Phosphates are also found in many foods. Medication to bind phosphate, known as phosphate binders, is taken by patients with high phosphate levels. Patients must take these medications with meals so they can bind with the phosphates and be eliminated in the stool. High phosphorus levels may cause severe itching, and patients may have open sores from scratching, placing them at risk for infections. Patients also may have muscle cramps and aches.

Disturbance of Removal of Waste Products

With azotemia (rapid accumulation of toxic wastes in the blood), the patient may show signs of weakness and fatigue, confusion, seizures, twitching movements of extremities (asterixis), nausea, vomiting, and lack of appetite and may report a metallic or bad taste in the mouth. There may be a smell of urine on the patient's breath. The patient may have yellowish pale skin and report itching due to urea crystals on the skin. Dialysis to remove excessive waste products in the blood is the only treatment for the underlying causes of these symptoms.

Disturbance in Maintaining Acid–Base Balance

Hydrogen ion excretion is affected, causing a disturbance in the acid–base balance that result in metabolic acidosis. Patients may report headache, fatigue, weakness, nausea, vomiting, and lack of appetite. As metabolic acidosis progresses, the patient shows signs of lethargy, stupor, and coma. Respirations become fast and deep as the lungs attempt to blow off carbon dioxide to correct the acidosis (Kussmaul's respirations). See Chapter 6 for a more detailed discussion of acid–base balance.

Disturbance in Hematologic Function

Anemia is seen mainly in CKD, which causes disturbances in blood cells over time. Damaged kidneys do not produce adequate erythropoietin, the hormone that stimulates RBC production. Nutritional deficiencies and blood loss during dialysis also contribute to anemia. Regular injections of epoetin (Epogen, Procrit), a synthetic form of erythropoietin, help restore RBC production and prevent anemia. A common side effect of erythropoietin is development of hypertension.

Impaired WBC and immune functions contribute to an increased risk for infection. The patient should be protected from potential sources of infection.

Impaired platelet function creates a risk for bleeding. The patient should be protected from injury, and signs of bleeding, such as blood in stool or emesis, are reported.

Therapeutic Measures for Kidney Disease

Kidney insufficiency and early kidney disease are treated based on symptoms with a restricted diet and fluid intake, medications, and careful monitoring for onset of serious problems that warrant initiation of dialysis. In later stages, dialysis is necessary to replace lost kidney function. A kidney transplant, when available, may return the patient to a nearly normal state of health.

Diet

Dietary recommendations are individualized by the dietitian and HCP based on the patient's needs. Calories are high to maintain weight and energy needs. Protein is usually restricted to limit nitrogen intake but is increased for a patient on dialysis because protein is lost during the dialysis process. Sodium is restricted to minimize sodium and fluid retention. Potassium is restricted, especially later in the disease when the kidneys are unable to eliminate it. Calcium may be increased or supplemented because of poor absorption related to faulty vitamin D activation. Phosphorus is restricted because of high blood levels related to hypocalcemia. Saturated fat and cholesterol are restricted for patients with hyperlipidemia. Fluids are restricted to prevent overload. Most patients are given iron, folic acid, vitamins, and minerals to supplement the restricted diet ("Nutrition Notes").

Because restrictions are complex, the diet may be a source of frustration for patients. The nurse should assist the patient to identify foods that are palatable yet within the diet plan. The dietitian should be consulted for instruction and assistance.

Medications

Early in the disease, diuretics are given to increase output, and ACE inhibitors, angiotensin receptor blockers, calcium channel blockers, or beta blockers may be used to control hypertension. Phosphate binders are given with meals to reduce phosphate levels. Calcium and vitamin D supplements are used to raise calcium levels. Both the active and storage forms of vitamin D should be considered to decrease fractures, cancer, and infection rates and improve cardiac function. Agents to lower potassium levels are used if needed. All drug therapy is closely monitored because diseased kidneys are unable to effectively remove medications from the body. The patient with diabetes needs less insulin because one of the functions of the kidneys is to break down insulin. Because it is not being broken down, it remains in the body longer, and therefore less is needed as the kidney disease progresses.

Dialysis

Dialysis is started when the patient develops symptoms of severe fluid overload, high potassium levels, acidosis, pericarditis, vomiting, lethargy, fatigue, or symptoms of uremia that are life threatening. Both peritoneal dialysis and hemodialysis involve the movement and diffusion of particles from an area of high concentration to an area of low concentration through a semipermeable membrane. Substances move from blood through the semipermeable membrane into the dialysate. Fluid and electrolyte imbalances can be corrected with dialysis. Dialysis can also be used to treat drug overdoses.

HEMODIALYSIS. Hemodialysis involves the use of an artificial kidney to remove waste products and excess water from the

Nutrition Notes

Understanding Dietary Changes in Renal Disease

Patients with impaired renal function require careful co-ordination of diet with current physiological status, which may change frequently, necessitating the services of a dietitian who specializes in renal treatment. The following principles are offered as general guidelines:

- Maintaining caloric intake is essential to avoid catabolism of tissue for energy.* Simple carbohydrates and monounsaturated and polyunsaturated fats are given freely because their end products, carbon dioxide and water, are less likely than protein to tax the kidney. Patients with diabetes and uremia may receive more sugar than usual because treatment of the uremia may take precedence over the diabetes; however, patients with type IV hypertriglyceridemia may have to limit carbohydrates.
- Protein may be restricted when the patient's kidneys are failing but increased when the patient is treated with dialysis to compensate for losses in the dialysate. Sometimes proteins of high biological value (e.g., eggs, meat, and dairy products) are prescribed because they are more easily converted to body protein than those of low biological value. In other situations, vegetarian diets may be given, with the plant proteins carefully selected to manage potassium and phosphorus serum levels.
- Sodium may be restricted, depending on blood pressure, edema, and laboratory findings.
- Potassium may be restricted for patients with oliguria. Salt substitutes are often potassium compounds that are to be avoided. Potassium content in foods varies with processing and preparation methods, so patients should choose from prescribed foods only.
- Fluid restriction may be altered daily according to output. Patients with renal insufficiency may receive 500 mL plus the amount of the previous day's output.

In short, renal diets are individualized for the patient's current condition. Nurses should not expect various patients to be served the same meals or even the same patient to require the same restrictions from one day to the next. Counseling and teaching patients to associate adherence to the diet and relief of symptoms is an important nursing task that encourages patients to persevere in managing their situation.

*Nepro (Abbott Laboratories) is a specially formulated oral supplement to meet the altered nutrition needs of patients on dialysis. Nepro blends carbohydrates to maintain steady glucose levels and increase albumin levels.

Source: Lutz, C. A., & Przytulski, K. R. (2014). *Nutrition and diet therapy* (6th ed.). Philadelphia: F.A. Davis.

patient's blood. During the dialysis procedure, the patient's blood and the dialyzing solution flow in opposite directions through the dialyzer across an enclosed semipermeable membrane. The dialysate contains electrolytes and water in a balanced mix that resembles blood plasma. On the other side is the patient's blood with metabolic waste products, excess water, and electrolytes. The waste products from the patient's blood move into the dialysate by diffusion through the membrane because of the difference in their concentrations. The dialysate solution carries the waste products away, and the cleansed blood is returned to the patient's body through another tube (Fig. 37.7). A hemodialysis treatment takes 3 to 4 hours and is usually done three or four times a week. Hemodialysis can be done at a hemodialysis center, at home, or in the hospital if the patient develops a complication and needs hospitalization (Fig. 37.8).

Hemodialysis provides a rapid and efficient way to remove waste products from the blood. It is also an excellent means to correct excessive fluid-overloaded states such as occur in heart failure.

Hemodialysis is not without side effects. After a treatment, the patient normally feels weak and fatigued, sometimes even too tired to eat. Sudden drops in blood pressure may cause the patient to become weak, dizzy, and nauseated. Cardiac dysrhythmias and angina may occur. Fluid and electrolyte levels drop rapidly and cause the patient to

FIGURE 37.7 Hemodialysis.

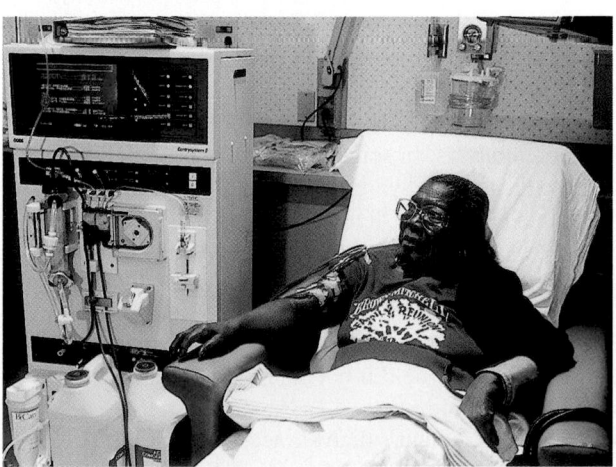

FIGURE 37.8 Patient undergoing hemodialysis at dialysis center.

feel lethargic and have muscle cramps. Patients are given large amounts of heparin, an anticoagulant, to keep the blood from clotting while it is in the artificial kidney; this may cause bleeding from the puncture sites, GI tract, nose, or other sites if injury occurs. Box 37-4 reviews nursing care for patients having hemodialysis.

Vascular Access. Hemodialysis requires a permanent way to access the bloodstream for blood removal and return to the body during dialysis. Typical permanent vascular access options are an arteriovenous (AV) fistula (considered to be the gold standard) or a vascular access graft. Fistulas or grafts are placed in the arm when possible.

 NURSING CARE TIP

It is important to save the veins of patients with CKD for possible future fistula creation. The non-dominant patient arm should not be used for IVs, blood draws, or blood pressure to avoid damage to the veins because it will likely be the arm used for the fistula. Early consultation with a nephrologist can identify which veins to protect.

Box 37-4 **Care for Hemodialysis**

1. Consult with the HCP about medications to hold before hemodialysis. Some medications, such as antihypertensives, can be harmful when they become effective during dialysis and can reduce blood pressure to dangerously low levels. Other medications are water-soluble and will be dialyzed out of the body, and thus are not effective.
2. Ensure that the patient is weighed both before dialysis in the morning and after dialysis to document weight loss as a result of fluid removal.
3. If the patient has laboratory tests ordered and blood needs to be drawn, coordinate this process with the dialysis nurse, who can obtain the blood samples and save the patient unnecessary needlesticks.
4. Try to get morning care done early and breakfast given before dialysis, if the patient tolerates eating before dialysis. In some patients, eating can cause hypotension by diverting blood flow to the gastrointestinal system for digestion during dialysis. After dialysis, patients are often exhausted and need rest.
5. When the patient returns from dialysis, weigh the patient, assess the access site for bleeding, and make sure the vital signs are stable. Administer medications that were held if not contraindicated and vital signs are stable.
6. Protect the patient's dialysis access as outlined in Box 37-5, *Care of Blood Access Fistula or Graft.*

Early referral to a nephrologist can allow for the establishment of vascular access so that it is matured (developed) before the need for dialysis. If this does not occur, then a temporary access is used until a fistula or graft is placed or usable. A central venous catheter with two or three ports (the third port can be used for medications by trained staff) is placed in a central vein for temporary access. Central catheters should not be used long term because of the risk of infection.

An AV fistula is made by sewing a vein and artery together under the skin (Fig. 37.9). AV fistulas may take several weeks to mature. The surgeon determines when the fistula is mature for use.

An AV graft uses a tube of synthetic material to attach to an artery and a vein. Needles are inserted into the graft to access the patient's blood. Traditional graft material is not self-sealing and requires time for tissue growth to serve as a plug for the hole that the needle makes before it can be used. This may take 1 to 2 weeks. The Vectra® vascular access graft is self-sealing and does not require tissue growth so it can be used almost immediately after surgical implantation. This self-sealing property also decreases postdialysis bleeding time and reduces the time required for the dialysis session.

Vascular Access Care. AV fistulas and grafts are regularly checked for patency by palpating for a thrill (a tremor) and auscultating for a bruit (swishing sound) at the site of the graft or fistula. Any decrease or cessation of bruit or thrill indicates occlusion. If a thrill or bruit is diminished or not present, the HCP is notified immediately. Special care of the access site must be taken because this is the patient's only way to eliminate waste products (Box 37-5). It is important for the site to be carefully monitored per institution policy to detect any clotting or problems. Early detection of clotting allows the

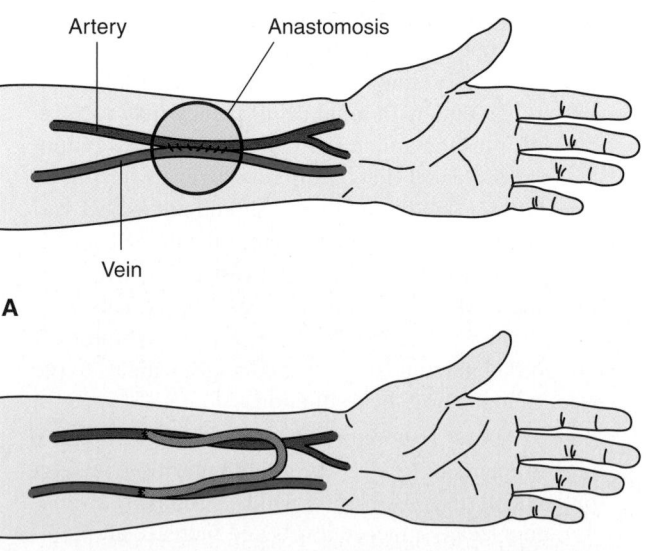

FIGURE 37.9 Hemodialysis access sites. (A) Arteriovenous fistula. (B) Arteriovenous graft.

Box 37-5 Care of Blood Access Fistula or Graft

These dialysis access sites should not be used for any purpose other than dialysis.

1. Watch for signs of bleeding or infection at the site.
2. Listen for a bruit at the site by placing the diaphragm of a stethoscope gently on the site. A bruit is a swishing sound made as the blood passes through the access site.
3. Gently palpate the site for a thrill, which is a buzzing or pulsing feeling that indicates good blood flow through the access site.
4. Do not take blood pressure, use a tourniquet, draw blood, or start any IV lines in the affected arm. Injections should be avoided if possible.
5. Many hospitals have the patient wear a red arm bracelet to signify that the arm should be protected. A sign above the bed may also be used.
6. Teach the patient to keep the site clean and not to bump or cut it.
7. Teach the patient to follow weight restrictions for lifting with the access arm.
8. Teach the patient to avoid wearing constrictive clothing or jewelry over the site.
9. Teach the patient to avoid prolonged bending or sleeping on the arm with an access.
10. Notify the HCP if signs of bleeding, reduced circulation, or infection occur in the access extremity: coldness, numbness, weakness, redness, fever, drainage, or swelling.

surgeon an opportunity to save the access by performing a declotting procedure rather than a total revision.

Postoperative Care. Initially, neurovascular checks are performed hourly for vascular surgery. Neurovascular checks include extremity movement and sensation, presence of numbness or tingling, pulses, temperature, color, and capillary refill (normally less than 3 seconds). Peripheral pulses are palpated to feel the thrill and auscultated to hear the bruit. If a pulse is absent or weak or the extremity is cool or dusky, the HCP is notified immediately. Dressings or incisions are checked, and any drainage, hematoma, or infection is documented and reported as needed. Vascular surgery pain is usually mild. Severe pain may indicate an occlusion of the graft. AV grafts can cause distal ischemia or "steal syndrome" because too much of the arterial blood is being "stolen" from the distal extremity. This is usually seen postoperatively and may require surgical correction to restore blood flow to the extremity.

Blood pressure readings and IVs should not be done in the extremity in which the access is placed. The extremity with the vascular access should be elevated postoperatively. Range-of-motion exercises should be encouraged. Patients are taught care of the access (see Box 37-5).

PERITONEAL DIALYSIS. **Peritoneal dialysis** provides continuous dialysis treatment and is done by the patient or family in the home. The peritoneal membrane is used as a semipermeable membrane across which excess wastes and fluids move from blood in peritoneal vessels into a dialysate solution that has been instilled into the peritoneal cavity. A peritoneal catheter is placed into the patient's peritoneal space between the two layers of the peritoneum below the waistline. This catheter is used to perform an exchange. The exchange process has three steps: (1) filling, (2) dwell time, and (3) draining.

The fill step involves instilling a bag of sterile dialyzing solution (dialysate) into the patient's peritoneal cavity through the catheter. The amount of solution is individualized but is often 1000 mL. The solution is left to dwell in the abdomen for several hours, allowing time for the waste products from the blood to pass through the peritoneal membrane into the dialysate solution (Fig. 37.10).

The solution is then drained out of the body and discarded. This process is repeated three or four times a day and is continuous for the patient. Several treatment plans use this exchange process. The treatment plan that best suits the patient's needs is determined by the patient and the dialysis team.

Continuous ambulatory peritoneal dialysis is the most commonly used treatment plan. Usually three exchanges are done during the day and one before bedtime. Other treatment plans allow for the use of a computerized machine called a cycler to regulate the exchanges during sleeping hours. Sometimes medications are added to the dialyzing solutions, such as heparin to prevent clotting of the catheter, insulin for the patient with diabetes, or antibiotics if there is infection.

Patient and family education is extremely important for peritoneal dialysis to be successful. The patient must be taught and be able to demonstrate that he or she is able to do a successful exchange. Sterile technique while performing the exchanges is imperative, and the exchanges should be done in a clean environment. A major complication is peritonitis (infection of the peritoneum), which can be life threatening. The major cause of peritonitis is poor technique when connecting the bag of dialyzing solution to the peritoneal catheter. The first sign of peritonitis is usually abdominal pain. (See Chapter 34 for additional signs and symptoms of peritonitis.) If any symptoms of peritonitis occur, the patient must contact the HCP immediately so antibiotic treatment can begin. The patient should be taught to care for the exit site (the site where the catheter comes out of the abdomen) and the need to inspect both the site and the dialysate solution for any signs of infection.

Dietary education is also important. A dietitian can assist the patient in making appropriate choices for adequate calories, protein, and potassium intake. The peritoneal dialysis patient typically has fewer dietary and fluid restrictions than the patient on hemodialysis because peritoneal dialysis is

• WORD • BUILDING •

peritoneal dialysis: peritoneal—peritoneum + dialysis— passage of a solution through a membrane

FIGURE 37.10 (A) Peritoneal dialysis works inside the body. Dialysis solution flows through a tube into the abdominal cavity, where it collects waste products from the blood. (B) Periodically the used dialysis solution is drained from the abdominal cavity, carrying away waste products and excess water from the blood.

continuous and maintains serum waste levels. Proteins are lost through the peritoneal membrane into the dialysate fluid, so increased dietary protein is needed. This loss increases with peritonitis, which further increases permeability.

LEARNING TIP

Differences among hemodialysis (HD), peritoneal dialysis (PD), and continuous renal replacement therapy (CRRT) include the following:

- **Patient access:** HD requires vascular access. PD requires insertion of a catheter into the peritoneal cavity. CRRT requires temporary vascular access such as a central line.
- **Equipment:** HD requires a specialized complex dialyzer. PD and CRRT do not require the specialized dialyzer, although machines are available for these therapies.
- **Training:** HD requires a skilled HD nurse. CRRT can be done by a non-HD nurse in a critical care setting. PD can be done by the patient.
- **Timing:** HD is intermittent. PD and CRRT are continuous.
- **Solute removal:** HD and PD use the principles of osmosis and diffusion, which require a dialysate solution. CRRT uses convection, so no dialysate is needed.
- **Cardiovascular effects:** HD may cause hypotension, which is a risk in the unstable patient. PD and CRRT have few cardiovascular effects. CRRT can be used for the unstable patient.

CRITICAL THINKING

Ms. Jackson

■ Ms. Jackson is a single, 56-year-old woman with a 20-year history of type 1 diabetes, hypertension, hyperlipidemia, chronic anemia, and a total knee replacement. She has been diagnosed with CKD. She was admitted to a medical unit for treatment of shortness of breath and CKD. Treatment will include hemodialysis. She has had increasing shortness of breath, has pitting edema, urine output of about 375 mL/day, and is having premature ventricular contractions (PVCs) as seen on the cardiac monitor. Her admitting laboratory values are Na 131, K 6, Cl 97, Ca 10, iron (Fe) 64, WBC 4000, RBC 3.12, Hgb 10.1, Hct 32, creatinine 7, BUN 30. Her blood glucose levels yesterday were as follows: 07:00, 154 mg/dL; noon, 122 mg/dL; 17:00, 188 mg/dL. She has sliding-scale insulin ordered. She is having an echocardiogram and chest x-ray done. She is having a two-tailed subclavian catheter placed for blood access. She is withdrawn and quiet.

1. What would be the first thing the nurse would address after getting the report?
2. What do Ms. Jackson's physical symptoms indicate and the laboratory values reflect?
3. What should the nurse say to Ms. Jackson in relation to her withdrawn behavior?
4. What should the nurse identify related to Ms. Jackson's understanding of self-care?
5. What teaching is needed for the diagnostic tests?
6. What nursing care is required for the blood access?
7. What type of insulin is used for sliding-scale insulin coverage? Why?
8. With what members of the health team would the nurse anticipate collaborating?

Suggested answers are at the end of the chapter.

Cultural Considerations

Because many Vietnamese people believe that the body must be kept intact even after death, they may object to removal of body parts or organ donation. Jewish law views organ transplantation from the recipient, the living donor, the cadaver donor, and the dying donor differently.

Kidney Transplantation

Kidney transplantation is another treatment for CKD and is extremely successful. An advantage of transplant compared with dialysis is that it reverses many of the physiological changes. The patient is also not dependent on dialysis and dietary restrictions.

A kidney transplant is a procedure in which a donor kidney is placed in the abdomen of a patient with CKD (Fig. 37.11). This healthy transplanted kidney functions as a normal kidney does. The donated kidney can come from a family member, a living, nonrelated donor, or a cadaver donor. Tissue and blood types must match so the body's immune system does not reject the donated kidney. Patients receive drugs to help prevent rejection, which must be taken for the rest of the patient's life. Sometimes even with these drugs, the body rejects the kidney, and the patient must go back on dialysis ("Cultural Considerations" and "Patient Perspective").

Clinical trials that give the same donor's bone marrow at the time of the kidney transplant to reduce rejection and the need for lifelong antirejection medications are in progress. Patients in the studies have been able to stop or greatly reduce their antirejection medications.

FIGURE 37.11 A transplanted kidney is placed in the abdomen. The patient's kidneys are usually left in place.

Diseased kidneys

Transplanted kidney

Transplanted ureter

Bladder

Patient Perspective

Kidney Transplantation: Pat

My experience with a kidney transplant spans three decades, but my overall renal illness experience also spans several years of illness and dialysis before the transplant. I think the biggest changes I have seen over the years are the involvement of patients in their own care options, as well as increased technical advances that allow transplantation to be very successful. Some of the feelings one experiences before transplantation are fear, uncertainty, and—if awaiting a donor—the guilt of knowing someone must die before you can live.

More than 30 years ago, there were no support groups and no one to talk to except family and doctors. Today, there are many support mechanisms in place for patients and families both before and after transplantation. As a nurse, you can help patients by knowing these support resources for referral. After a transplant, it is wonderful to feel better, almost immediately. However, as wonderful as transplantation is, the side effects of the antirejection medications may be felt immediately, while other problems take years to develop. Unfortunately, no one escapes the side effects of the medications. I have had breast cancer, osteoarthritis, cataracts, ulcers, skin cancer, anemia, weight gain, and other side effects of prednisone and Imuran (azathioprine). However, I can assure you that I feel this is much better than the alternative of dialysis.

Nursing Process for the Patient With Kidney Disease

Data Collection

Kidney disease progressively affects all body systems. If AKI is short term, fewer effects may be seen because some effects will not develop. In CKD, more effects are seen because the disease has time to progress. Data should be collected for signs and symptoms in all body systems. Family history of kidney disease and patient history of health problems such as hypertension, diabetes, systemic erythematous lupus, or urinary disorders are noted in the history. Also noted are medications the patient takes because they may be nephrotoxic and require adjustments. Recent changes in weight are documented.

Signs and symptoms vary depending on the severity of CKD and its cause. Common signs are hypertension, abnormal laboratory values (creatinine, BUN), or changes in urine. See signs and symptoms section for other effects.

Nursing Diagnosis, Planning, Intervention, and Evaluation

See the "Nursing Care Plan for the Patient With Chronic Kidney Disease."

NURSING CARE PLAN for the Patient With Chronic Kidney Disease

Nursing Diagnosis: *Excess Fluid Volume* related to kidney's inability to excrete water

Expected Outcomes: Fluid volume will be stable as evidenced by stable weight, absence of edema, lung sounds clear, and blood pressure within the patient's normal parameters.

Evaluation of Outcomes: Is weight stable? Is edema absent? Are lungs clear? Is blood pressure within the patient's normal parameters?

Intervention Monitor weight daily at same time; report gain of more than 2 pounds. **Rationale** Those retaining fluid will have weight gain. **Evaluation** Is weight stable? Should HCP be notified of change?

Intervention Monitor intake and output. **Rationale** This reveals degree of fluid retention. **Evaluation** Is output less than intake? Is this a change?

Intervention Monitor and report shortness of breath, tachycardia, crackles in lungs, frothy sputum, heart irregularities, hypotension, cold clammy skin. **Rationale** These are symptoms of heart failure that may accompany fluid overload. **Evaluation** Are symptoms of heart failure present?

Intervention Watch for new onset of jugular vein distention with patient's head raised to 30- to 45-degree angle. **Rationale** Fluid overload causes right-sided heart failure, resulting in distended jugular veins. **Evaluation** Are jugular veins distended? Is this a new finding?

Intervention Monitor vital signs, including orthostatic blood pressure. **Rationale** Blood pressure changes reflect fluid volume. **Evaluation** Is blood pressure increased?

Intervention Monitor for edema. **Rationale** Edema is a symptom of fluid overload. **Evaluation** Is edema present? Is this a change?

Intervention Monitor activity tolerance. **Rationale** Reduced activity tolerance may indicate heart failure related to fluid retention. **Evaluation** Is patient's tolerance of activity stable? Worsening?

Intervention Monitor serum protein and albumin levels. **Rationale** Low serum protein and albumin levels contribute to edema. **Evaluation** Are levels within normal limits?

Intervention Maintain sodium and fluid restrictions (often 600 mL plus the previous day's urine output) as ordered. Develop a plan with specific allotted amounts of fluid at each meal and for medications. Teach patient the importance of each. **Rationale** For those on dialysis, fluid intake is adjusted so that weight gains are no more than 1–3 kg between dialysis sessions. **Evaluation** Does patient understand and maintain sodium and fluid restriction?

Nursing Diagnosis: *Impaired Skin Integrity* related to dryness, excess fluid, crystal deposits

Expected Outcome: The patient will maintain intact skin.

Evaluation of Outcome: Does patient report no itching or dryness? Is patient's skin intact?

Intervention Observe skin for open areas and signs of infection. **Rationale** Detects early signs of problems. **Evaluation** Is skin intact?

NURSING CARE PLAN for the Patient With Chronic Kidney Disease—cont'd

Intervention Bathe with tepid water, oils, or oatmeal. **Rationale** Bathe regularly to reduce crystals with nondrying items to reduce itching and dryness and promote comfort. **Evaluation** Does patient report no itching or skin dryness?

Intervention Apply lotion to skin after bathing. **Rationale** Lotion is used for itching to reduce dry skin. **Evaluation** Is skin dry?

Nursing Diagnosis: *Activity Intolerance* related to anemia secondary to impaired synthesis of erythropoietin by the kidneys

Expected Outcome: The patient will be able to perform activities important to him or her.

Evaluation of Outcome: Does patient state satisfaction with level of activity tolerance?

Intervention Assess for pale mucous membranes and skin color, dyspnea, chest pain. **Rationale** These are signs and symptoms of anemia. **Evaluation** Does patient exhibit symptoms of anemia?

Intervention Monitor hemoglobin (Hgb), hematocrit (Hct). **Rationale** Low hemoglobin and hematocrit indicate anemia. **Evaluation** Are Hgb and Hct within normal limits?

Intervention Watch for signs of bleeding. **Rationale** Bleeding will worsen anemia. **Evaluation** Are signs of bleeding present?

Intervention Administer erythropoietin as ordered. Assist with blood transfusion as needed. **Rationale** Erythropoietin stimulates production of RBCs by bone marrow. **Evaluation** Are Hgb and Hct rising with use of erythropoietin?

Intervention Have patient space activities with rest periods. **Rationale** Rest periods decrease demand for oxygen. **Evaluation** Is patient able to tolerate activities with rest periods?

Nursing Diagnosis: *Risk for Injury* related to bleeding tendency from platelet dysfunction and use of heparin during dialysis, and from tendency for GI bleeding

Expected Outcomes: The patient will not experience bleeding. If bleeding occurs, it will be recognized and stopped quickly.

Evaluation of Outcomes: Are signs and symptoms of bleeding absent or recognized and reported quickly?

Intervention Observe for and report blood in stool or emesis, easy bruising, bleeding from mucous membranes or puncture sites, and report immediately if present. **Rationale** Bleeding must be recognized quickly to prevent complications. **Evaluation** Does patient have signs of bleeding?

Intervention Monitor Hgb, Hct, clotting studies, and platelets, and report results. **Rationale** Declining Hgb and Hct indicate blood loss. Declining platelet count or rising clotting times indicate increased risk of bleeding. **Evaluation** Are lab results stable?

Intervention Monitor vital signs. **Rationale** Falling blood pressure and rising pulse may indicate volume deficit from bleeding. **Evaluation** Are vital signs stable?

Intervention Avoid giving injections if possible. **Rationale** Injections can cause bleeding into tissue. **Evaluation** Can medications be given by another route?

Continued

NURSING CARE PLAN for the Patient With Chronic Kidney Disease—cont'd

Intervention If bleeding, apply gentle pressure to site if possible. **Rationale** Pressure promotes hemostasis. **Evaluation** Does pressure stop bleeding?

Intervention Teach patient to prevent injury to self and symptoms of bleeding to report. **Rationale** Injury can cause bleeding. Understanding symptoms of bleeding promotes early reporting. **Evaluation** Does patient verbalize understanding of need to prevent injury and report bleeding?

Intervention Protect patient from injury if confusion or seizures occur. **Rationale** Waste product accumulation or hyponatremia puts patient at risk of altered mental status or seizures. **Evaluation** Does patient require protection, such as seizure precautions? Is patient free from injury?

Nursing Diagnosis: *Risk for Infection* related to impaired immune system function

Expected Outcomes: The patient will not develop infection as evidenced by WBCs and temperature within normal limits, no signs and symptoms of infection.

Evaluation of Outcomes: Are WBCs and temperature within normal limits?

Intervention Monitor for signs and symptoms of infection, and report promptly to HCP. **Rationale** Early recognition of infection and prompt treatment help prevent complications. **Evaluation** Does patient have signs or symptoms of infection?

Intervention Protect patient from any source of infection, including infected roommates, visitors, or caregivers. **Rationale** Exposure to pathogens increases risk for infection. **Evaluation** Does anyone in contact with the patient have an infection?

Intervention Maintain skin integrity. **Rationale** Intact skin protects against infection. **Evaluation** Is skin intact?

Intervention Caregivers and patient practice good hand-washing technique. **Rationale** Hand washing helps control spread of infection. **Evaluation** Is good hand washing being practiced?

Intervention Culture any suspected site of infection as ordered by HCP. **Rationale** A culture identifies pathogens and guides treatment. **Evaluation** Is a culture needed?

Intervention Consult with HCP about influenza and pneumonia vaccines. **Rationale** Patients with impaired immune function are at risk for influenza and pneumonia. **Evaluation** Has the patient been vaccinated?

Intervention Teach patient and family signs and symptoms of infection to report to HCP. **Rationale** Early reporting of symptoms allows for prompt treatment. **Evaluation** Do patient and family verbalize understanding of symptoms to report?

Nursing Diagnosis: *Imbalanced Nutrition: Less Than Body Requirements* related to restricted diet, anorexia, nausea, and vomiting, and stomatitis secondary to effect of excessive urea on the GI system

Expected Outcomes: The patient will maintain ideal weight, and serum protein and albumin levels will be within normal limits.

Evaluation of Outcomes: Are weight and lab values at desired levels?

Intervention Monitor weekly weight and serum protein and albumin levels. **Rationale** Weight and laboratory results provide information about nutrition status. **Evaluation** Are weight and laboratory values stable?

NURSING CARE PLAN for the Patient With Chronic Kidney Disease—cont'd

Intervention Consult dietitian for low-protein diet planning and teaching. **Rationale** Low-protein diets decrease formation of waste products (urea, creatinine). **Evaluation** Does patient understand low-protein diet?

Intervention Initiate a calorie count—consult dietitian for assistance. **Rationale** A calorie count can provide information about the adequacy of the patient's diet. **Evaluation** Is patient receiving adequate calories?

Intervention Provide frequent oral care. **Rationale** Oral care enhances appetite and reduces urine taste in mouth. **Evaluation** Does oral care enhance appetite?

Intervention Offer frequent small feedings and dietary supplements. **Rationale** Smaller feedings are better tolerated and reduce risk of nausea. **Evaluation** Does patient tolerate small feedings?

Intervention Offer medications ordered for nausea before meals. **Rationale** Nausea reduces appetite and must be controlled. **Evaluation** Are antiemetics effective?

Intervention Ensure bowel movement daily or according to patient's usual pattern. **Rationale** Constipation can interfere with appetite. **Evaluation** Are patient's bowels functioning normally for him or her?

SUGGESTED ANSWERS TO

CRITICAL THINKING

■ Mrs. Milan

1. Sexual intercourse can be a predisposing factor to UTI, especially if the patient does not urinate after intercourse.

2. Mrs. Milan should be cautioned to always urinate after intercourse. (See also Box 37-1, "Patient Education").

3. The urinalysis will show WBCs, bacteria, RBCs, and positive nitrites.

4. Teaching should include the need to take all of the medication until it is gone even if she feels better. The reason for this is to ensure that the infection is completely resolved so it does not return due to some remaining bacteria. She should return for a urine culture after the therapy is complete.

■ Mr. Stevens

1. Weight, intake and output, blood pressure, and laboratory tests should be assessed as part of the morning evaluation.

2. BUN, serum creatinine, and potassium levels should also be checked.

3. Mr. Stevens should be taught that he needs to take antihypertensive medications, keep his follow-up visits to his HCP, follow a low-sodium diet, and restrict fluids if ordered.

■ Ms. Jackson

1. Collect data related to Ms. Jackson's breathing and respiratory status first. Then address the cardiovascular system to see how she is tolerating the dysrhythmia. Obtain Ms. Jackson's weight and intake and output to monitor fluid balance.

2. Shortness of breath and pitting edema related to fluid overload; urine output 375 mL/day is due to CKD; PVCs are due to elevated K. Na is low due to dilutional effect of excess fluid. K is retained due to CKD. WBC low due to CKD. RBC, Hgb, Hct low due to anemia. Creatinine and BUN are not excreted and are elevated due to CKD. Blood glucose is elevated due to diabetes.

3. Therapeutic conversation suggestions: "Ms. Jackson, would you like to talk about your diagnosis?" "How do you feel about your diagnosis?" "Do you have questions or concerns?" "What are your usual coping methods?" Provide explanations for procedures and interventions.

4. Determine Ms. Jackson's understanding of what CKD is, how it is treated, how to follow the renal diet and fluid restrictions, and the action and importance of medications. Identify barriers to self-care and her support systems.

5. Teaching includes that the chest x-ray and echocardiogram require no preparation and are not painful.

Continued

SUGGESTED ANSWERS TO—cont'd

6. A two-tail subclavian blood access is dedicated for hemodialysis. It is not used for any other purpose. Monitoring includes observing the site for signs of infection: redness, warmth, swelling, tenderness, drainage, and fever.
7. Regular insulin is used because a rapid acting insulin affects blood glucose levels now. Sliding scale insulin is ordered at intervals to monitor and treat the current blood glucose level. So only regular insulin is used for a sliding scale insulin order.
8. The registered nurse, licensed practical nurse/licensed vocational nurse, surgeon, nephrologist, dietician, pharmacist, and social worker.

REVIEW QUESTIONS

1. The nurse is planning a teaching session for a patient on preventing urinary tract infections. Which of the following information should the nurse include in the teaching plan? **Select all that apply.**
   1. Void frequently.
   2. Drink large amounts of citrus juices.
   3. Eat large amounts of vegetables.
   4. Wash the perineum every 8 hours.
   5. Void after sexual intercourse.
   6. Avoid drinking cranberry juice.

2. The nurse is planning care for a patient who is admitted to the hospital with a diagnosis of a kidney stone. Which of the following interventions would the nurse implement?
   1. Restrict fluids.
   2. Strain all urine.
   3. Increase calcium intake.
   4. Maintain bedrest.

3. The nurse is obtaining a history on a patient with a diagnosis of bladder cancer. Which of the following would the nurse expect to find in the patient's history?
   1. Tobacco use
   2. Vegetarian diet
   3. Caffeine use
   4. Alcohol use

4. While changing the pouch at the stoma site of an ileal conduit, the nurse notes the stoma is constantly spilling urine. Which of the following actions should the nurse take?
   1. Notify the physician of the constant spillage.
   2. Continue changing the pouch.
   3. Remove the overflow of urine with a straight catheter.
   4. Irrigate the stoma with a sterile solution of normal saline.

5. The nurse is contributing to the plan of care for a patient with glomerulonephritis. Which of the following interventions would the nurse recommend be included in the patient's plan of care?
   1. Increase fluid intake.
   2. Decrease sodium intake.
   3. Increase potassium intake.
   4. Decrease carbohydrate intake.

6. The nurse is caring for a postoperative patient who is receiving 0.9% normal saline IV at 125 mL/hour, morphine for pain control, and gentamicin (Garamycin) IV every 8 hours for 24 hours. The patient is allergic to iodine. Morning labs are WBC 8500, Hgb 12.4 g/dL, creatinine 2.2 mg/dL. Which of these findings is a priority for the nurse to report to the RN?
   1. WBC
   2. IV rate of 125 mL/hour
   3. Allergies
   4. Creatinine level

7. A patient with CKD who is on hemodialysis asks for a snack in the afternoon. The patient's potassium level is elevated. Which of the following foods could be given? **Select all that apply.**
   1. Banana
   2. Gelatin dessert
   3. Clear carbonated beverage
   4. Cranberry juice
   5. Nectarine

8. The nurse is checking patency of a new right arm AV fistula. What action does the nurse use to do this?
   1. Auscultate the right brachial pulse.
   2. Auscultate and palpate the right radial pulse.
   3. Measure blood pressure in the right arm.
   4. Palpate for thrill and auscultate bruit over the fistula.

9. A patient is returning to the medical unit after a dialysis session. The nurse notes bleeding from the patient's vascular access in the left arm. Which of the following is the nurse's first action?
   1. Call the physician.
   2. Notify the dialysis nurse.
   3. Apply pressure to access site.
   4. Take patient's blood pressure.

10. A patient is to receive 1600 mg of Renagel (sevelamer) orally with meals. Renagel 400-mg tablets are available. How many tablets should the nurse give?
    Answer: _____ tablets

Answers can be found in Appendix C.

References

American Cancer Society. (2013). *Key statistics about cancer.* Accessed January 26, 2014, at www.cancer.org/cancer /kidneycancer/detailedguide/kidney-cancer-adult-key-statistics

Dirkes, S. (2011). Acute kidney injury: not just acute renal failure anymore? *Critical Care Nurse, 31,* 37–50.

Isaac, S. (2012). Contrast-induced nephropathy: Nursing implications. *Critical Care Nurse, 32,* 41–48.

Jorgensen, A. (2013). Contrast-induced nephropathy: Pathophysiology and preventive strategies. *Critical Care Nurse, 33,* 37–46.

Pannu, N., James, M., Hemmelgarn, B. R., Dong, J., Tonelli, M., Klarenbach, S. (2011). Modification of outcomes after acute kidney injury by the presence of CKD. *American Journal of Kidney Disease, 58,* 206–213.

U.S. Renal Data System. (2013). *Annual data report: Atlas of CKD and end-stage renal disease in the United States.* Bethesda, MD: National Institute of Diabetes and Digestive and Kidney Diseases, National Institutes of Health.

 DavisPlus | For additional resources and information visit **davispl.us/medsurg5**

unit TEN

Understanding the Endocrine System

38

Endocrine System Function and Assessment

PAULA D. HOPPER AND
JANICE L. BRADFORD

KEY TERMS

affect (AF-feckt)
exophthalmos (EKS-off-THAL-mus)

LEARNING OUTCOMES

1. Identify the glands of the endocrine system.
2. Explain the function of each of the hormones in the endocrine system.
3. Describe the effects of aging on endocrine system function.
4. List data to collect when caring for a patient with a disorder of the endocrine system.
5. Plan nursing care for patients undergoing testing for an endocrine disorder.

NORMAL ENDOCRINE SYSTEM ANATOMY AND PHYSIOLOGY

The endocrine system consists of the endocrine (ductless) glands, which secrete hormones. Unlike other organ systems, the glands of the endocrine system are anatomically separate (Fig. 38.1). Their hormones are involved in fluid balance; metabolism, energy balance, growth, and development; contraction of smooth and cardiac muscle; glandular secretion; reproduction; and the establishment of circadian rhythms. Each hormone is secreted in response to a specific stimulus, is circulated by the blood, and affects target cells that have receptors for that hormone. Some hormones are secreted in response to hormones from other endocrine glands. Most hormone levels are regulated by negative feedback systems.

Pituitary Gland

The pituitary gland (hypophysis) is suspended by a short stalk from the hypothalamus in the brain (Fig. 38.2). There are two primary lobes or portions: anterior and posterior.

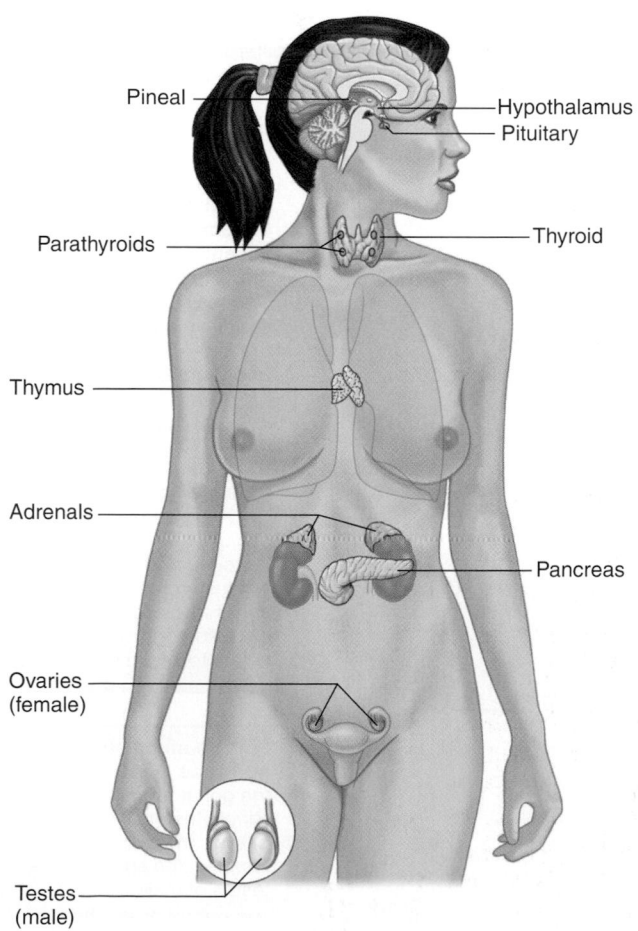

Pineal

Parathyroids

Thymus

Adrenals

Ovaries
(female)

Testes
(male)

Hypothalamus
Pituitary

Thyroid

Pancreas

FIGURE 38.1 Endocrine organs. From Thompson, G. S. (2013). *Understanding anatomy and physiology.* Philadelphia: F.A. Davis, p. 221.

Anterior Pituitary Gland

The anterior pituitary gland secretes its hormones in response to releasing hormones from the hypothalamus (Fig. 38.3). It is responsible for producing the hormones it releases.

Growth hormone (GH) increases cell division in tissues capable of mitosis. It also increases cellular uptake of amino acids for use in protein synthesis and releases fat from adipose tissue for energy production. Secretion of GH is regulated by growth hormone–releasing hormone (GHRH) and by growth hormone–inhibiting hormone (GHIH, or somatostatin), both from the hypothalamus. GHRH is produced during hypoglycemia or when there is a high blood level of amino acids. GHIH is secreted during hyperglycemia, when carbohydrates are available for energy production and the mobilization of fat is not needed.

Thyroid-stimulating hormone (TSH) stimulates growth and secretions of the thyroid gland. TSH secretion is stimulated by thyrotropin-releasing hormone (TRH) from the hypothalamus when the metabolic rate decreases.

Adrenocorticotropic hormone (ACTH) stimulates secretion of cortisol and related hormones from the adrenal cortex. Corticotropin-releasing hormone (CRH) from the hypothalamus stimulates the release of ACTH. CRH is produced during any type of stress such as injury, disease, exercise, or hypoglycemia.

See Figure 38.3 for other hormones of the anterior pituitary gland.

Posterior Pituitary Gland

The posterior pituitary gland stores and releases antidiuretic hormone (ADH; sometimes called vasopressin) and oxytocin (Fig. 38.4). Axon tracts from the hypothalamus transmit the hormones to the posterior pituitary and signal their release.

ADH increases water reabsorption by the kidney tubules, which decreases urine output. The water is reabsorbed back into the blood, thereby maintaining normal blood volume and pressure. In cases of great fluid loss, such as severe hemorrhage, the large amount of ADH secreted is especially important because it causes arteriole vasoconstriction, which increases blood pressure to homeostatic levels.

Oxytocin causes contractions of the myometrium to bring about delivery of a newborn and placenta. Release of oxytocin operates on a positive feedback loop. During breastfeeding, the subsequent release of oxytocin causes contraction of the smooth muscle cells around the mammary ducts. This release of milk is called milk ejection (or letdown).

Thyroid Gland

The thyroid gland consists of two lobes connected by a midpiece called the isthmus (Fig. 38.5). Three hormones are produced by the thyroid gland: triiodothyronine (T_3), thyroxine (T_4), and calcitonin.

T_3 and T_4 increase cellular respiration of glucose and fatty acids, which increases the metabolic rate—that is, energy and heat production. They are essential for normal physical growth, mental development, and reproductive maturation. Sufficient iodine intake is required for T_3 and T_4 production.

The direct stimulus for secretion of T_3 and T_4 is TSH from the anterior pituitary. A decrease in metabolic rate causes the

The tiny, pea-sized pituitary gland sits just underneath the hypothalamus. It lies cradled in the sella turcica, a cavity within the sphenoid bone.

Pituitary gland

Neurons within the hypothalamus synthesize various hormones. Some, called **releasing hormones**, stimulate the anterior pituitary to secrete its hormones. Others, called **inhibiting hormones**, suppress hormone secretion by the anterior pituitary.

Hypothalamus

Optic chiasm

Anterior pituitary

Posterior pituitary

A stalk called the *infundibulum* connects the hypothalamus and pituitary.

Despite its small size, the pituitary gland is actually two distinct glands: the **anterior pituitary**, or **adenohypophysis**, and the **posterior pituitary**, or **neurohypophysis**. These two glands are made of different tissue, excited by different types of stimuli, and secrete different hormones.

FIGURE 38.2 Pituitary gland and hypothalamus. From Thompson, G. S. (2013). *Understanding anatomy and physiology*. Philadelphia: F.A. Davis, p. 224.

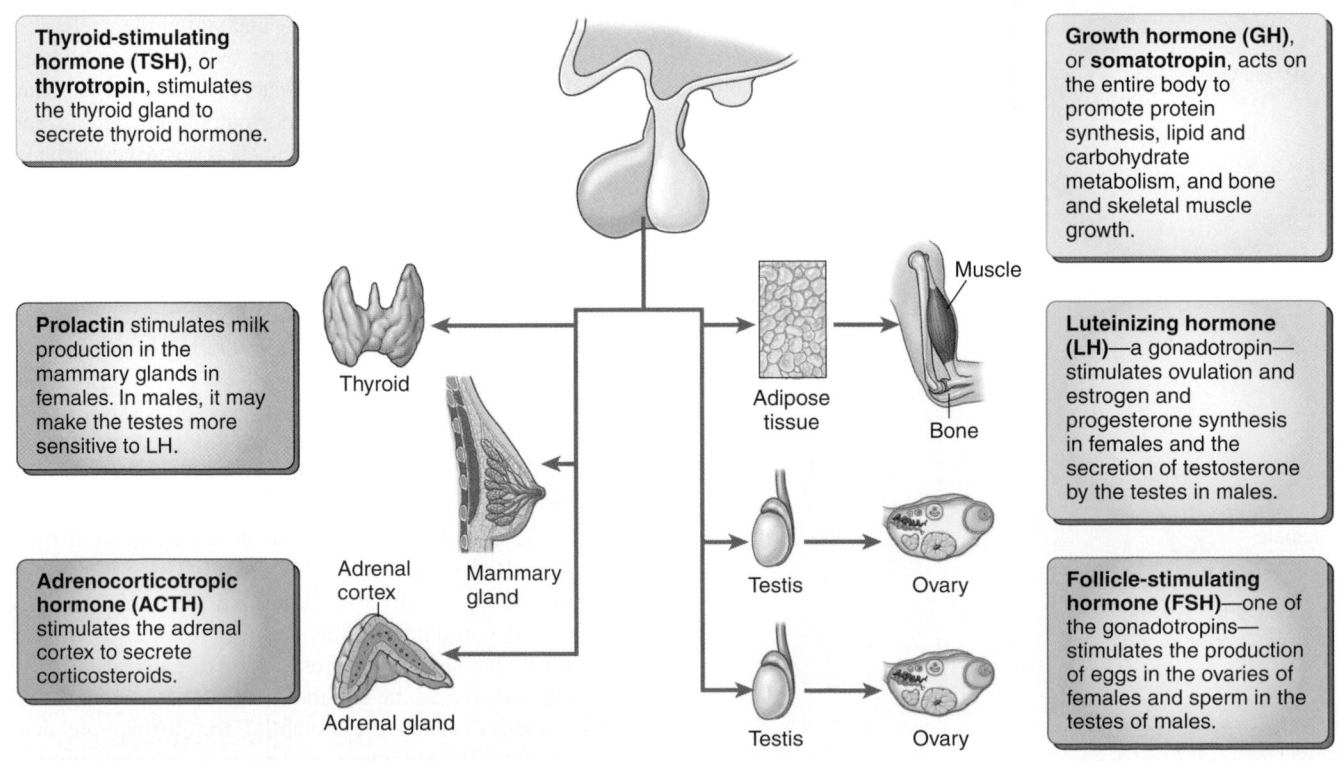

Thyroid-stimulating hormone (TSH), or **thyrotropin**, stimulates the thyroid gland to secrete thyroid hormone.

Growth hormone (GH), or **somatotropin**, acts on the entire body to promote protein synthesis, lipid and carbohydrate metabolism, and bone and skeletal muscle growth.

Prolactin stimulates milk production in the mammary glands in females. In males, it may make the testes more sensitive to LH.

Thyroid

Adipose tissue

Muscle

Bone

Luteinizing hormone (LH)—a gonadotropin—stimulates ovulation and estrogen and progesterone synthesis in females and the secretion of testosterone by the testes in males.

Adrenocorticotropic hormone (ACTH) stimulates the adrenal cortex to secrete corticosteroids.

Adrenal cortex

Mammary gland

Adrenal gland

Testis

Ovary

Testis

Ovary

Follicle-stimulating hormone (FSH)—one of the gonadotropins—stimulates the production of eggs in the ovaries of females and sperm in the testes of males.

FIGURE 38.3 Hormones of anterior pituitary. From Thompson, G. S. (2013). *Understanding anatomy and physiology*. Philadelphia: F.A. Davis, p. 225.

The nerve fibers that form the posterior pituitary originate in the hypothalamus.

The hypothalamic neurons synthesize hormones, which they send down to the posterior pituitary to be stored.

The posterior pituitary holds the hormones until stimulated by the nervous system to release them.

Oxytocin stimulates contraction of the uterus during childbirth. It also triggers the release of milk from the breasts during lactation.

Antidiuretic hormone (ADH) acts on the kidneys to reduce urine volume and prevent dehydration. ADH is also called **vasopressin**.

FIGURE 38.4 Posterior pituitary and hormones. From Thompson, G. S. (2013). *Understanding anatomy and physiology.* Philadelphia: F.A. Davis, p. 226.

Thyroid tissue is made of tiny sacs called **thyroid follicles**. Each follicle is filled with a thick fluid called **thyroid colloid**. The cells lining the sacs secrete the two main thyroid hormones: **T₃ (triiodothyronine)** and **T₄ (thyroxine)**. Unlike other glands, the thyroid gland can store the hormones for later use.

The thyroid gland resides in the neck, just below the trachea, where it is wrapped around the anterior and lateral portions of the trachea.

Larynx

Isthmus

Trachea

FIGURE 38.5 Thyroid. From Thompson, G. S. (2013). *Understanding anatomy and physiology.* Philadelphia: F.A. Davis, p. 229.

hypothalamus to secrete TRH. TRH stimulates the anterior pituitary to secrete TSH, which stimulates the thyroid to increase secretion of T_3 and T_4, which increase energy production and raise the metabolic rate. Negative feedback decreases the secretion of TRH from the hypothalamus until the metabolic rate decreases again.

The third thyroid hormone (TH), calcitonin, targets bone tissue and therefore is especially important during childhood when bone growth is accelerated. Calcitonin inhibits resorption of calcium and phosphate by osteoclasts, thereby lowering the blood levels of these minerals and retaining them in bones. This one function of calcitonin has two important results: the maintenance of normal blood levels of calcium and phosphate and the maintenance of a strong, stable bone matrix. The stimulus for secretion of calcitonin is hypercalcemia.

LEARNING TIP

Learning tip: Confused between resorption and reabsorption? Resorption breaks down bone tissue and releases calcium ions into circulation when PTH is secreted. Reabsorption is the process of absorbing a substance into the blood again, such as when ADH causes water to be reabsorbed from the kidney tubules back into the blood supply.

LEARNING TIP

An easy way to remember the function of calcitonin is to remember calciTONin TONes down serum calcium.

Parathyroid Glands

There are usually four parathyroid glands, two on the back of each lobe of the thyroid gland (Fig. 38.6). They produce parathyroid hormone (PTH), an antagonist to calcitonin. Besides bone, the target organs of PTH are the small intestine and kidneys. The overall effect of PTH is to raise the blood calcium level and lower the blood phosphate level.

Homeostasis of blood calcium level is regulated by calcitonin and PTH. (See animation on DavisPlus.) Calcium ion delivery through the blood is essential for normal excitability of neurons and muscle cells and for the process of blood clotting.

Adrenal Glands

The bilateral adrenal glands are located superior to each kidney. The inner adrenal medulla is surrounded by an outer adrenal cortex (Fig. 38.7).

Adrenal Medulla

The catecholamines (epinephrine and norepinephrine), released by the adrenal medulla, are sympathomimetic, meaning

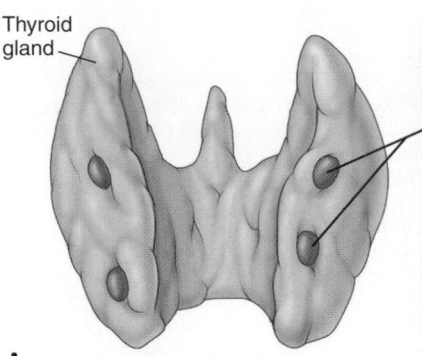

Thyroid gland

The parathyroid glands are embedded in the posterior corners of the lobes of the thyroid. Most people have four parathyroid glands, but the number of glands, as well as their locations, can vary.

A   **Posterior view**

PTH inhibits new bone formation while stimulating the breakdown of old bone, causing calcium (and phosphate) to move out of bone and into the blood.

PTH encourages the kidneys to reabsorb calcium—blocking its excretion into the urine—while promoting the secretion of phosphate. PTH also prompts the kidneys to activate vitamin D, necessary for intestinal absorption of calcium.

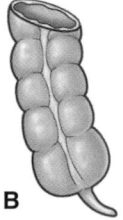

After it's activation by the kidneys, vitamin D allows the intestines to absorb calcium from food; the calcium is transported through intestinal cells and into the blood.

B

FIGURE 38.6 (A) Parathyroid. (B) Effectors/targets of parathyroid hormone. From Thompson, G. S. (2013). *Understanding anatomy and physiology.* Philadelphia: F.A. Davis, p. 230 (A), p. 231 (B).

they mimic the sympathetic nervous system. During stress, the hypothalamus stimulates their release to prolong the body's stress response.

Adrenal Cortex

The adrenal cortex secretes three types of steroid hormones: mineralocorticoids, glucocorticoids, and gonadocorticoids ("sex steroids").

Aldosterone is the most abundant of the mineralocorticoids, and its target organs are the kidneys. Aldosterone increases the reabsorption of sodium ions and the excretion of potassium ions by the kidney tubules. As sodium ions are reabsorbed, hydrogen ions may be excreted in exchange. This is one mechanism to prevent the accumulation of hydrogen ions that would lead to acidosis. Also, as sodium ions are reabsorbed, water follows; this is important for maintaining normal blood volume and blood pressure.

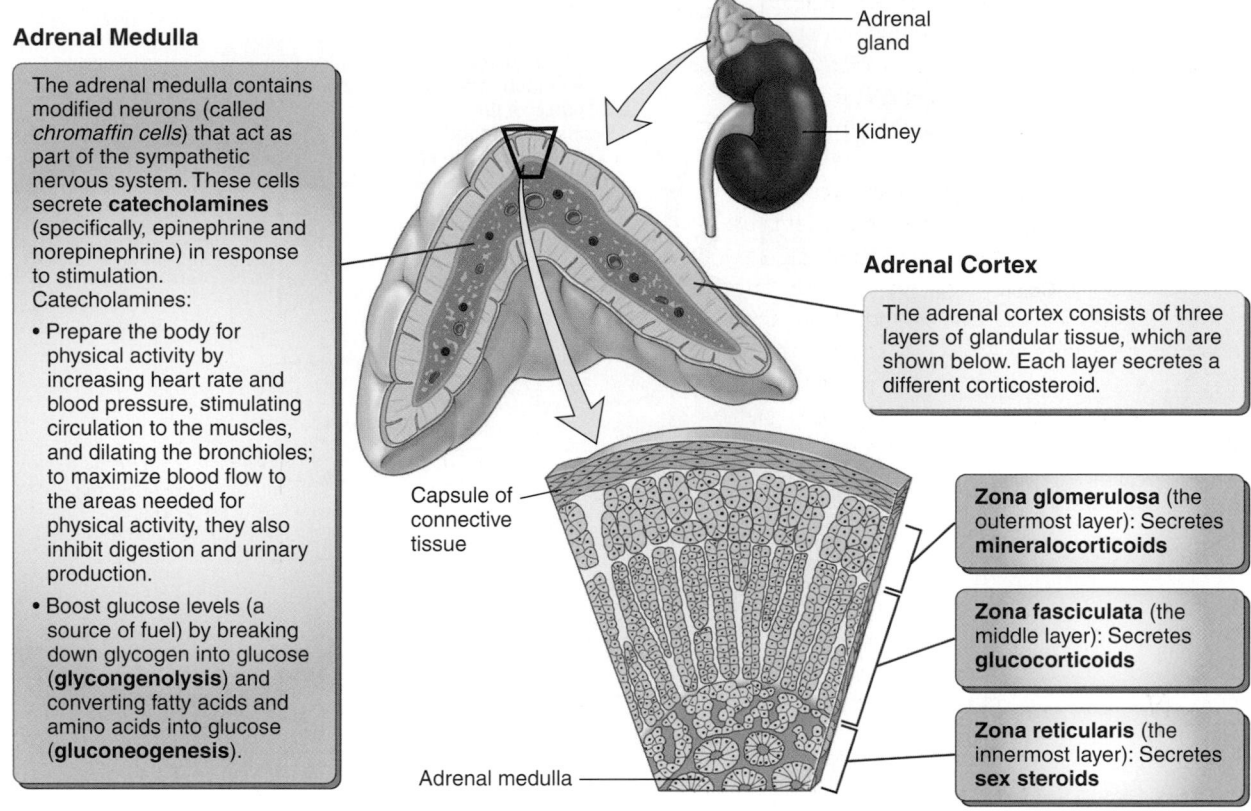

Adrenal Medulla

The adrenal medulla contains modified neurons (called *chromaffin cells*) that act as part of the sympathetic nervous system. These cells secrete **catecholamines** (specifically, epinephrine and norepinephrine) in response to stimulation.
Catecholamines:

- Prepare the body for physical activity by increasing heart rate and blood pressure, stimulating circulation to the muscles, and dilating the bronchioles; to maximize blood flow to the areas needed for physical activity, they also inhibit digestion and urinary production.
- Boost glucose levels (a source of fuel) by breaking down glycogen into glucose (**glycongenolysis**) and converting fatty acids and amino acids into glucose (**gluconeogenesis**).

Adrenal gland

Kidney

Adrenal Cortex

The adrenal cortex consists of three layers of glandular tissue, which are shown below. Each layer secretes a different corticosteroid.

Capsule of connective tissue

Zona glomerulosa (the outermost layer): Secretes **mineralocorticoids**

Zona fasciculata (the middle layer): Secretes **glucocorticoids**

Zona reticularis (the innermost layer): Secretes **sex steroids**

Adrenal medulla

FIGURE 38.7 Adrenal gland. From Thompson, G. S. (2013). *Understanding anatomy and physiology*. Philadelphia: F.A. Davis, p. 233.

Cortisol is the most abundant of the glucocorticoids and has many target tissues. It stimulates gluconeogenesis in the liver and increases lipolysis and protein catabolism for energy production. By providing energy sources to body tissues, cortisol ensures that glucose will be available for the brain (glucose-sparing effect).

Cortisol release is increased during response to stress. The hypothalamus causes secretion of ACTH by the anterior pituitary, which increases cortisol secretion by the adrenal cortex. The resultant increase in energy availability is necessary for stress-induced changes. Cortisol also has an anti-inflammatory effect. However, excess cortisol decreases the immune response and can delay healing of damaged tissue.

The gonadocorticoids are small amounts of male androgens. In females they are converted to estrogens and are the only source of estrogen after menopause. In both genders, they contribute to libido.

Pancreas

The pancreas is both an exocrine and endocrine gland. As an endocrine gland, the pancreas secretes insulin and glucagon for blood glucose homeostasis, and somatostatin, which inhibits both insulin and glucagon (Fig. 38.8).

Hypoglycemia stimulates alpha cells to release glucagon. Glucagon raises blood glucose, making it available to cells.

Hyperglycemia stimulates beta cells to release insulin. Insulin increases the uptake of glucose from the blood into cells, lowering blood glucose. Cells use glucose in cellular respiration to release energy.

Hyperglycemia occurs after meals, especially those high in carbohydrates. Insulin and glucagon function as antagonists; normal secretion of both hormones ensures a blood glucose level that fluctuates within normal limits (Fig. 38.9). Table 38.1 (see p. 880) reviews endocrine hormone function.

Aging and the Endocrine System

Most of the endocrine glands decrease secretion with age, but normal aging usually does not lead to serious hormone deficiencies or illness (Fig. 38.10). Unless specific pathological conditions develop, the endocrine system continues to function adequately in old age.

NURSING ASSESSMENT OF THE ENDOCRINE SYSTEM

Health History

When performing a health history, a number of questions can be asked to determine whether an endocrine problem exists. Often, however, you might be aware of a history of an endocrine disorder, such as diabetes or hypothyroidism. When a disorder exists or is suspected, you can do more focused data collection. Assessment of individual disorders is provided in Chapters 39 and 40. Table 38.2 offers general questions that can help you identify new problem areas. If the data reveal abnormalities, they should be reported to the registered nurse or health care provider (HCP).

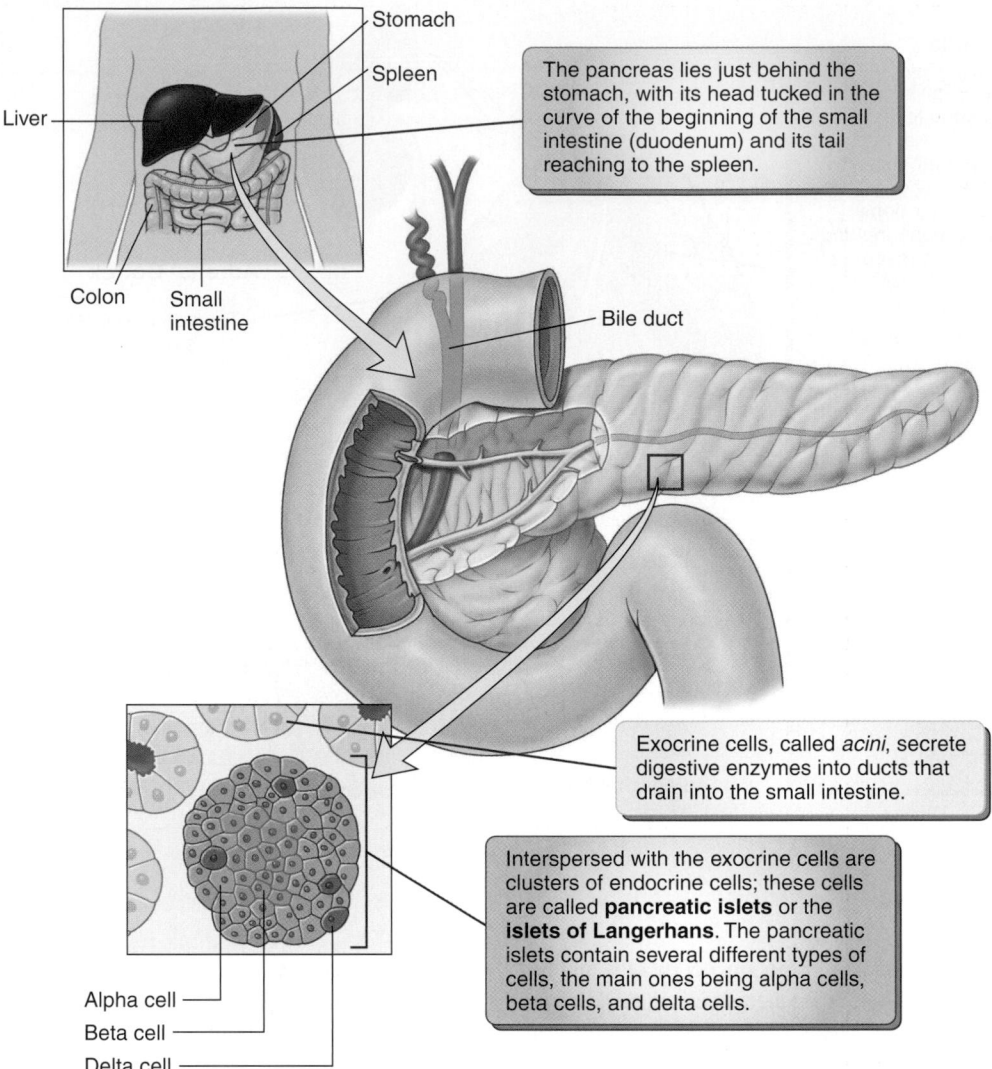

Stomach

Spleen

The pancreas lies just behind the stomach, with its head tucked in the curve of the beginning of the small intestine (duodenum) and its tail reaching to the spleen.

Liver

Colon   Small intestine

Bile duct

Exocrine cells, called *acini*, secrete digestive enzymes into ducts that drain into the small intestine.

Interspersed with the exocrine cells are clusters of endocrine cells; these cells are called **pancreatic islets** or the **islets of Langerhans**. The pancreatic islets contain several different types of cells, the main ones being alpha cells, beta cells, and delta cells.

Alpha cell
Beta cell
Delta cell

FIGURE 38.8 Pancreas. From Thompson, G. S. (2013). *Understanding anatomy and physiology.* Philadelphia: F.A. Davis, p. 235.

Physical Examination

The physical examination starts with height, weight, and vital signs. Compare findings with the patient's baseline assessment if available. Table 38.3 includes common endocrine-related causes of physical examination abnormalities.

Inspection

Observe the patient for mood and **affect** (emotional tone) throughout the physical assessment. Inspect the neck for thyroid enlargement. Look for eyes that bulge (**exophthalmos**). Note posture, body fat, and presence of tremor. Observe skin and hair texture and moisture. Note the presence of a moonlike face or "buffalo hump" on the upper back. Observe the lower extremities for skin and color changes that might indicate circulatory impairment. See Table 38.3 for the rationales for these observations.

Palpation

The thyroid gland is the only palpable endocrine gland. The licensed practical nurse/licensed vocational nurse may assist a physician or nurse practitioner (NP) to palpate the thyroid gland.

The practitioner stands behind or in front of the seated patient and palpates the gland while the patient swallows a sip of water. You can assist with positioning the patient, providing water, and instructing the patient to take a sip of water and hold it in his or her mouth until told to swallow. The thyroid gland should never be palpated in a patient with uncontrolled hyperthyroidism because this can stimulate secretion of additional TH.

Palpate all peripheral pulses. The posterior tibial and dorsalis pedis pulses may be diminished in patients with circulatory impairment. Palpate skin turgor by gently pinching a small piece of skin. The sternum is a good place to check. If a "tent" of skin remains in place, the patient may be dehydrated as a result of water loss, as in ADH deficiency.

Auscultation and Percussion

Auscultation and percussion are not usually part of an endocrine assessment.

• WORD • BUILDING •

exophthalmos: exo—outward + ophthalmos—relating to the eye

FIGURE 38.9 Regulation of blood glucose. From Thompson, G. S. (2013). *Understanding anatomy and physiology*. Philadelphia: F.A. Davis, p. 236.

DIAGNOSTIC TESTS FOR THE ENDOCRINE SYSTEM

Hormone Tests

Serum Hormone Levels

Many hormones can be measured from a simple blood specimen. This is useful in diagnosing hypofunctioning or hyperfunctioning gland states. See Table 38.4 for some commonly measured hormones.

Stimulation Tests

Stimulation tests may also help determine endocrine gland function. For this type of test, a substance is injected to stimulate a gland. The hormone secreted by that gland is then measured in the blood to determine how well it responded to the stimulation. For example, in a TRH stimulation test, TRH is injected. If the pituitary gland responds appropriately, TSH is secreted. If the thyroid gland responds appropriately to the TSH, T_3 and T_4 levels rise. Failure of TRH to stimulate TSH

TABLE 38.1 REVIEW OF ENDOCRINE FUNCTION

Hormone	Function(s)	Regulation of Secretion
Hormones of the Posterior Pituitary Gland		
Antidiuretic hormone (ADH or vasopressin)	Increases water reabsorption by the kidney tubules (water returns to the blood) Decreases sweating Causes vasoconstriction (in large amounts)	Decreased water content in the body stimulates secretion Alcohol inhibits secretion
Oxytocin	Promotes contraction of myometrium of uterus (labor) Promotes release of milk from mammary glands	Nerve impulses from hypothalamus, the result of stretching of cervix or stimulation of nipple Secretion from placenta at the end of gestation—stimulus unknown
Hormones of the Anterior Pituitary Gland		
Growth hormone (GH)	Increases rate of mitosis Increases amino acid transport into cells Increases rate of protein synthesis Increases use of fats for energy	GHRH (hypothalamus) stimulates secretion GHIH—somatostatin (hypothalamus) inhibits secretion
Thyroid-stimulating hormone (TSH)	Increases secretion of thyroxine and T_3 by thyroid gland	TRH (hypothalamus)
Adrenocorticotropic hormone (ACTH)	Increases secretion of cortisol by the adrenal cortex	CRH (hypothalamus)
Prolactin	Stimulates milk production by the mammary glands	PRH (hypothalamus) stimulates secretion PIH (hypothalamus) inhibits secretion
Follicle-stimulating hormone (FSH)	*In women:* Initiates growth of ova in ovarian follicles Increases secretion of estrogen by follicle cells *In men:* Initiates sperm production in the testes	GnRH (hypothalamus) stimulates secretion Inhibin (ovaries) inhibits secretion GnRH (hypothalamus) stimulates secretion Inhibin (testes) inhibits secretion
Luteinizing hormone (LH)	*In women:* Causes ovulation Causes the ruptured ovarian follicle to become the corpus luteum Increases secretion of progesterone by the corpus luteum *In men:* Increases secretion of testosterone by the interstitial cells of the testes	GnRH (hypothalamus) GnRH (hypothalamus)
Hormones of the Thyroid Gland		
Thyroxine and triiodothyronine (T_4 and T_3)	Increase energy production from all food types Increase rate of protein synthesis	TSH (anterior pituitary)
Calcitonin	Decreases the reabsorption of calcium and phosphate from bones to blood	Hypercalcemia

TABLE 38.1 REVIEW OF ENDOCRINE FUNCTION—cont'd

Hormone	Function(s)	Regulation of Secretion
Hormones of the Parathyroid Glands		
Parathyroid hormone (PTH)	Increases the reabsorption of calcium and phosphate from bone to blood Increases absorption of calcium and phosphate by the small intestine Increases the reabsorption of calcium and the excretion of phosphate by the kidneys; activates vitamin D	Hypocalcemia stimulates secretion Hypercalcemia inhibits secretion
Hormones of the Adrenal Medulla		
Epinephrine	Increases heart rate and force of contraction Dilates bronchioles Decreases peristalsis Increases conversion of glycogen in glucose in the liver Causes vasodilation in skeletal muscles Causes vasoconstriction in skin and viscera Increases use of fats for energy Increases the rate of cell respiration	Sympathetic impulses from the hypothalamus in stress situations
Norepinephrine	Causes vasoconstriction in skin, viscera, and skeletal muscles	
Hormones of the Pancreas		
Glucagon (alpha cells)	Increases conversion of glycogen to glucose in the liver Increases the use of excess amino acids and fats for energy	Hypoglycemia
Insulin (beta cells)	Increases glucose transport into cells and the use of glucose for energy production Increases the conversion of excess glucose to glycogen in the liver and muscles Increases amino acid and fatty acid transport into cells, and their use in synthesis reactions	Hyperglycemia
Somatostatin (delta cells)	Decreases secretion of insulin and glucagon. Slows absorption of nutrients.	Rising levels of insulin and glucagon
Hormones of the Adrenal Cortex		
Aldosterone	Increases reabsorption of Na^+ ions by the kidneys to the blood Increases excretion of K^+ ions by the kidneys in urine	Low blood Na^+ level Low blood volume or blood pressure High blood K^+ level
Cortisol	Increases use of fats and excess amino acids for energy	ACTH (anterior pituitary) during physiological stress

Continued

TABLE 38.1   REVIEW OF ENDOCRINE FUNCTION—cont'd

Hormone	Function(s)	Regulation of Secretion
	Decreases use of glucose for energy (except for the brain) Increases conversion of glucose to glycogen in the liver Anti-inflammatory effect: stabilizes lysosomes and blocks the effects of histamine	

Note. CRH = corticotropin-releasing hormone; GHIH = growth hormone–inhibiting hormone; GHRH = growth hormone–releasing hormone; GnRH = gonadotropin-releasing hormone; K+ = potassium; Na+ = sodium; PIH = prolactin-inhibiting hormone; PRH = prolactin-releasing hormone; TRH = thyrotropin-releasing hormone.

Source: Adapted from Scanlon, V. C., & Sanders, T. (2015). *Essentials of anatomy and physiology* (7th ed.). Philadelphia: F.A. Davis.

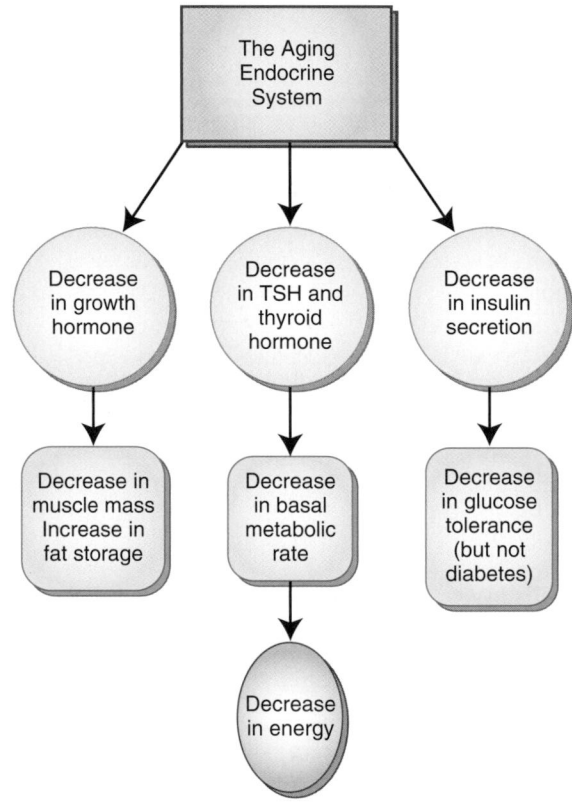

FIGURE 38.10 Effects of aging on the endocrine system.

Urine Tests

Sometimes it is helpful to measure the amount of hormone or hormone by-product excreted in the urine during a 24-hour period. Examples are cortisol and vanillylmandelic acid, a product of catecholamine metabolism. See DavisPlus for the procedure for collecting a 24-hour urine specimen.

Other Laboratory Tests

Some laboratory tests may indirectly reflect the function of an endocrine gland. For example, a serum calcium level helps indicate PTH or calcitonin secretion, and a blood glucose level reflects insulin secretion.

Nuclear Scanning
Thyroid Scan

A thyroid scan may be done to determine the presence of tumors or nodules. For this test, a radioactive material is given orally or by injection. The material is taken up by the thyroid gland. After a specified time, the thyroid gland is scanned with a scintillation camera. The scan will show hot spots (nodules), which are not malignant, or cold spots (areas that

and TH indicates a pituitary or thyroid condition. Further studies might be done to determine the cause.

Suppression Tests

Suppression tests are the opposite of stimulating tests. For this type of test, a substance is injected that is expected to suppress a hormone's release. For example, if dexamethasone (a steroid hormone) is injected, cortisol release from the adrenal cortex is expected to be suppressed via a negative feedback mechanism. If the cortisol level is not suppressed, adrenal cortex dysfunction is suspected.

TABLE 38.2   SUBJECTIVE DATA COLLECTION FOR THE ENDOCRINE SYSTEM

Category	Questions to Ask During the Health History	Rationale
Neuromuscular	Have you noticed muscle spasms or twitching?	These symptoms may be associated with excessive antidiuretic hormone secretion (SIADH) or calcium depletion resulting from hypoparathyroidism.
	Do you have numbness, tingling, or pain in your feet, legs, or hands?	These can be associated with neuropathy resulting from diabetes mellitus. Numbness and tingling can also indicate hypocalcemia related to hypoparathyroidism.
Nutrition/Fluid Balance	Have you gained or lost weight without trying?	Actual weight gain may be associated with hypothyroidism. Weight gain due to water retention may result from Cushing's syndrome or SIADH. Weight loss may result from uncontrolled diabetes or hyperthyroidism. Weight loss due to dehydration may be related to Addison's disease.
	Have you noticed excessive thirst or urination?	Excessive thirst and urination are classic symptoms of diabetes mellitus and diabetes insipidus.
	Have you noticed a change in your energy level?	Lack of energy may be associated with uncontrolled diabetes, hypothyroidism, hyperthyroidism, Addison's disease, or pituitary disorders.
Metabolic	Do you generally tolerate changes in environmental temperature?	Hypothyroidism can cause cold intolerance. Hyperthyroidism can cause heat intolerance.
Mood/Memory	Have you noticed a change in your mood or memory?	Mental function may be dull with hypothyroidism. Mood swings can occur with Cushing's syndrome. Agitation or confusion can result from hypoglycemia in a person with diabetes.
Family History	Does anyone in your family have a thyroid problem, diabetes, or another endocrine disorder?	Some disorders are hereditary.

Note. SIADH = syndrome of inappropriate antidiuretic hormone.

do not take up the radioactivity), which indicate malignancy. Cold spots can then be biopsied to confirm a diagnosis. Because such a small amount of radioactive material is used, the risk to the patient is minimal. The patient should be aware that the test takes approximately 30 minutes to complete.

Radioactive Iodine Uptake

A radioactive iodine uptake test is similar to a thyroid scan and is done to evaluate thyroid function. Several scans are taken over a 24-hour period after administration of radioactive iodine. The amount of iodine taken up by the thyroid indicates the

TABLE 38.3 ENDOCRINE-RELATED CAUSES OF ABNORMAL PHYSICAL EXAMINATION FINDINGS

Category	Abnormal Examination Finding	Possible Causes
Mood	Depressed mood or affect	Hypothyroidism
	Nervousness	Hyperthyroidism, pheochromocytoma
	Agitation	Low blood glucose level
Nutrition/Fluid Balance	Weight gain	Decreased metabolic rate in hypothyroidism, fluid excess
	Weight loss	Increased metabolic rate in hyperthyroidism; uncontrolled diabetes, dehydration
	Poor skin turgor	Dehydration due to water loss in Addison's disease, diabetes mellitus, diabetes insipidus
Integumentary	Hyperpigmentation of skin	Addison's disease
	Dry, scaly skin	Hypothyroidism
	Dusky lower extremities with weak peripheral pulses	Circulatory changes in diabetes mellitus
Vital Signs	Change in pulse rate or temperature	Elevated due to increased metabolic rate in hyperthyroidism
		Decreased due to slowed metabolic rate in hypothyroidism
	Elevated blood pressure	Increased catecholamine release in pheochromocytoma or fluid retention in Cushing's syndrome
	Decreased blood pressure	Sodium and water loss in Addison's disease
Neuromuscular	Tremor	Hyperthyroidism, hypoglycemia, or pheochromocytoma
Head and Neck	Exophthalmos (bulging eyes)	Fat deposits and edema behind the eyes in Graves' disease
	Fat pads on neck and shoulders ("buffalo hump"), round "moon" face	Accumulation of fat in Cushing's syndrome
	Enlarged thyroid gland	Excessive stimulation by thyroid-stimulating hormone in hypothyroidism or hyperthyroidism

TABLE 38.4 COMMON ENDOCRINE-RELATED LABORATORY TESTS

Test	Normal Values*	Significance of Abnormal Findings
Thyroid Tests		
Thyroid-stimulating hormone	0.4–4.2 microinternational units/mL	↑ in primary hypothyroidism ↓ in primary hyperthyroidism
Triiodothyronine (T_3), total	70–204 ng/dL	↓ in hypothyroidism ↑ in hyperthyroidism
Triiodothyronine (T_3), free	260–480 pg/dL	
Thyroxine (T_4), total	*Male:* 4.6–10.5 mcg/dL *Female:* 5.5–11 mcg/dL	↓ in hypothyroidism ↑ in hyperthyroidism

TABLE 38.4   COMMON ENDOCRINE-RELATED LABORATORY TESTS—cont'd

Test	Normal Values*	Significance of Abnormal Findings
Thyroxine (T$_4$), free	0.8–1.5 ng/dL	
Parathyroid Tests		
Parathyroid hormone	8–24 pg/mL	↑ in primary hyperparathyroidism ↓ in primary hypoparathyroidism, parathyroid trauma during thyroid surgery
Calcium, blood	8.2–10.2 mg/100 mL *Over age 90:* 8.2–9.6 mg/dL	↑ in some cancers, hyperparathyroidism ↓ in hypothyroidism
Phosphorus	2.5–4.5 mg/dL	↑ in hypoparathyroidism ↓ in hyperparathyroidism
Pituitary Tests		
Growth hormone	*Male:* 0–5 ng/mL *Female:* 0–10 ng/mL	↑ in acromegaly ↓ in small stature
Antidiuretic hormone (vasopressin)	0–4.7 pg/mL	↑ in SIADH ↓ in diabetes insipidus
Urine specific gravity	1.001–1.029	↓ in diabetes insipidus
Adrenocorticotropic hormone (ACTH)	9–52 pg/mL in a.m. *Women on oral contraceptives:* 5–29 pg/mL	↑ in Addison's disease ↓ in Cushing's syndrome, long-term corticosteroid therapy
Adrenal Tests		
Aldosterone	*Supine:* 3–16 ng/dL *Upright:* 7–30 ng/dL	↑ in heart failure, chronic obstructive pulmonary disease (COPD), hypovolemia ↓ in Addison's disease, hypoaldosteronism
Cortisol	5–25 mcg/dL at 0800 3–16 mcg/dL at 1600	↑ in Cushing's syndrome, stress ↓ in Addison's disease, steroid withdrawal
Vanillylmandelic acid (VMA; urine test)	1.4–6.5 mg/24 hr	↑ in pheochromocytoma
Pancreas Tests		
Fasting plasma glucose (FPG)	70–100 mg/dL	↑ in stress, Cushing's syndrome 101–125 mg/dL = pre-diabetes 126 mg/dL or greater = diabetes mellitus ↓ in hypoglycemia, Addison's disease
Fructosamine (glycated albumin)	174–286 micromol/L *Diabetes:* *Controlled:* 210–421 micromol/L *Uncontrolled:* 268–870 micromol/L	↑ in poor diabetes control ↓ in severe hypoproteinemia
Ketones, blood and urine	Negative	Positive in acidosis, fasting or starvation, diabetic ketoacidosis
Oral glucose tolerance test	Blood glucose level less than 140 mg/dL at 2 hr	140–199 mg/dL at 2 hr = prediabetes 200 mg/dL or greater at 2 hr = diabetes mellitus
Glycosylated hemoglobin	4%–6%	↑ in poor diabetes control

SIADH = syndrome of inappropriate antidiuretic hormone.

*All normal values are for a fasting test.

activity of the gland. This is especially helpful in diagnosing hyperthyroidism.

PET Scan

Positron emission tomography (PET) scanning is another type of scan that can be done to differentiate between benign and malignant endocrine tumors. PET scans are helpful because they can show metabolic changes in organs or tissues.

Radiographic Tests

A computed tomography (CT) scan or magnetic resonance imaging (MRI) may be done to locate a tumor or identify hypertrophy of a gland.

Ultrasound

Ultrasound may be done of the thyroid or parathyroid glands to determine if they are enlarged or to find masses.

Biopsy

Biopsy is done to obtain tissue to examine for possible cancerous cells. The thyroid gland can be biopsied either by needle aspiration under local anesthesia or using a surgical incision.

SUGGESTED ANSWERS TO

CRITICAL THINKING

■ *Ms. Hackworth*

1. "It's not your thyroid hormone that is high, it's your thyroid-stimulating hormone. That means your pituitary gland has to work extra hard to try to stimulate your thyroid gland."

2.
$$\frac{50 \text{ mcg}}{} \Bigg| \frac{1 \text{ mg}}{1000 \text{ mcg}} = 0.05 \text{ mg}$$

REVIEW QUESTIONS

1. Which hormones are secreted by the posterior pituitary gland? **Select all that apply.**
   1. Antidiuretic hormone
   2. Thyroid-stimulating hormone
   3. Growth hormone
   4. Luteinizing hormone
   5. Oxytocin
   6. Calcitonin

2. A patient is started on levothyroxine (Synthroid) to replace T_4 for a new diagnosis of hypothyroidism. What effect can the patient expect as the medication begins to work?
   1. Increased urination
   2. Improved blood sugar
   3. Lower blood pressure
   4. Increased energy

3. Which nursing action is appropriate when assisting an HCP with palpation of the thyroid gland during a routine physical examination?
   1. Ask the patient to take a deep breath.
   2. Give the patient a sip of water.
   3. Have the patient look up toward the ceiling.
   4. Help the patient to lie back on a pillow.

4. The nurse is doing an admission assessment on a new resident to an extended care facility. The patient's face and shoulders seem to have a lot of fat, but the patient's arms and legs are thin. Which of the patient's routine medications might be involved?
   1. Prednisone (Deltasone, a glucocorticoid)
   2. Calcitonin
   3. Insulin
   4. Thyroid hormone (levothyroxine/Synthroid)

5. When explaining a thyroid scan to a patient, which of the following statements is correct?
   1. "You will take a special pill, and then an ultrasound will be taken of your neck."
   2. "You will receive an injection of radioactive material, and then a special camera will take pictures of your thyroid gland."
   3. "You will be placed into a special machine, and x-rays will be taken of your neck. It may be noisy."
   4. "You will be given a special drink, and then magnetic energy is used to visualize the thyroid area."

Answers can be found in Appendix C.

 DavisPlus | For additional resources and information visit **davispl.us/medsurg5**

Nursing Care of Patients With Endocrine Disorders

PAULA D. HOPPER

LEARNING OUTCOMES

1. Identify disorders caused by variations in the hormones of the pituitary, thyroid, parathyroid, and adrenal glands.
2. Explain the pathophysiology of each of the endocrine disorders presented.
3. Describe the etiologies, signs, and symptoms of each of the endocrine disorders.
4. Describe current therapeutic measures used for each of the selected endocrine disorders.
5. List data to collect when caring for patients with each of the endocrine disorders discussed.
6. Plan nursing care for patients with each of the disorders.
7. Explain how you will know if nursing interventions have been effective.

KEY TERMS

amenorrhea (ay-MEN-uh-REE-ah)
ectopic (ek-TOP-ik)
euthyroid (yoo-THY-royd)
goitrogenic (GOY-troh-JEN-ik)
goitrogens (GOY-troh-jenz)
hyperplasia (HEYE-per-PLAY-zee-ah)
hypophysectomy (HEYE-pah-fi-SEK-tuh-mee)
myxedema (MIK-suh-DEE-mah)
nephrogenic (NEFF-roh-JEN-ik)
nocturia (nok-TYOO-ree-ah)
osmolality (ahs-moh-LAL-i-tee)
pheochromocytoma (FEE-oh-KROH-moh-sigh-TOH-mah)
polydipsia (PAH-lee-DIP-see-ah)
polyuria (PAH-lee-YOO-ree-ah)
tetany (TET-uh-nee)

The endocrine system is subject to a variety of disorders. Although the causes vary, the pathophysiology usually involves either too little or too much hormone activity. Insufficient hormone activity may be the result of hypofunction of an endocrine gland or insensitivity of the target tissue to its hormone. Excessive hormone activity may be the result of a hyperactive gland, **ectopic** hormone production, or self-administration of too much replacement hormone (Table 39.1). If you can remember the function of each hormone in the body, understanding the problems involved with an altered amount of each hormone becomes easier.

Most endocrine disorders are either primary or secondary. A primary disorder is a problem within the gland that is out of balance. Secondary disorders are caused by problems outside the gland, such as an imbalance in a tropic hormone, certain drugs, trauma, surgery, or a problem in the feedback mechanism. For example, if the thyroid gland is diseased and causing hypothyroidism, it would be considered a primary problem. Sometimes hypothyroidism is caused by a lack of thyroid-stimulating hormone from the pituitary gland, even though the thyroid gland is healthy. This would be considered a secondary problem.

LEARNING TIP

If you can remember what each hormone does in the body, it will be easier to remember what results from imbalances of that hormone. Most symptoms of hormone hyperactivity are the opposite of symptoms of that hormone's hypoactivity.

PITUITARY DISORDERS

Pituitary disorders often involve several hormone imbalances at once, caused by general hypopituitarism or hyperpituitarism. Problems involving all of the pituitary hormones at once, however, are rare. For simplicity, imbalances are considered separately here.

TABLE 39.1 CAUSES OF ENDOCRINE PROBLEMS

Insufficient hormone activity	Gland hypofunction
	Lack of tropic or stimulating hormone
	Target tissue insensitivity to hormone
Excess hormone activity	Gland hyperfunction
	Excess tropic or stimulating hormone
	Ectopic hormone production
	Self-administration of too much replacement hormone

Disorders Related to Antidiuretic Hormone Imbalance

Antidiuretic hormone (ADH; also called arginine vasopressin [AVP]) is synthesized in the hypothalamus and stored and secreted by the posterior pituitary gland. Recall that ADH is responsible for reabsorption of water by the distal tubules and collecting ducts in the kidneys. A decrease in ADH activity results in diabetes insipidus (DI). An increase in ADH activity is called syndrome of inappropriate antidiuretic hormone (SIADH). Table 39.2 compares DI and SIADH. Note how symptoms of too little ADH (water loss) are the opposite of symptoms of too much ADH (water retention).

Diabetes Insipidus

PATHOPHYSIOLOGY. DI is caused by a deficiency of ADH. If ADH is lacking, adequate reabsorption of water is prevented, leading to diuresis. In **nephrogenic** DI, there is enough ADH but the kidneys do not respond to it. Patients can urinate from 3 to 15 L per day. This leads to dehydration and increased serum **osmolality** (concentrated blood). The increased osmolality and decreased blood pressure normally trigger ADH secretion, which causes water retention and dilutes the blood; in patients with DI, this does not happen. Increased osmolality also leads to extreme thirst, which usually causes the patient to drink enough fluids to maintain fluid balance. In an unconscious patient or a patient with a defective thirst mechanism, however, dehydration can quickly occur if the problem is not recognized and corrected.

ETIOLOGY. DI has a variety of causes. Tumors, trauma, or other problems in the hypothalamus or pituitary gland can lead to decreased production or release of ADH. Surgery in the area of the pituitary and certain drugs, such as glucocorticoids or alcohol, can also cause DI. Nephrogenic DI is diagnosed when the kidneys do not respond to ADH. It can be triggered by certain drugs or neoplasms, or by damage to the kidneys from pyelonephritis, polycystic disease, or other causes. Primary DI, sometimes called primary polydipsia, can cause polydipsia and polyuria with no clear cause. Sometimes patients drink excessive amounts due to dry mouth.

SIGNS AND SYMPTOMS. The patient with DI urinates frequently **(polyuria)**, and nighttime urination **(nocturia)** is present. This results in high serum osmolality and low urine osmolality. Urine specific gravity is decreased, making the urine dilute and light in color.

The patient experiences extreme thirst **(polydipsia)**, and consumes large volumes of water. Often patients crave ice-cold water. If urine output exceeds fluid intake, dehydration occurs, with characteristic symptoms of hypotension, poor skin turgor, and weakness. Hypovolemic shock occurs if fluid

---

• WORD • BUILDING •

nephrogenic: nephro—kidney + genic—to produce
polyuria: poly—much + uria—urine
nocturia: noct—night + uria—urine
polydipsia: poly—much + dipsia—thirst

TABLE 39.2 ANTIDIURETIC HORMONE DISORDERS SUMMARY

	Insufficient ADH	Excess ADH
Disorder	Diabetes insipidus	Syndrome of inappropriate antidiuretic hormone
Signs and Symptoms	Polyuria, polydipsia, dehydration, dilute urine	Fluid retention, weight gain, concentrated urine
Diagnostic Tests	Urine specific gravity, urine and plasma osmolality, water deprivation test	Serum and urine sodium and osmolality; water load test
Therapeutic Measures	Synthetic ADH replacement	Treat cause
Priority Nursing Diagnoses	*Deficient Fluid Volume*	*Excess Fluid Volume*

balance is not restored. Dehydration and electrolyte imbalances result in a decrease in level of consciousness and death if the problem is not corrected.

The patient with DI may develop an enlarged bladder and kidney damage from constantly trying to "hold" too much urine.

DIAGNOSTIC TESTS. Diagnosis is based initially on a history of risk factors and reported symptoms. Urine specific gravity will be less than 1.001 (normal: 1.001–1.029) and can be monitored by laboratory tests or by using reagent strips at the bedside. Plasma and urine osmolality are measured and compared with each other. The actual amount of sodium in the blood may be normal, but it appears elevated in relation to the decreased amount of water. Computed tomography (CT) scanning or magnetic resonance imaging (MRI) are used to determine if a pituitary tumor is present.

A water-deprivation test may be done. For this test, the patient is deprived of water for up to 6 hours. Body weight and urine osmolality are tested hourly. If the urine continues to be diluted, even though the patient is not drinking and is losing weight as a result of volume depletion, DI is suspected. In the second stage of the test, the patient receives an injection of ADH, with a final urine test done 1 hour later. If the DI is nephrogenic, the kidneys will not respond to the injected ADH.

ADH levels can be measured in plasma or urine after administration of hypertonic saline or fluid restriction. The normal response would be elevated ADH; if it is not elevated, DI is suspected. The urine glucose level may also be checked to rule out diabetes mellitus.

THERAPEUTIC MEASURES. Hypotonic intravenous (IV) fluids such as 0.45% saline solution may be ordered to replace intravascular volume without adding extra sodium. IV fluids are especially important if the patient is unable to take oral fluids.

Medical treatment of DI involves replacement of ADH. In acute cases, vasopressin, a synthetic form of ADH, is given by the IV or subcutaneous route, along with IV fluid replacement. In patients who require long-term therapy, synthetic ADH (desmopressin, or DDAVP) can be administered orally, subcutaneously or intranasally. Thiazide diuretics may decrease urine flow in the absence of ADH (even though they usually are used to increase urine output!). ADH replacement won't help if the cause is nephrogenic; these patients may be placed on a low sodium diet and advised to drink plenty of water. Drugs such as chlorpropamide (Diabinese) can help the kidneys respond better to ADH. If a pituitary tumor is involved, treatment usually involves removal of the pituitary gland (**hypophysectomy**).

NURSING PROCESS FOR THE PATIENT WITH DIABETES INSIPIDUS.

Data Collection. When collecting data for a patient with DI, pay special attention to fluid balance. Daily weights are the most reliable method for monitoring the amount of fluid that is being lost. Taking accurate intake and output (I&O) measurements is also helpful. Skin turgor will be poor, and mucous membranes will be dry and sticky if the patient is becoming dehydrated. Monitor skin integrity because dehydration increases risk of breakdown. Monitor vital signs for signs of shock. Use a reagent strip (dipstick) or Urinometer to measure urine specific gravities. Monitor serum electrolytes and osmolality as ordered, and watch for changes in level of consciousness. Assess the patient's understanding of his or her disease and treatment. Once treatment is initiated, continue to monitor fluid balance, being especially alert to signs of fluid overload.

Nursing Diagnoses, Planning, and Implementation.
Deficient Fluid Volume related to failure of regulatory mechanisms
EXPECTED OUTCOME: The patient's fluid balance will be maintained as evidenced by urine specific gravity between

• WORD • BUILDING •

hypophysectomy: hypophysis—pituitary + ectomy—surgical removal

1.001 and 1.029, *skin turgor within normal limits, and stable daily weight.*

- Monitor daily weight, I&O, vital signs, and urine specific gravity. *Decreased weight, output greater than intake, low blood pressure, elevated pulse rate, and high urine specific gravity can all indicate fluid deficit.*
- Monitor patient for restlessness or weakness. *These can indicate significant fluid deficit.*
- Provide free access to oral fluids. If the patient's thirst mechanism is not intact, give the patient fluids every hour. *Oral fluids are essential to replace the excess lost in diuresis. If the patient is alert with an intact thirst mechanism, he or she can usually manage this independently.*
- Encourage the patient to participate in maintaining I&O records, monitoring weight, and checking urine specific gravity, if able. *This involves the patient and helps prepare him or her for self-monitoring at home.*
- Report a significant drop in blood pressure and a rising pulse to the registered nurse or physician *because these may be signs of hypovolemic shock.*
- Teach the patient the importance of monitoring daily weights at home; losses or gains of greater than 2 pounds in a day should be reported to the physician. *Weight loss or gain can indicate fluid imbalance and the need for a change in medication regimen.*
- Advise the patient to wear identification, such as a medical alert bracelet, that identifies the disorder. *Faster treatment can be initiated if emergency personnel are aware of a DI diagnosis.*

Evaluation. If treatment has been effective, signs of dehydration will be absent, and weight and vital signs will be stable.

Syndrome of Inappropriate Antidiuretic Hormone

PATHOPHYSIOLOGY. SIADH results from too much ADH in the body. This causes excess water to be reabsorbed by the kidney tubules and collecting ducts, leading to decreased urine output and fluid overload. As fluid builds up in the bloodstream, osmolality decreases, and the blood becomes diluted. Normally, a decreased serum osmolality inhibits release of ADH. In SIADH, however, ADH continues to be released, adding to the fluid overload.

ETIOLOGY. Some cancers, such as pancreatic cancer or some types of lung cancer, may be ectopic sites of production of an ADH-like substance. Drugs such as certain antidepressants, chemotherapy, or general anesthetic agents can increase ADH secretion. Neurologic problems such as central nervous system (CNS) infections or a brain tumor affecting pituitary function can also cause SIADH. It may also be a complication of DI treatment.

SIGNS AND SYMPTOMS. Symptoms of SIADH include symptoms of fluid overload, such as weight gain (usually without edema) and dilutional hyponatremia (Box 39-1). The actual amount of sodium in the blood may be normal

Box 39-1 Manifestations of Dilutional Hyponatremia
- Bounding pulse
- Elevated or normal blood pressure
- Muscle weakness
- Headache
- Personality changes
- Nausea
- Diarrhea
- Convulsions
- Coma

but appear to be low because of the diluting effect of the extra fluid. Serum osmolality is less than 275 mOsm/kg. The urine is concentrated because water is not being excreted. Electrolyte imbalance can cause muscle cramps and weakness. Because the osmolality of the blood is low, fluid can leak out of the vessels and cause brain swelling. If untreated, this results in lethargy, confusion, seizures, coma, and death.

DIAGNOSTIC TESTS. Serum sodium and osmolality are low, and urine sodium and osmolality are high. Serum ADH is high. Additional testing may be done to diagnose and locate an ADH-secreting tumor.

THERAPEUTIC MEASURES. Treatment is aimed at the underlying cause. If a tumor is secreting ADH, surgical removal may be indicated. Symptoms can be alleviated by restricting fluids to 800 to 1000 mL per 24 hours. Hypertonic saline fluids may be administered IV, and oral salt may be encouraged to maintain the serum sodium level. A loop diuretic such as furosemide (Lasix) increases water excretion. A vasopressin receptor antagonist such as conivaptan (Vaprisol) may be used to block the action of ADH in the kidney.

NURSING PROCESS FOR THE PATIENT WITH SAIDH.
Data Collection. Excess fluid volume with hyponatremia is the primary concern for the patient with SIADH. To monitor fluid balance, assess vital signs, daily weight, I&O, urine specific gravity, and skin turgor. Edema and pulmonary crackles are not typically present. Determine the patient's ability to maintain a fluid restriction. Assess level of consciousness and neuromuscular function. Monitor laboratory tests, including serum sodium level, as ordered by the physician. Assess the patient's understanding of the disease process and treatment.

Nursing Diagnoses, Planning, and Implementation.
Excess Fluid Volume related to compromised regulatory mechanism
EXPECTED OUTCOME: *The patient's fluid balance will be maintained as evidenced by weight, I&O, and serum sodium within normal limits.*

- Monitor daily weight, I&O, vital signs, and laboratory values. *Increased weight, intake greater than output, elevated blood pressure, bounding pulse, crackles, and low serum sodium may all indicate fluid overload.*

- Maintain fluid restriction as ordered *to reduce serum dilution and normalize serum sodium.*
- Offer small amounts of fluids high in sodium, such as broth, cola, or tomato juice, as ordered. *These may help correct dilutional hyponatremia.*
- Offer hard candy *to reduce sensation of thirst.*
- Provide ice chips (count as half the volume of fluid; that is, 100 mL of ice chips equal approximately 50 mL of water). *Ice chips take longer to consume than water and may be more satisfying to some patients.*
- Provide calibrated cups *to help the patient maintain the restriction independently if able.*
- Allow the patient to participate in planning the types and times of fluid intake. *Fluid restrictions are not pleasant for patients; patients who feel in control may be more likely to comply with restriction.*
- Report a change in level of consciousness immediately, and monitor the patient for seizures. *These are signs of serious fluid imbalance.*
- Instruct the patient to report any weight gain greater than 2 pounds in 1 day, a change in urine output, or acute thirst. *These are signs of fluid overload or risk for overload.*
- Encourage use of medical alert bracelet or other identification *so emergency personnel will have information if needed.*

Evaluation. Weight should stabilize at the pre-illness level once treatment is begun. Serum sodium level should be within normal limits.

CRITICAL THINKING

Mrs. Jackson

■ You are caring for Mrs. Jackson, a 78-year-old woman who has just returned to your unit after hip surgery. During the next 2 days, you notice that her weight increases from 118 to 124 pounds and she seems lethargic, but the nurse's report didn't indicate concern about it. You check her ankles and sacrum for edema but find none. In the afternoon, her son rushes out of the room and tells you she is becoming confused, adding that this is not like her at all.

1. What assessment should you do?
2. What do you suspect?
3. What should be your next steps?
4. Based on her weight gain, about how much water is Mrs. Jackson retaining?

Suggested answers are at the end of the chapter.

Disorders Related to Growth Hormone Imbalance

Growth hormone (GH), also called somatotropin, is responsible for normal growth of bones, cartilage, and soft tissue.

GH is synthesized and secreted by the anterior pituitary gland. An excess or deficiency of GH may be related to a more generalized problem with the pituitary gland or hypothalamus. A deficit of GH results in short stature if not corrected in childhood, and a variety of problems in adulthood. Excess GH results in gigantism (Fig. 39.1) or acromegaly.

Growth Hormone Deficiency

PATHOPHYSIOLOGY. When GH is deficient in childhood, a condition called short stature occurs. In the past, this was referred to as dwarfism (see Fig. 39.1). A deficiency of GH in adults does not affect growth, but in recent years, it has been found to have important functions even during adulthood.

ETIOLOGY. GH deficiency may be due to tumors, surgery, or trauma to the pituitary or hypothalamus. It may also be deficient in some cases of neglect or severe emotional stress. Malnutrition is the most common cause worldwide. Sometimes the cause is not known ("Cultural Considerations").

SIGNS AND SYMPTOMS. Children may grow to only 3 to 4 feet in height but have normal body proportions. Sexual maturation may be slowed, related to involvement of additional pituitary hormones. Short stature in children is sometimes accompanied by mental retardation.

FIGURE 39.1 Gigantism and dwarfism. From Tamparo, C. D., & Lewis, M. A. (2000). *Diseases of the human body (3rd ed.)*. Philadelphia: F.A. Davis, p. 247, with permission.

Cultural Considerations

Dwarfism, mostly related to a limited gene pool, often occurs among Amish communities. Ellis–van Creveld syndrome is prevalent among the Amish of Lancaster County, Pennsylvania. This syndrome is characterized by short stature and an extra digit on each hand, with some affected people having a congenital heart defect and nervous system involvement resulting in a degree of mental disability.

In adults, symptoms of GH deficiency include fatigue, weakness, excess body fat, decreased muscle and bone mass, sexual dysfunction, high cholesterol, and increased risk for cardiovascular and cerebrovascular disease. Headaches, mental slowness, and psychological disturbances may also occur. All of these signs and symptoms can lead to decreased quality of life.

DIAGNOSTIC TESTS. Growth hormone levels in the blood can be measured by a routine laboratory test, but the results may be unreliable because GH is not evenly secreted over the course of a day. A more reliable test is a growth hormone stimulation test that measures GH in response to induced hypoglycemia. An MRI scan can help determine the presence of a tumor; radiographic studies may be used to determine bone age. Genetic testing may also be done.

THERAPEUTIC MEASURES. Treatment of GH deficiency is administration of growth hormone. In the past, GH was derived from human pituitary glands, so treatment was expensive and risky. Now GH (somatotropin [Humatrope]) can be made in a laboratory using recombinant DNA technology, so it is more readily available to those who need it. It is administered by subcutaneous injection. Surgery may be indicated if a tumor is the cause.

NURSING PROCESS FOR THE PATIENT WITH GROWTH HORMONE DEFICIENCY.
Data Collection. Assessment of the adult with GH deficiency includes mental status, ability to cope with the effects of the disorder, and understanding of the treatment plan. Also assess for signs of cardiovascular disease and other complications of the disorder.

Nursing Diagnoses, Planning, and Implementation. If the problem has been present since childhood, most related problems will not be new to the patient. The priority for the nurse, then, is to approach the patient with respect while assessing current problems that may need attention. Nursing diagnoses in the adult with GH deficiency will depend on assessed needs. These may include diagnoses such as *Risk for Ineffective Self Health Management* (see below), *Fatigue, Knowledge Deficit, Imbalanced Nutrition, Risk for Injury,* or *Risk for Spiritual Distress.*

An excellent resource for people with short stature is the Little People of America organization, found at www .lpaonline.org.

Risk for Ineffective Self-Health Management related to knowledge deficit
EXPECTED OUTCOME: The patient will have requisite knowledge to be able to manage self-care as evidenced by statement and demonstration of self-care activities.

• Assess patient's understanding of his or her disease process and treatment. *Teaching should build on baseline knowledge.*
• Explain and demonstrate self-care measures as needed to the patient, including administration of GH injections. *The patient must understand the treatment to participate in it.*
• Help the patient explore the meaning of the disorder. *Talking about the disorder may help the nurse and patient identify needs that can be addressed.*

Evaluation. Nursing care has been effective if the patient is able to demonstrate self-administration of GH and describe plans for related self-care activities.

CRITICAL THINKING

Adoption

■ Three siblings were adopted to a loving home after having been in several foster homes. After a year in their new home, each child suddenly grew 6 to 8 inches. What do you think happened?
Suggested answers are at the end of the chapter.

Acromegaly

Acromegaly is a rare excess of GH that affects adults, usually in their 30s or 40s. If GH excess occurs in children, the condition results in gigantism.

PATHOPHYSIOLOGY. Acromegaly occurs as a result of overproduction of GH in an adult. Bones increase in size, leading to enlargement of facial features, hands, and feet. Long bones grow in width but not length because the epiphyseal disks are closed. Subcutaneous connective tissue increases, causing a fleshy appearance. Internal organs and glands enlarge. Impaired tolerance of carbohydrates leads to elevated blood glucose.

ETIOLOGY. Excess secretion of GH can be caused by pituitary **hyperplasia**, a benign pituitary tumor, or excess of GH-releasing hormone (GH-RH) due to hypothalamic dysfunction. Sometimes tumors in other parts of the body secrete ectopic GH or GH-RH.

SIGNS AND SYMPTOMS. Symptoms develop very slowly, and the disorder may be present for years before it is recognized. Often the first symptom noticed is a change in ring or shoe size. The nose, jaw, brow, hands, and feet enlarge (Fig. 39.2). The teeth may be displaced, causing difficulty chewing, or dentures may no longer fit. The tongue becomes thick, causing difficulty in speaking and swallowing (dysphagia). The patient may develop sleep apnea. Vertebral changes can lead to kyphosis. Visual disturbances can occur because of tumor pressure on the optic nerve. Headaches result from tumor pressure on the brain. Diabetes mellitus may develop because GH increases blood glucose and causes an increased workload for the pancreas. (see Chapter 40). Osteoporosis and arthritis may occur. Erectile dysfunction may occur in men and **amenorrhea** in women. With treatment, soft tissues reduce in size, but bone growth is permanent.

DIAGNOSTIC TESTS. Serum growth hormone levels are measured, and radiographs show abnormal bone growth. GH may also be measured after a large dose of oral glucose. Normally, glucose suppresses GH release. If it continues to be released even after a glucose load, acromegaly is suspected. A CT scan or an MRI is done to locate a pituitary tumor.

THERAPEUTIC MEASURES. Treatment is aimed at the cause. Lanreotide (Somatuline Depot) or octreotide (Sandostatin) are injectable medications that mimic the body's natural somatostatin and will decrease GH levels. Bromocriptine (Parlodel) is a pill that can lower GH. Pegvisomant (Somavert) blocks the effect of GH on receptor sites.

Hypophysectomy or radiation may be indicated if a tumor is the cause. If the pituitary is removed, lifelong replacement of thyroid hormone (TH), corticosteroids, and sex hormones is important to maintain homeostasis.

Pituitary Tumors

Most tumors of the pituitary gland are benign adenomas. However, even benign tumors in the brain can cause many symptoms, including visual disturbances, symptoms of increased pressure in the brain, and symptoms related to hormone imbalances, as described earlier. Treatment for pituitary tumors is usually hypophysectomy (surgical removal of the pituitary gland). Radiation may also be used, either alone or as an adjunct to surgery.

Nursing Care of the Patient Undergoing Hypophysectomy

Removal of the pituitary gland is called hypophysectomy. The procedure is most often done using minimally invasive endoscopic surgery, via the nose or a small incision just under the upper lip. This allows access through the sphenoid sinus to the pituitary gland, without disturbing brain tissue. Figure 39.3

• WORD • BUILDING •

hyperplasia: hyper—excessive + plasia—formation or deviation
amenorrhea: a—not + men—month + orrhea—flow

FIGURE 39.2 Patient with acromegaly. (A) Hands and (B) face. From Chanson, P., & Salenave, S. Acromegaly. (2008). *Orphanet Journal of Rare Disease, 3, 17.* Published online 2008 June 25, PMCID. © 2008 Chanson and Salenave, licensee BioMed Central Ltd.

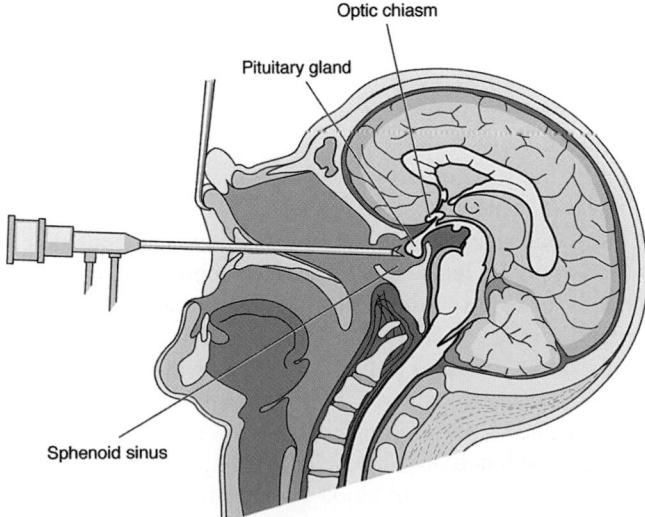

FIGURE 39.3 Transsphenoidal approach to pituitary gland for hypophysectomy.

shows the transsphenoidal approach to the gland through the upper lip. Some large tumors may need removal via transfrontal craniotomy (entry through the frontal bone of the skull).

PREOPERATIVE CARE. Make sure the patient understands the physician's explanation of surgery. Perform and document a baseline neurological assessment. Prepare the patient for what to expect following surgery. Explain that it will be important after surgery to avoid any actions that increase pressure on the surgical site, such as coughing, sneezing, nose blowing, straining to move bowels, or bending from the waist. Because coughing can raise intracranial pressure and is therefore contraindicated, instruct the patient in deep-breathing exercises or use of an incentive spirometer. Patients can usually expect to stay in the hospital about a day.

POSTOPERATIVE CARE. Perform routine neurologic assessments to monitor the patient for changes from the baseline assessment. Also be sure to check urine for specific gravity because DI can occur following pituitary surgery. If a patient has had transsphenoidal surgery, nasal packing and a "mustache dressing" will be present. These are left in place and not removed unless ordered by the physician. Monitor the dressing for signs of cerebrospinal fluid (CSF) leakage. CSF contains glucose, so glucose testing strips can be used to determine if drainage is actually CSF or just nasal discharge. Remind the patient to avoid any actions that increase pressure on the surgical site. The patient is placed on hormone replacement therapy after hypophysectomy. Pituitary hormones are difficult to replace, so target hormones are generally given. These may include TH, glucocorticoids, intranasal desmopressin, and sex hormones.

PATIENT EDUCATION. Instruct the patient before discharge according to agency guidelines. These usually include instructions to prevent increased pressure on the surgical site, as well as instructions on how to administer the hormones and side effects to report. Examples include:

- Expect a small amount of bloody or mucous drainage from your nose.
- If you must blow your nose, do so very gently. Blowing can injure the surgical site and cause bleeding or spinal fluid leakage.
- Take stool softeners as needed to prevent straining for bowel movements.
- Take cough suppressants as directed to prevent coughing.
- If an upper lip incision was used, wait until the incision line is healed to brush teeth with a toothbrush. Floss and mouth rinses can be used instead.
- Take all medications as prescribed. You will be on hormone therapy to replace the hormones made by your pituitary gland.
- Call immediately if you develop a fever, if you have more than a small amount of blood drainage from the incision site, if you have clear drainage, if you feel very thirsty or urinate more than usual (a sign of diabetes insipidus), or any other symptoms that concern you.

■ DISORDERS OF THE THYROID GLAND

Triiodothyronine (T_3) and thyroxine (T_4) are thyroid hormones secreted by the thyroid gland. These hormones may be collectively referred to as thyroid hormone (TH). Deficient secretion of TH results in hypothyroidism; excess TH results in hyperthyroidism. For more information on disorders of the thyroid gland, visit the American Thyroid Association at www.thyroid.org.

Hypothyroidism

Hypothyroidism occurs primarily in women over 50 years old. If hypothyroidism occurs in an infant, severe problems with growth and development occur. This is why all babies born in the United States are tested for hypothyroidism at birth.

Pathophysiology

Primary hypothyroidism occurs when the thyroid gland fails to produce enough TH even though enough thyroid-stimulating hormone (TSH) is being secreted by the pituitary gland. The pituitary responds to the low level of TH by producing more TSH. Secondary hypothyroidism is caused by low levels of TSH, which fail to stimulate release of TH. Tertiary hypothyroidism results from inadequate release of thyrotropin-releasing hormone (TRH), secreted by the hypothalamus. Most cases of hypothyroidism are primary (Table 39.3).

Because thyroid hormones are responsible for metabolism, low levels of these hormones result in a slowed metabolic rate, which causes many of the characteristic symptoms of hypothyroidism.

Etiology

Primary hypothyroidism may be a result of a congenital defect, inflammation of the thyroid gland, or iodine deficiency. Hashimoto's thyroiditis is an autoimmune disorder that eventually destroys thyroid tissue, leading to hypothyroidism. Secondary or tertiary hypothyroidism can be caused by a pituitary or hypothalamic lesion or by postpartum pituitary necrosis, a rare disorder in which the pituitary is destroyed after pregnancy and delivery. Treatment of hyperthyroidism, whether with medication or thyroidectomy, can lead to secondary hypothyroidism. Peripheral resistance to TH may also occur.

TABLE 39.3 THYROID HORMONE ABNORMALITIES

	Hyperthyroidism	Hypothyroidism
Primary	↑TH ↓TSH	↓TH ↑TSH
Secondary (pituitary cause)	↑TH ↑TSH	↓TH ↓TSH

Signs and Symptoms

Manifestations are related to the reduced metabolic rate and include fatigue, weight gain, bradycardia, constipation, mental dullness, feeling cold, shortness of breath, decreased sweating, and dry skin and hair ("Patient Perspective" and Table 39.4). Heart failure may occur because of decreased pumping strength of the heart. Altered fat metabolism causes hyperlipidemia, which can lead to cardiovascular disease. In advanced disease, **myxedema** develops, which is a nonpitting edema of the face, hands, and feet.

Complications

If the metabolic rate drops so low that it becomes life threatening, the result is myxedema coma. This usually occurs in patients with long-standing, untreated hypothyroidism and can be triggered by stress such as infection, trauma, or exposure to cold. The patient becomes hypothermic, with a temperature less than 95°F (35°C), and has a decreased respiratory rate, depressed mental function, and lethargy. Blood glucose drops. Cardiac output drops, which in turn can reduce perfusion of kidneys. Death can occur as a result of heart or respiratory failure. If you note changes in mental status or vital signs, contact the registered nurse (RN) or health care provider (HCP) immediately. Treatment of myxedema coma involves intubation and mechanical ventilation. The patient is slowly rewarmed with blankets. IV levothyroxine (Synthroid) is given, and the underlying cause is treated.

Diagnostic Tests

The levels of T_3 and T_4 are low, and the level of TSH may be high or low, depending on the cause. If the pituitary is

• WORD • BUILDING •

myxedema: myx—mucus + edema—swelling

Patient Perspective

Mary

When I turned 40-something, I began to notice a few changes in my body. I seemed to be easily fatigued, but I attributed that to moving our family across country and all the adjustments that needed to be made. I also noticed weight gain, most notably around my waist. Again, I thought, "Well, I *am* 40-something," but it seemed no matter how much I exercised and watched what I ate, I couldn't lose weight. Worse, I was gaining! One day a friend of mine pointed out that I always seemed tired. Each time she called to do something, my reply was always the same, "I'd love to, but not today. I'm just so tired."

Things started to get worse; I began losing hair by the handfuls each time I shampooed. It was so bad that every time I went to my hair stylist, she had to reassure me that I wasn't going bald. However, my hair just didn't seem as full as it once did. I began to notice dry skin (I thought it was just our hard water) and constipation (I thought I had irritable bowel syndrome). Finally, I went to the doctor for a physical, including laboratory tests, which included a TSH and free T_4. The diagnosis came back: I had hypothyroidism and was started on Synthroid. I noticed the effect on my energy almost immediately. Now I am able to exercise effectively. I have lost nearly all the weight I gained, and my husband no longer complains about having to clean out the drain in our shower every time I wash my hair. I am thankful for the diagnosis and treatment because I feel like myself again.

TABLE 39.4   SYMPTOMS OF THYROID DISORDERS

	Hypothyroidism	Hyperthyroidism
Cardiovascular	Bradycardia, decreased cardiac output, cool skin, cold intolerance	Tachycardia, palpitations, increased cardiac output, warm skin, heat intolerance
Neurologic	Lethargy, slowed movements, memory loss, confusion	Fatigue, restlessness, hyperactive reflexes, tremor, insomnia, emotional instability
Pulmonary	Dyspnea, hypoventilation	Dyspnea
Integumentary	Cool, dry skin; brittle, dry hair	Diaphoresis; warm, moist skin; fine, soft hair
Gastrointestinal	Decreased appetite, weight gain, constipation, increased serum lipid levels	Increased appetite, weight loss, frequent stools, decreased serum lipid levels
Skeletal	Increased bone density but poor bone quality and increased fracture risk	Reduced bone density, increased fracture risk
Reproductive	Decreased libido, erectile dysfunction	Decreased libido, erectile dysfunction, amenorrhea

functioning normally, TSH is elevated in an attempt to stimulate an increase in TH. Serum cholesterol and triglycerides are elevated. Antibodies are usually present in autoimmune disease.

Therapeutic Measures

Primary hypothyroidism is easily treated with oral thyroid replacement hormone. Most patients now take synthetic thyroid hormone (levothyroxine [Synthroid]). Doses are started low and are slowly increased to prevent symptoms of hyperthyroidism or cardiac complications.

Nursing Process for the Patient With Hypothyroidism

See the "Nursing Care Plan for the Patient With Hypothyroidism."

NURSING CARE PLAN for the Patient With Hypothyroidism

Nursing Diagnosis: *Activity Intolerance* related to fatigue

Expected Outcomes: The patient will be able to tolerate activity as evidenced by (1) reports of lessening fatigue after treatment initiated and (2) the ability to carry out usual activities of daily living (ADLs).

Evaluation of Outcomes: (1) Does patient report lessening fatigue? (2) Is patient able to carry out ADLs?

Intervention Assess level of fatigue. **Rationale** Assessment guides nursing care. **Evaluation** What is patient's fatigue level?

Intervention Assist patient with self-care activities. **Rationale** Patients with fatigue may have difficulty carrying out activities independently. **Evaluation** Are patient's self-care needs being met? Is assistance needed?

Intervention Allow for rest between activities. **Rationale** Rest periods will enable patient to conserve energy for activities. **Evaluation** Does patient state rest is adequate?

Intervention Slowly increase patient's activities as medication begins to be effective. **Rationale** As thyroid replacement therapy becomes effective, patient's fatigue will subside. **Evaluation** Does patient tolerate increases in activity?

GERIATRIC
Intervention When getting older patients up, watch for orthostatic hypotension. **Rationale** Orthostatic hypotension is common in older adults and may cause falls. **Evaluation** Does patient's blood pressure drop when changing positions?

Nursing Diagnosis: *Constipation* related to slowed gastrointestinal (GI) motility

Expected Outcome: Constipation will be resolved as evidenced by soft, formed stool passed at patient's pre-illness frequency.

Evaluation of Outcome: Are bowels movements soft and formed?

Intervention Monitor and record bowel movements. **Rationale** A record helps determine if a problem exists. **Evaluation** Does record show a problem?

Intervention Help patient follow usual pre-illness pattern (e.g., after morning coffee). **Rationale** A schedule allows bowel movement to occur before stool becomes hard and dry. **Evaluation** Is patient able to identify and implement usual self-care for bowels?

Intervention Increase fluids to eight 8-ounce glasses of water daily if cardiovascular status is stable. **Rationale** Adequate fluid intake helps prevent hard, dry stools. **Evaluation** Does patient take adequate fluids?

Intervention Add fiber to diet: fresh fruit, vegetables, bran. **Rationale** Fiber helps increase the number of bowel movements. **Evaluation** Does patient tolerate fiber? Is it effective?

Intervention Encourage regular ambulation. **Rationale** Activity increases peristalsis. **Evaluation** Is patient able to ambulate or engage in other activity?

NURSING CARE PLAN for the Patient With Hypothyroidism—cont'd

Intervention Use bedside commode or bathroom rather than bedpan. **Rationale** The sitting position aids in evacuation. **Evaluation** Is sitting position effective?

Intervention Obtain physician order for stool softener if needed. **Rationale** Soft stools are passed more easily. **Evaluation** Is stool softener needed? Is it effective?

Intervention If stool is impacted, break up stool digitally and gently remove. **Rationale** Breaking up stool eases evacuation. **Evaluation** Is stool impacted? Is digital disimpaction effective?

Intervention Avoid use of enemas. **Rationale** Enemas can cause fluid and electrolyte imbalances and can damage mucosa. **Evaluation** Does patient understand need to avoid enemas?

Nursing Diagnosis: *Risk for Impaired Skin Integrity* related to dry skin, inactivity

Expected Outcome: The patient's skin will remain intact as evidenced by soft moist skin without lesions

Evaluation of Outcome: Is skin soft, moist, and intact?

Intervention Assess skin daily for breakdown and risk for breakdown. **Rationale** Skin lesions are more effectively treated when identified early. **Evaluation** Is breakdown present? Is patient at risk?

Intervention Avoid use of soap on dry areas. Try bath oil. **Rationale** Soap is drying to skin. **Evaluation** Does use of bath oil help?

Intervention Use nondrying lotion following bath. **Rationale** Lotion helps trap moisture in skin. Some lotions contain alcohol, which is drying. **Evaluation** Does patient state relief with use of lotion?

Intervention Encourage/assist with position changes at least every 2 hours. **Rationale** Changing position enhances circulation to the skin, promoting healing and preventing breakdown. **Evaluation** Does patient change position at least every 2 hours? Are pressure areas prevented?

Nursing Diagnosis: *Imbalanced Nutrition: More Than Body Requirements* related to decreased metabolic rate

Expected Outcomes: (1) Nutrition will be balanced as evidenced by return to patient's pre-illness weight. (2) The patient will verbalize understanding of dietary recommendations.

Evaluation of Outcomes: (1) Is patient approaching pre-illness weight? (2) Is patient able to explain dietary recommendations and a plan for implementation?

Intervention Weigh weekly and record. **Rationale** Weekly weights record progress without the frustration of daily fluctuations. **Evaluation** Is patient approaching ideal weight?

Intervention Consult dietitian for therapeutic diet until hypothyroidism is controlled. **Rationale** The dietitian can provide food choices for gradual weight loss if necessary. **Evaluation** Does patient verbalize understanding of and ability to follow diet?

Intervention Encourage regular exercise within limits of fatigue. **Rationale** Exercise promotes weight control. **Evaluation** Does patient verbalize understanding of and ability to follow exercise plan?

Intervention Counsel patient that weight should normalize once hypothyroidism is controlled. **Rationale** Thyroid replacement hormone increases the metabolic rate, allowing return to normal weight. **Evaluation** Does patient verbalize understanding of instruction?

GERIATRIC
Intervention Allow patient to help determine acceptable diet modifications. **Rationale** Older patients may have long-standing dietary habits that are hard to change. **Evaluation** Is patient satisfied with weight loss plan?

CRITICAL THINKING

Mrs. Maino

■ Mrs. Maino is a 59-year-old woman who is tired all the time and has gained 16 pounds during the past year. Laboratory results show low T_3 and T_4 and elevated TSH levels. Her physician prescribes levothyroxine by mouth (PO).

1. Why is Mrs. Maino's TSH elevated?
2. What will happen to Mrs. Maino's caloric requirements as she begins treatment? Why?
3. The RN asks you to teach Mrs. Maino to check her pulse. Why is this important?
4. What team members are important to involve in Mrs. Maino's care?

Suggested answers are at the end of the chapter.

Patient Education

Instruct the patient in the importance of consistent use of thyroid replacement medication and regular blood tests to monitor TSH. The patient needs to be aware that too much TH will cause symptoms of hyperthyroidism. Such symptoms should be reported to the physician immediately. In addition, if the patient is experiencing mental status changes, discuss the need to avoid driving or operating machinery until symptoms are resolved.

EVIDENCE-BASED PRACTICE

Clinical Question
Is generic thyroid replacement hormone (levothyroxine) as good as brand name levothyroxine?

Evidence
A comparison of health care costs of patients who took a brand name of levothyroxine versus switching to a generic brand found that there was no cost benefit to using the generic form. Switching to generic form actually increased costs for other health care services.

Implications for Nursing Practice
While most generic formulations work as well as the brand names, the same may not be true for levothyroxine. As a nurse, you will take care of many older patients who take levothyroxine for hypothyroidism. Encourage patients to talk to their doctors and pharmacists about staying with the same brand of drug.

REFERENCE
Katz, M., Scherger, J., Conard S., Montejano, L., & Chang, S. (2010). Healthcare costs associated with switching from brand to generic levothyroxine. *Am Health Drug Benefits*, 3, 127–134.

Hyperthyroidism

Hyperthyroidism is most often diagnosed in women. Graves' disease, which is one cause of hyperthyroidism, is more common in young women. Multinodular goiter is more common in older women.

Pathophysiology

Hyperthyroidism results in excessive amounts of circulating TH (thyrotoxicosis). Primary hyperthyroidism occurs when a problem within the thyroid gland causes excess hormone release. Secondary hyperthyroidism occurs because of excess TSH release from the pituitary, causing overstimulation of the thyroid gland; tertiary hyperthyroidism is caused by excess TRH from the hypothalamus. A high level of TH increases the metabolic rate. It also increases the number of beta-adrenergic receptor sites in the body, which enhances the activity of epinephrine and norepinephrine. The resulting fight-or-flight response is the cause of many of the symptoms of hyperthyroidism.

Etiology

A variety of disorders can cause hyperthyroidism. Graves' disease is the most common cause; it is an autoimmune disorder in which thyroid-stimulating antibodies cause the thyroid gland to make too much TH.

Other causes include thyroid nodules that secrete excess thyroid hormone (multinodular goiter and toxic adenoma), inflammation of the thyroid (thyroiditis), or a thyroid tumor. A pituitary tumor can secrete excess TSH, which overstimulates the thyroid gland. Patients taking TH for hypothyroidism may take too much. Each of these problems can cause excess circulating TH and symptoms of hyperthyroidism.

Radiation exposure can predispose a patient to develop hyperthyroidism. Heredity may also play a role in autoimmune hyperthyroidism. Women who smoke nearly double their risk of Graves' disease.

Signs and Symptoms

Many signs and symptoms are related to the hypermetabolic state, such as heat intolerance, increased appetite with weight loss, and increased frequency of bowel movements. Nervousness, tremor, tachycardia, and palpitations are caused by the increase in sympathetic nervous system activity and may be more common in younger patients. Heart failure can occur because of tachycardia and the resulting inefficient pumping of the heart. See additional signs and symptoms in Table 39.4.

If treatment is not begun, the patient can become manic or psychotic. Additional signs that occur only with Graves' disease include thickening of the skin on the anterior legs and exophthalmos (bulging of the eyes; Fig. 39.4) caused by swelling of the tissues behind the eyes. Other eye changes include photophobia and blurred or double vision.

Older adult patients may not have the typical signs and symptoms of hyperthyroidism, so be especially alert for this. These patients may present with heart failure, atrial fibrillation, fatigue, apathy, and depression.

FIGURE 39.4 Exophthalmos caused by Graves' disease. From Tamparo, C. D., & Lewis, M. A. (2005). *Diseases of the human body* (4th ed.). Philadelphia: F.A. Davis, p. 339, with permission.

Complications

THYROTOXIC CRISIS. Thyrotoxic crisis (sometimes called thyroid storm) is a severe hyperthyroid state that can occur in hyperthyroid people who are untreated or who develop another illness or stressor. It also may occur after thyroid surgery in patients who have been inadequately prepared with antithyroid medication. Thyrotoxic crisis can result in death in as little as 2 hours if untreated. Symptoms include tachycardia, high fever, hypertension (with eventual heart failure and hypotension), dehydration, restlessness, and delirium or coma.

If thyrotoxic crisis occurs, treatment is first directed toward relieving the life-threatening symptoms. Acetaminophen is given for the fever. Aspirin is avoided because it binds with the same serum protein as T_4, freeing additional T_4 into the circulation. IV fluids and a cooling blanket may be ordered to cool the patient. A beta-adrenergic blocker such as propranolol is given for tachycardia and symptom control. Oxygen is administered and the head of the bed is elevated because the high metabolic rate requires more oxygen. Once symptoms are controlled and the patient is safe, the underlying thyroid problem is treated.

HYPOTHYROIDISM. Another complication of hyperthyroidism can be hypothyroidism. This can occur as a result of long-term disease or as a result of treatment. Patients with a history of hyperthyroidism should be monitored for recurrent hyperthyroidism or the onset of hypothyroidism.

Diagnostic Tests

Serum levels of T_3 and T_4 are elevated. TSH is low in primary hyperthyroidism or high if the cause is pituitary. A radioactive iodine uptake test or a thyroid scan can be done to determine hyperactivity of the gland or to locate a nodule or tumor. The thyroid gland may be enlarged; palpation of the thyroid in a patient suspected to be hyperthyroid should only be performed by a physician or an advanced practice nurse.

TSI (thyroid-stimulating immunoglobulin) is present in Graves' disease.

Therapeutic Measures

Several medications can be used to treat hyperthyroidism. Propylthiouracil and methimazole (Tapazole) inhibit the synthesis of TH, but they may take several months to be effective and must be continued for 12 to 18 months. Propranolol (Inderal) is a beta-blocking medication that relieves the sympathetic nervous system symptoms. High doses of oral iodine suppress the release of thyroid hormone. Calcium and vitamin D are given to protect bones.

Radioactive iodine (^{131}I or RAI) may be used to destroy a portion of the thyroid gland. The patient takes one oral dose of RAI. Dietary iodine normally goes to the thyroid gland, where it is used to make TH. When RAI is given, the radioactivity destroys some of the cells that make TH.

Sometimes medications or radioactive iodine alone control hyperthyroidism. If this does not occur, surgery is planned. If surgery is the treatment chosen, antithyroid medications are given to calm the thyroid before surgery. They help slow the heart rate and reduce other symptoms, making surgery safer. Iodine also reduces the vascularity of the thyroid gland, decreasing the risk of bleeding during surgery. Adequate preparation of the patient is important because a **euthyroid** state helps prevent a postoperative thyrotoxic crisis.

Thyroidectomy can be done with a traditional, open approach, or with newer minimally invasive techniques that use a combination of a tiny incision and an endoscope. Patients can usually go home the same day and have a faster recovery time with minimally invasive surgery. The surgeon may choose to leave some of the thyroid gland intact, to continue to secrete some hormone. Following surgery, the patient will likely be hypothyroid and will require thyroid replacement hormone (levothyroxine [Synthroid]). Nursing care of the patient undergoing a thyroidectomy is discussed later in this chapter.

If vision is impaired from exophthalmos, surgical orbital decompression can be done. Current endoscopic techniques have made this a safer option than in the past.

Nursing Process for the Patient With Hyperthyroidism

DATA COLLECTION. Monitor the patient with hyperthyroidism closely until normal thyroid activity is restored. Assess vital signs and lung sounds and report changes to the RN or HCP. Assess level of anxiety and ability to cope with symptoms. Monitor weight, bowel function, and ability to sleep. Assess eyes for risk for injury caused by exophthalmos, and note degree of muscle weakness. Never palpate the thyroid gland of a patient with hyperthyroidism because palpation can stimulate release of thyroid hormone and precipitate a thyrotoxic crisis.

• **WORD** • **BUILDING** •
euthyroid: eu—normal, healthy + thyroid

NURSING DIAGNOSES, PLANNING, AND IMPLEMENTATION.
Hyperthermia related to hypermetabolic state
EXPECTED OUTCOME: The patient's body temperature will be within normal limits.

• Monitor temperature. *Temperature may be elevated due to hypermetabolic state.*
• Administer acetaminophen as ordered (avoid aspirin) to reduce temperature. *Aspirin can cause an increase in circulating thyroid hormone.*
• Apply cooling blanket as ordered. *External cooling may be needed if acetaminophen is not effective.*
• If a cooling blanket is needed, set it to 1 to 2 degrees below the current temperature, and wrap the extremities with towels to prevent shivering, *which can further increase temperature.*
• Offer fluids *to replace fluids lost through diaphoresis.*

Diarrhea related to increase in peristalsis
EXPECTED OUTCOME: The patient will maintain fluid and electrolyte balance.

• Provide a low-fiber diet. *Fiber can increase peristalsis and stools.*
• Provide small, frequent meals of bland foods (bananas, rice, applesauce) *that are less likely to worsen diarrhea.*
• Monitor electrolytes, especially sodium and potassium. *Diarrhea can cause electrolyte loss.*
• Monitor for dehydration. *Diarrhea causes fluid loss.*
• Keep skin clean and dry; apply barrier cream *to protect skin from injury from stool.*

Imbalanced Nutrition: Less Than Body Requirements related to increased metabolism
EXPECTED OUTCOME: The patient will have balanced nutrition as evidenced by stable weight in proportion to height.

• Determine healthy weight for height, *so that the expected outcome is realistic for the patient.*
• Monitor weight weekly *to make sure interventions are working.*
• Consult dietician for high-calorie diet and supplements *to meet caloric requirements.*

Disturbed Sleep Pattern related to sympathetic stimulation
EXPECTED OUTCOME: The patient will have improved sleep as evidenced by stating feeling rested upon awakening.

• Provide a quiet, restful environment *to help the patient to fall asleep.*
• Ask the patient if music or earplugs are desired *to mask environmental noise.*
• Administer propranolol or sedative as ordered *to reduce sympathetic stimulation and calm patient.*

Anxiety related to sympathetic stimulation
EXPECTED OUTCOME: The patient will experience reduced anxiety as evidenced by patient statement that anxiety is controlled.

• Provide the patient with accurate information about the disorder and treatment, and explain that proper treatment will correct symptoms. *Fear of the unknown can produce anxiety.*
• Administer propranolol or antianxiety agent as ordered *to reduce sympathetic stimulation and calm patient.*
• Offer massage, music, or other relaxation techniques preferred by the patient. *These may promote relaxation.*

Risk for Injury related to hypermetabolic state and bone and eye involvement
EXPECTED OUTCOME: The patient will remain safe and without injury.

• Report changes in vital signs to RN or physician. *Prompt treatment can reduce complications.*
• Encourage all patients with Grave's disease to stop smoking if they are smokers. *Smoking is a risk factor for exophthalmos.*
• Administer lubricating saline eye drops as ordered to *protect eyes from drying.*
• Advise use of dark, tight-fitting glasses *to protect eyes from light and injury.*
• Gently tape eyes shut with nonallergic tape for sleeping. *Exophthalmos may prevent the patient from fully closing the eyes.*
• Elevate the head of the bed *to reduce edema behind the eyes.*
• Provide a low-sodium diet. *This may decrease edema behind the eyes.*
• Teach patient to notify the physician immediately if eye pain or vision changes occur. *These can be signs of pressure from edema on optic nerve, which can cause permanent damage if not corrected.*
• Protect from injury and falls. *Reduced bone density increases risk for fractures.*

PATIENT EDUCATION. Teach the patient about the disease and symptoms of hyperthyroidism or hypothyroidism to report. Also teach the patient how to take medications and the importance of routine follow-up laboratory testing.

EVALUATION. If the plan of care is effective, the patient will remain free from complications and injury. Vital signs will be within normal limits. Diarrhea will be controlled, and complications of diarrhea such as skin breakdown and dehydration avoided. The patient's weight should remain stable. The patient should report that he or she is rested on awakening and that anxiety is controlled.

Nursing Care of the Patient Receiving Radioactive Iodine

If radioactive iodine is used, it is usually given orally in one dose. If the dose is high, such as for the patient with thyroid cancer, the patient is hospitalized. Patients receiving lower doses may be treated as outpatients. You should limit time spent with the patient and maintain a safe distance when providing direct care (see Chapter 11). Pregnant caregivers should avoid caring for patients receiving radioactive iodine. Urine, vomitus, and other body secretions are contaminated and should be disposed of according to hospital policy. Flush the toilet twice after disposal of contaminated material. The radiation safety officer and hospital policy should be consulted for specific precautions.

At home, the patient is instructed to avoid close contact with family members and to use careful hand hygiene after urinating. Oral contact with others should be avoided, and eating utensils should be washed thoroughly with soap and water. Hospital teaching protocols should be used for specific patient teaching. The amount of time patients must avoid contact with others depends on the dose of radiation received. If the treatment is being administered for hyperthyroidism, inform the patient that symptoms should subside in about 6 to 8 weeks.

Side effects are rare, and can include sore throat, dry mouth or eyes, and nausea. Sore throat is easily treated with acetaminophen, and nausea can be reduced by taking the dose on an empty stomach. Dry eyes can be relieved with moisturizing eye drops. Encourage the patient to drink plenty of fluids and void frequently to help remove the radioactive iodine from the body and reduce radiation exposure to the bladder. In addition, the patient should be aware of symptoms of hypothyroidism to be reported because hypothyroidism can occur up to 15 years after the treatment.

Goiter

Pathophysiology and Etiology

Enlargement of the thyroid gland is called a goiter. The thyroid gland may enlarge in response to increased TSH levels, or sometimes in response to the autoimmune process that occurs in Graves' disease. TSH is elevated in response to low TH, iodine deficiency, pregnancy, or viral, genetic, or other conditions. When a goiter is caused by iodine deficiency or other environmental factors, it is called an endemic goiter.

Some foods and medications are **goitrogens**. These substances interfere with the body's use of iodine and include such foods as turnips, cabbage, broccoli, horseradish, cauliflower, and carrots ("Nutrition Notes"). Some **goitrogenic** medications include propylthiouracil, sulfonamides, lithium, and salicylates (aspirin).

A goiter can be associated with a hyperthyroid, hypothyroid, or euthyroid state. Goiter that occurs with hyperthyroidism is sometimes called a toxic goiter. Once the cause of the goiter is removed, the gland usually returns to normal size.

Signs and Symptoms

The thyroid gland is enlarged, and swelling may be apparent at the base of the neck (Fig. 39.5). Alternatively, the gland may enlarge posteriorly, which can interfere with swallowing or breathing. The patient may have a full sensation in the neck. Symptoms of hypothyroidism or hyperthyroidism may be present.

Diagnostic Tests

Serum TSH, T_3, and T_4 levels are measured to determine thyroid function. Ultrasound or a thyroid scan may be done to determine the cause or evaluate the size of the gland.

Nutrition Notes

Iodine Deficiency

Iodine deficiency is a global problem representing the most common preventable cause of mental retardation affecting about 200 to 300 million people worldwide. Inland areas of all continents have iodine-poor soils. People in developing countries with only local food sources are still subject to endemic goiter; however, addition of iodine to table salt has significantly reduced the occurrence of endemic goiter in developed countries.

Vegetables in the cabbage family contain goitrogens, substances that block the body's absorption or utilization of iodine, but the risk is small because cooking destroys the goitrogens. At higher risk of iodine deficiency are strict vegetarians who consume sea salt, which contains virtually no iodine, rather than iodized salt.

Iodine Excess

Saltwater fish, shellfish, and seaweed are naturally high in iodine. Seaweed has caused toxicity in Australian infants because of their mothers' excessive intake. Manifestations of excessive iodine can be either hyperthyroidism or hypothyroidism, sometimes producing "iodine goiter."

Reference

Emder, P. J., & Jack, M. M. (2011). Iodine-induced neonatal hypothyroidism secondary to maternal seaweed consumption: A common practice in some Asian cultures to promote breast milk supply. *Journal of Paediatric and Child Health, 47,* 750–752.

Therapeutic Measures

Treatment is aimed at the cause. If goitrogens are suspected, the patient is given a list of foods to be avoided. If iodine deficiency is a problem, it is added to the diet with supplements or iodized salt. Hypothyroidism or hyperthyroidism is treated if indicated. Levothyroxine (Synthroid) may be given to reduce TSH levels via negative feedback. Radioactive iodine therapy or thyroidectomy may be needed to treat hyperthyroid symptoms or if the enlarged gland is interfering with breathing or swallowing.

Nursing Care

Be careful to assess the effect of the goiter on breathing and swallowing. Stridor, a whistling sound, may be heard if the airway is obstructed. Stridor is an ominous sign and should be reported to the HCP immediately. If the patient experiences difficulty swallowing, notify the physician and collaborate

• WORD • BUILDING •

goitrogenic: goitro—goiter + genic—producing

FIGURE 39.5 Patient with unusually large goiter.

with the dietitian to provide soft foods that are easy to swallow. A swallowing study might be ordered, which can assist a speech pathologist or other expert to make specific recommendations for safe swallowing.

Cancer of the Thyroid Gland

Although thyroid cancer is rare, it is the most common cancer of the endocrine system. Women are affected more often than men. Most tumors of the thyroid gland are not malignant. See Chapter 11 for cancer pathophysiology.

Etiology

Thyroid hyperplasia can lead to thyroid cancer. Other causes include exposure to radiation ("Cultural Considerations"), iodine deficiency, and prolonged exposure to goitrogens. The tendency to develop some forms of thyroid cancer is inherited.

Signs and Symptoms

A hard, painless nodule may be palpable on the thyroid gland. Difficulty breathing or swallowing, persistent cough, or changes in the voice may occur if the tumor is near the esophagus and trachea. Most patients with cancer of the thyroid have normal TH levels.

Diagnostic Tests

A thyroid scan shows a "cold" nodule. This is because malignant tumors of the thyroid do not take up the radioactive iodine administered for the scan. A "hot" nodule indicates a benign tumor. A fine-needle aspiration biopsy confirms the diagnosis.

Therapeutic Measures

A partial or total thyroidectomy may be done. Chemotherapy, radioactive iodine therapy, or external beam radiation may also be used, alone or following surgery.

Nursing Care

Nursing care is determined by the symptoms the patient is experiencing. See Chapter 11 for care of the patient with cancer.

Nursing Process for the Patient Undergoing Thyroidectomy

Patients may undergo thyroidectomy for cancer of the thyroid, hyperthyroidism, or a goiter that is causing dyspnea or dysphagia. See Chapter 12 for general care of a patient having surgery.

A total thyroidectomy is usually performed if cancer is present. After a total thyroidectomy, lifelong replacement hormone must be taken. A subtotal (partial) thyroidectomy might be done for hyperthyroidism, leaving a portion of the thyroid gland to continue to secrete TH.

Preoperative Care

Before undergoing a thyroidectomy, the patient should be in a euthyroid state to avoid complications during and after surgery. This is accomplished with the use of antithyroid medication such as methimazole (Tapazole). A saturated solution of potassium iodide may also be administered to decrease the size and vascularity of the gland, reducing the risk of bleeding during surgery.

Cultural Considerations

Because of the Chernobyl nuclear disaster in Russia in 1986, Russian immigrants are at exceptionally high risk for developing pituitary, thyroid, and parathyroid disorders and cancers. The proximity of Estonia, Latvia, Lithuania, Poland, and other Eastern European countries to Russia places immigrants and long-term visitors from these countries at risk as well. The nurse needs to be alert for endocrine disorders among these populations and assist patients to arrange genetic counseling for those who desire it.

Perform a baseline assessment of vital signs and voice quality, so you can compare findings postoperatively. Explain what the patient can expect before, during, and after surgery. Preoperative teaching should include how to perform gentle range-of-motion exercises of the neck, how to support the neck during position changes, and how to use an incentive spirometer after surgery. See Chapter 12 for routine preoperative care.

Postoperative Care

DATA COLLECTION. Monitor vital signs, oxygen saturation, drain (if present), and dressing every 15 minutes initially, progressing to every 4 hours, as ordered. Decreased blood pressure with increased pulse should alert you to the possibility of shock related to blood loss. Tachycardia and fever, along with mental status changes, can indicate thyrotoxic crisis. Check the back of the neck for pooling of blood. Because of the location of the surgery, observe for signs of respiratory distress, including an increase in respiratory rate, dyspnea, or stridor. Ask the patient to speak to detect hoarseness of the voice, which can indicate trauma to the recurrent laryngeal nerve. Monitor the patient's serum calcium levels and watch for evidence of tetany (discussed later in this chapter). Report abnormal findings to the RN or physician immediately.

NURSING DIAGNOSES, PLANNING, AND IMPLEMENTATION.
Risk for Ineffective Airway Clearance related to edema at surgical site
EXPECTED OUTCOME: The patient will maintain a clear airway as evidenced by easy breathing without stridor.

- Notify physician about respiratory distress immediately; keep a tracheostomy set at the bedside. *Although not common, a tracheostomy may be needed in an emergency if edema obstructs the airway.*
- Maintain patient in semi-Fowler's position *to help reduce edema and promote comfort.*
- Monitor neck dressing. *If the dressing seems to get tighter, it may be a sign that the patient's neck is swelling, which could impair the airway.*
- Use room humidifier or humidified oxygen *to keep airways and secretions moist.*
- Remind the patient to do coughing and deep-breathing exercises every hour. *This keeps the airway clear of secretions.*
- Have suction equipment available *in case patient is unable to cough up secretions effectively.*
- Encourage the patient to use the incentive spirometer *to assist with deep breathing.*
- Assess the patient's swallowing and gag reflexes before offering clear liquids *to guard against aspiration.*

Risk for Injury (tetany, thyrotoxic crisis related to surgical procedure
EXPECTED OUTCOME: Complications will be recognized and treated quickly.

- Monitor patient for muscle spasms or numbness or tingling around the mouth, and report immediately if they

occur. *These are symptoms of tetany that must be treated immediately. Tetany is most likely to occur 24 to 72 hours postoperatively.*
- Monitor vital signs often, and report changes immediately. *Elevated vital signs may be signs of thyrotoxic crisis, which is most likely to occur up to 18 hours postoperatively.*

Acute Pain related to surgical procedure
EXPECTED OUTCOME: The patient's pain will be controlled as evidenced by patient stating pain rating is acceptable.

- Administer acetaminophen or opioids as ordered. Avoid aspirin products. *Aspirin binds to the same protein as thyroid hormone and can precipitate a thyrotoxic crisis.*
- Use pillows or sandbags to support the patient's head. *Unexpected movement may be painful.*

Risk for Ineffective Self Health Management related to knowledge deficit
EXPECTED OUTCOME: The patient will be able to effectively manage self-care needs as evidenced by (1) verbalizing understanding of follow-up care, (2) weight stabilizes at appropriate weight for height, and (3) TH levels are within normal limits.

- Teach the patient to do gentle range-of-motion exercises, avoiding hyperextension of the neck, which can cause strain on the incision line. *Avoidance of neck movement due to pain can result in contracture.*
- Consult dietitian to assist the patient with potential dietary changes needed following surgery. *With correction of metabolic alterations, dietary needs may be significantly altered.*
- Teach the patient the importance of follow-up care *to avoid complications:*
  - How to administer replacement hormone if ordered.
  - How to change the dressing and to report bleeding or signs of infection at the site.
  - Importance of immediately reporting unusual irritability, fever, palpitations, or signs of tetany.
  - Importance of follow-up lab work for thyroid function and medication adjustment.

EVALUATION. If the plan has been effective, complications caused by surgery will not occur or will be recognized and reported early. Pain will be prevented or controlled, and the patient will demonstrate understanding of postoperative self-care.

Complications

THYROTOXIC CRISIS. Thyrotoxic crisis can result from manipulation of the thyroid gland during surgery, with the subsequent release of large amounts of TH. This is a rare complication because the use of antithyroid drugs before surgery has become routine. For more information on thyrotoxic crisis, see the section on hyperthyroidism earlier in this chapter.

TETANY. **Tetany** is caused by low calcium levels and is characterized by tingling in the fingers and perioral area (around the mouth), muscle spasms, twitching, and cardiac dysrhythmias.

Muscle spasms in the larynx can lead to respiratory obstruction. Watch carefully for symptoms of tetany and report them immediately if they occur because if the problem is not recognized quickly, death can result.

Tetany can occur if the parathyroid glands are accidentally removed during thyroid surgery. Because of the proximity of the parathyroid glands to the thyroid, it is sometimes difficult for the surgeon to avoid them. In the absence of parathyroid hormone (PTH), serum calcium levels drop and tetany results. IV calcium gluconate is given to treat acute tetany.

 ## DISORDERS OF THE PARATHYROID GLANDS

Recall that the parathyroid glands secrete PTH in response to low serum calcium levels. PTH raises serum calcium levels by promoting calcium movement from bones to blood, increasing absorption of dietary calcium, and increasing resorption of calcium by the kidneys. Decreased PTH activity is called hypoparathyroidism. Increased PTH activity is called hyperparathyroidism.

Hypoparathyroidism
Pathophysiology

A decrease in PTH causes a decrease in bone resorption of calcium, a decrease in calcium absorption by the GI tract, and decreased resorption in the kidneys. This means that calcium stays in the bones instead of being moved into the blood, and more calcium is excreted from the body. The result is a decreased serum calcium level, called hypocalcemia. As calcium levels fall, phosphate levels rise.

Etiology

The most common causes of hypoparathyroidism are heredity and the accidental removal of the parathyroid glands during thyroidectomy or other neck surgeries. Hypoparathyroidism also occurs following purposeful removal of the parathyroid glands for hyperparathyroidism or cancer. Another cause is hypomagnesemia, which impairs secretion of PTH. Hypomagnesemia can occur with chronic alcoholism or certain nutritional problems.

Signs and Symptoms

Calcium plays an important role in nerve cell stability. Hypocalcemia causes neuromuscular irritability. In acute cases, tetany can occur, with numbness and tingling of the fingers and perioral area, muscle spasms, and twitching (Table 39.5). Positive Chvostek's and Trousseau's signs are early indications of tetany. See Figures 6.4 and 6.5 in Chapter 6 for illustrations of these tests.

Chronic hypocalcemia can lead to lethargy; calcifications in the brain, leading to psychosis; cataracts; and convulsions. Bone changes may be evident on x-ray examination. Electrocardiogram (ECG) changes, and heart failure can develop because of the importance of calcium to cardiac function. Death can result from laryngospasm if treatment is not effective.

Diagnostic Tests

Laboratory studies show decreased serum calcium and PTH levels and increased serum phosphorus. An ECG is done to evaluate cardiac function. Radiographs show bone changes.

Therapeutic Measures

Acute cases of hypoparathyroidism are treated with IV calcium gluconate. Long-term treatment includes a high-calcium diet (Box 39-2), with oral calcium and vitamin D supplements. Magnesium is given if hypomagnesemia is present.

Nursing Process for the Patient With Hypoparathyroidism

DATA COLLECTION.   The patient at risk for hypoparathyroidism should be closely monitored for symptoms of tetany.

TABLE 39.5   PARATHYROID DISORDERS SUMMARY

	Insufficient PTH	**Excess PTH**
Disorder	Hypoparathyroidism	Hyperparathyroidism
Signs and Symptoms	Hypocalcemia, neuromuscular irritability, tetany, positive Chvostek's and Trousseau's signs	Hypercalcemia, fatigue, pathological fractures
Diagnostic Tests	Serum PTH, calcium, and phosphate	Serum PTH, calcium, and phosphate
Therapeutic Measures	Calcium and vitamin D replacement; high-calcium, low-phosphorus diet	Calcitonin, parathyroidectomy
Priority Nursing Diagnoses	*Risk for Injury* related to tetany	*Risk for Injury* related to bone demineralization

Box 39-2 Dietary Sources of Calcium

- Milk
- Cheeses
- Yogurt
- Sardines
- Oysters
- Salmon
- Cauliflower
- Green leafy vegetables

See Chapter 6, Table 6.3, for a more detailed list.

If you suspect tetany, check for Chvostek's and Trousseau's signs. Monitor respirations closely for stridor, a sign of laryngospasm.

NURSING DIAGNOSES, PLANNING, AND IMPLEMENTATION.
Risk for Injury related to hypocalcemia and tetany
EXPECTED OUTCOME: The patient will remain free from injury; signs of tetany will be recognized and treated quickly.

- Monitor patient for signs of tetany, and report immediately to RN or physician *so that treatment can begin quickly.*
- Make sure a tracheostomy set, endotracheal tube, and IV calcium are available *for emergency use if laryngospasm occurs.*
- Consult a dietitian for high-calcium diet teaching. *The patient may need a lifelong high-calcium diet.*
- Teach the patient about the importance of long-term diet and medication therapy and follow-up laboratory testing. *The patient needs to understand self-care for follow-up at home.*

EVALUATION. Injury is prevented through early recognition and reporting of signs and symptoms of tetany. The patient should be able to describe correct treatment and self-care measures for home.

Hyperparathyroidism
Pathophysiology

Overactivity of one or more of the parathyroid glands causes an increase in PTH, with a subsequent increase in the serum calcium level (hypercalcemia). This is achieved through movement of calcium out of the bones and into the blood, absorption in the small intestine, and reabsorption by the kidneys. PTH also promotes phosphorus excretion by the kidneys.

Etiology

Hyperparathyroidism is usually the result of hyperplasia or a benign tumor of the parathyroid glands, or it may be hereditary. Parathyroid cancer is rare. Secondary hyperparathyroidism occurs when the parathyroids secrete excessive PTH

in response to low serum calcium levels. Serum calcium may be reduced in kidney disease because of the kidneys' failure to activate vitamin D, which is necessary for absorption of calcium in the small intestine.

Signs and Symptoms

Signs and symptoms of hyperparathyroidism are caused primarily by the increase in serum calcium level, although many patients are asymptomatic. Symptoms include fatigue, depression, confusion, increased urination, anorexia, nausea, vomiting, kidney stones, and cardiac dysrhythmias. The increased serum calcium level also causes gastrin secretion, resulting in abdominal pain and peptic ulcers. Because calcium is being removed from bones, bone and joint pain and pathological fractures can occur. Severe hypercalcemia can result in coma and cardiac arrest.

Diagnostic Tests

Laboratory studies include serum calcium, phosphorus, and PTH levels. Radiographs or bone density testing may show decreased bone density. A 24-hour urine test might be used to test how much calcium is being excreted in the urine. Nuclear scanning or ultrasound may be used to help locate the parathyroid glands if surgical removal is planned.

Therapeutic Measures

In acute situations, IV normal saline is given to hydrate the patient and lower the calcium level by dilution; furosemide (Lasix) is given to increase renal excretion of calcium. Alendronate (Fosamax) or calcitonin may be given to prevent calcium release from bones. For longer-term care, the patient is monitored for bone changes and decline in renal function. Oral calcium and vitamin D supplements are prescribed. Estrogen therapy might be used in women, although side effects must be considered.

If hypercalcemia is severe or if the patient is at risk for bone or kidney complications, surgery to remove the diseased parathyroid glands (parathyroidectomy) is performed. If possible, some parathyroid tissue is left intact to continue to secrete PTH. Minimally invasive radio-guided parathyroidectomy can be done under local anesthesia through a small incision.

Preoperative and postoperative care is similar to that of the patient undergoing thyroid surgery, with special attention paid to calcium and PTH levels. The patient will likely continue to be on calcium and vitamin D supplements following surgery.

Nursing Process for the Patient With Hyperparathyroidism

DATA COLLECTION. Assess the patient for symptoms related to hypercalcemia, including muscle weakness, lethargy, bone pain, anorexia, nausea, vomiting, behavioral changes, and renal insufficiency. Monitor serum calcium levels as ordered.

NURSING DIAGNOSES, PLANNING, AND IMPLEMENTATION.
Nursing diagnoses depend on assessment findings. Risk for injury usually takes priority.

Risk for Injury (fracture, complications of hypercalcemia) related to calcium imbalance

EXPECTED OUTCOME: The patient will remain free from injury.

• Monitor patient for signs or symptoms of calcium imbalance and report promptly. *Prompt treatment can prevent serious complications.*
• Encourage oral fluids *to prevent dehydration and kidney stones and help excrete calcium.*
• Encourage strengthening and weight-bearing exercises *to help keep calcium in the bones.*
• Provide a safe environment for ambulation; assist the patient with ambulation if needed. *A fall could result in fracture if bones are demineralized.*
• Encourage smoking cessation. *Smoking causes bone loss.*
• Teach patient symptoms to report and use of long-term medications *so that patient can manage self-care at home.*

EVALUATION. If the plan is effective, symptoms of hypercalcemia will be recognized and reported quickly, and complications and injury will be prevented.

DISORDERS OF THE ADRENAL GLANDS

Adrenal disorders can involve the adrenal medulla or the adrenal cortex. A rare tumor of the adrenal medulla, called a **pheochromocytoma**, causes hypersecretion of epinephrine and norepinephrine. Hyposecretion of epinephrine is rare and generally causes no symptoms. Hypersecretion of cortisol from the adrenal cortex results in Cushing's syndrome. Hypofunction of the adrenal cortex results in Addison's disease.

Pheochromocytoma
Pathophysiology

A pheochromocytoma is a rare tumor that arises from the chromaffin cells of the adrenal medulla. Occasionally, a pheochromocytoma occurs outside the adrenal gland, in the chest or abdomen. The tumor autonomously secretes catecholamines (epinephrine and norepinephrine) in excessive amounts. Most pheochromocytomas are benign.

Etiology

The cause of most cases of pheochromocytoma is unknown. About one-third of cases are hereditary.

Signs and Symptoms

Because norepinephrine is the fight-or-flight hormone, patients with a pheochromocytoma have exaggerated fight-or-flight symptoms. These might be fairly constant or occur in sporadic "attacks." Manifestations include hypertension, tachycardia (with heart rate greater than 100 beats per minute), palpitations, tremor, diaphoresis, feeling of apprehension, and severe pounding headache. Nausea and vomiting are occasionally present. Blood glucose may increase because catecholamines inhibit insulin release from the pancreas. Constipation may occur because catecholamines relax the bowel. The most prominent characteristic is intermittent unstable hypertension. Diastolic pressure may be greater than 115 mm Hg. If hypertension and tachycardia are not controlled, the patient is at risk for stroke, heart attack and failure, vision changes, seizures, psychosis, and organ damage. It is estimated that about 0.1% of cases of hypertension are caused by a pheochromocytoma.

Diagnostic Tests

Patients with a suspected pheochromocytoma will have a 24-hour urine test for metanephrines and vanillylmandelic acid (VMA). These are end products of catecholamine metabolism. A blood test for metanephrines may also be done. The patient should avoid caffeine and medications for 2 days before and during the test. Check institution policy for other dietary restrictions. If results are elevated, a CT scan or an MRI is done to locate the tumor.

Therapeutic Measures

Treatment for pheochromocytoma is surgical removal of one or both adrenal glands. Newer laparoscopic techniques make surgery safer than in the past. The patient must be stabilized before surgery. Calcium channel blockers and alpha blockers are used to control acute hypertension. Beta-blocking medication may be added to block beta-adrenergic receptors in the heart and lungs, reducing other fight-or-flight symptoms.

After surgery, the patient is at risk for hypotension, hypertension, and hypoglycemia. Monitor vital signs and blood glucose and report variations from normal. If both adrenal glands have been entirely removed, the patient will require lifelong replacement hormones. (See section on adrenalectomy later in this chapter.)

Nursing Process for the Patient With Pheochromocytoma

DATA COLLECTION. Monitor vital signs frequently, and report elevations promptly.

NURSING DIAGNOSES, PLANNING, AND IMPLEMENTATION.
Risk for Injury related to hypertensive crisis
EXPECTED OUTCOME: The patient will be free from injury related to hypertension.

• Monitor vital signs and report elevated pulse and blood pressure promptly. *Prompt treatment helps prevent complications.*
• Approach the patient calmly and maintain a quiet environment. *Stress may precipitate a hypertensive episode.*
• Administer medications as ordered *to control symptoms.*
• Teach the patient how the medications will reduce symptoms, and the importance of avoiding foods and beverages containing caffeine, *so that the patient can participate in self-care.*

 WORD • BUILDING •

pheochromocytoma: pheo—dark + chromo—color + cyt—cell + oma—tumor

• If patient has surgery, continue careful monitoring *because manipulation of tumor can increase catecholamine release.*

EVALUATION. If interventions have been effective, the patient's vital signs will be within normal limits, and complications will be avoided.

Adrenocortical Insufficiency/Addison's Disease

Adrenocortical insufficiency (AI) is the insufficient production of the hormones of the adrenal cortex. Primary AI is called Addison's disease.

Pathophysiology

AI is associated with reduced levels of cortisol, aldosterone, or both hormones. A deficiency in androgens may also exist. In primary disease, ACTH levels from the pituitary can be elevated in an attempt to stimulate the adrenal cortex to synthesize more hormone. In secondary disease, deficient ACTH fails to stimulate adrenal steroid synthesis. In most cases, the adrenal glands are atrophied, small, and misshapen and are unable to produce adequate amounts of hormone.

Etiology

Addison's disease is thought to be autoimmune; that is, the gland destroys itself in response to conditions such as tuberculosis, fungal infection, infection related to acquired immunodeficiency syndrome (AIDS), or metastatic cancer. It can also be associated with other autoimmune diseases, such as Hashimoto's thyroiditis. Bilateral adrenalectomy also results in AI.

Secondary AI may be caused by dysfunction of the pituitary or hypothalamus. In addition, prolonged use of corticosteroid drugs can depress ACTH and corticotropin-releasing hormone production, which in turn reduces steroid hormone production. A patient receiving long-term corticosteroid therapy is particularly at risk for AI if the drugs are abruptly discontinued. Because the pituitary has been suppressed for a prolonged period, it may take up to a year before ACTH is produced normally again.

NURSING CARE TIP

Always taper corticosteroid therapy slowly to avoid adrenal crisis.

Signs and Symptoms

The most significant sign of Addison's disease is hypotension. This is related to the lack of aldosterone. Remember that aldosterone causes sodium and water retention in the kidney and potassium loss. If aldosterone is deficient, sodium and water are lost and hypotension and tachycardia result. Low cortisol levels cause hypoglycemia, weakness, fatigue, weight loss, confusion, and psychosis. In primary AI, increased ACTH

may produce hyperpigmentation of the skin, causing the patient to have a tanned or bronze appearance. Anorexia, nausea, and vomiting may also occur, possibly as the result of electrolyte imbalances. Women may have decreased body hair because of low androgen levels. Patients may report craving salt.

Complications

If a patient is exposed to stress, such as infection, trauma, or psychological pressure, the body may be unable to respond normally with secretion of cortisol (our natural stress hormone), and an adrenal crisis can occur. Loss of large amounts of sodium and water and the resulting fluid volume deficit cause profound hypotension, dehydration, and tachycardia. Potassium retention can cause cardiac dysrhythmias. Hypoglycemia may be severe. Coma and death result if treatment is not initiated. Treatment of adrenal crisis involves rapidly restoring fluid volume and cortisol levels. IV fluids (containing glucose) and large doses of IV glucocorticoids are administered. Electrolytes are replaced as needed. The cause of the crisis should be identified and treated.

Diagnostic Tests

Serum and urine cortisol levels are measured. Blood glucose is low. Blood urea nitrogen (BUN) and hematocrit levels may appear to be elevated because of dehydration. Antibodies may be present in the blood in autoimmune disease. An ACTH stimulation test may help determine whether the adrenal glands are functioning. Serum sodium and potassium levels are monitored. A CT scan or an MRI may be done to evaluate the size of the adrenal glands or to locate a pituitary tumor in secondary disease.

Therapeutic Measures

Long-term treatment consists of replacement of glucocorticoids (hydrocortisone) and mineralocorticoids (fludrocortisone). Some patients also receive androgen therapy. Patients will need hormone replacement therapy for the rest of their lives. Hormones are given in divided doses, with two-thirds of the daily dose given in the morning and one-third in the evening to mimic the body's own diurnal rhythm. Remember that steroid hormones are our natural stress hormones and so are naturally elevated during times of stress. Therefore, during times of stress or illness, doses need to be increased to two to three times normal. The patient may also be placed on a high-sodium diet. If the patient is ill and can't tolerate oral medication, hormones must be injected.

Nursing Process for the Patient With Addison's Disease

DATA COLLECTION. The patient with Addison's disease should be assessed for understanding of and adherence to the treatment regimen. Monitor vital signs and daily weights or I&O to track fluid status. Monitor serum glucose levels and symptoms of hyperkalemia and hyponatremia. Report changes in mental status. If the patient is in crisis, monitor vital signs closely and report any signs of fluid volume deficit such as orthostatic hypotension or poor skin turgor to the HCP immediately.

NURSING DIAGNOSES, PLANNING, AND IMPLEMENTATION.
Risk for Deficient Fluid Volume related to deficient adrenal cortical hormones
EXPECTED OUTCOME: The patient's fluid volume will be stable as evidenced by stable weights and vital signs, and skin turgor within normal limits.

- Monitor vital signs, and report change promptly. *Hypotension and tachycardia indicate hypovolemia.*
- Monitor fluid status and report changes promptly to prevent complications of fluid deficit.
- *Administer steroid replacements as ordered* to maintain fluid and electrolyte balance.

Risk for Ineffective Self Health Management related to deficient knowledge about self-care of Addison's disease
EXPECTED OUTCOME: The patient will verbalize understanding of self-monitoring and self-medication at home.

- Assess patient's understanding of his or her disease process and treatment. *Teaching should build on baseline knowledge.*
- Teach the patient the importance of hormone replacement as ordered. *The patient who does not secrete endogenous adrenocortical hormones must rely on replacements for survival.*
- Help the patient identify the causes and symptoms of stress, and explain the need to increase medication dosage during times of stress or illness according to the physician's instructions. *Because these hormones are normally increased during times of stress, it is important that the patient understand how to increase the dose during stress to prevent adrenal crisis.*
- Advise patient he or she may need to increase salt intake in hot weather *because of fluid and salt losses.*
- Recommend medical alert identification. *A patient in adrenal crisis may not be able to provide a medical history to emergency personnel, and identification can prevent delay of treatment.*

- If ordered by the physician, teach the patient and significant other how to use an emergency intramuscular (IM) hydrocortisone injection kit. *IM medication may be needed during stress or times when the patient is unable to take oral medications.*

EVALUATION. If nursing care is effective, the patient's fluid status will be stable, and the patient and family will be able to carry out proper self-care of Addison's disease.

Cushing's Syndrome

Cushing's syndrome is caused by exposure to excess cortisol. This can occur because of an adrenal problem, a pituitary problem, or from treatment with exogenous corticosteroids. See Table 39.6 for a comparison of adrenal insufficiency and Cushing's syndrome.

Pathophysiology

Recall that cortisol, aldosterone, and androgens are the three steroid hormones secreted by the adrenal cortex. Cortisol is essential for survival and is normally secreted in a diurnal rhythm, with levels increasing in the early morning. Secretion is increased during times of stress. In Cushing's syndrome, cortisol is hypersecreted without regard to stress or time of day. When levels of cortisol are very high, effects related to excess aldosterone and androgens are also seen.

LEARNING TIP

An easy way to remember the hormones of the adrenal cortex is to think salt, sugar, and sex. Aldosterone promotes salt retention, cortisol affects sugar (carbohydrate) metabolism, and androgens are sex hormones.

TABLE 39.6   ADRENAL CORTEX HORMONE SUMMARY

	Hypofunction	Hyperfunction
Disorder	Adrenocortical insufficiency, Addison's disease	Cushing's syndrome
Signs and Symptoms	Sodium and water loss, hypotension, hypoglycemia, fatigue	Weight gain, sodium and water retention, hyperglycemia, buffalo hump, moon face
Diagnostic Tests	Serum and urine cortisol	Serum and urine cortisol
Therapeutic Measures	Glucocorticoid and mineralocorticoid replacement	Alter steroid therapy dose or schedule; surgery if tumor
Priority Nursing Diagnoses	*Risk for Deficient Fluid Volume*	*Risk for Excess Fluid Volume, Unstable Blood Glucose Level, Infection*

Etiology

Cushing's syndrome can be caused by the hypersecretion of ACTH by the pituitary. This is most often the result of a benign pituitary adenoma. Sometimes ACTH is produced by a tumor in the lungs or other organs. The high levels of ACTH cause adrenal hyperplasia, which in turn increases production and release of cortisol. A problem within the adrenal gland, such as an adrenal adenoma or carcinoma can also produce excess cortisol.

The most common cause of Cushing's syndrome is prolonged use of glucocorticoid medication (e.g., prednisone) for chronic inflammatory disorders such as rheumatoid arthritis, chronic obstructive pulmonary disease, and Crohn's disease. The use of smaller doses of glucocorticoids (in inhalers for asthma) or topical creams does not usually cause a problem.

Signs and Symptoms

Most signs and symptoms of Cushing's syndrome are related to excess cortisol levels. Weight gain, central obesity with thin arms and legs, fat pads on the upper back (buffalo hump), and a round, moon-shaped face result from deposits of adipose tissue at these sites (Fig. 39.6).

Cortisol also causes insulin resistance and stimulates gluconeogenesis, which results in glucose intolerance. Some patients develop secondary diabetes mellitus (see Chapter 40). Muscle wasting and thin skin with purple striae occur as a result of cortisol's catabolic effect on tissues. Catabolic effects on bone lead to osteoporosis, pathological fractures, and back pain from compression fractures of the vertebrae. Because cortisol has anti-inflammatory and immunosuppressive actions, the patient is at risk for infection. Hyperpigmentation of the skin may occur. About half of patients develop mental status changes, from irritability to psychosis (sometimes referred to as steroid psychosis). Sodium and water retention are related to the mineralocorticoid effect. As sodium is retained, potassium is lost in the urine, causing hypokalemia. (See Chapter 6 to review these electrolyte imbalances.) Androgen effects include acne, growth of facial hair, and amenorrhea in women.

Diagnostic Tests

Suspicion of Cushing's syndrome may initially be based on a cushingoid appearance and history of taking steroid medication. Plasma and urine cortisol and plasma ACTH are measured. A 24-hour urine test for cortisol may be collected. Levels of cortisol in the saliva may also be measured. A dexamethasone suppression test may be done. Serum potassium is measured. Additional tests to locate the cause of excess endogenous cortisol may be done.

Therapeutic Measures

If a pituitary or ACTH-secreting tumor is present, surgical removal or radiation therapy to the pituitary gland may be employed. If the adrenals are the primary cause of the problem, radiation or removal of the adrenal gland or glands may be

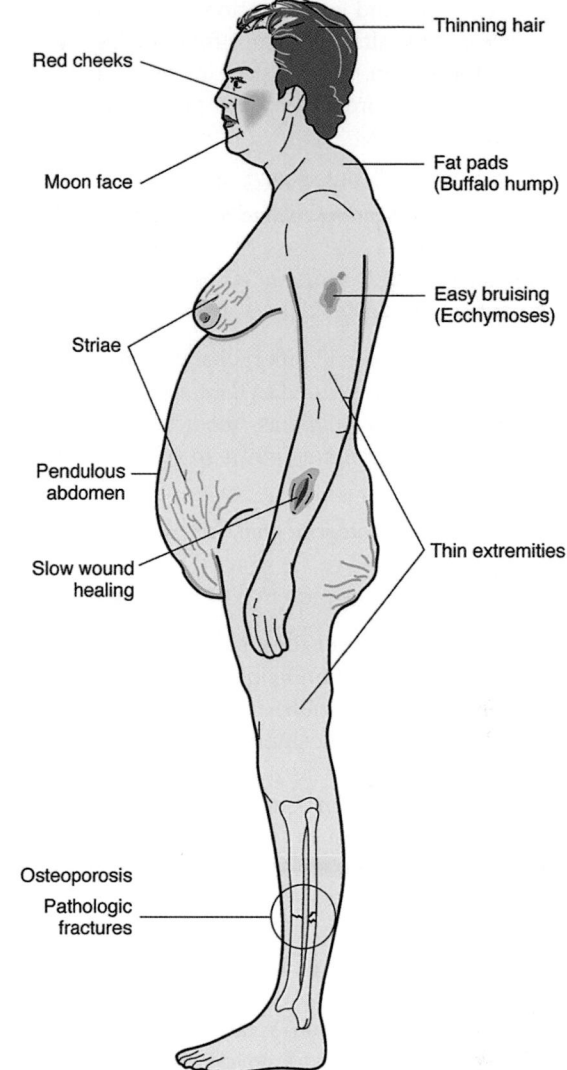

FIGURE 39.6 Physical manifestations seen in Cushing's syndrome.

performed. Minimally invasive surgeries have made surgery much safer. Drugs such as ketoconazole can be used to block production of adrenal steroids.

If the cause of Cushing's syndrome is administration of steroid medication, a lower dose, an every-other-day schedule, or once-a-day dosing in the morning may reduce side effects. Usually steroids are prescribed as a last resort for chronic disorders that are unresponsive to other treatment. The patient and HCP must weigh the risks and benefits of continuing the medication. The HCP may order a high-potassium, low-sodium, high-protein diet. Potassium supplements may be ordered. If the patient has high blood sugar, appropriate therapy for diabetes is instituted (see Chapter 40).

Nursing Process for the Patient With Cushing's Syndrome

DATA COLLECTION. When caring for the patient with Cushing's syndrome, assess the patient's medication history.

Monitor vital signs and complications related to fluid and sodium excess. Auscultate the lungs for crackles, and assess extremities for edema. Assess skin integrity, and monitor capillary glucose as ordered by the physician. Watch for signs of infection.

NURSING DIAGNOSES, PLANNING, AND IMPLEMENTATION.
Risk for Excess Fluid Volume related to sodium and water retention
EXPECTED OUTCOME: The patient's fluid volume will be stable as evidenced by stable daily weights.

• Monitor daily weights and report changes promptly *to prevent complications related to fluid excess.*
• Teach the patient ordered dietary modifications. *A low-sodium, high-potassium diet may help keep electrolytes in balance.*

Risk for Impaired Skin Integrity (thin, fragile skin) related to protein breakdown
EXPECTED OUTCOME: The patient's skin will remain intact.

• Observe skin, and monitor for breakdown with every position change. *Early recognition and treatment of a problem can prevent further breakdown.*
• Assist patient to change positions at least every 2 hours *to prevent pressure ulcers.*
• Use a lift sheet to move patient in bed *to prevent friction and shear.*
• Avoid harsh soaps and hot water. *These can dry skin and increase risk for injury.*
• Use moisturizing cream *to keep skin from drying.*
• Secure IVs and dressings without tape whenever possible. *Removal of tape can tear fragile skin.*
• Consider a specialty pressure-reducing mattress if the patient is very thin or unable to move *to reduce the risk of pressure ulcer.*
• Consult a dietitian if nutritional status is poor. *Poor nutrition further increases risk for skin breakdown and poor healing.*

Risk for Infection related to immune suppression
EXPECTED OUTCOME: The patient will be free from infection as evidenced by a white blood cell (WBC) count and temperature within normal limits.

• Monitor patient for signs of infection and report promptly *so appropriate treatment can be ordered.*
• Use good hand hygiene before and after patient care. *Hand washing is important in reducing exposure to pathogens.*
• Instruct the patient in good hand washing and in the importance of avoiding others who are ill. *A patient with an impaired immune system is more likely to contract illness from others.*
• Consult a dietitian if nutritional status is poor. *Poor nutrition further impairs immune function.*

• Encourage flu and pneumonia vaccinations *to help prevent illness in event of exposure.*

Risk for Unstable Blood Glucose Level related to impaired glucose tolerance
EXPECTED OUTCOME: The patient's blood glucose level will remain within normal limits.

• If glucose intolerance occurs, be prepared to administer insulin *because oral hypoglycemics are not usually effective.*
• Refer the patient and family to diabetes education classes *because diabetes is a complex disease that requires knowledge of self-care.*
• See Chapter 40 for care of the patient with diabetes.

Disturbed Body Image related to cushingoid appearance
EXPECTED OUTCOME: The patient will express feelings of acceptance of self.

• Approach patient with an attitude of acceptance and caring *to help develop trusting nurse–patient relationship.*
• Provide an opportunity for patient to verbalize feelings. *Expressing feelings may help reduce anxiety.*

EVALUATION. If care has been effective, complications of fluid overload will be recognized and treated early. The patient will have intact skin and be free from signs of infection. The patient will demonstrate skill in self-care of diabetes if indicated and will verbalize acceptance of self despite changes in appearance.

Nursing Care of the Patient Undergoing Adrenalectomy
Preoperative Care

Monitor the patient for electrolyte imbalance and hyperglycemia. Abnormalities must be corrected before surgery. To prevent adrenal crisis, glucocorticoids are administered because removal of the adrenals causes a sudden drop in adrenal hormones. Prepare the patient for adrenalectomy or hypophysectomy, depending on which surgery will be performed.

Postoperative Care

See care of the patient undergoing hypophysectomy earlier in this chapter. Following adrenalectomy, the patient receives routine postoperative care. In addition, the patient is closely monitored for changes in fluid and electrolyte balance and adrenal crisis. Patients who undergo bilateral adrenalectomy must take replacement glucocorticoid and mineralocorticoid hormones for the remainder of their life. If only one adrenal gland is removed, the remaining gland should eventually produce enough hormone to enable the patient to discontinue replacement hormone.

See Table 39.7 for a summary of endocrine disorders and Table 39.8 for a summary of medications used for endocrine disorders.

TABLE 39.7   SUMMARY OF ENDOCRINE DISORDERS

Hormone	Hypofunction	Hyperfunction
Antidiuretic hormone	Diabetes insipidus	Syndrome of inappropriate antidiuretic hormone
Growth hormone	Short stature	Acromegaly, gigantism
Thyroid hormone	Hypothyroidism	Hyperthyroidism
Epinephrine	Rare	Pheochromocytoma—hypertension
Parathyroid hormone	Hypoparathyroidism	Hyperparathyroidism
Cortisol	Addison's disease	Cushing's syndrome

TABLE 39.8   MEDICATIONS USED FOR ENDOCRINE DISORDERS

Medication Class	Examples/Action	Nursing Implications
Medications for ADH disorders	vasopressin (Pitressin): replaces antidiuretic hormone (ADH) desmopressin (DDAVP): replaces ADH conivaptan (Vaprisol): blocks action of ADH in the kidney. demeclocycline (Declomycin): reduces ADH release	Check daily weights and urine specific gravity. Do not give demeclocycline with dairy products or antacids.
Medications for growth hormone disorders	bromocriptine (Parlodel): reduces growth hormone (GH) release octreotide (Sandostatin) Lanreotide (Somatuline Depot) suppresses GH Pegvisomant (Somavert) blocks the effect of GH on receptor sites. somatotropin (Humatrope): replaces GH	Monitor blood pressure, serum GH. Teach patient self-administration. Monitor growth; teach patient self-administration.
Medications for thyroid disorders	levothyroxine (Synthroid): replaces T_4 propylthiouracil (PTU): inhibits synthesis of thyroid hormones methimazole (Tapazole): inhibits synthesis of thyroid hormones	Monitor vital signs and thyroid lab results. Monitor WBC and differential, thyroid function, liver function.
Medications for parathyroid disorders	calcium gluconate: replaces calcium alendronate (Fosamax): inhibits resorption of bone; keeps calcium in bones	Monitor vital signs and electrocardiogram during IV therapy. Do not take PO calcium with other medications. Do not take with calcium supplements or caffeine.
Medications for adrenal disorders	hydrocortisone: replaces cortisol in adrenal insufficiency fludrocortisone (Florinef): replaces aldosterone in adrenal insufficiency	Teach patient to take with food and not to discontinue abruptly. Monitor daily weights, vital signs, and serum potassium.

CRITICAL THINKING

Mrs. Tercini

■ Mrs. Tercini is a 62-year-old woman admitted to your unit in addisonian crisis. She is lethargic, with a blood pressure of 86/58 mm Hg, pulse 112, and respirations 18. While interviewing her daughter, you learn that Mrs. Tercini has a history of Cushing's syndrome treated with bilateral adrenalectomy 25 years ago. She has been taking 150 mcg fludrocortisone (Florinef) and 200 mg hydrocortisone daily ever since. Three days ago she developed the flu.

1. Why is an adrenalectomy done to treat Cushing's syndrome?

2. What is the most effective schedule for Mrs. Tercini's medication?
3. What might have precipitated this addisonian crisis?
4. Why is Mrs. Tercini's blood pressure low?
5. How could this crisis have been prevented?
6. Fludrocortisone is available as 0.1-mg tablets. How many should you administer?

Suggested answers are at the end of the chapter.

SUGGESTED ANSWERS TO

CRITICAL THINKING

■ *Mrs. Jackson*

1. Assess mental status and level of consciousness. Assess edema, lung sounds, and vital signs. Check intake and output during the past 2 days. Check recent lab work to see if her serum sodium is low. You also check a book on the unit and recall that anesthetics are possible causes of SIADH. Opioids, which Mrs. Jackson is likely taking after surgery, can also cause confusion.

2. Her weight gain is most likely caused by fluid retention, which can be a result of heart failure or SIADH, among other things.

3. Notify the registered nurse of your findings and suspicions. Be prepared to place Mrs. Jackson on a fluid restriction. Reassure her son that the physician is being notified of the changes he noted.

4. Remember "a pint's a pound." A pint is 2 cups for 480 mL.

$$\frac{6 \text{ pounds}}{} \frac{480 \text{ mL}}{1 \text{ pound}} = 2880 \text{ mL or almost 3 L}$$

■ *Adoption*

The children's growth hormone secretion was probably suppressed because of psychosocial stress. Once they felt secure in a loving environment, growth hormone levels returned to normal.

■ *Mrs. Maino*

1. Mrs. Maino's TSH is elevated because her pituitary gland is working overtime to try to stimulate the underactive thyroid gland.

2. Mrs. Maino's metabolism has been slow, so she has been burning fewer calories. When she starts on thyroid replacement hormone, her metabolic rate will return to normal, and she will need more calories. Intake of calories should be balanced with the possible need for weight loss.

3. If Mrs. Maino receives too much thyroid hormone, she will have symptoms of hyperthyroidism, including an increased pulse rate. She should know how to check her pulse and to call her HCP if it is elevated.

4. The nurse, HCP, and dietitian are essential. A physical therapist may be helpful if mobilization and exercise recommendations are needed. A social worker or discharge planner can help with discharge needs.

■ *Mrs. Tercini*

1. Cushing's syndrome is caused by too much cortisol. The adrenal cortex is responsible for secreting cortisol.

2. Mrs. Tercini should take two-thirds of her daily dose of hydrocortisone and fludrocortisone in the morning and one-third in the evening, or as ordered. This most closely mimics the body's natural corticosteroid secretion.

3. The flu probably triggered this crisis. Illness is a stressor, and normally the body secretes steroids during stress. Because Mrs. Tercini's body is unable to produce steroids, she experiences symptoms of hypoadrenalism during stressful times.

4. Mrs. Tercini's blood pressure is low because she has insufficient circulating mineralocorticoids. Without aldosterone, sodium and water are lost and blood pressure drops.

5. Mrs. Tercini should have taken extra medication when she became ill. Her HCP should provide guidelines for dosing during stress and illness.

6.

$$\frac{150 \text{ mcg}}{1000 \text{ mcg}} \bigg| \frac{1 \text{ mg}}{0.1 \text{ mg}} \bigg| 1 \text{ tab} = 1.5 \text{ tablets}$$

REVIEW QUESTIONS

1. Which assessment finding in a patient who has just returned from having a thyroidectomy should be immediately reported to the HCP?
   1. Neck discomfort
   2. Sore throat
   3. Tingling fingertips
   4. Sleepiness

2. A patient with SIADH asks the nurse why he has gained 10 pounds. Which response is best?
   1. "SIADH causes an increase in appetite. As soon as you are effectively treated, the weight should drop back to normal for you."
   2. "You are retaining a lot of sodium and potassium, and that causes you to gain water weight."
   3. "You have too much of a hormone in your system that causes you to retain water. The extra 10 pounds is likely water weight."
   4. "Your kidneys are not working correctly, so they can't get rid of extra water from your system."

3. Which assessment finding should the nurse expect to see in the patient with uncontrolled diabetes insipidus? **Select all that apply.**
   1. Edema
   2. Polyuria
   3. Heat intolerance
   4. Diarrhea
   5. Polydipsia
   6. Dehydration

4. Which of the following instructions should the nurse provide to the patient who is being discharged after a thyroidectomy?
   1. "You must take your thyroid replacement every day just as the physician prescribed."
   2. "You must weigh yourself daily and report any gain or loss of more than 1 pound."
   3. "You will need to return to the physician's office for a weekly blood pressure check."
   4. "You will need to restrict your sodium and potassium intake."

5. Which of the following nursing assessments is most important in the patient with hyperthyroidism and risk for thyrotoxic crisis?
   1. Intake and output
   2. Breath sounds
   3. Bowel sounds
   4. Vital signs

6. Which action by the nurse is most important following hypophysectomy?
   1. Performing a routine neurologic assessment
   2. Encouraging the patient to cough and deep breathe
   3. Monitoring for tracheal edema
   4. Assisting with use of an incentive spirometer

7. Which of the following statements by the patient with hypothyroidism indicates to the nurse that the plan of care has been effective?
   1. "I feel so much better now that my energy is returning."
   2. "I'm really glad the diarrhea has stopped."
   3. "I'm so glad I won't have to take medication for very long."
   4. "My fingers aren't tingling anymore."

Answers can be found in Appendix C.

 DavisPlus | For additional resources and information visit **davispl.us/medsurg5**

40

Nursing Care of Patients With Disorders of the Endocrine Pancreas

PAULA D. HOPPER

KEY TERMS

diabetes mellitus (DYE-ah-BEE-tis mel-EYE-tus)
endogenous (en-DAW-jen-uss)
gastroparesis (GASS-troh-puh-REE-sus)
glycosuria (GLY-kos-YOO-ree-ah)
hyperglycemia (HY-per-glye-SEE-mee-ah)
hypoglycemia (HY-poh-glye-SEE-mee-ah)
ketoacidosis (KEE-toh-as-ih-DOH-sis)
Kussmaul's respirations (KOOS-mahlz RESS-per-AY-shuns)
nephropathy (neh-FROP-uh-thee)
neuropathy (new-RAW-puh-thee)
nocturia (nok-TYOO-ree-ah)
polydipsia (PAH-lee-DIP-see-ah)
polyphagia (PAW-lee-FAY-jee-ah)
polyuria (PAH-lee-YOO-ree-ah)
postprandial (POHST-PRAN-dee-uhl)
preprandial (PREE-PRAN-dee-uhl)
retinopathy (RET-ih-NAW-puh-thee)

LEARNING OUTCOMES

1. Explain the pathophysiologies of type 1 and type 2 diabetes mellitus.
2. Identify risk factors for type 1 and type 2 diabetes mellitus.
3. Describe the signs and symptoms of diabetes mellitus.
4. Describe causes, signs and symptoms, and treatment of high and low blood glucose levels.
5. Discuss how diabetes increases risk of complications such as heart disease, blindness, and kidney failure.
6. Identify diagnostic tests used to diagnose and monitor diabetes mellitus and its complications.
7. Identify therapeutic measures to help patients with diabetes control blood glucose levels.
8. Differentiate the action of insulin and oral hypoglycemic agents in lowering blood glucose levels.
9. Plan nursing care and education for the patient with diabetes mellitus.
10. List measures to increase the safety of the patient with diabetes who is undergoing surgery.
11. Explain reactive hypoglycemia and its treatment.

914

DIABETES MELLITUS

Diabetes mellitus (be careful not to confuse this with diabetes insipidus) is a group of metabolic diseases in which defects in insulin secretion or action result in elevated blood glucose (**hyperglycemia**). According to the 2012 Centers for Disease Control and Prevention (CDC) data, approximately 29.1 million people or 9.3% of the population in the United States, have diabetes mellitus. Approximately 8.1 million people have diabetes and don't know it. Another 79 million have prediabetes. The direct and indirect cost (such as lost work time) of diabetes in the United States is about $245 billion per year. The incidence of diabetes mellitus varies by race and ethnicity. In the United States, Hispanic, African American, Native American, and Asian American populations have higher rates of diabetes than non-Hispanic white ethnic groups (CDC, 2012).

Diabetes is a serious disease that can cause complications such as blindness, kidney failure, heart attacks, and strokes. It is a leading cause of lower limb amputations in the United States. With good education and self-care, patients with diabetes can prevent or delay these complications and lead full, productive lives. Nurses play a major role in helping patients learn to care for themselves effectively.

Pathophysiology

Body tissues, and the cells that compose them, use glucose for energy. Glucose is a simple sugar provided by the foods we eat. When carbohydrates are eaten, they are digested into sugars, including glucose, which is then absorbed into the bloodstream. Carbohydrates provide most of the glucose used by the body; proteins and fats can indirectly provide smaller amounts of glucose. Glucose is able to enter the cells only with the help of insulin, a hormone produced by the beta cells in the islets of Langerhans of the pancreas (Fig. 40.1). When insulin comes in contact with the cell membrane, it combines with a receptor that allows activation of special glucose transporters in the membrane. By helping glucose enter the body's cells, insulin lowers the glucose level in the blood. Insulin also helps the body store excess glucose in the liver in the form of glycogen.

Another hormone, glucagon, is produced by the alpha cells in the islets of Langerhans. Glucagon raises the blood glucose when needed by releasing stored glucose from the liver and muscles. Insulin and glucagon work together to keep the blood glucose at a constant level.

Diabetes results from deficient production of insulin by the beta cells in the pancreas, or from inability of the body's cells to use insulin. When glucose is unable to enter body cells, it stays in the bloodstream; hyperglycemia results, and the cells are denied their energy source. Abnormal glucagon secretion may also play a role in type 2 diabetes. See Fig. 40.1.

Types and Causes

Type 1 Diabetes Mellitus

Type 1 diabetes (formerly called juvenile diabetes mellitus, insulin-dependent diabetes mellitus, or IDDM) is caused by destruction of the beta cells in the islets of Langerhans of the pancreas. When the beta cells are destroyed, they are unable to produce insulin. Insulin must then be injected for the body to use food for energy. See "Patient Perspective" for Dave's story about having type 1 diabetes. Only about 5% of people with diabetes have type 1 diabetes.

• WORD • BUILDING •
diabetes mellitus: diabetes—passing through + mellitus—sweet
hyperglycemia: hyper—excessive + glyc—glucose + emia—in the blood

Patient Perspective

Dave

I was diagnosed with type 1 diabetes mellitus at age 3 years. I remember being left in a children's ward of the hospital with the nuns (who were nurses) in their habits and looking into the parking lot as my parents got in the car and drove away. I remember the fear and horror of being left alone. Later, I remember my doctor teaching my mother and me about the diet and monitoring my urine for glucose and ketones. This was all we had in those days (the early 1960s). I was supposed to test my urine before meals and at bedtime, just like we monitor blood glucose today. Every time I saw my doctor, he would review and change my treatment based on the results. Insulin then was extracted from pig and cow cadavers.

I remember my life being pretty normal except at holidays. When my brothers and sisters were getting Halloween candy and Christmas candy canes, I felt odd and left out. My mom was really tough and observant, and I had to be sneaky to get away with stealing a treat or two left momentarily unobserved by those around me. I was thrilled when sugarless candy became available around age 10 or so and I could have my own candies to hoard for myself.

Hypoglycemic reactions were always a trauma-filled event at our house. They came at unexpected times, and my mom sometimes blamed herself. I can honestly say that my mom deserves more credit than I have ever given her for my good fortune with my diabetes. She did not have glucometers, glycohemoglobin tests, or even diabetes specialists and educators; she just had the desire of a mother who did everything she could to make sure I had and did everything right as far as she knew.

In my late teens I took everything my doctor and my mom had done for me and trashed them. I lived with reckless abandon: I did what I wanted, ate what I wanted, and didn't even think about the disease I lived with until I was about 30. I worked hard those years in construction, and the physical activity probably delayed the complications that might otherwise have occurred.

At age 35, I began to experience the inevitable effects of long-term hyperglycemia. I developed diabetic retinopathy, the leading cause of adult-onset blindness in the United States. My vision was restored in my left eye with laser surgery. It would take another surgery (vitrectomy) to bring the vision in my right eye back to the 20/60 it is now from the 20/2000 it was before the surgery.

It is believed that the pancreas may attack itself following certain viral infections or administration of certain drugs. This is called an autoimmune response. Almost 90% of patients newly diagnosed with type 1 diabetes have islet cell antibodies in their blood. These antibodies might be present for years before actual symptoms of diabetes develop. About 10% of people with type 1 diabetes cases also have a genetic predisposition to its development. The patient with type 1 diabetes is most often young and thin and is prone to develop ketoacidosis when blood glucose is elevated. Diabetic ketoacidosis is discussed later in this chapter. See Table 40.1 for a comparison of type 1 and type 2 diabetes. Research studies are ongoing to try to find ways to prevent type 1 diabetes once antibodies have been detected.

Type 2 Diabetes Mellitus

Ninety-five percent of people with diabetes have type 2 diabetes mellitus (formerly called adult-onset diabetes mellitus, non–insulin-dependent diabetes mellitus, or NIDDM). In type 2 diabetes mellitus, tissues are resistant to insulin. Insulin is still made by the pancreas but in inadequate amounts. Sometimes the amount of insulin is normal or even high, but because the tissues are resistant to it, hyperglycemia results. As the disease advances, the pancreas eventually wears out, and insulin production decreases. When this occurs, the patient will likely require insulin injections. Simply using insulin, however, does not make the person a type 1 diabetic. He or she is a type 2 diabetic who needs insulin to control the blood glucose level.

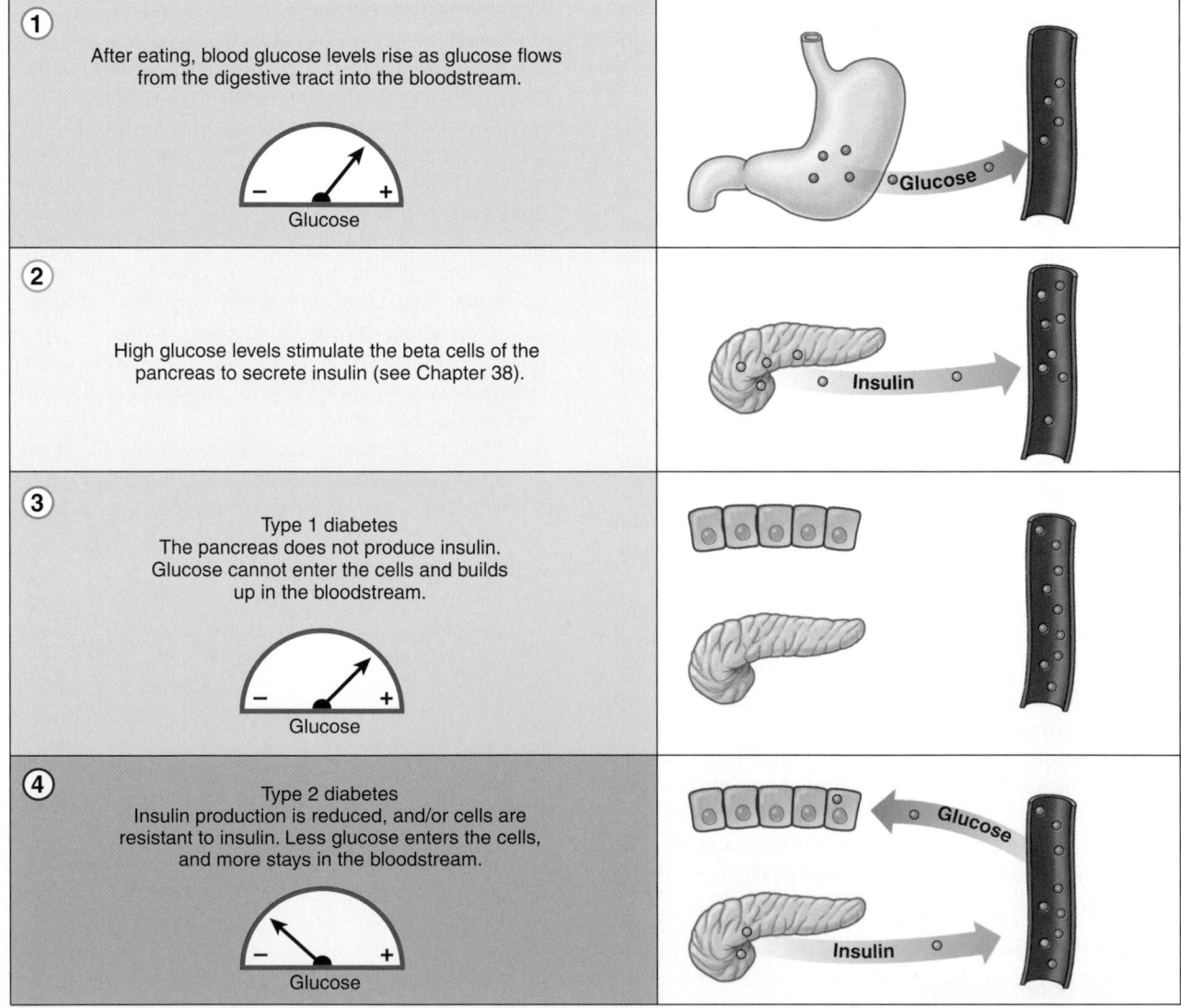

① After eating, blood glucose levels rise as glucose flows from the digestive tract into the bloodstream.

Glucose

Glucose

② High glucose levels stimulate the beta cells of the pancreas to secrete insulin (see Chapter 38).

Insulin

③ Type 1 diabetes
The pancreas does not produce insulin. Glucose cannot enter the cells and builds up in the bloodstream.

Glucose

④ Type 2 diabetes
Insulin production is reduced, and/or cells are resistant to insulin. Less glucose enters the cells, and more stays in the bloodstream.

Glucose

Glucose

Insulin

FIGURE 40.1 Regulation of blood glucose. Adapted from Thompson, G. S. (2013). *Understanding anatomy and physiology.* Philadelphia: F.A. Davis, p. 236.

TABLE 40.1   COMPARISON OF TYPE 1 AND TYPE 2 DIABETES

	Type 1	Type 2
Onset	Rapid	Slow
Age at onset	Usually younger than 40	Usually older than 40
Risk factors	Virus, autoimmune response, heredity	Heredity, obesity
Usual body type	Lean	Obese
High blood glucose complication	Ketoacidosis	Hyperosmolar hyperglycemic state; may develop ketoacidosis
Treatment	Diet, exercise; must have insulin to survive	Diet, exercise; may need oral hypo-glycemic agents or insulin to control blood glucose level

Heredity is responsible for up to 90% of cases of type 2 diabetes. Obesity is also a major contributing factor. Often the patient with a new diagnosis of type 2 diabetes is obese, relates a family history of diabetes, and has had a recent life stressor such as the death of a family member, illness, or loss of a job.

SELF-CARE TIP

Drink more water! Type 2 diabetes has been linked to drinking sweetened drinks. Now, research has also linked type 2 diabetes with consumption of diet drinks sweetened with artificial sweeteners. Water, unsweetened teas, and sparkling waters are healthier choices.

TYPE 2 DIABETES IN YOUTH. More and more children and adolescents are developing type 2 diabetes, which in the past only occurred in adults. This is related to increasing obesity and decreasing activity levels in children today. Earlier onset of diabetes increases the risk of early complications, including death from cardiovascular disease.

Gestational Diabetes

Gestational diabetes mellitus (GDM) occurs in 2% to 10% of pregnancies, especially in women with risk factors for type 2 diabetes. The extra metabolic demands of pregnancy trigger the onset of diabetes. Blood glucose usually returns to normal after delivery, but the mother has a 35% to 60% risk of developing type 2 diabetes within 10 to 20 years (CDC, 2011). If the mother with GDM is overweight, she should be counseled that weight loss and exercise will decrease her risk of developing diabetes. Mothers with GDM require specialized care and should be referred to an expert in this area.

Prediabetes

Prediabetes refers to blood glucose levels that are above normal but do not meet the criteria for diagnosing diabetes (Fig. 40.2). Prediabetes usually occurs before the onset of type 2 diabetes. It is diagnosed by evaluating fasting blood glucose levels, glucose tolerance tests (see tests of diabetes below), or HbA$_{1c}$. Those with prediabetes may be able to prevent the onset of diabetes with weight loss and exercise.

Other Types of Diabetes

Secondary diabetes can develop as a result of another chronic illness that damages the islet cells, such as pancreatitis or cystic fibrosis. Prolonged use of some drugs, such as steroid hormones, phenytoin (Dilantin), thiazide diuretics, and thyroid hormone, can also impair insulin action and raise blood glucose. Less common causes include pancreatic trauma and other endocrine disorders.

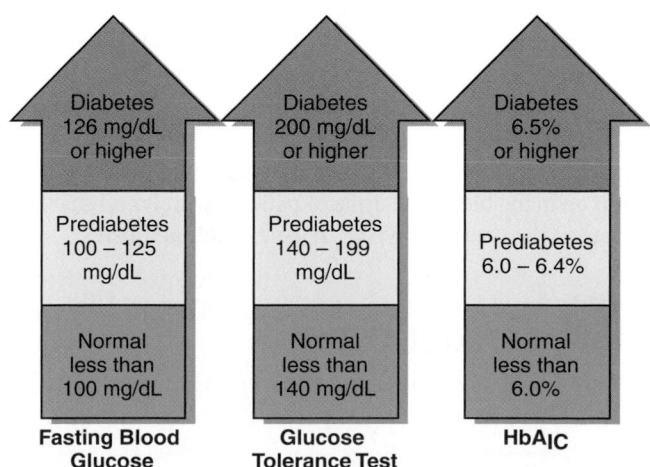

FIGURE 40.2 Prediabetes is the period between normal blood glucose levels and levels that are diagnostic for diabetes. Tests used to determine whether a patient has normal blood glucose levels, high-risk prediabetes, or diabetes include the fasting glucose level, glucose tolerance, and HbA$_{1c}$ tests.

Metabolic Syndrome

Prediabetes has been linked to a condition called metabolic syndrome or cardiometabolic syndrome. According to the American Heart Association and the National Heart, Lung, and Blood Institute, metabolic syndrome is diagnosed when at least three of the following criteria are met (American Heart Association, 2011):

1. Central or abdominal obesity (measured by waist circumference):
   • Men—greater than 40 inches
   • Women—greater than 35 inches
2. Fasting blood triglycerides greater than or equal to 150 mg/dL
3. Blood HDL cholesterol:
   • Men—less than 40 mg/dL
   • Women—less than 50 mg/dL
4. Blood pressure greater than or equal to 130/85 mm Hg
5. Fasting glucose greater than or equal to 100 mg/dL

Other risk factors include physical inactivity, aging, hormonal imbalance, and genetic predisposition. Hispanic Americans are at higher risk than Caucasians. A major factor is the growing obesity epidemic in the United States.

Any patient who fits this profile should be monitored closely for the onset of type 2 diabetes and heart disease. Patients should be counseled on the importance of a diet low in saturated fats and cholesterol, weight loss, physical activity, and control of blood pressure and cholesterol levels.

Signs and Symptoms

Classic symptoms of diabetes mellitus include **polydipsia** (excessive thirst), **polyuria** (excessive urination), and **polyphagia** (excessive hunger). The large amount of glucose in the blood causes an increase in serum concentration, or osmolality. The renal tubules are unable to reabsorb all the excess glucose that is filtered by the glomeruli, and **glycosuria** results. Large amounts of body water are required to excrete this glucose, causing polyuria, **nocturia** (nighttime urination), and dehydration. The increased osmolality and dehydration cause polydipsia. Because glucose is unable to enter the cells, the cells starve, causing polyphagia. High blood glucose can also cause fatigue, blurred vision, abdominal pain, and headaches. Ketones (acidic byproducts of fat breakdown) can build up in the blood and urine of patients with type 1 diabetes or late in the course of type 2 diabetes (**ketoacidosis**).

LEARNING TIP

Remember the classic symptoms of diabetes with the *Three Ps:* **p**olydipsia, **p**olyuria, and **p**olyphagia.

Diagnostic Tests

Fasting Plasma Glucose Level

Diagnosis of diabetes mellitus is based on plasma glucose levels measured by a laboratory. According to the American Diabetes Association (ADA, 2014), a normal plasma glucose level is less than 100 mg/dL. When the fasting plasma glucose (drawn after at least 8 hours without eating) is 126 mg/dL or greater, diabetes is diagnosed. A second test may be required if the first test is not clearly diagnostic. If the fasting plasma glucose is between 100 and 125 mg/dL, the patient has IFG and prediabetes.

Random Plasma Glucose

Sometimes it is not feasible to check a fasting plasma glucose. A random plasma glucose (RPG) is checked without regard to the last meal. Diabetes is diagnosed if the RPG is 200 mg/dL or greater, with symptoms of diabetes.

Oral Glucose Tolerance Test

Another test to diagnose diabetes is the oral glucose tolerance test (OGTT). An OGTT measures blood glucose at intervals after the patient drinks a concentrated carbohydrate drink. Diabetes is diagnosed when the blood glucose level is 200 mg/dL or greater after 2 hours. A result between 140 and 199 mg/dL at 2 hours leads to a diagnosis of impaired glucose tolerance and prediabetes.

Glycohemoglobin

The glycohemoglobin test (also called glycosylated hemoglobin, or HbA_{1c} [hemoglobin A1C]) is used to gather baseline data and to monitor the progress of diabetes control. In 2009, the ADA also changed its guidelines to include the HbA_{1c} as a diagnostic test for diabetes.

Glucose in the blood attaches to hemoglobin in the red blood cells, which live about 3 months. When the glucose that is attached to the hemoglobin is measured, it reflects the average blood glucose level for the previous 2 to 3 months. This is a helpful measurement when blood glucose levels fluctuate and a single measurement would be misleading. It also assists in determining the degree of effectiveness of a patient's treatment plan. A normal HbA_{1c} is 4% to 6%. An HbA_{1c} of 6.5% or higher is diagnostic for diabetes. An HbA_{1c} between 6% and 6.5% indicates high risk for developing diabetes (prediabetes).

Newer methods allow this test to be done in a physician's office while the patient waits. See Table 40.2 for average blood glucose levels based on HbA_{1c} results.

Glycohemoglobin testing might be inaccurate in some people, such as those with anemia. These patients may instead be tested for glycated serum protein (also called fructosamine), which is a similar test that indicates glucose levels over a period of 1 to 2 weeks instead of 3 months.

• WORD • BUILDING •

polydipsia: poly—many or much + dipsia—thirst
polyuria: poly—many or much + uria—urine
polyphagia: poly—many or much + phagia—to eat
glycosuria: glyc—glucose + uria—urine
nocturia: noc—by night + uria—urine
ketoacidosis: keto—ketones + acid—acidic + osis—condition

TABLE 40.2 CORRELATION BETWEEN HBA₁C AND MEAN FASTING PLASMA GLUCOSE

HbA$_{1c}$ (%)	Fasting Plasma Glucose (mg/dL)
6	126
7	154
8	183
9	212
10	240
11	269
12	298

Source: American Diabetes Association (2014).

Estimated Average Glucose

Some health care providers (HCPs) use a calculation to convert HbA$_{1c}$ results to estimated average glucose (eAG) numbers, which may be more meaningful to patients. The formula is:

$$28.7 \times HbA_{1c} - 46.7 = eAG.$$

Here is an example for a patient whose HbA$_{1c}$ is 8.6:

$$28.7 \times 8.6 - 46.7 = 200.12,$$ which can be rounded to 200 mg/dL.

Additional Tests

Because diabetes affects so many body systems, additional tests recommended for baseline data include a lipid profile, serum creatinine, and urine microalbumin levels to monitor kidney function, urinalysis, and electrocardiogram.

CRITICAL THINKING

Mr. McMillan

■ Mr. McMillan is a 50-year-old patient brought into the emergency department with extreme fatigue and dehydration. After the physician sees him, you ask Mr. McMillan some additional questions. Based on the patient's answers, you request that the physician add a glucose level to the laboratory tests ordered. The result is 1400 mg/dL.

1. What questions would you ask Mr. McMillan if you suspected diabetes?
2. Why was Mr. McMillan fatigued?
3. Why was he dehydrated?

Suggested answers are at the end of the chapter.

Prevention

Studies are ongoing to find ways prevent type 1 diabetes in people at risk. It is possible to prevent type 2 diabetes. Research studies have shown that patients at risk for type 2 diabetes, even those who already have impaired glucose tolerance or impaired fasting glucose (IFG), can prevent or delay the onset of diabetes with weight loss and regular exercise. On the basis of this research, the ADA (2014) recommends loss of 7% of body weight and moderate physical activity for 150 minutes per week. Use of the diabetes medication metformin can also help prevent diabetes in patients with prediabetes. Patients at risk should have their plasma glucose level checked regularly.

Therapeutic Measures

The only cure for diabetes is a pancreas (or islet cell) transplant. However, diabetes can be controlled. Treatment begins with diet and exercise. Insulin is added in patients with type 1 diabetes and insulin or oral hypoglycemic medication as needed in those with type 2 diabetes. Weight loss is essential for patients who have type 2 diabetes and are overweight or obese. Blood glucose monitoring and education are also important to good diabetes control.

To monitor the effectiveness of treatment, patients should have regular health care follow-up visits. See Box 40-1 for a summary of the diabetes goals and recommendations proposed by the ADA for 2014.

Box 40-1 Summary of Diabetes Goals and Recommendations for Adults

Target levels:*

• HbA$_{1c}$	Less than 7%
• Preprandial capillary glucose	70–130 mg/dL
• Peak postprandial capillary glucose	Less than 180 mg/dL
• Blood pressure	Less than 140/80 mm Hg

Blood lipids should be measured every 1 to 2 years, depending on risk. Target levels are as follows:

• Low-density lipoproteins	Less than 100 mg/dL
	Less than 70 mg/dL in patients with cardiovascular disease (CVD)
• Triglycerides	Less than 150 mg/dL
• High-density lipoproteins	Greater than 40 mg/dL (men)
	Greater than 50 mg/dL (women)

General recommendations:

• Yearly flu vaccine for all patients age 6 months and older
• One lifetime pneumococcal vaccine for patients older than age 2 years, with revaccination for patients older than age 65 years if first vaccine was more than 5 years earlier

Continued

Box 40-1 Summary of Diabetes Goals and Recommendations for Adults—cont'd

- Aspirin therapy, 75–162 mg/day, for patients at increased cardiovascular risk
- Statin therapy if history of myocardial infarction (MI) or if older than age 40 with CVD risk factors
- Avoidance of smoking and use of tobacco products
- Yearly comprehensive foot examination
- Dilated comprehensive eye examination within 5 years of onset of type 1 diabetes or at diagnosis of type 2 diabetes, and every 1 to 2 years thereafter.

---

* Target levels for blood glucose are different in hospitalized patients.

Source: Adapted from American Diabetes Association. (2014). Clinical practice recommendations 2014. *Diabetes Care, 37*(Suppl. 1).

Goals of Treatment

The ADA recommends that patients maintain a **preprandial** (premeal) plasma glucose level of 70 to 130 mg/dL, peak **postprandial** glucose less than 180 mg/dL, and glycohemoglobin level of less than 7% to prevent or delay complications of diabetes. Because of the risk for cardiovascular disease, they also recommend maintaining blood pressure of less than 140/80 mm Hg (ADA, 2014). All goals may be adjusted in individual circumstances. For example, the patient who is unable to feel symptoms of **hypoglycemia** (low blood glucose) might have a higher preprandial glucose goal to prevent undetected hypoglycemic episodes.

Medical Nutrition Therapy

The goal of medical nutrition therapy is to achieve and maintain blood glucose and lipid levels as near to normal as possible to prevent long-term complications. For some, especially those with type 2 diabetes, weight loss and cholesterol and blood pressure control may be additional goals of nutrition therapy.

Because the patient with diabetes has a limited amount of insulin, either **endogenous** (from within the body) or injected, it is important to eat an amount of food that will not exceed the insulin's ability to carry it into the cells. This requires a meal plan that includes consistent amounts of carbohydrates, proteins, and fats each day. Because carbohydrates contribute most to the blood glucose level, it is important that the amount of carbohydrates consumed is consistent from one day to the next. If a patient eats a small amount of carbohydrate one day and a large amount the next, the blood glucose will fluctuate, leading to complications. It is possible to relax nutrition restrictions somewhat if the patient is willing to test blood glucose frequently at home and adjust treatment accordingly.

The ADA recommends a complete assessment by a specially trained dietitian and an individualized nutrition therapy plan and teaching. The education of the patient with diabetes is a process that may take months and cannot be accomplished in a single visit or with a paper handout or referral to a website. Various meal plans are available, as shown in "Nutrition Notes." Because diabetes increases the risk of high serum cholesterol and triglycerides, all plans limit fat intake.

• WORD • BUILDING •

preprandial: pre—before + prandial—meal
postprandial: post—after + prandial—meal
hypoglycemia: hypo—deficient + glyc—glucose + emia—in the blood
endogenous: endo—within + genous—to produce

Nutrition Notes

Diabetic Meal Plans

Nutrition is integral to the management of diabetes and oftentimes the most challenging aspect of treatment for patients. No single approach is suitable for everyone but should be individualized based on the patient's health status and lifestyle, ability to learn, and willingness to change.

Overall goals and strategies differ by type of diabetes. In general:

- Patients with type 1 diabetes need to prevent wide swings in blood glucose levels through careful timing of meals and snacks in relation to insulin therapy and activity.
- Patients with type 2 diabetes use diet modifications with medication as needed to maintain near-normal glucose, blood pressure, and lipid levels and to lose weight as needed.

People with diabetes usually benefit from eating on a regular basis (every 4 to 5 hours while awake). Evidence has shown that the use of sucrose (table sugar) as part of the meal plan does not impair blood glucose control in individuals with diabetes.

A CDE can devise a meal plan based on the patient's abilities, past dietary habits, and commitment. Several meal-planning approaches are described next.

Create Your Plate

The ADA has devised a simple method of meal planning that divides a plate into one half and two quarters. Half the plate is filled with nonstarchy vegetables. One quarter is filled with starchy foods, such as whole grains and starchy vegetables. The last quarter is used for meats and meat substitutes. Finally, a serving of fruit and an 8-ounce glass of nonfat or low-fat milk completes the meal (Fig. 40.3).

Examples of foods suitable for each section of the plate are provided at www.diabetes.org/food-and-fitness/food/planning-meals/create-your-plate/?loc=ff-diabetesmealplans.

FIGURE 40.3 An example of the diabetes plate method.

National Institutes of Health Diabetes Pyramid

The National Diabetes Information Clearinghouse at the National Institutes of Health has developed extensive instructional materials on diabetes management. A diabetes food pyramid illustrates food groups and sample foods, including desirable methods of preparation. Categories of caloric needs by sex, weight, and activity levels are correlated with numbers of servings from each food group that could be used by the diabetic educator to individualize a patient's diet prescription. The site is not copyrighted, and reproduction of the printable sheets is encouraged. See http://diabetes.niddk.nih.gov/dm/pubs/eating_ez/#pyramid.

Exchange Lists

An exchange system is composed of six lists of foods (starch, vegetable, fruit, milk, meat, fat) plus a "free food" list. Foods in each list contain similar energy nutrients (carbohydrate, protein, and fat). For example, green peas are on the starch list rather than the vegetable list because they are closer in composition to a slice of bread than to green beans.

Individual food items within an exchange list are essentially equal to each other in nutrient composition and can thus be exchanged or swapped for each other. Exchanges were designed to be approximately equal in nutrients, not in volume; therefore, portion sizes vary widely. For instance, one fruit exchange is equal to 1¼ cup of whole strawberries but to only three dates.

To use this method correctly, for each meal, patients must choose the prescribed number of items from each appropriate list on their meal plan. A meal plan is a food guide that shows the number of choices or exchanges the patient should eat at each meal and snack, based on the total daily calories prescribed. Users of the exchange list system should weigh or measure their portions several times per week to avoid portion inflation. For more information, see www.eatright.org/search.aspx?search=Exchange%20lists.

Using Carbohydrate Counting

Because carbohydrate is the energy nutrient that has the greatest influence on blood glucose levels, the amount and timing of carbohydrate intake directly affect diabetes control. Only carbohydrates are counted with this system, but patients are counseled to eat about the same amount of protein each day and to choose low-fat foods. Reading labels is mandatory; some fat-free products are higher in carbohydrate than the items they replace.

Carbohydrate counting classifies all carbohydrates together, whether from starch, fruit, or milk (Table 40.3). This method offers more flexibility both in food choices within a day's meal plan and in insulin dosage than other systems and may achieve better control of blood glucose.

Despite those advantages, carbohydrate counting may entail the following:
- Weighing and measuring food
- Keeping food records
- Monitoring blood glucose before and after eating
- Controlling body weight.

This system does not permit carbohydrate intake as desired. Patients should maintain their carbohydrate intake at the same level each day to keep blood glucose as close to normal as possible. Carbohydrate counting is frequently inaccurate and associated with higher daily blood glucose

TABLE 40.3 EXAMPLE OF CARBOHYDRATE COUNTING

Meal	Prescribed Carbohydrate Choices (1200 to 1500 kilocalories/day)	Carbohydrate Selected*
Breakfast	3	3/4 cup dry cereal 8 ounces skim milk 1/2 cup unsweetened orange juice
Lunch	3	8 oz regular cola 1 cup melon 1 slice whole-wheat bread
Dinner	3	1/2 cup cooked potato 1/2 cup corn 1/2 cup regular ice cream
Snack	1	8 ounces skim milk

*Additional proteins and fats are added in moderate amounts but need not be counted. Each item selected is approximately 15 grams carbohydrate or 1 carb exchange.

Continued

variability. One study found that in adults with type 1 diabetes, patients' carb counting underestimated 63% of the 448 meals (Brazeau et al, 2013).

Glycemic Index

All carbohydrates are not metabolized identically. Foods containing equal amounts of carbohydrate affect blood glucose levels differently. The glycemic index is a classification of foods according to the speed and degree of change they produce in blood glucose levels. The standard is commonly set with glucose given a value of 100; other foods are then compared with glucose. For example, a sweet potato has a glycemic index of 54, and peanuts have a glycemic index of 14. The values are determined for the tested food only. Effects in a mixed meal may vary. Motivated patients have incorporated the glycemic index into the successful management of their disease.

Reference

Brazeau, A. S., Mircescu, H., Desjardins, K., Leroux, C., Strychar, I., Ekoé, J. M., Rabasa-Lhoret, R. (2013). Carbohydrate counting accuracy and blood glucose variability in adults with type 1 diabetes. *Diabetes Research and Clinical Practice, 99,* 19–23.

Patients who use fat replacers (in foods such as fat-free baked goods or ice cream) should be aware that they still have food value and calories, so they cannot be considered "free" foods. Simple sugars, which may raise blood glucose more than complex carbohydrates (they have a higher glycemic index), are used less but are not prohibited as they were in the past. Sodium intake is limited in individuals with hypertension. In the past, protein was limited in patients with any degree of kidney impairment; this is no longer recommended. Any meal plan should be chosen to fit the patient's lifestyle and food preferences. Patient preferences based on ethnic background should also be considered ("Cultural Considerations").

Many patients now use the carbohydrate counting method, which allows some degree of freedom for the patient who is able to learn to read labels and monitor carbohydrate intake (see Table 40.3). If the patient carefully counts carbohydrates, other foods do not need to be as tightly controlled, as long as general recommendations such as monitoring fat and sodium intake are followed. The success of medical nutrition therapy is evaluated by monitoring glucose levels, HbA_{1c}, lipids, weight, blood pressure, and kidney function.

Exercise

Exercise lowers blood glucose by improving the sensitivity of muscles to insulin, and the effects can last up to 48 hours. Exercise also improves blood lipid levels and circulation, which is important for the person with diabetes who already has an increased risk of cardiovascular disease. Patients are instructed to engage in moderate aerobic exercise at least 150 minute per week, spread over at least 3 days of the week. Resistance exercise also improves insulin sensitivity and is recommended (ADA 2014).

Patients with complications of diabetes must be careful in their exercise choices. For example, a patient with retinopathy should not do anything that causes straining. (See "Long-Term Complications" later in this chapter.) A patient with neuropathy or foot problems should limit weight-bearing exercise. The HCP or an exercise physiologist should be consulted for an individualized exercise plan.

Persons with diabetes who take insulin or medications that increase insulin secretion should check their blood glucose before exercise and always carry a quick source of glucose when exercising in case the blood glucose drops too low. They should also be cautious about exercising at the time of day when their blood glucose is at its lowest point (i.e., when insulin or medication action is peaking) and to have a carbohydrate snack before exercising if blood glucose is less than 100 mg/dL.

Caution patients to avoid exercise if they have ketones in their blood or urine. This indicates that insufficient insulin is available and glycogen may be released during exercise, further increasing the serum glucose.

Medication

INJECTED INSULIN. The person with type 1 diabetes has no endogenous insulin and therefore must inject insulin daily. At this time, insulin cannot be taken by mouth because it is a protein and is therefore digested, although oral and other forms of insulin are being developed. Insulin is typically given subcutaneously; fast-acting insulin may be ordered via the intramuscular or intravenous (IV) route in urgent situations. Several types of insulin are available with various schedules by which they may be given. The type and schedule are determined by the HCP in collaboration with the patient, based on the patient's lifestyle and willingness to spend time

Cultural Considerations

The "standard" diabetic diet may need significant adjustment for patients not of the dominant U.S. culture. Giving such a patient the typical food exchange list may prove unhelpful because it does not include the patient's usual foods. The patient may be considered to be nonadherent to therapy when, in reality, the HCP has been culturally insensitive. Helping the patient choose a meal plan that fits the appropriate cultural preference is important.

Some helpful websites include www.diabetes.org/espanol and www.eatright.org.

on injections. In general, more frequent injections lead to better glucose control.

Site Rotation. Insulin injections should be given in a different subcutaneous site with each dose to avoid tissue injury. A sample rotation chart is shown in Fig. 40.4. Because each area absorbs insulin at a slightly different rate, it is advisable to use one area for a week, then move on to the next area. Within that area, each injection should be spaced at least 1 inch from the previous injection. Some experts recommend using primarily the torso (abdomen and buttocks) to provide more uniform absorption. Aspirating for blood before injection and rubbing the site after injection are not recommended with insulin injections.

Insulin Pumps. Patients who desire tighter control of blood glucose levels and a more flexible lifestyle may choose to use an insulin pump (Fig. 40.5). A pump delivers subcutaneous insulin via a tiny catheter continuously in small (basal) amounts. The catheter is placed in subcutaneous tissue and remains in place for 2 to 3 days. The patient can then add a bolus of insulin with the push of a button before meals or snacks. This provides insulin

Rotation sites for injection of insulin.

FIGURE 40.4 Sample insulin rotation chart.

FIGURE 40.5 Patient wearing insulin pump.

levels that are more normal, like those of a person without diabetes. A pump typically is worn on the abdomen or buttocks. Some models receive input from continuous glucose monitors.

Insulin Sources. Insulin is synthetically produced in a laboratory and is either identical to human insulin, or one or two amino acids different (called insulin analogs). In the past, insulin was derived from cows and pigs; this is no longer available in the United States but may be available from other countries. Be careful to check the source when preparing insulin for injection (especially if you work in home care, where patients could purchase their insulin online from another country) because insulins from different sources may act slightly differently. Some people may be allergic to beef or pork preparations or may refuse them based on cultural practices.

Onset, Peak, and Duration. Once insulin is injected, a period elapses before it begins to lower blood glucose. This time is called the *onset of action.* The *peak action* occurs when the insulin is working at its hardest and the blood glucose is at its lowest point. It is during this peak time that the patient is most at risk for an episode of low blood glucose. *Duration of action* is the length of time the insulin works before it is used up. Onset, peak, and duration are determined by whether the insulin is short, intermediate, or long acting (Table 40.4). It is important for the individual with diabetes and the nurse to be aware of the onset, peak, and duration of any insulin given. This assists in making decisions such as when to give insulin in relation to meals, when to exercise, and when to be alert to low blood glucose symptoms.

Insulin Regimens. In the past, most patients with diabetes used an injection of intermediate-acting insulin before breakfast and possibly a second injection before supper. Many patients are now choosing to take more frequent injections of short-acting insulin before meals or a combination of short- and long-acting insulins to achieve better, "tighter" control. These patients are often taught to adjust their insulin dose based on blood glucose level and the amount of carbohydrates eaten. Although patients who choose tight control have to be more cautious about risk for hypoglycemia, it can significantly reduce the risk of long-term complications.

One regimen that is becoming more common because it mimics normal insulin secretion is sometimes called *basal-bolus insulin.* This consists of an injection of a basal insulin (such as Lantus) once a day, often at bedtime, to provide a constant small amount of insulin in the bloodstream. Then an injection of very short-acting insulin (such as Humalog) is given before meals to mimic the extra insulin that is secreted normally with meals.

Sliding-Scale Insulin. Some patients receive varying doses of short-acting insulin before meals based on their blood glucose reading. An example of a sliding scale might read as follows: "BG <140, 0 units; BG 141–170, 2 units; BG 171–200, 4 units; >200 call HCP." This is useful when the patient is ill and glucose levels are unstable, or when adjustments need to be made. However, routine use of sliding scale insulin is not recommended because although it corrects an already-high blood glucose, it is preferable to prevent hyperglycemia before it happens with routine insulin doses.

TABLE 40.4 ONSET, PEAK, AND DURATION OF INSULINS

Insulin Type	Example	Sample Brand Names	Onset	Peak	Duration
Very short acting	Insulin lispro	Humalog	5–15 min	30–90 min	5 hr or less
	Insulin aspart	NovoLog	10–20 min	1–3 hr	3–5 hr
	Insulin glulisine	Apidra	15–20 min	30–90 min	6 hr
Short acting	Regular	Humulin R, Novolin R	30 min	2–5 hr	5–8 hr
Intermediate acting	NPH	Humulin N, Novolin N	1–2 hr	6–12 hr	18–26 hr
Basal	Insulin glargine	Lantus AE	1–2 hr	No peak	Up to 24 hr
	Insulin detemir	Levemir	1 hr	No peak	Up to 24 hr

Note. A variety of premixed formulas are also available.

Mixing Insulins. When two insulins need to be given at the same time, they can often be mixed together to prevent having to give more than one injection. (See DavisPlus for procedure.) Preset mixtures of intermediate- and short-acting insulins are also available.

PROBLEMS REQUIRING INSULIN ADJUSTMENT. Two problems that can occur with glucose control are the *Somogyi effect* and the *dawn phenomenon.* The Somogyi effect may be at fault when the patient's blood glucose seems to be rising despite increasing insulin doses. If insulin levels are too high, the blood glucose may drop too low, stimulating release of counterregulatory hormones (epinephrine, glucagon, corticosteroids, growth hormone), which then elevate the blood glucose. The low glucose levels often occur during the night, and the patient may report night sweats or morning headaches. The high morning glucose is then interpreted as hyperglycemia, and the insulin dose may be further increased, compounding the problem.

The dawn phenomenon is thought to occur because of the natural release of growth hormone and cortisol during the early morning hours. This causes hyperglycemia on arising in the morning.

The patient might be asked to monitor blood glucose between 0200 and 0400 in addition to bedtime and morning testing to assess whether the Somogyi effect or the dawn phenomenon is occurring. Correction of the Somogyi effect involves reducing the insulin dose. The dawn phenomenon is treated with careful adjustment of meals and insulin so that insulin is peaking when the blood glucose is highest.

CRITICAL THINKING

Mrs. Evans

■ Mrs. Evans is a 78-year-old woman with type 2 diabetes who resides in the long-term care facility at which you

work. She is on 42 units of Lantus insulin every evening and 10 units of Humalog insulin before each meal.

1. What time should you administer her Lantus insulin? If she eats her meals at 0800, 1200, and 1700, when should her Humalog insulin be administered?
2. At what time of day should she be alert for symptoms of low blood glucose?
3. What could happen if Mrs. Evans feels ill and misses her lunch?
4. Mrs. Evans receives an apple with her meal but cannot eat it because her dentures do not fit well. She is on an ADA Exchange List diet. What should you do?

Suggested answers are at the end of the chapter.

ORAL HYPOGLYCEMIC MEDICATION. The patient with type 2 diabetes may be able to control blood glucose levels with medical nutrition therapy and exercise alone. If needed, oral hypoglycemic medication or insulin will also be prescribed. Oral hypoglycemic agents are not insulin pills but work in ways such as stimulating the pancreas to produce more insulin or making the tissues more sensitive to insulin. Because most oral hypoglycemic agents depend on at least a partially functioning pancreas, most are not useful for patients with type 1 diabetes. See Table 40.5 for a list of commonly used oral hypoglycemic agents and their mechanisms of action.

Most oral hypoglycemic agents should be administered before meals. Care should be taken to prevent passage of more than 30 minutes between medication administration and the meal because this may result in a hypoglycemic episode. Some must be taken with, rather than before, meals. Check individual drugs for specific timing.

If the blood glucose level is not controlled with an oral hypoglycemic agent, insulin may be needed for the person with type 2 diabetes. This does not mean the person has type 1 diabetes. Insulin may be needed to control blood glucose but unlike in the person with type 1 diabetes, insulin is not needed to sustain life.

TABLE 40.5 ORAL HYPOGLYCEMIC AGENTS

Medication Class/Action	Examples	Nursing Implications
Alpha-glucosidase inhibitors (AGIs) Lower postprandial glucose by reducing rate of carbohydrate digestion and absorption.	acarbose (Precose) miglitol (Glyset)	Give at start of each meal. No weight gain or hypoglycemia risk. Multiple dosing is less convenient. If used in combination with another drug and hypoglycemia occurs, treat with milk or glucose tablets, not table sugar.
DPP-4 inhibitor Inhibits DPP-4, an enzyme that breaks incretins. Incretins are hormones secreted by the GI system in response to food; they reduce glucagon secretion and increase insulin synthesis and release.	sitagliptin (Januvia) saxagliptin (Onglyza) linagliptin (Tradjenta)	Administer once a day. Only works when blood glucose is high so does not cause hypoglycemia when used alone. Watch for allergic reactions.
Biguanide Decreases glucose production by liver; increases glucose uptake by muscle.	metformin (Glucophage, Glucophage XR, Fortamet, Riomet, Glumetza)	Give with meals. May enhance weight loss. Withhold if patient is having tests involving contrast dye. Contraindicated in renal and hepatic disease and heart failure. Monitor serum creatinine level. Notify physician of early symptoms of lactic acidosis: hyperventilation, myalgia, malaise.
Thiazolidinediones (glitazones) Reduce insulin resistance in muscles. Improve blood lipids; may lower blood pressure and improve cardiovascular risk.	pioglitazone (Actos) rosiglitazone (Avandia)	Give with meal. Work well with obese patients. Avoid with liver disease; monitor liver enzymes. Monitor for heart failure. May alter effectiveness of some birth control pills.
Sulfonylureas Stimulate insulin secretion by pancreas, increase insulin receptor sensitivity.	glipizide (Glucotrol) glimepiride (Amaryl) glyburide (Micronase, Diabeta, Glynase Prestab)	Monitor patient for hypoglycemia. Teach patient to avoid alcohol.
Reduces reabsorption of glucose by kidneys, increasing glucose excretion in urine.	canagliflozin (Invokana) metformin and glyburide (Glucovance) metformin and rosiglitazone (Avandamet) glipizide and metformin (Metaglip)	Monitor for hypotension, hyperkalemia, and urinary tract infection. Monitor renal function. See individual agents.

INCRETIN MIMETIC AGENTS. A newer group of medications are the incretin mimetics. These are injectable drugs that were first isolated in the saliva of the Gila monster, a poisonous lizard native to the United States and Mexico. An incretin mimetic mimics natural incretins in the body. Incretins are hormones secreted by the gastrointestinal (GI) tract that (1) stimulate insulin release and (2) reduce glucagon release in response to nutrients in the intestine. Examples of incretin mimetics include exenatide (Byetta or Bydureon) and liraglutide (Victoza). These drugs can work in conjunction with oral hypoglycemic agents and stimulate insulin secretion, lower production of glucagon, slow gastric emptying, and promote weight loss.

Another injectable drug, pramlintide (Symlin), is used with insulin. It is a synthetic analog of amylin, a naturally occurring hormone that reduces glucose levels following meals. It may also promote weight loss in individuals who are overweight. Patients using Symlin have an increased risk of hypoglycemia.

NATURAL REMEDIES. Many herbs and other natural remedies have been promoted for diabetes treatment. If your patient wishes to try a natural remedy, it is essential to encourage a conversation with his or her HCP first. See the evidence about cinnamon in the "Evidence-Based Practice" feature.

Self-Monitoring of Blood Glucose

The ability to test blood glucose levels at home has been a major advance in diabetes care. Blood glucose can be better controlled because of the availability of monitoring at any time, in any place. A variety of blood glucose monitors are on the market at reasonable prices; one example is shown in Fig. 40.6. Most of the cost involved in monitoring is in the test strips that must be used. Health insurance programs may cover this cost.

Self-monitoring of blood glucose is usually done before meals and at bedtime by the person on insulin who wants to maintain tight control of blood glucose. Patients using multiple insulin injections should check capillary plasma glucose before meals and snacks, occasionally postprandially, at bedtime, before exercise, when experiencing low blood glucose, and before critical activities such as driving (ADA, 2014). Less frequent schedules may be prescribed for patients who are unable or unwilling to test four times a day or for patients not on insulin.

New devices are available that continuously monitor glucose via a small catheter inserted into the abdomen. The device records the glucose level every 5 minutes on a monitor that is worn like a pager on a belt. It can be set to alarm if the blood glucose level drops too low.

The diabetes provider should be consulted for desirable blood glucose ranges because these may differ for each patient. The ADA recommends a preprandial goal of 70 to 130 mg/dL for most patients. Patients who are prone to hypoglycemia or small children or older adults may have higher goal ranges, such as 100 to 150 mg/dL. Lower blood glucose levels for these populations could increase the risk of hypoglycemia.

An important aspect of blood glucose monitoring is the interpretation of results. Monitoring is useless if the results are not used to improve blood glucose control. The patient should be instructed to keep a diary of blood glucose levels (Fig. 40.7). Some patients have computer software that graphs results. The patient may be taught by a diabetes educator to interpret the trends in the results, or the diary may be taken on a regular basis to the HCP for interpretation and adjustment of the treatment plan.

EVIDENCE-BASED PRACTICE

Clinical Question
Does cinnamon lower blood glucose in patients with diabetes?

Evidence
Ten research studies were reviewed, involving 577 subjects with diabetes. There was no evidence that cinnamon was better than placebo in lowering blood glucose or HbA_{1c}.

Implications for Nursing Practice
Many patients look for natural remedies to replace or supplement prescribed therapies. It is important for nurses to encourage patients to find evidence to support their decisions, and to talk with their HCP before trying new treatments. They should never stop current treatment without consulting their HCP.

REFERENCE

Leach, M. J., Kumar, S. Cinnamon for diabetes mellitus. *Cochrane Database of Systematic Reviews* 2013, Issue 12. Art. No.: CD007170. DOI: 10.1002/14651858.CD007170.pub2

FIGURE 40.6 OneTouch Ultra glucose monitor. *Courtesy of LifeScan.*

Day		Break-fast	Lunch	Supper	Bedtime	Urine Ketones	Notes
Sunday	Time	7:00	11:30	6:00	11:00		
	Glucose	186	108	116	142		
	Insulin	10 units Humalog	10 units Humalog	10 units Humalog	32 units Lantus		
Monday	Time	7:30	12:00	6:00	10:30	6:00-neg	Ate cake at
	Glucose	171	97	302	180		Betty's party
	Insulin	10 units Humalog	10 units Humalog	10 units Humalog	32 units Lantus		at 3 pm-oops!
Tuesday	Time						
	Glucose						
	Insulin						
Wednesday	Time						
	Glucose						
	Insulin						
Thursday	Time						
	Glucose						
	Insulin						
Friday	Time						
	Glucose						
	Insulin						
Saturday	Time						
	Glucose						
	Insulin						

FIGURE 40.7 Sample diary of blood glucose results and insulin use.

Urine Glucose and Ketone Monitoring

Urine also may be tested for glucose and for ketones. Urine glucose testing was done routinely before the development of self-monitoring of blood glucose. A variety of dipsticks and tape products are available for urine testing. Glucose in the urine makes the patient aware that the blood glucose is elevated, but the actual level is unknown. Most people have glucose in their urine when their blood glucose is more than about 180 mg/dL, although this can be highly variable in patients with diabetes. It is difficult to base treatment on urine glucose levels, and so routine urine testing for glucose is no longer recommended.

Urine should be tested for ketones during acute illness or stress, when blood glucose levels are elevated in ketosis-prone patients, or when symptoms of ketoacidosis are present (see later in this chapter). If ketones are present, the patient knows an insulin deficiency is present and should notify the physician. Patients with type 1 diabetes are most at risk for developing ketoacidosis; however, it is wise for the patient with type 2 diabetes to test for ketones if risk factors are present. See Table 40.6 for a review of diabetes symptoms, diagnosis, and treatment.

Weight Loss

Weight loss can help the patient with type 2 diabetes control blood glucose, blood pressure, and blood lipid levels. Weight loss can even help prevent the need for medication in some patients. In obese patients who have difficulty losing weight with usual measures, bariatric surgery may be considered. There are several bariatric surgeries that may be effective; see Chapter 33 for more information.

TABLE 40.6 DIABETES SUMMARY

Signs and Symptoms	Polyuria Polydipsia Polyphagia Fatigue Blurred vision Headache Abdominal pain
Diagnostic Tests	Fasting plasma glucose HbA$_{1c}$ (glycosylated hemoglobin) Oral glucose tolerance test Additional testing for complications
Therapeutic Measures	Nutrition therapy Exercise Insulin Oral hypoglycemic medication Self-monitoring of blood glucose levels Education
Complications	Hypoglycemia, hyperglycemia Diabetic ketoacidosis, hyperosmolar hyperglycemia Long-term complications
Priority Nursing Diagnosis	*Risk for Unstable Blood Glucose Level*

Transplant

If the patient is evaluated to be an appropriate candidate, a pancreas transplant may be considered. This is especially beneficial in the patient with kidney disease, who can receive both a kidney and pancreas transplant at the same time. Another promising treatment is the implantation of pancreatic islet cells.

Acute Complications of Diabetes

A person with diabetes is at risk for a variety of complications. Acute complications related to high and low blood glucose levels are treatable and can be prevented with appropriate care.

Hyperglycemia

When calories eaten exceed insulin available or glucose used, high blood glucose (hyperglycemia) occurs. A common cause of hyperglycemia is eating more than the meal plan prescribes. Another major cause is stress. Stress causes the release of counterregulatory hormones, including epinephrine, cortisol, growth hormone, and glucagon. These hormones all increase the blood glucose level. In a person without diabetes, this is an adaptive function. However, the patient with diabetes is unable to compensate for the increased blood glucose with increased insulin secretion, and hyperglycemia results.

Patients must be able to recognize signs and symptoms of high blood glucose levels and know what to do if they occur (Table 40.7). For many patients, these are similar to the symptoms they experienced when they were first diagnosed with diabetes. Chronic high blood glucose levels can lead to long-term complications (discussed later in this chapter).

Hypoglycemia

Low blood glucose, or hypoglycemia, occurs when there is not enough glucose available in relation to circulating insulin. This is sometimes referred to as an *insulin reaction*. Hypoglycemia is usually defined as a blood glucose level below 70 mg/dL, although patients may feel symptoms at higher or lower levels. Occasionally, symptoms occur as a result of a rapid drop in blood glucose, even though the actual glucose level is normal or high. Causes of hypoglycemia may include skipping a meal, exercising more than usual, or accidentally administering too much insulin. An occasional hypoglycemic episode, treated promptly, should not lead to chronic complications. Repeated or extremely low blood glucose levels can cause neurologic damage because there is not enough glucose for brain function. It is therefore important to teach patients and families how to prevent and treat low blood glucose (see Table 40.7).

Symptoms of hypoglycemia include hunger, sweating, pallor, tremor, palpitations, and headache. These symptoms are caused by activation of the sympathetic nervous system. As hypoglycemia progresses, the brain is deprived of glucose (called neuroglycopenia) and neurologic symptoms such as irritability, confusion, seizures, and coma may occur.

TABLE 40.7   COMPARISON OF HIGH AND LOW BLOOD GLUCOSE LEVELS

	Hyperglycemia	Hypoglycemia
Causes	Overeating Stress Illness Too little insulin or medication	Undereating, skipping a meal Too much insulin or medication Exercise
Symptoms	Polyuria Polydipsia Polyphagia Blurred vision Headache Lethargy Abdominal pain Ketonuria Coma	Hunger Sweating Tremor Blurred vision Headache Irritability Confusion Seizures Coma
Treatment	Confirm hyperglycemia with glucose meter; if patient is at risk, check urine for ketones and increase fluid intake. Assess cause of hyperglycemia, and teach prevention. Return to prescribed treatment plan if applicable. Call physician for medication adjustment if indicated or if blood glucose exceeds 180 mg/dL for 2 days. Call physician if patient is ill or vomiting.	Confirm hypoglycemia with glucose meter (if able). Administer 15 g fast-acting carbohydrate. Recheck glucose in 15 minutes. If still low, re-administer carbohydrate. Continue cycle of checking glucose and administering fast sugar until hypoglycemia subsides. If symptoms worsen, call physician or emergency help. Administer glucagon subcutaneously or dextrose 50% IV if ordered. Assess cause of hypoglycemia, and teach prevention.

BE SAFE!

BE VIGILANT! You can prevent hypoglycemia in your patients by being aware of who is at risk, when they are most at risk, and monitoring for early symptoms. If you recognize early symptoms, such as shaking or hunger, and respond quickly, you can prevent a much more serious complication for your patient.

Box 40-2 **Fast Sugars**

- 4 oz orange juice
- 4 oz regular (not diet) soda
- 8 oz low-fat milk
- Miniature box of raisins
- Commercial glucose tablets or gel
- 6–8 Life Savers® (or other hard candies)

CRITICAL THINKING

Jeff

■ Jeff is a 16-year-old who is having trouble with repeated episodes of hypoglycemia. He says he has not had this trouble before, and it is interfering with his new job. What questions might you ask as you do your assessment to help him figure out how to prevent future episodes?

Suggested answers are at the end of the chapter.

To treat low blood glucose, administer a "fast sugar"—15 to 20 grams of carbohydrate that will enter the bloodstream quickly (Box 40-2). If the patient is not alert or is unable to safely swallow, subcutaneous glucagon can be given. If the patient is hospitalized, IV 50% dextrose can be administered by the registered nurse (RN). Recheck the blood glucose in 15 minutes. If it does not return to at least 70 mg/dL, repeat the procedure every 15 minutes until 70 mg/dL is reached—even if the patient is feeling better. Do not overtreat hypoglycemia with too much sugar because this may cause hyperglycemia and rebound hypoglycemia.

If you find someone with symptoms of altered blood glucose but are unable to identify whether it is high or low, do a blood glucose test. However, if the patient has neurologic symptoms, treat for low blood glucose immediately. The blood glucose may then be checked and further treatment provided as indicated.

NURSING CARE TIP

Avoid the temptation to add sugar to orange juice to treat hypoglycemia. Also be sure to avoid giving a form of sugar that has fat in it—this will slow down its digestion and delay recovery of the blood glucose level.

Once the hypoglycemic episode is resolved, the patient should eat a complex carbohydrate to prevent recurrence, unless the next meal is within a half hour. If symptoms worsen instead of improve, call 911, or contact the RN or HCP. Check hospital or agency policy for the specific protocol for treating hypoglycemic episodes.

Some older adult patients with poor autonomic nervous system function or patients taking beta-adrenergic blocking medication such as propranolol or atenolol (which block the sympathetic response) may not feel the symptoms of hypoglycemia. These patients should check glucose levels more often and keep the levels in a safe range to prevent hypoglycemic episodes.

All people with diabetes should be instructed to keep a fast sugar in their purse or pocket at all times. Fast sugars may also be stored in bedside tables, cars, and desks at work.

Diabetic Ketoacidosis

PATHOPHYSIOLOGY. Diabetic ketoacidosis (DKA) occurs when blood glucose levels become very high and insulin is deficient. This most commonly occurs in people with type 1 diabetes, but it may occur in type 2 diabetes when insulin deficiency exists, usually late in the disease process. DKA symptoms are often the reason a person with undiagnosed type 1 diabetes first seeks help. It may also be the result of stress or illness in a person with previously diagnosed type 1 (or rarely, type 2) diabetes. When there is insufficient insulin to allow glucose into cells, the cells starve. The body then breaks down fat to be used for energy. The fat breakdown releases an acid substance called ketones. As ketones build up in the blood, ketoacidosis occurs.

The body attempts to compensate for acidosis by deepening respirations to blow off excess carbon dioxide. Because carbon dioxide combines with water in the body to form carbonic acid, blowing off carbon dioxide is like blowing off acid. (See the section on metabolic acidosis in Chapter 6.) The deep, sighing respiratory pattern is called **Kussmaul's respirations**. The expired air has a fruity odor caused by the ketones and may be mistaken for alcohol. Some nurses have likened the odor to Juicy Fruit® chewing gum.

With such high blood glucose and the accompanying polyuria, the body becomes dehydrated very quickly. Tachycardia, hypotension, and shock can result. Acidosis also causes potassium to leave the cells and accumulate in the blood (hyperkalemia). Potassium is then lost in large amounts in the urine, which can lead to hypokalemia. The combination of dehydration, potassium imbalance, and acidosis causes the patient to develop flulike symptoms, including abdominal pain and vomiting. The patient loses consciousness and death occurs if DKA is not treated. The mortality rate for DKA is about 2%.

THERAPEUTIC MEASURES. Treatment includes IV fluids, IV insulin, and blood glucose monitoring, often initially in an intensive care unit setting. Glucose is added to the IV when the blood glucose drops to about 180 mg/dL to avoid hypoglycemia. Potassium should also be monitored closely because it is essential to have normal levels for cardiac function. Arterial blood gases help monitor acidosis. The cause of the DKA should be identified and treated.

Prevention of ketoacidosis involves careful monitoring of blood glucose levels at home. Teach at-risk patients to use a urine dipstick to check for ketones (Ketostix) if blood glucose is elevated. If ketones are present, the patient should drink water and recheck with the next urination. If ketones are still present, the physician should be notified. Instruct patients never to stop their insulin without a physician's supervision.

Hyperosmolar Hyperglycemic State

PATHOPHYSIOLOGY. Hyperosmolar hyperglycemic state (HHS, also called hyperosmolar hyperglycemic nonketotic syndrome, or HHNK) occurs mainly in type 2 diabetes, when blood glucose levels are high and the patient has reduced fluid intake as a result of stress or illness. Because the person with type 2 diabetes has some insulin production, cells do not starve, and DKA usually does not occur. HHS occurs more often in older adults.

As blood glucose level rises (hyperglycemia), polyuria causes profound dehydration, producing the hyperosmolar (concentrated) state. Blood glucose may rise as high as 1500 mg/dL, and electrolyte imbalances occur. Because ketoacidosis is not present, the patient may not feel as physically ill as the patient with DKA and may delay seeking treatment. Symptoms of HHS develop slowly and include extreme thirst, lethargy, and mental confusion. Shock, coma, and death occur if it is left untreated. The mortality rate for HHS is between 10% and 20%.

THERAPEUTIC MEASURES. Treatment includes IV fluids and insulin, and glucose monitoring. Electrolytes are closely monitored. The cause of HHS should be identified and treated. HHS can be prevented with careful monitoring of glucose levels at home. Instruct patients to drink plenty of fluids if blood glucose levels are beginning to rise, especially in times of stress and illness. They should also know when to call their physician with high blood glucose results.

NURSING CARE TIP

Government insurers (Medicare and Medicaid) consider DKA, HHS, and hypoglycemic coma to be preventable problems and will no longer pay hospitals for the extra expense of caring for patients who develop these conditions after they are in the hospital. You can help control costs by being vigilant for early signs and symptoms of these complications and reporting them promptly. The website that lists additional hospital-acquired conditions is www.cms.gov/HospitalAcqCond.

Long-Term Complications

Over time, chronic hyperglycemia causes a variety of serious complications in persons with diabetes. These involve the circulatory system, eyes, kidneys, skin, and nerves. Most of the complications involve either the large blood vessels in the body (macrovascular complications) or the tiny blood vessels, such as those in the eyes or kidneys (microvascular complications). The Diabetes Control and Complications Trial (DCCT), a large classic research study completed in 1993, showed that individuals with type 1 diabetes who maintain tight control of blood glucose experience fewer long-term microvascular complications than individuals who take traditional care of their diabetes (Diabetes Control and Complications Trial Research Group, 1993). Similarly, the United Kingdom Prospective Diabetes Study (UKPDS), completed in 1998, showed that individuals with type 2 diabetes who maintain an HbA_{1c} below 7% can significantly reduce complications. In fact, for every percentage of decrease in HbA_{1c}, there were 25% fewer deaths from diabetes-related complications (UK Prospective Diabetes Study Group, 1998). Unfortunately, tight control can be accompanied by an increased risk of hypoglycemia, and even tight control does not guarantee the prevention of all long-term complications.

Macrovascular Complications

CIRCULATORY SYSTEM. People with diabetes develop atherosclerosis and arteriosclerosis faster than the general population. They are more likely to have hypertension and elevated low-density lipoprotein cholesterol and triglyceride levels. High blood glucose can also affect platelet function, leading to increased clotting. These problems lead to a higher incidence of strokes, heart attacks, and poor circulation in the feet and legs. The risk of cardiovascular disease and strokes is two to four times more common in persons with diabetes than in the general population.

Control of blood glucose, blood pressure, and cholesterol levels is vital to help prevent these deadly complications. Patients should also avoid smoking, maintain normal weight, and exercise regularly. All patients should be evaluated by their HCP for treatment with aspirin or other antiplatelet medication, angiotensin-converting enzyme (ACE) inhibitor therapy, and statin therapy for control of blood lipids.

Microvascular Complications

EYES. Small blood vessels can become diseased, eventually leading to retinopathy in most patients with diabetes. **Retinopathy** involves damage to the tiny blood vessels that supply the eye. Small hemorrhages occur, which can cause blindness if not corrected. Diabetes is a leading cause of blindness in adults in the United States (CDC, 2014). Good control of blood glucose and blood pressure can reduce the risk of retinopathy. Newer laser surgery techniques may help improve vision after hemorrhages occur. Diabetes is also associated with a high incidence of cataracts. Patients with diabetes should have a yearly dilated eye examination.

• **WORD** • **BUILDING** •
retinopathy: retino—nervous tissue of the eye + pathy—illness

KIDNEYS. **Nephropathy** is caused by damage to the tiny blood vessels in the kidneys. Up to 40% of patients with diabetes develop some degree of nephropathy. Native Americans, Hispanics, and African Americans have the highest risk. A primary risk factor for diabetic nephropathy is poor control of blood glucose. If nephropathy occurs, the kidneys are unable to remove waste products and excess fluid from the blood. Diabetes is the leading cause of end-stage renal (kidney) disease (ESRD) in the United States. When the kidneys have lost most of their function, patients may have their blood cleansed artificially by either hemodialysis or peritoneal dialysis (see Chapter 37). The only cure for ESRD is a kidney transplant.

Patients should be taught the importance of blood glucose control to prevent or delay kidney disease. ACE inhibitor and angiotensin receptor blocker (ARB) medications have been shown to slow the development of kidney problems in patients with diabetes. Patients who have both diabetes and hypertension should be placed on an ACE inhibitor or ARB. Routine urine tests are done to check for albumin in the urine. A trained renal dietitian should work with the patient and physician to determine the best diet for the patient.

Nerve Complications

Another complication of diabetes is **neuropathy**, which is damage to nerves as a result of chronic hyperglycemia. Neuropathy can cause numbness and pain in the extremities, erectile dysfunction (impotence) in men, sexual dysfunction in women, **gastroparesis** (delayed stomach emptying), and other problems. Unfortunately, pain caused by neuropathy is difficult to treat with traditional analgesics. Some antidepressant and anticonvulsant drugs may be helpful, and in some cases, local injections of anesthetics may be used. Anticonvulsant agents gabapentin (Neurontin) and pregabalin (Lyrica) reduce painful nerve impulses in individuals with nerve pain. Improved control of blood glucose levels may also help.

Infection

Persons with diabetes are prone to infection for several reasons. If injuries occur, healing may be slow because of impaired circulation. There may not be enough blood supply to heal the wound or fight an infection. For the same reason, it may be difficult for IV antibiotics to reach an infected site, and topical antibiotics may be preferable. In the presence of hyperglycemia, white blood cells (WBCs) become sluggish and ineffective, further reducing the body's ability to fight infection.

The incidence of periodontal (gum) disease, caused by bacteria in plaque, is also increased in individuals with diabetes. Patients must be taught to maintain good oral hygiene and make regular visits to the dentist.

Foot Complications

The combination of macrovascular disease, neuropathy, and risk for infection makes patients with diabetes prone to foot problems. Consider the patient who has no feeling in his or her feet because of neuropathy. If the patient has a foot injury, it may not be felt right away. Vascular disease will prevent a good

blood supply from preventing infection and promoting healing. If infection sets in, it is slow to resolve and may progress to necrosis and gangrene. Pressure points on the feet may also break down (Fig. 40.8). One woman had a Bic pen in her shoe all day and did not realize it! Neuropathy can also lead to deformities of the feet, further increasing the risk of injuries.

NURSING CARE TIP

When you *do* your routine patient assessments, ALWAYS look carefully at your patients' feet. Remove shoes and socks, examine all skin surfaces, and look between toes. Report any redness, lesions, or other suspicious areas. You could make the difference between a small, treatable wound and an amputation!

For these reasons, diabetes is the leading cause of nontraumatic amputation of the lower extremities in the United States. Teach patients to protect their feet at all times by wearing well-fitting shoes and by washing, drying, and inspecting their feet daily (Box 40-3). If any sores are noted, the patient should not delay in seeking treatment. During routine visits to the physician, teach the patient to be sure to remove shoes and socks so the feet can be thoroughly examined. The physician or diabetes specialist can test sensation in the feet with tiny filaments. Loss of protective sensation is an early risk factor for amputation, so any reduction in sensation is a warning sign that extra care must

• WORD • BUILDING •
neuropathy: neuro—nervous system + pathy—illness
nephropathy: nephro—of the kidney + pathy—illness
gastroparesis: gastro—stomach + paresis—partial paralysis

FIGURE 40.8 Diabetic foot ulcer at site of amputated toe. From Goldsmith, L. A., Lazarus, G. S., & Tharp, M. D. (1997). *Adult and pediatric dermatology*. Philadelphia: F.A. Davis, p. 438, with permission.

Box 40-3 Foot Care Tips

- Wash and dry feet every day. Use warm (not hot) water to avoid burns.
- Apply lotion that does not contain alcohol, avoiding areas between toes.
- Inspect feet for sores or red areas daily (have a family member help if necessary).
- Report any abnormalities immediately.
- Wear leather shoes and white or light-colored cotton socks.
- Never go barefoot.
- Avoid garters and tight socks.
- Avoid crossing legs.
- Cut toenails to natural shape of nail—not into corners.
- See a podiatrist for calluses or problem toenails (avoid "bathroom surgery").
- Have feet checked at least once a year, preferably three to four times a year, for loss of sensation.

be taken. A podiatrist (foot doctor) can be consulted if problems occur. Specialized wound treatment centers have new healing techniques that have prevented many amputations. (See DavisPlus for "Ethical Considerations.")

 NURSING CARE TIP

Encourage patients to wear white or light-colored socks. One woman did not know she had a wound on her foot till she saw blood coming through her white cotton socks.

CRITICAL THINKING

Mr. Jones

■ Mr. Jones is a 54-year-old banker with type 2 diabetes admitted to your unit with a tiny red area on his right heel. His admitting blood glucose is 360 mg/dL. The lesion is so small you wonder what the fuss is about. While doing his assessment, you find that he wore a new pair of shoes to work all day about a month ago and has been avoiding seeing his physician about the resulting red area. He is placed on IV antibiotics, and within 3 days, the red area has broken open and has yellow drainage. He is sent home with topical antibiotics and crutches, to be followed by a visiting nurse. The wound takes 6 months to fully heal.

1. List three risk factors for foot problems.
2. Why did the sore take so long to heal?

3. Why do you think crutches are necessary?
4. Why might topical antibiotics work better than IV antibiotics?
5. The nurse documents the following description of Mr. Jones's wound: "Small red open area on heel, with yellow drainage on dressing." What is wrong with this charting? How can you improve it?
6. What team members should be involved with Mr. Jones's care?

Suggested answers are at the end of the chapter.

Special Considerations for the Patient Undergoing Surgery

Surgery is a stressor. The counterregulatory hormones released during stress cause the blood glucose to rise, even if the patient has been fasting. High blood glucose levels interfere with immune function and healing and can increase the patient's risk for infection. Some research studies have shown that tight blood glucose control during hospitalization and surgery can significantly reduce complications. Other studies have shown that tight control increases the risk of hypoglycemia and death. In 2009, the ADA and American Association of Clinical Endocrinologists determined that glucose levels in critically ill hospitalized patients should be maintained between 140 and 180 mg/dL, preferably with the use of IV insulin (Moghissi et al, 2009). See the "Nursing Care Plan for the Patient With Diabetes Mellitus" for goals for patients who are not critically ill.

Check with the physician for actual insulin orders. Often patients are placed on IV infusions of glucose and insulin during and immediately after surgery, in place of longer-acting insulins. Monitor blood glucose levels every 2 to 4 hours or as ordered, and monitor carefully for signs and symptoms of hypoglycemia or hyperglycemia. If a patient uses a pump at home, check with a diabetes resource nurse to determine if the patient can continue to use it during hospitalization.

Patients who were not previously on insulin may be placed on insulin during surgery and postoperatively. They can generally return to their presurgical treatment plan after the stress of surgery is past.

Nursing Process for the Patient With Diabetes Mellitus

Data Collection

A complete nursing history and physical examination should be carried out because diabetes affects every body system. Some areas on which to focus are shown in Table 40.8. It is especially important to assess each patient's knowledge of diabetes and its care so that appropriate teaching can be done.

Nursing Diagnoses, Planning, and Implementation

Because diabetes affects so many different areas, nearly any nursing diagnosis may be appropriate. See the "Nursing Care Plan for the Patient With Diabetes Mellitus" for an example of the diagnosis *Risk for Unstable Blood Glucose Level*. The

TABLE 40.8 DATA COLLECTION FOR THE PATIENT WITH DIABETES MELLITUS

Subjective Data	• Age and symptoms at onset • Understanding of diabetes (type 1 or type 2) and self-care • Current treatment plan (medication, nutrition therapy, exercise) and adherence to plan • Frequency of blood glucose self-monitoring, and pattern of blood glucose levels (check diary if patient has kept one) • History of diabetes-related complications • Involvement of family or other support systems
Objective Data	• Vital signs • Height, weight, body mass index • Skin: integrity, turgor, condition of injection sites • Feet: pulses, color, temperature, skin integrity, pressure points, sensation • Laboratory results: blood glucose, HbA$_{1c}$, creatinine, lipid profile, albuminuria, urine and serum ketones

actual presence of the defining characteristics should be confirmed with the patient before choosing any nursing diagnosis.

Once diagnoses have been identified, planning should be done with both the patient and family. Diabetes affects not only the person with the disease, but the entire family. The desired outcomes for the plan of care are for the patient to be knowledgeable about and able to care for his or her disease and to prevent complications. Consult the dietitian, social worker, certified diabetes educator, home care nurse, outpatient education programs, and other resources as needed ("Home Health Hints").

Home Health Hints

• Patients with newly diagnosed diabetes may be anxious and overwhelmed. Instruction may need to be repeated several times before they understand.
• Some home glucose monitoring devices have a memory that the nurse can access during the visit. It gives the date, time, and blood glucose result. This is a good indication of adherence with self-monitoring performed by patient or caregiver.
• Assist your patients in obtaining the necessary supplies to manage their diabetes. Many medical supply companies can deliver these supplies to the home. Work with your agency to identify reliable companies in your area.
• Remember to call the patient the day before performing a venipuncture for a fasting blood glucose and remind him or her not to eat after midnight.
• Older patients tend to skip meals. Assist them to identify easy but nutritious meals, such as frozen dinners that are low in sodium. Another option is Meals-on-Wheels, which is able to deliver meals that are tailored to special diets.
• If part of treatment is weight loss, encourage the patient to keep a food diary for three days to track areas in need of change.
• Prefilled syringes should be stored in the refrigerator flat or with needles pointing up. This prevents crystals from settling and clogging the needles. Allow syringes to come to room temperature before injecting.
• Patients can discard used syringes and needles in a hard plastic container such as a Clorox bottle with a screw top if red needle boxes are not available.
• If the patient has a visual or dexterity problem, suggest a syringe magnifier (check with the pharmacy) or a prefilled insulin pen.
• Help the patient learn to use a mirror to look at the bottom of the feet or have a family member examine the patient's feet.
• Instruct the patient on the importance of wearing comfortable shoes. The patient should avoid sandals, high heels, flip flops, or ill-fitting shoes. If necessary, the HCP can request a podiatry consult. A podiatrist can arrange for the patient to be measured and fitted with special shoes that properly fit his or her feet. Special shoes may be covered by Medicare.
• The patient should keep a pair of nonskid slippers at the bedside. If the patient needs to get up in the night to use the restroom, putting on secure slippers can help prevent the possibility of stepping on something and causing a foot injury.
• Due to decreased skin sensation in some persons with diabetes, hot water heaters should be set below 120°F (48.8°C).
• Even if patients have had diabetes for many years, observe them preparing and injecting their insulin. This provides an opportunity to praise good technique or correct bad habits.
• Diabetic patients with vision problems can become isolated and depressed. Assist your patient with obtaining vision aids that can help improve social outlets.

Evaluation

The best indicator of the success of a care plan for diabetes is controlled blood glucose and glycohemoglobin within target levels. The patient should also be without symptoms of hypoglycemia or hyperglycemia and be able to state what to do if they do occur. Long-term complications should be minimized. Another important indicator is the patient's statement of satisfaction and comfort with the plan and his or her ability to carry it out on a daily basis.

Diabetes Self-Management Education

The individual with diabetes must receive diabetes self-management education if at all possible. No amount of care from a physician or nurse can replace the self-care required of the person with diabetes. The involvement of family or significant others is also important for the successful treatment and well-being of the person with diabetes.

If the patient is hospitalized at diagnosis, the initial instruction is done in the hospital. However, hospital stays are so short, you cannot waste any time. Begin assessing baseline knowledge and teaching as soon as the patient is feeling physically well enough to learn. Depending on your state nurse practice act, this may be the responsibility of the primary or registered nurse, although aspects of the instruction may be delegated to the licensed practical nurse/licensed vocational nurse (LPN/LVN). Some hospitals have a certified diabetes educator who provides classroom or bedside instruction. The dietitian should be contacted to provide nutrition instruction.

Most hospitals have policies or management plans describing the instruction to be provided by the nurse. Generally this encompasses survival skills, which include the basic information the patient needs initially to survive at home. Survival skills include medication administration, glucose monitoring, meal plan basics, and what to do if high or low blood glucose levels occur. A variety of helpful aids, such as pamphlets and videos, are available. Diabetes equipment suppliers provide kits that are full of samples and information. These are a significant help when you are teaching a patient. Also advise the patient to purchase a medical alert bracelet or necklace.

It is difficult to know how to operate and teach glucose monitoring with the variety of glucose monitors available. Many drugstores and medical supply stores not only sell the monitors but also provide training for the patient and family. You can obtain this information by calling local medical suppliers or by contacting the certified diabetes educator or discharge planner at your institution.

After discharge, the patient should be referred to outpatient diabetes classes for further instruction. If classes are unavailable or if the patient is unable to leave home, a referral to a visiting nurse should be made. It is usually advisable to have a nurse present for the patient's first insulin injection at home. The ADA recommends that diabetes self-management education include information about the following:

- Disease process and treatment options
- Nutritional management
- Incorporating physical activity into lifestyle
- Using medications safely
- Monitoring blood glucose and using results
- Preventing, detecting, and treating acute complications
- Preventing, detecting, and treating chronic complications
- Personal strategies for psychosocial adjustment
- Personal strategies for health promotion and behavior change (ADA, 2014)

Two websites that might be helpful to both you and your patients are www.diabetes.org and www.lifeclinic.com/focus/diabetes/resources.asp.

Because many people with diabetes are older, it is important to be aware of their special needs ("Gerontological Issues").

Gerontological Issues

Diabetes care can be a challenge for many older adults.
- Syringe magnifiers and talking glucose meters are available for those with impaired vision.
- Family members can be taught to draw up a week's supply of insulin for the patient to store in the refrigerator. Family members should also be able to recognize signs and symptoms of hypo- and hyperglycemia.
- Home meal programs can help ensure an adequate diet.
- Older adults should also have an emergency call system in the home and regular contact with family members or other support people.

NURSING CARE PLAN for the Patient With Diabetes Mellitus

Nursing Diagnosis: *Risk for Unstable Blood Glucose Level*

Expected Outcomes: The patient will maintain at all times:
- HbA_{1c} less than 7%
- Premeal glucose 70–130 mg/dL
- Postmeal glucose less than 180 mg/dL.

NURSING CARE PLAN for the Patient With Diabetes Mellitus—cont'd

Critically ill, hospitalized patient treated with insulin will maintain:
• All blood glucose measurements between 140 and 180 mg/dL.

Noncritically ill, hospitalized patient treated with insulin will maintain:
• Premeal glucose less than 140 mg/dL
• Random glucose less than 180 mg/dL.

(Verify individual goals with physician.)

Evaluation of Outcomes: Are blood glucose levels within predetermined parameters? Does patient show understanding of diabetes self-care?

Intervention Assess knowledge of diabetes self-care. **Rationale** Teaching should be initiated only if a knowledge deficit exists. **Evaluation** Does patient exhibit knowledge of diabetes self-care?

Intervention Assist patient to collaborate with HCP to determine appropriate blood glucose levels and action to be taken if glucose levels are too high or too low. **Rationale** Appropriate blood glucose levels may be different for each patient. The patient should know what blood glucose levels require notification of the HCP. **Evaluation** Does patient state appropriate blood glucose levels and action to take if glucose is high or low?

Intervention Teach patient to assess glucose levels before meals and at bedtime or as ordered by HCP. Ensure that patient knows how to obtain glucose monitor and instruction for home use. **Rationale** Good blood glucose control depends on knowledge of glucose levels and trends. **Evaluation** Does patient demonstrate correct use of glucose monitor or state how monitor and instruction will be obtained?

Intervention In a hospitalized patient who is taking nothing by mouth (NPO) or on continuous feeding, check glucose level every 4–6 hours around the clock. Check patient on insulin drip every 1–2 hours. **Rationale** Regular blood glucose monitoring is needed for scale insulin administration and maintaining glucose levels within safe parameters. **Evaluation** Is blood glucose monitoring carried out on an appropriate schedule?

Intervention Teach patient how to administer insulin or oral hypoglycemic agent after evaluating blood glucose. Ensure that meals are timed appropriately with medications. Replace any uneaten foods to prevent hypoglycemia. **Rationale** If most medications are taken without food to supply calories, hypoglycemia can occur. Check individual medication for specific instructions. **Evaluation** Does patient state appropriate meal and medication schedule?

Intervention Teach technique for administering insulin if indicated. **Rationale** The patient and family will be administering insulin independently at home. **Evaluation** Does patient demonstrate correct injection technique?

Intervention Observe for symptoms of hypoglycemia and hyperglycemia, and treat as needed. Teach causes, prevention, recognition, and treatment of hypoglycemia and hyperglycemia. **Rationale** If the patient has a good understanding of hypoglycemia and hyperglycemia, most episodes can be prevented. If hypoglycemia or hyperglycemia does occur, prompt treatment is essential to prevent complications. **Evaluation** Does patient state causes, prevention, symptoms, and treatment of hypo and hyperglycemia? Does patient carry fast sugar at all times?

Intervention Administer 15–20 g glucose or carbohydrate if blood glucose level falls below 70 mg/dL, or according to institution hypoglycemia guidelines. Contact RN or HCP if blood glucose is above 180 mg/dL. **Rationale** A "fast sugar" provides prompt treatment of hypoglycemia to prevent complications. Glucose levels over 180 mg/dL are associated with poor outcomes. **Evaluation** Does "fast sugar" resolve hypoglycemic episode within 15 minutes? If not, repeat. Are glucose levels within safe range?

Intervention Consult with dietician for nutrition therapy instruction. **Rationale** The dietitian is trained to provide in-depth meal plan instruction. **Evaluation** Is patient able to state plan for obtaining appropriate meals?

Continued

NURSING CARE PLAN for the Patient With Diabetes Mellitus—cont'd

Intervention Teach patient on insulin to eat additional complex (not fast-acting) carbohydrate before exercise if glucose is less than 100 mg/dL. **Rationale** Exercise can further lower blood glucose. **Evaluation** Does patient state appropriate plan for eating additional carbohydrate?

Intervention Consult with social worker or case manager as needed. **Rationale** Some patients may not have the resources or support to carry out effective self-care. **Evaluation** Does patient state availability of adequate resources for self-care at home?

Intervention Provide patient with information regarding comprehensive diabetes education. Remind patient that only survival skills have been taught during initial instruction. **Rationale** Instruction provided in the hospital usually is not comprehensive. Outpatient diabetes classes can provide additional self-care and health promotion information. **Evaluation** Does patient state plan for obtaining further diabetes education after discharge?

Intervention Assist patient to obtain medical alert card or tag that identifies diabetes. **Rationale** If the patient is ever unresponsive for any reason, the HCP would need to be aware of diabetes condition. **Evaluation** Does patient state plan to carry or wear identification at all times?

GERIATRIC

Intervention Assess ability to see and manipulate syringe, glucose monitor, and other equipment. Obtain assistive devices as needed. **Rationale** The older adult patient may have poor eyesight or other sensory deficits. **Evaluation** Is patient able to manipulate equipment to safely care for self?

REACTIVE HYPOGLYCEMIA

Reactive hypoglycemia, also called postprandial hypoglycemia, occurs when the blood glucose drops below a normal level following meals, usually below 50 mg/dL. Hypoglycemia is most often a complication of diabetes treatment, but at times it may occur without the presence of diabetes. It may be a warning sign of impending diabetes.

Pathophysiology and Etiology

Low blood glucose can occur as an overreaction of the pancreas to eating. The pancreas senses the blood glucose level rising and produces more insulin than is necessary for the use of that glucose. As a result, the blood glucose drops to below normal. It may be due to abnormally low levels of glucagon, or alternatively, to high levels of insulin. Other causes include previous GI surgery, enzyme deficiencies, and pregnancy, among others. Some experts believe that reactive hypoglycemia is a rare condition and that many "hypoglycemic" episodes are instead related to activation of the sympathetic nervous system for other reasons, without true hypoglycemia.

Signs and Symptoms

Low blood glucose causes release of epinephrine, which in turn causes the blood glucose to rise. Epinephrine release causes a fight-or-flight reaction, which may produce shaking, sweating, and palpitations. Headache, chills, and confusion may also occur. Symptoms are the same as those described earlier related to hypoglycemia in diabetes.

Diagnosis

Diagnosis may be based on a 5-hour glucose tolerance test, with below-normal readings between 2 and 5 hours. However, with the availability of home glucose monitors, it is now preferable for patients to monitor blood glucose levels at home. Readings should be taken in the morning on arising, 2 hours after each meal, at bedtime, and during symptoms of hypoglycemia. These results may then be taken to the physician for interpretation.

Therapeutic Measures

Treatment includes frequent small meals and avoidance of fasting. Simple sugars are avoided because they can aggravate symptoms. High-fiber foods, complex carbohydrates, and proteins are recommended. See Table 40.9 for a sample diet.

TABLE 40.9 SAMPLE MEAL PLAN FOR HYPOGLYCEMIC DIET

Exchange Group	Sample Menu
Morning	
1 fruit	1/2 cup unsweetened orange juice
1 starch	3/4 cup whole-grain cereal
1 meat	1 oz low-fat cheese or meat
1/2 skim milk	1/2 cup skim milk
Free	Decaffeinated coffee
Midmorning	
1 meat	1 tbsp peanut butter
1 starch	4 whole-grain crackers
Noon	
Chef's salad:	
2–4 meat	2–4 oz lean meat
1 vegetable	Lettuce, tomatoes
1 fat	1 tbsp regular dressing
1 fruit	1 small piece fresh fruit
1 skim milk	1 cup skim milk
1 starch	2 breadsticks (4 (1/2 in.)
Midafternoon	
1 meat	1 oz low-fat cheese
1 starch	4 whole-grain crackers
Evening	
2–4 meat	2–4 oz lean meat
1 starch	1/2 cup potato or pasta
1 vegetable	1/2 cup vegetable
1 fat	Lettuce salad with 1 tbsp regular dressing
1 fruit	1 piece fresh fruit
Free	Decaffeinated coffee or tea
Bedtime	
1 starch and 1 meat	1/2 sandwich (1 slice whole-grain bread and 1 oz lean meat)
1 vegetable	Fresh vegetables
Free	Decaffeinated beverage

SUGGESTED ANSWERS TO

CRITICAL THINKING

■ Mr. McMillan

1. "Have you been eating or drinking more than usual? Have you been urinating more than usual? Do you get up at night to urinate? How is your appetite? Does anyone in your family have diabetes?"

2. Fatigue occurs because the glucose is unable to enter the cells without insulin, so they are starving.

3. Mr. McMillan is dehydrated because he is losing excessive amounts of urine as his kidneys lose excess glucose.

■ Mrs. Evans

1. Lantus insulin should be given the same time each day. Her order says each evening; any time in the evening is okay as long as it is consistent. Humalog is very fast acting so should be given no more than 15 minutes before eating—ideally when her food is ready to eat so no delay can occur.

2. She should be alert for low blood glucose 30 to 90 minutes after she receives her Humalog dose, the peak action time for Humalog. Eating her meal after her insulin dose should prevent hypoglycemia.

Continued

SUGGESTED ANSWERS TO—cont'd

3. If Mrs. Evans receives insulin and misses her meal, she will likely develop hypoglycemia. If you know she is not feeling well, it would be best to hold her insulin for that meal until you speak with the HCP.

4. She can eat another fruit of similar nutrient amount from the exchange list. Applesauce, canned sugar-free peaches or pears, or other soft fruits would be appropriate.

■ *Jeff*

What kind of new job is it? What schedule is he working? Is it more physically strenuous than his previous job? Does it interfere with his usual meal schedule? What other changes has he experienced in his life that may have affected his blood glucose?

■ *Mr. Jones*

1. Poor circulation, neuropathy, and slow wound healing place Mr. Jones at risk for problems.

2. Circulation to the foot may be poor, and WBCs are sluggish if the blood glucose is high.

3. Any pressure on the foot while walking may further impair circulation. He should not bear weight on the affected foot.

4. If circulation to the area is poor, IV antibiotics may not reach the sore.

5. "Small red open area on right posterior heel, 1 cm × 1.5 cm, 2 mm deep, 2-cm area of yellow drainage on dressing." In addition, many agencies are now taking instant photos of wounds to include in the chart. If no camera is available, a drawing of the size and shape is helpful.

6. Mr. Jones might benefit from involvement with a wound care nurse, dietitian, certified diabetes educator, and home care nurse. Assess for the need for a referral to a comprehensive diabetes education center.

REVIEW QUESTIONS

1. The nurse knows a patient with type 1 diabetes needs more education when the patient makes which of the following statements?
   1. "I must take insulin pills for the rest of my life."
   2. "I will count my carbohydrates at each meal and snack."
   3. "I will monitor my feet carefully every day."
   4. "I will try to keep my blood glucose between 70 and 130 mg/dL before meals."

2. Diabetes is diagnosed when the fasting blood glucose is greater than ____ mg/dL.

3. An obese older adult patient is admitted to the hospital with pneumonia. The nurse notes that the patient gets up four times during the night to urinate. Which action by the nurse is most important at this time?
   1. Offer a bedside commode to the patient.
   2. Request an order for a fasting blood glucose test.
   3. Contact the dietitian for weight-loss counseling.
   4. Provide thorough perineal care after voiding.

4. A nursing home resident with a long history of diabetes requests a heating pad for cold, numb feet. What is the best response by the nurse?
   1. "Let's soak your feet in hot water instead; that might be safer."
   2. "Let's elevate your feet to promote circulation and provide more warmth."
   3. "I will bring you a heating pad; it will help your circulation in your feet."
   4. "A heating pad can cause burns, but I can bring you some extra socks."

5. Which statement by the patient with a new diagnosis of diabetes best shows understanding of instruction related to leading a healthy life and preventing complications?
   1. "I should see my doctor for a complete checkup every 6 months."
   2. "I must check my feet daily."
   3. "I should aim to keep my premeal blood glucose readings under 130 mg/dL."
   4. "I will avoid all sweets and simple carbohydrates."

6. Which breakfast menu is most appropriate for a patient with diabetes?
   1. Two eggs, two strips bacon, orange juice, coffee
   2. Oatmeal with artificial sweetener, whole-grain toast, tea
   3. One half grapefruit, cranberry juice, bagel with sugar-free jelly
   4. One slice whole-grain toast with peanut butter, skim milk, orange juice

7. For which of the following blood glucose results would the nurse administer a "fast sugar"?
   1. 48
   2. 80
   3. 126
   4. 223

8. A patient who is preparing for surgery asks the nurse why the physician discontinued oral hypoglycemic agent orders and initiated sliding-scale insulin. Which response by the nurse is best?
   1. "It helps us maintain better control of your blood glucose during surgery. You will most likely be back on your pills before you go home."
   2. "The stress of surgery often exacerbates diabetes. We will teach you how to give insulin before you go home."
   3. "Oral hypoglycemics are ineffective during times of stress. Insulin is the only way to keep your blood glucose under control."
   4. "The oral agents must not be controlling your blood glucose any longer. I will check and see which insulin you will be going home on."

9. Which meal plan is best for the patient with reactive hypoglycemia?
   1. High-carbohydrate meals
   2. Small, frequent meals
   3. Avoidance of fats and proteins
   4. Three medium to large meals daily

Answers can be found in Appendix C.

References

American Diabetes Association. (2014). Standards of medical care in diabetes—2014. *Diabetes Care, 37*(Suppl. 1).

American Heart Association. (2011). Symptoms and Diagnosis of Metabolic Syndrome. Retrieved January 6, 2014, from www.heart.org/HEARTORG/Conditions/More /MetabolicSyndrome/Symptoms-and-Diagnosis-of -Metabolic-Syndrome_UCM_301925_Article.jsp

Centers for Disease Control and Prevention. (2012). *National diabetes fact sheet.* Retrieved January 5, 2014, from www.cdc.gov/diabetes/pubs/pdf/ndfs_2011.pdf

Diabetes Control and Complications Trial Research Group. (1993). The effect of intensive treatment of diabetes on the development and progression of long-term complications in insulin-dependent diabetes mellitus. *New England Journal of Medicine, 329,* 14.

Moghissi, E. S., Korytkowski, M. T., DiNardo, M., Einhorn, D., Hellman, R., Hris, I. B., . . . Umpierrez, G. E. (2009). American Association of Clinical Endocrinologists and American Diabetes Association consensus statement on inpatient glycemic control. *Endocrine Practice, 15,* 1–17.

UK Prospective Diabetes Study Group. (1998). Intensive blood-glucose control with sulphonylureas or insulin compared with conventional treatment and risk of complications in patients with type 2 diabetes. *Lancet, 352,* 837–853.

 For additional resources and information visit **davispl.us/medsurg5**

Understanding the Genitourinary and Reproductive System

41

Genitourinary and Reproductive System Function and Assessment

LAURA L. McCULLY,
MICHELLE JOHNSON,
AND JANICE L. BRADFORD

KEY TERMS

adnexa (ad-NECK-sah)
bimanual (by-MAN-yoo-uhl)
circumcised (SIR-kum-sized)
colposcopy (kul-PAHS-koh-pee)
conization (KOH-ni-ZAY-shun)
culdoscopy (kul-DOSS-kuh-pee)
curet (kyoo-RET)
cystic (SISS-tik)
ejaculation (ee-JACK-yoo-LAY-shun)
epispadias (EP-ih-SPAY-dee-ahz)
erection (ee-RECK-shun)
gravida (GRAV-vid-ah)
gynecomastia (JY-neh-koh-MASS-tee-ah)
hydrocele (HEYE-droh-seel)
hypospadias (HY-poh-SPAY-dee-ahz)
hysterosalpingogram (HISS-tur-oh-SAL-pinj-oh-gram)
hysteroscopy (HISS-tur-AW-skoh-pee)
insufflation (in-suff-LAY-shun)
libido (lih-BEE-doh)
mammography (mah-MAW-grah-fee)
menarche (meh-NAR-kee)
menopause (MEN-oh-pawz)
orgasm (OR-gazm)
para (PAR-ah)
salpingoscopy (SAL-ping-JOSS-koh-pee)
transillumination (TRANS-ih-loo-mih-NAY-shun)
varicocele (VAR-ih-koh-seel)

LEARNING OUTCOMES

1. Explain the normal structures and functions of the reproductive system.
2. Identify the effects of aging on the reproductive system.
3. List data you should collect when caring for a patient with a disorder of the reproductive system.
4. Identify commonly performed tests used to diagnose disorders of the reproductive system.
5. Plan nursing care for patients undergoing each of the diagnostic tests.

NORMAL GENITOURINARY AND REPRODUCTIVE SYSTEM ANATOMY AND PHYSIOLOGY

The male and female reproductive systems produce gametes (sperm and egg cells [ova]) and facilitate the union of gametes in fertilization following sexual intercourse. The uterus provides for the developing embryo/fetus until birth.

Female Reproductive System

The female reproductive system consists of paired ovaries and fallopian tubes, a single uterus and vagina, and external genitalia (Fig. 41.1). The mammary glands may be considered accessory organs to the system.

Ovaries

The ovaries are a pair of oval structures, about 5 cm long and 2.5 cm wide, located on either side of the uterus in the pelvic cavity. The ovarian ligaments and the broad ligament help keep the ovaries and uterus in position.

The ovaries produce egg cells by oogenesis (meiosis), which begins in the fetus, continues through puberty, and ends at menopause. This process is cyclical. Typically, one mature ovum with its 23 chromosomes is produced and released approximately every 28 days, under hormonal control. Ovarian follicles produce estrogen and later, as the corpus luteum, secrete progesterone as well.

Fallopian Tubes

Each fallopian (uterine) tube is about 10 cm in length and extends from near the ovary to the uterus. (Fig. 41.2) Its fimbriae draw an ovum into the tube, and ciliated epithelium transport either the ovum (or zygote if fertilized) toward the uterus.

Uterus

The uterus is a muscular organ about 8 cm long and 5 cm wide. Ligaments help keep the uterus in position, tilted anteriorly over the top of the bladder. During pregnancy, the uterus increases greatly in size and contains the placenta, which nourishes the fetus until birth. Rising oxytocin levels increases uterine contractions to bring about birth.

The uterus is divided into three layers: the external perimetrium, the myometrium, and the internal endometrium. The endometrium is a highly vascular mucous membrane, part of which is lost and regenerated with each menstrual cycle. During pregnancy, the endometrium helps form the maternal side of the placenta.

Vagina

The vagina extends from the uterine cervix to the vaginal orifice in the perineum. It lies between the urethra and the rectum.

After puberty, the vaginal mucosa is relatively resistant to infection. The normal bacterial flora of the vagina creates an acidic pH, which retards microbial growth. While present, the hymen provides mechanical protection.

External Genitalia

Also called the vulva, the female external genitalia include: the clitoris, mons pubis, and labia majora and minora (Fig. 41.3).

Mammary Glands

Enclosed within the breasts and surrounded by adipose tissue, the mammary glands produce milk after pregnancy (Fig. 41.4). During pregnancy, high levels of estrogen and progesterone prepare the glands for milk production. Prolactin causes the production of milk after pregnancy. Breastfeeding stimulates the release of oxytocin, which in turn stimulates the release of milk and contraction of the uterine muscle.

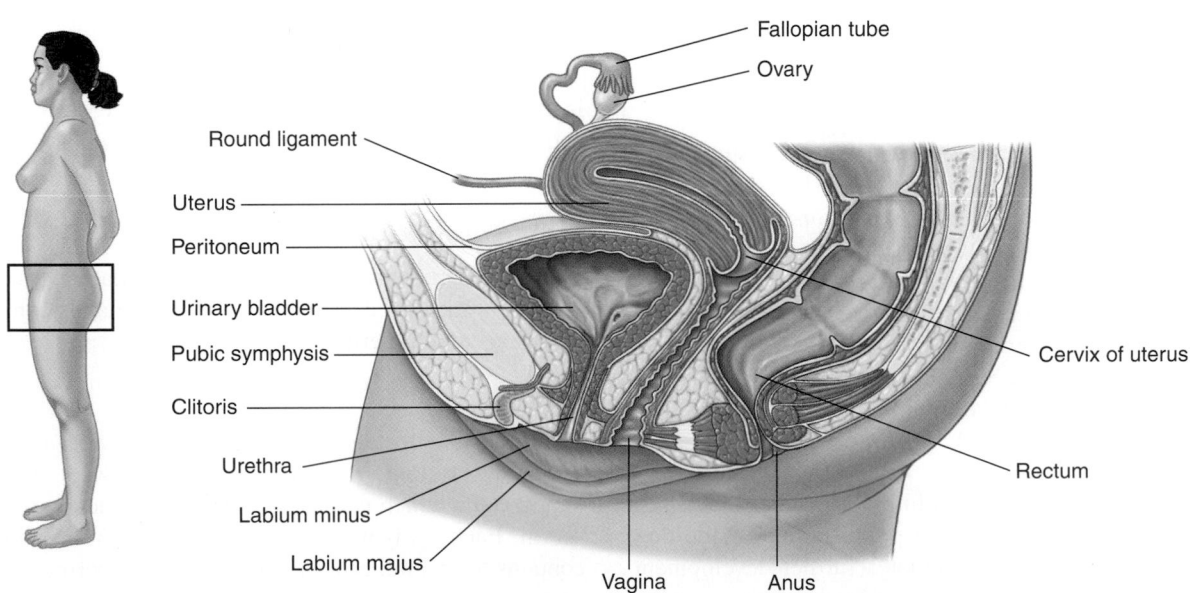

FIGURE 41.1 Female reproductive system in a midsagittal section. From Thompson, G. S. (2013). *Understanding anatomy and physiology.* Philadelphia: F.A. Davis, p. 425.

Fallopian Tubes

A narrow **isthmus** is the portion of the fallopian tube closest to the uterus.

The middle portion of the tube, called the **ampulla**, is the usual site of egg fertilization. Cilia line the inside of the tube. Their beating movements, combined with peristaltic contractions of the tube, propel an egg toward the uterus.

The distal funnel-shaped end of the fallopian tube is called the **infundibulum**. The fallopian tube does not attach directly to the ovary. Instead, finger-like projections called **fimbriae** fan over the ovary.

Uterus

The curved upper portion of the uterus is called the **fundus**. The upper two corners of the uterus connect with the fallopian tubes.

The central region of the uterus is the **body**.

The inferior end is the **cervix**. A passageway through the cervix, called the **cervical canal**, links the uterus to the vagina. Glands within the cervical canal secrete thick mucus; during ovulation, the mucus thins to allow sperm to pass.

Ovary

Endometrium
Myometrium

Fimbriae
Broad ligament
Cervical canal

Vagina

A muscular tube about 3 inches (8 cm) long, the **vagina** serves as a receptacle for the penis and sperm, a route for the discharge of menstrual blood, and the passageway for the birth of a baby. The smooth muscle walls of the vagina can expand greatly, such as during childbirth.

The lower end of the vagina contains ridges (**vaginal rugae**) that help stimulate the penis during intercourse and allow for expansion during childbirth.

A fold of mucous membrane called the **hymen** partially covers the entrance to the vagina. During the first intercourse, the hymen ruptures, sometimes producing blood. However, a number of things can tear the hymen before that time, including the use of tampons, vigorous exercise, and medical examinations.

The vagina extends slightly beyond the cervix, creating pockets called **fornices**.

FIGURE 41.2 Female internal genitalia. From Thompson, G. S. (2013). *Understanding anatomy and physiology*. Philadelphia: F.A. Davis, p. 426.

The Ovarian and Menstrual Cycles

The female reproductive cycles depend on follicle-stimulating hormone (FSH), luteinizing hormone (LH), estrogen, and progesterone (Table 41.1). These hormones bring about changes in the ovaries and uterus.

The menstrual cycle begins with the loss of the endometrium during menstruation, which lasts an average of 5 days. After the endometrium begins to proliferate again due to estrogen, FSH increases and several ovarian follicles begin to develop, although typically only one will dominate. The secretion of LH also increases, peaking to cause ovulation.

After ovulation, the ruptured follicle becomes the corpus luteum, which begins to secrete progesterone in addition to estrogen. Progesterone stimulates further development of the endometrium. If the ovum is not fertilized, the secretion of progesterone decreases. Without progesterone, the endometrium cannot be maintained and begins to slough off

in menstruation. FSH secretion begins to increase as estrogen and progesterone decrease, and the cycle begins again. An average cycle is 28 days.

Male Reproductive System

The male reproductive system consists of bilateral testes and a series of tubules, ducts, and glands. The glands contribute secretions to the sperm, producing semen.

Testes

The testes are located in the scrotum between the upper thighs, where the temperature is slightly lower than body temperature, which is necessary for the production of viable sperm. Each testis is about 5 cm long and 3 cm wide and contains the seminiferous tubules in which spermatogenesis (meiosis) takes place. In contrast to oogenesis, once started at puberty, spermatogenesis is a constant rather than cyclical process and usually continues throughout life. FSH initiates

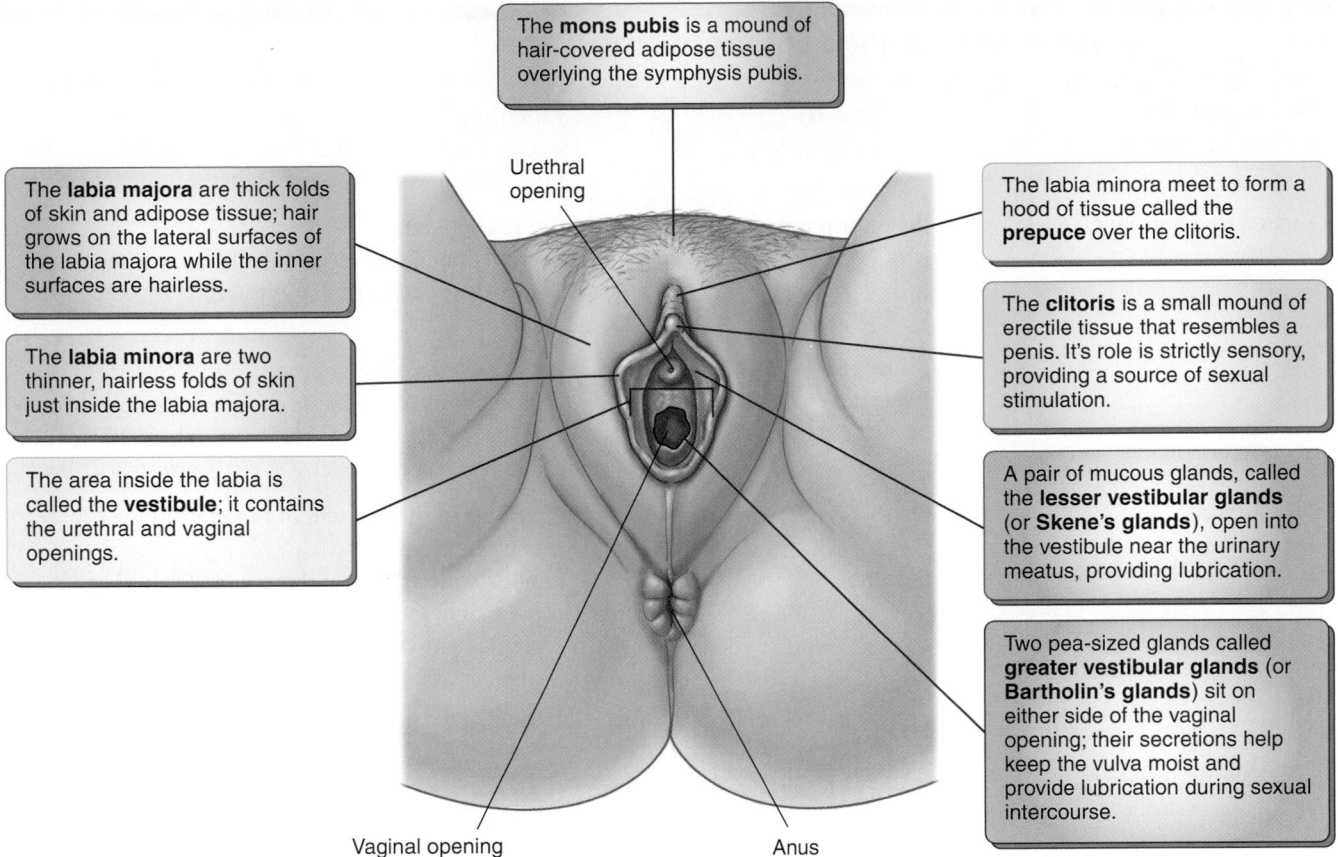

The **mons pubis** is a mound of hair-covered adipose tissue overlying the symphysis pubis.

Urethral opening

The **labia majora** are thick folds of skin and adipose tissue; hair grows on the lateral surfaces of the labia majora while the inner surfaces are hairless.

The **labia minora** are two thinner, hairless folds of skin just inside the labia majora.

The area inside the labia is called the **vestibule**; it contains the urethral and vaginal openings.

The labia minora meet to form a hood of tissue called the **prepuce** over the clitoris.

The **clitoris** is a small mound of erectile tissue that resembles a penis. It's role is strictly sensory, providing a source of sexual stimulation.

A pair of mucous glands, called the **lesser vestibular glands** (or **Skene's glands**), open into the vestibule near the urinary meatus, providing lubrication.

Two pea-sized glands called **greater vestibular glands** (or **Bartholin's glands**) sit on either side of the vaginal opening; their secretions help keep the vulva moist and provide lubrication during sexual intercourse.

Vaginal opening

Anus

FIGURE 41.3 Female external genitalia. From Thompson, G. S. (2013). *Understanding anatomy and physiology.* Philadelphia: F.A. Davis, p. 427.

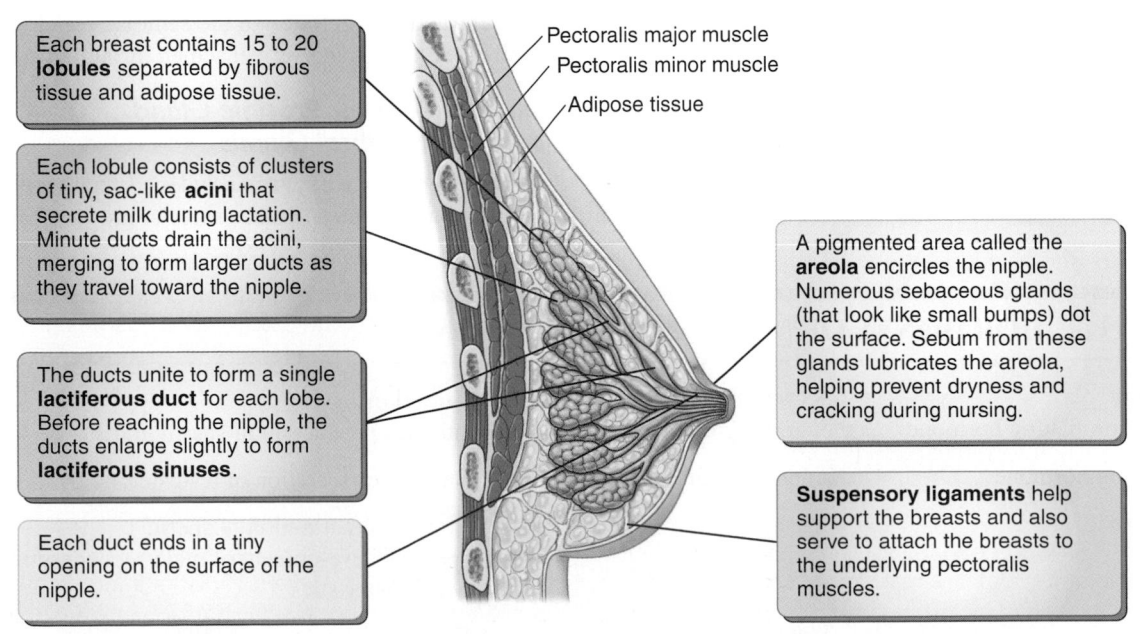

Each breast contains 15 to 20 **lobules** separated by fibrous tissue and adipose tissue.

Each lobule consists of clusters of tiny, sac-like **acini** that secrete milk during lactation. Minute ducts drain the acini, merging to form larger ducts as they travel toward the nipple.

The ducts unite to form a single **lactiferous duct** for each lobe. Before reaching the nipple, the ducts enlarge slightly to form **lactiferous sinuses**.

Each duct ends in a tiny opening on the surface of the nipple.

Pectoralis major muscle
Pectoralis minor muscle
Adipose tissue

A pigmented area called the **areola** encircles the nipple. Numerous sebaceous glands (that look like small bumps) dot the surface. Sebum from these glands lubricates the areola, helping prevent dryness and cracking during nursing.

Suspensory ligaments help support the breasts and also serve to attach the breasts to the underlying pectoralis muscles.

FIGURE 41.4 Breasts/mammary glands. From Thompson, G. S. (2013). *Understanding anatomy and physiology.* Philadelphia: F.A. Davis, p. 427.

TABLE **41.1** **HORMONES OF FEMALE REPRODUCTION**

Hormone	Secreted By	Functions
Follicle-stimulating hormone	Anterior pituitary	Initiates development of ovarian follicles Stimulates secretion of estrogen by follicle cells
Luteinizing hormone	Anterior pituitary	Causes ovulation Converts ruptured ovarian follicle into corpus luteum Stimulates secretion of progesterone by corpus luteum
Estrogen	Ovary (follicle) Placenta	Promotes maturation of ovarian follicles Promotes growth of blood vessels in endometrium Initiates development of secondary sex characteristics Promotes growth of duct system of mammary glands
Progesterone	Ovary (corpus luteum) Placenta	Promotes further growth of blood vessels in endometrium Inhibits contractions of the myometrium during pregnancy Promotes growth of secretory cells of mammary glands
Inhibin	Ovary (corpus luteum)	Decreases secretion of FSH toward end of cycle
Prolactin	Anterior pituitary	Promotes production of milk after birth
Oxytocin	Posterior pituitary	Promotes release of milk

Source: Scanlon, V. C., & Sanders, T. (2015). Essentials of anatomy and physiology (7th ed.). Philadelphia: F.A. Davis, with permission.

spermatogenesis. LH stimulates the secretion of testosterone, which contributes to the maturation of sperm. The secretion of inhibin is stimulated by testosterone; inhibin decreases the secretion of FSH, which helps keep the rate of spermatogenesis fairly constant. The functions of these hormones are summarized in Table 41.2.

Epididymis, Ductus Deferens, and Ejaculatory Ducts

A series of ducts lead sperm into and through the pelvic cavity where secretions are added; semen then exits the body via the urethra. The comma-shaped epididymis is a tube about 6 meters long that is coiled on the posterior side of a testis. Smooth muscle within its wall propels sperm from the testes into the ductus deferens. Also called the vas deferens, the ductus deferens extends from the epididymis in the scrotum to the ejaculatory duct within the pelvic cavity. Each of the two ejaculatory ducts receives sperm from the ductus deferens and the secretion of the seminal vesicle bilaterally. Both ejaculatory ducts propel semen through the urethra.

Seminal Vesicles, Prostate Gland, and Bulbourethral Glands

The male reproductive system includes bilateral seminal vesicles and bulbourethral glands, and a singular prostate (Fig. 41.5).

TABLE **41.2** **HORMONES OF MALE REPRODUCTION**

Hormone	Secreted By	Functions
Follicle-stimulating hormone	Anterior pituitary	Initiates production of sperm in the testes
Luteinizing hormone	Anterior pituitary	Stimulates secretion of testosterone by the testes
Testosterone	Testes	Promotes maturation of sperm Initiates development of male secondary sex characteristics
Inhibin	Testes	Decreases secretion of FSH to maintain a constant rate of spermatogenesis

Source: Scanlon, V. C., & Sanders, T. (2015). Essentials of anatomy and physiology (7th ed.). Philadelphia: F.A. Davis, with permission.

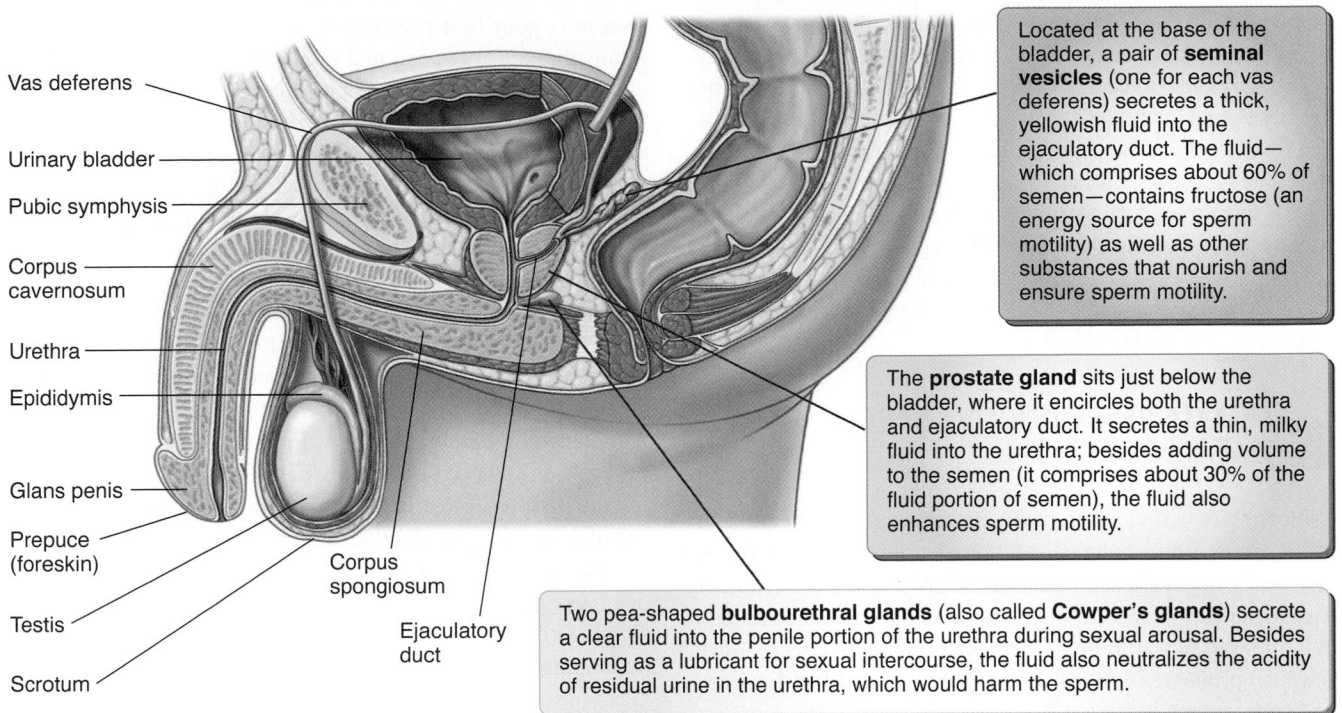

Vas deferens

Urinary bladder

Pubic symphysis

Corpus cavernosum

Urethra

Epididymis

Glans penis

Prepuce (foreskin)

Testis

Scrotum

Corpus spongiosum

Ejaculatory duct

Located at the base of the bladder, a pair of **seminal vesicles** (one for each vas deferens) secretes a thick, yellowish fluid into the ejaculatory duct. The fluid—which comprises about 60% of semen—contains fructose (an energy source for sperm motility) as well as other substances that nourish and ensure sperm motility.

The **prostate gland** sits just below the bladder, where it encircles both the urethra and ejaculatory duct. It secretes a thin, milky fluid into the urethra; besides adding volume to the semen (it comprises about 30% of the fluid portion of semen), the fluid also enhances sperm motility.

Two pea-shaped **bulbourethral glands** (also called **Cowper's glands**) secrete a clear fluid into the penile portion of the urethra during sexual arousal. Besides serving as a lubricant for sexual intercourse, the fluid also neutralizes the acidity of residual urine in the urethra, which would harm the sperm.

FIGURE 41.5 Male accessory glands. From Thompson, G. S. (2013). *Understanding anatomy and physiology*. Philadelphia: F.A. Davis, p. 420.

The mostly alkaline secretions of the male reproductive glands ensure that many sperm remain viable in the acidic environment of the vagina. The normal bacterial flora of the vagina create the acidic pH, but the pH of semen is about 7.4 and permits sperm to remain motile.

Urethra and Penis

The urethra is the last of the male reproductive ducts; its longest portion is within the penis. The penis is an external genital organ; its distal end is called the glans penis and when uncircumcised is covered with a fold of skin called the prepuce, or foreskin. Within the penis are three areas of erectile or cavernous tissue (Fig. 41.6).

When blood flow through these sinuses is minimal, the penis is flaccid (soft). Sexual stimulation causes the arterioles of the penis to dilate; the sinuses fill with blood, and the penis becomes erect and firm. This is brought about by parasympathetic impulses. The culmination of sexual stimulation is **ejaculation** (the expelling of semen from the urethra with force), which is brought about by peristalsis of the reproductive ducts and contraction of the prostate gland.

Spermatozoa

The head of the sperm cell contains 23 chromosomes. The midpiece connects the head to the flagellum. Sperm form in the seminiferous tubules of a testis and are stored in the epididymis.

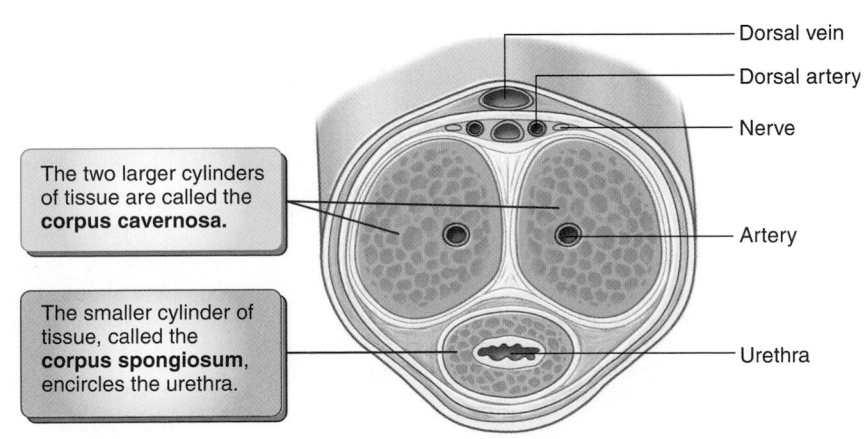

Dorsal vein

Dorsal artery

Nerve

Artery

Urethra

The two larger cylinders of tissue are called the **corpus cavernosa.**

The smaller cylinder of tissue, called the **corpus spongiosum**, encircles the urethra.

FIGURE 41.6 Penis—cross-section. From Thompson, G. S. (2013). *Understanding anatomy and physiology*. Philadelphia: F.A. Davis, p. 421.

Aging and the Reproductive Systems

For women, there is a definite end to reproductive capability; this is called **menopause** and is defined as having occurred when menses have ceased for 12 months. Menopause usually occurs between the ages of 45 and 55. Estrogen secretion decreases, and ovulation and menstrual cycles become irregular and finally cease. The decrease in estrogen has other effects as well. See Figure 41.7 for a concept map on the effects of aging.

For most men, testosterone secretion continues throughout life, as does sperm production, although both diminish with advancing age. Perhaps the most common reproductive problem for older men is enlargement of the prostate gland, called benign prostatic hyperplasia.

FEMALE REPRODUCTIVE SYSTEM DATA COLLECTION

Collecting data related to a women's reproductive health can seem challenging because of the complex relationship of physical and psychosocial factors. Hormones not only affect a multitude of body functions, they also can influence moods and mental functioning. Reproduction involves not only physical processes, but also relationships, role identification, and self-esteem issues.

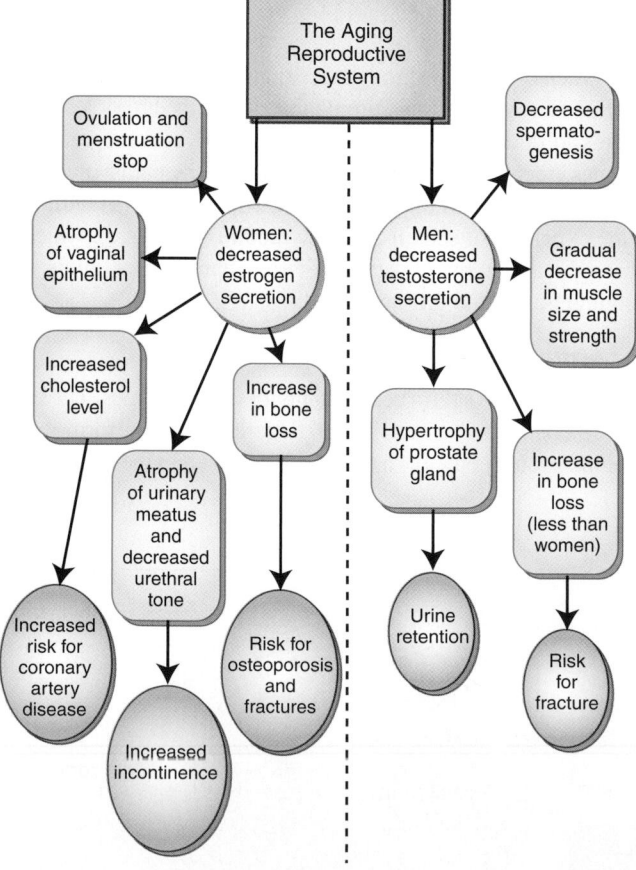

FIGURE 41.7 Aging and the reproductive system. This concept map shows the effects the aging process has on the reproductive system.

Normal Function Baselines

Knowing about expected functioning of the reproductive system is your best preparation for data collection. Regular, relatively pain-free shedding of an appropriate amount of the endometrial lining of the uterus (menstruation) is expected from puberty through midlife or later. Intercourse is normally expected to be free of pain and infection, to occur when desired by both partners, to be satisfying, and generally to result in pregnancy within a few months unless precautions are taken. A pregnancy is expected to last approximately 40 weeks and to produce a healthy child. Physical and psychological sexual characteristics and function including **libido** (sexual desire) are expected to be adequately maintained by hormones. Sexual functioning, desire, and fertility are expected to change throughout the process of aging. Although individuals may vary somewhat from these expected descriptions, these serve as a baseline for collecting data related to possible disorders. Chapter 42 further defines specific female reproductive system disorders.

Much of what happens in female reproductive system disorders occurs inside the body and may not show external signs. Skill in asking appropriate questions, documenting patient statements, and describing observations is essential. Descriptions of symptoms should be thorough and follow the **WHAT'S UP?** format described in Chapter 1. Because many signs and symptoms of reproductive system disorders occur in a cyclic fashion, you or the health care provider (HCP) may ask the patient to keep an accurate written record of occurrences, noting times and dates to identify patterns.

Health History

Subjective data related to the female reproductive system include general personal information as well as menstrual, obstetrical, gynecological, sexual, family, and psychosocial histories. See Table 41.3 for specific data to collect.

NURSING CARE TIP

It is helpful to have women retain a monthly calendar of their menstrual cycles and bring it to any appointment during which discussion of the cycle may take place.

An obstetrical history includes number of pregnancies, pregnancy outcomes, and complications. These are generally documented using abbreviations of Latin words: G = number of pregnancies (from the Latin word **gravida**); P = births, whether alive or stillborn (regardless of number of fetuses) after 20 weeks' gestation (from the Latin word **para**); A = abortions, whether spontaneous or therapeutic (from the Latin word *abortus;* a spontaneous abortion is sometimes

• **WORD** • **BUILDING** •
menopause: men—month + pause—stop

TABLE 41.3 SUBJECTIVE DATA COLLECTION FOR THE FEMALE REPRODUCTIVE SYSTEM

Category	Questions to Ask During the Health History	Rationale/Significance
Personal History	Have you ever been diagnosed or treated for any health problems?	Data may reveal general state of health, knowledge/practice of health promotion behaviors, meaning of health, expectations related to care.
	Have you had any recent weight changes? What type of change (if any)?	Weight changes may reflect physical or psychological pathology.
	Are you experiencing pain? (Use **WHAT'S UP?** questions if patient reports pain.)	Subjective indication of pain may indicate a variety of disorders.
	Do you have any allergies? (Agent/type of reaction?)	Allergy status should always be assessed to guide possible intervention should treatment be needed.
	Are you using any medications? (Include prescription, over-the-counter, and herbal remedies.) How much/how often do you take the medication?	A medication list may lead to health issues not yet revealed, and may guide possible interventions should treatment be needed.
	Do you smoke, consume caffeine, drink alcohol, or use recreational drugs? How much/how often?	Recreational behaviors can indicate risk of health disorders. Smoking increases risk of coagulation disorders with use of contraceptives containing estrogen in women over age 35.
	Do you exercise? What type of exercise do you do? How often?	Exercise is recognized as an activity that improves health status, in general, and for many disorders.
	How many hours of sleep do you get in a 24-hour period of time? Do you feel you get enough rest?	May indicate state of health or lead to discussion of social issues that lead to stress and, ultimately, physical disorders.
	Do you feel under stress? How do you deal with stress?	Can indicate social issues that may lead to physical disorders.
	Have you been hit, kicked, slapped, or made to do anything sexually against your will since your last visit?	Abuse screening should be considered during all primary care visits; may indicate need for intervention or guide care.
Menstrual History	At what age did you begin menstruating (**menarche**)? How often do you menstruate, and how long do your periods last? How heavy is your flow?	May reveal abnormalities of cycle and lead to a diagnosis of benign/malignant tumors, endometriosis, pregnancy, anemia, endocrine disorders.
	At what age did you enter menopause (if applicable)? If menopausal, has bone density screening been done? What is your calcium/vitamin D intake?	May determine need for bone density screening and teaching related to calcium and vitamin D intake.
Obstetric/ Gynecological History	How many pregnancies and deliveries have you had? Were they full term or preterm?	May indicate health of reproductive system, knowledge/meaning of health maintenance practice, and risk for disease.

Continued

• WORD • BUILDING •

menarche: men—month + arche—beginning

TABLE **41.3** SUBJECTIVE DATA COLLECTION FOR THE FEMALE REPRODUCTIVE SYSTEM—cont'd

Category	Questions to Ask During the Health History	Rationale/Significance
	Were your deliveries vaginal or by cesarean section? How much did your largest baby weigh? Did you have any complications following your deliveries?	
	Have you had previous treatment/surgery on your reproductive organs?	May indicate past health issues related to the reproductive organs and need for current evaluation related to issues.
	Have you had any itching of your perineum, or have you noted any unusual vaginal discharge (describe)?	Subjective report of itching or discharge may indicate disorder of inflammation or lead to diagnosis of sexually transmitted infection.
	When was your last Pap/pelvic exam? What were the results?	May reflect meaning of health and guide current care.
	Do you do breast self-examination? How often? Have you noticed any breast changes? When was your last mammogram (if applicable)?	If changes have been noted by the patient, they should be evaluated by the primary care provider for possible pathology.
	Did you breastfeed? How long?	Breastfeeding may offer some protection against breast cancer. If patient is currently breastfeeding, may help guide care and diagnosis.
Sexual History	Are you sexually active? How many partners do you have? Of what gender? What is your lifetime number of partners? Is your sexual activity satisfying?	May indicate risk of STIs, risk of unintended pregnancy, and indicate state of sexual satisfaction/intimacy.
	At what age did you become sexually active? What contraceptive method(s) do you use (if sexually active with a male)? How do you use them? How long have you used this method?	Early onset of sexual activity increases risk of STIs and cervical cancer. May reflect meaning of health, high-risk health behaviors, and risk for unintended pregnancy or STI. Asking length of use of a particular method allows assessment of need for replacement as in an intrauterine device, or need for a bone density exam.
	Have you ever been diagnosed with a STI? If so, when, what type, and how was it treated? That you are aware, was treatment successful?	May indicate high-risk sexual behavior patterns or potential for active disease and, therefore, indicate need for diagnostic testing and treatment.
Family History	Do you have a family history of cardiovascular problems, cancer, osteoporosis, diabetes, thyroid abnormalities?	May indicate underlying cause of or risk for sexual/physical abnormalities of the reproductive system.
Psychosocial History	Are you married or in a significant relationship? Is the relationship satisfying? Are you employed? Where?	Relevant to determine financial, social, and emotional support.

called a miscarriage). Roman numerals follow the letters to specify the number of each. For example, three pregnancies—twins, one single birth, and one spontaneous abortion—are recorded as GIII, PII, AI. This may also be written as G3P2A1. Some hospitals use additional notations such as number of premature or full-term births, number of living children, and number of therapeutic abortions. Be sure to follow your institution's documentation policy.

LEARNING TIP

Remember the word gravida by thinking of gravity and that a woman typically is heavier when pregnant.

Also ask about any tests, surgeries, or treatments done on the reproductive organs and excretory system. Medications the patient is taking (for whatever reasons), height-to-weight ratio, and marked changes in weight may also provide significant data for diagnostic and care planning purposes related to reproductive system disorders.

LEARNING TIP

There are many things to remember when asking health history questions. Make up an index card for your pocket or purchase a prepared one for a handy reference.

Many nurses feel awkward asking reproductive history questions, and patients may also feel some uneasiness with this line of questioning. A matter-of-fact attitude, an assurance of confidentiality, and an adequate explanation about why the information is needed tend to encourage patient comfort and cooperation.

Breast Examination

Palpation

Palpation is the most important technique for breast examination because it can be used to identify alterations from normal consistency, to confirm the presence of lumps, and to locate areas of tenderness. Even mammograms are not sensitive enough to detect a small percentage of masses that can be felt by the patient or HCP.

Breast Self-Examination

Self-palpation during breast self-examination (BSE), if done regularly and thoroughly, may be even more sensitive than physician or nurse palpation because the patient becomes so familiar with her own breasts that she is more likely to notice subtle changes that an infrequently visited HCP might overlook. Because recent studies of BSE have failed to show a reduction in cancer deaths, some HCPs are now simply urging women to

be familiar with their breasts and report changes, rather than teaching them to do monthly examinations. Other providers, however, continue to teach and recommend monthly BSE because they have seen it make a significant difference for many women. See Table 41.4 for additional objective data to collect.

Patient Education

If BSE is to be done monthly, a good time to perform it is 1 week after menses, when edema and swelling of normal breast tissue structures is at a minimum. For women who no longer have a regular menstrual period, any regular monthly schedule is fine. Although most women's breasts are not exactly the same size, marked differences between the breasts or a change in the size of one breast should be checked with a HCP. Puckering or dimpling of skin, asymmetrical movement, and different pointing position of the nipples should also be reported. Whether the breasts are examined in parallel lines, a spiral formation, or a wedge pattern is not important. It is important, however, for the examination to be methodical and cover all areas of the breast, including the tail of Spence, which extends into the axilla (Fig. 41.8).

NURSING CARE TIP

Some women do BSE the day their telephone bill (or other bill) arrives each month because it is a dependable monthly reminder.

CRITICAL THINKING

Jilli

■ Jilli, age 24, states, "Why should I do breast exams at my age? I probably won't get breast cancer until I'm older, if I get it at all."
What should your response to Jilli include?
Why would this be a good time to provide education about health maintenance?
Suggested answers are at the end of the chapter.

Diagnostic Tests of the Breasts

Ultrasound and Mammography

Ultrasound can determine the density of the tissues and map the breast structures. This is mainly useful for distinguishing fluid-filled (**cystic**) lumps from solid tumors but can also be used to guide a needle for fine-needle aspiration of cystic fluid or core needle biopsies.

Mammography is a radiographic (x-ray) examination of the breasts. A special machine is used that spreads and flattens

• WORD • BUILDING •
cystic: baglike
mammography: mammo—breast + graphy—recording

TABLE **41.4** **OBJECTIVE DATA COLLECTION FOR THE FEMALE REPRODUCTIVE SYSTEM**

Category	Physical Examination Findings	Possible Abnormal Findings/Causes
Clinical Breast Examination	Observe and palpate for presence of swelling, lumps, skin changes, nipple exudate.	Changes may indicate breast cancer, fibrocystic breast disease.
External Genitalia (mons pubis, clitoris, labia majora/minora, Bartholin's glands)	Observe for color, symmetry, hair distribution, lesions, swelling or exudate.	Changes may indicate vulvar cancer, developmental abnormalities, infection, or injury.
Vagina	Observe for shape, bulges, color changes, lesions, exudate.	Changes may indicate infection, structural abnormalities, or injury.
Internal Genitalia (uterus/cervix, fallopian tubes, ovaries; exam performed by trained personnel)	Palpate for tenderness, size, shape, mobility. Observe for color, lesions, exudate, bleeding.	Changes may indicate infection, structural abnormalities, cervical cancer, polyps, endometriosis, fibroid/malignant tumors, pregnancy, or injury.
Perineum	Observe for lesions, shape.	Abnormalities may indicate infection, structural abnormalities, or injury.
Anus	Observe for shape, color changes, lesions.	Abnormalities can indicate hemorrhoids or injury.
Inguinal Nodes	Palpate for swelling, tenderness.	May indicate infectious process or regional malignancy.

Note. A female physical examination is typically done by a physician or other trained provider.

Inspection

BREAST SELF-EXAMINATION
Palpation

FIGURE **41.8** Breast self-examination. From Venes, D. J. (Ed.). *Taber's cyclopedic medical dictionary (22nd ed.).* Philadelphia: F.A. Davis, p. 332, with permission.

the breast tissue to a thin layer to more effectively show benign and malignant growths, which might be hidden by breast structures on typical chest examination (Fig. 41.9). Generally, at least two radiographs are taken of each breast, with the machine compressing the breast top to bottom and side to side to give comparison views from more than one angle. If suspicious or unclear spots are seen, additional views may be taken. New digital technology is now available that may be more effective in detecting cancers in younger women and women who have dense breasts. The actual procedure is the same

FIGURE 41.9 Mammogram machine. Photo courtesy of Dinesh Patel, MD, Medical Oncology, Internal Medicine, Zanesville, OH.

for a digital mammogram, but the image is computerized, allowing the radiologist to look more closely at problem areas.

The American Cancer Society (2013) recommends the following for women:

- A screening mammogram at age 40 and yearly thereafter as long as they are in good health
- A clinical breast exam by a health professional every 3 years during the 20s and 30s, then yearly by a health professional at age 40 and thereafter
- Optional breast self-examination starting in the 20s; women should know how their breasts normally look and feel and report changes to their HCP
- Magnetic resonance imaging (MRI) and mammogram every year for women at high risk of breast cancer, such as women with *BRCA1* or *BRCA2* genetic mutations or strong family history

See Chapter 11 for more information.

PATIENT EDUCATION. Advise patients preparing for mammography to bathe and not to apply deodorant, powder, or any other substance to the upper body because these can cause false shadows on the test.

Thermography, Tomography, and MRI

Several other methods for diagnosis of breast disorders are available but are not commonly used. Thermography is a method of mapping the breast using photographic paper, which records temperature variations throughout the tissue in different colors. Computerized tomography (CT) or MRI can offer precise location of tumors without the displacement caused by flattening the breast for a mammogram.

Biopsy

If suspicious lesions are found, they may be further assessed with a biopsy. This may be done by surgically removing a portion of tissue or by aspirating fluid or cells through a needle that is placed into the lump or lesion.

Assessment of the patient's psychological condition during breast diagnosis procedures is essential. Most women know someone who has had breast cancer. Although breast cancer screening procedures can seem routine to health care workers, they can be a cause of much anxiety for patients and their families. An understanding and calm nurse who can explain the procedures can help the assessment phase to be less traumatic.

 BE SAFE!

BE VIGILANT! Use at least two patient identifiers when providing care, treatment, and services. Label containers used for blood and other specimens in the presence of the patient (Joint Commission's 2014 National Patient Safety Goals, © The Joint Commission, 2013. Reprinted with permission.).

Laboratory Tests

A blood test can be done to identify mutations in *BRCA1* and *BRCA2*, genes that are associated with breast and ovarian cancer. By reviewing a woman's family history, risk factors can be determined and testing can be offered. Women who test positive for either gene can discuss preventive treatments with their HCPs and also make their sisters and daughters aware of potential risk.

Bone Health Assessment

Bone health assessment is important for women of all ages. Teaching women early about the importance of good calcium and vitamin D intake will be of benefit later in life. Women of childbearing age produce estrogen, which helps prevent bone loss and works with calcium and other minerals to build bone. As women age and approach menopause, estrogen production slowly decreases, which decreases the processes of building and remodeling bone. Once a woman reaches menopause, her body is producing very little estrogen and therefore does not have the added benefit of bone protection. In fact, the body tends to break down more bone than it rebuilds. At this point in a woman's life, dietary calcium and vitamin D requirements increase unless the woman is on hormone replacement therapy.

There is current debate about calcium and vitamin D supplementation for menopausal women. The U.S. Preventive Task Force (USPTF) issued a statement in 2013, based on research, against supplementation with vitamin D of 400 IU or less and calcium of 1000 mg or less because of the increased kidney stone risk and no evidence of preventing fractures. More research is needed in this area, but for now women should aim to get recommended calcium and vitamin D amounts through diet. If a woman is diagnosed with osteoporosis, she should speak to her HCP about a treatment plan. See Table 41.5 for recommendations for calcium and vitamin D intake from the National Institutes of Health Office of Dietary Supplements. See Chapter 6 for the calcium content of selected foods.

TABLE 41.5   ADULT CALCIUM AND VITAMIN D RECOMMENDATIONS

Age (years)	Male	Female	Pregnant	Lactating
RDAs for Calcium				
14–18 years	1300 mg	1300 mg	1300 mg	1300 mg
19–50 years	1000 mg	1000 mg	1000 mg	1000 mg
51–70 years	1000 mg	1200 mg	—	—
71+ years	1200 mg	1200 mg	—	—
RDAs for Vitamin D				
14–18 years	600 IU (15 mcg)	600 IU (15 mcg)	600 IU (15 mcg)	600 IU (15 mcg)
19–50 years	600 IU (15 mcg)	600 IU (15 mcg)	600 IU (15 mcg)	600 IU (15 mcg)
51–70 years	600 IU (15 mcg)	600 IU (15 mcg)		
>70 years	800 IU (20 mcg)	800 IU (20 mcg)		

RDAs = recommended dietary allowances.
Source: From Office of Dietary Supplements, National Institutes of Health, Bethesda, MD. Retrieved August 6, 2013 from http://ods.od.nih.gov.

Diagnostic Tests of the Bones

In addition to recommending increasing the dietary intake of calcium and vitamin D, menopausal women older than age 50 who are not on hormone replacement therapy should be assessed for bone loss. The National Osteoporosis Foundation (www.nof.org) recommends bone density testing for all women over age 65 and for postmenopausal women under age 65 if they are at high risk (see Chapter 46).

The best test for bone density is a dual energy x-ray absorptiometry (DEXA) scan, which measures bone density at the hip or spine. This is a specialized x-ray that takes only 5 to 10 minutes to complete. A quantitative computed tomography (QCT) scan can also be done to determine bone density. Pharmacies or other outpatient facilities may offer tests of peripheral locations such as the heel. These are less sensitive but may still provide useful information that can be followed up with more extensive testing if indicated.

Additional Diagnostic Tests of the Female Reproductive System

Many tests are used to assess reproductive system function; this is currently an area of rapid change. The names of the individual procedures may also vary among institutions or according to particular methods used (e.g., a salpingoscopy is also called a falloposcopy, and a laparoscopy is the same as a peritoneoscopy). For this reason, this chapter is limited to general categories of procedures rather than an attempt to name all tests.

Hormone Tests

Hormone tests are commonly used to assess endocrine system function as it relates to reproduction. These tests may be used to measure potential fertility, to find reasons for abnormal menses, to assess hormone-producing tumors, and to determine whether treatments to adjust hormone levels have been effective. Some hormone tests are time-specific, so the samples can be rendered useless if not gathered within a certain time range.

NURSING CARE. Consult institution policy for specific instructions for each test. Explain the procedure to the patient and provide support. Women who are undergoing hormone tests may feel embarrassed, worried about their femininity and potential fertility, and depressed because of repeated tests. Some may fear loss of their spouse's love (and perhaps the relationship) if they are diagnosed with alterations in hormone levels or function that lead to infertility.

Pelvic Examination

The pelvic examination allows visual inspection of the vagina and cervix, as well as sampling of mucus, discharge, cells, and exudates. Palpation of portions of the reproductive system and some treatments may also be done as part of the procedure (Fig. 41.10).

NURSING CARE. Be prepared to assist the HCP with the examination. Explain the procedure as you set out the supplies according to policy or provider preference. Have the patient empty her bladder, then remove her clothing and change into a gown (socks can remain on, and often give a

FIGURE 41.10 Pelvic exam with Pap smear. From Dillon, P. M. (2007). *Nursing health assessment: A critical thinking case studies approach* (2nd ed.). Philadelphia: F.A. Davis, with permission.

woman a tiny bit of comfort!). When the HCP is ready, assist the patient into the lithotomy position, with her feet in stirrups. If the HCP is using a metal speculum, warm it under warm water to make it a little more comfortable for the patient. Have the patient take a deep breath and blow out as the speculum is being inserted, to help her relax. Being in lithotomy position may make some women feel embarrassed and exposed. Be sure to provide privacy. Ideally, the examination table faces away from the door.

Bimanual Palpation

Because much of the reproductive system is not visible even with a speculum, **bimanual** palpation is often done during a pelvic examination. One hand is placed on the abdomen and the other gloved hand is inserted deeply into the vagina. The uterus and **adnexa** are moved about between the two hands to feel the size, shape, and consistency of the uterus and adnexa and to check for any abnormal growths.

NURSING CARE. Explain the procedure, and support the patient. Some women may be fearful, embarrassed, or tense and may find the procedure uncomfortable (see "Patient Perspective—Thoughts From a Sexual Assault Nurse Examiner"). Active relaxation strategies may decrease discomfort.

• WORD • BUILDING •
bimanual: bi—two + manual—hands
adnexa: ad—together + nexa—to tie (usually refers to ovaries and tubes)

Patient Perspective

Thoughts From a Sexual Assault Nurse Examiner

When patients come in to see me, they are in crisis. They are unsure how or what to feel and whom to trust. They are very apprehensive. As patients give me the history of their assaults, they begin to trust me. They see someone who is interested in them and who believes them. By the time I actually start the head-to-toe physical examination, they know they are safe. Often, when I am performing the physical examination, I start small talk and take an interest in their lives that has nothing to do with the assault. When they are discharged from my care, they are more animated, talkative, and sometimes smiling.

The patient I remember the most was a child whose father was molesting her when her mother went to work. She was about 6 years old. When she came to the hospital, she wasn't talking to anybody, let alone a nurse in a scary hospital at midnight. I spent 4 hours with this child. We colored, played, and talked about her brothers. By the end of the night, she allowed me to examine her. And she trusted me enough to let the physician come in and look at her. Unfortunately, in her young life, she had a reason to be scared. Her life became much worse before it got better. Her father tried to kill her mother and himself as a result of this.

So many of us have grown up with pop culture television, and we think of forensic examiners as professionals working with dead people. In fact, forensic nursing is caring for patients as it applies to the law. As a sexual assault nurse examiner, I care for people who have experienced interpersonal violence. I care for this special population of patients through the nursing process. I not only care for their physical trauma but also for their spiritual needs; lastly, I collect evidence for the prosecution of a crime. I advocate for their safety needs, and I help provide for their physical needs. I provide a bridge to the legal and mental health systems.

I began forensic nursing years ago when the concept was still new. We were navigating uncharted waters and were unsure what the end result would bring. What we quickly learned is, when you deliver good nursing care to patients, the end result can be a positive change in their lives, and that is the reward of the job: making a positive difference in patients' lives, giving them some tools to help in their recovery process. Having the patient and family look at you and say "thank you for helping me" is what we all went into nursing for.

Becoming a sexual assault nurse examiner has made me become a more empathetic person, a more compassionate nurse, and a better citizen of my community.

Cytology

Cytology is the study of cells taken as tissue samples. Cells required for microscopic examination can be removed from the reproductive system in several ways. During a Papanicolaou (Pap) smear, one or more small samples of cells are gently scraped away from the surface of the cervical canal. They are then smeared or rolled onto microscope slides and sprayed with a fixative to preserve them for viewing, or placed into a fixative solution for later preparation and viewing in a laboratory. Cells may also be collected by **conization**, which involves removing a small cone-shaped sample from the cervical canal, or by punch biopsy, which removes a small core of cells. Endometrial biopsy specimens are samples of cells taken from the lining of the uterus by scraping with a small spoon-shaped tool called a **curet**, which is inserted through the cervix. Small biopsy specimens may also be taken by cutting or removing a suspicious lesion. Cells may be observed for changes indicative of hormonal secretion, cellular maturation, or abnormalities such as are seen with viral growths and cancerous or precancerous conditions. Results are reported simply as "normal, unclear, or abnormal."

NURSING CARE. Consult the procedure manual or HCP concerning specific types of instruments to set up for biopsies and Pap smears. Cells die and degrade rapidly once removed from the patient, so they must be packaged securely for transport to laboratory facilities. Always label specimens carefully.

Prepare the patient by explaining the procedure and providing support. The woman may be fearful of cancer or other abnormality. Removal of the sample may cause pain, bleeding, swelling, or, later, inflammation, so the patient is

monitored after the procedure and alerted to watch for and report these complications if they occur. After the procedure, document the woman's status on the chart and record that the sample was sent to the laboratory. Advise the woman that if results are unclear or abnormal, additional testing will be done. Assure her that abnormal results have many causes and typically do not mean a cancer diagnosis.

CRITICAL THINKING

Reproductive Assessment

■ How might the age of the patient change your approach, plans, and teaching for patients who have disorders of the reproductive system? Consider each of the following scenarios:
1. A 2-year-old child is brought into the clinic by her mother because she has a foul-smelling discharge coming from her perineal area and a slight yellowish discharge from her vagina.
2. A 21-year-old woman comes to the physician's office where you work to obtain a renewal of her yearly birth control pill prescription. Your employer enforces regular checks for cervical changes by renewing the prescription only after a Pap smear is done. As you start setting out the Pap smear materials, your patient expresses some reluctance to have it done today because she is so sore already.
3. Your 56-year-old patient comes in to "get things checked out" because she hurts every time that she and her husband have intercourse.

Suggested answers are at the end of the chapter.

Swabs and Smears

Swabs and smears are done to determine which microorganisms are causing infection, and consequently which antibiotics should be used.

NURSING CARE. If infection is suspected, add sample collection materials, including swabs, slides, and sterile saline in site-specific receptacles, and a gonorrhea/*Chlamydia* collection kit, to the pelvic examination equipment. *Chlamydia* samples are especially difficult to transport to laboratories, and special kits are available for this pathogen. Some microorganisms, such as yeasts and *Trichomonas,* can be identified well from smears on slides. Wet mounts are smears of discharge spread onto a slide. These must be taken to the microscope immediately after they are obtained. Sodium chloride and potassium hydroxide are dropped onto individual wet-mount slides before they dry to aid in identification of some microorganisms. Support the patient, who may be anxious about possible sexually transmitted infections (STIs) and effects on relationships.

• **WORD • BUILDING •**
conization: coniz—cone-forming + ation—process

Sonography

Ultrasound assessment (also called sonography) may be done to determine size, shape, development, and density of structures associated with the female reproductive system, as well as fetal measurements and some types of prenatal diagnoses. This procedure is especially useful for differentiating cysts from solid tumors and for locating ectopic pregnancies and intrauterine devices. Ultrasound may also be used to guide needles for obtaining samples of fluid or cells. Either external or vaginal transducers may be used to send and receive the signals for this procedure. Vaginal transducers are placed in a plastic sheath before insertion into the vagina. A full bladder may be required for some ultrasound tests.

NURSING CARE.   Explain the procedure and support the patient. The pressure of the transducer on the skin or in the vagina may be painful if the adjacent structures are inflamed or swollen, or if the bladder is very full.

Radiographic Procedures

Several radiographic procedures may be used for diagnosis of reproductive system problems. Computed tomographic (CT) scanning and MRI are used to locate tumors of the reproductive system. Structures of the female reproductive system may also be outlined by taking x-ray pictures of cavities that have been filled with a radiopaque substance. During a **hysterosalpingogram**, dye is injected into the uterus until it comes out the ends of the fallopian tubes. This test is useful for identifying congenital abnormalities in the shape or structure of the uterus and blockages of the fallopian tubes.

NURSING CARE.   Prepare the patient for a radiographic test according to agency policy, which may include a laxative, suppository, or enema. Ensure that the patient understands the procedure and that appropriate consents are signed as required. Ask about allergies to dye or iodine. Notify the supervisor immediately if the patient reports an allergy. After the procedure, assess for nausea, lightheadedness, and signs of allergic reaction and promote comfort, because some cramping can occur. Discharge teaching should include signs of infection and advice that the x-ray dye can stain clothing. Provide a perineal pad following the procedure and advise the patient to wear a perineal pad until vaginal drainage stops.

NURSING CARE TIP

No one is really allergic to iodine—iodine is an essential element in our bodies. But some people may be allergic to dyes that contain iodine. It is still important to ask about iodine allergy, because that is how some women identify an allergy to dye.

Endoscopic Examinations

Several types of endoscopic examinations are done to visually inspect internal areas to diagnose (and sometimes treat) reproductive system disorders. The names of the tests vary according to the area inspected, but all generally make use of a fiber-optic light and lens system, which is inserted through a tube called a cannula into a small incision. A laparoscopy is done to view the abdominal cavity and is useful for identifying problems such as endometriosis (Fig. 41.11). A **salpingoscopy** is performed to see the inside of the fallopian tubes and a **hysteroscopy** to see the inside of the uterus. A binocular microscope is used with an endoscope that is introduced into the vagina to closely study lesions of the cervix during a **colposcopy**. During **culdoscopy**, an endoscope is introduced into the vagina and through a small incision in the vagina into the cul-de-sac of Douglas, a cavity behind the uterus, to observe for abnormalities in this region (Fig. 41.12).

NURSING CARE.   Preoperatively the patient is prepared for an endoscopic examination according to agency protocol. This generally involves asking the patient whether she has fasted as instructed, assessing vital signs, recording the time of last voiding, helping the patient into a gown, and ensuring that the consent form has been signed. General anesthesia may be given for some endoscopic procedures. Explain what to expect and provide support for the woman. She may be anxious about possible disorders.

Postoperatively, provide comfort measures. These procedures produce almost no blood loss. The woman may experience pain in the neck, shoulders, and upper back if

• WORD • BUILDING •

hysterosalpingogram: hystero—womb + salpingo—tube + gram—record
salpingoscopy: salpingo—tube + scopy—looking
hysteroscopy: hystero—womb + scopy—looking
colposcopy: colpo—vagina + scopy—looking
culdoscopy: culdo—cul de sac + scopy—looking

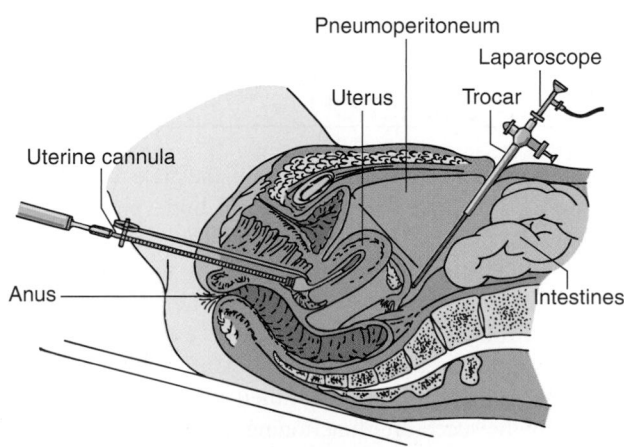

FIGURE 41.11 Laparoscopy. Modified from Cavanaugh, B. M. (2003). *Nurse's manual of laboratory and diagnostic tests* (4th ed.). Philadelphia: F.A. Davis, with permission.

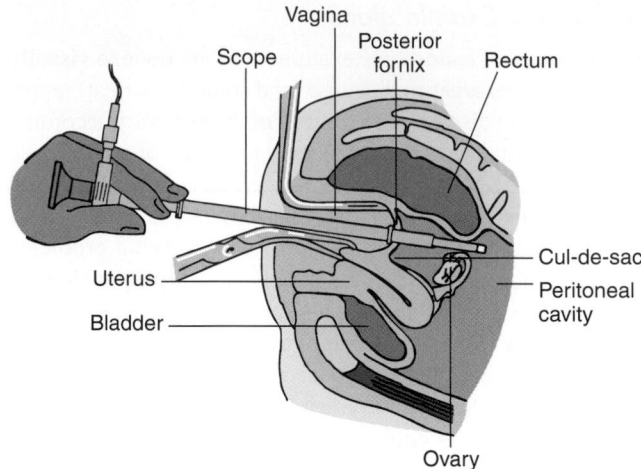

FIGURE 41.12 Culdoscopy. Modified from Cavanaugh, B. M. (2003). *Nurse's manual of laboratory and diagnostic tests* (4th ed.). Philadelphia: F.A. Davis, with permission.

carbon dioxide (CO_2) gas was pumped into the body compartment being examined. This is called **insufflation** and is done to increase the distance between structures, so that it is easier for the physician to visualize structures. The CO_2 remaining after completion of the examination travels to the highest level of the body before being absorbed, so lying flat for a few hours after the examination may decrease discomfort. If incisions were made through the abdominal wall for insertion of the endoscope and for insufflation, these are tiny and a Band-Aid or small dressing is applied.

PATIENT EDUCATION. Advise the patient to observe the incision sites for redness, bleeding, or drainage, seeking evaluation by the physician promptly if these should occur or otherwise seeing the physician as directed for suture removal. If the endoscopic procedure was done transvaginally, provide a perineal pad following the procedure and advise the patient to wear a pad until the drainage stops. Also instruct the patient to report any bright bleeding after the operative day and to report any fever or foul-smelling discharge. See Table 41.6 for a summary of diagnostic tests.

MALE REPRODUCTIVE SYSTEM DATA COLLECTION

As with the female reproductive system, the male reproductive system is a complex interaction of both physical and psychosocial factors. Unlike women, however, men may find it much more difficult in our society to talk about or admit to having problems related to reproductive health. From toilet training through adulthood, men are expected to have behaviors associated with maleness. Unfortunately, by the time some boys reach manhood, their male identity is often defined by the successful functioning of their sex organs.

One of the important first steps in obtaining a male reproductive assessment is to provide a comfortable, nonjudgmental, confidential atmosphere for discussion. This means you must

first be knowledgeable and comfortable with sexual issues. Although it may be challenging to ask questions about **erection** or ejaculation history, such questions may allow men to talk about difficulties they are experiencing. Be open and straightforward with all questions and answers. It may be necessary at times to use more commonly expressed sexual words instead of medical terminology. You will discover that many men do not know the function of their prostate gland or the difference between ejaculation and **orgasm**. Use the assessment as an opportunity to teach men the facts about their own sexual functioning.

Health History

Some basic questions to ask a male patient during a reproductive assessment are found in Table 41.7. As mentioned earlier, a professional, matter-of-fact attitude, along with an explanation as to why the questions are necessary, can put both you and the patient at ease while collecting data.

Physical Examination

The physical examination is generally performed by a physician or provider trained in physical assessments. The examination begins with the patient's general appearance. He is observed for male patterns of hair growth on the head, face, chest, arms, and legs. Normal male pubic hair pattern is in a triangular shape, with hair growth up toward the umbilicus. The patient's height and muscle mass are noted. Men are commonly taller than 5 feet, 6 inches tall, weigh more than 135 pounds, and have shoulders that are broader than their hips. The presence of excess breast tissue may indicate **gynecomastia**, from an excess of female hormones. Abnormal findings in either hair patterns or muscle mass often indicate a hormone imbalance.

The penis, scrotum, and testes (testicles) are examined by observation and palpation. On observation, the penis is normally flaccid (soft) and hanging straight down. The size can vary greatly and should not be a concern unless it is unusually small (microphallus) or edematous. The left testis typically hangs slightly lower in the scrotum than the right.

The penis is examined for warts, sores (evidence of STIs), swelling, curves, or lumps along the shaft. The examiner also makes sure the urethral opening is at the tip of the penis and not on the underside of the shaft (**hypospadias**) or on the dorsum of the shaft (**epispadias**). If the man is not **circumcised** (surgical removal of the foreskin), the foreskin should be pulled back carefully and the glans inspected for signs of inflammation or foul-smelling discharge. The provider should be sure to replace the foreskin in the forward position after the examination is completed.

The scrotum and testes are carefully examined and palpated. Both testes should be present and a normal size (approximately

---

• WORD • BUILDING •

insufflation: in—in + suffl—to blow + ation—process
gynecomastia: gyneco—female + mastia—breast
hypospadias: hypo—under + spadias—span, to draw
epispadias: epi—upon + spadias—span, to draw
circumcised: circum—around + cised—cut

TABLE 41.6 DIAGNOSTIC PROCEDURES FOR THE FEMALE REPRODUCTIVE SYSTEM

Procedure	Definition/ Normal Finding	Significance of Abnormal Findings	Nursing Management
Noninvasive			
Breast self-examination (BSE), clinical breast examination (CBE)	Assessment of breast tissue by patient (BSE) or HCP (CBE) through inspection and palpation	Abnormal physical exam may indicate pathology and does indicate need for further assessment.	Educate about appropriate technique and observe a return demonstration of BSE. Education about BSE may be demonstrated during CBE.
Ultrasound/sonography	High-frequency sound waves bounce off tissue to map tissue structure and determine tissue density. Also may be used to guide biopsy procedure.	May help to determine abnormal lesions, abnormalities of tissue structure, or presence of abnormal fluid volume.	Follow institutional guidelines for patient preparation and support, which may be determined by testing goals.
Mammography	Radiographic examination of tissue. X-ray may be used with dye contrast injected into body before procedure.	May help to determine abnormal lesions or abnormalities of normal tissue structure.	Educate patient not to apply lotions, powders or deodorant before test. If dye is used, inquire about past allergic reaction to dye and/or observe for allergic response.
Thermography, computed tomography (CT), magnetic resonance imaging (MRI)	Precise pictures of tissue using temperature (thermography), x-ray (computed tomography), or radiofrequency (MRI)	May help to determine abnormal lesions or abnormalities of normal tissue structure.	Ask patients about presence of metal or wire inside their bodies before MRI because the procedure may then be contraindicated.
Hormonal tests	Assessment of endocrine function related to reproduction	Abnormal hormone levels may reflect fertility potential, determine reasons for abnormal menses, identify hormone-producing tumors, or evaluate hormone replacement.	Explain procedure to patient and provide support.
Invasive			
Pelvic examination, bimanual examination	Inspection and palpation of external/internal reproductive organs by HCP	Abnormal physical examination may detect pathology or may indicate need for further testing.	Explain procedure to patient and provide support. Consult institutional policies for specific instructions.

Continued

TABLE 41.6 DIAGNOSTIC PROCEDURES FOR THE FEMALE REPRODUCTIVE SYSTEM—cont'd

Procedure	Definition/ Normal Finding	Significance of Abnormal Findings	Nursing Management
Biopsy, cytology, swabs, smears	Obtainment of body cells/tissue through aspiration or excision or by swabbing/scrapping of tissue/exudate	May diagnose pathology or infection.	Explain procedure to patient and provide support. Consult institutional policies for specific instructions.
Endoscopy, laparoscopy	Use of fiber-optic light and lens system to inspect internal structures	May help to determine abnormal lesions or abnormalities of normal tissue structure. Tissue biopsies may be taken during procedure.	Explain procedure to patient and provide support. Observe for postprocedure complications.

TABLE 41.7 SUBJECTIVE DATA COLLECTION FOR THE MALE REPRODUCTIVE SYSTEM AND SEXUAL HEALTH

Category	Questions to Ask During the Health History	Rationale/Significance
Medication	Are you using any medications? (Include prescription, over-the-counter, and herbal remedies.) How much/how often? (For medications that affect sexual desire, erection, or ejaculation, see Chapter 43.)	Loss of sexual desire, erection, ejaculation, orgasm, or fertility can occur as a result of some medication use.
Family History	Do you have a family history of genetically transmitted diseases (e.g., heart problems, hypertension, diabetes, cancer)? Did your mother use DES during pregnancy?	These conditions put men at high risk for circulation problems that interfere with erections, or congenital anomalies of reproductive organs.
Personal Habits and Health Promotion Behaviors	Do you smoke, consume caffeine, drink alcohol, use recreational drugs, or use steroids? How much/how often? Do you use hot tubs, engage in long-distance drives, or ride a bike? How much/how often? Do you use contraceptives? What type of contraceptives do you use? How do you use them? Do you do TSE? Have you noticed any changes in your testicles or other reproductive organs?	These habits may lead to decreased blood flow to penis, loss of erection; decreased testosterone (male hormone) interferes with erection and fertility; excessive heat decreases sperm production. Data will reveal knowledge/practice of health promotion behaviors, meaning of health, as well as history of changes or abnormalities.
Personal Health History	Did you have mumps during adolescence or have you recently had an infection or fever?	Some infectious processes may lead to decreased sperm production.

TABLE 41.7 SUBJECTIVE DATA COLLECTION FOR THE MALE REPRODUCTIVE SYSTEM AND SEXUAL HEALTH—cont'd

Category	Questions to Ask During the Health History	Rationale/Significance
Mental Health	Are you experiencing stress? How do you deal with stress? Are you having problems with a sexual partner? Have you ever or are you experiencing performance anxiety or depression?	Decreased sexual desire and ability to have an erection may result from mental and/or emotional stress.
Circulatory/Respiratory	Have you ever been diagnosed with or treated for heart problems/surgery, high blood pressure, sickle cell disease, lung disease, or sleep apnea?	Decreased circulation can lead to inability to have usable erection; decreased respiratory function can result in activity intolerance, loss of erection.
Gastrointestinal	Have you ever been diagnosed or treated for liver infection/disease or bowel problems?	Liver infections/disease can lead to decreased testosterone and increased estrogen production, and loss of erection; gastrointestinal/bowel problems can lead to pain, loss of desire; surgery may result in loss of blood flow or innervation.
Musculoskeletal	Do you have painful joints, pelvic/lower back pain, or nerve damage?	Pain, loss of desire; limited movement/positions, loss of erection, ejaculation, and orgasm may result from musculoskeletal problems.
Neurologic	Have you ever experienced a stroke or suffered from multiple sclerosis, Parkinson's disease, or other neurologic disorders?	Limited movement/positions, loss of sensations, and loss of control can result from neurologic problems.
Metabolic/Endocrine	Have you ever suffered from diabetes, obesity, or thyroid problems?	Diabetes mellitus can result in circulation problems, retrograde ejaculation, nerve damage; obesity can result in decreased male hormones, excess female hormones.
Genitourinary	Have you ever been diagnosed with a congenital deformity of the penis/testicles, suffered from prostate problems, or experienced erection/ejaculation problems? Have you ever been diagnosed with a sexually transmitted disease? When, what type, and how was it treated? That you are aware, was treatment successful? Do you have any lesions, pain, discharge, or swelling of the reproductive organs? Have you noticed any abnormalities/changes in size, shape, or color of your external reproductive organs? (Describe)	Difficulty with erection, penetration problems, retrograde ejaculation, or infertility may be associated with genitourinary abnormalities, stress, or medication use. Lesions, pain, discharge, swelling, or other abnormalities of the external reproductive organs may indicate infection, structural abnormalities such as varicocele, or other disease processes such as cancer.

Continued

TABLE **41.7** SUBJECTIVE DATA COLLECTION FOR THE MALE REPRODUCTIVE SYSTEM AND SEXUAL HEALTH—cont'd

Category	Questions to Ask During the Health History	Rationale/Significance
	For patients younger than age 40: "Do you practice monthly testicular self-examinations?" For patients older than age 40: "When was the last time you had a prostate examination?"	Men younger than age 40 should be encouraged to perform monthly testicular examinations as a cancer prevention measure. A digital rectal examination (DRE) should be a regular part of a man's routine physical after age 41. Prostate cancer is treatable when detected early.
Sexual Practices	Are you sexually active? How many partners do you have? Of what gender? How often do you have intercourse (including positions, timing with female ovulation cycle if heterosexual)? Is the amount/type of sexual activity satisfying? Do you masturbate or use lubricants?	Some sexual practices can lead to a decrease in quality and quantity of sperm that reach the female egg.

Note. DES = diethylstilbestrol; TSE = testicular self-examination.

2–4 cm). The testes are egg shaped and should feel smooth and rubbery when lightly palpated between the thumb and fingers. The epididymis can be felt along the top edge and posterior section of each testis. The testes and scrotum are palpated for any lumps, cysts, or tumors. If a fluid-filled mass (**hydrocele**) is found, further evaluation should be done.

A simple noninvasive test called **transillumination** is used to determine if a mass is fluid filled or solid. With the room lights out, a flashlight is held behind the scrotum. If the mass is fluid, a red glow appears; if it is solid, it appears opaque. Each spermatic cord (made up of veins, arteries, lymphatics, nerves, and the vas deferens) is palpated and should feel firm and threadlike. If a condition called a **varicocele** is present, the area feels like a bag of worms. A varicocele, which is swelling of the veins of the spermatic cord, is one of the most common problems associated with male infertility.

 BE SAFE!

Wrap the flashlight with clear plastic wrap to decrease the risk of contamination. Change the wrap between patients.

The male patient is also examined for inguinal hernias by pressing up through the scrotum into each of the inguinal rings while asking him to cough or bear down. Each side is examined separately while he is in the standing position. A hernia feels like a pulsation against the examiner's fingertips.

A digital rectal examination (DRE) may be done by an experienced practitioner. During DRE, the prostate gland is palpated by inserting a gloved, lubricated finger into the rectum while the man is in Sim's position or standing and bending at a right angle over the exam table. The entire posterior lobe of the gland can be felt this way. The gland should feel slightly firm and without any lumps. If the prostate gland feels very hard or soft, enlarged, or contains any lumps, a rectal ultrasound with needle biopsy is often ordered. A swollen, painful prostate generally indicates that an infection is present.

Remind all men older than age 40 that unless they have had a complete removal of the prostate gland, they still need a DRE every year. Many men are under the impression that any prostate surgery means the gland has been completely removed. When simple surgery is performed, prostate tissue is left in the body and will begin to regrow over time. This prostatic tissue can become cancerous and needs to be monitored with a yearly DRE. See Table 41.8 for a summary of objective data to collect for the male reproductive system.

Testicular Self-Examination

All men after puberty should do a monthly testicular self-examination (TSE) to detect any tumors or other changes in the scrotum (Figure 41.13). See Box 41-1 for instructions that can be used to teach a man how to examine his testicles.

• **WORD • BUILDING •**

hydrocele: hydro—water + cele—hernia
transillumination: trans—across + illumin—light + ation—process
varicocele: varico—twisted vein + cele—swelling

<table>
<tr><td>

CRITICAL THINKING

Tony

■ Tony is a 20-year-old who reports a "bump" on his right testicle. He comes into the health clinic and asks if he can take any medication for his "disease."

1. What would be the best action?
2. What should your health assessment include?

Suggested answers are at the end of the chapter.

</td></tr>
</table>

Breast Self-Examination

Although breast cancer in men is rare, it can occur. Men, like women, should be familiar with their breasts and report changes.

Diagnostic Tests of the Male Reproductive System
Ultrasound

An ultrasound may be done to diagnose or evaluate a variety of male reproductive or genitourinary problems. A transrectal ultrasound may be done to diagnose prostate cancer. For this procedure, a rectal probe transducer is inserted into the rectum and sound waves are used to evaluate the prostate gland.

TABLE 41.8 OBJECTIVE DATA COLLECTION FOR THE MALE REPRODUCTIVE SYSTEM

Category	Physical Examination Findings	Possible Abnormal Findings/Causes
Clinical Breast Examination	Observe and palpate for presence of swelling, lumps, skin changes, nipple exudates.	Changes may indicate breast cancer, although it is rare in males.
Glans of Penis	Observe for lesions, exudate, tenderness. Observe for placement of the urethra. If foreskin is present, attempt to reduce to observe for lesions, exudate, inflammation. (Be sure to replace when finished to prevent paraphimosis).	Lesions, exudate, tenderness can indicate presence of infective or disease process, injury. Epispadias/hypospadias may be noted when observing for placement of the urethra.
Shaft of Penis	Observe for lesions, tenderness, shape.	Lesions, exudate, tenderness can indicate presence of infectious or disease process, injury. Irregularity of shape may indicate structural abnormalities/disease.
Scrotum	Visualize and palpate for swelling, pain, lesions.	Inguinal herniation may be noted. Swelling may occur with heart or renal failure, local inflammation, injury.
Testes	Palpate for descent, pain, lesions, size, shape, consistency. Palpate for lesions/swelling of epididymitis.	Absence of palpated testes may indicate nondescent. Testicular lesion can indicate testicular cancer. Swelling, pain can indicate infectious process.
Spermatic Cord	Palpate for swelling, size, consistency, pain	Presence of swelling, pain can indicate infection or varicocele.
Inguinal Ring (exam performed by trained personnel)	Palpate for bulge, pain.	Bulge, pain may indicate inguinal hernia.
Inguinal Lymph Nodes	Palpate for swelling, pain.	Swelling, pain may indicate infectious process or regional malignancy.
Digital Rectal Exam (DRE; exam performed by trained personnel)	Observe external rectum for lesions, exudate. Palpate for pain, swelling, penile exudate.	Pain, swelling, exudate may indicate benign changes, infectious process, cancer, or injury.

Note. A male physical examination is typically done by a physician or other trained provider.

FIGURE 41.13 Testicular self-examination.

Box 41-1 **Guidelines for Monthly Testicular Self-Examination**

A testicular self-examination is easiest during or right after a warm shower or bath, when the scrotum is relaxed and the testicles are hanging low. Choose 1 day a month to always do the examination.

1. Raise the penis up out of the way and look for any difference in size or shape of each side of the scrotum (sac). The left side usually hangs a little lower than the right.
2. Using both hands, hold the scrotum in the palms. Begin, one at a time, to gently roll each testicle between the thumb and first three fingers, feeling for any lumps or hard spots.
3. Identify the parts. The testicles should feel round, smooth, and egg shaped. The epididymis along the top and back side should feel soft and a little bit tender. The spermatic cord is a tube that runs from the epididymis and usually feels firm, smooth, and movable.
4. See your physician immediately if you feel any lumps or unusual changes.

Pelvic or scrotal ultrasound helps evaluate and locate masses. Ultrasound may also be done to guide a needle during a fine-needle biopsy.

NURSING CARE. Explain the procedure to the patient. An enema may be ordered before the procedure. No special aftercare is needed.

Cystourethroscopy

A cystourethroscopy may be done to evaluate the degree of obstruction by an enlarged prostate gland. For this procedure, a Foley catheter is inserted, and a dye is injected into the bladder. Radiographs are taken with the dye in the bladder and while voiding after the catheter has been removed.

NURSING CARE. Explain the procedure to the patient and assess for allergy to dye. Instruct the patient to void before the procedure. A sedative or analgesic may be ordered to help the patient relax during the procedure. If an analgesic is used, the patient will need to have someone available to drive him home.

After the procedure, intake and output are measured for 24 hours and alteration from the patient's normal pattern, such as blood in the urine or absence of urination, is reported to the physician. Fluids are encouraged to promote excretion of the dye. A warm, moist cloth held over the urethra can assist with mild pain.

Laboratory Tests

PROSTATE-SPECIFIC ANTIGEN. Prostate-specific antigen (PSA) is a glycoprotein produced by prostate cells. The normal value of PSA is less than 4 ng/L. An elevated level indicates prostatic hypertrophy or cancer.

PROSTATIC ACID PHOSPHATASE. Prostatic acid phosphatase (PAP) is an enzyme that normally affects metabolism of prostate cancer cells. The normal value of PAP is less than 3 ng/mL. An elevated level indicates prostate cancer.

OTHER TESTS. If prostate cancer is suspected or diagnosed, additional tests may be done. Acid phosphatase may be elevated in metastatic prostate cancer. Alkaline phosphatase and serum calcium levels may be elevated if metastasis to the bone has occurred. See Table 41.9 for a summary of diagnostic procedures.

Tests for Infertility

Various hormone levels may be measured, including FSH, LH, testosterone, and adrenocorticotropic hormone (ACTH) to help determine causes of infertility in male patients.

Semen analysis may be done to provide information about causes of infertility or to evaluate whether a vasectomy has been effective. Semen may be analyzed for sperm count, motility, and shape. Other tests determine whether the semen contains adequate nutrients to support sperm, whether antibodies to the sperm are present, and the ability of the sperm to penetrate an ovum.

NURSING CARE. The patient is instructed to refrain from ejaculation for 3 days before collecting the semen sample to avoid altering findings. Generally, specimens are collected on three separate occasions over a period of 4 to 6 days. Masturbation and ejaculation directly into a sterile container are recommended to avoid loss of semen. Condoms and lubricants should be avoided. The sample should be taken to the laboratory within 1 hour of collection. Additional tests of the male reproductive system are discussed in Chapter 43.

TABLE 41.9 DIAGNOSTIC PROCEDURES FOR THE MALE REPRODUCTIVE SYSTEM

Procedure	Definition/ Normal Finding	Significance of Abnormal Findings	Nursing Management
Noninvasive			
Testicular self-examination (TSE)	Palpation of testes by patient.	Abnormalities may indicate pathology and require further evaluation.	Instruct patient on appropriate technique and witness a return demonstration.
Ultrasound	High-frequency sound waves bounce off tissue to map tissue structure and determine tissue density. Also may be used to guide biopsy procedure.	May help to determine abnormal lesions, abnormalities of tissue structure, or presence of abnormal fluid volume.	Follow institutional guidelines for patient preparation and support.
Hormonal tests, antigen level testing	Blood test to measure hormone or antigen levels.	Abnormal hormone levels may reflect fertility potential. Abnormal antigen levels may indicate pathology.	Consult institutional policies for specific instructions for each test. Explain procedure to patient and provide support.
Invasive			
Digital rectal examination	Palpation of internal reproductive organs, especially prostate gland, through rectum.	Abnormal physical exam may indicate pathology and indicates need for further testing.	Educate patient about procedure and provide support.
Cystourethroscopy	Insertion of a Foley catheter and dye into the bladder to evaluate for obstruction (usually an enlarged prostate) by radiography.	Obstruction may cause difficulty with urination.	Educate patient about the procedure and postprocedure care. Instruct patient to void before procedure. Measure intake and output for 24 hours following procedure. Observe for allergic reaction.

SUGGESTED ANSWERS TO

CRITICAL THINKING

■ *Jilli*

1. The answer should include basic breast health statistics and risks, as well as proper assessment practice and techniques as discussed in this chapter. She should be informed that although monthly BSE is not absolutely necessary, knowing her breasts and reporting changes is essential. Technique should be demonstrated and a return demonstration received during the visit.

2. Questions about breast health and self-assessment practices provide an opportunity for the nurse to educate a patient about health facts and technique. Patient questions can also be a cue to patient readiness and willingness to learn.

■ *Reproductive Assessment*

1. Calm fears. Explain simply. Allow the parent to stay with the child during the examination if appropriate. Consider whether it is possible that the child has been abused. If so, evidence needs to be collected and a report

Continued

SUGGESTED ANSWERS TO—cont'd

filed with the appropriate child protection authorities. Check with your supervisor if you believe this is a possibility. Teach the child that this is a normal part of the body that is to be protected and taken care of.

2. Assess knowledge and maturity. Prepare the patient for a Pap smear and for swabs and smears. Teach while getting supplies ready. Explain that vaginal soreness usually needs to be treated and that the physician must know more about the problem to do so effectively. Explain that inflammations can interfere with Pap smear results, so testing may have to be repeated after treatment. Explain culture and sensitivity testing. Teach about risk reduction and inform that oral contraceptives do not offer a barrier against sexually transmitted infections.

3. Try to put the woman at ease through general conversation. Set out supplies for a Pap smear (if needed) and for swabs and smears. Teach while getting supplies ready. Discuss aging and the effects of decreased estrogen in general and specifically on vaginal tissues. Inform her that there are several ways to deal with problems resulting from decreased estrogen, such as oral hormonal replacements, water-soluble vaginal lubricants, vaginal creams, estrogen patches, and estrogen receptor modulator medication.

■ *Tony*

1. Palpable scrotal changes can result from a variety of reproductive and/or genitourinary abnormalities. Before Tony's question can be answered, a complete history needs to be obtained and a clinical exam of the genitalia performed.

2. The history should explore:
   - If TSEs are regularly performed and if changes have been noted.
   - If Tony is sexually active and has, recently or in the past, been knowingly exposed to an STI.
   - If there has been pain associated with the "bump" or exudate noted from the penis.

   The assessment, done by a physician or primary care provider should include:
   - Visual inspection of the size, shape, symmetry, and color of the scrotum and its contents.
   - Palpation to assess for abnormalities and pain.
   - Cultures to rule out STIs.
   - An inguinal exam to rule out herniation.

   Ultimately, based on the patient's report, a testicular tumor should be ruled out.

REVIEW QUESTIONS

1. When obtaining the history of a 17-year-old male during a sports physical, what important screening practice should be discussed?
   1. Yearly DRE
   2. Monthly TSE
   3. Yearly PSA
   4. Bimonthly bimanual examination

2. A patient has just had a laparoscopy to investigate the causes of her infertility. Why should the nurse instruct her to lie flat in the bed for a few hours?
   1. She could rupture her abdominal incision.
   2. Her blood pressure will be low because of blood loss.
   3. The carbon dioxide left over from the test will travel upward and cause pain.
   4. Her uterus needs to be at the same level as her heart to prevent excessive swelling.

3. A 66-year-old woman is seen in an outpatient clinic for routine care. What teaching should the nurse provide related to bone health?
   1. "You should be taking in at least 1200 mg of calcium and 600 international units of vitamin D in your diet."
   2. "The benefit of eating red meat outweighs the risk as you age. You should eat 6 ounces three times a week."
   3. "Your bones are protected by the calcium you ate in your younger years; increasing intake now will not help your bones."
   4. "It is important to take a calcium and vitamin D supplement, because it is difficult to get enough in your diet."

4. How would the nurse document the reproductive history of a pregnant woman who is in her fourth pregnancy, has two living children ages 3 and 5, and had one miscarriage?
   1. P4G2M1
   2. G4P3P5M1
   3. P4G35A1
   4. G4P2A1

5. What is the role of the LPN/LVN in physical assessment of the male and female genitals?
   1. Perform a complete history and physical assessment of the genital area.
   2. Collect specimens under the supervision of the RN.
   3. Prepare the patient for what to expect during the practitioner's examination.
   4. The LPN/LVN does not have a role in assessment of the reproductive system.

Answers can be found in Appendix C.

References

American Cancer Society. (2013). *American Cancer Society Guidelines for the early detection of cancer.* Retrieved August 6, 2013, from www.cancer.org/healthy/findcancerearly /cancerscreeningguidelines/american-cancer-society -guidelines-for-the-early-detection-of-cancer

Joint Commission. (2013). *2014 national patient safety goals.* Retrieved August 6, 2013, from www.jointcommission.org /patientsafety/nationalpatientsafetygoals

 Davis*Plus* | For additional resources and information visit **davispl.us/medsurg5**

42

Nursing Care of Women With Reproductive System Disorders

LAURA L. McCULLY AND
DEBRA PERRY-PHILO

KEY TERMS

agenesis (ay-JEN-uh-sis)
amenorrhea (AY-men-oh-REE-ah)
anteflexion (AN-tee-FLEK-shun)
anteversion (AN-tee-VER-zhun)
augmentation (AWG-men-TAY-shun)
colporrhaphy (kohl-POOR-ah-fee)
contraceptive (KON-truh-SEP-tiv)
cryotherapy (KRY-oh-THER-uh-pee)
culdocentesis (KUL-doh-sen-TEE-sis)
culdotomy (kul-DOT-uh-mee)
cystocele (SIS-toh-seel)
dermoid (DER-moyd)
dilation and curettage (DIL-AY-shun and kyoor-e-TAHZH)
dysmenorrhea (DIS-men-oh-REE-ah)
dyspareunia (DIS-puh-ROO-nee-ah)
dysplasia (dis-PLAY-zee-ah)
fibrocystic (FIGH-broh-SIS-tik)
hypertrophy (high-PER-truh-fee)
hypoplasia (HEYE-poh-PLAY-zee-ah)
hysterectomy (HISS-tuh-REK-tuh-mee)
hysterotomy (HISS-tuh-RAH-tuh-mee)
imperforate (im-PER-foh-rate)
in vitro fertilization (in-VEE-troh FER-ti-li-ZAY-shun)
laparotomy (LAP-uh-RAH-tuh-mee)
leiomyoma (LYE-oh-my-OH-mah)
lumpectomy (lump-EK-tuh-mee)
mammoplasty (MAM-oh-PLAS-tee)
marsupialization (mar-SOO-pee-al-i-ZAY-shun)
mastalgia (mass-TAL-jee-ah)
mastectomy (mass-TEK-tuh-mee)
mastitis (mass-TIGH-tis)
mastopexy (MAS-toh-PEKS-ee)
myomectomy (MY-oh-MEK-tuh-mee)
oophorectomy (oo-fur-EK-tuh-mee)
perimenopause (PER-ee-MEN-oh-PAWS)
phytoestrogens (FY-toh-ES-troh-jenz)
postcoital (post-KOH-i-tal)
rectocele (REK-toh-seel)
retroflexion (RET-roh-FLEK-shun)

LEARNING OUTCOMES

1. Explain the pathophysiology of each of the disorders of the female reproductive system.

2. Describe the etiologies, signs, and symptoms of each disorder.

3. Identify tests used to diagnose female disorders.

4. Describe current therapeutic management for each disorder.

5. List data to collect when caring for patients with disorders of the female reproductive system.

6. Plan nursing care for female patients with reproductive disorders.

7. Explain how you will know if nursing interventions have been effective.

8. Compare different forms of contraceptives and their effectiveness.

KEY TERMS *continued*

retrograde (RET-roh-grayd)	**salpingectomy** (sal-pin-JEK-tuh-mee)	**vaginitis** (VAJ-in-EYE-tis)
retroversion (RET-roh-VER-zhun)	**teratoma** (ter-uh-TOH-muh)	**vaginosis** (VAJ-in-OH-sis)

Reproductive system disorders can be frightening, irritating, frustrating, embarrassing, and in some cases fatal. They involve not just body parts but also roles, relationships, and sense of identity and purpose in life. Nurses can play an important role in helping women with these disorders. Women's health is an area in which much research is being done. The Nurses' Health Study, conducted at Harvard Medical School, is a large ongoing study on many topics related to women's health. You can learn about it at www.nurseshealthstudy.org.

BREAST DISORDERS

Benign Breast Disorders

Much has been done in recent years to educate the general public concerning breast cancer. It is the most commonly diagnosed cancer in women (Centers for Disease Control and Prevention [CDC], 2011). Heightened awareness of the risks of breast cancer, however, sometimes results in excessive anxiety among women with benign breast conditions. The following section covers benign, or noncancerous, breast disorders.

Cyclic Breast Discomfort

PATHOPHYSIOLOGY, ETIOLOGIES, AND SIGNS AND SYMPTOMS. The most common breast symptoms result from cyclic variations in hormone levels. Swelling, tenderness, and sometimes pain (**mastalgia**) can be related to hormone-mediated changes within the breast tissues that prepare them for their potential role of breastfeeding.

TREATMENT. If persistent or severe, these symptoms can be treated with oral contraceptives that modify hormone levels or nonsteroidal anti-inflammatory drugs (NSAIDs) to control pain. Explaining that cyclic discomfort is temporary and not from a disease process helps to reduce fears.

Fibrocystic Breast Disease

Fibrocystic breast disease is common in women between the ages of 30 and 50. Many refer to it as simply "fibrocystic breast changes."

PATHOPHYSIOLOGY, ETIOLOGIES, AND SIGNS AND SYMPTOMS. Overresponsiveness of cells in the breasts to hormonal stimulation (especially estrogen) can cause long-term changes resulting in replacement of normal tissue with fibrous tissue, overdevelopment of cells, and blockage of ducts so that cysts form around trapped fluid. This makes the breasts feel somewhat hard and lumpy, and sometimes painful. These changes often occur during the reproductive years, and can respond to hormonal variations during the menstrual cycle. Fibrocystic changes usually subside with menopause.

DIAGNOSIS AND TREATMENT. Fibrocystic breast changes can be identified on palpation. A mammogram or ultrasound may be done to assist in diagnosis. A biopsy may be done to rule out cancer. Treatment for fibrocystic breast changes is based on patient symptoms. Often, no treatment is necessary. Analgesics, primarily NSAIDs, help reduce discomfort. Herbal remedies such as evening primrose oil, or supplemental vitamin therapy may offer symptomatic relief, but these therapies remain controversial. Limitation of dietary fat and caffeine and addition of oral contraceptive use may help control hormonal changes.

Although fibrocystic changes are not cancerous, more frequent mammography or ultrasound may be advised because fibrocystic changes can make it more difficult to feel early cancerous lumps during breast examination. Some types of breast cysts are associated with a higher cancer risk. Needle aspiration may be used to treat cystic lesions.

Mastitis

PATHOPHYSIOLOGY, ETIOLOGIES, AND SIGNS AND SYMPTOMS. Breast infection with inflammation (**mastitis**) occurs as a result of injury and introduction of bacteria into the breast. This condition most commonly occurs while breastfeeding. The breast becomes swollen, hot, red, and painful and can form an abscess.

TREATMENT. Mastitis can be treated either with antibiotics or by incision and drainage (I&D) of the abscessed area. NSAIDs, warm packs, and breast supports are often used to control pain and swelling.

NURSING CARE AND PATIENT EDUCATION. Teach the patient to wash her hands carefully to prevent the spread of infection. If the patient is breastfeeding, it is often continued to promote drainage of the breast, mother–infant bonding, and infant nutrition. The infant is often already colonized with the bacteria so further exposure is not thought to be detrimental.

• **WORD • BUILDING •**
mastalgia: mast—breast + algia—pain
fibrocystic: fibro—fibrous + cystic—saclike
mastitis: mast—breast + itis—inflammation

NURSING CARE TIP

To help prevent mastitis in a breastfeeding mother, recommend frequent changes in feeding positions to empty all portions of the breast, as well as good hand hygiene techniques when handling the breasts. Also recommend breastfeeding frequently, not restricting the length of feeds.

Malignant Breast Disorders

Pathophysiology and Etiology

Breast cancer is an abnormal growth of breast cells. It can arise from the milk-producing glands, the ductal system, or the fatty and connective tissues of the breast.

Research has identified factors that increase the risk of breast cancer: increasing age; personal or family history of breast, ovarian, or prostate cancer; a high-fat diet; high alcohol intake; treatment with estrogens (especially when used without progestins); early menarche; late menopause; and first pregnancy after age 25.

Signs and Symptoms

A lump or thickening of breast tissue, or a change in the shape or contour of a breast can indicate breast cancer. A tumor can also cause dimpling of the overlying skin or retraction of the nipple. Clear or bloody nipple discharge can occur. Swelling, tenderness, or discoloration of the breast can indicate inflammatory breast cancer, a rare but deadly form. Breast symptoms have many causes, but all should be investigated by a health care provider (HCP).

Prevention

Breast cancer risk can be reduced by exercising moderation in fat and alcohol consumption and using nonhormonal methods for birth control and menopausal symptoms. Breastfeeding may also reduce risk, even in women who have late first pregnancies (see "Evidence-Based Practice" box). However, many factors cannot be controlled, so the importance of early detection cannot be overemphasized. Recent research has discovered genes (*BRCA1* and *BRCA2*) that are linked with susceptibility to breast cancer. These findings offer the possibility of very early identification of women at the most risk of developing breast cancer (and also ovarian cancer for those with *BRCA1*). These women can then be monitored closely for breast changes and receive early treatment if cancer develops. Some women choose to have bilateral prophylactic (or risk-reducing) mastectomy.

Before any genetic testing, patients should be counseled by a professional who is qualified to explain and interpret the results. It is also important to review risk and benefits of doing testing before having testing done. Some insurance plans don't cover the expensive cost of such testing. More information regarding *BRCA* testing can be found at www.cancer.gov/cancertopics/factsheet/Risk/BRCA.

EVIDENCE-BASED PRACTICE

Clinical Question

Does breastfeeding reduce risk of breast cancer?

Evidence

A systematic review of 31 research studies was undertaken (Yang & Jacobsen, 2008). Eleven found that breastfeeding significantly reduces breast cancer risk, and 13 studies found a reduced risk only with extended lactation. Kotsopoulos et al (2012) found that breastfeeding protects against BRCA1- but not BRCA2-associated breast cancer.

Implications for Nursing Practice

There are many reasons to advise women to breastfeed their babies in addition to obvious benefits for the babies. Possible protection against breast cancer is one reason. Women with the BRCA mutation should be advised of the benefits of breastfeeding.

REFERENCES

Yang, L., & Jacobsen, K. H. (2008). A systematic review of the association between breastfeeding and breast cancer. *Journal of Women's Health, 17,* 1635–1645.

Kotsopoulos, J., Lubinski, J., Salmena, L., Lynch, H. T., Kim-Sing, C., Foulkes, W. D., . . . Narod, S. A. (2012). Breastfeeding and the risk of breast cancer in BRCA1 and BRCA2 mutation carriers. *Breast Cancer Research 14.* Retrieved July 17, 2013, from http://breast-cancer-research.com/content/14/2/R42

Diagnostic Tests

Breast self-examination (BSE) and clinical breast examinations play an important role in cancer identification. Cancerous growths tend to be harder, less mobile, less painful, more irregularly shaped, and have less clearly defined borders than benign growths. The prognosis is good for women who have breast cancers removed in the early stages but gets worse when treatment begins during later stages of the disease process. Teaching and encouraging regular use of BSE and appropriate use of mammography can save lives. See Chapter 41 for more about BSE and for explanations about diagnostic tests used to assist in determining whether tumors of the breast are malignant.

Staging

The spread (metastasis) of cancerous cells from the primary site to other areas of the body by way of the blood or lymph is denoted by staging classifications 0 to IV (see Chapter 11). Lower numbers indicate less cancer spread.

Therapeutic Measures

The five main treatment options for breast cancer are surgery, radiation therapy, chemotherapy, hormone therapy, and targeted therapy. These options may be used separately or in combination depending on the condition of the patient and the stage of the disease. Patients may also choose complementary and holistic therapies. Immunotherapy is a new and promising field of breast cancer treatment that uses the body's immune system to fight cancer. A number of immunotherapies are currently being studied, including the use of vaccines.

SURGERY. A **lumpectomy** removes just the tumor and a margin around it. A **mastectomy** may be partial (removing only part of the breast), simple (removing the breast tissue of one or both breasts), or radical (removing breast tissue, underlying muscle, and surrounding lymph nodes). The amount of tissue removed varies depending on the size, nature, and invasiveness of the cancer. Surgical practice has shifted from radical mastectomies to more breast-conserving surgeries with the addition of radiation therapy, resulting in survival rates similar to those for radical mastectomy. Surgeries to remove cancerous breast tissue can be disfiguring and have profound effects on a patient's body image and self-esteem.

RADIATION THERAPY. Radiation can be administered externally or internally to attack the rapidly dividing cells of a tumor. Although radiation affects all rapidly dividing cells in its path, including healthy cells, radiation to an area of the breast just surrounding the tumor bed reduces the incidence of side effects. It is usually used after surgery to reduce the risk of cancer recurrence or spread.

CHEMOTHERAPY. Chemotherapy kills all rapidly dividing cells, not just breast cancer cells, which leads to many side effects. This therapy may be used alone or in combination with other therapies. Newer chemotherapy options use higher doses over a shorter treatment period to reduce side effects (see Chapter 11).

HORMONE THERAPY. Hormone therapy may be used to deprive cancer cells of hormones that stimulate their growth. Because breast cancer cells are often estrogen sensitive, this may be accomplished by decreasing circulating estrogen levels with drugs or by blocking the use of estrogen by cancer cells. Interference with estrogen levels, however, may produce menopausal symptoms and increase the risk of osteoporosis and heart disease. Table 42.1 lists estrogen antagonists.

• WORD • BUILDING •
lumpectomy: lump + ectomy—excision
mastectomy: mast—breast + ec—away + tomy—cutting

TABLE **42.1** MEDICATIONS FOR DISORDERS RELATED TO HORMONAL ALTERATIONS (BREAST DISORDERS, MENSTRUAL DISORDERS, MENOPAUSE)

Medication Class/Action	Examples	Nursing Implications
Contraceptives Interfere with gonadotropin-releasing hormone, luteinizing hormone (LH), and follicle-stimulating hormone (FSH) release; maintain stable hormonal levels, relax uterus, limit endometrial proliferation	**Progesterone and estrogen:** Oral: norethindrone acetate/ethinyl estradiol (Loestrin); drospirenone/ethinyl estradiol (Yasmin, Yaz); levonorgestrel/ethinyl estradiol (Aviane); ethinyl estradiol/norgestimate (Ortho Tri-Cyclen) Patch: norelgestromin/ethinyl estradiol (Ortho Evra) Vaginal ring: etonogestrel/ethinyl estradiol (NuvaRing) **Progesterone only:** Norethindrone (Micronor); Medroxyprogesterone Acetate (Provera); levonorgestrel-releasing intrauterine system (Mirena)	Educate patient regarding use and side effects. (See ACHES side effects presented later in this chapter.) Smoking increases risk of blood clots; advise to stop smoking while on these medications.
Hormone Replacement Therapy (HRT) Interfere with gonadotropin-releasing hormone, luteinizing hormone (LH), and follicle-stimulating hormone (FSH) release; maintain stable hormonal levels, relax uterus, limit endometrial	**Progesterone and estrogen** conjugated estrogens and medroxyprogesterone (Prempro); estradiol/norethindrone acetate (Activella) **Estrogen only** conjugated estrogens (Premarin, Cenestin); estradiol (Estrace, Climara)	Educate patient regarding use and side effects. (See ACHES side effects presented later in this chapter.) Smoking increases risk of blood clots; advise to stop smoking while on these medications.

Continued

TABLE 42.1 MEDICATIONS FOR DISORDERS RELATED TO HORMONAL ALTERATIONS (BREAST DISORDERS, MENSTRUAL DISORDERS, MENOPAUSE)—cont'd

Medication Class/Action	Examples	Nursing Implications
proliferation, promote vasomotor stability, prevent bone loss.	**Vaginal preparations** conjugated estrogens (Premarin cream); Estradiol (Estrace Cream, Vagifem) **Progesterone only** norethindrone (Micronor); medroxyprogesterone acetate (Provera) **Estrogen and testosterone** Esterified estrogens/methyltestosterone (Estratest)	
NSAIDs Inhibit prostaglandin synthesis, therefore interrupt pain receptors and produce anti-inflammatory effect.	ibuprofen (Motrin, Nuprin, Advil) naproxen (Aleve) ketoprofen (Orudis) ketorolac (Toradol)	Avoid with aspirin allergy; administer with milk or food, caution about side effects, use during pregnancy, or use when on anticoagulant therapy.
Estrogen Antagonists Inhibit growth of estrogen-dependent tumors.	tamoxifen (Nolvadex) anastrozole (Arimidex) toremifene (Fareston) exemestane (Aromasin) letrozole (Femara) fulvestrant (Faslodex)	Report vaginal bleeding, leg cramps, shortness of breath, weakness. Promote use of nonhormonal contraceptives during use. Smoking increases the patient's risk of blood clots; advise patients to stop smoking during use.

TARGETED THERAPIES. Targeted therapies attack specific molecular agents or pathways involved in the development of cancer. Some targeted therapies are given to intensify positive body responses (e.g., stimulate the immune system) or to decrease negative body responses. Examples include biological response modifiers such as interferons, tumor necrosis factor, interleukins, and various experimental immunotherapy formulations. Two drugs that target the protein HER2, which is found in larger than normal amounts on the surface of breast cancer cells, are trastuzumab (Herceptin) and lapatinib (Tykerb). Another drug, bevacizumab (Avastin), works by blocking the growth of new blood vessels that cancer cells depend on to grow and function. Targeted therapy is an area of much research and is likely to expand greatly during the next few years.

Alternative therapies are also available for many cancers. See Chapter 5 for information about helping patients evaluate alternative and complementary therapies. The American Cancer Society and cancer treatment centers also have people who can answer questions about experimental and alternative therapies and discuss research findings. For more information about breast cancer, visit the American Cancer Society at www.cancer.org. Other helpful sites are www.breastcancer.org and ww5.komen.org.

Nursing Care

See the "Nursing Care Plan for the Patient Undergoing a Mastectomy." In addition to the diagnoses covered, the patient will need diagnoses for postoperative pain. See Chapters 10 and 12, respectively, for additional interventions for pain and postoperative patients.

CRITICAL THINKING

Julie

■ Julie, age 32, reports pain and grapelike "lumps" in her breasts, and her nurse practitioner diagnoses fibrocystic changes.

1. What questions would you ask to further assess Julie's symptoms?
2. What can you teach Julie to help her control her symptoms?
3. What can Julie do to remain vigilant for more concerning changes in her breasts?

Suggested answers are at the end of the chapter.

NURSING CARE PLAN for the Patient Undergoing a Mastectomy

Nursing Diagnosis: *Anxiety* related to uncertainty about diagnosis, prognosis, and treatments

Expected Outcomes: The patient will verbalize and demonstrate a decrease in anxiety.

Evaluation of Outcomes: Does the patient report a decrease in anxiety following education and explanation of the procedure? Do patient's vital signs, verbal, and nonverbal behavior suggest a decrease in anxiety?

Intervention Assess vital signs and observe verbal and nonverbal behavior. **Rationale** An increase in blood pressure, pulse, and respirations as well as observation of mild to severe agitation may indicate anxiety. **Evaluation** Are the patient's vital signs within normal range for the patient? Is verbal and nonverbal behavior consistent with anxiety?

Intervention Assess patient's current knowledge of the procedure and level of anxiety related to the procedure. **Rationale** Assessment of current knowledge provides a baseline for teaching. **Evaluation** What does the patient know?

Intervention Teach patient what to expect about the surgical experience based on patient's understanding, concerns, and willingness to learn. **Rationale** Knowledge dispels unreasonable fears and helps patient to prepare to cope with stressors. **Evaluation** Does patient evidence adequate understanding of the procedure and what to expect afterward?

Intervention Support and clarify the HCP's explanations, answer questions, and refer to knowledgeable sources. **Rationale** The patient may not remember or understand what the HCP said. **Evaluation** Does patient have accurate information? Are appropriate referrals made?

Nursing Diagnosis: *Risk for Ineffective Breathing Pattern* related to pain with chest movement

Expected Outcome: The patient will have an effective breathing pattern with clear lung sounds and Spo$_2$ of 95% or above.

Evaluation of Outcome: Are respirations regular, easy, and unlabored? Are respiratory rate and oxygen saturation within a normal range for the patient? Are lung sounds clear?

Intervention Assess patient's vital signs, oxygen saturation, pain level, and lung sounds. **Rationale** Pain contributes to shallow breathing, which can affect vital signs, Spo$_2$, and lung sounds. **Evaluation** Are the patient's vital signs and oxygen saturation within normal range for the patient? Does patient report pain at an acceptable level? Are lung sounds clear?

Intervention Medicate to relieve pain as necessary. **Rationale** Pain may inhibit deep breathing efforts. **Evaluation** Does patient evidence pain or guarding during chest movement? Does analgesic help?

Intervention Encourage deep breathing and coughing each hour. **Rationale** This helps to loosen secretions and to prevent atelectasis, pneumonia, and inadequate oxygenation of tissues. **Evaluation** Does chest sound clear? Are skin color and oxygen saturation adequate?

Intervention Encourage use of an incentive spirometer each hour when awake. **Rationale** To encourage deep breathing. **Evaluation** Does patient use spirometer correctly?

Nursing Diagnosis: *Risk for Ineffective Tissue Perfusion* related to damage to blood and lymph vessels and tension at surgical incision site

Continued

NURSING CARE PLAN for the Patient Undergoing a Mastectomy—cont'd

Expected Outcome: The patient's incision will heal by primary intention without excessive bleeding or swelling.

Evaluation of Outcome: Are edges of the incision well approximated, with scant bleeding/serous drainage, and mild edema/erythema?

Intervention Monitor vital signs and oxygen saturation according to agency policy and as necessary. **Rationale** Vital signs and oxygen saturation affect tissue perfusion and oxygenation. **Evaluation** Are vital signs and Spo_2 stable and within normal range? Are extremities pink and warm?

Intervention Avoid use of the affected arm for blood pressures, venipunctures, and injections. **Rationale** Restrictive and invasive procedures might further compromise tissue integrity of the affected arm. **Evaluation** Is the arm protected?

Intervention Assess incision for bleeding, amount and color of drainage, and swelling. Empty drain device prn. **Rationale** Excessive bleeding or swelling can compromise tissue perfusion. **Evaluation** Does incisional area look swollen, smooth, or shiny? Are drainage amount and color appropriate?

Intervention Measure circumference of arms daily and compare. Report changes. **Rationale** Swelling causes an increase in circumference and impairs circulation. **Evaluation** Is affected arm larger than unaffected arm?

Intervention Elevate affected arm if swelling occurs. **Rationale** Gravity aids fluid return to the heart. **Evaluation** Does elevation reduce swelling?

Intervention Place items where patient can easily reach them. **Rationale** Excessive movement of the affected arm may exert tension on incision and increase bleeding. **Evaluation** Can patient reach items without abducting the arm more than 90 degrees?

Intervention Encourage postmastectomy exercises of the affected arm according to agency policy. **Rationale** Appropriate exercise promotes circulation, preserves muscle and joint function, and increases self-care ability. **Evaluation** Is patient moving the arm appropriately and gradually increasing range of motion and self-care ability?

Intervention Teach postoperative self-care and signs and symptoms of ineffective healing to report. **Rationale** Early assessment and intervention help prevent the development of serious complications. **Evaluation** Does patient demonstrate and verbalize understanding of appropriate postoperative self-care?

Nursing Diagnosis: *Risk for Ineffective Coping* related to cancer threat and body image disturbance

Expected Outcomes: The patient will verbalize ability to cope and will seek help and support appropriately.

Evaluation of Outcomes: Does patient take an interest in care of condition? Does patient ask appropriate questions related to care and verbalize appropriate concerns?

Intervention Observe patient's interest in self-care, ability to problem solve, and level of family or other support. **Rationale** Poor self-care, problem-solving skills, and lack of support may indicate a risk for ineffective coping. **Evaluation** Does patient solve problems appropriately? Are family members or other support persons present? Is patient taking an active interest in her personal appearance?

Intervention Use therapeutic communication and listening skills to allow patient to share concerns. **Rationale** Loss of a breast disturbs many aspects of body image, and cancer threatens one's sense of security and stability in life. **Evaluation** Is patient able to share concerns?

Intervention Help patient remember previous successes in coping and strategies used. **Rationale** Memory of prior success can encourage hope for future success. **Evaluation** Does patient possess appropriate coping strategies?

NURSING CARE PLAN for the Patient Undergoing a Mastectomy—cont'd

Intervention Provide accurate information according to agency policy. **Rationale** Fear of the unknown can increase anxiety and reduce coping. **Evaluation** Does patient relate understanding of follow-up treatment?

Intervention Refer to appropriate agencies for further support as needed (e.g., American Cancer Society, Reach for Recovery, local support groups). **Rationale** Social support can assist individuals to meet their needs while developing effective coping skills and strategies. **Evaluation** Does patient have resources to call on as needed?

See Table 42.2 for a breast cancer summary.

Breast Modification Surgeries

Mammoplasty is surgical modification of the breast. This may be done to restore a normal shape after removal of cancerous tissues. Many women, however, undergo mammoplasty electively to reduce or increase the size or to improve the shape of their breasts. Because nurses are very aware of the dangers involved with surgery, psychosocial issues may seem to be a trivial reason to voluntarily assume such risks to life and health. However, body image is an important component of quality of life. Patients' informed decisions should be respected if they choose this surgery. It is essential that you present a caring and nonjudgmental attitude.

TABLE 42.2 BREAST CANCER SUMMARY

Signs and Symptoms	Swelling, tenderness, pain, redness Palpable lumps Leakage of fluid/blood from nipple Changes in contour of skin of breast/nipple
Diagnostic Tests and Findings	BSE/CBE Mammography Excisional/fine-needle biopsy
Therapeutic Measures	Lumpectomy/mastectomy/breast reconstruction Radiation Chemotherapy Hormone therapy Targeted therapy
Complications	Metastasis Significant treatment side effects Profound negative effect on patient's self-image.
Priority Nursing Diagnoses	*Anxiety* *Risk for Ineffective Breathing Pattern* *Risk for Ineffective Tissue Perfusion* *Risk for Ineffective Coping*

BSE = breast self-examination; CBE = clinical breast examination.

Breast Reduction and Mastopexy

Generally, in breast reduction operations the nipple is separated from the surrounding tissue except for a small section with the blood vessels and nerves that supply it (Fig. 42.1). A large wedge of tissue is removed from the bottom of the breast, the edges are sewn together, and the nipple is reimplanted in a

• WORD • BUILDING •
mammoplasty: mamm(o)—breast + plasty—to mold

A Area of skin to be removed

B Areas marked on breast

C Wedge of breast tissue removed, areola pulled up, gap closed

D Excess tissue removed, skin closed with stitches

E Post-operative appearance

FIGURE 42.1 Breast reduction. Modified from Love, S. M. (2000). *Dr. Susan Love's breast book (3rd ed.).* Cambridge, MA: Perseus Publishing, with permission.

higher position. This not only decreases the overall size of the breast, which may help with back, neck, and head pain, but it also corrects excessive sagging—a common problem for women with large breasts.

A **mastopexy** involves the removal of some skin and fat with subsequent resuturing so that the breast tissues are held higher on the chest to correct sagging breasts. This procedure usually does not remove as much tissue as a breast reduction.

Augmentation and Reconstruction Mammoplasty

Augmentation is a surgery to increase the size of the breasts. An implant—either a bag containing saline solution or silicone gel or a transplanted portion of the patient's own body tissues from another area—is inserted through an incision and positioned either under or over the pectoral muscles (Fig. 42.2).

For reconstructive mammoplasty, use of the patient's own tissues is generally safer than use of artificial implants because no foreign material is introduced into the body. For situations in which significant amounts of tissue are needed for reconstruction, a portion of tissue may be moved from one area of the body to another as a pedicle graft. Pedicle literally means "little foot" because the graft remains attached to a stalk (containing the blood vessels and nerves) somewhat resembling a little leg with a foot (the graft) attached.

Figure 42.3 shows two options for mastectomy graft repair. Tissue from the buttock area or the abdomen may also be grafted onto a mastectomy site without a pedicle.

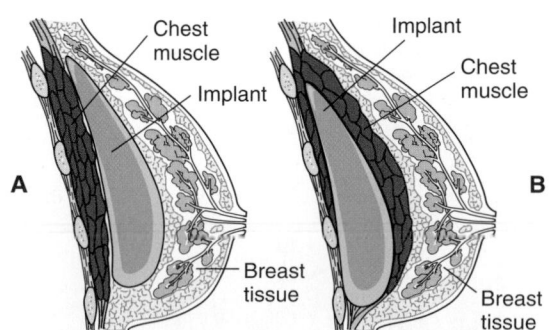

FIGURE 42.2 Breast implants. (A) Implant over muscle. (B) Implant under muscle. Modified from Love, S. M. (2000). *Dr. Susan Love's breast book* (3rd ed.). Cambridge, MA: Perseus Publishing, with permission.

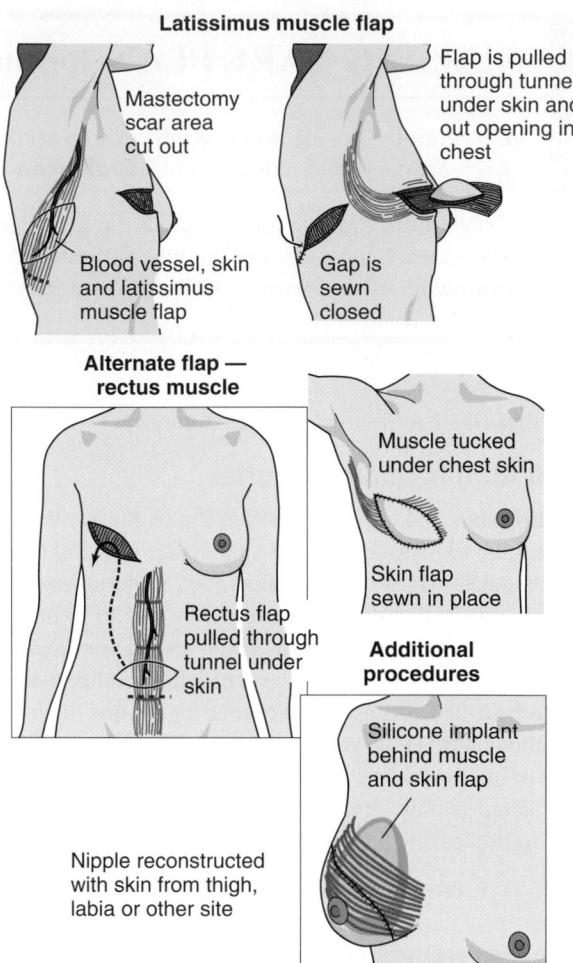

FIGURE 42.3 Mastectomy reconstruction. Modified from Love, S. M. (2000). *Dr. Susan Love's breast book* (3rd ed.). Cambridge, MA: Perseus Publishing, with permission.

Complications

Any surgery can be complicated by infection or impaired healing. The use of silicone implants has been less than satisfactory for many women. Some women have experienced hardening of breast tissues, and others have developed serious autoimmune problems after receiving silicone gel implants. Although actual etiologies of all the problems are uncertain, many surgeries have been undertaken recently to remove silicone implants, and saline implants are now more common.

Nursing Care and Patient Education

Carefully assess the healing process when changing dressings and explain to the patient how to assess healing, because not all tissues successfully attach at the new site. Failure of attachment can require surgical revision. Signs of poor attachment include unnatural color of the incision, graft, or surrounding tissues; swelling; drainage; gaping incision lines; and sloughing of the graft or edges of the site.

• WORD • BUILDING •
mastopexy: masto—breast + pexy—fixation

MENSTRUAL DISORDERS

Flow and Cycle Disorders

Pathophysiology, Etiologies, and Signs and Symptoms

There are many types of menstrual abnormalities (Table 42.3). Causes can include stress, pregnancy, hormonal imbalances, metabolic imbalances (such as obesity, anorexia nervosa, and loss of too much body fat through excessive exercise), tumors (both benign and malignant), infections, organ diseases (such as liver, kidney, or thyroid disease), blood or bone marrow abnormalities, and the presence of foreign bodies in the uterus (such as intrauterine devices, IUDs). Menstrual abnormalities can be distressing and can result in anemia, persistent fatigue, and sexual dysfunction. Establishment of a comfortable and open professional relationship between a woman and her HCP is essential for communication about such concerns.

Diagnostic Tests

Appropriate testing to determine the cause of menstrual abnormalities involves a thorough history and physical

TABLE 42.3 MENSTRUAL FLOW DISORDERS

Disorder	Description
Amenorrhea	Menses absent for more than 6 months or three of previous cycles Called primary amenorrhea when menarche has not occurred by age 17 Called secondary amenorrhea when menses are absent after menarche
Hypermenorrhea	Menses lasting longer than 7 days
Hypomenorrhea	Less than the expected amount of menstrual bleeding
Menometrorrhagia (also called metro-menorrhagia)	Overly long, heavy, and irregular menses
Menorrhagia	Passing more than 80 mL of blood per menses
Oligomenorrhea	Menstrual cycles of more than 35 days
Polymenorrhea (also called metrorrhagia)	Menses more frequently than 21-day intervals

examination. Papanicolaou (Pap) smear, cervical and vaginal cultures, laparoscopy, ultrasound, endometrial biopsy, pregnancy testing, urine testing, and blood testing may be done to screen for any of the disorders that can influence the menstrual cycle and flow.

Therapeutic Measures

Medical treatment of menstrual disorders often involves manipulation of hormone levels or use of NSAIDs. Surgical treatment can involve **dilation and curettage** (D&C), laser ablation of endometrial tissue, and **hysterectomy**. During D&C, the cervix is first dilated (opened wider) and then a curet—a sharp, spoonlike instrument—is inserted through the cervix and used to scoop out the inner lining of the uterus. Laser ablation involves targeted burning of endometrial tissue so that scar tissue forms that does not bleed. Hysterectomy (removal of the uterus), a last-resort treatment, is described later in this chapter.

Nursing Care

The only accurate way to estimate menstrual flow is to weigh used sanitary pads (sealed in a biohazard bag) and then subtract the weight of the original pads. A 1-g increase in pad weight equals approximately 1 mL of blood loss. Simply counting numbers of pads used is much less accurate, because women may change pads at different intervals. You may have to rely on a woman's report of blood loss. Be sure to document "patient estimate" after the quote.

D&C is typically done as an outpatient procedure. Women can expect some cramping and spotting or light bleeding for a few days afterward.

Dysmenorrhea

Pathophysiology, Etiologies, and Signs and Symptoms

Painful menstruation, or **dysmenorrhea**, is a common problem in women. Primary dysmenorrhea (menstrual cramps) is not pathological and is thought to be caused mainly by the action of endogenous prostaglandins that stimulate uterine contractions, producing cramping pain. Secondary dysmenorrhea is caused by a reproductive tract disorder such as endometriosis, pelvic infection, retroversion of the uterus, or fibroid tumors.

Diagnostic Tests

Hormonal tests such as estrogen and progesterone levels may be evaluated for primary dysmenorrhea. Additional tests such as laparoscopic examination, biopsies, or cultures may be required for investigation of secondary dysmenorrhea.

• WORD • BUILDING •
dilation and curettage: dilat(e)—to widen + ation—the process of + curet—scoop + tage—doing
hysterectomy: hyster—womb + ec—away + tomy—cutting
dysmenorrhea: dys—painful + men(o)—month + rrhea—flow

Therapeutic Measures

Primary dysmenorrhea can be treated with drugs that inhibit prostaglandin synthesis, such as aspirin and NSAIDs. Correction of secondary causes of dysmenorrhea may include such measures as hormonal adjustment, usually with oral contraceptives or hormone replacement therapy (HRT), D&C, or other surgical or medical intervention based on the cause.

Nursing Care and Patient Education

Aspirin or NSAIDs help reduce discomfort. A warm heading pad to the abdomen or a hot bath is also helpful. If dysmenorrhea is related to uterine retroversion, assuming a knee-to-chest position may relieve the discomfort. Sudden development of dysmenorrhea in a woman with no previous menstrual discomfort should always be investigated.

Premenstrual Syndrome and Premenstrual Dysphoric Disorder

Pathophysiology, Etiologies, and Signs and Symptoms

Premenstrual syndrome (PMS) is a recurrent problem for many women. Although the exact cause is not understood, ovarian hormones, aldosterone, and neurotransmitters such as monoamine oxidase and serotonin are believed to play a role. Symptoms include water retention; headaches; discomfort in joints, muscles, and breasts; changes in affect, concentration, and coordination; and sensory changes. Few women find PMS serious enough to interfere with work or relationships.

Premenstrual dysphoric disorder (PMDD) is a condition with symptoms of depression, irritability, and tension before menstruation more severe than PMS. Like PMS, the exact cause is unknown. Women with PMDD have at least five of the following symptoms, including one mood-related symptom (PubMed Health, 2012):

- No interest in daily activities and relationships
- Fatigue or low energy
- Feeling of sadness or hopelessness, possible suicidal thoughts
- Feelings of tension or anxiety
- Feeling out of control
- Food cravings or binge eating
- Mood swings with periods of crying
- Panic attacks
- Irritability or anger that affects other people
- Physical symptoms such as bloating, breast tenderness, headaches, and joint or muscle pain
- Problems sleeping
- Trouble concentrating

Therapeutic Measures

A variety of drugs have been given to combat PMS and PMDD with varying degrees of success. Some commonly used medications include drugs that affect prostaglandin production, hormonal balance, and neurotransmitter production and reuptake (such as antidepressants), as well as diuretics and supplements of calcium, magnesium, vitamin E, and vitamin B_6. Patients should be warned, however, that dosages of vitamins should not be increased without professional advice because vitamins are medications (as well as nutrients) and high doses of some vitamins can lead to physiological damage. Regular exercise and eating a healthy diet help to reduce symptoms as well.

Nursing Care and Patient Education

Being understanding and nonjudgmental is especially important. Some women who suffer from severe PMS or PMDD may have been treated as if they are psychologically impaired because of the interaction of hormones and neurotransmitters and because of outdated ideas concerning PMS or PMDD. You can help by providing educational materials on lifestyle measures, such as restriction of alcohol, caffeine, nicotine, salt, and simple sugars; participation in regular exercise; and development of stress management skills that may help to reduce symptoms. If the patient is experiencing severe depression, discuss the possibility of suicidal thoughts that can occur with increasing depression symptoms during the second half of the menstrual cycle. Counsel the patient to call 911 or seek medical care immediately if suicidal thoughts occur.

Endometriosis

Pathophysiology, Etiologies, and Signs and Symptoms

Endometriosis is a condition in which functioning endometrial tissue is located outside the uterus (Fig. 42.4). Several theories have been proposed to explain development of endometriosis, including faulty developmental differentiation of cells, transport of endometrial cells via blood and lymph to other parts of the body, and **retrograde** menstruation—a backward leakage of blood and tissue into the fallopian tubes during the menstrual period.

Endometriotic cells grow in areas of sufficient blood supply, extending into tissues such as intestinal walls, ovaries, and other abdominal structures. On a cyclic basis, mediated by ovarian hormones, these cells build up and slough just as

• WORD • BUILDING •
retrograde: retro—backward + grade—step

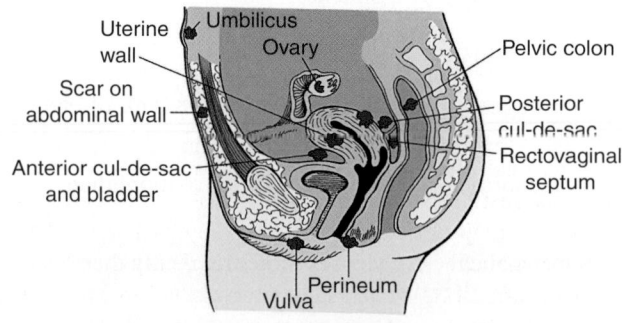

FIGURE 42.4 Possible sites of endometriosis.

they would in the uterus, but the sloughing and bleeding occur in the enclosed abdominal cavity or into the tissues that they have invaded. The buildup of the blood and cells can result in pain, swelling, damage to abdominal organs and structures, scar tissue development, and infertility.

Therapeutic Measures

Surgical intervention may be required, especially if scar tissue develops into tight bands that strangulate sections of bowel or ureters. Reduction of estrogen and prevention of ovulation either with medications or by surgical removal of the ovaries can be effective but results in infertility and menopausal symptoms. Analgesics may be required for pain.

Nursing Care and Patient Education

The severity and persistence of the pain of endometriosis can lead to reliance on pain medication, so it is important to teach patients alternative and complementary pain relief strategies such as relaxation exercises and application of heat to the abdomen or back.

Menopause
Pathophysiology and Signs and Symptoms

Menopause is the permanent cessation of menstrual cycles resulting from decreased hormone production. This is a natural part of aging, but related uncomfortable symptoms and conditions can occur. The climacteric (**perimenopause**) is the period of gradual decline in hormone production before the permanent end of menses and may last from a few months to several years. Perimenopausal physical symptoms vary widely and can include erratic menses, atrophy of urogenital tissues with a marked decrease in the amount of natural lubrication, a pH shift toward alkalinity (encouraging yeast overgrowth), and vasomotor instability (resulting in hot flashes and night sweats).

Estrogen protects women against several disease processes; the risk of heart disease and osteoporosis increases with declining estrogen production. Mental changes can occur because of the complex interplay of reproductive hormones and neurotransmitters. It is important to acknowledge symptoms such as irritability, anxiety, insomnia, memory problems, and mild depression as a normal, temporary result of hormonal changes, so that perimenopausal women do not doubt their sanity.

Therapeutic Measures

Hormone replacement therapy (HRT) is a controversial prevention and treatment for perimenopausal symptoms. Hormone replacement (see Table 42.1 for examples) may be prescribed for severe symptoms and can be administered orally, vaginally, or transdermally. The National Heart, Lung, and Blood Institute of the National Institutes of Health (NIH) conducted a major research project to study the risks and benefits of combined estrogen and progestin therapy for healthy women (NIH, 2002). The project was halted in July 2002, 3 years early, because of very worrisome results. Positive findings included a one-third reduction in hip fractures, a 24%

decrease in total fractures, and a 37% decrease in colorectal cancer with HRT. Disturbing findings, however, included a 26% increase in breast cancer, a 41% increase in strokes, a 29% increase in heart attacks, doubling of venous thromboembolism rates, and an overall 22% increase in cardiovascular disease. It is uncertain what to make of these data because there was no difference in total mortality when comparing women treated with HRT and those given a placebo. Long-term results will continue to be examined, but for now, the risks of HRT have been deemed too great to continue the study.

A 2013 Global Consensus Statement now states that benefits of HRT for menopause outweigh risks in some cases, such as in controlling vasomotor symptoms and osteoporosis-related fractures in women under 60 or within 10 years after menopause (deVilliers, 2013). Stay updated on the latest findings at www.nhlbi.nih.gov/health/women.

Dietary changes to include **phytoestrogens**, which are present in foods and herbs such as soy, tofu, flax seeds, black cohosh, and dong quai, may provide some of the benefits of estrogen replacement without HRT. However, even phytoestrogens have some risk. Women should discuss food and herb supplements with their HCP before using them.

Prevention of osteoporosis begins in early adulthood, long before perimenopause. Fair-skinned white women are at greatest risk for bone loss. Throughout life, adequate intake of calcium and vitamin D (preferably from foods) and regular weight-bearing exercise help to maximize bone mass. At menopause, some women may receive treatment with bone-building medications such as alendronate (Fosamax) to slow bone loss.

Complications

It is important to note that resumption of vaginal bleeding after menstruation has finally ceased can be a sign of an endometrial cell disorder caused by either benign changes, such as polyps, or malignant changes of internal reproductive organs. Any bleeding that occurs following previous cessation should always be investigated.

Nursing Care and Patient Education

Teach perimenopausal women that they can plan ahead for hot flashes by dressing in layers of clothing that may be removed. Not allowing hot flashes to interrupt activities is an important strategy, as is engaging in satisfying and calming activities that contribute to a sense of serenity. Vaginal symptoms can be treated with a water-soluble moisture restorer or lubricant, or with an estrogen cream (following prescription directions). Eating a healthy diet that is light in caffeine, sugar, and alcohol can help women better control their bodies and minds. Looking forward to new challenges rather than backward to the past may help to counteract hormone-related depressive tendencies. It is important to remind perimenopausal women that

• WORD • BUILDING •
perimenopause: peri—around + men(o)—month + pause—stopping
phytoestrogens: phyto—plant + estrogens—hormones

they may still be fertile even after several months of **amenorrhea**. To prevent conception, they need to continue to practice birth control until they receive confirmation from their HCP that menopause is complete.

See Table 42.4 for a summary of menstrual disorders.

CRITICAL THINKING

Lola

■ Lola, age 53, has been experiencing menopausal hot flashes during the afternoons as she works in her office.

1. What self-care measures can you suggest to help with her symptoms?
2. If she considers HRT, what information should you share with her?
3. With whom should you collaborate as you help Lola decide what to do?

Suggested answers are at the end of the chapter.

TABLE 42.4 MENSTRUAL DISORDERS SUMMARY

Signs and Symptoms	Increase or decrease in menstrual flow
	Increased pain with menses or generalized abdominal pain
	Fluid retention
	Headaches
	Breast pain/lesions/swelling
	Mood changes
Diagnostic Tests	Hormone levels
	Pregnancy test
	Pap smear
	Cervical/vaginal cultures
	Urine testing
	Ultrasound
	Laparoscopy
	Biopsy
Therapeutic Measures	Medication to stabilize hormone levels
	NSAIDs
	D&C, laser ablation, hysterectomy
	Treatment of underlying causes
	Vitamin/mineral supplements
	Diuretics/SSRIs/dietary changes
Priority Nursing Diagnoses	*Deficient Fluid Volume* related to increased bleeding
	Pain related to uterine cramping
	Deficient Knowledge related to self-care measures

D&C = dilation and curettage; NSAIDs = nonsteroidal anti-inflammatory drugs; SSRIs = serotonin reuptake inhibitors.

IRRITATIONS AND INFLAMMATIONS OF THE VAGINA AND VULVA

Various causative agents can irritate the vulva and the vagina. Signs and symptoms are often similar, but there are some differences in the discharge produced in response to the disorders. Table 42.5 lists common vaginal irritations and inflammations that are not generally sexually transmitted. See Chapter 44 for information on sexually transmitted infections.

Pathophysiology, Etiologies, and Signs and Symptoms

The normal vaginal environment is a balanced ecosystem with a pH of less than 4.2 as a result of lactic acid and hydrogen peroxide production by cells in the vagina. This acidic pH protects against the growth of many pathogenic microorganisms. A variety of normal resident microorganisms coexist unless the ecological balance is destroyed. Candidiasis, bacterial **vaginosis**, and cytolytic **vaginitis** are all instances of overgrowth of normally present, nonpathogenic microorganisms. Trichomoniasis also is included here because it can be transmitted nonsexually (on fomites, such as toilet seats), as well as sexually, and it grows well when the vaginal environment is disturbed.

Several conditions can predispose patients to an overgrowth of resident microbes: poor nutrition (especially diets high in simple sugars), inconsistent control of blood glucose levels in patients with diabetes, stress, pregnancy, marked hormonal fluctuations, pH changes, prolonged overheating of the genital area with little aeration (as happens with sitting still for long periods in restrictive clothing), and changes in the balance of vaginal flora types because of antibiotic treatment or douching. Patients who have a compromised immune system can experience frequent overgrowth of resident microbes, and, conversely, vaginal infections can make women more susceptible to sexually transmitted infections (STIs), such as gonorrhea and human immunodeficiency virus (HIV). Frequent and persistent yeast infections can be one sign of HIV infection. Vaginosis (overgrowth) and vaginitis (inflammation) can sometimes produce irritation and inflammation in the male sexual partner as well and may lead to urethritis, excoriation, and penile inflammation or lesions. A variety of anti-infective medications are used for these disorders (Table 42.6). If the male partner is not also treated, he may reactivate the problem for the woman. Therefore, several types of medication come in "partner packs" for both partners to use.

Nursing Care and Education of the Patient Undergoing Diagnostic Testing

The patient may feel embarrassed to talk about what is bothering her. A safe way to begin with most patients is, "Hello.

• WORD • BUILDING •

amenorrhea: a—without + men(o)—month + rrhea—flow
vaginosis: vagin—vagina + osis—condition
vaginitis: vagin—vagina + itis—inflammation

TABLE 42.5 COMMON VAGINAL IRRITATIONS AND INFLAMMATIONS

Disorder and Etiology	Signs and Symptoms	Discharge/ Examination	Diagnostic Tests	Usual Treatment
Candidiasis: *Candida albicans, glabrata,* or *tropicalis* overgrowth	Burning, itching, redness of vulva; burning on urination	White, cottage cheese appearance	Wet-mount slides (yeasts look like tiny, budding tree branches); may be cultured	Antifungal agents (drugs mostly ending in *-azole*)
Bacterial vaginosis: *Gardnerella vaginalis, Mycoplasma,* or anaerobe overgrowth	None or vulvar or vaginal irritation	White or gray, homogeneous, foul-smelling discharge; pH higher than 4.5	Wet-mount slides show "clue cells" or release fishy odor when potassium hydroxide is applied	Antibiotics
Trichomoniasis: *Trichomonas vaginalis* (may be transmitted by inanimate objects or sexually)	Itching, irritation, foul odor, redness, dysuria	Discharge may be frothy; pH higher than 4.5; "strawberry cervix" resulting from petechiae	Wet-mount slides treated with normal saline show motile cells with flagella (like tiny whips); may also be cultured	Metronidazole
Cytolytic vaginosis: *Lactobacilli* overgrowth, stress, some medications	Burning, irritation, pain with intercourse	Nonodorous, thick, white, pasty, or dry and flaking	Lower than normal pH as tested with pH indicator tape (or litmus strip); may be cultured	Depends on cause; alkaline douches may be prescribed
Contact vulvovaginitis: contact with allergens or irritating chemicals such as contraceptive creams or bubble baths	Itching, burning, redness	Generally no change from normal discharge, though may be increased	History and physical information, recent contact with chemicals	Avoidance of the offending substance; warm sitz baths or application of hydrocortisone cream
Atrophic vaginitis: estrogen levels too low to support estrogen sensitive vaginal tissues	Vulvovaginal irritation, dryness, dyspareunia, increased tendency for resident microbe overgrowth	May have little or increased discharge; discharge may be watery, yellow, or green; may be blood tinged	Maturation index may be determined during Pap test to identify atrophic cellular changes, but diagnosis is usually by history and physical information	Hormone replacement therapy (oral, patch, or vulvovaginal cream) or water-soluble lubricant replacing vaginal lubricants

What can I write on your chart as the reason for your visit today?" If embarrassment is evident, a comment that you need to know a bit about what materials to put out for examination purposes often defuses an uncomfortable situation. As you set up materials for a pelvic examination, you can explain that some information is needed to determine how to treat the problem (see Chapter 41). Often this is a good time to ask about vaginal discharge or other signs and symptoms using the **WHAT'S UP?** format (Chapter 1). Allow the patient privacy while she changes into a gown. Return to the room if requested as a chaperone, assistant, and support for the woman.

TABLE 42.6 MEDICATIONS FOR IRRITATIONS AND INFLAMMATIONS OF THE VAGINA AND VULVA

Medication Class/Action	Examples	Nursing Implications
Antibiotics Inhibit bacterial protein synthesis.	clindamycin (Cleocin)	Educate on correct use. Use as directed even if symptoms cease. Report change in symptoms.
Antifungals Believed to bind to sterol in fungal cell membrane, thereby altering cell permeability	fluconazole (Diflucan) miconazole (Monistat) terconazole (Terazol) clotrimazole (Gyne-Lotrimin)	Education on correct use; use as directed even if symptoms cease. Report side effects.
Antiprotozoal Enters cells of microorganisms that contain nitroreductase, interferes with DNA synthesis and causes cell death	metronidazole (Flagyl)	Teach patient to avoid alcohol use while on medication and for 48 hours after completion. Concurrent use of alcohol and metronidazole will induce severe nausea and vomiting. Use medication as directed, even if symptoms cease. Take with meals. Treat partner.

NURSING CARE TIP

If any wet-mount slides are made, these must be taken to the laboratory immediately while still wet. Use standard precautions to transport samples. Although samples may be taken for culture, the health care provider may prescribe medication before the results return because such irritations are so uncomfortable.

Nursing Care and Education of the Patient Undergoing Treatment

Vaginal inflammations and infections may require oral medication or local application of medication in cream, suppository, or medicated douche form. You may apply this for patients who cannot do so themselves, or you may teach patients to self-administer. Anatomically, the vagina slopes back toward the sacrum for about the length of an adult finger (although it can stretch longer). Application is easiest when the patient is lying down ready to sleep because vaginal medications tend to run out when the patient stands or sits. Medicated douches may be administered to a hospitalized patient sitting on a bedpan in bed in semi-Fowler's position.

Patients may self-administer while sitting on a toilet. Most vaginal medications come with an applicator that either injects a dose of creamy medication or pushes a firmer, shaped dose of medication off the end of the tube when the plunger is depressed. Consult the instructions supplied with the medication. Instruct patients to use all the medication as prescribed and to wear an absorbent pad to prevent possible staining of clothing.

TOXIC SHOCK SYNDROME

Pathophysiology, Etiologies, and Signs and Symptoms

Toxic shock syndrome (TSS), first identified in 1978, is mainly associated with superabsorbent tampon use during menstruation but can also occur with use of nasal packings, or in other individuals with no specific risk factors. It is a severe systemic infection with strains of *Staphylococcus aureus* that produce an epidermal toxin. The effect of the toxin on the liver, kidneys, and circulatory system makes TSS a life-threatening condition. A streptococcal infection can cause a similar syndrome.

Individuals with TSS may experience a sudden high fever with sore throat, headache, dizziness, confusion, redness of the palms and soles of the feet, rash, blisters, and petechiae, followed by peeling of the skin. Muscle pain and weakness, and gastrointestinal upset have also been reported. Signs and symptoms of TSS should be reported to a HCP immediately.

Prevention

Tampon makers have removed the highly absorbent fibers that were most often associated with the syndrome from their product lines, and TSS is now rare. Women can also reduce their risk of developing TSS by substituting sanitary pads for tampons at least part of the time, such as at night; changing tampons every 4 hours; washing hands carefully before inserting anything into the vagina; not leaving female barrier contraceptives in place for longer than needed; and not using tampons or female barrier contraceptives in the first 12 weeks after giving birth.

Nursing Care and Patient Education

All menstruating women should be taught measures to prevent TSS. They should also be taught to recognize symptoms of TSS because early identification and treatment can save lives.

DISORDERS RELATED TO THE DEVELOPMENT OF THE GENITAL ORGANS

Pathophysiology, Etiologies, and Signs and Symptoms

Several types of congenital malformations of the reproductive organs can affect the health of female patients. Genetic or environmental factors during pregnancy can cause these, and they may require medical or surgical treatment at some point in life. **Agenesis** of structures means that they never developed. **Hypoplasia** of reproductive tract portions means that they are underdeveloped. **Imperforate** means that expected openings do not exist. Blind pouches exist where cavities should meet but do not. The uterus can form in several configurations, including a double uterus.

Many malformations are discovered during childhood or early adolescence, but some are identified when patients seek medical help because of dysmenorrhea, **dyspareunia** (pain with intercourse), infertility, repeated spontaneous abortions (miscarriages), or preterm labor during pregnancy.

Diagnostic Tests

Procedures such as ultrasonography, hysterosalpingography, computed tomography (CT), magnetic resonance imaging (MRI), and endoscopy may be used to determine the type and extent of developmental defects.

Therapeutic Measures

Some defects can be repaired surgically; others cannot. Depending on the type and location of the defect, surgeries may be done by endoscopy or by surgical incision. Postoperatively the absence of hormone-producing tissue may be overcome by hormone replacements.

Nursing Care and Patient Education

Patients who have these problems may struggle with self-esteem issues, such as feeling that they are somehow incomplete or have been cheated of something they desire. You can show that you are willing to listen if and when the patient wishes to talk, while allowing her as much privacy as she desires.

DISPLACEMENT DISORDERS

Pathophysiology and Etiologies

The pelvic organs are suspended in the pelvis by ligaments and supported by muscles and fascia. The pubococcygeal muscle runs from the pubis to the coccyx and supplies support from below. Pregnancies (especially those producing large babies) and rapid or traumatic deliveries may result in stretching and injury of the supporting structures, which can cause displacement of the uterus, vagina, bladder, or bowel from a normal position.

The observation that some children have defective muscular support of the pelvic organs and that prolapse is more prevalent in some families seems to suggest that congenital defects and genetic inheritance may also influence displacement disorders even without pregnancy. Scarring from STIs also may be a factor. Aging generally increases the problem because the effects of gravity over time contribute to stretching, and lower estrogen levels weaken estrogen-dependent supportive tissues. Chronic constipation, obesity, and lack of exercise also worsen these problems.

Diagnostic Tests

Ultrasonography, hysterosalpingography, CT, MRI, and endoscopy may be used to determine the type and extent of displacement disorders.

Therapeutic Measures

A *pessary* is a supportive (usually ring-shaped) device that is placed in the proximal end of the vagina to help support the pelvic organs. A pessary is usually removed daily at bedtime for cleaning, but some types are designed to remain in the vagina for months at a time. When pessary use is begun, it is important that the woman return to the HCP for a recheck after an initial period of use to determine whether it is causing pressure damage to tissues. Because the pessary is a foreign object in the vagina, increased vaginal discharge can be expected. Discharge should not be pink, bloody, or purulent.

Nursing Care and Patient Education

Teach patients to eat a healthy diet to avoid obesity and constipation, and how to do Kegel exercises to keep the pubococcygeal muscle strong and able to support the organs in the pelvic cavity. One way to do Kegel exercises follows:

1. To find the pubococcygeal muscle, tighten while urinating so that the flow of urine stops.

• WORD • BUILDING •

agenesis: a—without + genesis—production
hypoplasia: hypo—little + plasia—shape (or form)
imperforate: im—not + perforate—pierced
dyspareunia: dys—painful or abnormal + pareunia—mating

2. Squeeze the muscle that stopped urinary flow tightly, holding for 10 seconds, and totally relaxing the muscle afterward. Repeat 15 times per day.

3. Practice controlling the muscle by contracting and relaxing it to move the pelvic floor upward and downward very slowly. Thinking of an elevator helps some women. Repeat this 15 times per day.

 NURSING CARE TIP

Teach women to do Kegel exercises while waiting in lines to use otherwise wasted time to promote their health. Another suggestion is to plan specific times of day or activities that would include Kegel exercises, such as while in a car or working at a computer. Kegel exercises can be done anywhere and are not apparent to anyone watching.

Cystocele
Pathophysiology, Etiologies, and Signs and Symptoms

Cystocele occurs when the bladder sags into the vaginal space because of inadequate support (Fig. 42.5A). A feeling of pelvic pressure and stress incontinence are common with this condition.

Therapeutic Measures

Kegel exercises or the use of a pessary may help. If these measures are ineffective, anterior **colporrhaphy**, which is a surgical repair of the anterior portion of the vagina, may be needed. Another possible surgical treatment involves resuspending the bladder.

Rectocele
Pathophysiology, Etiologies, and Signs and Symptoms

Rectocele occurs when a portion of the rectum sags into the vagina because of inadequate support (see Fig. 42.5B). A feeling of pelvic pressure, as well as fecal incontinence, constipation, and hemorrhoids, can result.

Therapeutic Measures

Kegel exercises can help strengthen the supporting muscles. The patient should maintain bowel regularity with a high-fiber diet to avoid further discomfort and sagging from bowel overdistention. Posterior colporrhaphy may be necessary to correct this problem.

Uterine Position Disorders
Pathophysiology, Etiologies, and Signs and Symptoms

The most common variations in position of the uterus are **anteversion**, **anteflexion**, **retroversion**, and **retroflexion** (Fig. 42.6). In anteversion, the uterus lies too far forward,

• **WORD** • **BUILDING** •

cystocele: cysto—bag (bladder) + cele—hernia
colporrhaphy: colpo—vagina + rrhaphy—suture
rectocele: recto—rectum + cele—hernia
anteversion: ante—front + version—turning
anteflexion: ante—front + flexion—bending
retroversion: retro—back + version—turning
retroflexion: retro—back + flexion—bending

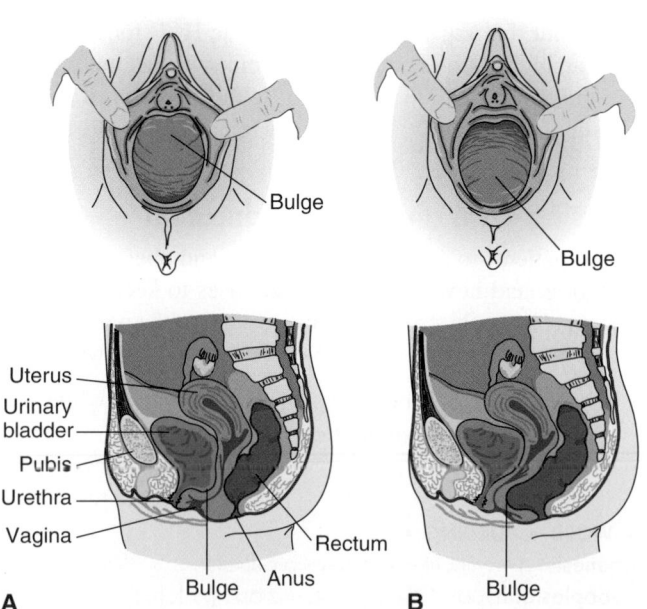

Uterus
Urinary bladder
Pubis
Urethra
Vagina
Rectum
Bulge   Anus
A   Bulge   **B**

FIGURE 42.5 (A) Cystocele. (B) Rectocele.

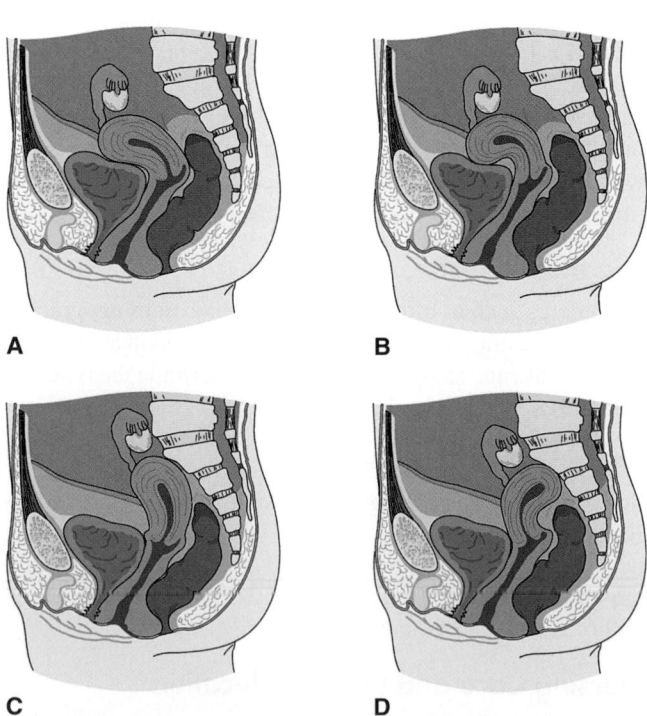

A   **B**

C   **D**

FIGURE 42.6 Uterine positions. (A) Anteversion. (B) Anteflexion. (C) Retroversion. (D) Retroflexion.

and in retroversion, it lies too far backward. In anteflexion, the upper portion of the uterus bends forward, and in retroflexion, it bends backward.

Symptoms that can result from these uterine displacements include painful menstruation and intercourse, infertility, and repeated spontaneous abortion.

Therapeutic Measures

A pessary may correct some positional problems. If infertility or recurrent spontaneous abortion is involved or the condition is very painful, surgery to correct the condition may be necessary.

Uterine Prolapse
Pathophysiology, Etiologies, and Signs and Symptoms

Uterine prolapse occurs when the uterus sags into the vagina (Fig. 42.7). The amount of sagging can vary and can increase over time as a result of the effects of gravity, poor pelvic support, and excessive lifting or straining. In first-degree prolapse, less than half the uterus sags into the vagina. In second-degree prolapse, the entire uterus sags into the vagina. In third-degree prolapse, the uterus sags outside the body.

Uterine prolapse can be very uncomfortable, resulting in back pain, pelvic pain, pain with intercourse (or inability to have intercourse), urinary incontinence, constipation, and development of hemorrhoids. Pressure on the uterus can compromise circulation, resulting in tissue necrosis. Vaginal vault prolapse can also occur in women who have had a hysterectomy, so that the vagina turns inside out and sags downward with similar signs and symptoms. This condition typically requires surgical resuspension.

Therapeutic Measures

Some minor uterine displacements may be treated with use of a pessary. Kegel exercises may be more effective in prevention of uterine prolapse than in treatment because, once the tissues become stretched sufficiently for the uterus to sag into the vagina, the continued weight of the uterus prevents adequate contraction of the muscles. Surgery may be done to correct this problem. Although the uterus can be resuspended by shortening the muscles and fascia, hysterectomy is the more common treatment unless further childbearing is desired.

See Table 42.7 for a summary of displacement disorders.

FERTILITY DISORDERS

Infertility is a complicated problem with many causes. Some couples with infertility may have multiple reproductive problems. Both male and female partners should be examined. (See Chapter 43 for greater detail on male reproductive system disorders.) Often the woman sees the HCP first and may be given a specimen container and advised to give the container to her partner for provision of a semen sample for analysis. See Table 42.8 for a summary of fertility disorders and diagnostic tests.

FIGURE 42.7 Uterine prolapse. (A) Normal uterus. (B) First-degree prolapse: descent within the vagina. (C) Second-degree prolapse. (D) Third-degree prolapse: vagina is completely everted.

TABLE 42.7   DISPLACEMENT DISORDERS OF THE GENITAL ORGANS SUMMARY

Signs and Symptoms	Pain with menses or sexual intercourse Infertility Spontaneous abortion or preterm labor Prolapse of uterus, bladder, or rectum into vagina or outside of body
Diagnostic Tests and Findings	Physical examination Ultrasound Hysterosalpingography CT or MRI scan Endoscopy
Therapeutic Measures	Kegel exercises Surgery Hormone supplements
Priority Nursing Diagnoses	*Acute* or *Chronic Pain* related to structural abnormality or surgery *Urinary Incontinence* or *Constipation* related to structural abnormalities *Sexual Dysfunction* related to disturbance in self-concept *Grief* related to absence or loss of reproductive status

CT = computed tomography; MRI = magnetic resonance imaging.

TABLE 42.8 FERTILITY DISORDERS

Disorder	Pathophysiology/Etiology	Diagnostic Tests
Male	Possible anatomic abnormalities, hormonal imbalances, genetic defects, inflammatory conditions, immune system disorders, difficulties with sexual function, psychological factors, or exogenous influences such as drug use, radiation or chemical exposure, trauma, and excessive testicular temperatures (may occur with prolonged hot tub use or tight clothing)	Semen analysis of number, condition, and movement of the sperm and composition of seminal fluid
Female Ovulation	Possible anatomic and physiological abnormalities of ovaries; hormonal imbalances related to hypothalamus, thyroid, or adrenal glands; polycystic ovary syndrome	Basal body temperature charting, midluteal serum progesterone blood levels, luteinizing hormone levels, blood or urine testing, ultrasound monitoring of a follicle for evidence of release of ovum, endometrial biopsy, observation of male hair distribution, other hormone testing as indicated
Tubal	Possible obstruction of the fallopian tubes resulting from anatomic variations, scarring, or adhesions; prior surgeries; inflammatory processes involving other abdominal tissues	Hysterosalpingography (see Chapter 41), laparoscopy
Uterine	Possible abnormalities in shape or blockages within the uterus (rare cause of infertility but a potential cause of pregnancy loss before maturity), menstrual disorders involving the endometrium	Hysteroscopy (see Chapter 41), removal of tissue samples using curet or endoscope
Other Sources	Possible reproductive environmental factors such as destructive antigen-antibody responses, inappropriate pH of seminal fluid for maximal sperm motility, or substances in female partner's genital tract fluids that disable sperm	Postcoital test: Couple is advised to have intercourse when luteinizing hormone and estrogen levels are high, then a specimen of cervical mucus is taken from the woman 2–12 hours later for analysis of reproductive environment

Nursing Care and Education of the Patient Undergoing Fertility Testing

An understanding attitude is very important because infertility can be a cause of low self-esteem, as well as relationship problems. Patients who have been undergoing diagnostic testing or treatment for infertility can become very discouraged with the process and the expense, especially if it has been ineffective. Having to plan your sexual activity around a HCP's directions can compromise feelings of spontaneity, enjoyment, and privacy. Extensive questioning by nurses can aggravate the situation, but avoiding conversation may convey a lack of caring. A friendly, "Which test shall I help you get ready for today?" may well be enough to get the needed information. Many women undergoing infertility testing are very well informed about the test they will be having and can tell you so that you know which equipment to prepare.

On the first infertility investigation visit, the nurse may teach or give a handout to the patient about keeping a precise record of her oral temperatures with a basal thermometer each morning on awakening, before any other activity. The first day of her menses is day 1 on the temperature chart. Changing levels of hormones result in slight temperature changes, which can be used to identify when ovulation seems to be occurring and when particular hormone levels should be tested. Because many factors can influence temperature and cycles, explain that it may take a few months of recording to clearly identify her pattern.

You may assist with office procedures such as endometrial biopsy, which can be done during a pelvic examination 2 or 3 days before menses is expected. A pregnancy test should be done before this procedure to avoid interfering with a pregnancy. The woman may receive pain medication and paracervical block anesthesia for the procedure. Assess pulse and blood pressure. A vasovagal reaction treatment kit containing epinephrine (or atropine, according to the health care provider's choice), a tourniquet, and a syringe should be available for injection if a vasovagal reflex occurs during the procedure. Vasovagal reflex is a reflex stimulation of the vagal nerve that can happen when the cervix, larynx, or trachea is manipulated and results in slowing of the heart rate and decreased cardiac output, so that the blood pressure drops markedly.

Therapeutic Measures

Treatment of infertility is designed to ensure that an adequate amount of sperm and an ovum can be in proximity in the most conducive environment for fertilization. Removal of barriers such as scar tissue may require surgery. Depending on the results of blood tests and the **postcoital** test (described in Table 42.8), adjustments of environmental factors may involve such actions as sperm washing to avoid destructive antigen–antibody responses, changing the pH of the seminal fluid to encourage sperm motility, treating the female partner to prevent substances in her genital tract fluids from disabling the sperm, or adjusting her hormone levels. The number of sperm or ova available can be increased through use of such fertility drugs as clomiphene citrate or various hormone preparations. Infertility treatments are quite complicated and expensive and change periodically as a result of ongoing research. For more information, check out www.cdc.gov/reproductivehealth /Infertility/index.htm.

Various methods can be used to bring the gametes into proximity. If the problem involves inability to get the sperm close enough to the ovum (as may happen with ejaculatory problems), the HCP may use intrauterine insemination (IUI) to place a semen sample from the male partner closer to the ovum via a small catheter. **In vitro fertilization** (IVF) involves bringing ova and sperm together outside the bodies of the participants. Ova may be harvested using a long needle or an endoscope after hormonal preparation of the woman. Sperm can be obtained through masturbation; intercourse with a nonlubricated, nonspermicidal condom; or electrical stimulation of ejaculation for patients with spinal cord injuries. Once fertilized, the ova are implanted in the woman's uterus.

For those whose sperm is unable to successfully penetrate the ovum, procedures involving gamete micromanipulation may be done. Under a microscope, an ovum from the female partner is partially opened by removing a portion of the outer covering to facilitate sperm penetration, or sperm may be injected into the ovum. This fertilized ovum is then reinserted into the woman's body.

When measures to improve the chances of conception using the partners' own gametes are unsuccessful, gametes from donors may be used. Artificial insemination by injecting another man's sperm into the woman's genital tract is the simplest of the donor procedures. Ova also may be harvested from a donor woman and used for in vitro fertilization using the male partner's sperm if possible. Both of these procedures allow for genetic inheritance from one member of the couple. If genetic inheritance is not possible or desirable (as with familial disease carriers), both donor sperm and ova may be used for in vitro fertilization to be transferred into the female patient. Surrogacy is a situation in which an embryo from one couple is placed into a "host" mother for growth of a baby for the couple and is a topic of much ethical debate.

Nursing Care and Education of the Patient Undergoing Treatment

Patients who are undergoing infertility treatment may experience many upsetting and distressing feelings. Feelings of inadequacy, frustration, depression, and anger are common. If the infertility was caused by something the patient perceives as avoidable, such as STI, guilt feelings may add to the psychological discomfort. Any or all of the previously described tests may be completed and some repeated many times without success in identifying an underlying etiology for infertility, and may result in repeated disappointments. The beginning of menses may signal a time of mourning for these couples. Depression may result after failed IVF attempts. Strained relationships may develop between marriage partners, especially if there is disagreement about the value of testing or the importance of having children.

In IVF, usually more than the desired number of embryos is implanted because it is expected that not all will survive and because this is more cost effective with less physical risk for the mother. However, this requires heart-wrenching decisions of whether to "reduce" (abort) extra pregnancies or to risk having more than the desired number of children at once as a result of the fertility treatments.

Offer a listening ear while being careful not to give advice about treatment modalities. Researchers and practitioners are engaging in ongoing debate as to the value of particular procedures; consequently, strategies may vary widely from one HCP to another. Encourage open communication among the patient, the HCP, and the patient's significant other, as well as informed decision making that is based on the patient's and her partner's values.

Many varieties of assistive reproductive technology are available, and the number is increasing with research. Most of the procedures are known by their acronyms. For example, *GIFT* means "gamete intrafallopian transfer" (gametes are placed together in the fallopian tube with the hope that fertilization will occur). *ZIFT* means "zygote intrafallopian transfer" (fertilization of gametes occurs outside of the body; the conceptus is then placed into a woman's fallopian tube to make the journey to the uterus). Acronyms can be useful shortcuts but can be confusing to patients. Most nurses probably do not need to know all acronyms or infertility treatments unless they work in a gynecologist's office or infertility clinic.

• **WORD • BUILDING** •
postcoital: post—after + coital—pertaining to intercourse
in vitro fertilization: in—inside + vitro—glass + fertiliz—fruitful + ation—process

REPRODUCTIVE LIFE PLANNING

Reproductive life planning is a more comprehensive term than *contraception* and implies reasoned decisions related to pregnancy timing and whether or not to have children. Nurses can contribute to the overall health and quality of life for women and families by helping them to find the information they need to make wise choices.

Many types of birth control are available, and several additional types are in developmental and testing stages. General categories of agents are discussed in this section. Understanding of how the different types of contraceptives work can assist the nurse in answering patients' questions or helping patients find additional information. The World Health Organization (2010) has put together a helpful publication called "United States Medical Eligibility Criteria for Contraceptive Use." This publication assigns an eligibility category of 1 (no restrictions) to 4 (unacceptable risk of a specific contraceptive method with a specified medical condition) to each contraceptive.

Methods are introduced in the order of usual effectiveness from most to least effective (with the exception that experimental methods are discussed at the end regardless of their efficacy). Consult your clinic or HCP for an approved, current comparison list of methods for distribution.

For some patients, the distinction of whether a birth control method actually prevents conception or only interferes with implantation or maintenance of a pregnancy is an important factor in their decision. If a patient believes life begins at conception, any action other than prevention of conception would be considered equivalent to abortion.

Oral Contraceptives

Oral **contraceptive** medications are among the most widely used forms of birth control in North America. Most contain an estrogen and a progestin in combination, although some (mini-pills) contain only a progestin. Some work to prevent conception by inhibiting ovulation or changing the environment of the reproductive tract so that activity of the sperm is inhibited. Others do not prevent conception but make implantation less likely and hasten the breakdown of the corpus luteum so that pregnancy-sustaining hormones are not produced. Many of the adverse effects that occurred in the past have been overcome by adjustment of dosage levels.

Oral contraceptives can also be used in some instances to regulate irregular menses, decrease menorrhagia or dysmenorrhea, or decrease the symptoms associated with endometriosis or cyclic breast changes. Oral contraceptives do not prevent STIs; advise women about the risks of contracting STIs and using condoms for the prevention of STIs while taking an oral contraceptive.

Advantages, Disadvantages, Side Effects, and Risks

Oral contraceptives are very effective. Improvement of dysmenorrhea, endometriosis, increased regularity of menses, and decrease in menstrual flow may occur; however, some women experience menstrual changes such as amenorrhea, irregular or prolonged menses, and intermenstrual spotting.

Oral contraceptives require a great deal of commitment because irregular use decreases their effectiveness. To encourage regular use, oral contraceptives are generally dispensed in containers labeled with the days of the week, and some companies include unmedicated pills in the package to be taken during the time of hormone cessation for menses, so that the woman only has to remember to take a daily pill, instead of timing the taking of the pills with her cycle. Some oral contraceptives are now available to be taken continuously. Women should speak to their care providers to determine which method is best for them.

Some women experience side effects such as acne, fluid retention, headaches, breast swelling and discomfort, midcycle bleeding, and sometimes depression. Use of an oral contraceptive also has some risks. Higher rates of blood clot formation, strokes, high blood pressure, heart attacks, and worsening of diabetes are rare occurrences with some hormonal contraceptives and are generally related to preexisting risk factors. Women who smoke or have diabetes, high blood pressure, heart disease, or a history of thrombophlebitis should receive information about the risks of oral contraceptives and alternative methods of contraception.

Oral contraceptives decrease the risk of endometrial and ovarian cancer, but there is debate about risk of breast cancer, and cervical **dysplasia** (cell changes that may become cancerous) sometimes occurs among oral contraceptive users. Women should definitely be advised to have regular Pap smears while taking oral contraceptives.

Many medications can alter the effectiveness of oral contraceptives, and women should be warned to always alert HCPs and pharmacists that they are using oral contraceptives when a new medication is started or a regular medication is discontinued. Use of hormonal contraceptives increases the risk of vitamin B deficiencies, so a healthy diet with good sources of B vitamins is advisable.

LEARNING TIP

Side effects of oral contraceptives can be serious. Teach your patient to watch for "ACHES" and to contact her primary care provider immediately if they occur. ACHES stands for:

    Abdominal pain
    Chest pain
    Headache
    Eye pain
    Severe leg pain

• WORD • BUILDING •

contraceptive: contra—against + ceptive—taking in (conceiving)

dysplasia: dys—painful or abnormal + plasia—shape or form

Contraceptive Implant and Injectable Medications

Contraceptive implants are small permeable tubes surgically implanted through a small incision under the skin; they slowly release hormones for long-term contraception. Implants have been used with varying success; an example is etonogestrel implant (Nexplanon).

Medroxyprogesterone acetate (Depo-Provera) is a contraceptive agent available in a slow-release depot form that can be injected intramuscularly. Medication is continuously released for 3 months.

Advantages, Disadvantages, Side Effects, and Risks

The main advantage of depot medications and implants is that the woman does not have to remember to take daily medication. Disadvantages are that the medications may not be immediately effective, so another method may be necessary for 1 to 2 weeks after the initial injection, and that fertility may not return for several months to 1 year after discontinuation.

Alterations in menstrual flow, especially amenorrhea, are the most commonly noted side effects with both depot medications and implants. Weight gain of 5 to 10 pounds is also common, which can lead to discontinuation of use. Other side effects and risks are similar to those encountered with oral contraceptives that contain progesterone only.

Estrogen-Progestin Contraceptive Ring

A newer method is an estrogen-progestin contraceptive ring (NuvaRing). It works in much the same manner as other hormonal contraceptives by slowly releasing hormones. The user inserts the ring into the vagina. The ring is left in place for 3 weeks; it is then removed for 1 week in order for menses to occur, after which a new ring is placed.

Advantages, Disadvantages, Side Effects, and Risks

Not having to remember daily medication can be an advantage to the contraceptive ring, but failing to remove it at the right time may disrupt the regularity of the menstrual cycles. With consistent use, it is very effective in preventing pregnancy. Because it does not provide a barrier over the cervix, there is less risk of infection than with a diaphragm or cervical cap. A common side effect is an increase in normal vaginal discharge. Other side effects and risks are similar to other low-dose hormonal contraceptives.

Transdermal Contraceptive Patch

A transdermal patch is now available that contains norelgestromin and ethinyl estradiol (Ortho Evra). It is placed on the abdomen, upper arm, or buttock after a menstrual period and left in place for 1 week. A new patch is placed on the body each week for 3 weeks. After 3 weeks, the patch is removed and not replaced for 1 week in order for menses to occur.

Advantages, Disadvantages, Side Effects, and Risks

The contraceptive patch has been found to be similar to oral contraceptives in effectiveness, side effects, and risks, without having to remember to take a pill each day. The patch will remain in place during bathing, swimming, and other activities.

Barrier Methods

Barrier methods of birth control are less effective in preventing pregnancy than most of the previously mentioned methods when used alone. Barriers are intended to prevent sperm from reaching the ovum. Used in combination, the effectiveness of barrier methods with spermicidal preparations comes close to that of oral contraceptives. Both may be purchased without a prescription.

Condoms

Condoms are barriers that are used once and then discarded into an appropriate waste receptacle. Most condoms come with spermicide/nonoxynol-9. Condoms used with contraceptive jelly or spermicide are most effective at decreasing risk of pregnancy. They should be stored in a cool, dry place before use and should not be stored where heat and continued pressure can weaken them. Storage in a wallet or glove compartment is not advisable. Petroleum-based substances, such as Vaseline, can also weaken condoms, so use of water-soluble lubricants (preferably spermicides) should be advised.

ADVANTAGES, DISADVANTAGES, SIDE EFFECTS, AND RISKS OF MALE CONDOMS. Male condoms have long been used for contraception because they are a relatively inexpensive, totally reversible method that men can control at the time of intercourse. They also provide some barrier protection against transmission of STIs. An electron microscopic study of a sample of nonlubricated latex condoms, however, found that most of those viewed had surface abnormalities, including cracking and melted areas. Patients should be informed that barrier methods can reduce risk but do not absolutely prevent transmission of STIs, especially in areas of contact not covered by the barrier.

The main disadvantages of condom use are interruption of foreplay for application, decreased sensation, and the possibility of slippage or breakage during intercourse. These disadvantages may be overcome by incorporating application of the condom by the female partner as a part of foreplay; using thinner, lubricated, or textured condoms to increase sensation; using the correct size condom with a reservoir or application that leaves about a half-inch at the tip of the condom loose enough to serve as a reservoir for semen (Fig. 42.8); and removal from the vagina before relaxation of the erection.

ADVANTAGES, DISADVANTAGES, SIDE EFFECTS, AND RISKS OF FEMALE CONDOMS. Female condoms are a more recent innovation that allows female initiation of contraception, as well as some barrier protection against STIs. Coverage of the labia by the condom may provide more of a barrier than male condoms (Fig. 42.9). Disadvantages are similar to those of male condoms; they are also more expensive than male condoms.

Diaphragms and Cervical Caps

Diaphragms and cervical caps work in the same manner as condoms, by blocking the entry of sperm through the cervix (Fig. 42.10). The barrier effect is enhanced by simultaneous

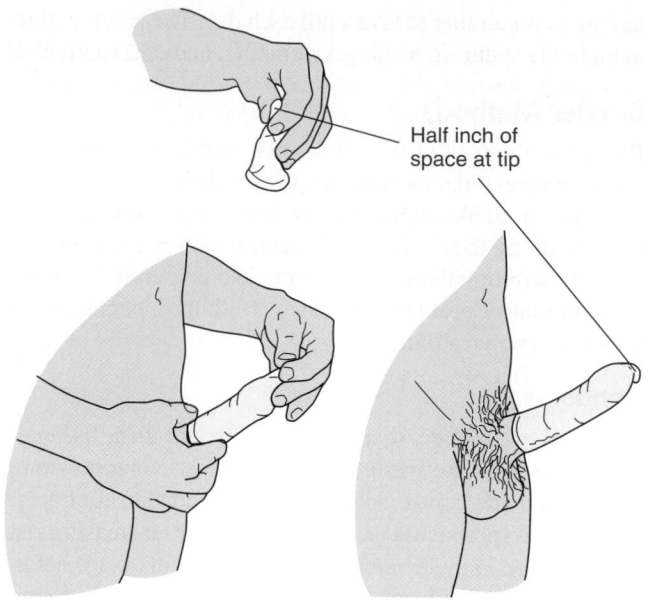

FIGURE 42.8 Correct application of a male condom.

use of a spermicide. Application of a spermicide to the edge of the device and placement of a small amount in the cup before use increases effectiveness.

ADVANTAGES, DISADVANTAGES, SIDE EFFECTS, AND RISKS.
These methods are relatively inexpensive, are female initiated, and work without systemic medication. Diaphragms and cervical caps require initial fitting and a prescription to buy them, may need to be refitted after childbirth and the loss or gain of weight, and can last for years. They should be replaced periodically based on manufacturer recommendations or whenever there is any evidence of hardening, cracking, or thin spots. They need to be washed with soap and water, dried, and stored in a case away from heat and sunlight between uses.

Women and their partners can experience irritation or allergic reaction to the spermicide or the contraceptive device material, which would require changing birth control methods. These types of methods require that the device be inserted before intercourse and left in place for several hours afterward. (See package inserts for specific recommendations.) An increase in incidence of urinary tract infection has been reported with use of the diaphragm, and risk of TSS increases with prolonged uninterrupted use of cervical barriers. Adequate fluid intake, voiding shortly after intercourse, and removal of the device as directed following intercourse all help to prevent these potential problems. If urinary tract infections are recurrent using the diaphragm, changing to a cervical cap may decrease the occurrence because there is less pressure against the bladder through the anterior vagina.

Spermicides

Spermicidal agents may be used alone, although use in combination with a barrier method is much more effective. They come in a variety of forms, such as creams, gels, foams, and suppositories, which kill or disable sperm so that fertilization does not occur.

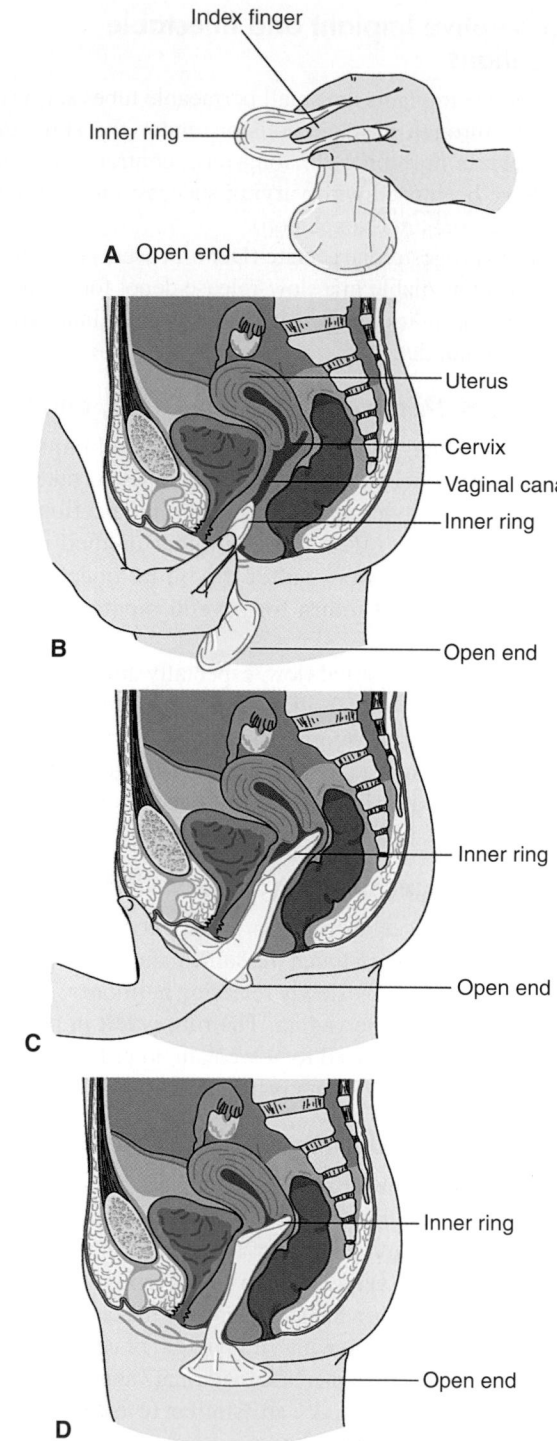

FIGURE 42.9 Female condom application. (A) Inner ring is squeezed for insertion. (B) Sheath is inserted similar to a tampon. (C) Inner ring is pushed up as far as it can go with index finger. (D) Condom in place.

Advantages, Disadvantages, Side Effects, and Risks

Spermicidal preparations are relatively inexpensive and can be male or female initiated. They do not produce systemic effects, and no hormones are involved. Spermicides require application before each act of intercourse and some patients

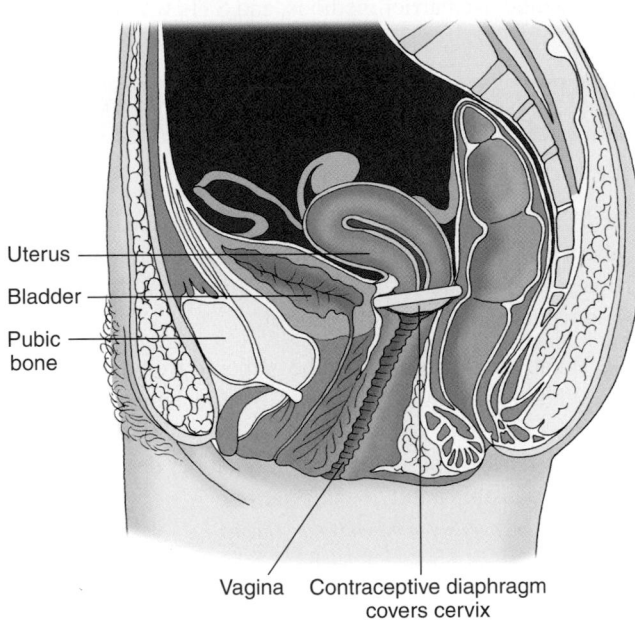

Uterus

Bladder

Pubic bone

Vagina   Contraceptive diaphragm covers cervix

FIGURE 42.10 Contraceptive diaphragm.

consider them to be somewhat messy. Many contain the same ingredient—nonoxynol 9. If genital irritation or a rash occurs with a spermicide, the patient should read labels carefully to avoid future contact with the same ingredient.

Intrauterine Devices

The presence of a foreign object in the uterus is thought to alter the environment so that implantation is less likely to occur. IUDs are generally made from a form of plastic and may contain copper wire (such as the ParaGard) or a supply of a progestin (for example, Mirena) that is slowly released into the system to further alter the uterine environment to hinder fertilization or implantation.

Advantages, Disadvantages, Side Effects, and Risks

The main advantage of an IUD is continuous contraception without the necessity of remembering to take medication and without the side effects associated with medications. The ParaGard is effective for 10 years, and the Mirena is effective for 5 years. Mirena may help lighten and potentially eliminate menstrual bleeding in women who have a history of anemia or heavy menstrual flow.

Disadvantages are changes in menstrual bleeding, cramping, and increased risk of pelvic inflammatory disease (PID). Rarely, an IUD has caused a uterine perforation. New research and changes in the medical eligibility criteria set up by the World Health Organization has shown that IUDs can be used by women who have never been pregnant because advantages far outweigh risks. IUDs should be avoided in women with uterine abnormalities, those with PID, and those who have current STIs. Expulsion or displacement of the IUD can occur, so women should be taught to feel for the presence of the external string before intercourse.

Insertion Procedure

Insertion of an IUD typically is done in a HCP's office, usually during the first 7 days of the menstrual cycle because the cervix is slightly dilated at this time. The IUD is inserted into the cervix through a tube that comes packaged with the IUD, which temporarily holds the IUD flat or folded for insertion. When the IUD is pushed out the end of the tube, it springs into a shape that helps to keep it inside the uterus. One potential danger of IUD insertion is vasovagal reflex stimulation (previously described in association with endometrial biopsy). Periodically assess pulse or blood pressure during the procedure and notify the HCP of slowing of the heart rate or a decrease in blood pressure.

Natural Family Planning

Periodic abstinence (natural family planning) is less effective than the previously described methods. It is a method by which couples control their fertility by restricting intercourse to "safe periods" during which risk of conception is low. Many signs can be assessed to determine "safe" days, including temperature changes, cervical consistency and mucus changes, calendar timing, and awareness of symptoms of fertility.

Slight body temperature changes can indicate ovulation. During the first half of the menstrual cycle, the temperature remains low, with a marked drop just before ovulation occurs. With ovulation the temperature rises and stays higher for the last half of the cycle. Women who use this assessment method should use a basal body temperature thermometer when they awaken, before doing anything else, and record it on a chart.

Cervical consistency and mucus changes can also help pinpoint ovulation. As hormone levels change, the consistency of cervical mucus changes. As ovulation approaches, there is an increase in the amount of mucus and the mucus becomes more clear, thin, slippery, and stretchable than at other times of the month. Around the time of ovulation, the cervix becomes softer to touch and more open than at other times of the cycle.

Following the calendar can work fairly well if a woman's menstrual periods are regular, but becoming aware of her pattern may take time. Symptoms such as breast tenderness and midcycle discomfort (*mittelschmerz*) can also help identify ovulation. Users of this method should be advised to abstain from intercourse for approximately 3 days before ovulation and 3 to 4 days after because the sperm and ovum can survive for a long period in the female genital tract.

Advantages and Disadvantages

The advantages of this method are that it requires no expense or medication, and it is the only birth control method currently approved by the Catholic Church. The disadvantages are that it requires the cooperation of both partners and may interfere with spontaneity of sexual expression. It is generally not very effective as a means of birth control. It may be difficult to accurately identify ovulation times because infectious and inflammatory processes can affect temperature readings, infections and feminine hygiene products can affect cervical mucus, and irregularity of flow and symptoms may make prediction difficult.

Less Effective Methods

Coitus Interruptus

Coitus interruptus involves removal of the penis from the vagina before ejaculation occurs.

ADVANTAGES, DISADVANTAGES, AND RISKS. Although this method requires no expense or preparation, it is not very effective. Excellent control of ejaculation is required, and even the small amount of sperm that may be present in pre-ejaculatory fluid can result in pregnancy.

Postcoital Douching

The intended purpose of postcoital douching is to wash sperm out of the reproductive tract or to kill or immobilize sperm that the douche solution contacts.

ADVANTAGES, DISADVANTAGES, AND RISKS. This is relatively inexpensive and female initiated, but it is not very effective. Sperm move very rapidly once deposited, and douching may actually push the sperm upward.

Lactational Amenorrhea Method (Breastfeeding)

Breastfeeding is sometimes used as a method of birth control because the high blood levels of prolactin that occur with breastfeeding may suppress ovulation. This may be effective in the first 6 months after delivery and requires "full or nearly full" breastfeeding, and that the woman has not experienced her first postpartum menses (any bleeding 56 days postpartum).

ADVANTAGES, DISADVANTAGES, AND RISKS. This method costs nothing but is not very effective. Prolactin levels can vary widely, and ovulation may resume at any time without any noticeable signs, resulting in pregnancy before even experiencing a menstrual period after the birth.

Ongoing Research: Future Possibilities for Contraceptive Choices

Many researchers have tried to develop effective and reversible male contraceptives. When taken orally a plant called *Tripterygium,* used in Chinese herbal medicine, yields substances that can limit numbers and mobility of sperm, but it also has active ingredients that suppress immunity somewhat, so further investigation is necessary. Reversible injection procedures to block the seminal vas deferens are also being investigated, as are reversible injection procedures to block the fallopian tubes. Reversible birth control vaccines are also being investigated for both men and women with the goal of causing an immune response to occur at some vital point in the process of conception.

Some questions related to contraceptive vaccines include the unknown long-term repercussions of stimulating the body to respond with immunity to itself and whether governments could use vaccines as a means to control populations without individuals' consent. Another frightening possibility is that with further removal of the threat of pregnancy, even fewer people would use barrier methods, and STIs would increase.

CRITICAL THINKING

Jessica

■ You have just observed a patient who appears to be about 13 years old announce loudly at the clinic reception desk that she is "ready to be a responsible adult" and would like some birth control.

1. What information should be gathered from her?
2. What do you think she needs to know before making a decision?
3. How can you base your teaching on her desire to be a responsible adult?

Suggested answers are at the end of the chapter.

Sterilization

Permanent sterilization can be accomplished by either interrupting the fallopian tubes or vas deferens (by vasectomy, as discussed in Chapter 43) or by removing the uterus (hysterectomy). Tubal interruption may be done by tying a suture or placing a ring or clip around each fallopian tube, by coagulating a section of the tubes, or by surgically removing a portion of the tube and suturing the ends. These procedures are usually done by laparoscope in an outpatient setting, as an additional procedure performed during a cesarean delivery, or within a few days after a vaginal delivery. A new nonsurgical procedure (Essure) uses an endoscope to implant a tiny insert into each fallopian tube to block patency.

Advantages, Disadvantages, Side Effects, and Risks

Although sterilization is not absolutely certain to be permanent, the failure rate is low and has been decreasing recently with newer surgical methods. After vasectomy, men must return to the HCP's office to supply at least two semen samples to ensure no sperm are present. Reversal is sometimes requested at a later time to reestablish fertility. This requires microsurgery with anesthesia and has a poor success rate.

Patient Education

Patients should be advised by their surgeon about the complications of the surgery and reversal before they sign a consent form for sterilization. If any uncertainty about the surgery is evident, the HCP should be notified promptly.

■ PREGNANCY TERMINATION

Termination of pregnancy (abortion) is a difficult topic. Discussions about it are often highly charged with emotion. Both prolife and prochoice advocates argue on the basis of human rights—the former based on rights of the fetus and the latter on rights of the mother—because of the humanity of each party. There are few people on either side of the philosophical argument, however, who would describe abortion as a healthy medical intervention. Most agree that abortion is a problematic solution to a difficult situation.

Types of Abortion

Therapeutic Abortion for Ectopic Pregnancy

An ectopic pregnancy is the implantation of a fertilized ovum in an area other than the uterus. This can occur because of an abnormally shaped uterus or fallopian tubes that are obstructed as a result of abnormal development, scarring from STIs or other inflammatory processes, or for unknown reasons. It is a life-threatening situation for the mother, and currently a therapeutic abortion is the only treatment.

Therapeutic Abortion for Prenatal Abnormalities

Development of a variety of prenatal testing methods has introduced the possibility of knowing many things about a baby before birth. Prenatal testing may be done using ultrasound, samples of fluid taken from the amniotic sac or the placental villi, or blood samples from the mother. From these tests, some genetic diseases and congenital deformities can be identified. After anomalies are diagnosed, some patients choose to abort the baby. This is a very difficult decision to consider even in instances in which the baby has a fatal defect that will not allow it to live outside the uterus. It is important to provide information about alternatives to abortion and possible treatments for their child when a patient has a serious prenatal diagnosis. No one should feel pressured to make the decision quickly to abort, but legal requirements and increasing risk for the mother may limit the time to decide. Abortion because of fetal abnormality may result in much grieving and guilt for the patient and her family.

Methods of Abortion

Several methods are available. The method is determined primarily by the length of the gestation and the goal of inflicting as little trauma to the mother's reproductive system as possible while still inducing pregnancy loss. Time periods for the different abortion methods and the allowable reasons for legal abortion vary according to the laws of the state, province, or country.

Chemical Agents

Emergency contraception, known as Plan B, is sometimes called the "morning-after pill." Treatment consists of postcoital administration of sufficient estrogen/progestin (levonorgestrel) to prevent ovulation and possibly to prevent fertilization if ovulation has already occurred. The drug also prevents a fertilized ovum from implanting in the uterine lining. If a fertilized ovum has already implanted when the patient takes the drug, the pregnancy will not be terminated. For this reason, there is some disagreement about whether Plan B is a form of contraception or a form of abortion.

Plan B is available at pharmacies without a prescription. Typically, it is used after unexpected, unprotected sexual intercourse (as with sexual assault) or with unexpected risk of conception (as with condom failure). For the medication to be effective, the initial dose typically is given within 72 hours after intercourse and preferably within the first 24 hours. Because no advance planning is required before intercourse, Plan B can be misused as a casual form of birth control. Patients who use it in this way need education about more appropriate birth control methods. Side effects of Plan B can include nausea, vomiting, headaches, and breast tenderness.

Another type of postcoital medication prevents the binding of progestins at their receptors, which causes a chemically induced abortion up to the 10th week of pregnancy. This is known as a medical abortion. Medication can be given orally and/or vaginally. You may recall the controversial RU-486 (mifepristone, marketed under the name Mifeprex). Mifepristone causes the blockage of progesterone from the uterine lining, causing the lining to break down. The patient is also then given a dose of misoprostol, which causes the uterus to empty. It must be used within 63 days after the first day of the woman's last period. Pregnancy must be confirmed along with how far pregnant a woman is before medical abortion. Nausea and cramping can accompany expulsion of the uterine contents.

There is much debate about whether mifepristone should be used at all or only within specific guidelines. The U.S. Food and Drug Administration approved mifepristone in 2000 in an accelerated drug-approval process, but legislative bills have been repeatedly introduced to stipulate prescribing regulations for HCPs. Undoubtedly mifepristone, as well as methotrexate (a chemotherapy medication) and misoprostol (a medication to prevent stomach ulcers), all of which can stimulate abortion, will continue to be the subject of much debate.

Abortion Methods for Early Pregnancy

Early in a pregnancy (during approximately the first 13 weeks), there are three primary means of pregnancy termination: menstrual extraction, vacuum aspiration, and D&C. Menstrual extraction is removal of the endometrial lining by manual suction and can be done during the first 7 weeks following the last menstrual period (LMP). This can be done without anesthesia and without cervical dilation by inserting a small cannula into the cervix and aspirating with a large syringe. Vacuum aspiration is a similar process that is used from confirmation of pregnancy through the first 13 weeks. It requires cervical dilation and usually is done with local anesthesia. The patient returns home 1 to 4 hours after the procedure. D&C also may be used during the first 13 weeks. In this procedure, the cervix is dilated and the uterine contents are scooped away with a curet. This is done as an outpatient procedure under general, regional, or local anesthesia.

Abortion Methods for Later Pregnancy

During the second trimester, the fetus is much larger, so more dilation is required. A dilation and evacuation (D&E) may be performed in much the same manner as a D&C. Dried laminaria (a type of seaweed) or some other absorbent substance is placed inside the cervical canal. This absorbs fluid and swells, thus gradually dilating the cervix. Prostaglandin may be administered either by suppository into the vagina or by injection into the amniotic sac; this usually induces uterine contractions and results in delivery a few hours later. Unfortunately, a live fetus too premature to survive may be born by this method and continue to breathe for a time until death.

An induction with either a saline or urea injection may be used for pregnancies beyond 16 weeks. A portion of amniotic fluid is removed and replaced with concentrated saline or urea solution, which kills the fetus and stimulates contractions. Sometimes saline and prostaglandins are used in combination to terminate a pregnancy.

Hysterotomy involves removal of the uterine contents through an abdominal incision in the same manner as a cesarean delivery. This procedure is rarely done for pregnancy termination.

Risks and Complications

Abortion involves risks. Some are the same risks inherent in childbirth, such as possible hemorrhage or introduction of infection, but there are additional risks related to the interruption of natural processes and the aggressiveness with which the products of conception are removed during abortion. During an uncomplicated childbirth, the uterine lining is not scraped or forcefully emptied by suction. Natural hormonal preparation for term childbirth contributes to uterine contraction after the birth, which decreases blood loss, but no such preparation occurs for abortion. Artificial dilation of the cervix may cause injury, as may introduction of the instruments used for abortion. Injured tissues can become sites for growth of microorganisms. Finally, the possibility of infertility as a result of complications related to abortion, although relatively uncommon, is a risk.

Some possible physical complications following therapeutic abortion are injuries to the uterus or cervix, excessive bleeding, infection, retention of some products of conception, and possible failure of abortion. Rarely, second-trimester abortions can be complicated by amniotic fluid embolism, in which amniotic fluid is absorbed into the uterine circulation because of disruption of placental attachments with instruments. Amniotic fluid in the mother's circulatory system can result in circulatory collapse and disseminated intravascular coagulation (DIC). DIC is a serious derangement of the body's blood clotting controls and, although rare, can be fatal.

Nursing Care and Patient Education

Care after abortion is very important. Patients rarely stay overnight, and complications can occur after they are discharged. Patients should be carefully assessed after the procedure for signs of bleeding. Instruct the patient that bleeding should not exceed that of a heavy period, that the passage of clots larger than a quarter may be a sign of complications, and that the discharge should not become foul smelling. Patients should be given a phone number to call 24 hours per day, 7 days per week if fever, chills, excessive bleeding, or foul-smelling discharge occur. The patient should be advised

to abstain from sexual intercourse for the time specified by the HCP (usually about 3 weeks).

A grief response may occur after a pregnancy termination, even if the baby was unwanted and the patient does not have strong beliefs against abortion. There is debate about frequency of postabortion syndrome or whether such a condition exists. However, loss and trauma have occurred in any case, and reorganization of the self takes time. Availability of psychological counseling for women after abortion is very important. Women should be given a number to call if they experience psychological discomfort. The need for birth control should be assessed.

Ethical Issues

Ethically, an individual nurse should not be required to assist in any treatment that demands he or she act in a way that contradicts personal moral beliefs. This would violate the nurse's rights. However, there is also an ethical duty to provide care to patients for whom the nurse is responsible. Therefore, it is wise for nurses who have moral objections to abortion to carefully choose their work setting. For example, choosing to work in day surgery in a hospital that performs abortions and refusing to care for abortion patients is not a legitimate option (see "Ethical Considerations" on DavisPlus). One way nurses can positively influence the abortion situation is by teaching about family planning, which may lower the number of requests for abortions. Another way might be to become involved with agencies that help pregnant women find viable alternatives to abortion.

TUMORS OF THE REPRODUCTIVE SYSTEM

Benign Growths
Fibroid Tumors

PATHOPHYSIOLOGY, ETIOLOGIES, AND SIGNS AND SYMPTOMS. Fibroid tumors, or **leiomyomas** (plural form is leiomyomata), are benign tumors made up of endometrial cells that have implanted on or within the walls of the uterus. These can grow very large and may cause pain or menstrual disorders, exert pressure on the bladder or bowel, cause necrosis because of pressure on the blood supply to tissues, and interfere with fertility. Although the exact cause is unknown, heredity and hormones play a role.

THERAPEUTIC MEASURES. Because fibroid tumors are estrogen sensitive, medical treatment may involve hormone suppression. Uterine artery embolization (also called fibroid embolization) involves introduction of tiny sponge-like particles into the artery that supplies the fibroid. This cuts off the blood supply to the tumor and causes it to shrink. Surgical options include myomectomy or hysterectomy. **Myomectomy** is re-

---

• WORD • BUILDING •

hysterotomy: hystero—womb + tomy—cutting
leiomyoma: leio—smooth + myom(a)—fibroid
myomectomy: myom(a)—fibroid + ec—away + tomy—cutting

moval of only the fibroid tumor and may be chosen to preserve fertility. Myomectomy may be done surgically through an abdominal or vaginal incision or with a laser introduced through a laparoscope. Hysterectomy may be necessary for very large fibroids or those that cause severe bleeding or discomfort.

Polyps

PATHOPHYSIOLOGY, ETIOLOGY, AND SIGNS AND SYMPTOMS. Polyps are benign growths that grow inside the uterus or on the cervix and may bleed after intercourse or between menstrual cycles. They are generally teardrop shaped and are attached by a stalk. Polyps develop most often after age 42. The cause is unknown, but estrogen plays a role in their development.

THERAPEUTIC MEASURES. Polyps are generally removed vaginally or transcervically by separating the stalk from the uterus and then stopping the bleeding by use of chemical, electrical, or laser cautery. Removal of polyps in the vagina can be done without anesthetic in an HCP's office. Removal of polyps transcervically requires cervical dilation and is more likely to be done in a hospital with anesthesia.

Reproductive System Cysts

PATHOPHYSIOLOGY, ETIOLOGIES, AND SIGNS AND SYMPTOMS. Several types of cysts can affect women's health. Cysts of the ovaries can develop associated with incomplete ovulation, **hypertrophy** of the corpus luteum after ovulation, or inflammation of the ovary. Most ovarian cysts will eventually shrink spontaneously and merely cause discomfort for a time. "Chocolate" cysts are formed when endometrial cells bleed into an enclosed space, as occurs with endometriosis. They are called chocolate cysts because they are filled with old blood that has become chocolate colored. Cystoadenomas are benign growths that can sometimes undergo cellular transformation and become cancerous. Any pelvic mass in a postmenopausal woman should be investigated for malignancy.

THERAPEUTIC MEASURES. Most cysts are not surgically removed, but excessive size, interference with fertility, and high cancer potential may make needle drainage, biopsy, laparoscopic surgery, or **laparotomy** advisable. If cysts are painful, application of heat to the abdomen or back can help promote comfort.

Polycystic Ovary Syndrome

PATHOPHYSIOLOGY AND ETIOLOGY. Polycystic ovary syndrome (PCOS) is a complex abnormality of endocrine balance of unknown etiology. Multiple cysts on the ovaries are a sign that was discovered early and for which the disease was named, but they are not present in all cases. There seem to be strong genetic links with such family history as too much or too little hair (especially for women), severe acne, diabetes, irregular menses, and infertility. Many of the symptoms of PCOS are a result of insulin resistance with excessive levels of insulin in the blood, which in turn stimulates secretion of androgens.

SIGNS AND SYMPTOMS. Women with PCOS often have infertility, obesity, and menstrual disturbances. They also may have masculinization because of the excess androgen secretion. They have an increased risk of diabetes mellitus, elevated blood pressure, coronary artery disease, and endometrial cancer.

DIAGNOSTIC TESTS. Diagnostic tests can include blood tests to rule out other causes of endocrine abnormality, tests to determine whether ovulation is occurring (such as midluteal progesterone levels and basal body temperature graphing), endometrial biopsies to determine the level of proliferation and to check for endometrial cancer, and blood tests to determine lipid levels and glucose tolerance.

THERAPEUTIC MEASURES. Medical treatments can involve blood pressure medications, lipid control medications, and oral hypoglycemic agents such as metformin (Glucophage). Diet and exercise may be recommended for weight reduction, control of lipid levels, and cardiac health. Oral contraceptives may be used to normalize hormone levels and protect the endometrium for those not desiring to conceive. Ovulation-inducing medication may be used for women who desire to conceive; treatment with metformin may also prompt ovulation.

If masculinization is a problem, antiandrogen medication such as spironolactone (Aldactone) may be prescribed. In severe cases, gonadotropin-releasing hormone (GnRH) agonists may be used to produce medical suppression of the ovaries, with results similar to removal of the ovaries. This is followed 6 months later with an estrogen-progestin combination to protect the bones from osteoporosis.

Bartholin's Cysts

PATHOPHYSIOLOGY, ETIOLOGY, AND SIGNS AND SYMPTOMS. Bartholin's cysts are actually infected Bartholin's glands at either side of the vaginal opening that occur due to obstruction of the glands. Excessive swelling of Bartholin's glands results in pain with sitting and with intercourse.

THERAPEUTIC MEASURES. Incision and drainage can alleviate the discomfort. If Bartholin's cyst formation occurs often, **marsupialization**—the surgical formation of a pouch around an opening made into a gland to facilitate drainage—may be needed. Sitz baths may be ordered to cleanse the area and to promote comfort and healing.

Dermoid Cysts

PATHOPHYSIOLOGY, ETIOLOGY, AND SIGNS AND SYMPTOMS. Rarely and for unknown reasons, a **dermoid** cyst (also called a cystic **teratoma**) may develop from a germinal

• WORD • BUILDING •
hypertrophy: hyper—too much + trophy—nourishment (growth)
laparotomy: laparo(o)—abdominal wall + tomy—cutting
marsupialization: marsupial—pouch + ization—process of making
dermoid: derm—skin + oid—form
teratoma: terat—monster + oma—growth

cell of an ovary. This cell divides and differentiates into various tissue types such as skin, teeth, bones, hair, and even extremities in a disordered arrangement. This type of cyst may grow quite large and may occur on both ovaries at the same time.

THERAPEUTIC MEASURES. Dermoid cysts are removed by laparoscopy or laparotomy. If the cyst contains glandular tissue that is secreting hormones, adjustment of hormone levels to normal may take some time. Although most teratomas are benign, some are malignant, especially in postmenopausal women, so a biopsy is generally done on the tissue.

NURSING CARE AND PATIENT EDUCATION. Growth of a dermoid cyst can be a frightening experience for a woman. Reassurance that this is a disordered group of cells identical to the other cells in her body, rather than a deformed baby, is important.

Malignant Disorders

It is difficult to distinguish benign growths from malignant growths without biopsy results, and some benign growths can become cancerous. Malignancies can occur in all parts of the reproductive system and at all ages. Although reproductive system cancers are more common in older age groups, ovarian tumors can occur even in young children. Both male and female children of women who were given diethylstilbestrol (DES) in the past to prevent premature delivery in high-risk pregnancies have experienced a high incidence of developmental defects and cancers of the reproductive organs.

This section presents a general overview of the most common cancers. If investigated and treated early enough, cure is often possible.

LEARNING TIP

"Three C" changes that may indicate cancer are changes in color, contour, and consistency of a tissue.

Vulvar Cancer

PATHOPHYSIOLOGY, ETIOLOGIES, AND SIGNS AND SYMPTOMS. Although vulvar cancer is not common, alertness to changes in visible parts of the reproductive system such as the vulva can result in early diagnosis, requirement of less drastic treatment, and end with more positive results. Persistent itching of the vulva or appearance of white or red patches, rough areas, skin ulcers, or wartlike growths should not be ignored; these can be signs of precancerous or cancerous changes. Risk factors for development of vulvar cancer are having an STI of any type, precancerous or cancerous changes of the anus or any of the genitalia, immune system depression, and smoking.

DIAGNOSTIC TESTS. Regular Pap smears and physical examinations can identify lesions. Biopsy of suspicious lesions is necessary to diagnose vulvar cancer.

THERAPEUTIC MEASURES. If discovered early, vulvar cancer may be treated with removal or destruction of cancerous cells. If not diagnosed early, it may require surgical removal of the entire vulva and associated lymph nodes (a radical vulvectomy) with subsequent skin grafting from other areas of the body for repair.

Cervical Cancer

PATHOPHYSIOLOGY, ETIOLOGIES, AND SIGNS AND SYMPTOMS. Changes in cervical cells seen with a Pap smear are called cervical dysplasia. Abnormal cells are most often caused by human papillomavirus (HPV). If abnormal cells are found on a biopsy of the cervix, then it is called cervical intraepithelial neoplasia. Without treatment, severe dysplasia can turn into invasive cancer. The severity of the dysplasia determines the treatment plan.

Some identified risk factors for development of cervical cancer include starting sexual activity at an early age, having multiple sexual partners, having several pregnancies, smoking, and being infected with HPV or herpes simplex virus type II (HSV-II). Use of oral contraceptives may also increase a woman's risk of developing cervical cancer, although some of the increase in incidence may be because women using oral contraceptives may not be using barrier protection against STIs. Although some women experience slight spotting or serosanguineous discharge with cervical cancer, many are asymptomatic until the cancer is widespread.

DIAGNOSTIC TESTS. Pap smears are the best method of screening for cervical cancer currently available, but some work is being done on self-tests that women can collect. A Pap smear determines the degree of cellular change, or dysplasia. Ranking systems vary, but Pap smear results are usually presented in categories that range from no atypical cells seen to invasive cancer evident (0 to IV). This procedure has significantly reduced the incidence of invasive cervical cancer over the years since its introduction because cellular changes can be identified early enough for treatment to begin before the cells become cancerous. Colposcopy is done to obtain more information following an abnormal Pap smear (see Chapter 41). New guidelines introduced in 2012 recommend Pap smears starting at age 21 and then every 3 years unless abnormalities develop (American Cancer Society, 2012). After a period of normal Pap smears, some HCPs advocate longer intervals for low-risk women.

THERAPEUTIC MEASURES. Treatments for preinvasive neoplasia include **cryotherapy** (freezing), laser therapy (burning), and surgical removal of the involved area with a loop excision instrument or by conization (Fig. 42.11). All of these procedures are done through the vagina, so there are no external incisions. After any of these treatments, the patient is advised not to douche, use tampons, or have intercourse for approximately 2 weeks to allow healing to take place. She should be advised to report immediately if fever,

• **WORD** • **BUILDING** •
cryotherapy: cryo—cold + therapy—treatment

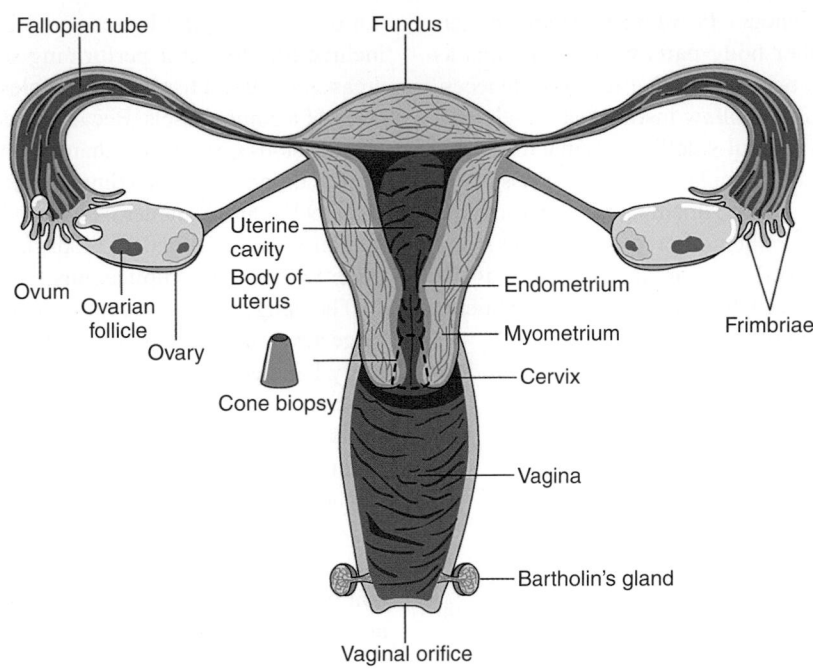

FIGURE 42.11 Conization.

bloody vaginal discharge, or foul-smelling vaginal discharge occurs. For invasive cancers, hysterectomy, radiation implant, or chemotherapy may be done.

PREVENTION. In 2006, a vaccination to help protect against HPV types 6, 11, 16, and 18 was introduced, known as Gardasil (human papillomavirus vaccine). Although there are many high-risk types of HPV, types 6 and 11 cause 90% of genital warts and types 16 and 18 cause 70% of cervical cancers. The vaccination is recommended for both males and females ages 9 to 26, regardless of sexually activity status or exposure to HPV. The vaccination consists of three injections over a 6-month period. The vaccination is still being studied for its longevity.

Endometrial Cancer

PATHOPHYSIOLOGY, ETIOLOGIES, AND SIGNS AND SYMPTOMS. Endometrial cancer is the most common type of uterine cancer. Most develop in response to relative estrogen excess. Abrupt changes in bleeding patterns, especially bleeding in a menopausal woman, can indicate endometrial cancer development. Estrogen excess can develop for many reasons. Estrogen levels fluctuate widely in the perimenopausal period. Obesity results in increased estrogen production that is not balanced by progestins. Estrogen replacement therapy for menopausal symptoms without the addition of progestins also has been associated with an increase in endometrial cancer, but addition of a progestin may decrease the risk of endometrial cancer to less than that of untreated women. Alcohol consumption may increase the risk of endometrial cancer by interfering with estrogen metabolism, but this is still a matter of debate. Some endometrial cancer is unexplained by any currently known risk factors.

DIAGNOSTIC TESTS. Diagnosis is generally done by endometrial biopsy, but MRI may be used to evaluate invasiveness and involvement of lymph nodes.

THERAPEUTIC MEASURES. Depending on the stage of endometrial cancer and metastasis, treatment with hysterectomy, radiation, or chemotherapy may be used.

Ovarian Cancer

PATHOPHYSIOLOGY, ETIOLOGIES, AND SIGNS AND SYMPTOMS. Ovarian cancer is an especially insidious killer because cellular changes in the ovaries often are asymptomatic until the cancer is advanced. Little is known about what prompts these cells to undergo malignant changes. Risk factors are not definitely identified, but some proposed factors include low fertility and number of children, late menopause, a family history of reproductive or colon cancers, and a diet rich in animal fats. Use of hormonal contraception may help prevent ovarian cancer because it results in less ovulation during a woman's lifetime.

DIAGNOSTIC TESTS. Identification of abnormal growths on the ovaries may begin with bimanual examination, so it is important for women, especially in the older age groups, to continue to have regular pelvic examinations even if they are not sexually active and even if they have had a hysterectomy. Various blood tests measuring tumor marker substances, ultrasonography, CT scanning, and MRI may also be used to assist in diagnosis.

THERAPEUTIC MEASURES. Treatment may involve surgical removal of the ovaries by laparoscopy or laparotomy. Sometimes the ovaries are removed to prevent the disease in women who have a high familial risk. Radiation and combination chemotherapy may also be used.

Nursing Care and Education of Patients With Malignant Disorders

Radiation therapy for cancers of the reproductive system may involve the placement of radioactive implants into the patient's body for 24 to 72 hours. Prevent inappropriate radiation of the patient's other body parts by such actions as maintaining patency of a urinary catheter to avoid unnecessary exposure of the bladder. Follow institutional guidelines for radiation precautions. A foul-smelling vaginal discharge is expected after radiation by implant because of tissue destruction caused by the radiation; document the amount and character of the discharge. Chemotherapy treatments often cause severe nausea, as well as anorexia and sores of the mouth, vagina, and anus. See Chapter 11 for care of patients receiving radiation or chemotherapy.

See Table 42.9 for a summary of tumors of the reproductive system.

 GYNECOLOGICAL SURGERY

Endoscopic Surgeries

Many of the surgeries performed on the reproductive system can be done using an endoscope. The endoscopes used contain

TABLE 42.9 TUMORS OF THE REPRODUCTIVE SYSTEM SUMMARY

Signs and Symptoms	Menstrual pain/dysfunction
	Infertility
	Constipation
	Vaginal bleeding
	Abdominal/perineal pain/swelling
	Androgen characteristics
	Obesity
	Diabetes
	Coronary artery disease
Diagnostic Tests and Findings	Physical examination
	Laparoscopy
	Ultrasound
	CT or MRI scan
	Biopsy
	Hormone levels
Therapeutic Measures	Surgery
	Chemical/electrical/laser cautery
	Oral contraceptives and medications
	Incision/drainage/marsupialization
	Chemotherapy
	Radiation therapy
Priority Nursing Diagnoses	*Acute* or *Chronic Pain* related to lesion/surgery
	Urinary Incontinence or *Constipation* related to lesion or surgery
	Disturbed Body Image related to body structure abnormality
	Sexual Dysfunction related to disturbance in self-concept

CT = computed tomography; MRI = magnetic resonance imaging.

not only magnifying lenses and a light source but may also include tiny tools for performing surgery, removal of small areas of diseased tissue and samples, suction, and cauterization of bleeding vessels. Because endoscopic surgeries require tiny incisions (usually less than 1 inch long), there is less tissue disruption and little bleeding compared with traditional surgical techniques. Smaller incisions also present less risk of infection than traditional methods, and recuperation is usually faster with fewer complications.

The danger to the patient is generally low for endoscopic surgeries; however, not all surgical situations can be satisfactorily handled in this way. The size of the cannula restricts the size of tissues that can be removed, unless they can be divided into smaller sections and then pulled out through the cannula. If affected areas are widespread, the endoscope may not be able to reach all sites. Traditional surgery still have may to be done when endoscopic surgery has been ineffective, and this can be frustrating to patients. However, information gained through the previous endoscopic surgery may decrease the time required for a traditional surgery.

Laparoscopies are the most common type of endoscopic surgical procedure used for women's reproductive system surgeries. This method can be used for access to the abdominal cavity and the anterior portions of the reproductive organs. Tubal ligations, tubal repairs, removal of ectopic pregnancy implantations, removal of small tumors, removal of endometriotic tissue, and aspiration of fluid-filled cysts can all be done by this method.

The newest method of surgery uses computers and robots and is minimally invasive (see Chapter 12). This method allows the surgeon to make a small number of 1- to 2-cm incisions to gain access and three-dimensional visualization into the pelvic cavity. Gynecologically, this method can be used for hysterectomy and myomectomy. The benefits of this method versus other surgical methods are a shorter hospital stay and less pain and scarring for the patient. There is also less risk of infection, less blood loss, fewer transfusions, faster recoveries, and quicker return to normal activities.

Culdoscopies may be done to access the area at the back of the uterus. A **culdotomy**, which is an incision into the upper posterior portion of the vagina, is necessary to insert the cannula. A **culdocentesis**, which is the removal of fluid from the cul-de-sac of Douglas, may be done during a culdoscopy. Aftercare is much the same as for a laparoscopy. The patient should be informed that a small amount of vaginal spotting may be expected from the incision but that heavy, purulent, or foul-smelling discharge should be reported because it could indicate infection.

Colposcopies typically are used to screen, diagnose, or treat problems of the cervix. The binocular microscope attached to the scope cannula, which is introduced into the vagina, allows the HCP to examine dysplastic cells while they

• WORD • BUILDING •
culdotomy: culdo—cul-de-sac + tomy—cutting
culdocentesis: culdo—cul-de-sac + centesis—puncturing

are still in their normal place and to treat cervical dysplasia as previously described.

Hysteroscopy may be used to treat problems within the uterus. Removal of polyps and other growths, modification of congenital malformations such as septa (walls of tissue where there should be none), and laser ablation of endometrial tissue may all be done during hysteroscopy. The endoscope may be inserted further into the fallopian tubes to perform a salpingoscopy, allowing surgical or laser opening of blocked tubes.

Nursing Care and Patient Education

Postoperative care involves careful assessment for signs of possible excessive internal bleeding, including assessment of vital signs, skin color and temperature, and pain. Women may experience pain because of carbon dioxide insufflation, which makes the internal organs easier to visualize and manipulate. Measures to reduce the related discomfort while the carbon dioxide is absorbed include instructing the patient to lie flat for a few hours, massaging the back and shoulders, and administering pain medication. Discharge teaching includes instruction about signs of complications to report, medications, and when and where to go for suture removal.

Hysterectomy

Removal of the uterus (hysterectomy) may be done for a variety of reasons, including abnormally heavy or painful menstruation, large fibroid or other benign tumors, severe uterine prolapse, and cancer of the uterus. It should not be done merely as a sterilization procedure because the risks involved in hysterectomy are much greater than the risks associated with tubal ligation. The surgery can be done through an abdominal incision (transabdominal hysterectomy, TAH), vaginally, laparoscopically, or robotically. The vagina is left intact and the proximal end (which had been attached to the uterus) is sutured, forming a blind pouch. Although less vaginal lubrication is present after hysterectomy, nerve routes are maintained, and satisfactory sexual intercourse is expected to continue.

There are three types of hysterectomy. *Total hysterectomy* is the removal of the uterus and cervix; *supracervical hysterectomy* (also known as partial or subtotal) removes just the upper part of the uterus while the cervix is left in place; and *radical hysterectomy,* which is the removal of the whole uterus, the tissue on the both sides of the cervix and the upper part of the vagina, done when cancer is present.

Sometimes the choice is made to remove the fallopian tubes and ovaries, which is known as a bilateral **salpingectomy** and **oophorectomy** (BSO). If the ovaries are removed, the woman undergoes immediate menopause and may suffer from symptoms associated with menopause, including the increased risks of cardiovascular disease and osteoporosis. If removal of the ovaries is done because of the presence of estrogen-dependent cancer, then estrogen replacement is not usually feasible. Extra care, comfort, and explanation from nurses is needed.

See the "Nursing Care Plan for the Patient Undergoing Hysterectomy." In addition to the nursing diagnoses covered, also assess for anxiety related to surgery, body image disturbance, and for ineffective coping. See Chapters 10 and 12, respectively, for additional interventions for pain and postoperative patients.

• WORD • BUILDING •
salpingectomy: salpingo—tubal + ec—from + tomy—cutting
oophorectomy: oophor—ovary + ec—from + tomy—cutting

NURSING CARE PLAN for the Patient Undergoing Hysterectomy

Nursing Diagnosis: *Risk for Ineffective Tissue Perfusion* related to surgical incision and removal of the uterus (and possibly the ovaries)

Expected Outcome: The patient's incision(s) will heal by primary intention without excessive bleeding.

Evaluation of Outcome: Is dressing dry and intact and/or does perineal pad show less than 3-cm stain every hour? Are edges of the incision well approximated, with scant bleeding/serous drainage, and mild edema/erythema (if applicable)?

Intervention Monitor vital signs and oxygen saturation according to hospital policy and as necessary. **Rationale** Vital signs and oxygen saturation reflect tissue perfusion status. **Evaluation** Are vital signs stable and within normal range?

Intervention Assess for bleeding or other discharge on perineal pad and on abdominal dressing (if applicable). **Rationale** Excessive bleeding may compromise tissue perfusion and slow healing. **Evaluation** Is pad or dressing dry? **Rationale** Vaginal discharge gives clues to healing of incision at the proximal end of the vagina. **Evaluation** Is discharge foul smelling?

Continued

NURSING CARE PLAN for the Patient Undergoing Hysterectomy—cont'd

Intervention Assess wound healing (if applicable) twice a day and as needed and report any evidence of infection or inadequate healing promptly. **Rationale** Early treatment of inadequate wound healing decreases postoperative complications. **Evaluation** Is incision area swollen, reddened, or draining purulent material?

Intervention Teach patient to report changes in incision site or excessive bleeding. **Rationale** Patients are discharged quickly and should know what to monitor at home. **Evaluation** Does patient verbalize understanding of instruction?

Nursing Diagnosis: *Risk for Urinary Retention* related to manipulation of the bladder and ureters during surgery, anticholinergic drugs, fluid intake changes, and fear of pain

Expected Outcome: The patient will void 30 mL/hr or more without difficulty.

Evaluation of Outcome: Is patient able to void and effectively empty bladder when voiding? Is patient voiding at least 30 mL/hr?

Intervention Assess urinary output after surgery. Report to RN or HCP if less than 30 mL/hr or unable to void. **Rationale** Inadequate urinary output can be an evidence of dehydration, low glomerular perfusion, kidney dysfunction, damage to ureter, or urinary retention. **Evaluation** Is output greater than 30 mL/hour? Is patient able to void without discomfort?

Intervention Assess bladder fullness using Doppler monitoring or scratch test (listening with a stethoscope, lightly scratch abdomen as you move downward from xiphoid until you hear change in sound indicating top of the bladder). **Rationale** Urine retention can cause infection and damage to kidneys, ureters, and bladder. The scratch test and Doppler monitoring cause less discomfort and pressure than palpation of the abdominal incision area. **Evaluation** Does patient feel she is emptying fully when voiding? Does Doppler or scratch test indicate residual urine after voiding?

Intervention Medicate for pain on a fixed schedule for operative day and first postoperative day (unless patient declines). **Rationale** Maintenance of a consistent blood level of medication in the immediate postoperative period provides relief of pain and promotes voiding without fear of discomfort. **Evaluation** Does patient state that she is comfortable?

Nursing Diagnosis: *Risk for Constipation* related to manipulation of the bowel during surgery, use of opioid analgesics and anticholinergic drugs, diet changes, less exercise than usual, and fear of pain when passing stool

Expected Outcome: The patient will pass soft, formed stool without excessive gas discomfort by third postoperative day.

Evaluation of Outcome: Are bowel sounds active in all four quadrants? Is patient passing gas without difficulty? Is patient able to have a soft, formed bowel movement within 3 days of surgery?

Intervention Assess for active bowel sounds in all four abdominal quadrants before giving anything orally. **Rationale** Manipulation of the bowel during surgery and anesthetics or other medications can interfere with bowel function. **Evaluation** Are bowel sounds within normal limits?

Intervention Encourage high fluid intake, and graduate diet toward a high-fiber, regular diet as soon as patient is able to tolerate it (or HCP orders prescribe). **Rationale** Adequate fluid and fiber in the diet softens the stool for easy passage. **Evaluation** Is patient able to tolerate fluids and high-fiber foods?

NURSING CARE PLAN for the Patient Undergoing Hysterectomy—cont'd

Intervention Encourage adequate exercise. **Rationale** Reasonable exercise promotes peristalsis and relieves gas discomfort. **Evaluation** Has patient dangled at bedside the day of surgery and then walked increasing amounts each following day?

Intervention Assess quantity and quality of pain. Control pain with analgesics, especially before administering a suppository or enema. **Rationale** The presence of pain may inhibit defecation. **Evaluation** Is pain controlled? Does patient express concern about pain with bowel movement?

Intervention Administer stool softeners, laxatives, suppositories, or enemas as ordered (check bowel protocol or standing orders). **Rationale** Soft stool is easier to pass. **Evaluation** Has patient passed soft, formed stool by the third day after surgery?

SUGGESTED ANSWERS TO

CRITICAL THINKING

■ Julie

1. Questions to further assess Julie's symptoms should include the following: How long have you been noticing the lumps? Do you do BSEs? Has there been a change in the characteristics of the lumps? Are the lumps mobile or fixed? Have you noticed any breast skin or nipple changes? Have you noticed any leakage of fluid or blood from your breasts? Are you breastfeeding or have you recently delivered an infant? Have you had a fever? Are the pain and lumps related to your menstrual cycle? Is there anything that makes the symptoms better or worse?

2. You can teach Julie to continue to do BSE because she is the best person to detect changes. Teach her that limiting fat and caffeine in her diet may help reduce symptoms. Reinforce any information or treatments provided by the nurse practitioner.

3. If Julie is doing BSE every month, then she knows her breasts better than anyone. She should be vigilant for changes that do not feel like her usual tissue.

■ Lola

1. Interventions that can help control Lola's discomfort related to hot flashes include possible HRT therapy, inclusion of phytoestrogens in her diet (with HCP direction), limiting caffeinated foods or beverages, dressing in layers so that some may be removed as needed, and lowering the thermostat as needed.

2. Information that should be shared with Lola concerning HRT includes the risks as well as benefits according to most recent studies. Risks include increased risk of stroke, cardiovascular disease, breast cancer, and thromboembolism. Benefits include symptomatic relief and decreased risk of complications from osteoporosis.

3. Collaborate with the HCP, because even herbal remedies can interact with medications and should be recommended by an HCP.

■ Jessica

1. Some important information from Jessica would include her true age (laws vary concerning birth control for minors), her intentions, her family situation, whether she is already sexually active, and what information she wants.

2. She needs to know that being sexually active involves more risks than just pregnancy. Discussion of STIs is vital. Early sexual activity may also be associated with abuse and psychological suffering. The choices of birth control should be explained, including the risks, effectiveness, disadvantages, and advantages of each method. Follow clinic protocol to determine your role in teaching the patient.

3. Potential scenarios can be presented for her "responsible" consideration, such as the following: What would she do if contraceptive failure resulted in a pregnancy? How would she feel if she contracted an incurable or permanently damaging STI that she might pass on to someone else? How would she react to a breakup with her partner after she has engaged in sexual intercourse? Ask about her goals and plans in life. Counseling that evidences concern for the individual at this stage may do a lot to postpone sexual activity until the patient is more mature. It is important for her to realize that choosing to delay sexual activity at this time may be the most responsible and health-promoting life decision she can make.

REVIEW QUESTIONS

1. A patient who is breastfeeding her baby says, "My doctor said I have mastalgia. What does that mean?" Which response by the nurse is best?
   1. "That means you may have an infection in your breasts."
   2. "Mastalgia is just the normal discomfort that is associated with breastfeeding."
   3. "The word mastalgia just means breast pain; it can occur with monthly cycles of hormone levels."
   4. "Mastalgia is the medical term for fibrocystic breast disease. It is important to have it treated promptly."

2. Which response by the nurse is most appropriate when a 60-year-old woman who has been menopausal for several years relates that she has begun having vaginal bleeding again?
   1. "Don't be concerned—it is perfectly normal."
   2. "Try taking some ibuprofen. That may reduce the bleeding."
   3. "You should see your health care provider to have that checked as soon as possible."
   4. "Give it time—bleeding after menopause usually goes away within a month."

3. During an endometrial biopsy, for which of the following signs and symptoms of vasovagal response should the nurse observe?
   1. Pain in the chest and abdomen
   2. Cramping and diaphoresis
   3. High blood pressure and tachycardia
   4. Bradycardia and falling blood pressure

4. Which of the following medications can be used to treat vasovagal response during gynecological procedures? Select all that apply.
   1. atropine
   2. morphine
   3. epinephrine
   4. metoprolol
   5. naproxen

5. The nurse is discharging a patient with endometriosis from an office visit. The patient says her medication helps but does not relieve all her discomfort. What other measures can the nurse recommend?
   1. "Check with the health food store. There are several herbal remedies that can be very effective."
   2. "Try using the relaxation exercises you learned in your childbirth classes. A warm compress to your abdomen might also help."
   3. "You can double up on your pain medication on occasion, but you shouldn't do it on a regular basis."
   4. "If the medications aren't effective, then it is time to talk to the physician about a hysterectomy."

6. The nurse enters the room of a patient who is 1-day postoperative left-sided mastectomy and notes a phlebotomist taking blood from her left antecubital space. What should the nurse do first?
   1. Nothing; the nurse is not the phlebotomist's supervisor.
   2. Nothing; blood pressures should be avoided in the affected arm, but blood draws are safe.
   3. Stop the phlebotomist and ask that the blood be drawn from the right arm.
   4. Notify the health care provider.

7. Following a total hysterectomy with bilateral oophorectomy (BSO), what should the nurse teach the patient to expect?
   1. Heavy bleeding for a week
   2. Symptoms of menopause
   3. Painful intercourse for approximately 6 months
   4. Monthly cramping but no menstrual flow

8. A patient who has just returned from a transabdominal hysterectomy is at risk for impaired urinary elimination. At least how many milliliters should be in her catheter bag 8 hours postoperatively? **Fill in the blank.**
   Answer: _____ mL

9. Which of the following is the least effective form of contraception?
   1. Douching
   2. Condom with spermicide
   3. Diaphragm with spermicide
   4. Oral contraceptive medication

Answers can be found in Appendix C.

References

American Cancer Society (2012). *Can cervical cancer be prevented?* Retrieved July 20, 2013 from www.cancer.org/cancer/cervicalcancer/detailedguide/cervical-cancer-prevention

Centers for Disease Control and Prevention. (2011). *Breast cancer statistics.* Retrieved July 16, 2013, from www.cdc.gov/cancer/breast/statistics

de Villiers, T. J., Gass, M. L. S., Haines, C. J., Hall, J. E., Lobo, R. A., Pierroz, D. D., & Rees, M. (2013). Global Consensus Statement on Menopausal Hormone Therapy. *Climacteric, 16,* 203–204.

National Institutes of Health. (2002). *NHLBI stops trial of estrogen plus progestin due to increased breast cancer risk, lack of overall benefit.* Retrieved November 20, 2009, from www.nhlbi.nih.gov/new/press/02-07-09.htm

PubMed Health. (2012). Premenstrual dysphoric disorder. Retrieved July 17, 2013, from www.ncbi.nlm.nih.gov/pubmedhealth/PMH0004461

World Health Organization. (2010). *United States Medical eligibility criteria for contraceptive use* (4th ed.). Retrieved July 20, 2013 from www.cdc.gov/reproductivehealth/UnintendedPregnancy/USMEC.htm

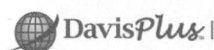 **DavisPlus** | For additional resources and information visit **davispl.us/medsurg5**

43

Nursing Care of Male Patients With Genitourinary Disorders

MICHELLE JOHNSON
AND DEBRA PERRY-PHILO

KEY TERMS

cryptorchidism (kript-OR-ki-dizm)
epididymitis (EP-i-DID-i-MY-tis)
erectile dysfunction (e-REK-tile dis-FUNK-shun)
hydrocele (HEYE-droh-seel)
orchiectomy (or-ki-EK-toh-mee)
orchitis (or-KY-tis)
paraphimosis (PAR-uh-fih-MOH-sis)
phimosis (fih-MOH-sis)
priapism (PRY-uh-pizm)
prostatectomy (PRAHS-tah-TEK-tuh-mee)
prostatitis (PRAHS-tuh-TY-tis)
retrograde (RET-roh-GRAYD)
suprapubic (SOO-pruh-PEW-bik)
urodynamic (YOO-roh-dy-NAM-ik)
urosepsis (YOO-roh-SEP-sis)
vasectomy (va-SEK-tuh-mee)

LEARNING OUTCOMES

1. Explain the pathophysiology associated with each male genitourinary and reproductive disorder discussed in this chapter.

2. Describe the etiologies, signs and symptoms, and treatments of prostate disorders.

3. Plan nursing care for men with genitourinary and reproductive disorders.

4. Describe disorders of the testicles and penis and how they affect sexual function.

5. List selected physical and emotional causes of erectile dysfunction.

6. Discuss the nurse's role in helping men cope with loss of sexual function.

7. Identify disorders of the male reproductive system that interfere with fertility.

8. List treatment options available for male infertility.

Problems affecting the male genitals and urinary system typically are difficult areas for both the patient and the nurse to deal with because of the sexual nature of the male anatomy. Nurses need to realize that sexuality is a natural part of each of us as human beings and should not be avoided when we provide care to patients. Often the nurse is an ideal person to provide important sexual health care teaching. If the patient is approached in a confident, confidential manner, discussions about sexual health can be positive learning experiences for both the patient and the nurse.

Some good general health guidelines for men can be found at the Agency for Healthcare Research and Quality's Put Prevention into Practice website at www.ahrq.gov/ppip /healthymen.htm.

 PROSTATE DISORDERS

The prostate gland sits at the base of the bladder and wraps around the upper part of the male urethra like a doughnut. The primary purpose of the prostate is to provide alkaline secretions to semen and to aid in ejaculation. The prostate does not contain any hormones; however, many men fear that prostate problems and treatment will cause problems with their erections or their sexual activities.

Prostatitis
Pathophysiology

Prostatitis, or inflammation of the prostate gland, can occur any time after puberty. The problem can be chronic or a single, acute episode. The inflammation causes the prostate gland to swell, resulting in pain, especially when standing. It can eventually lead to difficulty in passing urine as a result of an inward squeezing on the urethra and restricted urine flow.

Etiology

According to the National Institutes of Health, there are four basic types of prostatitis: (1) acute bacterial, (2) chronic bacterial, (3) chronic prostatitis/chronic pelvic pain syndrome, and (4) asymptomatic inflammatory prostatitis (National Kidney and Urologic Diseases Information Clearinghouse, 2012). Bacterial prostatitis is most common in older men. It results in edema and inflammation of all or part of the prostate gland.

Any bacteria that can cause a urinary tract infection can also cause infectious prostatitis. Common bacteria are organisms such as *Escherichia coli* and *Staphylococcus aureus*. Sexually transmitted infections (STIs) can also cause prostatitis. The prostate gland may become infected in the following ways:

- Bacteria ascending the urethra
- Infected urine refluxing from the bladder into the prostatic ducts
- Bacteria in the blood or lymph supply to the gland
- Surgical instrumentation or other forms of urethral trauma.

Prevention

Ways to avert prostatitis are regular and complete emptying of the bladder to prevent urinary tract infection (UTI), avoiding excess alcohol (more than 2 to 3 oz per day—alcohol is a bladder irritant), and avoiding high-risk sexual practices, such as multiple partners.

Signs and Symptoms

The most common symptoms are those that occur with any UTI: urgency, frequency, hesitancy, dribbling, and dysuria. Because of the location and function of the prostate gland, the patient may report low-back, perineal, and postejaculation pain. He may also have a fever and chills.

Complications

One complication of acute bacterial prostatitis is urinary retention. If the prostate is extremely swollen, the bladder cannot be completely emptied. Another complication may be a temporary problem with erections. Ascending infections, prostatic abscess, epididymitis, and prostatic calculi (stones) are some of the more serious and rare complications of prostatitis.

Diagnostic Tests

Initial diagnosis is based on symptoms. The first test performed is a careful, gentle, digital rectal examination of the prostate. The prostate gland is examined by the health care provider (HCP) by insertion of a gloved finger into the rectum. The examiner may find a warm, irregular, swollen, and painful prostate gland. A urine culture generally is positive for bacteria. The examiner may also gently massage the prostate gland and order an expressed prostate secretion test that reveals bacteria and a large number of white blood cells. Cystoscopy also may be done.

Therapeutic Measures

Acute bacterial prostatitis is treated with antibiotic therapy. Additional treatments may include anti-inflammatory agents, stool softeners, warm sitz baths, prostatic massage, and dietary changes such as decreasing spicy foods and alcohol. Alpha-adrenergic blockers such as alfuzosin (Uroxatral) can help relax the bladder neck and reduce the pain on urination (Table 43.1). In some cases, prostate surgery is needed to remove the obstruction.

 BE SAFE!

BE VIGILANT! Patients with prostate disorders should avoid alpha-adrenergic agonist and anticholinergic medications, which can cause urine retention.

• WORD • BUILDING •
prostatitis: prostat—prostate gland + itis—inflammation

TABLE 43.1 MEDICATION USED TO TREAT DISORDERS OF THE MALE REPRODUCTIVE ORGANS

Medication Class	Medication/Action	Nursing Implications
Testosterone suppressing/ blocking agents	leuprolide (Lupron) *Initially stimulates and then inhibits follicle-stimulating and luteinizing hormones (FSH and LH) to suppress testosterone.* goserelin (Zoladex) *Analogue to luteinizing-releasing hormone; works on pituitary to decrease FSH to decrease sex hormones.* flutamide (Eulexin) *Inhibits androgen uptake and/or binding in tissues.*	Store drug at room temperature and protect from light. Instruct patient that signs and symptoms may increase initially. Monitor for side effects. Inject into upper abdominal wall. Do not aspirate syringe. Teach patient that medication may increase testosterone initially and thus also increase signs and symptoms. Instruct patient that urine color changes to amber/yellow-green. Teach patient to avoid excess exposure to sun and to promptly report side effects. Monitor hepatic function tests.
Alpha-adrenergic antagonists and alpha-reductase inhibitors	tamsulosin (Flomax) terazosin (Hytrin) alfuzosin (Uroxatral) doxazosin (Cardura) *Alpha-adrenergic antagonists. Relax smooth muscle; produce vasodilatation.* finasteride (Proscar) dutasteride (Avodart) *Alpha reductase inhibitors. Inhibit enzyme responsible for formation of potent androgen from testosterone.*	Warn patient dizziness may occur with onset of use. Urge him to report side effects. Monitor blood pressure/pulse. Tell patient not to crush or chew tablets. Caution against driving or use of heavy machinery. Do not chew or crush tablets. Obtain baseline PSA and DRE before use. Instruct patient on side effects. Caution with liver dysfunction.
Vasodilators, smooth muscle relaxers, hormone replacement	sildenafil (Viagra) tadalafil (Cialis) vardenafil (Levitra) *Relaxes smooth muscle; produces vasodilation.* alprostadil (Caverject injection or Muse suppository) prostaglandin E1 *Relaxes smooth muscle; produces vasodilation.* Yohimbine *Herbal vasodilator* testosterone transdermal (Testoderm, Androderm) testosterone cypionate (Depo-testosterone injection) *Testosterone replacement; produces androgen effects.*	Take about 1 hour before sexual activity (may be taken 1/2 to 4 hours before). Assess cardiovascular status before use; may be contraindicated. Avoid use when taking nitroglycerin preparations. If erection lasts more than 4 hours, seek emergency care. Monitor vital signs. Inform patient erection should occur in 2 to 5 minutes and not last more than 4 hours. Instruct patient to report side effects immediately. Assess for other medical conditions before use. Monitor blood pressure and renal and hepatic function. Rule out cancer before use. Monitor hepatic function and red blood cell count Instruct patient to report side effects, prolonged erection or difficulty urinating.

Note. CNS = central nervous system; GI = gastrointestinal; MI = myocardial infarction.

Nursing Process for the Patient With Prostatitis

DATA COLLECTION. Begin the assessment by asking the patient to describe signs and symptoms that indicate evidence of a UTI, such as sudden fever, chills, and reports of urgency, frequency, hesitancy, dysuria, and nocturia. The patient may also have pain in the lower back, the perineum, or after ejaculating. Ask the patient if he has ever had a UTI or prostate infection in the past. Care must be taken to assess urinary retention resulting from obstruction. Obtain a urine culture and assist with collection of the expressed prostate secretion (EPS) specimen, if requested, as part of the patient assessment.

NURSING DIAGNOSES, PLANNING, AND IMPLEMENTATION.
Urinary Retention related to obstruction as evidenced by residual urine in bladder after voiding
EXPECTED OUTCOME: The patient will be able to void effectively as evidenced by residual urine of less than 25% of bladder capacity.

- Evaluate patient's medications for urinary retention as a side effect. *Many medications, especially those with anticholinergic effects, can cause urinary retention.*
- If suspicion of urine retention is present, determine residual urine volume by catheterizing patient (according to HCP order) or obtaining a bladder ultrasound immediately after voiding. *Incomplete emptying of the bladder may lead to increased discomfort or ascending infection.*
- Have the patient complete a bladder log including patterns of elimination and related symptoms, as well as volume/type of fluid consumed for 3 to 7 days. *This will provide for an objective verification of intake and output volumes and aid in determination of urinary retention.*
- Educate patient about avoidance of risk factors for urine retention (e.g., alpha-adrenergic agonists, anticholinergic agents, overfilling of the bladder). *These are modifiable variables that may limit retention of urine.*
- Report urine retention to registered nurse (RN) or HCP. *Catheterization may be needed to empty bladder and prevent complications.*

Deficient Knowledge About Cause, Treatment, and Prevention of Prostatitis
EXPECTED OUTCOME: The patient will verbalize understanding of disorder and demonstrate appropriate self-care.

- Determine patient's current knowledge and understanding about cause and treatment of prostatitis. *This will allow for additional and/or correct information to be provided about the disorder for appropriate understanding.*
- Provide patient with additional and/or correct information about the cause and treatment of prostatitis. *This will allow the patient to have a full understanding of the etiology and care related to the disorder and increase likelihood of patient adherence to treatment.*
- Teach avoidance of risk factors such as urinary catheterization, poor hygiene, risky sexual practices, and excessive intake of bladder irritants such as alcohol, caffeine, or citrus juices. *Avoiding risk factors is important to resolving or preventing prostatitis.*

- Encourage the patient to wash his hands and sitz bath equipment before and after each treatment *to prevent infection.*
- Encourage the patient to empty his bladder every 2 to 3 hours even if he does not feel the urge to urinate. *An overstretched bladder increases risk of infection.*
- Encourage fluids such as water and cranberry juice up to 2500 to 3000 mL/day unless contraindicated by heart failure or other chronic illness. *Fluids help flush the bladder and prevent infection.*
- Include patient's partner in care. *Some treatment options may also include treatment of the partner (e.g., STIs such as gonorrhea, chlamydiosis, or trichomoniasis; see Chapter 44).*
- Explain use of antibiotics as directed, and advise patient to take complete course of medication *to best treat infection and prevent development of antibiotic-resistant bacteria.*

Acute Pain related to swelling and irritation of the prostate gland as evidenced by pain rating
EXPECTED OUTCOME: The patient's pain will be controlled as evidenced by patient statement that comfort is at an acceptable level.

- Use a culturally appropriate pain scale to help patient identify comfort level. *This will aid in understanding comfort level as defined by the patient and aid in guiding appropriate interventions.*
- Encourage appropriate use of anti-inflammatory medication as ordered. *This will decrease inflammation and promote comfort.*
- Encourage use of comfort measures such as warm sitz baths, sitting on a pillow, or prostatic massage, as needed, *to decrease swelling and promote comfort.*
- Teach patient to avoid spicy and acidic foods, alcohol, and caffeine. *These can exacerbate symptoms.*
- Consult HCP about need for stool softeners. *Firm stool will further irritate the prostate during defecation and increase discomfort.*

Anxiety related to sexual concerns as evidenced by patient statement
EXPECTED OUTCOME: The patient will identify presence of anxiety and verbalize concerns about sexuality.

- Identify source of concern related to sexual activity and meaning assigned to disorder as described by patient. *This will help in guiding appropriate interventions.*
- Explore coping skills previously used by patient to relieve anxiety; reinforce these skills and explore other outlets for stress management. *Coping mechanisms that have been helpful in the past can aid patient in dealing with current stressors that result in anxiety.*
- Encourage patient to discuss possible complications and questions about sexual practices with his HCP. *In some cases, sexual intercourse is encouraged as a means of relieving prostatic congestion; in other situations, it may be contraindicated.*

EVALUATION. A clean urine culture with absence of all symptoms of prostatitis is the desired outcome. If interventions have been effective, the patient will have an acceptable comfort level, understand the cause and treatment plan, and verbalize concerns related to the disorder. Prevention of chronic prostatitis can generally be achieved with patient education.

Benign Prostatic Hyperplasia

Enlargement of the prostate gland is a normal process in older men. It begins around age 50 and exists in 75% of men older than age 70. Benign prostatic hyperplasia (BPH) is a nonmalignant growth of the prostate that gradually causes urinary obstruction. According to current studies, BPH does not increase a man's risk of developing cancer of the prostate.

Pathophysiology

A slow increase in the number of cells in the prostate gland is generally the result of aging and the male hormone dihydrotestosterone. As the size of the prostate gland increases, it begins to compress or squeeze the urethra. Narrowing of the urethra means that the bladder must work harder to expel the urine. More effort and a longer time is needed to empty the bladder. Eventually the narrowing causes obstruction and can lead to urine retention or eventually distention of the kidney with urine (hydronephrosis).

The location of the enlargement, rather than the size, determines symptoms. A small growth in the prostate gland closest to the urethra can cause more problems with urination than a growth the size of an orange in the outer portion of the gland.

Etiology

There is no known cause of BPH other than normal aging. Some men think they may have caused the problem by certain sexual practices; however, there is no scientific proof of that at this time. Some factors that are being investigated in research studies are high-fat diet and ethnic background.

Prevention

Because there is no known cause, there is no proven method to prevent enlargement of the prostate gland. Many new treatments are aimed at slowing down the enlargement process. One such treatment that is being researched is the herbal supplement saw palmetto.

Signs and Symptoms

Symptoms of BPH are usually identified in two ways: problems related to obstruction or problems related to irritation. Symptoms related to obstruction include a decrease in the size or force of the urinary stream, difficulty in starting a stream, dribbling after urination is complete, urinary retention, and a feeling that the bladder is not empty. The patient may also experience overflow incontinence or an interrupted stream, where the urine stops midstream and then starts again.

Symptoms related to irritation include nocturia, dysuria, and urgency. HCPs may use a standardized symptom score index tool with patients to assess symptoms and determine treatment options.

Complications

When BPH is untreated and obstruction is prolonged, serious complications can occur. Urine that sits in the bladder for too long can back up into the kidneys, causing hydronephrosis, renal insufficiency, or **urosepsis**; it can also damage the bladder walls, leading to bladder dysfunction, recurrent UTIs, or calculi (stones). Acute urine retention with total inability to urinate can occur; this is a medical emergency that requires catheterization.

Diagnostic Tests

The first test is usually digital rectal examination of the prostate to assess for enlargement and whether the gland is hard, lumpy, or "boggy." Additional tests include urinalysis, blood urea nitrogen (BUN), serum creatinine, and prostate-specific antigen (PSA). Secondary tests include **urodynamic** flow studies, which may show a decreased urine flow rate. Transrectal ultrasound of the prostate and cystoscopy can reflect structural abnormalities.

Therapeutic Measures

If the patient has no symptoms or mild symptoms, the most current medical approach is "watchful waiting." The HCP watches for any increase in symptoms that suggest the urethra is becoming obstructed. Treatment of symptoms may include use of a catheter (indwelling or intermittent), encouraging oral fluids, and antibiotics for UTI.

Conservative medical treatment includes the use of medication to either relax the smooth muscles of the prostate and bladder neck or block the male hormone to prevent or shrink tissue growth. Alpha-adrenergic antagonists, such as tamsulosin (Flomax), are medications that relax the smooth muscles. These medications are also used to treat high blood pressure; therefore, patients need to work closely with their HCPs to avoid overdose or the negative side effects of postural hypotension (see Table 43.1).

The most commonly used medications to block the action of the male hormone in the prostate gland are finasteride (Proscar) and dutasteride (Avodart). These medications must be taken on a long-term, continuous basis to achieve results. Conservative measures are used initially unless the patient is experiencing recurring infections, repeated gross hematuria, bladder or kidney damage, evidence of cancer, or unsatisfactory lifestyle changes.

Nonsurgical invasive treatments, some of which are experimental, are available in some areas of the country in addition to surgical options. These include transurethral microwave therapy, which involves heat applied directly to the gland to inhibit growth; transurethral needle ablation; and high-intensity focused ultrasound, which uses radio or sound waves to destroy parts of the gland. Prostatic stents may be used to open the passageway for urine to flow more freely.

• **WORD** • **BUILDING** •

urosepsis: uro—urine + sepsis—systemic infection
urodynamic: uro—urine + dynamic—force

Surgical Treatment

Because so many other treatments are available now, surgery is not needed as often. When symptoms are severe enough to require surgery, several types are available, as described next.

TRANSURETHRAL RESECTION OF THE PROSTATE. Called TURP, this is the surgical treatment used most often to relieve obstruction caused by an enlarged prostate (Fig. 43.1). Several other transurethral options also exist. Transurethral incision of the prostate (TUIP) uses surgical incisions into the gland to relieve obstruction. Transurethral ultrasound-guided laser-induced prostatectomy uses a laser to relieve obstruction.

For TURP, the patient is anesthetized, and the surgery is performed using an instrument called a resectoscope. The resectoscope is inserted into the urethra, and the prostate gland is "chipped" away a piece at a time. Special surgical instruments are used to "vaporize" or "microwave" the pieces and cut down on the amount of bleeding during surgery. During routine TURP, the "chips" are flushed out using an irrigating solution and are sent to the laboratory to be analyzed for possible evidence of cancer. The prostate gland is not completely removed but peeled away like the rind of an orange. The prostatic tissue that remains eventually grows back and can cause obstruction again at a later time. Patients need to be reminded to continue having yearly prostate examinations.

As the tissue is removed during TURP, bleeding occurs. A Foley catheter is left in place with 30 to 60 mL of sterile water inflating the balloon. The balloon is overfilled and may be secured tightly to the leg or abdomen to tamponade (compress) the prostate area and stop the bleeding. Irrigation solution generally flows continuously (Fig. 43.2); manual irrigation may be done for the first 24 hours to help remove clots and chips and maintain catheter patency. The Foley catheter is removed after the danger of hemorrhage has passed.

FIGURE 43.2 Bladder irrigation.

You may need to save "serial urines" to monitor for bleeding. To do this, each time the patient urinates or the catheter bag is emptied, save a sample of urine in a transparent cup. Place it in a safe place, such as on a shelf in the bathroom. With each subsequent urination, place the new cup to the right of the previous cup. When five or six cups are lined up, you can start over at the left side, replacing the oldest cup with the newest one. This allows the nurse or HCP to examine the urine for progressively less blood with each void.

Complications associated with prostate surgery depend on the type and extent of the procedure performed. The main medical complications include clot formation, bladder spasms, and infection. Less common complications are urinary incontinence, hemorrhage, and erectile dysfunction (see the "Nursing Care Plan for the Postsurgical Patient Having Transurethral Resection of the Prostate for Benign Prostatic Hyperplasia").

Retrograde ejaculation is a common result of prostate surgery. When any of the prostate gland is removed, there is a decrease in the amount of semen produced and a part of the ejaculatory ducts may be removed. This results in less semen being pushed outside the body, and instead it "falls back" into the bladder. This causes no harm; the semen is simply passed during the next urination.

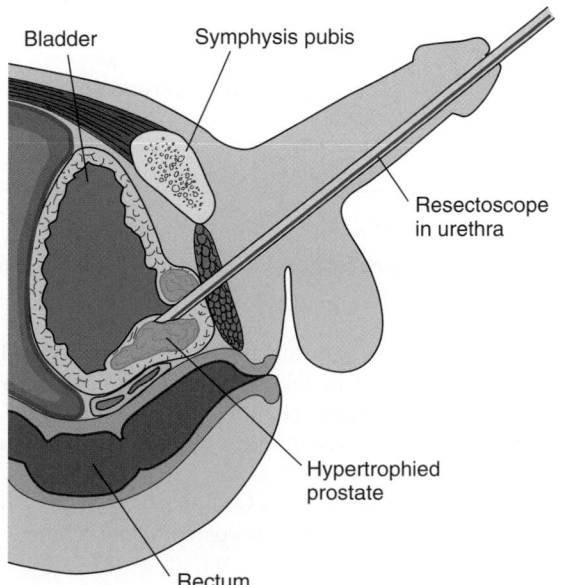

FIGURE 43.1 Transurethral resection of the prostate.

• WORD • BUILDING •
retrograde: retro—backward + grade—step

NURSING CARE PLAN for the Postsurgical Patient Having Transurethral Resection of the Prostate for Benign Prostatic Hyperplasia

Nursing Diagnosis: *Risk for Bleeding* related to surgical intervention

Expected Outcome: The patient's bleeding will be minimal, as evidenced by urine becoming progressively more clear.

Evaluation of Outcome: Is urine clearing? Is bleeding reported promptly?

Intervention Closely monitor urinary output in terms of amount, color, and presence of clots at least every hour for the first 24 to 48 hr postoperatively. Monitor serial urines. **Rationale** Careful monitoring and reporting of changes can help prevent major complications. **Evaluation** Is urine becoming progressively less bloody and more clear with each void?

Intervention Explain to patient that some bloody urine is normal after a TURP, as long as it does not suddenly get much worse. Also explain that a little blood mixed with irrigating fluid in a Foley bag may look worse than it actually is. **Rationale** Seeing the catheter bag filled with bloody drainage may be upsetting to a patient or his family. **Evaluation** Is patient aware of what to expect in Foley bag?

Intervention Encourage patient to drink up to 2500 mL/day (unless contraindicated by other medical conditions) of water, noncitrus juices, and other noncaffeinated, nonalcoholic beverages. **Rationale** Increasing urine flow can help flush blood from bladder. **Evaluation** Is patient drinking adequate amounts?

Intervention Teach patient to avoid constipation (suggest stool softener, fluids, prune juice) and heavy lifting. **Rationale** These can increase pressure in the abdomen and increase risk of bleeding. **Evaluation** Does patient verbalize understanding of instructions?

Intervention Advise patient to lie down if urine becomes bright red or has large clots. **Rationale** Activity can increase bleeding. **Evaluation** Does patient reduce activity if bleeding increases?

Intervention Teach patient to avoid aspirin and nonsteroidal antiinflammatory drugs (NSAIDs) until risk of bleeding is over. **Rationale** Aspirin and NSAIDs inhibit platelet function and increase risk of bleeding. **Evaluation** Does patient verbalize understanding?

Nursing Diagnosis: *Acute Pain* related to bladder spasms, obstruction, or surgical process as evidenced by patient pain rating

Expected Outcome: The patient's pain will be controlled as evidenced by patient statement of lower pain rating.

Evaluation of Outcome: Does patient state that pain is decreased to acceptable level?

Intervention Monitor pain on an appropriate scale every 2 to 4 hr for first 48 hr and within 30 minutes after any intervention. **Rationale** A pain scale is the most accurate measure of pain. **Evaluation** Does patient verbalize pain as increasing or decreasing on the scale?

Intervention Monitor for signs of pain related to bladder spasms, obstruction, or surgical process, such as facial grimaces, irrigation solution that does not flow into bladder, urinating around catheter, multiple clots. **Rationale** Relief of mechanical cause of pain promotes comfort, rest, and healing. **Evaluation** Is patient free from signs of pain related to bladder spasms, obstruction, or surgical process?

Intervention Administer prescribed medication (analgesics, antispasmodics such as B&O suppository) and monitor response. **Rationale** B&O suppositories relieve bladder spasms. **Evaluation** Does patient state relief when medications are given?

NURSING CARE PLAN for the Postsurgical Patient Having Transurethral Resection of the Prostate for Benign Prostatic Hyperplasia—cont'd

Intervention Irrigate catheter as ordered. **Rationale** Irrigation promotes removal of clots to reduce spasms and pain. **Evaluation** Does irrigating solution flow in and out easily?

Intervention Educate patient regarding nonpharmacological methods to control pain such as relaxation and deep-breathing techniques. **Rationale** Relaxation calms spasms and relieves pain. Nonpharmacological measures should be used with, not in place of, medication. **Evaluation** Are clots being removed? Is patient able to relax?

Nursing Diagnosis: *Urge Urinary Incontinence* related to poor sphincter control as evidenced by inability to control urination

Expected Outcome: The patient will be able to prevent incontinence.

Evaluation of Outcome: Is incontinence prevented?

Intervention Teach Kegel (pelvic floor) exercises (see Chapter 42)—to be practiced every time patient urinates and throughout the day. **Rationale** Kegel exercises strengthen muscle tone to hold urine after catheter is removed. **Evaluation** Is patient able to start and stop urine stream?

Intervention Discuss use of condom catheter or penile pads. **Rationale** These can keep patient dry until incontinence can be controlled. **Evaluation** Does patient indicate an informed choice of incontinence products?

Intervention Instruct patient to continue drinking 2000 to 4000 mL of noncaffeinated, nonalcoholic beverages each day. **Rationale** Adequate nonirritating fluid intake is important for healing and preventing UTI. **Evaluation** Does patient drink adequate fluids even though he dribbles?

Intervention Encourage patient to discuss long-term (longer than 6 months) incontinence problems with HCP. **Rationale** Patient may need to learn self-catheterization or try medication. **Evaluation** Does patient verbalize understanding of what to do if incontinence continues?

Intervention Refer patient to national incontinence support group if indicated. **Rationale** Support groups can provide information and emotional support. **Evaluation** Does patient show interest in a support group?

Nursing Diagnosis: *Deficient Knowledge* related to lack of experience with postoperative restrictions and care

Expected Outcomes: The patient will avoid activities that increase intra-abdominal pressure resulting in excessive bleeding. The patient will verbalize understanding of how to prevent postoperative infection.

Evaluation of Outcomes: Does patient verbalize understanding of how to prevent bleeding? Is infection prevented?

Intervention Teach patient to avoid lifting heavy objects (more than 10 lbs), stair climbing, driving, strenuous exercise, constipation, straining during bowel movements, and sexual activities until approved by HCP (about 6 weeks). **Rationale** Heavy lifting or straining can disrupt the healing process and result in tissue damage or excess bleeding. **Evaluation** Does patient verbalize understanding of reasons for limitation of heavy lifting and straining?

Intervention Instruct patient on proper catheter care if patient will be discharged with catheter. Include the following information: • Keep catheter tubing secured to abdomen or thigh and keep bag below bladder. • Wash catheter/meatus junction with soap and water once daily. • Use clean technique with good hand hygiene to change from leg bag to night drainage bag. • Report signs and symptoms of UTI to HCP immediately. • Encourage oral fluids. **Rationale** UTIs are extremely dangerous and can cause death following genitourinary surgery in an older patient. **Evaluation** Can patient give a return demonstration of proper catheter care? Is patient free from signs and symptoms of infection?

Continued

NURSING CARE PLAN for the Postsurgical Patient Having Transurethral Resection of the Prostate for Benign Prostatic Hyperplasia—cont'd

Intervention Teach all patients to report bleeding that is not stopped with resting; fever; swelling; or difficulty urinating to HCP promptly. **Rationale** These are signs of complications that may require prompt medical intervention. **Evaluation** Does patient verbalize understanding of signs and symptoms to report?

Nursing Diagnosis: *Anxiety* related to concerns over loss of sexual functioning following prostate surgery as evidenced by patient statement

Expected Outcomes: The patient will verbalize normal sexual changes that happen after prostate surgery. The patient will identify available support systems if needed.

Evaluation of Outcomes: Is patient able to verbalize understanding of expected body function after prostate surgery? Does the patient access support systems?

Intervention Explain to patient that he will probably have retrograde ejaculation into bladder after surgery. It is not harmful and semen will come out when he urinates. **Rationale** Removal of the prostate gland often results in retrograde ejaculation. **Evaluation** Does patient understand what will happen when he ejaculates?

Intervention Instruct patient to talk with urologist if erection problems occur. **Rationale** Urologists who specialize in treatment of erectile dysfunction can provide information and treatment. **Evaluation** Is patient aware of local support services?

Note. B&O = belladonna and opium; NSAIDs = nonsteroidal anti-inflammatory drugs; TURP = transurethral resection of the prostate; UTI = urinary tract infection.

It is important to understand that erection, ejaculation, and orgasm are all separate actions. Erection means the penis becomes hard, ejaculation is the release of semen, and orgasm is felt as pulsations along the urethra. Unless additional problems are present, the patient continues to have erections and orgasmic sensations but decreased or no ejaculation.

RADICAL PROSTATECTOMY. When the prostate gland is very large, is causing obstruction, or is cancerous, a radical **prostatectomy** may be performed to remove the entire prostate gland.

Open Prostatectomy. Several approaches may be taken during traditional radical surgery (Fig. 43.3). In the **suprapubic** approach, an incision is made through the lower abdomen into the bladder. The gland is removed, and the urethra is reattached to the bladder. The retropubic approach is similar except there is no incision into the bladder. A perineal prostatectomy involves making an incision between the scrotum and anus to remove the gland. This procedure is rarely done because of the increased risk of contamination of the incision (close to the rectum), and risk of urinary incontinence, erectile dysfunction, or injury to the rectum.

An open prostatectomy means a longer hospital stay compared with other BPH surgeries. The presence of a suprapubic catheter and care for an abdominal incision increase the length of stay and risk for complications. Follow-up home care for wound and catheter care is important for these patients.

Minimally Invasive Prostatectomy. Newer techniques use laparoscopy and tiny robot arms to perform radical prostatectomy through five small "porthole" incisions in the abdomen. The surgeon makes all the decisions about the surgery while guiding the robotic arms. The robotic arms allow more precision and maneuverability, especially in small areas. Because robotic surgery is so much less invasive, patients experience better results with less postoperative bleeding and incontinence and shorter hospital stays.

Nursing Process for the Patient With BPH Who Undergoes a TURP Procedure

DATA COLLECTION. Begin by asking the patient if he has ever had treatment or surgery for prostate trouble. Assess amount and type of fluid intake per day and whether the patient has noticed any of the symptoms of BPH. Monitor output, and, if he is not catheterized, ensure that urine retention is being managed appropriately.

NURSING DIAGNOSES, PLANNING, AND INTERVENTIONS. For nursing care of the patient following TURP, see the "Nursing Care Plan for the Postsurgical Patient Having

• WORD • BUILDING •
prostatectomy: prostat—prostate gland + ectomy—excision
suprapubic: supra—above + pubic—pubic bone

A Suprapubic prostatectomy

B Retropubic prostatectomy

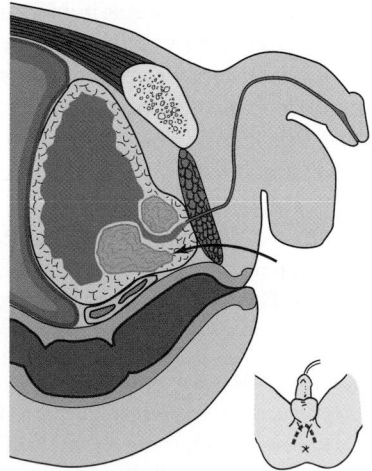

C Perineal prostatectomy

FIGURE 43.3 (A) Suprapubic prostatectomy. (B) Retropubic prostatectomy. (C) Perineal prostatectomy.

Transurethral Resection of the Prostate for Benign Prostatic Hyperplasia." In addition, each patient experiences individual responses and needs. Care plans must be individualized, keeping in mind that the majority of these patients are older and have secondary medical problems such as cardiovascular disease.

EVALUATION. A patient should be discharged home with a minimum of bladder discomfort, light pink to clear urine, no evidence of UTI, and knowledge related to self-care at home. Home care nursing may be required if the patient lives alone or does not have the capacity to provide for meals, toileting, or transportation for the follow-up visit. Table 43.2 provides a summary of BPH.

CRITICAL THINKING

Mr. Atkinson

■ Mr. Atkinson is a 68-year-old African American farmer with an enlarged prostate gland. He lives on a 75-acre farm with his wife and one son. He is scheduled for a TURP in 6 weeks.

1. Mr. Atkinson is currently taking terazosin (Hytrin), and his HCP wants him to increase his dose from 2 to 5 mg daily until surgery. He has a bottle at home of 2-mg tablets. How should you instruct him to take his medication? What side effect should he be advised to watch for?
2. What special postoperative instructions should he be given because of his occupation?
3. What should you tell him if he asks about how the surgery will affect his "nature" (sexual activities)?
4. What other health team members can you collaborate with and anticipate Mr. Atkinson might need while in the hospital or when he goes home?

Suggested answers are at the end of the chapter.

Cancer of the Prostate

Cancer of the prostate is the most common cancer in American men. Most prostate cancers grow very slowly and often do not cause a major threat to health or life. Many treatment options are available, and the prognosis is often very good.

Pathophysiology

Prostate cancer depends on testosterone to grow. The cancer cells are usually slow growing and begin in the posterior (back) or lateral (side) part of the gland. The cancer spreads by one of three routes. If it spreads by local invasion, it will move into the bladder, seminal vesicles, or peritoneum. The cancer may also spread through the lymph system to the pelvic nodes and may travel as far as the supraclavicular nodes. The third route is through the vascular system to bone, lung, and liver. Prostate cancer is staged or graded based on the growth or spread.

TABLE 43.2 BENIGN PROSTATIC HYPERPLASIA (BPH) SUMMARY

Signs and Symptoms	**Related to obstruction:** Decrease in size/force of stream, difficulty in starting stream, dribbling, interrupted stream, urinary retention, overflow incontinence **Related to irritation:** Nocturia, dysuria, urgency
Diagnostic Tests	**Primary:** DRE, urinalysis, BUN, serum creatinine, prostate-specific antigen (PSA) **Secondary:** Urodynamic flow studies, transrectal ultrasound, cystoscopy
Therapeutic Measures	**Conservative:** Alpha-blockers, testosterone blockers **Nonsurgical:** Transurethral microwave antenna (TUMA), prostatic balloon, prostatic stents **Transurethral:** Transurethral incision of the prostate (TUIP), transurethral ultrasound-guided laser-induced prostatectomy (TULIP), transurethral resection of the prostate (TURP) **Radical prostatectomy:** Suprapubic, retropubic, perineal, laparoscopic, or robotic resection
Complications	Ascending or localized infection Injury to surrounding tissues during surgery Impaired sexual function related to tissue injury
Priority Nursing Diagnoses	*Impaired Urinary Elimination* related to obstruction

Etiology

Age is the primary risk factor. Prostate cancer is found most often in men older than age 65 and is rare in men younger than age 40. Other risk factors are higher levels of testosterone, high-fat diet, and immediate family history.

Prostate cancer rates are highest in African American men and lowest in American Indian and Native Alaskan men (American Cancer Society, 2012). Occupational exposure to cadmium (e.g., welding, electroplating, alkaline battery manufacturing) has been identified as an added risk factor.

Signs and Symptoms

Symptoms are rare in the early stage of prostate cancer. Later stages include symptoms of urinary obstruction, hematuria, and urinary retention. Advanced (metastatic) stage symptoms can include pain in the back or hip from metastasis to the bone, anemia, weakness, weight loss, and overall tiredness.

Complications

Early complications of prostate cancer are related to bladder problems, such as difficulty urinating, and bladder or kidney infection. Erectile dysfunction can occur as a result of the cancer or its treatment (see "Evidence-Based Practice" box).

If the cancer metastasizes, the patient may develop problems such as pain, bone fractures, weight loss, and depression; eventually death can occur if treatment is not successful.

EVIDENCE-BASED PRACTICE

Clinical Question
What interventions are available for men with sexual dysfunction after treatment for prostate cancer?

Evidence
Two Cochrane reviews have looked at treatments for erectile dysfunction. The first found that focused group therapy was as effective as local injection or vacuum devices, and that group therapy combined with drug therapy (sildenafil [Viagra]), was more effective than drug therapy alone (Melnik, Soares, & Nasello, 2008). The second found that PDE5 inhibitors (such as sildenafil [Viagra] and tadalafil [Cialis]) are effective following treatment for prostate cancer (Miles et al, 2012).

Implications for Nursing Practice
Nurses can play a role in assessing men's knowledge of interventions for erectile dysfunction related to treatment for prostate cancer. Although specific intervention is beyond the scope of practice of the licensed practical nurse/ licensed vocational nurse (LPN/LVN), it is appropriate to advise men that medications, local injections, vacuum devices, and group therapy have all been shown to help, and refer them to their HCPs for further assistance.

REFERENCES

Melnik, T., Soares, B., & Nasello, A. G. (2008). Psychosocial interventions for erectile dysfunction. *Cochrane Database of Systematic Reviews 2008*, Issue 4 (Art. No. CD004825; DOI: 10.1002/14651858.CD004825.pub2).

Miles, C. L., Candy, B., Jones, L., et al (2012). Interventions for sexual dysfunction following treatments for cancer. *Cochrane Database of Systematic Reviews 2012* (8) Retrieved August 6, 2013, from www.bibliotecacochrane .com/pdf/CD005540.pdf

Diagnostic Tests

A routine digital rectal examination of the prostate is the first test; often the examiner finds a hard lump or hardened prostate lobe. Blood tests looking for high levels of PSA or PAP may be done. When there is a palpable tumor, the HCP may order a transrectal ultrasound and biopsy to help confirm the diagnosis. Bone scans and other tests may be ordered to determine if the cancer has spread outside the prostate gland.

In the past, the PSA test was used to screen men for prostate cancer, but more recently, the American Cancer Society withdrew this recommendation because routine screening has not been found to save lives. Instead, many slow-growing, noninvasive cancers were discovered and treated. Although aggressive cancers require treatment, many prostate cancers are not aggressive, and the treatment may be worse than the disease. Patients with elevated PSA levels may now have additional testing to determine how aggressive the cancer is, so that appropriate treatment decisions can be made.

Therapeutic Measures

Prostate cancer in the early stages may be treated with testosterone-suppressing medications, such as leuprolide (Lupron) or goserelin (Zoladex), or drugs that block testosterone's action on the prostate gland, such as bicalutamide (Casodex). Surgery, such as TURP or radical prostatectomy, or a combination of medication and radiation therapy may be done. In later stages, the treatment is usually a radical prostatectomy, radiation therapy, or implantation of radioactive "seeds" into the prostate (brachytherapy). A new vaccine, sipuleucel-T (Provenge) that will slow the growth and aggressiveness of some prostate cancers is currently being tested.

Metastatic prostate cancer treatment involves relief of symptoms or blocking testosterone by bilateral **orchiectomy**, administration of antiandrogen (flutamide [Eulexin]), or use of agents such as leuprolide and goserelin. Sometimes chemotherapy is used to help relieve symptoms resulting from spread of the cancer.

Unfortunately, any therapy that reduces androgen activity in a man can cause side effects, such as hot flashes, breast tenderness and growth, osteoporosis, and loss of muscle mass. These in turn can cause significant concerns with body image.

Brachytherapy, external-beam radiation therapy, and radical prostatectomy combinations are showing favorable results in the treatment of advanced cancer. Gene therapy and immune-based interventions are also under investigation.

RADICAL PROSTATECTOMY. A radical prostatectomy (described earlier in this chapter) is done for patients with cancer of the prostate or when the gland is too large to resect using a less invasive method.

The patient returns from surgery with a large indwelling catheter in the urethra and may also have a suprapubic catheter. A drain is often placed to remove fluids from the abdominal cavity and allow the wound to heal from the inside outward. Special care must be taken to keep the incision and drain sites clean and dry. Dressings should be changed according to institution policy using sterile technique.

Radical prostatectomy has more complications associated with it than any other treatment option. The major complications are hemorrhage, infection, loss of urinary control, and erectile dysfunction.

Patient Education

All men older than age 40 should be encouraged to have a yearly digital rectal examination of the prostate. Prevention and early detection are the best ways to fight prostate cancer.

PENILE DISORDERS

Problems of the penis, aside from those caused by STIs, are fairly rare but may cause great concern and worry for the patient. Many men have difficulty seeking help for such a personal problem. It is important to be sensitive when assessing or providing care for these patients.

Peyronie's Disease

Peyronie's disease gives the penis a curved or crooked look when it is erect. Fibrous bands or plaques form mainly on the dorsal (top) part of the layer of tissue that surrounds one of the corpora cavernosa of the penis. The plaque may be caused by injury or inflammation of the penile tissue, or it may come and go spontaneously. If the plaque is thick enough, it can cause curvature, painful erection, difficulty in vaginal penetration, and erectile dysfunction. When conservative treatments such as oral vitamin E, colchicine, or potassium aminobenzoate do not work, surgery may be needed to remove the plaque. Another option is injections into the scar tissue to break it down. Patients need to be reassured that the problem is not life threatening and can be treated.

Priapism

Priapism is a painful erection that lasts longer than 4 hours. If not relieved, it can become a medical emergency. The small veins in the corpora cavernosa spasm, so blood cannot drain back out of the penis as it should. When the blood cannot drain, penile tissue does not get oxygen, and permanent tissue damage can result. There may be a complete loss of erection ability after the priapism episode. Prolonged priapism can also prevent the patient from passing urine, which can lead to painful bladder and kidney problems. Some causes of priapism are sickle cell anemia, leukemia, widespread cancer, spinal cord injury or tumors, and use of medications to manage erectile dysfunction (such as sildenafil [Viagra]) or recreational drugs such as crack cocaine. Treatment in the emergency department may include ice packs, sedatives, analgesics, injection of medications directly into the penis to relax the vein spasms, needle aspiration, and irrigation of the corpora. Surgery to implant a shunt that reroutes blood flow can also be done.

• WORD • BUILDING •
orchiectomy: orchi—testicles + ectomy—excision
priapism: priap—phallus + ism—condition of

Phimosis and Paraphimosis

Phimosis is the term used to describe a condition in which the foreskin of an uncircumcised male becomes so tight that it is difficult or impossible to pull back away from the head of the penis. It may make it impossible to clean the area underneath. Smegma, a cottage cheese–like secretion made by the glands of the foreskin, becomes trapped under the foreskin and is an excellent place for the growth of bacterial and yeast infections. Antibiotics and warm soaks may be ordered if infection is present. Topical steroid ointment and stretching exercises for the foreskin may be prescribed. A circumcision may be recommended if the problem continues. Phimosis is generally prevented by teaching uncircumcised males to pull the foreskin back carefully, wash with mild soap and water daily, and replace the foreskin to its normal position.

Paraphimosis occurs when the uncircumcised foreskin is pulled back, during intercourse or bathing, and not immediately replaced in a forward position. This causes constriction of the dorsal veins, which leads to edema and pain. Moderate to severe paraphimosis is a medical emergency and requires immediate care by a HCP. The longer the problem continues, the greater the risk of circulation problems and possible gangrene. Prevention through daily cleaning and replacing the foreskin to its normal place is important.

Cancer of the Penis

Cancer of the penis has been found in men who were not circumcised as infants or adolescents, or have acquired the human papillomavirus (HPV). The tumor is typically a squamous cell carcinoma and may look like a small round raised wart, induration, or red area. This form of cancer can be spread to a sexual partner. Several research studies have found a link between cancer of the penis and cancer of the uterine cervix. Cancer of the penis may be treated with minor surgery, such as a circumcision or laser removal of the growth. If the cancer has spread, sections of the penis may be surgically removed. Penile reconstruction can be done if necessary after surgery. Radiation or chemotherapy may also be done. Finding and treating any lesion in its earliest stages is an important part of patient education, as is education about circumcision of infants as a preventive measure.

 TESTICULAR DISORDERS

Cryptorchidism

Cryptorchidism (undescended testicles) is a congenital condition in which an infant boy is born with one or both of his testicles not in the scrotum. The testicles normally drop down (descend) into the scrotum in the last 1 to 2 months before the boy is born. Often, undescended testicles descend into the scrotum on their own in the first few months of life. If they do not descend by that time, surgery should be done to correct the problem, typically before age 1. Testicles that are not brought down into the scrotum decrease a man's chances of producing a child, because excessive body heat damages sperm production in the

testicles. Also, the risk of testicular cancer is higher if the condition is not corrected before the child reaches his teen years.

Hydrocele

A **hydrocele** is a collection of fluid in the scrotal sac. Hydroceles are not dangerous and generally do not cause pain. The cause is not known, and they can happen at any point during the lifetime. No treatment is necessary unless the hydrocele is so large that it causes discomfort or embarrassment or is a threat to the blood supply to the testicles. If treatment is needed, the HCP can perform a needle aspiration, or surgically drain the fluid.

Varicocele

A varicocele is a condition sometimes called varicose veins of the scrotum. The main blood supply to the testicles travels along the spermatic cord. The veins become dilated, and when the man is standing, the area in the scrotum begins to feel like a "bag of worms." The patient may report a pulling sensation, a dull ache, or scrotal pain. The sensations are most often felt when standing up. Most varicoceles occur on the left side because of the way the scrotal vein enters at a sharp angle from the left renal vein.

A varicocele is often not discovered until a couple is unable to conceive. It is believed that the varicose veins may increase the temperature of the testicles and cause damage to the sperm. The most successful treatment is surgical repair of the varicose veins.

Epididymitis

The epididymis is a small tube along the back of the testicles where sperm is matured for its last 10 to 12 days before it is ready to be ejaculated. **Epididymitis** is inflammation or infection of the epididymis that can be caused by bacteria, viruses, parasites, chemicals, or trauma. Risk factors include sexual or nonsexual contact, STI, a complication of some urological procedures, or reflux (backflow) of urine. The problem can also be associated with prostate infections and is usually painful, with the scrotal skin being tender, red, and warm to the touch.

Epididymitis is treated with antibiotics; the partner is also treated if it was sexually transmitted. Depending on the severity of the pain, the patient may be placed on bedrest with the scrotum elevated, possibly on ice packs, and given analgesics. The pain and tenderness usually go away in about a week, although the swelling may last for several weeks. Complications include chronic epididymitis, abscess formation, and sterility.

• **WORD • BUILDING** •

phimosis: phimo—muzzling + osis—condition
paraphimosis: para—abnormal + phimo—muzzling + osis—condition
cryptorchidism: crypt—hidden + orchid—testicle + ism—condition
hydrocele: hydro—water + cele—swelling
epididymitis: epididymis + itis—inflammation

Orchitis

Orchitis is a rare inflammation or infection of the testicles. The problem may be caused by trauma or infection from epididymitis, UTI, STI, or systemic diseases such as influenza, infectious mononucleosis, tuberculosis, gout, pneumonia, or mumps (after puberty). The patient has swollen, extremely tender testicles, red scrotal skin, and a fever. Interventions are basically the same as for epididymitis and include bedrest, scrotal support, antibiotics, and medication to relieve pain and fever. Complications such as sterility as a result of orchitis caused by mumps can be prevented by giving boys the mumps vaccine at an early age.

Cancer of the Testicles
Pathophysiology and Etiology

Cancer of the testicles is the most common cancer in men between ages 15 and 34 in the United States. The etiology of testicular cancer is unknown. Some of the known risk factors are cryptorchidism, family history, white race, and high socioeconomic status. Some older studies showed a link between a mother's use of DES (diethylstilbestrol, an estrogen preparation once used to prevent spontaneous abortion) while pregnant, but current research has not shown this risk to be significant. The tumors are mostly a germ cell type of cancer formed during normal embryo development.

Prevention

The best prevention is early detection with a monthly testicular self-examination (TSE). The American Cancer Society does not necessarily recommend monthly TSE for all men, because not enough studies have been done to show that it reduces death. However, men should be aware of what is normal for them, so they can recognize changes if they occur. The TSE procedure is simple and easy to learn, and it makes sense to teach it to all men until more data are available. See Chapter 41 for instructions on TSE.

Signs and Symptoms

Early warning signs of cancer can include a small, usually painless lump on the testicle. The patient may also notice that the scrotum is swollen and feels heavy. Some tumors produce hormones that cause breast enlargement and tenderness.

Complications

Emotional complications can range from fear of cancer and death to feelings of loss of masculine body image and sexual function. Physical complications may involve dealing with pain and the effects of metastasis to areas such as the lungs, abdomen, or lymph nodes. Other less common areas of cancer spread are the liver, brain, and bone.

Diagnostic Tests

When a lump is found, several laboratory and radiographic tests are done. An ultrasound of the testicles is done first, to differentiate a possible tumor from a hydrocele or other noncancerous condition. Blood is drawn to look for tumor markers. An example of a tumor marker for testicular cancer is human chorionic gonadotropin (HCG). A surgical biopsy or removal of the testicle is done to determine the stage of the tumor. If cancer is confirmed, a chest x-ray examination is done to look for spread to the lungs. A scan of the lymph nodes, liver, brain, and bones also may be ordered.

Testicular tumors may be staged or classified in several ways. The simplest way to stage a testicular tumor is as follows:

• Stage I—tumor only in the testicles
• Stage II—tumor spread to abdominal lymph nodes
• Stage III—tumor spread past lymph nodes, usually to the lungs, liver, bones, and/or brain.

Therapeutic Measures

Intervention depends on the stage of the cancer. All treatment begins with complete removal of the cancerous testicles, spermatic cord, and local lymph nodes. Based on the stage of the cancer, radiation or chemotherapy may be done in addition to surgery. If the cancer is found in the beginning stages, the chances for complete recovery are very good. All patients should have regular follow-up testing.

Nursing Care

Nursing care is directed first at prevention, by teaching young men to practice monthly TSE and to see their HCP if they notice any changes. If a diagnosis of cancer has been made, provide emotional support for the patient. If he wants to have children, he should be encouraged to make deposits in a sperm bank before any surgery or treatment is started. The patient and his partner may have many questions about sexual activities as they go through treatment. Encourage them to talk with their HCP or a sex therapist about ways to express love and tenderness toward one another. Helping patients deal with pain and the side effects of chemotherapy or radiation therapy are also important nursing interventions for these men. See Chapter 11 for care of the patient with cancer.

CRITICAL THINKING

Mr. Cunningham

■ Mr. Cunningham is a 23-year-old college student engaged to be married next spring. While taking a shower one day, he discovers a lump on his left testicle.

1. What should he do?
2. What are the treatment options if Mr. Cunningham has testicular cancer?
3. How can you help Mr. Cunningham cope with the diagnosis?

Suggested answers are at the end of the chapter.

• WORD • BUILDING •
orchitis: orch—testicle + itis—inflammation

SEXUAL FUNCTIONING

Vasectomy

A **vasectomy** uses tiny clamps or cauterization to seal off the vas deferens to prevent sperm from reaching the outside of the body (Fig. 43.4). This 15- to 30-minute surgery is done through a small puncture in the upper part of the scrotum. It is performed as a permanent birth control method for men. The patient should carefully discuss the surgery with his physician, so there is a clear understanding of the results following the procedure.

After the procedure, the testicles continue to produce sperm and the male hormone testosterone. The prostate gland, along with the seminal vesicles, still ejaculates semen, but the semen does not contain sperm. There should be no major change in the way the ejaculate looks or feels after the procedure. The patient should be encouraged to continue using another birth control method for about 3 months after surgery to be sure there are no sperm left in the tract above the surgical site. A semen sample should be evaluated for the absence of sperm before the procedure is considered successful. Sperm continue to be produced in the testicles but are absorbed by the body.

Vasectomy Reversal

Sometimes a man may decide he wants to have more children and asks to have a vasectomy reversed. The surgical procedure to reverse a vasectomy is called a vasovasostomy. Using microscopic instruments, the surgeon reconnects the vas deferens. If this is not possible, the surgeon may reconnect the vas deferens to the epididymis. During the surgery the physician typically tries to determine whether the testicles are still producing good sperm. Vasectomy reversal is more successful if it is done soon after the vasectomy. Success rates drop as the period of time between vasectomy and reversal grows longer.

Erectile Dysfunction

A problem getting or keeping an erection can happen at any age and has been a concern of men and their partners for centuries. It is a unique problem because it affects not only the man but his partner as well. Most men experience a temporary erection problem at some time during their lives. It is often caused by stress, illness, fatigue, or an excessive use of alcohol or drugs. When the problem becomes persistent, it is time to seek medical help.

Before the 1980s, 90% of men who went to their HCPs for help were told the problem was emotional, not physical. As a result of improved testing methods, however, researchers now believe that 80% to 90% of erection problems have a physical cause.

Pathophysiology

The term *impotence* means powerlessness. This term is being replaced with the more accurate term **erectile dysfunction** (ED), which describes a physical condition. Erectile dysfunction means that a man cannot obtain or keep a usable erection that is firm enough and long-lasting enough for satisfactory

• WORD • BUILDING •
vasectomy: vas—vas deferens + ectomy—excision

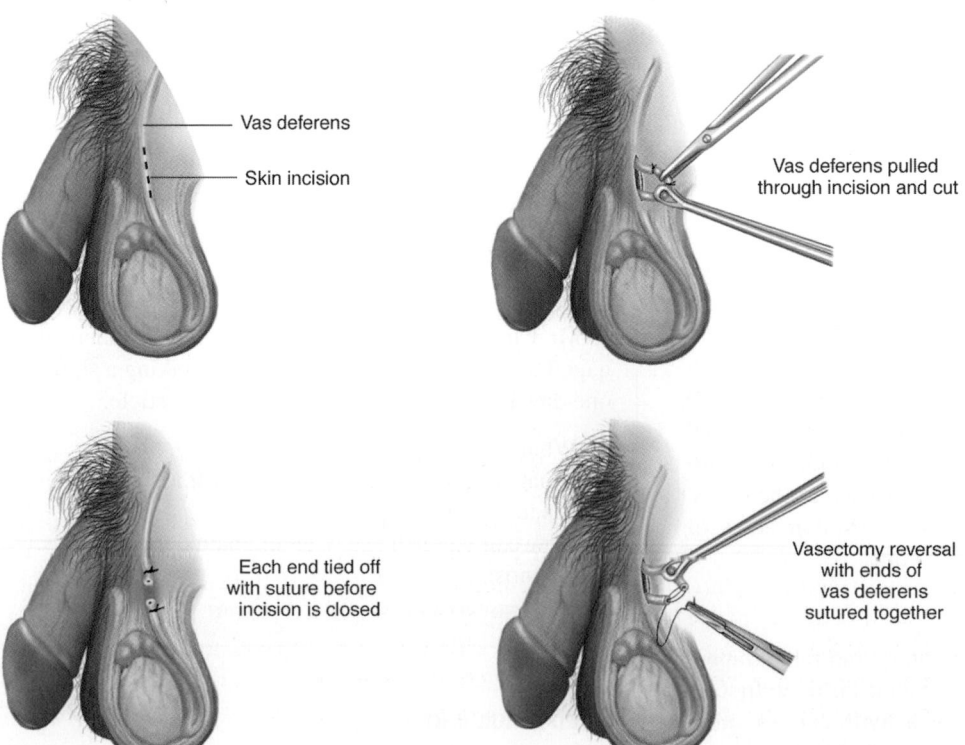

Vas deferens
Skin incision

Vas deferens pulled
through incision and cut

Each end tied off
with suture before
incision is closed

Vasectomy reversal
with ends of
vas deferens
sutured together

FIGURE 43.4 Vasectomy and reversal.

sexual intercourse. For a man to have a usable erection, several conditions must be met:

1. *Circulatory system.* The blood supply coming into the penis from the arteries must be sufficient to fill the corpus cavernosa (spongy erectile tissue inside the penis), causing the penis to become rigid. The veins in the penis must then be able to constrict to trap the blood in the corporal bodies to keep the penis erect. The most common cause of erectile dysfunction is failure in the circulatory system.
2. *Nervous system.* Both the sympathetic and parasympathetic nerves are involved in the erection, ejaculation, orgasm, and resting phases of the penile response cycle. There are many nerve receptors and transmitters in the spinal cord and the penis that must be intact for a usable erection. Spinal cord injury is the most common neurologic cause of erectile dysfunction.
3. *Hormonal system.* There are three basic male hormones involved with an erection. The most important hormone, testosterone, affects a man's sex drive and desire. Luteinizing hormone stimulates testosterone production, and prolactin in large amounts may block testosterone.
4. *Limbic system.* This is the center in the brain that affects how we feel emotionally. It works with our five senses to stimulate the desire for sex.

All of these systems can be influenced by physical, emotional, and chemical factors. A good assessment is important to determine the cause of erectile dysfunction.

Etiology

ED has many psychological and physical causes. It can also be caused by many medications and chemicals that interfere with desire, blood supply, or nerve transmission (Table 43.3). The most common types of medications that cause problems are those prescribed for high blood pressure and cardiovascular disease. Recently, obstructive sleep apnea has been found to be related to ED, but it is unclear which condition might come first.

Diagnostic Tests

In the first step of the assessment process, the HCP obtains a history, including medical-surgical history; use of medications, including any substance abuse; lifestyle patterns; and sexual history. During physical examination, the provider looks for evidence of genital disorders, hormonal imbalance (such as hair patterns or enlarged breasts), surgical interventions, decreased circulation, and lack of nerve sensation. Blood tests evaluate glucose levels; testosterone; evidence of liver, heart, or kidney disorders; signs of infection; or blood disorders. Some HCPs may use intracorporeal injection of vasoactive medications that can create an erection to test the blood flow in the penis. A psychosocial evaluation may be recommended to rule out relational or emotional problems that may contribute to erectile dysfunction or affect the treatment outcome.

TABLE 43.3 CAUSES OF ERECTILE DYSFUNCTION

Psychological	Stress Anxiety Depression Fatigue
Urological	Peyronie's disease Kidney failure Treatment for prostate disease
Endocrine	Low testosterone levels Diabetes mellitus
Respiratory	Obstructive sleep apnea
Cardiovascular	Heart disease Atherosclerosis Metabolic syndrome Stroke
Neurologic	Spinal cord injury Parkinson's disease Multiple sclerosis
Lifestyle	Tobacco use Alcohol use Drug use (marijuana, cocaine, others) Excessive caffeine use
Medications*	Antianxiety agents Antidepressants Antihistamines Antineoplastic agents Angiotensin-converting enzyme inhibitors Beta blockers Diuretics Estrogens Histamine (H_2) antagonists Muscle relaxants Nonsteroidal anti-inflammatory drugs Opioids Drugs for Parkinson's disease

Note: Not all drugs in a category cause erectile dysfunction.

A second level of testing may involve the use of sophisticated vascular flow studies to locate areas where either the blood vessels are narrowed or the veins allow the blood to drain out of the penis too rapidly. Another area of testing monitors erections during sleep. A healthy man typically has erections every 60 to 70 minutes while he sleeps. Absence of erections during sleep indicates a physical cause for erectile dysfunction. Because of the expense of vascular flow studies and sleep studies, they are used on a limited basis.

Therapeutic Measures

One of the most important treatment options begins with the couple being able to share intimate communication. No matter what is causing the problem, if the patient and his partner are not touching, talking, and sharing feelings with one another, treatment options are going to have limited success.

When the problem has clearly been identified as psychological, counseling therapy is the treatment of choice. If long-term therapy has been tried with only limited success, the addition of oral medication or even intracorporeal injection therapy may be added to provide a boost in confidence and self-esteem. Medical treatment for physical erection problems begins with conservative, nonsurgical treatment and then progresses to surgical options if needed. See Table 43.1 for additional information on medications.

MEDICATION CHANGES.   Sometimes all that is needed to correct the problem is a change in medication. It is important for the patient to talk with the HCP before stopping any medication. Some men have stopped taking their blood pressure medication and risked a stroke or heart attack because it interfered with their sexual activity.

ORAL MEDICATIONS.   Oral medications (sildenafil [Viagra], tadalafil [Cialis], and vardenafil [Levitra]) are now the first line of therapy used to treat erectile dysfunction. These medications cause the arterioles and cavernous tissue to relax, allowing more blood to flow into the penis in response to sexual stimulation. The pill is usually taken 30 to 60 minutes before anticipated sexual intercourse. Men using nitrate medication (antianginal agents) should avoid using the pills because of risk for severe low blood pressure.

HORMONE TREATMENT.   If the testosterone level is low, replacement hormone may be needed. The HCP should first examine the patient carefully for any evidence of prostate cancer because testosterone replacement can cause the cancer to grow and spread. Testosterone replacement can be given by intramuscular injection, topical gel, or transdermal patch. Testosterone levels must be monitored closely for both positive and negative side effects.

HERBAL REMEDIES.   Several herbal remedies may be effective, including yohimbine, dehydroepiandrosterone (DHEA, a steroid hormone), ginseng, ginkgo, and others. Herbal remedies have side effects, just like prescription medications, and should not be taken without a HCP's recommendation.

INJECTED MEDICATION.   After careful evaluation, a patient or his partner may be taught how to inject a medication into the penis using a 26- or 27-gauge needle on a tuberculin syringe or a prefilled autoinjector. The injections are nearly painless and produce a natural erection in 10 to 15 minutes. The most serious side effect is priapism, which requires immediate reversal in a physician's office or emergency room.

TRANSURETHRAL SUPPOSITORY.   To facilitate medication dispersion and absorption, a patient may choose to use a suppository. The patient is instructed to urinate before use of the suppository. A tiny pellet (microsuppository) is inserted into the urethra using a specialized single-dose applicator. The medication usually begins to work in 5 to 10 minutes, and the effects last for about 30 to 60 minutes.

OTHER NONSURGICAL TREATMENTS.
Sexual Devices and Techniques.   A variety of mechanical sexual aids can be considered by patients who do not want or cannot afford expensive medical treatment. Men should be encouraged to talk with a HCP or qualified sex therapist before trying these alternatives.

Suction devices are another nonsurgical treatment option. This is an external cylinder vacuum device that fits over the penis and draws the blood up into the corporeal bodies, causing an erection. A penile ring is then slipped onto the base of the penis. Once the cylinder is removed, sexual intercourse can begin. Special care must be taken to remove the penile ring within 15 to 20 minutes to prevent tissue damage.

SURGICAL TREATMENTS.
Penile Implants (Prostheses).   Penile implants are a pair of solid or fluid-filled chambers that are surgically placed into the corporeal bodies in the penis to produce an erection. There are two basic types of implants—noninflatable and inflatable (Fig. 43.5).

FIGURE 43.5 Penile implants. (A) Inflatable penile implant. Inflatable cylinders are implanted in the penis, the small hydraulic pump in the scrotum, and the fluid-filled reservoir in the lower abdomen. Sterile radiopaque saline from the reservoir fills the cylinders to provide an erection. (B) Malleable penile implant. Malleable rods are implanted into the penis. The penis is always firm, but the rods can be bent close to the body when erection is not desired.

Vascular Surgery. If a younger man has an erection problem caused by poor blood flow into the penis or from blood leaking out of the penis, rapidly causing the loss of the erection, corrective surgery may be performed. A bypass graft may be done to increase blood flow into the penis or to go around a blockage (as occurs, for example, with Peyronie's disease).

Nursing Process for the Patient With Erectile Dysfunction

DATA COLLECTION. Your role as a nurse may vary based on your work setting. It is always appropriate to ask a man if he has any concerns related to sexual health. It may open the door for him to talk further. It is important to provide privacy and ensure confidentiality. Ask history questions about possible psychosocial causes, including use of medications, street drugs, alcohol, or nicotine. If a problem is identified, alert the HCP, who will continue a more thorough assessment.

NURSING DIAGNOSES, PLANNING, AND IMPLEMENTATION. *Readiness for Enhanced Self Health Management related to treatment of sexual dysfunction*

Expected Outcome: The patient will verbalize understanding of the cause and treatment options for erectile dysfunction.

- Determine patient and partner's current knowledge and understanding about cause and treatment of the disorder. *This will allow for additional and/or correct information to be provided about sexual dysfunction for appropriate understanding.*
- Provide patient and partner with additional and/or correct information about cause and treatment of disorder. *This will allow the patient to have a full understanding of the etiology and care related to the disorder, and increase likelihood of patient adherence to and success of treatment.*
- Refer patient and partner (as appropriate) for medical treatment, psychological treatment, or counseling. *An individualized treatment plan (determined by the etiology) is needed to move toward restoration of sexual functioning.*

EVALUATION. The best indicator of a positive outcome is restoration of erectile function with a verbal account of understanding the disorder and satisfaction with the treatment process. Sometimes the physical problem is easier to correct than the emotional scars that the problem has created. It is important to evaluate both the physiological and emotional outcomes of treatment.

PATIENT EDUCATION. The nurse plays an important role in public education related to erectile dysfunction. Men need to know that they are not alone with their problem. More than 30 million men in the United States experience ongoing problems with erections. Usually, the cause is physical, and help is available through HCPs who specialize in treating erectile dysfunction. See Table 43.4 for a summary of male sexual dysfunction.

TABLE 43.4 MALE SEXUAL DYSFUNCTION SUMMARY

Signs and Symptoms	Report of problems with obtaining and keeping an erection Reported dissatisfaction with sexual performance
Diagnostic Tests	Primary: History and physical Secondary: Vascular flow evaluation, sleep studies
Therapeutic Measures	Counseling Medication to increase blood flow to the penis Surgical implants or repair of structural disorders
Priority Nursing Diagnosis	*Readiness for Enhanced Self-Health Management*

CRITICAL THINKING

Mr. Kittle

■ Mr. Kittle presents to the clinic saying that he is not able to sustain an erection long enough for sexual intercourse that is satisfactory for himself and his partner.

1. You have never had a patient tell you his sexual problems, and you feel a little uncomfortable. How should you respond?
2. What will your assessment include?
3. What is an appropriate role for the LPN/LVN in helping Mr. Kittle?

Suggested answers are at the end of the chapter.

Infertility

A growing number of couples in the United States are having difficulty conceiving children. Several factors can interfere with a man's ability to father a child.

Physiology

A number of conditions must be present in the man for conception to occur. Endocrine function, autonomic nervous system function, and male reproductive structures must all be functioning properly. Normal healthy sperm in a concentration of at least 20 million per milliliter of semen are needed.

Etiology

The factors related to infertility are divided into three general categories: pretesticular, testicular, and post-testicular.

PRETESTICULAR (ENDOCRINE) FACTORS. The first factor involves the proper functioning of the hypothalamus, the pituitary gland, and the testicles. These endocrine functions are complex and are a rare cause of infertility. Examples of endocrine causes might be pituitary or adrenal tumors, thyroid problems, or uncontrolled diabetes.

TESTICULAR FACTORS. The two most common causes of male infertility are varicoceles (40%–50%) and idiopathic causes (40%). It is believed that a varicocele lowers the sperm count by raising the blood flow and temperature in the testicles. Sperm cannot live if the temperature is too high or too low.

Congenital anomalies such as Klinefelter's syndrome (a chromosomal defect) or cryptorchidism result in absent or damaged testicles. Certain disease or inflammatory processes may cause damage to the storage area (epididymitis) or to the testicles themselves (mumps orchitis). Any high fever or viral infection can interfere with the production of sperm for up to 3 months.

Medications, radiation, substance abuse, environmental hazards, and lifestyle practices have all been identified as possible factors that can interfere with spermatogenesis (sperm production). Excessive use of hot tubs and saunas, wearing tight jeans, and long-haul truck driving have all been identified as raising the temperature level in the scrotum to the extent that sperm production is decreased.

POST-TESTICULAR FACTORS. The most common factor in post-testicular infertility is the result of surgery or injury along the pathway from the testicles to the outside of the man's body. Examples of surgical causes are vasectomy, bladder neck reconstruction, pelvic lymph node removal, or any surgery that causes retrograde ejaculation. Congenital anomalies and various types of infections may also cause infertility problems.

Prevention

Prevention involves possible lifestyle changes to avoid excessive heat to the scrotum, substance abuse, exposure to toxins, and environmental hazards. Problems related to medication or infections should be discussed with the HCP.

Signs and Symptoms

A couple is considered infertile if they have been unsuccessful at becoming pregnant after at least 1 year of unprotected intercourse. If pregnancy has occurred during the year but there was

no delivery, the problem usually is considered a female rather than a male factor.

Diagnosis

Diagnosis begins with a detailed history and physical examination that looks for known male causes of infertility.

HISTORY. Initial assessment includes frequency of intercourse, timing (according to ovulation cycle), use of contraceptives, problems with premature ejaculation, and erection problems. Use of hot tubs or saunas; tight jeans; use of nicotine, caffeine, alcohol, or marijuana; and the desire for children on the part of the man are all assessed. High stress, long periods of sitting, and exposure to environmental toxins are determined. The patient also may be questioned about STIs, endocrine problems, congenital urinary problems, serious illnesses or groin injuries, cancer, and treatment with chemotherapy or radiation.

PHYSICAL EXAMINATION. The HCP will observe for normal hair pattern and growth, muscle development, size of testicles, and any evidence of a varicocele or hydrocele.

DIAGNOSTIC TESTS. Analysis is done on several semen specimens to see if they contain the right amount and type of healthy sperm needed for a pregnancy. Infection should be ruled out. Several other tests may be done, including hormone tests, genetic testing, ultrasound, and others, depending on the level of desire and the financial resources of the couple. Many insurance companies do not pay for testing or treatment for infertility.

Therapeutic Measures

Treatment may be as simple as making a change in sexual or lifestyle practices. Surgery to correct a varicocele or obstruction may be done. If the couple is able to handle the emotional and financial strain, they may try a variety of in vitro fertilization (IVF) procedures. IVF is very costly, and success rates vary. Another option that may be presented to the couple is adoption.

You can play an important role in the emotional support a couple needs during infertility studies. It is important that the couple feel comfortable in communicating their feelings and frustrations with one another and their HCP. It also may help them to attend a support group designed for couples experiencing infertility.

SUGGESTED ANSWERS TO

CRITICAL THINKING

■ *Mr. Atkinson*

1.
$$\frac{5 \text{ mg}}{} \frac{1 \text{ tablet}}{2 \text{ mg}} = 2.5 \text{ tablets}$$

2. Mr. Atkinson should be alert for signs of hypotension, such as dizziness or lightheadedness on arising. He

should not drive until effects and side effects of the medication are known.

3. Mr. Atkinson should be instructed not to lift anything heavier than 10 lb for the first 6 weeks, and he will not be able to plow or drive for the first 6 weeks. It is important that his son understand his father's limitations and how important it is for him or someone else to help out with the farm chores.

SUGGESTED ANSWERS TO—cont'd

4. Mr. Atkinson will notice a change in his ejaculation (either very little ejaculate or none at all). If he could have an erection before surgery, the chances are very good that he will continue to be able to have intercourse; however, he will not ejaculate.

5. A home health nurse can assist Mr. Atkinson with care at home, such as catheter care and removal, possible dribbling postsurgery and reinforcement of activity level. A dietitian can help with dietary instructions related to foods high in dietary fiber and fluids to avoid such as caffeine, citrus juices, and alcohol beverages.

■ *Mr. Cunningham*

1. Mr. Cunningham should be encouraged to see his HCP immediately for an evaluation to rule out testicular cancer.

2. Depending on the stage of the cancer, he will have the cancerous testicle, cord, and lymph nodes removed. He may need chemotherapy or radiation treatments as well.

3. Mr. Cunningham should be encouraged to make deposits at a certified sperm bank before any treatments. It is also important to include his future wife and his family in the decision-making process and encourage them to share their feelings and concerns

with one another. Cancer support groups may also be helpful to Mr. Cunningham.

■ *Mr. Kittle*

1. It is okay to "pretend" here! Act like you are perfectly comfortable and that you hear this sort of thing every day. (Of course, you would never pretend to know something you don't—it is always okay to say you don't know.) Have a matter-of-fact communication style. If you get nervous and forget what questions you should ask, start with something general such as, "Can you tell me more about your symptoms?"

2. Begin a psychosocial assessment to identify presence of stress, fear, depression, fatigue, or problems with interpersonal relationships; also ask about medication, alcohol, and nicotine use. Assure him you will alert the HCP to follow up with further assessment.

3. After alerting the HCP, encourage Mr. Kittle to share openly so that an accurate diagnosis can be made. Reassure Mr. Kittle that many men have the same problem and that he is not alone. Let him know there are many treatments available and that his HCP will work with him to find what is best for him.

REVIEW QUESTIONS

1. A patient with benign prostatic hyperplasia expresses concern that he has cancer. Which response by the nurse is best?
   1. "Don't worry; prostatic hyperplasia is not the same thing as cancer."
   2. "Since it is called benign, you don't have to worry about it. No treatment should be necessary; you will just need to have it watched."
   3. "Hyperplasia means your prostate is growing too many cells. They are not cancerous, but they could interfere with your ability to urinate, so it is important to have it treated."
   4. "You are correct, it is a form of cancer, but it is very slow growing and very treatable. Your doctor will recommend treatments for you."

2. A nurse is discharging a man from the emergency department after treatment for priapism. Which statement by the patient shows understanding of instructions?
   1. "I should use hot packs three times a day for the next three days."
   2. "I should be seen immediately if I have another erection lasting more than 2 hours."
   3. "The Viagra I took may have caused this problem."
   4. "I should avoid having sex for one month."

3. A patient who is 1-day post–transurethral resection of the prostate says he is having pain in his bladder, and the nurse notices urine leakage around his catheter. Which of the following responses by the nurse is best?
   1. "Bladder spasms are common after your surgery. Take some deep breaths while I get a B&O suppository."
   2. "You should not be experiencing spasms. I will notify the RN right away."
   3. "Spasms can be very painful. Would you like an injection of Demerol?"
   4. "Your catheter is leaking; we will need to replace it right away."

4. A nurse working in a nursing home notes that it is difficult but not impossible to retract the foreskin for washing on an older gentleman. Which action is correct?
   1. Avoid retracting the foreskin for cleaning to prevent paraphimosis.
   2. Gently retract the foreskin for cleaning, then replace it and notify the HCP.
   3. Retract the foreskin for cleaning, and leave it retracted to prevent infection.
   4. Retract the foreskin and leave it retracted until the HCP can evaluate it.

5. Which statement by a patient shows the need for more education about erectile dysfunction?
   1. "I may have blood flow problems that are causing the dysfunction."
   2. "I can try some herbal remedies such as ginseng before consulting my physician."
   3. "Some men inject drugs into their penis to cause an erection."
   4. "My sleep apnea could be a factor in erectile dysfunction."

6. A patient is admitted to a medical unit for complications of diabetes. The nurse asks if he is satisfied with his level of sexual functioning, and he becomes tearful. Which initial response by the nurse is best?
   1. "You seem upset with my question. Are you having a problem you would like to talk about?"
   2. "Impotence is common with diabetes. Don't let it worry you."
   3. "What kind of sexual dysfunction are you experiencing?"
   4. "I am sorry you are having problems with your sexual functioning. Would you like a referral to a sex therapist?"

7. What are common complications of varicocele? **Select all that apply.**
   1. Infertility
   2. Infection
   3. Erectile dysfunction
   4. Pain
   5. Priapism
   6. Cancer

8. Which of the following should the nurse anticipate teaching about when caring for a man with infertility?
   1. Penile implants
   2. Prostatectomy
   3. TURP
   4. Decrease in nicotine and alcohol use

Answers can be found in Appendix C.

References

American Cancer Society. (2012). *Cancer incidence and mortality rates by site, race, and ethnicity, US, 2005–2009.* Retrieved May 31, 2013, from www.cancer.org/acs/groups/content /@epidemiologysureilance/document/document /acsps-036845.pdf

National Kidney and Urologic Diseases Information Clearinghouse. (2012). Prostatitis: Disorders of the prostate (NIH Pub. No. 08-4553). Retrieved May 31, 2013, from http:// kidney.niddk.nih.gov/kudiseases/pubs/prostatitis

 Davis*Plus* | For additional resources and information visit **davispl.us/medsurg5**

44

Nursing Care of Patients With Sexually Transmitted Infections

LAURA L. McCULLY AND
DEBRA PERRY-PHILO

LEARNING OUTCOMES

1. Identify the pathogens involved with each of the common sexually transmitted infections (STIs).
2. Describe the signs and symptoms of each of the common STIs.
3. Plan teaching to promote STI prevention.
4. Describe treatment options for common STIs.
5. Plan nursing care for patients with STIs.
6. Explain how you will know if your nursing interventions have been effective.

KEY TERMS

cervicitis (SIR-vih-SY-tiss)
chancre (SHANK-er)
condylomata acuminata (KON-dih-LOH-mah-tah ah-KYOOM-in-AH-tah)
condylomatous (KON-dih-LOH-mah-tus)
conjunctivitis (kon-JUNK-tih-VY-tis)
cytotoxic (SY-toh-TOK-sick)
electrocautery (ee-LEK-troh-CAW-tur-ee)
electrocoagulated (ee-LEK-troh-coh-AG-yoo-LAY-ted)
endometritis (EN-doh-meh-TRY-tiss)
epidemiological (EP-ih-DEE-mee-ah-LAH-jih-kuhl)
gummas (GUH-mahs)
hepatosplenomegaly (heh-PAT-oh-SPLEH-noh-MEG-ah-lee)
herpetic (her-PET-ik)
lymphadenopathy (lim-FAD-deh-NAW-puh-thee)
mucopurulent cervicitis (MYOO-koh-PYOO-ruh-lent SIR-vih-SY-tiss)
ophthalmia neonatorum (awf-THAL-mee-ah NEE-oh-nuh-TOR-uhm)
proctitis (prok-TY-tiss)
puerperal (pyoo-UR-pur-uhl)
sacral radiculopathy (SAY-krul ra-DIK-yoo-LAW-puh-thee)
salpingitis (SAL-pin-JY-tiss)
serological (SEAR-uh-LAW-jih-kuhl)
urethritis (YOO-reh-THRY-tiss)
verrucous (veh-ROO-kuss)
vesicular (veh-SIK-yoo-lur)
vulvovaginitis (VUL-voh-VAJ-ih-NY-tiss)

Sexually transmitted infections (STIs) are infections that can be transmitted through intimate contact with the genitals, mouth, or rectum of another individual. Some STIs can also be spread by other routes such as blood or body fluids. A nurse's best protection against catching diseases from blood and body fluids of infected patients is the strict practice of standard precautions and maintaining his or her own healthy, intact skin.

Physically, STIs can cause tremendous suffering through pain, scarring of genitourinary structures, damage to other body organs, infertility, birth defects, nervous system damage, development of cancer, and even death of infected patients and sometimes their children. Psychologically and socially, these infections also have profound effects on individuals, families, and relationships. Guilt about passing on an incurable infection to a loved one or feelings of betrayal because of being infected as a result of someone else's choices are some of the emotional consequences of STIs.

Changing social values have been associated with increasing incidence of almost all types of STIs, including some previously rare infections related to anal intercourse. Coexistence of more than one STI in an individual is also occurring more often. Many infections and syndromes are associated with STIs; the more common ones are discussed here. Human immunodeficiency virus (HIV) and acquired immunodeficiency syndrome (AIDS) are discussed separately in Chapter 20.

One of the most important ways you can help those who experience STIs is by being kind, nonjudgmental, and sensitive to the patient's communication. Maintaining an open posture and eye contact that is appropriate for the patient's culture relays a sense of openness and willingness to talk and preserves the possibility of continuing health promotion with these individuals in the future.

DISORDERS AND SYNDROMES RELATED TO SEXUALLY TRANSMITTED INFECTIONS

Vulvovaginitis

Vulvovaginitis is an inflammation of the vulva and vagina and can be asymptomatic or involve redness, itching, burning, excoriation, pain, swelling of the vagina and labia, and discharge. A variety of sexually and nonsexually transmitted infectious agents can cause vulvovaginitis. The odor, consistency, and color of the discharge vary with the different microbes involved. Nonsexually transmitted vaginitis, vulvovaginitis, and vaginosis are described in Chapter 42. Some microorganisms may be acquired either by sexual or nonsexual routes, so they are also mentioned in this chapter. Bartholin's glands can develop abscesses as a result of infection with nonsexually transmitted microbes or STIs such as gonorrhea and chlamydia.

Urethritis

Both STIs and nonsexually transmitted microorganisms can cause **urethritis** in men and women. In men, inflammation of the urethra, prostate, and epididymis can result in difficult,

painful, and frequent urination and a urethral discharge, which may be clear, cloudy, or yellow. Female partners of men with urethritis may also suffer from urethritis, and they may also develop **mucopurulent cervicitis** (MPC) and a variety of other symptoms of the particular infection. Some causative agents for urethritis include *Neisseria gonorrhoeae, Chlamydia trachomatis, Ureaplasma urealyticum, Trichomonas vaginalis, Candida albicans,* and herpes simplex. Often this infection category is divided into gonococcal urethritis caused by *N. gonorrhoeae* and nongonococcal urethritis.

Mucopurulent Cervicitis

MPC is an inflammation of the cervix that may produce a mucopurulent yellow exudate on the cervix or may have no noticeable symptoms. MPC during pregnancy can result in **conjunctivitis** and pneumonia in newborn infants, as well as **puerperal** infection of the mother. MPC can be caused by such organisms as *C. trachomatis, N. gonorrhoeae, T. vaginalis, C. albicans,* and herpes simplex. MPC may spread to become pelvic inflammatory disease (PID).

Proctitis and Enteritis

Proctitis is inflammation of the rectum and anus that may be due to either nonsexually transmitted microbes or to STIs. This is especially prevalent among those who practice heterosexual or homosexual anal intercourse. Enteritis, which is inflammation of the lining of the intestine, may occur as a result of contamination during anal intercourse. Infection with *Campylobacter* species, *Shigella* species, and *Giardia lamblia* can be a problem for gay men. Care of patients who have gastrointestinal disorders is discussed in Unit 8.

Genital Ulcers

Genital ulcers are formed when papules or macules erode and leave painful, raw, pitted, or excoriated areas on or around the genitals. Not all genital ulcers are caused by STIs—injury, some

* **WORD • BUILDING •**

vulvovaginitis: vulvo—vulva + vagin—vagina + itis—inflammation

urethritis: ureth—urethra + itis—inflammation

mucopurulent cervicitis: muco—involving mucus + purulent—involving pus + cervic—cervix + itis—inflammation

conjunctivitis: conjunctiv(a)—lining of the eyelids and sclera of the eye + itis—inflammation

puerperal: childbirth

proctitis: proc—anus + itis—inflammation

non-STI viruses, some types of drug reactions, radiation, and some forms of cancer can also produce genital ulcers. STIs that can produce genital ulcers include syphilis, herpes, and HIV. Although the ulcerations can look similar in these STIs, a distinctive difference is that a syphilitic ulcer is painless. Genital ulcers from one type of disease may increase the risk of infection with other STIs during sexual activity because the open areas present an easy portal of entry for the infecting organism.

Cellular Changes

Cellular changes can also be caused by STIs, including **condylomatous** (wartlike) growths and dysplasia or neoplasia, which may result in precancerous or cancerous conditions. Herpes viruses, HIV, and human papillomavirus (HPV) have all been linked to the development of cancer.

Pelvic Inflammatory Disease
Pathophysiology and Etiology

PID is an infection of the upper genital tract that can cause chronic pelvic pain due to inflammation. The primary sources of infection include *C. trachomatis* and *N. gonorrhoeae,* but it may result from any organism that is associated with a STI. These organisms can invade the endocervical canal, resulting in **cervicitis**, and move upward resulting in infection of the endometrium (**endometritis**), fallopian tubes (**salpingitis**), and pelvic cavity. The chronic inflammation results in extensive scarring and adhesions, which can cause infertility and increase the risk of ectopic pregnancy. Increased risk for PID occurs with a history of multiple sexual partners, STIs, substance abuse, frequent vaginal douching, and insertion of an intrauterine device (IUD). Testing for STIs and treatment before insertion of an IUD greatly reduces the risk of PID.

Signs and Symptoms

Some women with PID are asymptomatic or have minimal symptoms. Other women present with lower abdominal pain and tenderness, purulent vaginal discharge or vaginal bleeding, pain with sexual intercourse, fever, nausea and vomiting, and pain with urination. Findings during physical examination include adnexal tenderness upon palpation, and pain in the uterus and cervix when moved during a bimanual examination.

Diagnostic Tests

Laboratory tests may reveal a positive culture of the causative organism(s) and leukocytosis. Urinary tract infection may need to be ruled out.

Therapeutic Measures

With serious infection, hospitalization and intravenous (IV) antibiotics may be indicated. IV therapy can be changed to oral therapy after 48 hours if status improves. Outpatient therapy with oral antibiotics is used with minor infections. Laparoscopic surgery may be done to release adhesions and reduce complications. Testing and treatment for other STIs should be considered for both the patient and her partner. Education on the cause of the infection and prevention of future episodes is essential.

SEXUALLY TRANSMITTED INFECTIONS

Chlamydia
Etiology and Signs and Symptoms

Chlamydia is the most commonly diagnosed STI in the United States (see Table 44.1 for a summary of this and other common STIs). It can be transmitted sexually and by blood and body fluid contact. There are several strains of the bacteria *C. trachomatis*. Chlamydia is often asymptomatic (a "silent" STI) in women, but it can cause urethritis, MPC, and conjunctivitis. Fitz-Hugh-Curtis syndrome, a surface inflammation of the liver, can also be caused by *C. trachomatis*. This inflammation can cause nausea, vomiting, and sharp pain at the base of the ribs that sometimes refers to the right shoulder and arm. Chlamydia is a frequent cause of pelvic inflammatory disease (PID) and infertility, and it increases the risk of ectopic pregnancy. The infection can be passed from mother to baby during birth, resulting in neonatal pneumonia and conjunctivitis. It also increases the risk of HIV infection.

Lymphogranuloma venereum (LGV) is also caused by some strains of *C. trachomatis* but is more commonly seen in tropical climates or among people who emigrated from tropical areas. This disease also causes urethritis and proctitis, and it inflames lymph nodes that drain the pelvic area, resulting in draining sores and fistula development. Scarring from this disease can complicate vaginal deliveries.

Diagnostic Tests

Several tests for chlamydia are available. Samples are gathered in a special collection tube to send to a laboratory for culture. Culturing is difficult and expensive and generally requires 2 to 6 days for results. A newer type of testing, called nucleic acid amplification testing, identifies the presence of chlamydial DNA or RNA in urine, cervical, or urethral specimens. Because this disease is so common, it is wise to set out an unopened *Chlamydia* collection kit within easy reach of the health care provider (HCP) for each pelvic examination. The Centers for Disease Control (CDC) recommends that all sexually active females under the age of 25 and women over age 25 who are at risk should be tested annually for *Chlamydia* (CDC, 2013a).

Therapeutic Measures

Antibiotics are typically given to treat chlamydia in adults (Table 44.2). Erythromycin or azithromycin is used during pregnancy because other antibiotics may pose a risk to the fetus. Use of an ophthalmic ointment or solution containing silver nitrate, erythromycin, or tetracycline is recommended as treatment of the neonate shortly after birth for the prevention

---

• **WORD** • **BUILDING** •

condylomatous: condyl—rounded projection + oma(t)—growth + ous—like

cervicitis: cervic—cervix + itis—inflammation

endometritis: endo—inside + metr—womb + itis—inflammation

salpingitis: salping—tube + itis—inflammation

TABLE 44.1 COMMON SEXUALLY TRANSMITTED INFECTIONS SUMMARY

	Chlamydia	Gonorrhea	Syphilis	Trichomoniasis	Herpes Simplex	Condylomata (HPV)
Signs and Symptoms	Conjunctivitis; in men, urethritis, epididymitis, prostatitis; in women, MPC, urethritis	In men, urethritis, penile discharge, epididymitis, prostatitis; in women, MPC, urethritis, abnormal menses	Primary syphilis, chancre; secondary syphilis, flulike symptoms, rashes, condylomatous growths	Genital redness, swelling, itching, burning, foul discharge; in men, urethritis, prostatitis; in women, "strawberry cervix"	Vesicles/ ulcerations in mouth, genitals; flu-like symptoms, lymphadenopathy, urethritis, cystitis, MPC	Fleshy tumors, primarily on genitalia
Diagnostic Tests	NAT culture, urine	NAT culture, urine	VDRL, ELISA, RPR, FTA-ABS	Microscopic examination	Culture, Western blot, ELISA	Colposcope examination biopsy, visualization of lesions
Therapeutic Measures	Antibiotics (see Table 44.2)	Antibiotics (see Table 44.2)	Penicillin	Metronidazole, tinidazole	Antiviral medication (see Table 44.2)	Wart removal, interferon therapy
Complications	Fitz-Hugh–Curtis syndrome, increased susceptibility to HIV infection; PID, infertility, transmission to baby at birth; co-infection with gonorrhea	PID, disseminated gonococcal infection, Fitz-Hugh–Curtis syndrome, transmission to baby at birth, co-infection with chlamydia	Tertiary syphilis, gumma damage to heart, circulatory system, nervous system; transmission to fetus during pregnancy	Preterm delivery, infertility, increased risk of HIV transmission	Lifelong infection, disseminated infection, nervous system invasion, increased risk of cervical cancer, transmission to baby at birth	Cancers of the reproductive organs and anus, including cervical cancer; transmission to fetus during pregnancy

Note. ELISA = enzyme-linked immunosorbent assay; FTA-ABS fluorescent treponemal antibody absorption; HPV = human papillomavirus; MPC = mucopurulent cervicitis; NAT = nucleic acid amplification testing; PID = pelvic inflammatory disease; RPR = rapid plasmin reagin; VDRL = Venereal Disease Research Laboratory.

of conjunctivitis. This is done regardless of whether the mother is diagnosed with chlamydia because asymptomatic or undiagnosed chlamydia is common, and this simple treatment can prevent serious complications later. Institutional policies and state regulations determine the type of eye preparation to be used and whether administration of the medications requires specific consent of the parents.

Gonorrhea
Etiology and Signs and Symptoms

According to the CDC (2013b), 321,849 new cases of gonorrhea were reported to the CDC in 2011 (the most recently available statistics). It is caused by the bacterium *N. gonorrhoeae* and can be transmitted vaginally, rectally, orally, or

TABLE 44.2 MEDICATIONS USED TO TREAT SEXUALLY TRANSMITTED INFECTIONS

Medication Class	Examples/Action	Nursing Implications
Chlamydia **Antibiotics**	*Macrolides:* erythromycin azithromycin *Inhibit bacterial protein synthesis.* *Tetracyclines:* doxycycline *Inhibits protein synthesis by binding to ribosomes.* amoxicillin *Binds to bacterial cell wall, causing cell death.* *Fluoroquinolones:* ofloxacin levofloxacin *Inhibit cell wall synthesis.*	Administer on empty stomach. Do not administer with antacids. Use caution with hepatic disorders. Do not administer during pregnancy due to bone/teeth effects. Do not give with antacids or dairy products. Administer on empty stomach. Avoid unnecessary exposure to sunlight. Safety under age 18 not established. Do not administer with antacids. Use caution with other medications and with renal, hepatic, or CNS disorders.
Gonorrhea **Antibiotics**	*Cephalosporins:* ceftriaxone cefixime *Inhibit cell wall synthesis.*	Use caution with penicillin allergies or renal or hepatic dysfunction. Avoid excess sun exposure.
Syphilis **Antibiotics**	*Penicillin:* penicillin G *Inhibits cell wall synthesis.* *Tetracyclines:* tetracycline doxycycline *(See information above)*	Administer deep IM or slow IV. Apply ice packs to injection site as needed. Administer PO on empty stomach. Instruct patient to report fever/rash. Avoid tetracycline in children and pregnant women.
Trichomoniasis **Amebicides/** **antiprotozoals**	Metronidazole, tinidazole *Bind to DNA to inhibit synthesis and cause cell death.*	Administer with food. Avoid alcohol; abstain for a minimum of 48 hr following treatment to prevent severe flu-like reaction. Treat partner as well as patient.
Herpes **Antivirals**	acyclovir valacyclovir famciclovir *Inhibit DNA synthesis.*	Use systemic preparations cautiously with CNS, hepatic, or renal disorders. Infuse IV slowly. Maintain hydration. Caution patient that viral transmission can still occur during treatment. Some patients take daily as suppressive therapy.
Genital Warts **Antimitotics** **and acidic agents**	Podophyllin/trichloroacetic acid (TCA)/bichloracetic acid (BCA)	Instruct patient to return for repeated applications as needed. Avoid medication contact with eyes or tissue surrounding lesion.

Continued

TABLE **44.2** **MEDICATIONS USED TO TREAT SEXUALLY TRANSMITTED INFECTIONS—cont'd**

Medication Class	Examples/Action	Nursing Implications
Antimitotic agent	podofilox solution (Condylox)	Can be applied by patient at home with cotton-tipped applicator. Instruct patient to apply to warts only and allow to dry completely, or as ordered by provider.
Antiviral/immune response modifier	imiquimod (Aldara)	Can be applied by patient at home. Instruct patient to apply thin film to clean dry skin at bedtime, as ordered by provider. May take up to 16 weeks to completely clear warts.

Note. CNS = central nervous system; GI = gastrointestinal; IM = intramuscular; IV = intravenous; PO = by mouth.

via contact with other mucous membranes, or through contact with blood and body fluids. It can produce a variety of signs and symptoms. Men may be asymptomatic or may have urethritis with a yellow urethral discharge. Women who have gonorrhea may have either no noticeable symptoms or have a sore throat, MPC, urethritis, or abnormal menstrual symptoms such as bleeding between periods. Many cases of PID are caused by gonorrhea. Intercourse with an infected partner during menstruation may be especially risky for development of PID because removal of the cervical mucous barrier can promote the growth of the gonococcus in the higher reproductive tract. Gonorrhea can also cause Fitz-Hugh-Curtis syndrome. Fever, nausea, vomiting, and lower abdominal pain may be present. Gonorrhea may also infect the throat and the rectum and may cause disseminated gonococcal infection, resulting in inflammation of the joints, skin, meninges, and lining of the heart.

Newborns born to mothers who have gonorrhea can develop **ophthalmia neonatorum**, which involves inflammation of the conjunctivae and deeper parts of the eye and can, ultimately, result in blindness. The newborn may also experience a gonorrheal infection at other sites following birth. Abscesses may develop where fetal scalp monitors were attached during labor, and infection of the nose, lungs, and rectum may occur.

Diagnostic Tests

Diagnosis is done by microscopic examination of smears and cultures of the discharge or identification of bacterial DNA (nucleic acid testing) in the urine. More than one test may be done to verify the diagnosis.

Therapeutic Measures

Development of antibiotic resistance by *N. gonorrhoeae* and co-infection with other microorganisms, such as *C. trachomatis,* is making treatment more complicated. Cephalosporin antibiotics are recommended for the treatment of gonorrhea (see Table 44.2). It is also recommended that the patient be treated

for chlamydia because co-infection is common. Ophthalmia neonatorum can be prevented by use of antibiotic eye preparations that contain silver nitrate, erythromycin, or tetracycline. It is recommended, as with prophylactic treatment of chlamydial conjunctivitis, that all infants be treated shortly after birth regardless of diagnostic status of the mother. The treatment is simple and may prevent a devastating outcome for the newborn. Institutional policies and state regulations determine the type of eye drops to be used and whether administration of the drops requires specific consent of the parents.

CRITICAL THINKING

Mrs. Miller

■ Mrs. Miller delivered an infant boy 1 hour ago. The nurse is currently applying erythromycin ointment to the infant's eyes bilaterally. Mrs. Miller asks if the medication is necessary.

1. How will you respond?
2. Should all infants receive prophylactic eye treatment at birth?

Suggested answers are at the end of the chapter.

Syphilis
Pathophysiology, Etiology, and Signs and Symptoms

Syphilis is an ancient infection that has not disappeared, although it is overshadowed by more commonly occurring

• WORD • BUILDING •

ophthalmia neonatorum: ophthalmia—eye disease + neonatorum—of the newborn infections such as chlamydia. It occurs in stages. The primary stage of syphilis begins with the entry of the *Treponema pallidum* spirochete through the skin or mucous membranes. Between 3 and 90 days later, a papule develops at the site of entry, then sloughs off, leaving a painless, red, ulcerated area called a **chancre** (Fig. 44.1). Chancres can also develop in other areas of the body at this time. Chancre formation typically is the only symptom of this stage of syphilis. The chancre eventually heals, but the spirochete remains active in the infected individual and can be passed on to others.

Secondary syphilis begins 2 to 8 weeks later and affects the body more generally, causing such problems as flulike symptoms, joint pain, hair loss, skin rashes (primarily on the soles of the hands and feet), mouth sores, and condylomatous growths in moist areas of the body.

Serious damage can occur if syphilis is untreated in the early stages. About 15% of infected individuals will progress to the tertiary (or late) stage, up to 10 to 20 years later. At this stage, it can involve any organ system of the body. The spirochete can form **gummas**, which are tumors of a rubbery consistency that can break down and ulcerate, leaving holes in body tissues. The gummas can damage the heart, circulatory system, and nervous system (called neurosyphilis). Ulceration of gummas can destroy areas of vital tissue and lead to mental and physical disability or early death.

Syphilis can be passed on to the unborn children of women who carry the spirochete, resulting in **hepatosplenomegaly**, increase in bilirubin, destruction of red blood cells, birth defects (especially of the face), **lymphadenopathy**, and a baby who can transmit the spirochete through nasal drainage. If left untreated, syphilis during pregnancy can cause lesions in various organs of the unborn baby and result in higher rates of spontaneous abortion, stillbirth, and premature birth.

Diagnostic Tests

Several tests for syphilis exist, and a combination may be used for accurate diagnosis. Cultures may be done but are difficult to grow. **Serological** (blood) tests include the venereal disease research laboratory (VDRL) test, the rapid plasma reagin (RPR) test, and the automated reagin test (ART). These tests indirectly check for syphilis by detecting the presence of antibodies that the body forms in response to *Treponema* and, unfortunately, in response to some other disorders, so false-positive results can occur. Diagnosis of neurosyphilis is even more difficult because some testing of cerebrospinal fluid may result in false-negative results. Treponemal enzyme-linked immunosorbent assay (ELISA), fluorescent treponemal antibody absorption (FTA-ABS), and polymerase chain reaction (PCR) tests for treponemal DNA are some newer methods that reduce the risk of false results.

Therapeutic Measures

Penicillin G is the treatment of choice for patients diagnosed with syphilis (see Table 44.2). For those who are allergic to penicillin, doxycycline and tetracycline are treatment options. When HIV and syphilis are diagnosed in the same individual, symptoms of neurosyphilis are more likely to occur.

Trichomoniasis
Pathophysiology and Etiology

Trichomoniasis is an STI caused by a protozoan parasite. It can be also be transmitted through nonsexual contact with infected articles because it can survive for a long time outside the body. Carriers of *Trichomonas vaginalis* can be asymptomatic for several years until changes in vaginal or urethral conditions encourage an outbreak of the infection. A decrease in resident bacteria, injuries to the vaginal tissues, and development of lesions from other STIs or from some forms of cancer can activate the organism.

Signs and Symptoms

Symptoms include redness, swelling, itching, and burning of the genital area; pain with intercourse and voiding; and a frothy, foul-smelling discharge that can be clear, white, yellowish, or greenish. Men with trichomonal infection can develop prostatitis and infertility. Men who are also infected with HIV are more likely to transmit HIV to others, and women with *Trichomonas vaginalis* are more susceptible to HIV infection if exposed. Women who are pregnant risk preterm delivery and low birth weight babies.

Diagnostic Tests

A Papanicolaou (Pap) test can be used to diagnose trichomoniasis. Visualization of the cervix during pelvic examination shows a characteristic "strawberry cervix." When wet-mount slides of discharge are viewed under a microscope, the

FIGURE 44.1 Syphilis chancre. From Reeves, J. R. T., & Maibach, H. (1991). *Clinical dermatology illustrated: A regional approach.* Philadelphia: F.A. Davis, p. 88.

• WORD • BUILDING •
chancre: hard ulceration
gummas: from the word meaning "rubber"—rubbery tumors
hepatosplenomegaly: hepato—liver + spleno—spleen + megaly—enlargement
lymphadenopathy: lymph—lymph nodes + adeno—node + pathy—disorder
serological: sero—blood + logical—science

organisms can be identified by their motility and whiplike flagella. Because trichomoniasis can produce abnormal Pap smear readings, more frequent Pap smears must be done to provide adequate surveillance of cellular changes.

Therapeutic Measures

Antiparasitic agents metronidazole (Flagyl) or tinidazole (Tindamax) are used to treat trichomoniasis (see Table 44.2). Because some people carry the organism without symptoms, sexual partners should also be treated regardless of symptoms.

CRITICAL THINKING

Kerri

■ Kerri presents to the health clinic with a report of generalized redness, swelling, itching, and burning of her external genitalia. Following history, physical, and microscopic examination, trichomoniasis is diagnosed. Kerri is upset, stating she has been in a monogamous relationship for 2 years.

1. What should your response to Kerri include?
2. Kerri is placed on metronidazole (Flagyl), but you are not comfortable with the dose prescribed, so you look it up. How do you approach the HCP with what appears to be an error?
3. What patient education is important for Kerri?

Suggested answers are at the end of the chapter.

Herpes
Pathophysiology, Etiology, and Signs and Symptoms

Herpes infection is caused by the herpes simplex virus types 1 and 2 (HSV-1 and HSV-2). Herpes viruses have an affinity for tissues of the skin and nervous system and can lie dormant in nervous system tissues and then reactivate periodically when the body undergoes stress, fever, or immune system compromise. Both HSV-1 and HSV-2 can cause "fever blisters" of the mouth (Fig. 44.2), as well as genital lesions. However, HSV-1 is more frequently associated with oral lesions and HSV-2 with genital lesions.

Genital HSV-2 outbreaks are more severe than genital HSV-1 outbreaks. After infection, vesicles develop, spontaneously rupture, and produce painful ulceration of the underlying skin tissues. Asymptomatic latent periods are generally interspersed between the **vesicular** outbreaks. Although not as common, the virus may still be transmitted even during latent periods.

An initial outbreak following infection with the herpes virus occurs 2 days to 2 weeks after exposure and can produce a flulike condition. Urethritis, cystitis, and MPC with vaginal discharge can also occur. Infection of the spinal nerve roots by HSV can result in **sacral radiculopathy** (damage of

FIGURE 44.2 Herpes simplex. From Reeves, J. R. T., & Maibach, H. (1991). *Clinical dermatology illustrated: A regional approach.* Philadelphia: F.A. Davis, p. 64.

the sacral spinal nerves), causing retention of urine and feces. Although rare, disseminated herpes infection can result in inflammation of the spinal cord, meninges, nerve pathways, and lymph nodes; urethral strictures; and increased risk for development of cervical cancer in women.

It is estimated that one in five of all pregnant women carry herpes, although most of their babies do not develop **herpetic** disease. If infected, the baby's skin, eyes, mucous membranes, and nervous system can be involved, and death from disseminated herpes infection is possible. The greatest risk of herpes transmission from mother to child during pregnancy occurs if the mother has an active genital lesion at the time of delivery.

Diagnostic Tests

Testing for HSV requires special viral collection kits for swabbed or scraped specimens from lesions. Follow the directions on the viral collection kit as well as institutional policies. Blood tests are used to test specifically for HSV-1 or HSV-2 antibodies.

Therapeutic Measures

There is currently no known cure for herpes infection, although antiviral medications may be given to decrease the severity of symptoms (see Table 44.2). Pregnant women with a history of HSV are treated prophylactically with antiviral medication during the last 36 weeks of pregnancy (CDC, 2013b). If an active genital lesion is present when a woman is close to the time of delivery, a cesarean delivery is likely to be performed. However, an active lesion at any time during pregnancy poses a risk for transmission. See the "Nursing Care Plan for the Patient With an STI" later in this chapter.

• **WORD** • **BUILDING** •

vesicular: vesicul—blister + ar—type
sacral radiculopathy: sacral—sacrum + radiculo—root + pathy—disorder or disease
herpetic: herpet—herpes + ic—pertaining to

Genital Warts

Signs and Symptoms

Condylomata acuminata (genital warts) is a common sexually transmitted viral infection, and its incidence is increasing rapidly. Infection with human papillomavirus (HPV) produces the condylomata—soft, raised, **verrucous** fleshy tumors, which may also have finger-like projections and resemble cauliflower (Fig. 44.3). Lesions most commonly develop on the external genitalia and perineum, as well as on the internal vaginal wall and cervix in women. However, lesions can also develop on other areas of the body after contact with the virus. Some people remain asymptomatic, but can still transmit the infection.

More than 100 types of HPV have been identified, and several have been closely linked to the development of cancers of the reproductive organs and anus in both males and females. The latent period from the time of exposure to development of the warts can be as long as 3 years.

HPV can be passed on from a pregnant woman to her fetus, resulting in the growth of genital warts on the baby, HPV infection of the baby's respiratory tract, and a possible future increased risk of cancer development. HPV infection during pregnancy can cause particularly difficult problems. Genital warts tend to grow more rapidly in pregnant women and to bleed more easily with injury than in nonpregnant women.

Diagnostic Tests

Diagnosis can be made by applying dilute acetic acid (vinegar) to the skin of the external genital area, vagina, cervix, and anus and then closely examining with a colposcope for areas that turn a lighter color. Biopsy specimens of the suspicious areas can be sent for further study of the cells. Other tests to diagnose HPV include an antigen test and the Southern and dot blot tests, which use radioactive probes. Cancerous changes stimulated by the virus may be identified on Pap smears.

FIGURE 44.3 Condylomata, commonly known as genital warts. From Lemone, P., & Burke, K. M. (1996). *Medical-surgical nursing: Critical thinking in client care.* Menlo Park, CA: Addison-Wesley, p. 2079, with permission.

Therapeutic Measures

There is currently no known cure for papillomavirus infection. The warts can be treated by freezing, burning, or chemically destroying them or by manipulating the patient's immune system to attack the virus. Cryotherapy (freezing) of the warts can be done by touching each wart with a cryoprobe or a liquid nitrogen–soaked swab. Warts may also be burned or **electrocoagulated** with an **electrocautery** or a laser. Heat causes the proteins to coagulate, resulting in death of the wart tissue. Several topical agents are also available (see Table 44.2).

Some treatment options are not appropriate for use during pregnancy because of their **cytotoxic** effects, which might damage the fetus, but cryosurgery and laser destruction of wart tissue can be done during pregnancy. All treatments may require multiple applications and generally result in a great deal of discomfort as the warts degenerate, ulcerate, and slough over a long period. Wart removal does not cure the infection, and new wart growth can occur after treatment.

Various types of immunotherapy have been used against HPV. Interferons are proteins produced by the body that can inhibit viral growth. Several types of interferons have been used to combat HPV. These substances can be applied topically, injected into the condyloma, or administered systemically. Interferons can produce side effects of flulike symptoms, a drop in the number of white blood cells, and changes in liver function. Systemic interferon treatment, however, may offer the advantage of being able to attack warts all over the body at the same time, rather than individually as with topical treatments, thus speeding the process of treatment.

Research to develop vaccines against HPV strains is ongoing, but the multitude of varieties makes this difficult. The Gardasil vaccine was introduced in 2006 for the prevention of four types of HPV. Gardasil protects against the low-risk types of HPV, 6 and 11, which cause 90% of genital warts. Gardasil also protects against high-risk types 16 and 18, which are known to cause 70% of cervical cancers. Women and men ages 9 through 26 receive three doses of the vaccine, starting with the initial dose, then again at 2 and 6 months after the initial dose. The vaccine does not prevent many of the other types of both high- and low-risk HPV.

Home Care

Patients who have genital warts (condylomata acuminata) burned off need to recuperate at home. Multiple areas may be

---

• **WORD** • **BUILDING** •

condylomata acuminata: condyl—rounded projection + oma—growth + ta—pluralizes the word (singular form is condyloma) + acuminata—genital growths

verrucous: verruc—wart + ous—like

electrocoagulated: electro—electrical + coagul—curdled or hardened + ated—process completed

electrocautery: electro—electrical + cautery—branding iron

cytotoxic: cyto—cell + toxic—poison

treated. If the burns are near the urethra or rectum, the patient may need a Foley catheter inserted to avoid contamination and irritation of the lesions after treatment. Also, the patient is instructed to increase dietary roughage and fluids to prevent constipation. Consult the health care provider for care of the burns. Use sterile technique for dressing changes, and premedicate the patient for pain control as needed for dressing changes.

Hepatitis B

Pathophysiology and Etiology

Hepatitis B is an infection of the liver caused by the hepatitis B virus (HBV). There are several hepatitis viruses, but this section deals only with hepatitis B virus, which is generally considered within the STI category because it can be transmitted through sexual contact with blood and body fluids. During pregnancy, hepatitis B virus may be transmitted to the unborn baby, which can result in acute hepatitis and the possibility of becoming a chronic carrier of HBV. (See Chapter 35 for a full discussion on hepatitis.)

Prevention

Prevention is better than treatment and can be accomplished by using HBV vaccine. This is especially important for health care workers who come in contact with blood and body fluids. Standard precautions should be used when contact with any body fluids is expected. All infants now receive HBV vaccine at birth before discharge from the hospital, again at 1 to 2 months, and a final dose at age 24 weeks or older.

Infants whose mothers are HBV-positive will receive HBV immune globulin and HBV vaccine within 12 hours of birth (CDC, 2012). After two additional doses of the vaccine, these infants should be tested for the hepatitis B surface antigen.

Signs and Symptoms

Early signs of hepatitis are loss of appetite, rashes, malaise, muscle and joint pain, headaches, nausea, and vomiting. Because the virus affects the liver, the urine may darken and the stool color may lighten (as a result of changes in bile excretion), liver enzymes may rise, and jaundice may appear. Enlargement of the spleen, enlargement and tenderness of the liver, necrosis of liver cells, cirrhosis, coma, and death may follow if the disease is severe. Chronic asymptomatic carrier status can follow hepatitis virus infection, with an increased risk of liver cancer.

Diagnostic Tests

Diagnosis of hepatitis is generally made using a variety of blood tests based on antigen and antibody responses. A blood test for liver enzymes and liver biopsy may be done to determine the extent of liver damage.

Therapeutic Measures

If a person is aware of being exposed to HBV, hepatitis B immune globulin can be injected within 24 hours to provide passive immunity. Supportive medical care with avoidance of drugs that require liver metabolism may help the patient through the active stage of the disease. Interferon-alpha therapy and antiviral agents are also available for patients with chronic hepatitis B. In severe cases, liver transplant may be needed.

Genital Parasites

Etiology and Signs and Symptoms

Genital parasites are not a true STI, but they may be transmitted during close body contact. The two most commonly seen parasites are pubic lice (*Phthirus pubis,* commonly called "crabs" because of the shape of the lice) and scabies (*Sarcoptes scabiei*). These parasites cause itching, redness, and, for scabies, tracks under the skin where the females burrow to lay their eggs.

Diagnostic Tests

History, physical examination, and direct visualization or magnified view of the parasites aid in diagnosis.

Therapeutic Measures

Parasites are treated with topical insecticides such as permethrin (Elimite, Acticin, for scabies) or malathion (Ovide, for pubic lice). Advise the patient to refer to package inserts for application instructions and precautions to avoid reinfection.

 ## REPORTING OF SEXUALLY TRANSMITTED INFECTIONS

The nurse may be required to facilitate the reporting and public health follow-up of STIs by filling in patient information on an STI reporting form and placing the form in the patient's chart for completion by the HCP. The requirements for reporting STIs may vary for different states, provinces, and countries. In some areas, laboratories are also required to submit a report form for positive reportable STI results. Laboratory reports that are not followed by an HCP's report may result in investigation by an STI investigator. Generally, the report form has spaces for listing of sexual contacts that should be notified of possible STI exposure. Depending on the laws of the state, province, or country, HCPs may notify identified sexual contacts, or patients may do so themselves. Contacts may also be notified by a public health authority that they have been listed as a sexual contact by an anonymous person who has tested positive for an STI.

 ## NURSING PROCESS FOR SEXUALLY TRANSMITTED INFECTIONS

Data Collection

STIs are usually assessed, diagnosed, and treated in HCPs' offices and in clinics. It is important to evaluate the patient's reason for seeking health care with every outpatient visit. Sometimes patients visit clinics or HCPs' offices for stated reasons other than STIs, yet their real concern is an STI.

If a patient presents with signs and symptoms that could lead to an STI diagnosis, inquire about whether he or she currently has any irritation, pain, lesions, or discharge in the genital region. Explaining to the patient the need to know what examination supplies to prepare for an appropriate assessment, may allow him or her to share concerns and true reasons for the visit. Establishing rapport and conveying acceptance may also facilitate communication. Often the nurse is present during the examination to assist the HCP and to serve as a chaperone or patient support person.

STIs may also be discovered in hospitalized patients. Nurses are often the ones who bathe and provide perineal care to patients. It is important to be aware of signs and symptoms in older adults as well as younger people ("Gerontological Issues"). Unusual discharge, redness, blisters, swollen areas, ulcers, and evidence of parasites in the genital area may be observed during patient care. STI awareness can also sensitize you to the possible significance of patient reports of persistent pelvic pain, dysuria, discharges, and rectal soreness. Such problems should be accurately documented and reported, so that further investigation and possible treatment can take place.

Gerontological Issues

Older adults retain interest in and are capable of engaging in sex. Do not assume that because an older adult is single or widowed that he or she is not sexually active. Older adults who have enjoyed active and fulfilling sex lives with a previous spouse or partner may seek that in new relationships. Older adults who engage in high-risk sexual behaviors (multiple partners, genital-anal sex, no use of barriers during sexual intercourse) are also at risk for STIs.

NURSING CARE TIP

Neighbors, friends, or family members may seek information from you because they know nurses are educated about health issues. Such questions may be stated in indirect terms, such as "I have a friend who is having a problem. . . ." You can provide accurate information and stress the importance of diagnosis and treatment to prevent the serious consequences of untreated STIs, without asking probing or embarrassing questions.

TABLE 44.3   BARRIER METHODS FOR SAFER SEX

Barrier	Related Information
Male condoms	• Latex condoms are less likely than other types to break during intercourse. • Lubrication decreases the chance of breakage during use. Only water-soluble lubricants should be used because substances such as petroleum jelly (Vaseline) may weaken the condom. • Condoms should never be inflated to test them; doing so can weaken them. • Condoms should be applied only when the penis is erect. • Condoms should have a reservoir tip or should be applied while holding about 1/2 inch of tip flat between the fingertips to allow room for ejaculate; otherwise, the condom might break. • The penis should be withdrawn after ejaculation and before the erection begins to subside while holding the condom securely around the penis to avoid spillage. • Condoms should never be reused and should be discarded properly after use so that others will not come in contact with contents.
Female condoms	• Female condoms should be applied before any penetration occurs; even pre-ejaculation fluid can contain microorganisms. • Lubrication decreases the chance of breakage during use, but only water-soluble lubricants should be used because substances such as petroleum jelly (Vaseline) may weaken the condom. • Female condoms should never be reused and should be discarded properly after use so that others will not come in contact with contents.
Cervical caps or diaphragms	• These may provide some protection for the cervix only. They are not effective barriers against STIs.
Rubber gloves, rubber dental dams, split (opened) male condoms	• These may provide some barrier protection for manual and oral sex. Although some groups suggest that male condoms may be split down one side and opened or rubber dental dam material may be taped over areas that have lesions to avoid direct contact with blood and body fluid, especially during sadomasochistic sexual activity, this very high-risk behavior is not recommended.

Continued

TABLE 44.3 BARRIER METHODS FOR SAFER SEX—cont'd

Barrier	Related Information
Double condoms	• Anal intercourse is a very high-risk activity for transmission of many types of STIs, as well as many intestinal organisms, and is not recommended. Gay and lesbian networks advise wearing double condoms and using water-soluble lubricants, preferably containing nonoxynol-9, to decrease risk somewhat if engaging in this type of sexual activity.

NURSING CARE PLAN for the Patient With Genital Herpes

Nursing Diagnosis: *Acute Pain* related to inflammation and skin lesions as evidenced by patient pain rating

Expected Outcome: The patient will experience relief as evidenced by a decrease in pain rating to a level that is acceptable to patient.

Evaluation of Outcome: Does patient state relief of pain level is acceptable?

Intervention Assess pain using the **WHAT'S UP?** format. **Rationale** Assessment of the characteristic of the pain assists the nurse in providing appropriate relief measures. **Evaluation** Can patient describe the pain characteristics?

Intervention Recommend pain relief measures appropriate to the type and location of the pain (both alternative measures, such as heat, ice, and change of position, and medication may be offered). **Rationale** Not all types of pain respond well to the same treatment. **Evaluation** Does patient express satisfactory relief of pain? Does patient move and rest without evidence of pain?

Intervention Document results of pain relief measures. **Rationale** Documentation alerts other caregivers about what works and does not work, thus providing more consistent, effective pain relief. **Evaluation** Have you gained sufficient information from patient to document results?

Intervention Instruct patient about self-care for pain and STI treatment at home. **Rationale** Most STIs are treated at home. **Evaluation** Does patient verbalize understanding of self-care measures?

Nursing Diagnosis: *Risk for Infection,* transmission to others, related to lack of knowledge about transmission, symptoms, and treatment

Expected Outcome: The patient will verbalize understanding of measures to prevent transmission to others.

Evaluation of Outcome: Does patient verbalize understanding of transmission prevention? Does patient practice preventive behaviors?

Intervention Assess patient's understanding of transmission, symptoms, complications, and treatment of STIs. **Rationale** New instruction should be based on patient's previous knowledge. **Evaluation** Is patient's current understanding accurate? What teaching is needed?

Intervention Assess whether patient is engaging in high-risk behaviors. **Rationale** If patient is continuing to engage in high-risk behaviors, the risk for infection of others is high. **Evaluation** Is patient protecting self and others appropriately?

Intervention Use standard precautions and strict aseptic technique for all procedures involving blood and body fluids. **Rationale** The health team, in addition to other patient contacts, must be protected. **Evaluation** Are standard precautions observed?

Intervention Instruct patient in appropriate strategies to reduce risk of infecting others: • Abstinence • Monogamy (if no active infection) • Use of barrier methods and spermicides • Adherence to treatment regimen. **Rationale** These measures may help prevent transmission of infection to others. **Evaluation** Does patient verbalize understanding of methods to prevent transmission and intent to practice them?

NURSING CARE PLAN for the Patient With Genital Herpes—cont'd

Intervention Teach patient signs and symptoms of STIs to report immediately. **Rationale** Prompt treatment of patient and partners further reduces risk of transmission of infection. **Evaluation** Does patient verbalize understanding of signs and symptoms to report?

Intervention Explain importance of follow-up evaluation. **Rationale** Follow-up is essential to affirm that treatment was successful. **Evaluation** Does patient make a follow-up appointment?

Nursing Diagnosis: *Fear* related to diagnosis of an incurable illness and effects on sexual relationships and reproduction as evidenced by patient statement

Expected Outcomes: The patient will relate accurate knowledge and control of excessive fear.

Evaluation of Outcomes: Does patient relate accurate knowledge? Is fear manageable?

Intervention Assess patient's fears. **Rationale** Fear is a normal response and may be appropriate. **Evaluation** What specifically does the patient fear?

Intervention If fear is based on misconceptions, provide factual information. **Rationale** When fear is based on misconceptions, they should be corrected. **Evaluation** Are fears based on factual information?

Intervention Allow patient to verbalize feelings. Be empathetic, but do not offer false hope. **Rationale** Sharing fears may help patient gain insight into dealing with them. **Evaluation** Is patient able to verbalize feelings?

Intervention Explain all procedures and treatments. **Rationale** Unfamiliar procedures or treatments may contribute to fear. **Evaluation** Does patient understand procedures and treatments?

Intervention Help patient identify support systems and coping strategies that have worked in the past. **Rationale** Methods that have worked for patient before are likely to be helpful again. **Evaluation** Does patient have effective coping skills and support systems?

Nursing Diagnosis: *Readiness for Enhanced Self-Health Management* related to lack of knowledge about STIs as evidenced by patient requesting information

Expected Outcome: The patient will verbalize realistic and accurate information about disease prevention.

Evaluation of Outcome: Does patient relate accurate knowledge and plans for prevention?

Intervention Assess the patient's health beliefs and correct misconceptions. **Rationale** Many myths about sexual activity are sincerely believed by some patients (see Table 44.4). **Evaluation** Does patient have an accurate understanding of STI prevention?

Intervention Explain the importance of patients knowing the sexual and lifestyle history of any potential partner before sexual activity has occurred. **Rationale** Having a sexual relationship with someone is the **epidemiological** equivalent of engaging in sexual activity with all of that person's previous partners. **Evaluation** Can patient relate a plan to approach this subject with a potential partner?

Intervention Provide pamphlets or other materials. (Make sure the patient is able to read.) **Rationale** Written materials can reinforce teaching. **Evaluation** Is patient observed viewing materials offered?

Intervention Explain that abstinence or lifelong monogamy of both sexual partners in a relationship is the only sure prevention against STIs. **Rationale** These practices eliminate risk of exposure. **Evaluation** Does patient relate understanding of monogamy?

• WORD • BUILDING •

epidemiological: epi—on + demio—people + logical—study of

NURSING CARE PLAN for the Patient With Genital Herpes—cont'd

Intervention Educate the patient that consumption of alcohol or other psychoactive drugs can reduce inhibitions and may result in unintended sexual encounters, which can transmit STIs. **Rationale** Avoiding or limiting alcohol and other drug consumption when with potential partners may help prevent STI infection from occurring. **Evaluation** Does patient relate a plan to limit the effect of substances on sexual encounters?

Nursing Diagnosis: *Ineffective Sexuality Pattern* related to infection and risk for transmission of infectious organism

Expected Outcome: The patient will describe acceptable, alternative sexual practices and safer sex practices.

Evaluation of Outcome: Does patient relate safer sex practices?

Intervention Provide privacy and be verbally and nonverbally nonjudgmental when allowing patient and patient's partner to express concerns about sexual practice. **Rationale** Treatment success rates are generally higher when a rapport is established with the health care provider and the partner is included in the decision-making process. **Evaluation** Do the patient and partner express concerns?

Intervention When teaching patients, use *safer sex* terminology. **Rationale** *Safer* sex practices may decrease the risk of (but not absolutely prevent) transmission of STIs (Table 44.3). Safe sex and STI prevention are misnomers, since no practices provide absolute protection. **Evaluation** Does patient exhibit understanding of the concept of safer sex?

Intervention Discuss alternative means of sexual expression, as appropriate. **Rationale** This may allow for intimacy when the desired sexual expression is not recommended, such as during treatment. **Evaluation** Can patient identify some acceptable (to patient) alternative means of sexual expression?

Intervention Support realistic expectations about treatment and outcomes. **Rationale** Unrealistic expectations may lead to additional undesired issues related to sexuality pattern. **Evaluation** Does patient have realistic expectations?

For more information on STIs, visit www.cdc.gov/std/healthcomm/fact_sheets.htm and www.ashastd.org.

TABLE 44.4 COMMON MYTHS ABOUT SEXUALLY TRANSMITTED INFECTIONS

Myth	Factual Data
People who have STIs are easily identifiable.	Inspection of the potential partner's genitals before sexual activity may decrease the risk (if one does not participate in sexual activity with a person who has visible lesions), but: • Not all people who are infected have visible symptoms. • There is no standard personality or physical profile for people who can be infected with STIs—anyone can be and may be infected.
Avoiding persons who have a history of engaging in casual sex, IV drug use, homosexual activity, bisexual activity, or a previous sexual relationship with persons who engage in these high-risk practices effectively protects one from infection with STIs.	Avoiding people with these types of history may decrease risk, but: • Not everyone is honest when responding to questions about sexual history. • Not everyone is aware of their previous partners' histories or the histories of others with whom their previous partners have had sexual relationships. • Asking such questions is difficult and may be avoided until it is too late.

TABLE **44.4** **COMMON MYTHS ABOUT SEXUALLY TRANSMITTED INFECTIONS—cont'd**

Myth	Factual Data
STIs never happen the first time.	Only one contact with one microorganism is needed for infection.
Intact genital skin is impervious to the pathogens (and gentle sexual activity does no harm).	Intact skin is the body's first line of defense, but: • Some microorganisms can be transmitted without a noticeable tissue injury. • Minor injuries can occur during many types of sexual activity, including vaginal intercourse.
Condoms prevent the spread of all STIs.	Condoms can greatly decrease the risk of STIs, but: • Condoms can have tiny channels in the latex or other material that can allow microorganisms to pass through. • Condoms can break, slip off, or be applied improperly. • Petroleum-based lubricants may weaken latex condoms. • Condoms do not provide a barrier for any area other than the penis and most of the vagina or anus. Some STIs may still be transmitted by contact with surrounding uncovered tissues.
The female condom prevents all transmissions of STIs.	It does cover more surface area, but it may have problems similar to male condoms (see previous entry).
Manual, oral, and anal stimulation cannot transmit STIs.	Contact of hands to genitals can allow for transmission of microorganisms through breaks in the skin. Oral sex can transmit some STI-causing microorganisms. Anal intercourse is a very high-risk activity for transmission of STIs because anal tissues are easily injured and the gastrointestinal tract can be a reservoir for many microorganisms.
Nonoxynol-9 spermicide kills all STI germs.	Nonoxynol-9 can reduce the risk of transmission of STIs, but: • *Nonoxynol-9 is not guaranteed to kill all microorganisms.*
People get AIDS only by homosexual sexual activity or by blood transfusion.	Homosexual activity may result in a higher incidence of transmission of HIV, but: • *HIV can be transmitted during heterosexual activity.*
A woman cannot transmit HIV to a man. *A man cannot transmit HIV to a woman.*	Gender does not protect a person from being infected with HIV.
Sexual activity during menstruation is less likely to result in STIs.	Sexual activity during menstruation is more likely to result in transmission of some microorganisms that cause STIs because of the vulnerability of the lining of the uterus caused by sloughing of the outer layers of cells and because blood and cellular debris may serve as a nutritious medium for growth of microorganisms.
Lesbian sexual activity cannot transmit STIs.	Transmission of microorganisms can occur by contact with mouth, anus, genital tissues, or fomites (inanimate objects, such as vibrators and other sex paraphernalia) that have been contaminated with microorganisms from an infected person—regardless of the original source of the infection.
Those who have not been infected after sexual activity with several people are naturally immune to STIs.	There is no known natural immunity to STIs. The person may not yet have had contact with someone who has an active STI.

Continued

TABLE 44.4 COMMON MYTHS ABOUT SEXUALLY TRANSMITTED INFECTIONS—cont'd

Myth	Factual Data
Those who have had an STI and have been cured of it by taking medicine are now immune to that infection.	Infection that has been eradicated by medication does not confer immunity.
People can be certified free of all STIs by having a blood test and taking a simple medication if an infection is present.	Testing of those who suspect they may have contracted an STI and treatment (if possible) may decrease the spread of STIs, but: • No one test identifies all STIs. Some are identified by examination, and not all infected people show symptoms. • Some STIs do not show positive test results for long periods yet may be transmitted by the person while the tests are still negative. • People may be infected with more than one agent at a time, and each must be treated (if possible). One STI may obscure the symptoms of other concurrent STIs, so that one or more types may go unnoticed and untreated or may not be evident until other STIs have been treated. • There are no known cures for some STIs.
Oral contraceptive pills give protection against STIs.	Oral contraceptives are not antibiotics—they provide only some protection against conception. Use of a barrier method with spermicide along with the oral contraceptive can decrease risk of STIs and pregnancy.

CRITICAL THINKING

Stephanie

■ As you seat a young woman in an examining room of the clinic where you work, she comments, "I am new to this area, and I've heard that there are three guys in this town who have syphilis and are spreading it around. Is that true?"

1. What are some concerns this question might reflect?
2. You find out that Stephanie knows very little about syphilis. List in outline form a teaching plan that includes the information that is important for Stephanie to know about syphilis.

Suggested answers are at the end of the chapter.

SUGGESTED ANSWERS TO

CRITICAL THINKING

■ *Mrs. Miller*

1. You can educate Mrs. Miller about the possibility of neonatal infections from *C. trachomatis* or *N. gonorrhoeae*, especially of the eyes. Institutional and governmental policies related to treatment should be explained. Care should be taken to explain to Mrs. Miller that treatment is widely used, so as not to make her feel she has a condition she has not been told about.
2. Because the benefits of prophylactic eye treatment of the neonate for *C. trachomatis* and *N. gonorrhoeae* exposure are generally seen as greater than the risks, it is recommended by governmental agencies and supported by most institutional policies to treat all newborns, regardless of known exposure, shortly after birth.

■ *Kerri*

1. Explain to Kerri the fact that trichomoniasis is often an STI, but that the organism that causes the infection can be transmitted through infected articles during nonsexual contact, can survive a long time outside the body, and that one can be asymptomatic for many

SUGGESTED ANSWERS TO—cont'd

years following exposure to the organism before an outbreak occurs. Her partner could also have an undiagnosed infection.

2. You don't want to assume the HCP is wrong. An approach might sound something like, "I noticed in the drug guide that the usual dose is 2 grams, but I see you have written for 4 grams."

3. Teach Kerri that treatment should be provided to her partner regardless of symptoms. Also, reinfection may occur if both partners are not treated. Teach her how the infection is spread and how to avoid it in the future. She and her partner should use condoms or remain abstinent until treatment is effectively completed. Be sure to tell her that she should abstain from alcohol while on metronidazole and for at least 48 hours following its completion. Patients who drink alcohol while taking it are very likely to vomit.

■ *Stephanie*

1. Concerns might include (a) a wish to speak with a health care worker, (b) uncertainty about whether patient information will be kept confidential (give assurance that if you knew about anyone with syphilis, it would be your professional responsibility to keep it confidential), (c) fear that she might have become infected through heterosexual contact, (d) a desire to protect herself by avoiding those who have syphilis, and (e) a desire for information about syphilis and its transmission routes.

2. The teaching plan might include information about (a) the spirochete that causes syphilis, (b) signs and symptoms, (c) diagnostic tests, (d) means of transmission, (e) strategies for risk reduction, (f) treatment, (g) research, and (h) rights and responsibilities of those who have the disease.

REVIEW QUESTIONS

1. What signs and symptoms of STIs should nurses assess for in all patients? **Select all that apply.**
   1. Itching
   2. Discharge
   3. Dysuria
   4. Genital ulcers
   5. Genital warts
   6. Rectal pain

2. A young woman is seen at a walk-in clinic and is diagnosed with an STI. She says, "How could I have an STI? I only have sex with my boyfriend. I don't sleep around!" Which of the following responses by the nurse is best?
   1. "You are right, that should have kept you safe. There just are no guarantees."
   2. "If your boyfriend is not infected, then it is apparent that you have had sex with someone else."
   3. "You or your boyfriend could be infected from past sexual encounters. He should also be tested at this time for STIs."
   4. "Even lifelong monogamy cannot prevent many STIs."

3. A home care nurse is preparing to change a dressing on a patient who had genital warts removed the previous day. Which intervention should be completed first?
   1. Clean the wounds.
   2. Remove the old dressing.
   3. Assess for drainage.
   4. Administer an analgesic.

4. An older man is admitted to the hospital with mental status changes. As the nurse begins the shift assessment, the patient begins to cry and says his doctor thinks his problems stem from an untreated syphilis infection when he was in the military as a young man. Which response by the nurse is best?
   1. "Why didn't you have it treated when it occurred?"
   2. "What's done is done; it's unfortunate that treatment is too late now."
   3. "That must be upsetting for you. Do you want to talk about it?"
   4. "Don't cry; I am sure there is treatment that can help now."

5. A nurse has completed instruction related to STI risk reduction with a 17-year-old woman. Which statement by the patient indicates that teaching has been effective?
   1. "I should avoid drinking alcohol when I will be in situations with potential sex partners."
   2. "If I make sure my partners wear condoms, I will be protected from STIs."
   3. "Use of a barrier method of birth control will prevent infection with an STI."
   4. "As long as I know my partner well, I am safe."

Answers can be found in Appendix C.

References

Centers for Disease Control and Prevention (2013a). *Chlamydia—CDC fact sheet*. Retrieved August 13, 2013, from www.cdc.gov/std/Chlamydia/STDFact-Chlamydia.htm

Centers for Disease Control and Prevention. (2013b). *Gonorrhea—CDC fact sheet*. Retrieved August 13, 2013, from www.cdc.gov/std/gonorrhea/stdfact-gonorrhea.htm

Centers for Disease Control and Prevention. (2012). *Hepatitis B information for health professionals*. Retrieved August 13, 2013, from www.cdc.gov/hepatitis/hbv/perinatalxmtn.htm

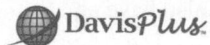 DavisPlus | For additional resources and information visit **davispl.us/medsurg5**

unit TWELVE

Understanding the Musculoskeletal System

45

Musculoskeletal Function and Assessment

SHARON GORDON
AND JANICE L. BRADFORD

KEY TERMS

arthrocentesis (AR-throw-sen-TEE-siss)
arthroscopy (ar-THROSS-scuh-pee)
articular (ar-TIK-yoo-lar)
bone (BOWN)
bursae (BURR-sah)
crepitation (crep-ih-TAY-shun)
gout (GOWT)
hemarthrosis (heem-ar-THROW-siss)
joint (JOYNT)
muscle (MUH-suhl)
resorption (ree-SORP-shun)
synovitis (sin-oh-VY-tiss)
vertebrae (VER-teh-bray)

LEARNING OUTCOMES

1. Explain the normal anatomy and function of the musculoskeletal system.
2. Describe the effects of aging on the musculoskeletal system.
3. List subjective data that are collected when caring for a patient with a disorder of the musculoskeletal system.
4. List the objective data that are collected when caring for a patient with a disorder of the musculoskeletal system.
5. List areas included in a neurovascular assessment that relate to the musculoskeletal system.
6. Identify diagnostic tests for musculoskeletal problems.
7. Describe the nursing care provided for patients undergoing diagnostic tests of the musculoskeletal system.

NORMAL MUSCULOSKELETAL SYSTEM ANATOMY AND PHYSIOLOGY

The skeletal and muscular systems can be considered as one system because together they move the body. The skeleton is the framework of the body to which the voluntary **muscles** are attached. The framework includes the **joints**, or articulations, between **bones**. Contraction of a muscle stabilizes or changes the angle of a joint. Movement would not be possible without the proper functioning of the nervous, cardiovascular, and respiratory systems. Voluntary muscles require nerve impulses to contract, a continuous supply of blood provided by the circulatory system, and oxygen provided by the respiratory system.

SKELETAL SYSTEM TISSUES AND THEIR FUNCTIONS

The tissues that make up the skeletal system are primarily bone tissue, **articular** cartilage, and fibrous connective tissue that forms the ligaments (that connect bone to bone) and other structures within joints. The tissues of the muscular system include skeletal muscle tissue and fibrous connective tissues. The fibrous connective tissue forms tendons (which connect muscle to bone) and fasciae (the strong membranes enclosing individual muscles).

Besides its role in movement, the skeleton has other functions. It protects organs and tissues from mechanical injury. In particular, the brain is protected by the skull, and the heart and lungs are protected by the thoracic cage. Flat and irregular bones as well as the ends of long bones contain red bone marrow, the hematopoietic (blood-forming) tissue. The bones also store excess calcium, which may undergo **resorption** (bone broken down with minerals including calcium released into blood) for blood calcium homeostasis. Calcium in the blood is needed for blood clotting and for the proper functioning of nerves and muscles.

Although the primary function of the muscular system is to move or stabilize the skeleton, the voluntary muscles collectively contribute significantly to heat production, which maintains normal body temperature. Another important function of the muscular system is to aid in the return of blood from the legs through muscular compression on the leg veins.

Bone Tissue and Bone Growth

Bone tissue is composed of bone cells, called osteocytes, within a strong, nonliving matrix made of calcium salts and the protein collagen. In compact bone, the osteocytes and matrix are in precise, densely structured arrangements called osteons. In spongy bone, the arrangement of cells and matrix is more irregular and sparse, giving the bone a spongy appearance. Compact bone forms the diaphyses (shafts) of the long bones, covers the spongy bone of the epiphyses of long bones, and covers the spongy bone that forms the bulk of short, flat, and irregular bones.

Osteoblasts produce bone matrix during growth and replace matrix during normal remodeling or in repair of fractures. Other cells called osteoclasts resorb bone matrix when more calcium is needed in the blood, or during repair when excess bone must be removed as bone changes shape.

The growth of bone from fetal life until final adult height depends on many factors. Proper nutrition (particularly vitamins and minerals) provides the raw material to produce bone matrix, comprising calcium, phosphorus, and protein. Vitamin D is essential for the efficient absorption of calcium and phosphorus in the small intestine. Vitamins A and C are required for the production process of bone matrix. Hormones directly needed for growth include growth hormone (GH) from the anterior pituitary gland, thyroxine from the thyroid gland, and insulin from the pancreas. GH increases mitosis and protein synthesis; thyroxine stimulates osteoblasts and also increases energy production. Insulin is essential for the efficient use of glucose to provide energy. If a child is lacking any of these hormones, growth is slower, and the child may not reach his or her genetic potential for height.

Bone is not a fixed tissue, even when growth in height has ceased. Calcium and phosphate are constantly being removed and replaced (remodeled) to maintain normal blood levels of these minerals. Parathyroid hormone, secreted by the parathyroid glands, increases the removal of calcium and phosphate from bones; the hormone calcitonin from the thyroid gland promotes the retention of calcium in bones.

Structure of the Skeleton

The 206 bones of the human skeleton are in two divisions: the axial and appendicular skeleton. (Fig. 45.1; axial in white, appendicular in turquoise). The axial bones are flat or irregular bones and contain red bone marrow (hematopoietic tissue). Within the appendicular skeleton, the limbs consist of long bones (except the carpals, tarsals, and patella). All long bones have the same general structure: a central diaphysis, or shaft, with two ends called epiphyses.

Skull

The skull consists of 8 cranial bones and 14 facial bones, and also contains the 3 auditory bones found in each middle ear cavity. All of the joints between the cranial bones and those between most of the facial bones are immovable joints called sutures.

Vertebral Column

The vertebral column (or spinal column) is made of individual bones called **vertebrae** (Fig. 45.2). *Atlas*, the first cervical vertebra, articulates with the occipital bone of the skull and forms a pivot joint with the *axis*, the second cervical vertebra. The thoracic vertebrae articulate with the posterior ends of the ribs. The lumbar vertebrae are the largest and strongest. The *sacrum* articulates with the *os coxae* at the sacroiliac joints. The coccyx serves as an attachment point for some muscles of the perineum.

The vertebrae as a unit form a flexible backbone that supports the trunk and head and contains and protects the

Anterior view

Posterior view

Skull
- Frontal bone
- Maxilla
- Mandible

Pectoral Girdle
- Clavicle
- Scapula

Thoracic Cage
- Sternum
- Ribs
- Costal cartilages

- Vertebral column

Pelvis
- Os coxae
- Sacrum
- Coccyx

- Carpals
- Metacarpal bones
- Phalanges

- Patella

- Tarsals

- Parietal bone
- Occipital bone
- Mandible
- Clavicle
- Scapula
- Humerus

- Os coxae
- Ulna
- Radius

- Femur

- Fibula
- Tibia

- Metatarsal bones
- Phalanges

FIGURE 45.1 Adult skeleton—anterior and posterior views. From Thompson, G. S. (2013). *Understanding anatomy and physiology.* Philadelphia: F.A. Davis, p. 95.

spinal cord. Spinal nerves and vessels exit via intervertebral foramina. Intervertebral discs cushion and permit movement of the column.

Thoracic Cage

The thoracic cage consists of 12 pairs of ribs and the sternum. The thoracic cage protects the heart and lungs, as well as upper abdominal organs such as the liver and spleen, from mechanical injury. During breathing, the flexible thoracic cage is pulled upward and outward by the external intercostal muscles to expand the chest cavity and bring about inhalation.

Synovial Joints

The primary joints of the appendicular skeleton are summarized in Table 45.1. All freely movable joints (diarthroses) are synovial joints (Fig. 45.3). Many synovial joints also have **bursae** (small

sacs of synovial fluid between the joint and structures that cross over the joint). Bursae lessen wear in areas of friction.

MUSCLE STRUCTURE AND ARRANGEMENTS

One muscle can consist of thousands of skeletal muscle cells (fibers), which are specialized for contraction. When a muscle contracts, it shortens and exerts force on a bone. Each muscle fiber receives its own motor nerve ending, and the numbers of fibers that contract depend upon the workload. Muscles are anchored to bones by tendons, which are made of fibrous connective tissue. A muscle usually has at least two tendons, each attached to a different bone. The more stationary muscle attachment is called its origin; the more movable attachment is the insertion. The muscle itself crosses the joint formed by

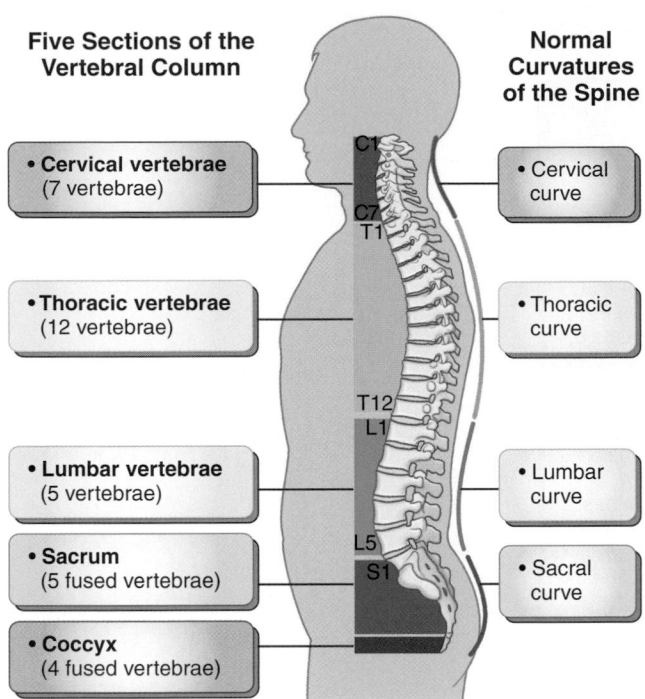

Five Sections of the Vertebral Column

- **Cervical vertebrae** (7 vertebrae)
- **Thoracic vertebrae** (12 vertebrae)
- **Lumbar vertebrae** (5 vertebrae)
- **Sacrum** (5 fused vertebrae)
- **Coccyx** (4 fused vertebrae)

Normal Curvatures of the Spine

- Cervical curve
- Thoracic curve
- Lumbar curve
- Sacral curve

FIGURE 45.2 Vertebral column. From Thompson, G. S. (2013). *Understanding anatomy and physiology*. Philadelphia: F.A. Davis, p. 102.

TABLE 45.1 JOINTS OF THE APPENDICULAR SKELETON

Type of Joint and Description	Examples
Symphysis—disk of fibrous cartilage between bones	Between vertebrae Between pubic bones
Ball and socket— movement in all planes	Scapula and humerus (shoulder) Pelvic bone and femur (hip)
Hinge—movement in one plane	Humerus and ulna (elbow) Femur and tibia (knee) Between phalanges (fingers and toes)
Combined hinge and planar	Temporal bone and mandible (lower jaw)
Pivot—rotation	Atlas and axis (neck) Radius and ulna (distal to elbow)
Gliding—side-to-side movement	Between carpals (wrist)
Saddle—movement in several planes	Carpometacarpal of thumb

Source: Modified from Scanlon, V. C., & Sanders, T. (2015). *Essentials of anatomy and physiology* (7th ed.). Philadelphia: F.A. Davis, with permission.

the two bones to which it is attached, and when the muscle contracts, it pulls on the insertion moving the bone in a particular direction. The muscle causing this particular action is termed the agonist.

There are approximately 700 skeletal muscles in the body (Fig. 45.4). The general type of arrangement is the agonist with opposing antagonists and the cooperative synergists. Without synergism, maintaining balance or having fine motor control for writing or talking would be difficult if not impossible.

 ROLE OF THE NERVOUS SYSTEM

Skeletal muscles are voluntary: conscious control initiates nerve impulses to cause contraction. Nerve impulses originate in the motor areas of the frontal lobes of the cerebral cortex. The coordination of voluntary movement is a function of the cerebellum. Neurons in the central nervous system (CNS) also act involuntarily to regulate muscle tone, the state of slight contraction usually present in muscles. Healthy muscle tone is important for posture and coordination.

Neuromuscular Junction

Each of the fibers in a muscle has its own motor neuron ending. The neuromuscular junction is the termination of the motor neuron at the muscle fiber. The neuron releases the neurotransmitter acetylcholine (Ach), which signals muscle contraction (Fig. 45.5).

1. An action potential travels along the motor neuron, reaching the synaptic end bulb.
2. Acetylcholine is exocytosed (process in which a cell releases a large molecule) from vesicles into the synaptic cleft and bonds with receptors on the motor end plate.
3. An action potential initiates and travels along the sarcolemma and into the transverse tubules, transferring to the sarcoplasmic reticulum.
4. Calcium ions released from the sarcoplasmic reticulum bond to troponin of the thin filament, exposing bonding sites on actin for myosin heads. Myosin of the thick filament attaches and pulls the thin filament, shortening the sarcomeres and thus the muscle fiber.

If a muscle has little work to do, few of its many muscle fibers contract; but if the muscle has more work to do, more of its muscle fibers contract.

AGING AND THE MUSCULOSKELETAL SYSTEM

The amount of calcium in bones depends on several factors (Fig. 45.6). Good nutrition is certainly one factor, but age is another, especially for women. One function of estrogen (or testosterone) is the maintenance of a strong bone matrix. For women after menopause, bone matrix loses more calcium than is replaced. Osteoporosis may result in bone fractures. The loss can be offset by weight-bearing physical exercise, which stimulates bone matrix deposition, increasing bone density.

Bone

Periosteum

Joint capsule: Extending from the periosteum of each of the articulating bones is a sheet of connective tissue that encloses the joint cavity.

Synovial membrane: This moist, slippery membrane lines the inside of the joint capsule, where it secretes synovial fluid.

Joint cavity: This small space between the bones allows for freedom of movement. It also contains **synovial fluid**, a slippery, viscous fluid that has the consistency of an egg white. Synovial fluid lubricates the joint, nourishes the cartilage, and contains phagocytes to remove debris.

Articular cartilage: A thin layer of hyaline cartilage covers the bone surfaces. In combination with synovial fluid, the articular cartilage permits friction-free movement.

Ligaments: Tough cords of connective tissue help bind the bones more firmly together.

FIGURE 45.3 Synovial joints. From Thompson, G. S. (2013). *Understanding anatomy and physiology.* Philadelphia: F.A. Davis, p. 116.

Weight-bearing joints are also subject to damage after many years. Often the articular cartilage wears down and becomes rough, leading to pain and stiffness.

Muscle strength declines with age as protein synthesis decreases. Such loss of strength need not be exaggerated because aging muscles also benefit from regular exercise. Furthermore, maintenance of muscle strength reduces falls and accidents (see "Evidence-Based Practice").

EVIDENCE-BASED PRACTICE

Clinical Question
What are the risk factors of falls in patients with cognitive impairment?

Evidence
An observational study of residential care patients older than 60 years, with cognitive impairment, who had a life expectancy of at least 6 months and were not bed bound or recently discharged from the hospital revealed the following risk factors: medications (especially antidepressants), functional impairment, poor gait and balance,

impulsivity, dementia, attention and orientation impairment, and poor memory. Factors that especially put residents at risk were poor attention and orientation, increased postural sway with eyes closed, anxiety, and use of antidepressants.

Implications for Nursing Practice
Attention to fall risk factors can guide care planning in high-risk populations of dementia patients.

REFERENCE
Whitney, J., Close, J., Jackson, S., & Lord, S. (2012). Understanding risk of falls in people with cognitive impairment living in residential care. *Journal of American Medical Directors Association, 13,* 535–540.

NURSING ASSESSMENT OF THE MUSCULOSKELETAL SYSTEM

Initial assessment of the patient begins with a history that includes the effects the condition is having on the patient's life. It then proceeds to a physical and psychosocial assessment (Table 45.2). Frequent neurovascular assessments may be

Temporalis
Orbicularis oculi
Zygomaticus
Orbicularis oris

Deltoid

Brachialis
Biceps brachii
Rectus abdominis
Brachioradialis
External oblique
Internal oblique
Transversus abdominis

Iliopsoas

Adductor longus
Adductor magnus

Quadriceps femoris
    Rectus femoris
    Vastus lateralis
    Vastus medialis

Tibialis anterior
Fibularis longus

Frontalis

Masseter
Sternocleidomastoid

Pectoralis major
Teres minor
Teres major
Serratus anterior

Linea alba

Gluteus medius
Gluteus maximus

Sartorius

Adductor magnus
Gracilis

Anterior

Trapezius

Deltoid

Triceps brachii

Latissimus dorsi

External abdominal oblique

Biceps femoris
Semitendinosus
Semimembranosus
} Hamstring group

Gastrocnemius

Soleus

Achilles tendon (calcaneal tendon)

Posterior

FIGURE 45.4 Superficial muscles. From Thompson, G. S. (2013). *Understanding anatomy and physiology*. Philadelphia: F.A. Davis, pp. 136–137.

Motor neuron

Vesicles of acetylcholine

Synaptic cleft

ACh receptors

Sarcolemma   T tubule

Sarcoplasmic reticulum

Myofilaments

Ca+

Sarcomere

FIGURE 45.5 How muscle fibers contract. From Thompson, G. S. (2013). *Understanding anatomy and physiology*. Philadelphia: F.A. Davis, p. 129.

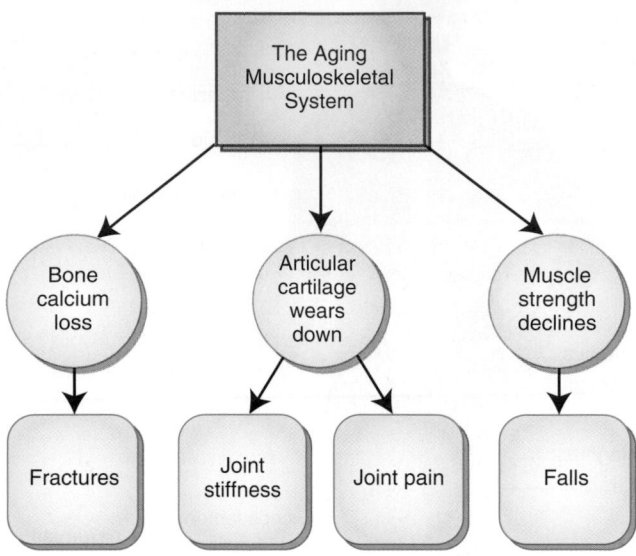

FIGURE 45.6 Aging and the musculoskeletal system. This concept map shows the effects the aging process has on the musculoskeletal system.

needed if there is a risk of circulation impairment, such as might happen if the patient has a fracture or has had musculoskeletal surgery (Table 45.3).

Health History

The patient's history should include the following:

• For an injury, how and when it happened
• Risk factors for musculoskeletal problems and family history of musculoskeletal problems (to detect hereditary factors)
• Diet history (including whether calcium and vitamin D intake are adequate to ensure proper bone and muscle maintenance and repair)
• Occupation and activities, including sports and other physical activities
• Information specific to the patient's musculoskeletal problems.

Patients with musculoskeletal problems frequently report pain or related stiffness and tenderness as a major concern. The pain may be acute or chronic and may limit the patient

TABLE 45.2 DATA COLLECTION FOR THE MUSCULOSKELETAL SYSTEM

Category	Questions to Ask During the Health History	Rationale/Significance
Subjective Data Collection **Demographic**	Age, gender, socioeconomic status	Increased age, being female, and lower socioeconomic status increase risk of musculoskeletal injury/problems.
	Occupation	Enables nurse to begin planning for discharge teaching if the patient has to alter his or her employment.
Previous Health History	Allergies	Prevents exposure to medication or compounds used in diagnostic tests, treatments, and therapies.
	Activities patient participates in	Provides information regarding the level of activity the patient had before the concern.
	Risk factors for musculoskeletal problems	Smoking and a sedentary lifestyle are risk factors for musculoskeletal problems.
	Diet history	Dietary intake such as calcium and vitamin D influences some musculoskeletal disorders.
	Family history	Some musculoskeletal conditions have genetic and familial tendencies.
History of Injury or Present Concern	History of the injury (if there was one)	Provides information that helps in the diagnosis of the problem, as well as making you aware of possible complications of the injury.
	Pain (use pain assessment scale)	Provides information about severity of the condition and effectiveness of the treatment and therapy.
Psychosocial Assessment	Determine if deformities, changes in body image, self-concept, socialization, or employment are present.	The patient may need assistance with strategies to cope with the stress of a possible chronic musculoskeletal condition.
	Determine coping skills.	Some musculoskeletal conditions require lifestyle alterations that can cause increased stress and difficulties in coping.

TABLE 45.2   DATA COLLECTION FOR THE MUSCULOSKELETAL SYSTEM—cont'd

Category	Questions to Ask During the Health History	Rationale/Significance
Objective Data Collection **Physical Examination**	Inspect, palpate, and observe range of motion (ROM) of affected areas.	Altered gait, tone, size, shape, posture, contractures, deformities, ROM, pain, and effects on activities of daily living (ADLs) can be determined.
	Assess color, warmth, circulation, and movement of affected areas.	Nerve function, sensation, movement, weakness, and the potential development of compartment syndrome can be determined.
	Palpate all pulses below involved area.	Alterations may indicate altered vascular integrity (and therefore tissue integrity) of affected area or demonstrate developing compartment syndrome.

TABLE 45.3   NEUROVASCULAR DATA COLLECTION

Monitor	Report
Color	Pallor, cyanosis, redness, or discoloration
Temperature	Unusual coolness or warmth
Pain	Pain that is worse on passive motion; pain that no longer responds to analgesics
Movement	Alterations in movement
Sensation	Alterations in feeling; tingling or paresthesias
Pulses	Diminished or absent distal pulses
Capillary refill	Nailbed that does not blanch in 3–5 seconds

in everyday life. Assessment includes previous diagnoses, pain severity, medications, treatments, and procedures the patient uses to alleviate the pain. The **WHAT'S UP?** model can be used to assess the patient's pain (see Chapter 1).

Physical Examination

Three areas of musculoskeletal data collection are important: inspection, palpation, and range of motion (ROM). If the patient can walk, inspect posture and gait, noting poor posture or alterations in movement, such as limping. Note the use of mobility aids, such as a cane or walker. Document other gross deformities, such as unequal limbs, malalignment, or contractures. Spinal deformities are especially significant because they can compromise breathing and balance. Inspect the joints and muscles of the arms, hands, legs, and feet for deformity, redness, swelling, or **crepitation** (grating sound

as joint or bone moves). Also note the patient's general nutritional status (e.g., normal, obese, emaciated).

After inspection, gently palpate for warmth and tenderness in the areas of swelling, and areas where the patient reported pain (being careful to minimize the pain this may cause). For example, reddened joints should be palpated for **synovitis** (swollen synovial tissue within the joint) or the presence of bony nodes. In some cases, joints and muscles may seem healthy but are tender when palpated.

Next, observe joint mobility. Stabilize the body area proximal to the joint being moved. Observe the patient's ROM for performing independent activities of daily living (ADLs). Pay particular attention to the hands and observe movement in finger joints. For a quick and easy check of ROM in the hands, ask the patient to touch each finger, one by one, to the thumb (known as opposition) and then to make a fist.

Also note the size, shape, strength, and tone of muscles. Evaluate bilateral muscle strength by asking the patient to grip your hands. This enables you to feel the strength and equality. Pushing an extremity against your hand provides a general indication of muscle strength. More specific evaluation is performed by a physical therapist (PT) or an occupational therapist (OT). Using a scale of 0 to 5 (0 paralysis and 5 moving a muscle against resistance), the PT or OT measures the strength of each muscle group and rates it as a fraction. For example, 5/5 means that the patient reached 5 out of a possible 5 on the muscle strength scale.

Psychosocial Data Collection

Deformities resulting from arthritis or other musculoskeletal disorders can affect a patient's body image and self-concept and result in social withdrawal (see Chapter 46). Chronic pain may keep the patient from working or socializing. Data collection should include questions related to the psychological effects of the musculoskeletal disorder.

• **WORD** • **BUILDING** •
synovitis: synovia—joint + itis—inflammation

Patients may experience psychological stress from the withdrawal from friends and family, pain, and loss of income. Determine the patient's ability to cope, asking what coping strategies have been used in the past for other life stressors and support systems for the patient. As needed, consult the appropriate member of the health care team (social work, clergy, support groups) to ensure that the patient's psychosocial needs are being met.

CRITICAL THINKING

Mrs. O'Donnell

■ Mrs. O'Donnell, age 80, is brought to the emergency department with a fractured left hip. She is positioned for comfort while you collect data.

1. What subjective and objective data should you look for in Mrs. O'Donnell's history?
2. What should be assessed in Mrs. O'Donnell's physical examination?

Suggested answers are at the end of the chapter.

DIAGNOSTIC TESTS FOR THE MUSCULOSKELETAL SYSTEM

Diagnosis of musculoskeletal problems is assisted by laboratory tests and diagnostic imaging (Table 45.4 and Table 45.5). Specific tests for connective tissue diseases are described in Chapter 46.

Laboratory Tests
Calcium and Phosphorus

Bone disorders commonly cause changes in calcium and phosphorus (or phosphate) levels. In a healthy person, calcium and phosphorus have an inverse relationship. This means that when serum calcium increases, serum phosphorus decreases, and vice versa. Some disorders, however, cause an increase in both values or a decrease in both values. Calcium and phosphorous levels are regulated by calcitonin from the thyroid gland and parathyroid hormone from the parathyroid glands. When these glands are not functioning properly, alterations in calcium and phosphorous levels can occur.

Serum calcium tends to decrease in patients with osteoporosis or in people who consume inadequate amounts of calcium

TABLE 45.4 DIAGNOSTIC LABORATORY TESTS FOR THE MUSCULOSKELETAL SYSTEM

Test	Normal Value	Significance of Abnormal Findings
Calcium	8.5–10.5 mg/dL	Hypercalcemia—may be related to metastatic bone disease or extended immobilization. Hypocalcemia—may be due to poor dietary intake. Can ultimately lead to rickets in a child or osteomalacia (bone softening) or osteoporosis in older adults.
Phosphorus	2.6–4.5 mg/dL	Usually evaluated with serum calcium. A number of disorders can be associated with high or low serum phosphorus.
Alkaline phosphatase (ALP)	*Male:* 45–115 units/L *Female:* 30–100 units/L	ALP increases may indicate bone abnormality (examples: Paget's disease, metastatic bone cancer). ALP is increased when new bone is formed.
Myoglobin	50–120 mcg/mL	Increased myoglobin can indicate myocardial infarction or skeletal muscle destruction.
Creatine kinase (CK)	*Male:* 60–400 units/L *Female:* 40–150 units/L	Intramuscular injections can cause increase in CK.
Isoenzyme CK3 (MM)	95%–100%	High levels indicate need for further testing for muscle disease. Can be used as a screening test for malignant hyperthermia. Will be increased in rhabdomyolysis.
Uric acid	*Male:* 4.4–7.6 mg/dL *Female:* 2.3–6.6 mg/dL	Elevated serum levels indicate gout.

TABLE 45.5 DIAGNOSTIC PROCEDURES FOR THE MUSCULOSKELETAL SYSTEM

Procedure	Definition	Significance of Abnormal Findings	Nursing Management (if applicable)
Noninvasive			
X-Rays	Visualization of skeletal abnormality or deformity. Can also be used to visualize dense or inflamed tissues and joints.	Aids in treatment plan and provides additional information for care. *Example:* Broken ribs demand increased attention to respiratory system.	Inform patient of what to expect during ordered procedures.
Computed Tomography	Radiographic "slices" of bone or soft tissue. Provides a better image.		Check for allergies to contrast medium. Patient should have nothing by mouth (NPO) for 4 hours before test.
Magnetic Resonance Imaging (MRI)	Electromagnets provide a three-dimensional visualization of the area. Produces the best image available.		Screen for contraindications to MRI such as metal in body. Inform patient of what to expect during ordered procedures.
Ultrasonography	Visualizes bone or soft tissue using sound waves.		Inform the patient that the jelly-like conducting substance will feel cold when applied.
Nerve Conduction Studies	Electromyography (EMG) is the electrical testing of nerves and muscles.	Alterations usually indicate a problem with the nerves or the muscles.	Explain that there may be some discomfort during nerve and muscle stimulation as well as when the needles are inserted (if needed).
Invasive			
Arthrography	Air or a contrast medium is injected into a synovial joint which is then x-rayed.	Aids in the diagnosis of joint abnormalities.	Inform patient that the test is uncomfortable during injection. Joint swelling is common after the procedure. Apply ice and elevate limb. Discourage physical activity for 12 to 24 hours after procedure.
Myelogram	Visualizes the spine and spinal cord. May use injection of a contrast medium.	Identifies spinal problems.	Assess for headache and nausea postprocedure. Maximum head raise is 45 degrees for at least 3 hours postprocedure (or as ordered).

Continued

TABLE 45.5 DIAGNOSTIC PROCEDURES FOR THE MUSCULOSKELETAL SYSTEM—cont'd

Procedure	Definition	Significance of Abnormal Findings	Nursing Management (if applicable)
Nuclear Medicine Scans	A radioisotope is injected to help visualize bone and other soft tissue abnormalities.	Finding a "hot spot" usually indicates metastases or bone infection.	Inform patient that the test is not dangerous. Inform patient that the test may take up to 90 minutes.
Gallium/ Thallium Scans	A radioactive element is injected that migrates to bone, and inflammatory tissue.	Gallium concentrates in areas of tumors, inflammation, and infections. Thallium detects osteosarcoma.	Check if your facility recommends that children and pregnant women stay a few feet away from the patient for the first 48 hr.
Arthroscopy	Provides direct visualization of a joint and its capsule using an instrument inserted into the joint space.	Identifies joint abnormalities.	Assess color, warmth, circulation, and movement often. Monitor patient for complications. Apply ice, and keep limb elevated to minimize swelling (if ordered).
Arthrocentesis	Involves the withdrawal of synovial fluid from a joint space. Used for analysis of synovial fluid or reduction of excess fluid pressure.		Monitor patient for infection, inflammation, or hemarthrosis.
Bone or Muscle Biopsy	Involves needle aspiration (closed) or surgical extraction (open) of bone or muscle tissue.		Monitor site of biopsy for bleeding. Provide normal wound care for open biopsy. Perform neurovascular assessments as needed.

in their diets. Serum calcium levels increase in patients with bone cancer, particularly those with metastatic disease.

Alkaline Phosphatase

Alkaline phosphatase (ALP) is an enzyme that increases when bone or liver tissue is damaged. In metabolic bone diseases and bone cancer, ALP increases to reflect osteoblast (bone-forming cell) activity.

Myoglobin

Myoglobin is a protein found in striated (skeletal or cardiac) muscle. It is what causes the red color of muscle. When skeletal or cardiac muscle is damaged, myoglobin levels rise in the blood.

Muscle Enzymes

When muscle tissue is damaged, a number of serum enzymes are released into the bloodstream, including skeletal muscle

creatine kinase (CK-MM [CK3]), aldolase (ALD), aspartate aminotransferase (AST), and lactate dehydrogenase (LDH).

RHABDOMYOLYSIS. Rhabdomyolysis is a very serious and potentially fatal condition associated with muscle destruction due to an injury (such as crush syndrome), high fever, convulsions, or prolonged muscle compression. The patient's creatine kinase (CK) levels can be five times greater than normal. If the patient has muscle destruction, look for elevated CK, myoglobin, and serum potassium levels to monitor for rhabdomyolysis. Also observe for dark urine, muscle weakness, and myalgia (muscle pain). The goal of treatment is to restore normal fluid and electrolyte balance.

Uric Acid

Uric acid is normally found in blood. When uric acid levels rise in the serum, a condition called **gout** can occur (Chapter 46).

Other Diagnostic Tests

X-Rays

An x-ray examination can determine bone density, texture, changes in alignment and bone relationship, erosion, swelling, and intactness. In addition, x-ray examinations can be useful in identifying certain soft tissue damage (e.g., ligaments and tendons) because of alterations in bone position and spacing.

Computed Tomography

Tomograms can show a particular slice of bone or soft tissue, such as ligaments and tendons. Computed tomography (CT) is especially helpful for diagnosing problems of the joints or vertebral column (Fig. 45.7). It may be used with or without contrast med, which is given orally or intravenously (IV).

Bone Density Screening

A bone density test measures both bone strength and weight-bearing abilities. A special x-ray process, dual-energy x-ray absorptiometry (DEXA), measures bone density. It is used to diagnose osteoporosis (Chapter 46).

Arthrography

An x-ray examination of any synovial joint can be performed for patients with suspected joint trauma. The most common joints tested are the knee and shoulder.

Myelogram

During a myelogram, a contrast medium is injected into the subarachnoid space so that the spine and spinal cord can be visualized. Inform patients that they may be positioned head down for a short period to allow the contrast medium to flow up to the level of the neck. This test is usually reserved for those patients unable to have a CT or magnetic resonance imaging (MRI) scan or for complicated spinal surgery revisions.

Magnetic Resonance Imaging

MRI, with or without contrast medium, is a commonly performed test to diagnose musculoskeletal problems, especially those involving soft tissue ("Patient Perspective"). MRI is more accurate than CT for diagnosing many problems of the vertebral column (Fig. 45.8). If the patient has had previous spinal surgery, a contrast medium is used (see Chapter 36 for contrast-induced nephropathy).

Patient Perspective

Emily: Undergoing an MRI

After a traumatic injury, I had an MRI and was instructed on the procedure. I had seen MRI scanners on TV, but didn't know much about them. I knew I had to lie still and not move. I knew if I opened my eyes, I would start getting scared, so I kept them closed. I did take a peek, and saw a part of the machine just inches from my face. I closed my eyes, and repeated in my head, "Inhale, exhale, relax. Inhale, exhale, relax," a mantra I had learned in yoga class. I could feel myself going in and out of consciousness, but when I was conscious I repeated my mantra, the only thing that helped me hang on to reality. I didn't feel any pain, so I thought I was OK. Before I knew it, the test was over and I felt relieved. My personal coping techniques really helped me through the MRI so that I could complete the test. Providing information to patients on what to expect during the test, as well as coping methods to use, can help them successfully complete an MRI.

BE SAFE!

Check with the facility where the MRI will take place for all contraindications for metal implants within a person's body to prevent injury to the patient.

FIGURE 45.7 Computed tomography scan of fifth cervical vertebra showing a burst fracture of the vertebral body (top arrow) and both laminae (bottom arrows). From McKinnis, L. N. [2005]. *Fundamentals of musculoskeletal imaging* (2nd ed.). Philadelphia: F.A. Davis, p. 164, with permission.

Nuclear Medicine Scans

Several tests are performed using radioactive material, which is not harmful to the patient, to help visualize bone and other tissues. A bone scan allows visualization of the entire skeleton. The patient is injected with a radioisotope 2 to 3 hours before the scan. The radioisotope is attracted to bone and therefore travels to bone tissue. If the bone scan is ordered to assess for bone infection (osteomyelitis), a picture will be taken immediately after the first injection. Then a second series is done 2 to 3 hours later, once the radioisotope has collected in the bone.

FIGURE 45.8 *Magnetic resonance image of a normal cervical spine. (A) Cerebellum. (B) Spinal cord. (C) Marrow of C2 vertebral body. (D) C4–5 intervertebral disk. From McKinnis, L. N. (1997). Fundamentals of orthopedic radiology. Philadelphia: F.A. Davis, p. 26, with permission.*

For an accurate test, the patient must be able to lie still for up to 90 minutes during scanning. Patients who are older adults, restless, agitated, or in pain may therefore find this test uncomfortable. Sedatives or analgesics may have to be administered before or during the procedure. Patients need to be instructed to remove all jewelry before testing.

The health care provider (HCP) looks for "hot spots" on the test results. Hot spots are created because increased circulation occurs in abnormal bone areas, resulting in increased amounts of the radioactive substance being transported to the abnormal area by the circulation. These hot spots indicate bone disease.

Gallium/Thallium Scans

A gallium or thallium scan is similar to a bone scan but is more specific and sensitive as a diagnostic test. Gallium concentrates in areas of tumors, inflammation, and infections. Traditionally used for heart problems, thallium is now used for evaluation of bone cancers. Thallium is best for detecting osteosarcoma.

Arthroscopy

An arthroscope allows the surgeon to directly visualize a joint. The knee and shoulder are the joints most often evaluated. Because **arthroscopy** is an invasive procedure performed under local or light general anesthesia, the patient is treated as a surgical candidate in a same-day surgery setting.

The surgeon makes several small incisions and distends the joint with injected saline. The scope is inserted and the joint is visualized from different angles. The joint is moved through range of motion, so tears, defects, or other soft tissue damage can be assessed and/or repaired through the scope using special instrumentation. Depending on the extent of the procedure, a bulky or small dressing wrapped with an elastic bandage may be applied.

The perianesthesia care nurse monitors the neurovascular status of the surgical limb frequently (see Table 45.3). If the patient had a diagnostic arthroscopy and no surgical repair, the perianesthesia care nurse encourages the patient to exercise the leg, including straight-leg raises. A mild analgesic usually relieves pain, and the patient returns to regular activities in 24 to 48 hours. If a surgical repair was performed, the patient may have activity restriction and need a stronger analgesic.

Although complications are not common, teach the patient the signs to report to the surgeon for the following:

- Thrombophlebitis (blood clot and vein inflammation)
- Infection (fever or warmth, pain, redness, swelling at surgical site)
- Increased joint pain.

If a repair was done during the surgery, the patient is seen by the surgeon in 1 week to check for complications and progress. The patient may need crutches for the first week to limit weight bearing, depending on the surgical procedure performed. Physical or occupational therapy may be ordered (see "Home Health Hints").

Home Health Hints

- When visiting a patient at home, the nurse needs to determine if the patient is homebound. Patients are considered homebound if
  1. they are bedbound or require maximum assistance to ambulate while using a walker or to transfer,
  2. they can ambulate with only moderate assistance while using a cane to negotiate uneven surfaces, or
  3. they can leave home only for periods of relatively short duration or when in need of medical treatment.
- If it is determined that the patient is not homebound, then services such as physical and occupational therapy can be performed in an outpatient setting.
- When testing strength, extend two or three fingers and ask the patient to squeeze the fingers. Deficits in arm strength can be easily detected using this simple method.
- Observe patients moving around a room or bed. If they are clumsy or have involuntary movement, make efforts during that visit and later visits to protect them from potential injury. Research has shown that pain or fear of falling may prevent a patient from moving and functioning to maximum potential.
- Use sand or cat box filler on icy steps to increase traction, preventing slips and falls.

• WORD • BUILDING •

arthroscopy: arthro—joint + scopy—to examine

Mrs. Gardenio

■ Mrs. Gardenio, 84 years old, fell when using a step-stool in her home. She was taken to the hospital, where it was determined that she had a femoral neck fracture of her left hip.

1. What data should you obtain from Mrs. Gardenio?
2. What possible condition may be the cause of her fracture?
3. What tests may be performed to identify the condition creating her problem?
4. Mrs. Gardenio is to receive morphine 4 mg by intramuscular injection now. You have available morphine 5 mg/mL. How many milliliters will you give?

Suggested answers are at the end of the chapter.

Bone or Muscle Biopsy

Bone or muscle tissue can be surgically extracted for microscopic examination to confirm cancer, infection (bone biopsy), inflammation, or damage (muscle biopsy). Muscle can also be biopsied to diagnose malignant hyperthermia, a genetic disorder (see Chapter 12). Two techniques are used to retrieve muscle tissue: a needle (closed) biopsy or an incisional (open) biopsy.

A closed biopsy can be performed in the patient's room or special procedures area. After local or general anesthesia, the physician inserts a long needle into the tissue for extraction of a sample.

The open biopsy is performed in the operating suite under general anesthesia. A small incision is made and a section of bone or muscle is removed. A sterile pressure dressing is applied because bone is highly vascular.

The nurse inspects the biopsy site for bleeding, swelling, and hematoma formation. Increased pain that is unresponsive to analgesic medication may indicate bleeding in the soft tissue. Vital signs and neurovascular assessments are monitored (see Table 45.3).

Ultrasonography

Sound waves are used to detect osteomyelitis (bone infection), soft tissue disorders, traumatic joint injuries, and surgical hardware placement.

Arthrocentesis

Arthrocentesis is a diagnostic or therapeutic procedure in which synovial fluid is aspirated from a joint for analysis or to relieve pressure (pain) from effusion. This fluid buildup often occurs secondary to an inflammatory process such as bursitis. Analysis of the synovial fluid can also aid in the diagnosis of noninflammatory conditions, septic arthritis, crystal detection, and **hemarthrosis** (blood in the joint cavity). In addition, the removal of fluid will decrease pain and improve mobility.

Using aseptic technique, the physician provides local anesthetic and then uses a needle to aspirate the contents of the joint space. The fluid can then be sent to the lab to evaluate for infection and/or inflammation. If required, the physician will also instill medications such as a corticosteroid, an anti-inflammatory, or an antibiotic. The site is covered with a sterile dressing to prevent infection.

Nursing considerations following the test include monitoring the injection site for increased bruising, bleeding, redness, and warmth.

Nerve Conduction Studies

Electromyography (EMG) measures a muscle's electrical impulses. This aids in the diagnosis of muscle diseases or nerve damage, which may follow a traumatic injury. An indication of nerve damage is limited return of muscle function following injury resolution. Inform the patient what will occur, and instruct the patient to not apply lotions before the test and to remove all jewelry. Occasionally, slight discomfort and bruising occurs at the site where the study occurred. Warm compresses or mild analgesics can be offered for pain relief (see Table 45.5).

CRITICAL THINKING

■ Mrs. O'Donnell

1. Determine if Mrs. O'Donnell has any allergies, how and when the injury occurred, if she has had any previous surgeries, what medications she takes, her medical history, and any past problems with anesthesia (in Mrs. O'Donnell or her family).

2. Inspect her left leg in comparison with her right leg, including limb length, deformity, pain, loss of range of motion, edema, and ecchymosis. Perform neurovascular checks, including movement, sensation (numbness/tingling), presence of pulses, skin temperature, color, and capillary refill.

■ Mrs. Gardenio

1. Assess Mrs. Gardenio's age, her diet (does she have a low-calcium or vitamin D–deficient diet?), what she was doing at the time of the break, whether anything like this has happened before, whether anything similar has happened to any of her relatives, her pain level, when she ate last, her medications, her medical history, whether she smokes, and whether she has any allergies.

2. Mrs. Gardenio may have osteoporosis that has resulted in a pathological fracture from decreased bone density. This is common in postmenopausal women.

Continued

SUGGESTED ANSWERS TO—cont'd

3. X-ray examinations, bone scans, bone density tests, and laboratory tests such as serum calcium, phosphorus, acid phosphatase, thyroid, and vitamin D levels are tests that might be performed.

4. Unit analysis method:

$$\frac{4\ \text{mg}}{} \begin{array}{|c} 1\ \text{mL} \\ \hline 5\ \text{mg} \end{array} = \frac{4\ \text{mL}}{5} = 0.8\ \text{mL}$$

REVIEW QUESTIONS

1. The nurse is assigned to care for a patient who has been diagnosed with a musculoskeletal disease that causes decreased bone density. Which data collection questions are most appropriate by the nurse? **Select all that apply.**
   1. "Do you have any broken bones?"
   2. "Has your doctor informed you not to exercise so you will not break a bone?"
   3. "What forms of physical activity are you able to participate in?"
   4. "Do any of your spouse's relatives have problems with their bones?"
   5. "Do you exercise regularly?"
   6. "What is typically included in your daily diet?"

2. The nurse is caring for a patient with a fractured left leg. Which of the following findings during a neurovascular assessment of the lower extremities would the nurse recognize as a priority to report to the health care provider?
   1. Strong bilateral left leg post tibial pulse
   2. Right foot capillary refill less than 2 seconds
   3. Bilateral dorsal flexion
   4. Pallor of the left leg

3. A patient is scheduled for an MRI of the pelvis. Which of the following actions would the nurse take if during data collection it was revealed that the patient had had a previous surgery for heart problems?
   1. Ask if there is any metal in the patient's body.
   2. Obtain an order for a chest x-ray
   3. Cancel the MRI.
   4. Inform the physician.

4. The nurse is caring for a patient who has undergone an arthroscopy. Two hours after the procedure, the patient's pedal pulses are diminished compared with the previous assessment. What action should the nurse take?
   1. Take vital signs.
   2. Notify the surgeon.
   3. Perform neurovascular assessment in 30 minutes.
   4. Change the dressing and rewrap the elastic wrap.

5. The nurse is caring for a patient who is undergoing an arthroscopy of the knee with ligament repair. Which of the following would be included in nursing preoperative care for the patient the morning of surgery? **Select all that apply.**
   1. A soft breakfast
   2. No food after midnight
   3. Explaining the surgical procedure
   4. Explaining the anesthetic agents
   5. Reinforcing how to perform coughing and deep-breathing exercises
   6. Teaching the patient to perform straight-leg raises

Answers can be found in Appendix C.

 DavisPlus | For additional resources and information visit **davispl.us/medsurg5**

Nursing Care of Patients With Musculoskeletal and Connective Tissue Disorders

SHARON GORDON

LEARNING OUTCOMES

1. Explain the pathophysiology, signs and symptoms, and complications of fractures.
2. Plan nursing interventions for a patient in a cast, traction, or external fixation.
3. Describe the causes and prevention of osteomyelitis.
4. Plan nursing care for osteomyelitis.
5. Describe risk factors, pathophysiology, treatment, and nursing care for osteoporosis.
6. Describe pathophysiology, signs and symptoms, treatment, and nursing care for Paget's disease.
7. Describe the pathophysiology, treatment, and nursing care for gout.
8. Compare the care for osteoarthritis and rheumatoid arthritis.
9. Plan care for the patient with a fractured hip.
10. Plan care for a patient undergoing a total joint replacement.
11. Explain the patient education that would be included for a patient with a lower extremity amputation and prosthesis.

KEY TERMS

arthritis (ar-THRYE-tiss)
arthroplasty (AR-throw-PLAS-tee)
avascular necrosis (a-VAS-cue-lar neh-KROW-siss)
fasciotomy (fash-ee-OTT-oh-mee)
hemipelvectomy (heh-mee-pell-VEC-tuh-mee)
hyperuricemia (HYE-purr-yoor-eh-SEE-mee-ah)
osteomyelitis (AWS-tee-oh-my-eh-LEYE-tiss)
osteosarcoma (AWS-tee-oh-sar-KOH-mah)
replantation (ree-plan-TAY-shun)
rhabdomyolysis (wrab-DOE-my-o-LEYE-sis)
synovitis (sin-oh-VYE-tiss)

BONE AND SOFT TISSUE DISORDERS

A variety of injuries and diseases can affect bone, soft tissue, or both and are discussed here.

Strains

A strain is a soft tissue injury that occurs when a muscle or tendon is excessively stretched. Causes of strains include falls, excessive exercise, and lifting heavy items. A mild strain causes minimal inflammation; swelling and tenderness are present. A moderate strain involves partial tearing of the muscle or tendon fibers. Pain and inability to move the affected body part result. The most severe strain occurs when a muscle or tendon is ruptured, with separation of muscle from muscle, tendon from muscle, or tendon from bone. Severe pain and disability result from this injury.

RICE is an acronym for *R*est, *I*ce, *C*ompression, and *E*levation, which is the therapy for strain injuries. Immediately after a strain, the injured area should be Rested to protect it. Ice should be applied to decrease pain, swelling, and inflammation. Applying an elastic bandage for Compression and Elevating the affected area (if appropriate) provide support and minimize swelling. After inflammation subsides, heat application (15–30 minutes four times a day) brings increased blood flow to the injured area for healing. Activity is limited until the soft tissue heals, and nonsteroidal anti-inflammatory drugs (NSAIDs) are prescribed. Muscle relaxants may also be used. Exercise may begin as early as 2 to 5 days after the injury depending on the severity of the injury; in some cases, it may take 1 to 3 weeks of immobility before exercise can begin. For more severe strains, ambulatory surgery to repair the tear or rupture may be needed.

Sprains

A sprain is excessive stretching of ligaments from twisting movements during a sports activity, exercise, or fall. A mild sprain involves tearing of a few ligament fibers that causes tenderness. RICE and NSAIDs are used for several days until swelling and pain diminish. In a moderate sprain, more fibers are torn, but the stability of the joint is not affected. Moderate sprains may need immobilization with a brace or cast. A moderate sprain is uncomfortable, especially with activity. A severe sprain causes instability of the joint and usually requires surgical intervention for tissue repair or grafting. Pain and inflammation restrict mobility.

Dislocations

A dislocation is a common injury in which the ends of the bones are forced from their normal position. This is usually caused by trauma as in falls or contact sports or by a disease such as rheumatoid **arthritis**. Any joint, large or small, may become dislocated. Severe pain along with lost range of motion (ROM) of the joint and joint deformity occurs. Immediate medical treatment is required to preserve function. Splint the extremity as it is found, apply ice, and seek help. Do not move the extremity because blood vessels, muscles, and nerves could be damaged.

BE SAFE!

For patients with disease processes that could result in a dislocation or fracture, careful moving is essential. Use lifting devices such as draw sheets and mechanical devices when moving a patient rather than pulling on the patient's arms to avoid patient injury. Follow institutional policy for moving patients to avoid patient injury and liability for a patient's injury.

Bursitis

Bursae (fluid-filled sacs) cushion tendons during movement to prevent friction between the bone and tendon. Several joints have bursae (shoulder, elbow, hip, knee, ankle, heel). Inflammation of a bursa, called bursitis, occurs from arthritis, gout, repetitive movement, or sleeping on one's side, which compresses the shoulder bursa. Prevention is key because bursitis may become harder to cure over time. To protect the bursae and prevent compression, teach patients to stretch and strengthen muscles, move frequently, avoid repetitive movements for long periods, use cushioned seats, and avoid leaning on the elbows.

Symptoms of bursitis include achy pain, stiffness, or burning pain over the joint area that worsens with activity. Usually pain decreases in about a week. The condition can become chronic if it lasts more than 6 months. Treatment includes resting the joint, application of ice 20 minutes several times per day until joint warmth is gone, then switching to heat, elevating the joint, ultrasound, massage, NSAIDs, or physical therapy.

Rotator Cuff Injury

Short tendons that are connected to muscles around the shoulder form the rotator cuff. The cuff covers the top, front, and back of the shoulder. Muscle contraction causes these tendons to tighten and move or rotate the shoulder. Various cuff injuries can occur. With chronic impingement syndrome, the top tendon of the cuff (supraspinatus tendon) and bursae become impinged in the narrow space under the acromion bone. This causes inflammation when the arm is repeatedly moved forward, and pain results. Over time the tendon can tear from the bone.

Symptoms of rotator cuff injury include shoulder aching, increased pain with lifting the arm, pain that is greater at night, weakness, and sometimes limited ROM. Magnetic resonance imaging (MRI) diagnoses the injury. For minor injury, resting the shoulder, ice, NSAIDs, and physical therapy are recommended. For a severe injury, arthroscopic and/or small-incision surgery relieves the impingement or repairs the tear. A sling or special brace is worn after surgery. Physical therapy is ordered for rehabilitation.

• WORD • BUILDING •
arthritis: arthr(on)—joint + itis—inflammation

Carpal Tunnel Syndrome

Pathophysiology

Carpal tunnel syndrome results in the compression of the median nerve within the carpal tunnel when there is swelling in the tunnel. The swelling can result from edema, trauma, rheumatoid arthritis, or repetitive hand movements (repetitive motion injury) used in some occupations such as typing or factory work.

Signs and Symptoms

Carpal tunnel syndrome usually results in slow-onset finger, hand, and arm pain and numbness. Painful tingling and paresthesia may also be present. Eventually, fine motor deficits and then muscle weakness may develop.

Diagnostic Tests

Diagnosis is based on signs and symptoms and patient history. A positive Phalen's test (numbness with wrist flexion) indicates carpal tunnel syndrome. Electromyography is used to detect nerve abnormalities.

Therapeutic Measures

Treatment aims to relieve the inflammation and rest the wrist. A splint can be ordered for the patient to wear. Anti-inflammatories such as aspirin and NSAIDs or cortisone injection into the tunnel are used to reduce inflammation and pain.

For some patients, endoscopic or open incision surgery can be needed. The median nerve is released from compression during the surgery, thus correcting the problem of the nerve and the surrounding area becoming inflamed. Physiotherapy helps in the recovery of function.

Nursing Care

Educate the patient on methods to prevent carpal tunnel syndrome, such as frequent short breaks during the workday, alternating nonrepetitive tasks with repetitive movements throughout the day, and using ergonomically appropriate devices to minimize the pressure placed in the area of the wrist.

Manage pain as ordered. After surgery, elevate the patient's hand and instruct the patient on use of a splint as ordered for up to 2 weeks. Lifting is restricted for several weeks. Teach the patient to report signs and symptoms of neurovascular compromise, such as numbness and tingling, coolness, lack of pulse, pale skin or nailbeds, or limited movement. The patient may need family assistance with activities of daily living (ADLs).

Fractures

A fracture is a break in a bone that can be minor and treated on an ambulatory basis or complex with surgical intervention and rehabilitation.

Pathophysiology

Bone is a dynamic, changing tissue. When it is broken, the body immediately begins to repair the injury (Fig. 46.1). For an adult, within 48 to 72 hours after the injury, a hematoma (blood clot) forms at the fracture site because bone has a rich blood supply. Various cells that begin the healing process are attracted to the damaged bone. In about a week or so, a nonbony union called

FIGURE 46.1 Fracture healing phases.

a callus develops and can be seen on x-ray examination. As healing continues, osteoclasts (bone-destroying cells) resorb any necrotic bone, and osteoblasts (bone-building cells) make new bone as a replacement. This process is referred to as bone remodeling. Young, healthy adult bone completely heals in about 6 weeks; however, it can take up to a year before the whole process of remodeling is complete. An older person takes longer to heal.

Adequate nutrition that includes vitamins, minerals, and protein is essential to heal fractures and keep the musculoskeletal system healthy (see Chapter 45).

Etiology and Types

The major reason for a fracture is trauma from a fall, an accident (usually motor vehicle), or a crushing injury. Bone disease (such as osteoporosis and metastatic bone cancer), malnutrition, and regular drinking of carbonated beverages with added phosphoric acid (which may interfere with calcium absorption) can lead to fractures. Side effects from medications can cause a decrease in bone density, resulting in fracture. When fractures result from disease, they are referred to as pathological fractures. Hip fracture is a commonly occurring fracture in middle-aged and older women who have osteoporosis (irreversible bone loss).

In a complete fracture, the bone is broken into two separate pieces. Complete fractures have the potential to be life threatening because sharp bone fragments can sever blood vessels and nerves. In an incomplete fracture, the bone does not divide into two pieces. With a displaced fracture, the bone sections are out of alignment. In a closed fracture, the bone does not disrupt the skin. In an open fracture, the bone breaks the skin. Open fractures are more likely to become infected than closed fractures. Fractures can be described by the way the bone breaks (spiral or oblique; Fig. 46.2). There are many types of fractures: avulsion, comminuted, impacted, greenstick, interarticular, displaced, pathological (also called neoplastic), spiral, longitudinal, oblique, stress, transverse, and depressed (Table 46.1).

| Avulsion | Comminuted | Impacted | Greenstick |

| Interarticular | Displaced | Pathologic | Spiral |

| Longitudinal | Oblique | Stress | Transverse |

FIGURE 46.2 Types of fractures.

TABLE 46.1 TYPES OF FRACTURES

Fracture Type	Description
Avulsion	Piece of bone is torn away from the main bone while still attached to a ligament or tendon.
Comminuted	Bone splintered or shattered into numerous fragments. Often occurs in crushing injuries.
Impacted	Bone is forcibly pushed together, resulting in bone being pushed into bone.
Greenstick	Bone is bent and fractures on the outer arc of the bend. Often seen in children.
Interarticular	Fracture involves bones within a joint.
Displaced	Bone pieces are out of normal alignment. One or more pieces may be out of alignment.
Pathological (also called neoplastic)	Caused when bone is weakened either by pressure from a tumor or an actual tumor within the bone.
Spiral	Fracture curves around the shaft of the bone.
Longitudinal	Fracture occurs along the length of the bone.
Oblique	Fracture occurs diagonally or at an oblique angle across the bone.
Stress	Results in the bone being fractured across one cortex. This is an incomplete fracture.
Transverse	Bone fractured horizontally.
Depressed	Bone pushed inward. Often seen with skull and facial fractures.

Signs and Symptoms

This section focuses on fractures of upper and lower extremities. If the patient sustains a hairline (microscopic) fracture, the signs and symptoms are not readily observable. The patient may report tenderness over the site of the injury or more severe pain when moving the affected part of the body. The patient with a hip fracture usually experiences pain either in the groin area (the hip is a deep joint) or at the back of the knee (referred pain). If the fracture is complete, the limb is often shortened because of contraction of the muscles pulling on the bone sections.

In addition to pain, patients with more complex fractures experience limb rotation or deformity and shortening of the limb (if a limb bone is broken). ROM is decreased. If the

affected part is moved, a continuous grating sound (crepitation) caused by bone fragments rubbing on each other may be heard. The extremity should not be moved (to try and reposition the bone alignment) if crepitation is present.

Inspect the skin for intactness. A patient with a closed fracture may have ecchymosis (bruising) over the fractured bone from bleeding into the soft underlying tissue. Ecchymosis may not develop for several days after the injury. Swelling may also be present and can impair blood flow, causing marked neurovascular compromise. In an open fracture, one or more bone ends pierce the skin, causing a wound, thus increasing the possibility of infection.

Diagnostic Tests

An x-ray examination can visualize bone fractures, showing bone malalignment or disruption. Computed tomography (CT) detects fractures of complex areas, such as the hip and pelvis. MRI determines the extent of associated soft tissue damage.

For patients with moderate to severe bleeding, a hemoglobin and hematocrit level is obtained. If soft tissue damage is extensive, the erythrocyte sedimentation rate (ESR) usually is elevated, indicating the expected inflammatory response. The health care provider (HCP) might order a serum calcium level to determine baseline values because bone repair requires a sufficient amount of calcium and other minerals.

Emergency Treatment

A patient with a suspected fracture often has injuries elsewhere in the body. Observe the patient for respiratory distress, bleeding, and head or spine injury. If any of these problems occurs, emergency treatment is provided before concern is given to extremity or other fractures to prevent possible life-threatening complications. Box 46-1 describes emergency interventions for the patient with an extremity fracture.

 LEARNING TIP

For emergency care of a suspected fracture, do not try to reposition the limb. Remember: Splint it as it lies. Also, ensure that the limb is secured above and below the break to minimize movement and bone grating (crepitation).

Fracture Management

The goals of fracture management are reduction, or realignment, of bone ends; immobilization of the fractured bone (with bandages, splints, casts, traction, or fixation device); preservation or restoration of surrounding soft tissue structures such as vessels, tendons, ligaments and muscles; prevention of deformity or further injury; preservation or restoration of function; promotion of early healing; and pain relief.

CLOSED REDUCTION. Closed reduction is the most common treatment for simple fractures. While manually pulling on the bone (limb), the HCP manipulates the bone ends into realignment.

Box 46-1 Urgent Management of Fractures

1. Immediately immobilize affected limb. If movement is required before splinting, support limb above and below fracture.
2. Unless there is bleeding, apply splints and padding above and below the fracture site, directly over the clothing. If bleeding is present, visualization may be needed before pressure can be applied where bleeding is originating. Keep patient covered to preserve body heat.
3. If the fractured extremity is a leg bone, the unaffected extremity can be used as a splint by bandaging both legs together. An arm can be bandaged to the chest or put into a sling to minimize further tissue damage.
4. Assess color, warmth, circulation, and movement (CWCM) of the limb distal to the fracture.
5. For an open fracture, the protruding bone should be covered with a clean (sterile preferred) dressing.
6. Do not attempt to straighten or realign a fractured extremity. Move the affected limb as little as necessary.
7. Transport to an emergency department as soon as possible.

Analgesia and/or conscious sedation is given before the procedure. An x-ray is done to confirm that the bone ends are aligned before the area is immobilized by a cast or splint.

BANDAGES AND SPLINTS. For some areas of the body, such as the clavicle or wrist, an elastic or muslin bandage or a splint may be used to immobilize the bone during the healing phase. Splints can be used when the fracture has some associated soft tissue damage that needs care or if there is an expectation of swelling. It is important for the splint to be well padded, thereby preventing skin breakdown or unnecessary pressure. Perform neurovascular assessments hourly (or as ordered) to monitor adequate blood flow to the area until the concern for swelling has passed, then typically every 2 to 4 hours (see Chapter 45).

CASTS. Casts provide a strong support for fractured bones, thereby aiding in early mobility and decreased pain. They are also used to correct deformities and to support weak joints while restricting movement. The type of cast used depends on the reason the cast is applied. For more extensive fractures or for weight-bearing areas, a rigid and durable cast is used for immobilization. When bone healing is complete, the cast is removed.

Several types of materials are used for casts, including the traditional plaster of Paris (anhydrous calcium sulfate) and a variety of synthetic products such as fiberglass. Plaster is used for large casts and for weight-bearing areas. Because of a chemical reaction that occurs when the plaster is wet, the cast feels hot when applied for about 30 minutes and then feels cool, taking anywhere from 24 to 72 hours to completely dry. The cast is dry when it feels hard and firm, is odorless, and is shiny white. Keep the wet cast open to air, and turn the patient about every 2 hours to expose all sides of the cast to the air to aid in drying and to prevent mold growth. A wet cast should be handled with the palms of the hand ("palming the cast") to prevent indentations or a change in the shape of the cast (Fig. 46.3). This prevents the possibility of pressure points forming inside the cast. Unlike plaster of Paris, synthetic material casts such as fiberglass harden quickly and dry in less than 2 hours.

A casted limb is elevated for 24 to 48 hours, and ice can be applied over the injury to reduce swelling. Observe the cast for dryness, tightness, drainage, and odor. A serious complication of a cast being too tight is *compartment syndrome* (discussed later). If the cast becomes too tight, the HCP orders it to be cut (bivalved) with a cast cutter to relieve pressure and prevent pressure necrosis of the underlying skin (Fig. 46.4). If a wound is present or an odor is detected, a window opening into the cast is created to treat the underlying skin problem, often an infected area. The cast window should always be taped in place when wound care is not being provided to prevent the skin from "popping up" through the window and developing pressure points and ischemia. Box 46-2 describes nursing interventions for a patient with a cast.

FIGURE 46.3 A wet plaster cast is moved with the palms of the hand to prevent making indentations in the plaster that could become pressure points.

FIGURE 46.4 Bivalving a cast with a cast saw.

Box 46-2 Nursing Interventions for a Patient With a Cast

1. Assess color, warmth, circulation, and movement (CWCM) every 1 to 2 hours for 24 hours and then qid and prn.
   a. Assess cast for tightness (ask patient) and for rough or frayed edges (can interfere with skin integrity).
   b. Make sure patient can move (wiggle) all digits distal to the cast.
2. With newly applied casts (wet):
   a. Never grasp a wet cast to hold or move it, and do not place it on any surface that can cause an indentation. Use only the palms of the hands, because finger pressure on a wet cast can cause pressure points on the inside surface.
   b. Make sure patient is turned every 1 to 2 hours to prevent flattening of cast surface during drying.
   c. With hip spicas or any cast with an abductor bar, do not use bar to move limb or to help with turns.
   d. Inform patient that plaster casts give off heat when drying. Make sure cast air dries (may require 24 to 72 hours for complete drying). Do not cover cast or use drying aids such as blow dryers. Place cast on absorbent surfaces, not plasticized pillows.
   e. Protect skin integrity by ensuring rough edges of cast are properly covered.
   f. Make sure patient knows to keep cast dry during bathing by covering with plastic and preventing water from seeping into cast ends.
   g. Synthetic casts (e.g., fiberglass) can be exposed to water (e.g., for hydrotherapy) as needed but require complete drying afterward.
3. Maintain tissue integrity within the cast.
   a. When assessing CWCM, assess visible skin for signs of impaired integrity.
   b. Cast edges can be smoothed and covered with stockinettes or gauze and tape (make sure there are no tape allergies) to prevent rubbing of skin.
   c. Monitor for signs and symptoms of infection, such as foul odor, heat, redness, and pain.
   d. Do not use skin products on affected limb.
   e. Monitor visible blood on the surface of the cast. Outline area with a pen to observe for increasing size. Shadowing of blood not quite reaching the surface of the cast is fairly common but also should be circled and monitored.
   f. Never place any object inside the cast, and instruct patient not to do so. Explain the risk of skin damage.

TRACTION. Traction is the application of a pulling force to part of the body to position and hold bone fragments in correct alignment. Advances in orthopedic surgery have decreased the use of traction.

Skin Traction. Buck's traction is skin traction that is used for patients with hip fractures who are not candidates for early surgery. It is commonly applied for comfort to relieve muscle spasms and to prevent further injury while the patient waits for surgery. With skin traction, the amount of weight that can be applied directly on the skin is about 5 to 10 lbs (2.2–4.5 kg).

Skeletal traction. Skeletal traction uses pins, wires, or tongs inserted into the bone for bone alignment as the fracture heals (Fig. 46.5). Heavier weights from 20 to 40 lb (9–18 kg) are used. Skeletal traction must be maintained with weights hanging freely at all times. Neurovascular and skin checks are done regularly. Pin site care is discussed later.

OPEN REDUCTION WITH INTERNAL. One of the most common indications for this surgical procedure is a fractured hip. Hip fractures involve the proximal femur and affect older adults more than any other age group. Open reduction with internal fixation of the hip allows early mobilization while the bone is healing.

As the name implies, the bone ends are realigned (reduced) by direct visualization through a surgical incision (open reduction). The bone ends are held in place by internal fixation devices such as metal plates and screws or by a prosthesis with a femoral component similar to that used for total joint replacement (Fig. 46.6). For hip surgery, the internal fixation device is not removed after the fracture heals. For ankle or long-bone surgery, the hardware may be removed after healing due to loosening or pain (see the "Nursing Care Plan for the Patient After Open Reduction With Internal Fixation of the Hip").

EXTERNAL FIXATION. External fixation (EF) is used when bone damage is severe, as in crushed or splintered fractures, or if the bone has numerous breaks. After the fracture is reduced, the surgeon inserts pins into the bone. The pins are held in place by an external metal frame to prevent bone movement (Fig. 46.7). EF allows visualization of soft tissue damage that also requires treatment. Pin sites are monitored for infection. Pin-site care varies by agency. The main principle is to ensure that strict aseptic technique is always maintained because the pin is a pathway for microorganisms to directly enter bone tissue and cause **osteomyelitis** (see the "Nursing Care Plan for the Patient With External Fixation of the Lower Extremity").

• WORD • BUILDING •
osteomyelitis: osteo—bone + myel—bone marrow + itis—inflammation

FIGURE 46.5 Skin traction: Buck's (boot) traction.

FIGURE 46.6 Internal fixation. (A) Intertrochanteric fracture of the hip with fracture fixation via a side plate and screw combination device. (B) Side plate and screw fixation of radial fracture. From McKinnis, L. N. (1997). *Fundamentals of orthopedic radiology.* Philadelphia: F.A. Davis, p. 230 (A) and p. 381 (B), with permission.

FIGURE 46.7 External fixation for complex fractures and wound care.

NURSING CARE PLAN for the Patient After Open Reduction With Internal Fixation of the Hip

Nursing Diagnosis: *Pain* related to surgical incision

Expected Outcome: The patient will state that pain relief is satisfactory.

Evaluation of Outcome: Does patient state that pain is absent or at a tolerable level (pain rated 0 to 2 on pain assessment scale)?

Intervention Assess pain level every 2–4 hours or as needed and with each interaction. **Rationale** Frequent pain assessment provides baseline and ongoing data and allows for timely interventions. **Evaluation** Does patient indicate pain or pain relief?

Intervention Give analgesics as needed; anticipate need for pain relief. **Rationale** Analgesics relieve pain, especially if given before pain is severe. **Evaluation** Does patient state pain is relieved?

Intervention Give analgesics before activity (e.g., session with physical therapist). **Rationale** Increased activity can cause pain. **Evaluation** Is patient restless or agitated during activity?

Intervention Use pain relief measures, such as distraction, guided imagery, other relaxation techniques. **Rationale** Analgesic therapy is enhanced with complementary pain relief measures. **Evaluation** Does patient report pain relief with music or relaxation?

Intervention Use fracture bedpan. **Rationale** Fracture bedpans are more comfortable and easier to position for patients. **Evaluation** Is patient able to use fracture pan with comfort?

NURSING CARE PLAN for the Patient After Open Reduction With Internal Fixation of the Hip—cont'd

Nursing Diagnosis: *Impaired Physical Mobility* related to surgical pain

Expected Outcome: The patient will maintain desired level of activity.

Evaluation of Outcome: Does patient maintain activity desired?

Intervention Observe level of physical mobility with each interaction, and as needed. **Rationale** Early and frequent data collection provides baseline data and allows for timely interventions. **Evaluation** Is the patient able to transfer and ambulate? With or without assistance?

Intervention Reinforce transfer and ambulation techniques. **Rationale** Activity is restricted because of hip precautions and weight-bearing limitations. **Evaluation** Does patient use trapeze bar for movement in bed with less pain?

Intervention Monitor patient for and take measures to prevent complications of immobility: • Turn patient every 2 hours and check skin. • Keep heels off bed. • Teach patient to deep breathe and cough every 2 hours. • Teach use of incentive spirometer. **Rationale** Immobility complications can occur if preventive measures are not used. **Evaluation** Does patient experience complications of immobility?

Intervention Apply thigh-high elastic stockings or sequential compression device to unaffected limb as ordered. Remind patient to practice leg exercises. Give anticoagulants as ordered. Get patient out of bed as soon as ordered. Ambulate patient as early as possible. **Rationale** These precautions and activities help prevent blood clots. **Evaluation** Is patient free from blood clots?

NURSING CARE PLAN for the Patient With External Fixation of the Lower Extremity

Nursing Diagnosis: *Risk for Infection* related to open skin at pin site

Expected Outcome: The patient does not develop an infection.

Evaluation of Outcome: Does patient remain free from infection?

Intervention Inspect dressings, wounds, pin sites for signs and symptoms of infection (warmth, redness, heat, edema, drainage, pain). **Rationale** Early and frequent inspection allows for timely intervention to prevent infection. **Evaluation** Are any wounds infected?

Intervention Monitor color, odor and amount of pin site drainage. **Rationale** Pin site drainage color and amount can indicate infection. **Evaluation** Does pin site have purulent drainage?

Intervention Provide pin site care per agency policy using aseptic technique. **Rationale** Use of aseptic technique reduces risk of infection. Pin sites should be free of crusting, which promotes infections. **Evaluation** Are pin sites clean with no crusting?

Intervention Monitor blood pressure, pulse, and temperature frequently. **Rationale** Increases in blood pressure, pulse, and temperature can indicate infection. **Evaluation** Are vital signs within baseline findings?

Continued

NURSING CARE PLAN for the Patient With External Fixation of the Lower Extremity—cont'd

Nursing Diagnosis: *Impaired Physical Mobility* related to the limb injury

Expected Outcome: The patient will maintain desired level of mobility/activity.

Evaluation of Outcome: Has patient maintained desired level of mobility and activity?

Intervention Assess patient's mobility with EF device in place. **Rationale** Assessment provides data concerning patient's abilities and allows for timely nursing interventions. **Evaluation** Can patient transfer and ambulate with or without assistance?

Intervention Reinforce transfer and ambulation techniques. **Rationale** Depending on severity of fracture and size of EF device, there may be special needs to transfer and ambulate. **Evaluation** Does patient transfer and ambulate as instructed?

Intervention Place overhead frame and trapeze bar on bed. Teach patient how to use them. **Rationale** Patient mobility is increased and pain decreased with use of trapeze bar for movement. **Evaluation** Does patient use trapeze bar for movement with less pain?

Intervention Teach patient how to move limb using EF device. **Rationale** Provide patient with instruction on moving the extremity promotes independence and minimizes pain. **Evaluation** Does patient move the extremity using EF device?

Intervention Assess patient for and take measures to prevent complications of immobility. Promote early ambulation to minimize complications. **Rationale** Immobility complications can occur if preventive measures are not used. **Evaluation** Does patient have any complications of immobility?

Intervention Include other disciplines such as the physiotherapist in promoting and teaching about ambulation. **Rationale** Physiotherapy can provide initial teaching or reinforce education needed to promote ambulation (e.g., with crutch walking). **Evaluation** Has patient used information learned from other disciplines to aid ambulation?

Nursing Diagnosis: *Disturbed Body Image* related to external fixation device appearance.

Expected Outcome: The patient will demonstrate acceptance of body image while EF device is in place.

Evaluation of Outcome: Does patient adjust to new image resulting from EF device?

Intervention Prepare patient preoperatively for what EF device will look like. **Rationale** Preparing patient increases the likelihood of acceptance and minimizes anxiety. **Evaluation** Was patient able to verbalize why device is to be used and what device will look like?

Intervention Observe patient's reaction to external fixation device. **Rationale** Determining patient's reaction will guide further nursing responses. **Evaluation** How does patient react to EF device?

Intervention Reinforce the idea that the EF device will decrease discomfort and allow for earlier ambulation. **Rationale** Promoting early ambulation and increased comfort enhance acceptance. **Evaluation** Did patient understand benefit of EF device allowing for early ambulation and increased comfort?

Intervention Provide psychological support and an environment of acceptance. **Rationale** Accepting the patient and allowing for discussion of concerns promote a sense of well-being and acceptance of EF device. **Evaluation** Did patient feel comfortable expressing concerns related to body image?

CRITICAL THINKING

Mrs. Martinez

■ Mrs. Martinez, a care-center resident, was found lying on her left side, moaning and holding her left leg at 1000. She cried out with any movement, and said she fell and broke her leg. The supervisor notified paramedics and Dr. Haas. Vital signs are blood pressure 150/84 mm Hg, pulse 100 beats per minute, and respirations 20 per minute. Her left leg is noticeably shorter than her right leg. The licensed practical nurse (LPN) remained with Mrs. Martinez and instructed her not to move until help arrived. The LPN got blankets and a pillow for her head. The paramedics took Mrs. Martinez to nearby Memorial Hospital, where she was diagnosed as having an incomplete femoral neck (hip) fracture. Dr. Haas ordered 5 pounds of Buck's traction until surgery the next morning.

Later, Mrs. Martinez is restless and picking at her bedcovers when the nurse arrives to assess her at the beginning of the nurse's shift.

1. How should the LPN document the incident of Mrs. Martinez's fall at the care center?
2. What is the purpose of Buck's traction for Mrs. Martinez?
3. What are the nursing responsibilities while caring for Mrs. Martinez?
4. What might explain Mrs. Martinez's restlessness?

Suggested answers are at the end of the chapter.

CRITICAL THINKING

Frank Schnell

■ Frank, age 18, was in a motor vehicle accident that resulted in a fractured pelvis and an open right femoral fracture.

1. Identify four priority nursing diagnoses related to Frank's care
2. What are nursing interventions and rationales for these diagnoses?
3. How can the constipating effects of opioids be balanced with the benefits of pain relief to manage bowel elimination (see Chapter 10)?

Suggested answers are at the end of the chapter.

NONUNION MODALITIES. Although most bones heal properly with the correct treatment, some patients experience malunion (malalignment of healed bone) or nonunion (delayed or no healing). Several factors influence how a bone heals, including age, nutritional status, and diseases that alter the healing process,

such as diabetes mellitus. Identification of the reason for nonunion allows appropriate treatment selection. Treatment methods for nonunion can include electrical bone stimulation, bone grafting or external fixation.

NURSING CARE TIP

When moving a limb that has an external fixation device, grasp the device and lift, raise, or move the limb as needed. By grasping the device, there is less movement of the healing bone and therefore less trauma to the healing site and less pain with movement. Care must be taken not to loosen any fasteners holding the pins in place.

Complications of Fractures

Monitor the patient for possible complications, such as impaired neurovascular status, hemorrhage, infection, and thrombi. Although rare, acute compartment syndrome and fat embolism syndrome (more common with fractures of long bones) can be life-threatening complications of fractures.

NEUROVASCULAR STATUS. Neurovascular checks are done as needed to detect abnormalities. Decreased or absent pulses, cool skin temperature, and dusky color indicate circulation alterations. Numbness and tingling, decreased sensation, and mobility indicate neurologic alterations. These findings should be reported to the HCP immediately.

HEMORRHAGE. Bone is highly vascular, and damage to or surgery on bone (particularly the large long bones of the extremities) can cause bleeding. Check for bleeding and monitor vital signs carefully. Hypovolemic shock may result from severe hemorrhage (see Chapter 9).

INFECTION. Trauma predisposes the body to infection, especially when the skin, the body's first line of defense, is disrupted. Wound infections, pin-site infections, drainage tube infections, and osteomyelitis (bone infection) are common.

VENOUS THROMBOEMBOLITIC COMPLICATIONS. Deep venous thrombosis (DVT) or pulmonary embolus (PE; see Chapter 31) can develop in patients who are immobile because of trauma or surgery. Thromboembolitic complications are the most common problems of lower extremity surgery or trauma and the most fatal complication of musculoskeletal surgery, particularly in the older adult. Leg exercises, early ambulation, and prophylactic anticoagulant therapy such as with dalteparin (Fragmin), enoxaparin (Lovenox), fondaparinux (Arixtra), or rivaroxaban (Xarelto), help prevent these problems.

ACUTE COMPARTMENT SYNDROME. Compartments are sheaths of fibrous tissue that support and partition nerves, muscles, and blood vessels, primarily in the extremities (Fig. 46.8). Each extremity has several compartments. Acute compartment syndrome is a limb-and life-threatening condition

Fascia surrounds
each compartment

Fibula

Tibia

A

Fascia surrounds
each compartment

Fibula

Tibia

B

FIGURE 46.8 (A) Lower leg compartments. Each compartment contains muscles, an artery, a vein, and a nerve. (B) Compartment syndrome. Increased pressure in a compartment compresses structures within the compartment.

in which pressure in one or more limb compartments increases, causing reduced circulation to the compartment's muscles and nerves. An EF device such as a cast or bulky dressing can increase pressure when there is tissue swelling or compression in the area. The early symptom of acute compartment syndrome is the patient's report of severe, increasing pain that is not relieved with opioids and occurs more in active movements than passive movements. Decreased sensation follows before ischemia becomes severe. In severe acute compartment syndrome, the patient has the six *P*s:

1. *P*ain (severe, unrelenting, and increased with passive stretching)
2. *P*aresthesia (painful tingling or burning)
3. *P*aralysis (late symptom)
4. *P*allor (but there may be warmth or redness over the area)
5. *P*ulselessness (late and ominous sign)
6. *P*oikilothermia (temperature matches environment; i.e., the extremity is cool to touch).

Relief of pressure is the goal. It may be accomplished by removing the source of pressure, such as by bivalving a cast, or by performing a **fasciotomy**, which is an incision into the fascia that encloses the compartment. This incision allows the compartment tissue to expand and relieves the pressure. If more than one compartment has increased pressure, multiple fasciotomies are required. These surgical wounds remain open until the pressure decreases. Then they are closed and could require skin grafting. If this condition continues without pressure relief, tissue necrosis, infection, Volkmann's contracture (permanent flexion of hand/wrist), **rhabdomyolysis** (muscle break down releases myoglobin which is harmful to the kidneys), or renal failure may result.

FAT EMBOLISM SYNDROME. Fat embolism syndrome (FES) is another serious complication of fractures in which small fat droplets are released from yellow bone marrow into the bloodstream (Table 46.2). The droplets then travel to the lung fields, causing respiratory insufficiency, which can lead to respiratory failure. This process occurs with long bone fractures (especially the femoral shaft) and perhaps when the patient has multiple fractures. The older adult patient with a fractured hip is also at a high risk for FES. This condition can occur up to 72 hours after the initial injury.

The three primary manifestations of FES are respiratory failure, cerebral involvement, and skin petechiae. Pulmonary

• WORD • BUILDING •
fasciotomy: fascia—fibrous tissue + otomy—opening into
rhabdomyolysis: rhabdo—striped + myo—muscle + lysis—break down

TABLE 46.2 FAT EMBOLISM SYNDROME VS. PULMONARY EMBOLISM

	Fat Embolism Syndrome	Pulmonary Embolism
Signs and Symptoms	Gradual onset with tachycardia, dyspnea, and cyanosis.	Sudden onset, shortness of breath and chest pain
Origin	Multiple small fat droplets	Large clot or fat globule
Cause	Long bone fractures. Surgical fracture repair. Multiple fractures. Hip fracture.	Complication of deep vein thrombosis

dysfunction is the earliest sign and includes tachypnea, dyspnea, and cyanosis. Cerebral changes are often seen and include confusion or drowsiness. A petechial (red, measle-like) rash on the chest, neck, axilla, and conjunctiva appears in some patients. Other signs include tachycardia, fever, and retinal changes. If a fat embolism is suspected, these actions should be taken as ordered:

1. Notify the HCP immediately.
2. Promote oxygenation by administering oxygen at 2 L/min via nasal cannula, and apply a pulse oximeter.
3. Place the patient in high-Fowler's position or raise the head of the bed as tolerated.
4. Maintain bed rest, and minimize movement of the extremity.
5. Obtain arterial blood gas (ABG).
6. Initiate venous access, then administer IV.
7. Administer corticosteroids.
8. Prepare patient for a chest x-ray and an MRI of the brain.
9. Provide emotional support and calm environment.

Nursing Process for the Patient With a Fracture

Caring for the patient with a fracture requires coordinated teamwork with other health team members.

DATA COLLECTION. The most important aspect of monitoring the patient with a fracture is frequent checking of neurovascular status (circulation, sensation, mobility) distal to the fracture site to detect problems (see Chapter 45).

Pain is managed by both medications and complementary therapies. Bone pain can be excruciating and must be treated aggressively. For the patient who cannot report pain, such as a patient who is cognitively impaired or comatose, ensure that pain relief is maintained by regularly scheduled analgesic administration.

NURSING DIAGNOSES, PLANNING, AND IMPLEMENTATION. Determination of the appropriate nursing diagnosis depends on the type of fracture. See the "Nursing Care Plan for the Patient After Open Reduction Internal Fixation of the Hip."

Acute Pain related to fractured bone
EXPECTED OUTCOME: The patient will report relief from pain using a pain assessment scale.

- Identify pain level on a 0 to 10 pain scale *to establish baseline for further interventions.*
- Provide analgesics and anti-inflammatories as ordered *to relieve pain and swelling.*
- Ensure proper positioning and alignment *to promote pain relief and future functioning.*
- Monitor for compartment syndrome if patient has a cast in place *to prevent neurovascular complications.*
- Apply ice as ordered *to decrease swelling and pain.*
- Teach alternative methods for pain relief *to maximize relief of pain.*

Impaired Physical Mobility related to bone fracture
EXPECTED OUTCOME: The patient will demonstrate increased mobility.

- Observe patient's mobility to provide baseline assessment data.
- Encourage independence *to promote mobility.*
- Utilize other disciplines such as occupational and physiotherapy *to encourage and promote patient mobility.*
- Provide equipment and resources such as crutches and wheelchairs *to improve mobility.*

Risk for Peripheral Neurovascular Dysfunction related to increased tissue volume or restrictive envelope
EXPECTED OUTCOME: The patient will maintain peripheral pulses, warm skin, sensation, and ability to move extremity.

- Assess often for compartment syndrome *to promote prompt reporting.*
- Assess for swelling of affected limb (especially if patient has a cast or tight dressing) *to detect complications.*
- Keep limb elevated above heart *to minimize edema.*
- Administer anti-inflammatory agents as ordered *to reduce pain and swelling.*
- Monitor for increasing pain even after analgesic administration *to detect complications.*

 NURSING CARE TIP

- A patient who is confused or comatose may not be able to report pain, which can be problematic because the most reliable indicator of pain is the patient's report. Nonverbal indicators (e.g., grimacing, restlessness, elevated blood pressure and heart rate) are not reliable for pain assessment and should not be used to assume the absence of pain.

- Prevent pain by anticipating it and treating it in advance. This can be done by recognizing causes of pain and understanding that the effects of mild but repetitive pain (as in turning several times a day) can adversely affect the patient (e.g., by leading to exhaustion).
- Causes of pain include conditions or diseases (such as fractures, trauma, or cancer), procedures (such as surgery, turning, or wound care), and biomedical devices (such as orthopedic fixation devices, wound drains, urinary catheters, nasogastric tubes, and chest tubes).
- With few patients being medicated before painful procedures, some of which may be done several times a day (turning), patients who are confused or comatose are at greater risk for lack of pain relief. To keep patients comfortable, provide analgesics as ordered before painful procedures and on a regular basis when pain is assumed to be present. For anticipated pain, use the acronym APP (assume pain present).
- Use pain assessment tools designed for those who are cognitively impaired to ensure that their pain is adequately relieved. The Pain Assessment IN Advanced Dementia (PAINAD) tool, for example, was developed for this purpose. Share pain research findings with institution administrators to establish policies that support proactive pain management for all patients.

Box 46-3 Extremity Care After Cast Removal

- Make sure skin is properly cleansed. Soak rather than rub skin to remove dry scales.
- The extremity likely will be weak, with decreased ROM. Move it gently, and provide analgesics as needed.
- When extremity is not in use, provide support with pillows or orthotic device until strength and movement return.
- Ensure active and passive ROM are performed as recommended by physical therapist and as patient tolerance will allow.
- Lower extremity swelling can be prevented with elastic support stockings.

EVALUATION. The outcome is met if the patient reports or demonstrates that pain is within tolerable levels on a pain assessment scale, demonstrates increased physical mobility, and maintains peripheral pulses, warm skin, sensation, and ability to move extremity.

PATIENT EDUCATION. If the patient has a cast, review appropriate instructions for cast care (see Box 46-2). Health teaching is also important for care of the extremity after cast removal (Box 46-3). If the patient has a wound, teach patient and caregiver how to assess and dress the wound, including pin care if needed, and when to report changes, such as signs and symptoms of infection. Teach the importance of adequate protein, calories, vitamins, and minerals in healing.

Osteomyelitis

Osteomyelitis is an infection of bone that can be either acute (lasts less than 4 weeks) or chronic (lasts more than 4 weeks).

Pathophysiology

Bone infection results from invasion of bacteria into the bone and surrounding soft tissues. Inflammation occurs, followed by ischemia (decreased blood flow; Fig. 46.9). Bone tissue then becomes necrotic (dies), which retards healing and causes more infection, often as a bone abscess.

Etiology

Pathogens enter bone in several ways. Injury to the body allows the offending microbes direct access to bone tissue. An open fracture is an example of that process. Infection beginning in another part of the body can migrate to a bone. For instance, a patient with a total hip replacement may acquire osteomyelitis from a urinary tract infection. The most common pathogen causing osteomyelitis is *Staphylococcus aureus.*

Signs and Symptoms

The patient with acute osteomyelitis has fever, as well as local signs of inflammation, such as tenderness, redness, heat, pain, and swelling. Pain (particularly over the area of infection), may be the only apparent patient concern. Ulceration, drainage, and localized pain are typical signs and symptoms of chronic osteomyelitis.

Diagnostic Tests

The patient with osteomyelitis typically has an elevated white blood cell (WBC) count, an elevated ESR, positive bone biopsy for infection, and possibly a positive blood culture. MRIs, x-rays, and CT scans show infected areas.

Therapeutic Measures

Long-term antibiotic therapy (4–6 weeks) is the treatment of choice for patients with osteomyelitis. Infection in bone tissue is difficult to resolve. Surgery to remove necrotic bone tissue or replace it with healthy bone tissue can also be needed. Amputations are reserved for patients who have massive infections that have not responded to one or more of the conventional treatments.

Nursing Care

Patients receive the IV antibiotics at home. Patients and caregivers require teaching about side effects, toxicity, interactions,

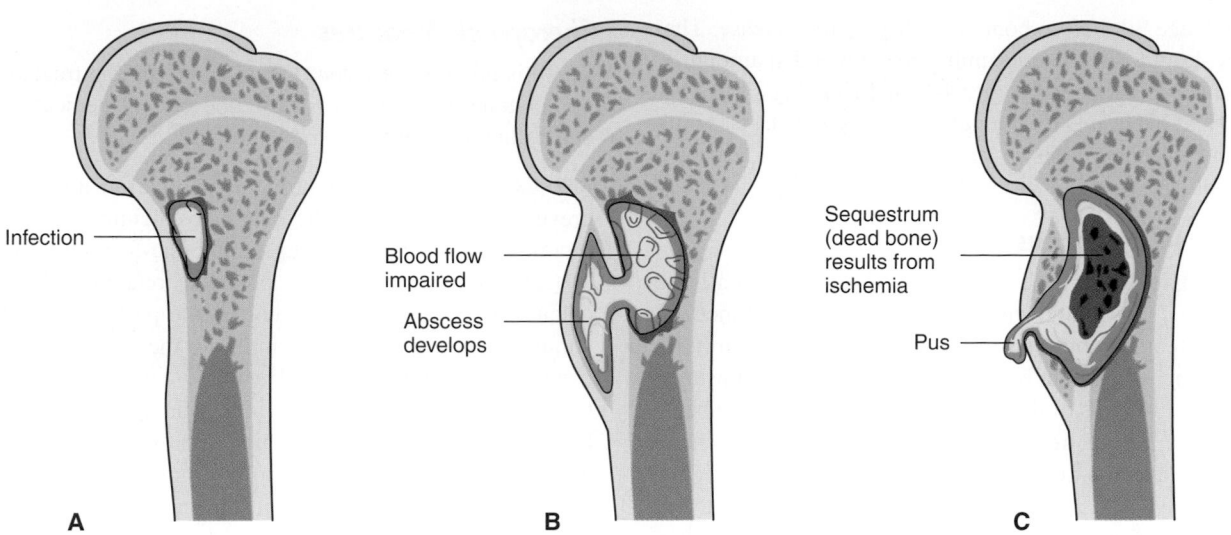

FIGURE 46.9 Sequence of osteomyelitis development. (A) Infection begins. (B) Blood flow is blocked in the area of infection. An abscess with pus forms. (C) Bone dies within the infection site, and pus formation continues.

and precautions for antibiotic therapy. A home health nurse often assists the patient.

If a soft tissue wound is present, ensure that sterile technique is used for dressing changes. The home health nurse teaches the patient and family how to perform dressing changes, the importance of hand hygiene before dressing changes, and how to avoid the spread of pathogens.

Osteoporosis

Osteoporosis (porous bone) is a metabolic disorder in which there is low bone mass and deterioration of bone structure, resulting in fragile bones that are prone to fracture. The spine, wrist, and hip are most commonly involved although all bones can be affected.

Prevalence

More than 57 million people have osteoporosis, or low bone density (National Osteoporosis Foundation, 2013). Women are at greatest risk because their bones are smaller than men's bones. As the U.S. population ages, the incidence and cost of osteoporosis will rise. By 2020, half of all Americans over age 50 may have weak bones. This is significant because hip or vertebral fractures are associated with reduced quality of life, increased disability, and increased risk of death, especially within the year after the fracture.

Pathophysiology

Bone is living tissue that is resorbing (breaking down) old bone tissue (osteoclast cells) and constantly building new bone tissue (osteoblast cells). Normally, this bone remodeling process is balanced. In osteoporosis, an imbalance results. Bone density (mass) peaks between ages 30 and 35. After these peak years, the rate of bone breakdown exceeds the rate of bone buildup. For postmenopausal women, decreased estrogen appears to slow the absorption of calcium, leading to increased bone loss.

Types and Risk Factors

Osteoporosis is categorized as either primary or secondary. Primary osteoporosis is the most common and is not associated with another disease. Some risk factors for primary osteoporosis can be controlled but others cannot. Those that are not controllable include the following:

• Female gender
• Aging
• Caucasian or Asian
• Small boned, petite body build
• Postmenopausal status
• Low testosterone and estrogen in men
• Family history of osteoporosis or fractures
• History of fractures

Risk factors related to lifestyle that are controllable include:

• Cigarette smoking
• Excessive alcohol consumption
• Anorexia nervosa
• Nutrition: low calcium or vitamin D intake, excessive caffeine, protein, or sodium intake
• Sedentary lifestyle

For a Personal Bone Profile Questionnaire, visit www.niams.nih.gov/Health_Info/Bone/Optool/index.asp.

Secondary osteoporosis results from an associated medical condition or procedure, such as hyperparathyroidism; renal dialysis; drug therapy with steroids, certain antiseizure drugs, sleeping medications, aluminum-containing antacids, hormones for endometriosis, or cancer drugs; and prolonged immobility, such as that seen with patients who have a spinal cord injury.

Prevention

To protect against osteoporosis, practicing healthy lifestyle and nutritional habits that build bone are especially important through age 30, before bone mass begins to decrease. These habits should include consuming recommended amounts of calcium (1000 mg/day for ages 4–8, and 1300 mg/day for ages 9–18) and vitamin D (600 mg/day for ages 4–18); performing weight-bearing and muscle-strengthening exercises, especially in childhood; avoiding alcohol; and not smoking.

Signs and Symptoms

Most people do not realize they have osteoporosis until they fracture a bone falling, sustaining a mild bump, or sneezing. With vertebral compression fractures, a decrease in height (up to 6 inches), severe back pain, and the classic "dowager's hump," or kyphosis of the spine, is present as the spine begins to collapse. The patient may be embarrassed by the change in body image and may have curtailed social activities. Some patients have difficulty finding clothes that fit comfortably.

General effects of the disease go beyond the obvious bone deformities. Quality of life can be affected. Acute or chronic pain may occur. Physiological effects can include decreased respiratory capacity due to spinal deformities. It can be difficult to expand the lungs because of curvature of the spine or painful vertebral fractures. This can increase fatigue and the risk of pneumonia. Osteoporosis can be associated with chronic obstructive pulmonary disease (COPD) because of limited activity related to dyspnea and corticosteroid therapy (which breaks down bone).

Functional abilities (ADLs and instrumental activities of daily living [IADLs]) may be limited, which increases the patient's dependence. Emotional effects can relate to body image changes, depression, or anxiety from fear of breaking a bone including during intimacy. Socialization may be reduced because of activity limitations or fear of injury. Because these effects are interrelated, the whole person, not just the disease, needs to be assessed and treated to improve quality of life.

Diagnostic Tests

Dual-energy x-ray absorptiometry (DEXA) is the standard screening tool to measure bone density ("Gerontological Issues"). This noninvasive scan is a low-dose x-ray and takes about 5 minutes to perform while the patient lies on a table. A DEXA scan identifies low bone density at the hip and spine. It can show response to treatment.

Serum calcium and vitamin D values can be decreased, and serum phosphorus may be increased. With severe bone loss, alkaline phosphatase levels may be elevated, confirming bone damage.

Gerontological Issues

Bone mineral density testing can be helpful in assessing the risk of fractures for residents in extended care. Providing treatment for osteoporosis can reduce the risk of hip fractures.

Therapeutic Measures

There is no cure for osteoporosis, but it can be treated. The cornerstone of treatment for osteoporosis is medication and controlling risk factors to prevent bone loss.

MEDICATION.   Supplements and medication are used for prevention or treatment. These include calcium supplements, vitamin D, antiresorptive drugs, and bone-forming drugs.

Calcium is important to prevent bone loss. If serum calcium falls below normal levels, the parathyroid glands stimulate bone to release calcium into the bloodstream. The result is demineralized bone. Therefore, calcium supplements to maintain normal levels are important. The patient should be taught to drink plenty of fluids to prevent calcium-based urinary stones. Vitamin D supplementation, to aid calcium absorption, also may be needed, especially for patients who have reduced exposure to sunlight (residents of extended care facilities or northern geographical areas, for example) or who cannot metabolize vitamin D.

Antiresorptive Medications.   Bisphosphonates are used to prevent or slow the progress of osteoporosis. They bind to bone and suppress osteoclast activity to prevent or reduce the breakdown process. They include alendronate (Fosamax, Fosamax Plus D), ibandronate (Boniva), risedronate (Actonel), and zoledronic acid (Reclast). Bisphosphonates have been shown to be effective for at least 10 years. However, over time bone loss still continues.

Side effects of bisphosphonates include bone, muscle, or joint pain; gastrointestinal (GI) upset; gastric ulcers; and rarely osteonecrosis (bone death) of the jaw. Teach the patient specifically how to take each medication to reduce side effects. Typically, the tablet or solution form is taken in the morning after awakening on an empty stomach. It is followed by a full glass of water (only water) with nothing else to eat or drink for up to 1 hour. The patient should not lie down for at least 30 minutes to 1 hour after taking the drug.

Calcitonin (Fortical, Miacalcin) is a synthetic thyroid hormone and treats osteoporosis by decreasing bone loss. It is used for women who have been menopausal for 5 years. Denosumab (Prolia) is a monoclonal antibody that inhibits the protein that signals bone removal. Raloxifene (Evista) is a selective estrogen receptor modulator (SERM) that increases bone mass by 2% to 3% each year. SERM drugs are designed to mimic estrogen in some parts of the body while blocking its effects elsewhere.

Estrogen therapy may be used to prevent the bone loss that occurs with menopause as estrogen levels fall. However, other treatments should be considered first due to risk factors associated with estrogen therapy.

Anabolic (Bone-Forming) Medications.   Teriparatide (Forteo) is used for men and women at great risk for fracture. Teriparatide increases bone mass by increasing the action and number of osteoblasts that form bone. It should not be taken for more than 2 years.

DIET.   Increasing calcium and vitamin D intake are the main dietary considerations. Generally, calcium intake should be

1000 mg/day for those ages 18 to 49 and 1200 mg for those over age 50. Teach patients which foods are high in calcium, such as dairy products (yogurt and skim milk may have low levels) and dark green, leafy vegetables.

EXERCISE.   Exercise in childhood is essential in preventing osteoporosis. Weight-bearing exercise, especially walking, stimulates bone building. The patient should wear well-supporting, nonskid shoes at all times and avoid uneven surfaces that could contribute to falls. Resistance exercise such as weight training is also beneficial ("Gerontological Issues").

Fall Prevention

Osteoporotic bone may cause a pathological fracture, in which the hip breaks before the fall. For other patients, a fall can cause a hip or other fracture. Therefore, fall prevention programs in hospitals and extended care facilities are important.

In collaboration with the physical or occupational therapist, case manager, or discharge planner, assess the patient's home environment. Patient and family are taught how to create a hazard-free environment, such as avoiding scatter rugs and slippery floors. Walking paths in the home must be kept free of clutter to prevent falls. If needed, a walker or cane provides additional support.

Nursing Care

Nursing care for osteoporosis focuses on education for prevention, providing pain relief and support for symptoms, and medication teaching. For more information, visit the National Osteoporosis Foundation at www.nof.org.

Paget's Disease

Paget's disease is a metabolic bone disease in which there is increased breakdown and formation of bone that results in abnormally formed, weak bones, causing deformities, bone pain and fractures, and osteoarthritis (www.paget.org). Paget's disease affects mainly older adults and men. The most common areas involved are the spine, femur, skull, and pelvis. X-rays show bones with punched-out areas. Bone scan shows how widespread the disease is. An increased serum alkaline phosphatase level occurs due to osteoblast activity. Pain is a major symptom in many. Other symptoms based on the bone affected include limping, joint stiffness, and a pinched nerve with numbness and tingling.

There is no cure for Paget's disease, but medications are used to relieve pain and promote quality of life. NSAIDs are given for pain control, bisphosphonates reduce bone resorption and calcitonin (Fortical, Miacalcin), a synthetic thyroid hormone, decreases bone loss. Exercise maintains bone health and joint mobility. For uncontrolled pain, surgery such as joint replacement can be done. Nursing care aims to provide pain relief, supportive symptom care and education.

Bone Cancer

Bone tumors may be benign or malignant. Malignant tumors may be either primary (originating in the bone) or metastatic, originating from another location and migrating to bone. Metastatic lesions are more common and most often affect older adults.

Primary Malignant Tumors

Osteosarcoma, or osteogenic sarcoma, is the most common primary malignant bone tumor as well as being the most fatal bone tumor. It is a fairly large tumor that typically metastasizes to the lung within 2 years of diagnosis and treatment. It usually affects young people between ages 10 and 25, and boys are twice as likely to develop the disease. Long bones of the legs (particularly around the knees), and arms are most often the sites of origin but it can be found in other bones. Older patients with Paget's disease also may develop these lesions. The disease itself is relatively rare, with an occurrence rate of about 2 per million people.

Pain and swelling in an arm or leg that worsens with exercise or at night are some of the manifestations of osteosarcoma. A lump in the area or an unexplained limp also may be cause for further investigation. X-rays, bone biopsy, CT scan, bone scan, and MRI are helpful in diagnosing the malignancy. Chemotherapy and surgical excision of the affected bone with bone grafting, or amputation of the affected limb are the treatments most commonly used for osteosarcomas.

Ewing's sarcoma is the most malignant bone tumor. In addition to local pain and swelling, systemic signs and symptoms, including low-grade fever, leukocytosis, and anemia, are common. The pelvis and legs are most often affected in children and young men.

Patients with a *chondrosarcoma* (cancer of cartilaginous cells) have a better prognosis than those with the previously described types of bone cancer. This type of cancer occurs in middle-aged and older people.

METASTATIC BONE DISEASE.   Primary malignant tumors that occur in the prostate, breast, lung, and thyroid gland are called bone-seeking cancers because they migrate to bone more than any other primary cancer. Once cancer has metastasized, multiple sites in the bone are typically seen. Pathological fractures and severe pain are major concerns in managing metastatic disease (see Chapter 11).

Signs and Symptoms

Primary tumors cause local swelling and pain at the site. A tender, palpable mass is often present. Metastatic disease is not

Gerontological Issues

Falls become more common as people age. Exercise is one way of reducing falls in older adults. It should focus on these activities: strength, balance, agility, and coordination. Exercise such as yoga, hiking, weight training, and bicycling can be done in groups or individually.

• WORD • BUILDING •
osteosarcoma: osteo—bone + sarc—flesh + oma—tumor

as visible, but the patient reports diffuse severe pain, eventually leading to marked disability.

Diagnostic Tests

Diagnosis of bone cancer is made by x-ray, CT scan, bone scan, bone biopsy, or MRI (see Chapter 45). Patients with metastatic disease have elevated alkaline phosphatase levels and possibly an elevated ESR, indicating secondary tissue inflammation.

Therapeutic Measures

Management of bone cancer depends on the type and extent of the tumor. The treatment of primary bone tumors is usually surgery, often combined with chemotherapy or radiation. The surgeon attempts to salvage the limb and performs a resection of the tumor. For patients with Ewing's sarcoma or early osteosarcoma, external radiation may be the treatment of choice to reduce tumor size and pain.

Care of the postoperative patient is similar to that for any patient undergoing musculoskeletal surgery. Monitoring the neurovascular status of the operative limb is a vital nursing intervention (see Chapters 12 and 45).

For metastatic bone disease, surgery is not appropriate. External radiation is given, primarily for palliation. The radiation is directed toward the most painful sites in an attempt to shrink them and provide more comfort for the patient.

Nursing Care

Nursing care for the patient with bone cancer is not unlike that for patients with any other type of cancer. Help the patient adjust to the diagnosis, and refer the patient to resources such as the American Cancer Society and support groups (www.cancer.org). Chapter 10 describes the nursing care associated with chemotherapy and radiation therapy.

CONNECTIVE TISSUE DISORDERS

Connective tissue disorders comprise a group of more than 100 diseases in which the major signs and symptoms result from joint involvement. Some connective tissue diseases affect only one part of the body; others affect many body organs and systems. Several disorders are discussed here, including gout, osteoarthritis, and rheumatoid arthritis.

Gout

Gout is an easily treated systemic connective tissue disorder from the buildup of uric acid. Men, especially those middle aged and older, are more often affected than women. Patients with gout are seldom hospitalized for their disease.

Pathophysiology

Uric acid is a waste product resulting from the breakdown of proteins (purines) in the body. Urate crystals are formed because of excessive uric acid buildup (**hyperuricemia**) and are deposited in joints and other connective tissues, causing severe inflammation. When an "attack" of gout occurs, the patient has severe pain and inflammation in one or more small joints, usually the great toe. The inflammation may resolve in several days, with or without treatment. Months or years may pass between attacks, and the patient may have no signs or symptoms of joint inflammation between episodes. Urate deposits (tophi) occasionally appear under the skin (outer ear commonly; Fig. 46.10) or in the kidneys or urinary system, causing stone (calculi) formation (see Chapter 37).

Etiology and Types

Primary gout is the most common type of gout and is caused by an inherited problem with purine metabolism. Uric acid production is greater than the kidneys' ability to excrete it. Therefore, the amount of uric acid in the blood increases. Acute attacks of gout may be triggered by stress, alcohol consumption, illness, trauma, dieting, or certain medications.

Patients with secondary gout also experience hyperuricemia, but the increase is the result of another health problem, such as renal insufficiency, or medications, such as diuretic therapy and certain chemotherapeutic agents.

Signs and Symptoms

ACUTE GOUT. Patients with acute gout have one or more severely inflamed joints due to the uric acid crystals, usually small joints, often in the joint of the great toe. The joint is swollen, red, hot, and usually too painful to be touched.

CHRONIC GOUT. Patients with chronic gout may not have obvious signs and symptoms. Renal stones can develop from elevated uric acid.

Diagnostic Tests

Diagnosis of gout is based on an elevated serum uric acid level. Joint fluid aspiration analysis can also identify uric acid crystals in the synovial fluid.

• WORD • BUILDING •

hyperuricemia: hyper—excessive + uric—uric acid + emia— in blood

FIGURE 46.10 Gout: subcutaneous nontender lesions near joints. From Goldsmith, L. A., Lazarus, G. S., Tharp, M. D., et al (1997). *Adult and pediatric dermatology.* Philadelphia: F.A. Davis, p. 405, with permission.

Therapeutic Measures

MEDICATION. Drug therapy is the first-line treatment for primary gout. Treatment for secondary gout involves management or removal of the underlying cause. For an acute gout episode an NSAID, colchicine (Colcrys) or steroids are prescribed until the joint inflammatory response to the urate crystals subsides. If these medications are not tolerated or effective, pegloticase (Krystexxa) by IV infusion can be given every 2 weeks.

Uricosuric agents (medications used to decrease uric acid) are the drug of choice to prevent increased serum uric acid levels. Febuxostat (Uloric) and allopurinol (Zyloprim) decrease uric acid production. The patient must take these drugs every day to keep the uric acid level within the normal range. Probenecid (Benemid) may also be used temporarily to increase renal excretion of uric acid. Serum uric acid level is monitored periodically.

DIET. Certain foods should be avoided or consumed in moderation (Box 46-4). Aspirin, diuretics, and alcohol (especially beer) should be avoided because they can trigger a gout attack. Increasing daily fluid intake helps prevent kidney stones.

Osteoarthritis

Osteoarthritis (OA) is the most common type of connective tissue disorder, affecting more than 20 million people in

---

Box 46-4 Health Promotion for Patients With Gout

- Avoid high-purine (protein) foods, such as organ meats, shellfish, and oily fish (e.g., sardines).
- Avoid alcohol.
- Drink plenty of fluids, especially water.
- Avoid all forms of aspirin and drugs containing aspirin.
- Avoid diuretics.
- Avoid excessive physical or emotional stress.

---

the United States. It is also referred to as degenerative joint disease.

Pathophysiology

OA occurs when the articular cartilage and bone ends of joints slowly deteriorate due to "wear and tear," a normal result of aging (Table 46.3). The joint space narrows, bone spurs develop, and the joint may become somewhat inflamed. The body's repair process is not able to overcome the loss of cartilage and bone, resulting in pain, swelling and stiffness. Weight-bearing joints (hips and knees), hands, and the vertebral column are most often affected (Fig. 46.11).

TABLE 46.3 OSTEOARTHRITIS AND RHEUMATOID ARTHRITIS SUMMARY

	Osteoarthritis	Rheumatoid Arthritis
Pathophysiology	Articular cartilage and bone ends deteriorate. Joint is inflamed.	Inflammatory cells cause synovitis. Synovium becomes thick and fluid accumulates, causing swelling and pain. Joint becomes deformed.
Etiology	*Primary (idiopathic):* • Cause unknown. • Risk factors include age, obesity, activities causing joint stress. *Secondary:* • Causes include trauma, sepsis, congenital abnormalities, metabolic disorders (Paget's disease), rheumatoid arthritis.	Periodontal disease may be a cause. Autoimmune disease. Can occur at any age (including juvenile rheumatoid arthritis). Familial history possible.
Signs and Symptoms	Joint pain and stiffness. Pain increases with activity and decreases with rest. Nodes on joints of fingers (Heberden's nodes, Bouchard's nodes).	Symptoms vary according to disease process. *Early symptoms:* • Bilateral and symmetrical joint inflammation • Redness, warmth, swelling, stiffness, pain • Stiffness after resting (morning stiffness) • Activity decreases pain and stiffness

Continued

TABLE 46.3   OSTEOARTHRITIS AND RHEUMATOID ARTHRITIS SUMMARY—cont'd

	Osteoarthritis	Rheumatoid Arthritis
		• Low-grade fever, weakness, fatigue, anorexia (mild weight loss) • Organ system involvement. *Late symptoms:* • Joint deformity • Secondary osteoporosis.
Therapeutic Measures	Medication • Nonsteroidal anti-inflammatory drugs (NSAIDs) • Acetaminophen • Muscle relaxants. Balanced rest and exercise. Splinting of joint to promote rest. Heat and cold. Diet for weight loss. Complementary therapies. Surgery for total joint replacement.	Medication • Antibiotics • NSAIDs • Biological response modifier • Prednisone • Disease-modifying antirheumatic drug (DMARD) • T-cell modulators. Heat and cold. Balanced rest and activity. Surgery for total joint replacement.
Priority Nursing Diagnoses	*Chronic Pain* *Impaired Physical Mobility* *Disturbed Body Image*	*Chronic Pain* *Self-Care Deficits* *Ineffective Health Maintenance*

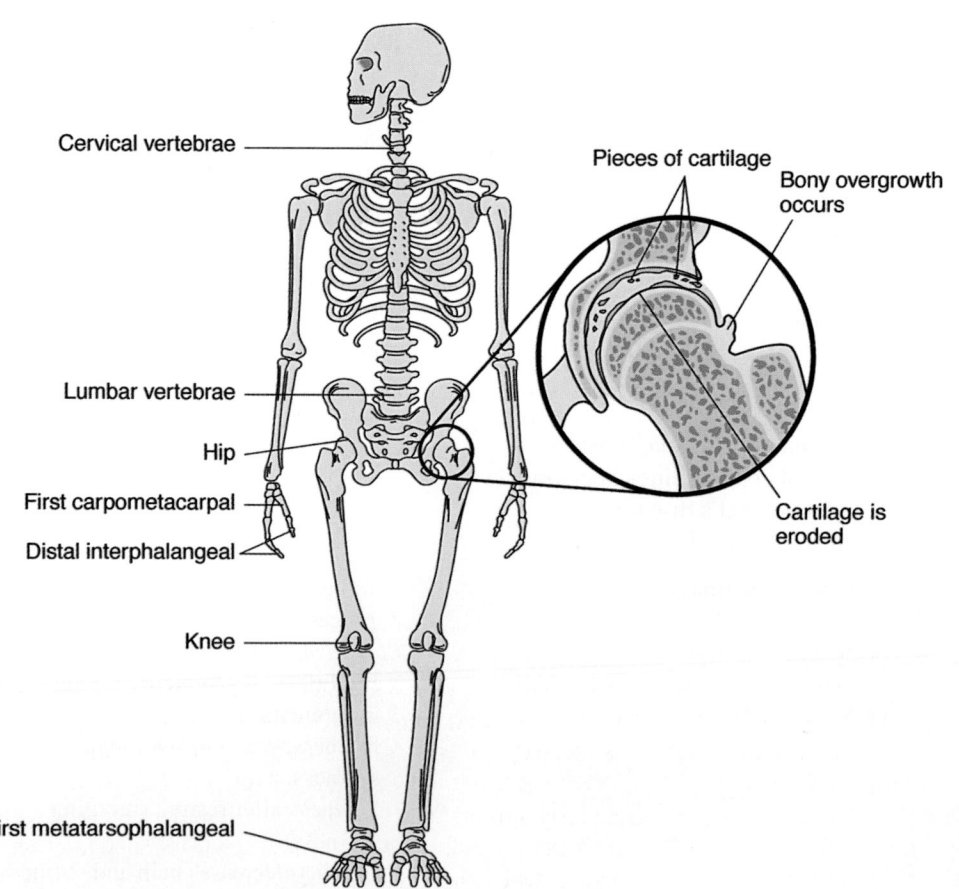

FIGURE 46.11 Common joints affected by osteoarthritis and the changes that result in the joint.

Etiology and Types

The most common type of OA is primary (idiopathic) osteoarthritis. The cause of OA is unknown, but several risk factors have been identified. Aging, obesity, and physical activities that create mechanical stress on synovial joints are major risks. Most people over age 60 have some degree of symptomatic joint degeneration. Native Americans are affected more often than other groups. The reason for this is unknown.

Patients with secondary OA develop joint degeneration as a result of trauma, sepsis, congenital anomalies, certain metabolic diseases (such as Paget's disease), or systemic inflammatory connective tissue disorders such as rheumatoid arthritis.

Signs and Symptoms

The patient usually seeks medical attention when joint pain and stiffness become severe or the patient has problems with everyday activities. One or more joints may be affected, most commonly in the hands, hips, knees, spine, and feet. Joint pain intensifies after physical activity but lessens following rest. If the vertebral column is involved, the patient reports radiating pain and muscle spasms in the extremity innervated by the area affected.

About half of patients with OA have bony nodes on the joints of their fingers, called Heberden's and Bouchard's nodes. Women tend to have them more often than men. They can be painful. The nodes have a familial tendency and often are a cosmetic concern to female patients.

Diagnostic Tests

X-ray examinations are useful in outlining joint structure and detecting bone changes. A CT scan or MRI is used to diagnose joint involvement. Analysis of synovial fluid can aid in the diagnosis of OA while ruling out other pathological joint conditions.

Therapeutic Measures

There is no cure for OA. Pain control is the focus of treatment, which is accomplished by drug therapy, other pain relief measures, or ultimately surgery. An interdisciplinary approach is needed to prevent decreased mobility and preserve joint function.

 EVIDENCE-BASED PRACTICE

Clinical Question
Does acetaminophen work as well or better than NSAIDs when administered for the pain of arthritis?

Evidence
A systematic review of 273 studies looked at the comparative effectiveness, benefits, and adverse effects of analgesics used for osteoarthritis. It was found that acetaminophen does not reduce arthritis pain quite as well as NSAIDs. Each drug class is not without risks. NSAIDS carry GI and cardiovascular risks. Acetaminophen can be toxic to the liver. Topical NSAIDS are effective but can have skin side effects.

Implications for Nursing Practice
Each patient should be encouraged to develop an effective individualized treatment plan with their HCP based on health factors, concurrent medications, family history, body mass index (BMI), age, disease advancement, and effectiveness of pain medication. Adverse effects to report should be taught by the nurse.

REFERENCE
Smith, A., Workman, T., Braun, U., & Fordis, M. (2011). Comparative effectiveness and safety of analgesics for osteoarthritis: An update of the 2006 comparative effectiveness review, comparative effectiveness (Review No. 38), prepared by the Oregon Evidence-based Practice Center under Contract No. HHSA-290-2007-10057-I for the Agency for Healthcare Research and Quality.

Synvisc-One® (one injection) or SYNOVISC® (three injections) are injected directly into osteoarthritic knees to act like healthy, cushioning synovial fluid (www.synviscone.com). Pain is relieved and flexibility restored when the knee joint is again lubricated and cushioned.

CRITICAL THINKING

Mr. Finn

■ Mr. Finn a 59-year-old hardware store manager, is 5'11" and weighs 250 pounds. He visits his HCP because of knee pain. He has noticed that it is becoming increasingly difficult to bend to pick up heavy boxes. The HCP suspects osteoarthritis.

1. What data collection questions should be included in this patient's history?
2. What risk factors does the patient have?
3. What other signs and symptoms might Mr. Finn have?
4. What are patient-centered care interventions for Mr. Finn?
5. What health care team members can provide collaborative care?

Suggested answers are at the end of the chapter.

MEDICATION. Drug therapy is commonly used to reduce pain in patients with OA (see "Evidence-Based Practice"). Often, it is combined with other pain-reducing therapies. The most commonly used drugs are NSAIDs (Table 46.4). These drugs have analgesic and anti-inflammatory effects. Common side effects include GI distress and bleeding, which can be severe; and sodium and fluid retention. They also may increase the risk of cardiovascular events, such as myocardial infarction or stroke. Older patients taking NSAIDs on a routine basis should

TABLE 46.4 COMMON DRUGS USED TO TREAT CONNECTIVE TISSUE DISEASES: OSTEOARTHRITIS, RHEUMATOID ARTHRITIS, AND OTHERS

Medication Class/Action	Examples	Nursing Implications
Biological Response Modifiers Interleukin-1 inhibitors that reduce inflammation and cartilage degradation.	anakinra (Kineret)	Monitor neutrophils.
Corticosteroids Reduce inflammation and swelling.	prednisone (Deltasone, Orasone)	Take daily weight. Monitor intake and output. Assess for infection. Give with food/milk. Recommend patient obtain medic alert ID. Not used for osteoarthritis.
Disease-Modifying Antirheumatic Drugs (DMARDs) For rheumatoid arthritis, ankylosing spondylitis.		Slow-acting drugs may take months for effect.
Reduce symptoms, prevent joint damage, and preserve joint function by suppressing immune or inflammatory systems.		Other drugs used to control symptoms until effective. Effect ends when drug stopped.
Pyrimidine synthesis inhibitors	leflunomide (Arava)	Screen for tuberculosis before starting. Monitor blood pressure, complete blood count, liver function. Teach patient to report rash promptly.
Gold preparations	auranofin (Ridaura) aurothioglucose (Solganal)	Lab testing for gold toxicity effect recommended.
Immunosuppressives	azathioprine (Imuran) cyclophosphamide (Cytoxan) cyclosporine (Sandimmune, Neoral) leflunomide (Arava; rheumatoid arthritis only) methotrexate (Mexate) d-penicillamine (Cuprimine, Depen).	Protect from infection. Monitor for infections.
Tumor necrosis factor inhibitors	adalimumab (Humira) etanercept (Enbrel)	Screen for tuberculosis.
Antimalarials	chloroquine (Aralen) hydroxychloroquine (Plaquenil)	Report vision problems. Promote safety due to dizziness.
Nonsteroidal Anti-Inflammatory Drugs (NSAIDs) Block activity of enzyme cyclooxygenase (COX-1, COX-2),	acetylsalicylic acid (aspirin) diclofenac sodium (Voltaren)	Those with asthma at higher risk for allergic reaction.

TABLE 46.4   COMMON DRUGS USED TO TREAT CONNECTIVE TISSUE DISEASES: OSTEOARTHRITIS, RHEUMATOID ARTHRITIS, AND OTHERS—cont'd

Medication Class/Action	Examples	Nursing Implications
which makes prostaglandins that produce inflammation, fever, pain; support platelets; and protect stomach lining (COX-1 only).	diflunisal (Dolobid) etodolac (Lodine; osteoarthritis only) fenoprofen (Nalfon) flurbiprofen (Ansaid) ibuprofen (Motrin) indomethacin (Indocin) ketoprofen (Orudis) naproxen (Aleve, Naprosyn) oxaprozin (Daypro) piroxicam (Feldene) nabumetone (Relafen) sulindac (Clinoril) tolmetin (Tolectin)	Teaching: Risk of gastrointestinal bleeding.
T-Cell Modulators Reduce activation of T cells in the inflammatory process.	abatacept (Orencia)	Screen for tuberculosis. Use silicone-free syringe only. Infused over 30 minutes. Monitor for serious infections.

be carefully monitored for heart failure and hypertension from fluid retention. Over-the-counter topical creams such as capsaicin (ArthriCare) can be applied to the joints.

REST AND EXERCISE. Joint pain from OA tends to decrease with rest; therefore, pain is less severe in the morning. Activities should be scheduled at this time. A severely inflamed joint may be splinted by the OT or PT to promote rest to a selected joint. However, rest must be balanced with exercise to prevent muscle atrophy from disuse. Exercise has been identified as a means to maintain general health and weight, ROM, and muscle strength, while decreasing anxiety and depression. To minimize muscle atrophy and to stabilize and protect arthritic joints, patients should be encouraged to perform exercises to strengthen their quadriceps if they have OA of the knee.

Joints should always be placed in their functional position—that is, a position that does not lead to contractures. For example, only a small pillow should be placed under the head when sleeping to prevent excessive neck flexion.

HEAT AND COLD. The patient with OA usually prefers heat therapy unless the joint is acutely inflamed. Hot packs, warm compresses, warm showers, moist heating pads, and paraffin dips provide sources of heat. Cold therapy minimizes inflammation while altering cutaneous pain receptors, thereby decreasing pain. Cold packs should be applied for no longer than 20 minutes at a time.

DIET. Obese or overweight patients benefit from losing weight to decrease stress on weight-bearing joints and thereby reduce pain. If the patient is on medications that can alter fluid volumes (corticosteroids), a diet low in sodium may be appropriate.

COMPLEMENTARY AND ALTERNATIVE THERAPIES. The popularity of complementary and alternative therapies to reduce pain and stress has grown tremendously. Imagery, music therapy, acupressure, acupuncture, and other holistic modalities that foster the mind-body-spirit connection work well for many people.

SURGERY. If the patient's pain cannot be managed successfully, a total joint replacement (TJR) may be indicated. TJR is the most common type of **arthroplasty** (see later section on musculoskeletal surgery).

Nursing Process for the Patient With Osteoarthritis

DATA COLLECTION. The patient's report of pain is noted and affected joints observed for signs of inflammation or deformity. Also examined are joint function, alterations in ADLs, and mobility ("Gerontological Issues").

• **WORD • BUILDING •**
arthroplasty: arthro—joint + plasty—creation of

Gerontological Issues

OA affects millions of Americans. Because of the large number of people with this condition, it is recommended that nurses check for OA even when it is not the admitting diagnosis to help identify functional deficits and treatment needs.

OA treatment focuses on pain management and functional ability. In addition, interventions that have been shown to help a hospitalized older adult patient after discharge include:
• Identifying a social support system
• Teaching medication side effects as well as interactions that may cause bleeding
• Encouraging participation in occupational and physical therapy
• Referring to a nutritionist for weight loss if indicated
• Referring for cognitive-behavioral therapy for pain management and coping as prescribed.

NURSING DIAGNOSES, PLANNING, IMPLEMENTATION, AND EVALUATION.

Chronic Pain related to chronic inflammatory disease

EXPECTED OUTCOME: The patient will state that pain is within tolerable levels on a pain assessment scale of 0 to 10.

• Ask patient to rate pain on a scale of 0 to 10 *to determine level of pain and need for pain relief.*
• Provide analgesics as ordered *to help alleviate painful sensations.*
• Collaborate with interdisciplinary team such as pain clinic *to explore alternative pain relief measures.*
• Consider alternative methods of therapy such as guided imagery, distraction, acupuncture, and biofeedback *to use all possible methods of pain control.*

Activity Intolerance related to pain

EXPECTED OUTCOME: The patient will participate in ADLs as tolerated.

• Monitor pain during activity *to provide baseline data for future assessments.*
• Encourage as much independence as possible *to promote activity.*
• Assist with ADLs as needed *to ensure that patient does not become exhausted.*
• Provide pain relief measures before activity *to enable an increase in activity level.*
• Ensure nursing interventions are grouped together *to minimize patient exertion.*
• Collaborate with interdisciplinary team (e.g., occupational therapy, home health physiotherapy) *to utilize their resources and knowledge.*

Chronic Sorrow related to altered body image, altered role, pain, and ongoing losses

EXPECTED OUTCOME: The patient will verbalize improvement in feelings of sorrow.

• Observe patient's affect and mood connected to pain and loss *to provide baseline data.*

• Allow time to discuss feelings and anticipate trigger events *to ensure the patient is aware of what may increase feelings of sorrow.*
• Encourage use of interdisciplinary team such as social worker, psychologist, clergy, or spiritual adviser *to provide alternate methods of dealing with sorrow.*
• Encourage use of support groups *to enable the patient to discuss concerns with others experiencing the same problems.*

Disturbed Body Image related to changes in joint function and structure

EXPECTED OUTCOME: The patient will demonstrate acceptance of changes in body image.

• Encourage patient to discuss feelings and concerns *so patient knows that nurse understands what patient is experiencing.*
• Provide information and clarify misconceptions *to ensure that patient is aware of expected problems and concerns.*
• Encourage socialization *to improve the patient's perceptions of how he or she appears to others.*

Impaired Physical Mobility related to altered joint function and pain

EXPECTED OUTCOME: The patient will demonstrate improved physical mobility.

• Observe mobility capabilities *to provide baseline data.*
• Administer analgesics and anti-inflammatory agents as ordered *to improve joint function and decrease pain.*
• Encourage active range-of-motion exercises *to prevent or minimize further alteration in joint function.*
• Ensure proper positioning and alignment *to promote joint function and decrease pain.*
• Use interdisciplinary team such as physiotherapy and occupational therapy *to utilize resources and knowledge from other sources.*

Self-Care Deficit related to chronic degenerative joint disease

EXPECTED OUTCOME: The patient will be able to provide own self-care.

• Observes patient's self-care abilities *to gather baseline data for planning care.*
• Encourage independence *to decrease feelings of despair about being unable to care for self.*
• Assist when necessary *to minimize frustration when patient cannot perform self-care.*
• Teach patient about assistive devices to help with activities of daily living *to promote self-care.*
• Collaborate with interdisciplinary team such as home care, occupational therapy, or physiotherapy *to acquire assistive devices and use alternate resources.*

EVALUATION. The outcomes are met if patient reports pain is within tolerable levels on a pain assessment scale of 0 to 10, is able to participate in ADLs, verbalizes improvement in feelings of sorrow, demonstrates acceptance of changes in body image, demonstrates improved physical mobility, and is able to provide own self-care.

PATIENT EDUCATION. A vital function of each member of the health care team is health teaching. The patient with OA is seldom admitted to the hospital for treatment of OA unless surgery is scheduled. However, many patients with OA are admitted for other reasons, and their arthritis needs must also be considered in the comprehensive plan of care. Most patients residing in extended care facilities also have OA, which can affect their participation in recreational activities, as well as ADLs.

Patients can be taught ways to protect their joints and conserve energy. For educational materials and self-help courses, visit the Arthritis Foundation at www.arthritis.org.

Rheumatoid Arthritis

Rheumatoid arthritis (RA) is a chronic, progressive, systemic inflammatory disease that destroys synovial joints and other connective tissues, including major organs.

Pathophysiology

Inflammatory cells and chemicals cause **synovitis**, an inflammation of the synovium (the lining of the joint capsule). As the inflammation progresses, the synovium becomes thick and fluid accumulation causes joint swelling and pain. A destructive pannus (new synovial tissue growth infiltrated with inflammatory cells) erodes the joint cartilage and eventually destroys the bone within the joint (Fig. 46.12). Ultimately the pannus is converted to bony tissue, resulting in loss of mobility. Joint deformity and bone loss are common in late RA (see Table 46.3).

Any connective tissue may be affected in RA, including blood vessels, nerves, kidneys, pericardium, lungs, and subcutaneous tissue. Dysfunction or failure of the organ or system can occur. Death can result if the disease does not respond to treatment.

Many patients experience spontaneous remissions and exacerbations (flare-ups) of RA. Symptoms may disappear without treatment for months or years. Then the disease flares up just as unpredictably often due to physical or emotional stress.

Etiology

Oral pathogens might be a cause of RA. Studies have shown that the symptoms of RA improve with antibiotic treatment (Ogrendik, 2013). In RA, an autoimmune response occurs that affects the synovial membrane of the joints. Antibodies (called rheumatoid factor) are often found in patients with RA. It is suggested that these antibodies join with other antibodies and form antibody complexes. These complexes lodge in synovium and other connective tissues, causing local and systemic inflammation, and may be responsible for the destructive changes of RA in body tissues.

RA affects people with a family history of the disease two to three times more often than the rest of the population.

Signs and Symptoms

Signs and symptoms vary because the disease progresses differently in patterns and rates from person to person. In general, the signs and symptoms can be divided into early and late manifestations.

The typical pattern of joint inflammation is bilateral and symmetrical. The disease usually begins in the upper extremities and progresses to other joints over many years (Fig. 46.13). Affected joints are slightly reddened, warm, swollen, stiff, and painful. The patient with RA often has morning stiffness lasting for up to an hour, and those with severe disease may report experiencing stiffness all day. Generally, activity decreases pain and stiffness.

Because of the systemic nature of RA, the patient may have a low-grade fever, malaise, depression, lymphadenopathy, weakness, fatigue, anorexia, and weight loss. As the disease worsens, major organs or body systems are affected. Joint deformities occur as a late symptom, and secondary osteoporosis (bone loss) can lead to fractures.

Several associated syndromes are seen in some patients with rheumatoid arthritis. For example, Sjögren's syndrome is an inflammation of tear ducts (causing dry eyes) and salivary glands (causing dry mouth). Felty's syndrome is less common and is characterized by an enlarged liver and spleen and leukopenia (decreased WBC count).

FIGURE 46.12 Rheumatoid arthritis.

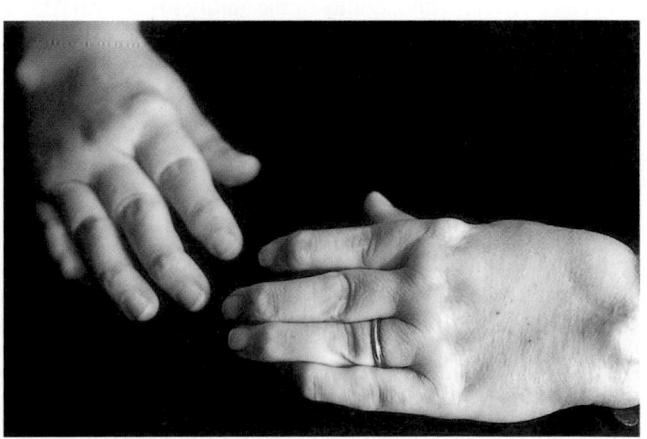

FIGURE 46.13 Joint abnormalities in hands of patient with rheumatoid arthritis.

Diagnostic Tests

No specific diagnostic test confirms RA. An increase in WBCs and platelets is typical, unless the patient has Felty's syndrome. Immunological tests findings for patients with RA usually include the following:

- Presence of rheumatoid factor (RF) in serum
- Decreased red blood cell (RBC) count
- Decreased C4 complement
- Increased erythrocyte sedimentation rate (ESR)
- Positive antinuclear antibody (ANA) test
- Positive C-reactive protein (CRP) test.

RF can indicate the aggressiveness of the disease. However, it is not specific to RA. The ESR test screens for inflammation. It measures the amount of time it takes for RBCs to settle to the bottom of a test tube. In the presence of inflammation, RBCs settle faster in the tube. Therefore, the ESR increases with the presence of inflammation. It also evaluates the effectiveness of treatment. If the disease responds to treatment, the ESR decreases.

LEARNING TIP

Avoid shaking hands with people who have RA. A simple "Nice to meet you" or a fist bump can be more appropriate at times and will avoid the pain of even a weak handshake.

X-ray examination and MRI detect joint damage and bone loss, especially in the vertebral column. A bone or joint scan assesses the extent of joint involvement throughout the body. For some patients, an arthrocentesis may be performed; the synovial fluid is cloudy, milky, or dark yellow with inflammatory cells present.

Therapeutic Measures

Antibiotics may improve the symptoms of RA. Chronic joint pain can interfere with mobility or the ability to perform ADLs. Drug therapy can relieve or reduce pain as well as to slow the progression of the disease. Disease-modifying antirheumatic drugs can prevent joint destruction, deformity, and disability with early single or combination drug use; NSAIDs; and corticosteroids (see Table 46.4). Many of these medications have potentially serious side effects, such as severe infection, and must be monitored carefully.

Complementary therapies that may help decrease inflammation or pain include capsaicin cream, fish oil, and antioxidants such as vitamin C, vitamin E, and beta carotene (see Chapter 5).

HEAT AND COLD. Heat applications or hot showers help decrease joint stiffness and make exercise easier for the patient. For acutely inflamed, or "hot," joints, cold applications are preferred. A program that balances rest and exercise is most beneficial for the patient.

SURGERY. If nonsurgical approaches are not effective in relieving arthritic pain, the patient may have a total joint replacement (discussed later).

Nursing Process for the Patient With Rheumatoid Arthritis

DATA COLLECTION. A complete history and physical examination are needed for the patient with RA because the disease can involve every system of the body. In addition to assessing physical signs and symptoms, assess the patient for psychosocial, functional, and vocational needs.

After having the disease for approximately 15 years, fewer than half of RA patients are totally independent in their ADLs. These limitations may place a burden on family members, who must be included in the care of the patient with RA. Many patients with the disease are young or middle-aged. RA can impair their ability to work, depending on the type of job they have. The health care team assesses the patient's work skills to determine the need for changes in the workplace or a need to train for a new type of work.

NURSING DIAGNOSES, PLANNING, AND IMPLEMENTATION.

Acute Pain related to chronic disease process
EXPECTED OUTCOME: The patient will report relief from pain within 30 minutes of pain relief intervention.

- Ask patient to rate pain on a scale of 0 to 10 *to determine level of pain and need for pain relief.*
- Provide analgesics as ordered *to relieve pain.*
- Ensure proper positioning and alignment *to minimize discomfort and promote pain relief.*
- Teach alternative measure of pain relief *to maximize means to relieve pain.*
- Encourage maintenance of normal weight *to prevent excess wear and tear on joints.*

Disturbed Body Image related to changes resulting from disease process
EXPECTED OUTCOME: The patient will come to accept alterations in body.

- Encourage patient to discuss feelings and concerns *to provide the nurse with an understanding of what the patient is experiencing.*
- Provide information and clarify misconceptions *to ensure that the patient is aware of the expected problems and concerns.*
- Encourage socialization *to improve on the patient's perceptions of how he or she "looks" to others.*
- Encourage sharing with support groups *so that the patient discusses his or her concerns with others experiencing the same problems.*

Fatigue related to chronic pain and limited mobility
EXPECTED OUTCOME: The patient will have decreased episodes of fatigue.

- Monitor levels of fatigue throughout the day *to determine the patient's reaction to various activities.*
- Ensure regular rest periods throughout the day *to not overexert the patient.*

- Assist as required *to minimize the amount of energy the patient needs to use.*
- Teach patient the need to delegate *to avoid overexertion.*
- Teach energy conservation techniques *to reduce workload.*

Self-care Deficit related to chronic degenerative disease process

EXPECTED OUTCOME: The patient will be able to provide own self-care.

- Observe patient's ability to care for self *to determine level of ability and adjust patient's plan of care.*
- Encourage independence *to decrease feelings of despair about being unable to care for self.*
- Assist when necessary *to minimize frustration when patient is unable to perform self-care function.*
- Teach patient about assistive devices *to help with activities of daily living and promote self-care.*
- Collaborate with interdisciplinary team such as home care and occupational or physical therapy *to acquire assistive devices and use alternate resources.*

Impaired Physical Mobility related to chronic inflammation of joints

EXPECTED OUTCOME: The patient will have improved physical mobility.

- Administer analgesics and anti-inflammatory agents *to reduce pain and increase mobility.*
- Administer heat and cold therapy *to aid in joint function and movement.*
- Encourage continued mobilization *to minimize complications of immobility.*
- Collaborate with other disciplines *to help with maintaining mobility.*

EVALUATION. The outcomes are met if the patient reports pain is within acceptable levels on a pain assessment scale of 0 to 10, demonstrates acceptance of changes in body image, has decreased episodes of fatigue, is able to provide own self-care, and demonstrates improved physical mobility.

CRITICAL THINKING

Mrs. Harris

■ Mrs. Harris is a 48-year-old nurse who has had upper extremity joint pain and swelling for about 4 years. She was recently diagnosed with RA but has no systemic involvement other than extreme fatigue at this time. She is concerned that she will have to give up providing direct patient care on a busy medical unit in the local hospital.

1. What questions might the nurse ask her at this time about her illness?
2. What should the nurse discuss with Mrs. Harris about pain management?

Suggested answers are at the end of the chapter.

PATIENT EDUCATION. The patient with RA needs extensive patient education regarding the disease process, medication management, and the comprehensive plan of care. In collaboration with health team members, help the patient plan a daily schedule that balances rest and exercise. Child care responsibilities and other day-to-day activities need to be scheduled. A vocational counselor may be necessary for job training if the patient needs to pursue a different occupation. Patients who are unable to work may be able to qualify for disability benefits through the federal Social Security program. Inform the patient about community resources such as support groups (www.arthritis.org).

 MUSCULOSKELETAL SURGERY

Some health problems cannot be managed conservatively and require surgery. The most common orthopedic surgeries are discussed here.

Total Joint Replacement

Total joint replacement (TJR) is most often performed for patients who have some type of connective tissue disease in which their joints become severely deteriorated. TJR may also be done for patients on long-term steroid therapy, such as patients with systemic lupus erythematosus (SLE) or asthma. Long-term use of steroids, trauma, and complications of joint replacement can cause **avascular necrosis**, a condition in which bone tissue dies (usually the femoral head) as a result of impaired blood supply. Advanced avascular necrosis is very painful and usually does not respond to conservative pain relief measures. The primary goal of TJR is to relieve severe chronic pain and improve ability to carry out ADLs when no other treatment is successful.

The most common surgeries are the total hip replacement (THR) and total knee replacement (TKR) surgeries, although any synovial joint can be replaced, including finger joints. Another term used for joint replacement is *arthroplasty.* The replacement devices, sometimes referred to as prostheses, are made of metal, ceramic, plastic, or a combination of these materials. Some prostheses are held in place by cement. Others are secured by the patient's bone as it grafts and connects to the prosthesis. Bone substitutes, also called biologics, are used when the amount of available bone is insufficient to provide a good base of support for the replacement devices.

Total Hip Replacement

A THR uses two components: an acetabular cup that is inserted into the pelvic acetabulum and a femoral component that is inserted into the femur to replace the femoral head and neck (Fig. 46.14). A THR lasts 15 years to a lifetime.

PREOPERATIVE CARE. TJR is an elective procedure and scheduled far enough in advance to allow ample time for preoperative

• WORD • BUILDING •
avascular necrosis: a—without + vascular—blood + necrosis—death

FIGURE 46.14 Total hip arthroplasty of arthritic right hip. From McKinnis, L. N. (1997). *Fundamentals of orthopedic radiology.* Philadelphia: F.A. Davis, p. 233, with permission.

teaching and screening. A case manager (registered nurse or social worker) may be assigned to assess the patient's needs and the support systems that are available postoperatively. It is important for the patient to have a caregiver who can assist the patient after surgery.

In addition to the normal preparations for preoperative care (see Chapter 12), the orthopedic patient requires preoperative baseline assessments. The nurse assesses the neurovascular status (circulation, sensation, mobility) of the extremity to be operated on as well as the patient's level of pain preoperatively. Preoperative mobility is noted to assist in determining the effectiveness of the surgery. The patient is taught about the surgery and what to expect postoperatively. Some patients are scheduled to meet with the PT to learn postoperative exercises and how to ambulate with a walker or crutches.

Depending on the amount of blood loss during surgery, some patients receive postoperative blood transfusions. Because TJR is an elective procedure, the HCP may order autologous blood donation by the patient. The patient donates blood before surgery per guidelines (e.g., time frames specified, hemoglobin levels normal), which is then available for reinfusion postoperatively as needed. This predeposited blood donation is cost-effective and reassures patients who are concerned about receiving blood from other donors.

Patients are often admitted to the hospital the morning of surgery. A prophylactic antibiotic preoperatively is given just before surgery to minimize the chance of an infection (especially osteomyelitis) developing. The patient's length of stay varies but is about 2 to 5 days, depending on the patient's age and progress. Some hospitals have joint camp programs where a group of patients undergoing joint replacements are admitted on the same day, undergo their surgery, and then recover together during activities such as physical therapy with each other for support.

POSTOPERATIVE CARE. Care for the patient having a total hip replacement is interdisciplinary. The patient usually gets out of bed and into a chair the night of surgery or early the next day. Ensure that the patient does not adduct or hyperflex the surgical hip during transfer to the chair. The chair should have a straight back and be high enough to prevent excessive flexion. The toilet seat should also be raised for the same purpose. Permitted amounts of weight bearing depend on the type of prosthesis used. In general, weight bearing as tolerated or full weight bearing is used for cemented prostheses. If an uncemented device is used, the patient may be restricted to toe-touch, partial weight bearing, or featherweight bearing.

Because patients undergoing total hip replacement are in chronic pain preoperatively, some patients report that they have less pain postoperatively than they had before surgery. Initially, pain typically is managed by epidural analgesia, patient-controlled analgesia (PCA), or injections with analgesics. After the first postoperative day, the patient usually progresses to an oral analgesic.

Early ambulation helps prevent postoperative complications such as atelectasis and deep vein thrombosis (DVT). The PT works with the patient for ambulation, a walker or crutches. After 4 to 6 weeks, the patient progresses to a cane. The patient does not need an ambulatory device if there is no limping.

Because of restrictions in hip flexion, patients are instructed not to bend forward to tie shoes or put on pants. The OT provides adaptive or assistive devices, such as dressing sticks and long-handled shoe horns, to assist the patient in being independent in ADLs.

In addition to providing the general postoperative care that all patients undergoing general or epidural anesthesia require, plan and implement interventions to help prevent the following common complications of THR (see Chapter 12).

Hip Dislocation. The most common postoperative complication for the patient having a total hip replacement is subluxation (partial dislocation) or total dislocation. Dislocation occurs when the femoral component becomes dislodged from the acetabular cup. Often, if a dislocation occurs, there is an audible "pop" followed by immediate pain in the affected hip. In addition to pain, the patient experiences shortening of the surgical leg and possibly internal rotation of the surgical leg. If any of these signs and symptoms occur, notify the surgeon immediately and keep the patient in bed. Additional analgesics may be ordered until the patient can be taken to the operating room. Under anesthesia, the surgeon manually manipulates the hip back into alignment and immobilizes the leg until healing occurs.

Prevention of dislocation is a major nursing responsibility. Correct positioning of the surgical leg is critical. The primary goals are to prevent hip adduction (across the body's midline) and hyperflexion (bending forward more than 90 degrees). To accomplish these goals, place the patient returning from the perianesthesia care unit (PACU) in a supine position with the head slightly elevated. A trapezoid-shaped abduction pillow (sometimes called a triangular pillow), splint, wedge, or regular bed pillows may be placed between the legs to prevent adduction. The patient can be turned to the side specified by the HCP (even the operative side if the patient is comfortable enough), with hip adduction avoided. The patient is turned with the abductor pillow or three regular pillows (one proximal and two distal) in place between the legs. When turning, it is important to turn the hip and legs simultaneously to minimize the chance of dislocation. Support for the leg and abductor pillow is also required when the patient is turned on his or her side to decrease the chance of dislocation.

To prevent hyperflexion, some surgeons initially allow the patient to sit at no more than a 60-degree angle in a reclining chair. The patient's position is progressed to 90 degrees, the maximum allowed to prevent hyperflexion (Fig. 46.15). While the patient is on bedrest, the use of a fracture bedpan is recommended when helping the patient with toileting needs to minimize discomfort and to prevent the possibility of dislocation.

Skin Breakdown. Because most patients having total joint replacements are older, skin breakdown prevention is a major part of postoperative care. Turning the patient at least every 2 hours (more often if high risk) and keeping the heels off the bed help prevent pressure ulcers. Heels, elbows, and the sacrum are vulnerable and can break down in 24 hours. A reddened area that does not blanch is a stage 1 pressure ulcer and must be treated aggressively to prevent progression to other stages. Prophylactic application of cushioning dressings and the use of heel protectors help to decrease the chance of skin breakdown of the heels.

Patients who are incontinent must be kept clean and dry. Assisting the patient to use the toilet every 2 hours and using a protective barrier cream also help prevent skin problems related to incontinence. Adequate diet and hydration are also important to prevent skin breakdown. Box 46-5 describes additional nursing interventions that meet the needs of postoperative patients recovering from THR.

Infection. Orthopedic surgery patients are at an increased risk for infection because of the nature of the surgery and age. In addition to a preoperative prophylactic IV antibiotic, the surgeon can irrigate the incision with antibiotics intra-operatively, place antibiotic beads in the incision, or continue IV antibiotics for 24 hours postoperatively.

Depending on institution policies, the surgeon may be the one who removes the initial dressing. Regardless of who removes the dressing, meticulous aseptic care of the surgical wound is important to minimize the chance of infection. Care

of the incision, as well as exit sites for drains, is performed aseptically. When performing dressing changes, observe the incision for signs and symptoms of infection (redness, swelling, warmth, odor, pain, or yellow, green, or brown-tinged drainage). Monitor temperature. An older patient with an infection might not experience a fever, but may exhibit confusion due to the infection.

Infection may not occur during the patient's hospital stay but can occur 1 or more years later. If this late infection does not respond to antibiotics, the prosthesis may be removed and replaced.

Box 46-5 Nursing Interventions Following Total Hip Replacement

- Ensure the hip is not allowed to become adducted. Can use abductor pillow or pillows.
- Turning patient requires abduction to be maintained. Turn patient as a whole, not allowing hip or legs to fall forward or backward. Use pillows to support raised limb.
- Monitor for skin integrity of the opposite heel, which often is used to help mobilize in bed and so is prone to friction and pressure sores. Apply protective devices for heels.
- Make sure limb remains in abduction when moving patient out of bed.
- Prevent postoperative pneumonia by encouraging deep breathing and coughing and use of incentive spirometer.
- Pain control is of utmost importance. Provide regularly scheduled analgesics, and make sure breakthrough analgesia is provided as needed. Decreased pain allows for earlier mobilization and fewer complications of immobility.
- Monitor level of consciousness and orientation. Many older patients have alterations in mental status after surgery because of anesthetics, analgesics, blood loss, and environmental changes.

Correct hip flexion   Incorrect hip flexion

≤90°   >90°

FIGURE 46.15 Hip flexion after total hip replacement should be 90 degrees or less to prevent dislocation.

CRITICAL THINKING

Mrs. Adam

■ Mrs. Adam is 78 years old and had a left total hip replacement 3 days ago. When changing her dressing, the nurse notices a purulent discharge. Cefaclor (Ceclor) 500 mg by mouth every 8 hours is ordered. It is available as a 375-mg/5-mL suspension. How many milliliters should Mrs. Adam be given?

Suggested answers are at the end of the chapter.

Bleeding. In TJR, up to two-thirds of any blood loss can occur postoperatively. The patient might have a surgical drain (e.g., Hemovac or Jackson-Pratt) that is emptied every 8 to 12 hours as ordered for the first day or two, although the use of drains has decreased to prevent infection. Monitor dressings for drainage and report large or unexpected amounts. Reinforce it as needed. On the second or third postoperative day, the patient's hemoglobin and hematocrit may decrease to the point that blood transfusion is needed. The patient might receive autologous blood or salvaged operative or postoperative blood. By using an orthopedic patient autotransfusion (such as OrthoPAT®) during surgery, about 50% of blood that is lost can be recovered and saved for reinfusion into the same patient. Postoperatively, blood can be replaced by collecting shed blood via suction into a reservoir, then filtering and reinfusing it within 6 hours of collection. Monitoring for blood loss and signs of shock is an important nursing action.

Neurovascular Compromise. For any musculoskeletal surgery or injury, frequent neurovascular checks for circulation (color, warmth, pulses), sensation, and movement are performed distal to the surgical procedure or injury (and compared with the unaffected side) when vital signs are checked. The procedure and significance of these assessments are described in Chapter 45.

Venous Thromboembolic Complications. Patients having hip surgery are at the greatest risk for DVT or pulmonary embolus. Older adult patients, obese patients and those with a history of thromboembolic problems are also at a high risk for potentially fatal problems. Thigh-high elastic stockings and intermittent pneumatic compression devices may be used while the patient is hospitalized (see Chapter 12). Anticoagulant medication is given to help prevent clot formation.

 NURSING CARE TIP

When giving anticoagulant medications such as enoxaparin (Lovenox) or dalteparin (Fragmin), follow manufacturer's instructions for administration. The air bubble should not be removed from the prefilled syringe before administration to ensure the whole dose is given.

Because most DVTs occur in the lower extremities, leg exercises are started in the immediate postoperative period and continued until the patient is fully ambulatory. The PT teaches the patient how to perform foot and ankle exercises such as heel pumping, foot circles, and straight-leg raises. The patient also performs quadriceps-setting exercises (quad sets) by straightening the legs and pushing the back of the knees toward the bed. Remind the patient to do several sets of these exercises each day to improve muscle tone and to help prevent blood clots in the leg.

If the patient is medically stable, he or she is discharged home for rehabilitation or to a subacute care unit, rehabilitation unit, or nursing home for short-term rehabilitation, lasting a week or less. The rehabilitation program that began in the hospital continues after discharge until the patient is independent in ambulation and self-care.

Before hospital discharge, the interdisciplinary team provides patient education for home care, including hip precautions that need to be used until the surgeon reevaluates the patient at the 6- to 8-week follow-up visit (Box 46-6).

Total Knee Replacement

The knee is the second most commonly replaced joint. It requires three components for total replacement: a femoral component, a tibial component, and a patellar button (Fig. 46.16).

Box 46-6 Patient Education After Total Hip Replacement

Follow these safety measures to prevent hip dislocation:

- Keep legs abducted (away from center of body) with pillows.
- Sleep with pillows between legs until HCP states otherwise.
- Bend at the waist (hip) no more than 90 degrees.
- Get up from a sitting position by pushing straight up off of the chair or bed without leaning forward.
- Use a walker, if desired, to assist walking.
- Physiotherapy and occupational therapy can provide equipment that aids in putting on socks and shoes.
- Sexual activity can be started when tolerated, provided hip safety measures are followed.

FIGURE 46.16 Knee joint replacement. From Richardson, J. K., & Iglarsh, Z. A. (1994). *Clinical orthopaedic physical therapy.* Philadelphia: W.B. Saunders, p. 651, with permission.

For patients who do not yet need a total replacement, partial knee resurfacing is available.

Care for the patient with a TKR is similar to that required for a patient with a hip replacement except that dislocation, and therefore preventive positioning, are not a concern. Postoperatively, a bulky dressing and possibly a surgical drain are in place. Once again, it is important to monitor for bleeding along with the usual postoperative interventions. Medical complications described for THR, such as DVT, may be seen in the patient undergoing knee replacement (see Box 46-5).

Amputation

An amputation is the removal of a body part, which can be as limited as removing part of a finger or as devastating as removing nearly half the body. Amputations may be *surgical* as a result of disease or *traumatic* as a result of an accident.

Surgical Amputation

The main indication for surgical amputations is ischemia from peripheral vascular disease (PVD) in the older adult. The rate of lower extremity amputation is much higher in the diabetic patient than in the nondiabetic patient (see diabetes in Chapter 40). Surgical amputations may also be done for bone tumors, thermal injuries (frostbite, electric shock), crushing injuries, congenital problems, or infections.

Traumatic Amputation

Traumatic amputations occur from accidents, often in young and middle-aged adults. Industrial machinery, motor vehicles, lawn mowers, chain saws, and snow blowers are common causes of accidental amputation.

Because in these patients the amputated part is usually healthy, attempts at **replantation** can occur. One of the most common replantations is one or more fingers. Prehospital care of the severed body part includes rinsing if dirty and wrapping in a clean, moist cloth that is placed in a sealed plastic bag. The bag should then be placed into ice cold water until the body part is transported to the hospital. The surgical procedure is performed by specialists who operate using a microscope. Nerves, vessels, and muscle must be reattached.

Levels of Amputation

The most common surgical amputation site is the lower extremity. The loss of the great toe affects balance and gait. Midfoot amputations are preferred over below-the-knee amputations for patients with peripheral vascular disease. The more proximal the amputation, the more disability is present.

If the lower leg is amputated, a below-the-knee amputation is preferred over an above-the-knee amputation to preserve joint function. The higher the level of amputation, the more energy required for ambulation. Hip disarticulation (removal through the hip joint) and **hemipelvectomy** (removal through part of the pelvis) are reserved for young patients who have cancer or severe trauma. Rarely, a hemicorporectomy (hemipelvectomy plus a translumbar amputation) is performed as a last resort for young patients with cancer. This radical surgery removes nearly half of the body and requires both bowel and urinary diversion surgeries (ostomies) as well.

Upper extremity amputations are usually more significant than lower extremity amputations and more often result from trauma. The arms and hands are necessary for performing ADLs. Early replacement with a prosthesis is crucial for the patient with an upper extremity amputation.

Preoperative Care

Patients who are scheduled for elective amputations have the advantage of time for preoperative teaching, prosthesis fitting, and adjustment to the loss of part of their bodies. Preoperative teaching is started in the surgeon's office. Postoperative and rehabilitative care is reviewed with the patient and family or significant other. Those patients experiencing a traumatic amputation have no opportunity to prepare for the significant changes that will result from the accident. Preoperative care will not only involve physical needs being met, but significant psychological and emotional concerns also have to be addressed (this also continues postoperatively).

Preoperatively, the patient should be referred to a certified prosthetist-orthotist to begin plans for replacing the removed body part with a prosthesis.

Disturbed Body Image is a common nursing diagnosis for the patient having an amputation. If possible, it is helpful for the preoperative patient to meet with a rehabilitated amputee. Assess the patient's reaction to having an amputation with the expectation that the patient will experience many of the stages of loss and grieving. Support systems and coping mechanisms are identified that can help the patient through the surgery and postoperative period. Ensure that appropriate support is provided by other disciplines such as social work and clergy.

Postoperative Care

In addition to the general postoperative care described here, plan and implement interventions to help prevent postoperative complications, including hemorrhage and infection (see Chapter 12).

PREVENTION OF HEMORRHAGE AND INFECTION. When a patient loses part of the body, because of either surgery or trauma, blood vessels are severed or damaged. The patient returns from surgery with a large pressure dressing that is secured with an elastic wrap. Assess the closest proximal pulse between the heart and the amputated body part for strength and compare findings with the nonsurgical extremity. Assess the bulky dressing for bloody drainage. If blood is on the dressing when the patient is admitted to the PACU or the surgical unit, circle, date, and time the area of drainage and closely monitor for enlargement. If bleeding continues, the surgeon is notified immediately. A tourniquet should be readily available in case severe hemorrhage occurs.

After the dressing is removed, observe for adequate perfusion to the skin flap at the end of the residual limb, referred to as the stump. The skin should be pink in a light-skinned

• WORD • BUILDING •

replantation: re—again + plant—to plant + ation—process
hemipelvectomy: hemi—half + pelv—pelvis + ectomy—removal of

patient and not discolored (lighter or darker than other skin pigmentation) in a dark-skinned patient. The residual limb temperature to touch should be warm but not hot.

Infection of the wound can be problematic, especially if the infection enters the bone (osteomyelitis). Inspect the wound for intense redness or drainage. Localized infections usually do not cause an increase in body temperature. If temperature is elevated, it could indicate a serious wound infection, a systemic infection, or some other type of infection. Traumatic amputations are at risk for developing infection due to the nature of the injury and the likelihood of exposure to environmental pathogens from the source of the amputation.

PAIN CONTROL. Phantom pain arises from the spinal cord and brain. The patient reports severe pain usually distal to the removed body part. The pain may be described as intense burning, cramping, shooting, stabbing, or throbbing. Phantom pain can be triggered by touching the residual limb, fatigue, emotional stress, or weather changes. It can improve over time.

Never doubt that a patient is experiencing phantom pain. Phantom sensation is different from phantom pain in that the patient feels as if the limb is still present rather than being painful. Treat phantom pain with prescribed medication and complementary and alternative therapies. Medications used include anticonvulsants, such as gabapentin (Gralise, Neurontin) or pregabalin (Lyrica), beta-blocking agents, such as propranolol (Inderal), and antidepressants like amitriptyline (Elavil). To complement traditional therapy, a number of alternative therapies may be useful, including biofeedback, nerve stimulation, myoelectric prosthesis, massage, mirror box (watch unaffected limb while moving), imagery, acupuncture, spinal cord or brain stimulation (small electric current used). Future therapy involves virtual reality goggles (appears as if no amputation occurred).

MOBILITY AND AMBULATION. To reduce surgical swelling, cold application may be ordered. Alternately, the residual limb may be elevated on a pillow for 24 hours or less. Continued use of a pillow for elevation can lead to flexion contractures, especially for patients with a below-the-knee or above-the-knee amputation. If the hip becomes contracted, using a prosthesis will not be possible because the patient will not be able to walk. Check the limb periodically to ensure that it lies completely flat on the bed. The patient should avoid positions of flexion such as sitting for long periods. If the patient is able, lying prone (on the stomach) for 30 minutes four times daily helps prevent hip contracture (abnormal shortening of muscle or scar tissue).

Postoperative care after amputation is interdisciplinary, often requiring an extensive rehabilitation program in a subacute unit, an extended care facility, or on an ambulatory basis. The PT teaches the patient muscle-strengthening exercises that help with ambulation and transfers and prevent flexion contractures. A trapeze bar on an overhead bed frame aids in strengthening the arms and helps the patient move around in bed.

PROSTHESIS CARE. The residual limb must be prepared for wearing the prosthesis. A temporary prosthesis may be worn until the swelling subsides.

The residual limb is wrapped at least every 8 hours using an elastic wrap (such as an Ace wrap) in a figure-of-eight

fashion (Fig. 46.17). It is important to perform neurovascular checks and assess the residual limb for infection and alterations in tissue integrity at each rewrapping. Begin with the most distal portion and proceed proximally until the bandage is secured to the most proximal joint. The bandage should be tighter at the distal end.

The prosthesis requires special care, which the patient should be taught:

• Clean the prosthesis socket with mild soap and water and then dry it.
• Clean inserts and liners regularly.
• Use garters to keep socks in place.
• Grease parts as instructed.
• Replace shoes when they wear out, with same height and type of shoe.

LIFESTYLE ADAPTATION. The patient may feel that life will be markedly changed as a result of the amputation. If the case manager thinks it is needed, a job analysis may be conducted by a vocational analyst or specialized case manager. With technological advances in prostheses, most patients who worked before surgery are able to return to their jobs after surgery. Many patients with amputations are able to bowl, ski, hike, and continue with all of the recreational hobbies that they were able to do before surgery.

A supportive family or significant other is vital to help the patient adjust to body image change. Consider the need for a sexual counselor or psychologist if indicated. For any patient with an amputation, help the patient set realistic expectations.

For the patient who is not a candidate for a prosthesis, home adaptations for a wheelchair may be needed. The patient must have access to toileting facilities and areas necessary for self-care. Structural changes in the living environment may be needed before the patient can be discharged from rehabilitation.

FIGURE 46.17 Application of elastic wraps on an above-the-knee amputation helps mold the stump for a prosthesis.

Home Health Hints

- If equipment or modifications to the home are needed following hospitalization for an orthopedic adaptation, it is best if they can be arranged or obtained before discharge.
- Physical and/or occupational therapy are often ordered for the orthopedic patient discharged from the hospital to help with ambulation, ADLs, and obtaining and use of assistive devices: raised toilet seats, handheld reachers, walkers, canes, wheelchairs, and hand rails.
- Physical and/or occupational therapy can also be ordered to help the patient regain strength following surgery. The home health nurse can work with the therapist to educate the patient on the prescribed exercises.
- Patients who use walkers can get pressure ulcers on their palms. One way to relieve the pressure is to wear padded cycling gloves that leave the fingers free.
- A patient on crutches can use the crutch to prop a casted leg or foot.
- Research has shown that pain or fear of falling may prevent a patient from moving and functioning to maximum potential. Encourage patients to wear flat, sturdy, rubber-soled shoes to prevent slipping, tripping, or turning an ankle.
- Encourage the patient to remove all throw rugs, unnecessary furniture, and other possible fall hazards in the home.

- The risk of DVT after hip or knee surgery is highest by the fifth postoperative day, and the risk persists for up to 12 weeks. Be alert for such signs as warmth, redness, edema, positive Homans' sign, and protective behavior of the affected leg.
- Patients who are having a difficult time putting on compression stockings can be shown how to slip them on easily. Using a plastic grocery bag, instruct the patient to tie a knot on the closed end. Slip the bag over the foot, and then put the stocking on over the bag. Once the stocking is on over the heel, the patient or caregiver can pull the bag out using the knot that was tied.
- Aids are available for putting on compression stockings such as the Doff N' Donner, a rubberized device filled with water, that slides up the leg unrolling the stocking in place (www.doffanddonner.com).
- Many times the patient is discharged home still requiring medication injections to prevent DVT formation. The nurse will educate the patient on how to administer the injection. If the patient cannot do this and no one is available to teach him or her, the home health nurse can make visits to administer the injection.
- Instruct the patient with rheumatoid arthritis to rest during acute inflammations and to stop activity if pain develops.
- Home health nurses frequently remove staples and sutures. Always have several of each type of removal device on hand. Remember staples, scissors, or other items that are "sharp" need to be disposed of in a biohazard container.

SUGGESTED ANSWERS TO

CRITICAL THINKING

■ *Mrs. Martinez*

1. When documenting, answer the questions what, why, where, who, and how to make the charting complete.

    What = Patient found on the floor on her left side, moaning and holding her left leg, crying out with any movement.

    Why = fall

    When = Date/Time: 1000

    Where = day room

    Who = Mrs. Martinez (patient)

    How = unknown, was not witnessed.

    Date: 1000. Found on floor in day room lying on left side, moaning and holding left leg, crying

out with any movement. Stated, "I fell. I think my leg is broken." Supervisor immediately notified paramedics and Dr. Haas notified. BP 150/84, P 100, R 20. Left leg shorter than right. Remained with patient and instructed not to move until paramedics arrived. Blankets applied and pillow under head. Taken to Memorial Hospital by ambulance at 1000. I. Smith, LPN

2.

  A. Risk for vascular trauma related to possible hip fracture.

  B. Pain, related to fall, as evidenced by patient moaning and holding her leg, crying with movement.

  C. Fear related to pain at left hip as evidenced by anxiety.

Continued

SUGGESTED ANSWERS TO—cont'd

■ *Frank Schnell*

1. Possible priority nursing diagnoses include:

   a. *Pain* related to injury and immobility

   b. *Risk for constipation* related to opioids and immobility

   c. *Risk for Impaired Skin Integrity* related to extended recovery time

   d. *Risk for Social Isolation* related to hospitalization

   e. *Deficient Diversional Activity* related to extended need for bedrest

2. Nursing interventions may include:

   a. Monitor pain level, provide analgesics as ordered, check pain relief. Check position for comfort. Provide backrubs prn.

   b. Ensure Frank's diet includes fiber and adequate hydration (1.5–2 L/day); give stool softener as ordered; monitor daily bowel movements.

   c. Ensure Frank does the exercises recommended by occupational and physical therapists; reposition him every 2 to 3 hours; have trapeze bar set up for Frank to use; use skin assessment tool to determine risk for skin breakdown; check for pressure points and signs and symptoms of skin breakdown.

   d. Encourage Frank's family and friends to alternate visits; have an occupational therapist assess Frank's social needs.

   e. Encourage Frank to listen to music; encourage visitors; and ensure access to hobbies, videos, books, magazines, and comics.

3. Because opioids are an essential part of pain management and can cause constipation when used long term, planning is necessary to prevent it. Monitor daily bowel movements. Give medications to prevent opioid constipation as ordered such as AMITIZA (lubiprostone), or opioid antagonists like methylnaltrexone. Be proactive in ensuring normal elimination. Report lack of bowel movements promptly for intervention. Reduce opioid dosage and move to nonopioids promptly as pain relief allows.

■ *Mr. Kardos*

1. Data collection should include the following:

   a. Perform a neurovascular check.

   b. Perform a further pain assessment.

   c. Asking Mr. Kardos to flex the muscles in his limb to see if the pain worsens.

   d. Take his vital signs.

   e. Check for the six Ps: pain, paresthesia, paralysis, pallor, pulselessness, and poikilothermia.

2. He might be experiencing compartment syndrome.

3. Interventions may include the need for a bivalved cast or a possible fasciotomy.

■ *Mr. Finn*

1. a. "What is your typical day on the job like?"

   b. "Do certain activities increase joint pain?"

   c. "When is your pain worse, after activity or after rest?"

   d. "How long have you experienced joint pain?"

   e. "What relieves the joint pain?"

2. Risk factors include that he is overweight, is in late middle age, and has a physically demanding job.

3. Other signs and symptoms may include bony nodules on his fingers (such as Heberden's nodes) and secondary inflammation causing joint swelling.

4. Pain management pain, weight loss, restoring and maintaining functional ability: bending ability for work.

5. HCP, pharmacist, nurse, physical therapist, occupational therapist.

■ *Mrs. Harris*

1. Ask:

   a. The nature of her pain

   b. If it is worse after activity or rest

   c. If she experiences joint stiffness and, if so, when.

   Follow the **WHAT'S UP?** method of pain assessment.

2. Teach the following:

   a. Balance rest with exercise.

   b. Use ice for very hot, swollen joints.

   c. Use heat to decrease stiffness.

■ *Mrs. Adam*

Unit analysis method:

$$\frac{500 \text{ mg}}{} \frac{5 \text{ mL}}{375 \text{ mg}} = 6.7 \text{ mL}$$

REVIEW QUESTIONS

1. The nurse is caring for a patient being transferred into bed who has just had a plaster long-leg cast applied and reports pain of 6 on a scale of 0 to 10. Place the nursing interventions in order of priority.
   1. Expose cast to air dry.
   2. Administer ordered analgesic.
   3. Check circulation, sensory, and mobility status.
   4. Palm cast while position on pillow.
   5. Obtain vital signs.

2. The nurse is caring for a patient with an external fixation device. Which of the following actions should the nurse implement? **Select all that apply.**
   1. Avoid touching the pins.
   2. Follow agency protocol for pin care.
   3. Cleanse pins with hydrogen peroxide four times daily.
   4. Loosen screws holding the pins during cleaning.
   5. Monitor pin insertion sites daily.

3. The nurse is caring for a patient with an open fracture. Which of the following actions are essential for the nurse to perform to help prevent osteomyelitis? **Select all that apply.**
   1. Perform hand hygiene before dressing change.
   2. Wear a protective gown.
   3. Wear a mask.
   4. Wear goggles.
   5. Wear sterile gloves to apply new dressing.

4. The nurse is caring for a patient who is postmenopausal, has osteoporosis, lost 2 inches of height, is thin, and has never exercised regularly. Which of these interventions should be included in the plan of care to prevent further bone loss?
   1. Decrease participation in activities of daily living.
   2. Avoid weight-bearing activities.
   3. Encourage regular exercise.
   4. Encourage weight gain.

5. The nurse is contributing to the plan of care for a patient with Paget's disease. Which of these is a priority nursing diagnosis for this patient?
   1. Pain
   2. Deficient Knowledge
   3. Excess Fluid Volume
   4. Deficient Fluid Volume

6. The nurse is caring for a male patient with gout. Which of the following lab values would the nurse expect in this patient?
   1. White blood cell count 6.2 cells/mL
   2. Potassium 5 mEq/L
   3. Uric acid 10.2 mg/dL
   4. Ammonia 34 μmol/L

7. A patient with osteoarthritis who had a right total knee replacement tells the nurse that the other knee is becoming painful. Which of the following is the most appropriate instruction to help the patient preserve function of the left knee?
   1. Reduce dietary purines.
   2. Maintain ideal body weight.
   3. Maintain normal uric acid levels.
   4. Begin a jogging program.

8. A patient is scheduled for a right total hip replacement. The nurse should teach which of the following postoperative leg positions?
   1. Maintain legs in adduction.
   2. Maintain legs in abduction.
   3. Maintain internal leg rotation.
   4. Maintain more than 90-degree hip flexion.

9. The nurse is caring for a patient immediately after a below-the-knee amputation. Which of these assessments should the nurse consider a PRIORITY?
   1. Sacral edema
   2. Mobility
   3. Stump dressings
   4. Blood sugar level

10. The nurse is collecting and reviewing data on a patient with a left tibia fracture. Which of the following findings would indicate a complication of this fracture?
    1. Increased red blood cell count.
    2. Decreased body temperature.
    3. Decreased lymphocyte count.
    4. Absent left pedal pulse.

11. A patient who has a 36-hour-old fractured femur had morphine 5 mg intramuscularly 1 hour ago and is now reporting severe unrelieved pain. Which nursing action is most appropriate?
    1. Administer an analgesic.
    2. Apply Buck's traction.
    3. Reposition with head of bed up.
    4. Notify the health care provider.

12. A patient who had a total knee replacement is to receive Toradol 15 mg intramuscularly every 6 hours as needed for pain. The Toradol comes as 30 mg/mL. How many milliliters should the nurse give?
    Answer: _____ mL

Answers can be found in Appendix C.

References

American Academy of Orthopedics. (2013). Retrieved November 18, 2013, from www.aaos.org

National Osteoporosis Foundation. (2013). Retrieved November 18, 2013, from www.nof.org/hcp/clinicians-guide

Ogrendik, M. (2013). Rheumatoid arthritis is an autoimmune disease caused by periodontal pathogens. *International Journal of General Medicine, 7,* 43–47.

 DavisPlus | For additional resources and information visit **davispl.us/medsurg5**

unit THIRTEEN

Understanding the Neurologic System

47

Neurologic System Function, Assessment, and Therapeutic Measures

DEBORAH L. WEAVER
AND JANICE L. BRADFORD

KEY TERMS

anisocoria (an-ih-suh-KOR-ee-ah)
aphasia (ah-FAY-zee-ah)
cerebrovascular (sur-EE-broh-VASS-kyoo-lur)
contractures (kon-TRAK-churs)
decerebrate (dee-SER-eh-brayt)
decorticate (dee-KOR-tih-kayt)
dysarthria (diss-AR-three-ah)
dysphagia (diss-FAYJ-ee-ah)
electroencephalogram (ee-LEK-troh-en-SEFF-uh-loh-gram)
myelogram (MY-eh-loh-gram)
nystagmus (nih-STAG-mus)
paresis (puh-REE-sis)
paresthesia (PAR-es-THEE-zee-ah)
subarachnoid (SUB-uh-RAK-noyd)

LEARNING OUTCOMES

1. Describe the normal structures and functions of the nervous system
2. Identify the effects of aging on the nervous system.
3. List data to collect when caring for a patient with a disorder of the nervous system.
4. Identify tests used to diagnose disorders of the nervous system.
5. Plan nursing care for patients undergoing each of the diagnostic tests for disorders of the nervous system.
6. Describe common therapeutic measures that are used for patients with disorders of the nervous system.

NORMAL NEUROLOGIC SYSTEM ANATOMY AND PHYSIOLOGY

The nervous system has two divisions: the central nervous system (CNS), which consists of the brain and spinal cord, and the peripheral nervous system (PNS), which includes the nerves of the autonomic nervous system (ANS). Electrical impulses are transmitted through the nervous system to permit sensory, motor, and integrative activity. Actions are either automatic by reflex or a result of gathering, organizing, and processing data.

Nerve Tissue

Nerve tissue consists of neurons and support cells called neuroglia (Table 47.1). There is diversity in neurons; including unipolar, bipolar, and multipolar anatomy. Most common is the multipolar neuron with multiple dendrites and a singular axon (Fig. 47.1).

Myelination of axons increases their conduction speed. The level of myelination correlates to the necessity of speed. For example, neurons involved in protective reflexes are heavily myelinated, whereas processing neurons of the CNS lack myelin.

Types of Neurons

Functional classification of neurons considers their position and direction of signal: a neuron is sensory (afferent), motor

TABLE 47.1 NEUROGLIA OF THE CNS

Name	Function
Oligodendrocytes	• Produce the myelin sheath to electrically insulate neurons of the central nervous system.
Microglia	• Capable of movement and phagocytosis of pathogens and damaged tissue.
Astrocytes	• Contribute to the blood–brain barrier, which prevents potentially toxic waste products in the blood from diffusing out into brain tissue. • Disadvantage: Some useful medications cannot cross the blood–brain barrier, which becomes important during brain infection, inflammation, or other disease.
Ependyma	• Line the ventricles of the brain. • Many of the cells are ciliated. • Involved in production and circulation of cerebrospinal fluid.

(efferent), or an interneuron (between the afferent and efferent neurons, Fig. 47.2). Receptors are specialized to detect external or internal changes and then generate electrical impulses. Sensory neurons, from receptors in the skin, skeletal muscles, and joints, are called somatic. Those sensory neurons from receptors in internal organs are called visceral sensory neurons. Motor neurons that innervate skeletal muscle are called *somatic;* those to smooth muscle, cardiac muscle, and glands are called *visceral.*

LEARNING TIP

To remember the difference between *afferent* and *efferent,* try these clues:

- **A**fferent: A is for affect or sense.
- **E**fferent: E is for effect (action).
- Or, think of the alphabet—**A** before **E**: You have to feel or sense (afferent) a stimulus before you can take action (efferent).

Nerve Impulses

A nerve impulse, which is also called an *action potential,* is an electrical change brought about by the movement of ions across the neuron cell membrane. When a neuron is at rest, it is polarized with a positive charge outside the membrane and a relatively negative charge inside the membrane. A threshold stimulus will cause a reversal in charge (action potential). A wave of depolarization travels the length of the neuron as a positive feedback loop. Immediately after is repolarization, restoring the positive charge outside and the negative charge inside. After a *refractory period* (the brief time after being stimulated when a nerve still can't react to another stimulus), the neuron is polarized again and ready to respond to another stimulus. A myelinated neuron is capable of transmitting hundreds of impulses per second and at speeds of more than 100 meters per second.

Synapses

Neurons typically work in a circuit. When the axon of a neuron must transmit an impulse to the dendrite or cell body of another neuron, the impulse must cross a small gap called a *synapse.* An electrical impulse is incapable of crossing this microscopic space, so when an impulse reaches the synapse, impulse transmission becomes chemical.

At chemical synapses, impulse transmission is one way because the neurotransmitter is released only by the presynaptic neuron; the impulse cannot go backward. This is important for the normal activity of functional neurons. The relative complexity of synapses also makes them a potential target for the actions of medications. For example, some antidepressants block the reuptake (reabsorption) of serotonin, a neurotransmitter, back into the proximal nerve endings, increasing the mood-elevating serotonin levels in the synapse.

The **cell body** (also called the **soma**) is the control center of the neuron and contains the nucleus.

Dendrites, which look like the bare branches of a tree, receive signals from other neurons and conduct the information to the cell body. Some neurons have only one dendrite; others have thousands.

The **axon**, which carries nerve signals away from the body, is longer than the dendrites and contains few branches. Nerve cells have only one axon; however, the length of the fiber can range from a few millimeters to as much as a meter.

The axons of many (but not all) neurons are encased in a **myelin sheath**. Consisting mostly of lipid, myelin acts to insulate the axon. In the peripheral nervous system, Schwann cells form the myelin sheath. In the CNS, oligodendrocytes assume this role.

Gaps in the myelin sheath, called **nodes of Ranvier**, occur at evenly spaced intervals.

The end of the axon branches extensively, with each axon terminal ending in a **synaptic knob**. Within the synaptic knobs are vesicles containing a neurotransmitter.

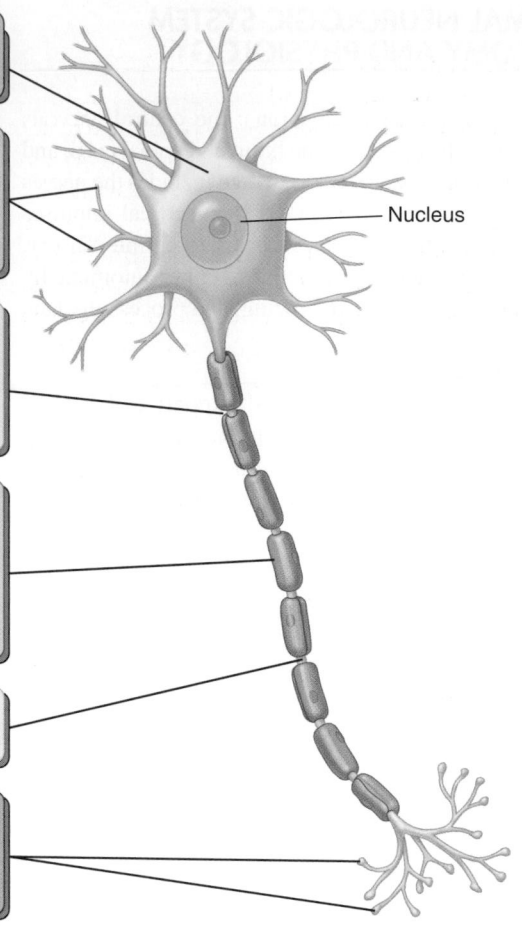

Nucleus

FIGURE 47.1 Multipolar neuron structure. From Thompson, G. S. (2013). *Understanding anatomy and physiology.* Philadelphia: F.A. Davis, p. 157.

Interneurons

Interneurons, which are found only in the CNS, connect the incoming sensory pathways with the outgoing motor pathways. Besides receiving, processing, and storing information, the connections made by these neurons make each of us unique in how we think, feel, and act.

Sensory neurons

Sensory (afferent) neurons detect stimuli—such as touch, pressure, heat, cold, or chemicals—and then transmit information about the stimuli to the CNS.

Motor neurons

Motor (efferent) neurons relay messages from the brain (which the brain emits in response to stimuli) to the muscle or gland cells.

FIGURE 47.2 Neurons: sensory, interneurons, motor. From Thompson, G. S. (2013). *Understanding anatomy and physiology.* Philadelphia: F.A. Davis, p. 156.

Nerves and Nerve Tracts

A nerve (whether cranial, spinal, or peripheral) is a group of axons with blood vessels, wrapped in connective tissue. Most nerves are mixed; that is, they contain both sensory and motor neurons. Some, however, are not mixed. For example, the optic nerve for vision is sensory only; and the autonomic nerves are purely motor.

A nerve tract is a group of thickly myelinated neurons within the CNS; such tracts within white matter appear white due to the myelin sheaths. A nerve tract within the spinal cord carries either sensory or motor impulses; those within the brain may have sensory, motor, or integrative functions.

Spinal Cord

The spinal cord transmits impulses to and from the brain and is the integrating center for spinal cord reflexes. The spinal cord is within the vertebral canal formed by the vertebrae of the skeleton and extends from the foramen magnum of the occipital bone to the intervertebral disk between the first and second lumbar vertebrae. The spinal nerves emerge from the intervertebral foramina.

In cross-section, the spinal cord is oval shaped; internally it has an H-shaped mass of gray matter surrounded by white matter (Fig. 47.3). Each spinal nerve attaches to the cord by two roots: dorsal and ventral. Meninges (three concentric, external layers of connective tissue) and circulating cerebrospinal fluid (CSF) offer further protection to the spinal cord.

Spinal Nerves

There are 31 pairs of spinal nerves, named according to their respective vertebrae: 8 cervical pairs, 12 thoracic pairs, 5 lumbar pairs, 5 sacral pairs, and 1 coccygeal pair. These nerves are often referred to by letter and number: the second cervical nerve is C2, the tenth thoracic is T10, and so on (Fig. 47.4).

Spinal Cord Reflexes

A reflex is a fast, involuntary, automatic, and predictable response to a stimulus. A spinal cord reflex uses a neural circuit, independent of the brain, called a spinal reflex arc. Sensory input elicits motor output (Fig. 47.5).

The somatic spinal cord reflexes include stretch reflexes and flexor reflexes. In a stretch reflex, a muscle that is stretched automatically contracts; an example is the familiar patellar reflex, but all skeletal muscles have such a reflex. Because gravity exerts a constant force on the body, the purpose of these reflexes is to keep the body upright without requiring conscious processing. They also avoid potential injury from overstretching a muscle. Flexor reflexes may also be called withdrawal reflexes: the stimulus is painful trauma to tissue and the response is to pull away from it. Again, this occurs without the need for conscious thought; the brain is not directly involved.

The clinical testing of spinal cord reflexes provides a way to assess the functioning of their reflex arcs. For example, if the patellar reflex is absent, the problem might be in the quadriceps femoris muscle, the femoral nerve, or the spinal cord itself. If the reflex is present, it indicates that all parts of the reflex arc are functioning normally.

Brain

The brain consists of many parts that function as an integrated whole. The four principle areas are the cerebrum, the diencephalon (thalamus and hypothalamus), the brainstem (midbrain, pons, and medulla oblongata), and the cerebellum (Fig. 47.6).

Meninges

The meninges are the three layers of connective tissue that cover the CNS. Where they enclose the brain, they are referred to as cranial meninges.

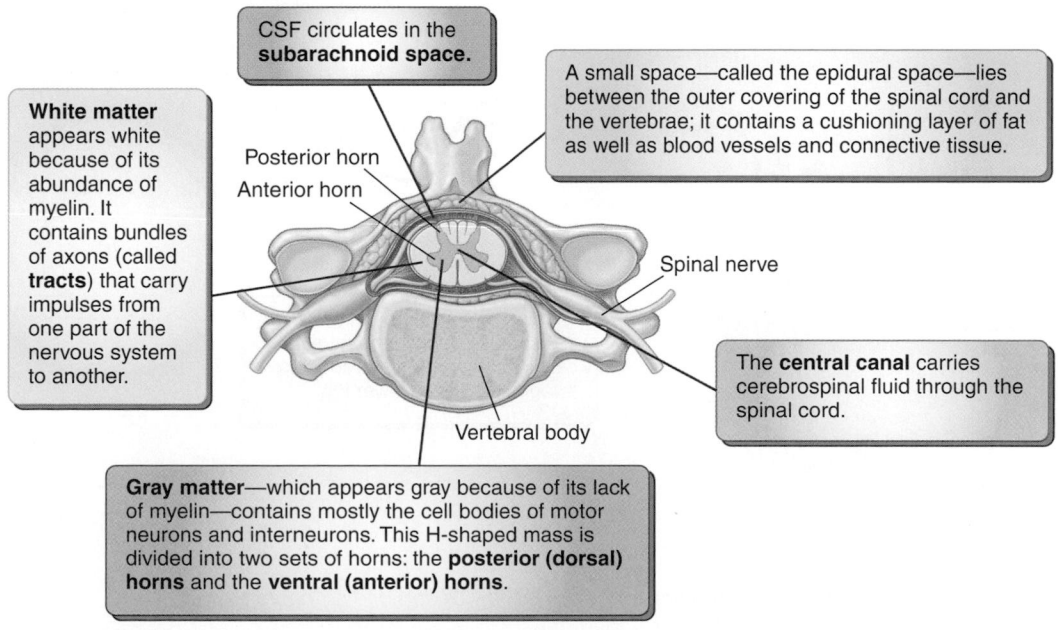

CSF circulates in the subarachnoid space.

White matter appears white because of its abundance of myelin. It contains bundles of axons (called **tracts**) that carry impulses from one part of the nervous system to another.

Posterior horn
Anterior horn

A small space—called the epidural space—lies between the outer covering of the spinal cord and the vertebrae; it contains a cushioning layer of fat as well as blood vessels and connective tissue.

Spinal nerve

The **central canal** carries cerebrospinal fluid through the spinal cord.

Vertebral body

Gray matter—which appears gray because of its lack of myelin—contains mostly the cell bodies of motor neurons and interneurons. This H-shaped mass is divided into two sets of horns: the **posterior (dorsal) horns** and the **ventral (anterior) horns**.

FIGURE 47.3 Spinal cord—internal anatomy, cross-section, superior view. From Thompson, G. S. (2013). *Understanding anatomy and physiology.* Philadelphia: F.A. Davis, p. 165.

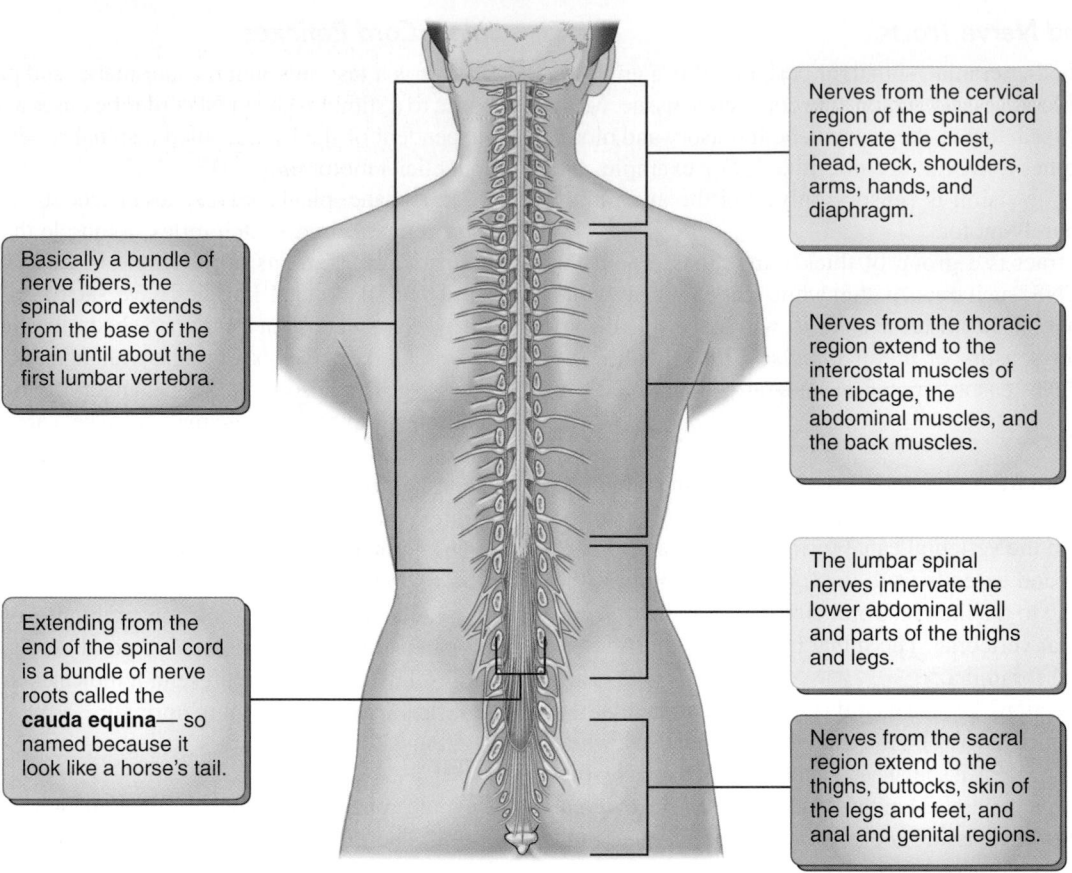

Nerves from the cervical region of the spinal cord innervate the chest, head, neck, shoulders, arms, hands, and diaphragm.

Nerves from the thoracic region extend to the intercostal muscles of the ribcage, the abdominal muscles, and the back muscles.

The lumbar spinal nerves innervate the lower abdominal wall and parts of the thighs and legs.

Nerves from the sacral region extend to the thighs, buttocks, skin of the legs and feet, and anal and genital regions.

Basically a bundle of nerve fibers, the spinal cord extends from the base of the brain until about the first lumbar vertebra.

Extending from the end of the spinal cord is a bundle of nerve roots called the **cauda equina**— so named because it look like a horse's tail.

FIGURE 47.4 Spinal cord—full length, posterior view. From Thompson, G. S. (2013). *Understanding anatomy and physiology*. Philadelphia: F.A. Davis, p. 164.

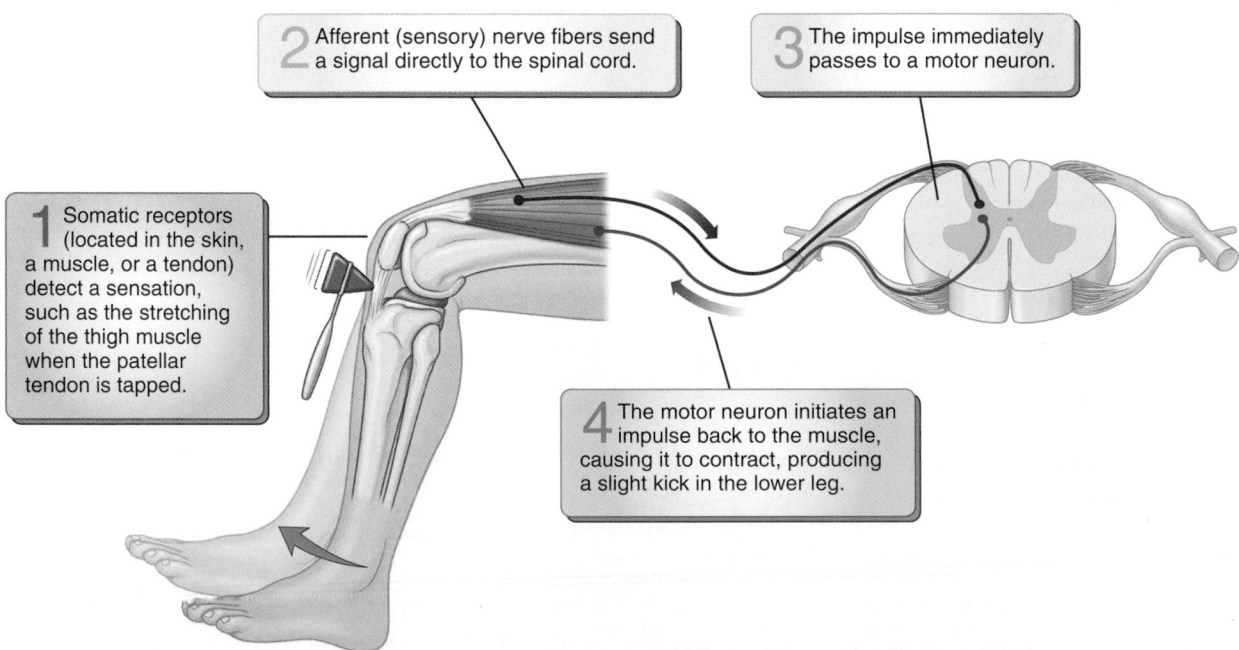

2 Afferent (sensory) nerve fibers send a signal directly to the spinal cord.

3 The impulse immediately passes to a motor neuron.

1 Somatic receptors (located in the skin, a muscle, or a tendon) detect a sensation, such as the stretching of the thigh muscle when the patellar tendon is tapped.

4 The motor neuron initiates an impulse back to the muscle, causing it to contract, producing a slight kick in the lower leg.

FIGURE 47.5 Somatic spinal reflex. From Thompson, G. S. (2013). *Understanding anatomy and physiology*. Philadelphia: F.A. Davis, p. 169.

Gyri   Sulci

The **cerebrum** is the largest portion of the brain. It's surface is marked by thick ridges called **gyri** (singular: **gyrus**). Shallow grooves called **sulci** (singular: **sulcus**) divide the gyri. Deep sulci are called **fissures**.

The **diencephalon** sits between the cerebrum and the midbrain.

The **cerebellum** is the second largest region of the brain.

The **brainstem** makes up the rest of the brain. It consists of three structures:
• Midbrain
• Pons
• Medulla oblongata

FIGURE 47.6 General structures of the brain—external, left lateral view. From Thompson, G. S. (2013). *Understanding anatomy and physiology.* Philadelphia: F.A. Davis, p. 170.

Ventricles and Cerebrospinal Fluid

The ventricles are four cavities within the brain: two lateral ventricles are located within the cerebral hemispheres, the third ventricle lays midline within the thalamus, and the fourth ventricle is midline between the brainstem and cerebellum. Cerebrospinal fluid is formed from capillaries of the choroid plexus within, and circulates through the four ventricles. Circulation of CSF moves inferiorly within the CNS, into the **subarachnoid** space, and ultimately superiorly to drain into the dural venous sinuses. Cerebrospinal fluid permits the exchanges of nutrients and wastes between the blood and CNS neurons. It also acts as a cushion or shock absorber for the CNS. The pressure and constituents of CSF may be determined by means of a lumbar puncture (spinal tap) and may be helpful in the diagnosis of diseases such as meningitis.

Brainstem: Midbrain, Pons, and Medulla Oblongata

Primarily a reflex center, the midbrain regulates visual reflexes (coordinated movement of the eyes), auditory reflexes (turning the ear toward a sound), and righting reflexes that keep the head upright and contribute to balance. Within the pons are two respiratory centers that work with those in the medulla to produce a normal breathing rhythm. The medulla lies just superior to the spinal cord. It regulates the most vital life functions.

Cerebellum

The cerebellum is posterior to the brainstem. The functions of the cerebellum include the involuntary aspects of voluntary movement: coordination, appropriate direction and endpoint of movements, and the maintenance of posture and balance. For the maintenance of balance, the cerebellum uses input from vision, proprioceptors, and equilibrium

receptors in the inner ear to detect movement and changes in position.

Diencephalon: Thalamus and Hypothalamus

Deep beneath the cerebral hemispheres, the diencephalon consists primarily of the thalamus and hypothalamus. Above the brainstem, the thalamus acts as a gateway for nearly every sensation traveling to the cerebral cortex. The thalamus filters sensory input, permitting the cerebrum to concentrate on more important sensations with less distraction. The hypothalamus suspends the pituitary gland from a stalk called the infundibulum; they are anatomically and physiologically connected.

Cerebrum

The two cerebral hemispheres form the largest part of the human brain. The right and left hemispheres are connected primarily by the corpus callosum, a band of about 300 million nerve fibers. The cerebral cortex is folded extensively into convolutions (or gyri) that create more surface area for neurons. The deep grooves between the folds are called fissures; shallow grooves are called sulci. The cerebral cortex is divided into lobes, whose functions have been extensively mapped (Fig. 47.7).

Collectively, the cerebral cortex has areas that enable learning, memory, and thought. It also helps form our individual personalities with complex behaviors that require integration of several cerebral and lower brain areas.

Deep within the white matter of the cerebral hemispheres are masses of gray matter called the basal nuclei (*ganglia*).

• **WORD** • **BUILDING** •

subarachnoid: sub—below + arachnoid—middle layer of the meninges

Frontal Lobe
- Central sulcus forms the posterior border
- Contains the motor areas that generate impulses that bring about voluntary movement
- Each motor area controls movement on the opposite side of the body
- Usually prominent in the left hemisphere, Broca's motor speech area controls the movements involved in speaking
- Personality aspects include: initiative, emotion, judgment, reasoning, conscience

Occipital lobe
- Contains the visual areas that receive and interpret sight

Parietal lobe
- Central sulcus forms the anterior border
- Receives, perceives, and interprets the somatic senses and taste (gustation)

Temporal lobe
- Separated from the parietal lobe by the lateral sulcus
- Contains sensory areas for hearing and olfaction (smell)
- Visual recognition
- Also in the temporal and parietal lobes, usually only on the left side, is Wernicke's area where comprehension of speech occurs.

Precentral gyrus — Central sulcus — Postcentral gyrus — Lateral sulcus

FIGURE 47.7 Cerebrum—lobes, left lateral view. From Thompson, G. S. (2013). *Understanding anatomy and physiology.* Philadelphia: F.A. Davis, p. 176.

Their functions are concerned with certain subconscious aspects of voluntary movement: regulation of muscle tone, inhibiting tremor, and use of accessory movements such as arm swinging when walking.

Cranial Nerves

The 12 pairs of cranial nerves emerge from the brainstem with the exception of pair one, which originates from the temporal lobe and pair two from the occipital lobe. Some are purely sensory nerves, whereas others are mixed nerves. The impulses for sight, smell, hearing, taste, equilibrium, and somatic senses of supplied areas are all carried by cranial nerves to their respective sensory areas in the brain. Other cranial nerves carry motor impulses to muscles of the face, neck, shoulders, and tongue, or to glands. Cranial nerves III, VII, IX, and X contain axons of both the somatic and autonomic nervous systems. The functions of all the cranial nerves are summarized in Table 47.2.

Autonomic Nervous System

Autonomic nervous system (ANS) motor output provides dual innervation to effectors, that is, smooth muscle, cardiac muscle, and glands that produce the response (effect). These two divisions (sympathetic and parasympathetic) function in opposition to one other and their activity is integrated by the hypothalamus.

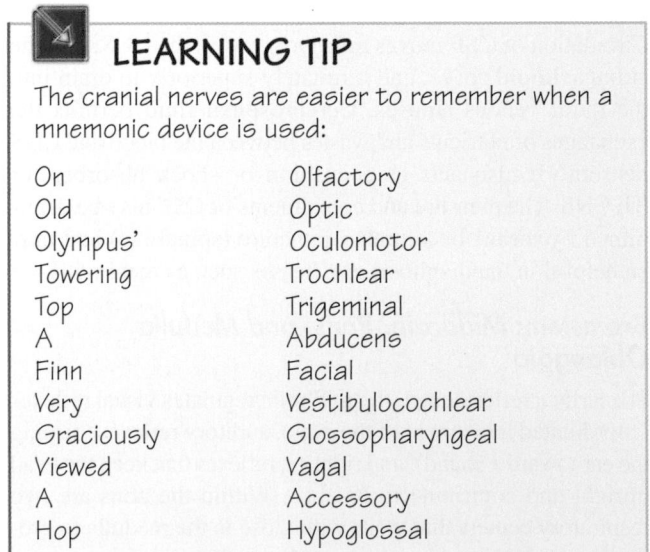

LEARNING TIP

The cranial nerves are easier to remember when a mnemonic device is used:

On	Olfactory
Old	Optic
Olympus'	Oculomotor
Towering	Trochlear
Top	Trigeminal
A	Abducens
Finn	Facial
Very	Vestibulocochlear
Graciously	Glossopharyngeal
Viewed	Vagal
A	Accessory
Hop	Hypoglossal

Sympathetic Division

The cell bodies of the sympathetic preganglionic neurons are thoracolumbar (in the thoracic and lumbar segments of the spinal cord, Fig. 47.8). The sympathetic division is dominant in stressful situations such as fear, anger, anxiety, excitement, and exercise. The responses prepare the body for physical activity,

TABLE 47.2   CRANIAL NERVES

Number	Name	Function
I	Olfactory	• Sense of smell
II	Optic	• Sense of sight
III	Oculomotor	• Movement of eyeball • Constriction of pupil for bright light or near vision
IV	Trochlear	• Movement of eyeball
V	Trigeminal	• Sensation in face, scalp, and teeth • Contraction of chewing muscles
VI	Abducens	• Movement of eyeball
VII	Facial	• Sense of taste • Contraction of facial muscles • Secretion of saliva
VIII	Vestibulocochlear	• Sense of hearing • Sense of equilibrium
IX	Glossopharyngeal	• Sense of taste • Secretion of saliva • Sensory input for cardiac, respiratory, and blood pressure reflexes • Contraction of pharynx
X	Vagus	• Sensory input in cardiac, respiratory, and blood pressure reflexes • Sensory and motor input to larynx (speaking) • Decreased heart rate • Contraction of alimentary tube (peristalsis) • Increased digestive secretions
XI	Accessory	• Contraction of neck and shoulder muscles • Motor input to larynx (speaking)
XII	Hypoglossal	• Movement of the tongue

whether or not it is actually needed. Heart rate increases, vasodilation in skeletal muscles increases oxygen and glucose supply, bronchioles dilate to take in more air, and the liver converts glycogen to glucose to provide energy. The neurotransmitters of the sympathetic division are acetylcholine and norepinephrine. Acetylcholine is released by sympathetic preganglionic neurons; its inactivator is acetylcholinesterase. Norepinephrine is released by most sympathetic postganglionic neurons at the synapses with the effector cells; its inactivator is catechol-*O*-methyltransferase (COMT) or monoamine oxidase (MAO). Table 47.3 summarizes both ANS divisions.

Parasympathetic Division

The cell bodies of the parasympathetic preganglionic neurons are craniosacral (in the brainstem and the sacral segments of the spinal cord, Fig. 47.9). The parasympathetic division dominates during relaxed, nonstressful situations to promote normal functioning of several organ systems. Digestion proceeds normally, with increased secretions and peristalsis; defecation and urination may occur, and the heart beats at a normal resting rate (see Table 47.3). Acetylcholine is the neurotransmitter at all parasympathetic synapses, both preganglionic and postganglionic; it is inactivated by acetylcholinesterase.

CRITICAL THINKING

Mrs. Stevens

■ Mrs. Stevens receives albuterol treatments for her chronic obstructive pulmonary disease. The medication opens her airways effectively, but after her treatments, she often reports that her heart is racing. What part of the PNS do you think this medication affects?

Suggested answers are at the end of the chapter.

Aging and the Nervous System

With age, the brain loses neurons, but this is only a small percentage of the total and is not the usual cause of mental

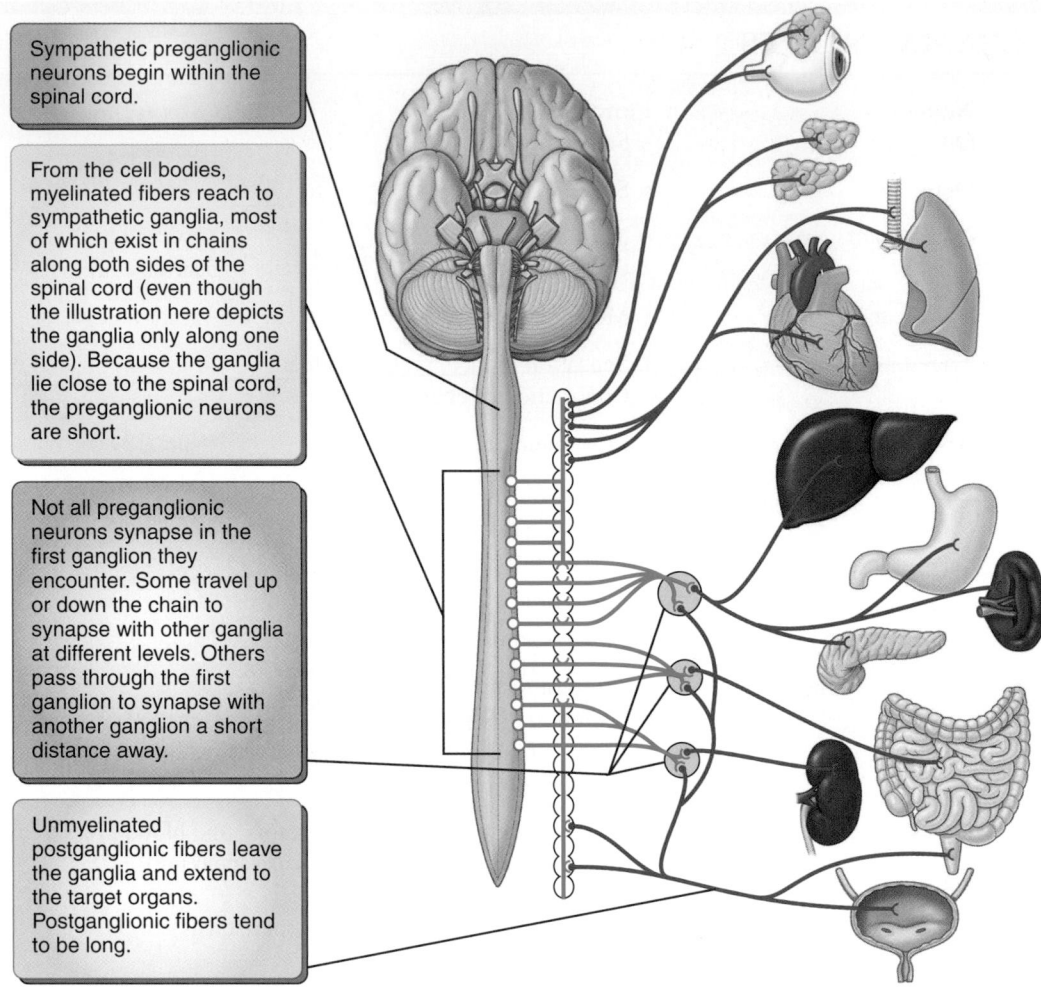

Sympathetic preganglionic neurons begin within the spinal cord.

From the cell bodies, myelinated fibers reach to sympathetic ganglia, most of which exist in chains along both sides of the spinal cord (even though the illustration here depicts the ganglia only along one side). Because the ganglia lie close to the spinal cord, the preganglionic neurons are short.

Not all preganglionic neurons synapse in the first ganglion they encounter. Some travel up or down the chain to synapse with other ganglia at different levels. Others pass through the first ganglion to synapse with another ganglion a short distance away.

Unmyelinated postganglionic fibers leave the ganglia and extend to the target organs. Postganglionic fibers tend to be long.

FIGURE 47.8 Sympathetic nervous system. From Thompson, G. S. (2013). *Understanding anatomy and physiology.* Philadelphia: F.A. Davis, p. 188.

impairment in older adults; far more common causes of mental changes include depression, malnutrition, infection, hypotension, and the side effects of medications. Some forgetfulness is to be expected, as is a decreased ability for problem solving (Fig. 47.10).

LEARNING TIP

Sympathetic—S is for STRESS RESPONSE: The sympathetic response is referred to as the fight-or-flight response. When thinking of the sympathetic nervous system, imagine getting away from a lion. You need dilated pupils to see the path better, copious production of sweat to lose heat through evaporation, increased rate and force of heart contraction to ensure that enough blood gets to the extremities so you can run faster, dilated bronchioles to get more oxygen to your muscles, decreased digestion because that would be wasted energy, decreased urine output so you won't have to stop for the restroom, and increased mental alertness so you are always aware of where the lion is.

Parasympathetic—P is for PEACEFUL: The parasympathetic nervous system brings the body back to balance and rest. It is sometimes referred to as the rest-and-digest response. Think, "There is no longer a lion. Now my body can go back to normal and start digesting and urinating again!"

NURSING ASSESSMENT OF THE NEUROLOGIC SYSTEM

The focus of a nursing neurologic assessment is to establish the present function of the patient's neurologic system and to detect changes from previous assessments. A complete neurologic assessment, intended to determine the

TABLE 47.3 FUNCTIONS OF THE AUTONOMIC NERVOUS SYSTEM

Organ	Sympathetic Response	Parasympathetic Response
Heart (cardiac muscle)	Increase rate	Decrease rate (to normal)
Bronchioles (smooth muscle)	Dilate	Constrict (to normal)
Iris (smooth muscle)	Pupil dilates	Pupil constricts (to normal)
Salivary glands	Decrease secretion	Increase secretion (to normal)
Stomach and intestines (smooth muscle)	Decrease peristalsis	Increase peristalsis for normal digestion
Stomach and intestines (glands)	Decrease secretion	Increase secretion for normal digestion
Internal anal sphincter	Contract to prevent defecation	Relax to permit defection
Urinary bladder (smooth muscle)	Relax to prevent urination	Contract for normal urination
Internal urethral sphincter	Contract to prevent urination	Relax to permit urination
Liver	Change glycogen to glucose	None
Sweat glands	Increase secretion	None
Blood vessels in skin and viscera (smooth muscle)	Constrict	None
Blood vessels in skeletal muscle (smooth muscle)	Dilate	None
Adrenal glands	Increase secretion of epinephrine and norepinephrine	None

Source: From Scanlon, V. C., & Sanders, T. (2015). *Essentials of anatomy and physiology* (7th ed.). Philadelphia: F.A. Davis, with permission.

existence of neurologic disease, is performed by a health care provider (HCP). A baseline neurologic assessment should be performed on every patient admission (Box 47-1). In addition to providing valuable information about the current functioning of the patient's neurologic system, the assessment provides baseline data for later comparison. This is especially important if the patient has chronic neurologic deficits on admission.

Consider a patient admitted for surgery who has had a previous **cerebrovascular** accident resulting in **paresis** (weakness or partial paralysis) of the right arm. A complete neurologic assessment would document that the right arm is weaker than the left. If during the postoperative course you assess that both arms are equal in strength, you would want to notify the physician so the patient could be further assessed for possible causes of weakening of the left arm.

The results of the baseline assessment are invaluable in planning and implementing safe care. For example, a patient who has a history of seizures needs a safe environment and careful monitoring, and all staff members who interact with such patients should be aware of how to respond to a seizure. Patients with **dysphagia** (difficulty

swallowing) may need to have restrictions placed on the types of food or fluids they can have. This information must be consistently communicated to all staff involved in the patient's care.

The frequency of neurologic assessments depends on the patient's admitting diagnosis, the presence of any chronic neurologic disorders, and the current functioning of the patient's neurologic system. Orders for neurologic assessments vary from every 15 minutes for an acutely ill or injured patient, to every 8 hours for a patient who is close to being discharged, to every 24 hours for a resident living in long-term care. It is always appropriate to assess a patient more often than ordered, based on observed changes in the patient's condition, and to communicate the findings of those assessments to the HCP. Rapid detection and intervention may mean the difference between chronic dysfunction and recovery or even between life and death for the patient.

• WORD • BUILDING •

cerebrovascular: cerebro—brain + vascular—vessels
paresis: partial paralysis
dysphagia: dys—difficult + phagia—eating

Parasympathetic fibers leave the brainstem by joining one of the following cranial nerves:

- **Oculomotor nerve (III):** Parasympathetic fibers carried in this nerve innervate the ciliary muscle, which thickens the lens of the eye, and the pupillary constrictor, which constricts the pupil.
- **Facial nerve (VII):** These parasympathetic fibers regulate the tear glands, salivary glands, and nasal glands.
- **Glossopharyngeal nerve (IX):** The parasympathetic fibers carried in this nerve trigger salivation.
- **Vagus nerve (X):** This nerve carries about 90% of all parasympathetic preganglionic fibers. It travels from the brain to organs in the thoracic cavity (including the heart, lung, and esophagus) and the abdominal cavity (such as the stomach, liver, kidneys, pancreas, and intestines).

Parasympathetic fibers leave the sacral region by way of pelvic nerves and travel to portions of the colon and bladder.

Unlike the ganglia of the sympathetic division, the ganglia of the parasympathetic division reside in or near the target organ. As a result, the preganglionic fibers of the parasympathetic division are long while the postganglionic fibers are short.

Because the ganglia are more widely dispersed, the parasympathetic division produces a more localized response than that of the sympathetic division.

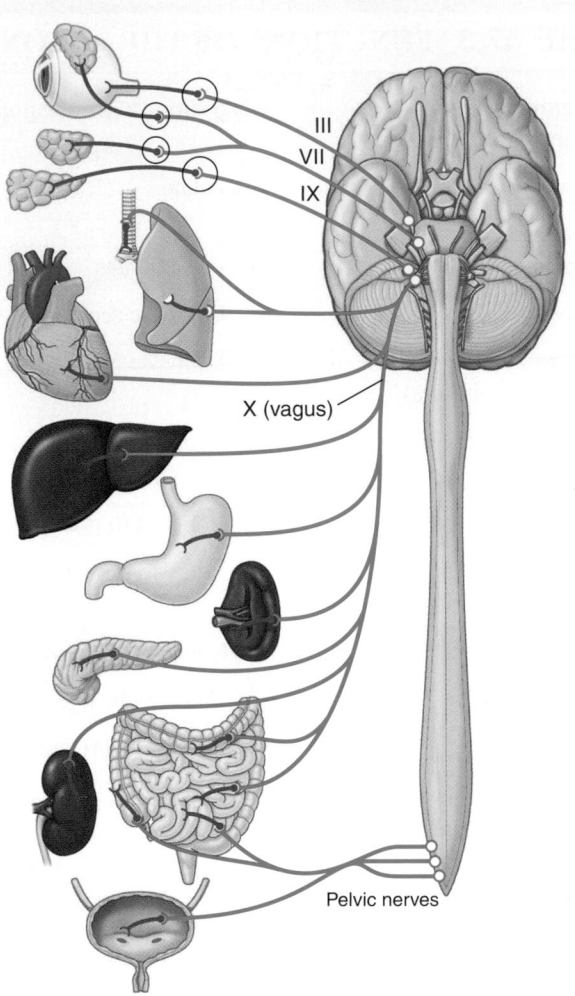

FIGURE 47.9 Parasympathetic nervous system. From Thompson, G. S. (2013). *Understanding anatomy and physiology.* Philadelphia: F.A. Davis, p. 189.

Health History

To understand the patient's neurologic status, ask about past and current symptoms, use of prescription and over-the-counter medications, use of recreational drugs, past surgeries, treatments, and risk factors such as family history, diet, exercise, sedentary lifestyle, caffeine intake, and recent stressors. Assessment of symptoms, as with other body systems, includes asking the **WHAT'S UP?** questions.

You should also obtain a history of the patient's general health and then focus on any neurologic symptoms. Symptoms of neurologic disorders vary in type, location, and intensity. It is important to remember that some neurologic disorders can affect the patient's ability to think, remember, speak, or interpret stimuli. It may be necessary to question significant others about duration and severity of symptoms. Some patients may not be able to recognize their own neurologic deficits. In such cases, the significant other usually initiates contact with the health care system and provides the medical and social history. See Table 47.4 for sample questions to ask if the patient has a change in mental status.

In addition to questioning the patient, the nurse observes the patient during the health history. Is he or she shifting positions and exhibiting signs of discomfort? Is the patient able to move about freely? Is he or she able to carry on a coherent conversation?

Physical Examination

The physical examination begins when you first meet the patient and evaluate the patient's mental and physical status. The neurologic system is assessed using inspection, palpation, and percussion (with a reflex hammer). When conducting the mental status and cognitive portions of the examination, be aware that fatigue, illness, or medications can alter findings. When interpreting neurologic findings, be sure to consider the patient's age, educational background, and cultural background.

Level of Consciousness

Level of consciousness exists along a continuum from full wakefulness, alertness, and cooperation to unresponsiveness to any form of external stimuli. A fully conscious patient responds to questions spontaneously. As consciousness becomes impaired, a patient may show irritability, a shortened attention span, or an inability to cooperate. The level of consciousness should be the first thing assessed

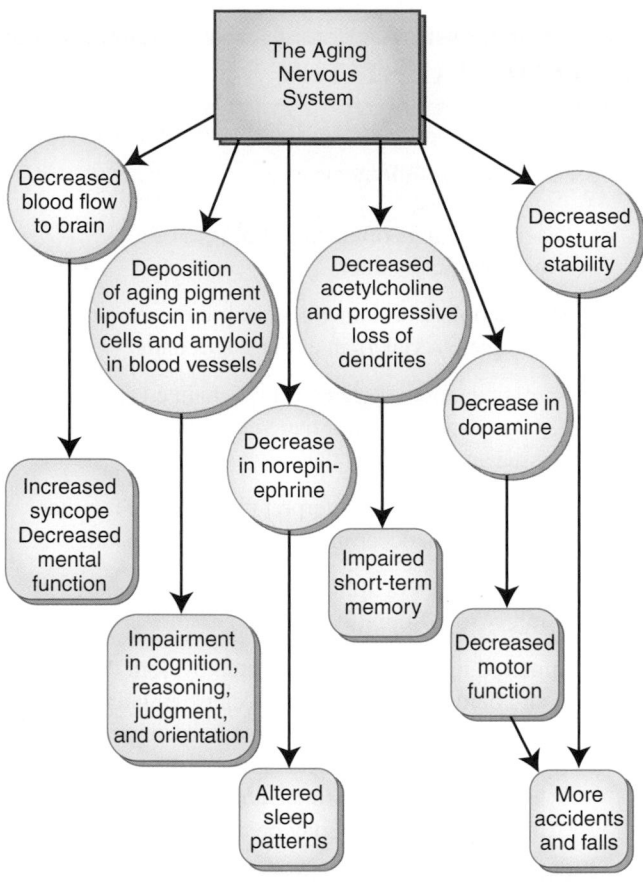

FIGURE 47.10 Aging and the neurologic system. This concept map shows the effects the aging process has on the neurologic system.

Box 47-1 Basic Neurologic Assessment

Assess level of consciousness (patient's response to verbal or tactile stimulation) and orientation.

Obtain vital signs (specifically blood pressure, pulse, and respirations).

Check pupillary response to light.

Assess strength and equality of hand grip and movement of extremities.

Determine ability to sense touch or pain in extremities.

during a neurologic examination because the information obtained can be used to modify the remainder of the examination if necessary. Keep in mind that a decrease in the level of consciousness can be caused by problems such as hypoxia, hypoglycemia, or intoxication, not just dysfunction of the neurologic system.

Many health care institutions use the Glasgow Coma Scale (GCS), which is an international scale used to assess level of consciousness (LOC) and document findings (Table 47.5). The GCS is used to evaluate patients who have a potential for

rapid deterioration in consciousness. When assessing LOC, consider the patient's physical ability to respond, taking into consideration trauma, medical condition, and medications. For example, a patient who cannot open his or her eyes because of facial trauma may still have an intact neurologic system.

Motor response is scored in the GCS based on following commands, responding to pain, or displaying abnormal postures. Abnormal postures includes **decorticate** and **decerebrate**. In decorticate, or flexion, posturing, the patient's arms are flexed at the elbow, the hands are raised toward the chest, and the legs are extended (Fig. 47.11A). This posture indicates significant impairment of cerebral functioning. In decerebrate, or extension, posturing, both the arms and legs are extended and the arms are internally rotated (Fig. 47.11B). This abnormal posturing indicates damage in the area of the brainstem.

The total possible score on the GCS ranges from 3 to 15. A score of less than 7 indicates a comatose patient and a score of 15 indicates the patient is fully alert and oriented. When used to score the effects of a head injury, a score of 13 or 14 indicates mild head injury, 9 to 12 indicates moderate injury, and any score of 8 or below indicates severe head injury. For all categories of the GCS, the type of painful stimuli required to elicit a response should be documented. Deterioration in the patient's condition (i.e., a lowering of the GCS score) should be reported to the physician promptly. See "Evidence-Based Practice."

EVIDENCE-BASED PRACTICE

Clinical Question

Is the Glasgow Coma Scale (GCS) the best tool for neurologic assessment?

According to a recent study by Sadaka, Patel, and Lakshmanan (2012), there has been a known problem with the GCS when used with intubated patients. A new scale has been developed, known as the Full Outline of Unresponsiveness scale (FOUR). Both scales were used to assess level of consciousness and predict the patient outcome after a traumatic brain injury. A high degree of consistency was found between the two scales. The conclusion was that the FOUR scale is an accurate predictor of outcome for TBI patients and had an advantage over the GCS when assessing an intubated patient. The FOUR evaluates four components: eye and motor responses, brainstem reflexes and respiration.

Source: Sadaka, F., Patel, D., & Lakshmanan, R. (2012), The FOUR score predicts outcome in patients after traumatic brain injury. *Neurocritical Care, 16*, 95–101 doi: 10.1007/s12028-011-9617-5.

• WORD • BUILDING •

decorticate: de—down + corticate—cerebral cortex
decerebrate: de—down + cerebrate—cerebrum

TABLE 47.4 COLLECTION OF DATA RELATING TO MENTAL STATUS

Category	Questions to Ask During the Health History	Rationale/Significance
Mental Status	What is your name? What is the month? Year? Where are you now?	Disorientation is often an initial sign of a neurologic disorder.
Intellectual Function	Subtract 7 from 100, then 7 from that answer, and so on (serial 7s).	Most people with intact neurologic function can complete serial 7s in about 90 seconds.
Thought Content	What would you do if you smelled smoke? Where would you put milk?	Assessment of the patient's ability to interpret information and act appropriately is an important safety issue and activity of daily living.
Perception	Show patient pencil and pen and ask what each is.	Agnosia (inability to interpret or recognize familiar objects) can occur in stroke and brain lesions.
Language Ability	Read the following sentence: ____.	Different types of aphasia can result from injury to different parts of the brain.
Memory	Repeat these four or five words: ____. Repeat them again in 5 minutes.	Impaired memory can be affected by both delirium and dementia. Delirium can cause impaired immediate and short-term memory, whereas dementia not only affects immediate and short-term memory but also the ability to learn new information. It also may be related to stroke.
Pain	On a scale of 0 to 10 with 0 as no pain and 10 as the worst you have ever had, what is your pain level?	Pain perception may be altered or impaired by spinal injury, medications, alcohol, stress, and level of consciousness. Some spinal injuries may be critical, but the patient will not report pain.

TABLE 47.5 GLASGOW COMA SCALE

Eye opening	Spontaneous	4
	To verbal stimulus	3
	To painful stimulus	2
	No response	1
Verbal response	Normal conversation	5
	Confused conversation	4
	Inappropriate words	3
	Incomprehensible sounds	2
	No response	1
Motor response	Obeys commands	6
	Localizes pain	5
	Withdraws from pain*	4
	Abnormal flexion	3
	Abnormal extension	2
	No response	1

Note. This scale is for adults only. Criteria specific to children should be used for pediatric cases.

*To elicit pain, place pressure on a nailbed or on the trapezius muscle. Be sure to apply the stimulus long enough to elicit a response.

The *Full Outline of UnResponsiveness (FOUR)* is a newer tool that has been introduced into many critical care and emergency department areas and has been shown to be as effective if not better than the GCS. A major benefit of using the FOUR is that no evaluation of verbal response is necessary, which is a problem when using the GCS with intubated patients. The FOUR uses four categories: eye response, motor movement, reflexes, and breathing pattern. A maximum of four points can be earned in each of the four areas. The terms *decorticate* and *decerebrate* are not used when assessing the motor response to prevent confusion. In addition, the brainstem is evaluated using both pupillary reflexes and corneal reflexes along with the cough reflex. Once each of the components is assessed and assigned a numerical value, the components are totaled. In general, the lower the FOUR Score is, the worse the patient is neurologically and the poorer the prognosis. Conversely, the higher the score, the better the prognosis (see Fig. 47.12).

Mental Status

Mental status can be affected not only by the aging process but by a variety of neurologic disorders and injuries. A traumatic brain injury can result in memory impairment, delayed amnesia, affective (mood) disorders, and dementia. To assess

Wrists and fingers flexed

Feet plantar flexed   Legs internally rotated   Elbows flexed   Arms adducted

A Decorticate posturing

FIGURE 47.11 Abnormal posturing.
(A) Decorticate posturing. (B) Decerebrate
posturing.

Feet plantar flexed   Wrists and fingers flexed   Arms adducted

Forearms pronated   Elbows extended

B Decerebrate posturing

Eye response
 4 = eyelids open or opened, tracking,
    or blinking to command
 3 = eyelids open but not tracking
 2 = eyelids closed but open to loud voice
 1 = eyelids closed but open to pain
 0 = eyelids remain closed with pain

Motor response
 4 = thumbs-up, fist, or peace sign
 3 = localizing to pain
 2 = flexion response to pain
 1 = extension response to pain
 0 = no response to pain or
    generalized myoclonus status

Brainstem reflexes
 4 = pupil and corneal reflexes present
 3 = one pupil wide and fixed
 2 = pupil or corneal reflexes absent
 1 = pupil and corneal reflexes absent
 0 = absent pupil, corneal, and cough reflexes

Respiration
 4 = not intubated, regular breathing pattern
 3 = not intubated, Cheyne-Stokes
    breathing pattern
 2 = not intubated, irregular breathing
 1 = breathes above ventilator rate
 0 = breathes at ventilator rate or apnea

FIGURE 47.12 FOUR Score Coma Scale. From Wijdicks, E. F. M., Bamlet, W. R., Marmatton,
B. V., Manno, E. M., & McClelland, R. L. (2005). Validation of a new coma scale: The FOUR Score.
Annals of Neurology, 58, 585–593. DOI: 10.1002/ana.20611. Figure 1 and Table 1. Used
with permission. © Mayo, 2005.

for cognitive impairment, the Mini-Mental State Examination (MMSE) or Confusion Assessment Method can be used. The Confusion Assessment Method uses the following criteria to help diagnose delirium (Waszynski, 2007):

• Acute onset and fluctuating course
• Inattention
• Disorganized thinking
• Altered level of consciousness

Find more about the Confusion Assessment Method at the Hartford Institute for Geriatric Nursing (http://consultgerirn.org), an excellent collaborative website that provides best practice information related to older adults. A change in mental status should be taken seriously, especially when the patient takes multiple medicines or has had a recent change in medicines. A primary cause of delirium and acute states of confusion is adverse effects from medications.

When you assess cognitive function, you are evaluating the patient's thinking capacity. You want to determine the length of attention span, ability to concentrate, judgment, memory, orientation, perception, problem-solving ability, and motor function.

You can learn a great deal about a patient's mental capacities and emotional state by simply interacting with the patient. Behavior, mood, hygiene, grooming, and choice of dress reveal pertinent information about mental status. Mental status examinations can be performed to determine patients' cognitive functioning, thought processes, and perceptions by observing the patient's verbal and nonverbal responses to questions and specific requests. Table 47.4 includes some ways to assess these areas.

Orientation refers to the patient's ability to comprehend himself or herself in relation to person, location (place), and time. A patient who is fully oriented is often referred to as "oriented times three." Typical questions include, "What is your name? Where are you? What day is it?" (Keep in mind that we all forget the date from time to time!) You can also ask if the person knows what season it is (spring, fall, etc.). A resident of a long-term care facility who says he is "at home" may consider the facility his home and is not necessarily disoriented. Be sure your question is appropriate to the patient's age, culture, living conditions, lifestyle, and medical condition. If the patient is unable to speak because of a stroke (expressive **aphasia**) or being intubated, do not rule out the possibility that the patient is oriented. Give expressively aphasic patients yes-or-no questions such as "Are you in a grocery store? Are you in a bowling alley? Are you in a hospital?" Patients may be able to answer with a shake of the head, eye blinks, or hand squeezes as instructed.

Examination of the Eyes

Examination of the pupils is an important part of the neurologic assessment and cranial nerve evaluation. The size of the pupils at rest is documented in millimeters (Fig. 47.13). If the patient's pupils are unusually large or small, determine whether the patient has had any medications that can affect pupil size. If the patient's pupils are unequal in size **(anisocoria)**, without a correlating diagnosis or symptoms,

Pupil gauge (mm)

2   3   4   5   6   7   8   9

FIGURE 47.13 Assessment of pupil size.

ask the patient or significant others if the patient normally has unequal pupils. Anisocoria may be congenital; it can also be caused by cataract surgery. Development of unequal pupils in a patient who previously had equal pupils is an emergency and should be reported to the physician immediately. Any deviation from the normal round shape of the pupils is documented.

Once the resting size of the pupils has been noted, the next step is to assess their response to light. In a darkened room, a light source (such as a flashlight) is directed at the pupil from the lateral aspect of the eye. This allows the examiner to see the direct and the consensual response to the light. A consensual response means that when one pupil is exposed to direct light, the other pupil also constricts. Absence of a consensual response may indicate a pathological condition in the area of the optic chiasm. Typically, the speed of the reaction to light is described as brisk, sluggish, or absent. Differences in the speed or size of constriction between the two pupils should be reported to the practitioner.

Accommodation is the process of visual focusing from far to near. To evaluate for accommodation, have the patient focus on an object at a distant point and then refocus on the object at a near point. Pupils should constrict with the adjustment to the near object and the eyes should converge. Upon completion of the assessment of the pupils, document your findings. PERRLA is a commonly used abbreviation to note that *p*upils are *e*qual, *r*ound, and *r*eactive to *l*ight and *a*ccommodation. Note, if you have not assessed for accommodation, then do not include the A in the acronym.

You will also evaluate for range of motion and for smoothness and coordination of movements. Eyes that move in the same direction in a coordinated manner are said to have a *conjugate* gaze. Conversely, a *dysconjugate* gaze is movement of the eyes in different directions. Some patients may be unable to move one or both eyes in a specific direction; this is called *ophthalmoplegia*. It is often documented as "limited extraocular movements." Always document what the limitation is (e.g., "Patient is unable to look laterally with left eye"). This allows colleagues to compare their findings with yours and detect any changes.

Nystagmus is involuntary movement of the eyes. Nystagmus varies in the speed of the movement and the direction. Horizontal nystagmus is the most common. Common causes

• WORD • BUILDING •
aphasia: a—absence + phasia—speech
anisocoria: aniso—unequal + coria—pupil

of nystagmus are phenytoin (Dilantin) toxicity and injury to the brainstem.

Examination of Muscle Function

Examine muscle groups systematically in the upper extremities and then the lower extremities, comparing right to left. Compare muscle groups for symmetry of size and strength. Keep in mind the patient's age and general physical condition when evaluating muscle strength. You would not expect the same amount of strength from a 75-year-old woman as from a 20-year-old man. If the patient has chronic neurologic deficits, ask if the results of the assessment are different from his or her usual level of function.

Many HCPs use a 5-point scale to document muscle strength. A score of 5 describes a patient who is able to move the extremity against gravity and the resistance of the examiner, displaying normal muscle strength. If the examiner is able to provide more resistance than the patient can overcome with active movement, the score is 4. If the patient can move the extremity only against gravity, but not resistance, the score is 3. If gravity must be eliminated by having the examiner support the extremity to allow the patient to move the extremity, the score is 2. A score of 1 is given if there is no active movement of the extremity, but a minimum muscular contraction can be palpated. If the examiner is unable to detect any muscular function, a score of 0 is given.

To test the deltoid muscles, ask the patient to raise his or her arms at the shoulder. Have the patient resist as you push down on the upper arms. The biceps are tested by having the patient flex the arm at the elbow and bring the palm toward the face, then resist as you attempt to straighten the arm by pulling on the forearm. With the arm similarly flexed, ask the patient to straighten the arm while you resist the movement.

Hand grasps are tested by having the patient squeeze your fingers. Remember to cross your index and middle fingers to prevent the patient from hurting your fingers. If the patient does not release the grasp when told to, it is a reflex grasp, not a response to command. A reflex palmar grasp may indicate a pathological condition of the frontal lobe.

Assess for arm drift by asking the patient to hold both arms straight in front with the palms upward while keeping the eyes closed. A downward drift of the arm or rotation so that the palm is down indicates impairment of the opposite side of the brain. If a pathological condition is present, arm drift may be apparent before differences in muscle strength can be detected.

Assessment of leg muscle strength begins with the iliopsoas muscle. Place your hand on the patient's thigh and ask the patient to raise the leg, flexing at the hip. Hip adductors are tested by having the patient bring his or her legs together against your hands. The hip abductors and gluteus medius and minimus are tested by having the patient move the legs apart against resistance. Hip extension by the gluteus maximus is tested by placing the hand under the thigh and having the patient push down with the leg. The quadriceps femoris extends the knee and is tested by having the patient attempt to straighten the leg at the knee. The hamstrings are responsible for knee flexion and are evaluated by having the patient attempt to keep the heel of the foot against the bed or chair rung. Dorsiflexion is tested by having the patient pull the toes toward the head against resistance. Plantar flexion is tested by having the patient push against the examiner's hand with the ball of the foot.

Babinski's reflex is tested by firmly stroking the sole of the foot. Normal response is flexion of the great toe. If the great toe extends and the other toes fan out, neurologic dysfunction should be suspected if the patient is more than 6 months old. Deep tendon reflexes are not usually part of a routine nursing assessment. The patient's gait should be assessed to detect any neurologic dysfunction and also to assess ability to ambulate safely. Patients who stagger, weave, or bump into objects may need assistance with walking.

Romberg's test is performed by having the patient stand with feet together and eyes closed. Be sure to stand close to the patient, especially if he or she is an older adult, to prevent falling. A negative Romberg's test means that the patient experiences minimal swaying for up to 20 seconds. A patient who experiences swaying or who leans to one side is said to have a positive Romberg's test. A positive Romberg's test may be seen in cerebellar dysfunction.

BE SAFE!

A positive Romberg's test in an older adult is expected as a result of normal aging changes in the cerebellum. Be sure to protect the patient with a positive result from falls. A gait belt may be helpful when assisting the patient with ambulation.

Examination of Cranial Nerves

The cranial nerves are usually not examined in depth during a routine bedside neurologic assessment. Testing requires a patient who is able to cooperate with the examiner. Table 47.6 provides basic testing techniques that offer a basic assessment of cranial nerve function.

Summary of Examination Findings

In all cases, the findings of the neurologic examination should be correlated with the remainder of the physical examination findings. A decreased level of consciousness, coupled with a decreased oxygen saturation on pulse oximetry, point to hypoxia as a cause. Correlation of vital signs with neurologic signs is particularly important. Bradycardia, increasing systolic blood pressure with widening pulse pressure, and irregular respirations, commonly referred to as Cushing's triad, are late indications of increasing intracranial pressure. These findings, in conjunction with a unilateral dilated pupil, may indicate impending herniation of the brain (discussed further in Chapter 48).

TABLE 47.6   COLLECTION OF DATA RELATED TO CRANIAL NERVE FUNCTION

Nerve	Test
Olfactory nerve	Ask patient to identify common scents, such as cinnamon and coffee.
Optic nerve	Ask patient to read something or tell how many fingers you are holding up.
Oculomotor nerve	Check pupils for reaction to light and accommodation.
Oculomotor, trochlear, and abducens nerves	Ask patient to follow your finger while moving it in front of his or her eyes in the positions of a clock: 1, 3, 5, 7, 9, and 11 o'clock.
Trigeminal nerve	Ask patient to identify touch on different parts of the face with eyes closed.
Facial nerve	Ask patient to frown, smile, wrinkle forehead; check for symmetry.
Vestibulocochlear nerve	Have patient identify whisper close to each ear. Observe gait for balance.
Glossopharyngeal and vagus nerves	Watch for uvula and palate to rise when patient says "ahh." Touch back of throat with cotton-tipped applicator to elicit gag reflex.
Spinal accessory nerve	Ask the patient to turn head and shrug the shoulders against resistance.
Hypoglossal nerve	Ask the patient to stick out the tongue and move it from side to side.

CRITICAL THINKING

Tim Thompson

■ You are caring for Tim, a 78-year-old man admitted with heart problems. As you enter his room with his afternoon medications, you find Tim confused. He thinks he is at home, that the year is 1968, and he does not understand who you are or why you are there. He recognizes his wife, who is at his bedside, and he knows his own name.

1. How would you describe and document his mental status?
2. What additional data do you need to decide how to proceed?
3. What may have contributed to his confusion?
4. What members of the health team can you collaborate with in caring for Tim?

Suggested answers are at the end of the chapter.

DIAGNOSTIC TESTS FOR THE NEUROLOGIC SYSTEM

Laboratory Tests

Specific diagnostic blood tests do not exist for neurologic disorders. However, depending on the history and physical examination, the HCP may include laboratory tests to look for underlying causes of symptoms: thyroid hormone levels, vitamin B_{12}, complete blood count (CBC), electrolytes, creatine kinase and isoenzymes (CK), venereal disease research lab (VDRL) test (for syphilis), liver function, and renal function. Measurement of erythrocyte sedimentation rate (ESR) and white blood cell (WBC) count may indicate an infection, such as meningitis. Hormone levels, such as prolactin or cortisol, may indicate dysfunction of the pituitary gland related to a brain tumor. Anticholinesterase testing and antibody titers are useful in diagnosing myasthenia gravis. Research is ongoing to develop a blood test for Alzheimer's disease.

Lumbar Puncture

Cerebrospinal fluid (CSF) may be obtained via lumbar puncture and evaluated for glucose and protein levels, the presence of bacteria and WBCs, levels of immunoglobulin, antibodies, and culture and sensitivity. See Appendix A for nursing care of a patient undergoing lumbar puncture.

NURSING CARE TIP

The idea of a needle being introduced into the spinal canal is frightening to many people. Give simple, clear directions to the patient; help the patient maintain his or her position; and provide emotional support throughout the procedure.

X-Ray Examination

Spinal x-ray examinations are done to determine the status of individual vertebrae and their relationship to one another. If the patient experiences pain with certain movements, he or she may be asked to flex and extend the area of the spine being examined while the radiographs are taken. This allows detection of abnormal movement of the vertebrae. If the patient may have sustained trauma to the spine, particularly the cervical spine, radiographs are taken before the immobilizing devices are removed. Skull radiographs may be taken to detect skull fractures or foreign bodies. No special nursing care is required.

Computed Tomography

A computed tomography (CT) scan is used for diagnosing neurologic disorders of the brain or spine. Some of the disorders that can be detected by CT are hemorrhage, altered ventricle size, cerebral atrophy, tumors, skull fractures, and abscesses. CT is used when magnetic resonance imaging (MRI) is contraindicated because of metal aneurysm clips or other metal implants.

The scan may be performed with or without radiopaque contrast material to enhance the clarity of the images. Contrast material is most commonly used if a tumor is suspected or following surgery in the area to be scanned. CT scans are commonly used in emergency evaluations because they can be done quickly, an important consideration if the patient is ventilated or unstable.

Nursing Care

During the CT scan, the patient must lie still on a movable table. Noncontrast scans take about 10 minutes; contrast scans take 20 to 30 minutes. Patients who are receiving dye should be warned that they may feel a sensation of warmth following the injection; warmth in the groin area might make them feel as though they have been incontinent of urine. Nausea, diaphoresis, itching, or difficulty breathing can indicate allergy to the dye and should be reported immediately to the physician or nurse practitioner. Sedation may be required for patients who are agitated or disoriented. Patients who are in pain may need pain medication before the examination. See Appendix A for nursing care of a patient undergoing a CT scan.

Magnetic Resonance Imaging

MRI is used for diagnosis of degenerative diseases such as multiple sclerosis, arteriovenous malformations, small tumors, hemorrhages, and cerebral and spinal cord edema. An MRI of the mediastinal cavity will determine if the thymus gland is enlarged and facilitate diagnosis of myasthenia gravis. It is a longer procedure and may be difficult for unstable, disoriented, or ventilated patients. As with a CT scan, the MRI can be done with or without contrast material. Some facilities have the capability to perform magnetic resonance angiograms (MRAs). This test allows visualization of blood vessels and assessment of blood flow without being as invasive as a traditional angiogram. See Appendix A for nursing care of a patient undergoing MRI.

Angiogram

An angiogram provides information about the structure of specific vessels, as well as overall circulation to an area. See Appendix A for nursing care of a patient undergoing an angiogram.

Myelogram

A **myelogram** is an x-ray examination of the spinal canal and its contents after injection of contrast material. Compression of nerve roots, herniation of intravertebral disks, and blockage of cerebrospinal fluid circulation can all be detected by myelogram. See Appendix A for nursing care of a patient undergoing a myelogram.

Electroencephalogram

Electrical activity of the brain is evaluated by use of an **electroencephalogram** (EEG). Analysis of the tracing can identify areas of abnormality, such as a seizure focus or areas of slowed activity.

THERAPEUTIC MEASURES FOR THE NEUROLOGIC SYSTEM

Moving and Positioning

Patients who have pain may need help changing positions and ambulating. Use of heat, cold, or analgesics may allow the patient to be more independent in mobility.

If the patient has sensory loss, make sure that no part of the body is inadvertently compressed (e.g., a hand caught under a hip or the scrotum compressed between the legs). Pressure ulcers are a primary concern with the patient who is unable to move independently. Collaborate with the physical therapist to determine positioning techniques that maximize the chance of useful recovery.

Patients with paresis, paralysis, or **paresthesia** (abnormal sensation such as burning or tingling) may be partially or completely dependent in moving and positioning. Take care to maintain the body in functional positions when routine position changes are made. This means keeping the trunk, extremities, hands, and feet in usable positions—for example, hands can be splinted to keep the thumb and fingers opposed, or tennis shoes can be used to keep the feet in an appropriate position for standing or walking.

Contractures and footdrop are complications that are often associated with neurologic disorders. Contractures are permanent muscle contractions with fibrosis of connective tissue that occur from lack of use of a muscle or muscle group. They cause permanent deformities and prevent normal functioning of the affected part. Footdrop occurs when the feet are not supported in a functional position and become contracted in a position of plantar flexion (Fig. 47.14). Use

• WORD • BUILDING •

myelogram: myelo—referring to the spinal cord + gram— picture
electroencephalogram: electro—electrical activity + encephalo—referring to the brain + gram—picture
paresthesia: para—beside + asthesia—sensations

FIGURE 47.14 Contractures, footdrop. From Hegner, B. (1998). *Assisting in long term care* (3rd ed.). Albany, NY: Delmar, with permission.

footboards, high-top tennis shoes, and splints to help prevent footdrop. Splints are commonly used to prevent contractures of the upper and lower extremities and to keep the affected parts in a functional position. If splints are used, the patient must be evaluated for and protected from discomfort and skin breakdown at the splint site.

Mobilization should begin as soon as a patient is medically stable. Initially this may involve the use of a cardiac chair if the patient is unable to bear weight. Transfer of the patient to a bedside chair or use of ambulation aids may require a multidisciplinary approach. Be careful to recognize any physical or cognitive deficits that might affect safety and adjust the environment to protect the patient. This includes communicating any safety concerns to unlicensed personnel who interact with the patient.

Activities of Daily Living

The effects of neurologic disorders on activities of daily living (ADLs) can range from an inconvenience to complete dependence. Patients may have trouble bending over to put on their shoes and socks, lifting a full cooking pot, or caring for an infant. A quadriplegic patient may be completely unable to perform ADLs but can be taught to direct his or her own personal care. Encourage patients to use strategies they learned in occupational or physical therapy.

Assessment of a hospitalized patient should include a discussion of the strategies the patient normally uses at home to accomplish ADLs. Every attempt should be made to continue to use these strategies. This is particularly true if the patient is admitted to a long-term care facility. Patients who have intact cognitive function should be included in care planning and encouraged to work collaboratively with caregivers. If the strategies the patient uses during ADLs must be changed (e.g., if the patient's transfer technique is unsafe), be sure to explain the rationale for the changes to the patient and significant others. If patients have impaired cognitive function, try to maintain a specific routine that is as close to their normal environment as possible. Normalizing routines may help patients adapt to a change in environment and maximize their ability to function.

Communication

The communication problems associated with neurologic disorders have a variety of etiologies. Some neurologic disorders cause difficulty speaking (**dysarthria**). Dysfunction of the lips, tongue, or jaw makes speech difficult or impossible to understand. When dysarthric individuals know what they want to say but cannot be understood, they can become very frustrated. This frustration is compounded if the patients are treated as if they have cognitive deficits merely because they have difficulty communicating.

Patients who have had a stroke can experience different types of aphasia. Expressive aphasia is difficulty or inability to verbally communicate with others. The patient may be able to speak in sentences but inappropriately substitute words, such as "The sky is dish." Word-finding difficulty is another type of expressive aphasia. These patients may tell you "I want a . . ." and then be unable to complete the sentence. In severe cases of aphasia, the patient may make sounds that resemble words or may only utter sounds. For individuals with no intelligible speech or with word-finding difficulty, a picture board with commonly used items may facilitate communication. (See an example of a picture board in Chapter 49.) Keep in mind that patients with expressive aphasia may answer yes to all questions rather than just those for which yes is correct. The same is true of answering no. This is one reason why a nurse should never ask a patient, "Are you Mrs. Gonzalez?" An aphasic patient may say yes even if that is not her name. Instead, ask the patient to state her name. Always check the identification band.

For patients who substitute words, simply correct the substitution and continue the conversation. Patients with expressive aphasia are often very aware of and frustrated by their difficulty communicating. Give them time to try to express themselves. If you cannot understand them, offer possibilities based on the situation. If the patient is sitting in the chair, ask if he or she wants to go back to bed or wants to use the bathroom. If the patient is restless, ask if he or she is in pain.

Some patients use the same word in response to all questions, and for a few patients, that word is a profanity. This is very difficult for significant others to deal with, particularly if swearing is not something the patient normally did. Make it clear to the family that you understand that this behavior is part of the patient's illness.

Receptive aphasia affects the patient's ability to understand spoken language. Again, the severity of the aphasia varies.

• **WORD** • **BUILDING** •

dysarthria: dys—dysfunctional + arthria—movement of the joints used in speech

Some patients may understand simple directions such as "sit down" or "squeeze my fingers." In other cases, the nurse may need to pantomime the action the nurse wants the patient to perform, such as showing the patient pills and then mimicking taking the pills and drinking water.

BE SAFE!

If the patient has receptive aphasia, assume that he or she cannot understand or follow safety instructions, such as "Do not stand up until I get back." Even going around the corner to get water can give a patient enough time to try to stand up and subsequently fall.

Nutrition

Alterations in the ability to maintain an adequate nutritional intake can have many causes. The level of consciousness may be depressed enough that the patient does not recognize that she or he is hungry or thirsty. Decreased level of consciousness or cranial nerve dysfunction may impair the patient's ability to swallow safely. Severe weakness may limit the patient's ability to take in enough food to meet the body's requirements. These conditions are often compounded by the increased metabolic rate that accompanies neurologic injury or illness.

If there is any question of the patient's ability to swallow, a swallowing evaluation should be performed by a speech therapist. Some institutions use a radiological examination to evaluate the ability to swallow. A small amount of barium is added to food or fluid, and fluoroscopy is used while the patient swallows. This allows visualization of the path of the food or fluid. Patients with swallowing difficulty (dysphagia) may have better success with foods or thick liquids rather than thin fluids. Liquids may be thickened with special thickening agents to allow easier swallowing. All patients should be positioned as upright as possible while eating or drinking, and patients who have difficulty swallowing should be monitored during eating and not left alone.

If weakness or fatigue is the cause of decreased nutritional intake, several modifications are possible. Serving small portions of food more frequently can increase intake. Using high-protein, high-calorie foods and supplements increases the nutritional content of small amounts of foods.

For patients who cannot swallow or who cannot swallow enough food, enteral tube feedings may be needed. If enteral feedings are anticipated to be for a short duration, a nasogastric tube may be used. The disadvantages of nasogastric tubes include impairment of the integrity of nasal skin and the risk of aspiration. The risk of aspiration in neurologically impaired patients who have cognitive impairments is increased because these patients may pull out the nasogastric tube due to their lack of understanding the purpose of the tube. If long-term enteral feedings are anticipated, a gastrostomy tube may be placed directly through the abdominal wall into the stomach. This feeding method has the advantage of reducing the risks of aspiration and eliminating nasal skin breakdown.

Family

When working with patients who have a neurologic deficit, whether acute or chronic, in the hospital, extended care facility, or at home, the family should be included in their care and rehabilitation. Depending on the patient's diagnosis and prognosis, the family will need support from staff. It is rewarding to see the patient who has had an accident recover with rehabilitation, but it is also rewarding to promote quality of life for the patient with Alzheimer's disease and his or her family. Communication with the family regarding patient improvements and information about the illness is extremely important. Include the family in the patient's care, such as bathing, feeding, and grooming. Suggest that the family participate in physical, occupational, and speech therapy sessions. Education is of vital importance, especially if the patient is going to be discharged home. Direct the patient and family to support groups and case managers for information regarding financial assistance and community resources during rehabilitation.

SUGGESTED ANSWERS TO

CRITICAL THINKING

■ *Mrs. Stevens*

Albuterol is an adrenergic agonist (sometimes called a sympathomimetic), which is given to stimulate the sympathetic nervous system, resulting in open airways in patients with respiratory disease. However, it can also stimulate the cardiac system and cause a rapid heart rate and increased blood pressure. Be sure to monitor vital signs in patients receiving medications that affect the autonomic nervous system.

■ *Tim Thompson*

1. He is alert but confused, oriented to person only.
2. The nurse should ask his wife if this has ever happened before, check his medical history for any disorders that may contribute to neurologic dysfunction, do a quick neurologic examination to determine if any additional deficits exist, check vital signs and pulse oximetry if available, and notify the physician immediately if the symptoms are a new finding.
3. Some possible explanations to explore include hypoxemia, stroke, worsening heart problems causing inadequate flow of blood to the brain, hypoglycemia, or even confusion (delirium) related to a sudden transition from home to an unfamiliar environment.
4. Consider based on further assessment (as noted in #2 and 3) if there may be a need to contact the HCP for evaluation. Involve a respiratory therapist, electrocardiogram technician, or others based on assessed needs.

REVIEW QUESTIONS

1. What assessments are included in the FOUR Score coma scale? **Select all that apply.**
   1. Eye response
   2. Motor response
   3. Brainstem reflexes
   4. Respiration
   5. Verbal response

2. Which instruction would the nurse provide for the patient when testing the trigeminal nerve?
   1. "Stick out your tongue."
   2. "Turn your head side to side."
   3. "I am going to shine a light into your eyes and observe your pupils."
   4. "Close your eyes and tell me where you feel the cotton touching your face."

3. Which of the following is a symptom of increasing intracranial pressure that should be reported immediately to the primary care provider? .
   1. Constricted pupils
   2. Decreasing level of consciousness
   3. Narrowing pulse pressure
   4. Bradypnea

4. What are the normal effects of aging on the CNS? **Select all that apply.**
   1. Increased postural stability
   2. Reduced blood flow to the brain
   3. Impaired short-term memory
   4. Sleep disturbances
   5. Loss of deep tendon reflexes
   6. Decrease in acetylcholine

5. The nurse knows the patient understands teaching about an angiogram when the patient makes which of the following statements?
   1. "A small needle will be inserted into my spinal column to withdraw fluid for examination."
   2. "I will be in a large machine that uses magnetic energy to create images; it has a noisy knocking sound."
   3. "Electrodes will be placed on my head to monitor electrical activity in my brain."
   4. "A catheter will be placed in an artery in my groin, and dye will be injected that will make my vessels show up on x-ray."

6. A patient has returned from having a CT scan with contrast. Which of the following should be a priority in the hours after the scan?
   1. Ambulation
   2. Drinking fluids
   3. Turning side to side
   4. Coughing and deep breathing

7. Which of the following nursing interventions should be included in the plan of care for a patient at risk for footdrop?
   1. Position the patient in the left lateral position.
   2. Provide daily foot massage.
   3. Apply high-top tennis shoes.
   4. Maintain the patient in an upright position as much as possible.

Answers can be found in Appendix C.

Reference

Waszynski, M. (2007). How to try this: Detecting delirium. *American Journal of Nursing, 107,* 50–59.

 Davis*Plus.* | For additional resources and information visit **davispl.us/medsurg5**

48

Nursing Care of Patients With Central Nervous System Disorders

DEBORAH L. WEAVER

KEY TERMS

akinesia (AH-kin-EE-zee-uh)
ataxia (ah-TAK-see-ah)
bradykinesia (BRAY-dee-kin-EE-zee-ah)
contralateral (KON-truh-LAT-er-uhl)
craniectomy (KRAY-nee-EK-tuh-mee)
cranioplasty (KRAY-nee-oh-plas-tee)
craniotomy (KRAY-nee-AHT-oh-mee)
delirium (de-LEER-ee-um)
dementia (dee-MEN-cha)
dysreflexia (DIS-re-FLEK-see-ah)
encephalitis (en-SEFF-uh-LYE-tis)
encephalopathy (en-SEFF-uh-LAHP-ah-thee)
hemiparesis (hem-ee-puh-REE-sis)
hydrocephalus (HEYE-droh-SEF-uh-luhs)
ipsilateral (IP-si-LAT-er-uhl)
laminectomy (LAM-i-NEK-toh-mee)
meningitis (MEN-in-JIGH-tis)
neurodegenerative (new-roh-de-JEN-er-uh-tiv)
nuchal rigidity (NEW-kuhl re-JID-i-tee)
paraparesis (PAR-ah-puh-REE-sis)
paraplegia (PAR-ah-PLEE-jee-ah)
photophobia (FOH-tuh-FOH-bee-ah)
postictal (pohst-IK-tuhl)
prodromal (proh-DROH-muhl)
quadriparesis (KWA-dri-puh-REE-sis)
quadriplegia (KWA-dri-PLEE-jee-ah)
turbid (TERR-bid)

LEARNING OUTCOMES

1. Explain causes, risk factors, and pathophysiology of central nervous system infections, including meningitis and encephalitis.

2. Plan nursing interventions for a patient with a central nervous system infection.

3. Differentiate between the various types of headaches.

4. Identify teaching you will provide for a patient experiencing headaches.

5. List the causes and types of seizures.

6. Describe appropriate interventions for an individual experiencing a seizure.

7. Recognize a patient who is developing increased intracranial pressure.

8. Identify nursing interventions that can help prevent increased intracranial pressure.

9. Explain the causes, risk factors, and pathophysiology of injuries to the brain and spinal cord.

10. Plan nursing care for a patient with an injury to the brain or spinal cord.

11. Explain causes, risk factors, and pathophysiology associated with neurodegenerative disorders such as Parkinson's, Huntington's, and Alzheimer's diseases.

12. Plan nursing care for a patient with a neurodegenerative disorder.

13. Plan nursing interventions for the patient with dementia.

Disorders of the central nervous system (CNS) include problems originating in the brain and spinal cord. Because the CNS is the control center for the entire body, disorders in this system can cause symptoms in any part of the body, ranging from pain to confusion, paralysis, and coma. This chapter presents nursing care of patients with these disorders. Care of patients with cerebrovascular disorders is covered in Chapter 49.

 CENTRAL NERVOUS SYSTEM INFECTIONS

Infectious agents can enter the CNS via a variety of routes (Table 48.1). Anything that depresses the patient's immune system such as steroid administration, chemotherapy, radiation therapy, or malnutrition can make the patient more vulnerable to infection.

Meningitis
Pathophysiology and Etiology

Meningitis is an inflammation of the meninges that surround the brain and spinal cord. It can be caused by either bacterial or viral infection. Any microorganism that enters the body can result in meningitis. Bacterial meningitis is a serious infection that is spread by direct contact with discharge from the respiratory tract of an infected person. Viral meningitis, also called aseptic meningitis, is more common and rarely serious. It usually presents with flulike symptoms, and patients recover in 1 to 2 weeks.

The most common bacteria causing meningitis include *Neisseria meningitidis, Streptococcus pneumoniae,* and *Haemophilus influenzae* type b (Hib). With current immunization standards in the United States, *H. influenzae* type b has decreased in recent years. *N. meningitidis,* the cause of meningococcal meningitis, and *S. pneumoniae,* the cause of pneumococcal meningitis, are the major causes of bacterial meningitis. Bacterial infection generally begins in another area, such as the upper respiratory tract, enters the blood, and

invades the CNS, causing the meninges to become inflamed and intracranial pressure (ICP) to increase. Vessel occlusion and necrosis of areas in the brain can occur. Cranial nerve function can be transiently or permanently affected by meningitis. Some of the effects are listed in Table 48.2.

Prevention

Vaccines are available against some pathogens. Hib vaccinations are begun during infancy. A vaccine against *S. pneumoniae* is recommended for people over age 65 and those who have a chronic medical condition. Currently the Centers for Disease Control and Prevention (CDC) recommends 2 doses of meningococcal vaccine (MCV4) for adolescents, one at age 11 or 12 and a booster at age 16. Other groups at increased risk who should be vaccinated are college freshmen living in dormitories, U.S. military recruits, anyone with compromised immunity, laboratory personnel, and those traveling to areas of the world where meningococcal disease is common.

Chemoprophylaxis is recommended for those who have had significant exposure to anyone currently infected with meningitis. To destroy the organism from the nasopharynx, antimicrobials such as rifampin, quinolones, or sulfonamides are used.

Signs and Symptoms

The most common symptom of meningitis is a severe headache, caused by tension on blood vessels and irritation of the pain-sensitive dura mater. A high fever and stiff neck are present, and the patient may experience **photophobia** (light sensitivity). The patient with meningococcal meningitis usually presents with petechiae on the skin and mucous membranes.

Nuchal rigidity (pain and stiffness when the neck is moved) is caused by spasm of the extensor muscles of the neck. Positive Kernig's and Brudzinski's signs are often seen in patients suffering from meningitis. Both signs are caused by inflammation of the meninges and spinal nerve roots. To elicit Kernig's sign, the examiner flexes the patient's hip to

TABLE 48.1 ROUTES OF ENTRY FOR CENTRAL NERVOUS SYSTEM INFECTIONS

Route of Entry	Examples
Bloodstream	Insect bite
	Otitis media
Direct extension	Fracture of frontal or facial bones
Cerebrospinal fluid	Dural tear
	Poor sterile technique during procedure
Nose or mouth	Meningococcus meningitis
In utero	Contamination of amniotic fluid
	Rubella
	Vaginal infection

TABLE 48.2 CRANIAL NERVES AFFECTED BY MENINGITIS

Cranial Nerve Affected	Manifestation
III, IV, VI	Ocular palsies
	Unequal and sluggishly reactive pupils
VII	Facial weakness
VIII	Deafness and vertigo

90 degrees and tries to extend the patient's knee. The sign is positive if the patient experiences pain and spasm of the hamstring. Brudzinski's sign is positive when flexion of the patient's neck causes the hips and knees to flex (Fig. 48.1). Nausea and vomiting associated with meningitis are caused by direct irritation of brain tissue and by increased ICP.

Encephalopathy refers to the mental status changes seen in patients with meningitis. These are manifested as short attention span, poor memory, disorientation, difficulty following commands, and a tendency to misinterpret environmental stimuli. Late signs of meningitis include lethargy and seizures.

Complications

Resolution of meningitis depends on how quickly and effectively the disease is treated. Viral meningitis usually has no lasting effects; however, bacterial meningitis can be fatal. Cranial nerve damage can leave the patient blind or deaf. Seizures can continue to occur even after the acute phase of the illness has passed. Cognitive deficits ranging from memory impairment to profound learning disabilities can occur.

Diagnostic Tests

A lumbar puncture is the most informative diagnostic test for a patient with suspected meningitis (see Chapter 47). Viral meningitis is characterized by clear cerebrospinal fluid (CSF) with normal glucose level and normal or slightly increased protein level. No bacteria are seen, but the white blood cell (WBC) count is usually increased. In contrast, the CSF of an individual with bacterial meningitis is **turbid**, or cloudy, because of the elevated number of white blood cells. Bacteria are identified by Gram stain and culture, and a sensitivity test is done to identify the most effective antibiotic. The bacteria use the glucose normally found in CSF, thereby lowering the glucose level. The amount of protein in the CSF is elevated. A magnetic resonance image (MRI) or computed tomographic (CT) scan can be done to evaluate for complications.

Therapeutic Measures

Antibiotics such as penicillin G, vancomycin, and cephalosporins are administered for bacterial meningitis. It is important to note the sensitivity report when it is complete to confirm the antibiotic in use is the best choice because there has been an increase in antibiotic/antimicrobial-resistant strains. Symptom management is the same for viral or bacterial meningitis. Antipyretics such as acetaminophen are used to control the fever; a cooling blanket also can be used. Care should be taken to avoid cooling the patient too much because shivering increases the metabolic demand for oxygen and glucose. Analgesics are given to lessen head and neck pain. Corticosteroids and anti-inflammatory agents are given to decrease swelling. Nausea and vomiting are controlled with antiemetic medications. The patient with meningococcal meningitis should be placed in isolation for at least the first 24 hours of medication administration to prevent transmission to others.

Patients can become agitated. A quiet, dark environment lessens the stimulation of a patient who has a headache or photophobia and who is agitated, disoriented, or at risk for seizures. An important aspect of nursing care focuses on keeping patients from harming themselves. It is very upsetting to families to see a loved one acting agitated or disoriented. Therefore, it is important to teach the family about symptoms and treatment goals for the patient (Table 48.3).

Encephalitis
Pathophysiology

Encephalitis is an inflammation of brain tissue. Nerve cell damage, edema, and necrosis cause neurologic findings localized to the specific areas of the brain affected. Hemorrhage in the brain can occur in some types of encephalitis. Increased ICP can lead to herniation of the brain (see later section on increased ICP).

Etiology

Viruses are the most common cause of encephalitis. They can be specifically related to a particular time of year or geographic location. Some viruses, such as West Nile virus, are carried by ticks or mosquitoes. Others are systemic viral infections, such as infectious mononucleosis or mumps, which spread to the brain. Parasites, toxic substances, bacteria, vaccines, and fungi are other potential causes of encephalitis.

Herpes simplex is the most common non–insect-borne virus to cause encephalitis. The majority of individuals harbor herpes simplex virus type 1 in a dormant state. This is the virus responsible for sores on the oral mucous membranes, commonly called cold sores. Communicable diseases, fever, and emotional stress are possible reasons for the virus becoming active, but the exact mechanism is not known.

A   Kernig's sign

B   Brudzinski's sign

FIGURE 48.1 (A) Kernig's sign. (B) Brudzinski's sign.

• WORD • BUILDING •
encephalopathy: encephalo—brain + pathy—illness
encephalitis: encephalo—brain + itis—inflammation

TABLE 48.3   MENINGITIS SUMMARY

Signs and Symptoms	Nuchal rigidity Positive Kernig's and Brudzinski's signs Fever Photophobia Petechial rash on skin and mucous membranes Encephalopathy
Diagnostic Tests	Lumbar puncture with CSF analysis, culture and sensitivity (C&S) Complete blood count C&S nose and throat
Therapeutic Measures	Antimicrobials (if bacterial) Seizure precautions Antipyretics Pain management Reduction of environmental stimuli Education
Complications	Seizures Increased ICP Hearing loss Vision impairment Cognitive defects
Possible Nursing Diagnoses	*Hyperthermia* *Acute Pain* related to nuchal rigidity *Risk for Injury* related to positive culture in CSF

CSF = cerebrospinal fluid; C&S = culture and sensitivity; ICP = intracranial pressure.

Signs and Symptoms

As with many viruses, there is a period of headache, general malaise, nausea and vomiting, and fever. These symptoms usually develop over a period of several days. Additional symptoms include nuchal rigidity, confusion, decreased level of consciousness, seizures, photophobia, **ataxia** (lack of muscle coordination), abnormal sleep patterns, and tremors. The patient may also have **hemiparesis** (slight paralysis or weakness on one side of the body).

The patient with herpes encephalitis develops edema and necrosis (sometimes associated with hemorrhage), most commonly in the temporal lobes. This significant cerebral edema causes increased ICP and can lead to herniation of the brain. If the patient becomes comatose before treatment is begun, the mortality rate can be as high as 70% to 80%. The first 72 hours is the most likely time for death to occur due to the cerebral edema.

Complications

Patients who have had encephalitis are often left with cognitive disabilities and personality changes. Ongoing seizures,

motor deficits, and blindness can also occur. Deterioration in cognition and personality changes are particularly stressful for significant others. The patient's behavioral control is a major factor in determining discharge plans. You can assist significant others to realistically assess the patient's functional level and the family's ability to care for the patient. In-home care, outpatient therapy, and adult day care are options to explore. For some severely impaired individuals, custodial care may be the only feasible and safe discharge option.

Diagnostic Tests

CT scan, MRI, lumbar puncture to obtain CSF, and electroencephalogram (EEG) are used to diagnose encephalitis. CSF analysis typically reveals increased WBC count and protein level and normal glucose levels. Breakdown of blood after cerebral hemorrhage results in yellow-colored CSF. Viral serology can be useful to identify the type of virus and guide treatment options.

Therapeutic Measures

No specific treatment is currently available for insect-borne encephalitis. Careful neurologic assessment and treatment of symptoms can help prevent complications and improve survival. Anticonvulsants, antipyretics, and analgesics are administered to reduce seizures, fever, and headache. Corticosteroids are used to decrease swelling from inflammation. Sedatives may be given for irritability. Antiviral medications such as acyclovir (Zovirax) may also be used, especially for herpes simplex.

INCREASED INTRACRANIAL PRESSURE

Pathophysiology and Etiology

Any patient with a pathological intracranial condition is at risk for increased ICP. ICP is the pressure exerted inside the cranial cavity by its components (blood, brain, and CSF). Normal ICP is 0 to 15 mm Hg. This pressure fluctuates with normal physiological changes, such as arterial pulsations, changes in position, and increases in intrathoracic pressure (e.g., coughing or sneezing). Common causes of increased ICP include brain trauma, intracranial hemorrhage, and brain tumors. Prompt detection of changes in neurologic status indicating increased ICP allows intervention aimed at preventing permanent brain damage.

The skull is a rigid compartment containing three components: brain, blood, and CSF. If an increase in one component is not accompanied by a decrease in one or both of the other components, the result is increased ICP (Fig. 48.2). The consequences of increased ICP depend on the degree of elevation and the speed with which the ICP increases. Patients with slow-growing tumors can have significantly increased ICP before they develop symptoms. Conversely, patients with a subarachnoid hemorrhage can sustain a sudden sharp increase in ICP.

• WORD • BUILDING •

hemiparesis: hemi—one side + paresis—partial paralysis

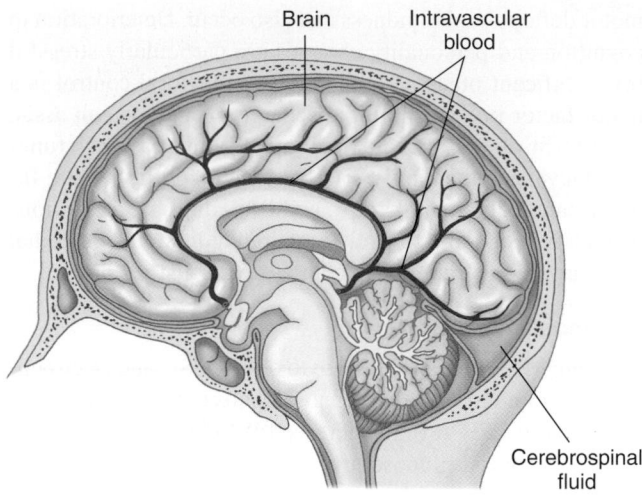

FIGURE 48.2 Any increase in brain tissue, blood, or cerebrospinal tissue can increase intracranial pressure.

The normally functioning body has several methods of compensating for increased ICP. CSF can be shunted into the spinal subarachnoid space. Hyperventilation can trigger constriction of cerebral blood vessels, decreasing the amount of blood within the cranial vault. These compensatory mechanisms are temporary and not particularly effective if the increase in ICP is sudden or severe.

Signs and Symptoms

Initial symptoms of increased ICP include restlessness, irritability, and decreased level of consciousness because cerebral cortex function is impaired. If not intubated, the patient can hyperventilate, causing vasoconstriction as the body attempts to compensate. As the pressure increases, the oculomotor nerve can be compressed on the side of the impairment. Compression of the outermost fibers of the oculomotor nerve results in diminished reactivity and dilation of the pupil. As the fibers become increasingly compressed, the pupil stops reacting to light. If the compression continues and the brain tissue exerts pressure on the opposite side of the brain from the injury, both pupils become fixed and dilated.

Vital sign changes are a late indication of increasing ICP. Cushing's triad is a classic late sign of increased ICP and is characterized by bradycardia, irregular respirations, and arterial hypertension (increasing systolic blood pressure while diastolic blood pressure remains the same), resulting in widening pulse pressure. By the time these symptoms appear, the ICP is significantly increased and interventions may not be successful.

Monitoring

ICP monitoring allows for early detection of changes in the pressure on the brain, before changes in symptoms are seen. The most common method of monitoring ICP in adults is by placing a catheter in the ventricle of the brain, in the cerebral parenchyma, or in the subdural or subarachnoid space. This can be done at the bedside or in surgery. Each

of these methods requires anesthetizing the scalp and drilling a hole, called a burr hole, into the skull.

Placement of a catheter into one of the lateral ventricles is referred to as external ventricular drainage (Fig. 48.3). This method allows for pressure monitoring as well as drainage of CSF to reduce ICP. Disadvantages to this method include difficulty in locating the ventricle for insertion of the catheter and clotting of the catheter by blood in the CSF.

To allow communication with the subarachnoid space, a subarachnoid bolt can be tightly screwed into the burr hole after the dura has been punctured (Fig. 48.4). The advantage of a subarachnoid bolt is ease of placement. Disadvantages include occlusion of the sensor portion of the bolt with brain tissue and inability to drain CSF. An intraparenchymal monitor is placed directly into brain tissue. Some physicians believe that this most accurately reflects the actual situation within the skull. These monitors cannot be used to drain CSF and can become occluded by brain tissue.

Patients with ICP monitors are cared for in an intensive care unit (ICU) and require aggressive nursing care to prevent complications. These patients are often mechanically ventilated and may be pharmacologically paralyzed and sedated. In addition to meeting the patient's physiological needs and preventing complications, education and emotional support for significant others is important.

Nursing Process for the Patient With a Communicable or Inflammatory Neurologic Disorder

Data Collection

Collaborate with the registered nurse (RN) to obtain a complete history from the patient, if feasible, and from significant others. Pay particular attention to exposure to risk factors. The physical examination must include all body systems because neurologic impairment affects the entire person. Following the initial examination, serial neurologic assessments continue to be important to detect and report changes promptly. You can assist with monitoring pupil response, level of consciousness (LOC), and vital signs for signs of increased ICP (Box 48-1). Monitor headache on a pain scale if the patient is able to participate. The Glasgow Coma Scale

FIGURE 48.3 Ventricular drain. A catheter into the ventricle allows intracranial pressure monitoring and cerebrospinal fluid drainage.

Scalp
Skull
Dura mater
Arachnoid
Subarachnoid space

Syringe

Three-way stopcock

Transducer

Subarachnoid screw

Close-up of placement into subarachnoid space

FIGURE 48.4 Subarachnoid bolt monitor.

or the FOUR Score, presented in Chapter 47, are valuable tools to monitor level of consciousness.

Nursing Diagnoses, Planning, and Implementation

The licensed practical nurse/licensed vocational nurse (LPN/LVN) collaborates with the RN in implementing care. For additional interventions for patients with communicable or inflammatory disorders, see the "Nursing Care Plan for the Patient With a Brain Tumor or Injury."

Patient Education

The nature and focus of teaching depend on the patient's level of consciousness and cognitive status. When appropriate, both the patient and significant others should be included in the education process. If the patient is not able to participate, the significant others become the focus of teaching.

NURSING CARE PLAN for the Patient With a Brain Lesion or Injury

Nursing Diagnosis: *Hyperthermia* related to infectious process

Expected Outcome: The patient will not exhibit evidence of hyperthermia.

Evaluation of Outcome: Is temperature controlled?

Intervention Assess temperature every 4 hours and as needed (prn). **Rationale** An elevated temperature can increase risk for seizures. **Evaluation** Is temperature controlled?

Continued

NURSING CARE PLAN for the Patient With a Brain Lesion or Injury—cont'd

Intervention Administer acetaminophen or aspirin as ordered. **Rationale** Antipyretic agents reduce fever. **Evaluation** Are antipyretics effective?

Intervention Provide a cooling mattress or tepid sponge baths as necessary. **Rationale** A cooling mattress may be necessary to reduce fever. These are uncomfortable for the patient. Comfort can be increased and shivering reduced by cooling the patient gradually and wrapping extremities in bath blankets during cooling mattress therapy. **Evaluation** Is cooling mattress or tepid bath effective? Is patient comfort maintained?

Nursing Diagnosis: *Risk for Acute Confusion* related to cerebral edema and increased intracranial pressure

Expected Outcomes: The patient will be oriented to person, place, and time; if this is not possible, patient's safety will be maintained.

Evaluation of Outcomes: Is patient oriented to self, place, and time and able to ask for help appropriately to prevent injury?

Intervention Assess level of consciousness (LOC) using Glasgow Coma Scale or the FOUR Score. **Rationale** Change in LOC can indicate increased intracranial pressure and should be reported. **Evaluation** Is patient alert and responsive? Is LOC stable?

Intervention Monitor orientation and reorient as needed. **Rationale** Giving correct information to patient will assist in orientation. **Evaluation** Can patient identify who he/she is, location, and month, year, or season?

Intervention Observe patient's reaction to simple commands such as "raise your hand." **Rationale** This helps distinguish between reflexes and purposeful movement. **Evaluation** Is patient able to follow simple commands?

Intervention Monitor patient's capabilities as activities increase. **Rationale** Patient can experience dizziness, imbalance, and confusion; the patient will need assistance with mobilization until stable. **Evaluation** Can patient sit up and ambulate to chair without dizziness?

Intervention If patient is not able to be reoriented, assess for safety and implement appropriate safety measures. **Rationale** Depending on the patient's prognosis, orientation may not be a realistic goal. **Evaluation** Is patient's safety maintained?

Nursing Diagnosis: *Self-Care Deficit,* dressing/feeding/toileting, related to mental status changes and inability to perform ADLs independently

Expected Outcome: The patient will maintain as much independence with ADLs as possible.

Evaluation of Outcome: Is the patient able to participate in self-care at an appropriate level?

Intervention Assess what the patient was able to do before admission/injury. **Rationale** The patient's potential for participation will depend on what he or she was able to do before injury. **Evaluation** What was the patient able to do? How does that compare with what he or she can do now?

Intervention Provide all supplies and equipment needed to carry out ADLs. **Rationale** Assembling equipment for the patient reserves energy for performing self-care. **Evaluation** Is the patient able to perform the majority of bath and hygiene tasks with appropriate setup?

Intervention Encourage the patient to perform activities at own pace. **Rationale** The patient may need more time to perform activities. **Evaluation** Does the patient gradually increase performance of self-care in a timely fashion?

NURSING CARE PLAN for the Patient With a Brain Lesion or Injury—cont'd

Intervention Teach and encourage family to participate with care. **Rationale** Including the family in the patient's care promotes support and family interaction. **Evaluation** Is the family involved? Is the patient accepting of their assistance?

Intervention Refer to occupational therapy if indicated. **Rationale** An occupational therapist is trained to assist patients to manage ADLs within health limitations. **Evaluation** Is occupational therapist able to assist patient with strategies to maintain independence?

Nursing Diagnosis: *Acute/Chronic Pain* related to cerebral edema and headache as evidenced by patient pain rating or evidence of painful behaviors

Expected Outcomes: Patient's pain is controlled as evidenced by statement that pain level is acceptable, or decrease in painful behaviors.

Evaluation of Outcomes: Does patient state pain level is acceptable? Are pain behaviors reduced?

Intervention Assess pain using a scale of 0 to 10 or PAINAD scale (see Chapter 10). **Rationale** The patient's self-report is the best measure of the patient's pain. **Evaluation** Is the patient able to rate pain? Is there evidence that pain is present?

Intervention Monitor vital signs. **Rationale** Pulse and blood pressure can be elevated in acute pain. **Evaluation** Are vital signs elevated?

Intervention Administer appropriate pain medication as ordered. **Rationale** Nonnarcotic medications are preferred because they do not alter the level of consciousness. If these are not effective, codeine preparations, which have a minimal effect on LOC, may be prescribed. **Evaluation** Does patient state pain has decreased? Is sedation minimized?

Intervention Implement measures to reduce ICP. See Table 48.4 for measures and rationales. **Rationale** Increased intracranial pressure can increase pain. **Evaluation** Do measures to reduce ICP help prevent pain?

Intervention Provide alternative comfort measures such as dim lights, a quiet environment, and positioning for comfort. **Rationale** Decreasing stimuli in the room by dimming lights and decreasing noise can have a calming effect. **Evaluation** Is patient resting quietly, with no evidence of pain?

Nursing Diagnosis: *Risk for Injury Secondary to Impaired Sensory Perception* related to brain injury and cranial nerve involvement as evidenced by alterations in response to stimuli

Expected Outcome: The patient will be kept safe from injury related to reduced sensation.

Evaluation of Outcome: Is patient safe? Is skin intact?

Intervention Monitor patient's ability to perceive stimuli. **Rationale** Changes in patient's perceptions must be incorporated into the plan of care. **Evaluation** What can the patient feel?

Intervention Turn patient and assess skin at least every 2 hours while in bed; provide moisturizer as needed. Protect bony prominences. **Rationale** If the patient cannot determine pressure or dryness, the nurse must evaluate and act to prevent skin breakdown. **Evaluation** Is skin intact, pink, warm, dry, and without redness?

Intervention Assist the patient out of bed and into a different environment. **Rationale** This can help prevent sensory deprivation and social isolation. **Evaluation** How does patient respond to being in a chair or wheelchair and taken to sunroom or common area?

Continued

NURSING CARE PLAN for the Patient With a Brain Lesion or Injury—cont'd

Intervention Teach the patient to monitor own position and skin, and to direct position changes. **Rationale** This provides a way for the patient to maintain some control over his body and to take part in preventing complications. **Evaluation** Is patient able to direct care activities effectively?

Nursing Diagnosis: *Impaired Physical Mobility* related to motor deficits as evidenced by weakness, inability to change position

Expected Outcomes: The patient will maintain maximum mobility and be free from complications of immobility.

Evaluation of Outcomes: Is patient kept mobile without contractures? Is skin intact?

Intervention Assess degree of mobility limitation. **Rationale** A good assessment can help determine how much the patient can actively participate in a plan for mobilization. **Evaluation** How much can patient do independently? Is physical/occupational therapy evaluation indicated?

Intervention Turn patient every 1 to 2 hours; if postoperative, avoid positioning on the operative site unless specifically permitted by the surgeon. **Rationale** Turning helps prevent skin and respiratory complications. **Evaluation** Is a turning schedule maintained? Is skin free from redness and breakdown?

Intervention Position patient in correct body alignment. High-top tennis shoes, trochanter rolls, and slings can be used to keep the body in alignment. **Rationale** This keeps the patient in functional position in case function is regained in the future. **Evaluation** Are all joints maintained in correct alignment?

Intervention Perform range-of-motion (ROM) exercises; consult physical therapy as ordered. **Rationale** ROM exercises help prevent contractures. **Evaluation** If patient unable to perform active ROM exercises, are passive ROM exercises provided on a regular schedule?

Intervention Consult occupational therapist to assist the patient in learning to perform ADLs. **Rationale** The patient may be able to participate in self-care with assistive devices. **Evaluation** Do assistive devices help patient mobilize and maintain independence?

Nursing Diagnosis: *Risk for Injury* related to seizures

Expected Outcome: The patient will remain free of injury if a seizure occurs.

Evaluation of Outcome: Is safety maintained? Is skin intact, without bruising or discoloration?

Intervention Observe the patient's behavior and time the length of the seizure. When patient is alert following seizure, determine if an aura occurred, and what it was. **Rationale** Observing the seizure can provide clues for teaching the patient to recognize the warning signs of a future seizure and how to maintain safety. **Evaluation** What did the patient experience? What can be taught to help keep patient safe in the future?

Intervention If patient loses consciousness during the seizure, lay patient on his or her side or turn head to the side. **Rationale** This helps prevent oral secretions from being aspirated. **Evaluation** Did patient maintain a patent airway without respiratory distress?

Intervention Remove objects from patient's surroundings to prevent injury during a seizure. If the patient must have side rails, pad them with blankets or foam (see also Table 48.6, later in chapter). **Rationale** During a tonic-clonic seizure the patient can be harmed by hitting furniture or other objects. **Evaluation** Is patient protected from objects that could cause injury during a seizure?

TABLE 48.4 MEASURES TO PREVENT INCREASED INTRACRANIAL PRESSURE

Preventive Measures	Rationale
Keep head of bed elevated 30 degrees unless contraindicated.	Head elevation reduces ICP in some patients.
Avoid flexing the neck; keep head and neck in midline position.	Neck flexion can obstruct venous outflow.
Administer antiemetics and antitussives as necessary to prevent vomiting and cough.	Coughing and vomiting can increase ICP.
Administer stool softeners.	Straining for bowel movement can increase ICP.
Minimize suctioning. If absolutely necessary, oxygenate first and limit suction passes to one or two.	Suctioning can increase ICP.
Avoid hip flexion.	Hip flexion can increase intra-abdominal and thoracic pressure, which can increase ICP.
Prevent unnecessary noise and startling the patient.	Noxious stimuli can increase ICP in some patients.
Space care activities to provide rest between each disturbance.	Clustering care activities can increase ICP.

ICP = intracranial pressure.

Describing the brain as in control of body functions can help significant others to understand some of the symptoms of neurologic disorders. The spinal cord can be compared to a telephone cord, with hundreds of tiny individual wires (nerves) making up the cord. The specific wires affected by disease determine the symptoms the patient experiences.

CRITICAL THINKING

Mr. Chung

■ Mr. Chung is an 18-year-old Asian college student. He comes to the emergency department with a headache, stiff neck, and fever. On physical assessment, you notice a petechial rash on his legs and torso. The physician diagnoses meningococcal meningitis.

1. What tests are likely to be performed?
2. What patient education should be planned for Mr. Chung?
3. What infection control practices should be instituted?
4. What comfort measures might you offer to Mr. Chung?
5. What concerns do you have about how Mr. Chung contracted his illness?

Suggested answers are at the end of the chapter.

HEADACHES

As mentioned throughout this chapter, headache is a common symptom of neurologic disorders. However, most headaches are transient events and do not indicate a serious pathological condition. If headaches are recurrent, persistent, or increasing in severity, the patient should undergo a neurologic evaluation. This section addresses the most common types of headache.

Types of Headaches

Headaches are divided into three major types: (1) primary, (2) secondary, and (3) cranial neuralgias, central and primary facial pain and other headaches. Primary headaches are discussed in this section. Secondary headaches are caused by trauma, infection, or other disorders. Cranial neuralgias are discussed in Chapter 50. For more information visit the International Headache Society at http://ihs-classification .org/en. Because the causes, signs and symptoms, pathophysiology, and treatment of headaches vary based on the type of headache experienced, these subjects are discussed separately for each type of headache.

Migraine Headaches

One long-held theory is that a migraine headache is caused by cerebral vasoconstriction followed by vasodilation. The vasoconstriction can be due to a response triggered by the trigeminal nerve, which stimulates release of substance P, a pain transmitter, into the vessels or by the release of amines such as serotonin, norepinephrine, and epinephrine. A migraine may or may not begin with an aura (visual phenomena, such as a flashing light that precedes an attack). The tendency to develop migraine headaches is often hereditary; they frequently begin in childhood or adolescence and are more common in women. Commonly used descriptors of migraine pain include *throbbing, boring, vise-like,* and *pounding.* The pain is usually on one side of the head. Noise and light tend to worsen the headache, leading patients to seek a dark, quiet environment. Triggers for the headache include hormones (menses-related), changes in barometric pressure, specific foods, noise, bright light, alcohol, and stress.

There are two major types of migraine: migraine with aura and migraine without aura. There are four phases generally associated with migraine headaches: prodromal, aura, headache, and resolution. The preheadache phase **(prodromal)** can include visual disturbances, difficulty speaking, and/or numbness or tingling. The headache that follows is often accompanied by nausea and sometimes vomiting and can last for hours to days.

Treatment of migraine may be prophylactic or directed at an acute episode. Prophylactic treatment is usually reserved for those patients experiencing one or more migraine headaches per week. Dietary restrictions can be helpful if precipitating foods or beverages can be identified.

Several types of medications are available to treat acute migraine headaches. Nonsteroidal anti-inflammatory drugs (NSAIDs) such as naproxen (Naprosyn, Aleve) may be tried first. Ergot (Cafergot), a vasoconstrictor, is effective only if taken before the vessel walls become edematous, usually within 30 to 60 minutes of headache onset. Triptans such as sumatriptan (Imitrex) and zolmitriptan (Zomig) work at the serotonin receptor sites and have a vasoconstricting action. Treximet combines naproxen and sumatriptan. Opioids are habit forming and are used only as a last resort. The potentially additive effects of multidrug regimens requires careful monitoring.

Tension or Muscle Contraction Headaches

Persistent contraction of the scalp and facial, cervical, and upper thoracic muscles can cause tension headaches. A cycle of muscle tension, muscle tenderness, and further muscle tension is established. This cycle may or may not be associated with vasodilation of cerebral arteries. Headaches of this type can be associated with premenstrual syndrome or psychosocial stressors such as anxiety, emotional distress, or depression. Symptoms typically develop gradually. Radiation of pain to the crown of the head and base of the skull, with variations in location and intensity, is common. *Pressure, aching, steady,* and *tight* are some of the words patients use to describe the pain of tension headaches.

Care must be taken to thoroughly rule out physical causes before attributing the headache to psychosocial origins. Symptom management may include the use of relaxation techniques, massage of the affected muscles, rest, localized heat application, nonopioid analgesics, and appropriate counseling.

Cluster Headaches

Vascular disturbance, stress, anxiety, and emotional distress are all proposed causes of cluster headaches. As indicated by the name, these headaches tend to occur in clusters during a time span of several days to weeks. Months or even years can pass between episodes. Alcohol consumption may worsen the episodes.

The patient may state that the headache begins suddenly, typically at the same time of night. *Throbbing* and *excruciating* are often the adjectives used by the patient. The headache tends to be unilateral, affecting the nose, eye, and forehead. A bloodshot, teary appearance of the affected eye is common.

Because of the brief nature of cluster headaches, treatment is difficult. A quiet, dark environment and cold compresses can lessen the intensity of the pain. NSAIDs or tricyclic antidepressants may be prescribed.

Diagnosis of Headaches

Most headaches are diagnosed based on the patient's history and symptoms. MRI, CT, skull x-ray, arteriogram, EEG, cranial nerve testing, and lumbar puncture to test CSF may be done to rule out other causes for the headaches.

Nursing Process for the Patient With a Headache

Data Collection

The **WHAT'S UP?** mnemonic is particularly useful in helping the patient provide useful information regarding the headache:

W—Where is the pain? Does it remain in one place or radiate to other areas of the head? Does the headache consistently start in one place?

H—How does the headache feel? Is it throbbing, steady, dull, bandlike, or does it have other qualities?

A—Aggravating or alleviating factors should be assessed. Some aggravating factors include red wine, caffeine, chocolate, and foods containing nitrates or monosodium glutamate (MSG). Other factors include particular stages of the menstrual cycle, emotional stress, and tension. Alleviating factors might include lying down in a dark room, cold compresses, or medications.

T—Timing can be a factor for a patient who experiences headaches just before or during her menstrual period. For other patients, there may be no predictive timing. Also ask how long the headache lasted.

S—Ask the patient to rate the severity on a scale of 0 to 10. Is the severity consistent or does it vary from headache to headache?

U—Ask about other useful data. For example, are there associated symptoms, such as nausea, vomiting, or bloodshot eyes?

P—Determine the patient's perception of the headache. Does it interfere with the patient's life? If so, how? Has the patient had a previous evaluation of headaches?

• WORD • BUILDING •
prodromal: pro—before + dromos—running

Nursing Diagnoses, Planning, and Implementation

Acute Pain (Headache) related to lack of knowledge of pain prevention and control techniques as evidenced by patient's pain rating

EXPECTED OUTCOME: Headache will be prevented or controlled as evidenced by patient statement of no pain or acceptable pain rating.

• Assist the patient to identify and reduce or eliminate aggravating factors. This can be accomplished by keeping a headache diary for a time, recording the time of day the headache occurs, foods eaten or other aggravating factors, description of the pain, identification of associated symptoms such as nausea or visual disturbances, and other factors related to headache symptoms. *Identification of triggers can help the patient lessen the frequency and intensity of attacks.*

• Encourage the patient to use alleviating techniques such as biofeedback or stress reduction. *This helps the patient participate in the treatment of the headache and provides a sense of control over his or her illness.*

• Teach the patient to use relaxation exercises and warm or cool moist compresses. *These interventions may be helpful for tension headaches.*

• Provide a dark room and rest *to reduce stimulation during a migraine headache.*

• Teach the patient about medications, appropriate dosage, expected action, side effects, and consequences of misuse. *The patient will need to understand medication administration for appropriate use at home.*

Evaluation

If interventions have been effective, the patient will understand self-care to prevent and treat headaches and be able to report a reduction in headache pain and occurrences.

 SEIZURE DISORDERS

Seizures/Epilepsy

A seizure can be a symptom of epilepsy or of other neurologic disorders such as a brain tumor or meningitis. Epilepsy is a chronic neurologic disorder characterized by recurrent seizure activity.

Pathophysiology

The normal stability of the neuron cell membrane is impaired in individuals with epilepsy. This instability allows for abnormal electrical discharges to occur. These discharges cause the characteristic symptoms seen during a seizure.

Seizures can be classified as partial or generalized. Partial seizures begin on one side of the cerebral cortex. In some cases, the electrical discharge spreads to the other hemisphere and the seizure becomes generalized. Generalized seizures are characterized by involvement of both cerebral hemispheres.

Etiology

Epilepsy can be acquired or idiopathic (unknown cause). Causes of acquired epilepsy include traumatic brain injury and anoxic events. No cause has been identified for idiopathic epilepsy. The most common time for idiopathic epilepsy to begin is before age 20. New-onset seizures after this age are most commonly caused by an underlying neurologic disorder. As the population ages, more older adults are having first-time seizure as a result of bleeding or bruising in the brain related to a fall. Multiple medications in the elder population and untreated hypertension can increase the risk of falls, as well as brain injury after a fall.

Signs and Symptoms

Symptoms of seizure activity correlate with the area of the brain where the seizure begins. Some patients experience an aura or sensation that warns that a seizure is about to occur. An aura can be a visual distortion, a noxious odor, or an unusual sound. Patients who experience an aura may have enough time to sit or lie down before the seizure starts, thereby minimizing the risk of injury.

PARTIAL SEIZURES. Repetitive, purposeless behaviors, called automatisms, are the classic symptom of partial seizures. The patient appears to be in a dreamlike state while picking at his or her clothing, chewing, or smacking his or her lips. Patients may be labeled as mentally ill, particularly if automatisms include unacceptable social behaviors such as spitting or fondling themselves. Patients are not aware of their behavior or that it is inappropriate. If the patient does not lose consciousness, the seizure is labeled as simple partial and usually lasts less than 1 minute. Older terms for simple partial seizures include *Jacksonian* and *focal motor.* If consciousness is lost, it is called a complex partial seizure or psychomotor seizure, and can last from 2 to 15 minutes.

Partial seizures arising from the parietal lobe can cause paresthesias on the side of the body opposite the seizure focus. Visual disturbances are seen if the seizure originates in the occipital lobe. Involvement of the motor cortex results in involuntary movements of the opposite side of the body. Typically, movements begin in the arm and hand and can spread to the leg and face.

The **postictal** period is the recovery period after a seizure. Following a partial seizure, the postictal phase may be no more than a few minutes of disorientation.

GENERALIZED SEIZURES. Generalized seizures affect the entire brain. Two types of generalized seizures are absence seizures and tonic-clonic seizures. Absence seizures, sometimes referred to as petit mal seizures, occur most often in children and are manifested by a period of staring that lasts several seconds.

Tonic-clonic seizures are what most people envision when they think of seizures; they are sometimes called grand mal

• WORD • BUILDING •
postictal: post—after + ictal—seizure

seizures or convulsions. Tonic-clonic seizures follow a typical progression. Aura and loss of consciousness may or may not occur. The tonic phase, lasting 30 to 60 seconds, is characterized by rigidity, causing the patient to fall if not lying down. The pupils are fixed and dilated, the hands and jaws are clenched, and the patient can temporarily stop breathing. The clonic phase is signaled by contraction and relaxation of all muscles in a jerky, rhythmic fashion. The extremities can move forcefully, causing injury if the patient strikes furniture or walls. The patient is often incontinent. Biting the lips or tongue can cause bleeding.

The postictal period is usually longer after a tonic-clonic seizure. Patients may sleep deeply for 30 minutes to several hours. Following this deep sleep, patients may report headache, confusion, and fatigue. Patients may realize that they had a seizure but not remember the event itself.

Diagnostic Tests

An EEG is the most useful test for evaluating seizures. An EEG can determine where in the brain the seizures start, the frequency and duration of seizures, and the presence of subclinical (asymptomatic) seizures. Sleep deprivation and flashing light stimulation may be used to evaluate the seizure threshold. See Chapter 47 for more information on EEGs.

Therapeutic Measures

If an underlying cause for the seizure is identified, treatment focuses on correcting the cause. If no cause is found or if the seizures continue despite treatment of concurrent disorders, treatment focuses on stopping or preventing the seizure activity.

Numerous anticonvulsant medications are available, each with specific actions, therapeutic ranges, and potential side effects (Table 48.5). Typically, the patient is started on one drug, and the dosage is increased until therapeutic levels are attained or side effects become troublesome. If seizures are not controlled on a single drug, another medication is added. Many anticonvulsants require periodic blood tests to monitor serum levels as well as kidney and liver functions. Most of these medications can cause drowsiness, so teach the patient to avoid driving or operating machinery until the effects of the drug are known. Driving is also contraindicated until seizures are under control.

If a patient must discontinue an anticonvulsant, it should be tapered slowly according to manufacturer directions. Stopping an anticonvulsant abruptly can result in status epilepticus, discussed later. If seizures continue despite anticonvulsant therapy, surgical intervention may be considered.

TABLE 48.5 ANTICONVULSANT MEDICATIONS

Medication Class/Action	Examples	Nursing Implications
Suppress abnormal discharge of neurons, suppress spread of seizure activity from focus to other parts of brain.	carbamazepine (Tegretol)	Monitor CBC. Therapeutic level 6–12 mcg/mL. Do not crush SR form.
	ezogabine (Potiga)	Monitor for urinary retention.
	gabapentin (Neurontin)	Blood levels not necessary
	lacosamide (Vimpat)	Injectable form available. May increase risk of suicidal ideation.
	levetiracetam (Keppra)	May need reduced dose for older adults. Assess WBC, RBC, and liver function tests.
	lamotrigine (Lamictal)	Discontinue therapy and notify health care practitioner if rash appears. Monitor blood levels.
	topiramate (Topamax)	Blood levels not necessary.
	phenytoin (Dilantin)	Regular dental care essential Therapeutic level is 10–20 mcg/mL. Binds to tube feedings—hold tube feeding 1 hr before and 2 hr after dose.
	phenobarbital (Luminal)	Monitor vital signs.
	valproic acid (Depakote)	Therapeutic level 15–40 mcg/mL. Therapeutic level 50–100 mcg/mL. Do not crush SR form.
Emergency Agents		
Potentiate GABA, an inhibitory neurotransmitter in the CNS.	lorazepam (Ativan) diazepam (Valium, Diastat)	Given to stop a seizure that has not resolved within 5 minutes. Given IM or IV push by emergency personnel. Rectal Diastat may be given at home.

Note. RBC = red blood cell; SR = sustained release; WBC = white blood cell.

Surgical Management

The success of surgical intervention for epilepsy depends on identification of an epileptic focus within nonvital brain tissue. The surgeon attempts to resect the area affected to prevent spread of seizure activity. In some cases, seizures can be cured, but in others, the goal is to reduce the frequency or severity of the seizures. If no focus is identified or if it is in a vital area such as the motor cortex or speech center, surgery is not feasible.

The preoperative assessment for epilepsy surgery is an extensive multistage process. Thorough assessment and teaching are essential. To adequately identify seizure foci, the patient is weaned off anticonvulsant therapy. Increasing the frequency of seizures with weaning is anxiety provoking for patients and significant others.

Emergency Care

Emergency care is required when a seizure occurs. The prime objective is to prevent injury during a seizure. Side rails, if used, should be padded to prevent injury if the patient strikes his or her extremities against them. If the patient falls to the floor, move furniture out of the way. Maintain a patent airway and, if possible, turn the patient on his or her side to prevent aspiration if vomiting occurs. Do not force an airway or anything else into the patient's mouth once the seizure has begun. Do not restrain the individual because this can also increase the risk of injury. Observe and document the patient's behavior during the seizure: which part of the body was first involved, progression of the seizure, and the length of time the seizure lasted (see "Patient Perspective"). After the seizure, assess the patient for breathing, suction if necessary, and, in rare cases, initiate rescue breathing or cardiopulmonary resuscitation (CPR) as indicated.

Patient Perspective

Mrs. Rowley

I have had seizures for 35 years and, as a result of falling during seizures, have experienced cuts, bruises, and a broken bone. I usually have an aura that lets me know a seizure is about to occur. This is helpful if I can get myself to a safe place to prevent falling or being injured. When a patient is having a seizure you can best help by using padding such as pillows or blankets for protection, talking calmly, and using gentle touch to prevent injury. You should not sit on or hold down someone during a seizure. I have had the frightening experience of waking up with a nurse sitting on me and holding down my arms. After you have protected the patient, let the person come out of the seizure naturally. When the seizure is over, I usually want to sleep because seizures are exhausting.

Status Epilepticus

Status epilepticus is characterized by at least 30 minutes of repetitive seizure activity without a return to consciousness. This is a medical emergency and requires prompt intervention to prevent irreversible neurologic damage. Abrupt cessation of anticonvulsant therapy is the usual cause of status epilepticus.

Seizure activity precipitates a significant increase in the brain's need for glucose and oxygen. This metabolic demand is even greater during status epilepticus. Irreversible neuronal damage can occur if cerebral metabolic needs cannot be fulfilled. Adequate oxygenation must be maintained, if necessary, by intubating and mechanically ventilating the patient. These patients are also at significant risk for aspiration. Therefore, it is important that the nurse assist in airway maintenance and suction as needed to prevent hypoxia and aspiration pneumonia.

Intravenous (IV) diazepam (Valium) or lorazepam (Ativan) is given to stop active seizures. Diazepam can also be given rectally. Because both of these drugs can cause respiratory depression, careful airway management is required. After obtaining serum drug levels, anticonvulsant therapy is adjusted to achieve therapeutic levels.

If seizures remain resistant to treatment, a barbiturate coma may be induced with IV pentobarbital. The last line of treatment for status epilepticus is general anesthesia or pharmacological paralysis. Both of these therapies require intubation, mechanical ventilation, and management in an ICU setting. Continuous EEG monitoring is used to verify that the seizures have actually stopped. A patient treated with neuromuscular blockade drugs can still be seizing but have no visible manifestations.

For more information on seizures, visit the Epilepsy Foundation of America at www.efa.org.

Psychosocial Effects

Finances can be a major concern to patients with seizure disorders. Some patients with epilepsy experience hiring discrimination, or they may not qualify for some jobs in which safety is a concern. Remind patients that falsifying information on job applications may be grounds for dismissal. Refusal of health insurance coverage can create financial hardships for patients on long-term medications. Most patients whose seizures are controlled can work and lead productive lives. A social worker can help explore options for financial assistance if needed.

Patients with poorly controlled seizures should not operate motor vehicles. In today's society, a driver's license is a sign of adulthood and independence, and patients who cannot drive can experience lowered self-esteem. Job opportunities may be limited for patients who depend on public transportation. Encourage the patient to obtain a state identification card. This can be used in place of a driver's license for identification.

Patients may limit interpersonal relationships out of fear of having a seizure. The involuntary movements, sounds, and possible incontinence that occur with seizures are embarrassing to patients and can be frightening to laypeople.

Role-playing may help the patient determine when and how to confide in others.

Nursing Process for the Patient With Seizures

Data Collection

Perform a general neurologic examination of the patient with a history of seizures. Determine the type of seizure manifestations and type of aura if any. Assess the patient's knowledge of the disease and its treatment. It is important to assess whether the patient has the resources to purchase prescribed anticonvulsant medications and whether the medication regimen is adhered to. Drug levels can help determine degree of adherence to therapy.

Nursing Diagnoses, Planning, and Implementation

Risk for Injury related to seizure activity

EXPECTED OUTCOME: The patient will remain free from injury.

- Instruct the patient with generalized seizures to recognize an aura and to get to safety if it occurs. This may mean lying down away from furniture or other objects. *This helps prevent injury during involuntary movements.*
- Institute seizure precautions for the patient admitted to a health care institution. See Table 48.6 for precautions and interventions *to prevent injury.*
- Encourage all patients to wear medical alert jewelry or other identification *to alert others to the presence of seizure disorder.*
- Assist patients to identify conditions that trigger seizures. Hypoglycemia, hypoxia, and hyponatremia are all potential triggers of hypersensitive neurons. Teach the patient the importance of a consistent schedule of eating and sleeping. *The patient may be able to prevent seizures by avoidance of triggers.*

Risk for Ineffective Self Health Management related to complex regimen and possible lack of resources

EXPECTED OUTCOME: The patient will follow medication regimen as evidenced by therapeutic drug levels and controlled seizure activity.

- Assess patient's ability to obtain and pay for medication. *Stopping a medication suddenly can result in status epilepticus.*
- Refer patient to a case manager or social worker, if needed, *to assist with obtaining resources for medications.*
- Teach the patient about medication action, dose, side effects, schedule, and the importance of not stopping treatment suddenly. *Patients with seizures can have several medications to take several times each day. Patients who understand their regimens are more likely to comply.*
- Teach the patient about the importance of regular blood tests if required. *Therapeutic blood levels help prevent seizures (too low) and toxicity (too high).*

Evaluation

Successful care of a patient with epilepsy is manifested by a decrease in seizures to the lowest possible frequency. Patient verbalization of understanding of needed lifestyle changes is another indication of success. Patients should be able to state measures to prevent injury if a seizure should occur and should verbalize understanding of all medications and their administration schedules. Therapeutic drug levels can be measured to evaluate adherence to the medication regimen.

TRAUMATIC BRAIN INJURY

Traumatic brain injury is a major cause of death and disability in adults. Young men make up a large proportion of brain injury victims.

Pathophysiology

Traumatic brain injury is a complex phenomenon with results ranging from no detectable effect to a persistent vegetative state. Trauma can result in hemorrhage, contusion or laceration of the brain, and damage at the cellular level. In addition to the primary insult, the brain injury can be compounded by cerebral edema, hyperemia, or hydrocephalus.

Etiology

Motor vehicle accidents account for the largest percentage of traumatic brain injuries. Falls, sports-related injuries, and violence are also common causes of traumatic brain injury.

The brain is susceptible to various types of injury that can be classified in several ways. The term *closed head injury* or *nonpenetrating injury* is used when there has been rapid back and forth movement of the brain that causes bruising and tearing of brain tissues and vessels, but the skull is intact. An *open head injury* or *penetrating injury* refers to a break in the skull. *Acceleration injury* is the term used to describe a moving object hitting a stationary head. An example of this type

TABLE 48.6　INTERVENTIONS FOR SEIZURES

Seizure Precautions
- Pad side rails of hospital bed with commercial pads or bath blankets folded over and pinned in place.
- Keep call light within reach.
- Assist patient when ambulating.
- Keep suction and oral airway at bedside.

Nursing Care During a Seizure
- Stay with patient.
- Do not restrain patient.
- Protect from injury (move nearby objects).
- Loosen tight clothing.
- Turn to side when able to prevent occlusion of airway or aspiration.
- Suction if needed.
- Monitor vital signs when able.
- Be prepared to assist with breathing if necessary.

of injury is a patient who is hit in the head with a baseball bat. A *deceleration injury* occurs when the head is in motion and strikes a stationary surface. This type of injury is seen in patients who trip and fall, hitting their head on furniture or the floor.

A combination of acceleration-deceleration injury occurs when the stationary head is hit by a mobile object and the head then strikes a stationary surface. A soccer player who sustains a blow to the head and then hits the ground with his or her head can sustain an acceleration-deceleration injury.

Rotational injuries have the potential to cause shearing damage to the brain, as well as lacerations and contusions. Rotational injuries can be caused by a direct blow to the head or can occur during a motor vehicle accident in which the vehicle is struck from the side. Twisting of the brainstem can damage the reticular activating system, causing loss of consciousness. Movement of the brain within the skull can result in bruising or tearing of brain tissue where it comes in contact with the inside of the skull.

Types of Brain Injury and Signs and Symptoms

Concussion

Cerebral concussion is considered a mild brain injury. If there is a loss of consciousness, it is for 5 minutes or less. Concussion is characterized by headache, dizziness, or nausea and vomiting. The patient may describe amnesia of events before or after the trauma. On clinical examination, there is no skull or dura injury and no abnormality detected on CT or MRI.

Contusion

Cerebral contusion is characterized by bruising of brain tissue, possibly accompanied by hemorrhage. There can be multiple areas of contusion, depending on the causative mechanism. Severe contusions can result in diffuse axonal injury. The symptoms of a cerebral contusion depend on the area of the brain involved.

Brainstem contusions affect level of consciousness. Decreased level of consciousness can be transient or permanent. Respirations, pupil reaction, eye movement, and motor response to stimuli can also be affected. The autonomic nervous system can be affected by edema or by hypothalamic injury, causing rapid heart rate and respiratory rate, fever, and diaphoresis.

Hematoma

SUBDURAL HEMATOMA. Subdural hematomas are classified as acute or chronic based on the time interval between injury and onset of symptoms. Acute subdural hematoma is characterized by appearance of symptoms within 24 hours following injury. The bleeding is typically venous in nature and accumulates between the dura and arachnoid membranes (Fig. 48.5). About 24% of patients who sustain a severe brain injury develop an acute subdural hematoma. Damage to the brain tissue can cause an altered level of consciousness. Therefore, it can be difficult to recognize a subdural hematoma on the basis of clinical examination alone. As the

subdural hematoma increases in size, the patient may exhibit one-sided paralysis of extraocular movement, extremity weakness, or dilation of the pupil. Level of consciousness can deteriorate further as ICP increases.

Older adults and people with alcoholism are particularly prone to chronic subdural hematomas. Atrophy of the brain, common in these populations, stretches the veins between the brain and the dura. A seemingly minor fall or blow to the head can cause these stretched veins to rupture and bleed. Often there are no other injuries associated with the trauma. Because a chronic subdural hematoma can develop weeks to months after the injury, the patient may not remember an injury occurring.

The patient with a chronic subdural hematoma may be forgetful, lethargic, or irritable or may report a headache. If the hematoma persists or increases in size, the patient can develop hemiparesis and pupillary changes. The patient or significant other may not associate the symptoms with a previous injury and therefore may delay seeking medical care.

EPIDURAL HEMATOMA. About 10% of patients with severe brain injuries develop epidural hematomas. This collection of blood between the dura mater and skull is usually arterial in nature and is often associated with skull fracture (see Fig. 48.5). Arterial bleeding can cause the hematoma to become large very quickly. Patients with epidural hematoma typically exhibit a progressive course of symptoms. The patient loses consciousness directly after the injury; he or she then regains consciousness and is coherent for a brief period. The patient then develops a dilated pupil and paralyzed extraocular muscles on the side of the hematoma and becomes less responsive. If there is no intervention, the patient becomes unresponsive. Seizures or hemiparesis can occur. Once the

FIGURE 48.5 (A) A subdural hematoma is usually venous and forms between the dura and the arachnoid membranes. (B) An epidural hematoma is usually from an arterial bleed and forms between the dura mater and the skull.

patient has symptoms, the deterioration can be rapid. Airway management and control of ICP must be instituted immediately. If ICP is not controlled, the patient will die.

Diagnostic Tests

CT scan is usually the first imaging test performed on a patient with a brain injury. It is faster and more accessible than MRI. This is particularly important for unstable patients or those with multiple injuries. It is easier to identify skull fractures on CT than on MRI. MRI can be used later to identify damage to the brain tissue.

Neuropsychological testing by a trained specialist can be useful in assessing the patient's cognitive function. This information helps direct rehabilitation placement, discharge planning, and return to work or school. Neuropsychological testing identifies problems with memory, judgment, learning, and comprehension. Patients may be able to learn compensation strategies based on the results.

Therapeutic Measures

Surgical Management

Surgical treatment of hematomas is discussed under intracranial surgery later in this chapter.

Medical Management

Medical management of traumatic brain injury involves control of ICP and support of body functions. Patients with brain injuries can be partially or completely dependent for maintenance of respiration, nutrition, elimination, movement, and skin integrity.

A variety of techniques are used to control ICP in the patient with moderate or severe brain injury. The first step is to insert an ICP monitor to allow measurement of the ICP. Refer to the section on increased ICP earlier in this chapter for further information.

If ICP remains elevated despite drainage of CSF, the next step is use of an osmotic diuretic. The most commonly used drug is IV mannitol (Osmitrol). Mannitol uses osmosis to pull fluid from the brain into the intravascular space and eliminate it via the renal system. Serum osmolarity and electrolytes must be carefully monitored when mannitol is being administered. Some patients experience a rebound increase in ICP after the mannitol wears off.

Mechanical hyperventilation may be used if the patient is still experiencing increased ICP. Hyperventilation is effective in lowering ICP because it causes cerebral vasoconstriction. Vasoconstriction allows less blood into the cranium, thereby lowering ICP. Research has demonstrated, however, that aggressive hyperventilation, particularly within the first 24 hours after injury, can induce ischemia in the already compromised brain. Therefore, hyperventilation is now reserved for increased ICP that does not respond to other treatments.

High-dose barbiturate therapy may be used to induce a therapeutic coma, which reduces the metabolic needs of the brain during the acute phase following injury. These patients are completely dependent for all of their needs and care. They will be mechanically ventilated and cared for in an ICU

setting. Vasopressors may be required to maintain blood pressure, and the patient's temperature should be kept as normal as possible.

Complications

Brain Herniation

If interventions to control ICP are unsuccessful, the patient can experience uncontrolled edema or herniation of brain tissue (Fig. 48.6). Herniation is displacement of brain tissue out of its normal anatomical location. This displacement prevents function of the herniated tissue and places pressure on other vital structures, most commonly the brainstem. Herniation usually results in brain death.

Patients who experience brain death may be suitable organ donor candidates. For some significant others, the opportunity to donate their loved one's organs provides some sense of purpose in the death (Table 48.7).

Diabetes Insipidus

Edema or direct injury that affects the posterior portion of the pituitary gland or hypothalamus can result in inadequate release of antidiuretic hormone, causing diabetes insipidus.

A

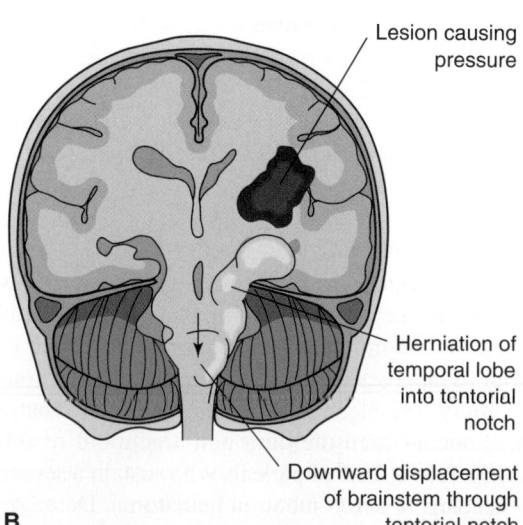

B

Lesion causing pressure

Herniation of temporal lobe into tentorial notch

Downward displacement of brainstem through tentorial notch

FIGURE 48.6 Herniation of the brain. (A) Normal brain. (B) Herniation of brain tissue into tentorial notch.

TABLE 48.7   TRAUMATIC BRAIN INJURY SUMMARY

Signs and Symptoms	Loss or decrease in level of consciousness, depending on severity and type of injury Loss of memory before or after the injury Increased ICP Headache, dizziness Nausea and vomiting Unequal pupils Tachycardia, tachypnea Diaphoresis Hemiparesis
Diagnostic Tests	CT scan, MRI Skull x-rays Routine laboratory tests (hemoglobin, electrolytes, coagulation studies, type and crossmatch) Neuropsychological testing
Therapeutic Measures	Control intracranial pressure Surgical management of hematoma Maintain respiratory function Maintain diet/nutrition Maintain skin integrity Prevent complications Education
Complications	Increased intracranial pressure Diabetes insipidus Acute hydrocephalus Post-traumatic syndrome Cognitive and personality changes
Possible Nursing Diagnoses	*Acute Confusion* related to cerebral edema or increased intracranial pressure *Self-Care Deficit* related to increased intracranial pressure *Pain* related to cerebral edema

This results in polyuria and, if the patient is awake, polydipsia. Fluid replacement and IV vasopressin are used to maintain fluid and electrolyte balance. See Chapter 39 for more information on diabetes insipidus.

Acute Hydrocephalus

Cerebral edema can interfere with cerebrospinal fluid circulation, causing **hydrocephalus**. Initial treatment is use of an external ventricular drain, followed by a ventriculoperitoneal shunt if necessary. A shunt drains excess CSF into the peritoneum, where it is reabsorbed into circulation and excreted.

Labile Vital Signs

Direct trauma to or pressure on the brainstem can cause fluctuations in blood pressure, cardiac rhythm, or respiratory pattern. Treatment is aimed at control of ICP.

Post-Traumatic Stress Disorder

Patients who sustain a concussion can experience ongoing, somewhat vague symptoms. They may report headache, fatigue, difficulty concentrating, depression, or memory impairment. Symptoms can be severe enough to interfere with work, school, and interpersonal relationships. Neuropsychological testing can provide objective evidence of cognitive dysfunction and establish the need for cognitive rehabilitation for posttraumatic stress disorder, or PTSD (see Chapter 57 for more about PTSD). Symptoms can take 3 to 12 months to resolve.

Cognitive and Personality Changes

Alterations in personality and cognition may be the most difficult long-term complication for patients and significant others to adjust to. The patient can have significant short-term memory impairment. This limits his or her ability to learn new information and can interfere with ability to function at work or school. Impaired judgment can make the patient a safety risk to self or others. It also affects social functioning.

Emotional lability, loss of social inhibitions, and personality changes may occur. These consequences of traumatic brain injury have a profound effect on the patient and significant others. Spouses may state, "This is not the person I married." If behavior is violent, bizarre, or profane, children may be unwilling to bring their friends home and can become socially isolated. Young children, in particular, have difficulty understanding why a parent is behaving so differently. Disintegration of relationships is not uncommon following traumatic brain injury.

Neuropsychological testing objectively identifies problems. These deficits can then be addressed with cognitive rehabilitation. Individual and family counseling can be of benefit. Support groups for patients and significant others are often helpful.

Motor and speech impairment are additional possible long-term complications of traumatic brain injury. Intensive rehabilitation provides the best opportunity for maximizing recovery. For more information, visit the Brain Injury Association at www.biausa.org.

Nursing Process for the Patient With Traumatic Brain Injury

Acute care is presented here. Also see the "Nursing Care Plan for the Patient With a Brain Tumor or Injury."

Data Collection

After stabilization in the emergency department, care of the patient with a severe traumatic brain injury is in the

---

• **WORD • BUILDING** •

hydrocephalus: hydro—water + cephalus—head

intensive care setting, where ICP can be carefully monitored. Frequent data collection is essential, including a Glasgow Coma Scale score or the FOUR Score (see Chapter 47), pupil responses, muscle strength, and vital signs. Review Box 48-1, "Signs and Symptoms of Increased Intracranial Pressure," for additional signs of increased ICP for which to monitor. Once the patient is stabilized, neurologic damage is assessed. Identification of deficits guides nursing care. Assessment of discharge needs should begin as soon as possible. The patient may require extensive rehabilitation, and early referral can speed transfer to an appropriate facility.

Nursing Diagnoses, Planning, and Implementation

Risk for Ineffective Cerebral Tissue Perfusion related to increased ICP

EXPECTED OUTCOME: Changes in cerebral tissue perfusion will be prevented or recognized and reported promptly.

- Monitor vital signs for widening pulse pressure or irregular respirations. *These are signs of increased ICP and should be reported promptly.*
- Monitor Glasgow Coma Scale or FOUR Score and report worsening status promptly. *Decreasing level of consciousness (LOC) can indicate increased ICP and may necessitate emergency intervention.*
- Implement measures *to prevent increased ICP.* See Table 48.4 for preventive measures and rationale.

Ineffective Airway Clearance related to reduced cough reflex and decreased level of consciousness as evidenced by adventitious lung sounds and dropping SpO₂.

EXPECTED OUTCOME: The patient will maintain a clear airway as evidenced by clear breath sounds and SpO₂ of 90% or above.

- Monitor airway and breath sounds. *If the patient has excess secretions and is unable to cough effectively, suctioning may be necessary.*
- Limit suction passes to one or two at a time for a maximum of 5 to 10 seconds each time. *Suctioning can increase ICP.*
- Keep head of bed elevated 20 to 30 degrees *to reduce risk of aspirating oral secretions and reduce ICP.*
- Turn the patient frequently *to help mobilize secretions and prevent other complications of immobility.*

Risk for Ineffective Breathing Pattern related to pressure on respiratory center

EXPECTED OUTCOME: The patient will maintain SpO₂ of 90% or above.

- Monitor respiratory rate and depth, arterial blood gases (ABGs), and SpO₂ and report changes. *If respiratory status is deteriorating, mechanical ventilation may be necessary.*
- Elevate head of bed 20 to 30 degrees *to allow chest expansion and ease work of breathing.*
- Administer oxygen as ordered and needed *to prevent hypoxia. Hypoxia promotes brain death.*

Evaluation

The plan of care has been successful if the patient shows no unexpected worsening of neurologic function and injuries and complications are prevented. The patient's airway should be clear and SpO₂ level should be 90% or above. The patient is kept comfortable, and self-care needs are met.

Rehabilitation

Once the patient is stabilized, evaluation for discharge to a rehabilitation facility is completed. The patient must be able to physically tolerate the rehabilitation program, in which the patient will be taught to function as independently as possible. The family must be prepared for changes in the patient's ability to function and possible changes in personality. It can take months to years before the patient reaches his or her maximum potential. In some cases of severe brain damage or continued comatose state, rehabilitation is not feasible and the patient is discharged to home or a long-term facility for custodial care.

CRITICAL THINKING

Mr. Evans

■ Mr. Evans is a 24-year-old white male who was involved in a motor vehicle crash. His blood alcohol level was 0.24. Mr. Evans has no preexisting medical problems. Emergency medical services personnel report that Mr. Evans was unconscious on their arrival at the scene and then became alert and combative. His CT scan shows a left-sided epidural hematoma. Mr. Evans is admitted to your unit for observation.

1. What symptoms would you expect to see if Mr. Evans' hematoma increases in size?
2. What emergency preparations should you have ready?
3. What psychosocial data should you collect?
4. What other members of the health team should be consulted?

Suggested answers are at the end of the chapter.

BRAIN TUMORS

Brain tumors are neoplastic growths of the brain or meninges. Brain tumors can be characterized by vague symptoms such as headache or visual changes or by focal neurologic deficits such as hemiparesis or seizures.

Pathophysiology and Etiology

Brain tumors cause symptoms by either compressing or infiltrating brain tissue. Tumors can arise from CNS cells or can metastasize from other locations in the body. Primary brain tumors rarely metastasize; however, if they do, it is to the spine.

There is no established cause for primary brain tumors. It is unclear what causes the cells to begin reproducing in an uncontrolled fashion. Risk factors include age (45 and older), exposure to radiation or industrial chemicals, and family history. Whites are more likely to be diagnosed with a brain tumor than other racial or ethnic groups.

Brain tumors can be classified in several ways. The traditional distinction of benign and malignant is less helpful when classifying brain tumors than when classifying other cancers. A benign tumor in the brainstem can be fatal, whereas a malignant tumor in the frontal lobe may not be. Location of the tumor can be just as important a factor in outcome as the cell type.

Primary tumors are those arising from cells of the CNS. Intra-axial tumors are those that arise from the glial cells within the cerebrum, cerebellum, or brainstem. These tumors infiltrate and invade brain tissue. Extra-axial tumors arise from the skull, meninges, pituitary gland, or cranial nerves; they place pressure on the brain.

Most brain tumors are secondary; that is, they have metastasized from a primary malignancy somewhere else in the body (Fig. 48.7). These tumors commonly spread via the arterial system. If untreated, they cause increased ICP. This can be the cause of the patient's death rather than the primary malignancy.

Signs and Symptoms

The symptoms of a brain tumor are directly related to the location of the tumor in the brain and to the rate of growth. Slow-growing types of tumors such as meningiomas (a tumor arising from the meninges; Fig. 48.8) can get to be quite large before causing symptoms. Conversely, glioblastoma multiforme or metastatic tumors can abruptly cause seizures or hemiparesis. Other types of tumors include oligodendroglioma, astrocytoma, and acoustic neuroma. The suffix *-oma* refers to tumor. The prefix denotes the type of cell from which the tumor arises.

FIGURE 48.7 Metastatic brain tumor. This patient's primary cancer was in the lung.

FIGURE 48.8 Meningioma.

The most common early symptom of a brain tumor is fatigue. Other symptoms depend on tumor size and location and can include seizures, motor and sensory deficits, nausea and vomiting, headaches, personality changes, confusion, and speech and vision disturbances. If the pituitary gland is involved, additional symptoms related to changes in hormone secretion occur, such as abnormal growth or fluid volume imbalances.

Diagnostic Tests

MRI gives the clearest images of a brain tumor. If the tumor appears to be highly vascular or in proximity to major blood vessels, an angiogram may be performed. It is now possible to do a magnetic resonance angiogram, which involves the IV administration of contrast material and is much less invasive than a traditional angiogram. If the tumor is in the region of the pituitary gland, serum hormone levels are evaluated. Biopsy may be done during surgical removal of the tumor, or using needle aspiration. Additional tests may be carried out to find a primary cancer site.

Therapeutic Measures

Surgery

Surgical treatment involves removal of the tumor or as much of the tumor as possible. Care of the patient undergoing intracranial surgery is discussed later in this chapter.

Medical Treatment

Medical treatment is aimed at controlling symptoms. Patients who have a seizure are placed on anticonvulsants. If significant cerebral edema is noted on the MRI or if the patient is suffering from headaches or other symptoms, a steroid such as dexamethasone (Decadron) may be prescribed to lessen the edema and reduce symptoms. Typically, patients do not require narcotics for pain relief.

Radiation Therapy

External beam radiation therapy is standard treatment for many patients with a brain tumor. The therapy is typically given 5 days a week for 6 weeks. Some clinicians use a hyperfractionated schedule, in which the patient has therapy twice a day for less time. Brachytherapy is a means of delivering radiation therapy directly to the tumor. Small catheters are implanted in the tumor, and then tiny radioactive particles are inserted into the catheters. The treatment typically takes 3 to 5 days. During this time the patient is confined to a private room and interaction with visitors and staff is kept to a minimum because of the radioactivity. This therapy is not appropriate for confused individuals because they may not be able to cooperate with restrictions.

Stereotactic radiosurgery is a technique that uses small amounts of radiation directed at the tumor from different angles. A metal frame is affixed to the patient's skull, and the tumor is visualized within the framework on a CT or MRI. A computer plan is generated to direct the radiation. Because multiple small sources are used, the normal brain tissue receives very little radiation, while the majority of the radiation accumulates in the tumor.

Chemotherapy

The blood–brain barrier is a protective mechanism that prevents many injurious substances from reaching brain tissue. Unfortunately, it is also effective in preventing most chemotherapy agents from reaching the brain. To penetrate the blood–brain barrier, large doses of chemotherapy may be required. These doses may not be well tolerated by other body systems. New treatments are currently being investigated. Some clinicians place chemotherapy substances in the cavity left by surgical resection. Others disrupt the blood–brain barrier with mannitol (an osmotic diuretic) and then deliver intra-arterial chemotherapy under general anesthesia. Another newer treatment, called targeted drug therapy, uses a drug such as bevacizumab (Avastin), which stops formation of new blood vessels that support the tumor. Gene therapy is also being used in an effort to kill malignant cells.

Complementary and Alternative Therapies

The rate of success for treatment of brain tumors is not as high as treatment of other neoplasms. Patients may be drawn to nontraditional therapies both as cures and for treatment of symptoms. Encourage patients to look at each option in a rational manner. Some questions they should ask themselves include the following:

- Will this interfere with any of my other treatments or medications?
- What is the cost?
- What are the side effects?
- Is there any objective information (research) available?
- What does my physician think of this?

Additional information on evaluation of complementary and alternative therapies is found in Chapter 5.

Acute and Long-Term Complications

It is difficult to distinguish between symptoms of a brain tumor and complications of treatment. Seizures, headaches, memory impairment, cognitive changes, and ataxia can be symptoms of the tumor or the result of surgery or radiation therapy. Patients can experience hemiparesis or aphasia following surgery. If the tumor continues to grow despite treatment, the patient will experience further decline in function. Gradually the patient becomes more lethargic and unresponsive. Once the patient becomes comatose, death occurs within a matter of days, particularly if artificial nutrition and hydration are not administered.

Nursing Process for the Patient With a Brain Tumor

Nursing care of the patient with a brain tumor is similar to that for the patient with a brain injury because both experience neurologic deficits. See the "Nursing Care Plan for the Patient With a Brain Lesion or Injury."

■ INTRACRANIAL SURGERY

The primary purpose of intracranial surgery is to remove a mass lesion. These types of lesions include hematomas, tumors, arteriovenous malformations, and, occasionally, contused brain tissue. Other indications for surgery include elevation of a depressed skull fracture, removal of a foreign body, debridement of a wound, or resection of a seizure focus. The term **craniotomy** refers to any surgical opening in the skull. A burr hole is an opening into the cranium made with a drill. **Craniectomy** is the term used to describe removal of part of the cranial bone. **Cranioplasty** refers to repair of bone or use of a prosthesis to replace bone following surgery.

The goal of intracranial tumor surgery is gross total resection of the tumor. This involves removal of all visible tumor, called *debulking*. Even with the use of an operative microscope, viable tumor cells can be left behind that can give rise to recurrence. If the entire tumor cannot be removed, the surgeon debulks as much as possible, thereby giving radiation therapy or chemotherapy less of a burden to combat. In some cases, it is not feasible to attempt more than a biopsy of the tumor. Location of the tumor or the patient's age or medical condition may not allow the patient to tolerate a full craniotomy. The biopsy may be done under local or general anesthesia, depending on the patient's condition. The goal of a biopsy is to obtain tissue that allows pathological diagnosis of the tumor, which then guides any further treatment.

• WORD • BUILDING •
craniotomy: crani—skull + otomy—incision
craniectomy: crani—skull + ectomy—excision, removal
cranioplasty: cranio—skull + plasty—to form

Intracranial surgery is usually performed under general anesthesia. Occasionally, a procedure requires that the patient be awake and cooperative.

Preoperative Care

Preoperative care of the patient undergoing intracranial surgery is similar to that of patients having other surgeries (see Chapter 12). The patient undergoes a laboratory workup and anesthesia evaluation. If the patient has cognitive impairments, it is important that a significant other be available to provide information and sign consents. A thorough baseline neurologic assessment should be documented.

Patient education is important preoperatively. The extent of education depends on the patient's ability to absorb new information, which is influenced by the disease process, cognitive functioning, anxiety, and educational level. Significant others are involved as needed. Information about the disease process and surgery is provided by the surgeon. The nurse can play an important role in reinforcing and clarifying the information presented.

Anxiety is also a significant concern before surgery. The patient is anticipating serious surgery, as well as an unknown outcome. Allow time for the patient and significant others to express their fears and ask questions. Honest and accurate information should be provided.

Significant others should be prepared for how the patient will look after surgery. A preoperative visit to the intensive care unit may help prevent some anxiety postoperatively. Significant others should be accompanied on this visit by a knowledgeable nurse who can explain what they are seeing.

Surgery can last 2 hours for a biopsy to 12 hours or longer for more involved procedures. Patients and significant others should be prepared for the idea that some or all of the patient's hair will be shaved off. Some people prefer to have all their hair shaved rather than just part. The patient should be prepared to see his or her face swollen after surgery, particularly around the eyes; the periorbital region may be bruised. Many patients wish to wear a scarf or scrub cap after the dressing is removed.

Nursing Process for the Postoperative Care of the Patient Having Intracranial Surgery

Acute care of the postoperative patient is presented here. Also see the "Nursing Care Plan for the Patient With a Brain Tumor or Injury."

Data Collection

After intracranial surgery, the patient will be cared for in an ICU. Plan to assist the RN with frequent neurologic assessments in addition to routine postoperative monitoring. Patients should have their neurologic status assessed every hour for the first 24 hours or as ordered by the health care provider (HCP). Many patients undergo a CT scan within the first 24 hours following surgery to assess cerebral edema. Also assess the patient's response to changes in body image and the patient's knowledge base related to care that will be required following discharge.

Nursing Diagnoses, Planning, and Implementation

The primary goal after intracranial surgery is prevention of complications. Once the patient is stabilized, goals can change to longer-term outcomes such as acceptance of changes in body image and understanding of self-care following discharge. If the patient has severe deficits following surgery, rehabilitation or long-term care may become necessary. A consultation with a social worker can help with planning for this transition. Priority nursing diagnoses are discussed next.

Risk for Ineffective Cerebral Tissue Perfusion related to edema of the operative site

EXPECTED OUTCOME: The patient will have adequate cerebral tissue perfusion as evidenced by stable or improving neurologic assessments.

- Monitor neurologic status as ordered. Report changes promptly. *Deteriorating status can signify increased ICP.*
- Implement measures *to prevent increased ICP.* See Table 48.4 for preventive measures and rationales.
- Position patient with the head of the bed at 30 degrees or higher, unless ordered otherwise, *to promote venous drainage and minimize increases in ICP.* The exception to this is patients who have had a chronic subdural hematoma removed; these patients must remain flat. Patients can turn from side to side or lie on their back but should not lie on the operative side.
- Implement seizure precautions *because the patient is at risk for seizures due to cerebral edema.*
- Use caution to protect the many monitoring systems being used. The patient may have an intracranial monitor in place following surgery *to monitor ICP.* Some patients may also have central venous pressure catheters or pulmonary artery catheters *to monitor fluid status.* Urinary catheters are used during the immediate postoperative period *to accurately monitor fluid balance.*
- Monitor dressings for drainage. *Drainage that is blood tinged in the center with a yellowish ring around it can be CSF leakage. A suspected CSF leak should be reported to the RN or physician immediately.*

Risk for Infection related to surgical procedure

EXPECTED OUTCOME: The patient will remain free from infection as evidenced by temperature and white cell count within normal limits and incision sites clean and dry.

- Monitor patient for rise in temperature, purulence at incision site, and increase in white cell count. *These are signs of infection and should be reported immediately.*
- Use strict aseptic technique for all care of the incision, dressing, and monitoring equipment sites *to reduce risk of infection.*
- Use appropriate hand hygiene *to reduce risk of transmitting infection.*

Disturbed Body Image related to changes in appearance or function as evidenced by patient statement of disturbance or unwillingness to observe changes

EXPECTED OUTCOME: The patient will display an accepting attitude toward change in appearance, as evidenced by willingness to look in mirror and/or be seen by others.

- Offer a turban, scarf, or hat if the patient desires *to help conceal a shaved head.*
- Portray an accepting attitude toward the patient. *Patients are likely aware of nurses' nonverbal behavior.*
- Allow the patient to express his or her feelings if desired. *Talking may help the patient work through feelings, but it should not be forced.*

Deficient Knowledge related to change in treatment regimen after surgery as evidenced by patient statement

EXPECTED OUTCOME: The patient and significant others will verbalize correct information for follow-up care at home. They will state they have the resources to manage care effectively.

- Teach the patient and family or significant other home management, including medication regimen, wound care, and ordered activity restrictions, including driving. Have the patient and significant others verbalize the signs of infection or other possible complications to report. *The patient and family will assume responsibility for care after discharge, unless the patient is being transferred to another facility.*
- Teach patient and family seizure precautions and the importance of taking anticonvulsants as ordered. *The patient may be on anticonvulsants to prevent seizures after surgery. If seizure free for 1 year, the physician may discontinue anticonvulsants.*
- Consult social worker or case manager for resources if needed. *The patient may need discharge planning if transfer to another facility is planned. If discharge home is expected, the patient and family will benefit from visiting nurse follow-up. Assistance with obtaining medications can also be provided if necessary.*

Evaluation

Interventions have been effective if the patient's neurologic status is stable and infection and other complications have been prevented. The patient might be able to look in the mirror and begin to show evidence of acceptance of changes in body image, although this may not happen until after discharge from the hospital. The patient or significant others should be able to demonstrate appropriate follow-up care.

SPINAL DISORDERS

Herniated Disks

Herniated intravertebral disks are a common health problem. They are characterized by pain and paresthesias that follow a radicular (nerve path) pattern. It is not uncommon for patients to have more than one herniated disk or to have herniated disks in different areas of the spine.

Pathophysiology

When the disk between two vertebrae herniates, it moves out of its normal anatomical position. In most cases, the annulus fibrosus, the tough outer ring of the disk, tears. This allows escape of the nucleus pulposus, the soft inner portion of the disk. Displacement of the disk compresses one or more nerve roots, causing the characteristic symptoms (Fig. 48.9).

Etiology

In some cases, a specific event can be correlated with a herniated disk. The patient may describe a fall, lifting a heavy object, or a motor vehicle accident. In other instances, the patient cannot identify a triggering incident.

Signs and Symptoms

Cervical disk herniation causes pain and muscle spasm in the neck. The patient may have decreased range of motion secondary to pain. Hand and arm pain is unilateral (one sided) and follows the distribution of the spinal nerve root. Patients often report numbness or tingling in the extremity. Asymmetrical weakness and atrophy of specific muscle groups may be detected. If weakness involves the entire extremity, it is unlikely that disk herniation is the etiology. The severity of the pain or paresthesia does not correlate directly with the severity of the nerve compression. However, weakness and atrophy are indicators of significant nerve compression.

Thoracic herniated disks are not common. This portion of the spine is the least mobile; therefore, less stress is exerted on the disks. Patients with herniated thoracic disks may report pain in the back. It is uncommon to detect muscular weakness.

A herniated lumbar disk is typically characterized by low back pain, pain radiating down one leg, paresthesias, and weakness. The patient may limp on the affected leg or may have difficulty walking on his or her heels or toes. Muscle

Spinous process

Lamina

Nerve root

Nucleus pulposus herniates and compresses nerve root

FIGURE 48.9 A herniated disk places pressure on a spinal nerve root.

spasm is often present. Pain and muscle spasm can limit the patient's range of motion. Depending on the disk affected, the knee or ankle deep tendon reflex may be decreased or absent. A severely herniated L5–S1 disk can affect bowel or bladder continence. This is an emergency situation and should be reported immediately.

The **WHAT'S UP?** mnemonic can be used to assess symptoms of herniated disks at any level:

W—Where is the pain? Does it radiate into an extremity? In what distribution?

H—How does it feel? Sharp, stabbing, burning?

A—Do certain positions or activities alleviate or aggravate the pain? Holding the affected arm above the head can alleviate cervical pain. Sitting places pressure on disks and aggravates lumbar pain. Lying down may relieve it.

T—Is there a correlation between time and pain? Some patients have more pain at the end of the day. Is the pain constant or intermittent?

S—Ask the patient to rate the severity of the pain on a scale of 0 to 10. Which is the most painful, the spine or the extremity?

U—Ask the patient to identify other useful data, such as symptoms of numbness, tingling, or weakness.

P—What is the patient's perception of the pain? Is it interfering with work or other aspects of the patient's life?

Diagnostic Tests

An MRI will detect herniation of a disk and compression or abnormality of the spinal cord. If the patient has previously had surgery in the area of the suspected herniation, the MRI is done with and without contrast to differentiate between scar tissue and a herniated disk.

If the patient cannot tolerate an MRI or if the MRI does not provide enough information, a myelogram can be done. Refer to Appendix A for a description of both tests.

Therapeutic Measures

Most HCPs and patients prefer to try conservative medical therapy before performing surgery for a herniated disk.

MEDICAL TREATMENT.

Rest. In the past, bedrest was advised as part of conservative management. The current recommendation is 1 or 2 days of bedrest, followed by a careful, gradual increase in activity.

Physical Therapy. Physical therapy can be very useful for some patients. A gradually progressive course of exercise strengthens the muscles. This is particularly important in the lumbar area, where the muscles help stabilize the spine. Techniques such as ultrasound, electrical stimulation, heat, ice, and deep massage can decrease pain and muscle spasm and allow for increased ROM. Instructions in proper body mechanics and strategies for avoiding reinjury are important components of physical therapy.

Traction. Cervical traction is a noninvasive technique sometimes used by physical therapists for patients with herniated cervical disks. The patient's head is placed in a halter-like device. A series of ropes and pulleys connect the halter to a weight. This gently pulls the head away from the shoulders. The rationale is that this traction slightly separates the vertebral bodies and can allow the disk to return to its proper position. If it is effective in relieving the patient's pain, cervical traction can be done at home on an as-needed basis. Traction is discontinued immediately if it increases the patient's pain. Lumbar traction is not particularly effective because the lumbar paraspinal muscles are large and strong. The amount of traction needed to overcome the muscular resistance can cause injury.

Medication. Muscle relaxants are often prescribed as a short-term therapy for patients who are experiencing muscle spasms. These medications decrease pain by decreasing the spasm, helping the patient increase range of motion and activity. Muscle spasm is actually a protective mechanism. Muscles tighten and become painful, causing the patient to limit movement. This lessens the chance that the disk will be further injured. However, chronic spasm can cause tearing and scarring of the muscles. Patients should be warned that drowsiness is a common side effect of many muscle relaxants. They should be cautioned against driving or operating machinery until they determine how well they tolerate the medication. Diazepam is an effective muscle relaxant; however, it has a strong potential for addiction, so it is usually used only if muscle spasm cannot be adequately treated with other medications.

Inflammation of the nerve root is caused by compression and irritation from the herniated disk. NSAIDs can be effective in reducing this inflammation, but there is no way to predict response to a given drug. It may be necessary for the patient to try several NSAIDs before an effective one is found. Because several of these drugs are now available without prescription, the patient should be cautioned not to use a nonprescription NSAID at the same time as a prescription NSAID. Patients should be instructed to report any stomach upset to the clinician because NSAIDs can cause gastric bleeding. Occasionally, oral steroids are used on a short-term basis for patients with severe inflammation that does not respond to other treatments. A rapidly tapering dose of steroid over 1 week is often prescribed. Steroids can also cause gastric upset, in addition to elevated serum glucose levels. Instruct patients with diabetes to monitor glucose levels closely and consult a physician if the levels are outside their normal parameters.

Epidural injections may be tried for patients who have no relief with more conservative measures. A mixture of medications, typically a steroid, long-acting anesthetic, and long-acting pain reliever, is injected into the epidural space. The anesthetic provides immediate relief, while the steroid reduces swelling for a longer lasting effect. If relief is obtained, the injection can be repeated every 3 to 4 months.

The use of opioid pain medication is a subject of concern in the treatment of patients with herniated disks. Opioids generally are appropriate for short-term treatment of acute pain. However, if treatment is not effective, the pain can become chronic. In that circumstance, the physician and patient must discuss the potential complications of long-term opioid use, such as constipation, tolerance, and dependence. A referral to a pain clinic for alternative strategies may be appropriate.

Some alternatives to long-term use of opioids include topical lidocaine patches or NSAID patches, or use of agents for neuropathic pain such as pregabalin (Lyrica) or amitriptyline (Elavil).

Complementary and Alternative Therapy. A transcutaneous electrical nerve stimulator (commonly called a TENS unit) is a noninvasive pain-relief technique. Small electrodes are placed on the skin around the area of the pain. The device then transmits a low-voltage electrical current through the skin. The patient feels a tingling or buzzing sensation, which can help block the pain impulses. A physical therapist or pain specialist teaches the patient where to place the electrodes and how to operate the unit. The patient decides when to use it and at what settings. This allows the patient to actively participate in his or her care and have some control over the pain level.

SURGICAL MANAGEMENT. Surgeries are less common today than in the past, because conservative measures have been found to be successful for most patients. If surgery is indicated, several options are available. A **laminectomy** removes one of the laminae, the flat pieces of bone on each side of a vertebra. This may be done to relieve pressure or to gain access for removal of a herniated disk. A diskectomy removes the entire disk. A spinal fusion uses a bone graft to fuse two vertebrae together if the area is unstable. Surgery can be done through a microscope for less scarring and faster recovery. Most patients are discharged within 24 hours of surgery.

A diskectomy is generally done for a herniated cervical disk. This can be accomplished via an anterior or posterior approach. Most surgeons use the anterior approach for cervical herniations because the muscles in the front of the neck are much smaller and more mobile than those in the back of the neck. Therefore, there is less pain and muscle spasm following surgery. It is also safer than the posterior approach, which involves more maneuvering around the spinal cord.

Most surgeons replace the disk with bone or another material. This prevents collapse of the disk space and creates a spinal fusion. If bone is used, it may be harvested from the patient's iliac crest or donated from a cadaver. Mobility of the spine is lost in the area of a fusion. Spinal fusions may also be done to correct instability of the spine from other causes, such as scoliosis or degenerative disorders.

A posterior approach is used for a herniated lumbar disk. Typically, the vertical incision is 1 to 2 inches long. It is necessary to pull some of the muscle away from the bone, which accounts for some of the postoperative pain that patients experience. A laminectomy is done, and the herniated portion of the disk is resected. The remainder of the disk continues to provide a cushion between the intravertebral bodies. The surgeon removes any free fragments and any disk material that appears unstable.

Percutaneous diskectomy involves insertion of a large needle into the disk under local anesthesia to aspirate herniated disk material. This technique is not used for severely herniated disks. Laser disk surgery may be used to disintegrate the herniated tissue. Laparoscopic techniques may also be used.

In 2004, the U.S. Food and Drug Administration approved an artificial disk for use with selected patients. It is made of two plastic disks designed to slide so that mobility is not impaired as with spinal fusion. The artificial disk is attached to the vertebra above and below after the damaged disk is removed. This alternative to spinal fusion has been effective for those with single-disk problems.

Complications After Surgery

HEMORRHAGE. As with any surgery, intraoperative hemorrhage is possible, although it is not common in disk surgery. If a postoperative hemorrhage occurs in a patient who has had an anterior cervical diskectomy, the airway can become occluded. The patient is monitored for bleeding from the incision and respiratory distress.

NERVE ROOT DAMAGE. If the nerve root is severed during surgery, the patient experiences loss of motor and sensory functions in that nerve's distribution area. This can result in decreased use of the extremity. If the nerve root is damaged or excessive scarring occurs, the patient can experience pain, weakness, or paresthesias. In some cases, physical therapy and NSAIDs may be effective in improving function and reducing pain.

REHERNIATION. Lumbar disks can reherniate. This can occur anywhere from 1 week to several years after the initial surgery. If the reherniation occurs within a few weeks to months after the first surgery, the patient usually undergoes another microdiskectomy. Reherniation of a cervical disk does not occur because the entire disk is removed.

HERNIATION OF ADJACENT DISK. Fusion of the cervical spine results in loss of movement at that motion segment. This can place increased stress on the disks above and below the fusion. This can increase the risk of another herniated disk, especially if the patient already has degeneration of other disks. The patient should be instructed to maintain an exercise program and to frequently move the spine through ROM exercises.

Nursing Process for the Patient Having Spinal Surgery
Preoperative Care

Routine preoperative care is appropriate for the patient undergoing spinal surgery. In addition to routine teaching, instruct the patient in how to logroll following surgery. This procedure involves keeping the body in alignment and rolling as a unit, without twisting the spine, to prevent injury to the operative site.

• WORD • BUILDING •
laminectomy: lamin—posterior portion of the vertebra + ectomy—surgical removal of

Postoperative Care

DATA COLLECTION. In addition to routine postoperative data collection, monitor extremities for changes in circulation, movement, and sensation. Monitor color, warmth, and presence of pulses in the extremities. Assess movement by asking the patient to move the extremities. Assess sensation by gently touching the patient's extremity and asking if feeling is present. Report any changes immediately to the physician because this can indicate nerve or circulatory damage.

Monitor pain frequently. The pain that necessitated surgery should be relieved, but the patient can still have muscular and incisional pain. Reassure the patient that it will gradually subside. Monitor the surgical dressing and drain (if present) for CSF drainage or bleeding. Any sign of CSF drainage or significant bleeding should be reported to the physician immediately. If bone was taken from a separate donor site, this site must also be monitored. Intake and output are measured to ensure that the patient is able to void. Notify the physician if the patient has difficulty voiding.

NURSING DIAGNOSES, PLANNING, AND IMPLEMENTATION. Goals of nursing are to keep the patient safe and free from injury or complications, and free from pain. Gradual return to normal physical activity is expected. Possible postoperative diagnoses are discussed next.

Acute Pain related to surgical procedure as evidenced by patient's pain rating

EXPECTED OUTCOME: The patient will verbalize an acceptable pain level.

- Monitor pain following surgery using an appropriate pain scale. *The patient's self-report is the most reliable method for assessing pain.*
- Administer muscle relaxants, analgesics, and NSAIDs as ordered. If a local anesthetic was injected into the surgical site during surgery, the patient may not have pain immediately postoperatively. *Medications to relieve pain help the patient to mobilize following surgery, which helps prevent complications.*
- Position the patient in bed in correct body alignment. If ordered, keep the patient flat for 6 to 8 hours. *Correct alignment avoids twisting and injury to the operative site.*
- Place a pillow between the legs when lying on the side *to promote alignment and comfort.*

Risk for Impaired Urinary Elimination related to effects of surgery

EXPECTED OUTCOME: The patient will be able to empty bladder without assistance.

- Monitor urine output for retention. *Patients may have difficulty voiding following lumbar surgery because of anesthesia, immobility, or occasionally because of nerve damage related to surgery.*
- If activity orders allow, assist the patient to get up to urinate (or to stand for men). *This may help the patient urinate.*
- If unable to void, try running warm water over the perineum, or taking a warm bath or shower. *This may stimulate voiding.*

- If difficulty urinating occurs, contact the physician for an order for intermittent catheterization until the problem resolves. *Urine retention that is not resolved can lead to bladder rupture. Intermittent catheterization is a safe way to empty the bladder.*

Risk for Impaired Physical Mobility related to neuromuscular impairment

EXPECTED OUTCOME: The patient will be able to ambulate and prevent complications of immobility after surgery.

- Assess mobility of affected extremities following surgery. *A reduction in expected mobility following surgery indicates nerve damage in surgery and should be reported immediately.*
- Assist the patient to logroll to get out of bed and ambulate on the first postoperative day, as ordered. If spinal fusion has been done, the fused area of the spine will be immobile. *Early mobilization after surgery helps prevent complications.*
- Apply a soft cervical collar to the patient with a cervical laminectomy as ordered *for neck support.*

EVALUATION. The patient is expected to be free of complications and pain, be able to urinate, be able to move all extremities, and return gradually to preillness activity level.

Spinal Stenosis

Spinal stenosis is a condition in which the spinal canal compresses the spinal cord (Fig. 48.10). Arthritis is a major cause of spinal stenosis. The facet joints of the spine become

FIGURE 48.10 Stenosis of the cervical spine (left). Compare with normal spinal column (right).

inflamed and enlarged, narrowing the diameter of the spinal canal and compressing the spinal cord. Patients may report pain and weakness. Compression of the cervical portion of the spinal cord can result in hyperreflexia and weakness of the legs and arms.

A laminectomy may be done to relieve pressure on the spinal cord. The size of the incision depends on the number of vertebrae involved. These patients are often older and may have concurrent illnesses. They may require inpatient rehabilitation before returning home.

 SPINAL CORD INJURIES

Injuries to the spinal cord affect people of all ages but take their greatest toll on young people. These injuries are characterized by a decrease or loss of sensory and motor functions below the level of the injury.

Pathophysiology

The spinal cord is made up of nerve fibers that allow communication between the brain and the rest of the body. Damage to the spinal cord results in interference with this communication process. Damage may be caused by bruising, tearing, cutting, edema, or bleeding into the cord. The damage can be caused by external forces or by fragments of fractured bone.

Etiology and Types

The causes of spinal cord injury are similar to those of traumatic brain injury. It is not uncommon for a patient to have both a spinal cord injury and traumatic brain injury. Motor vehicle accidents are the most common causes of spinal cord injury in the United States. Females are more often injured by falls and males are more often injured during acts of violence or contact sports. Assaults can cause cord injury if a knife or bullet penetrates the spinal cord. Diving into shallow water is a common cause of cervical cord injury.

Spinal cord injuries can be classified by location or by degree of damage to the cord. A complete spinal cord injury means that there is no motor or sensory function below the level of the injury. With an incomplete lesion, some function remains. This does not necessarily mean that the remaining function will be useful to the patient. Some patients find that having areas where sensation is intact may be more painful than useful.

The cervical and lumbar portions of the spine are injured more often than the thoracic or sacral segments. This is because the cervical and lumbar areas are the most mobile portions of the spine.

Signs and Symptoms
Cervical Injuries

Signs and symptoms depend on the level at which the cord is damaged (Fig. 48.11). Cervical cord injuries can affect all four extremities, causing paralysis and paresthesias, impaired respiration, and loss of bowel and bladder control. Paralysis of all four extremities is called **quadriplegia**; weakness of all extremities is called **quadriparesis**. If the injury is at C3 or above, the injury is usually fatal because muscles used for breathing are paralyzed. An injury at the fourth or fifth cervical vertebra affects breathing and may necessitate some type of ventilatory support. Such patients typically need long-term assistance with activities of daily living.

Thoracic and Lumbar Injuries

Thoracic and lumbar injuries affect the legs, bowel, and bladder. Paralysis of the legs is called **paraplegia**; weakness of the legs is called **paraparesis**. Sacral injuries affect bowel and bladder continence and may affect foot function. Individuals with thoracic, lumbar, and sacral injuries can usually learn to perform activities of daily living independently.

Spinal Shock

Spinal cord injury has a profound effect on the autonomic nervous system. Immediately after injury, the cord below the injury stops functioning completely. This causes a disruption of sympathetic nervous system function, resulting in vasodilation, hypotension, and bradycardia—called neurogenic shock or spinal shock. Dilation of the blood vessels allows more blood flow just beneath the skin. This blood cools and is circulated throughout the body, causing hypothermia. The patient is unable to maintain control of body temperature. In addition, all reflexes below the level of the injury are lost, and retention of urine and feces occurs. Spinal shock can last from a week to many weeks in some patients.

Complications
Infection

Impaired respiratory effort, decreased cough, mechanical ventilation, and immobility all predispose a patient with a spinal cord injury to pneumonia. Urinary catheterization, whether indwelling or intermittent, places patients at risk for urinary tract infection.

Deep Venous Thrombosis

Lack of movement in the legs inhibits normal blood circulation. Compression stockings, sequential compression devices, and subcutaneous heparin or enoxaparin may be used to reduce the risk of deep venous thrombosis.

Orthostatic Hypotension

Most patients with spinal cord injuries no longer have muscular function in their legs to promote venous return to the heart. They also have impaired vasoconstriction. This leads to pooling of the blood in the legs when the patient moves from a supine to a sitting position. If the movement is sudden, the patient can become dizzy or lightheaded. Gradual elevation

• WORD • BUILDING •

quadriplegia: quad—four + plegia—paralysis
quadriparesis: quad—four + paresis—partial paralysis
paraplegia: para—beside + plegia—paralysis
paraparesis: para—beside + paresis—partial paralysis

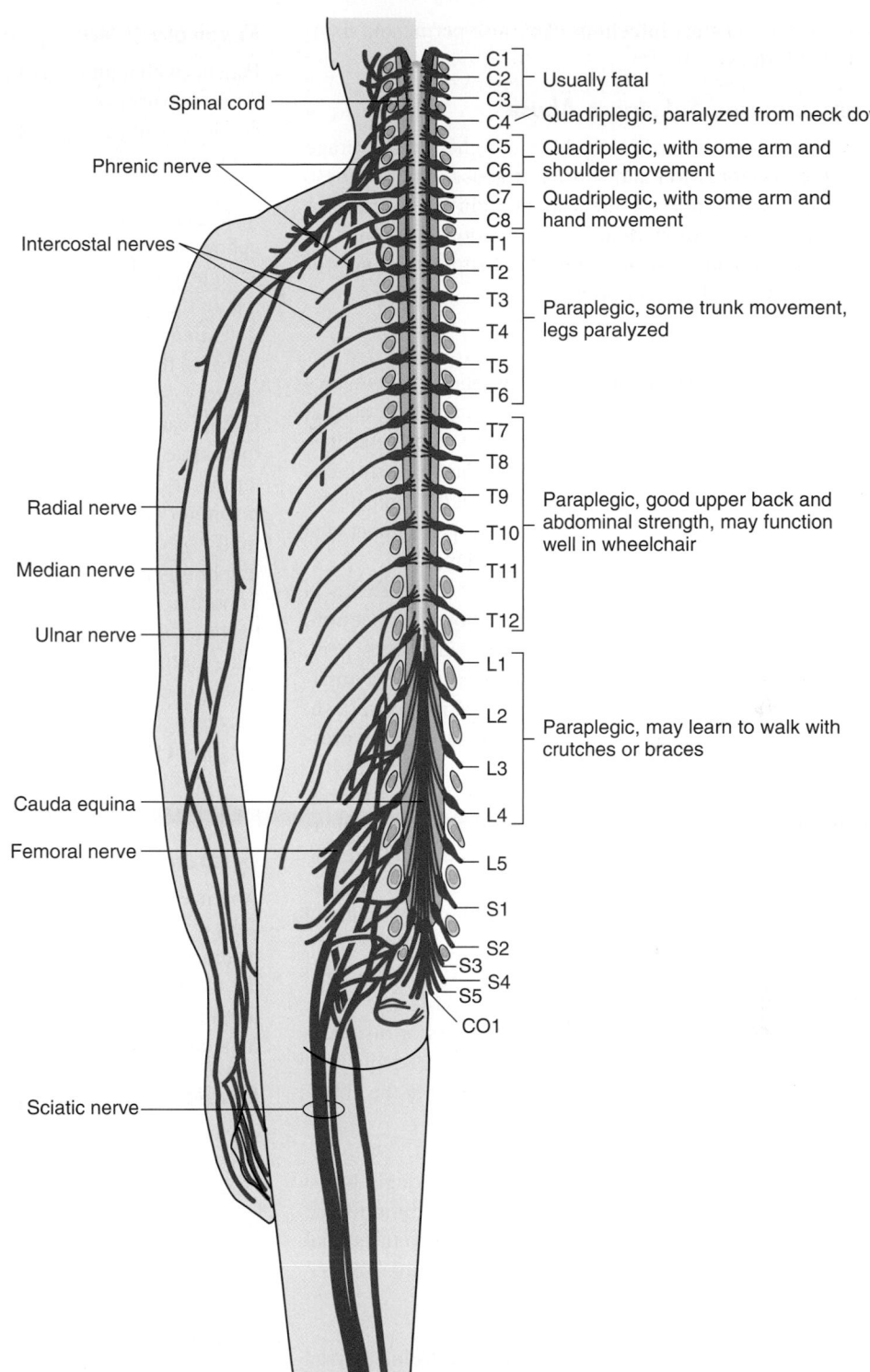

C1
C2 } Usually fatal
C3
C4 — Quadriplegic, paralyzed from neck down
C5 } Quadriplegic, with some arm and
C6   shoulder movement
C7 } Quadriplegic, with some arm and
C8   hand movement
T1
T2
T3 } Paraplegic, some trunk movement,
T4   legs paralyzed
T5
T6
T7
T8
T9 } Paraplegic, good upper back and
T10   abdominal strength, may function
       well in wheelchair
T11
T12
L1
L2 } Paraplegic, may learn to walk with
L3   crutches or braces
L4
L5
S1
S2
S3
S4
S5
CO1

Spinal cord
Phrenic nerve
Intercostal nerves
Radial nerve
Median nerve
Ulnar nerve
Cauda equina
Femoral nerve
Sciatic nerve

FIGURE 48.11 Spinal cord injury—quadriplegia versus paraplegia. Modified from Scanlon, V. C., & Sanders, T. (2007). *Workbook for essentials of anatomy and physiology* (5th ed.). Philadelphia: F.A. Davis, p. 163, with permission.

of the head, use of elastic stockings, and a reclining wheelchair help lessen this response.

Skin Breakdown

Patients or their caregivers must be diligent about relieving pressure on the skin by position changes and cushioning of bony prominences. It is important to realize that the patient may not be able to feel pain and therefore may not ask for position changes. Development of pressure ulcers can lead to infection and loss of skin, muscle, or bone. Treatment of pressure ulcers is time-consuming and expensive and can interfere with work or school.

Renal Complications

Urinary tract infections are an ongoing concern for patients with spinal cord injuries. Caregivers as well as the patient need to be taught to observe the color, clarity, and odor of urine and to report changes promptly. Both urinary reflux and untreated urinary tract infections can cause permanent damage to the kidneys.

Depression and Substance Abuse

Patients with spinal cord injury have a higher than average incidence of depression and substance abuse. Both of these factors can interfere with the patient's ability to care for himself or herself. Individual or family counseling may be helpful. Some rehabilitation centers have support groups for patients with spinal cord injuries.

Autonomic Dysreflexia

This life-threatening complication occurs in patients with injuries above the T6 level. The spinal cord injury impairs the normal equilibrium between the sympathetic and parasympathetic divisions of the autonomic nervous system. If a noxious stimulus below the spinal cord injury causes activation of the sympathetic system, it will continue unchecked because the parasympathetic responses cannot descend past the spinal cord injury.

The most common cause of autonomic **dysreflexia** is bladder distention. Other causes include bowel impaction, urinary tract infection, ingrown toenails, pressure ulcers, pain, and labor in a pregnant woman. Stimulation of the sympathetic nervous system results in cool, pale skin, gooseflesh, and vasoconstriction below the level of the injury. Blood pressure can rise as high as 300 mm Hg systolic. The parasympathetic response results in vasodilation, causing flushing and diaphoresis above the lesion, and bradycardia as low as 30 beats per minute. The patient reports a pounding headache and nasal congestion secondary to the dilated blood vessels.

Care of the patient with autonomic dysreflexia is discussed in the care plan later in this section.

Diagnostic Tests

Plain radiographs are done to identify fractures or displacement of vertebrae. A CT scan is also useful for identifying fractures. An MRI can demonstrate lesions within the cord.

Therapeutic Measures

Patients with spinal cord injuries typically are brought to the emergency department. They should be kept immobilized until they are assessed by a physician. If injury to the spinal cord is detected, the patient needs to remain immobilized.

Emergency Management

Emergency management involves careful monitoring of vital signs and airway and keeping the patient immobilized. Intubation and mechanical ventilation may be necessary, especially with cervical spine injuries. IV normal saline may be used for fluid replacement and provision of an access site for medication administration. The physician does not rely on fluid administration alone to correct hypotension. It is possible to administer enough fluid to cause pulmonary edema and not correct the hypotension. Vasoactive drugs may be required. The use of various medications to reduce the extent of injury, including IV methylprednisolone (a steroid), is routine. Often treatment is started by emergency medical services (EMS) personnel before arrival at the emergency department.

Respiratory Management

Patients with injuries above C4–C5 have some degree of respiratory impairment. The patient may require a tracheostomy and continuous mechanical ventilation or require a ventilator only at night or when fatigued. Some patients are able to breathe by using a phrenic nerve stimulator. This device, similar to a pacemaker, artificially stimulates the phrenic nerve, causing the diaphragm to contract. These patients use a mechanical ventilator at night to lessen the stress on the phrenic nerve and remove the risk of the system failing while the patient is asleep.

Patients can be breathing independently when they first arrive in the emergency department and then experience respiratory compromise as the spinal cord becomes edematous. Edema can compress the spinal cord above the lesion, leading to symptoms at a higher level. This deterioration is usually temporary. Fatigue of the accessory muscles can also cause respiratory compromise. The intercostal muscles are not normally of major importance in respiration. However, if the diaphragm is paralyzed, the intercostal muscles become very important. As these muscles fatigue, the patient's breathing becomes shallow and rapid. Elective intubation and mechanical ventilation protect the patient from expending huge amounts of energy trying to breathe. Feeling their breathing becoming more labored is terrifying to these patients, and they need to be reassured that it is probably a temporary setback. As the edema recedes and the accessory muscles become stronger, the patient may be weaned from the ventilator.

Gastrointestinal Management

Absence of bowel sounds is a common finding on examination. Oral or enteral feedings are not started until bowel function resumes. The metabolic needs of the patients are influenced by the work of breathing and the extent of other injuries. If positioning or paralytic ileus precludes oral or enteral feedings, IV hyperalimentation is begun.

Genitourinary Management

An indwelling urinary catheter is placed to prevent bladder distention and protect skin integrity until spinal shock resolves. Once it is determined what degree of hand function the patient will have, a bladder management program is devised.

Immobilization

The cervical spine can be immobilized with skeletal traction such as Crutchfield or Gardner-Wells tongs (Fig. 48.12). Some patients have a halo brace, a device that attaches to the skull with four small pins. The skull ring attaches to a rigid plastic vest by four poles (Fig. 48.13). This device keeps the head and neck immobile while fusion and healing take place. The advantage over traction is that the patient is not confined to bed.

Surgical Management

The goal of surgery following spinal cord injury is to stabilize the bony elements of the spine and relieve pressure on the

• WORD • BUILDING •
dysreflexia: dys—abnormal + reflexia—reflex activity

FIGURE 48.12 Skeletal traction for cervical injuries. (A) Crutchfield tongs. (B) Gardner-Wells tongs.

FIGURE 48.13 Halo brace.

Research is being conducted now with stem cells to help with nerve regeneration. Stem cells can be harvested and then processed in a laboratory before reinjection into the body. The goal is improvement in mobility and/or sensation.

Nursing Process for the Patient With a Spinal Cord Injury

Patients with spinal cord injury need ongoing evaluation of all body systems. Frequent neurologic and respiratory assessments are essential. Early assessment of the patient's support systems can help with discharge and rehabilitation planning. Initial goals for the patient include maintenance of safety and prevention of complications. Long-term goals include rehabilitation and maximizing remaining function.

See the "Nursing Care Plan for the Patient With a Spinal Cord Injury," "Gerontological Issues," and Table 48.8.

spinal cord. Surgery may or may not improve functional outcome. Stabilization of the spine allows for earlier mobilization of the patient. This decreases the risk of complications from immobility and speeds the transition to a rehabilitation setting. Patients who have been in cervical traction before surgery may be placed in a halo brace postoperatively.

Unstable thoracic and lumbar fractures may also be treated with surgical implantation of rods to stabilize the spine. It is more difficult to stabilize these areas in the postoperative recovery period. Patients may wear a supportive corset, a rigid brace, or occasionally a body cast to supplement the support provided by the internal fixation devices. For more information, visit the Spinal Cord Injury Information Network at www.spinalcord.uab.edu.

Gerontological Issues

Aging With Spinal Cord Injury

Individuals aging with a spinal cord injury have an increased risk for developing complications in the following areas:

- Blood pressure control
- Abnormalities in carbohydrate and lipid metabolism related to immobilization
- Cardiovascular disease
- Respiratory complications
- Osteoporosis
- Bladder infections
- Skin ulcers
- Chronic pain

NURSING CARE PLAN for the Patient With a Spinal Cord Injury

Nursing Diagnosis: *Impaired Gas Exchange* related to respiratory muscle weakness as evidenced by SpO_2 less than 90%, abnormal ABGs

Expected Outcome: The patient will maintain oxygenation as evidenced by SpO_2 of 90% or greater, PaO_2 of 75 mm Hg or greater, $PaCO_2$ of 45 mm Hg or less.

Evaluation of Outcome: Are ABGs and SpO_2 within normal limits?

Intervention Monitor respiratory rate, effort, ABGs, and SpO_2. **Rationale** These are indicators of respiratory function. The patient may have difficulty maintaining normal respiration if diaphragm or accessory muscles are weak related to injury. **Evaluation** Are ABGs and SaO_2 within normal limits? Does patient appear distressed?

Intervention Notify physician immediately if SpO_2 or PaO_2 drops, or if $PaCO_2$ rises. **Rationale** If patient is unable to maintain blood gases, mechanical ventilation may be needed. **Evaluation** Are changes recognized and reported promptly?

Nursing Diagnosis: *Ineffective Airway Clearance* related to ineffective cough and decreased muscle control as evidenced by adventitious breath sounds, SpO_2 less than 90%

Expected Outcome: The patient will maintain a clear airway as evidenced by clear breath sounds and SpO_2 of 90% or greater.

Evaluation of Outcome: Are breath sounds clear? Is SpO_2 90% or greater?

Intervention Monitor cough and lung sounds. **Rationale** Patient may not have adequate muscle strength to cough effectively. **Evaluation** Is patient able to cough up secretions? Is there evidence that secretions are retained?

Intervention Suction patient prn if unable to cough effectively. **Rationale** To keep the airway clear. **Evaluation** Is suctioning effective in clearing airway?

Intervention Once the patient is stable, try assisting him or her to cough to clear secretions. Gently push upward and inward on the patient's chest while he or she coughs as strongly as possible. **Rationale** This can help the patient clear secretions without invasive suctioning. This is similar to the Heimlich maneuver but not as forceful. **Evaluation** Does the assisted cough technique help the patient to clear the airway?

Intervention Provide humidified air and oral or enteral fluids. **Rationale** Humidification helps keep secretions thin and mobile. **Evaluation** Are secretions thin and easily expectorated?

Nursing Diagnosis: *Risk for Autonomic Dysreflexia* related to stimuli below the level of injury

Expected Outcomes: The patient will not demonstrate signs of autonomic dysreflexia as evidenced by stable vital signs. If dysreflexia occurs, it is recognized and corrected promptly.

Evaluation of Outcomes: Is patient free of signs or are signs recognized and promptly treated?

Intervention Monitor for signs of autonomic dysreflexia: sudden high blood pressure, bradycardia, headache, pale skin below the injury, gooseflesh. Remember that patients with spinal cord injury are typically hypotensive, so a finding of even mild hypertension can represent a dramatic increase from their baseline blood pressure. **Rationale** Autonomic dysreflexia must be recognized quickly to remove cause and prevent complications such as seizures, intracerebral hemorrhage, or death. **Evaluation** Are signs of dysreflexia present?

NURSING CARE PLAN for the Patient With a Spinal Cord Injury—cont'd

Intervention If you suspect autonomic dysreflexia, immediately take the patient's blood pressure and continue to monitor it every 5 minutes. **Rationale** Blood pressure must be continually monitored until it is under control, to prevent complications. **Evaluation** Is blood pressure higher than normal for patient? Are emergency interventions warranted?

Intervention Place the patient in high-Fowler's position. Remove elastic stockings or any other garment that could prevent blood from pooling in the periphery. **Rationale** High-Fowler's position uses the effect of orthostasis to control blood pressure. Allowing blood to pool in periphery can help reduce blood pressure. **Evaluation** Does position change reduce blood pressure?

Intervention Evaluate the indwelling catheter for patency. If it is not patent or a catheter is not in place and the bladder is full, obtain an order to insert a catheter immediately. Monitor blood pressure during catheterization. **Rationale** A full bladder can be the cause of the stimuli causing the dysreflexia. **Evaluation** Is catheter patent? Is bladder full? Does emptying bladder resolve dysreflexia?

Intervention Perform a rectal examination to determine if an impaction is present. Apply anesthetic ointment to the rectum before disimpaction. Simultaneously monitor blood pressure and stop disimpaction if the blood pressure increases. **Rationale** Fecal impaction can be the stimulus causing the dysreflexia. Anesthetic is used because further rectal stimulation can exacerbate symptoms. **Evaluation** Is impaction present? Does removal resolve dysreflexia?

Intervention If bowel or bladder distention is not present, examine the patient for other causative mechanisms. If a cause cannot be identified, or removal of the cause does not relieve hypertension, notify the physician immediately. **Rationale** If the cause cannot be found and removed, an antihypertensive agent may be ordered. **Evaluation** Are other causes identifiable? Is an antihypertensive agent ordered?

Intervention If hypertension is treated with medication, continue to carefully monitor blood pressure. **Rationale** Blood pressure can decrease rapidly once the cause of the autonomic dysreflexia is corrected. **Evaluation** Is blood pressure stabilized?

Intervention Once the acute episode is past, work with patient and significant others to devise a plan to prevent reoccurrence. Teach the patient how to direct caregivers in treating autonomic dysreflexia. **Rationale** Episodes of dysreflexia can recur, and most can be prevented. **Evaluation** Do patient and caregivers verbalize understanding of how to prevent and treat future episodes of dysreflexia?

Nursing Diagnosis: *Reflex Urinary Incontinence* related to spinal cord damage and no sensation to void as evidenced by inability to control flow of urine

Expected Outcomes: The patient's skin will be dry and free of urine; urine elimination will be controlled.

Evaluation of Outcomes: Is patient clean and dry at all times?

Intervention Assess patient's ability to control urination. **Rationale** If patient has some control, a bladder training program may be effective. **Evaluation** Is patient able to sense need to urinate? Is any degree of control present?

Intervention Implement a bladder training program, using set times for voiding. **Rationale** Following a voiding schedule can help reduce incontinence. **Evaluation** Is patient able to avoid incontinence with regular voiding?

Intervention Use bladder ultrasound to scan bladder for residual urine. **Rationale** Incomplete voiding can increase risk for urinary tract infection. **Evaluation** Is patient effectively emptying bladder?

Intervention Teach the patient or caregiver self-catheterization as ordered, if bladder training is not effective. **Rationale** Intermittent self-catheterization is associated with fewer complications than an indwelling catheter. **Evaluation** Is patient able to perform self-catheterization correctly?

Continued

NURSING CARE PLAN for the Patient With a Spinal Cord Injury—cont'd

Intervention Monitor appearance of urine, temperature, and white cell count. **Rationale** Cloudy urine, and an increase in temperature and white cell count indicate urinary tract infection. **Evaluation** Is urine clear, and temperature and white blood cell count within normal limits?

Intervention Consult with physician regarding indwelling Foley catheter if patient is not a candidate for intermittent self-catheterization. **Rationale** An indwelling catheter can increase risk for infection, but may be necessary as a last resort for some patients. **Evaluation** Is Foley catheter necessary? Are signs of infection avoided?

Nursing Diagnosis: *Constipation* related to immobility and nerve damage as evidenced by passage of hard, dry, or infrequent stools

Expected Outcome: The patient will return to preinjury bowel pattern.

Evaluation of Outcome: Does patient pass soft stool at regular intervals?

Intervention Assess previous and current bowel pattern and continence. **Rationale** Decreased or absent sphincter tone, inability to detect the need to defecate, and immobility put the patient at risk for incontinence and constipation. **Evaluation** What was previous pattern? How can it be maintained for the patient?

Intervention Monitor bowel sounds and abdominal distention. **Rationale** These are indicators of bowel function. **Evaluation** Are bowel sounds present? Is abdomen soft?

Intervention Institute a bowel management program as soon as oral feedings are resumed. Include a suppository on a scheduled daily or every-other-day basis as ordered. **Rationale** A management program including stool softeners and routine suppository use can help to restore regular defecation. **Evaluation** Does management program keep bowel movements soft and regular and maintain continence?

Intervention If possible, have patient sit on a toilet or bedside commode to move bowels. **Rationale** Sitting allows gravity to help evacuate the bowel. **Evaluation** Does sitting help patient move bowels?

Intervention Provide a high-fiber diet with adequate fluid intake. **Rationale** Fiber and fluids help keep stool soft. **Evaluation** Is patient receiving adequate fiber and fluids?

Nursing Diagnosis: *Impaired Physical Mobility* related to hemorrhage, ischemia, and edema of cord as evidenced by paresis or paralysis

Expected Outcomes: The patient will maintain maximum mobility and be free from complications of immobility.

Evaluation of Outcomes: Is patient kept mobile without contractures? Is skin intact? Can patient complete ADLs with assistance?

Intervention Determine patient's ability to move independently. **Rationale** Assessment should guide interventions. **Evaluation** What can patient do independently?

Intervention Assess patient's ability to feel pressure and pain. **Rationale** If the patient is unable to feel pain or pressure, it will be even more important to monitor skin and prevent prolonged pressure. **Evaluation** Can patient feel pressure and pain?

Intervention Reposition every 2 hours, using supportive devices. **Rationale** Unrelieved pressure on the skin, especially bony prominences, will result in ischemia and necrosis. **Evaluation** Is skin intact without redness?

Intervention Change positions slowly; have patient sit at side of bed before standing (if able) or getting up to a chair. **Rationale** Patients with cervical spine injuries or patients remaining immobile for long periods are prone to orthostatic hypotension. **Evaluation** Does patient become dizzy when getting up?

NURSING CARE PLAN for the Patient With a Spinal Cord Injury—cont'd

Intervention Perform active or passive ROM exercises at least once every 8 hours. If patient has arm mobility, teach patient to participate in doing as much ROM as possible. **Rationale** ROM exercises maintain mobility and prevent contractures. **Evaluation** Is patient able to perform ROM exercises with minimal difficulty?

Intervention Teach patient importance of repositioning self at least every 2 hours. **Rationale** Patients with some mobility can learn to reposition themselves; this helps prevent total dependence on caregivers. **Evaluation** Does patient demonstrate correct repositioning every 2 hours?

Intervention Teach patient to direct own care, if unable to reposition independently. **Rationale** This allows the patient some control over his or her situation. **Evaluation** Does patient direct own care and prevent complications of immobility?

Nursing Diagnosis: *Self-Care Deficit* related to paralysis

Expected Outcome: The patient's self-care needs will be met by self or caregivers.

Evaluation of Outcome: Are patient's needs met? Does patient verbalize satisfaction with care?

Intervention Determine patient's level of function and ability to perform ADLs. **Rationale** The patient should be encouraged to be as independent as possible. **Evaluation** What is patient able to do? Is it incorporated into plan of care?

Intervention Explain the rationale for nursing activities, and encourage the patient and significant others to participate in hands-on care as much as possible. **Rationale** This will help prepare the patient and significant others to assume responsibility for care at home. **Evaluation** Do patient and significant others verbalize understanding of care? Are they able to demonstrate procedures correctly?

Intervention If the patient will not be able to perform self-care, assist him or her to learn to direct care. **Rationale** This allows the patient some control over his or her care. **Evaluation** Does patient participate by directing care?

Intervention Consult with physical and occupational therapists. **Rationale** Physical and occupational therapists can help the patient learn to adapt to physical limitations; they can provide a wheelchair or other mobility aids. **Evaluation** Is patient adapting to limitations with help?

Intervention Discuss discharge to a rehabilitation facility with patient, physician, and discharge planner. **Rationale** A rehabilitation facility can teach the patient to function independently. Some patients may require long-term care. **Evaluation** Is the patient a candidate for rehabilitation?

Intervention Assist patients and caregivers to determine contingency plans. These include what to do in the event of a power failure, fire, or illness of the caregiver. **Rationale** Planning ahead what to do in an emergency can mean the difference between life and death for an immobile patient. **Evaluation** Do patient and caregivers have a plan to keep the patient safe?

Intervention Encourage the patient to establish a relationship with a primary practitioner who is familiar with spinal cord injury. **Rationale** Patients with spinal cord injuries experience the same basic health care needs as individuals without injuries. **Evaluation** Does patient have a primary care practitioner who understands his or her unique needs?

Nursing Diagnosis: *Risk for Impaired Skin Integrity* related to immobility and possible paresthesias

Expected Outcome: The patient's skin will remain intact without redness or breakdown.

Evaluation of Outcome: Is patient's skin intact?

Continued

NURSING CARE PLAN for the Patient With a Spinal Cord Injury—cont'd

Intervention Monitor skin frequently. When permitted by the physician, turn the patient frequently and assess bony prominences for redness. **Rationale** The patient who does not have sensation is at increased risk of developing pressure ulcers. **Evaluation** Is the patient turned and repositioned at least every 2 hours? Is skin intact?

Intervention Start preventive measures in the emergency department by being sure to remove anything between the patient and the backboard. **Rationale** Patients have developed pressure ulcers from lying on keys or other objects in their pockets. **Evaluation** Are skin surfaces protected from pressure?

Intervention Use a pressure-reducing mattress. **Rationale** Specialty mattresses or beds can reduce pressure, but do not reduce the need to turn the patient. **Evaluation** Is the patient on an appropriate mattress?

Intervention If on a self-turning bed, make sure the patient is not sliding as the bed turns. Avoid pulling and friction on skin when repositioning patient in bed. **Rationale** Sliding can cause friction and shearing damage to the skin. **Evaluation** Is friction damage to skin avoided?

Intervention Ensure that the patient's extremities do not get caught in side rails or wheelchair spokes. **Rationale** The patient may not be aware this is happening, and a pressure ulcer can result. **Evaluation** Are all patient's body parts accounted for and safe?

Intervention If a patient is in traction or a halo brace, assess pin sites frequently. Keep the sites clean and dry, and report any sign of infection. **Rationale** Skin sites are at risk for infection and breakdown. **Evaluation** Are pin sites clean and dry?

Intervention Monitor temperature of bath water (no more than 102 degrees F). **Rationale** Patient may not be able to feel burning if water is too hot. **Evaluation** Are burns prevented?

Nursing Diagnosis: *Risk for Ineffective Role Performance* related to effects of injury

Expected Outcome: The patient will identify new ways to carry out essential roles.

Evaluation of Outcome: Is patient able to identify ways to carry out roles?

Intervention Allow the patient to verbalize concerns about his or her roles if desired. **Rationale** This can help to clarify potential role problems for the patient, and begin the process of developing a plan. **Evaluation** Is patient able to identify roles he or she has filled in the past that will be difficult to carry out due to injury?

Intervention Help patient and family to identify resources. **Rationale** Interpersonal relationships can be significantly stressed by spinal cord injury. Friends, family, and members of the patient's religious affiliation can provide emotional and physical help. **Evaluation** Does patient have adequate support systems in place to provide help?

Intervention Consult a social worker to help the patient gain access to appropriate physical and financial assistance. **Rationale** Loss of income can be temporary or permanent and can add to the burden of spinal cord injury. Not all insurance policies cover the extensive inpatient rehabilitation needed by patients with spinal cord injuries. Adaptive equipment is expensive and may not be covered by insurance. **Evaluation** Is patient able to access appropriate financial assistance if needed?

Intervention Provide information about area support groups. **Rationale** Individuals who have been through similar experiences can provide support and information for the patient and family. **Evaluation** Is patient willing to contact support groups?

Nursing Diagnosis: *Risk for Sexual Dysfunction* related to autonomic nervous system dysfunction

Expected Outcome: The patient will state he or she has an acceptable means for sexual expression.

Evaluation of Outcome: Does patient state satisfaction with sexual function?

NURSING CARE PLAN for the Patient With a Spinal Cord Injury—cont'd

Intervention If a male patient has an erection during a bath or catheterization, discontinue the procedure and continue at a later time if possible. Maintain a matter-of-fact attitude. **Rationale** Male patients with quadriplegia may develop an erection during any penile stimulation. **Evaluation** Is patient's dignity maintained during personal care?

Intervention Allow patient to voice concerns about sexual function if desired. **Rationale** Male patients with paraplegia can have difficulty achieving and maintaining an erection. **Evaluation** Is patient able to voice concerns? Is a consult with a urologist or other specialist needed?

Intervention Encourage the patient and partner to explore alternative methods of sexual expression. **Rationale** Closeness and touching may be a satisfying alternative. **Evaluation** Is patient able to discuss alternative methods with partner?

Intervention If a male patient wishes to have children, encourage a consult with a fertility specialist or urologist. **Rationale** Men with spinal cord injuries may not ejaculate in the normal manner. A specialist can provide some help for conception if desired. **Evaluation** Is patient given information about conception if desired?

Intervention Advise women who wish to become pregnant to seek an obstetrician familiar with spinal cord injuries. **Rationale** A specialist may be needed to meet the unique needs of these patients. **Evaluation** Is the patient interested in pregnancy? Does she have the information needed related to pregnancy with spinal cord injury?

Intervention If the patient does not wish to become pregnant, provide information about contraception. See Table 48.9 for contraception for women with spinal cord injuries. **Rationale** Spinal cord injury does not impair female fertility. **Evaluation** Does the patient have information and resources to prevent pregnancy if desired?

Intervention Encourage partners to verbalize feelings about caregiving activities such as catheterizations and make alternative arrangements for care if possible. Some patients with the financial resources to do so may choose to hire an attendant rather than rely on significant others for personal care. **Rationale** Performing tasks such as catheterization or bowel care may interfere with feelings of intimacy between partners. **Evaluation** Are patient and partner able to discuss feelings about caregiving activities and find alternate arrangements if desired?

Nursing Diagnosis: *Anxiety* related to change in health status as evidenced by behavioral changes such as insomnia, poor eye contact, and irritability

Expected Outcomes: The patient will participate in rehabilitation activities. The patient will be able to verbalize fears, concerns, and expectations.

Evaluation of Outcomes: Is the patient able to participate in rehabilitation? Does patient verbalize that anxiety is controlled?

Intervention Allow patient to voice feelings of fear and anxiety. **Rationale** Communication is vital to assess the patient's coping abilities. **Evaluation** Is the patient able to verbalize anxiety?

Intervention Provide information about what is happening to the patient physiologically and about procedures. **Rationale** Understanding of what is happening can help the patient cope with changes. **Evaluation** Does patient verbalize understanding of what is happening? Does information help keep patient less fearful?

Intervention Consult a social worker, pastoral care, and/or support groups. **Rationale** A social worker or pastor can help provide emotional and spiritual support. Discussing rehabilitation with patients and their families who have had similar experiences can provide insight and encouragement. **Evaluation** Does patient state talking with support persons helps reduce anxiety?

Intervention Encourage the patient to participate in physical and occupational therapy. **Rationale** Seeing progress toward becoming independent can help reduce anxiety and fear about the future. **Evaluation** Does patient participate in therapies? Is anxiety lessening?

TABLE 48.8 SPINAL CORD INJURY SUMMARY

Signs and Symptoms	Flaccid paralysis and paresthesias (depending on level of the lesion) Loss of reflex activity below the level of the lesion Spinal shock initially Risk for autonomic dysreflexia (injuries above sixth thoracic vertebra)
Diagnostic Tests	Radiograph CT scan MRI
Therapeutic Measures	Immobilization Maintenance of airway and respiratory status Bowel and bladder training Nutrition/diet Activity/rehabilitation Prevention of dysreflexia Prevention of skin breakdown Sexual counseling Education
Complications	Infection Deep venous thrombosis Paralysis Orthostatic hypotension Pressure ulcers Depression
Priority Nursing Diagnoses	*Impaired Gas Exchange* *Ineffective Airway Clearance* *Risk for Autonomic Dysreflexia* *Reflex Urinary Incontinence* *Constipation* *Impaired Physical Mobility*

TABLE 48.9 BIRTH CONTROL ISSUES FOR PATIENTS WITH SPINAL CORD INJURY

Method	Comments
Oral contraceptives	Contraindicated because of the risk of deep venous thrombosis
Diaphragm	May be difficult to insert for a patient with poor hand function
Intrauterine device	Patient may not feel device move out of position Patient may not feel perforation of uterus
Implantable device	No contraindications
Condom	No contraindications

on management of the illness, education related to prevention and treatment of complications, and referrals to support groups or case managers. As patients decline, many families will come to a time when they can no longer care for their loved one in their homes and must consider care in a long-term facility.

Dementia

Dementia is not a disease but rather a symptom of a number of neurocognitive disorders. According to the National Institute of Neurological Disorders and Stroke (2013), "People with dementia have significantly impaired intellectual functioning that interferes with normal activities and relationships. They also lose their ability to solve problems and maintain emotional control, and they may experience personality changes and behavioral problems, such as agitation, delusions, and hallucinations. While memory loss is a common symptom of dementia, memory loss by itself does not mean that a person has dementia." Some patients can have mild mental status changes that do not interfere significantly with day-to-day functioning. This is sometimes referred to as mild cognitive impairment, or MCI. However, patients with MCI are more likely to go on to develop Alzheimer's disease than those without MCI.

Etiology and Pathophysiology

There are many causes of dementia, including Huntington's, Parkinson's, and Alzheimer's diseases, which are discussed later in this chapter. Multiple "mini-strokes" (multi-infarct dementia or vascular dementia) are another common cause. Chronic alcoholism, neurologic infections, head injuries, and many medications (Box 48-2) also can cause changes

NEURODEGENERATIVE AND NEUROCOGNITIVE DISORDERS

Neurodegenerative is a term that can apply to any nervous system disorder that causes degeneration, or wasting, of the neurons in the nervous system. The disorders discussed in this section are some of the most common neurodegenerative disorders. Neurocognitive is the term used to describe acquired neurological disorders that cause cognitive decline. By 2030, it is estimated that 150 million Americans will have one or more chronic conditions. Management of chronic conditions does not focus on the short-term stay in the hospital due to a exacerbation of the disease process but rather on the long-term goal of facilitating the patient and family to cope with the disease process and maintain the patient's independence for as long as possible. Nursing care involves providing information

• **WORD • BUILDING •**

neurodegenerative: neuro—nervous system + degenerative—deteriorating

dementia: de—down or from + mental—the mind

in mental status leading to dementia. Although aging is associated with more frequent dementia diagnoses, dementia is not a normal part of aging. Pathophysiologies vary depending on the cause. In general, thinking is affected by changes in the brain that result from reduced blood flow or from structural changes related to disease states.

Much research has been done to determine factors related to dementia; such knowledge helps in its prevention. Some studies indicate that patients who have more education, have higher socioeconomic status, and engage in stimulating intellectual and leisure activities are less likely to develop dementia. Some experts believe these individuals develop a sort of cognitive reserve that keeps them functioning at a high level, even when changes in their brains on autopsy indicate dementia. People with less education, fewer leisure activities, and less intellectual stimulation are more likely to develop symptoms of Alzheimer's disease.

Signs and Symptoms

Have you ever forgotten something important? Most people have occasional memory lapses. Students may have memory lapses during examinations, but they do not generally have dementia. In patients with dementia, recent memories are usually affected first. Patients may have difficulty recalling whether they ate breakfast or may accuse a family member of not calling when in reality they called just a few hours earlier. This same patient, however, may easily recall an event or even a phone number from childhood.

As patients become more forgetful, they may ask the same questions repeatedly. They can get lost driving or walking in a familiar neighborhood. They can become disoriented to time, and not be aware of the year. Patients might say that Eisenhower is president, for example, because they remember that as true when they were younger. Later, they may not recognize where they are, and last, they can lose recognition of even their own family members.

Later in the course of the dementia, remote memory can be lost. Patients can forget how to perform simple tasks, such as doing the dishes or making a phone call. They may wander and become lost. Safety is a significant issue with a wandering patient—patients have been found wandering in their nightclothes in the middle of a road, unaware of what they

are doing. Patients can develop aphasia and become unable to communicate their needs or follow simple instructions. This can become frustrating to both the family and nursing caregivers. Behavioral problems may necessitate admission to a long-term care facility. In very late stages, the patient becomes totally dependent on caregivers.

Diagnostic Tests

Diagnosis of dementia is twofold: First, dementia must be identified, and then the focus moves to finding the cause of the mental status change. Early diagnosis is essential, because some causes of MCI may be reversible, and early treatment may delay progression. Neuropsychological testing can determine the degree of memory, personality, and behavior changes. The Mini-Mental State Examination is commonly used. The patient should also be tested for depression, which can cause mental status changes but is often easily treated. A review of medications by a knowledgeable nurse, physician, or pharmacist may reveal a medication that is contributing to the mental changes. MRI, CT scan, positron emission tomographic (PET) scan, and blood tests help diagnose underlying causes.

Therapeutic Measures

Medical interventions depend on the cause of the dementia. See Table 48.10 for medications that can be used to delay progression of Alzheimer's dementia. If medical treatment cannot alter the course of the disease, the focus will shift to delaying progression of symptoms and maintaining patient safety. Excellent nursing care becomes essential for both the patient and family at this point. An important aspect of care in early dementia is determination of the patient's wishes while the patient is still able to make decisions. Some difficult decisions relate to the patient's continued ability to drive and live alone. Other decisions related to resuscitation, guardianship, and powers of attorney for health care and finances are essential to discuss.

Nursing Process for the Patient With Dementia

See the "Nursing Care Plan for the Patient With Dementia."

Delirium

Whereas dementia is chronic and progressive, **delirium** is a mental disturbance that is temporary and can have either a rapid or gradual onset. Delirium is considered to be a medical emergency and should be diagnosed and treated promptly. Delirium is characterized by disorganized thinking and difficulty staying focused and is seen most commonly in older adults when experiencing an illness. Patients who are severely ill or who have a history of hypertension, alcoholism, or preexisting dementia are most at risk. Many times response to medications is the cause (see Box 48-2). The disturbance can also be the result of anything that is a stressor to the person's body, such as pain, oxygen deficiency, urinary catheters, fluid and electrolyte imbalances, a change in environment, or nutritional deficiency. Often the most effective nursing intervention is

TABLE 48.10 MEDICATIONS USED TO TREAT ALZHEIMER'S DEMENTIA

Medication Class/Action	Examples	Nursing Implications
Cholinesterase Inhibitors Inhibit cholinesterase, to improve function of acetylcholine in central nervous system. May improve cognitive function but will not alter course of disease.	donepezil (Aricept) tacrine (Cognex) rivastigmine (Exelon) galantamine (Reminyl)	Must be taken regularly; patient may need reminders to take, or family member may need to assist. Monitor for weight loss and report to health care provider.
NMDA Antagonist Reduces binding of glutamate, an excitatory neurotransmitter.	memantine (Namenda)	Teach patient and family that improvements may take months.

to have a family member present to assist with orientation and reassurance. Additionally, it is beneficial to have continuity in nursing personnel when possible.

NURSING CARE TIP

Patients with delirium or dementia must be kept safe, and interventions are similar for both. One important difference, however, is in how you respond to confusion. If a patient is experiencing delirium, reorient him or her to the present time and situation. If a patient with dementia is chronically confused, however, reorientation may not be effective. In this case, validate their feelings. An example would be comforting a patient who is calling for a long-lost parent, rather than reminding the patient the mother has been gone for 30 years.

It is essential that delirium not be mistaken for dementia. If an older adult is hospitalized and exhibits new-onset confusion, consider that it might be delirium. Correcting electrolyte levels, controlling pain, changing medications, or administering oxygen can be helpful in reversing delirium. See the "Nursing Care Plan for the Patient With Dementia" for nursing interventions.

EVIDENCE-BASED PRACTICE

Clinical Question
How can delirium be managed in the acute care setting?

Evidence
Delirium is associated with increased mortality in the ICU setting, prolonged ICU and hospital stays, and higher incidence of confusion following an ICU stay. The Agency for Healthcare Research and Quality evidence-based guideline addresses management of pain, agitation, and delirium in the critical care setting. Early mobilization and exercise, attention to risk factors for delirium, promotion of sleep, routine monitoring of delirium, and sedation if necessary have been found to be effective in managing delirium. It is also important to restart psychotropic medications if the patient has been treated with them before admission.

Implications for Nursing Practice
Be vigilant about (1) identifying patients at risk for delirium, (2) getting patients up and moving as soon as possible, (3) advocating for administration of preadmission psychotropic medications, and (4) allowing the patient time for sleep.

REFERENCE

Agency for Healthcare Research and Quality National Guideline Clearinghouse. (2013). Clinical practice guidelines for the management of pain, agitation, and delirium in the intensive care unit. Retrieved August 25, 2013, from www.guideline.gov/content.aspx?id=43903&search=2013+confusion

Parkinson's Disease

Parkinson's disease (PD) is a chronic degenerative movement disorder that arises in the basal ganglia in the cerebrum. PD has typically been considered a disease of older adults; however, there are many people with young-onset Parkinson's. An example is Michael J. Fox (actor and founder of the Michael J. Fox Foundation for Parkinson's Research), who was diagnosed at age 30. The disease is

NURSING CARE PLAN for the Patient With Dementia

Nursing Diagnosis: *Risk for Injury* related to impaired memory, thought processes, and judgment

Expected Outcome: The patient will remain free from injury.

Evaluation of Outcome: Is patient safe and free from injury? Is environment safe?

Intervention Monitor patient's ability to maintain safety. **Rationale** As dementia worsens, the patient's needs change. **Evaluation** Is patient able to make decisions and negotiate the environment safely?

Intervention Keep environment simple and familiar; label doors and objects. Keep patient in familiar environment as long as possible. **Rationale** Change can result in confusion; even a minor change in furniture arrangement can result in falls. **Evaluation** Is patient able to remain in the home with minimum confusion and without injury?

Intervention Remove harmful objects (scissors, matches); store medicines in locked cabinet; remove knobs from stoves. **Rationale** Impaired judgment can make safety a major concern for patients who live at home. **Evaluation** Is the environment safe for the patient?

Intervention Make sure patient has eyeglasses and hearing aids if necessary. **Rationale** Impaired sensory perception can increase confusion and risk for falls. **Evaluation** Is patient able to see and hear effectively?

Intervention Use nightlights; remove throw rugs; use safety gates on stairs. **Rationale** These can reduce the risk for falls. **Evaluation** Is environment set up to reduce risk for falling?

Intervention Have identification bracelet on patient and ID tags sewn into clothes, and locks on doors to prevent leaving. **Rationale** Patients can wander, making them prone to injury. **Evaluation** Is wandering confined to a monitored area? Is environment set up to allow movement within a safe area?

Intervention Provide daily walks or exercise. **Rationale** Exercise can decrease wandering. **Evaluation** Does exercise reduce wandering?

Nursing Diagnosis: *Imbalanced Nutrition: Less Than Body Requirements* related to impaired thought processes and lack of interest in eating or refusal to eat

Expected Outcomes: The patient will maintain adequate food intake and weight within normal limits for height.

Evaluation of Outcomes: Does patient maintain appropriate weight?

Intervention Monitor intake, weight, and serum albumin. **Rationale** Loss of weight or a serum albumin level of less than 3.5 indicates poor nutrition. **Evaluation** Are weight and serum albumin level stable and within normal limits?

Intervention Develop meal plan to include likes and dislikes, snacks, and protein supplements as necessary. **Rationale** Using the patient's favorite foods will encourage eating. **Evaluation** Is patient consuming majority of meals?

Intervention Offer larger meal when patient has the greatest appetite or serve small meals five to six times a day. **Rationale** A lot of food at one time can feel overwhelming to the patient. **Evaluation** Is patient eating meals that are served?

Intervention Offer one food at a time if patient is not successful with a whole plate full. **Rationale** Too many choices on a plate can feel overwhelming to the patient. **Evaluation** Does patient eat more if one food at a time is offered?

Intervention Offer finger foods. **Rationale** Utensils can be difficult for the patient to use and can discourage eating. **Evaluation** Does patient eat more when finger foods are offered?

For additional information, see also "Nutrition Notes."

Continued

NURSING CARE PLAN for the Patient With Dementia—cont'd

Nursing Diagnosis: *Chronic Confusion* related to dementia

Expected Outcome: The patient will function at optimal cognitive level.

Evaluation of Outcome: Is patient maintaining optimum cognitive function?

Intervention Monitor changes in thought processes. **Rationale** As cognitive function declines, care plan will need to be revised. **Evaluation** Is patient able to correctly identify objects, remember tasks, speak clearly, identify person, place, and time?

Intervention Provide a box of safe, familiar items, such as empty thread spools, or pretty handkerchiefs for women. **Rationale** Patients often rummage through drawers, closets, or boxes. These patients may not recognize the difference between their own possessions and those of others. Keeping them occupied with a box of safe items may decrease their need to look for things. **Evaluation** Does a box of items keep patient occupied and content?

Intervention Place calendars, clocks, personal items, and seasonal decorations in patient's environment. **Rationale** These provide orientation to the present. **Evaluation** Can patient identify the season or year?

Intervention If patient hallucinates or has delusions, do not attempt to correct. Focus instead on the feelings related to the hallucinations, such as "Do you feel frightened?" **Rationale** Having feelings validated can help develop trust, while not validating the hallucination. **Evaluation** Does patient respond to refocusing on feelings?

Intervention Reduce stressors such as fatigue, overstimulation, or pain. **Rationale** Stress may increase dysfunctional behaviors. **Evaluation** Are stressors eliminated as much as possible? Is patient's behavior calm?

Intervention Maintain patient's usual routines as much as possible. **Rationale** Familiar routines such as sleeping or eating habits are more comfortable for patients. Change can be stressful. **Evaluation** Are routines organized around the patient rather than the staff?

Intervention Communicate clearly. Make eye contact, speak slowly and directly to the patient, use nonverbal gestures. Use a tone of voice conveying respect and sincerity. **Rationale** Unclear communication can increase confusion and stress. Research indicates that the tone of voice plays a role in the ability of the patient to cooperate (Barnes & Brannelly, 2008). **Evaluation** Do all staff members communicate clearly and respectfully with the patient?

Intervention Involve family in care planning and implementation. **Rationale** The family knows the patient's preferences and routines best. **Evaluation** Does family presence help patient stay calm and function at optimum level?

Intervention Provide video or audiotapes of patient's family members. **Rationale** Familiar sounds and pictures can reduce agitation when family is not present. **Evaluation** Do video or audiotapes help calm the patient?

Nursing Diagnosis: *Risk for Caregiver Role Strain* related to demands of caring for patient with declining mental status while balancing other demands

Expected Outcomes: The caregiver will have support needed to safely manage care of patient. The caregiver will be able to identify when the patient is too difficult to care for and requires more structured observation.

Evaluation of Outcomes: Is caregiver managing demands of caring for patient? Is patient safe? Is additional support or a change in environment for patient indicated?

Intervention Allow caregiver to verbalize concerns related to burden of caring for patient. **Rationale** An assessment of caregiver concerns and challenges can help the nurse plan appropriate support. **Evaluation** Does the caregiver share concerns? What are the caregiver's current support systems?

NURSING CARE PLAN for the Patient With Dementia—cont'd

Intervention Observe for signs of depression or stress in the caregiver. **Rationale** A stressed or depressed caregiver may have difficulty providing safe care for the patient. **Evaluation** Are signs of stress present? Does patient care appear to be suffering?

Intervention Encourage caregiver to identify family and friends that can provide support. If they are involved in a local church or religious organization, encourage caregiver to make his or her needs known. **Rationale** There are often resources in the family or community that can be accessed without cost and are able to help if they know the need exists. **Evaluation** Can caregiver identify potential resources to contact?

Intervention Refer for assistance with caregiving and/or day care utilizing Alzheimer's support groups and resources. **Rationale** Formal support systems in the community may be available to help relieve some of the caregiver's burden. **Evaluation** Is caregiver able to obtain support and take some time for himself or herself?

Intervention Encourage caregiver to use support systems identified to allow him or her time to care for self; encourage to take care of own health needs, and enjoy some respite time doing something enjoyable on a regular basis. **Rationale** If the caregiver becomes ill due to the stress of caregiving, he or she will no longer be able to assist the patient. **Evaluation** Does caregiver maintain own physical and emotional health?

Intervention Allow the caregiver to grieve over the losses he or she is experiencing: losses in the patient as well as loss of control over his or her own life. **Rationale** As the disease progresses, the patient gradually loses awareness of the neurologic deterioration. Occasional lucid moments can be very difficult for patient and caregiver as they realize what has been lost. **Evaluation** Is the caregiver able to identify feelings of grief, anger, or sorrow?

Intervention Discuss progression of the disease process and the possibility of transferring the patient to an extended care facility. **Rationale** The caregiver may feel guilt over not being able to care for the patient and may need permission to consider placement at an extended care facility. **Evaluation** Is caregiver able to identify when home care is too demanding, and choose an alternative arrangement?

---

characterized by tremors, changes in posture and gait, rigidity, and slowness of movements. Approximately 50,000 to 60,000 new cases of PD are diagnosed each year in the United States; it ranks 14th in causes of death according to the Centers for Disease Control and Prevention (National Parkinson Foundation, 2013).

Pathophysiology

The substantia nigra is a group of cells located within the basal ganglia, which is situated deep in the brain. These cells are responsible for the production of dopamine, an inhibitory neurotransmitter. Dopamine facilitates the transmission of impulses from one neuron to another. Parkinson's disease is caused by destruction of the cells of the substantia nigra, resulting in decreased dopamine production. Loss of dopamine function results in impairment of semiautomatic movements. Parkinson's disease is sometimes referred to as an extrapyramidal disorder because the extrapyramidal tracts in the spinal cord that contain motor neurons are affected.

Acetylcholine, an excitatory neurotransmitter, is secreted normally in individuals with Parkinson's disease. The normal balance of acetylcholine and dopamine is interrupted in these patients, causing a relative excess of acetylcholine, which results in the tremor, muscle rigidity,

and akinesia (loss of muscle movement) characteristic of Parkinson's disease.

Etiology

The etiology of Parkinson's disease is unknown. It was first described in 1817 by London surgeon James Parkinson. Although scientists now know that the symptoms are caused by death of dopamine-producing cells in the substantia nigra, they do not know what causes the cells to die. There may be a genetic component, especially in younger patients. Certain environmental toxins can also play a role. Parkinson's disease–like symptoms, referred to as parkinsonism, can be associated with use of certain drugs, such as phenothiazines. Parkinsonism was also linked to an outbreak of encephalitis in the 1920s.

Signs and Symptoms

The onset of symptoms in patients with Parkinson's disease is usually gradual and subtle. A substantial percentage of the dopamine-producing cells are nonfunctional before the

• WORD • BUILDING •

akinesia: a—not + kinesia—movement

Nutrition Notes

Nutrition Issues in Dementia

Efforts are ongoing to identify influences that might delay or mitigate dementia. Preliminary evidence on the role of nutrients in cognitive aging and dementia is fairly strong for protective associations of vitamin E from food, vitamin B_{12} and folate, DHA (the omega-3 fatty acid found in fish), and a high ratio of polyunsaturated to saturated fats (Morris, 2012). In patients with Alzheimer's disease, synapse loss is the structural change that correlates most strongly with cognitive impairment. Experimental use of a medical food containing factors promoting synthesis of neuronal membranes improved memory in patients with *very mild* Alzheimer's disease (de Wilde, Kamphuis, Sijben, & Scheltens, 2011).

For caregivers of the 4.5 million people in the United States already affected with dementia, the immediate problem may be providing the patient with sufficient nutrients. Most commonly, patients with dementia demonstrate a slowing of the swallowing process that may increase time required to finish a meal. They also often have difficulties self-feeding. Both situations increase the risk for malnutrition (Sura, Madhavan, Carnaby, & Crary, 2012). (See Chapter 49, Box 49-2, for dysphagia interventions.)

Dining rooms should be quiet and have adequate lighting. Occupying the same chair for every meal lends familiarity. Serving one course at a time and providing necessary but not extraneous flatware, with large handles if needed, limits distractions. Dishes with high sides enable the patient to scoop the food onto a spoon or fork. Finger foods that the patient can manage may increase intake with minimal staff assistance.

Patients with dementia must be reminded of the steps involved in self-feeding:
- Putting the food on the spoon
- Directing it to the mouth
- Chewing
- Swallowing

Use of verbal cues or guiding the patient's hand to start the necessary movement helps the process. Common courtesies model social expectations and help maintain a person's dignity:
- Introducing the patient to the other persons at the table
- Providing a cup rather than a carton for milk
- Offering foods separately rather than mixing them all together.
- Providing color contrast between foods and plate
- Ensuring use of eyeglasses if needed
- Ascertaining favorite foods, especially aromatic ones, to tempt poor eaters
- Playing music with a slow tempo to relax the patient and mask distracting noises

Nearly all patients with advanced dementia develop feeding problems. Health care providers may advise families that high caloric supplements, perhaps in combination with assisted feeding, foods modified in taste or texture, and appetite stimulants can promote weight gain for several months. Given the progressive nature of dementia, families should be counseled not to expect improvements in function or survival with any available form of feeding (Hanson, Ersek, Gilliam, & Carey, 2011).

References

Chang, C. C., & Roberts, B. L. (2011). Strategies for feeding patients with dementia. *American Journal of Nursing, 111,* 36–44.

de Wilde, M. C., Kamphuis, P. J., Sijben, J. W., & Scheltens, P. (2011). Utility of imaging for nutritional intervention studies in Alzheimer's disease. *European Journal of Pharmacology, 668*(Suppl 1):S59–S69.

Hanson, L. C., Ersek, M., Gilliam, R., & Carey, T. S. (2011). Oral feeding options for patients with dementia: A systematic review. *Journal of the American Geriatric Society, 59,* 463–472.

Morris, M. C. (2012). Nutritional determinants of cognitive aging and dementia. *Proceedings of the Nutrition Society, 71,* 1–13.

Sura, L., Madhavan, A., Carnaby, G., & Crary, M. A. (2012). Dysphagia in the elderly: Management and nutritional considerations. *Clinical Interventions in Aging, 7,* 287–298.

patient becomes symptomatic. Symptoms may be mistakenly attributed to aging or fatigue. In retrospect, patients and their significant others often identify a long period in which symptoms were present but not identified as symptoms of Parkinson's disease.

The primary symptoms of Parkinson's disease are muscular rigidity, **bradykinesia** (slow movement) or akinesia, changes in posture, and tremors. The brain is no longer able to direct the muscles to perform in the usual manner. This lack of communication between the brain and the muscles can have a profound impact on the patient's ability to ambulate safely, perform ADLs and job functions, or enjoy leisure activities. The symptoms may also have a significant negative impact on the patient's self-esteem.

The patient may have difficulty initiating movement; this can be particularly apparent when the patient tries to start walking, rise from a sitting position, or begin dressing. Because considerable effort is required to move the rigid muscles, the patient performs voluntary movements very slowly. At times, the patient can experience freezing of gait and be unable to initiate ambulation or negotiate a turn during ambulation.

• WORD • BUILDING •
bradykinesia: brady—slow + kinesia—movement

The extensor muscles are more affected by Parkinson's disease than the flexor muscles. This impaired function of the extensor muscles results in the stooped posture typical of patients with Parkinson's disease (Fig. 48.14). Flexion of the hips, knees, and neck shifts the center of gravity forward. The gait is characterized by shuffling, short steps that may increase in speed once the patient finally gets walking. Once in motion, the patient may have difficulty stopping. The patient maintains a broad base when making turns to try to compensate for imbalance. These changes place patients at high risk for falls. Slowness of movement and stiff muscles make it much harder for patients to catch themselves if they start to fall or to relax the muscles to minimize injury.

Tremors typically begin in the hand and then progress to the **ipsilateral** foot. In most patients, the tremor then moves to the **contralateral** side. Many patients identify one side of the body as being more affected by the tremor than the other. Tremor of the hand has been described as a pill-rolling tremor; the thumb typically moves back and forth across the fingers and looks like the patient is rolling a pill. Tremors typically lessen or disappear during movement and are more noticeable when the extremity is at rest or when trying to hold an object still (this is called a resting tremor). The tremors disappear when the patient is asleep. The inability to hold an object still can make simple acts such as drinking a glass of water or reading a book nearly impossible. The signs and symptoms of Parkinson's disease tend to increase in severity when the patient becomes fatigued. Another type of tremor, a benign familial (or essential) tremor, can sometimes be mistaken for Parkinson's disease. Treatment is different for each. See Table 48.11 for differentiation of these tremors.

TABLE 48.11 SYMPTOMS OF PARKINSON'S DISEASE VERSUS ESSENTIAL TREMOR

Disease	Parkinson's Tremor	Benign Familial Tremor
Resting tremor	Yes	No
Intention tremor (with movement)	No	Yes
Pill-rolling tremor	Yes	No
Head/voice tremor	No	Yes
Relieved with beta-blocking medication (propranolol)	No	Yes
Relieved with anti-Parkinson's medications	Yes	No

The secondary symptoms of Parkinson's disease include generalized weakness, muscle fatigue and cramping, and difficulty with fine motor activities. This fine motor dysfunction can make it difficult for the patient to button a shirt or tie shoes. Handwriting typically deteriorates as the disease progresses. A soft, monotone voice and masklike facial expression can make the patient appear to be lacking in emotional responses. It may be necessary to ask patients about their emotional status and help them develop ways to express their emotions. The normal blink response is diminished, so the patient and significant others must be educated about eye care to prevent corneal abrasions.

Dysfunction of the autonomic system can cause diaphoresis, constipation, orthostatic hypotension, drooling, dysphagia, seborrhea, and frequent urination. Patients who experience seborrhea and diaphoresis need frequent attention to personal hygiene. Drooling and dysphagia can make the patient reluctant to appear in public. Slowness in initiating walking, balance problems, and frequent urination place the patient at risk for urinary incontinence, which can also increase the patient's reluctance to leave home.

Late in the disease, mental function may become slowed, and the patient may develop dementia. This is compounded by the side effects of many anti-Parkinson's drugs. Death is usually from complications of immobility.

Complications

The most typical acute complications of Parkinson's disease are related to the patient's difficulties with mobility and balance.

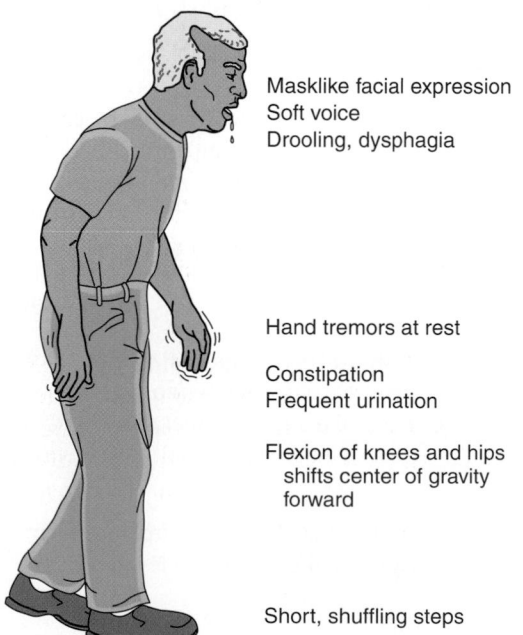

Masklike facial expression
Soft voice
Drooling, dysphagia

Hand tremors at rest

Constipation
Frequent urination

Flexion of knees and hips shifts center of gravity forward

Short, shuffling steps

FIGURE 48.14 *Manifestations of Parkinson's disease.*

• WORD • BUILDING •
ipsilateral: ipsi—same + lateral—side
contralateral: contra—opposite + lateral—side

Patients are prone to falls, which can result in injuries ranging from bruises or fractures to head or spinal cord injuries. Constipation is common because of decreased activity, diminished ability to take in food and fluids, and side effects of anticholinergic medications. Patients are encouraged to increase fiber and fluids in their diets. If constipation is not alleviated by dietary modifications, the patient may need to use stool softeners.

Muscular rigidity and bradykinesia contribute to joint immobility, which decreases patients' ability to ambulate and care for themselves. Position changes can be painful for patients. A turning sheet and adequate personnel are necessary when turning a patient in bed to prevent stress on the joints. Tremors interfere with ADLs, consume immense amounts of energy, and can prevent the patient from working or performing leisure activities. Swallowing can become so impaired that enteral (tube) feeding is required. Depression is a common complication at any stage of Parkinson's disease and may compromise communication, ability to learn, and performance of ADLs. Patients may require counseling or antidepressants.

Diagnostic Tests

No specific tests are used to diagnose Parkinson's disease. The diagnosis is based on the history given by the patient and a thorough physical examination. An MRI may be done to rule out alternative causes of the patient's symptoms.

Therapeutic Measures

There is no cure for Parkinson's disease. Treatment is aimed at controlling symptoms and maximizing the patient's functional level. Drugs used to control symptoms are listed in Table 48.12.

TABLE 48.12 MEDICATIONS USED TO TREAT PARKINSON'S DISEASE

Medication Class/Action	Examples	Nursing Implications
Cholinergic Blockers Blocks the action of acetylcholine to control tremor and salivation.	trihexyphenidyl (Artane), benztropine (Cogentin)	Monitor I&O for urinary retention. Teach patient not to discontinue abruptly. Implement measures to prevent constipation.
Dopamine Agonist Facilitates release of dopamine.	amantadine (Symmetrel)	Use caution with alcohol and other CNS agents.
Dopamine Agonists Convert into dopamine in the brain.	levodopa (L-dopa) levodopa/carbidopa combination (Sinemet). Carbidopa prevents peripheral breakdown of levodopa so more is available in the CNS.	Teach patient to take food shortly after (not before or with) each dose to prevent gastric irritation. May discolor urine and sweat. Teach patient to take ATC to control symptoms.
Dopamine Agonists Stimulates dopamine receptors in the brain.	pramipexole (Mirapex) ropinirole (Requip)	Patients can fall asleep suddenly; caution patient to avoid driving until effects known. Giving with meals may reduce nausea. Caution about drowsiness and sleep attacks (falling asleep during activities that require alertness).
Monoamine Oxidase B Inhibitor Blocks metabolism of central dopamine, increasing dopamine in CNS.	selegiline (Eldepryl, Zelapar), rasagiline (Azilect)	Can slow progression of Parkinson's disease. Administer daily at noon to prevent insomnia. Can cause dangerous interaction with meperidine (Demerol), alcohol, CNS depressants.
COMT Inhibitor Blocks the enzyme COMT to prevent breakdown of levodopa, prolonging levodopa action. For use with Sinemet.	entacapone (Comtan)	Report elevated temperature, muscular rigidity, altered LOC, elevated CPK.

Note. With all anti–Parkinson's disease agents, teach patient to check with physician before taking over-the-counter medications, especially cold preparations. Teach to rise slowly to prevent orthostasis. ATC = around the clock; COMT = catechol-*O*-methyltransferase; CNS = central nervous system. CPK = creatine phosphokinase; I&O = input and output; LOC = level of consciousness.

Many patients with Parkinson's disease experience fluctuations in motor function related to their drug therapy. This is referred to as the on–off phenomenon. Patients may experience a decreased response to levodopa, or off period, particularly as the dose is wearing off. As the disease progresses, patients may notice that the off periods become less predictable and occur more rapidly. The patient may have a delayed or absent response to the next dose of levodopa, resulting in the patient being stuck in the off stage and being significantly disabled for that period. Fluctuations in motor function can be accompanied by other symptoms, such as pain, diaphoresis, anxiety attacks, hallucinations, or mood swings. These symptoms significantly increase the disability associated with the episodes.

Patients who are taking maximum doses of medication for Parkinson's disease symptoms may benefit from a "drug holiday." During a drug holiday, patients are taken off all drugs for a time, then restarted on lower doses. Hospitalization may be necessary during this time to maintain patient safety.

Surgical Treatments

Pallidotomy may be an option for patients whose rigidity, tremor, and bradykinesia are uncontrollable by medical management. During this stereotactic procedure, a destructive lesion is placed in the basal ganglia. The surgery is only performed on one side of the brain. The patient remains awake during the surgery to make sure that the lesion is being placed in the appropriate location. These patients need a great deal of education and support before and during the surgery.

Deep-brain stimulation is another surgical treatment, in which a tiny electrode is placed into brain tissue. A generator is then implanted under the skin on the chest, and is connected to the electrode. The generator delivers electrical pulses to the electrode, which may help control symptoms.

Some centers have experimented with implanting stem cells into the brain to develop into dopamine-producing cells; research into gene therapies is also ongoing. These therapies are only experimental at this time. For more information, visit the National Parkinson Foundation at www.parkinson.org.

Nursing Process for the Patient With Parkinson's Disease

DATA COLLECTION.   Ask the patient about symptoms of Parkinson's disease and their effect on level of functioning. Observe ability to move, walk, and perform ADLs safely. Determine risk for injury related to immobility or falls. Assess nutritional status and condition of skin. Identify presence of confusion and side effects of medications. Psychosocial assessment includes the patient's and caregiver's responses to the disease, coping strategies, and support systems.

NURSING DIAGNOSES, PLANNING, AND IMPLEMENTATION. The patient with Parkinson's disease is at risk for many problems. Priority diagnoses are addressed below. If confusion is present, also see the "Nursing Care Plan for the Patient With Dementia."

Impaired Physical Mobility related to muscle stiffness and tremor

EXPECTED OUTCOME: The patient will maintain optimal mobility and ability to ambulate as long as possible.

- Assist patient to plan daily activities based on anticipated response to medications. *Certain times of day may be less troublesome than others.*
- Consult with physical and occupational therapists to provide assistive devices *to help maintain mobility and provide diversional activities.*
- Provide assistance with ROM exercises *to maintain flexibility of muscles.*
- Teach patients who have difficulty initiating walking to pick up one foot as though attempting to step over something to take the first step. It may also help to take several steps in place before starting to walk. *This may help overcome freezing of gait.*

Self-Care Deficit related to reduced mobility

EXPECTED OUTCOME: The patient's self-care needs will be met as evidenced by patient statement

- Encourage the patient to participate in ADLs as much as possible. *This helps the patient maintain independence and self-esteem.*
- Consult occupational therapist *to assist with devices and strategies for maintaining independence.*
- Instruct the patient or family to provide clothing without buttons and supply shoes with adherent fasteners, rather than shoelaces, *to help maintain independence.*
- Assist the patient and family to make decisions about long-term care. Consult a social worker as needed for assistance. *As the patient ages, so do the significant others who are providing care. The point may be reached at which the caregiver is no longer able to meet the increasing needs of the patient. The decision to place the patient in a skilled nursing facility is extremely difficult and emotional.*

Risk for Injury related to reduced mobility and balance

EXPECTED OUTCOME: The patient will remain safe and without injury.

- If the patient is in the hospital or extended care facility, keep the call light within reach at all times. Remind the patient to request assistance with ambulation. *The patient is at risk for injury from falls related to problems with mobility.*
- Maintain bed in the low position, with side rails raised if appropriate (side rails may be prohibited in some institutions). *Maintaining the bed in a low position reduces the risk for injury or fall when getting out of bed. Side rails can increase the risk for injury, and must be used carefully.*
- Use an alarm system that alerts the staff that the patient is getting up *so that staff can assist the patient to get up and ambulate.*
- Avoid use of restraints. *Restraints can increase the risk for injury.*

• Keep environment free from clutter, throw rugs, or other items *that can cause a patient to trip.*
• Provide walkers and other assistive devices *to provide support and prevent falls.*

EVALUATION. The care of the patient with Parkinson's disease has been successful if the patient remains as mobile and independent as possible. Self-care needs should be met by the patient or others, and the patient should remain safe from injury.

CRITICAL THINKING

Ms. Simpson

■ Ms. Simpson is a 47-year-old Caucasian woman. She has had Parkinson's disease for the past 5 years, and the symptoms are becoming progressively worse. She is now admitted for a urinary tract infection.

1. What problems do you foresee when caring for Ms. Simpson?
2. What safety measures should you implement?
3. Ms. Simpson is receiving IV fluids of 5% dextrose in 0.45% saline, 1000 mL over 12 hours. The RN on duty is accountable for her IV, but as you are bathing her you notice that the bag is nearly full and it has been hanging for 4 hours. How many milliliters should still be in her IV bag after 4 hours?
4. What members of the health team should you collaborate with in providing Ms. Simpson's care?

Suggested answers are at the end of the chapter.

Huntington's Disease

Huntington's disease is a progressive, hereditary, degenerative, incurable neurologic disorder. It was first described in 1872 by George Huntington, a general practitioner in New York. The uncontrolled movements associated with Huntington's disease caused some sufferers in the 17th century to be accused of and executed for witchcraft. Many of the cases around the world can be traced back to specific individuals.

Pathophysiology and Etiology

Huntington's disease (also known as Huntington's chorea) is inherited in an autosomal dominant manner, which means that each offspring of an affected parent has a 50% chance of inheriting the disorder. A mutation in a specific gene has been identified, however, the cause of the mutation is not known. According to a study completed recently at Johns Hopkins in Baltimore, Maryland, a protein called *rhes* may be responsible for the activation of a mutant protein that causes destruction of the cells in the corpus striatum (Saey, 2009). Destruction also occurs in the caudate nucleus and other deep nuclei of the brain and portions of the cerebral

cortex. This degeneration results in progressive loss of normal movement and intellect. The rate of disease progression varies from person to person.

Signs and Symptoms

Signs and symptoms usually begin in middle age and develop slowly, becoming progressively more apparent. Cognitive signs can be noticed before movement problems. Patients who are not aware of their hereditary risk for Huntington's disease may be incorrectly diagnosed as being mentally ill.

The patient can display personality changes and inappropriate behavior. The patient may be euphoric or irritable and can rapidly alternate between moods. Paranoia is common, and behavior can become violent as dementia worsens. The patient eventually progresses to the point at which he or she is incontinent and totally dependent on others for care. These symptoms are difficult for family and friends as well as professional caregivers to cope with. The disease progression and associated symptoms are particularly devastating for offspring, who may or may not know whether they have inherited the disease.

Physical symptoms also develop slowly. Huntington's disease is characterized by involuntary, irregular, jerky, dancelike (choreiform) movements. Initially these symptoms can take the form of mild fidgeting and facial grimacing. In the early stages of the disease, the patient may try to cover the movements by incorporating them into a voluntary movement such as crossing the arms or scratching. The involuntary movements usually start in the arms, face, and neck and progressively involve the remainder of the body. Patients display hesitant speech, eye blinking, irregular trunk movements, abnormal tilt of the head, and constant motion (Fig. 48.15). The gait is wide, and the patient may appear to be dancing. Emotional upset, stress, or trying to perform a voluntary task can significantly increase the severity and rate of the abnormal movements; the movements typically diminish or disappear during sleep. Dysphagia can significantly impair the patient's nutritional status.

Depression and suicide are common in the earlier stages of the disease, when the patient still has the cognitive ability to carry out a suicidal act. As the disease progresses, the patient becomes more and more dependent. Aspiration resulting in respiratory failure is the primary cause of death. Life span following diagnosis is about 10 to 30 years.

Diagnostic Tests

Huntington's disease has typically been diagnosed based on the clinical examination and a family history of the disease. MRI or CT may be helpful. Genetic testing is available for prenatal use and to determine if an individual has Huntington's disease before he or she becomes symptomatic. This is important because Huntington's disease does not become symptomatic until patients are in their 30s or 40s, when they may already have children who could be affected (see "Patient Perspective").

FIGURE 48.15 A 47-year-old patient with Huntington's disease. Note constant fidgety movement. From Spillane, J. D. (1968). *An atlas of clinical neurology.* New York: Oxford University Press, p. 219, with permission.

Patient Perspective

Betty

I was born the second of six children. My mom was diagnosed with Huntington's chorea (an old name for Huntington's disease) after she had all of us. My brother was diagnosed with Huntington's disease at the age of 60. He started out with terrible mood swings and a bad temper, but eventually he had a lot of movement problems, including pronounced facial and tongue movements.

By the time we knew the disease had affected our family, many of us had children and grandchildren of our own. My kids wanted me to be tested. It is a hereditary disease and you have a 50/50 chance of having it if a parent has it. If I had Huntington's, then my kids would have a 50/50 chance of having it. If I tested negative, then they and their children would not be at risk.

I was very nervous and afraid of being tested. When I went for the initial visit at the University of Michigan, they observed my movements, how I walked and talked, and my facial movements. They made me go to a psychologist to see if I could handle the results if they did the blood test that would tell for sure. I understand the suicide rate is kind of high for people with Huntington's. After talking for an hour and a half, they decided I could handle the results.

At my next visit, they just drew blood, which was sent out for testing. I had to return to the university 6 weeks later for the results. When I went back, I was a nervous wreck. A friend went with me. When the technician came in, she said the doctor would be with me soon. I immediately had bad thoughts. Then when the technician and doctor came back, they were both smiling and had tears in their eyes—I had tested negative. So my friend, the doctor, the technician, and I all hugged and cried.

It is a very hard disease to live with, whether you or another family member has it. My brother has it very bad. Out of my five siblings, four have it for sure, and we think the fifth has it because of mood swings we have observed.

I am the only one of the six who tested clear. I felt very guilty at first that they all had it and I didn't. I'm starting to get over that, but when I see one of them having a bad time with talking, or temper, or movement, the guilt starts to kick in again.

Therapeutic Measures

Because there is no cure, treatment of Huntington's disease focuses on minimizing symptoms and preventing complications. Antipsychotic, antidepressant, and antichoreic drugs may be used to treat both the involuntary movements and behavioral outbursts. A new medication, tetrabenazine (Xenazine), may help reduce involuntary movements by increasing dopamine in the brain. Physical and occupational therapy can help keep the patient mobile and independent for as long as possible. Research has been done on the benefits of transplanting stem cells into the brains of patients with Huntington's disease, but this is still experimental at this time.

Nursing Care

Patients with Huntington's disease are typically cared for on an outpatient basis. When a patient with Huntington's disease is admitted to an inpatient facility, it is important to obtain as much information as possible about that person's response to medication, daily routine, and emotional and cognitive functioning from the caregivers. For example, knowing that a certain patient is intensely afraid of bathtubs but willingly takes showers can prevent unnecessary struggles and outbursts. Providing some objects from home can make the new environment seem less threatening. The caregivers may relate that the patient has better cognitive functioning at a particular time of day. As the dementia progresses, the patient responds less to attempts at reasoning. Giving directions in a calm but firm tone may help the patient cooperate with activities. The environment should be modified to keep the patient safe. Keep in mind that forceful, involuntary movements of the patient's extremities can happen at any time and should not be misinterpreted as an attempt to harm caregivers.

Difficulty swallowing typically begins toward the middle of the disease course. Patients exhibit trouble swallowing liquids in particular. At this stage, it may still be possible to teach the patient to hold the chin down to the chest while swallowing, which lessens the chance of aspiration. Have patients sit straight upright while eating. Thickening agents can be added to thin liquids to help prevent aspiration. Adaptive devices can prolong the patient's ability to eat independently. Soft foods that are easily manipulated in the mouth are most suitable. These patients may have difficulty taking in adequate calories to maintain a normal body weight, even if a caregiver assists with feeding them. One of the many ethical issues faced by these patients and their significant others is whether artificial feeding should be used and, if so, for how long. Patients and their significant others should be encouraged to discuss end-of-life decisions early in the course of the disease.

Also see the "Nursing Care Plan for the Patient With Dementia."

Alzheimer's Disease

Alzheimer's disease (also called dementia of the Alzheimer's type [DAT]) is the most common of several types of dementia. Dementia is a progressive loss of mental functioning that interferes with memory, ability to think clearly and learn, and eventually ability to function (see discussion of dementia earlier in this chapter).

Alois Alzheimer, a German neurologist, first described the disease in 1907. He described pathological changes, now referred to as neurofibrillary tangles and neuritic plaques, that he discovered while performing an autopsy on a patient with dementia. Alzheimer's disease is a progressively degenerative disease that is inevitably fatal. The incidence of Alzheimer's disease is more common in women than men and doubles for every 5 years a person lives beyond age 65.

Etiology and Pathophysiology

Many etiologies have been theorized for Alzheimer's disease, including viral or bacterial infection and autoimmune dysfunction. Markers associated with Alzheimer's disease can be found on several chromosomes. Chromosome 21 in particular has been associated with Alzheimer's disease, and is also the location of the genetic abnormality responsible for Down syndrome. Patients older than age 40 who have Down syndrome usually develop Alzheimer's disease. The exact correlation between the two disorders is still being studied. Lifestyle factors that increase risk of Alzheimer's disease include hypertension, hypercholesterolemia, and poorly controlled diabetes.

Although the exact cause of Alzheimer's disease is unknown, the structural changes associated with it have been well documented. An abnormality exists within the protein of the cell membrane of a neuron. As the axon terminals and dendrite branches disintegrate, they collect in neuritic plaques. Inside the normal brain is a precise arrangement of filaments and tubules that are responsible for cell integrity. Individuals with Alzheimer's disease develop neurofibrillary tangles instead of the normal orderly arrangement. Instead of remaining a small area of abnormality, these neuritic plaques and neurofibrillary tangles spread via axons to other areas of the brain. In addition, patients tend to have a deficiency of acetylcholine in the cerebral cortex. Remember that acetylcholine is a neurotransmitter important for nervous system function.

Advancement of neurofibrillary tangles and neuritic plaques typically affects the hippocampus first, resulting in short-term memory dysfunction. As the tangles and plaques spread to the temporal lobe, the memory impairment becomes more severe. It may be at this point that the patient accesses the health care system. Personality changes and incontinence are inevitable results of Alzheimer's disease. These symptoms can be attributed to the spread of plaques and tangles to the frontal lobes of the brain.

It is believed that the younger the patient is at the time of onset, the faster the neurofibrillary tangles and neuritic plaques spread. Therefore, these patients tend to deteriorate faster, require complete care earlier, and have a shorter life span.

One area of the brain that is left relatively untouched by Alzheimer's is the subcortical area. This structure is responsible for our subconscious urge to survive. The needs for basic requirements such as shelter, food and water, security, and reproduction are controlled by the subcortical area, as are emotional responses to situations. The patient with Alzheimer's disease may experience hunger but no longer know how to meet that basic need. Left to their own devices, these individuals would starve.

Signs and Symptoms

The signs and symptoms of Alzheimer's disease are typically broken down into three stages.

ALZHEIMER'S STAGE 1. The early stage, stage 1, lasts from 2 to 4 years and is characterized by increasing forgetfulness. At this stage, the patient may attempt to cope by using lists and reminders. Interest in day-to-day activities, acquaintances, and surroundings tends to diminish. The patient is reluctant to take on tasks because of uncertainty in how to perform them. If the patient is still working, his or her performance deteriorates and can result in being terminated from the job.

ALZHEIMER'S STAGE 2. The middle stage, stage 2, is the longest in duration, lasting 2 to 12 years. Progressive cognitive deterioration causes difficulty doing simple calculations or answering questions. Patients may become irritable, particularly when asked to perform a task that they know they should be able to perform but cannot. It may help the patient to break down the task into manageable steps. Depression is common. Aphasia and the resulting inability to make themselves understood can exacerbate patients' irritability. It is during the middle stage, as cognitive function significantly deteriorates, that the patient may become more physically active. The normal sleep–wake cycle is disrupted, and the patient tends to wander aimlessly, particularly at night. The patient may become lost in familiar surroundings, which compounds the anxiety that typically develops during this stage. Hallucinations and seizures can occur. Management of day-to-day activities such as feeding a pet or paying bills becomes overwhelming. Personal hygiene deteriorates, as does appropriate social behavior. Patients may make up stories to cover for deficits, saying that possessions they misplaced were stolen. Some patients hoard food or money.

ALZHEIMER'S STAGE 3.   The third stage of Alzheimer's disease is characterized by progression to complete dependency. The patient loses the ability to converse or control bowel or bladder function. If the patient is still mobile, constant supervision is required to protect from wandering and avoid injury. Emotional control and the ability to recognize significant others are lost. This lack of recognition is particularly devastating for family members. Eventually the patient is unable to move independently, swallow, or express needs. Death usually occurs from complications of immobility.

The duration of the final stage of Alzheimer's disease, characterized by complete dependence, depends in part on the physical stamina and general health of the individual. The healthier the patient, the longer the body will continue to function. Another factor is the decisions that have been made regarding artificial feeding and respiratory support. Few significant others or HCPs advocate intubation and mechanical ventilation for patients with Alzheimer's disease. The issue of enteral (tube) feedings, however, is an emotional one with few easy answers. The use of enteral feedings can prolong the patient's life, despite the absence of cognitive functioning. As with patients suffering from Huntington's disease, every effort should be made to determine the patient's wishes before cognitive impairment makes that impossible. See Table 48.13 for a comparison of the symptoms of Parkinson's, Huntington's, and Alzheimer's diseases.

Diagnostic Tests

The only absolute method of confirming a diagnosis of Alzheimer's disease is by pathological examination at autopsy. In actuality, the disease is diagnosed on the basis of clinical examination, history, and elimination of other possible causes of the symptoms. MRI can reveal the presence of the classic neurofibrillary tangles and neuritic plaques. Positron emission tomography (PET) and single photon emission computed tomography (SPECT) scans show areas of neuronal inactivity. A recent study by Roe et al (2013) found biomarkers that can predict the risk of Alzheimer's disease using brain imaging and spinal-fluid testing. It is also thought that these biomarkers may be able to be used to test new treatments for efficacy in controlling the onset of the disease.

Therapeutic Measures

There is no known cure for Alzheimer's disease. Treatment has traditionally focused on minimizing the effects of the disease and maintaining independence as long as possible. Acetylcholinesterase (AChE) inhibitors such as donepezil (Aricept) or rivastigmine (Exelon) are thought to inhibit the breakdown of the neurotransmitter acetylcholine (see Table 48.10). Increased levels of acetylcholine in the brain allow better functioning of the remaining neurons. They appear to be most effective for those patients who exhibit mild to moderate symptoms of Alzheimer's disease. It can take some time to notice any effects of the drugs. Use of AChE inhibitors diminishes the amount of medical care and social service interventions required and delays admission to skilled nursing facilities. This delay in institutionalization can result in significant positive impact on quality of life, as well as financial savings for the patient and family.

Another class of medications, NMDA (N-methyl-D-aspartate) antagonists, can prevent overexcitation of NMDA

TABLE 48.13   COMPARISONS OF PARKINSON'S DISEASE, HUNTINGTON'S DISEASE, AND ALZHEIMER'S DISEASE

Symptom	Parkinson's Disease	Huntington's Disease	Alzheimer's Disease
Tremors	Present	Absent	Absent
Bradykinesia/akinesia	Present	Absent	Absent
Muscle rigidity	Present	Absent	Absent
Memory dysfunction	Late	Early	Late
Cognitive dysfunction	Late	Early	Present
Inability to perform ADLs	Progressive	Progressive	Progressive
Involuntary movements	Absent	Absent	Present
Depression	Present	Present	Present

receptors in the brain and allow more normal function. Memantine (Namenda, Axura) is the only drug currently available in this class. These drugs can be given at any stage of Alzheimer's disease and, like AChE inhibitors, simply slow the patient's decline.

Antidepressants, antipsychotics, and antianxiety drugs can be used as a last resort to control symptoms of depression and behavioral disturbances, but they do not treat the dementia. Patients should be carefully monitored for drug interactions and side effects. For more information, visit the Alzheimer's Association at www.alz.org.

Nursing Process for the Patient With Alzheimer's Disease

See the earlier discussion of dementia and the "Nursing Care Plan for the Patient With Dementia."

CRITICAL THINKING

Mrs. Johnson

■ Mrs. Johnson has just become a resident at the Valley Bend extended care facility. She is diagnosed with Alzheimer's disease and is in the second stage with some signs of stage 3 disease. When you check on her during the evening, you find her walking around her room, talking to herself. What other signs and symptoms are typical for stage 2 and stage 3 Alzheimer's disease? How should you address her behavior?

Suggested answers are at the end of the chapter.

Home Health Hints

To assess a patient's neurologic status at home:
- Note whether the patient's clothes are matched and properly fastened. Is the patient clean and well groomed?

- Observe the patient during bathing, grooming, or dressing to assess motor function and coordination.
- Assess energy level by noting if the patient makes frequent requests to sit or lie down.
- Observe the patient's gait for steadiness.

To help the patient perform ADLs more easily at home:
- Ask permission to move furniture and small rugs to provide a clear path for ambulation.
- Position frequently used items such as a comb, glass of water, eyeglasses, books, tissues, and phone where they are easily accessible.
- Recommend shoes with Velcro closures.
- Use chairs with armrests—the patient can use the armrests to push against to stand.
- Keep the patient cleaner at meals with a clip-on bib such as those used at the dentist's office. Attach clips from suspenders to a piece of elastic and place around the back of the patient's neck. Attach a clean napkin or washcloth for each meal.

To help the patient with Alzheimer's disease who has perceptual deficits:
- Have things used together the same color (e.g., toothbrush and toothpaste).
- Contrast colors in the environment to help patients function independently—slipper color should be different from the floor, a dark-colored placemat can be used under light dishes, and the first and last steps of a stairway can be painted a contrasting color.
- Use a bath or shower seat, handheld showerhead, and soothing music to help the patient feel safe and oriented to the task while bathing.
- Cover doorknobs with a piece of cloth to keep the patient from wandering away, or have a caregiver purchase inexpensive child safety devices that can fit over doorknobs and/or cabinet latches.
- Family members may require respite care and homemaker services. Discuss with the registered nurse or physician about having social services complete a visit to assist the family with access to community resources.

SUGGESTED ANSWERS TO

CRITICAL THINKING

■ Mr. Chung

1. Be prepared to assist with a lumbar puncture.
2. You should use short, simple sentences because he may be very anxious or disoriented. Involve his family. Further education can be provided when he is feeling better.

3. Because meningococcal meningitis is contagious, he should be placed in isolation. Gloves, gowns, and masks should be used. Explain the need for these practices to Mr. Chung and his visitors.
4. Comfort measures include tepid baths, a quiet, dark environment, and minimal stimulation. Administer acetaminophen and analgesics as ordered.

SUGGESTED ANSWERS TO—cont'd

5. The health service at his college should be notified of his diagnosis. Close contacts may require prophylactic treatment. If Mr. Chung lives at home rather than at college, his family members should be advised to see their HCP and begin prophylactic treatment.

■ *Mr. Evans*

1. You might expect to see impaired speech, right-sided weakness, and a rapid decrease in consciousness if Mr. Evans' hematoma is enlarged.

2. Intubation equipment, mannitol, and IV access should be ready. He should be given nothing by mouth (NPO) and the results of laboratory tests should be ready in the event of emergency surgery. The location of Mr. Evans' next of kin must be known.

3. Who are Mr. Evans's support people? Was this drinking episode an isolated incident or a chronic problem that should be addressed if he is discharged safely?

4. Health team members needed for Mr. Evans depend on the extent of his injury and include a social worker; physical, occupational, and speech therapists; neuropsychologist; dietitian; and others.

■ *Ms. Simpson*

1. Urinary tract infection is often accompanied by urinary urgency. Ms. Simpson may have difficulty getting to the bathroom quickly and safely.

2. Keep a bedside commode nearby if the bathroom is not close. Assist Ms. Simpson to the bathroom or commode at regular intervals to prevent urgency. Remind her to ask for help if she needs to get up. Make sure that her call light is within reach.

3.

$$\frac{1000 \text{ mL}}{12 \text{ hours}} \quad \bigg| \quad 4 \text{ hours} = 333 \text{ mL}$$

After 4 hours: 1000–333 mL = 667 mL should remain in the bag. Because it is still nearly full, the RN should be notified.

4. Occupational, physical, and speech therapy may be involved in Ms. Simpson's care. Speech therapy can help with swallowing problems. Work with nursing assistants to be sure she is mobilized and protected from falls.

■ *Mrs. Johnson*

Being admitted to a new and unfamiliar facility can increase confusion. Signs of second-stage Alzheimer's disease include memory loss, wandering at night, sleeplessness, irritability, loss of way in familiar surroundings, losing possessions and searching for them, and neglect of personal hygiene. During the third stage of the disease, the patient will lose weight, recognize hunger but be unable to eat, be unable to communicate verbally or in writing, lose ability to recognize family, become incontinent of urine and feces, and eventually lose ability to stand and walk. Address Mrs. Johnson by her name and ask her what she needs. Reorient her to where she is and assure her that she is safe and being cared for.

REVIEW QUESTIONS

1. A college student is admitted to the hospital with a severe headache. Which finding in the student's history is consistent with the diagnosis of meningitis?
   1. A sore throat for 3 days
   2. A family history of migraine headaches
   3. A muscle injury in the neck
   4. A recent motor vehicle accident

2. A patient with meningitis has photophobia and a severe headache. Which nursing interventions will be most helpful to relieve symptoms?
   1. Administer antibiotics as ordered, and prepare the patient for a lumbar puncture.
   2. Darken the room and administer analgesics.
   3. Administer acetaminophen as ordered and maintain isolation.
   4. Check level of consciousness with the Glasgow Coma Scale and monitor vital signs.

3. A patient makes an appointment to see a primary care practitioner for recurrent severe headaches. Which instruction by the nurse will help gather the best additional data before the appointment?
   1. "Try relaxation and warm moist compresses for your headaches and document your response."
   2. "Call and come in the next time you have a headache so you can be examined."
   3. "Keep track of how many headaches you have before you come in."
   4. "Keep a diary of your headaches, recording symptoms, timing, and headache triggers."

4. A patient who has had a generalized tonic-clonic seizure is sound asleep 30 minutes after the seizure. Meals are about to be delivered. Which nursing action is most appropriate?
   1. Wake the patient because nourishment is essential following a seizure.
   2. Wake the patient to do a neurologic assessment before the meal.
   3. Let the patient sleep during the postictal state, and keep the meal warm.
   4. Do not attempt to wake the patient because of the risk of a repeat seizure.

5. A patient with a history of seizures reports experiencing an aura and is concerned about an impending seizure. Place the nurse's interventions in the correct order.
   1. Protect the patient from injury during the seizure.
   2. Document the events of the seizure.
   3. Help the patient lie down in a safe place.
   4. Turn the patient on his or her side to sleep.

6. Which patients should be closely monitored by the nurse for symptoms of increased intracranial pressure? **Select all that apply.**
   1. The patient who has a history of epilepsy
   2. The patient admitted with a high fever and severe headache
   3. The patient in the postanesthesia care unit following craniectomy
   4. The patient with a brain tumor who is admitted for radiation therapy
   5. The patient with a history of migraine headaches, admitted for orthopedic surgery
   6. The patient with Alzheimer's disease admitted with a urinary tract infection

7. Which of the following actions should the nurse take to help prevent increased intracranial pressure in a patient following a traumatic brain injury?
   1. Cluster care so the patient can have long periods of rest.
   2. Keep the head of the bed elevated at 30 degrees.
   3. Suction frequently to keep the airway clear.
   4. Do not give anything by mouth.

8. A patient is admitted following a T4 spinal injury. When taking morning vital signs, the nurse notes that the patient appears restless and the blood pressure is elevated. Which of the following actions by the nurse is appropriate?
   1. Recheck the patient's blood pressure in 30 minutes.
   2. No action is necessary. This is an expected finding.
   3. Check for a full bladder or bowel.
   4. Encourage the patient to express any anxiety.

9. Which nursing interventions are appropriate for the patient with a neurodegenerative disorder who has difficulty swallowing?
   1. Have the patient tuck his or her chin down during swallowing.
   2. Provide clear to full liquids; avoid solid foods.
   3. Place the patient in semi-Fowler's position for eating.
   4. Provide adaptive eating utensils.

10. A resident of an extended care facility who has Alzheimer's disease is sitting in a corner, crying loudly that no one is paying attention. Several staff members have tried to find out what's wrong, but the patient won't answer, and just keeps rocking back and forth and crying. Which approach by the nurse might best help the patient?
    1. Say in a quiet voice, "What is wrong? We can't help you if you don't tell us what's wrong."
    2. Sit quietly by the patient and say, "I'm here; you aren't alone."
    3. Say in a firm voice, "Several staff members have asked what you need. Now it is time to stop crying."
    4. Ignore the continued crying. Continuing to respond will encourage the behavior.

Answers can be found in Appendix C.

References

Barnes, M., & Brannelly, T. (2008). Achieving care and social justice for people with dementia. *Nursing Ethics, 15*, 384–395.

International Headache Society. (2005). *International classification of headache disorders* (2nd ed., 1st revision). Retrieved June 12, 2013, from www.ihs-headache.org/frame_non_members.asp

National Institute of Neurological Disorders and Stroke. (2013). NINDS dementia information page. Retrieved June 20, 2013, from www.ninds.nih.gov/disorders/dementias/dementia.htm

National Parkinson Foundation. (2013). Parkinson's disease overview. Retrieved June 23, 2013, from www.parkinson.org/parkinson-s-disease.aspx

Saey, T. H. (2009, July 4). Huntington's protein may have a crony. *Science News, 176*(1). Retrieved July 29, 2009, from www.sciencenews.org

Roe, C. M., Fagan, A. M., Grant, E. A., Hassenstab, J., Moulder, K. L., Maue Dreyfus, D., . . . Morris, J. C. (2013). Amyloid imaging and CSF biomarkers in predicting cognitive impairment up to 7.5 years later. *Neurology, 80*, 1784–1791. (See more at www.nia.nih.gov/newsroom/announcements/2013/06/biomarkers-can-predict-risk-alzheimers-several-years-symptoms-appear#sthash.IXI6fLWl.dpuf)

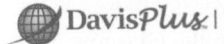 For additional resources and information visit **davispl.us/medsurg5**

49

Nursing Care of Patients With Cerebrovascular Disorders

DEBORAH L. WEAVER AND JOHN STURTEVANT

LEARNING OUTCOMES

1. Describe the causes, risk factors, and pathophysiology of transient ischemic attack, ischemic stroke, and hemorrhagic stroke.
2. Identify emergency interventions for transient ischemic attack, ischemic stroke, and hemorrhagic stroke.
3. Plan therapeutic measures for transient ischemic attack, ischemic stroke, and hemorrhagic stroke.
4. Identify outcomes that can be expected for a stroke victim.
5. Plan nursing care for a patient with a cerebrovascular disorder.

KEY TERMS

aphasia (uh-FAY-zhuh)
ataxia (ah-TAK-see-ah)
diplopia (dip-LOH-pee-ah)
dysphasia (dis-FAY-zhah)
embolic (em-BOL-ik)
embolism (EM-buh-lizm)
endarterectomy (end-AR-tur-EK-tuh-mee)
hemiplegia (HEM-ee-PLEE-jee-ah)
hemorrhagic (hem-uh-RAH-jik)
intracerebral (IN-trah-sur-EE-brul)
ischemic (i-SKEE-mik)
penumbra (puh-NUM-brah)
thrombolytic (throm-buh-LIT-ik)
thrombosis (throm-BOH-sis)
thrombotic (throm-BOT-ik)

Cerebrovascular disorders occur when the supply of blood and oxygen to brain cells is inadequate, allowing brain tissue to die, and causing a cerebrovascular accident (stroke). The most common cerebrovascular disorders include transient ischemic attack, ischemic stroke, and hemorrhagic stroke.

TRANSIENT ISCHEMIC ATTACK

A transient ischemic attack (TIA) is a temporary blockage of blood to the brain that causes a transient (brief) neurologic impairment. The episode typically lasts minutes to hours, and the patient recovers completely. The risk factors, causes, and symptoms of a TIA are identical to those of a cerebrovascular accident (CVA), commonly known as a stroke. Indeed, if the blockage that causes a TIA does not reverse, an area of the brain is permanently damaged, and the event is a stroke. About 15% of all strokes are preceded by a TIA (American Stroke Association, 2013). Urgent evaluation of a TIA is essential to decrease the risk of stroke.

Treatment of a TIA is focused on preventing a full stroke. The cause of the TIA may be discovered with diagnostic tests, which can then guide treatment. However, there may be no clear etiology of the TIA. Treatment, therefore, is mostly centered on minimizing the patient's risk factors for a stroke.

STROKE (CEREBROVASCULAR ACCIDENT)

A stroke is caused by the disruption of blood flow to the brain, resulting in death of brain cells. In most cases, permanent disability results. A stroke is more likely to happen as one ages; about 795,000 people of all ages are affected each year. Because of their increased longevity, 60,000 more women have strokes each year than men. Stroke is our nation's number four cause of death and the leading cause of disability. African Americans, Hispanic Americans, American Indian/Alaska Natives, and multiracial people are at higher risk than non-Hispanic whites (American Heart Association [AHA], 2013). There is also a higher incidence of stroke in people with lower levels of education, lower socioeconomic status, and those living in the southeastern United States.

Pathophysiology

Cerebral function depends on oxygen and glucose delivery to neurons in the brain. The brain cannot store oxygen or glucose, so it relies on a constant supply of these nutrients. If the supply of oxygen and glucose is stopped, brain tissue dies. When a stroke occurs, brain cells begin dying immediately. There is an area of brain tissue surrounding the damage, called the **penumbra**, which contains brain cells that are "stunned" and can be revived if the brain is reperfused quickly. However, they will die if the blood supply is not restored.

The particular vessel or vessels involved determine the area of the brain affected and the symptoms that result. The duration of ischemia determines whether the symptoms are transient or permanent. TIA symptoms generally resolve within 24 hours; however, a TIA can be a warning of an impending stroke.

Etiology

Strokes are classified as either ischemic or hemorrhagic. Ischemic strokes are more common, accounting for about 87% of all strokes (AHA, 2013). Hemorrhagic strokes account for the remaining 13% of strokes.

Ischemic Stroke

Ischemic stroke occurs when the blood supply to the brain is blocked or significantly slowed. It can be one of two major types: thrombotic or embolic (Fig. 49.1).

THROMBOTIC STROKE. **Thrombotic** strokes occur when an occlusion builds up in an artery until it significantly decreases or stops blood flow to the brain. Thrombotic strokes most often occur in the internal or common carotid arteries.

EMBOLIC STROKE. An **embolic** stroke is typically caused by a blood clot that is created somewhere in the body, often within the heart, and travels through the arteries until it becomes trapped in a smaller vessel, preventing the passage of blood. Typically, the embolism will travel and become lodged in the middle, anterior, or posterior cerebral arteries.

Risk Factors

Risk factors for ischemic stroke are classified as modifiable or nonmodifiable (Box 49-1). Nonmodifiable risk factors are those that cannot be altered, such as age or gender. Modifiable risk factors are those that can be changed with treatment, such as high blood pressure. Women have additional risks due to hormone changes in pregnancy and menopause. Children with sickle cell disease, cardiac anomaly, and hyperlipidemia are also at risk for stroke. Minimizing or eliminating these modifiable risk factors can significantly lower risk of a stroke. See Fig. 49.2, Stroke Risk Scorecard, to find out your risk for stroke.

NURSING CARE TIP

Print the Stroke Risk Scorecard from DavisPlus and keep it in your pocket for patient teaching opportunities.

Hemorrhagic Stroke

Hemorrhagic strokes are caused by the rupture of a cerebral blood vessel that allows blood to escape into brain tissue and not travel beyond the point of the rupture. It can be further classified into two major types: subarachnoid hemorrhage and **intracerebral** hemorrhage.

• WORD • BUILDING •
penumbra: healthy tissue surrounding infarct
ischemic: isch—to hold back + emia—blood
thrombotic: thrombus—clot + ic—relating to
embolic: embolism—to throw (as in clot or other debris) + ic—relating to
hemorrhagic: blood loss
intracerebral: intra—within + cerebral—cerebrum

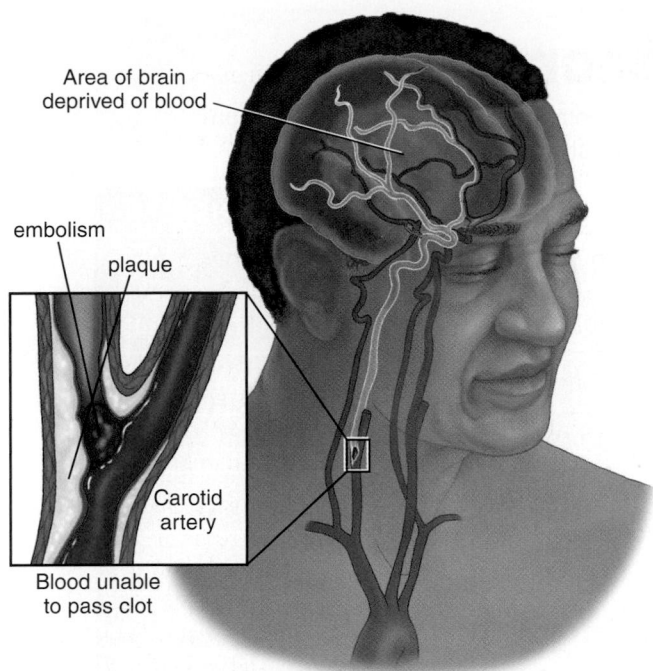

Area of brain
deprived of blood

embolism

plaque

Carotid
artery

Blood unable
to pass clot

FIGURE 49.1 Embolism and thrombosis.

Box 49-1 Modifiable Risk Factors for Stroke

Men and Women

- Cigarette smoking
- High blood pressure
- Diabetes mellitus
- Cardiovascular disease
  - High total cholesterol
  - Low high-density lipoprotein cholesterol
  - Dyslipidemia
- Atrial fibrillation
- Asymptomatic carotid stenosis
- Sickle cell anemia
- Obesity
- Excessive alcohol intake
- Poor diet (high sodium, high fat, low potassium)
- Physical inactivity

Women

- Pregnancy
- Oral contraceptives
- Hormone replacement therapy
- High triglycerides
- History of migraines
- Thick waist

SUBARACHNOID HEMORRHAGE. This type of stroke occurs on the surface of the brain and is most often the result of a ruptured cerebral aneurysm (covered later in this chapter). Strokes caused by subarachnoid hemorrhage usually are

very serious and require surgery to correct. They are often fatal.

INTRACEREBRAL HEMORRHAGE. This type of stroke occurs in the deeper tissues of the brain and usually is caused by uncontrolled hypertension. Patients can experience multiple undetected intracerebral hemorrhages, with minimal deficits noted. However, damage will eventually accumulate and the patient will develop major deficits. Maintaining blood pressure below 120/80 mm Hg should be the goal for these patients. (More specific information related to special care of patients with hemorrhagic strokes will be addressed later in the chapter.)

Warning Signs of Any Type of Stroke

Patients and family members should be taught to recognize signs and symptoms and how to activate emergency medical services (EMS) if these signs occur. There is evidence that if treatment begins within 1 hour of the onset of symptoms, permanent loss of function can be avoided or minimized.

The acronym FAST can be used to teach emergency triage nurses, first responders, nonlicensed personnel, and community members to recognize a stroke and respond quickly. Time is extremely important to preserve brain cells. Quick access to the EMS system is of particular importance. Research has shown that patients arriving by ambulance are admitted to an emergency department (ED) and evaluated faster than those who "walk in" on their own. Those arriving by ambulance are also more likely to arrive within 2 hours of symptom onset (Table 49.1).

In addition to FAST, the following five signs or symptoms recognized by the American Heart Association and American Stroke Association require immediate EMS activation:

- Sudden numbness or weakness of face, arm, or leg, especially on one side of the body
- Sudden confusion or trouble speaking or understanding
- Sudden trouble seeing in one or both eyes
- Sudden trouble walking, dizziness, loss of balance, or coordination
- Sudden severe headache with no known cause (American Stroke Association, 2013).

Women have other unique symptoms such as sudden onset of

- Nausea
- Facial and limb pain
- General weakness
- Chest pain
- Shortness of breath
- Hiccups
- Palpitations (Ennen, 2013)

 NURSING CARE TIP

When teaching a stroke victim and family, repetition is very important. Besides the anxiety and stress they may be feeling, the patient's ability to process information can also be altered by the stroke.

Stroke Risk Scorecard

Each box that applies to you equals 1 point. Total your score at the bottom of each column and compare with the stroke risk levels on the back.

RISK FACTOR	HIGH RISK	CAUTION	LOW RISK
Blood Pressure	■ >140/90 or unknown	☐ 120-139/80-89	■ <120/80
Atrial Fibrillation	■ Irregular heartbeat	☐ I don't know	■ Regular heartbeat
Smoking	■ Smoker	☐ Trying to quit	■ Nonsmoker
Cholesterol	■ >240 or unknown	☐ 200-239	■ <200
Diabetes	■ Yes	☐ Borderline	■ No
Exercise	■ Couch potato	☐ Some exercise	■ Regular exercise
Diet	■ Overweight	☐ Slightly overweight	■ Healthy weight
Stroke in Family	■ Yes	☐ Not sure	■ No
TOTAL SCORE	☐ High Risk	☐ Caution	☐ Low Risk

Risk Scorecard Results

High Risk ≥3: Ask about stroke prevention right away.

Caution 4-6: A good start. Work on reducing risk.

Low Risk 6-8: You're doing very well at controlling stroke risk!

Ask your healthcare professional how to reduce your risk of stroke.

To reduce your risk:

1. Know your blood pressure.
2. Find out whether you have atrial fibrillation.
3. If you smoke, stop.
4. Find out if you have high cholesterol.
5. If diabetic, follow recommendations to control your diabetes.
6. Include exercise in your daily routine.
7. Enjoy a lower-sodium (salt), lower-fat diet.

Act FAST and CALL 9-1-1 IMMEDIATELY at any sign of a stroke:

F **FACE:** Ask the person to smile. Does one side of the face droop?

A **ARMS:** Ask the person to raise both arms. Does one arm drift downward?

S **SPEECH:** Ask the person to repeat a simple phrase. Is their speech slurred or strange?

T **TIME:** If you observe any of these signs, call 9-1-1 immediately.

1-800-STROKES (787-6537) • www.stroke.org

FIGURE 49.2 Stroke Risk Scorecard. From the National Stroke Association, © 2013. Reprinted by permission of National Stroke Association. Please visit www.stroke.org for stroke education resources.

TABLE 49.1   AVERAGE TIME FROM SYMPTOM ONSET TO TREATMENT

Mode of Transportation	Average Time to Treatment
Emergency medical system (911)	1.4 hours
Walk-in to emergency department	3.5 hours
Physician's office	4.5 hours

Source: American Association of Neuroscience Nurses, 2008.

Acute Signs and Symptoms

Most patients with stroke symptoms present with sudden or rapidly evolving symptoms. Symptoms are varied and depend on the area of the brain affected (Table 49.2). Common symptoms include visual disturbances, language disturbances, weakness or paralysis on one side of the body, and difficulty swallowing (dysphagia). Signs and symptoms are generally the same for both ischemic and hemorrhagic stroke. Patients may have drowsiness and a severe headache, often described as "the worst headache of my life."

TABLE 49.2   POSSIBLE SYMPTOMS OF STROKE ACCORDING TO ARTERY AFFECTED

Artery Affected	Paralysis	Sensory Loss	Mental Status	Visual Changes	Speech
Carotid artery	Contralateral face, arm, leg Dysphagia	Contralateral face, arm, leg	Confusion Amnesia, Personality changes	Same side hemianopsia Temporary blindness	If dominant hemisphere is involved
Anterior cerebral artery	Contralateral face, arm, leg Dysphagia	Contralateral foot and leg			
Middle cerebral artery	Contralateral face, arm Dysphagia	Contralateral face, arm	Unilateral neglect if right hemisphere is affected	Contralateral hemianopsia	Difficulty reading, writing, and calculating if left hemisphere is affected
Posterior cerebral artery	Tremor		Memory deficits Perseveration	Hemianopsia	Dyslexia
Posterior inferior cerebellar artery	Unsteady gait Vertigo	Contralateral pain, temperature, balance		*Same sided:* conjugate gaze paralysis, nystagmus *Bilateral:* visual defects	Dysarthria
Vertebrobasilar/ cerebellar artery	Dysphagia Hemiplegia/ hemiparesis or quadriplegia or quadriparesis Dysphagia	Same side—face	Vertigo Clumsiness Ataxia	Diplopia Hemianopsia Conjugate gaze paralysis	Mutism Dysarthria
Brainstem/ cerebellum arteries	*Motor loss:* all limbs, gait ataxia	All limbs		Bilateral visual defects Nystagmus Dysconjugate gaze	Dysarthria

Source: American Association of Neuroscience Nurses, 2008.

Language Disturbances

Difficulty with language is commonly associated with a TIA and stroke. **Aphasia** refers to the absence of language; **dysphasia** refers to difficulty with speech and is not as severe as aphasia. The patient may experience trouble selecting the correct words, use incomprehensible or nonsense speech, have trouble understanding others' speech, and have trouble writing or reading. Aphasia can be *expressive,* in which the patient knows what he wants to say but cannot speak or make sense, or *receptive,* with an inability to understand spoken and/or written words. When both expressive and receptive aphasia are present, it is called *global aphasia.* Slurred or indistinct speech because of a motor problem (lack of coordination) is referred to as dysarthria. This speech impairment is often the cause of delay in treatment and emphasizes the importance of observation of symptoms by others.

Motor Disturbances

Motor disturbances include paralysis, weakness, and numbness. Sometimes the first evidence of paralysis or weakness is clumsiness or a feeling of heaviness in a limb. The onset will be sudden and typically involves one side of the body—the side opposite the damaged area of the brain. Deficits can appear on both sides of the body if the patient has had a brainstem or vertebrobasilar stroke.

Most commonly, paralysis or weakness affect the arm and face together. Some patients present with complete hemiparesis, with one entire side of the body flaccid. **Ataxia** may be present, which is poor balance or a stumbling, staggering gait. This can be related to damage to the cerebellum or to poor coordination due to weakness or paralysis. If the swallowing muscles are affected, the patient will have trouble swallowing (dysphagia).

BE SAFE!

BE VIGILANT! Before giving a patient with a suspected stroke anything to eat or drink, including medications, the patient should pass a swallow (dysphagia) screening test to prevent possible aspiration. Evaluate the patient's facial features and, if there is any apparent weakness or asymmetry, stop and do not give the patient anything by mouth. If no weakness is evident, have the patient swallow about 30 mL of water. If the patient coughs, has difficulty swallowing, or has a wet or gurgly voice afterward, keep the patient NPO (nothing by mouth) until evaluated and cleared by a physician or speech and language pathologist.

Visual Disturbances

Visual field disturbances are also a common symptom of a stroke. The vision loss is painless and can involve loss of all or part of the vision in one eye. Patients often describe the change as a curtain dropping, as fog, or as a gray-out or blackout of vision. The involved eye is on the same side as the diseased artery. Potential visual field abnormalities are shown in Figure 49.3. When you are assessing the patient, stop talking and keep moving across the room. If the patient's eyes do not follow you, there is a good chance he or she has a deficit in that visual field.

Diagnostic Tests

On arrival at the ED, a computed tomographic (CT) scan will be performed immediately. The purpose of the CT scan is to identify whether symptoms are caused by a hemorrhagic stroke so that the health care provider (HCP) can determine the appropriate course of treatment. Ischemic stroke changes will not be visible on a CT until several days after the event. Interventions for hemorrhagic strokes are different than for ischemic strokes. Care for hemorrhagic strokes is discussed later in this chapter.

After the CT scan, patients may have an electrocardiogram (ECG) to determine if atrial fibrillation is present. An echocardiogram may be done to determine the presence of other heart disease that increases the risk of thrombus formation. Other tests that may be performed in the ED include complete blood count (CBC), blood glucose level, metabolic panel, blood typing, prothrombin time (PT), international normalized ratio (INR), and serum pregnancy, if indicated. Stools and emesis may be checked for blood if indicated. The patient will be placed on a cardiac monitor and pulse oximeter. The ED nurse will complete a dysphagia screen before the patient consumes anything.

ED staff may complete the National Institutes of Health Stroke Scale (NIHSS) to determine the patient's neurologic deficit level. This 11-point scale determines the severity of a stroke. Nurses can be specially trained and certified to use it. Find out more about the NIHSS at www.nihstrokescale.org.

Once the patient is stabilized, additional tests can be done. Carotid Doppler testing uses ultrasound to detect stenosis of the carotid arteries. Carotid angiography can be done to further determine degree of blockage and help guide treatment.

Therapeutic Measures

Initial emergency care is supportive while test results are pending. ABCs (airway, breathing, and circulation) are monitored. Oxygen is administered if oxygen saturation is less than 92% and the patient's level of consciousness (LOC) is reduced. Vital

• WORD • BUILDING •
aphasia: a—absent + phasia—speech
dysphasia: dys—difficult + phasia—speech

Normal vision

Bitemporal hemianopsia

Left homonymous hemianopsia

Right homonymous hemianopsia

Horizontal defect

Quadratic defect

FIGURE 49.3 Visual deficits in stroke.

signs and heart rhythm are monitored. A temperature greater than 99.6°F is treated because hyperthermia is associated with poorer outcomes. If intravenous (IV) fluids are needed, only solutions without glucose, such as normal saline solution, are used to prevent hyperglycemia. When test results verify whether the stroke is hemorrhagic or ischemic, therapeutic interventions are begun.

Some hospitals have a stroke team that evaluates all patients who arrive at the hospital within 2 hours of symptom onset. The stroke team will assess the patient within the first 15 minutes of arrival and have lab tests, ECG, and CT scans done with results back within 45 minutes after assessment. The HCP will make a decision regarding **thrombolytic** therapy within 1 hour of arrival.

Patients suffering from a stroke can develop increased intracranial pressure (ICP), which further adds to brain damage. Stroke patients are also at risk for repeated strokes. Careful serial neurologic assessments and vital signs are needed to promptly detect and report changes.

Thrombolytic Therapy

Some patients with ischemic stroke may be candidates for thrombolytic therapy. This is a "clotbuster" medication (alteplase [tissue plasminogen activator; tPA]) that can dissolve a clot and potentially completely reverse stroke symptoms. tPA works best when administered within 4.5 hours of symptom onset, so it is only an option if the patient arrives at the ED quickly after symptoms begin. Some patients awaken after a night's sleep to discover they have had a stroke; their symptom onset is considered the time they went to bed, so they are not candidates for thrombolytic therapy.

Thrombolytic agents can lyse (disintegrate or break down) a thrombus by causing conversion of plasminogen to plasmin. Plasmin is the enzyme that causes thrombi to break down. Patients treated effectively with tPA may be able to leave the hospital within 1 or 2 days with no residual effects from the stroke. Thrombolytics are associated with a significant

• WORD • BUILDING •
thrombolytic: thrombo—clot + lytic—causing breakdown

LEARNING TIP

Remember: Time lost is brain lost. This means the faster the patient with a stroke receives treatment, the more brain (and brain function) can be saved. Teaching your patients to recognize the signs and symptoms of a stroke and encouraging them to call 911 if needed could mean the difference between leading a normal life and total disability. **Act FAST!**

risk of hemorrhage, so all risk of bleeding must be ruled out before these drugs will be considered. They are used very cautiously.

Pharmacological Management

Blood pressure control is vital for the stroke patient. Because of the lack of perfusion to certain areas of the brain, the body's response is to increase the systolic blood pressure to force blood into the affected areas. If the patient will receive tPA, the blood pressure must be maintained below 185/110 mm Hg to reduce the risk of bleeding. This is often done through the use of a beta blocker (labetalol) or calcium channel blocker (nicardipine), because of their fast-acting effects and ability to be given IV. See Table 49.3 for medications commonly used for cerebrovascular disorders.

If tPA is not being given, the HCP may allow the blood pressure to remain high for a period of time to help salvage brain tissue, depending on the source of the stroke and the location of the clot. This "permissive hypertension" helps blood travel through collateral blood vessels in the brain to reach the affected area. Antihypertensive agents should be given if the systolic pressure exceeds 220 mm Hg or the diastolic pressure exceeds 120 mm Hg.

Postemergent Care

Once emergent treatment is completed, medical management focuses on controlling the cause of the TIA or stroke. The results of the diagnostic tests assist HCPs in determining the course of treatment. If the patient has residual physical deficits, the HCP will order physical, occupational, and speech therapy consultations to evaluate the patient's functional status and make recommendations for further treatment.

The American Stroke Association recommends that patients who have a TIA or stroke receive an antiplatelet drug such as clopidogrel (Plavix), aspirin/dipyridamole (Aggrenox), or aspirin within 24 hours of symptom onset. Decreasing platelet aggregation lessens the likelihood of thrombus formation. The patient in atrial fibrillation may also receive an anticoagulant to prevent clot development.

Cholesterol-lowering medication, preferably a statin, will be ordered for patients who have a low-density lipoprotein (LDL) cholesterol level greater than 100 mg/dL. This will also help minimize the development of atherosclerotic plaques. Statins also may have a neuroprotective effect and may further decrease risk of a stroke.

Deep vein **thrombosis** (DVT) is of concern when caring for patients who have had a stroke. The decrease in movement, confinement to a hospital bed, and hypercoagulable state all increase risk of DVT. Not only can DVTs cause severe pain and complications in the affected leg, but the blood clot can dislodge and travel to the lungs and cause a pulmonary **embolism**, or to the brain and cause a repeat stroke. Prevention involves anticoagulant medication, or nondrug treatments such as sequential compression devices and elastic stockings.

Patients are at risk for respiratory complications for several reasons, such as an increase in intracranial pressure. Patients with stroke are prone to aspiration because of a decreased level of consciousness and possibly impaired swallowing ability. Patients should be suctioned as needed to keep the airway clear. A patient who vomits should be turned to the side to reduce the risk of aspiration. Oral feedings should be started carefully and progressed slowly and only after the patient is alert and the ability to swallow safely has been determined by an appropriate swallowing evaluation.

• WORD • BUILDING •
thrombosis: thromb—clot + osis—condition
embolism: embol—to throw + ism—condition

TABLE 49.3   MEDICATIONS USED IN CEREBROVASCULAR DISORDERS

Medication Class/Action	Examples	Nursing Implications
Dissolve existing clots.	tissue plasminogen activator (tPA)	Must be administered within 3 hr of symptom onset.
Prevent formation of clots.	aspirin clopidogrel (Plavix) aspirin/dipyridamole (Aggrenox)	Monitor patient for bruising, change in level of consciousness, prolonged bleeding time.
Prolong time to form clots; prevent new clots.	warfarin (Coumadin) heparin	Monitor patient for bruising, change in level of consciousness, prolonged bleeding time. For warfarin, monitor international normalized ratio frequently until therapeutic, then monthly.
Reduce cholesterol level.	simvastatin (Zocor), pravastatin (Pravachol), atorvastatin (Lipitor), lovastatin (Mevacor)	Patient should notify prescriber if muscle pain or weakness occur.

Surgery

Patients with warning signs of stroke or patients who have been stabilized after a stroke may be candidates for surgery. In patients with significant carotid artery occlusion, a carotid **endarterectomy** may be performed. This involves a small incision in the neck and surgical removal of the occlusion from the artery.

Alternatively, a patient who is at high risk for complications with a carotid endarterectomy may have a carotid stent placed. This is placed during a carotid angiogram procedure. A catheter is advanced to the carotid artery, where a balloon is inflated to open the artery by pushing on the plaque. Then a stent (a tiny metal or polymer-based tube) is expanded inside the artery to keep it open and allow better blood flow to the brain.

CRITICAL THINKING

Mr. Jankowski

■ You are caring for Mr. Jankowski, a 56-year-old man who has been admitted to your orthopedic unit after knee surgery. As you listen to his lungs at the start of the shift, you notice that his lung sounds are diminished. You ask if he is a smoker and find that he has smoked for 40 years. You realize this will place Mr. Jankowski at risk for stroke.

1. What further data should you collect?
2. What preventive measures can you provide?
3. What resources can you provide to support smoking cessation?
4. What other interdisciplinary team members should you work with regarding your respiratory assessment?

Suggested answers are at the end of the chapter.

Prevention of Stroke

The incidence of stroke can be lessened by reducing risk factors (refer back to Box 49-1). Keeping hypertension, cholesterol level, weight, and diabetes controlled can go a long way toward preventing strokes. Smoking cessation is essential. Emboli may be prevented with warfarin in people at high risk from atrial fibrillation. Aspirin or other antiplatelet agents help prevent abnormal clotting.

It is important to educate all patients about new treatments for stroke and the potential for reversal of symptoms with the use of thrombolytic agents. Patients must be educated about risk factors for a stroke, warning signs, and the importance of immediate EMS transport if symptoms occur.

Long-Term Effects of Stroke
Impaired Motor Function and Sensation

Paresthesias and paralysis are common long-term effects of strokes that were not treated with a thrombolytic agent. The side

of the body opposite the side of the cerebral infarct (the contralateral side) is affected because nerve fibers cross over as they pass from the brain to the spinal cord (Fig. 49.4). Paralysis on one side of the body is called **hemiplegia** (Fig. 49.5). The affected limbs may be weak or totally paralyzed (flaccid). The

• WORD • BUILDING •
endarterectomy: endo—inside + arter—artery + ectomy—surgical removal of
hemiplegia: hemi—one side + plegia—paralysis

Left-side infarct — Right-side infarct

Right-sided weakness or paralysis
Aphasia (in left–brain-dominant clients)
Depression related to disability common

Left-sided weakness or paralysis
Impaired judgment/safety risk
Unilateral neglect more common
Indifferent to disability

FIGURE 49.4 The side opposite the infarct is affected by a stroke.

FIGURE 49.5 Note the left-sided weakness in this man's smile as result of a stroke.

arm or the leg may be weaker, depending on the artery affected. These patients are particularly prone to contractures, which cause permanent immobility of a muscle or joint from fibrosis of connective tissue. Adaptation or assistance with activities of daily living (ADLs) is required.

Motor involvement also often affects swallowing and control of urination and bowel function. Patients should be mobilized within 24 hours if possible to prevent complications of immobility. Physical and occupational therapy are provided to maximize functioning and to progress the patient toward a return to baseline functioning.

Sensation changes may prevent the patient from being aware of pressure, temperature, or injuries on the affected side. Patients must be taught to be aware of these changes and protect the involved limbs.

APHASIA. If a stroke affects the temporal lobe region, especially on the dominant side, the speech center will likely be affected. Aphasia may be expressive, receptive, or global, as described earlier. Patients may be able to say words but be unable to form coherent speech, such as the patient who picks up a fork but calls it a comb. If a patient does not understand what is said, avoid the temptation to speak louder to try to help the patient understand. Remember that it is not the patient's hearing that is affected. You need to be patient and understanding as the patient tries to communicate with you. Speech therapy can help the patient relearn to communicate. See the "Nursing Process for the Patient With a Cerebrovascular Disorder" section for interventions for the aphasic patient.

Emotional Lability

Emotional lability, or instability, is a common consequence of stroke. Patients may move rapidly from profound sadness to an almost euphoric state and back again. Laughing or crying may have no relationship to the patient's situation at any given moment. Families can be upset by this behavior because they do not understand why a once happy person is now crying all the time or why the patient laughs inappropriately. You can help by explaining that these responses probably do not reflect how the patient is feeling but rather are caused by the stroke damage.

Impaired Judgment

All patients who have had a stroke, in particular those with right-sided lesions, present a high safety risk. Patients may have poor understanding of their own limitations and believe that they are capable of performing tasks they did before the stroke. Those with left-sided lesions are more likely to be hesitant even to try performing ADLs. These generalizations may be the opposite if the individual is predominantly left-handed. Precautions must be taken to protect the patient from injury.

If the frontal lobes are involved, learned social behaviors may be lost. The patient may undress in public, use profanity, or make inappropriate sexual advances. These behaviors are extremely difficult for significant others to cope with. Education and emotional support of significant others are essential. Allowing them to talk about their frustration and anger may facilitate coping. Distracting the patient from inappropriate behavior may help. The patient should never be reprimanded or punished because he or she no longer has the cognitive ability to control the behaviors.

Unilateral Neglect

The phenomenon of unilateral neglect is seen predominantly in patients who have right hemisphere infarcts. It has been estimated to affect up to 30% of all patients who have had a stroke. These patients do not acknowledge the left side of their environment and may not even be aware of their own body on the affected side. Safety is a primary consideration. Essential items such as the call light and telephone should be placed on the patient's right side. Position the bed so the patient's right side is toward the door. Treatment should focus on providing stimuli to all senses on the patient's affected side and teaching the patient to focus on the left side. This involves teaching the patient to purposefully check where the left limbs are positioned and to look for safety risks. The patient can learn to turn his or her head and scan the environment. Patients may also need reminders to accomplish simple tasks such as turning their plates during meals to recognize the food on the left side of the plate.

Other Long-Term Effects

The stroke patient may experience other complications after the acute phase of the stroke has passed. These include pneumonia, deep venous thrombosis, pulmonary embolism, pressure ulcers, malnutrition, and depression. For the homeward-bound patient, education for the patient and family regarding prevention and recognition of these complications will assist the patient in a successful recovery. If a patient needs to receive rehabilitation in a skilled nursing facility, prevention of these issues will be a part of the care plan at the facility. For more information, visit the National Stroke Association at www.stroke.org or the American Stroke Association at www.strokeassociation.org.

CEREBRAL ANEURYSM, SUBARACHNOID HEMORRHAGE, AND INTRACRANIAL HEMORRHAGE

A cerebral aneurysm is a weakness in the wall of a cerebral artery. It may be congenital, traumatic, or the result of disease. If the aneurysm ruptures, the result is often a subarachnoid hemorrhage. It is unknown what causes the formation of congenital aneurysms or what causes them to rupture. Unruptured aneurysms are typically asymptomatic. The exception is a very large aneurysm, which can cause symptoms similar to a brain tumor. Aneurysms often affect children and young, otherwise healthy adults.

Pathophysiology and Etiology

Aneurysms can occur in any of the cerebral arteries, although most occur in the circle of Willis. The most common site is at the bifurcation of an artery. It is theorized that increased turbulence at the bifurcation can cause an outpouching of a congenitally weak arterial wall.

Subarachnoid hemorrhage is the collection of blood beneath the arachnoid mater following aneurysm rupture. Rupture of an arteriovenous malformation or head trauma may also result in subarachnoid hemorrhage (Fig. 49.6). The presence of blood outside the blood vessels is very irritating to brain tissue. It is believed that irritation from blood breakdown is the major cause of vasospasm, a common complication of subarachnoid hemorrhage.

It is unclear what causes an aneurysm to rupture. Some people develop a subarachnoid hemorrhage while performing Valsalva's maneuver, engaging in sexual activity, or physically exerting themselves. For others, the aneurysm ruptures during a quiet, inactive period. If the aneurysm rupture is associated with a particular activity, the patient may be very frightened of engaging in that activity again. This may have a negative effect on the patient's interpersonal relationships if the associated activity was sexual in nature. The patient's partner may feel guilty or responsible for the hemorrhage. Education, emotional support, and confidentiality are essential to help both the patient and significant other.

Signs and Symptoms

Some patients experience a small hemorrhage before diagnosis of subarachnoid hemorrhage. This leakage of blood may cause a mild headache, vomiting, or disorientation. The symptoms may be attributed to a flulike syndrome. Patients may dismiss the symptoms and not seek medical care.

The most common presentation of rupture of an aneurysm is sudden onset of a severe headache. Typically, a patient will state, "I have never had a headache this bad in my life." Patients may hold their heads and moan or cry in pain. Sensitivity to light is a common finding. This may make patients reluctant to cooperate with pupil examinations.

LOC varies based on the severity of the hemorrhage. Patients may be alert and coherent, may lose consciousness immediately, or may gradually become less responsive. The decreased LOC is caused by ICP and impairment of cerebral blood flow. Patients may experience generalized seizures.

Blood in the subarachnoid space causes meningeal irritation. The patient may exhibit nuchal rigidity. The most commonly affected cranial nerves are III and VI. This is manifested as an enlarged pupil or abnormal gaze. Motor dysfunction may involve one or both limbs on the side opposite the hemorrhage.

Diagnostic Tests

Because of the severe nature of the symptoms, patients with subarachnoid hemorrhage almost always come to the ED rather than seeking care from a primary HCP. A CT or an MRI scan is done to identify and locate a hemorrhage. Precise diagnosis of an aneurysm requires a cerebral angiogram. The contrast material fills the aneurysm if one exists. For a patient with a severe headache and facing a life-threatening illness, this test can be very frightening. If the patient's neurologic status does not allow him or her to cooperate, sedation may be required before and during the examination.

Therapeutic Measures

Patients with subarachnoid hemorrhage are cared for in an intensive care unit (ICU) setting. They typically have an arterial line and a central venous pressure monitoring catheter. Blood pressure is carefully monitored because high pressures increase the risk of rerupture of the aneurysm and low pressures can be associated with ischemia. Values outside parameters identified by the HCP are reported. Typically, the systolic blood pressure is kept between 120 and 160 mm Hg. Vasoactive drugs may be required to maintain blood pressure within the prescribed parameters.

There is no cure for subarachnoid hemorrhage. Treatment consists of correcting the cause of the hemorrhage if possible. Preventing or managing complications and providing supportive care are important aspects of nursing care.

Surgical Management

Definitive treatment of the aneurysm involves performing a craniotomy and exposing the aneurysm. If the aneurysm has a neck (berry aneurysm), it is identified and clamped with a metal clip (Fig. 49.7). An aneurysm without a neck

FIGURE 49.6 Arteriovenous malformation. Note tangled vessels.

FIGURE 49.7 Surgical management of aneurysms.

may be wrapped with a sterile plastic or muslin wrap. This provides stability to the aneurysm walls, lessening the chance of rupture. In some situations, it is possible to clamp the artery on either side of the aneurysm, removing that portion of the vessel, and the aneurysm, from the circulation. After the removal, the ends are reconnected to maintain blood flow.

Nonsurgical Management

Nonsurgical intervention may be provided for aneurysms that are inoperable because of size, configuration, or the patient's medical status. A foreign material such as a metallic or polymer-based coil may be introduced into the aneurysm. A thrombus develops around the foreign body and, if the treatment is successful, occludes the aneurysm. The goal is to fill the aneurysm enough to prevent blood flowing into it, without causing rupture.

Complications
Rebleeding

Recurrent rupture of a cerebral aneurysm carries significant morbidity and mortality rates. Patients are at risk for rebleeding until the aneurysm is surgically repaired. If the aneurysm is wrapped or embolized, there is a risk of rebleeding, but risk is much lower than if the aneurysm is left untreated.

Hydrocephalus

Blood in the ventricular system interferes with the circulation and reabsorption of cerebrospinal fluid (CSF), and hydrocephalus can develop. Early in the course of subarachnoid hemorrhage, an external ventricular drain may be used to treat hydrocephalus.

About 25% of patients with subarachnoid hemorrhage require placement of a ventriculoperitoneal shunt to treat hydrocephalus (Fig. 49.8). This surgical procedure involves placement of a catheter into a ventricle in the brain. The catheter is then connected to a valve, which regulates the rate of CSF drainage. Another catheter connects to the valve and is passed down to the peritoneal cavity. The CSF drains out of the peritoneal catheter and is absorbed into the peritoneal cavity.

Vasospasm

Vasospasm is responsible for most long-term complications of subarachnoid hemorrhage. Vasospasm causes a blood vessel's diameter to narrow. Although it typically begins in the vessel giving rise to the aneurysm, vasospasm may spread to other vessels. This explains why the ischemia or infarct caused by vasospasm can be so widespread and devastating.

The long-term complications of subarachnoid hemorrhage are similar to those of stroke.

Rehabilitation

If the patient can tolerate intensive therapy, discharge from the hospital may be to a rehabilitation center. Rehabilitation and long-term care are similar whether the patient has had an aneurysm, intracerebral bleed, or an ischemic stroke.

CRITICAL THINKING

Mrs. Washington

■ Mrs. Washington is a 68-year-old African American woman and retired office worker. She was admitted to your unit after a right-sided intracerebral hemorrhage. Her daughter states that Mrs. Washington has taken antihypertensive medication for the past 20 years. However, she states that her mother has been forgetful lately, and that there are five more pills in the medicine bottle than expected. On admission, Mrs. Washington is oriented only to person and has hemiparesis.

1. What may have precipitated Mrs. Washington's stroke?
2. On which side do you expect Mrs. Washington's extremities to be affected?
3. List two safety concerns and strategies to promote patient safety.
4. List at least two educational needs for Mrs. Washington and her daughter.
5. What health care providers are important in the interdisciplinary team caring for Mrs. Washington? What is the role of nursing on this team?

Suggested answers are at the end of the chapter.

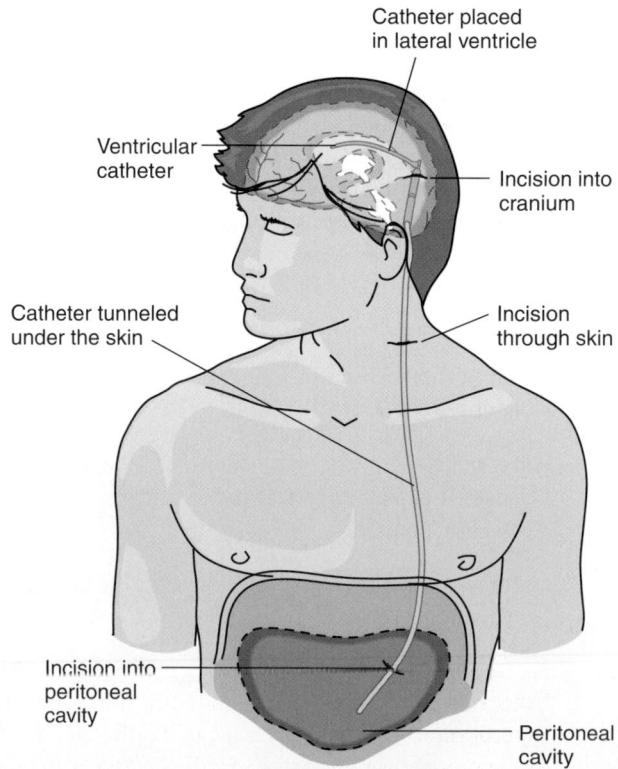

FIGURE 49.8 A ventriculoperitoneal shunt drains cerebrospinal fluid into the peritoneal cavity.

Nursing Process for the Patient With a Cerebrovascular Disorder

Data Collection

Observe the patient for signs and symptoms of decreased cerebral tissue perfusion: decreased level of consciousness, irritability or restlessness, dizziness, syncope, blurred or dimmed vision, **diplopia** (double vision), change in visual fields, unequal pupils or a sluggish or absent pupillary reaction to light, paresthesias, motor weakness, paralysis, or seizures. Reassess frequently and report any decline. Monitor vital signs and oxygen levels. Monitor laboratory tests: CBC, lipid profile, and INR/PT if the patient takes warfarin (Coumadin). Perform a routine respiratory assessment. Monitor lung sounds for adventitious sounds or a change in breath sounds. Assess pain level. Assess swallowing ability before offering oral intake. Promptly report any changes in vital signs, laboratory values, respiratory function, or neurologic status.

Nursing Diagnoses, Planning, and Implementation

See the "Nursing Care Plan for the Patient With Stroke" for nursing diagnoses during acute care. Possible postacute nursing diagnoses are listed next with outcomes and interventions.

• WORD • BUILDING •
diplopia: diplo—double + opia—sight

NURSING CARE PLAN for the Patient With Stroke

Nursing Diagnosis: *Ineffective Cerebral Tissue Perfusion* related to interruption of blood supply

Expected Outcomes: The patient will experience improved cerebral tissue perfusion as evidenced by:

• Absence of or reduction in dizziness, syncope, visual disturbances
• Improved level of consciousness
• Pupils equal and reactive to light
• Improved motor and sensory function.

Evaluation of Outcomes: Are the patient's symptoms of ineffective perfusion improving?

Intervention Monitor neurologic status at least every 30 minutes initially and then every 4 hours or as ordered. Report changes. **Rationale** A change in status could indicate decreased perfusion. **Evaluation** Is there a change in neurologic status since the previous documented assessment?

Intervention Assess vital signs every 30 minutes initially and then every 4 hours or as ordered. **Rationale** High or low blood pressure can lead to decreased tissue perfusion and recurrent stroke. Temperature above 99.6°F can worsen ischemic injury to brain tissue. **Evaluation** Are vital signs within normal limits? Are changes reported?

Intervention Monitor oxygen saturation and administer oxygen as ordered for SpO_2 less than 92%. **Rationale** Hypoxemia can increase brain damage. **Evaluation** Is SpO_2 92% or greater?

Intervention Monitor blood glucose as ordered and report value greater than 140 mg/dL. **Rationale** Elevated glucose is associated with worsening of infarct and hemorrhage. **Evaluation** Is glucose level greater than 140 mg/dL? Was HCP notified?

Intervention Keep head of bed elevated 20 to 30 degrees. Keep neck in neutral position. **Rationale** This facilitates venous return and reduces risk of cerebral edema. **Evaluation** Is head of bed elevated? Is neck in neutral position?

Intervention Monitor medication for therapeutic and nontherapeutic effects. Monitor coagulation studies if appropriate. **Rationale** Anticoagulant therapy must be closely monitored to make sure it is at a therapeutic level and not increasing risk for bleeding. **Evaluation** Are coagulation studies within normal or therapeutic ranges? Are signs of bleeding present?

Continued

NURSING CARE PLAN for the Patient With Stroke—cont'd

Nursing Diagnosis: *Ineffective Airway Clearance* related to stasis of secretions associated with decreased mobility and poor cough effort and airway obstruction resulting from tongue falling back in throat

Expected Outcome: The patient will maintain an open airway as evidenced by respirations quiet and unlabored, 12 to 20 per minute, SpO_2 greater than 92%.

Evaluation of Outcome: Are respirations quiet, 12 to 20 per minute, with SpO_2 greater than 92%?

Intervention Monitor lung sounds, cough, and respirations. **Rationale** Assessment provides the basis for intervention. **Evaluation** Are lung sounds clear? Is cough effective? Are respirations quiet and easy?

Intervention Position the patient to maintain an open airway. **Rationale** Side lying may keep tongue from obstructing airway. **Evaluation** Is patient positioned to keep airway clear?

Intervention Consult with RN or HCP about an oral airway if airway is not clear. **Rationale** An oral airway will keep tongue from obstructing airway if needed. **Evaluation** Is an airway indicated?

Intervention Encourage patient to deep breathe and cough if able. **Rationale** Coughing and deep breathing will help clear secretions from airway and prevent atelectasis. **Evaluation** Is patient able to deep breathe and cough? Is cough effective?

Intervention If cough is ineffective, suction as needed. **Rationale** Suctioning may be needed if patient is unable to swallow secretions or cough effectively. **Evaluation** Is suctioning indicated? Is airway clear after suctioning?

Nursing Diagnosis: *Risk for Injury* related to seizure, repeat stroke, or hemorrhage secondary to thrombolytic therapy

Expected Outcome: The patient will remain free from injury.

Evaluation of Outcome: Is patient free from injury? Are problems recognized and reported quickly?

Intervention Monitor neurologic status frequently and report changes promptly. **Rationale** Prompt recognition of a repeat stroke is essential. **Evaluation** Are neurologic checks within normal limits? Are changes reported promptly?

Intervention Monitor for signs of hemorrhage for 24 to 36 hours following thrombolytic therapy. **Rationale** Hemorrhage is the most common side effect of thrombolytic therapy. **Evaluation** Are signs of hemorrhage present? Are they reported promptly?

Intervention Administer anticonvulsant agent as ordered. **Rationale** Patient is at increased risk for seizures following a stroke. **Evaluation** Is patient seizure free?

Intervention Implement seizure precautions (see Chapter 48). **Rationale** Precautions help protect patient in event of a seizure. **Evaluation** Are precautions in place and patient protected? Is patient assisted with mobility?

Intervention Assist with transfers and ambulation. **Rationale** Patient is at risk for falls because of motor and sensory deficits and impaired judgment. **Evaluation** Is patient able to call for help when needed?

Impaired Physical Mobility related to decreased motor function

EXPECTED OUTCOME: The patient will maintain physical mobility as evidenced by maximum physical mobility within limitations of deficits. Patient will not experience complications related to immobility.

• Consult physical and occupational therapists *to assess the patient's abilities and make specific recommendations related to mobility.*
• Discuss use of constraint therapy with physical and occupational therapists. *Constraint therapy forces the use of the affected limbs by restraining the unaffected side.*
• Maintain the patient in correct body alignment *to prevent contractures and promote comfort.*
• Support affected extremities with pillows *to prevent dislocation injuries and promote comfort.*
• Perform range-of-motion exercises as prescribed by the physical therapist *to prevent contractures and atrophy.*
• Follow physical/occupational therapy recommendations for being up in chair or ambulation. *Prolonged bedrest is associated with complications and poor outcomes.*
• If patient is unable to get out of bed, turn and reposition at least every 2 hours *to prevent skin, respiratory, and musculoskeletal complications.*

 EVIDENCE-BASED PRACTICE

Clinical Question
Is there benefit to having a comprehensive stroke unit?

Evidence
A study using Cochrane Library and Medline evidence from 1980 through 2010 looked at different types of stroke care delivery, different types of stroke unit models, and improvement in patient recovery. It was found that comprehensive stroke units were associated with reduced length of stay, lower mortality, and improved functional outcomes.

Implications for Nursing Practice
The creation of a comprehensive stroke unit should be considered in acute care and rehabilitation settings in both metropolitan and rural areas to reduce the economic burden of stroke care.

REFERENCE
Chan, D. K., Cordato, D., O'Rourke, F., Chan, D. L., Pollack, M., Middleton, S., & Levi, C. (2013). Comprehensive stroke units: A review of comparative evidence and experience. *International Journal of Stroke, 8,* 260–264. doi: 10.1111/j.1747-4949.2012.00850.x.

Imbalanced Nutrition, Less Than Body Requirements, related to impaired swallowing and motor deficits

EXPECTED OUTCOME: The patient will maintain adequate nutrition without aspiration as evidenced by stable weight at appropriate level for height, and no signs of aspiration.

• Keep patient NPO until swallowing can be evaluated *to prevent aspiration.*
• Perform dysphagia screening. *This quick assessment can identify problems before a complete evaluation can be done.*
  • Observe for facial weakness or inability to completely close mouth.
  • Ask patient to stick out tongue and move it side to side.
  • Observe for drooling.
• If swallowing appears to be intact, have patient swallow a sip of water from a cup before offering other foods or fluids. Observe for coughing, choking, or noisy lung sounds. *These are signs of difficulty swallowing.*
• Request speech pathologist evaluation if indicated *to diagnose specific swallowing problems and make recommendations.*
• Implement measures to prevent aspiration. *Aspiration can lead to pneumonia, which will greatly complicate the patient's recovery.*
  • Stay with patient during meals.
  • Ensure that patient is fully alert before feeding.
  • Place the patient in high-Fowler's position or chair for meals.
  • Avoid use of straws.
  • Use a thickening agent if swallowing study recommends.
  • Place food on unaffected side of mouth.
  • Teach the patient to swallow twice after each bite.
  • Check the patient's mouth for pocketing of food.
  • Have suction equipment available.
• Notify primary care provider if patient is unable to take in adequate oral calories. *A feeding tube may be needed if the patient cannot take in enough calories to maintain nutrition. Advance directives should be consulted before a feeding tube is placed.*
• Assist with insertion and care of feeding tube if needed. *If patient cannot swallow effectively, a feeding tube may be needed to maintain nutrition.*
• See "Nutrition Notes" and Chapter 47 for additional interventions.

Disturbed Sensory Perception related to CNS damage

EXPECTED OUTCOME: The patient will adapt to sensory-perceptual deficits as evidenced by avoidance of injury to affected areas.

• Assist occupational therapist to assess for visual and/or spatial deficits and decreased sensory perception: heat and cold, position of body parts, pressure. *Identification of specific deficits is the first step in creating a plan of care.*
• Teach patient to scan the environment *to compensate for a visual deficit.*
• Implement plans for skin integrity and mobility *to protect patient from complications related to sensory deficits.*

Nutrition Notes

Feeding Patients With Swallowing Disorders

Dysphagia affects up to 68% of older adult nursing home residents, up to 30% of older adults admitted to the hospital, up to 64% of patients after stroke, and 13% to 38% of independently living older adults. It also has been associated with increased mortality and morbidity (Sura, Madhavan, Carnaby, & Crary, 2012). In settings with a systematic dysphagia screening program, however, significantly better patient outcomes are seen with a 55% reduction in pneumonia and reduced hospitalization time (Kaspar & Ekberg, 2012). EAT-10, a self-administered screening tool, is available at www.nestlenutrition-institute.org/Documents/test1.pdf.

Suggestions for persons who have difficulty swallowing include the following:
- Sit up straight while eating.
- Eat slowly.
- Avoid distractions while eating.
- Do not drink with a straw.
- Do not talk while eating.
- Use a teaspoon, taking only half a teaspoonful at a time.
- Swallow completely between bites or sips.

Possible nursing interventions to aid a person with a swallowing disorder include the following:
- Remove loose dentures.
- Position the head correctly. A speech therapist can help determine the optimum head position. A hemiplegic patient often benefits from turning the head toward the weak side.
- When spoon-feeding a patient with hemiplegia, place the food on the unaffected side of the tongue.
- A speech therapist may be able to design strengthening exercises, particularly for stroke patients, to increase the patient's swallowing ability.
- Consult a dietitian concerning appropriate textures for liquids and solids.

A multidisciplinary assessment may be needed to tailor the diet prescription to the patient's strengths and weaknesses. Foods with mixed textures such as vegetable soup are frequently problematic. Often thicker substances are better managed than liquids. Although infant cereal can be an effective thickener, it may be refused on a psychological basis in favor of instant potato flakes, unflavored gelatin, or a commercial thickener.

Be aware that thickening agents may:
- Cause food to become thicker over time
- Add significant calories to foods
- React differently in different foods
- Affect the palatability of the thickened item leading to its rejection
- Result in inadequate fluid intake and consequent dehydration

REFERENCES

Kaspar, K., & Ekberg, O. (2012). Identifying vulnerable patients: Role of the EAT-10 and the multidisciplinary team for early intervention and comprehensive dysphagia care. *Nestle Nutrition Institute Workshop Series, 72,* 19–31.
Sura, L., Madhavan, A., Carnaby, G., & Crary, M. A. (2012). Dysphagia in the elderly: Management and nutritional considerations. *Clinical Interventions in Aging, 7,* 287–298.

Risk for Impaired Skin Integrity, Irritation or Breakdown, related to immobility and incontinence
EXPECTED OUTCOME: The patient's skin integrity will be maintained as evidenced by absence of redness or breakdown.

- Examine the skin often for redness or breakdown, especially around bony prominences, dependent areas, and perineum. *Any signs of breakdown must be treated immediately to prevent further damage.*
- Thoroughly cleanse and dry the perineal area after each episode of incontinence. *Urine and feces can be very irritating to the skin.*
- If incontinence is unavoidable, use a barrier cream such as zinc oxide *to protect skin.*
- Turn and position the patient at least every 2 hours, or more often if the patient experiences breakdown. *Pressure impairs circulation and increases risk of breakdown.*
- Use a lift sheet to move patient in bed *to avoid damage from friction and shear.*
- Consider the use of a pressure-reducing mattress if patient cannot be out of bed for long periods. *This helps reduce pressure but does not eliminate the need to reposition the patient every 2 hours.*
- If breakdown occurs, contact the HCP or wound care specialist *to obtain treatment recommendations.*

Incontinence related to loss of voluntary control of elimination
EXPECTED OUTCOME: Episodes of incontinence are avoided, or if unavoidable, they will be cleaned up quickly and skin complications avoided.

- Monitor for incontinence of bowel or bladder *so patient can be cleaned promptly and skin protected.*
- Determine usual pattern of urinary and bowel elimination. *Keeping the patient on his or her regular prehospitalization pattern may help prevent incontinence.*
- Provide assistance with toileting according to the patient's usual schedule. *The patient who is unable to get up unaided may wait too long for help or try to get up alone and be injured.*
- Respond quickly to requests for assistance with toileting *to avoid accidental incontinence.*

Self-Care Deficit related to impaired motor function, spatial-perceptual alterations, and fear of injury

EXPECTED OUTCOME: Self-care will be accomplished as evidenced by patient's ADL needs being met and patient becoming increasingly independent.

- Determine the patient's ability to perform ADLs. *Good baseline data will guide development of a care plan.*
- Work with the patient to create a plan for meeting daily physical needs. *The patient will be more likely to participate in a plan if he or she participated in creating it.*
- Encourage the highest level of independence possible; facilitate patient's ability to do ADLs. *Providing too much assistance can promote dependence and further loss of mobility.*
  - Place objects within reach and within visual field.
  - Place food/fluids within patient's visual field.
  - Encourage use of assistive devices.
- Assist patient with learning to use nondominant side of body. *If dominant side is affected, the patient may have to use the nondominant side.*
- Provide positive feedback *to help reduce discouragement with slow progress.*
- Provide education for family members and significant others regarding patient's deficits and recovery plan. *The family can assist the patient with mobility if they understand what needs to be done.*

Impaired Verbal Communication, Dysarthria, related to loss of motor function of the muscles of speech articulation, or aphasia or dysphasia related to ischemia of the dominant hemisphere

EXPECTED OUTCOME: Communication will be effective as evidenced by the patient communicating needs and desires effectively and by avoidance of frustration.

- Listen for difficulties in verbal communication (difficulty speaking, articulating or incorrect ordering of words, inability to find or name words and objects). *Good baseline data will guide planning of care.*
- Consult a speech pathologist for assistance in determining types of aphasia or dysphasia and need for follow-up treatment. *A speech pathologist is specially trained to diagnose and treat communication problems and can work with nursing staff to develop a plan of care.*
- Implement measures to facilitate communication. *These measures help ensure the patient has his or her immediate needs met while learning to adapt to communication impairment.*
  - Answer call light in person rather than over an intercom.
  - Assess needs frequently.
  - Listen carefully: avoid interrupting patient and allow ample time for communication.
  - When patient is tired, ask questions that require short answers.
  - Provide appropriate aids to communication (picture board, magic slate, pencil and paper). See Figure 49.9.
- Provide education to family members and significant others regarding communication problems and interventions *so they can communicate with patient and participate in care.*

- If the patient is unable to communicate, do not assume that he or she cannot hear and understand. Make every effort to speak to the patient and to keep conversation appropriate when it is within the patient's range of hearing. *The patient may understand exactly what is being said, even if he or she is unable to respond.*
- Contact HCP if impairment increases. *This may be a sign of stroke extension.*

Acute or Chronic Confusion related to cerebral ischemia

EXPECTED OUTCOME: The patient's thought processes will be as clear as possible within limitations of brain damage as evidenced by responses appropriate to situation; the patient's safety will be maintained and patient will feel calm and safe.

- Observe patient for thought process impairment such as shortened attention span, impaired memory, confusion, slowed or quick and impulsive responses, and aggressive and/or inappropriate responses. *Disturbed thinking can be manifested in a variety of ways. See Chapter 48 for interventions for patients with disturbed thought processes.*

Risk for Falls related to changes in mobility, sensation, or confusion

EXPECTED OUTCOME: The patient will remain safe and free from falls.

- Perform a fall risk assessment according to agency policy *to identify patients at risk.*
- Instruct the patient and family to call for help before the patient gets up *so staff can assist.*
- Keep call light and other essential items within patient's reach *to prevent falls while trying to access needed items.*
- Provide frequent toileting. *Patients often fall while getting up to use the toilet.*
- Avoid restraints if at all possible. *Restraints are associated with injuries.*

Deficient Knowledge related to diagnosis and treatment

EXPECTED OUTCOME: The patient and family will have the necessary knowledge to make decisions and assist with care.

- Explain what has happened to the patient. Explain tests, procedures, and care activities. *The patient and significant others are likely to be very frightened about what is happening. Providing correct information about what a stroke is, tests and procedures, and rationale for care activities helps reduce anxiety.*
- Present information in small amounts and as simply as possible. *The patient may have difficulty managing large amounts of information while acutely ill or if confusion is present.*
- Orient the patient and family to the ICU or other setting and the constant monitoring provided. *This can help reduce anxiety and reassure the patient and significant others that the patient is receiving competent care.*
- If the patient is to be discharged to home, make sure information is provided related to medications, treatments, and follow-up care. *The patient and family need to know how to provide appropriate care at home.*

FIGURE 49.9 Picture board.

• Evaluate the need for home nursing, physical therapy, and occupational therapy, and request appropriate referrals. *The patient will likely need continued therapy after discharge to regain as much function as possible.*

Risk for Caregiver Role Strain related to changes in roles, responsibilities, finances, and intimacy

EXPECTED OUTCOME: The caregiver will be comfortable with role as evidenced by statement that she or he understands how to care for the patient and has the needed resources to do so. The caregiver will maintain her or his own health.

• Work with caregiver to identify how the patient's functional level will affect their lives. *Assumption of roles or responsibilities previously fulfilled by the patient may be very stressful to significant others. If the caregiver can anticipate the impact, he or she can plan ahead regarding how to make sure needs are met.*
• Encourage patient and caregiver to identify support systems and make use of community resources.

• Provide a list of resources. *If support is in place before discharge, they are more likely to use it after the patient goes home.*
• Consult social worker or case manager. *These individuals have access to many resources and can help the patient and caregiver identify appropriate sources of assistance, including a caregiver support group.*
• Provide support if transfer to a skilled nursing facility is needed. *This can be a very difficult decision for a patient and caregiver.*

Evaluation

If interventions have been effective, the patient will not experience increased deficits due to decreased perfusion of brain cells. The patient will recover as much physical ability as possible and adjust to remaining deficits to meet self-care needs. Basic needs, including safety, elimination, nutrition, and skin integrity, will be met by the patient or caregiver. The patient will be able to communicate effectively and have needs and desires understood. Caregivers will identify support systems available to help (Table 49.4).

Home Health Hints

- Work with a physical therapist, occupational therapist, and speech therapist to assist the patient with rehabilitation.
- Provide assistive devices to aid the patient to function independently.
- Keep home environment clutter-free to prevent falls.
- Offer frequent praise for all achievements.
- Keep regularly used items close by. If the patient is using a walker, have him or her tie a small bag to the top to store these items.
- If the patient does not have a portable phone, encourage the purchase of one. Instruct the patient to keep it near at all times in case of an emergency.
- If necessary, assist the patient with obtaining a medical alert device. If the patient falls, he or she can access an emergency medical service by pushing a button.
- Assist with obtaining homemaker or respite care for caregivers if necessary.
- Patients on a pureed diet can make their own food at home using a food processor. Baby food can also be purchased to meet swallowing guidelines.
- Patients with one-sided paralysis following a stroke can be taught to wear clothes that are easy to get on and off. Examples include pants with elastic waists, shoes with Velcro closures or slip-on shoes, and pullover shirts without buttons.
- If the patient has difficulty speaking (dysarthria), try using magnetic alphabet letters. Ask questions that require a yes or no answer. The patient can respond with the letter Y or N. You can also help the patient and caregiver develop a communication board of frequently used words and objects.
- Keep bedside commode lids up with patches of Velcro attached to the seat and the frame.

TABLE 49.4 STROKE SUMMARY

Signs and Symptoms	Dizziness Syncope Visual disturbances Irritability, restlessness, confusion Decreased level of consciousness Unequal pupils Paresthesias Motor weakness Paralysis Seizures Difficulty swallowing, understanding language, speaking
Diagnostic Tests	CT, MRI Scan Electrocardiogram Carotid Doppler Echocardiogram Cerebral angiogram Laboratory: INR/PT, metabolic panel, glucose, complete blood count, PTT, serum pregnancy (if appropriate), oxygen saturation
Therapeutic Measures	Oxygen for Spo$_2$ less than 92% Antiplatelet, anticoagulant, or thrombolytic medication Physical, occupational, speech therapy Carotid endarterectomy or stent Knee-high antiembolism stockings
Complications	Stroke evolves, causing more deficits, aspiration pneumonia, skin breakdown, urinary tract infection, malnutrition
Priority Nursing Diagnoses	*Ineffective Cerebral Tissue Perfusion* *Ineffective Airway Clearance* *Risk for Injury*

INR/PT = international normalized ratio/prothrombin time; PTT = partial thromboplastin time; Spo$_2$ = peripheral oxygen saturation.

SUGGESTED ANSWERS TO

CRITICAL THINKING

■ *Mr. Jankowski*

1. Ask Mr. Jankowski about other risk factors for stroke, such as his dietary and alcohol habits. Check his chart for history of diabetes, hypertension, or heart disease. Check his weight and cholesterol levels if drawn. Educate him about risk factors for stroke and how they can be modified. Use the Stroke Risk Scorecard and teach him the FAST acronym (see Fig. 49.2). As a nurse, you will be in a position to recognize risks and help patients modify risk factors for many problems before they occur.

2. Discuss use of an anticoagulant agent or sequential compression device with the RN or HCP.

3. Provide written or audiovisual information on stroke prevention and smoking cessation. Ask the HCP about use of a nicotine patch or other medication for smoking cessation, if Mr. Jankowski is willing.

4. Involve a dietitian for dietary counseling if indicated. Consult the smoking cessation coordinator at your agency if one is on staff.

■ *Mrs. Washington*

1. Uncontrolled hypertension, in the presence of a preexisting aneurysm, might have precipitated Mrs. Washington's stroke.

2. Her left extremities will be affected.

3. Mrs. Washington is disoriented. Her room should be as close to the nurse's station as possible. Reorient her to her surroundings and condition frequently. Keep side rails up when Mrs. Washington is alone. Mrs. Washington also has hemiparesis. Obtain a commode because Mrs. Washington will probably not be able to walk to the bathroom. Place the call light and telephone on her right side. Assist Mrs. Washington with positioning to prevent injury to her affected limbs.

4. If Mrs. Washington will be going back to her home, you should teach her and her daughter about the relationship of uncontrolled hypertension to intracranial hemorrhage; options for inpatient, outpatient, and in-home therapy; and memory strategies to prevent missed medication doses (e.g., weekly pill box, keeping medications with breakfast food, or an alarm clock or watch).

5. The HCP directs the medical care, but often it is the nurse (typically an RN) who oversees the multidisciplinary team and ensures that everything is being done as ordered. Other important team members include the case manager or discharge planner, dietitian, physical, occupational, and speech therapists, and pastoral care if the patient desires.

REVIEW QUESTIONS

1. Which of the following are modifiable risk factors that should be taught to patients at risk for stroke? *Select all that apply.*
   1. Heredity
   2. Age
   3. Diabetes
   4. Race
   5. High cholesterol
   6. Obesity

2. What interventions can help prevent aspiration in a poststroke patient with dysphagia? *Select all that apply.*
   1. Ensure that patient is fully alert before feeding.
   2. Place the patient in high-Fowler's position or chair for meals.
   3. Use straws for thin liquids.
   4. Use a thickening agent.
   5. Place food on affected side of mouth.

3. How soon after symptom onset must a person who has had a stroke receive thrombolytic treatment?
   1. 30 minutes
   2. 1 hour
   3. 2 hours
   4. 4.5 hours

4. How should the nurse communicate with the patient experiencing receptive aphasia?
   1. Be patient as the patient tries to speak
   2. Listen carefully, while making eye contact
   3. Speak loudly toward the patient's good side
   4. Use gestures, standing where the patient can see

5. A nurse is caring for a patient who is recovering from an ischemic stroke. Upon entering the room to pick up the supper tray, the nurse notes that the patient has only eaten food on the left side of the tray. What should the nurse do?
   1. Turn the plate 180 degrees and observe the patient's response.
   2. Remove the tray and do not comment.
   3. Encourage the patient to eat the rest of the meal.
   4. Assist the patient by providing finger foods and feeding the patient items that require a utensil.

6. A nurse is doing an afternoon assessment on a patient transferred to a medical unit from intensive care following a subarachnoid hemorrhage. The patient was alert and oriented during the morning assessment but reported being very tired. Now the patient is difficult to arouse. What action should the nurse take?
   1. Let the patient sleep; transferring from the ICU can be very strenuous.
   2. Reassess the patient in an hour. If the sleepiness continues, notify the RN.
   3. Call the RN immediately.
   4. Call a code.

Answers can be found in Appendix C.

References

American Association of Neuroscience Nurses. (2008). *AANN clinical practice guidelines series. Guide to the care of the hospitalized patient with ischemic stroke* (2nd ed.). Glenview, IL: Author.

American Heart Association. (2013). Heart disease and stroke statistics—2013 update. A report from the American Heart Association Statistics Committee and Stroke Statistics Subcommittee. *Circulation, 127,* 143–152.

American Heart Association/American Stroke Association. (2013). Spot a stroke F.A.S.T. Retrieved June 23, 2013, from StrokeAssociation.org/WarningSigns

Ennen, K. A. (2013). Taking a second look at stroke in women. *American Nurse Today, 8,* 12–15.

 Davis*Plus* | For additional resources and information visit **davispl.us/medsurg5**

50

Nursing Care of Patients With Peripheral Nervous System Disorders

DEBORAH L. WEAVER

KEY TERMS

amyotrophic (ay-MY-oh-TROH-fik)
anticholinesterase (AN-tee-KOH-lin-ESS-ter-ays)
atrophy (AT-troh-fee)
demyelination (dee-MY-uh-lin-AY-shun)
fasciculation (fah-SIK-yoo-LAY-shun)
neuralgia (new-RAL-jee-ah)
neuropathies (new-ROP-uh-thees)
neurectomy (new-REK-tuh-mee)
plasmapheresis (PLAZ-mah-fer-EE-siss)
ptosis (TOH-sis)
remyelination (ree-MY-uh-lin-AY-shun)
rhizotomy (rye-ZOT-uh-mee)
sclerosis (skleh-ROH-sis)

LEARNING OUTCOMES

1. Identify disorders that are caused by disruption of the peripheral nervous system.
2. Explain the pathophysiology, major signs and symptoms, and complications of selected peripheral nervous system disorders.
3. Identify therapeutic measures used for selected peripheral nervous system disorders.
4. List common nursing diagnoses associated with peripheral nervous system disorders.
5. Plan prioritized nursing interventions for patients with peripheral nervous system disorders.
6. Evaluate the effectiveness of nursing care.

The peripheral nervous system (PNS) consists of all nervous system structures outside the central nervous system (CNS). A variety of disorders affect the PNS. Some of these disorders become chronic and cause degeneration of body systems. Some other disorders are more temporary. Two common types of PNS disorders are discussed in this chapter. Neuromuscular disorders compose one group and can include motor or sensory disorders or both. The second group includes cranial nerve disorders. Both types of disorders present a challenge to the nurse caring for the patient and family.

NEUROMUSCULAR DISORDERS

This group of neurologic conditions is chronic and degenerative in nature. Neuromuscular disorders involve a disruption of impulse transmission between neurons and the muscles they stimulate. This breakdown in transmission results in muscle weakness. If the muscles of the respiratory system are affected, deadly complications can develop, including pneumonia and respiratory failure. Common neuromuscular disorders include multiple sclerosis, myasthenia gravis, amyotrophic lateral sclerosis, and Guillain-Barré syndrome.

Multiple Sclerosis
Pathophysiology

Multiple **sclerosis** (MS) is a chronic progressive degenerative disease that affects the myelin sheath of the neurons in the CNS. Myelin is responsible for the smooth transmission of nerve impulses. Muscles contract when nerve impulses stimulate the muscle tissue. In MS, the myelin sheath begins to break down (degenerate; Fig. 50.1) as a result of activation

of the body's immune system. The nerve becomes inflamed and edematous, which interrupts impulses to the muscles. As the disease progresses, sclerosis or scar tissue damages the nerve. Nerve impulses become completely blocked, causing permanent loss of muscle function in that area of the body.

Etiology

The cause of MS is not really understood. Damage to the myelin sheath is thought to be from an autoimmune process; however, the disease can be related to viral infections, heredity, and other unknown factors. Some research indicates that there is an inherited tendency to develop MS, and the manifestations of the disease only appear in the presence of environmental triggers. The disease usually starts between ages 15 and 50. Women are 2 to 3 times more likely to develop MS than men and are more likely to have relapses (National MS Society, 2013). Smokers and those with vitamin D deficiency have a higher risk of MS. Caucasians have a higher incidence of MS than those of African descent (Multiple Sclerosis Association of America [MSAA], 2013). The course of the disease is unpredictable, and there are many variations in symptoms, depending on which nerves are affected. Some individuals have mild illness, while others suffer permanent disability or rapid decline and death.

Signs and Symptoms

The patient with MS presents with muscle weakness, tingling sensations, and numbness. Other common symptoms include visual disturbances, usually in one eye at a time. These disturbances may be accompanied by pain with eye movement. Symptoms may begin slowly over weeks to months or start suddenly and dramatically. MS affects many body systems

A   B   C

FIGURE 50.1 The myelin sheath breaks down in multiple sclerosis, interrupting transmission of nerve impulses. (A) Normal myelin sheath. (B) Myelin beginning to break down. (C) Total myelin disruption. Modified from Scanlon, V. C., & Sanders, T. (2014). *Workbook for essentials of anatomy and physiology* (7th ed.). Philadelphia: F.A. Davis, with permission.

(Box 50-1). Many factors can trigger the onset of symptoms or aggravate the condition, including extreme heat and cold, fatigue, infection, and physical and emotional stress. Hormonal changes after pregnancy can also cause symptom onset or exacerbation.

Periods of exacerbation and remission lead patients with MS to be uncertain about when the disease will flare up and what body system will be affected. Intense fatigue is common; therefore, immobility can become a problem. Accidents and falls are common because of muscle weakness or numbness of the trunk and limbs. Some people with MS experience symptoms such as muscle spasticity, bowel or bladder dysfunction, or paralysis. Difficulty with concentration or forgetfulness can also be problematic. Pneumonia can occur from immobility and from weakness of the diaphragm and intercostal muscles. Death, often resulting from respiratory infection, typically occurs 20 to 35 years after diagnosis.

Diagnostic Tests

Diagnosis is based on the patient's history and signs and symptoms. Analysis of cerebrospinal fluid (CSF) may show an increase in oligoclonal immunoglobulin G (IgG). Magnetic resonance imaging (MRI) can be helpful in diagnosis because sclerotic plaques can be detected. A new blood test, gMS DX, is now available to help identify people likely to have identifying antibodies associated with MS. Evoked potential tests may be done to determine slow transmission of impulses.

Therapeutic Measures

MS has no cure. Many people with MS do well with no medication at all, although early treatment can delay progression of the disease. Interferon therapy with beta-interferons such as Betaseron or Avonex can reduce exacerbations and delay disability. Steroids such as adrenocorticotropic hormone (ACTH) and prednisone are given to decrease inflammation and edema of the neurons, which can relieve some symptoms. Immunosuppressant drugs such as azathioprine (Imuran) and cyclophosphamide (Cytoxan) may be given to suppress the immune system. In 2012, oral teriflunomide (Aubagio) was added to the Food and Drug Administration–approved medications, and in 2013, dimethyl fumarate (Tecfidera) was added (MSAA, 2013). Clinical trials have shown that these medications can reduce the number and severity of relapses, reduce the number of new lesions shown on MRI, and for some, delay disease progression and disability. Each of these medications has serious side effects.

Anticonvulsants such as carbamazepine (Tegretol) or duloxetine (Cymbalta) help relieve neuropathic pain. Valium (Diazepam), baclofen (Lioresal), tizanidine (Zanaflex), and physical therapy assist in controlling muscle spasms. Bladder problems are treated with parasympathetic agents such as bethanechol (Urecholine) and oxybutynin (Ditropan). Fatigue can be treated with antidepressants or an antiviral agent such as amantadine (Symmetrel). Table 50.1 reviews additional medications used to treat PNS disorders.

For those who suffer sudden severe attacks or who do not respond to high doses of steroids, plasma exchange or **plasmapheresis** may be used to remove from the blood antibodies that are attacking the myelin (Box 50-2). New research is focusing on treatments to regenerate myelin.

Rehabilitation after an acute episode includes physical, speech, and occupational therapies. Rehabilitation therapy helps the patient and family adapt the home environment to the patient's special needs. Assistive devices such as braces, canes, wheelchairs, and splints allow the patient increased mobility and independence. Patients who develop speech difficulties benefit from speech therapy. Exercise also can be beneficial (see "Evidence-Based Practice").

Box 50-1 Problems Associated With Multiple Sclerosis

- Weakness/paralysis of limbs, trunk, or head
- Diplopia (double vision)
- Slurred speech
- Spasticity of muscles
- Numbness and tingling
- Patchy blindness (scotomas)
- Blurred vision
- Vertigo
- Tinnitus
- Impaired hearing
- Nystagmus
- Ataxia
- Dysarthria
- Dysphagia
- Constipation
- Spastic (uninhibited) bladder
- Flaccid (hypotonic) bladder
- Sexual dysfunction
- Anger, depression, euphoria

 EVIDENCE-BASED PRACTICE

Clinical Question
What is the effect of physical activity and self-efficacy on the quality of life of persons with MS?

Evidence
A sample of 269 persons with relapsing–remitting MS was studied for 1 year. Exercise strategies were implemented with individuals who believed they could be successful in the treatment plan. Physical activity and self-efficacy were associated with improvements in reported quality of life.

• WORD • BUILDING •
plasmapheresis: plasma—liquid of blood + pheresis—removal

Implications for Nursing Practice

As nurses we can support individuals in their efforts to manage their chronic illness by encouraging them to embrace their ability to be successful along with a reasonable exercise regimen. Fewer exacerbations can mean improved quality of life as well as fewer complications.

REFERENCE

Motl, R. W., McAuley, E., Wynn, D., Sandroff, B., & Suh, Y. (2012). Physical activity, self-efficacy, and health-related quality of life in persons with multiple sclerosis: Analysis of associations between individual-level changes over one year. *Quality of Life Research.* Retrieved June 29, 2013, from http://link.springer.com/article/10.1007/s11136 -012-0149-z#page-1

Nursing Care

See the "Nursing Care Plan for the Patient With a Progressive Neuromuscular Disorder."

In addition to reviewing routine care, instruct the patient to avoid factors that can exacerbate symptoms. This includes avoiding stressful situations as much as possible. Rest, exercise, and a balanced diet are important self-care steps to control symptoms. In addition, avoiding extreme temperature changes, especially heat, and avoiding infection and illness are important. Any infection, especially respiratory, should be reported immediately to the health care provider (HCP). Two excellent sources of information on MS are the National Multiple Sclerosis Society at www.nationalmssociety.org and the Multiple Sclerosis Foundation at www.msfocus.org.

TABLE 50.1 MEDICATIONS USED TO TREAT PERIPHERAL NERVOUS SYSTEM DISORDERS

Medication Class/Action	Examples	Nursing Implications
Cholinesterase Inhibitors Increase acetylcholine at synapses.	neostigmine (Prostigmin) pyridostigmine (Mestinon) edrophonium chloride (Tensilon, used in diagnosis of MG)	Atropine is antidote.
Glucocorticoids Reduce inflammation.	prednisone prednisolone prednisolone acetate or sodium phosphate	Provide calcium supplement. Avoid crowds and others with infections. Monitor fluid balance. May need to treat blood sugar with insulin while on medication.
Immunosuppressants Suppress immunity and antibody formation.	azathioprine (Imuran) cyclophosphamide (Cytoxan)	Monitor blood counts. Protect from bleeding and infection. Administer with meals to reduce nausea.
Antispasmodics/Muscle Relaxants Relax muscles, reduce pain.	dantrolene (Dantrium) baclofen (Lioresal) diazepam (Valium) tizanidine (Zanaflex)	Avoid operating machinery or driving until effects are known. Monitor patient for respiratory depression.
Anticonvulsants Treat nerve pain.	phenytoin (Dilantin) carbamazepine (Tegretol) gabapentin (Neurontin) duloxetine (Cymbalta)	Teach good oral hygiene with soft bristle brush, floss, and gum massage (phenytoin). Monitor for fall risk. Monitor blood counts.

Continued

TABLE 50.1 MEDICATIONS USED TO TREAT PERIPHERAL NERVOUS SYSTEM DISORDERS—cont'd

Medication Class/Action	Examples	Nursing Implications
Glutamate Antagonist Delays progression of ALS.	riluzole (Rilutek)	Rest, monitor for respiratory depression. Give on empty stomach. Avoid large quantities of caffeine. Avoid charcoal-broiled foods. Monitor liver function laboratory values.
Biologic Response Modifiers Reduce relapses in relapsing-remitting MS	teriflunomide (Aubagio) dimethyl fumarate (Tecfidera)	Monitor liver enzymes, blood pressure, potassium level, and signs of infection. Monitor CBC and signs of infection.

Note. ALS = amyotrophic lateral sclerosis; CBC = complete blood count; MS = muscular sclerosis.

Box 50-2 Plasmapheresis

Plasmapheresis, also known as plasma exchange therapy, is a procedure that removes the plasma component from whole blood and replaces it with fresh plasma. The goal is to remove antibodies through plasma exchange, suppressing the immune response and inflammation.

Preprocedure Nursing Care

- Teach patient about the procedure and what to expect, including what the machine looks like (similar to but smaller than a dialysis machine), the need for arterial and venous access sites, and the length of the procedure (2 to 5 hours).
- The HCP may order medications held until after the procedure. Some patients may require premedication, especially if they have experienced complications in the past.
- Assess baseline vital signs and weight.

- Assess complete blood cell count (CBC), platelet count, and clotting studies.
- Check blood type and crossmatch for replacement blood products.

Postprocedure Nursing Care

- Observe the patient for signs of hypovolemia, such as dizziness and hypotension.
- Apply pressure dressings to the access sites.
- Monitor the patient for infection and bruits at the access site.
- Monitor electrolytes and signs of electrolyte loss. Report imbalances, and administer replacement electrolytes as ordered.
- Compare preprocedure and postprocedure laboratory data, such as CBC, platelet count, and clotting times.

NURSING CARE PLAN for the Patient With a Progressive Neuromuscular Disorder

Nursing Diagnosis: *Ineffective Airway Clearance* related to respiratory muscle weakness, with impaired cough and gag reflexes

Expected Outcomes: The patient will maintain a patent airway as evidenced by clear lung sounds and freedom from signs and symptoms of respiratory distress.

Evaluation of Outcomes: Is patient's airway patent and are lung sounds clear? Is patient free of signs and symptoms of respiratory distress?

NURSING CARE PLAN for the Patient With a Progressive Neuromuscular Disorder—cont'd

Intervention Monitor respiratory rate and depth, breath sounds, oxygen saturation (Spo_2), and arterial blood gases (as ordered). Report deterioration. **Rationale** Increasing respiratory distress indicates progressing muscle weakness that may require mechanical ventilation or end-of-life decisions. **Evaluation** Is patient's respiratory rate status stable or is intervention indicated?

Intervention Encourage patient to cough and deep breathe every 2 hours. **Rationale** Effective coughing helps keep airway clear. **Evaluation** Does patient have the strength to cough effectively?

Intervention Observe patient for breathlessness while speaking. **Rationale** Inability to speak without breathlessness indicates declining respiratory function. **Evaluation** Is patient able to finish sentences without needing to take a breath?

Intervention Elevate head of bed. **Rationale** Fowler's position improves lung expansion, decreases work of breathing, improves cough efforts, and decreases risk for aspiration. **Evaluation** Does elevation of head of bed help relieve dyspnea and prevent aspiration?

Intervention Evaluate cough, swallow, and gag reflexes frequently. Notify HCP if absent. **Rationale** Frequent evaluation of reflexes is needed to prevent aspiration, respiratory infections, and respiratory failure. **Evaluation** Is patient able to cough effectively? Is gag reflex intact?

Intervention Suction secretions as needed, noting color and amount of secretions. **Rationale** Muscle weakness can result in inability to clear airway. **Evaluation** Does patient require suctioning to clear airway? What color are secretions?

Nursing Diagnosis: *Impaired Physical Mobility* related to muscle weakness

Expected Outcomes: The patient will maintain optimum mobility and activity level, identify measures to help maintain mobility, and perform exercises that help maintain current mobility.

Evaluation of Outcomes: Is optimum activity level maintained? Can patient identify measures that will help maintain mobility? Does patient perform exercises that help maintain mobility?

Intervention Determine preillness and current level of mobility. **Rationale** Assessment guides care planning. **Evaluation** Do assessment findings help determine goals and interventions?

Intervention Identify factors that affect ability to be mobile and active. **Rationale** Some factors that interfere with mobility can be modified. **Evaluation** Are interfering factors modified effectively?

Intervention Encourage patient to perform self-care to maximum ability. **Rationale** Promotes sense of control and independence for patient. **Evaluation** Does patient perform self-care activities? Is assistance required?

Intervention Consult physical therapist or occupational therapist to provide assistive devices for walking (canes, braces, walker, wheelchair) and other activities. **Rationale** Assistive devices decrease fatigue and promote independence, comfort, and safety. **Evaluation** Does patient use assistive devices safely during activities? Do they help keep patient active?

Intervention Reposition frequently when patient is immobile. **Rationale** Prevents skin breakdown and stasis of pulmonary secretions. **Evaluation** Is patient free from complications of immobility?

Intervention Provide active/passive range-of-motion (ROM) exercises on a regular basis. **Rationale** Prevents contractures and disuse atrophy. **Evaluation** Does patient have any contractures or atrophy?

Intervention Plan activities with a balance of frequent rest periods. **Rationale** Rest decreases fatigue. **Evaluation** Is fatigue controlled?

Continued

NURSING CARE PLAN for the Patient With a Progressive Neuromuscular Disorder—cont'd

Intervention Administer medications as ordered. **Rationale** Medications can slow progress of disease and reduce symptoms that limit mobility. **Evaluation** Are symptoms controlled?

Nursing Diagnosis: *Risk for Imbalanced Nutrition: Less Than Body Requirements* related to weakness or lack of coordination of muscles for chewing and swallowing

Expected Outcome: The patient will maintain body weight within normal limits for height and frame.

Evaluation of Outcome: Is patient's weight stable and within normal limits?

Intervention Evaluate cough, swallow, and gag reflexes frequently. Notify HCP if absent. **Rationale** If patient is unable to swallow, a feeding tube may be indicated, depending on patient's wishes. **Evaluation** Does patient eat and drink without aspirating?

Intervention Offer soft foods that are easy to chew and swallow. **Rationale** Soft foods require less effort to chew and are less fatiguing. **Evaluation** Is patient able to chew and swallow without excessive fatigue?

Intervention Request speech therapist and dietitian consultations as indicated. **Rationale** Speech therapist can help evaluate swallowing and make recommendations. Dietitian can recommend appropriate foods. **Evaluation** Are consults indicated? Are recommendations implemented?

Intervention Institute swallowing precautions as needed. **Rationale** Swallowing precautions help prevent aspiration and allow patient to maintain oral intake as long as possible. **Evaluation** Do precautions prevent aspiration?

Nursing Diagnosis: *Impaired Verbal Communication* related to impaired respiratory and muscle function

Expected Outcome: The patient will be able to communicate needs.

Evaluation of Outcome: Does patient indicate that needs are met with a minimum of frustration?

Intervention Assess ability to speak and communicate. **Rationale** Assessment is essential to planning appropriate communication interventions. **Evaluation** Can patient speak or communicate needs?

Intervention Request referral to speech therapist for assistance if indicated. **Rationale** Speech therapist can recommend appropriate alternative communication techniques. **Evaluation** Is speech therapy referral indicated? Is referral completed?

Intervention Assess for nonverbal signs of pain or distress, such as restlessness, agitation, grimacing. **Rationale** Patient may not be able to tell you if he or she is in pain or distress. **Evaluation** Are signs of pain or distress present? Are they attended to?

Intervention Use picture board or paper and pencil. Ask questions that require a yes or no answer. **Rationale** These do not require the patient to speak to communicate. **Evaluation** Do alternative methods help patient communicate needs?

Intervention Use nonhurried, calm, and caring approach while providing care. **Rationale** This will help decrease anxiety and provide emotional support to patient and family. **Evaluation** Do patient and family appear anxious? Does calm approach help?

Intervention Explain all procedures. **Rationale** Patient can still hear and needs to know what is happening. **Evaluation** Does patient indicate understanding?

Myasthenia Gravis

Pathophysiology

Myasthenia gravis (MG) means "grave muscle weakness," or weakness of the voluntary or skeletal muscles of the body. MG is a noncommunicable (chronic) disease of the neuromuscular junction (Fig. 50.2). Normally, at the neuromuscular junction, the neuron releases the chemical neurotransmitter acetylcholine (ACh), which crosses the synaptic cleft. Receptors on the muscle tissue take up ACh and contraction of the muscle results. In MG, the body's immune system is activated, producing antibodies that attack and destroy ACh receptors at the neuromuscular junction. Therefore, ACh cannot stimulate muscle contraction because the number of ACh receptors has been reduced, resulting in loss of voluntary muscle strength.

Etiology

MG is a chronic autoimmune process. No specific cause has been found for MG. However, current thought is that a virus or bacteria may initiate the autoimmune process. Genetic

A

B

FIGURE 50.2 Myasthenia gravis. (A) Normal neuromuscular junction. (B) Note damaged acetylcholine receptor sites in myasthenia gravis. Modified from Scanlon, V. C., & Sanders, T. (2014). *Workbook for essentials of anatomy and physiology* (7th ed.). Philadelphia: F.A. Davis, with permission.

susceptibility may also play a role. Disorders of the thymus gland are often associated with MG. Thymomas or tumors on the thymus gland can account for the malfunction of the immune system that initiates the autoimmune process. All ethnic groups and both genders can develop this disease. Peak age of onset in women is ages 20 to 30. Men are affected more often after age 60. MG occurs slightly more often in women than men.

Signs and Symptoms

MG results in progressive extreme muscle weakness. The classic sign of MG is increased muscle weakness during activity and improvement in muscle strength after rest. Muscles are strongest in the morning, when the person is rested. Activities affected by MG include eye and eyelid movements, chewing, swallowing, speaking, and breathing, as well as skeletal muscle function. Patients often present with drooping of the eyelids (**ptosis**). Facial expressions become masklike. After long conversations, the patient's voice can fade. Falls occur because of weakness of the arm and leg muscles. Patients with MG experience periods of exacerbation and remission of symptoms, similar to patients with MS. Exacerbations can be caused by emotional or physical stress such as menses, illness, trauma, extremes in temperature, pregnancy, electrolyte imbalance, surgery, and drugs that block action at the neuromuscular junction.

Complications

Major complications associated with MG result from weakness of muscles that assist with swallowing and breathing. Aspiration, respiratory infections, and respiratory failure are the leading causes of death. Sudden onset of muscle weakness in patients with MG resulting from not enough medication is called a myasthenic crisis. Overmedication with **anticholinesterase** (anti-ACh) drugs causes a cholinergic crisis (Table 50.2). Both crises require immediate medical attention.

 LEARNING TIP

Symptoms of cholinergic crisis can be remembered with the acronym **SLUDGE**: **s**alivation, **l**acrimation, **u**rination, **d**iarrhea, **g**astrointestinal (GI) cramping, and **e**mesis. A severe crisis has been described as "liquid pouring out of every body orifice."

Diagnostic Tests

Diagnosis of MG is based on history of symptoms and physical examination of the patient. A simple test involves the patient looking upward for 2 to 3 minutes. Increased droop of the eyelids (ptosis) occurs if MG is present. After a brief rest, the eyelids can be opened without difficulty. Another test is done by injecting edrophonium (Tensilon, an anticholinesterase

• **WORD • BUILDING** •
anticholinesterase: anti—against + cholinesterase—chemical that breaks down acetylcholine

TABLE 50.2 COMPARISON OF MYASTHENIC CRISIS AND CHOLINERGIC CRISIS

	Myasthenic Crisis	Cholinergic Crisis
Cause	Too little medication	Too much medication
Signs and Symptoms	Ptosis	Increasing muscle weakness
	Difficulty swallowing	Dyspnea
	Difficulty speaking	Salivation
	Dyspnea	Lacrimation
	Weakness	Incontinent urination
		Abdominal cramping, diarrhea
		Nausea, emesis
		Increased bronchial secretions
		Sweating
		Miosis (constriction of pupils)

Box 50-3 Medications That Can Exacerbate Symptoms of Myasthenia Gravis

- Antibiotics (some)
- Alpha interferon
- Anticholinergic agents
- Beta blockers
- Botulinum toxin
- Calcium channel blockers
- Chloroquine
- Lithium
- Magnesium
- Neuromuscular blocking agents (such as those used during surgery)
- Penicillamine
- Prednisone
- Procainamide
- Quinidine

drug) intravenously (IV). If muscle strength improves dramatically (e.g., the patient can suddenly open the eyes wide), MG is diagnosed. However, improvement is only temporary. An increased number of anti-ACh receptor antibodies in the blood are present in 90% of patients with MG. Electromyography (EMG) may be done to rule out other conditions. Pulmonary function tests may be done to predict potential myasthenic crisis leading to respiratory failure.

Therapeutic Measures

No cure is currently available for MG. Treatment is aimed at controlling symptoms. Removal of the thymus gland (thymectomy) can decrease production of ACh receptor antibodies and decrease symptoms in most patients. Medications used to treat MG include the anticholinesterase drugs neostigmine (Prostigmin) and pyridostigmine (Mestinon). These drugs improve MG symptoms by destroying the acetylcholinesterase that breaks down ACh. Remember that ACh causes muscles to contract. If ACh is allowed more time to attach to muscle tissue receptors, the muscle contracts and strength is increased. Steroids such as prednisone and immunosuppressants are used to suppress the body's immune response. Plasmapheresis can be used to remove antibodies from the patient's blood (Box 50-3). Use of immune globulin is being researched.

Nursing Process for the Patient With Myasthenia Gravis

DATA COLLECTION. Determine the patient's baseline muscle strength. Ask how much activity is tolerated before fatigue and muscle weakness occur. Identify the patient's support systems and determine whether the patient's needs are being met. Assess the knowledge base of the patient and family. Check respiratory function and swallowing ability.

NURSING DIAGNOSES, PLANNING, AND IMPLEMENTATION. *Activity Intolerance related to muscle weakness*
EXPECTED OUTCOME: The patient will improve activity tolerance as evidenced by ability to carry out necessary activities.

- Schedule anticholinesterase drugs so that peak action occurs at times when increased muscle strength is needed *so the patient has strength for activities such as meals and physical therapy.*
- Teach the patient to schedule activities such as grocery shopping or errands at times when medication is at peak action, *so that muscle strength is adequate for the activity.*
- Be aware of symptoms and treatment of myasthenic and cholinergic crises, *so quick intervention can be carried out to prevent worsening symptoms.*
- Teach the patient and significant others signs and symptoms of crisis conditions *because both crises constitute medical emergencies and require immediate medical attention* (see Table 50.2).
- Teach methods to conserve energy, such as sitting down to do grooming and housekeeping activities whenever possible. *This helps the patient conserve energy to manage ADLs.*
- Teach the patient to rest between activities *to allow time for muscle strength to be restored.*

- Teach the importance of avoiding people with infections and exposure to cold *to minimize risk for respiratory infections, which can exacerbate symptoms and increase risk for ineffective airway clearance.*
- Instruct the patient to eat nutritious, well-balanced meals *to maintain strength and resistance to infections, which can exacerbate symptoms.*
- Teach the patient to only use medications that are prescribed by the HCP. If multiple providers are used, all medications should be checked with the provider who is treating the MG. *Many medications can exacerbate muscle weakness* (Box 50-3).
- Provide information about support groups *that can provide encouragement and assistance to patients and their families.*

EVALUATION.   If the plan of care has been effective, the patient's activity and self-care needs will be met, either by the patient or by other support individuals.

Also see the "Nursing Care Plan for the Patient With a Progressive Neuromuscular Disorder." More information can be found at the Myasthenia Gravis Foundation of America website at www.myasthenia.org.

CRITICAL THINKING

Jamie

■ Jamie is referred to a neurologist because of muscle weakness.

1. What history can help differentiate between MS and MG?
2. What physical examination can be done to differentiate between MS and MG?
3. The neurologist prepares to do a Tensilon test and asks you to prepare 2 mg of Tensilon for IV injection. It is supplied as 10 mg per milliliter. How much should you draw up?
4. In preparing for a case management meeting for a patient with a neuromuscular disease, which other HCPs should be invited?

Suggested answers are at the end of the chapter.

Amyotrophic Lateral Sclerosis
Pathophysiology and Etiology

Amyotrophic lateral sclerosis (ALS, also called Lou Gehrig's disease) is a progressive, degenerative condition that affects motor neurons responsible for the control of voluntary muscles. In the brain and spinal cord, upper and lower motor neurons begin to degenerate and form scar tissue or die, blocking transmission of nerve impulses. Without stimulation, muscles **atrophy**, and muscle strength and coordination decrease. As the disease progresses, more muscle groups, including muscles controlling breathing and swallowing, become involved. The heart and GI tract are controlled involuntarily, and so are not affected by ALS. The ability to think and reason also is not affected.

ALS can occur at any age but usually does not appear until adulthood. The cause of ALS is not known, but it is believed to have a genetic component.

Signs and Symptoms

Symptoms are vague early in the course of ALS. Primary symptoms include progressive muscle weakness and decreased coordination. This can begin in the arms, legs, or muscles of speech and swallowing. Atrophy of muscles and **fasciculations** (twitching) also occur. Muscle spasms can cause pain. Difficulty with chewing and swallowing place the patient at a risk for choking and aspiration as the disease progresses. Inappropriate emotional outbursts of laughing and crying can occur. Speech becomes increasingly difficult. Bladder and bowel functions remain intact, yet problems such as constipation, urinary urgency, hesitancy, or frequency can occur.

Late in the disease, communication becomes limited to moving and blinking the eyes in response to questions. Pulmonary function becomes severely compromised to the point of requiring mechanical ventilator assistance if the patient chooses. Other complications can include extreme malnutrition, falls, pulmonary emboli, and congestive heart failure. ALS eventually leads to death from respiratory complications such as atelectasis, respiratory failure, and pneumonia.

Diagnostic Tests

Diagnosis is made based on clinical symptoms. Additional tests such as CSF analysis, electroencephalogram (EEG), nerve biopsy, nerve conduction velocity (NCV), or EMG may be done to rule out other conditions. Blood enzymes can be increased as a result of muscle atrophy.

Therapeutic Measures

There is no cure for ALS, and treatments are palliative in nature. Goals of treatment are aimed at improving function as long as possible and emotionally supporting the patient and family through the illness. Baclofen (Lioresal) and diazepam (Valium) may be given to relieve muscle spasticity. Quinine may be used for muscle cramps. Riluzole (Rilutek) slows the progression of the disease and can prolong life by 3 to 4 months. New treatments are constantly being researched.

Nonpharmacological measures such as physical therapy, massage, position changes, and diversional activities can help control pain. Tube feedings via a surgically placed gastrostomy tube help provide adequate nutrition. Prevention of infections, such as pneumonia and urinary tract infection (UTI), is vital. Meticulous skin care minimizes the incidence of pressure ulcers. Physical, occupational, and speech therapies allow the patient to maximize function and control for as long as possible. Therapy can also decrease the occurrence of complications such as aspiration, falls, and contractures.

• WORD • BUILDING •
amyotrophic: a—without + myo—muscle + trophic—nourishment
atrophy: a—without + trophy—nourishment

Patients with speech problems may benefit from the use of augmentative alternative communication. A variety of such systems are available; most involve laptop computers that patients can use to type in words or symbols to generate speech. Medicare pays at least a portion of the cost for the equipment. Support groups and counseling provide emotional support for the patient and family.

Nursing Care

See the "Nursing Care Plan for the Patient With a Progressive Neuromuscular Disorder."

PATIENT EDUCATION. Reinforce information given by the HCP to the patient and family about ALS and its prognosis. Support groups can provide emotional support as the patient and family deal with the likely reality of untimely death. Assistive devices and exercises help prevent complications. Teaching family members how to perform physical therapy and other health care activities allows the patient to spend as much time as possible at home. Teach the patient to avoid exposure to persons with infections because an infection can be deadly to a patient with a debilitating disease. Request a consultation with a palliative care specialist or other resource person at your institution to help the patient and family develop an advance directive.

NURSING CARE TIP

When planning care, remember that a person with ALS has an intact mind—it is the body that is deteriorating.

CRITICAL THINKING

Mr. Miller

■ Mr. Miller has been having difficulty swallowing. He is diagnosed with ALS.

1. What are the priority nursing diagnoses for Mr. Miller?
2. How can the patient and his family be supported in coping with this disease?
3. What other team members should be consulted for his care?

Suggested answers are at the end of the chapter.

Guillain-Barré Syndrome
Pathophysiology

Guillain-Barré syndrome (GBS) is a rare neuromuscular disease affecting only 1 in every 100,00 persons. Both men and women in the United States are affected equally. Onset is usually between 30 and 50 years of age. GBS is an inflammatory disorder characterized by abrupt onset of symmetrical paresis (weakness) that progresses to paralysis. The myelin sheath

of the spinal and cranial nerves is destroyed by a diffuse inflammatory reaction. The peripheral nerves are infiltrated by lymphocytes, which leads to edema and inflammation. Segmental **demyelination** causes axonal atrophy, resulting in slowed or blocked nerve conduction. Typically, the demyelination begins in the most distal nerves and ascends in a symmetrical fashion. **Remyelination**, which is a much slower process, occurs in a descending pattern and is accompanied by a resolution of symptoms.

There are four recognized variants of GBS; however, only the most common type, ascending GBS, is addressed in this chapter. It is characterized by progressive weakness and numbness that begins in the legs and ascends up the body. The numbness tends to be mild, but the muscle weakness usually progresses to paralysis. The paralysis can ascend all the way to the cranial nerves or stop anywhere between the legs and head. Deep tendon reflexes are either depressed or absent. Respiratory function becomes compromised in approximately 50% of patients with ascending GBS.

Etiology

GBS is believed to be caused by an autoimmune response to some type of viral infection or to certain vaccines, although the exact cause is not known. Usually the viral illness affects the respiratory or GI system, and occurs within 2 weeks before onset of neurologic symptoms. The most common organism found to be associated with GBS is *Campylobacter jejuni*, a common cause of gastroenteritis.

Signs and Symptoms

GBS is divided into three stages.

STAGE 1, ONSET OF SYMPTOMS. The first stage starts with the onset of symptoms and lasts until the progression of symptoms stops. This stage can last from 24 hours to 3 weeks and is characterized by abrupt and rapid onset of muscle weakness and paralysis, with little or no muscle atrophy. Many patients give a history of a recent viral illness or vaccination, supporting the theory that the cause is autoimmune in nature. The degree of respiratory involvement correlates to the type of GBS and the level of paralysis. Patients with ascending GBS may gradually notice a reduced ability to take deep breaths or carry on conversations and may feel short of breath. These patients are terrified that they will not be able to breathe and may require intubation and artificial ventilation.

The autonomic nervous system is often affected by GBS. Patients can experience labile blood pressure, cardiac dysrhythmias, urine retention, or paralytic ileus. Patient reports of discomfort range from annoying numbness and cramping to severe pain. The discomfort is exacerbated by the patient's inability to move voluntarily.

• WORD • BUILDING •

demyelination: de—down or from + myelin—sheath surrounding neurons + ation—process

remyelination: re—repeat + myelin—sheath surrounding neurons + ation—process

STAGE 2, PLATEAU. The second stage is the plateau stage, when symptoms are most severe but progression has stopped. It can last from 2 to 14 days. Patients may become discouraged if no improvement is evident.

STAGE 3, RECOVERY. Axonal regeneration and remyelination occur during the third state, recovery. This stage lasts from 6 to 24 months and symptoms slowly improve. Most patients with GBS recover completely within a few months to a year. A few patients experience chronic disability.

Complications

Complications that can occur include respiratory failure, infection, and depression. Fatigue and paralysis of the respiratory muscles lead to insufficient respiratory effort. Some patients with impending respiratory failure attempt to convince the staff that they are not in distress and do not need to be intubated. It is important to discuss the possible need for intubation early in the patient's illness. The decision to intubate in GBS is different from that with other PNS disorders because GBS patients are expected to recover. It is important to be vigilant in monitoring pulse oximetry, respiratory rate and depth, and dyspnea to predict the need for intervention and maintain the patient's safety.

Patients with GBS are prone to pneumonia and UTIs. Maintaining infection control practices and maximizing the patient's nutritional status help decrease the likelihood of infection. Immobility leads to such problems as skin breakdown, pulmonary embolus, deep venous thrombosis, and muscle atrophy. Patients with GBS have little time to adjust to their illness and deterioration, and often fear they will not recover function. Calm, supportive reassurance is important.

Diagnostic Tests

A lumbar puncture is performed to obtain CSF. The CSF analysis shows a normal cell count with an elevated protein level. Electromyographic and nerve conduction velocity tests are done to evaluate nerve function. Pulmonary function testing helps confirm impending respiratory problems.

Therapeutic Measures

During the initial stages, patients are partially or completely dependent for all needs. They are often frightened and anxious. Oxygen and mechanical ventilation may be required. Plasmapheresis may be used to remove the patient's plasma and replace it with fresh plasma. This procedure is thought to lessen the body's immune response. To be most effective, plasmapheresis should begin 7 to 14 days from the onset of symptoms. Immunoglobulin therapy may help reduce the severity of the disease. Steroid hormones, although used in the past, are not effective and may be harmful. Supportive interventions include anticoagulants to prevent deep vein thrombosis, and analgesics for pain.

During the plateau phase, patients can become discouraged because they are not getting any better. Emotional support is important during this phase. Axonal regeneration and remyelination occur during the recovery phase. Intensive rehabilitation helps the patient regain function during this phase.

Nursing Process for the Patient With Guillain-Barré Syndrome

See the "Nursing Care Plan for the Patient With a Progressive Neuromuscular Disorder." In addition, be prepared to teach the patient and family about the disease and treatment.

DATA COLLECTION. Assess the patient's vital signs, ABGs, and SpO_2 to monitor respiratory status. Assess gag, corneal, and swallowing reflexes to determine whether safety measures are needed to prevent aspiration or injury to the eyes. Assess the patient's and family's knowledge about the disease and treatment.

NURSING DIAGNOSES, PLANNING, AND IMPLEMENTATION.
Deficient Knowledge related to new diagnosis and treatment
EXPECTED OUTCOME: The patient and family will verbalize understanding of what to expect as disease progresses, how treatments will help, and how to participate in care.

• Explain all procedures to the patient and family. *Patients and family members who understand the rationale for assessments or interventions are more likely to cooperate and assist.*
• Educate the patient and family about the need for frequent respiratory assessments and possible need for temporary respiratory support. *Patients may deny respiratory difficulty because of a fear of intubation and mechanical ventilation.*
• Teach and encourage use of diversional activities such as visits from family and friends, listening to music or relaxation tapes, and watching television or videos. *Recovery can be prolonged, and diversional activities can help alleviate boredom, loneliness, and depression.*
• As the patient begins to regain function, assist in teaching patient and family how to participate in patient care and therapies. Encourage family members to attend therapy appointments. *Participation in patient care activities and therapies can provide a sense of control over the situation and helps prepare the patient and family for discharge.*
• Provide information about the disease, treatments, and recovery. *Recovery can take months or years; most of that time will be spent at home.*

EVALUATION. If interventions have been effective, the patient and family will demonstrate understanding of the disease process and participate in care appropriately. Table 50.3 summarizes and compares MS, MG, ALS, and GBS.

Postpolio Syndrome
Pathophysiology and Etiology

Postpolio syndrome is a condition that affects survivors of polio 20 to 40 years after they have recovered from infection caused by the poliomyelitis virus. Up to 40% of patients who previously had polio develop this syndrome. The severity of the syndrome depends on the degree of residual weakness and disability left from the initial illness.

Signs and Symptoms

Postpolio syndrome involves a further weakening of the muscles that were affected with the first involvement with

TABLE 50.3 SUMMARY OF PERIPHERAL NERVOUS SYSTEM DISORDERS

	Multiple Sclerosis	Myasthenia Gravis	Amyotrophic Lateral Sclerosis	Guillain-Barré Syndrome
Signs and Symptoms	Muscle weakness Muscle paralysis Visual disturbances Fatigue	Progressive severe muscle weakness of voluntary muscles Muscles regain strength with rest Masklike face	Progressive muscle weakness Decreased coordination Muscle twitching Muscle spasms Pain Emotional outbursts Difficulty with speech Intact thought processes	Three stages: 1. Ascending paralysis 2. Plateau 3. Descending resolution Pain, cramping or numbness
Diagnosis	CSF analysis MRI gMS DX (blood test)	Ptosis test Tensilon test EMG	CSF analysis EEG Nerve biopsy NCV	CSF EMG NCV
Therapeutic Measures	Interferon therapy Steroids Immunosuppressants Plasmapheresis Anticonvulsants Antiviral agents Muscle relaxants Physical therapy Assistive devices for ADLs Speech therapy	Plasmapheresis Thymectomy Anticholinesterase agents Steroids	Antispasmodics/ quinine Riluzole (Rilutek) Physical therapy Massage Muscle relaxants Diversional activities Tube feeding Alternative communications devices	Plasmapheresis Ventilation support Physical therapy
Complications	Falls Muscle spasms Bowel and bladder problems, risk for UTI Forgetfulness Extreme fatigue	Aspiration Respiratory infections Respiratory failure Myasthenic crisis or cholinergic crisis	Communication problems Risk for aspiration Pain Respiratory failure	Respiratory infection Respiratory failure Depression Fatigue UTI Complications of immobility
Priority Nursing Diagnoses	*Ineffective Airway Clearance* *Impaired Physical Mobility* *Risk for Imbalanced Nutrition: Less Than Body Requirements* *Impaired Communication*			

CSF = cerebrospinal fluid; EEG = electroencephalography; EMG = electromyography; MRI = magnetic resonance imaging; NCV = nerve conduction velocity; UTI = urinary tract infection.

the poliovirus. Symptoms range from fatigue to progressive muscle weakness and atrophy. Sleeping problems, joint pain, scoliosis, and respiratory compromise can occur. Some people suffer great debilitation; others have fewer problems.

Diagnostic Tests

Observation and history and excluding other problems are most important in diagnosis of this syndrome.

Therapeutic Measures

No interventions have been found to be effective at this time. Symptoms seem to be best controlled by rest and moderate exercise without pushing the limits of tolerance.

CRANIAL NERVE DISORDERS

Cranial nerves are the peripheral nerves of the brain. There are 12 pairs of cranial nerves. Areas that the cranial nerves innervate include the head, neck, and special sensory structures (see Chapter 48). Cranial nerve problems are classified as peripheral **neuropathies**. Disorders can affect the sensory, motor, or both branches of a single nerve. Causes of cranial nerve disorders include tumors, infections, inflammation, trauma, and unknown causes. Two common cranial nerve problems are trigeminal neuralgia (tic douloureux) and Bell's palsy.

Trigeminal Neuralgia
Pathophysiology and Etiology

Trigeminal **neuralgia** (TN), sometimes called tic douloureux, involves the fifth cranial (trigeminal) nerve. This cranial nerve has three branches that include both sensory and motor functions. The branches innervate areas of the face, including the forehead, nose, cheek, gums, and jaw. TN affects only the sensory portion of the nerve. Irritation or chronic compression of the nerve is suspected to initiate symptoms. This condition is seen more often in women and usually begins around age 50 to 60.

Signs and Symptoms

Intense recurring episodes of pain, described as sudden, jabbing, burning, or knifelike, characterize this condition. Episodes of pain begin and end suddenly, lasting a few seconds to minutes. Attacks can occur in clusters up to hundreds of times daily. However, some patients have only a few attacks per year. Pain is felt in the skin on one side of the face. A slight touch, cold breeze, talking, or chewing can trigger attacks of pain. The areas of the face where pain is triggered are referred to as trigger zones. Areas affected include the lips, upper or lower gums, cheeks, forehead, or side of the nose (Fig. 50.3). Sleep provides a period of relief from the pain. Therefore, persons with trigeminal neuralgia may sleep most of the time to avoid painful attacks. They also may refrain from activities such as talking, face washing, teeth brushing, shaving, and eating to prevent pain. Frequent blinking and tearing of the eye on the affected side also occur.

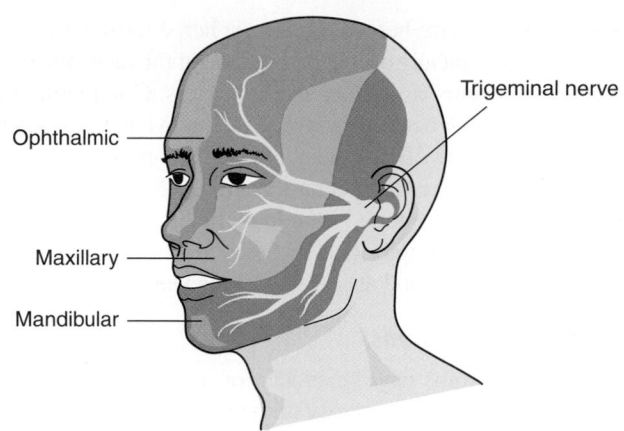

FIGURE 50.3 Areas innervated by the three main branches of the trigeminal nerve (cranial nerve V) are affected in trigeminal neuralgia.

Diagnostic Tests

History of symptoms and direct observation of an attack confirm diagnosis. Radiological studies, including computed tomography (CT) and MRI, may be used to rule out other causes of the pain.

Therapeutic Measures

Initial management includes the use of anticonvulsants such as phenytoin (Dilantin), gabapentin (Neurontin), or carbamazepine (Tegretol) to reduce transmission of painful nerve impulses. Baclofen or clonazepam may also be effective in controlling symptoms. If medications are not effective, a nerve block using a local anesthetic may be performed. This option offers 8 to 16 months of relief. If medications and nerve blocks do not provide relief, a **rhizotomy** can be done to destroy selected nerve fibers. A **neurectomy** may be done if no vessel is found to be compressing the nerve. Surgical options leave the patient with varying degrees of numbness. Complementary and alternative therapies such as acupuncture, electrical stimulation, vitamin and nutritional therapy may be used with varying success.

PATIENT EDUCATION POSTPROCEDURE. The patient will need to learn to protect anesthetized areas of the face after nerve block or ablation. If corneal sensation is lost, goggles and sunglasses should be used as needed to protect the affected eye. An eye patch may be needed at night to prevent injury during sleep. Artificial tears may also be needed to prevent corneal damage.

Bell's Palsy
Pathophysiology and Etiology

In Bell's palsy, the facial nerve (cranial nerve VII) becomes inflamed and edematous, causing interruption of nerve impulses. The cause is thought to be nerve trauma from a viral infection

---

• WORD • BUILDING •

neuropathies: neuro—nerve + pathies—disease
neuralgia: neur—nerve + algia—pain
rhizotomy: rhiz-nerve root + otomy—incision, excision
neurectomy: neur-nerve + ectomy—excision

such as Epstein-Barr, herpes simplex, or herpes zoster. Loss of motor control typically occurs on one side of the face; bilateral facial palsy occurs in less than 1% of cases. Contracture of facial muscles can occur if recovery is slow. Men and women are affected equally. Bell's palsy is more common in women in the third trimester of pregnancy, in people with immune disorders such as human immunodeficiency virus (HIV) infection, and in people with diabetes. It occurs in all ages (including children) and at all times of the year.

Signs and Symptoms

Onset of symptoms may be sudden or may progress over a 2- to 5-day period. The severity of the paralysis usually peaks within several days of onset of symptoms. Pain behind the ear may precede the onset of facial paralysis. Other vague initial symptoms are dry eye or tingling around the lips with progression to the more recognizable symptoms of Bell's palsy. The patient may be unable to close the eyelid, wrinkle the forehead, smile, raise the eyebrow, or close the lips effectively. The mouth is pulled toward the unaffected side (Fig. 50.4). Drooling of saliva occurs, and the affected eye has constant tearing. Sense of taste is lost over the anterior two-thirds of the tongue. Speech difficulties occur. Fifty percent of patients will have complete recovery in a short period of time. Thirty-five percent will experience full recovery in less than 1 year ("Patient Perspective—Angela, Bell's Palsy").

Forehead not wrinkled

Eyeball rolls up, eyelid does not close

Flat nasal labial fold, paralysis of lower face

A

B   Facial nerve

FIGURE 50.4 Bell's palsy. (A) Note weakness of affected side of face. (B) Distribution of facial nerve.

Patient Perspective

Angela, Bell's Palsy

I woke up that Thursday morning with the same intense pain in my forehead that I had been experiencing for the past week. When I rolled out of bed, I realized that I didn't have morning breath (or so I thought). Knowing that I had not brushed my teeth yet, I proceeded to do so and noticed that I could not taste the toothpaste. The fruit cup I ate for lunch tasted like Clorox. I chomped up and down on each bite, then carefully attempted to swallow. It was like I had been injected with several shots of Novocain. My throat felt like it had closed up, and each swallow took a concentrated effort. Over the course of eating my fruit, I managed to bite my tongue three times.

I was 35 weeks pregnant and on strict bedrest due to pregnancy-induced hypertension and severe edema (which later spiraled into toxemia). We attributed the numbness in my mouth to the edema. I had already swollen up like a balloon and had experienced intense numbness in my extremities since the 12th week of pregnancy. As the afternoon progressed, I grew more and more concerned. I knew something was not quite right. By 5:30 that evening, I had lost control of the entire left side of my face. I called my obstetrician, and she said to get to the ER because I was either having a stroke or had developed Bell's palsy. The doctor at the ER confirmed that I had Bell's palsy and prescribed Valtrex and prednisone to treat it.

The symptoms of Bell's that I experienced were severe pain in my forehead, not being able to breathe out of the left side of my nose, and difficulty chewing, swallowing, and saying most consonants. I completely lost the ability to smile, blink, close my eye, raise my eyebrow, or use a straw or blow. My eyesight in the left eye blurred, and I could not go out at night due to the intense pain behind my eye triggered by headlights and having to use eyedrops every 5 to 20 minutes.

I delivered my baby (after induction, 2 days of labor, 2 hours of pushing, and emergency C section) 2 weeks after being diagnosed with Bell's palsy. During labor, I continuously asked for my eyedrops and the pain in my head was so fierce that it overshadowed the contractions.

After delivery, I was desperate for my face to be "fixed." I tried everything that anyone suggested: herbal supplements, chiropractic, facial massage, laser treatments, facial exercise, shock treatments, a neurologist consultation, and physical therapy. The only thing that has worked for me is time (and lots of it)!

For the first 15 weeks after being diagnosed, I wanted to hide from the world. However, here it is

7 months later, and I have come to terms with it. I am constantly aware of it, though I have regained a tremendous amount of the muscle control. I still have not shared a "real smile" with my daughter and do not blink my left eye. Covering my mouth when I smile or laugh so others do not see has become almost like a reflex now.

Diagnostic Tests

History of the onset of symptoms is used to diagnose Bell's palsy. Observation of the patient confirms the diagnosis. EMG may be done. The possibility of a stroke must be ruled out.

Therapeutic Measures

Prevention of complications is the goal of treatment. Prednisone may be given over 7 to 10 days to decrease inflammation. Antiviral agents such as acyclovir may be used to fight the virus and can shorten the course of the disease. Analgesics are given for pain control. Moist heat and gentle massage to the face and ear also ease pain. A facial sling can be used to aid in eating and support of facial muscles.

Nursing Process for the Patient with a Cranial Nerve Disorder (Trigeminal Neuralgia and Bell's Palsy)

DATA COLLECTION. Assess attacks using the **WHAT'S UP?** format, being sure to include factors that trigger pain. Are sensory or motor problems associated with the pain? Assess the effect of the disorder on the patient's life, including nutritional status, general and oral hygiene, behavior, and emotional state. Carefully document all findings.

NURSING DIAGNOSES, PLANNING, AND IMPLEMENTATION.
Acute Pain related to inflammation or compression of the nerve
Expected Outcome: The patient will state pain is controlled at an acceptable level.

- Assess pain level and response to interventions as needed. *Assessment guides intervention.*
- Administer medications as needed for pain. Anticonvulsant and antidepressant agents used to treat neuropathic pain must be given routinely to prevent pain. *Medications prevent or decrease pain and increase comfort.*
- Discuss and implement alternative and complementary pain relief measures *to complement medications and increase patient's control over pain.*
  - Biofeedback
  - Diversional activities
- Plan hygiene activities when pain relief is at its peak *to decrease discomfort with activities.*
- Provide alternative communication methods. *The patient may not be able to speak clearly or want to speak due to pain.*
  - Paper and pencil/pen
  - Dry erase board
  - Communication board
  - Pain scales for pointing to level of pain.

- Teach the patient to chew on the opposite side of the face *to avoid triggering pain and injury.*
- Encourage use of an electric razor rather than blades *to prevent injury to numb areas.*
- Provide measures for trigeminal neuralgia *to reduce pain triggers.*
  - Provide soft cloths for facial hygiene using lukewarm water.
  - Avoid touching the patient's face.
  - Provide a soft bristle toothbrush for oral care.
  - Teach patient to protect face from cold or wind.
- Provide measures for Bell's palsy *to reduce pain and prevent muscle atrophy.*
  - Provide warm, moist compresses prn.
  - Massage face.
  - Assist with facial exercises as prescribed by physical therapy.
  - Provide a facial sling.

Imbalanced Nutrition: Less Than Body Requirements, related to fear of triggering pain as evidenced by poor intake, weight loss
Expected Outcome: The patient will maintain sufficient nutrition as evidenced by stable weight.

- Weigh patient twice weekly and record *to monitor weight loss or gain.*
- Provide small, frequent meals *to promote nutrition without increasing pain.*
- Provide soft, easy-to-chew foods at lukewarm temperature *to prevent triggering pain.*
- Provide a high-protein and high-calorie diet. *Protein and calories are needed for cellular repair.*
- Avoid hot or cold foods and drinks. *Temperature extremes can trigger pain. If foods are associated with pain, the patient may avoid them.*
- Encourage oral hygiene after each meal and at bedtime *to prevent gum and tooth disease as triggers for pain.*
- Insert a feeding tube as ordered on unaffected side if nutrition is severely impaired *to provide means for nutrient intake while avoiding painful nerve areas.*

Risk for Injury to Eyes related to inability to blink (Bell's palsy)
Expected Outcome: The patient's cornea will remain intact and without injury.

- Administer eyedrops or eye ointment as ordered by the HCP *to protect the eye.*
- Teach patient to use a patch over the affected eye *to protect the eye.*
- Advise patient to wear glasses or goggles, especially when outside or in areas with particles in the air, *to protect the eyes.*

EVALUATION. Nursing care has been successful if the patient reports that pain is controlled, nutrition is maintained with no inappropriate weight loss, and the eyes are intact and without injury. Table 50.4 summarizes and compares trigeminal neuralgia and Bell's palsy.

TABLE 50.4 SUMMARY OF CRANIAL NERVE DISORDERS

	Trigeminal Neuralgia	Bell's Palsy
Cranial Nerve Involved	5th sensory	7th motor
Signs and Symptoms	Intense pain on one side of face: • Sudden onset • Jabbing, burning, knifelike Sensitive to temperature, air flow, and touch Pain exacerbated by talking or chewing Frequent blinking or tearing of the eye on affected side	Loss of motor control, paralysis on one side of face Variable onset of symptoms Facial droop and inability to close affected eye Drooling Loss of taste over anterior tongue Speech difficulties
Diagnosis	History CT MRI	History EMG
Therapeutic Measures	Anticonvulsants Antispasmodics Nerve block with local anesthetic Surgical radio-frequency ablation	Prednisone Analgesics Moist heat Gentle massage Facial sling
Complications	Corneal damage Poor nutrition Depression	Corneal damage Poor nutrition Depression
Priority Nursing Diagnoses	*Acute Pain* *Imbalanced Nutrition: Less Than Body Requirements* *Risk for Injury* to eye (Bell's palsy)	

CT = computed tomography; EMG = electromyography; MRI = magnetic resonance imaging.

LEARNING TIP

Remember! TN (cranial nerve V) is a sensory disorder; Bell's palsy (cranial nerve VII) is a motor disorder.

Home Health Hints

• If a homebound patient has difficulty speaking (dysarthria), try using magnetic alphabet letters. Ask questions that require a yes or no answer. The patient can respond with the letter Y or N.
• Keep bedside commode lids up with patches of Velcro attached to the seat and the frame.
• Do a thorough nutritional assessment for patients with a history of trigeminal neuralgia to identify if there is a risk for malnutrition.
• Patients with trigeminal neuralgia may benefit from using a small spoon and softer foods for eating during periods of mild to moderate pain.

SUGGESTED ANSWERS TO

CRITICAL THINKING

■ *Jamie*

1. Muscle weakness caused by myasthenia gravis improves with rest.

2. Have Jamie look up for 2 to 3 minutes. If ptosis occurs, have her close her eyes for several minutes. If she can open her eyelids and look up, myasthenia gravis is likely.

3.
$$\frac{2 \text{ mg}}{} \frac{1 \text{ mL}}{10 \text{ mg}} = 0.2 \text{ mL}$$

4. Team: nurse, OT, PT, neurologist, pharmacist, dietitian, and primary HCP for other health issues.

■ *Mr. Miller*

1. Priority nursing diagnoses include *Ineffective Airway Clearance* related to muscle weakness and *Risk for Aspiration* related to muscle weakness. If a patient's respiratory system is compromised by a disease, nursing care should be focused on maintaining pulmonary function to preserve life.

2. Providing compassionate care to the patient and providing information about the disease and its prognosis to the patient and family establish an honest and supportive relationship. Support groups provide resources and emotional support.

3. Team: RN, respiratory therapy, speech pathologist, neurologist, dietitian. In addition, find out who at your institution helps patients make end-of-life decisions. A palliative care specialist or social worker can help the patient and family work through some difficult decisions and develop an advance directive.

REVIEW QUESTIONS

1. A patient with trigeminal neuralgia asks the nurse why carbamazepine (Tegretol) has been ordered. Which response is best?
   1. "It will help decrease the inflammation in your nervous system."
   2. "It will depress your immune system, which can slow the progression of the disease."
   3. "Carbamazepine is used to help relieve nerve pain."
   4. "It is an anticonvulsant to prevent seizures."

2. A patient with amyotrophic lateral sclerosis (ALS) expresses concern about not having enough breath to sing anymore. Which explanation by the nurse is best?
   1. "ALS can damage the nerves to your bronchi and bronchioles, causing constriction and reduced airflow."
   2. "The demyelination of your nerves caused by ALS causes confusion in the impulses to your lungs."
   3. "ALS can affect your vocal cords, making it difficult to form sounds as you speak or sing."
   4. "ALS may be affecting the nerves that go to your respiratory muscles, making them weak."

3. A patient who is newly diagnosed with ALS says to the nurse, "I do not want to be kept alive on machines." Which nursing action is best in response?
   1. Ask the patient whether advance directives have been prepared and provide information if indicated.
   2. Reassure the patient that decisions about machines will not have to be made for a long time.
   3. Inform the patient that individuals with ALS are not candidates for artificial ventilation.
   4. Explain to the patient that a ventilator will be necessary to maintain respiratory function as the disease progresses.

4. When caring for a patient admitted with Guillain-Barré syndrome, which nursing diagnosis should take priority?
   1. Anxiety
   2. Imbalanced Nutrition
   3. Impaired Gas Exchange
   4. Impaired Mobility

5. Which nursing interventions are appropriate for the patient with Bell's palsy? **Select all that apply.**
   1. Administer moisturizing eyedrops.
   2. Apply an eye patch.
   3. Avoid touching the patient's face.
   4. Apply warm compresses.
   5. Provide facial massage.
   6. Teach the patient to protect the face from cool breezes.

6. Which meal would be the best choice for a patient with myasthenia gravis?
   1. Baked chicken sandwich, fresh carrots, apple
   2. Meatloaf, mashed potatoes, canned green beans
   3. Steak, baked potato, green salad
   4. Tacos, fresh vegetables, sliced peaches

7. How will the visiting nurse caring for a patient with myasthenia gravis and severe muscle weakness know if interventions have been effective?
   1. The patient verbalizes satisfaction with the plan of care.
   2. The patient states understanding of the medication regimen.
   3. The patient and family state that no further home visits are needed.
   4. The patient is able to perform ADLs with Sao_2 remaining at 95%.

Answers can be found in Appendix C.

References

Karadimas, C. L., Vu, T. H., Holve, S. A., Chronopoulou, P., Quinzii, C., . . . Hirano, M. (2006). Navajo neurohepatopathy is caused by a mutation in the MPV17 gene. *American Journal of Human Genetics, 79,* 544–548. Retrieved on June 30, 2013, from www.ncbi.nlm.nih.gov/pmc/articles/PMC1559552/

Multiple Sclerosis Association of America. (2013). Long-term treatments for MS. Retrieved June 29, 2013, from http://mymsaa .org/about-ms/treatments/long-term

National Multiple Sclerosis Society. (2013). *About MS.* Retrieved June 29, 2013, from www.nationalmssociety.org/about-multiple -sclerosis/index.aspx

 For additional resources and information visit **davispl.us/medsurg5**

unit FOURTEEN

Understanding the Sensory System

51

Sensory System Function, Assessment, and Therapeutic Measures: Vision and Hearing

KEY TERMS

accommodation (ah-KOM-uh-DAY-shun)
arcus senilus (AR-kuss seh-NILL-uss)
cochlear implant (KOK-lee-ur IM-plant)
consensual response (kon-SEN-shoo-uhl ree-SPONS)
electroretinography (ee-LEK-troh-RET-in-AW-gruh-fee)
esotropia (ESS-oh-TROH-pee-ah)
exotropia (EKS-oh-TROH-pee-ah)
hearing aid (HEER-ing AYD)
hypotropia (HYE-poh-TROH-pee-ah)
nystagmus (nye-STAG-mus)
ophthalmologist (AWF-thal-MAW-luh-jist)
ophthalmoscope (awf-THAL-muh-skohp)
optician (awp-TISH-uhn)
optometrist (awp-TOM-uh-trist)
otalgia (oh-TAL-jee-ah)
otorrhea (OH-toh-REE-ah)
ototoxic (OH-toh-TOK-sik)
ptosis (TOH-sis)
Rinne test (RIH-nee TEST)
Romberg's test (RAHM-bergs TEST)
Snellen's chart (SNEL-enz CHART)
tropia (TROH-pee-ah)
Weber test (VAY-ber TEST)

LAZETTE V. NOWICKI
AND JANICE L. BRADFORD

LEARNING OUTCOMES

1. Describe the normal anatomy of the sensory system.
2. Explain the normal function of the sensory system.
3. List data to collect when caring for a patient with a disorder of the sensory system.
4. Identify diagnostic tests commonly performed to diagnose disorders of the sensory system.
5. Plan nursing care for patients undergoing diagnostic tests for sensory disorders.
6. Describe therapeutic measures for patients with disorders of the sensory system.

Our eyes and ears provide us with a great deal of sensory information. It is difficult to imagine what it would be like not to see or hear the world around us. Nurses have an important role in assessing vision and hearing. Patients depend on health care personnel to assist them in maintaining these primary senses. To learn more about ways to promote vision and hearing health, visit http://web.health.gov/healthypeople.

VISION

Normal Anatomy and Physiology of the Eye
External Structures

Several structures protect the eye from debris and desiccation (extreme dryness; Figs. 51.1 and 51.2).

Eyebrow: Perhaps the most significant role of the eyebrows is to enhance facial expressions, aiding in nonverbal communication. They also help keep perspiration out of the eye and shield the eye from glare.

Eyelashes: These hairs along the edges of the eyelids help keep debris out of the eye. Touching the eyelashes stimulates the blink reflex.

Eyelids (palpebrae): Formed primarily by the orbicularis oculi muscle covered with skin, the eyelids protect the eye from foreign bodies and block light when closed to allow for sleeping. Periodic blinking also helps moisten the eyes with tears and wash out debris.

Conjunctiva: The conjunctiva is a transparent mucous membrane that lines the inner surface of the eyelid and covers the anterior surface of the eyeball (except for the cornea). It secretes a thin mucous film to help keep the eyeball moist. It is very vascular, which becomes apparent when eyes are "bloodshot," a result of dilated vessels in the conjunctiva.

Lateral canthus

Medial canthus

Palpebral fissure: This is the opening between the lids.

Tarsal glands: These glands, which lie along the thickened area at the edge of the eye (called the **tarsal plate**), secrete oil to slow the evaporation of tears and help form a barrier seal when the eyes are closed.

FIGURE 51.1 Accessory structures of the eye. From Thompson, G. S. (2013). *Understanding anatomy and physiology.* Philadelphia: F.A. Davis, p. 209.

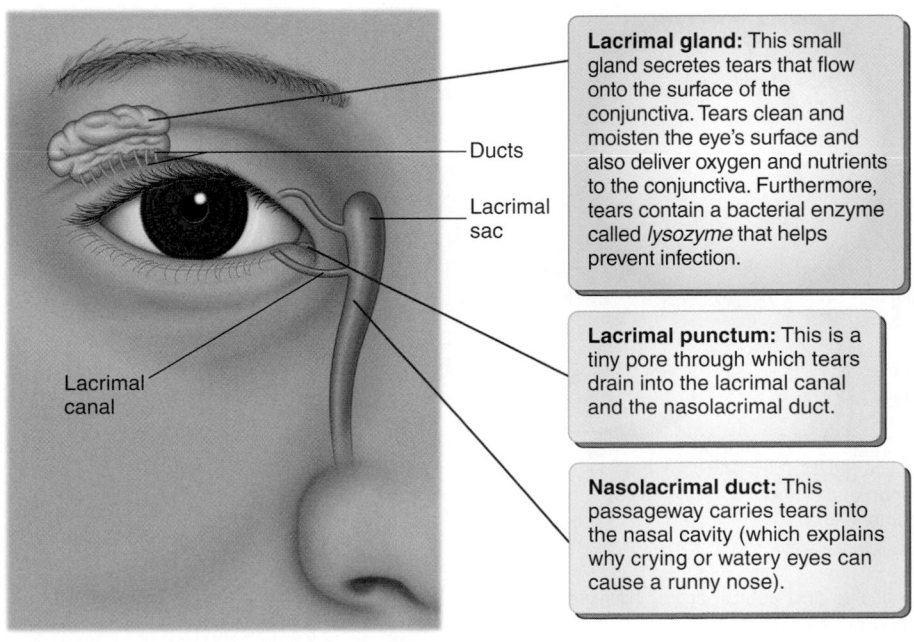

Lacrimal gland: This small gland secretes tears that flow onto the surface of the conjunctiva. Tears clean and moisten the eye's surface and also deliver oxygen and nutrients to the conjunctiva. Furthermore, tears contain a bacterial enzyme called *lysozyme* that helps prevent infection.

Ducts

Lacrimal sac

Lacrimal punctum: This is a tiny pore through which tears drain into the lacrimal canal and the nasolacrimal duct.

Lacrimal canal

Nasolacrimal duct: This passageway carries tears into the nasal cavity (which explains why crying or watery eyes can cause a runny nose).

FIGURE 51.2 Lacrimal apparatus. From Thompson, G. S. (2013). *Understanding anatomy and physiology.* Philadelphia: F.A. Davis, p. 209.

Structure of the Eyeball

Most of the eyeball is within the orbit, the bony socket that protects the eye from trauma. The six extrinsic muscles that move the eyeball are attached to the orbit and to the outer surface of the eyeball. There are four rectus muscles that move the eyeball side to side or up and down, and two oblique muscles that rotate the eye. The cranial nerves that innervate these muscles are the oculomotor, trochlear, and abducens (third, fourth, and sixth cranial nerves, respectively). Actions of the six extrinsic eye muscles not only allow voluntary control of movement but also will be innervated by the autonomic nervous system to perform convergence, an alignment of the visual axis of each eye on the same field of view.

The wall of the eyeball has three layers: the outer fibrous tunic (sclera and cornea), the middle vascular tunic (choroid, ciliary body that suspends the lens, and iris), and the inner nervous tunic (retina; Fig. 51.3). The lens divides the interior of the eye into two main cavities: anterior cavity and posterior cavity (Fig. 51.4). Anterior to the lens is the ring-shaped curtain called the iris, which divides the anterior cavity into two chambers: anterior chamber and posterior chamber.

The retina lines the posterior two-thirds of the eyeball and contains the photoreceptors (rods and cones). Rods detect only the presence of light, whereas cones respond to photons of differing wavelengths. The fovea centralis is a small depression in the macula lutea of the posterior retina, directly behind the center of the lens, and contains only cones. It

is, therefore, the area of most acute color vision. Rods are proportionately more abundant toward the periphery of the retina, and for this reason night vision is best at the sides of the visual field.

Neurons called ganglion cells transmit the impulses generated by the rods and cones. These neurons all converge at the optic disc and pass through the wall of the eyeball as the optic nerve. The optic disc may also be called the blind spot because no rods or cones are present.

Physiology of Vision

Vision involves the focusing of light rays on the retina and the transmission of the subsequent nerve impulses to the visual areas of the cerebral cortex.

The refractive structures of the eye are, in order, the cornea, aqueous humor, lens, and vitreous humor. The lens is the only adjustable part of this focusing system. When the eye shifts focus to an object that is near, accommodation of the lens occurs (Fig. 51.5). Also, the pupil will constrict in near vision to force photons through the thickness of the lens (Fig. 51.6). Accommodation and pupil constriction increase the number of photons that strike the fovea centralis.

When photons strike the retina, they stimulate chemical reactions in the rods and cones. Resultant changes generate a nerve impulse for transmission. Rods generate an action potential in dim light but only allow shades of gray vision. The cones are specialized to respond to a portion of the visible

Fibrous Outer Layer

The **sclera**—formed from dense connective tissue— is the outermost layer of the eye. Most of the sclera is white and opaque; it forms what is called "the white of the eye." Blood vessels and nerves run throughout the sclera.

The **cornea** is a transparent extension of the sclera in the anterior part of the eye. It sits over the iris (the colored portion of the eye) and admits light into the eye. It contains no blood vessels.

Vascular Middle Layer

The **iris** is a ring of colored muscle; it works to adjust the diameter of the pupil (the central opening of the iris) to control the amount of light entering the eye.

The **ciliary body** is a thickened extension of the choroid that forms a collar around the lens. It also secretes a fluid called aqueous humor.

The **choroid** is a highly vascular layer of tissue that supplies oxygen and nutrients to the retina and sclera.

Neural Inner Layer

The **retina** is a thin layer of light-sensitive cells.

Exiting from the posterior portion of the eyeball is the **optic nerve** (cranial nerve II), which transmits signals to the brain.

FIGURE 51.3 Eye tissue layers—fibrous, vascular and neural. From Thompson, G. S. (2013). *Understanding anatomy and physiology.* Philadelphia: F.A. Davis, p. 211.

The space between the lens and the cornea is the **anterior cavity**. This cavity is further divided into an *anterior chamber* (anterior to the iris) and a *posterior chamber* (posterior to the iris but anterior to the lens). A clear, watery fluid called **aqueous humor** fills the anterior cavity.

The **lens** is a transparent disc of tissue just behind the pupil, between the anterior and posterior cavities. The lens changes shape for near and far vision.

Anterior chamber
Canal of Schlemm
Posterior chamber

The **posterior cavity** is the larger cavity lying posterior to the lens. It is filled with a jelly-like substance called **vitreous humor**. This semi-solid material helps keep the eyeball from collapsing.

The ciliary body secretes aqueous humor that fills the anterior cavity. The fluid flows from the posterior chamber, through the pupil, and into the anterior chamber. It then drains into a blood vessel called the **canal of schlemm**.

FIGURE 51.4 Chambers and fluids. From Thompson, G. S. (2013). *Understanding anatomy and physiology*. Philadelphia: F.A. Davis, p. 212.

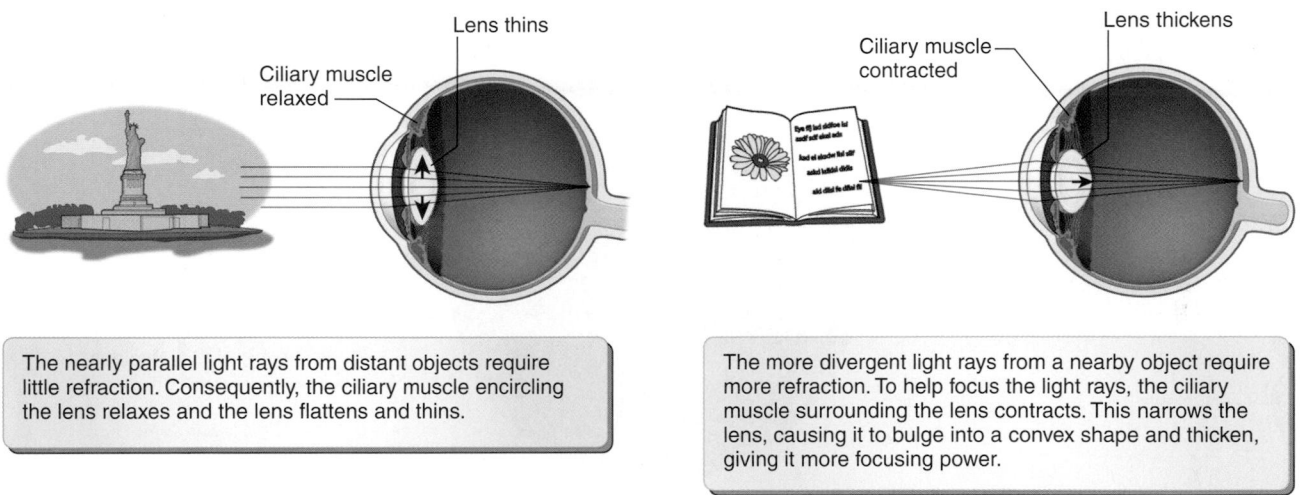

Lens thins
Ciliary muscle relaxed

Ciliary muscle contracted
Lens thickens

The nearly parallel light rays from distant objects require little refraction. Consequently, the ciliary muscle encircling the lens relaxes and the lens flattens and thins.

The more divergent light rays from a nearby object require more refraction. To help focus the light rays, the ciliary muscle surrounding the lens contracts. This narrows the lens, causing it to bulge into a convex shape and thicken, giving it more focusing power.

FIGURE 51.5 Accommodation of the lens. From Thompson, G. S. (2013). *Understanding anatomy and physiology*. Philadelphia: F.A. Davis, p. 215.

light spectrum; there are red-absorbing, blue-absorbing, and green-absorbing cones. Differing combinations of three cone types allow interpretation of color (Fig. 51.7).

Refraction inverts the image onto the photoreceptors in the retina. The impulses from the rods and cones are transmitted to the ganglion neurons, which converge at the optic disc and become the optic nerve. The optic nerves from both eyes converge at the optic chiasma, just in front of the pituitary gland. Here, the medial fibers of each optic nerve cross to the other side. This crossing permits each visual area to receive impulses from both eyes, which is important for binocular vision.

The visual areas are in the occipital lobes of the cerebral cortex. It is here that the upside-down retinal images are

righted and the slightly different pictures from the two eyes are integrated into one image; this is binocular vision, which also provides depth perception.

Aging and the Eye

The most common changes in the aging eye are those in the lens (Fig. 51.8). With age, the lens may become partially or totally opaque. The lens also loses its elasticity with age; most people become farsighted as they age and by 40 years begin to need corrective lenses. Peripheral vision losses may occur. Depth perception decreases and glare intensifies, both of which can affect safety. Color vision fades with lesser discrimination of blue, green, and violet colors. Red, yellow, and orange colors are best visible.

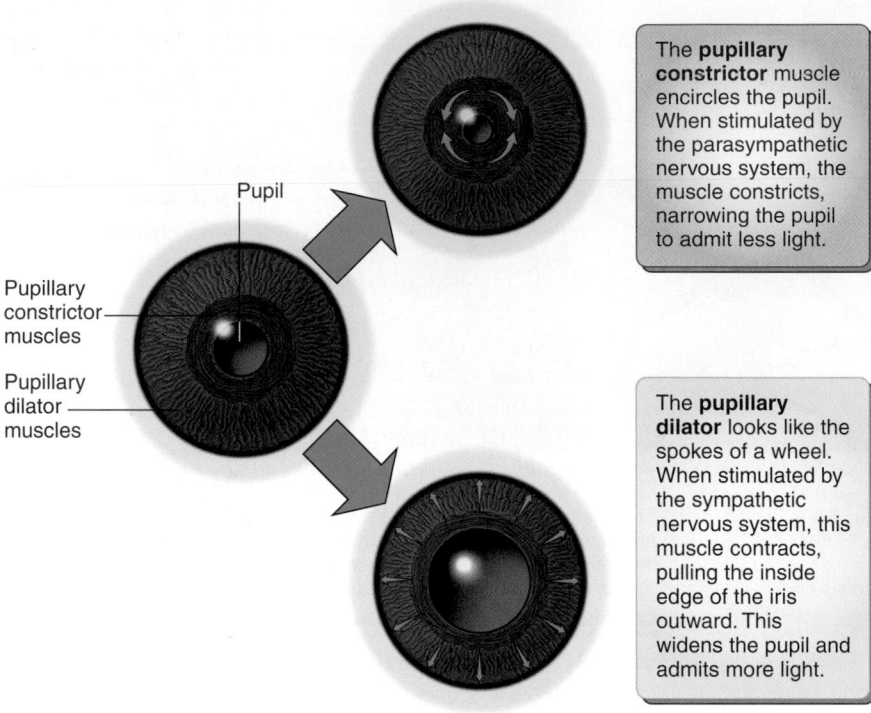

The **pupillary constrictor** muscle encircles the pupil. When stimulated by the parasympathetic nervous system, the muscle constricts, narrowing the pupil to admit less light.

The **pupillary dilator** looks like the spokes of a wheel. When stimulated by the sympathetic nervous system, this muscle contracts, pulling the inside edge of the iris outward. This widens the pupil and admits more light.

FIGURE 51.6 Constriction of the pupil. From Thompson, G. S. (2013). *Understanding anatomy and physiology.* Philadelphia: F.A. Davis, p. 215.

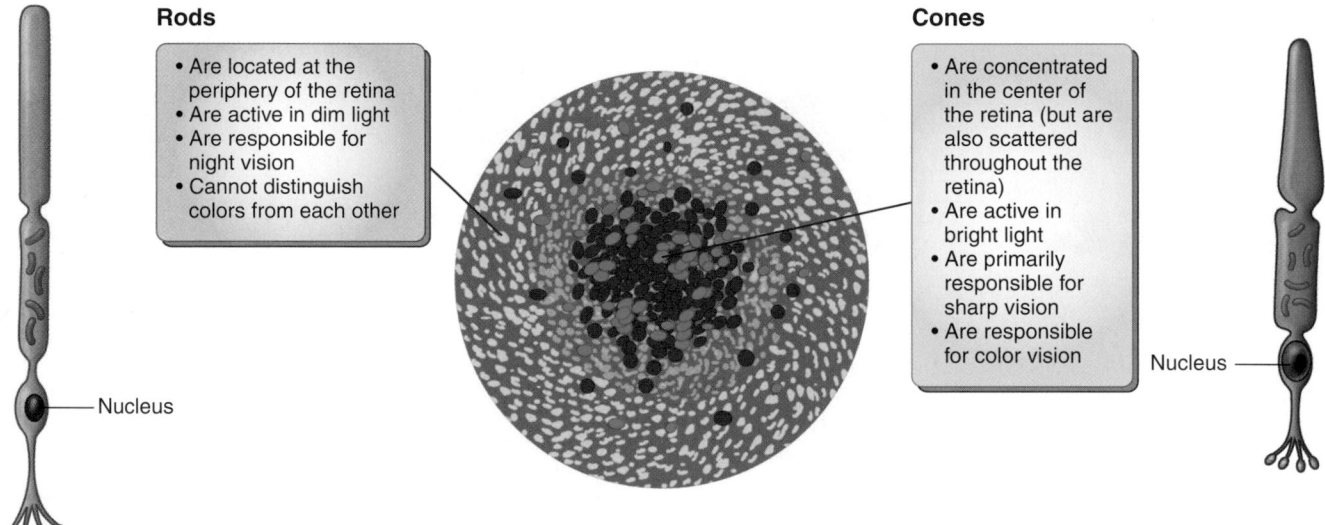

Rods
- Are located at the periphery of the retina
- Are active in dim light
- Are responsible for night vision
- Cannot distinguish colors from each other

Cones
- Are concentrated in the center of the retina (but are also scattered throughout the retina)
- Are active in bright light
- Are primarily responsible for sharp vision
- Are responsible for color vision

Nucleus

Nucleus

FIGURE 51.7 Action of photoreceptors. From Thompson, G. S. (2013). *Understanding anatomy and physiology.* Philadelphia: F.A. Davis, p. 216.

Nursing Assessment of the Eye and Visual Status

Nursing assessment of the eye begins with the collection of subjective data, then moves to observation and testing, and finally, a more invasive physical examination. Licensed practical nurses/licensed vocational nurses (LPN/LVNs) usually assist the health care provider (HCP) in conducting invasive data collection.

Health History

The nurse asks about family history that may affect vision, particularly glaucoma, diabetes, blindness, and cataracts. Many eye disorders are genetically transmitted, so this information alerts the nurse to potential alterations in eye health. Patients are asked about their general health and diseases such as diabetes and hypertension. A patient medication review looks for any ocular (eye) effects. Then, the nurse asks the patient about any changes in visual acuity or symptoms of abnormality (Table 51.1).

Physical Examination

VISUAL ACUITY. Objective data collection begins by checking the patient's visual acuity (Table 51.2). Visual acuity is measured in a variety of ways but usually starts with the use of **Snellen's chart**, an E chart, or a handheld visual acuity chart (Rosenbaum's card) to test near and far vision. Snellen's chart

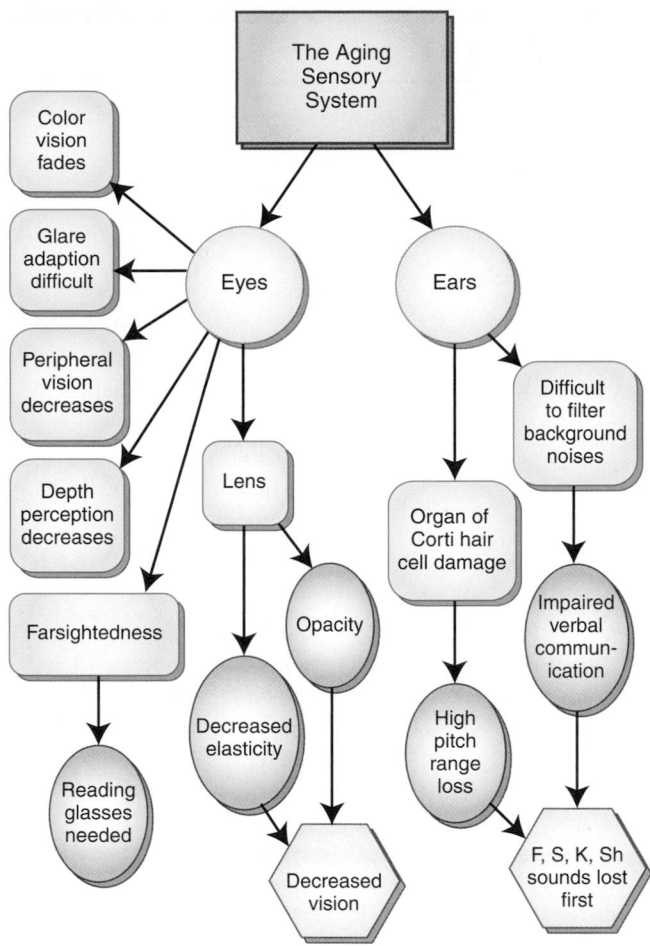

FIGURE 51.8 Aging and the sensory system.

has alphabetical letters graduating in size from the smallest on the bottom to the largest on the top (Fig. 51.9). The examiner measures 20 feet and marks the distance on the floor. The examiner then asks the patient to cover one eye with a 3 × 5 card or eye cover and then read out loud an indicated line of letters. The lowest line on the chart that the patient is able to read accurately is used to indicate visual acuity for that eye. Normal vision is 20/20, which means the patient can read at 20 feet what the normal eye can read at 20 feet.

Low vision occurs at 20/70 and legal blindness at 20/200 or less in the best eye with the best possible correction. An example of visual findings is the patient who identifies all of the letters correctly on the line marked 30; this patient has a visual acuity of 20/30. This means that the patient can see at 20 feet what the average individual can see at 30 feet. The examination is conducted on both eyes separately, then together, and documented as follows: "oculus dexter (OD) [right eye] 20/30, oculus sinister (OS) [left eye] 20/20, oculus uterque (OU) [both eyes] 20/20."

In addition to identifying the eye tested, the examiner conducts the examination with and without the patient's corrective lenses, if applicable. When corrective lenses are used, documentation reflects this as "OD 20/100 without correction, OD 20/20 with correction." The E chart is used for patients who have literacy issues. The patient is asked to indicate the direction of the E-shaped figure. The handheld

visual acuity chart is used to indicate visual acuity by having the patient hold the card approximately 14 inches from the eyes. The test is conducted and documented in the same way as the Snellen's and E chart examinations.

Visual Fields by Confrontation. The examiner also tests peripheral vision, which is the ability of the eye to see objects peripherally while the eye is fixed or kept in one position. This is also known as testing visual fields by confrontation. To do this, the examiner compares his or her own ability to see peripheral objects with that of the patient. This test should be done with an examiner who has normal peripheral vision. The examiner stands 2 feet in front of, and facing, the patient and instructs the patient to cover one eye. The examiner covers his or her own corresponding eye (the eye that is aligned with the patient's eye; e.g., if the patient's right eye is covered, the examiner's left eye is covered). The examiner uses the arm opposite the covered eye, extends it to the space midway between the patient and the examiner, and brings it toward the eye from three directions: superior, inferior, and temporal (middle). The examiner wiggles the finger while moving the arm. The examiner asks the patient to look straight ahead and indicate at what point he or she is able to see the examiner's finger. One eye is tested and then the other. The patient has full visual fields if the point at which the patient sees the finger matches that at which the examiner sees it. The examiner documents the results as "visual fields equal to examiner," "full visual fields," or, if abnormal, "visual fields unequal to examiner in. . ." (identify position, e.g., left superior).

MUSCLE BALANCE AND EYE MOVEMENT. The examiner tests extraocular muscle balance and cranial nerve function by instructing the patient to look straight ahead and follow the examiner's finger movement without moving his or her head. As with the confrontation test, the patient and examiner face each other either standing or sitting. The examiner moves his or her finger in the six cardinal fields of gaze, coming back to the point of origin between each field of gaze (Fig. 51.10). If the patient's eyes are able to follow the examiner's finger in all fields of gaze without nystagmus, the patient is assessed to have adequate extraocular muscle strength and innervation. Nystagmus is an involuntary, cyclical, rapid movement of the eyes in response to vertical, horizontal, or rotary movement.

The corneal light reflex test assesses muscle balance. This test is conducted by shining a penlight toward the cornea while the patient is staring at an object straight ahead. The light reflection should be at exactly the same place on both pupils. If the eyes lack symmetry, muscle weakness could be present.

The cover test is used in conjunction with an abnormal corneal light reflex test to evaluate muscle balance. The patient is asked to look straight ahead at a far object. The examiner covers one of the patient's eyes with a 3 × 5 card. The uncovered eye should have a steady gaze; if it moves, there may be muscle weakness. Next, the cover is quickly removed and the action of this eye is observed. If this eye moves to fixate on the light instead of staring straight ahead, it indicates a drifting of the eye when it was covered, which is a sign of muscle weakness. This deviation of the eye away

TABLE **51.1** SUBJECTIVE DATA COLLECTION FOR THE EYE

Category	Questions to Ask During the Health History	Rationale/Significance
Family History	Do you have any family members with a history of diabetes? Hypertension? Cataracts? Glaucoma? Blindness? Diabetes mellitus? Do any family members wear glasses or contact lenses? Is their vision corrected with the lens?	Many eye disorders are genetically transmitted.
Patient's General Health	How would you describe your general health? What health problems do you currently have? How are they treated? What health problems have you had in the past? Have you ever had trauma to your eyes? What medications do you take? How often do you have eye examinations? When was the last time you had an eye examination?	Some metabolic disorders are precursors to eye disorders, such as diabetes and hypertension. Assess for ocular effects of systemic medications. Assess preventive practices.
Visual Acuity	Do you wear glasses or contact lenses? Have you had any changes in vision such as difficulty seeing distances, difficulty seeing close up, difficulty seeing at night? Do you see things double? Do you have clouded vision? Do you see halos around lights? Does it look like you are looking through a veil or web? Is there sensitivity to light? Is there pain? Itching? Tearing? Burning? Do you have headaches? If so, what are the precipitating events?	Any of these signs and symptoms could indicate visual disorders/disturbances.

TABLE **51.2** OBJECTIVE DATA COLLECTION FOR THE EYE

Category	Physical Examination Findings	Possible Abnormal Findings/Causes
Visual Acuity	Normal vision is 20/20.	Hyperopia, myopia, presbyopia, blurred or cloudy vision Possible causes: refractive error, opacity, or disorder of pathway
Visual Fields	Full peripheral fields	Peripheral field loss
Muscle Balance and Eye Movement	Movement in all six cardinal fields of gaze Corneal light reflex test (Light is at the same place on both pupils.) Cover test–steady gaze	Nystagmus Inability to move in all six fields can indicate cranial nerve impairment Asymmetry could mean muscle weakness Drifting eye indicates muscle weakness
Pupillary Reflexes	Pupillary light reflex Accommodation	Dilated, fixed, or constricted pupils Absence of constriction or convergence
External Structures	Inspection and palpation of eyebrows, orbital area, eyelids, palpebral fissure, medial canthus, irises, corneal clarity, anterior chamber	Ptosis (drooping of eyelid) usually indicates nerve dysfunction. Opaque whitening of outer rim of cornea can indicate arcus senilis. Corneal opaqueness can be from cataract or trauma.

FIGURE 51.9 Using Snellen's chart to assess visual acuity.

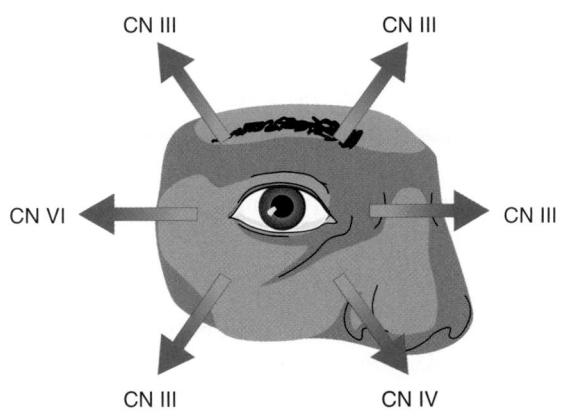

FIGURE 51.10 Six cardinal fields of gaze.

from the visual axis is known as **tropia**. Deviation of the eye toward the nose is known as **esotropia**, movement laterally is known as **exotropia**, and downward deviation is **hypotropia**.

PUPILLARY REFLEXES. When observed, the pupils should be round, symmetrical, and reactive to light. To test pupillary response to light, both consensual and direct examinations should be completed. A slightly darkened room works best. The patient is asked to look straight ahead, and the size of the pupil is noted. A penlight is shone toward the pupil from a lateral position, and the movement of the pupil is observed. The pupil should quickly constrict. The size of the pupil is noted when it constricts. This is known as direct response.

To conduct a consensual pupil examination, observe the eye just tested for reaction while shining the penlight into the other eye. The observed pupil should constrict. This is known as **consensual response**. Then repeat the procedure for the opposite eye.

The examiner proceeds to test for **accommodation**, which is the ability of the pupil to respond to near and far distances.

The patient is told to focus on an object far away. The size and shape of the pupils are observed. The examiner continues to observe the pupils as the patient focuses on a near object (the examiner's penlight or finger) held approximately 5 inches from the patient's face. Normally, the patient's eyes turn inward and the pupils constrict. These responses, convergence and constriction, are called accommodation ("Gerontological Issues—Age-Related Changes in Vision and Hearing"). Examiners use the acronym PERRLA to indicate pupils equal, round, reactive to light, accommodation. If accommodation is not tested along with the other tests, the examiner may use the acronym PERRL.

• WORD • BUILDING •

esotropia: eso—inward + tropia—movement of the eye
exotropia: exo—out + tropia—movement of the eye

Gerontological Issues

Age-Related Changes in Vision and Hearing
Vision

Older adults commonly have the following changes in their vision:

• Presbyopia, an inability to focus up close because of decreased elasticity in the ocular lens
• Narrowing of the visual field and more difficulty with peripheral vision
• Decreased pupil size and responsiveness to light
• Difficulty with vision in dimly lit areas or at night (requires more light to see adequately)
• Increased opacity of the lens, which causes sensitivity to glare, blurred vision, and interference with night vision
• Yellowing of the lens, which reduces ability to differentiate low-tone colors of blues, greens, and violets (yellow, orange, and red hues are more clearly visible)
• Distorted depth perception and difficulty correctly judging the height of curbs and steps
• Decreased lacrimal secretions

Because visual accommodation decreases with aging, older adults have an increased risk of falling. An older person has difficulty making a visual adjustment when moving from a well-lit room into the evening darkness, for example, or when stepping out of a dark area into the sunlight.

The increased time needed to accommodate to near and far, dark and light, is often the reason that older adults do not drive at night. Usually they say that light from oncoming traffic blinds them or that their eyes do not focus properly.

One of the simplest and most effective ways to improve vision for older adults is to ensure that eyeglasses are clean.

Hearing

Presbycusis is an age-related change in which progressive hearing loss is caused by loss of hair cells and decreased blood supplying the ear, resulting in a decreased ability to hear high-frequency sounds. Deafness or decreased hearing acuity is one of the main reasons that older adults withdraw from social activities. The loss of high-pitched hearing causes the older adult to hear distracting background noises more clearly than conversation.

Older adults who are deaf may need adaptive equipment in their home for safety. The use of a hearing aid can increase hearing for those who do not have nerve damage deafness. The use of flashing lights instead of buzzers or alarms increases the safety of an older adult who is not able to hear a smoke detector or fire alarm.

INSPECTION AND PALPATION OF EXTERNAL STRUCTURES. The extraocular structures are inspected beginning with the eyebrows. The presence of eyebrows, symmetry, hair texture, size, and extension of the brow are noted. The examiner inspects and palpates the orbital area for edema, lesions, puffiness, and tenderness. Then the eyelids are inspected for symmetry, presence of eyelashes, eyelash position, tremors, flakiness, redness, and swelling. The patient is asked to open and close the eyelids. When open, the eyelid should cover the iris margin but not the pupil. The distance between the upper and lower eyelid, known as the palpebral fissure, is inspected; it should be equal in both eyes. If the palpebral fissure is nonsymmetrical, observe for **ptosis**, a drooping of the eyelid, which is commonly seen in stroke patients. Next the medial canthus of the lower lid is gently palpated and observed for exudate. The eyelids are palpated for nodules while the eye is palpated for firmness over the closed eyelid.

The lower eyelid is pulled down, and the patient is asked to look upward. The conjunctiva and sclera are inspected for color, discharge, and pterygium (thickening of the conjunctiva). To inspect the upper eyelid, the upper lid is everted (turned inside out) over a cotton-tipped applicator. The patient blinks to return the eyelid to its resting position when the inspection is complete.

The external eyes are inspected for color and symmetry of the irises, clarity of the cornea, and depth and clarity of the anterior chamber. Shining a light obliquely across the cornea assesses the clearness of the cornea. The cornea should be transparent without cloudiness. In individuals older than 40 years, there may be bilateral opaque whitening of the outer rim of the cornea known as **arcus senilus**. It is caused from lipid deposits and is considered normal. It does not affect vision. The anterior chamber (the area between the cornea and the iris) of the eye is inspected using oblique light. The anterior chamber should be clear when the light shines on it.

INTERNAL EYE EXAMINATION. Examination of the internal eye is done by the advanced practitioner. The LPN/LVN may be required to explain the procedure to the patient and to assist the practitioner in the examination. To perform the internal eye examination, specialized equipment must be used. It is useful, but not always necessary, to have the pupil dilated for the internal eye examination. Having a dark room allows the pupil to dilate, as does the application of anticholinergic mydriatic (causing dilatation) eyedrops.

The handheld instrument with a light source used to examine the internal eye is called an **ophthalmoscope**. The ophthalmoscope magnifies the internal structures of the eye, so the examiner can visualize the retina, optic nerve, blood vessels, and macula. The patient is asked to hold the head still with the eyes focused on a distant object and informed that the bright light might be uncomfortable. The **ophthalmologist** can also examine the internal eye using a stationary device called a slit-lamp microscope. For this, the patient is seated and rests the chin on a support while a microscope and light source are directed into the eye.

Intraocular Pressure. Estimation of intraocular pressure is measured by using one of several types of tonometer. Often, the procedure is performed with anesthetic drops being instilled. One type of tonometer testing uses a puff of air to make an indentation in the cornea to measure intraocular pressure. Readings above the normal range may indicate glaucoma.

Diagnostic Tests for the Eye

There are a number of diagnostic tests for the eye, including bacterial culture, digital imaging, optical coherence tomography, fluorescein or indocyanine green angiography, electroretinography, ultrasonography, and other imaging tests.

Eye Culture

If exudate from any portion of the eye or surrounding structure is present, an eye culture may be ordered. Results of the culture determine if anti-infective treatment is necessary.

Digital Imaging

Digital imaging is a newer way of viewing the retina without requiring the use of dilating eyedrops. The instrument takes a digital picture of the retina in 2 seconds. The majority of the retina is viewable and assists in early detection of eye disease. It provides a permanent photographic reference for the retina.

Optical Coherence Tomography (OCT)

OCT takes a picture of the retina. It is safe, fast, and does not have the risks associated with the use of dye. Light beams are shone into the eye at various angles and the amount of interference is measured creating a detailed image of the depth of the retina.

Fluorescein or Indocyanine Green Angiography

Angiography with dye is a test using special cameras to find leaking or damaged blood vessels in the retinal or deeper choroidal circulation. Fluorescein is a yellow dye that glows in visible light and is useful for showing the retinal circulation, and indocyanine green is a green dye that shows up with invisible infrared light to highlight the choroidal circulation.

The patient is assessed for dye allergies (indocyanine green contains iodine) before the procedure. Then the pupil is dilated and the dye is injected into the patient's venous system where it travels to the eye's circulation to make the blood vessels there visible. Fluorescein is used in diabetic retinopathy and retinal vascular disease. Indocyanine green is useful for the wet form of macular degeneration when blood is present in the macula.

Electroretinography

Electroretinography is useful in diagnosing diseases of the rods and cones of the eye. The procedure evaluates differences in the electrical potential between the cornea and retina in response to light wavelengths and intensity. The test is conducted by placing contact lenses with electrodes directly on the eye.

Ultrasonography

Ultrasound is useful when the internal eye cannot be visualized directly because of obstructions such as corneal opacities or bloody vitreous. The eye is anesthetized with instillation of anesthetic drops, and a transducer probe is placed on the eye to perform the ultrasound.

Imaging Tests

X-ray films show bone structure and tumors. Computed tomography (CT) and magnetic resonance imaging (MRI) visualize ocular structures and abnormalities of the eye and surrounding tissues.

Therapeutic Measures for the Eye and Vision

Nurses have an important role in screening and educating individuals, families, and the community about the care for healthy eyes and prevention of disease. To learn more about ways to promote vision health, visit www.lighthouse.org. For resources to help those persons who are blind, visit the American Foundation for the Blind at www.afb.org or the National Federation of the Blind at www.nfb.org.

Regular Eye Examinations

People who are not known to have visual deficits and do not have diseases associated with visual loss, such as diabetes, should have their eyes examined at regular intervals throughout their life. Screening tests usually are done during an annual physical examination to detect gross visual deficits. Patients who wear corrective lenses or have disease processes that place them at risk for visual loss should have their eyes examined by an eye care provider at least yearly.

Eye care providers include the ophthalmologist and **optometrist**. An ophthalmologist is a physician who specializes in the comprehensive care of the eyes and visual system, including diagnosing and treating eye diseases. An optometrist specializes in eye examinations to identify visual defects, diagnosis problems, prescribe corrective lenses or other treatments, and refer for medical treatment. The optometrist is not a physician but is identified as a doctor of optometry. An **optician** is a person trained to grind and fit lenses according to prescriptions written by the ophthalmologist or optometrist.

Eye Hygiene

It is important to keep debris out of the eyes to prevent scratching of the eye's delicate surfaces. When a foreign object gets into the eye, such as dirt or an eyelash, the person should be taught not to rub the eye but to allow tears to wash out the object. This can be done by pulling the eyelid down over the eye for a brief time. When wiping the eyes, the nurse should wipe from the inner canthus to the outer canthus.

Nutrition for Eye Health

Adequate nutrition is important for eye health ("Nutrition Notes"). Eye disorders related to inadequate vitamin intake include corneal damage and night blindness from lack of vitamin A and optic neuritis as a result of vitamin B deficiency.

Eye Safety and Prevention of Injury

Many people in the United States suffer eye injuries each year. Common household activities are responsible for the majority of injuries. Activities such as microwave cooking, lawn care, and shooting rubber bands and BB guns all contribute to eye injury. Many of these injuries could be prevented with education and implementation of safety measures (Table 51.3).

Eye Irrigation

If it is necessary to irrigate foreign bodies or chemical substances out of the eye, the nurse prepares the patient by explaining the

Nutrition Notes

Nutrition and Eye Disease

In some developing countries, vitamin A deficiency is a leading cause of preventable blindness and the leading cause of childhood blindness. In developed countries, antioxidants have been investigated in relation to cataracts and age-related macular degeneration (AMD), two conditions that can also lead to severely impaired vision. Little evidence supports a role for antioxidants in preventing cataracts, and further research efforts along that line are discouraged. Research on AMD is ongoing. Evidence suggests that antioxidant vitamin and mineral supplementation may delay the progression of AMD in people already diagnosed with the disease. Other risk factors for AMD are modifiable obesity-related risk factors, notably low physical activity and serum lipid levels.

Recommendations

The value of specific foods or nutrients in preventing eye disease has not been proven. If a person chooses to take supplements, a multivitamin and multimineral product at recommended dietary allowance levels is advocated rather than separate preparations of individual nutrients. Other choices should be made in consultation with the patient's HCP.

TABLE 51.3 EYE SAFETY AND INJURY PREVENTION

To Protect From	Use These Eye Safety Measures
Foreign objects	Wear safety goggles. Avoid mowing over rocks or sticks. Always wear safety goggles when using lawn edging yard devices.
Chemical splashes	Use splash shields when working with chemicals such as cleaning solution or body fluids. Close eyes to avoid getting hair spray in them.
Corneal lens abrasions/infections from contact lenses	Follow manufacturer's or eye care professional's directions for length of use and cleaning procedures. Do not overwear lenses.
Ultraviolet light (UV)	Wear ultraviolet-protected sunglasses when outdoors. Instruct patients to wear sunglasses with side shields after administration of mydriatics. Wear a hat to shield sun.
Visual deficits in adult with corrective lenses	Update prescription of glasses yearly. Glasses should fit properly, be clean, and be free of scratches.
Eye strain from computer usage	The position of the bottom of the monitor should be 20 degrees below the line of sight and should be positioned 13 to 18 inches from the eyes. The light in the room should prevent glare. Increase the font size on the screen if letters appear too small. If dry eyes are a problem while using a computer, adjust the monitor to a lower level so the eyes do not have to open as wide, which increases evaporation.
Eye injury from sports	Wear protective eyewear with polycarbonate lenses. Wear facemasks or helmets while participating in any high-contact or high-impact sports.

procedure. An isotonic solution is usually used. It is delivered onto the eye using intravenous (IV) tubing or a Morgan lens (Box 51-1 and Fig. 51.11).

Guide Dogs for the Blind and Visually Impaired

Special guide dogs are trained to lead blind and visually impaired people around obstacles. Generally they are allowed in places where animals are banned such as stores or restaurants. While the dogs are working, they should not be approached, touched, or fed without their owner's permission.

Medication Administration

A variety of drugs are available for eye application. Most are applied as drops, ointments, or irrigations. The nurse must know the usual dosage and strength, desired action, side effects, and contraindications of the medication being administered to prevent harm to the patient. Systemic adverse reactions can occur, and diseases can be exacerbated from the administration of eye medications. Older adults are especially susceptible to this because they have more chronic diseases, as well as use ophthalmic agents long term. These agents can interact with other medications the patient is taking. So the nurse observes patients for possible reactions.

Chapter 52 discusses specific ophthalmic medications and their uses. To identify the steps in the application of eye medications, see Boxes 51-2 and 51-3. Whenever eye medications, especially eyedrops, are administered, the punctum (tear duct) of the eye should have pressure applied to it by either the nurse wearing gloves or the patient, if able, for at least 1 minute or longer as directed. This reduces systemic absorption of the medication through the punctum. Some eye medications can have serious cardiac or respiratory effects, and patients have had life-threatening reactions to them. The nurse should teach the patient the proper instillation of eye medications to reduce these reactions.

 NURSING CARE TIP

Older patients, when instilling their own eyedrops, may not feel the drops go in. Teaching patients to refrigerate the drops, if not contraindicated, for 15 to 30 minutes before instillation helps them feel if the drops go into the eye or on the face.

Box 51-1 Eye Irrigation

1. Explain procedure to patient.
2. Perform hand hygiene.
3. Gather equipment. For low-volume irrigation, a prefilled squeezable bottle is used. For large-volume irrigation, an IV bag of isotonic solution such as normal saline or lactated Ringer's solution is used. Attach IV tubing to the bag and flush the line.
4. Apply anesthetic drops, if ordered.
5. Place a basin by side of patient's head and pad area with towels to absorb irrigant.
6. Apply gloves.
7. Eye may be irrigated by holding distal end of IV tubing at inner canthus of the eye, or a Morgan lens may be attached (see Fig. 51.11). Lens is placed directly on the anesthetized eye, and tubing is connected to IV bag tubing. Proceed with irrigation using a slow, steady stream of irrigant. Generally, use of the Morgan lens is more comfortable for patients because eyelids do not need to be held open.
8. Assess patient's tolerance to the procedure.
9. Remove Morgan lens if used.
10. Remove gloves. Perform hand hygiene.
11. Document assessment, type and amount of irrigant, and patient's tolerance of procedure.

EYE PATCHING. After treating an injured or infected eye, the physician may order the eye to be patched. The nurse applies ointment or drops if ordered, asks the patient to keep the eyelid shut, and then places a disposable, cotton gauze eye patch over the depression of the eye socket. If the patient has a deep eye socket, the nurse may need to place two pads over the socket

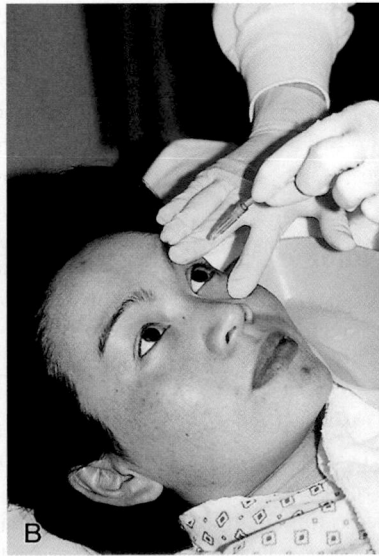

FIGURE 51.11 (A) Morgan lens is used for eye irrigation. (B) Irrigation of eye.

Box 51-2 Administration of Eyedrops

1. Explain procedure to patient. Contact lenses should be removed. They should not be worn if eyes are reddened, and for 10 minutes after drops have been instilled or as directed.
2. Assess allergies, and check medication dosage, strength, side effects, contraindications, and expiration date. Do not use if solution is cloudy.
3. Perform hand hygiene and apply gloves.
4. Avoid touching tip of dropper to anything to avoid contamination that could cause an eye infection. Do not wash or rinse dropper.
5. Instruct patient to tilt head backward and look up toward the ceiling.
6. Gently pull lower lid down and out to form a pocket to catch eyedrop.
7. Approach patient's eye from the side and instill prescribed amount of medication into the pocket. It is helpful (including for patient who is self-administering eyedrops) to use the forehead as a stabilizing area for the hand administering the drop.
8. Release lower eyelid. Have patient close eye.
9. Apply gentle pressure with a tissue to the punctum (over the tear duct) for at least 1 to 5 minutes to keep medication from being systemically absorbed. Nurse or patient can do this.
10. Wipe excess medication off eyelids or cheek.
11. If another eyedrop is to be given, wait 5 to 10 minutes before administering.
12. Remove gloves. Perform hand hygiene.
13. Document medication administration and patient's tolerance of procedure.

Box 51-3 Administration of Eye Ointment

1. Explain procedure to patient.
2. Check medication for dosage, strength, side effects, contraindications, and expiration date.
3. Perform hand hygiene and apply gloves.
4. Instruct patient to tilt head backward and look up toward the ceiling.
5. Gently pull lower lid down to form a pocket into which ointment is placed.
6. Express ointment directly into exposed palpebral conjunctiva, moving from inner to outer canthus. Be careful not to touch patient's eye or surrounding structure with tip of ointment tube. The tip of the ointment tube must remain sterile.
7. Release lower eyelid over the ointment.

Continued

Box 51-3 Administration of Eye Ointment—cont'd

8. Instruct patient to gently close eyes.
9. Remove gloves. Perform hand hygiene.
10. Explain that vision may be blurred while ointment is in the eye.
11. Document medication administration and patient's tolerance of procedure.

to help the eyelids remain closed. The purpose of eye patching is to protect the eye from further damage by keeping the lids closed. Sometimes an additional metal shield is placed over the soft pads to protect the eye from external injury. The patch is taped in place and the patient instructed to rest the eyes. The nurse should suggest quiet activities, such as listening to music or an audio book, or sleeping. Watching television or reading is not recommended because the patched eye follows the movement of the unpatched eye.

HEARING

Normal Anatomy and Physiology of the Ear

The ear consists of three areas: the outer ear, the middle ear, and the inner ear. The inner ear contains the receptors for the senses of hearing and equilibrium.

Outer Ear

The outer ear consists of the auricle and the auditory canal (Fig. 51.12).

Middle Ear

The middle ear is an air-filled cavity in the temporal bone. Vibrations of the tympanic membrane caused by sound are transmitted through the three auditory bones (ossicles). The stapes then transmits vibrations to the fluid-filled inner ear at the oval window.

Inner Ear

The inner ear is a cavity in the temporal bone called the bony labyrinth, lined with membranes called the membranous labyrinth. The fluid between bone and membrane is called perilymph, and that within the membrane is called endolymph. The structures of the bony labyrinth include the semicircular canals, vestibule, and cochlea (Fig. 51.13).

The process of hearing involves the transmission of vibrations and the generation of nerve impulses. When sound waves enter the auditory canal, vibrations are transmitted by the following structures: tympanic membrane, malleus, incus, stapes, oval window of the inner ear, perilymph and endolymph within the cochlea, and hair cells of the organ of Corti. When the hair cells bend, they generate impulses that are carried by the eighth cranial nerve to the brain. The auditory areas, for both hearing and interpretation, are in the temporal lobes of the cerebral cortex.

The inner ear also has receptors for equilibrium: dynamic equilibrium receptors are within the semicircular canals whereas static equilibrium receptors are within the vestibule (Fig. 51.14). Within the utricle and saccule of the vestibule, the hair cells bend in response to gravity on the otoliths as the position of the head changes. The impulses generated are carried by the vestibular branch of the eighth cranial nerve to the cerebellum, medulla, and pons. The cerebellum sends this information continuously to the cerebral motor cortex. The cerebellum and brainstem use this information to maintain equilibrium at a subconscious level; the cerebrum interprets the conscious awareness of the position of the head.

When the head moves, movement of the endolymph will bend the cupula within the ampulla. The bending of the hair cells at its base generates impulses carried by the vestibular branch of the eighth cranial nerve to the cerebellum and brainstem, and then impulses are sent to the cerebral cortex. These impulses are interpreted as directional acceleration or deceleration; this information is used to maintain equilibrium during movement.

Aging and the Ear

In the ear, cumulative damage to the hair cells in the organ of Corti usually becomes apparent sometime after the age of 60 (see Fig. 51.8). Damaged hair cells cannot be replaced. Ability to hear high frequencies is usually lost first (presbycusis), whereas hearing may still be adequate for lower pitched ranges. The high-pitched sounds *f*, *s*, *k*, and *sh* are common losses. Also, it becomes more difficult to filter out background noises, so busy, loud environments make it difficult to hear conversations.

 LEARNING TIP

Presbycusis is the loss of hearing high-pitched sounds (pitch = cycles per second; loudness = decibels [dB]). Because the ability to hear pitch is lost rather than loudness, it is not helpful to talk louder to a patient with this type of hearing loss. In fact, talking louder can make it more difficult to discriminate sounds. It is important to know the type of hearing loss a patient has.

Nursing Assessment of the Ear and Hearing

A quiet environment is helpful for collecting accurate hearing data. Document the patient's behavior because it may provide information related to hearing loss.

Health History

The patient's self-appraisal of his or her hearing or related symptoms is obtained during the health history. Data collection regarding symptoms includes asking the **WHAT'S UP?** questions: where it is, how it feels, aggravating and alleviating factors, timing, severity, useful data for associated symptoms, and perception of the problem by the patient. Symptoms related to the ear that may be reported include decreased

Outer Ear

The **auricle (pinna)** is the visible part of the ear. Shaped by cartilage, this part of the ear funnels sound into the auditory canal.

The **auditory canal** leads through the temporal bone to the eardrum. (The opening of the auditory canal to the outside of the body is called the **external acoustic meatus.**) Glands lining the canal produce secretions that mix with dead skin cells to form cerumen (ear wax). Cerumen waterproofs the canal and also traps dirt and bacteria. The cerumen usually dries and then, propelled by jaw movements during eating and talking, works its way out of the ear.

Ossicles:
Malleus
Incus
Stapes
Semicircular canals
Vestibular nerve
Cochlear nerve
Cochlea
Round window
Eustachian tube

Outer ear   Middle ear   Inner ear

Middle Ear

Auditory ossicles: The three smallest bones in the body connect the eardrum to the inner ear; they are named for their shape:
• **Malleus** (hammer)
• **Incus** (anvil)
• **Stapes** (stirrup)
The stapes fits within the **oval window** of the vestibule, which is where the inner ear begins.

Tympanic membrane (or eardrum): This membranous structure separates the outer ear from the middle ear; it vibrates freely in response to sound waves.

Oval window

The **auditory** or **eustachian tube** is a passageway from the middle ear to the nasopharynx. Its purpose is to equalize pressure on both sides of the tympanic membrane. Unfortunately, it can also allow infection to spread from the throat to the middle ear.

FIGURE 51.12 Outer and middle ear. From Thompson, G. S. (2013). *Understanding anatomy and physiology.* Philadelphia: F.A. Davis, p. 205.

hearing or loss of hearing, **otorrhea** (discharge), **otalgia** (ear pain), itching, fullness, tinnitus (ringing, buzzing, or roaring in the ears), or vertigo (dizziness).

Information about current and past medications is obtained. Many medications are potentially toxic to the ear and can cause hearing loss or decreased hearing. Pay particular attention to any exposure to medications that are potentially **ototoxic**, such as certain antibiotics or diuretics (see Chapter 52).

Ask about **hearing aids** or assistive hearing devices, surgeries, treatments, allergies, sodium and alcohol intake (which can affect the amount of endolymph in the inner ear), and childhood illnesses including mumps, measles, or scarlet fever. Also ask about recent upper respiratory infections, history of infections, injury to the ear, hospitalizations, swimming habits, exposure to pressure changes (flying or diving), medical diseases, and any recent or past exposure to any loud noises.

Family history related to ear disorders includes any hearing problems or hearing loss and family members with Ménière's disease. Significant findings are recorded, including the patient's relationship to the family member with the problem.

Information about the patient's care of the ears is also gathered. It is important to assess what preventive measures the patient practices and what the patient's learning needs are concerning care and protection of the ears. Determine how the patient cleans the ears, any exposure to loud noises during

• WORD • BUILDING •

otorrhea: oto—related to the ear + rrhea—to flow
otalgia: ot—related to the ear + algia—signifying pain
ototoxic: oto—related to the ear + toxic—poison

Inner Ear

Semicircular canals: These structures are crucial for the maintenance of equilibrium and balance.

Vestibule: This structure, which marks the entrance to the labyrinths, contains organs necessary for the sense of balance.

Cochlea: This snail-like structure contains the structures for hearing.

Vestibular nerve

Cochlear nerve

Perilymph

Cochlear duct (with endolymph)

Oval window

Round window

The spirals of the cochlea are divided into three compartments. The middle compartment is a triangular duct (called the **cochlear duct**) filled with endolymph; the outer two compartments are filled with perilymph.

Resting on the floor (called the **basilar membrane**) of this duct is the **organ of Corti**, the hearing sense organ.

Hairs

Tectorial membrane

Supporting cells

Basilar membrane

Fibers of cochlear nerve

The organ of Corti consists of a layer of epithelium (composed of sensory and supporting cells). Thousands of hair cells project from this epithelial layer and are topped with a gelatin-like membrane called the **tectorial membrane**. Nerve fibers extending from the base of the hairs eventually form the cochlear nerve (cranial nerve VIII).

FIGURE 51.13 Inner ear. From Thompson, G. S. (2013). *Understanding anatomy and physiology.* Philadelphia: F.A. Davis. p. 206.

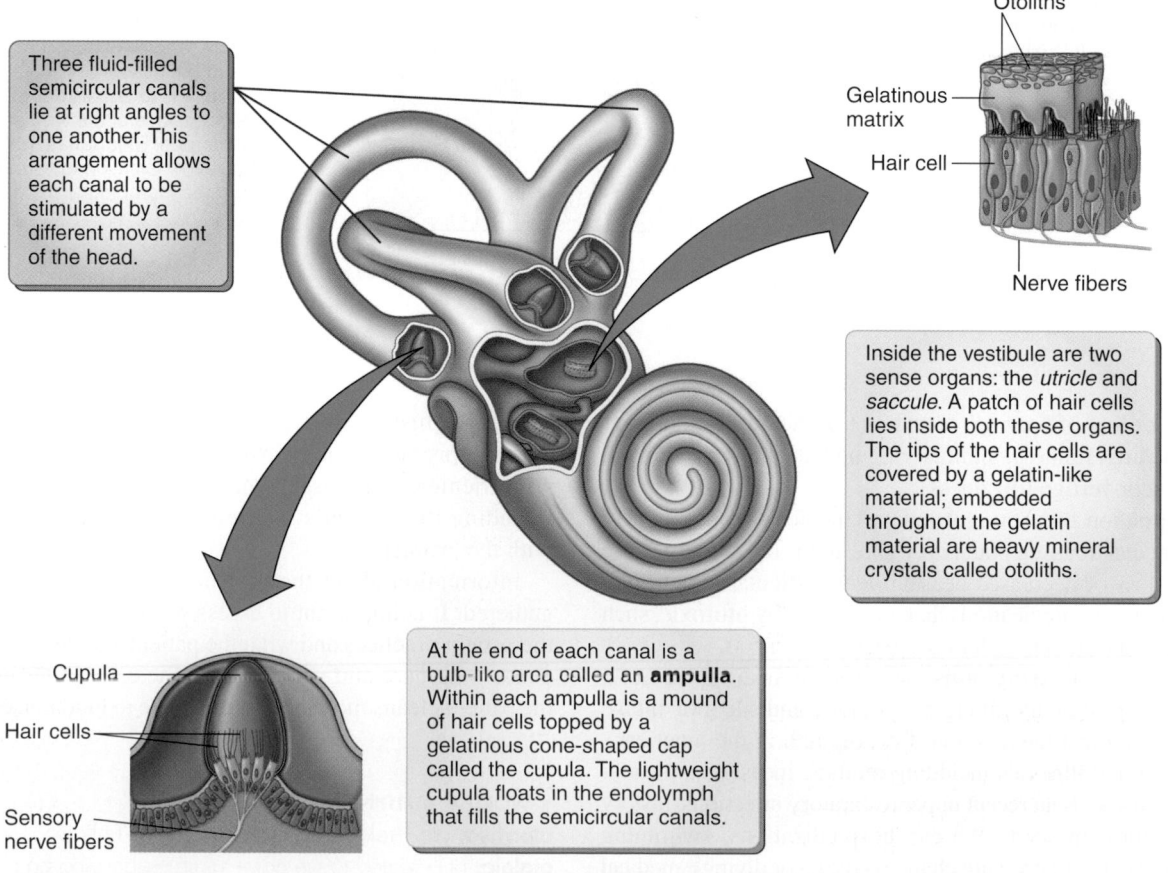

Three fluid-filled semicircular canals lie at right angles to one another. This arrangement allows each canal to be stimulated by a different movement of the head.

Otoliths

Gelatinous matrix

Hair cell

Nerve fibers

Inside the vestibule are two sense organs: the *utricle* and *saccule*. A patch of hair cells lies inside both these organs. The tips of the hair cells are covered by a gelatin-like material; embedded throughout the gelatin material are heavy mineral crystals called otoliths.

Cupula

Hair cells

Sensory nerve fibers

At the end of each canal is a bulb-like area called an **ampulla**. Within each ampulla is a mound of hair cells topped by a gelatinous cone-shaped cap called the cupula. The lightweight cupula floats in the endolymph that fills the semicircular canals.

FIGURE 51.14 Balance. From Thompson, G. S. (2013). *Understanding anatomy and physiology.* Philadelphia: F.A. Davis, p. 208.

recreational or work activities, any changes in ability to hear, and any exposure to ototoxic medications. Determine if the patient has had a hearing evaluation and if there is a history of ear problems (Table 51.4). On the basis of these findings, instruct the patient in ways to care for the ears and maintain ear health.

Physical Examination

Physical examination of the ear begins by observing the behaviors of the patient (Box 51-4). Note how the patient communicates. Observe how the patient talks, noting any slurred speech or words. Examination of the ear includes inspection, palpation, testing auditory acuity, balance testing, and, for the advanced practitioner, otoscopic examination (Table 51.5).

INSPECTION AND PALPATION OF THE EXTERNAL EAR. Inspection of the external ear begins with examining the auricle. The external ear should be inspected for size, symmetry, configuration, and angle of attachment. Note any obvious deformities or scars. The skin should be smooth and without

breaks, particularly behind the ear in the crevice. The color should be uniform, without signs of inflammation. To inspect the external ear canal, tip the adult patient's head to the side and use a penlight or otoscope to inspect the canal. Note any drainage or cerumen (wax), including the color, odor, and clarity of the drainage. The skin should be smooth and without inflammation, edema, or breaks. There should be no lesions, foreign bodies, erythema, or edema in the external ear canal. Inspection of the external ear canal should be completed before obtaining an infrared ear temperature because the presence of cerumen can alter the accuracy of the reading.

Next the auricles are palpated and any tophi, lesions, or masses noted. Tophi are deposits of uric acid crystals that appear as small, hard nodules in the helix (external ear margin); they may also occur in gout. The auricle should be nontender when it is palpated; tenderness can indicate an external ear infection. A downward protrusion of the helix, called Darwin's tubercle, is a normal finding. The mastoid process should be smooth and hard when palpated. The mastoid process can be of different sizes but should not be tender or swollen.

TABLE 51.4   SUBJECTIVE DATA COLLECTION FOR THE EAR

Category	Questions to Ask During the Health History	Rationale/Significance
Family History	Has any family member had any hearing problems or loss? Has any family member had Ménière's disease?	This may give information about the patient's current ear problem.
Patient Health History	What medications are you currently taking?	Many medications are ototoxic and can cause hearing loss (see Chapter 52).
	Have you had any surgeries or trauma to the ear?	Recent trauma or surgeries can affect hearing.
	Do you have any allergies to food, medications or other substances? Have you had any recent upper respiratory infections? Do you have a history of upper respiratory infections or ear infections?	Can cause nasal congestion leading to middle ear congestion and/or infections.
	Do you have any discharge from the ear (otorrhea), ear pain (otalgia), itching, fullness, tinnitus, or vertigo? Do you have a fever, nausea, or vomiting?	May indicate outer, middle, or inner ear infections. May indicate ototoxicity or other ear diseases.
	Are you exposed to pressure changes such as with flying or diving?	Barotrauma may occur due to pressure changes.
	Have you had any recent or past exposure to loud noises? If so, what type and for how long?	Can indicate hearing loss and the cause of hearing loss. Further assessment needed.
Hearing Impairment	Have you noticed any hearing loss? If so, has it been gradual or sudden? Do you have difficulty understanding certain words or entire conversations? Do you have difficulty hearing when there is a lot of background noise?	Could indicate hearing loss and further assessment is needed. Patient already may have hearing loss in one or both ears.

Continued

TABLE 51.4 SUBJECTIVE DATA COLLECTION FOR THE EAR—cont'd

Category	Questions to Ask During the Health History	Rationale/Significance
	Do you hear better out of one ear than the other?	
	Have your friends or family commented on your decreased hearing?	
	Do you wear a hearing aid or other assistive device?	
	If so, what is the device and for which ear is it used?	
	How does your hearing loss affect your daily life?	Hearing loss can cause social isolation.
	Do you feel embarrassed or frustrated because of your hearing loss?	
	How do your friends and family react to your hearing loss?	
	Are you exposed to loud noises, such as with your current or past job, busy traffic, machinery, or loud music?	Can cause damage to the ear leading to hearing loss over time.
Self-Care Behaviors	Have you had your hearing checked? If so, when?	Provides information about patient's ear self-care and health.
	How do you clean your ears?	
	How do you protect your ears from loud noises?	

Box 51-4 Behaviors Indicating Hearing Loss

Adults with hearing loss may show any or all of the following behaviors:

- Turns up volume on the television or radio.
- Frequently asks, "What did you say?"
- Leans forward or turns head to one side during conversations to hear better.
- Cups hand around ear during conversation.
- Mentions that people are talking softly or mumbling.
- Speaks in an unusually quiet or loud voice.
- Answers questions inappropriately or not at all.
- Has difficulty hearing high-frequency consonants.
- Avoids group activities.
- Shows loss of sense of humor.
- Has strained or serious look on face during conversations.
- Appears to ignore people or is aloof; does not participate.
- Is irritable or sensitive in interpersonal relations.
- Reports ringing, buzzing, or roaring noise in the ears.

AUDITORY ACUITY TESTING. Auditory function can be grossly evaluated using three assessment tests. The whisper voice test is one test to check hearing function in each ear. The patient occludes one ear with a finger, and the nurse stands 1 to 2 feet away on the opposite side. The nurse whispers two-syllable words toward the unoccluded ear. The patient restates the whispered words. The nurse should be by the patient's side to prevent the patient from lip reading. The nurse's voice can be increased from a soft, medium, or loud whisper to a soft, medium, or loud voice. The process is repeated on the other ear. The patient is asked if hearing is better in one ear than in the other ear. The patient should be able to hear a soft whisper equally well in both ears. Findings of one ear hearing better than the other or an inability to hear a soft whisper can be indicative of hearing impairment. Results of the test are documented.

A second acuity test is the **Rinne test**. This test is performed with a tuning fork and is useful for differentiating between conductive and sensorineural hearing loss. To perform the test, strike the tuning fork and place it on the patient's mastoid process (Fig. 51.15). Verify that the patient is able to hear the tuning fork, and then instruct the patient to say immediately when the sound is no longer heard. When the patient indicates that the sound is not heard, place the vibrating tuning fork 2 inches in front of the ear (see Fig. 51.15). Ask the patient if he or she hears the tuning fork and then to indicate when the sound is no longer heard. Normally, air conduction (AC) is heard twice as long as bone conduction (BC). The patient reports this by hearing the tuning fork when placed in front of the ear (AC) after no longer hearing it when placed on the mastoid process (BC). Normal results are recorded as "AC greater than BC." The test is repeated on the other ear and findings recorded. Abnormal findings can indicate conduction or sensorineural problems (Table 51.6).

TABLE 51.5   OBJECTIVE DATA COLLECTION FOR THE EAR

Category	Physical Examination Findings	Possible Abnormal Findings/Causes
Inspection and Palpation of the External Ear	Ears should be symmetrical in size, configuration, and angle of attachment.	Asymmetrical size and placement could indicate congenital deformities.
	Skin covering the ear should be intact, smooth, and without edema, erythema, or inflammation.	Discharge, breaks in skin, or inflammation can be caused by trauma, external ear infections, poorly fitting hearing aid or skin disorders.
	Canal should have minimal or no cerumen.	Excessive cerumen may be found. This can alter hearing and cause inaccurate tympanic temperature readings. Excess cerumen may need to be removed.
	No lesions, tophi, or masses should be palpated. No tenderness of auricle when palpated. No odor detected.	Tophi may be present in the patient with gout. Tenderness and odor could indicate an external ear infection.
Auditory Acuity Testing	Patient can hear whispered words at 1–2 feet away. Rinne's and Weber's tests normal (see Table 51.6). Able to understand and converse with examiner.	Patient may have indications of conductive, sensorineural, mixed, or neural hearing loss.
Balance Testing	Patient can sit and walk without difficulty. Patient can complete Romberg's test with minimal swaying.	Difficulty sitting and/or walking. Increased swaying or falling with Romberg's test due to balance difficulties. May be due to inner ear infection or disorder.
Otoscopic Examination	Ear canal should be smooth and empty, without redness, scaliness, swelling, drainage, excessive cerumen, or foreign objects.	Ear canal may be reddened and swollen; drainage may be present; excessive cerumen or foreign object may be present. Caused by infection, improper care, or excessive cerumen production.
	Internal otoscope examination is completed by experienced practitioner and should reveal a slightly conical, shiny, smooth, pearly gray eardrum.	Eardrum may be dull, bulging or retracted, reddened if caused by middle ear infection or blockage.
Other	Observe the patient's position and posture during the interview and physical exam. Does the patient watch the examiner's mouth or lean toward the examiner?	Behaviors may indicate hearing loss and the patient's effort to compensate. The patient may be unaware of the behaviors.

The **Weber test** is a third test to assess hearing acuity. The Weber test is also performed using a tuning fork. Place the vibrating tuning fork on the center of the patient's forehead or head (Fig. 51.16). Verify that the patient can hear the tuning fork. If the patient gives a positive answer, ask the patient if the sound is heard better in the left ear, better in the right ear, or the same in both ears. It is important to give the patient three choices from which to choose. Normally, the patient hears the sound the same in both ears (see Table 51.6).

BALANCE TESTING.   When the patient reports dizziness, nystagmus, or problems with equilibrium, simple tests can be performed to assess vestibular function. The first test is simply to observe the patient's gait by having the patient walk away from the examiner and then walk back. Note the

FIGURE 51.15 Rinne test. (A) Bone conduction. (B) Air conduction.

TABLE 51.6   AUDITORY ACUITY TUNING FORK TESTS

Test	Expected Results	Conductive Hearing Loss	Sensorineural Hearing Loss
Rinne Test	Air conduction heard longer than bone conduction	Bone conduction heard longer than air conduction in affected ear	Air conduction heard longer than bone conduction in affected ear (may be less than 2:1 ratio)
Weber Test	Tone heard in center of the head; no lateralization	Sound heard louder in affected ear	Sound heard louder in better ear

FIGURE 51.16 Weber's test.

patient's balance, posture, and movement of arms and legs. The patient should be able to walk in an upright position with no difficulties in balance or movement.

Romberg's test, or falling test, is another simple test to assess vestibular function. Instruct the patient to stand with feet together, first with eyes open and then with eyes closed. Normally, the patient has no difficulty maintaining a standing position with only minimal swaying. If the patient has difficulty maintaining balance or loses balance (a positive Romberg test), the patient may have an inner ear problem. If a fall appears likely, be prepared to support the patient to prevent injury.

OTOSCOPIC EXAMINATION. An otoscope is an instrument consisting of a handle, a light source, a magnifying lens, and an optional speculum for inserting in the ear. Some otoscopes have a pneumatic device for injecting air into the canal to test the eardrum's mobility and integrity. The otoscope is used to visualize the external ear, ear canal, and tympanic membrane. Otoscopic examination is completed to identify specific disorders or infections, remove wax, or remove foreign bodies. Examination of the ear canal should be completed during insertion and removal of the speculum. The ear canal should be smooth and empty. There should be no redness, scaliness, swelling, drainage, nodules, foreign objects, or excessive wax (see "Evidence-Based Practice"). The internal otoscopic examination is conducted to examine the eardrum and is done by the HCP. The eardrum should appear slightly conical, shiny, and smooth and be a pearly gray color.

EVIDENCE-BASED PRACTICE

Clinical Question
Does cerumen removal affect cognition?

Evidence
Three cerumenolytic agents were compared for removal of cerumen, and the effect of cerumen removal on cognition was assessed. Thirty-eight older-adult subjects (mean age: 78 years) were treated. A statistically significant difference between the Raven's standard progressive matrices (measures test takers reasoning ability) score before and after the removal of cerumen was found.

Implications for Nursing Practice
Ensuring that the ear canal is kept clear of cerumen is important to the well-being of older adults.

REFERENCE
Oron, Y., Zwecker-Lazar, I., Levy, D., Kreitler, S., & Roth, Y. (2011). Cerumen removal: Comparison of cerumenolytic agents and effect on cognition among the elderly. Archives of Gerontology & Geriatrics, 52, 228–232.

Diagnostic Tests for the Ear and Hearing
Audiometric Testing

Audiometric testing is used as a screening tool to determine the type and degree of hearing loss. An audiologist conducts the hearing tests in a soundproof booth. The audiometer produces a stimulus that consists of a musical tone, pure tone, or speech. To test air conduction, the patient is placed in the booth, wears earphones, and signals the audiologist when and if the tone is heard. Each ear is tested separately as the patient is exposed to sounds of varying frequency or pitch (hertz) and intensity (decibels). By varying the levels of the sound, a hearing level is established (Table 51.7). The use of earphones measures air conduction, level of speech hearing, and understanding of speech. During bone conduction testing, a vibrator is placed on the mastoid process and the earphones are removed. Testing proceeds as with air conduction.

A patient with normal hearing should have the same air conduction as bone conduction hearing levels. Alterations in testing air and bone conduction hearing can provide information about the location and type of hearing loss.

Tympanometry

Tympanometry is a test used to measure compliance of the tympanic membrane and differentiate problems in the middle

TABLE 51.7 COMMON NOISE LEVELS

Human hearing threshold	**0–25 dB**
Quiet room	30–40 dB
Conversational speech	60 dB
Heavy traffic	70 dB
Telephone	70 dB
Alarm clock	80 dB
Vacuum cleaner	80 dB
Unsafe noise levels begin	**90 dB**
Circular saw	100 dB
Rock music	120 dB
Jet planes	120–130 dB
Pain threshold	**130 dB**
Firearms	140 dB

ear. Varying amounts of pressure are applied to the tympanic membrane, and the results create a distinctive response recorded on a graph called a tympanogram. The test is useful in determining the amount of negative pressure within the middle ear. The patient is informed that the tympanometry may cause transient vertigo. The patient should report any nausea or dizziness experienced during the test.

Caloric Test

The caloric test is used to test the function of the eighth cranial nerve and to assess vestibular reflexes of the inner ear that control balance. The test is performed first on one ear and then the other. Warm (112°F [44.5°C]) or cold (86°F [30°C]) water is instilled into the ear canal. This stimulates the endolymph of the semicircular canals, which stimulates movement of the head. Nystagmus is a normal response. The patient may also feel dizzy. No nystagmus is seen if the patient has a disease of the labyrinth such as Ménière's disease. The test is contraindicated if the patient has a perforated tympanic membrane. Otoscopic examination should be completed before this test to assess for excessive cerumen or perforated tympanic membrane.

Electronystagmogram

The electronystagmogram is used to diagnose the causes of unilateral hearing loss of unknown origin, vertigo, or ringing in the ears. It is similar to the caloric test. The test is usually completed in a darkened room. Five electrodes are taped to the patient's clean face at certain positions around the eye. The electrodes measure nystagmus in response to vestibular stimulation. Measurements are taken at rest, looking at different objects, with eyes open and closed, in different positions, with water of different temperatures, and with air. Usually tranquilizers, alcohol, stimulants, and antivertigo agents are held for 1 to 5 days before the test. The patient should also avoid tobacco and caffeine on the day of the test. The test is contraindicated in patients who have pacemakers. The patient may experience nausea, vertigo, or weakness following the test.

Computed Tomography

CT is useful for visualizing the temporal and mastoid bones, the middle and inner ears, and the eustachian tube.

Magnetic Resonance Imaging

MRI allows the membranous organs, nerve, and blood vessels of the temporal bone to be examined for disease.

Laboratory Tests

EAR CULTURE. Culture of drainage from the ear canal or surgical incision is important in diagnosis and treatment of acute infections. Identifying the organism responsible for the infection allows the appropriate antibiotic to be used. Often with chronic infections, the culture is less helpful because Gram-negative bacilli cover up the original pathogen. Drainage from the external ear is collected using a sterile cotton-tipped or polyester-tipped swab. Samples should be taken to the laboratory immediately.

PATHOLOGY EXAMINATION. Pathology examination of tissue obtained during surgery is completed to rule out a malignancy and identify any unusual problems. A cholesteatoma (cyst of epithelial cells and cholesterol found in the middle ear) is usually documented by a pathology examination.

Therapeutic Measures for the Ear and Hearing
Medications

The medications most often used to treat ear disorders include anti-infectives, anti-inflammatories, antihistamines, decongestants, cerumenolytics, and diuretics. Anti-infectives can be administered systemically or as a topical solution. Ear medications are generally in a liquid form for ease in administration as drops (Box 51-5 and Fig. 51.17). Anti-inflammatories, antihistamines, and decongestants are used with acute infections to reduce nasal and middle ear congestion. Cerumenolytics are used to soften cerumen and remove it from the ear canal. Diuretics are used with some inner ear disorders to reduce pressure caused by fluids.

CRITICAL THINKING

Mr. Frank

■ At a physician's office visit, Mr. Frank's wife expresses concern about his changing behavior during the last 6 months. She reports that Mr. Frank no longer enjoys talking to neighbors or visiting with friends in their church group, is irritable, has lost his sense of humor, and does not always answer her questions appropriately.

1. What do you suspect is happening with Mr. Frank?

2. What examination techniques or tests might you use to gather data related to Mr. Frank's signs and symptoms?
3. What would be the expected findings of these tests?
4. What other members of the health care team might be involved in Mr. Frank's care?
5. What teaching for these symptoms and their effect on Mr. Frank's lifestyle would be helpful?
6. What safety issues should Mr. Frank be taught to address?

Suggested answers are at the end of the chapter.

Box 51-5 Administration of Eardrops

1. Explain procedure to patient.
2. Check medication for dosage, strength, side effects, contraindications, and expiration date. Make sure medication is at room temperature.
3. Perform hand hygiene and apply gloves.
4. Position patient sitting up with head tilted toward unaffected side or lying down on the unaffected side.
5. For a child, pull auricle down and back. For an adult, pull auricle up and back.
6. Instill prescribed number of drops, being careful not to touch tip of dropper to anything to prevent contamination.
7. Have patient remain in position for 2 to 3 minutes.
8. A small cotton plug may be inserted to prevent medication from running out of ear.
9. Remove gloves. Perform hand hygiene.
10. Document eardrop administration and patient's tolerance of procedure.

FIGURE 51.17 Eardrop administration.

Ear Health Maintenance

Safe routine cleaning and care of the ears should be taught to all patients (Fig. 51.18). Patient education should include prevention of trauma, prevention of hearing loss, and early detection of hearing loss. All patients can benefit from this type of education, as found in Table 51.8.

Assistive Hearing Devices

Hearing aids are instruments that amplify sound (see Chapter 52). Certain hearing aids may be designed to amplify sounds and attenuate certain portions of the sound signal. A small battery serves as the energy source. Digital hearing aids contain computers that convert sound waves into numerical codes, before amplifying. This provides clearer and crisper sound that is programmable to each person's hearing loss. Digital hearing aids are more expensive than analog (convert sound waves into electrical signals for amplifying) hearing aids. Three types of hearing aids are commonly used today:

1. The in-the-ear aid fits into the ear. It is small and unobtrusive to the wearer and others.

FIGURE 51.18 Ear drum perforation. Avoid putting things into the ear canal for cleaning to prevent injury.

2. The canal aid fits into the ear canal and is nearly unseen.
3. New technology for assistive devices is being used or developed that involves the use of Bluetooth and smart phones. Several amplification apps are available.

To care for a hearing aid, ensure that it is turned off and the battery is removed when it is not in use. This reduces battery expense for the patient, who may be on a fixed income. When turning the hearing aid on, the volume should be turned up just until it squeals and then turned down until the patient indicates it is at the appropriate level for hearing. At least weekly, clean the hearing aid mold portion with either a dry cloth or a damp, soapy cloth and rinse with a damp cloth. A brush may come with the hearing aid for cleaning, or a cotton-tipped swab can be used to clean the small tip that fits into the ear.

Other types of assistive hearing devices are middle ear implants and **cochlear implants**. The middle ear implant (see www.vibrant-medel.com) is for those with a sensorineural hearing loss. It provides sound perception by enhancing the normal middle ear hearing function. A person who is profoundly deaf and has lost all hearing may use a cochlear implant, which is placed surgically. Cochlear implants feature a microelectronic processor for converting the sound into electrical signals, a transmission system to relay signals to the implanted parts, and a long, slender electrode placed in the cochlea to deliver the electrical stimuli directly to the fiber of the auditory nerve.

Safety products are available to help people with hearing impairments. These include visual-alarm smoke detectors, such as a flashing light, or alarms that vibrate the bed as a means to alert a person with a hearing impairment of a fire.

Guide Dogs for the Deaf and Hearing Impaired

Hearing ear dogs are trained to respond to sounds that the person who is hard of hearing cannot hear. Examples include a crying baby, oven timer, and smoke alarm. These dogs provide a valuable service that enriches the lives of those with hearing problems.

TABLE 51.8 PREVENTION OF EAR PROBLEMS

Activity	Patient Education	Rationale
Care of external ear	Wash external ear with soap and water only.	Keeps external ear clean.
	Do not routinely remove wax from the ear canal.	The ear is generally self-cleaning. Wax is normally removed during showering. Wax serves as a protective mechanism to lubricate and trap foreign material.
Preventing ear trauma	Avoid inserting any objects or solutions into the ear. Avoid swimming in polluted areas.	Prevents traumatizing the ear and tympanic membrane or exposing the ear to infection.

Continued

TABLE **51.8** **PREVENTION OF EAR PROBLEMS—cont'd**

Activity	Patient Education	Rationale
	Avoid flying when the ear or upper respiratory system is congested.	Prevents barotrauma due to pressure changes.
Preventing damage from noise pollution	Avoid exposure to excessive occupational noise levels. Avoid other causes of excessive noise such as use of firearms and high-intensity music. Use protective earplugs or earmuffs if exposure to noise cannot be avoided. Instruct adults to have hearing checked every 2–3 years.	Normal speech is 60 dB; heavy traffic is 70 dB. Above 80 dB is uncomfortable. If there is ringing in the ear, damage may be occurring. Occupational noise is the primary cause of hearing loss. Hearing loss can occur due to exposure to loud noises. Protects ears from hearing loss by decreasing exposure to loud noises. Degenerative changes occur in the ear with aging.
Early detection of hearing loss	Monitor for side effects of ototoxic drugs. Instruct patient to report any dizziness, decreased hearing acuity, or tinnitus when taking ototoxic medications. Caution older patients who use aspirin that it is ototoxic. Instruct patient to report to physician any prolonged symptoms of ear pain, swelling, drainage, or plugged feeling. Instruct patient to blow nose with both nostrils open during upper respiratory infections (colds).	Prevents side effects of medications from causing hearing loss. Older patients may have hearing loss and not be able to hear the tinnitus. Many medical problems can be prevented with prompt treatment. Prevents infected secretions from moving up the eustachian tubes into the middle ear.

SUGGESTED ANSWERS TO

CRITICAL THINKING

■ *Mr. Frank*

1. He is exhibiting behaviors of hearing loss.

2. Ear inspection, a whisper voice test, a Rinne test, and a Weber test might be performed.

3. For inspection of ear, cerumen impaction may be found. For a whisper voice test, the whisper is not heard in affected ear. For a Rinne test, bone conduction is heard longer than air conduction in affected ear. For a Weber test, sound is heard louder in affected ear.

4. Audiologist.

5. Explaining to Mr. and Mrs. Frank symptoms of hearing loss will help them understand Mr. Frank's behaviors. Explore with them the effects of these symptoms in daily life to develop plans for coping with the hearing loss until an intervention is implemented.

6. Mr. Frank may not hear telephones or alarms such as smoke or carbon monoxide detectors, so alternatives such as visual alarms could be considered. If he drives, he may not hear car horns or emergency vehicles of which he should be aware so he can compensate.

REVIEW QUESTIONS

1. In what order does a beam of light pass through the refractive structures in the eye? (Use all items, and place them in the correct order.)
   1. Aqueous humor
   2. Cornea
   3. Lens
   4. Vitreous humor

2. The nurse is asked to assist with the assessment of a patient's visual fields. Which assessment method does the nurse anticipate will be used?
   1. Inspection using an ophthalmoscope
   2. Fluorescein angiography
   3. Vision test using Snellen's chart
   4. Comparison of the patient's visual fields with the nurse's own

3. Which patient behavior would the nurse expect to find in the health history of a patient who has a hearing loss?
   1. Turns volume lower on the television.
   2. Is irritable or sensitive in interpersonal relations.
   3. Answers questions appropriately.
   4. Mentions that people talk too loudly

4. The nurse is collecting data during a patient's clinic visit. Which question will best collect data about a patient's preventive ear health?
   1. "What symptoms are you having?"
   2. "Tell me about your ear pain."
   3. "When was your last hearing evaluation?"
   4. "What medications do you take?"

5. The nurse is assisting with a Romberg's test. What is the most important nursing intervention during the Romberg's test?
   1. Ensure patient safety.
   2. Whisper softly into each ear.
   3. Ensure a quiet environment.
   4. Remove all cerumen from ear canal.

6. The nurse teaches a patient about ear care. Which patient statement indicates to the nurse that the patient understands the ear care teaching?
   1. "I should insert a cotton swab into my ear canal for cleaning."
   2. "I should not get my external ear wet during bathing."
   3. "I should block one nostril when blowing my nose."
   4. "Aspirin can be toxic to the ears."

7. The nurse prepares to provide an eye irrigation to a patient with a methicillin-resistant *Streptococcus aureus* (MRSA) infection. Contact precautions are ordered. Which of the following protective items will the nurse need while performing this procedure? **Select all that apply.**
   1. Gloves
   2. Gown
   3. Goggles
   4. Mask
   5. Shoe protectors
   6. Sterile gloves

8. A patient is taking aspirin. Which finding would indicate to the nurse that the patient is experiencing a toxic effect related to the medication?
   1. Halos around lights
   2. Decreased night vision
   3. Tinnitus
   4. Vertigo

Answers can be found in Appendix C.

References

American Academy of Ophthalmology: www.aao.org
American Foundation for the Blind: (800) 232-5463 or www.afb.org
American Speech-Language-Hearing Association: http://asha.org
National Association for Visually Handicapped: (212) 889-3141 or www.navh.org
National Library Service for the Blind and Physically Handicapped: (800) 424-8567 or www.loc.gov/nls

Lighthouse International: (800) 334-5497 or www.lighthouse.org
National Eye Institute: (301) 496-5248 or www.nei.nih.gov
Prevent Blindness America (800) 331-2020 www.preventblindness.org

 For additional resources and information visit **davispl.us/medsurg5**

52

Nursing Care of Patients With Sensory Disorders: Vision and Hearing

KEY TERMS

astigmatism (uh-STIG-mah-TIZM)
blepharitis (BLEF-uh-RIGH-tis)
blindness (BLYND-ness)
carbuncle (KAR-bung-kull)
cataract (KAT-uh-rakt)
chalazion (kah-LAY-zee-on)
conductive hearing loss (kon-DUK-tiv HEER-ing LOSS)
conjunctivitis (kon-JUNK-ti-VIGH-tis)
enucleation (ee-NEW-klee-AY-shun)
external otitis (eks-TER-nuhl oh-TIGH-tis)
furuncle (FYOOR-ung-kull)
glaucoma (glaw-KOH-mah)
hordeolum (hor-DEE-oh-lum)
hyperopia (HIGH-per-OH-pee-ah)
macular (MAK-yoo-lar)
Ménière's disease (ma-NEARS di-ZEEZ)
miotics (my-AH-tiks)
myopia (my-OH-pee-ah)
myringoplasty (mir-IN-goh-PLASS-tee)
myringotomy (MIR-in-GOT-uh-mee)
otosclerosis (OH-toh-skle-ROH-sis)
photophobia (FOH-toh-FOH-bee-ah)
presbycusis (PREZ-by-KYOO-sis)
presbyopia (PREZ-by-OH-pee-ah)
retinopathy (ret-i-NAH-puh-thee)
sensorineural (SEN-suh-ree-NEW-ruhl)
stapedectomy (stuh-puh-DEK-tuh-mee)

LEARNING OUTCOMES

1. Explain the pathophysiology of each of the disorders of the sensory system.

2. Define blindness and the refractive errors of vision.

3. Explain the etiologies, signs, and symptoms of each sensory disorder.

4. Plan nursing care for patients undergoing tests for sensory disorders.

5. Identify therapeutic measures for each sensory disorder.

6. Identify medications contraindicated for patients with acute angle-closure glaucoma.

7. List three ototoxic drugs.

8. List data to collect when caring for patients with disorders of the sensory system.

9. Plan nursing care for patients with disorders of the eye or ear.

10. Plan nursing care interventions for the patient with a hearing impairment.

11. Discuss how to know if nursing interventions for sensory disorders have been effective.

VISION DISORDERS

Early detection of visual problems can reduce their impact. Nurses play an important role in assisting the patient with visual problems (Table 52.1).

Infections and Inflammation

Infections and inflammation of the eye and surrounding structures can be bacterial or viral in origin. The eye may become aggravated by allergens, chemical substances, or mechanical irritation, leading to infection by microorganisms. Mechanical irritation may be caused by sunburn or bacterial infection. Inflammation results from allergies to environmental substances or by irritation of chemical irritants found in perfumes, makeup, sprays, or plants. Viral agents that cause infection include herpes simplex virus, cytomegalovirus, and human adenovirus. Bacterial agents that infect the eye include *Staphylococcus* and *Streptococcus* ("Cultural Considerations").

Conjunctivitis

Conjunctivitis is inflammation of the conjunctiva caused by either a virus or a bacterium. Viral conjunctivitis occurs more commonly than bacterial conjunctivitis and is highly contagious. The virus is usually transmitted via contaminated eye secretions on the hand that then touches or rubs an eye, infecting that eye. The virus is hardy and may live on dry surfaces for 2 weeks or more. Viral conjunctivitis lasts 2 to 4 weeks. Bacterial conjunctivitis (commonly called pinkeye) usually is due to staphylococcal or streptococcal bacteria and is also highly contagious. Conjunctivitis can also be caused by the organisms *Haemophilus influenzae*, *Chlamydia trachomatis,* and *Neisseria gonorrhoeae*. Conjunctivitis is commonly transmitted among children and then to family members. Signs and symptoms of conjunctivitis include conjunctival redness and crusting exudate

• WORD • BUILDING •

conjunctivitis: conjunctive—joining membrane + itis—inflammation

TABLE 52.1 EYE DISORDER SUMMARY

Signs and Symptoms	Visual disturbances Pain Redness, secretions, itchiness Sensation of pressure in eyes
Diagnostic Tests and Findings	Visual acuity Ophthalmoscopic examination of internal and external eye Amsler grid (identifies visual field disturbances) Slit-lamp examination (identifies abnormalities on cornea and sclera) Tonometry (identifies intraocular pressure)
Therapeutic Measures	Medications: reduce intraocular pressure, treat infections, anesthetize the eye Surgery
Complications	Worsening vision or loss of vision Acute pain
Priority Nursing Diagnoses	*Anxiety* related to visual-sensory deficit *Risk for Injury* *Deficient Knowledge*

 ## Cultural Considerations

Vision

Trachoma, a form of conjunctivitis, is a common, chronic disease that affects millions of people worldwide. It is primarily seen among low-income persons in the Mediterranean, Africa, Brazil, and the Far East. Trachoma is caused by a viral strain of *Chlamydia trachomatis* that is highly contagious. Following the acute conjunctivitis phase, the eyelids shrink as a result of scarring. The shrinking tends to pull the eyelashes inward (entropion), which may scratch the cornea. In addition, granulations form on the inner eyelids. This painful condition may eventually lead to corneal ulceration and blindness. Trachoma is medically treated with topical and oral erythromycin or tetracycline.

on the lids and in the corners of the eyes, itching, pain, and excessive tearing.

Viral conjunctivitis is treated by supportive measures, which seek to keep the patient comfortable until the infection resolves on its own. Treatment includes eyewashes or eye irrigations, which cleanse the conjunctivas and relieve the inflammation and pain. Bacterial conjunctivitis is treated with antibiotic eye drops or ointments (Table 52.2). Adults generally prefer eye drops because they do not impair vision. Ointments are commonly used when the eye is resting (at night) or in children, who may squeeze their eyes shut and cry when ocular medications are applied, thus expelling the medication. With either type of conjunctivitis, hand hygiene is the best means of preventing the spread of the disease.

Blepharitis

Blepharitis, an inflammation of the eyelid margins, is a chronic inflammatory process. The cause may include staphylococcal infection, seborrhea (dandruff), rosacea (a chronic disease of the skin usually affecting middle-aged and older adults), dry eye, or abnormalities of the meibomian glands and their lipid secretions. There are two types of blepharitis: seborrheic blepharitis and ulcerative blepharitis. Seborrheic blepharitis is characterized by reddened eyelids with scales and flaking at the base of the lashes. Ulcerative blepharitis produces crusts at eyelashes, reddened eyes, and inflamed corneas. Eyelids chronically infected with *Staphylococcus* may become thickened, and eyelashes may be lost. Treatment requires a commitment to long-term daily cleansing with cotton-tipped swabs dipped in

TABLE 52.2 OPHTHALMIC MEDICATIONS

Medication Class/Action	Examples	Nursing Implications
Diagnostic Aids **Fluorescein Sodium** Staining of eye. Lesions of foreign objects pick up bright yellow-orange stain so abnormality can be detected.	fluorescein (AK-Fluor)	Stain needs to be irrigated out of eye when examination is complete. Stain is colorfast, so caution should be used when irrigating.
Topical Anesthetics Provide local anesthesia to area, making examination painless. Also used to reduce pain of injury.	tetracaine (Pontocaine)	Eye must be protected because blink reflex is temporarily lost. Lid should be kept closed to keep eye moist after examination and treatment.
Antiangiogenetics **Antivascular Endothelial Growth Factor** Inhibits growth of new blood vessels and slows progression of wet age-related macular degeneration	pegaptanib (Macugen)	Monitor for 1 week after to detect infection early.
Eye Allergy Symptom Relief Relieves red, itchy eyes caused by allergies	nedocromil (Alocril) azelastine (Astelin) naphazoline (Naphcon) olopatadine (Patanol)	See Box 51-4. Caution patient not to wear soft contact lenses while eyes are red.
Anti-Infectives **Antibiotics** Treat bacterial eye infections.	ciloxan (Cipro)	Give on an empty stomach. Encourage fluids. Urge patient to take with full glass of water.
	gatifloxacin (Zymar)	See Boxes 51-4 and 51-5.

TABLE 52.2 OPHTHALMIC MEDICATIONS—cont'd

Medication Class/Action	Examples	Nursing Implications
	polymyxin B and trimethoprim ophthalmic (Polytrim) tobramycin (Tobrex) sulfacetamide (Bleph-10, Isopto Cetamide, Sodium Sulamyd)	
Antivirals Treat viral eye infections.	trifluridine (Viroptic)	See Box 51-4.
Antifungals Treat fungal eye infections.	natamycin (Natacyn)	Follow instructions for instillation.
Anti-Inflammatories Reduce inflammation of conjunctiva, cornea, or eyelids due to infection, edema, allergic reaction, cataract surgery or burns.		
Steroidal	dexamethasone (Decadron) May be combined with antibiotic, as in TobraDex (tobramycin and dexamethasone)	See Box 51-4.
Nonsteroidal	ketorolac (Acular) bromfenac (Xibrom)	See Box 51-4 Use only as prescribed. Reduces ocular inflammation and pain following cataract surgery usually within 2 days of bid treatment.
Lubricants Moisten eyes in healthy and ill persons.	artificial tears (Lacri-Lube, Tears Plus)	Explain that ointment distorts vision.
Miotics Lower intraocular pressure by stimulating papillary and ciliary sphincter muscles.	pilocarpine (Pilocar) physostigmine (Isopto Eserine)	See Box 51-4. Expect to see a smaller than normal pupil with little if any reaction to light.
Carbonic Anhydrase Inhibitors Reduce intraocular pressure by reducing aqueous humor formation. Used for glaucoma when other miotics have been unsuccessful.	acetazolamide (Diamox)	Check for sulfa allergy. Instruct patient to avoid excess sun exposure.
Osmotics Reduce intraocular pressure in acute open-angle glaucoma.	mannitol (Osmitrol)	Monitor for headache, nausea, vomiting, and confusion.
Beta-Adrenergic Blockers Reduce intraocular pressure by reducing aqueous humor formation and increasing its outflow.	timolol (Timoptic) betaxolol (Betoptic)	See Box 51-4. Monitor for bradycardia, heart block, and wheezing.

Continued

TABLE 52.2 OPHTHALMIC MEDICATIONS—cont'd

Medication Class/Action	Examples	Nursing Implications
Mydriatics Dilate pupils for examination or surgical procedures.	atropine	See Box 51-4 Dilated pupils cannot protect eye from bright light, so dark glasses are needed until drug effects have worn off. Monitor for side effects.
Cycloplegics Paralyze muscles of accommodation for examination or surgical procedures.	cyclopentolate	Contraindicated in patients with glaucoma because of increase in intraocular pressure.

diluted baby shampoo or sterile eyelid cleanser solutions to prevent infection. If infection occurs, antistaphylococcal antibiotic ointment (bacitracin, erythromycin) is applied to the lid margins one to four times a day after the eyelids have been cleansed. Warm compresses may also be used.

Hordeolum and Chalazion

Another type of eyelid infection is a **hordeolum**. An external hordeolum (sty) is a small staphylococcal abscess in the sebaceous gland at the base of the eyelash (either the glands of Zeis or glands of Moll). Styes are small, raised, reddened areas. Use of cosmetics on the eyes may contribute to hordeolum formation. A second type of abscess, a **chalazion** (internal hordeolum), may form in the connective tissue of the eyelids, specifically in the meibomian glands. A chalazion is larger than an external hordeolum. Styes may be tender; however, a chalazion often puts pressure on the cornea, causing more discomfort. Hordeolums usually form and heal spontaneously within a few days and require no treatment. Chalazions may require surgical incision and drainage (I&D) if they do not drain spontaneously. If either type of abscess persists, administration of oral antibiotics may be prescribed along with application of warm compresses to aid healing.

Keratitis

PATHOPHYSIOLOGY AND ETIOLOGY. Keratitis is inflammation of the cornea and may be acute or chronic and superficial or deep. The depth of keratitis is determined by the layers of the cornea that may be affected. Keratitis may be associated with bacterial conjunctivitis, a viral infection such as herpes simplex, a corneal ulcer, or diseases such as tuberculosis and syphilis. Herpes simplex keratitis is the most common corneal infection in developed countries, with bacterial and fungal infections being more prevalent throughout the rest of the world. People who have dry eyes, wear contact lenses and practice poor contact lens hygiene, have decreased corneal sensation, or are immunosuppressed are at increased risk of keratitis.

SIGNS AND SYMPTOMS. The cornea has many pain receptors, so any inflammation of the cornea is painful. This pain increases

with movement of the lid over the cornea. Other symptoms of keratitis include decreased vision, **photophobia** (sensitivity to light), tearing, and blepharospasm (spasm of the eyelids). The conjunctiva often appears reddened. In advanced cases, the cornea may appear opaque (cloudy).

DIAGNOSTIC TESTS. Assessment of keratitis or corneal ulcer is made by use of a slit lamp or a handheld light. The cornea is examined by shining the light source obliquely (diagonally) across the cornea to show opacity in the cornea. Fluorescein stain may also be used to outline the area of involvement. When the stained area is viewed with a blue light, the disruption in the corneal surface shows up clear. If the patient is having pain from blepharospasm (contraction of the orbicularis oculi muscle), the examiner may instill a topical ophthalmic anesthetic such as proparacaine.

THERAPEUTIC MEASURES. Therapeutic interventions may include topical antibiotics, topical corticosteroids, topical interferons, antiviral medications for herpes simplex, cycloplegic agents (to keep the iris and ciliary body at rest), and warm compresses. If the cornea is severely damaged, corneal transplant may be required. The eye may be patched to decrease the amount of eyelid movement over the cornea during healing.

COMPLICATIONS. Corneal infections are usually serious and often threaten eyesight. The corneal tissue may become thin and susceptible to perforation. Untreated, keratitis can cause permanent scarring of the cornea, resulting in permanent loss of vision.

Nursing Process for the Patient With Inflammation and Infection of the Eye

DATA COLLECTION. Table 52.3 reviews the subjective data that is collected. Objective data collection includes the condition of the conjunctiva, eyelids, and eyelashes; the presence of exudate, tearing, any visible abscess on the palpebral border, or a palpable abscess in the eyelid; opacity of the cornea; and visual acuity testing comparing unaffected and affected eyes.

• WORD • BUILDING •

photophobia: photo—light + phobia—fear of

TABLE 52.3 SUBJECTIVE DATA COLLECTION FOR EYE INFLAMMATION AND INFECTION CONDITIONS

W Where is it?	What part of the eye is affected? Eyelid, conjunctiva, cornea?
H How does it feel?	Pressure? Itchy? Painful? No pain? Irritated? Spasm?
A Aggravating and alleviating factors	Is it worse when rubbing eyes or blinking? Is there photosensitivity?
T Timing	Was there exposure to a pathogen? Previous infection or irritation? How long have symptoms persisted?
S Severity	Is there visual impairment? Does pain affect activities of daily living?
U Useful data for associated symptoms	Is patient infected with lice? Immunosuppression? Do other members of the family or peer group have symptoms? Are eyedrops used? Is there exudate? Are the eyelids stuck together on awakening? Does patient wear contact lenses, soft contact lenses overnight, disposable contact lenses? Does patient have dry eyes? Is patient infected with tuberculosis, syphilis, HIV? What is typical eye hygiene?
P Perception of the problem by the patient	What does patient think is wrong?

HIV = human immunodeficiency virus.

NURSING DIAGNOSES, PLANNING, AND IMPLEMENTATION.
Acute Pain related to inflammation or infection of the eye or surrounding tissues
EXPECTED OUTCOME: The patient's pain will be decreased or absent as evidenced by lower rating on a pain scale.

• Assess the patient for pain. *Use of dark glasses, rubbing the eye, squinting, and avoiding light may be indicators of pain that should be assessed.*
• Administer eye medications (topical anesthetic drops or ointments, antibiotics, anti-inflammatory agents, or analgesics) as ordered *to relieve eye pain.*
• Apply warm or cool packs as ordered *to assist in soothing the eye.*
• Patching of the affected eye may help reduce pain *by decreasing the movement of the eye across the eyelid.*
• Explore additional methods of pain reduction, *such as guided imagery, relaxation techniques, music, or distraction.*

Risk for Injury related to visual impairment
EXPECTED OUTCOME: The patient will not experience injury as a result of visual impairment.

• Assess and plan for visual impairments that may be present *to promote safety.*
• Advise patient with one eye patched not to drive *to prevent injury because depth perception is altered.*
• Teach caution when ambulating and reaching for things *to prevent injury because inflamed eyes often do not focus well and may have exudate, tearing, or ointment present, which can interfere with vision.*

Deficient Knowledge related to eye disease process, prevention, and treatment from lack of previous experience
EXPECTED OUTCOME: The patient will be able to explain the disease process, prevention, and treatment measures. The patient will demonstrate the treatment regimen correctly, such as administration of eye drops.

• Teach patient prevention, care of the affected eye, medication administration, and safety issues *for understanding and adherence to therapeutic plan.*
• Have patient demonstrate the administration of ointments or drops after teaching has occurred *to evaluate understanding.*
• Teach patient and family how to prevent spreading infection *if it is contagious.*
• Teach patient proper eye hygiene *to prevent further complications.*
• Teach contact lens hygiene *to prevent reinfection of the eye.*
• Teach not to wear contact lenses when the eye or surrounding structure is inflamed *to prevent irritation.*

EVALUATION. The therapeutic measures have been successful if pain is reduced to an acceptable rating, vision improves or returns to preillness level, injury does not occur as a result of visual impairment, infection does not occur as a result of poor eye hygiene or wearing of contact lenses, patient explains disease process, prevention, or treatment regimen accurately, or prescribed treatment is stated or demonstrated correctly (e.g., administering eye drops or ointments).

Refractive Errors

Pathophysiology and Etiology

Refraction refers to the bending of light rays as they enter the eye. *Emmetropia,* or normal vision, means that light rays are bent to focus images precisely on the macula of the retina. *Ametropia* is a term used to describe any refractive error. When an image is not clearly focused on the retina, refractive error is present. Ametropia occurs when parallel light rays entering the eye are not refracted to focus on the retina. Refractive errors account for the largest number of impairments in vision. There are four common ametropic disorders: **hyperopia**, **myopia**, **astigmatism**, and **presbyopia**.

HYPEROPIA. Hyperopia (farsightedness) is caused by light rays focusing behind the retina (Fig. 52.1). People who are hyperopic see images that are far away more clearly than images that are close. Physiologically, the globe or eyeball is too short from the front to the back, causing the light rays to focus beyond the retina. Hyperopia is corrected with convex lenses.

MYOPIA. Myopia (nearsightedness) is caused by light rays focusing in front of the retina. The eyeball is elongated, and thus the light rays do not reach the retina. Distance vision is blurred but items close up are clear. Myopia is corrected with concave lenses (Fig. 52.1).

ASTIGMATISM. Astigmatism results from unequal curvatures in the shape of the cornea. When parallel light rays enter the eye, the irregular cornea causes the light rays to be refracted to focus on two different points. This can result in either myopic or hyperopic astigmatism. The person with astigmatism has blurred vision with distortion. The corneal irregularities can be caused by injury, inflammation, corneal surgery, or an inherited autosomal dominant trait.

PRESBYOPIA. Presbyopia is a condition in which the crystalline lenses lose their elasticity, resulting in a decrease in ability to focus on close objects. The loss of elasticity causes light rays to focus beyond the retina, resulting in hyperopia. This condition usually is associated with aging and generally occurs after age 40. If an individual has preexisting hyperopia, the onset of presbyopia may occur earlier than age 40. Likewise, if a person has myopia, presbyopia may correct the myopia by projecting the light rays directly on the retina. Because accommodation for close vision is accomplished by lens contraction, people with presbyopia exhibit the inability to see objects at close range. They often compensate for blurred close vision by holding objects to be viewed farther away. Reports of eyestrain and mild frontal headache are common. These symptoms are relieved with eye rest and corrective lenses.

Signs and Symptoms

People with refractive errors commonly report difficulty reading or seeing objects. Often, the eyestrain that occurs as one attempts to improve visual acuity causes headache.

• WORD • BUILDING •
presbyopia: presby—old age + opia—concerning vision

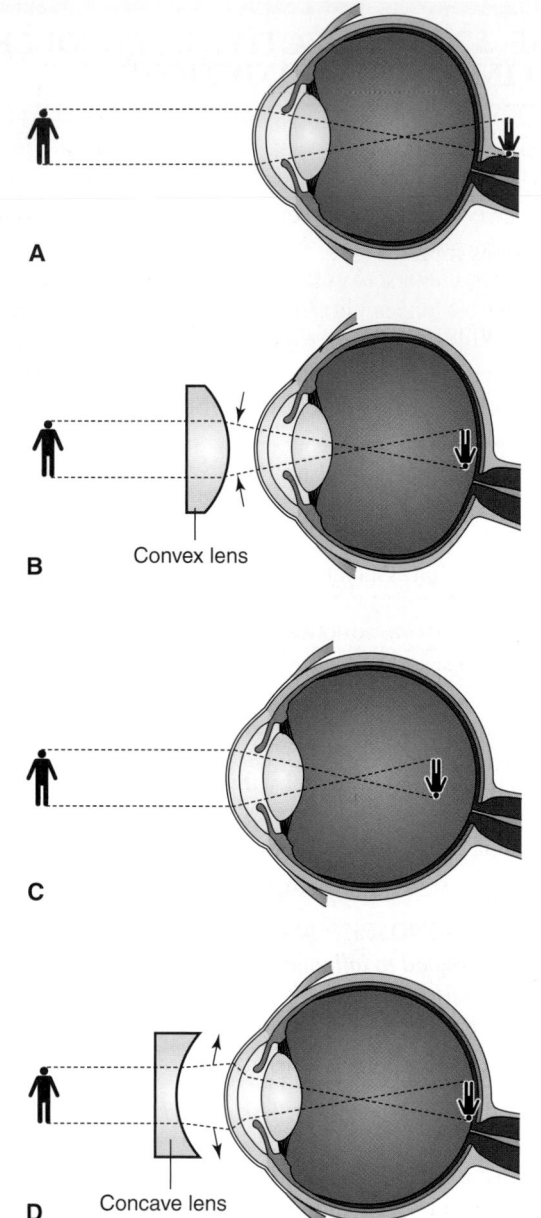

FIGURE 52.1 Refractive disorders. (A) Hyperopia (farsighted). The eyeball is too short, causing the image to focus beyond the retina. (B) Corrected hyperopia. (C) Myopia (nearsighted). A long eyeball causes the image to focus in front of the retina. (D) Corrected myopia.

LEARNING TIP

To remember the type of vision a person has, use this saying: *You are what you say.* For example, if you say you are farsighted, this means that you have clear vision of far away images, but difficulty seeing images that are nearer. If you say you are nearsighted, this means that you have clear vision of near images, but difficulty seeing images that are farther away.

Diagnostic Tests

A refractive error can be roughly estimated by use of Snellen's chart. For definitive refractive error measurement, a retinoscopic examination is needed. Before this examination, a cycloplegic drug is often instilled (see Table 52.2). A cycloplegic drug dilates the pupil and temporarily paralyzes the ciliary muscle, thus preventing accommodation. During the examination, an ophthalmologist or optometrist examines the internal and external eye and uses trial lenses via a retinoscope to assess the type of lens best suited to correct the refractive error, which may differ in each eye. If a cycloplegic agent has been used, patients need to be told that blurred vision might be present and sunglasses worn until the agent wears off. In addition, the patient should be instructed that driving and reading might not be possible until the effect of the cycloplegic drug is gone.

Therapeutic Measures

Refractive errors are commonly treated with either eyeglasses or contact lenses. The corrective lenses bend the parallel light rays so that they converge on the macular portion of the retina. Laser-assisted in situ keratomileusis (LASIK) and photorefractive keratectomy (PRK) are surgical procedures also used to correct refractive error. With LASIK and PRK, laser energy is applied to reshape the cornea. The cornea is made flatter for individuals with myopia and more cone shaped for those with hyperopia.

Blindness

Blindness is the complete or almost complete absence of the sense of sight. Some people consider the terms *blind* and *partially sighted* to be negative and prefer the term *visually impaired* to describe their condition.

Pathophysiology and Etiology

Blindness in adults is caused by a variety of factors, including trauma, complications from various diseases such as hypertension and diabetes and conditions such as **cataracts** and **glaucoma**. Blindness is produced when the rays of light on their way to the optic nerve are obstructed, or by disease of the optic nerve or tract of the part of the brain connected with vision. Blindness may be permanent or transient, complete or partial, or may occur only in darkness (night blindness).

Signs and Symptoms

Aside from a general loss of vision, patients may describe their visual image as blurred, distorted, or absent in specific areas of the visual field. Objects may appear dark or absent around the peripheral field in glaucoma or retinitis pigmentosa. Retinitis pigmentosa is a degeneration of the pigmented layer of the retina. The center of the visual field may appear dark for individuals with diabetic **retinopathy** or **macular** degeneration. Half the visual field may be impaired in patients with hemianopia. This results from a defect in the optic pathways in the brain and is often seen with stroke. Patients may report that the visual field appears blurry or hazy in corneal visual problems, cataracts, diabetic retinopathy, or refractive errors (Fig. 52.2).

Diagnostic Tests

Diagnostic tests may include a visual field examination, tonometry, and slit-lamp microscope examination. Retinal angiography is used to follow blood flow through the retinal vessels and to detect vascular changes. Ultrasonography may be used to visualize changes in the posterior eye that cannot be directly examined because of other pathological conditions, such as a cloudy cornea, a bloody vitreous, or an opaque lens.

Therapeutic Measures

Therapeutic interventions for blindness center on treating the underlying condition and preventing further impairment. Treatment may include medications, surgical intervention, corrective eyewear, and referral to supportive services.

Nursing Process for the Patient With Visual Impairment

What do you think some of the challenges would be for a person who is blind?

DATA COLLECTION. Table 52.4 reviews the collection of subjective data. Collection of objective data involves observing the patient. Is there squinting? Rubbing of eyes? Is the patient using compensatory measures—magnifying glass, sitting close to television, using large-print reading materials, avoiding reading, using eyeglasses?

Psychosocial data are important because a blind person may be withdrawn or socially isolated, have low self-esteem or poor coping mechanisms, or have poor interpersonal skills as a result of the visual impairment.

NURSING DIAGNOSES, PLANNING, AND IMPLEMENTATION. Nursing care begins by understanding how to interact with a patient who has a visual impairment (Box 52-1). A patient's level of independence must be included in the planning phase. If patients have minimal visual impairment or have attended rehabilitation, they may be able to function independently. If a patient has recently become visually impaired, he or she may be completely dependent until alternative ways of coping with this impairment have been learned.

Planning focuses on meeting self-care needs, keeping the patient safe from injury, supporting the grieving process, and helping the patient acquire knowledge of agencies, services, and devices that allow maintenance of independence. Families must be included in the planning phase because they need to understand and be supportive

• WORD • BUILDING •

retinopathy: retino—having to do with the retina + pathy—
   illness, disease, or suffering

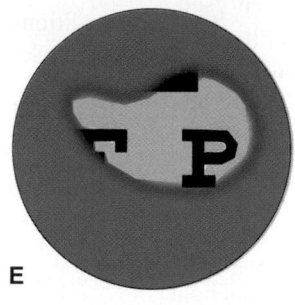

FIGURE 52.2 Visual field abnormalities. (A) Normal vision. (B) Diabetic retinopathy. (C) Cataracts. (D) Macular degeneration. (E) Advanced glaucoma.

TABLE 52.4 SUBJECTIVE DATA COLLECTION FOR VISUAL DISORDERS

W Where is it?	What part of the visual field is affected? If there is vision, what are the characteristics of what can be seen? Blurry? Hazy? Dark? Halos around lights?
H How does it feel?	Is there associated pain with the visual impairment? Headaches? How does it make the patient feel? Fearful? Anxious? Depressed? Helpless? Hopeless? Accepting?
A Aggravating and alleviating factors	Is it worse when reading? Is it worse when watching TV? Does it affect the patient only at night? Is vision better at distances or close up?
T Timing	When did the symptoms start? Do they come and go? Is the impairment progressively getting worse? Was onset sudden?
S Severity	Does the impairment affect the patient's activities of daily living? If so, how severely? Does the patient need assistance to cook, dress, bathe, read mail, pay bills, access health care, obtain transportation, maintain household, shop?
U Useful data for associated symptoms	Does the patient have diabetes, hypertension, a family history of retinitis pigmentosa, a history of eye infection, or eye trauma? Has the patient recently traveled out of the country?
P Perception of the problem by the patient	What does the patient think is wrong? How severe does the patient perceive the impairment to be?

of the self-image and role performance changes that may occur (see the "Nursing Care Plan for the Patient With Visual Impairment"). Referral to organizations that enhance the independence of people with visual impairments is helpful.

EVALUATION. The outcomes for a patient with a visual impairment are met if the patient demonstrates the ability to complete activities of daily living (ADLs) with increasing independence, remains free of injury, and demonstrates the ability to assess agencies and services for those with visual impairments.

Box 52-1 Interacting With a Patient Who Has a Visual Impairment

- People entering a room and at each contact with the patient should identify themselves.
- Post a sign on the door or over the bed that identifies the patient's visual status so that others can interact appropriately.
- Remember that the individual is not having hearing problems, so use a normal tone of voice and do not yell.
- Ask patients with visual impairments what their needs are; do not assume they need help with everything.
- Talk directly to the patient, not through a companion.
- At mealtime, explain the location of items on the tray by comparing their position to the numbers on a clock (e.g., milk is at 2 o'clock, peas are at 7 o'clock).
- Explain any activity going on in the room or within the patient's auditory range.
- Explain procedures before beginning them. Speak to the patient before touching.

- When walking with the patient, allow the patient to grasp an arm and walk a half step behind. Be aware of obstacles on either side when walking.
- When seating a patient, place the patient's hand on the arm of the chair.
- Tell the patient when leaving the room or area so the patient does not continue conversation in an empty room, which may cause embarrassment.
- When orienting the patient to the hospital room, explain the location of items the patient may need, such as the water pitcher, call light, bed controls, urinal, and tissues. Attempt to keep these items in the same place at all times.
- If the patient has a seeing eye dog, do not play with the dog, pet it, or feed it without consulting the patient—the dog is working! Make sure the patient's dog is near the bed, on a mat provided especially for the dog, preferably on the side of the bed that is less likely to be used by staff. Instruct staff and visitors about the seeing eye dog.

NURSING CARE PLAN for the Patient With Visual Impairment

Nursing Diagnosis: *Dressing and Feeding Self Care Deficit* related to altered vision.

Expected Outcome: The patient will demonstrate ability to perform ADLs, with assistance if necessary.

Evaluation of Outcome: Patient is able to perform ADLs as independently as possible.

Intervention Identify patient's ability to perform activities of daily living such as dressing and feeding. **Rationale** Determines patient's ability to adequately dress and feed self. **Evaluation** Can patient dress and feed self independently? If not, what level of assistance is required?

Intervention Provide assistance with dressing and grooming as required such as pre-matching coordinated clothing for easy selection or selecting and laying coordinated clothing out for patient to dress. **Rationale** Ensures patient's dressing and grooming needs are met. **Evaluation** Is patient able to dress and groom self adequately?

Intervention Provide assistance with preparing food and feeding as required such as for severe vision loss use the face of a clock for referencing location of foods on a plate. **Rationale** Ensures patient's feeding needs are met. **Evaluation** Is patient able to eat as desired?

Nursing Diagnosis: *Risk for Injury* related to altered vision

Expected Outcome: The patient will remain safe from injury.

Evaluation of Outcome: The patient remains injury free.

Continued

NURSING CARE PLAN for the Patient With Visual Impairment—cont'd

Intervention Provide for optimal care of assistive appliances such as eyeglasses, including maintenance of proper prescription, fit, and cleaning. **Rationale** Improperly fitting or dirty eyeglasses may impair vision even further. Older adults should have their eyeglass prescription checked yearly. **Evaluation** Do eyeglasses fit properly? Are lenses clean? Is prescription current?

Intervention Structure environment to compensate for visual loss by adding color and contrast (e.g., chairs and carpeting should be in contrasting colors, bright tape or paint on stairs, medicine bottles color coded with colored dot stickers). **Rationale** Makes the environment easier to visualize and interpret and assists in depth perception and identifying medications. **Evaluation** Does the environment have clearly delineated walkways, sitting areas, and doorways? Are areas with changes in elevation clearly identified using contrasting tape or paint? Is there a way for patient to safely self-administer medications?

Intervention Structure environment to compensate for visual loss by use of large-print directional signs and arrows, well-lit areas, nonglare surfaces, consistent placement of objects, traffic areas free of clutter. **Rationale** Large directional signs assist the patient in maintaining orientation. Shiny floors or areas with bright window glass can impair vision. Traffic areas free of clutter assist in preventing injury. **Evaluation** Can the patient identify locations such as bathroom, dining room, and office areas? Can the patient ambulate freely without safety hazards?

Intervention Introduce other assistive devices such as handheld magnifying glasses, tableside magnifiers, television magnifiers, large-print items, and phone dial covers with large numbers, talking watches, alarm clocks, and calculators. **Rationale** Patients may not be aware of assistive devices that could help them adapt to vision loss and continue previous activities, such as watching TV or reading letters and magazines. Allows people to rely on hearing rather than vision. **Evaluation** Is patient aware of assistive devices that allow participation in previously enjoyed activities such as TV or reading? Is the patient able to pay bills? Read mail? Communicate on the telephone?

Nursing Diagnosis: *Deficient Knowledge*

Expected Outcome: The patient will understand resources that will allow maintenance of independence.

Evaluation of Outcome: The patient will identify resources that can be used to support independence.

Intervention Refer to specialized clinician such as ophthalmologist or occupational therapist or to specialized resources such as American Federation for the Blind or Prevent Blindness America. **Rationale** Specialized clinicians can provide detailed examination and treatment for the disorder. Specialized resource groups have networks in place to assist people in coping with loss and assisting with maximizing abilities. **Evaluation** Does patient know who to call for detailed examination and treatment of problems? Does patient know that there are specialized clinicians and resource groups to help with the visual impairment? Does patient know how to access these specialists?

Diabetic Retinopathy
Pathophysiology and Etiology

Retinopathy is a disorder in which vascular changes occur in the retinal blood vessels. It is most common in persons with diabetes. The pathological changes in diabetic retinopathy are related to excess glucose, changes in the retinal capillary walls, formation of microaneurysms, and constriction of retinal blood vessels. Three stages of diabetic retinopathy have been identified: background retinopathy, preproliferative retinopathy, and proliferative retinopathy.

Background retinopathy is the earliest stage, in which microaneurysms form on the retinal capillary walls. These microaneurysms may leak blood into the central retina or macula. If the leakage causes edema, the patient may notice a decrease in color discrimination and visual acuity.

The second stage, preproliferative retinopathy, is characterized by swollen and irregularly dilated veins, which results in sluggish or blocked blood flow. Patients generally are not aware of this stage because there are no symptoms.

Proliferative retinopathy, the third stage, is characterized by the formation of new blood vessels growing into the retinal and optic disc area in an attempt to increase the blood supply to the retina. The newly formed blood vessels are fragile and often leak blood into the vitreous and retina. In addition to leaking, the newer vessels may grow into the vitreous, which causes a traction effect, pulling the vitreous away from the retina and subsequently pulling the retina away from the choroid. This condition is called retinal detachment (discussed later).

Signs and Symptoms

There may be a reduction in central visual acuity or color vision as a result of macular edema (see Fig. 52.2). Many patients with diabetic retinopathy have no symptoms until the proliferative stage, at which point vision is lost. Visual loss at the last stage usually cannot be restored.

Complications

Early treatment for diabetic retinopathy is highly successful in preventing further visual loss; however, existing visual loss cannot be reversed. For this reason, it is very important for patients with diabetes to have a comprehensive eye examination through dilated pupils at least once each year or as directed by their health care provider (HCP). Careful control of diabetes during the first 5 years after diagnosis reduces occurrence and delays onset of diabetic retinopathy.

Diagnostic Tests

Diabetic retinopathy, as well as the other retinopathies, can be diagnosed only on examination of the internal eye. The examination is conducted with an ophthalmoscope following dilation of the pupil with a cycloplegic agent. The examination may be enhanced by use of retinoangiography. In the initial stages, vessels may appear swollen and tortuous (twisted).

Therapeutic Measures

Treatment of diabetic retinopathy focuses on stopping the leakage of blood and fluid into the vitreous and retina. The leaking microaneurysm is sealed by use of laser photocoagulation. Lasers can also be used to shrink the abnormal blood vessels. If blood has already leaked into the vitreous, a vitrectomy is performed. During a vitrectomy, the vitreous humor is drained out of the eye chamber and replaced with saline or silicon oil (oil often removed months later). The replacement fluid is necessary to support the structures of the eyeball until healing can occur. Use of intravitreal corticosteroids is beneficial.

Nursing Process for the Patient With Diabetic Retinopathy

DATA COLLECTION. Nursing data collection for diabetic retinopathy includes risk factors associated with the incidence of the disease. The patient may not have any symptoms. If people with diabetes do have changes in perceptions of visual acuity or color discrimination, they should immediately contact their HCP.

NURSING DIAGNOSIS, PLANNING, AND IMPLEMENTATION. The planning phase of the nursing process for diabetic retinopathy focuses on prevention of visual loss by early detection and treatment. If the patient has entered phase three and is already visually impaired, the "Nursing Care Plan for the Patient With Visual Impairment" is used. Nursing diagnosis,

goal, and intervention for diabetic retinopathy include but is not limited to the following:

Risk for or Actual Ineffective Self Health Management

EXPECTED OUTCOME: The patient will state ability to manage therapeutic regimen.

- Determine whether the patient with a visual impairment who is diabetic can monitor blood glucose and draw up and administer the correct amount of insulin. *Specialty devices are available that can be preset to draw up the correct amounts of insulin. Family members may have to assist the patient.*
- Teach patient the importance of yearly comprehensive eye examinations *to detect visual changes for treatment.*

EVALUATION. Patient goals are met if the patient is able to manage the therapeutic regimen.

Retinal Detachment
Pathophysiology and Etiology

Retinal detachment is a separation of the retina from the choroid layer beneath it (see Fig. 51.1), allowing fluid to enter the space between the layers. The three causes of retinal detachment are a hole or tear in the retina that allows fluid to flow between the two layers, fibrous tissue in the vitreous humor that contracts and pulls the retina away from its normal position, or fluid or exudate accumulation in the subretinal space that separates the retinal layers.

Signs and Symptoms

Patients experiencing a retinal detachment report a sudden change in vision. Initially, as the retina is pulled, patients report seeing flashing lights and then *floaters*. The flashing lights are caused by vitreous traction on the retina, and floaters are caused by hemorrhage of vitreous fluid or blood. When the retina detaches, patients commonly describe it as "looking through a veil" or "cobwebs" and finally "like a curtain being lowered over the field of vision," with darkness resulting. There is no pain because the retina does not contain sensory nerves. On visual examination, the patient typically has a loss of peripheral vision when the visual fields are tested and a loss of acuity in the affected eye.

Diagnostic Tests

Indirect ophthalmoscopy allows the examiner to visualize the retina, which may be pale, opaque, and in folds with retinal detachment to diagnose the type of detachment. If there are lesions in the eye, the slit-lamp examination allows the examiner to magnify the lesions.

Therapeutic Measures

Immediate medical treatment must be sought to help protect vision. The degree of vision restoration varies and depends on the affected area. One or more procedures may be performed to treat retinal tears, or detachment: laser surgery, cryopexy, scleral buckling, and pneumatic retinopexy.

LASER SURGERY. Laser surgery focuses a laser beam at the torn area of the retina, causing a controlled burn, which scars around the tear and reattaches the retina to surrounding tissue.

CRYOPEXY. Cryopexy is the placement of a supercooled probe on the sclera over the affected area. The probe freezes and scars the tear or hole, a principle similar to the laser procedure.

SCLERAL BUCKLING. Scleral buckling is a surgical procedure for retinal detachment that involves placing a silicon implant in conjunction with a beltlike device around the sclera to bring the choroid in contact with the retina. Cryosurgery or laser surgery is used before the buckling procedure to seal the tear and form a scar that helps adhere the retina and choroid layers together. Vitrectomy is often done as well.

PNEUMATIC RETINOPEXY. Pneumatic retinopexy, done for retinal detachment, is a procedure that can be conducted in the health care provider's office but is time-consuming for the patient. This procedure involves injecting air or gas into the chamber to hold the retina in place. The patient must be extremely compliant with the treatment regimen, reclining for about 16 hours before the procedure to allow the retina to fall back toward the choroid. Because air rises, the patient must maintain a position that keeps the air bubble against the detached area for up to 8 hours a day for 3 weeks.

Complications

With any of the retinal procedures there is risk of increased intraocular pressure (IOP), tears and recurrent detachment.

Nursing Process for the Patient With Retinal Detachment

DATA COLLECTION. Subjective data collected include patient observation of the loss of peripheral vision, any change in visual acuity, and the presence of floaters, flashing lights, cobwebs, or veil-like visual impairments. There should be an absence of pain. Objective data collected include the patient's visual acuity, visual fields, ability to perform ADLs, and level of anxiety.

NURSING DIAGNOSES, PLANNING, IMPLEMENTATION, AND EVALUATION. The nursing process for patients with retinal detachment can be found in the "Nursing Process for the Patient Having Eye Surgery" section later in this chapter.

CRITICAL THINKING

Mr. Samuel

■ Mr. Samuel, age 65, is working in the yard when a branch strikes his right eye. He sees flashes of light and then a short time later a dark shadow out of the right eye.

1. What should Mr. Samuel do?
2. After having a scleral buckling procedure, Mr. Samuel reports nausea. What action should the nurse take?
3. Ondansetron (Zofran) 4 mg intramuscular (IM) now is ordered. Available is ondansetron 2 mg/mL in 2 mL/vial. How many milliliters should be given?

Suggested answers are at the end of the chapter.

Glaucoma

Glaucoma is a group of diseases characterized by damage to the optic nerve, the structure responsible for transmitting visual information from the eye to the brain. The damage is silent, progressive, and irreversible until the end stages, when loss of peripheral vision occurs, followed by reductions in central vision and eventually blindness (see Fig. 52.2). Sometimes there is abnormal pressure within the eyeball that damages the optic nerve, but not always. Normal tension glaucoma is now known to exist. There is no cure for glaucoma, so treatment plans must be followed to prevent further vision loss.

Pathophysiology

The most common form of glaucoma, called primary, consists of two types: primary open-angle glaucoma (POAG) and acute angle-closure glaucoma (AACG). Secondary glaucoma may be caused by infections, tumors, or injuries. A third form, congenital glaucoma, is due primarily to developmental abnormalities.

AACG occurs in people who have an anatomically narrowed angle at the junction where the iris meets the cornea. When nearby eye structures such as the iris protrude into the anterior chamber, the angle is occluded, which blocks the flow of aqueous fluid. This is considered a medical emergency and results in partial or total blindness if not treated. POAG occurs when the drainage system of the eye, the trabecular meshwork and Schlemm's canal, degenerate and subsequently block the flow of aqueous humor.

Etiology and Prevention

The incidence of AACG is highest among Asians, women older than age 45, and people who are nearsighted. POAG incidence increases in those older than age 40 (over age 50 for European Americans, over age 35 for African Americans), in people with diabetes, and in those with a family history of glaucoma, and is four to five times more prevalent in African Americans than European Americans. Those over age 60 or in high-risk groups should have yearly eye examinations for glaucoma detection.

Signs and Symptoms

An ophthalmic emergency, AACG typically has a unilateral, rapid onset. The patient may report severe pain over the affected eye, blurred vision, rainbows around lights, and photophobia and have eye redness, a steamy-appearing cornea, and tearing. Increased IOP can cause nausea and vomiting.

POAG develops bilaterally. The onset is usually gradual and painless, so the patient may have no noticeable symptoms or, after time, may experience mild aching in the eyes, headache, halos around lights, or frequent visual changes that are not corrected with eyeglasses.

Diagnostic Tests

Measuring IOP and identifying optic nerve damage and visual loss are done to diagnose glaucoma. Tonometry detects increased IOP (normal: 12–20 mm Hg), which may be present in about 50% of glaucoma cases. In AACG, IOP may exceed 50 mm Hg. The GDx Access, a laser device, detects nerve damage long before the patient has symptoms of glaucoma. Additionally, a visual field examination looks for loss of peripheral vision, distance vision is assessed, and corneal thickness is measured. With gonioscopy, a special lens is used to determine if glaucoma is open-angle or angle-closure.

Therapeutic Measures

The first-line treatment for glaucoma focuses on opening the aqueous flow by administering cholinergic agents (**miotics**) such as carbachol (Isopto) or pilocarpine (Pilocar) to constrict the pupil. When the pupil is constricted, the iris pulls away from the drainage canal so the aqueous fluid can flow freely. A second medication may be given to slow the production of aqueous fluid that includes carbonic anhydrase inhibitors such as acetazolamide (Diamox), adrenergic agonists such as dipivefrin (Propine), and beta blockers such as timolol (Timoptic). Slowing the production of aqueous fluid helps decrease IOP. Additionally, steroid eyedrops may be ordered to reduce inflammation. The patient experiencing an acute attack of AACG is given these types of medications and mannitol, a hyperosmolar agent, to rapidly reduce IOP, as well as analgesics, and is on complete bed rest.

Patients with glaucoma need lifelong use of eye drop medications twice or more daily. In the absence of symptoms, adherence to treatment is often an issue. Other factors that contribute to nonadherence to treatment include the patient's age, inability to afford the medication, and lack of understanding of the disease process. Patients should carry medical alert identification for their glaucoma and medications. This can help prevent administration of medications in emergency situations that are contraindicated for glaucoma.

There are medications, regardless of their route, that are contraindicated in AACG that can result in blindness if given to a patient with AACG. These medications include anticholinergics such as atropine, antihistamines such as diphenhydramine (Benadryl), or hydroxyzine (Vistaril) because they are mydriatics. Before a medication is given, the nurse should determine that it is not contraindicated in AACG, to prevent blindness from occurring.

Surgical Management

When medication is no longer able to control the flow of aqueous humor or reduce the IOP, surgical intervention may become necessary. Surgery focuses on creating an area where the aqueous humor can flow freely, thus preventing increased IOP (Fig. 52.3). For AACG, laser peripheral iridotomy or surgical iridectomy is performed. Laser iridotomy is a noninvasive procedure using a laser to remove a portion of the iris, thus allowing aqueous fluid to flow through the area. Prophylactic iridotomy may be performed on the other eye to prevent AACG. POAG is treated with laser trabeculoplasty (noninvasive laser beam creates openings in trabecular meshwork), trabeculectomy (part of iris and trabecular meshwork removed), or cyclocryotherapy (cryoprobe destroys part of ciliary body).

LEARNING TIP

- Mydriatic medications are contraindicated in acute angle-closure glaucoma because they can cause an acute episode of increased IOP by dilating the pupil and pushing the iris back, blocking the outflow of aqueous humor.
- Miotic medications constrict the pupil and so may be given to patients with acute angle-closure glaucoma.
- To remember what miotic medications and mydriatic medications do, so that the appropriate medication is given and contraindicated ones are never given, remember the following:

D = **d**ilate = my**d**riatic = **d**o not give.
No D = constricts = miotic = okay to give.

Nursing Process for the Patient With Glaucoma

DATA COLLECTION. The patient should be monitored for pain, loss of central and peripheral vision, understanding of disease and adherence to treatment regimen, and ability to conduct ADLs.

NURSING DIAGNOSES, PLANNING, AND IMPLEMENTATION. The goal of nursing care for the patient with glaucoma is to prevent further visual loss and to promote comfort if the patient is experiencing pain with acute glaucoma. See the "Nursing Process for the Patient With Visual Impairment and Nursing Process for the Patient Having Eye Surgery" sections for additional nursing diagnoses.

Pain related to increased intraocular pressure
EXPECTED OUTCOME: The patient will report that pain is relieved.

- Give analgesics as needed for acute glaucoma *to relieve pain.*

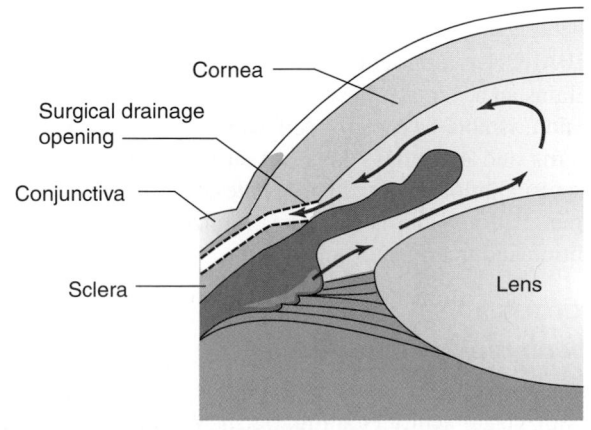

FIGURE 52.3 Flow of aqueous humor after trabeculoplasty (arrows).

Self-Care Deficit related to decreased vision
EXPECTED OUTCOME: The patient will be able to care for self with assistance if needed.

• Assist with self-care as needed *to ensure ADLs are met.*

Anxiety related to partial or total visual loss
EXPECTED OUTCOME: The patient will state that anxiety is reduced.

• Encourage patient to verbalize concerns about glaucoma *to allow questions to be answered.*

Risk for Injury related to decreased vision
EXPECTED OUTCOME: The patient will not suffer injury as a result of the visual impairment.

• Refer patient to support services that *provide adaptive visual devices.*
• Teach patient and family not to rearrange furniture without patient knowledge *to prevent falls or injury.*

Deficient Knowledge related to medical regimen, disease process due to no prior experience
EXPECTED OUTCOME: The patient will demonstrate correct instillation of eye medications and be able to verbalize understanding of condition and treatment.

• Teach need for regular eye examinations through dilated pupils *to monitor disease and detect complications.*
• Teach how to administer medications with a return demonstration *to ensure that eye drops are administered properly.*
• Teach the patient to rest his or her hand on the forehead *if the patient has trouble keeping the hand steady when administering eye drops.*
• Consider large-print labels or audiotaped directions *if the patient is unable to see the label on the eye drop bottle.*
• Consider placing large, multicolored dot stickers on medication bottles and on corresponding instruction cards *for patients with multiple medications.*
• Advise family members that they are at increased risk of developing glaucoma and should have regular eye examinations *because glaucoma can be hereditary.*

EVALUATION.   Interventions are successful if the patient maintains an acceptable level of comfort, has no further loss of vision, is able to care for self with assistance, expresses concerns and anxieties, does not suffer injury as a result of the visual impairment, demonstrates correct instillation of eye medications, and is able to verbalize understanding of condition and treatment.

Cataracts
Pathophysiology and Etiology
A cataract is an opacity in the lens of the eye that may cause a loss of visual acuity (see Fig. 52.2). Vision is diminished because the light rays are unable to get to the retina through the clouded lens.

Factors that contribute to cataract development may include age, ultraviolet radiation (sunlight), diabetes, smoking, steroids, nutritional deficiencies, alcohol consumption, intraocular infections, trauma, and congenital defects.

Signs and Symptoms
Cataracts are painless. Symptoms of cataract formation may include halos around lights, difficulty reading fine print or seeing in bright light, increased sensitivity to glare such as when driving at night, double or hazy vision, and decreased color vision.

Diagnostic Tests
Cataracts are diagnosed with an eye examination. Visual acuity is tested for near and far vision. The direct ophthalmoscope and slit-lamp microscope are used to examine the lens and other internal structures.

Surgical Management
When cataracts begin to interfere with daily living and quality of life, treatment is recommended. One eye is treated at a time with outpatient surgical removal of the cloudy lens. Implantable lenses, which come in various types, are typically inserted after lens removal. Eyeglasses or contact lenses are needed if no lens is reinserted. Eyeglasses may also be needed with some of the lens implants. With the no-stitch cataract operation, there are no postoperative activity restrictions, and vision improves in about 1 to 2 days.

Complications
Complications of cataract surgery are rare but include inflammation, increased IOP, macular edema, retinal detachment, vitreous loss, hyphema, endophthalmitis, and expulsive hemorrhage.

Nursing Process for the Patient With Cataracts
DATA COLLECTION.   The patient is monitored for visual deficits to assist care planning, as well as knowledge needs about the disease process, surgical intervention, postoperative care, and medical regimen. The majority of patients undergoing cataract surgery have same-day surgery and then go home. So the home situation, the ability of the patient or family member to follow the medical regimen, and transportation to and from the hospital for the patient are evaluated.

NURSING DIAGNOSES, PLANNING, IMPLEMENTATION, AND EVALUATION. Preoperative and postoperative nursing care is the primary nursing responsibility for the patient with cataracts, as discussed next.

Nursing Process for the Patient Having Eye Surgery
DATA COLLECTION. Table 52.5 reviews subjective data to be collected. Objective data may include visual acuity and peripheral field measurements. Visual acuity should be tested with and without any corrective lenses. Eye tearing, redness, or swelling is noted.

TABLE 52.5   SUBJECTIVE DATA COLLECTION FOR PATIENTS HAVING EYE SURGERY

W Where is it?	Where is the visual disturbance? Is it centrally located? Peripherally? Throughout the entire visual field? Unilateral? Bilateral?
H How does it feel?	How does it feel? Painful? Is there an absence of pain?
A Aggravating and alleviating factors	Is it worse in bright light or at night? Better when resting eyes or with head of bed elevated?
T Timing	Was there a sudden onset? Gradual onset?
S Severity	Does it affect activities of daily living? Does it affect close-up work?
U Useful data for associated symptoms	Does the patient suffer from hypertension? Diabetes? Has there been trauma? Vascular disease? What is the level of anxiety? Is the patient older than age 50?
P Perception of the problem by the patient	Will the visual disturbance impair ability to carry out activities of daily living? Ability to comply with medical regimen? Ability to manage home maintenance?

Nursing Diagnoses, Planning, and Implementation

Risk for Injury related to altered visual acuity

EXPECTED OUTCOME: The patient will remain free of injury.

- Explain that depth perception may be affected by eye surgery, which can result in falls, *to help prevent injury.*
- Ambulate with assistance and use clearly marked stairs *to prevent injury.*
- At home, beverages can be poured and stored in the refrigerator in single-serving glasses *to prevent spills and slippery floors.*

Deficient Knowledge related to preoperative and postoperative eye care

EXPECTED OUTCOME: The patient will verbalize preoperative and postoperative care directions.

- Teach disease process, surgical intervention, use of correct technique for administering eye medications, need to report for medical follow-up as instructed, and need to protect the eye from further injury *to increase patient knowledge.*
- Patients are told to seek medical treatment if they experience sudden, worsening pain, an increase in watery or bloody discharge, or sudden loss of vision *because these are signs of hemorrhage or problems.*

Anxiety related to visual alteration and surgery

EXPECTED OUTCOME: The patient will report reduced anxiety.

- Give patients the opportunity to discuss their feelings about vision loss and surgery *to reduce anxiety.*

EVALUATION. The patient goals have been met if the patient is free of injury, verbalizes preoperative and postoperative directions, and reports reduced anxiety.

Macular Degeneration
Pathophysiology and Etiology

Age-related macular degeneration (AMD) is the leading cause of visual impairment in U.S. residents older than age 50. It involves deterioration and scarring within the macula, the area on the retina where light rays converge for the sharp, central vision needed for reading and seeing small objects. The macula is also responsible for color vision (Fig. 52.4). There are two types of AMD: dry (atrophic) and wet (exudative). In dry AMD, photoreceptors in the macula fail to function and are not replaced because of advancing age. This accounts for 70% to 90% of cases. In the wet form, retinal tissue degenerates, allowing vitreous fluid or blood into the subretinal space. New fragile blood vessels form (angiogenesis) and compromise the macular tissue, causing subretinal edema. Eventually, fibrous scar tissue forms, severely limiting central vision.

People at risk of developing macular degeneration include those older than age 60, those with a family history of macular degeneration, persons with diabetes, people who smoke, those frequently exposed to ultraviolet (UV) light, and Caucasian people.

NURSING CARE TIP

Most damaging exposure to UV light occurs before age 18. So it is important for everyone of all ages to use adequate UV protective eyewear.

FIGURE 52.4 Macular degeneration. The macula is a small area of the retina responsible for central and color vision.

Prevention

A healthful lifestyle and a diet that includes dark green leafy vegetables (kale, collard greens, lettuce, spinach), and orange (peppers) and yellow (corn) color fruits and vegetables is important. Measuring macula pigment optical density is an important preventative tool. Taking the retinal carotenoids lutein and zeaxanthin and zinc supplementation for a low macula pigment optical density (less than 44) can be beneficial in raising the macula pigment optical density over time and preventing progression of some macular degeneration.

Signs and Symptoms

AMD of the dry type is characterized by slow, progressive loss of central and near vision (see Fig. 52.2). Although people usually have the condition in both eyes, each eye may be affected in varying degrees. AMD of the wet type has the same loss of central and near vision, but the onset is sudden and results in more severe vision loss. The loss can occur in one or both eyes. This vision loss is described as blurred vision, distortion of straight lines, and a dark or empty spot in the central area of vision. Some patients may have a decreased ability to distinguish colors.

Diagnostic Tests

Examination of the patient begins with visual acuity for near and far vision and an examination of the internal eye structures with an ophthalmoscope. The examiner uses an Amsler grid (Fig. 52.5) to detect central vision distortion and a color vision test to evaluate color differentiation. Patients are given an Amsler grid to look at on a regular basis to monitor vision

changes. If any of the grid lines look crooked or disappear, the patient should contact the HCP. Digital imaging, optical coherence tomography retinal scan (similar to a computed tomography scan) or intravenous fluorescein (dye) angiography can also be used to evaluate blood vessel leakage or abnormalities in the eye.

Therapeutic Measures

Unfortunately, there is no treatment for the dry type of AMD, so prevention is important when possible. Most patients with dry AMD do not lose peripheral vision or become totally blind, but most are classified as legally blind (less than 20/200 vision with correction). Low-vision telescopic glasses can enhance remaining vision. A telescope implant for those

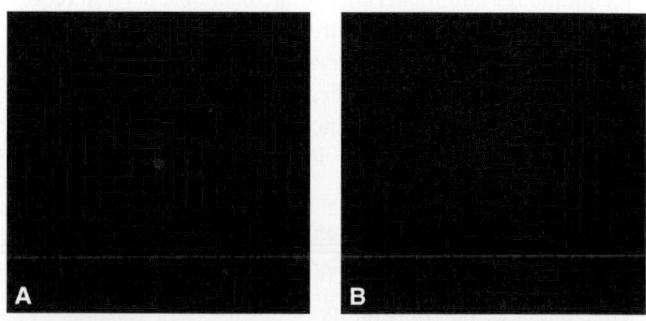

FIGURE 52.5 An Amsler grid is used for self-assessment to identify central vision blind spots or distortions. (A) Normal Amsler grid. The red on black grid was developed to increase better accuracy with the test. (B) Abnormal Amsler grid with distortion and small area of central vision loss.

with advanced AMD, done in one eye after the lens in the eye is removed, can help restore central vision. Visit www.CentraSight.com for more information.

The newer evidence-based treatment option for wet type AMD is intermittent injection into the eye of an antiangiogenesis medication (e.g., ranibizumab [Lucentis]). Drugs that are antiangiogenetic prevent the formation of new fragile blood vessels that can become leaky and bleed. Treatment options that are not used as much as in the past due to the availability of antiangiogenesis drugs include laser photocoagulation that seals the leaking blood vessels or photodynamic therapy. If the patient receives laser photocoagulation, there is a small, permanent blind spot at the point of laser contact with the macula. Clinical trials are ongoing with an eye drop to treat wet AMD (Squalamine Lactate Ophthalmic Formulation 0.2%) that prevents angiogenesis. Another treatment in development is the VEGF Trap Eye, a biologically produced protein that will also prevent angiogenesis. With either type of AMD, patients have significant visual loss and must adapt to it.

Nursing Process for the Patient With Macular Degeneration

See the "Nursing Process for the Patient With Visual Impairment" section.

Trauma

Emergencies and trauma of the eye must be assessed immediately so that proper treatment can be initiated. Injuries to the eye include foreign bodies, chemical burns, ultraviolet, or direct heat sources, abrasions, lacerations from dragging something across the eye, and penetrating wounds, which are the most serious eye injury and increase the risk for infection and blindness.

Signs and Symptoms

Foreign bodies produce pain when the eyeball or eyelid moves. Usually the eye tears excessively in an attempt to irrigate the noxious substance out of the eye. Injuries that irritate or penetrate layers of the cornea range from mild to severe pain. With corneal abrasions, the pain sensation may be delayed for several hours. Other symptoms that may be seen with abrasions, lacerations, and foreign bodies include conjunctival redness, photosensitivity, decreased visual acuity, erythema, and pruritus. Acute pain and burning are characteristic symptoms of a burn to the eye. Penetrating wound symptoms depend on the area of the eye involved and the extent of the damage.

Diagnostic Tests

Visual acuity is tested. It is important to establish baseline acuity to evaluate effectiveness of treatment, although many patients resist acuity testing because of the discomfort. Testing includes examination by slit-lamp microscope and direct ophthalmoscope. Fluorescein staining is used to evaluate abrasions.

Therapeutic Measures

Foreign bodies are treated with a normal saline flush to irrigate the object out of the eye or to a point where it can be removed with a swab. Topical antibiotic ointment is prescribed to prevent infection. Chemical burns must be treated immediately with a 15- to 20-minute irrigation of either tap water at the work site or sterile solution at the medical facility. Topical antibiotic ointments are usually prescribed. Burns from heat or UV radiation are not irrigated.

Abrasions and lacerations usually are treated with anti-infective ointments or drops after cleansing the eye with normal saline.

An eye specialist treats penetrating wounds. Upon initial injury, both eyes should be covered to prevent ocular movement. If there is a protruding object, it should be stabilized but not removed until the HCP can assess the patient.

Complications

If the eye cannot be saved with medical treatment, it may be necessary to surgically remove the eye. This procedure is called **enucleation** (entire eyeball removal).

Nursing Process for the Patient With Eye Trauma

DATA COLLECTION AND EMERGENCY INTERVENTION.

Foreign Bodies. The eye is inspected for foreign bodies, which may be visible on the eyeball. The lids should be everted to examine the surface. Then the eye is irrigated.

Burns. Assessment of the type of burn is done because treatment options vary. Immediate irrigation of the eyes is performed once it has been established that a chemical burn has taken place unless contraindicated for the chemical. Medication and eye patching are applied as indicated.

Abrasions and Lacerations. The eye is assessed for visible lacerations and then cleansed, medicated, and patched as indicated.

Penetrating Wounds. The patient is kept calm and relaxed to minimize eye movement and increased IOP. If a protruding object is present, the object is stabilized with tape or other supports.

NURSING DIAGNOSES, PLANNING, AND IMPLEMENTATION.

Acute Pain related to inflammatory process and injury
EXPECTED OUTCOME: The patient's pain level will be within an acceptable range for the patient.

- Administer analgesics as ordered *to reduce pain.*
- Assist patient in remaining calm and relaxed *to reduce pain.*

Risk for Infection related to eye trauma
EXPECTED OUTCOME: The patient will remain free of infection.

- Use sterile technique when irrigating the eye, when applying medications, and during examination *to prevent infection.*

Anxiety related to visual-sensory deficit
EXPECTED OUTCOME: The patient will verbalize a reduction in anxiety.

- Encourage the patient to verbalize feelings about visual impairment *to reduce anxiety.*
- Reassure patient as appropriate *to reduce anxiety.*

• WORD • BUILDING •
enucleation: e—removed from + nuclear—center

Deficient Knowledge related to medical regimen due to lack of previous experience
EXPECTED OUTCOME: *The patient will be able to verbalize care of the eye.*

• Teach patient about interventions and follow-up care *to inform patient.*

EVALUATION. Patient goals have been met if pain level is within an acceptable range for the patient, patient remains free of infection, patient is able to verbalize a reduction in anxiety, and patient is able to verbalize care of the eye.

 HEARING DISORDERS

Hearing Loss

Hearing loss is the most common disability in the United States and can be acquired or congenital. Hearing impairment ranges from difficulty understanding words or hearing certain sounds to total deafness (Table 52.6). Hearing impairment can affect communication, social activities, and work activities and can diminish quality of life. Nurses have a responsibility to communicate with patients with hearing impairments and provide needed information regarding health care.

Conductive Hearing Loss

Conductive hearing loss, a mechanical problem, is interference with the conduction of sound impulses through the external auditory canal, the eardrum, or the middle ear to the inner ear. The inner ear is not involved in a pure conductive hearing loss. Causes of conductive hearing loss include cerumen, foreign bodies, infection, perforation of the tympanic membrane, trauma, fluid in the middle ear, cysts, tumor, and **otosclerosis**. Many causes of conductive hearing loss, such as infection, foreign bodies, and impacted cerumen, can be corrected. Hearing devices may improve hearing for conditions resulting in conductive hearing loss that cannot be corrected, such as scarred tympanic membrane or otosclerosis.

Sensorineural Hearing Loss

Sensory hearing loss originates in the cochlea and involves the hair cells and nerve endings. Neural hearing loss originates in the nerve or brainstem. **Sensorineural** hearing loss results from disease or trauma to the sensory or neural components of the inner ear. Some of the causes of nerve deafness are complications of infections (such as measles, mumps,

• WORD • BUILDING •
otosclerosis: oto—ear + sclerosis—hardening

TABLE 52.6 HEARING LOSS SUMMARY

Signs and Symptoms	Difficulty understanding words or certain sounds Total deafness Changes in social and work activities, turns up volume on TV, asks "What did you say?" Reports people are talking softly, speaks in a quiet or loud voice, answers questions inappropriately. Avoids group activities, loss of sense of humor, appears aloof Reports ringing, buzzing, or roaring noise in ears
Diagnostic Tests and Findings	Abnormal Rinne and Weber tests Audiometric testing indicates hearing loss
Therapeutic Measures	Cerumenolytics Anti-infectives Anti-inflammatories Assistive devices (hearing aids, implantable middle ear hearing devices, cochlear implants)
Complications	Safety issues related to not hearing Withdrawal from social activities and relationships related to hearing loss
Priority Nursing Diagnoses	*Impaired Verbal Communication* related to impaired hearing *Impaired Social Interaction* related to impaired hearing and decreased communication skills *Disturbed Body Image* related to impaired hearing and use of assistive hearing devices *Ineffective Coping* related to difficult communication *Deficient Knowledge* related to care of hearing aid due to lack of prior experience

and meningitis), ototoxic drugs (Table 52.7), trauma, noise, neuromas, arteriosclerosis, and the aging process.

Presbycusis is hearing loss caused by the aging process that results from degeneration of the organ of Corti. This degenerative process often begins in the fifth decade of life. The individual develops an inability to decipher high-frequency sounds (consonants *s, z, t, f,* and *g*). This interferes with the person's ability to understand what is being said, especially in noisy environments. The older adult commonly has more difficulty understanding higher pitched female voices than lower pitched male voices.

Other Types of Hearing Loss

Mixed hearing loss occurs when an individual has both conductive and sensorineural hearing loss. This can be caused by a combination of any of the disorders previously mentioned. Central hearing loss occurs when the central nervous system cannot interpret normal auditory signals.

TABLE 52.7   OTOTOXIC DRUGS

Aminoglycoside antibiotics	Amikacin
	Gentamicin
	Neomycin
	Streptomycin
	Tobramycin
Other antibiotics	Erythromycin
	Minocycline
	Vancomycin
Diuretics	Bumetanide
	Furosemide
	Hydrochlorothiazide
Other drugs	Cisplatin
	Indomethacin
	Methotrexate
	Salicylates

This condition occurs with such disorders as cerebrovascular accidents and tumors. Functional hearing loss is a hearing loss for which no organic cause or lesion can be found. It is also called psychogenic hearing loss and is precipitated by emotional stress.

Therapeutic Measures

The goal of medical management is to improve the patient's hearing. With any permanent hearing loss, the use of a hearing aid should be considered (Chapter 51, Fig. 52.6). Surgical intervention may be available for patients whose hearing is not improved with hearing aids. Implantable middle ear hearing aids can improve sound perception for patients with moderate-to-severe sensorineural hearing loss. Cochlear implants can restore up to half of the patient's hearing (Chapter 51).

Nursing Process for the Patient With Hearing Impairment

DATA COLLECTION. Nursing care includes identifying those patients at risk for hearing impairment (Table 52.8). Patients with renal or hepatic disease, using two or more ototoxic drugs, or previously having used ototoxic drugs are at risk for developing hearing impairment. If your patient is taking ototoxic medications, assess for tinnitus, sensorineural hearing loss, or vestibular dysfunction, which could indicate ototoxicity. The medications should be discontinued if signs of ototoxicity are present. Monitor for signs of vertigo, horizontal nystagmus, nausea, vomiting, and spinning or rocking sensation while sitting still. To collect data for the patient with hearing impairment, ask family members, as well as the patient, questions related to the patient's hearing status.

Objective data collection should start with normal conversation with the patient. Observe the patient for any difficulty understanding conversation or questions. Clarity of the patient's speech is also determined. Physical examination includes the whisper voice, Rinne, and Weber tests (see Chapter 51). Test results provide an estimate of conductive or sensorineural hearing loss. The patient should be assessed for the underlying cause of the problem to determine if it is an external, middle,

FIGURE 52.6 Hearing aids. (A) Behind-the-ear hearing aid. (B) In-the-ear hearing aid.

TABLE 52.8   SUBJECTIVE DATA COLLECTION FOR HEARING DISORDERS

W Where is it?	Are both ears affected? Is one side worse than the other?
H How does it feel?	Are certain words unclear, or entire conversations? Are high-frequency sounds (consonants *s, t, z, f, g,* and female voices) unclear or difficult to understand? Is any pain associated with the hearing loss? Any tinnitus or vertigo?
A Aggravating and alleviating factors	Is hearing worse in large groups or when there is a lot of background noise? Is hearing improved in a quiet environment or when speaking only to an individual? Is it easier to understand someone when seeing the person's lips move? Does the patient own or use any assistive hearing devices? Are they effective? What type is used?
T Timing	When did the hearing loss start? Was it gradual or sudden? Is the hearing loss associated with any illness or traumatic event? Is it associated with any recent flying? Any history of ototoxic drug use?
S Severity	Does it cause communication impairment? How much? Does it affect activities of daily living? Does it affect or limit usual social activities? Have family or friends commented on decreased hearing? Does patient avoid communication or social activities because of difficulty hearing? Is patient having difficulties hearing telephone voices, radio, television, or movies?
U Useful data for associated symptoms	Is there any fever, nausea, vomiting, or dizziness? Is there any history of occupational or environmental exposure to loud noises? What are the usual ear self-care habits? Any history of impacted cerumen? Has patient ever had cerumen removed from ears?
P Perception of the problem by the patient	What does the patient feel is wrong? Does the patient think that he or she has a hearing problem? How does the patient feel about hearing assistive devices? How does the patient perceive the hearing loss, and how is it influencing the patient's life?

or inner ear problem. Examination of the external ear may reveal an external ear problem. The HCP may examine the ear canal for impacted cerumen or a tympanic membrane problem. Any assistive hearing devices should be noted and inspected for proper functioning. The results of the examination are documented and communicated to other health team members (see "Evidence-Based Practice" box).

EVIDENCE-BASED PRACTICE

Clinical Question
Is hearing loss associated with hospitalizations and burden of disease?

Evidence
A recent study analyzed data from 2005–2006 and 2009–2010 of the National Health and Nutrition Examination Survey (NHANES), an ongoing epidemiological study designed to assess the health and functional status of the civilian, noninstitutionalized U.S. population.

Results demonstrated that hearing loss was independently associated with hospitalization and poorer self-reported health over the past 12 months.

Implications for Nursing Practice
Additional research is needed to investigate whether hearing rehabilitative therapies could help reduce hospitalizations and improve self-reported health in older adults with hearing loss. Nurses can implement interventions to ensure that older adults optimize their ability to hear. Improved hearing positively affects communication and other areas of self-reported health and might possibly decrease hospitalizations.

REFERENCE
Genther, D., Frick, K., Chen, D., Betz, J., & Lin, F. (2013). Association of hearing loss with hospitalization and burden of disease in older adults. *JAMA: The Journal of the American Medical Association, 309,* 2322–2324. doi:10.1001/jama.2013.5912

NURSING DIAGNOSES, PLANNING, AND IMPLEMENTATION.
Planning focuses on helping the patient optimize hearing, promoting communication, and promoting adjustment to impaired hearing (Box 52-2 and Box 52-3). Nursing management for the patient with hearing impairment focuses on enhancing communication and quality of life (see the "Nursing Care Plan for the Patient With Hearing Impairment"). Families should be included in discussions about therapeutic hearing devices and their care, enhancing communication, and limiting isolation.

EVALUATION.   The patient's goals are met if the patient communicates effectively, engages in usual social activities, uses assistive hearing device, copes with emotional

---

Box 52-2 Communicating with a Person Who Has a Hearing Impairment

- Get the person's attention before beginning to speak.
- Face and stand close to the person being spoken to and maintain eye contact.
- Avoid standing in the glare of bright sunlight or other bright lights.
- Speak clearly, at a normal rate and volume. Do not shout or overarticulate.
- Inform the listener of topics to be discussed and when a change of topic occurs. Stick to a topic for a while and avoid quick shifts.
- Use short sentences and assess for understanding. If the listener does not understand after the message is repeated, rephrase the message. If the listener has difficulty with high-pitched sounds, lower the voice pitch.
- Allow extra time for the listener to respond and do not rush the listener.
- Ensure an optimum environment by reducing background noises: turn off television and radio, close the door, or move to a quieter area.
- Encourage nonverbal communication such as touch or gestures as appropriate.
- If the listener uses a hearing device, ensure that it is operational and in place before beginning to communicate. Give the person time to adjust the hearing device before speaking.
- Do not smile, chew gum, or cover the mouth when talking.
- Use active listening with attentive body posture, pleasant facial expressions, and a calm, unhurried manner.
- Do not avoid conversation with a person who has hearing loss.
- Use written communication if unable to communicate verbally.

Box 52-3 Care of Hearing Aids

- Insert hearing aid while over a soft surface such as a pillow to prevent damage if the hearing aid is dropped during insertion.
- Remove hearing aid before showering or bathing. Do not immerse in water.
- Turn the hearing aid off when not in use to conserve battery.
- Do not expose the hearing aid to extreme heat or cold.
- Clean the hearing aid daily with a dry, soft cloth. Clean earmold with small brush or toothpick to keep free of earwax.
- Turn off the hearing aid and turn the volume down before inserting. Turn hearing aid on and increase volume once it is inserted.
- Minimize whistling noise by ensuring that the volume is not too high, the aid fits securely, and the aid is free from earwax.
- Check battery or lower the volume if sound is not clear or is intermittent. Buzzing noise may indicate that the battery door is not completely closed.
- Do not expose the hearing aid to hair or medicinal sprays by applying sprays before inserting hearing aid.

---

reaction to hearing impairment, and demonstrates care of hearing aid.

External Ear

Infections

PATHOPHYSIOLOGY AND ETIOLOGY.   Infection is the most common disorder of the external ear, with **external otitis** being the most common infection. Exposure to moisture, contamination, or local trauma provides an ideal environment for pathological growth in the external ear, which results in external otitis. It may be caused by bacterial or fungal pathogens. Staphylococci are the most common causative organism. *Pneumocystis* infections have been seen in patients who have human immunodeficiency virus (HIV). A bacterial or fungal external otitis that occurs when water is left in the ear and washes away protective earwax, often after water exposure or trauma, is known as swimmer's ear. External otitis occurs more often in the summer months but can be seen year-round in patients who swim indoors.

A localized infection called ear canal **furuncle** or abscess results when a hair follicle becomes infected. A **carbuncle** forms when several hair follicles are involved in forming the abscess. Most furuncles and carbuncles erupt and drain spontaneously. Otomycosis is an infection caused by fungal growth and is typically seen after topical corticosteroid or antibiotic use. Otomycosis occurs more often in hot weather. An infection of the auricle is called perichondritis, which can result in necrosis of cartilage.

NURSING CARE PLAN for the Patient With Hearing Impairment

Nursing Diagnosis: *Impaired Verbal Communication* related to impaired hearing

Expected Outcome: Patient will use effective communication techniques.

Evaluation of Outcome: Patient is able to communicate effectively to have needs met and reduce social isolation.

Intervention Begin assessment of hearing by inspecting ear canals for mechanical obstruction. If cerumen is found, use of a softening product is recommended to assist in wax removal. If canal is clear, continue assessment by using a tuning fork, loud ticking clock, or verbal cues to determine auditory ability at various distances. **Rationale** Hearing loss may result from buildup of cerumen in the auditory canal. Determination of hearing ability assists nurse in developing interventions appropriate to patient's hearing level. **Evaluation** Is ear canal free of mechanical obstruction? Is patient able to hear verbal input? If not, how severe is the impairment?

Intervention Enhance hearing by giving auditory cues in quiet surroundings. **Rationale** The presence of background noise such as television, radio, or large numbers of people makes hearing more difficult. **Evaluation** Are auditory cues being delivered in an environment free of extraneous background noises?

Intervention Enhance understanding of auditory cues in well lit area but not in front of window causing glare by getting patient's attention before speaking, speaking slowly with careful enunciation of words, adding hand gestures, speaking face to face with the person with the impairment, and adjusting the voice pitch downward without increasing volume. **Rationale** Hearing is enhanced when additional cues assist the person in understanding the message. Use of hand gestures to point, lip-reading, facial expression, and lower pitch all assist communication. **Evaluation** Are auditory cues being understood by patient? Are instructions given in step-by-step format with written cues?

Intervention Structure environment to compensate for hearing loss by adding visual indicators to telephone ringer, doorbell, smoke detectors, and other emergency sounds. **Rationale** Assists in communication and safety. **Evaluation** Is patient able to receive input in ways other than auditory?

Intervention Provide for optimal care of assistive appliances such as hearing aids by making sure that cerumen has been cleaned from the device, that batteries are charged, and that the appliance is placed correctly in ear. **Rationale** Appliances that are not functioning properly will not assist patient in hearing. **Evaluation** Is patient's hearing aid in place correctly? Is cerumen blocking sound conduction? Do batteries work?

Intervention Introduce assistive devices such as hearing amplifiers, telephone amplifiers, telephones with extra-loud bells, written communication, and sign language. **Rationale** Patients may not be aware of assistive devices that could help them adapt to hearing loss and continue previous activities, such as talking on the telephone or listening to television. **Evaluation** Is patient aware of assistive devices that will allow him or her to continue to verbally communicate with others? Is patient able to use the devices to compensate for auditory impairment?

Intervention Refer to specialized clinician such as an audiologist or occupational therapist or to specialized resources such as the National Association of the Deaf or American Speech, Language and Hearing Association. **Rationale** Specialized clinicians can provide detailed examination and treatment. Specialized resource groups have networks in place to help people cope with loss and maximize abilities. **Evaluation** Does patient know whom to call for detailed examination and treatment? Does patient know that there are specialized clinicians and resource groups to help with hearing impairment? Does patient know how to access these specialists?

SIGNS AND SYMPTOMS. The most common sign of infection of the external ear is pain (Table 52.9). An early indication of infection is pain with gentle pulling on the pinna. The patient may also experience pain when moving the jaw or when the otoscope is inserted into the ear canal. Pruritus (itching) is also a common symptom and can be an early sign of infection. Signs of inflammation are present on the external ear. The ear canal may become swollen or occluded, and as a result hearing may be diminished. Redness, swelling, and drainage can be observed during otoscopic examination. If drainage is present, it usually starts out clear and becomes purulent as the disease progresses. The patient may also be febrile.

DIAGNOSTIC TESTS. A complete blood cell count (CBC), with elevated white blood cell (WBC) counts, and cultures of discharge help diagnose infections. Culture and sensitivity tests isolate the specific infective organism and determine which antibiotics would be most effective to treat the infection. The Rinne and Weber tests can indicate conductive hearing impairment.

Impacted Cerumen

PATHOPHYSIOLOGY AND ETIOLOGY. Normally, the ear is self-cleaning. However, cerumen (wax) may become impacted, blocking the ear canal. People with large amounts of hair in the ear canal or who work in dusty or dirty areas are prone to cerumen impaction. Improper cleaning can also result in cerumen impaction. The older adult is at risk to develop impacted cerumen. This occurs because the amount of cerumen secreted is decreased and because of increased amounts of keratin. These two factors cause the cerumen to be drier, harder, and more easily impacted. Patients with hearing aids tend to have problems with impacted cerumen. Patients with bony growths secondary to an osteophyte or osteoma are at risk for cerumen impaction.

SIGNS AND SYMPTOMS. The patient may experience hearing loss, a feeling of fullness, or blocked ear if cerumen has become impacted (see Table 52.6). Otoscopic examination reveals cerumen blocking the ear canal.

DIAGNOSTIC TESTS. Audiometric testing reveals conductive hearing loss in the affected ear. Hearing acuity can be decreased by 45 decibels because of impacted cerumen. Whisper voice, Rinne, and Weber tests also indicate conductive hearing loss.

Masses

PATHOPHYSIOLOGY AND ETIOLOGY. Benign masses of the external ear are usually cysts resulting from sebaceous glands. Other benign masses are lipomas, warts, keloids, and infectious polyps. Infectious polyps usually arise from the

TABLE 52.9 EXTERNAL EAR DISORDERS SUMMARY

Signs and Symptoms	Pain Pruritus, swelling, redness Drainage Lacerations, contusion, hematomas, abrasion Erythema, blistering Hearing loss Foreign body
Diagnostic Tests and Findings	Complete blood count with elevated white blood cells with infections audiometric, Rinne, Weber, and whisper voice tests (indicate conductive hearing loss with impacted cerumen and trauma) Imaging studies to indicate extent of trauma
Therapeutic Measures	Cerumenolytics to remove earwax Anti-infectives and anti-inflammatory medications (to treat infection) Debridement, surgical repair, or application of protective covering with trauma to external ear
Complications	Spread of infection to other parts of the ear Disfigurement Loss of hearing Scarring
Priority Nursing Diagnoses	*Acute Pain* related to inflammation or trauma *Risk for Injury* related to self-cleaning of external ear *Deficient Knowledge* related to care of hearing aid due to lack of prior experience

middle ear and enter the external ear through a hole in the tympanic membrane. Actinic keratosis is a precancerous lesion that can be found on the auricle and may be seen in older adults. Malignant tumors such as basal cell carcinoma on the pinna and squamous cell in the ear canal may develop and can spread.

SIGNS AND SYMPTOMS. Changes in the appearance of the skin can occur with benign or malignant masses. Usually, impaired conductive or sensorineural hearing loss occurs with masses. Pain is another symptom and is usually described as deep pain radiating inward on the affected side. Ear drainage may be present. As the condition progresses, facial paralysis may occur. Visualization of the mass may be observed during otoscopic examination.

DIAGNOSTIC TESTS. A biopsy may be obtained to determine if the mass is benign or malignant. Imaging studies are also used to diagnose tumors. Audiometric studies reveal any hearing impairment.

Trauma

PATHOPHYSIOLOGY AND ETIOLOGY. Injuries to the external ear are commonly caused by a blow to the head, automobile accidents, burns, foreign bodies lodged in the ear canal, or cold temperatures. Cotton ball pieces and insects are the most common foreign bodies found in adults.

SIGNS AND SYMPTOMS. Lacerations, contusions, hematomas, abrasions, erythema, and blistering are signs seen with thermal or physical trauma. Repeated trauma to the ear can cause swelling, also known as cauliflower ear. This is common among boxers, rugby players, martial artists, and wrestlers. Conductive hearing loss can occur if the ear canal is partially or totally blocked. Patients who have contusions or hematomas commonly report numbness, pain, and paresthesia of the auricle. Symptoms associated with foreign bodies may include decreased hearing, itching, pain, and infection. Care is taken during otoscopic examination not to push the foreign body further into the ear canal.

DIAGNOSTIC TESTS. Imaging studies may be needed to determine the extent of the trauma. Audiometric, whisper voice, Rinne, and Weber tests may demonstrate conductive hearing loss.

Complications of External Ear Disorders

If not treated, infections can spread, causing cellulitis, abscesses, middle ear infection, and septicemia. Metastasis can occur if malignant tumors are not treated. Infection, trauma, and malignant tumors may cause temporary or permanent hearing loss, disfigurement, discoloration, and scarring.

Therapeutic Measures for External Ear Disorders

For external ear infections topical antibiotics are given. Systemic antibiotics are used for severe infections that are localized or have spread to surrounding tissues. Analgesics are used to control pain. Topical or systemic steroids may be used to treat inflammation. The ear is thoroughly cleaned before starting any topical treatment. If the external ear canal has drainage or is swollen shut, a wick may be inserted. The wick serves to aid in removing drainage or to aid in administering medication into the ear canal. Cerumen may be removed with irrigation by a trained clinician (Fig. 52.7; see "Evidence-Based Practice"). Irrigation is not used if the patient has a history of perforated tympanic membrane (eardrum) or other contraindications. Débridement, surgical repair, or application of a protective covering may be done when trauma occurs to the external ear. Surgical management consists of incision and drainage of abscesses. Excision of cysts or cutaneous carcinomas may also be required.

A Pull ear back and down to straighten ear canal in a child

B Pull ear up and back to straighten ear canal in an adult

C Irrigation – Fluid is aimed off top of ear canal wall behind impacted cerumen

FIGURE 52.7 Ear irrigation. (A) Child. (B) Adult. (C) Irrigation.

EVIDENCE-BASED PRACTICE

Clinical Question
Can isopropyl alcohol be used to reduce cerumen build up in the ear canal?

Evidence
A crossover study looked at safety and efficacy of using 70% isopropyl alcohol as a weekly ear irrigant to reduce cerumen buildup. Participants instilled the alcohol weekly using a squeeze bottle. Alcohol rinses and removal of the cerumen in the physician's office were alternated. The results demonstrated that weekly rinses with the 70% isopropyl alcohol was safe and reduced the amount of cerumen that accumulated in the external ear canal.

Implications for Nursing Practice
Nurses can help educate patients with recurring cerumen accumulation that safe options exist. Patients can be encouraged to discuss weekly ear rinses with isopropyl alcohol with their HCP to reduce accumulation of ear wax. This can help prevent pain, hearing difficulties and unnecessary HCP visits.

REFERENCE
Silverstein, H., Wycherly, B. J., Alameda, Y., & Van Ess, M. J. (2012). A prospective study to evaluate the efficacy of isopropyl alcohol irrigations to prevent cerumen impaction. *ENT: Ear, Nose & Throat Journal, 91*, E25–E28.

Nursing Process for the Patient With External Ear Disorders

DATA COLLECTION. Subjective data obtained in a patient history include reports of pain, fullness, previous cerumen impaction, itching, or hearing loss, as well as onset, duration, and severity of symptoms. Additional data include patient's occupation, previous ear problems, use of a hearing aid, and typical ear hygiene. Observation for objective data includes redness, swelling, drainage, furuncles, carbuncles, lesions, abrasions, lacerations, growths, cerumen, scaliness, or crusting. The patient may report pain when the ear is palpated. Basic hearing acuity tests are conducted to evaluate hearing loss (see Chapter 51).

NURSING DIAGNOSES, PLANNING, AND IMPLEMENTATION. Possible nursing diagnoses include the following.

Acute Pain related to inflammation or trauma
EXPECTED OUTCOME: The patient's pain will be decreased or absent as evidenced by a lower rating on a pain scale.

• Assess for nonverbal signs of ear pain *to identify pain.*
• Identify with the patient an optimum analgesic schedule *to promote comfort.*
• Implement nonpharmacological methods, such as relaxation, massage, music, guided imagery, or distraction techniques *to relieve pain.*

• Apply heat as ordered to the area *to promote comfort.*
• Offer liquid or soft foods *to relieve pain when chewing.*

Risk for Injury related to self-cleaning of external ear
EXPECTED OUTCOME: The patient will explain or demonstrate prescribed treatment.

• Explain ear care (Box 52-4) *to prevent injury.*
• Teach patient treatment regimen *to ensure completion of treatment.*

Deficient Knowledge related to lack of information on preventive ear care
EXPECTED OUTCOME: The patient will explain or demonstrate procedures to maintain wellness of the external ear.

• Explain procedure before removal of cerumen *to decrease anxiety.*
• If a wick is inserted into the ear canal, explain to patient that it is used *to monitor for drainage and report excessive drainage to HCP.*
• Teach patient how to use topical antibiotics, oral antibiotics, and/or anti-inflammatory medications *to promote healing.*
• Teach the patient how to complete the prescribed treatment and maintain ear health (see Box 52-4). Include how to administer eardrops or ointments, keep the ear clean and dry, and use cotton with petroleum jelly or earplugs *to avoid getting water in the ears during an infection.*

Box 52-4 Ear Care

1. Cleanse the external ear with a wet washcloth. Gently cleanse the helix.
2. The ear has an effective self-cleaning system that continually moves protective earwax outward to prevent buildup. Cleaning attempts such as with swabs can impact the wax. Never insert anything into the ear canal, including, cotton-tipped applicators, hair pins, matchsticks, safety pins, toothpicks, paper clips, or fingers. The thin skin of the ear canal is very fragile and can become abraded and then infected from being touched with these objects.
3. A person with a history of ear infections, perforated tympanic membrane, or swimmer's ear should prevent moisture from entering the ear canal and should avoid swimming in contaminated water. Moisture or water in the ear canal can be prevented by using special earplugs.
4. For frequent swimming use: an ear conditioner to prevent ear dryness, an ear dryer after swimming, swim earplugs (custom or over the counter).
5. Avoid home remedies for ear care without consulting a HCP.
6. A person with an upper respiratory infection should gently blow the nose with both nares open to prevent microbes from being forced up the eustachian tubes.

EVALUATION. The outcomes for the patient are met if patient indicates pain is decreased or absent as evidenced by a lower rating on a pain scale, hearing improves or returns to preillness level, states or demonstrates prescribed treatment (e.g., administering ear drops or ointments) without injury, and explains or demonstrates measures to maintain wellness of the external ear.

Middle Ear, Tympanic Membrane, and Mastoid Disorders

Infections

PATHOPHYSIOLOGY AND ETIOLOGY. Otitis media is the most common disease of the middle ear. Otitis media is a general term for inflammation of the middle ear, mastoid, and eustachian tube. Inflammation of the nasopharynx causes most cases of otitis media. As inflammation occurs, the nasopharyngeal mucosa becomes edematous and discharge is produced. When fluid, pus, or air builds up in the middle ear, the eustachian tube becomes blocked, and this impairs middle ear ventilation.

There are several types of otitis media in which inflammation can occur alone, with infective drainage, or with noninfective drainage. The first type of otitis media is otitis media without effusion. This is an inflammation of the middle ear mucosa without drainage. The second type of otitis media occurs when there is a bacterial infection of the middle ear mucosa. This is called acute otitis media, suppurative otitis media, or purulent otitis media. The infected fluid becomes trapped in the middle ear. If the infection continues longer than 3 months, chronic otitis media results. The third type of otitis media is otitis media with effusion. Other names include serous otitis media, nonsuppurative otitis media, and glue ear. With this type of otitis media, noninfective fluid accumulates within the middle ear.

SIGNS AND SYMPTOMS. Acute otitis media commonly follows an upper respiratory infection. A fever, earache, and feeling of fullness in the affected ear are common symptoms (Table 52.10). As purulent drainage forms, pain and conductive hearing loss occur. Nausea and vomiting may also be present. Purulent drainage may be evident in the external ear canal if the tympanic membrane ruptures. Mastoid tenderness indicates that the infection may have spread to the mastoid area. Otoscopic examination reveals a reddened, bulging tympanic membrane.

Symptoms of otitis media with effusion may go undetected in adults because there are no signs of infection. The patient may report fullness, bubbling, or crackling in the ear. The patient may have a slight conductive hearing loss or allergies or be a mouth breather. Otoscopic examination can reveal a bulging tympanic membrane with a fluid level, but the eardrum is not reddened.

COMPLICATIONS. A perforation may occur with an acute or chronic infection. Buildup of fluid and pressure in the middle ear can cause a spontaneous perforation of the tympanic membrane. The patient usually experiences pain before the rupture and relief of pain after the rupture. The fluid in the

TABLE 52.10   MIDDLE EAR DISORDERS SUMMARY

Signs and Symptoms	Fever, earache, and feeling of fullness in affected ear following upper respiratory infection Nausea, vomiting Mastoid tenderness Reddened, bulging tympanic membrane Progressive hearing loss Vertigo Disorientation
Diagnostic Tests	Complete blood count Ear drainage culture Audiometric, Rinne, Weber, and whisper voice tests
Therapeutic Measures	Antibiotics Analgesics Myringotomy Myringoplasty Stapedectomy
Complications	Perforation of tympanic membrane Cholesteatoma Tympanosclerosis Mastoiditis Permanent hearing loss
Priority Nursing Diagnoses	*Acute Pain* *Deficient Knowledge* *Risk for Infection*

middle ear moves through the perforation into the ear canal, relieving the pressure and pain. A tympanic membrane perforation causes hearing loss. The location and size of the perforation determine the extent of hearing loss. Damage to the ossicles can also occur with perforation.

Repeated infections in the middle ear or mastoid can cause a cholesteatoma, which is an epithelial cystlike sac that fills with debris such as degenerated skin and sebaceous material. The cholesteatoma starts in the external ear canal and spreads to the middle ear through a perforation in the tympanic membrane. Damage occurs in the middle ear structures as a result of pressure necrosis. The cholesteatoma causes conductive hearing loss. As the disease progresses, facial paralysis and vertigo may occur.

Tympanosclerosis is another complication of repeated middle ear infections. Tympanosclerosis consists of deposits of collagen and calcium on the tympanic membrane. The condition can slowly progress over time to the area around the middle ear ossicles. These deposits appear as chalky white plaques on the tympanic membrane and contribute to conductive hearing loss.

Mastoiditis can occur if acute otitis media is not treated. The infection spreads to the mastoid area, causing pain. The use of antibiotics has resulted in acute mastoiditis becoming relatively uncommon. Chronic mastoiditis is still seen with repeated middle ear infections.

DIAGNOSTIC TESTS. An elevated WBC count may be seen and cultures on ear drainage identify the specific infective organism. Conductive hearing loss is usually present on audiometric studies and Rinne, Weber, and whisper voice tests. Imaging studies may be done to diagnose infection.

THERAPEUTIC MEASURES. Bacterial infections are treated with topical and systemic antibiotics. Topical antibiotics may contain steroids to help with inflammation. Oral analgesics are given to control pain.

A modified Politzer ear device can be used to help equalize pressure in the middle ear and aid fluid drainage. The device, also known as the ear popper (www.earpopper.com), emits a stream of air into the nasal cavity that gently opens the eustachian tubes. This relieves negative pressure and allows pressure to equalize and fluid to drain.

Surgical intervention includes several techniques. Paracentesis may be performed with a needle and syringe. The tympanic membrane is punctured with the needle, and the fluid is drained from the middle ear. A **myringotomy** may also be performed. During this procedure, an incision is made in the tympanic membrane and fluid is allowed to drain out or is suctioned out of the middle ear. Another technique is laser-assisted myringotomy, which vaporizes the tympanic membrane. Various types of transtympanic tubes may be inserted to keep the incision open. The transtympanic tube keeps the incision in the tympanic membrane open, equalizes pressure, and prevents further fluid formation and buildup. The transtympanic tubes are left in place until the infection is cured. Most tubes spontaneously extrude in 3 to 12 months and rarely have to be removed.

Reconstructive repair of a perforated tympanic membrane is called a **myringoplasty**. One technique involves placing Gelfoam over the perforation. A graft from the temporal muscle behind the ear or tissue from the external ear is then placed over the perforation and Gelfoam. The Gelfoam is absorbed, and the graft repairs the perforation.

A mastoidectomy involves incision, drainage, and surgical removal of the mastoid process if the infection has spread to the mastoid area.

Otosclerosis

PATHOPHYSIOLOGY AND ETIOLOGY. Otosclerosis, or hardening of the ear, results from the formation of new bone along the stapes. With the new bone growth, the stapes becomes immobile and causes conductive hearing loss. The formation of the new bone growth begins in adolescence or early adulthood and progresses slowly. Hearing loss is most apparent after the fourth decade of life. Otosclerosis is more common in women than in men. The disease usually affects both ears. Although the exact cause of otosclerosis is not known, most patients have a family history of the disease. It is therefore thought to be a hereditary disease.

SIGNS AND SYMPTOMS. The primary symptom of otosclerosis is progressive hearing loss. The patient usually experiences bilateral conductive hearing loss, particularly with soft, low tones. Usually, medical treatment is sought when the hearing loss interferes with the patient's ability to hear conversations. The patient may also experience tinnitus. Otoscopic examination reveals a pinkish orange tympanic membrane because of vascular and bony changes in the middle ear.

DIAGNOSTIC TESTS. Audiometric testing indicates the type and extent of the hearing loss. Imaging studies indicate the location and the extent of the excessive bone growth. The whisper voice test and normal conversation show decreased hearing. The patient hears best with bone conduction in the Rinne test, whereas lateralization to the most affected ear occurs with the Weber test.

THERAPEUTIC MEASURES. There is no cure for otosclerosis, but hearing aids may be used to improve hearing for the patient. Although total restoration of hearing is not possible, reconstruction of necrotic ossicles is done to restore some of the patient's hearing. Various methods are used to reposition and replace some or all of the ossicles. Unfortunately, the surgeries are not always successful over time. Ossiculoplasty is the reconstruction of the ossicles. Prostheses made of plastic, ceramic, or human bone are used to replace the necrotic ossicles. Total or partial ossicular replacement prosthesis may be used.

Stapedectomy is the treatment of choice for otosclerosis. Either part or all of the stapes is removed and replaced with a prosthesis. The prosthesis is placed between the incus and the oval window. Advances in surgical treatment include the use of lasers for improved visualization, less trauma, and greater precision during surgery. The goal is to restore vibration from the tympanic membrane to the oval window and allow sound transmission. Many patients experience improved hearing immediately, others not until swelling subsides. Complications of ossiculoplasty and stapedectomy include extrusion of the prosthesis, infection, hearing loss, dizziness, and facial nerve damage.

NURSING CARE. The operative ear is positioned upward when lying in bed. An earplug may be used to help keep the area aseptic; the proximity of the brain makes this necessary to prevent brain infection. Activity orders may vary. The patient may be dizzy and experience nausea. Antiemetics should be given promptly to prevent vomiting. The patient's safety should be ensured if dizziness occurs. To prevent dislodgment or damage to the prosthesis, patients are instructed not to cough, sneeze, blow their nose, vomit, fly in an airplane, lift heavy objects, or shower. If the patient develops a cold, the HCP should be contacted.

• **WORD** • **BUILDING** •

myringoplasty: myringo—tympanic membrane + plasty—surgical repair

stapedectomy: stape(s)—stirrup + ectomy—excision of

CRITICAL THINKING

Mrs. Springhorn

■ Mrs. Springhorn is an 83-year-old woman who is scheduled to be discharged from the hospital after a stapedectomy. She lives alone at home and is able to care for herself.

1. How would you communicate with Mrs. Springhorn to ensure that she understands the discharge instructions?
2. What teaching methods would you use to enhance communication?
3. What ear care instructions would you give her?

Suggested answers are at the end of the chapter.

Trauma

ETIOLOGY AND PHYSIOLOGY.

Trauma such as a blasting force, a blunt injury to the side of the head, or sudden changes in atmospheric pressure can cause the tympanic membrane to perforate and middle ear ossicles to fracture. Blast injuries cause injury from the direct pressure on the ear. Blunt injury to the head can cause temporal skull fractures and trauma to both the middle and inner ear. Barotrauma caused by sudden changes in atmospheric pressure in the ears can occur during scuba diving and airplane takeoffs and landings. Pressure changes can occur during normal atmospheric conditions such as nose blowing, heavy lifting, and sneezing. During these rapid changes of pressure, the eustachian tube does not ventilate because of occlusion or dysfunction and a negative pressure develops in the middle ear. The resulting pressure can cause the tympanic membrane to rupture or cause damage to the middle and inner ear.

SIGNS AND SYMPTOMS. Pain and hearing loss are the most common symptoms associated with trauma. Other signs and symptoms of barotrauma include fullness of the ears, vertigo, nausea, disorientation, edema of the affected area, and hemorrhage in the external or middle ear. In severe cases of barotrauma when scuba diving, these symptoms can cause drowning or cerebral air embolism from an overly rapid ascent. Otoscopic examination may reveal a retracted, reddened, and edematous tympanic membrane.

DIAGNOSTIC TESTS. Audiometric studies are completed to determine the hearing loss. Imaging studies may be done to determine the extent of middle and inner ear damage. Conductive or sensorineural hearing loss may be evident, depending on the extent and location of the damage.

Nursing Process for the Patient With Middle Ear, Tympanic Membrane, and Mastoid Disorders

DATA COLLECTION. Table 52.11 reviews the subjective data that should be collected. The external ear should be inspected and palpated to obtain objective data. Pain with palpation is indicative of external ear problems, not middle ear problems. Pain over the mastoid area can indicate a mastoid problem.

TABLE 52.11   SUBJECTIVE DATA COLLECTION FOR MIDDLE EAR, TYMPANIC MEMBRANE, AND MASTOID DISORDERS

W Where is it?	Are both ears affected? Is it deep within the head?
H How does it feel?	Is there pressure? Fullness? Is it painful; if so, is it sharp, dull, continuous, intermittent, throbbing, localized? No pain?
A Aggravating and alleviating factors	Is it worse with change of position? Worse with movement? Is there relief after drainage? Relief with change of position? Relief with heat or analgesics?
T Timing	When did it start? Has there been any recent upper respiratory infection, airline travel, scuba diving, trauma, or weight lifting? Was it a gradual or sudden onset? How long have symptoms persisted? Has there been a change in symptoms?
S Severity	Does it cause hearing impairment? How much? Does it affect activities of daily living?
U Useful data for associated symptoms	Is there any fever, drainage from the ear canal, nausea, vomiting, dizziness? Is there a family history of otosclerosis? Any previous ear problems or ear surgeries? Any occupational or recreational risk factors, such as scuba diving, weight lifting, or frequent airline travel?
P Perception of the problem by the patient	What does the patient think is wrong? Has problem occurred before? If so, what was the same and what was different?

The middle ear and mastoid cavity cannot be visualized directly. The tympanic membrane is the only middle ear structure that can be directly visualized with an otoscope. Objective assessment also includes vital signs, noting any elevation in temperature. Any drainage from the ear should be noted and described. Hearing acuity is screened with the whisper voice, Rinne, and Weber tests.

NURSING DIAGNOSES, PLANNING, AND IMPLEMENTATION.

Risk for Infection related to broken skin, pressure necrosis, chronic disease, or surgical procedure

EXPECTED OUTCOME: The patient will have no signs of infection (no drainage from ear, no tenderness over mastoid, negative culture, afebrile).

• Explain to patient not to blow nose by pinching off nares *to prevent spread of upper respiratory infections up the eustachian tube.*
• Teach patient not to insert anything into ear canal *to prevent ear damage* (see Box 52-4).
• Teach patient how to correctly remove cerumen from ear *to prevent infection or damage.*

Acute Pain related to fluid accumulation, inflammation, or infection

EXPECTED OUTCOME: The patient will indicate pain is decreased or absent as evidenced by a lower rating on a pain scale.

• Monitor pain using a pain scale, and determine optimum analgesic schedule with patient *to maximize pain control.*
• Use nonpharmacological measures such as heat, distraction, and relaxation techniques *for pain reduction.*
• Teach patient how to administer eardrops or ear ointment *to help resolve infection and decrease pain.*
• Instruct patient to take all prescribed antibiotics, even after symptoms are relieved, *to ensure that infection is completely resolved.*

Deficient Knowledge Regarding Hearing Loss and Lack of Information or Surgery related to lack of exposure to information due to no prior experience

EXPECTED OUTCOME: The patient will state an understanding of methods for preventing problems in the middle ear, tympanic membrane, and mastoid process or impending surgery.

• Teach patient to avoid trauma to the ear, loud noise exposure, and environmental or occupational conditions *to prevent damage to the ear.*
• Teach patient to yawn or perform jaw-thrust maneuver (opening mouth wide and moving jaw) *to equalize ear pressure, which helps maintain ear health.*
• Teach patient methods of effective communication *to compensate for hearing loss* (see the "Nursing Care Plan for the Patient With Hearing Loss").
• Ask about patient's knowledge regarding surgery *to determine learning needs.*
• Include family in teaching sessions *to enhance learning and assist with retention of information.*

• Provide preoperative and postoperative instructions *to promote patient understanding* (Box 52-5).
• Teach patient to avoid getting water in ear postoperatively *to prevent moisture from reaching surgical site.*

Box 52-5 Preoperative and Postoperative Nursing Interventions for the Patient Having Ear Surgery

Preoperative Care

Nursing care for the patient undergoing ear surgery begins as soon as the decision to have surgery is made. The nurse collects data, determines if the patient understands the events, notes the patient's mental readiness, and obtains baseline physiological data.

• Ask understanding of the surgery and whether local or general anesthesia will be used.
• Help alleviate the patient's fear by encouraging the patient to ask questions. Ensure that all questions are answered before the surgery by appropriate person.
• Explain the type of pain, any packing or dressings that may be in place postoperatively, and any other postoperative restrictions that may be needed.
• Establish baseline vital signs and document findings.
• Ensure that the operative permit is signed.
• Determine current medications the patient is taking and document in the patient's record.
• Determine if the patient understands that surgery does not always correct impaired hearing.
• Leave any hearing devices in place as long as possible before the surgery.

Postoperative Care

Postoperatively the nurse is responsible for assessing the patient's physiological status. The nurse is also responsible for ensuring that the patient and family members understand discharge instructions.

• Some degree of pain may be expected, even with minor procedures. Explain how and when to take pain medication when the patient is discharged.
• Monitor postoperative vital signs and return to presurgical baseline.
• Tell patients that if an occlusive dressing is in place, hearing may be decreased until the dressing is removed.
• Instruct patients with tubes to avoid getting water in the ear. A shower cap or earplugs may be used.
• Instruct the patient to seek medical attention if excessive bleeding or drainage occurs. If a cotton plug is to be left in place, instruct the patient to change it daily.

Continued

Box 52-5 Preoperative and Postoperative Nursing Interventions for the Patient Having Ear Surgery—cont'd

- Teach the patient, unless contraindicated, to blow the nose very gently one side at a time for the first week after surgery. Instruct the patient to sneeze or cough with the mouth open for 1 week after surgery.
- Avoid airplane flights for 1 week after surgery. For sensations of ear pressure, hold nose, close mouth, and swallow to equalize pressure.
- The patient should avoid strenuous work for several weeks. The patient may return to work in a few days, depending on the type of surgery and the type of work the patient does.
- Tell the patient to take prescribed medication and antibiotics as ordered.
- Have the patient arrange for a follow-up appointment by calling HCP's office.

EVALUATION. The goals for the patient are met if there is no ear drainage or pain over mastoid and if the patient has negative culture and remains afebrile, states that no pain is present or pain is decreased, verbalizes care of ears and methods to prevent further infection, describes signs requiring medical attention, and verbalizes the rationale and outcome for any upcoming surgery as well as preoperative and postoperative instructions.

Inner Ear
Labyrinthitis

PATHOPHYSIOLOGY AND ETIOLOGY. Labyrinthitis is an inflammation or infection of the inner ear and can be caused by either viral or bacterial pathogens. The bacterium or virus enters the inner ear from the middle ear, meninges, or bloodstream. Serous labyrinthitis is a type of acute labyrinthitis that sometimes follows drug intoxication or overindulgence in alcohol. It can also be caused by an allergy. Diffuse suppurative labyrinthitis occurs when acute or chronic otitis media spreads into the inner ear or after middle ear or mastoid surgery. Destruction of soft tissue structures from the infection can cause permanent hearing loss.

SIGNS AND SYMPTOMS. Vertigo, tinnitus, and sensorineural hearing loss are the most common symptoms. Vertigo, or dizziness, occurs when the vestibular structures are involved. Tinnitus, or ringing in the ear, occurs when the infection is located in the cochlea. Sensorineural hearing loss can be caused by infections in the cochlea or vestibular structures. Nystagmus on the affected side may occur. Other signs and symptoms include pain, fever, ataxia, nausea, vomiting, and beginning nerve deafness.

DIAGNOSTIC TESTS. A CBC is done to diagnose infection. A hearing evaluation by an audiologist may reveal mild to complete hearing loss. Rinne and Weber tests indicate conductive or sensorineural hearing loss.

THERAPEUTIC MEASURES. Antibiotics are used to treat bacterial inner ear infections. Viral infections usually run their course in about 1 week. Mild sedation may help the patient relax. Although there is no specific medicine to relieve dizziness, antihistamines can be used if they prove helpful on an individual basis. Patients may be placed on bed rest.

NURSING CARE. Nursing management includes helping the patient manage symptoms and self-care, and educating the patient about safety issues while on bed rest and sedatives to prevent falls and injury. The patient should avoid turning the head quickly to help alleviate vertigo. The patient is assisted to cope with anxiety that may be present because of the frustration surrounding hearing loss or loss of work.

Neoplastic Disorders

PATHOPHYSIOLOGY AND ETIOLOGY. Inner ear tumors can be benign or malignant. Acoustic neuroma, a tumor of the eighth cranial nerve, is the most common benign tumor. It is slow growing, occurs at any age, and usually occurs unilaterally. As it spreads, it compresses the nerve and adjacent structures. Malignant tumors arising from the inner ear are rare. Squamous and basal carcinomas arise from the epidermal lining of the inner ear.

SIGNS AND SYMPTOMS. Early symptoms of an acoustic neuroma include progressive unilateral sensorineural hearing loss of high-pitched sounds, unilateral tinnitus, and intermittent vertigo. Headache, pain, and balance disorders may also be present. Symptoms progress as the tumor spreads to other structures. Most malignant tumors grow quickly. The symptoms vary depending on the area of the ear that is involved.

DIAGNOSTIC TEST. Neurologic, audiometric, and vestibular testing are used to diagnose neuroma. Auditory brainstem-evoked response and electronystagmography are completed. Examination of the cerebrospinal fluid shows increased protein. Computed tomography (CT) and magnetic resonance imaging (MRI) are used to determine size and location of the tumor.

THERAPEUTIC MEASURES. The preferred method of treatment involves surgical removal of the tumor. The labyrinth is destroyed, with a resulting permanent hearing loss. Steroids and radiation may be used to decrease the size of the tumor or for inoperable tumors.

NURSING CARE. Nursing care focuses on preparing the patient for surgery and adjusting to the diagnosis and the resulting hearing loss (see Box 52-5).

Ménière's Disease

PATHOPHYSIOLOGY AND ETIOLOGY. **Ménière's disease** is a balance disorder. Its cause is unknown. With the disease, there is a dilation of the membranous labyrinth resulting from a disturbance in the fluid physiology of the endolymphatic system. The exact etiology is unknown but is thought to stem from hypersecretion, hypoabsorption, deficit membrane permeability, allergy, viral infection, hormonal imbalance, or mental stress. The disease usually develops between ages 40 and 60. The symptoms range from vague to severe and debilitating.

SIGNS AND SYMPTOMS. A triad of symptoms of vertigo, hearing loss, and tinnitus characterizes Ménière's disease. Recurring episodic bouts of the incapacitating triad of symptoms and nausea and vomiting occur with Ménière's disease. The attacks may occur suddenly, or the patient may experience warning signs such as headache or fullness in the ears. During an acute episode, the patient experiences vertigo that lasts 2 to 4 hours. The vertigo is usually accompanied by nausea and vomiting, followed by dizziness and unsteadiness. The patient is uncoordinated and has gait changes when walking. Hearing loss is often described as a fluctuating fullness in the ears. Tinnitus is present. Irritability, depression, and withdrawal are common. Vital signs usually remain normal. It takes several weeks for symptoms to resolve, and hearing loss in the affected ear remains. The patient then enters a stage of remission until the next attack. The acute episodes occur two to three times yearly. Eventually the patient has complete remission with some degree of permanent hearing loss.

DIAGNOSTIC TESTS. Audiometric studies identify the type and magnitude of the hearing loss. Neurologic testing and radiographic studies are done to rule out other pathological conditions. A caloric stimulation test may demonstrate a difference in eye movement.

THERAPEUTIC MEASURES. Medical treatment consists of symptomatic treatment for acute attacks and prophylactic treatment between attacks. Tranquilizers and vagal blockers may be needed during acute attacks. Salt-restricted diet,

diuretics, antihistamines, and vasodilators are used during prophylactic treatment. The patient should avoid alcohol, caffeine, and tobacco use. The patient may be placed on bed rest during acute attacks. The goals of medical treatment are to preserve hearing and reduce symptoms. Some patients who do not respond to treatment may be placed on low doses of methotrexate.

Surgical treatment is used only when medical management has failed. When involvement is unilateral, a labyrinthectomy can be performed. This causes complete loss of hearing in that ear. Another surgical intervention establishes a shunt from the inner ear to the subarachnoid space. This procedure helps drain the fluid and prevent future hearing loss. Another surgical treatment is intratympanic gentamicin injection, which is usually done in the HCP's office.

NURSING CARE. Nursing management focuses on managing the patient's symptoms and providing safety during the acute attacks. Because of the unpredictability of Ménière's disease, the nursing care focuses on emotional support for the patient during periods of remission. Provide emotional support and resources to help the patient cope with the unpredictable nature of the disease and the physical impairments associated with the disease.

Nursing Process for the Patient With Inner Ear Disorders

DATA COLLECTION. Table 52.12 reviews subjective data to be collected. Objective data include examination of gross hearing, the whisper voice, Rinne, and Weber tests, a physical examination, and lab data. The patient should be assessed for any nutritional deficiencies, including dehydration, weight loss, or weight gain. An unsteady gait or temperature is also noted.

TABLE 52.12   SUBJECTIVE DATA COLLECTION FOR INNER EAR DISORDERS

W Where is it?	Are both ears affected?
H How does it feel?	Is there pressure? Fullness? Vertigo? Tinnitus? Is it painful; if so, is it sharp, dull continuous, intermittent, throbbing, localized? No pain?
A Aggravating and alleviating factors	Is it worse with change of position? Worse with movement? Is there relief with medications? Is the patient taking current medications? Are there any allergies?
T Timing	When did it start? Was it a gradual or sudden onset? How long have symptoms persisted? Do symptoms progress in a set timing pattern? Do symptoms occur together or separately? Has there been a change in symptoms?
S Severity	Does it cause hearing impairment? How much? Does it affect activities of daily living, nutritional intake, work, or leisure?
U Useful data for associated symptoms	Any fever, nausea, vomiting, or dizziness? Any previous ear problems or ear surgeries? Headache?
P Perception of the problem by the patient	What does the patient think is wrong? Has patient had this problem before? If so, what was the same and what was different?

NURSING DIAGNOSES, PLANNING, AND IMPLEMENTATION.
Planning focuses on helping the patient maintain a normal lifestyle, remain free of injuries, cope with the illness or hearing loss, and maintain adequate nutrition and hydration. The major nursing diagnoses and interventions for internal ear disorders include those discussed next.

Anxiety related to unpredictability of sudden and severe acute attacks

EXPECTED OUTCOME: The patient will state that anxiety is decreased.

• Encourage patient to express concerns about hearing loss and the unpredictability of acute attacks *to identify causes of anxiety.*
• Assess for signs of anxiety such as fidgeting, restlessness, apprehension, shakiness, and increased heart rate *to determine if anxiety is present.*
• Explore with patient techniques that have and have not worked in the past *to determine which techniques to use to reduce anxiety.*
• Use a calm reassuring approach *to help instill confidence.*
• Provide quiet environment and diversional activities *to calm patient.*
• Provide factual information regarding diagnosis and treatment *to promote understanding and reduce anxiety.*

Risk for Injury related to impaired equilibrium

EXPECTED OUTCOME: The patient will not be injured from falling due to alterations in equilibrium.

• Institute fall precautions *to help prevent injury.*
• Ensure that environment is safe and free of obstacles (throw rugs, electrical cords in walkways, and poor lighting) *to prevent falls.*
• Monitor for signs of headache or fullness in the ears *to detect oncoming Ménière's disease attack.*
• Instruct patient to avoid sudden movement of the head during periods of vertigo *to prevent increasing symptoms.*
• Instruct patient on correct dosage and administration of medications *to help ensure resolution of symptoms.*
• Instruct patient to avoid use of alcohol, caffeine, and tobacco *to decrease disruptions of equilibrium.*

CRITICAL THINKING

Mrs. Belmont

■ Mrs. Belmont is a 48-year-old woman diagnosed with Ménière's disease. She is currently in a state of remission. She states that she is fearful that the next attack will occur during her daughter's upcoming wedding.

1. What information would you ask of Mrs. Belmont about her attacks?
2. What instructions can you provide her regarding treatment during her attacks?
3. How will you handle Mrs. Belmont's fears about future attacks?

Suggested answers are at the end of the chapter.

• Instruct patient to call for assistance when ambulating *to minimize risk of falling.*
• If indicated, instruct patient to remain on bed rest until symptoms are relieved *to prevent injury.*

Nutrition: Less Than Body Requirements related to nausea and vomiting

EXPECTED OUTCOME: The patient will experience adequate nutrition and hydration with relief of nausea and vomiting.

• Monitor for signs of nausea, vomiting, and inadequate hydration *to determine baseline information.*
• Instruct patient to use deep breathing, voluntary swallowing, and eating slowly *to suppress the vomiting reflex.*
• Medicate as ordered *to relieve symptoms and prevent episodes of nausea and vomiting.*
• Institute salt-restricted diet, if ordered, and instruct patient on low- and high-sodium foods *to reduce fluid retention.*

EVALUATION. The goals for the patient have been met if signs of anxiety are decreased and if the patient remains free from injury and maintains weight within normal range with no signs of dehydration.

SUGGESTED ANSWERS TO

CRITICAL THINKING

■ *Mr. Samuel*

1. Mr. Samuel should seek assistance, patch both eyes, and have someone take him to receive medical treatment immediately.

2. Ensure that an antiemetic is ordered postoperatively on the patient's return to the unit. When Mr. Samuel reports nausea, the antiemetic should be given promptly.

3. Did you recognize that the concentration is 2 mg/ 1 mL, and the volume of the vial is 2 mL? The concentration is what is needed to calculate the dose:

$$\frac{4 \text{ mg}}{} \left| \frac{1 \text{ mL}}{2 \text{ mg}} \right. = 2 \text{ mL}$$

■ *Mrs. Springhorn*

1. Gain her attention, face and stand in her visual field, avoid glare, speak clearly, inform her of topics to be discussed, assess for understanding, allow extra time, reduce background noises, use nonverbal communication, and do not cover your mouth when talking.

2. Use active listening. Use written communication to enhance spoken words. Use demonstration and return demonstration. Allow questions. Do not hurry. Provide information in short segments. Reassess understanding at each session.

3. Place the operative ear upward when lying in bed. Use earplug as ordered. Do not cough, sneeze, blow nose, vomit, fly in an airplane, lift heavy objects, or shower. If a cold develops, call the HCP. If dizzy, be careful when standing up.

■ *Mrs. Belmont*

1. You would ask Mrs. Belmont about specific signs she may have before attacks, such as headache or fullness in the ears. You should also ask her specifically what symptoms she has during attacks. Common symptoms include the triad of vertigo, hearing loss, and tinnitus. She may also have nausea, vomiting, and unsteady gait.

2. Discuss treatment that Mrs. Belmont has used with previous attacks. Ask her which treatments seemed to help. Common treatments you can recommend include taking recommended medication such as tranquilizers and vagal blockers; instruct her to maintain adequate fluid and nutritional intake during attacks; ambulate with assistance; limit salt in diet; avoid alcohol, caffeine, and tobacco use.

3. Discuss with Mrs. Belmont prophylactic treatment such as salt-restricted diet, diuretics, antihistamines, and vasodilators. Discuss the normal progress of the disease. Provide emotional support and discuss methods to help her cope with the disease, such as counseling and relaxation techniques.

REVIEW QUESTIONS

1. The nurse is caring for a patient who is diagnosed with otosclerosis. The patient asks the nurse what this disease is. Which is the most appropriate response by the nurse?
   1. "Infection of the external ear commonly caused by moisture."
   2. "Tumor of the eighth cranial nerve."
   3. "Hardening of the stapes due to new bone growth."
   4. "Inflammation of the inner ear caused by pathogens."

2. The nurse is caring for a patient who is diagnosed with a refractive error. The patient asks the nurse what this means. What would be the appropriate explanation by the nurse?
   1. "You will lose your vision and become blind."
   2. "You will need corrective lenses in order to see clearly."
   3. "The pressure in your eyes is higher than normal."
   4. "Your vision is 20/20."

3. A patient comes to the health clinic for a suspected ear infection. Which of the following data collection findings does the nurse expect with an external ear infection?
   1. Pain
   2. Fullness in ears
   3. Fever
   4. Dizziness

4. A patient has been prepped for an internal eye examination. Anesthetic drops and a mydriatic drug have been administered. Which of the following should the patient be taught for eye safety following the examination?
   1. "Wear sunglasses after the exam."
   2. "Rub your eye hourly to increase blood circulation."
   3. "You may reapply contact lenses when the eye exam is completed."
   4. "Flush your eye with water to remove the eye drops."

5. The nurse cares for patients after eye surgery. Which of the following patients would the nurse provide specific positioning instructions to after eye surgery to prevent complications?
   1. 19-year-old after removal of congenital cataract
   2. 30-year-old woman after pneumatic retinopexy
   3. 52-year-old man after trabeculectomy
   4. 82-year-old man after corneal transplant

6. The nurse is caring for a patient with a history of acute angle-closure glaucoma. The nurse is preparing to administer the patient's medications. Which medications should the nurse question before administration?
   1. Morphine
   2. Cefazolin (Kefzol)
   3. Atropine
   4. Ranitidine (Zantac)
   5. Hydroxyzine (Vistaril)
   6. Warfarin (Coumadin)

7. The nurse is assisting with discharge instructions for a patient. For which of the following medications would the nurse teach the patient that the medication can cause hearing loss?
   1. Furosemide (Lasix)
   2. Acetaminophen (Tylenol)
   3. Warfarin (Coumadin)
   4. Penicillin (Pen-Vee K)

8. The nurse is caring for a patient with macular degeneration. During data collection, which symptom would the nurse anticipate the patient to report?
   1. Loss of peripheral vision
   2. Sudden darkness
   3. Dull ache in the eyes
   4. Loss of central vision

9. The nurse is contributing to the plan of care for a patient with Ménière's disease. What is the primary goal for a patient with Ménière's disease that the nurse should recommend to include in the plan of care?
   1. Prevent dehydration
   2. Decrease pain
   3. Prevent injury
   4. Preserve hearing

10. The nurse is caring for a patient with presbycusis. Which technique is *most* important for the nurse to use to increase communication with this patient?
    1. Talk in a very loud voice.
    2. Lower voice pitch.
    3. Do not smile or chew gum when talking to the patient.
    4. Allow extra time for patient to respond.

11. A patient with acute angle-closure glaucoma reports use of the following medications. The use of which of these medications indicates to the nurse that the patient requires further instruction?
    a. Acetaminophen
    b. Cefazolin (Kefzol)
    c. Ranitidine (Zantac)
    d. Diphenhydramine (Benadryl)

Answers can be found in Appendix C.

 For additional resources and information visit davispl.us/medsurg5

unit FIFTEEN

Understanding the Integumentary System

53

Integumentary System Function, Assessment, and Therapeutic Measures

KEY TERMS

alopecia (AH-low-PEE-she-ah)
ecchymosis (EK-ih-MOH-siss)
erythema (AIR-ih-THEE-mah)
petechiae (peh-TEE-kee-eye)
turgor (TUR-gur)

RITA BOLEK TROFINO,
MARTY KOHN, AND
JANICE L. BRADFORD

LEARNING OUTCOMES

1. Explain the normal structures and functions of the integumentary system.
2. Identify the effects of aging on the integumentary system.
3. List data to collect when caring for a patient with an integumentary system disorder.
4. Identify laboratory and diagnostic tests commonly performed to diagnose integumentary disorders.
5. Describe therapeutic measures that are used for patients with integumentary disorders.

NORMAL INTEGUMENTARY SYSTEM ANATOMY AND PHYSIOLOGY

The skin, its accessory structures, and the subcutaneous tissue form the integumentary system, the covering of the body that separates the living internal environment from the external environment. The skin itself is considered an organ and consists of two layers: the outer epidermis and the inner dermis (Fig. 53.1).

Epidermis, Dermis, and Hypodermis

The epidermis has up to five epithelial layers. The innermost epidermal layer is called the stratum germinativum, where mitosis occurs to produce new epidermal cells. The rate of mitosis is fairly constant, but increases from chronic abrasion to the skin, as in callus formation. The new cells, keratinocytes, produce the protein keratin and a water-repelling sealant. As they are pushed to the surface of the skin, they die and become the stratum corneum, the outermost of the epidermal layers. These cells resist abrasion and water entry and exit.

The stratum corneum consists of many layers of dead, keratinized cells. An unbroken stratum corneum is an effective barrier against pathogens and most chemicals, although even microscopic breaks are sufficient to permit their entry. As dead cells are worn off the surface of the skin (which contributes to the removal of pathogens), they are continuously replaced by cells from beneath. Loss of large portions of the stratum corneum, as with extensive third-degree burns, greatly increases the risk for infection and dehydration.

Melanocytes are cells in the lower epidermis that produce the protein melanin. The amount of melanin is a genetic characteristic and gives color to skin and hair. When the skin is exposed to ultraviolet (UV) rays from the sun or artificial lighting, production of melanin increases, and it is incorporated into the epidermal cells making the cells darker. Melanin is a pigment barrier to prevent further exposure of living cells in the stratum germinativum to UV rays. UV rays are mutagenic; that is, they are capable of damaging the DNA in cells and causing mutations that can result in malignancy.

Also in the epidermis are Langerhans cells, a type of macrophage that presents foreign antigens to immune cells. This is the first step in the destruction of pathogens that penetrate the epidermis.

Extensive collagen fibers in the dermis give the skin its strength as an organ. Elasticity results from widespread elastic fibers and allows stretched skin to return to its proper position.

The hypodermis is areolar and adipose tissue. This subcutaneous adipose tissue cushions, insulates, and stores energy as triglyceride. The subcutaneous tissue contains

The **epidermis**—the outermost layer—consists of stratified squamous epithelial tissue. It contains no blood vessels; instead, it obtains oxygen and nutrients by diffusion from the dermal layer beneath it.

The **dermis**—the inner, deeper layer—is composed of connective tissue. It contains primarily collagen fibers (which strengthen the tissue), but it also contains elastin fibers (which provide elasticity) and reticular fibers (which bind the collagen and elastin fibers together).

The dermis contains an abundance of blood vessels in addition to sweat glands, sebaceous glands, and nerve endings. Hair follicles are also embedded in the dermis. Finger-like projections, called **papillae**, extend upward from the dermis. These projections interlock with downward waves on the bottom of the epidermis, effectively binding the two structures together.

Beneath the skin is a layer of subcutaneous tissue called **hypodermis.** Made of loose connective (areolar) tissue and adipose tissue, the hypodermis binds the skin to the underlying tissue. Hypodermis that's composed mostly of adipose tissue is called subcutaneous fat. This layer of fat helps insulate the body from outside temperature changes; it also acts as an energy reservoir.

Dermal papilla
Sweat pores
Hairs
Sensory nerve fibers
Pressure receptor
Sebaceous gland
Hair follicle
Hair bulb
Apocrine sweat gland
Arrector pili muscle
Motor nerve fibers
Cutaneous blood vessels
Eccrine sweat gland

FIGURE 53.1 Structure of the skin. From Thompson, G. S. (2013). *Understanding anatomy and physiology.* Philadelphia: F.A. Davis, p. 69.

abundant leukocytes that destroy pathogens that enter through broken skin.

Hair

Human hair with significant function includes the eyelashes and eyebrows, which keep dust and sweat out of the eyes, and nostril hair, which filters air entering the nasal cavities. Hair on the head provides thermal insulation (Figure 53.2).

Nails

Nail roots are found at the ends of the fingers and toes; growth of nails is similar to growth of hair. Mitosis in the nail root is a continuous process to produce new, keratinized cells. As these cells die, they form the visible nail. Nails protect the ends of the digits from mechanical injury and are useful for picking up small objects.

Receptors

Sensory receptors for the cutaneous senses reside in the dermis. Receptors for heat, cold, and pain are free nerve endings; encapsulated nerve endings are specific for touch and pressure. The sensitivity of an area of skin is determined by the density of receptors present.

Glands

Cutaneous exocrine glands lie within the dermis and secrete to the surface of the skin through ducts. These include sudoriferous glands (both eccrine and apocrine), sebaceous glands, ceruminous glands (cerumen), and ciliary glands (tears) (Figure 53.3).

Water lost to eccrine gland secretion, at minimum, is about 500 mL per day through insensible perspiration. Excessive loss can rise to a liter per day in extreme heat or during vigorous exercise. Such dehydration and electrolyte loss must be replaced to avoid potential imbalances.

Blood Vessels

Blood vessels in the dermis serve the usual function of tissue nourishment, but the arterioles are also involved in maintaining body temperature. Blood carries heat produced by active organs and distributes it throughout the body. In a warm environment, dilation of blood vessels in the dermis increases blood flow and loss of heat to air. Constriction of blood vessels in a cold environment decreases blood flow to the skin and conserves body heat.

Stressful situations also cause vasoconstriction in the dermis, which allows blood to circulate to more vital organs, such as the heart, liver, brain, or muscles.

Other functions of the skin are the formation of vitamin D from cholesterol when the skin is exposed to the UV rays of the sun, and the excretion of small amounts of ammonia, urea, and sodium chloride in sweat.

Aging and the Integumentary System

The effects of age on the integumentary system are often quite visible. Figure 53.4 summarizes the effects of aging.

The **shaft** is the part of the hair that extends above the skin's surface.

Each hair lies within a sheath of epidermis called a **hair follicle**. Hair follicles have a rich nerve and blood supply.

Buried in the dermis is the hair **bulb** or **root**; this is the lowest part of the hair and is where growth occurs.

At the base of the hair is a cluster of connective tissue and blood vessels called the **papilla** that nourishes each hair.

Attached to each hair follicle is a small bundle of smooth muscle called the **arrector pili** muscle. Cold temperatures, or emotions such as fear, cause the muscle to contract. When it does, the hair becomes more upright, sometimes called "standing on end."

Sebaceous gland

Apocrine gland

Epidermis

Dermis

Subcutaneous layer

FIGURE 53.2 Hair. From Thompson, G. S. (2013). *Understanding anatomy and physiology*. Philadelphia: F.A. Davis, p. 73.

Eccrine glands

- Contain a duct that leads from a secretory portion (consisting of a twisted coil in the dermis), through the dermis and epidermis, and onto the skin's surface
- Are widespread throughout the body, but are especially abundant on the palms, soles, forehead, and upper torso
- Produce a transparent, watery fluid called sweat, which contains potassium, ammonia, lactic acid, uric acid, and other wastes
- Sweat plays a chief role in helping the body maintain a constant core temperature and also helps the body eliminate wastes.

Sebaceous glands

Sebaceous glands, which open into a hair follicle, secrete an oily substance called sebum. Sebum helps keep the skin and hair from drying out and becoming brittle. Sebum has a mild antibacterial and antifungal effect. Under the influence of sex hormones, sebum production increases during adolescence. When excess sebum accumulates in the gland ducts, pimples and blackheads can form. (When the accumulated sebum is exposed to air, it darkens, forming a blackhead. A pustule results if the area becomes infected by bacteria.)

Apocrine glands

- Contain a duct that leads to a hair follicle (as opposed to opening onto the skin's surface)
- Are located mainly in the axillary and anogenital (groin) regions
- Are scent glands that respond to stress and sexual stimulation
- Begin to function at puberty
- Sweat produced by these glands does not have a strong odor unless it accumulates on the skin; when this occurs, bacteria begins to degrade substances in the sweat, resulting in body odor

FIGURE 53.3 Glands. From Thompson, G. S. (2013). *Understanding anatomy and physiology.* Philadelphia: F.A. Davis, p. 75.

NURSING ASSESSMENT OF THE INTEGUMENTARY SYSTEM

Health History

Skin problems are a fairly common reason for a patient to enter the health system. Many factors can influence the integumentary system. A skin problem may be the only problem the patient has, or it may be a manifestation of an underlying systemic condition or psychological stress. Most important, the skin can visibly communicate the patient's health. Therefore, questions that are posed to the patient are important in determining if the skin problem is a disease entity of its own or a sign of a more systemic disorder. Table 53.1 provides examples of general questions that can be asked of the patient to gather information.

If further assessment of a particular problem area is needed, the **WHAT'S UP?** line of questioning can be used. For example, if the patient has a rash, you can respond by pursuing the following information:

- **W**here is it? Is that the only area where you have a rash?
- **H**ow does it feel? Does it itch? Burn? Hurt?
- **A**ggravating and alleviating factors. Does scratching aggravate it? Does anything else aggravate it, such as soaps and detergents? What relieves it? How have you treated it in the past?
- **T**iming. How long have you had this problem? Does it recur?
- **S**everity. How bad is the discomfort on a scale of 0 to 10, with 0 being comfortable and 10 being unable to touch the area?
- **U**seful other data. Do you have other symptoms besides the rash?
- **P**atient's perception. What do you think is causing your rash?

Physical Examination

Examination of the skin involves not only the entire skin area, but also the hair, nails, scalp, and mucous membranes. The main techniques used in physical examination of the skin are inspection and palpation. Make sure the patient is undressed but adequately draped in a well-lighted and warm environment. Use a handheld magnifying glass or penlight to see small details and light the area being inspected.

Normally the skin is intact, with no abrasions, and is smooth, dry, well hydrated, and warm. Skin **turgor** (tension) is firm and elastic. The skin surface is flexible and soft. Skin color ranges from light to ruddy pink or olive in

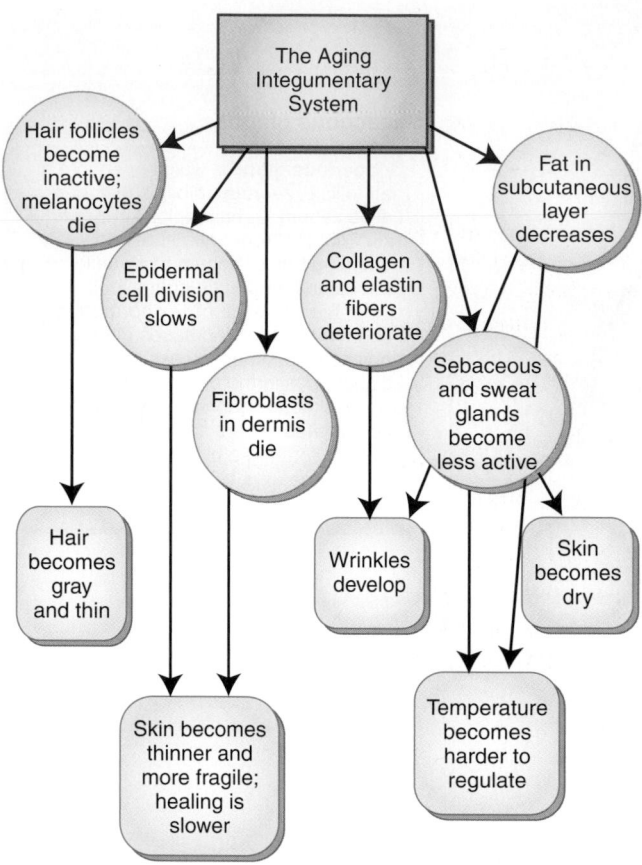

FIGURE 53.4 Aging and the integumentary system.

white-skinned patients and light brown to deep brown in dark-skinned patients.

Be aware of normal developmental changes when performing an examination. The skin of the neonate is very thin and friable (easily broken). During adolescence, the skin becomes thicker, with active sebaceous, eccrine, and apocrine glands. Body hair also changes during adolescence as a result of hormonal influences. In older patients, the skin loses some of its elasticity and moisture. There is decreased activity of sebaceous and sweat glands. The older patient's skin is thinner, more fragile, and more wrinkled.

Inspection

Inspect each area of the skin, including nails, hair, scalp, and mucous membranes, for color, moisture, lesions, edema, intactness, vascular markings, turgor, and cleanliness. This examination should be done in an orderly sequence, such as hair, scalp, nails, buccal mucosa, and then the general skin surface from head to toe.

COLOR. Skin color can be influenced by many factors, including the temperature of the patient, oxygenation, blood flow, exposure to UV rays, and positioning. Because skin color can differ genetically from very light to very dark, skin assessment can be difficult for the novice practitioner.

Commonly noted alterations can include pallor, **erythema** (redness), jaundice, cyanosis, and brown color. Pallor is paleness or decrease in color and can be caused by vasoconstriction, decreased blood flow, or decreased hemoglobin levels

TABLE 53.1   SUBJECTIVE DATA COLLECTION FOR THE INTEGUMENTARY SYSTEM

Category	Questions to Ask During the Health History	Rationale
History	Do you (or does anyone in your family) have a history of dryness, rashes, itching, skin disease, psoriasis, eczema, dermatitis, asthma, hay fever, hives, or allergies?	These conditions may be hereditary.
Risk Factors	Have you noticed any changes in your skin, such as a sore that does not heal, rashes, lumps, or a change in an existing mole?	Sores that do not heal, moles that change color, or lumps may indicate cancer. Slow healing can also be associated with diabetes. Brown staining of the skin in the lower legs is associated with venous stasis.
	Have you had any recent trauma to your skin? Do you have a tendency to sunburn easily? Do you use sunblock? Do you go to tanning salons or use a sun lamp?	A break in skin integrity can lead to infection. Repeat sunburns and tanning are a risk factor for skin cancer.
Hair	Do you wear a wig or hairpiece?	Adequate examination of the scalp requires permission for removal of a wig or hairpiece.
	Have you noticed a change in the growth or loss of your hair?	Hair loss can result from systemic illness or treatment or sometimes from infections or hair care products.
Nails	Have you experienced recent trauma or changes in your nails? Do you wear artificial nails?	Nail changes may be caused by circulatory problems. Artificial nails may mask changes.

TABLE 53.1   SUBJECTIVE DATA COLLECTION FOR THE INTEGUMENTARY SYSTEM—cont'd

Category	Questions to Ask During the Health History	Rationale
Medications	What medications do you take every day (prescription or nonprescription)?	The patient may be taking medication for a skin disorder. Many medications cause skin reactions, from hives and photosensitivity to serious inflammatory conditions.
	What medications did you take most recently? When did you take your last dose?	This might help pinpoint the cause of a new reaction.
Exposures	What is your occupation?	Occupational exposures can lead to skin problems.
	How often do you bathe or shower?	Frequent bathing can cause dry skin.
	What kind of soap do you use?	Some soap may cause allergic reactions.
	What recreational activities do you participate in?	Skin disorders can be caused by gym equipment that was not cleaned properly. Poison ivy may result from being in wooded areas.
	Do you or any members of your immediate family or your coworkers have recent skin issues?	Some skin disorders are contagious.
	Have you traveled recently?	This could help to pinpoint causes of suspicious skin changes.
	Is there anything in your current environment, at home or work, that may be causing any skin problems (e.g., animals, plants, chemicals, infections, new carpeting, or new soaps or detergents)?	Various environmental factors cause contact dermatitis; release of some chemicals can cause skin disorders.
	Is there anything that touches your skin that causes a rash?	This may help pinpoint causes of contact dermatitis

from anemia. Pallor is best assessed on the face, conjunctivae, nailbeds, and lips. Erythema, or red discoloration, can be caused by vasodilation or increased blood flow to the skin from fever or inflammation. Erythema is best assessed on the face or in an area of trauma.

Jaundice, a yellow-orange discoloration, can result from liver disease. Although skin is affected by jaundice, the best place to inspect for jaundice is in the sclera of the eye. Cyanosis, or bluish discoloration, can indicate a cardiac, pulmonary, or perfusion problem. The best places to inspect for cyanosis are the lips, nailbeds, conjunctivae, and palms. People of Mediterranean descent normally have a bluish tone to their lips; this is not cyanosis.

A brown color in an otherwise light-skinned patient may be caused by increased melanin production and can indicate chronic exposure to sunlight, or pregnancy. This is best assessed on areas exposed to the sun; changes in pregnancy can be seen on the face, areolae, and nipples. A brownish color also may result from chronic peripheral vascular disease, especially noted on the lower legs.

LESIONS. A lesion is any change or injury to tissue. Assessment of skin lesions helps determine the cause of a skin disorder. Lesions are described as primary or secondary. Primary lesions are the initial reaction to a disease process. Secondary lesions are changes that take place in the primary lesion because of trauma, scratching, infection, or various stages of a disease. Lesions are further described according to type and appearance in Figure 53.5.

When assessing and documenting skin lesions, note the color or colors of the lesion and the size (usually in centimeters), location, distribution, and configuration. Configuration refers to the pattern of the lesions, as shown in Figure 53.6. Also note any exudate, including amount, color, and odor, and any accompanying symptoms. Gently stretching the skin over the affected area makes lesions stand out more for further assessment.

In general, healthy patients with naturally dark skin have a reddish undertone, with pinkish buccal mucosa, tongue, nails, and lips. If a dark-skinned patient is pale, the mucous membranes have an ash-gray color, lips and nailbeds appear paler

PRIMARY LESIONS

Macule:
Flat, nonpalpable change in skin color, with different sizes, shapes, color; usually smaller than 1 cm (e.g., rubella, scarlet fever, freckles)

Papule:
Palpable solid raised lesion that is less than 1 cm in diameter due to superficial thickening in the epidermis (e.g., ringworm, wart, mole)

Nodule:
Solid elevated lesion that is larger and deeper than a papule (e.g., fibroma, intradermal nevi)

Vesicle:
A small, blisterlike raised area of the skin that contains serous fluid, up to 1 cm in diameter (e.g., poison ivy, shingles, chickenpox)

Bulla:
A fluid-filled vesicle or blister larger than 1 cm (e.g., burns, contact dermatitis)

Pustule:
Small elevation of skin or vesicle or bulla that contains lymph or pus (e.g., impetigo, scabies, acne)

Wheal:
Round, transient elevation of the skin caused by dermal edema and surrounding capillary dilatation; white in center and red in periphery (e.g., hives, insect bites)

Plaque:
A patch or solid, raised lesion on the skin or mucous membrane that is greater than 1 cm in diameter (e.g., psoriasis)

Cyst:
A closed sac or pouch which consists of semisolid, solid, or liquid material (e.g., sebaceous cyst)

SECONDARY LESIONS

Scale:
Dry exfoliation of dead epidermis that may develop as a result of inflammatory changes (e.g., very dry skin, cradle cap, psoriasis)

Crust:
A scab formed by dry serum, pus, or blood (e.g., infected dermatitis, impetigo)

Excoriation:
Traumatized abrasions of the epidermis or linear scratch marks (e.g., scabies, dermatitis, burns)

Fissure:
A slit or cracklike sore that extends into dermis, usually due to continuous inflammation and drying (e.g., athlete's foot, anal fissure)

Ulcer:
An open sore or lesion that extends to the dermis (e.g., pressure sores)

Lichenification:
Thickening and hardening of skin from continued irritation such as from intense scratching

Scar:
A mark left in the skin due to fibrotic changes following healing of a wound or surgical incision

FIGURE 53.5 Description of skin lesions.

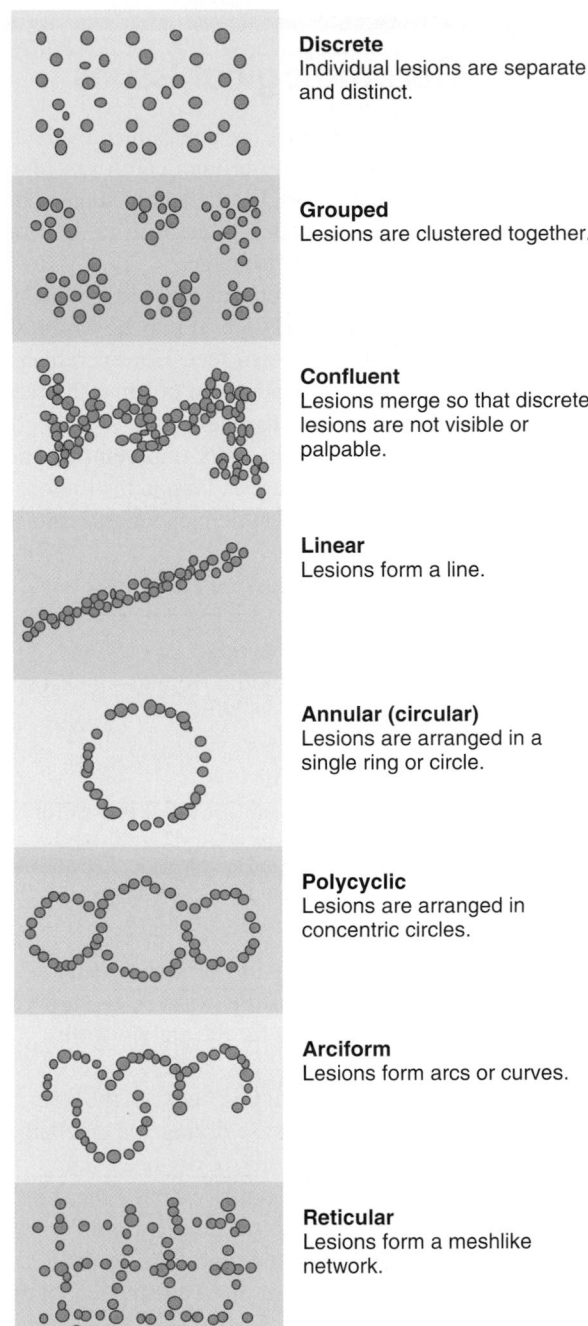

Discrete
Individual lesions are separate and distinct.

Grouped
Lesions are clustered together.

Confluent
Lesions merge so that discrete lesions are not visible or palpable.

Linear
Lesions form a line.

Annular (circular)
Lesions are arranged in a single ring or circle.

Polycyclic
Lesions are arranged in concentric circles.

Arciform
Lesions form arcs or curves.

Reticular
Lesions form a meshlike network.

FIGURE 53.6 To assess configuration, observe the relationship of the lesions to each other. Then characterize the configuration by choosing one of the patterns illustrated in the chart.

than usual, and the skin appears yellow-brown to ash gray. Erythema presents as a purplish gray color. Cyanosis presents as a gray cast to the skin. The nailbeds, palms, and soles may have a bluish cast. Jaundice can be noted in the oral mucosa (particularly the hard palate) and in the sclerae closest to the cornea.

MOISTURE/DRYNESS. Assessment of moisture provides clues to the patient's level of hydration. Observe the skin for dryness, moisture, scales, and flakes. Moisture may be found in skinfold areas. The skin is normally smooth and dry. Flaking and scaling of the skin can indicate dry skin, or an inflammatory disorder.

EDEMA. Edema occurs because of a buildup of fluid in the tissues. Edema can cause the skin to become stretched, dry, and shiny. Examine and document the location, distribution, and color of edematous areas. If edema is unilateral, compare it with the opposite side of the body. Measure edematous extremities to track improvement or worsening of the condition. Dependent edema is edema that occurs in the part of the body that is at the lowest point, typically noted in the feet and ankles or in the sacrum if the patient is lying down.

VASCULAR MARKINGS. Vascular markings can be classified as normal and abnormal. Two common abnormal vascular changes are **petechiae** and **ecchymosis** (see Figures 28.1 and 28.5 in Chapter 28). Petechiae are reddish purple hemorrhagic spots that are smaller than 0.5 mm in diameter. In the darker skinned patient, petechiae are usually not visible on the skin but can be visualized in the conjunctivae and oral mucosa. Ecchymosis is a bruise that changes color from blue-black to greenish brown or yellow over time.

GENERAL INTEGRITY AND CLEANLINESS. Examine the integrity of the skin. Older adults have thin, fragile skin that is easily broken or torn. Be sure to check between toes and skinfolds and under a pendulous abdomen or breasts. Check over bony prominences for signs of pressure. Note general cleanliness and odors.

Palpation

Palpation is used with inspection. Use the dorsum (back) of the hand to palpate temperature because this part of the hand is most sensitive to changes in temperature. Use the fingertips to gently palpate over the skin to determine size, contour (flat, raised, depressed), and consistency (soft or indurated) of lesions. If a lesion is moist or draining, wear gloves to protect against the spread of infectious organisms. Note the degree of pain or discomfort associated with light palpation of lesions.

Examine for turgor and observe the texture of the skin. Skin turgor is a measure of the amount of skin elasticity. To assess for turgor, pinch the skin on the back of the forearm or over the sternum between the thumb and forefinger and then release. Normally, the skin lifts easily and then quickly returns to its normal state. Poor skin turgor is indicated by "tenting" of the skin, with more gradual return to its normal state. Poor skin turgor can indicate dehydration. Normal aging of skin produces some loss of skin elasticity; the preferred place to check skin turgor in older adults is over the sternum.

If edema is suspected, palpate those areas to assess for tenderness, mobility, and consistency. Press the edematous area (against bone, if possible) with your thumb for 5 seconds and then release. When pressure from your fingers leaves an indentation, this is called pitting edema. If the edema is in an

• **WORD** • **BUILDING** •
ecchymosis: ec—out + cchymos—juice + is—condition

extremity, measure and record the circumference in centimeters, and monitor it for increase or decrease in size.

Inspect and/or palpate over the entire body for hair color, quantity, thickness, and texture. Note any areas of **alopecia** (hair loss). Determine any recent changes in color and growth pattern. Note cleanliness, redness, scaling, flakes, and tenderness. If lesions or lice are suspected, use disposable gloves to avoid spread of infection.

Terminal hair is the hair on the scalp, eyebrows, axillae, and pubic areas and on the face and chest of men. Vellus hairs are the soft, tiny hairs covering the body. Normally, body hair has a uniform distribution. Note male or female pubic hair distribution. Scalp hair can normally be thick, thin, coarse, smooth, shiny, curly, or straight. Describe scalp hair distribution and cleanliness.

Nails can reflect the patient's general health. Examine fingers and nails for color, shape, texture, thickness, and abnormalities. Normally, the nails appear pink, smooth, hard, and slightly convex (160-degree angle), with a firm base. The nails of older adults may have a yellowish gray color, thickening, and ridges. Brown or black pigmentation between the nail and nail base is normal in dark-skinned patients. Abnormal findings include clubbing, which may indicate hypoxia, and spoon nails (concave nails, also called koilonychia), which can be associated with anemia. Thick nails may indicate fungal infection. Palpate for nail consistency, and observe for redness, swelling, or tenderness around the nail area. Table 53.2 describes other nail abnormalities.

Describe any abnormal skin conditions in detail. Include findings such as color of lesion, pain, swelling, redness, location, size, drainage (including amount, color, and odor), and eruption patterns. If equipment is available, an excellent way to supplement documentation is by photographing the area; serial photographs can be mounted in the chart to document healing progression. "Gerontological Issues" describes assessment and care specific to older adults.

TABLE 53.2 ABNORMALITIES OF THE NAILS

Physical Examination Finding	Description	Possible Causes
Beau's lines	Transverse depressions in the nails	Systemic illnesses or nail injury
Splinter hemorrhages	Red or brown streaks in the nailbed	Minor trauma, subacute bacterial endocarditis, or trichinosis
Paronychia	Inflammation of the skin at the base of the nail	Local infection or trauma

Gerontological Issues

In acute care settings, priorities are determined by medical diagnoses and often center around cardiovascular, respiratory, nutrition, comfort, or other immediate concerns. The feet may be forgotten in the rush to care for the patient and plan a timely discharge.

Feet are also viewed by some as dirty, and washing the feet may be seen as a lowly job. It may be assumed that people take care of their own feet. However, many older people are unable to bend down or bring the feet up high enough to see or care for them.

For these reasons it is especially important for the nurse to assess and care for the feet, both in institutional settings and at home. General guidelines for assessment include the following:

• Inspect feet for redness or pressure ulcers over bony prominences.
• Inspect feet for dryness or cracking.
• Inspect between toes for cracking, wounds, or excess moisture.
• Inspect and palpate for calluses.
• Inspect toenails for thickening.
• Palpate dorsalis pedis and posterior tibial pulses for circulatory status.
• Assess patient's sensation using a wisp of cotton, monofilament, or light touch.

Hints to promote healthy feet:

• Soak the patient's feet briefly in warm water and wash using a gentle soap. Test the water to be sure it is not too warm, especially for the patient with reduced sensation.
• Thoroughly dry the feet, including between the toes. Water left to evaporate can cause drying and cracking.
• Use a pumice stone to help remove dry dead skin over heels or calluses. Work gently, rubbing the stone in one direction only and removing only a small amount of dead skin at any one time.
• Use a cream or lotion that does not contain alcohol to moisturize the feet. *Do not* apply between toes. Apply it with gentle massage while moving the patient's feet through range-of-motion exercises. To prevent falls, never apply lotion before the patient steps into the tub or shower.
• Use gauze or a commercially made pad to decrease pressure and friction in areas between toes that cross or other areas where breakdown is likely.
• Encourage the patient to wear cotton or dry weave socks that allow feet to stay dry with perspiration.
• Encourage the patient to wear comfortable leather shoes or hard-soled slippers to avoid injury to the feet and prevent falls. Patients with diabetes should be encouraged to wear closed-toe shoes.
• Take extra care to assess and care for feet in patients with diabetes because of their increased risk for injury and slow healing.

DIAGNOSTIC TESTS FOR THE INTEGUMENTARY SYSTEM

Laboratory Tests

Cultures

Skin cultures are done to determine the presence of fungi, bacteria, and viruses. When a fungal infection is suspected, gently scrape scales from the lesion into a Petri dish or other indicated container. The specimen is then treated with a 10% potassium hydroxide solution to make fungi more prominent. The specimen can remain at room temperature until sent to the laboratory.

NURSING CARE TIP

When scraping scales for culture, position the patient so that the skin lesion is vertical. Place the slide against the skin below the lesion. Be sure to wear gloves when collecting specimens, and perform hand hygiene before and after.

If a viral culture is ordered, the fluid is expressed (gently squeezed) from an intact vesicle, collected with a sterile cotton swab, and placed in a special viral culture tube. If the lesion has crusts, they are removed or punctured before swabbing. The viral culture tube must be kept in ice and sent to the laboratory as soon as possible.

Bacterial cultures may be collected with a sterile swab or wound culture kit. Box 53-1 gives specific instructions.

Skin Biopsy

A skin biopsy is indicated for deeper infections, suspicious lesions, or for evaluation of current treatment. A biopsy is an excision of a small piece of tissue for microscopic examination. Three common types of skin biopsies are punch, shave, and incisional.

A punch biopsy uses a small round cutting instrument, called a punch, to cut a cylinder-shaped plug of tissue for a

Box 53-1 Steps in Culturing a Wound

1. Use sterile saline to remove excess drainage and debris from the wound. Purulent material may have different bacteria than those actually causing the infection.
2. Using a sterile calcium alginate swab in a rotating motion, swab wound and wound edges 10 times in a diagonal pattern across the entire surface of the wound.
3. Do not swab over eschar or slough.
4. Place swab in culture tube, label, and send to lab.

full-thickness specimen. A shave biopsy removes just the area that has risen above the rest of the skin. An incisional biopsy is performed with a scalpel to make a deep incision and almost always requires sutures for closure. For all biopsies, explain the procedure, assist in preparing a sterile field, calm and comfort the patient during the procedure, and assist in dressing the site following the procedure. The most uncomfortable part of the procedure is usually the injection of the local anesthetic. Explaining the procedure and calming the patient can make the procedure less traumatic.

Other Diagnostic Tests

Wood's Light Examination

Wood's light examination involves the use of UV rays to detect fluorescent materials in the skin and hair present in certain diseases such as tinea capitis (ringworm). This examination is performed with a handheld black light in a darkened room.

Skin Testing

Patch and scratch tests are performed when allergic contact dermatitis is suspected. These are usually done by a dermatologist on uninvolved skin, such as the upper back or arms. Any hair in the area must first be shaved.

For the scratch test, the skin is superficially scratched or pricked with an allergen for an immediate reaction. If a reaction such as a wheal occurs, the test is positive for that allergen. Resuscitation equipment should be in the immediate vicinity in the event of a severe allergic (anaphylactic) reaction.

With the patch test, allergens are applied under occlusive tape patches; a delayed hypersensitivity reaction develops in 48 to 96 hours. For this test, the skin should be free of oils to promote patch adhesion, so cleanse the skin first with alcohol. The test site must remain dry and free from moisture. The patch is removed in 2 days. Any reaction is noted, with a final reading in 2 to 5 days.

THERAPEUTIC MEASURES FOR THE INTEGUMENTARY SYSTEM

Open Wet Dressings

Wet compresses may be ordered for acute, weeping, crusted, inflamed, or ulcerated lesions. The purpose of wet dressings is to decrease inflammation, cleanse and dry a wound, and promote drainage of infected areas. They may be ordered either sterile or clean, depending on the risk for infection. The solutions commonly consist of room temperature to cool tap water or normal saline solution, aluminum acetate solution (Burow's solution), or magnesium sulfate. The dressing is saturated with the solution before it is applied. Wet dressings usually are applied every 3 to 4 hours for 15 to 30 minutes.

Wet dressings should not be prescribed for more than 72 hours because the skin may become too dry or macerated. If cool compresses are used, they should be reapplied every 5 to 10 minutes because they become too warm from body heat. If warm compresses are used, monitor the skin closely to prevent burns.

NURSING CARE TIP

To prevent chilling, no more than one-third of the body should be treated with a wet dressing at one time. Keep the patient warm during wet dressing treatment.

Balneotherapy

Balneotherapy (therapeutic bath) is useful in applying medications to large areas of the skin, as well as for débridement, or removing old crusts; for removing old medications; and to relieve itching and inflammation. The temperature of the water should be kept at a comfortable level, avoiding hot baths. The bath should last for 15 to 30 minutes, while maintaining its warmth. Fill the tub half full. Keep the room warm to minimize chilling. Advise the patient to wear loose clothing after the bath.

Water and saline solution are utilized for weeping, oozing, and erythematous lesions. Colloidal baths (such as oatmeal or Aveeno) are used for widely distributed skin lesions, for drying, and for relief of itching. Medicated tar baths, such as Almar-Tar or Balnetar, are used for chronic eczema and psoriasis. Any loose skin crusts can be removed after the bath. The room should be well ventilated because tars are volatile.

To increase hydration after the bath, a lubricating agent is applied to damp skin if prescribed. Bath oils, such as Alpha-Keri and Lubath, are used for lubrication and to relieve itching.

NURSING CARE TIP

A bath mat should be used for treatment baths because some of the treatments may make the tub slippery.

Topical Medications

Many types of topical medications are used to treat skin conditions. These include lotions, ointments and creams, powders, gels, pastes, and intralesional therapy. Systemic medications may be given for more serious conditions.

Lotions tend to cool the skin through water evaporation. They also may have a protective effect and may be antipruritic (anti-itch). Lotions are usually applied with cotton, gauze, gloves, or a soft brush.

Ointments and creams have a varied base (greasy, non-greasy, or penetrating), depending on the drug applied. These medications can protect the skin, provide lubrication, and prevent water loss. They are used for localized or chronic skin conditions. Ointments and creams can cause some reduction in blood flow to the skin. They are applied with a gloved hand or wooden tongue depressor.

Powders usually have a zinc oxide, talc, or cornstarch base and are used to absorb moisture and reduce friction. Powders are usually applied with a shaker top. Avoid use of powders in patients with respiratory disease or tracheostomies.

NURSING CARE TIP

Avoid applying too much powder in skinfold areas. Dermatitis can occur with too much powder in these areas. Products with a cornstarch base can provide a good medium for growth of microorganisms.

Gels, or semisolid emulsions, become liquid with topical application. They are usually greaseless and do not stain. Many topical steroids are prescribed in this manner.

Pastes are semisolid substances comprising ointments and powders. They are used for inflammatory disorders. Mineral oil can facilitate removal of pastes.

Topical corticosteroids are used to reduce or relieve pain and itching by decreasing inflammation. Steroids should be used sparingly and according to package directions. Overuse of topical steroids can cause thinning of the skin. Caution is needed when used on the face to prevent glaucoma, cataracts, and perioral dermatitis. Some clinicians use steroid inhalers (usually used for patients with asthma) to apply a fine mist of medication to affected areas.

Intralesional therapy may be used for anti-inflammatory action. This procedure uses a sterile suspension of a corticosteroid injected just below the lesion with a tuberculin syringe. Local atrophy may occur if the injection is made into subcutaneous tissue. Common conditions that are treated with this therapy include psoriasis and keloids.

CRITICAL THINKING

Mr. Evans

■ Mr. Evans comes to the doctor's office with atrophic skin (thin, shiny, pink, with visible vessels) at the area of psoriasis where he is applying his corticosteroid ointment. He says that he has been applying a thick layer of ointment four times a day.

1. What should you teach Mr. Evans about his treatment?
2. What should you include when you document his skin condition?

Suggested answers are at the end of the chapter.

Dressings

Dressings may be used to enhance absorption of topical medications, promote retention of moisture, prevent evaporation of medication, and reduce pain and itching. Occlusive dressings (for sealing a wound) are commonly used for skin disorders. For an occlusive dressing, an airtight plastic film is applied directly over the topical agent. Corticosteroids are also available in a special plastic surgical tape that can be cut to size. See the "Nursing Care Plan for the Patient With an Occlusive Dressing."

Proper application of a plastic wrap dressing includes washing the area, lightly patting it dry, applying the medication to moist skin, covering the medicated area with plastic wrap, and covering with a dressing to seal the edges. Wet dressings and ointments should only be applied to affected areas, not to healthy intact skin, because this can cause maceration of good skin. Plastic wrap dressings should be used for no more than 12 hours a day.

NURSING CARE TIP

Continued use of occlusive dressings can cause skin atrophy, folliculitis, maceration, erythema, and systemic absorption of the medication. To prevent some of these complications, the dressing is removed for at least 12 of every 24 hours.

Hydrocolloid dressings (e.g., DuoDERM, Tegasorb THIN) can help protect areas exposed to pressure and treat pressure ulcers in early stages. Gels, pastes, and granules can be used to fill in deep wounds to promote granulation and aid healing. See Chapter 54 for dressings used specifically for pressure ulcers. Skin tears should be covered with a nonadherent dressing such as Xeroform and wrapped with gauze. Table 53.3 summarizes various types of wound dressings.

Other items commonly used with topical treatments for skin conditions include gauze or cotton cloth held in place with:

• Small, stretchable tubular material (e.g., Surgitube, tube gauze) for fingers, toes, and extremities
• Disposable polyethylene gloves sealed at the wrist for hands
• Cotton socks or plastic bags for the feet
• Disposable diapers or cotton diapers for the groin and perineal areas
• Cotton cloth held in place with dress shields for the axillae
• Cotton or light flannel pajamas for the trunk
• A shower cap for the scalp
• A facemask made from gauze and stretchable dressings with holes cut out for eyes, nose, mouth, and ears.

The patient's HCP or a wound care specialist should specify the type of dressing and particular materials needed.

TABLE 53.3 COMMON DRESSINGS

Dressing Type	Description	When Used	Examples
Alginates	Derived from brown seaweed; absorbent and conform to the shape of the wound.	When packed into wound, absorb exudate and form a soft gel to maintain a moist environment for wound healing.	Kaltostat SeaSorb Tegagen
Antimicrobial dressings	Topical dressings derived from such agents as silver, iodine, and polyhexamethylene biguanide.	Intended for use in draining, nonhealing wounds that have bacterial contamination, such as burns, surgical wounds, diabetic ulcers, pressure ulcers, and leg ulcers.	Acticoat Aquacel Ag Silversorb gel Tegaderm Ag mesh
Collagen dressings	Collagen is the most abundant protein in the body; its fibers are found in connective tissues, skin, bone, ligaments, and cartilage.	Stimulate new tissue development.	CellerateRX gel BGC Matrix dressing Fibracol plus collagen
Promogran matrix	Oxidized regenerated cellulose and 55% collagen. Binds metalloproteases, which protect growth factors.	Used for diabetic foot ulcers, venous leg ulcers, and surgical wounds.	Prisma
Composite dressings	Combine two or more distinct products into a single dressing.	May absorb and also cover a wound, for example.	Alldress Covaderm
Contact layers	Nonadherent dressing layers often used with other products.	Used to allow exudate to flow through to a secondary dressing; protects wound.	Mepitel Wound veil Profore

Continued

TABLE 53.3   COMMON DRESSINGS—cont'd

Dressing Type	Description	When Used	Examples
Foam dressings	Absorbent; some have a film coating and adhesive border.	Used to provide a moist environment and thermal insulation.	Allevyn Mepilex Foam Lyofoam Biatain adhesive dressing PolyMem and PolyMax
Honey	Medical grade honey used in a variety of dressing types	Used for colonized wounds; antimicrobial and anti-inflammatory properties.	Medihoney—various forms Therahoney
Hydrocolloid dressings	Occlusive or semiocclusive dressings made of pectin, gelatin, and carboxymethylcellulose.	Used when a moist environment is needed that allows clean wounds to granulate; provides autolytic debriding.	DuoDERM Tegaderm Absorbent Tegasorb THIN Comfeel Plus
Hydrogels	Water or glycerine-based amorphous gels, impregnated gauzes, or sheet dressings	Used when a moist healing environment is needed to promote granulation and epithelialization and facilitate autolytic débridement.	DuoDERM gel Saf-Gel Amerigel AquaSite CarraDres Curage Silvasorb
Impregnated gauze	Woven or nonwoven material impregnated by the manufacturer with substances such as iodinated agents, petrolatum, zinc, bismuth tribromophenate, chlorhexidine gluconate, crystalline sodium chloride, or aqueous saline.	Used for a variety of conditions, depending on the agent added to the dressing.	Mesalt Xeroform Xeroflo Adaptic Curity nonadherent dressing Dermagran Vaseline petroleum gauze Iodoform packing AMD gauze
Transparent films	Adhesive semipermeable polyurethane membrane dressings that are waterproof and impermeable to bacteria and contaminants yet permit water vapor to cross the barrier.	Used when a moist healing environment is needed, promoting formulation of granulation tissue and autolysis of necrotic tissue.	Bioclusive Transparent Dressing Tegaderm CarraFilm OpSite Mefilm Adhesive Dressing Polyskin II Transparent Dressing
Wound fillers	Sterile products that absorb exudate and conform to the shape of the wound bed.	Used when wound has exudate and would benefit from débriding.	FlexiGel strands Absorbent wound dressing Iodosorb gel Iodoflex pads

NURSING CARE PLAN for the Patient With an Occlusive Dressing

Nursing Diagnosis: *Impaired Skin Integrity* related to open lesions

Expected Outcome: The patient will experience improved skin integrity as evidenced by reduction in size of lesion.

Evaluation of Outcome: Is there a decrease in wound size?

Intervention Assess areas of lesions for changes in size, color, swelling, and drainage three times a day or as ordered. **Rationale** Areas of redness, swelling, pain, and drainage may indicate infection. **Evaluation** Are lesions free of redness, swelling, pain, and drainage?

Intervention Assess lesions for presence or absence of dead tissue and exudates. **Rationale** Appearance indicates areas of healing and infection. **Evaluation** Are lesions free of exudates and dead tissue?

Intervention Cleanse wound as prescribed. Lightly pat dry. **Rationale** Cleansing helps provide a healthy granulation area for healing. **Evaluation** Is wound clean and free of debris, crusts, and exudate?

Intervention Apply prescribed topical agent to moist skin as ordered. Apply sparingly or as directed. **Rationale** Rationale depends on agent and reason prescribed. **Evaluation** Does area exhibit signs of healing (e.g., decrease in size and numbers of lesions, free from infection, less itching)?

Intervention Cut plastic film to size and apply. Cover with an appropriate dressing to seal edges. **Rationale** Film enhances absorption of medication and helps retain moisture. **Evaluation** Is the topical agent adherent to the skin?

Intervention Remove dressing for 12 of 24 hours. **Rationale** Continued use may cause skin atrophy, folliculitis, erythema, and systemic absorption of medication. **Evaluation** Are there signs of healthy granulation tissue? Is skin pink? Are there fewer open areas? Is dressing removed for at least 12 hours every 24 hours?

Nursing Diagnosis: *Disturbed Body Image* related to presence of lesions or wound

Expected Outcomes: The patient will verbalize acceptance of condition. The patient will be willing to participate in care of lesion or wound.

Evaluation of Outcomes: Does patient verbalize acceptance of condition? Does patient participate in care of lesions?

Intervention Assess patient's feelings regarding condition. **Rationale** Assessment provides a baseline for care. If patient denies condition, he or she may not comply with care. **Evaluation** Does patient state willingness to follow care instructions?

Intervention Care for patient with an accepting attitude. **Rationale** Patient will be aware of nuances in nurse's behavior. **Evaluation** Does patient allow nurse to partake in care of lesion or wound?

Intervention Allow opportunities for patient to verbalize concerns about condition. **Rationale** Verbalization allows patient to begin to accept changes and problem solve. **Evaluation** Does patient verbalize feelings appropriately?

Intervention Provide referrals to support groups and counselors as appropriate. **Rationale** Patient may benefit from talking to others with similar condition or to another professional for objective evaluation. **Evaluation** Is patient receptive to appropriate referrals?

Intervention Assist patient in concealing lesion or wound in a safe and appropriate manner. **Rationale** Long sleeves and long pants may help conceal and protect lesions, and prevent further skin damage. **Evaluation** Is patient accepting of appearance of lesions? Are lesions or wounds visible?

Continued

NURSING CARE PLAN for the Patient With an Occlusive Dressing—cont'd

Nursing Diagnosis: *Self-Care Deficit: Bathing/Hygiene* related to presence of lesions or wound and discomfort

Expected Outcomes: The patient will verbalize the importance of good hygiene. The patient will participate in bathing/hygiene.

Evaluation of Outcomes: Does patient verbalize importance of good hygiene? Is patient's skin clean and dry?

Intervention Assess patient's level of hygiene. **Rationale** Assessment provides a baseline for care. **Evaluation** Is patient's level of hygiene at an acceptable level?

Intervention Instruct patient in appropriate bathing/hygiene: • Avoid strong detergents and soaps; use gentle emollient soaps or prescribed soaps. • Gently stroke areas of lesions. • Pat dry; avoid friction. • Maintain a little moisture on skin. • Maintain comfortable environmental temperature. • Have temperature of bath at a comfortable level to patient but not too hot. **Rationale** Patient needs to be able to properly cleanse lesions to prevent infection. Avoidance of friction and strong soaps prevents further trauma to skin. Patient will not shiver in comfortable temperatures. **Evaluation** Does patient demonstrate good bathing techniques? Are lesions free of infection?

SUGGESTED ANSWERS TO

CRITICAL THINKING

■ *Mr. Evans*

1. Teach Mr. Evans to apply the ointment in a thin layer and usually only twice daily (as ordered). He may be sensitive or allergic to the medication. Most likely, he is applying too much, too often.

2. Note the size (usually in centimeters), location, color, distribution, and configuration of lesions. Describe exactly what you see, avoiding judgments about what you think it is. Document any teaching you provided related to how his medication should be applied.

REVIEW QUESTIONS

1. When is the best time for the nurse to apply prescribed ointment to a patient with an inflamed skin rash?
   1. In the morning before the patient dresses
   2. When the patient will be resting for at least an hour
   3. After the patient bathes
   4. In the evening before bed

2. Which nursing interventions are essential to achieve maximum benefit for the patient receiving balneotherapy for widespread dermatitis? **Select all that apply.**
   1. Maintain the bath water at the hottest temperature tolerated by the patient.
   2. Keep the patient in the water for 15 to 30 minutes.
   3. Keep the tub room warm.
   4. Dry the skin vigorously following the bath.
   5. Use gentle or emollient soaps.

3. Which term should the nurse use to document a raised, fluid-filled lesion smaller than 1 cm?
   1. Macule
   2. Papule
   3. Vesicle
   4. Wheal

4. What equipment is most important to have readily available when a patient is undergoing skin testing for allergies?
   1. Resuscitation equipment
   2. Flashlight
   3. Measuring device
   4. Alcohol and cotton swabs

5. Which nursing intervention is essential to protecting the patient's skin integrity when applying occlusive dressings?
   1. Make sure all skin surfaces are covered.
   2. Remove the dressings for 12 of every 24 hours.
   3. Apply a thick layer of prescribed ointment before applying the dressings.
   4. Apply a gauze dressing next to the skin, underneath the plastic film.

Answers can be found in Appendix C.

 DavisPlus | For additional resources and information visit **davispl.us/medsurg5**

54

Nursing Care of Patients With Skin Disorders

MARTY KOHN AND
RITA BOLEK TROFINO

KEY TERMS

cellulitis (sell-yoo-LYE-tis)
comedo (KOH-meh-doh)
dermatitis (DER-mah-TYE-tiss)
dermatomycosis (DER-mah-toh-mye-KOH-siss)
eschar (ESS-kar)
lichenified (lye-KEN-i-fyde)
onychomycosis (ON-ih-koh-my-KOH-siss)
pediculosis (peh-DIK-yoo-LOH-siss)
pemphigus (PEM-fih-guss)
pruritus (proo-RYE-tuss)
psoriasis (suh-RYE-ah-siss)
purulent (PURE-you-lent)
pyoderma (PYE-oh-DER-mah)
seborrhea (SEB-uh-REE-ah)

LEARNING OUTCOMES

1. Explain the pathophysiology of each of the skin disorders listed in this chapter.

2. Describe the etiologies, signs, and symptoms of each of the skin disorders.

3. Describe current therapeutic measures that are used for each of the skin disorders.

4. List data to collect when caring for patients with disorders of the integumentary system.

5. Plan nursing care for patients with each of the skin disorders.

6. Explain how you will know if your nursing interventions have been effective.

Skin disorders cover a wide array of diseases and conditions. They can be generalized or localized, acute, chronic, or traumatic. This chapter discusses common skin disorders encountered by nurses. An excellent resource on skin disorders is available at www.nlm.nih.gov/medlineplus/skinconditions .html. The American Academy of Dermatology can be accessed at www.aad.org.

 PRESSURE ULCERS

Pathophysiology and Etiology

Patients often refer to pressure ulcers with old terms such as *bedsores, decubitus ulcers,* or *pressure sores.* Essentially, a pressure ulcer is a lesion caused by prolonged pressure against the skin. This may result from spending a prolonged period in one position, causing the weight of the body to compress the capillaries against a bed or chair, especially over bony prominences. Pressure ulcers are the result of tissue anoxia and begin to develop within 20 to 40 minutes of unrelieved pressure on the skin. Other causes include pressure from a tight splint or cast, traction, or other device. Those at risk are immobile patients, those with decreased circulation, and those with impaired sensory perception or neurologic function.

Mechanical forces (pressure, friction, and shear) lead to the formation of pressure ulcers. The pressure level that closes capillaries in healthy people is 25 to 32 mm Hg. When pressure applied to the skin is greater than the pressure in the capillary bed, the blood supply to the tissues is decreased, which impairs cellular metabolism. This eventually causes tissue ischemia. This reduction in blood flow causes the skin to *blanch,* or lose color. The longer the pressure lasts, the greater the risk of skin breakdown and the development of a pressure ulcer.

Friction is the rubbing of the skin surface with an external mechanical force. Also referred to as "sheet burns," this can happen when the patient is dragged or pulled across bed linens instead of being lifted.

Shearing occurs when the patient slides down in bed when the head of the bed is raised, or when being pulled or repositioned without being lifted off the sheets. With shearing, the skin and subcutaneous tissue remain stationary, and the fat, muscle, and bone shift in the direction of body movement. As a result, damage occurs deep within the tissues.

Any patient experiencing prolonged pressure is at risk for a pressure ulcer. Older adult patients have increased risk because of normal aging changes of the skin. Because thin patients have little padding when pressure is present, they have the greatest pressure applied to their capillaries. Obesity also is a contributing factor because adipose tissue is poorly vascularized and is therefore more likely to develop ischemic changes. Impaired peripheral circulation also makes the skin more susceptible to ischemic damage. See Chapter 24 for more information on problems caused by poor circulation.

Prevention

There are many interventions for the prevention of pressure ulcers (see "Evidence-Based Practice").

USE A VALIDATED ASSESSMENT TOOL. Use an assessment tool such as the Braden or Norton scale to assess patients for physical condition, mental status, activity, mobility, and incontinence to determine the risk for pressure ulcers. Advanced age, low diastolic blood pressure, elevated body temperature, and inadequate current intake of protein are all risk factors associated with the development of pressure ulcers. See Table 54.1 for the Braden instrument.

CLEANSE THE SKIN. Gently cleanse the skin daily with tepid water and mild soap to prevent drying. To reduce friction, pat the skin dry rather than rubbing it dry. After bathing, daily lifelong lubrication of the skin with moisturizers is important to prevent dryness. Thoroughly dry skin-to-skin surfaces, such as under the breasts, skinfolds (especially in the groin and abdominal folds), and between the toes, to prevent prolonged exposure to moisture.

PREVENT DAMAGE FROM INCONTINENCE. If incontinence is a problem, clean the skin promptly with tepid water and mild soap, pat dry, and apply a moisture barrier to prevent breakdown.

AVOID MASSAGING BONY PROMINENCES. Avoid massaging bony prominences or reddened skin areas; blood vessels are damaged by massage when ischemia is present or when they lie over a bone.

MAINTAIN MOBILITY. Maintain the highest possible level of mobility, as follows:

- Teach patients to shift their weight every 15 minutes if possible when lying or sitting.
- Provide frequent active or passive range-of-motion exercises, as well as turning according to a written repositioning schedule. If patients are on bedrest, turn and reposition them at least every 2 hours, but preferably more often because ischemia development begins after 20 to 40 minutes of pressure.
- When positioning patients on their side, place them at a 30-degree angle or less and not directly on the trochanter because this area is especially sensitive to pressure and can quickly break down. If patients are placed on the trochanter, they usually become restless and squirm around to get off the trochanter.
- If the patient is seated in a chair, repositioning every hour is important. A mobility program specific to the patient must be developed.

REDUCE PRESSURE, FRICTION, AND SHEAR DAMAGE. Avoid elevating the head of the bed more than 30 degrees to reduce pressure on the coccyx and friction and shear damage from sliding down in the bed. Use a sheet to lift and move patients; provide an overbed trapeze to assist patients to move themselves.

ELEVATE HEELS AND AVOID PRESSURE ON CALVES. Elevate heels off the bed with pillows placed lengthwise under the calf or with heel elevators. Take care so pressure is not applied on the calves from the pillows.

TABLE 54.1   BRADEN SCALE FOR PREDICTING PRESSURE SORE RISK

Patient's Name
Evaluator's Name
Date of Assessment

SENSORY PERCEPTION ability to respond meaningfully to pressure-related discomfort	1. Completely Limited Unresponsive (does not moan, flinch, or grasp) to painful stimuli, due to diminished level of consciousness or sedation OR Limited ability to feel pain over most of body	2. Very Limited Responds only to painful stimuli. Cannot communicate discomfort except by moaning or restlessness OR Has a sensory impairment which limits the ability to feel pain or discomfort over 1/2 of body	3. Slightly Limited Responds to verbal commands, but cannot always communicate discomfort or the need to be turned OR Has some sensory impairment which limits ability to feel pain or discomfort in 1 or 2 extremities	4. No Impairment Responds to verbal commands. Has no sensory deficit which would limit ability to feel or voice pain or discomfort.
MOISTURE degree to which skin is exposed to moisture	1. Constantly Moist Skin is kept moist almost constantly by perspiration, urine, etc. Dampness is detected every time patient is moved or turned.	2. Very Moist Skin is often, but not always moist. Linen must be changed at least once a shift.	3. Occasionally Moist Skin is occasionally moist, requiring an extra linen change approximately once a day.	4. Rarely Moist Skin is usually dry, linen only requires changing at routine intervals.
ACTIVITY degree of physical activity	1. Bedfast Confined to bed	2. Chairfast Ability to walk severely limited or nonexistent. Cannot bear own weight and/or must be assisted into chair or wheelchair.	3. Walks Occasionally Walks occasionally during day, but for very short distances, with or without assistance. Spends majority of each shift in bed or chair.	4. Walks Frequently Walks outside room at least twice a day and inside room at least once every two hours during waking hours
MOBILITY ability to change and control body position	1. Completely Immobile Does not make even slight changes in body or extremity position without assistance	2. Very Limited Makes occasional slight changes in body or extremity position but unable to make frequent or significant changes independently	3. Slightly Limited Makes frequent though slight changes in body or extremity position independently	4. No Limitation Makes major and frequent changes in position without assistance
NUTRITION usual food intake pattern	1. Very Poor Never eats a complete meal. Rarely eats more than 1/3 of any food offered. Eats 2 servings or less of protein (meat or dairy	2. Probably Inadequate Rarely eats a complete meal and generally eats only about 1/2 of any food offered. Protein intake includes only 3 servings of	3. Adequate Eats over half of most meals. Eats a total of 4 servings of protein (meat, dairy products) per day. Occasionally will refuse a meal, but	4. Excellent Eats most of every meal. Never refuses a meal. Usually eats a total of 4 or more servings of meat and dairy products.

TABLE 54.1 BRADEN SCALE FOR PREDICTING PRESSURE SORE RISK—cont'd

	products) per day. Takes fluids poorly. Does not take a liquid dietary supplement OR Is NPO and/or maintained on clear liquids or IVs for more than 5 days	meat or dairy products per day. Occasionally will take a dietary supplement. OR Receives less than optimum amount of liquid diet or tube feeding	will usually take a supplement when offered. OR Is on a tube feeding or TPN regimen which probably meets most of nutritional needs	Occasionally eats between meals. Does not require supplementation.
FRICTION AND SHEAR	**1. Problem** Requires moderate to maximum assistance in moving. Complete lifting without sliding against sheets is impossible. Frequently slides down in bed or chair, requiring frequent repositioning with maximum assistance. Spasticity, contractures, or agitation leads to almost constant friction.	**2. Potential Problem** Moves feebly or requires minimum assistance. During a move skin probably slides to some extent against sheets, chair, restraints, or other devices. Maintains relatively good position in chair or bed most of the time but occasionally slides down.	**3. No Apparent Problem** Moves in bed and in chair independently and has sufficient muscle strength to lift up completely during move. Maintains good position in bed or chair.	

© Copyright Barbara Braden and Nancy Bergstrom, 1988. Reprinted with permission.
Note. IV = intravenous; NPO = nothing by mouth; TPN = total parenteral nutrition.

Total Score

INTERVENTIONS FOR SPECIFIC RISK LEVEL	**SPECIFIC CONDITION MANAGEMENT**
AT RISK (15–18)*	**MANAGE MOISTURE**
FREQUENT TURNING	USE COMMERCIAL MOISTURE BARRIER
MAXIMAL REMOBILIZATION	USE ABSORBANT PADS OR DIAPERS THAT
PROTECT HEELS	WICK & HOLD MOISTURE
MANAGE MOISTURE, NUTRITION, AND FRICTION AND SHEAR	ADDRESS CAUSE IF POSSIBLE
PRESSURE-REDUCTION SUPPORT SURFACE IF BED- OR CHAIRBOUND	OFFER BEDPAN/URINAL AND GLASS OF WATER IN CONJUNCTION WITH TURNING SCHEDULES
*If other major risk factors are present(advanced age, fever, poor dietary intake of protein, diastolic pressure below 60 mm Hg, hemodynamic instability) advance to next level of risk.	
MODERATE RISK (13–14)*	**MANAGE NUTRITION**
TURNING SCHEDULE	INCREASE PROTEIN INTAKE
USE FOAM WEDGES FOR 30° LATERAL POSITIONING	INCREASE CALORIE INTAKE TO SPARE PROTEINS
PRESSURE-REDUCTION SUPPORT SURFACE	SUPPLEMENT WITH MULTIVITAMIN (SHOULD HAVE VITAMINS A, C, & E)
MAXIMAL REMOBILIZATION	ACT QUICKLY TO ALLEVIATE DEFICITS
PROTECT HEELS	CONSULT DIETITIAN
MANAGE MOISTURE, NUTRITION,	

Continued

TABLE 54.1 BRADEN SCALE FOR PREDICTING PRESSURE SORE RISK—cont'd

AND FRICTION AND SHEAR *If other major risk factors present, advance to next level of risk.	
HIGH RISK (10–12) INCREASE FREQUENCY OF TURNING SUPPLEMENT WITH SMALL SHIFTS PRESSURE REDUCTION SUPPORT SURFACE USE FOAM WEDGES FOR 30° LATERAL POSITIONING MAXIMAL REMOBILIZATION PROTECT HEELS MANAGE MOISTURE, NUTRITION, AND FRICTION AND SHEAR	**MANAGE FRICTION AND SHEAR** ELEVATE HOB NO MORE THAN 30° USE TRAPEZE WHEN INDICATED USE LIFT SHEET TO MOVE PATIENT PROTECT ELBOWS & HEELS IF BEING EXPOSED TO FRICTION
VERY HIGH RISK (9 or below)* ALL OF THE ABOVE USE PRESSURE-RELIEVING SURFACE IF PATIENT HAS INTRACTABLE PAIN OR SEVERE PAIN EXACERBATED BY TURNING OR ADDITIONAL RISK FACTORS *Low-air-loss beds do not substitute for turning schedules.	**OTHER GENERAL CARE ISSUES** NO MASSAGE OF REDDENED BONY PROMINENCES NO DONUT TYPE DEVICES MAINTAIN GOOD HYDRATION AVOID DRYING THE SKIN

© Barbara Braden, 2001.

PROTECT BONY PROMINENCES FROM PRESSURE. Be sure also to protect the patient's elbows, sacrum, scapulae, ears, and occipital area from pressure.

PREVENT ISCHEMIA. Avoid the use of donut-shaped cushions. They create a circle of pressure that cuts off the circulation to the surrounding tissue, promoting ischemia rather than preventing it.

PROTECT SKIN CONTACT SURFACES. Pad skin contact surfaces, especially bony prominences, so they do not press against each other. (For example, place a small pillow between the knees when the patient is in a side-lying position.)

USE PRESSURE-REDUCING MATTRESSES AND CUSHIONS. Provide an appropriate pressure-relieving or pressure-reducing mattress and chair cushion for immobile patients.

PREVENT MALNUTRITION AND DEHYDRATION. Prevent malnutrition and dehydration by ensuring an adequate intake of protein, calories, and fluid; provide 2500 mL of fluid each day if not contraindicated by other medical problems.

"Gerontological Issues" summarizes additional preventive measures.

Signs and Symptoms

A developing pressure ulcer begins with a reddened area, usually over a bony prominence, that does not blanch with pressure. You have learned to check for capillary refill by pressing on a fingertip and watching it turn white, then red

Gerontological Issues

Interventions to Prevent Skin Breakdown

• Avoid use of soap and water on dry skin areas. Use a moisture barrier cream or ointment on dry skin before bathing to protect the skin from the drying effects of water.

• Regularly wash and dry between toes.

• Toilet patient often, and institute a bowel program to prevent incontinence.

• Use perineal cleansing products to cleanse urine and feces residue from the perineum and anal area. These products are specially designed to break down and facilitate the complete removal of urine and feces without irritating the skin.

• Use moisturizing creams that have no alcohol or perfume, which can irritate the skin.

• Avoid pressure, especially over bony areas, by assisting the older adult to change positions on a regular schedule.

• Remind the patient to change position or shift weight frequently while sitting in a chair to avoid prolonged pressure.

• Examine skin for areas of redness. If redness occurs, the positioning schedule should be more frequent.

- Keep fingernails short to avoid scratching.
- Use pillows and pads to help maintain alignment with position changes. Use specialized mattresses and chair cushions designed to decrease pressure. Keep the patient's heels off the bed with pillows under the calves for support and to prevent pressure.
- Encourage the older adult to be out of bed and active throughout the day. Remember to assess skin and reposition frequently even when out of bed because areas of pressure occur whether the patient is in or out of bed.
- Provide a high-protein, vitamin-rich diet if not contraindicated.
- Assess for dehydration and encourage fluids if not contraindicated.
- Make sure bed linens are kept dry and unwrinkled.

EVIDENCE-BASED PRACTICE

Clinical Question
What are best practices for preventing pressure ulcers?

Evidence
Researchers at both the Joanna Briggs Institute and the Agency for Research and Quality evaluated studies to determine which interventions are most effective for preventing pressure ulcers. Recommendations for assessment include regular skin inspection and use of the Braden Scale (Table 54.1) to predict pressure ulcer risk. Interventions to reduce pressure ulcer risk include good skin care with warm (not hot) water and use of lotion after bathing, avoidance of massage over bony prominences, protection of skin from incontinence or other body fluids with barrier products, individualized repositioning schedules based on patient condition, and use of pressure reducing devices or mattresses.

For at-risk patients, follow nutritional guidelines for hydration (1 ml/kcal of fluid per day) and calories (30–35 kcal/kg of body weight per day), protein (1.25–1.5 g/kg per day). Give high-protein supplements or tube feedings in addition to the usual diet in persons at nutritional and pressure ulcer risk (Agency for Health Care Research and Quality, 2013).

Implications for Nursing Practice
Use a valid risk assessment tool such as the Braden Scale according to agency policy. Use a pressure-reducing mattress and administer oral nutritional supplements and fluids to the at-risk patient (Braden Scale score 18 or less). Keep skin clean and dry and reposition the patient

frequently. See www.guideline.gov/content.aspx ?id=43935 for additional recommendations.

REFERENCE

Agency for Healthcare Research and Quality, National Guideline Clearinghouse. (2013). Pressure ulcer prevention. In Evidence-based geriatric nursing protocols for best practice. Retrieved November 23, 2013, from www.guideline .gov/content.aspx?id=43935

Joanna Briggs Institute (2008). Pressure ulcers: Prevention of pressure related damage. Best Practice, 12(2), 1–4. Retrieved November 23, 2013, from http://connect .jbiconnectplus.org/ViewSourceFile.aspx?O=428

NURSING CARE TIP

Implement all preventive measures possible, and be sure to document with photographs all pressure ulcers present on admission to the hospital. Pressure ulcers are classified as serious reportable events because they can be prevented, and therefore hospitals will not be paid by Medicare for care of stage III, IV, or unstageable pressure ulcer acquired during hospitalization.

again. If redness returns within 3 seconds, then capillary refill is considered to be adequate. A pressure ulcer stays red and does not blanch. If pressure is not relieved and healing does not occur, it can progress to an open, ulcerated area. Stages of ulcers are discussed in the section on data collection.

The most common sites for pressure ulcers are the sacrum, heels, elbows, lateral malleoli, greater trochanters, ischial tuberosities, base of the skull, scapulae, and ears. Most patients experience pain at the ulcer site. A report of pain requires continual monitoring, documentation, and treatment.

LEARNING TIP

Pressure ulcers may be described according to a three-color system:

- *Black* wounds indicate tissue necrosis.
- *Yellow* wounds have slough, which is a layer of dead tissue surrounding living tissue. It is usually yellow, creamy, or tan in color. It may have exudate and may be infected.
- *Red* wounds are pink or red and are in the healing stage.

A wound may contain a mixture of black, yellow, and red colors. Necrotic wounds are the worst because they contain dead tissue. Beefy red wounds are desired because they are healing wounds. It is important to consider treating the worst color present first, or healing will be delayed. For example, if a wound is both yellow and black, the dead tissue must be removed first before the infection can be effectively treated. This color system is a helpful system for patients and families to use to describe wounds to the home care nurse because colors are easily recognized and understood by most people.

Complications

Wound infection is a common complication. New ulcers can also appear, and the present ulcer can progress to a deeper wound. Some wounds take a prolonged time to heal or never heal.

Diagnostic Tests

All open pressure ulcers are considered to be colonized with bacteria. This means that bacteria are present, but the wound is not necessarily infected. In most cases, adequate cleansing and débridement can prevent bacterial colonization from advancing to clinical infection. Swab cultures and culture and sensitivity tests may be done to identify the causative organism in suspected infection sites. (See Chapter 53 for instructions for obtaining a culture.) Results need to be interpreted to distinguish between true wound infection and bacterial colonization. If the wound is healing by secondary intention, it becomes colonized by bacterial flora from the skin and from the environment. If, however, the wound is extensive, bacterial growth may exceed the defenses of the local tissue, and a true wound infection will result.

If the wound does not show signs of healing or if an ischemic ulcer is suspected, noninvasive (such as Doppler studies) or invasive (such as arteriogram) arterial blood supply studies are recommended. Biopsies may be performed for large, extensive unhealing wounds to be sure a cancer is not a complicating factor.

Therapeutic Measures

Treatment varies according to the size, depth, and stage of the pressure ulcer; the special needs of the patient; and health care provider preference. All pressure must be removed from the affected area for healing to occur. Cleanliness must be maintained. Basic treatment includes débridement, cleansing, and dressing of the wound to provide a moist and healing environment.

LEARNING TIP

The epidermis "skates" on moisture, so wounds must be kept moist to heal.

Débridement

Débridement is the removal of dead or nonviable tissue from a wound to help clean the wound and facilitate formation of granulation tissue. It may be done with or without surgery.

Nonsurgical débridement includes mechanical, enzymatic, and autolytic methods. Surgical débridement is used only if the patient has sepsis or **cellulitis** or to remove extensive **eschar**. Eschar is a black or brown hard scab or dry crust, or thick, black, leather-like tissue that forms from necrotic tissue. It may hide the true depth of the wound and must be removed for the wound to heal.

MECHANICAL DÉBRIDEMENT. Scissors and forceps can be used for mechanical débridement to selectively remove nonviable tissue. Dextranomer beads, another method of mechanical débridement, can be sprinkled over the wound to absorb exudate and all other products of tissue breakdown, as well as surface bacteria. Whirlpool baths and wet-to-dry saline gauze dressings may also be used for mechanical débridement. For wet-to-dry dressings, the wet gauze is placed directly on the wound (avoiding surrounding healthy tissue) and allowed to dry completely. The drying process causes the gauze to adhere to the wound; when it is pulled off, tissue is pulled off with it. This results in nonselective débridement because viable tissue may also be removed in this process. These methods are painful, so the patient should be premedicated for pain and assessed often.

ENZYMATIC DÉBRIDEMENT. Enzymatic débridement involves application of a topical enzyme débriding agent. These agents vary as to application methods, so careful reading of instructions is necessary. Most débriding agents are proteolytic enzymes that selectively digest necrotic tissue. Be careful to apply them only to the wound and to avoid contact with healthy tissue.

AUTOLYTIC DÉBRIDEMENT. Autolytic débridement is the use of a synthetic dressing or moisture-retentive dressing over the ulcer. The eschar then self-digests via the action of the enzymes that are present in the fluid environment of the wound. This method is not used for infected wounds, because the infection would worsen.

SURGICAL DÉBRIDEMENT. Surgical débridement involves the removal of devitalized tissue, slough, or thick, adherent eschar with a scalpel, scissors, or other sharp instrument. Slough is loose, yellow to tan stringy necrotic tissue. Slough, like eschar, can be tightly adhered to the wound bed.

Depending on the amount of débridement to be done, this may be performed in the operating room, a treatment room, or the patient's room. Following surgical débridement, grafting may be required to close the wound. This becomes necessary if it is a full-thickness ulcer, if there is loss of joint function, or for cosmetic purposes. For procedures performed without anesthesia, be sure to premedicate the patient for pain. Continually monitor for pain during the procedure, especially if there is a donor site for grafting.

• **WORD** • **BUILDING** •

cellulitis: cellu—cell + itis—inflammation
eschar: eschara—scab

Wound Cleansing

The ulcer should be thoroughly cleansed using a whirlpool, a handheld showerhead, or an irrigating system with a pressure between 4 and 15 pounds per square inch (psi). A 30-mL syringe with an 18-gauge needle works well for this purpose. Pressure less than 4 psi does not adequately cleanse the wound, and pressure greater than 15 psi may damage tissue. If an irrigating system is used, 250 mL of normal saline solution (or sometimes tap water for home care) should be used to thoroughly cleanse the wound. If the wound is red, gentle irrigation with a needleless 30- to 60-mL syringe should be used to prevent trauma and bleeding. However, if the wound has been diagnosed as being infected, flushing with a 30- to 60-mL syringe and an 18-gauge needle provides the pressure needed to help remove bacteria.

   LEARNING TIP

Dilution is the solution to wound pollution!

Once the wound has been cleansed and débrided, apply a dressing. Wounds heal more rapidly in a moist environment, with minimal bacterial colonization and a healing temperature. This takes 12 hours to occur after the wound is covered with an occlusive dressing. If a dressing is frequently removed, the wound may not reach its healing temperature, and healing may be impaired. When possible, the dressing should be left in place for extended periods. Draining wounds may require frequent dressing changes.

Wound Dressings

Dressings vary according to size, location, depth, stage of ulcer, and preference of the ordering practitioner. Commonly used dressing materials include hydrogel dressings, polyurethane films, hydrocolloid wafers, biological dressings, alginates, and cotton gauze. See Chapter 53 for more information on dressing types. The use of an appropriate dressing promotes an optimum healing environment. Hypoallergenic tape should be used to secure dressings if tape is necessary. Protective paste may be applied to protect unaffected tissue from topical agents. In all cases, pressure should be kept off the wound. No treatment will be effective if pressure continues to damage the tissue.

Negative Pressure Wound Therapy

Negative pressure wound therapy (NPWT) may be effective for healing large open pressure ulcers (Fig. 54.1). In NPWT, a wound is packed loosely with a sterile sponge and then covered with an occlusive dressing. A vacuum source is placed in the wound, and gentle negative pressure is applied. The negative pressure allows excess drainage and infectious material to be removed, which reduces pressure on delicate new tissue. With small vessels decompressed, circulation

FIGURE 54.1 Negative pressure wound therapy. (A) Occlusive dressing is applied to wound with tubing to vacuum source. (B) Vacuum source exerts gentle negative pressure.

is increased, and healing is accelerated. NPWT also maintains a moist environment for optimal healing. Evidence strongly supports NPWT for nonischemic diabetic foot ulcers; it is also effective for pressure ulcers and other deep wounds (Vig et al, 2011). Risks of NPWT include bleeding in patients at risk, such as those on anticoagulant therapy.

Other Therapies

Much research is ongoing in the field of wound healing. Some success has been shown with the following therapies: biological or biological skin equivalent dressings, collagen application, platelet-rich plasma application, platelet-derived growth factor application, silver-based products, hyperbaric oxygen therapy, and ozone-oxygen treatments.

Nursing Process for the Patient With a Pressure Ulcer

Data Collection

Collaborate with the registered nurse (RN) to evaluate the status of the pressure ulcer often, as well as underlying causes and barriers to healing. Monitor for risk factors for impaired healing, such as prolonged immobility, incontinence, and inadequate nutrition and hydration. Also monitor intact skin to prevent development of new pressure ulcers.

Use transparency film or a disposable ruler to measure the diameter of the ulcer in centimeters. Imagine a clock superimposed over the wound with 12 o'clock at the head and 6 o'clock at the feet. Measure in centimeters from 12 to 6 o'clock, and from 9 to 3 o'clock. Depth can be measured with a cotton-tipped applicator. Also, gently probe a cotton-tipped applicator under the skin edges to detect tunneling and measure lateral tissue destruction.

Several staging systems are available for pressure ulcers based on the depth of tissue destroyed. Most staging systems categorize wounds from stage I to stage IV. Additional categories may include deep tissue injury and unstageable (Fig. 54.2).

- *Deep tissue injury:* The National Pressure Ulcer Advisory Panel (NPUAP, 2007) defines deep tissue injury as a "purple or maroon localized area of discolored intact skin or blood-filled blister due to damage of underlying soft tissue from pressure and/or shear. The area may be preceded by tissue that is painful, firm, mushy, boggy, warmer, or cooler as compared to adjacent tissue." Deep tissue injury is considered unstageable because it is impossible to determine how deep the tissue damage is. This stage can progress quickly to a stage III or IV ulcer, even with appropriate treatment.
- *Stage I:* The skin is still intact, but the area is red and does not blanch when pressed. There may also be warmth, hardness, and discoloration of the skin. A stage I ulcer may be difficult to detect on a dark-skinned person.
- *Stage II:* There is a break in the skin, with partial-thickness skin loss of epidermis, dermis, or both. The ulcer may appear as an abrasion, a shallow crater, or a blister. Stage II ulcers do not contain slough (yellow fibrous tissue).
- *Stage III:* There is full-thickness skin loss, which extends to the subcutaneous fat but not to the fascia. The ulcer

looks like a deep crater and may have undermining of adjacent tissue. Bone, tendon, and muscle are not visible.
- *Stage IV:* There is full-thickness skin loss with exposed muscle, bone, or support structures such as tendons. Slough or eschar may be present. There may be undermining and sinus tracts (tunneling).
- *Unstageable:* The base of the ulcer is covered by slough or eschar so that the depth cannot be evaluated. The wound bed must be debrided before staging and treatment can take place. One exception, according to NPUAP (2007), is stable, dry, intact eschar on the heels. It serves as the body's natural (biological) cover and should not be removed.

Observe wound exudate. Two common types of wound exudate are serosanguineous and **purulent**. Serosanguineous exudate is fluid consisting of serum and blood. It is blood-tinged, amber-colored fluid. Purulent fluid is a fluid that contains pus. It can vary in color and have different odors, depending on which bacteria are present. Creamy yellow pus may indicate *Staphylococcus*. Beige pus that has a fishy odor may suggest *Proteus*. Green-blue pus with a fruity odor may indicate *Pseudomonas*. Brown pus with a fecal odor may suggest *Bacteroides*. The wound must be cultured to accurately identify bacteria.

Gently palpate the wound with a gloved hand to determine the texture of granulations. Granulation tissue has a budding appearance from the development of tiny new capillaries. If the granulations are healthy, they have a slightly spongy texture.

Document all findings carefully in the medical record, so all health team members can monitor progress of healing. Many institutions have specific forms for drawing pictures of the locations and sizes of wounds and for photographs to monitor the healing process. Follow policy at the institution where you work.

Nursing Diagnoses, Planning, Implementation, and Evaluation

See the "Nursing Care Plan for the Patient With a Pressure Ulcer."

- WORD • BUILDING •
purulent: purulentus—pus

Stage I   Stage II   Stage III   Stage IV

FIGURE 54.2 Stages of pressure ulcers include deep tissue injury, stages I through IV, shown here, and unstageable, as described in the text. From Dillon, P. M. (2007). *Nursing health assessment* (2nd ed.). Philadelphia: F.A. Davis, p. 239, with permission.

NURSING CARE PLAN for the Patient With a Pressure Ulcer

Nursing Diagnosis: *Impaired Skin Integrity* related to pressure on skin surface, reduced circulation, or immobility

Expected Outcomes: The patient's skin integrity will be improved as evidenced by decrease in wound size and depth, no development of additional pressure ulcers.

Evaluation of Outcomes: Is there a decrease in wound size? Are there any new pressure ulcers?

Intervention Monitor status of pressure ulcer according to stage, color, exudate, texture, size, and depth. **Rationale** Provides data on which care is based. **Evaluation** What stage is ulcer? Is it improving or worsening?

Intervention Determine and remove cause of pressure (e.g., immobility, friction, shearing). **Rationale** Allows for correction and also prevents further trauma. **Evaluation** What is the cause of the ulcer? Is cause removed?

Intervention Cleanse wound gently with warm water; rinse; pat dry gently with gauze. Do not rub the area. **Rationale** Reduces number of bacteria. Drying prevents maceration of skin. Gentle handling prevents further trauma. **Evaluation** Is wound clean and dry?

Intervention Débride or assist with débridement of wound as prescribed (method depends on patient's condition and goals of care). **Rationale** Débridement removes drainage and wound debris. Permits granulation of tissue. **Evaluation** Does wound look clean and free of debris?

Intervention Apply topical agents and/or dress wound as prescribed. Make sure dressing stays intact with movement and edges do not roll, causing more pressure. **Rationale** Protects underlying wound and helps promote healing. **Evaluation** Is dressing applied appropriately?

Intervention Position patient off the ulcer. **Rationale** Prevents further pressure and trauma on ulcer. **Evaluation** Is patient positioned off the ulcer?

Intervention If a leg ulcer, provide for frequent rest periods with leg elevated; if immobile, reposition every 2 hours. **Rationale** Prevents further tissue breakdown. **Evaluation** Is leg elevated? Is patient repositioned every 2 hours?

Nursing Diagnosis: *Risk for Infection* related to open wound

Expected Outcomes: The patient will not experience wound infection or systemic sepsis as evidenced by clean wound bed and by temperature and white blood cell count within normal limits. (Total elimination of bacteria is impossible because of the nature of the condition.)

Evaluation of Outcomes: Is patient free from signs and symptoms of local and systemic infection?

Intervention Examine ulcer at every dressing change. Check for areas of tenderness, swelling, redness, heat, and drainage. Report changes. **Rationale** Allows for early recognition of infection and response to treatment. **Evaluation** Are signs of infection present? Are they reported promptly?

Intervention Monitor temperature at least every 12 hours. **Rationale** Elevated body temperature is one sign of infection. **Evaluation** Is patient afebrile?

Intervention Provide meticulous wound care (see Impaired Skin Integrity). **Rationale** Helps decrease the level of contamination and prevent infection. **Evaluation** Is wound showing signs of healing without purulent drainage?

Intervention Use thorough hand hygiene techniques. Use sterile technique for dressing changes. **Rationale** Prevents cross-contamination. **Evaluation** Does nurse take proper precautions?

Continued

NURSING CARE PLAN for the Patient With a Pressure Ulcer—cont'd

Nursing Diagnosis: *Pain* related to ulcer and treatments as evidenced by pain rating on 0-to-10 scale

Expected Outcomes: The patient will be as comfortable and as pain free as possible as evidenced by statement of decreased pain and ability to sleep at night.

Evaluation of Outcomes: Does patient express comfort? Does patient express a decrease in pain? Is patient able to sleep?

Intervention Assess level of pain with pain scale and by observing facial expressions and positioning of body. **Rationale** Monitors level of pain and response to therapy. **Evaluation** At what level is pain? Is it better or worse with treatment?

Intervention Offer analgesics as prescribed. Request order for topical analgesics as needed with dressing changes and cleaning of the wound. **Rationale** Analgesics help relieve pain. **Evaluation** Are analgesics effective?

Intervention Decrease anxiety with relaxation techniques (e.g., distraction, music). **Rationale** Relaxation can lessen pain intensity. **Evaluation** Is patient less anxious? Does patient verbalize less pain?

Intervention Maintain a comfortable environment: provide for privacy; position in good alignment and comfortably; and maintain a comfortable room temperature. **Rationale** Relaxes patient and lessens intensity of discomfort. **Evaluation** Does patient express an increase in comfort?

NURSING CARE TIP

Many institutions now have nurses who have been specially trained in wound care. Consult one of these nurses for expert wound assessment and treatment recommendations.

CRITICAL THINKING

Mr. Russ

■ Mr. Russ is an 84-year-old man who was admitted from home to the medical-surgical unit after a fall that fractured his femur. He has a history of type 2 diabetes. He had an open reduction and internal fixation of his femur and is now in a brace. He is 6 feet tall and weighs 160 pounds. His appetite is poor; his wife states he has lost 15 lb in the past 3 months. He is occasionally incontinent of urine.

1. How can you be vigilant in identifying risks and preventing skin breakdown in Mr. Russ?
2. What other members of the health team might you collaborate with when planning care for Mr. Russ?

Suggested answers are at the end of the chapter.

INFLAMMATORY SKIN DISORDERS

Dermatitis

Pathophysiology and Etiology

Dermatitis is inflammation of the skin and is characterized by itching, redness, and skin lesions, with varying borders and distribution patterns. There are three common types of dermatitis: contact dermatitis, atopic dermatitis, and seborrheic dermatitis. Contact dermatitis is caused by exposure to an allergen or irritant such as soap, perfume, or poison ivy. Atopic dermatitis tends to be hereditary and is associated with allergies, asthma, and hay fever. Seborrheic dermatitis occurs most often on the scalp, usually in individuals with oily skin. All types tend to be chronic and respond well to treatment but are prone to recur. See Table 54.2 for common types of dermatitis.

Prevention

The patient should prevent irritation to the skin by avoiding irritants, allergens, and excessive heat and dryness and by controlling perspiration. Baths should be short, in tepid water. Deodorant soaps should be avoided; mild superfatted soaps are recommended instead. Dry skin can be lubricated with creams, oils, or ointments as appropriate.

• **WORD** • **BUILDING** •
dermatitis: derma—skin + itis—inflammation

TABLE 54.2 COMMON TYPES OF DERMATITIS

Type	Description
Contact	Acute or chronic condition; caused by contact with irritant or allergen
Irritant contact	Caused by direct contact with an irritating substance, such as soap, detergent, strong medication, astringent, cosmetic, or industrial chemical
Allergic contact	From contact with an allergen, such as perfume, tanning lotion, medication, hair dye, poison ivy, poison oak; contact results in cell-mediated immune response
Atopic	Chronic inherited condition; may be associated with respiratory allergies or asthma; can vary between bright red maculas, papules, oozing, and **lichenified** or hyperpigmented areas
Seborrheic	Chronic, inflammatory disease usually accompanied by scaling, itching, and inflammation; **seborrhea** is excessive production of sebaceous secretions; found in areas with abundant sebaceous glands (scalp, face, axilla, groin) and where there are folds of skin; can appear as dry, moist, or greasy scales, yellow or pink-yellow crusts, redness, and dry flakiness; can be associated with emotional stress; genetic predisposition may exist

Contact dermatitis caused by nail polish.

Contact dermatitis caused by topical anesthetic.

Seborrheic dermatitis.

Itching and scratching should be prevented as much as possible.

Signs and Symptoms

Itching and rashes or lesions are the main clinical manifestations of dermatitis. The lesions vary depending on the type and location of dermatitis. Rashes and lesions may present as dry, flaky scales, yellow crusts, redness, fissures, macules, papules, and vesicles. (These are described in Chapter 53.) Scratching can make any of these lesions worse.

NURSING CARE TIP

Itching and scratching can occur during sleep, causing the rash to worsen. Have the patient wear cotton gloves at night to prevent scratching. Oatmeal baths may also help.

Complications

The lesion or rash worsens with continued irritation, exposure to offending agents, or scratching. Infections of the skin are common and may be due to the many open areas and breaks in the skin, as well as the patient's reluctance to properly wash the affected area because of pain from the lesions. Some infections can also become systemic.

Diagnostic Tests

Diagnosis is usually based on history, symptoms, and clinical findings. If infection is suspected, cultures of the lesions may be ordered to identify the infecting agent.

Therapeutic Measures

Treatment varies according to symptoms. Basic treatment objectives are to control itching, alleviate discomfort and pain,

• WORD • BUILDING •
lichenified: leichen—scaly growth + facere—to make
seborrhea: sebum—tallow + rhoia—flow

decrease inflammation, control or prevent crust formation and oozing, prevent infection, prevent further damage to the skin, and heal the lesions as much as possible.

Itching (**pruritus**) and discomfort can be somewhat relieved by antihistamines, analgesics, and antipruritic medications as ordered. Colloidal oatmeal preparations added to baths may also help.

Steroids such as hydrocortisone or methylprednisolone may be used to suppress inflammation. They can be administered as topical, intralesional, or systemic agents. The specific type used depends on the type of lesion, the body area involved, and the extent of the lesion. Topical administration is preferred if possible because systemic steroids can cause serious side effects, including adrenal suppression.

Tub baths and wet dressings help control oozing and prevent further crust formation; they also serve to loosen exudates, scales, and other wound debris, providing a clean area for topical application of medication. Protect the skin by lightly patting dry, avoiding friction, and avoiding hot water. Advise the patient to use a sunscreen agent when outdoors.

Nursing Process for the Patient With Dermatitis

DATA COLLECTION.   You can use the **WHAT'S UP?** format to assess the rash, as described in Chapter 53. Also refer to Chapter 53, Table 53.1, for specific questions to ask. Observe the rash or lesions for character, distribution, description, tenderness, signs of scratching, and other associated problems.

NURSING DIAGNOSES, PLANNING, AND IMPLEMENTATION.
Impaired Skin Integrity related to rash, lesions, and scratching
EXPECTED OUTCOME: The patient's skin integrity will improve as evidenced by reduction in lesions and absence of signs or symptoms of infection.

- Monitor skin condition regularly *to determine if treatment is working.*
- Cleanse the area as ordered by health care provider (HCP), taking care not to irritate the skin further, *to keep area clean and prevent infection.*
- Provide cool moist compresses, dressings, or tepid tub baths *to help relieve inflammation and itching, débride lesions, and soften crusts and scales.*
- Pat the skin dry rather than rubbing *to prevent further trauma.*
- Apply topical agents as ordered *to help suppress inflammation and itching.*
- Provide skin care at bedtime *to help promote comfortable sleep. Many antihistamines also have a sedative effect.*
- Encourage patient to eat a high-protein diet to promote healing and replace lost protein. *If lesions are generalized, protein can be lost through oozing of serum.* Confirm appropriateness of high-protein diet with primary care provider.
- Encourage use of gloves or mitts, especially at night, *to help prevent scratching.*
- Advise the patient to keep fingernails short *to prevent scratching.*
- Teach the patient that application of slight pressure with a clean cloth *may help relieve itching.*

- Teach relaxation exercises *to help the patient cope with distressing symptoms.*

Disturbed Body Image related to visible rash or lesions
EXPECTED OUTCOME: The patient will have improved body image as evidenced by a statement of acceptance of the condition and ability to socialize with others.

- Allow patients to verbalize concerns if they wish to do so. *Talking about concerns may help the patient to begin to work through feelings about body image but should not be forced.*
- Refer to a support group, if available, *to receive support from others in similar circumstances.*
- Display an accepting attitude while caring for skin lesions. *The patient will be quick to pick up your reaction to the lesions, especially if it is negative.*
- Encourage the patient to participate in skin care *to allow more control over the situation.*
- Encourage the patient to wear long sleeves or other appropriate covering if the patient desires *to make the lesions less noticeable.*

Deficient Knowledge related to disease and treatment
EXPECTED OUTCOME: The patient will verbalize understanding of the condition and demonstrate ability to perform self-care measures.

- Determine patient's baseline knowledge of condition and treatment. *Teaching should build on baseline understanding.*
- Instruct the patient in application of topical agents and dressings. *Overuse of medications can further traumatize skin; be sure to follow package or prescription directions.*
- Instruct the patient in how to recognize changes, improvement, or flare-ups of the disorder and what symptoms to report to the health care provider. *Because most skin conditions are cared for at home, it is important for the patient to have the skills needed to monitor the condition and carry out treatment appropriately.*
- Advise the patient to avoid overexposure to sun and to use sunscreen agents when outdoors *to prevent skin damage.*
- Encourage use of a humidifier in the home *to help maintain hydration of skin and control itching during dry weather, especially in winter.*
- Teach the patient measures to prevent future flare-ups if possible. *Flare-ups may be avoided if the patient understands what triggers them.*

NURSING CARE TIP

Teach patients that when applying topical medications, more is not better!

• **WORD** • **BUILDING** •
pruritus: prur—itch + itis—condition

EVALUATION. If medical and nursing care have been effective, the lesions will be controlled or in remission, the patient will state that itching and other discomforts are controlled, the patient will be able to socialize without undue difficulty, and the patient will be able to describe and demonstrate self-care measures.

Psoriasis

Pathophysiology and Etiology

Psoriasis is a chronic inflammatory skin disorder in which the epidermal cells proliferate abnormally fast. Usually, epidermal cells take about 27 days to shed. With psoriasis, the cells shed every 4 to 5 days. The abnormal keratin forms loosely adherent scales with dermal inflammation.

The exact cause is not known; however, it is autoimmune in nature, with T cells attacking healthy skin cells, causing an increase in skin cell, T-cell, and white cell production. Often there is a family history of psoriasis. The average age at onset is 27 years, although it can begin at any age. The condition can be severe if the onset is in childhood.

Psoriasis is characterized by exacerbations and remissions. Many factors influence the suppression and outbreak of lesions, which varies from individual to individual. Sun and humidity may suppress lesions. Aggravating factors include streptococcal pharyngitis, emotional upset, stress, hormonal changes, cold weather, skin trauma, smoking, alcohol, and certain drugs (e.g., antimalarial agents, lithium, beta blockers).

Prevention

Because the exact etiology is not known, measures to prevent exacerbation of symptoms are specific to the patient's circumstances. General preventive measures include avoidance of upper respiratory infections, especially streptococcal infections; avoidance of or coping with emotional stress; avoidance of skin trauma, including sunburns; and avoidance of medications that can precipitate a flare-up.

Signs and Symptoms

Signs and symptoms vary according to the patient and the particular type of psoriasis. Lesions are red papules that join to form plaques with distinct borders (Fig. 54.3). Silvery scales develop on untreated lesions. Areas most often affected are the elbows and knees, scalp, umbilicus, and genitals. Other signs and symptoms include nail involvement, involvement in the gluteal fold (called intergluteal pinking), itching, and dry or brittle hair.

Complications

Because of the nature of the disease with its lesions and itching, secondary infections can occur. Psoriatic arthritis can develop after the psoriasis has developed, with nail changes and destructive arthritis of large joints, the spine, and interphalangeal joints. If the psoriasis becomes severe and widespread, fever, chills, increased cardiac output, and benign lymphadenopathy can result.

Diagnostic Tests

Testing depends on the severity of the psoriasis. Usually, diagnosis is based on physical assessment alone. Skin biopsy

FIGURE 54.3 Psoriasis. Note bright red scaly plaque with silvery scales. From Goldsmith, L. A., Lazarus, G. S., & Tharp, M. D. (1997). *Adult and pediatric dermatology.* Philadelphia: F.A. Davis, p. 258, with permission.

or other diagnostic tests may be performed to rule out concurrent disease or secondary infection.

Therapeutic Measures

Treatment varies according to the type and extent of the disease, as well as patient preference. Psoriasis is a chronic disease with remissions and exacerbations. Basic treatment objectives are to decrease the rapid epidermal proliferation, inflammation, and itching and scaling. The patient may be instructed to bathe daily in a tub, using a soft brush to assist in the removal of scales.

A variety of topical and systemic agents are used to treat psoriasis. Topical corticosteroids may be used for their anti-inflammatory effect. Occlusive dressings are commonly used to enhance penetration of medications (see Chapter 53). Keratolytic ointments or gels enhance the effects of salicylic acid to loosen or remove scales. Synthetic vitamin D cream slows the proliferation of skin cells. Fish oil supplements may reduce inflammation in some patients.

Tar preparations may be prescribed along with corticosteroids. The tar acts as an antimitotic, slowing the epidermal cell division. Occlusive dressings are not used with tars. Anthralin is a substance extracted from coal tar that suppresses mitotic activity. The anthralin may be mixed with salicylic acid in a stiff paste. The patient must be closely observed because anthralin is a strong irritant and can cause chemical burns. It is usually applied for no longer than 2 hours. Both coal tar and anthralin are commonly used in combination with ultraviolet (UV) light and are usually administered in inpatient settings or specialized outpatient clinics.

• **WORD • BUILDING** •

psoriasis: psor—itch + iasis—inflammation

Topical preparations for the scalp are used in shampoo form. Teach the patient to read package instructions; these preparations generally need to be left in the hair for a period of time to work.

UV light may be designated as UVB, shorter wavelength, or UVA, longer wavelength. UVA is from an artificial source, such as special mercury vapor lamps. The amount of exposure depends on the patient's condition, pigmentation, and susceptibility to burning. The patient must wear eye guards during treatments. Oral psoralen tablets (a photosensitizing agent) followed by exposure to UVA is called PUVA therapy. PUVA therapy temporarily inhibits DNA synthesis, which is antimitotic. Because psoralen is a photosensitizing agent, the patient must wear dark glasses not only during the treatment period but also for the entire day after a treatment. The long-term safety of PUVA therapy is still unknown. Possible side effects include increased skin carcinomas, premature skin aging, and actinic keratosis (premalignant lesions of the skin). The patient should be observed closely for redness, tenderness, edema, and eye changes. Initial and follow-up eye examinations, skin biopsies, urinalysis, and blood tests may be ordered.

Retinoids are oral agents such as acitretin (Soriatane) that promote skin cell differentiation and inhibit malignancies from forming in the skin. They may be used in combination with UV therapy.

Antimetabolites, usually used for cancer chemotherapy, are reserved for the most severe cases. Methotrexate is the most common agent given. Because of its hepatotoxicity, it is contraindicated in patients with liver disease, alcoholism, renal disease, and bone marrow suppression. Other systemic agents, such as cyclosporine and etanercept (Enbrel) work by altering the immune system.

Nursing Care

Nursing care for the patient with psoriasis is the same as nursing care for the patient with dermatitis. Teach the patient how to use prescribed medications and how to identify and avoid triggers. Explain that drinking alcohol can interfere with some treatments. In addition, consult with the physician about recommending small amounts of sunlight to help improve skin lesions.

INFECTIOUS SKIN DISORDERS

A variety of infections can affect the skin. The most common disorders are discussed in this section. See Table 54.3 for a summary of additional skin infections.

TABLE 54.3 INFECTIOUS SKIN DISORDERS

Type	Description	Complications	Treatment/Nursing Care
Impetigo Contagiosa Impetigo on the face Impetigo Contagiosa.	Common contagious, infectious, inflammatory skin disorder usually caused by *Streptococcus* or *Staphylococcus aureus;* sources of infection include swimming pools, pets, dirty fingernails, beauty and barber shops, and contaminated clothing, towels, sheets; may occur secondary to scrapes, cuts, insect	Glomerulonephritis—may occur up to 6–7 weeks after infection. Lesions may spread. Lesions may persist if not permitted to dry. Secondary **pyoderma**, or acute inflammatory purulent dermatitis, can occur if lesions are unresponsive to treatment.	Administer systemic antibiotics as prescribed. Apply topical antibiotics after crust removal. Wash gently with a mild soap, or soak with warm, moist compresses to aid in removal of crusts and debris, and to provide a clean bed for topical therapy.

• WORD • BUILDING •
pyoderma: pyo—pus + derma—skin

TABLE 54.3   INFECTIOUS SKIN DISORDERS—cont'd

Type	Description	Complications	Treatment/Nursing Care
	bites, burns, dermatitis, poison ivy. Rash appears as oozing, thin-roofed vesicle that rapidly grows and develops a honey-colored crust; crusts are easily removed, and new crusts appear; lesions heal in 1 to 2 weeks if allowed to dry. Rash is contagious until all lesions are healed.		Keep fingernails short and clean, and use gloves or hand mitts as necessary to prevent scratching. Teach proper disposal or washing of any material that comes in contact with lesions.
Furuncles and Carbuncles Furuncles and carbuncles.	Furuncle: small, tender boil that occurs deep in one or more hair follicles and spreads to surrounding dermis; usually caused by *Staphylococcus;* usually on body areas prone to excessive perspiration, friction, and irritation (e.g., buttocks, axillae); can recur; eventually comes to a soft yellow, black, or white head with localized pain and surrounding cellulitis; lymphadenopathy may be present. Carbuncle: an abscess of skin and subcutaneous tissue; deeper than a furuncle; usually caused by *Staphylococcus;* usually appears where skin is thick, fibrous, and inelastic (e.g., back of neck, upper back, and buttocks); associated symptoms may include fever, pain, leukocytosis, prostration.	Furuncles may progress to more severe carbuncles. Carbuncles may progress to infection of bloodstream. Further spread of infection can occur to self and others.	Administer antibiotics as ordered. Prevent trauma; avoid squeezing or irritation. Cleanse surrounding skin with antibacterial soap, followed by application of antibacterial ointment. Surgical incision and drainage may be performed. Cover draining lesions with dressings. Follow standard precautions to prevent cross-contamination. Cover mattress and pillows with plastic and wipe daily with a disinfectant. Wash all linens, towels, and clothing after each use. Properly discard razor blades after each use.

Herpes Simplex
Pathophysiology and Etiology

Herpes simplex virus (HSV) infection is a common viral infection that tends to recur repeatedly. There are two types of herpes simplex: that caused by type 1 virus (HSV-1), which occurs above the waist and causes a fever blister or cold sore (Fig. 54.4), and that caused by type 2 virus (HSV-2), which occurs below the waist and causes genital herpes. See Chapter 44 for information on genital herpes.

The primary infection occurs through direct contact, respiratory droplet, or fluid exposure from another infected person. Following the initial infection, the virus lies dormant in nerve ganglia near the spinal column, where the immune system cannot destroy it. The patient is asymptomatic at this time.

FIGURE 54.4 Herpes simplex. From Goldsmith, L. A., Lazarus, G. S., & Tharp, M. D. (1997). *Adult and pediatric dermatology.* Philadelphia: F.A. Davis, p. 306, with permission.

Recurrence of symptomatic infection can happen spontaneously or may be triggered by a stressor such as fever, sunburn, illness, menses, fatigue, or injury. The secondary lesion may appear isolated or as groups of small vesicles or pustules on an erythematous base. Crusts eventually form, and the lesions heal in about 1 week. The lesions are contagious for 2 to 4 days before dry crusts form.

Prevention

Avoidance of contact with a known infected lesion during the blistering phase can prevent the primary lesions. Patients should also be taught to avoid sharing contaminated items such as toothbrushes, lipsticks, and drinking glasses. This disease can recur spontaneously. Avoidance of stressors, such as sunburn, injury, and fatigue, may delay a recurrence. The use of sunscreens, especially on the lips, may be helpful.

Signs and Symptoms

Some patients may have a prodromal phase of burning or tingling at the site for a few hours before eruption. The area becomes erythematous and swollen. Vesicles and pustules erupt in 1 to 2 days. There may also be redness with no blistering. Lesions can burn, itch, and be painful. The attacks vary in frequency but diminish with age. The patient is contagious with each outbreak until scabs are formed.

Complications

If herpes simplex is present in the vagina at childbirth, the newborn may be infected (meningoencephalitis or a panvisceral infection may occur). If the person touches the affected area and then rubs the eyes, the eyes can become severely infected. Secondary bacterial infection of lesions can occur. Rarely, herpes encephalitis can occur. This is deadly if not treated promptly.

Diagnostic Tests

Cultures of the lesions provide a definitive diagnosis. Most lesions are diagnosed on the basis of history, signs, and symptoms.

Therapeutic Measures

There is no complete cure for herpes simplex. Recurrences will happen. Topical acyclovir (Zovirax) ointment is the drug of choice for primary lesions, to suppress the multiplication

of vesicles. Docosanol (Abreva) is an over-the-counter topical antiviral agent that may be effective. Oral antivirals (acyclovir, famciclovir, or valacyclovir) may be recommended for severe or frequent attacks (six or more attacks per year) or for patients who are immunosuppressed. Various lotions, creams, and ointments may be prescribed to accelerate drying and healing of lesions (e.g., camphor, phenol, alcohol). Antibiotics may be indicated for secondary infections.

Herpes Zoster (Shingles)
Pathophysiology and Etiology

Herpes zoster, or shingles, is an acute inflammatory and infectious disorder that produces a painful vesicular eruption on bright red edematous plaques along the distribution of nerves from one or more posterior ganglia. This eruption follows the course of the cutaneous sensory nerve and is almost always unilateral (one sided; Fig. 54.5).

Herpes zoster is caused by the varicella zoster virus—the same virus that causes chickenpox. After a case of chickenpox, the virus remains dormant in nerve tissue near the brain and spinal cord. Herpes zoster is a reactivation of this latent varicella virus. The incubation period of herpes zoster is 7 to 21 days. Vesicles appear in 3 to 4 days. Eruption usually occurs posteriorly and progresses anteriorly and peripherally along the dermatome. The total duration of the outbreak can vary from 10 days to 5 weeks.

This disease occurs most commonly in older adults or in those who have a diminished resistance, such as the patient with acquired immunodeficiency syndrome (AIDS), the patient on immunosuppressant agents, or the patient with a malignancy or injury to the spine or a cranial nerve.

FIGURE 54.5 Herpes zoster (shingles). From Goldsmith, L. A., Lazarus, G. S., & Tharp, M. D. (1997). *Adult and pediatric dermatology.* Philadelphia: F.A. Davis, p. 307, with permission.

Prevention

Avoidance of persons with herpes zoster during the contagious phase (a few days before eruption until vesicles dry or scab) is the best prevention. Varicella vaccine (Varivax) in children and adults who have not had chickenpox can reduce the risk of becoming infected with varicella. Another newer vaccine, Zostavax, is recommended for all patients over age 60 who have had chickenpox. It reduces the risk of shingles outbreak, and reduces the severity if it does occur.

Signs and Symptoms

In addition to the vesicles and plaques, there may be irritation, itching, fever, malaise, and, depending on the location of lesions, visceral involvement. Lesions may be very painful; the incidence of pain increases with age.

Complications

Postherpetic neuralgia, persistent dermatomal pain, and hyperesthesia are common in older adults and can last for weeks to months after the lesions have healed. The incidence and severity of these complications increase with age.

Ophthalmic herpes zoster affects the fifth cranial nerve and can be a serious complication. Consultation with an ophthalmologist is essential because this complication can affect eyesight. Other complications can occur with facial and acoustic nerve involvement, including hearing loss, tinnitus, facial paralysis, and vertigo. Full-thickness skin necrosis and scarring can occur if lesions do not heal properly; systemic infection can occur from scratching, causing the virus to enter the bloodstream.

Diagnostic Tests

Diagnosis is usually confirmed by history and physical examination of the patient and associated signs and symptoms. Cultures may be ordered if secondary bacterial infections are suspected.

Therapeutic Measures

Treatment is aimed at controlling the outbreak, reducing pain and discomfort, and preventing complications. Mild cases may heal without medication. Antiviral agents such as acyclovir are used for more severe cases and are most effective if started within 72 hours of the onset of the rash. Analgesics may be prescribed for pain and discomfort. Anticonvulsants (gabapentin/Neurontin) or antidepressants (amitriptyline/Elavil) may also be effective for neuropathic pain.

Use of corticosteroids is controversial, but they may help reduce discomfort and improve quality of life when used with antiviral agents. Topical steroids should not be applied if a secondary infection is present because they suppress the immune system. Antihistamines can be administered to control itching. Antibiotics are prescribed for secondary bacterial infections.

In addition to medications, cool compresses or baths may help with pain and itching. Topical agents containing calamine or lidocaine may also be helpful.

Fungal Infections
Pathophysiology and Etiology

Dermatomycosis, or a fungal infection of the skin, occurs when there is an impairment of the skin integrity in a warm, moist environment. This infection occurs through direct contact with infected humans, animals, or objects. *Tinea* is the term used to describe fungal skin infections; the name used after tinea indicates the body area affected. For example, tinea capitis is a fungal infection of the scalp, and tinea pedis is the term used for athlete's foot. The term *candidiasis* is used when *Candida* is the infecting organism. Common fungal infections and treatments are described in Table 54.4.

Cellulitis
Pathophysiology and Etiology

Cellulitis is inflammation of the skin and subcutaneous tissue resulting from infection, usually with *Staphylococcus* or *Streptococcus* bacteria. Methicillin-resistant *Staphylococcus aureus* (MRSA) is becoming a common cause and is resistant to many antibiotics. Cellulitis can occur as a result of skin trauma; as a secondary bacterial infection of an open wound, such as a pressure ulcer; or it may be unrelated to skin trauma. It most often occurs in the extremities, especially the lower legs.

Prevention

Good hygiene and prevention of cross-contamination are important. If an open wound is present, preventing infection and promoting healing are critical.

Signs and Symptoms

The initial sign of cellulitis is a localized area of inflammation that may become more generalized if not treated promptly. Common clinical manifestations include warmth, redness, localized edema, pain, tenderness, fever, and lymphadenopathy. The infection can worsen rapidly and become systemic if not treated properly.

Diagnostic Tests

Culture and sensitivity testing of any pustules or drainage is necessary to identify the infecting organism. Blood cultures may also be indicated to rule out bacteremia.

Therapeutic Measures

Topical and systemic antibiotics are prescribed according to culture and sensitivity test results. Débridement of nonviable tissue is necessary if an open wound is present. Systemic antibiotics are indicated if fever and lymphadenopathy are present.

Elevation of the extremity can reduce pain and swelling. Monitor vital signs and report hypotension and tachycardia, because such changes can indicate systemic infection. Measure the extremity daily and document to monitor progress.

• WORD • BUILDING •
dermatomycosis: derma—skin + myco—fungus + osis—condition

TABLE 54.4 FUNGAL INFECTIONS

Type	Description	Treatment/Nursing Care
Tinea Pedis (Athlete's Foot)	Common fungal infection, most frequently seen in those with warm, diaphoretic feet; occlusive shoes; or friction/trauma to the feet Four types: interdigital (between the toes), chronic hyperkeratotic (chronic plantar erythema and scaling), inflammatory/vesicular (vesicles on plantar surface), and ulcerative (vesicular lesions and ulcers between toes and on plantar surface).	Administer topical antifungal agents as ordered; may be oral in more severe or unresponsive cases. Apply topical agents in a thin layer; treat for time specified, even after apparent clearing. Wet dressings or vinegar soaks may be ordered to dry blisters. Teach patient prevention measures: keep feet dry; dry carefully between toes; apply foot powder and wear cotton socks to absorb perspiration; if weather permits, use perforated shoes or sandals; avoid plastic or rubber-soled shoes; wear water shoes in public showers and near swimming pools.
Tinea Capitis (Ringworm of Scalp) Tinea capitis (ringworm of scalp). *From Taber's 22e, p. 2326.*	Contagious fungal infection of the scalp; commonly causes hair loss in children. Appears as scattered round, red, scaly patches; small papules or pustules may be evident at edges of patches; hair is brittle at site, breaks off, and temporary areas of baldness result; mild itching, tenderness, and pain may be present. Kerion is a severe inflammation of the scalp with resulting alopecia that sometimes occurs with tinea capitis.	Administer systemic antifungals as prescribed; relapse rate is high with topical agents. Oral corticosteroids are indicated for kerion inflammation to help prevent alopecia. Instruct family on contagious aspect of disease; assess other family members and pets for organism. Teach prevention measures: never share combs, brushes, pillowcases, or headgear.
Tinea Corporis (Tinea Circinata, Ringworm of Body)	Fungal infection of the body that appears as an erythematous macule; progresses to rings of vesicles or scale with a clear center that appears alone or in clusters; usually occurs on exposed areas of body; can be moderately to intensely itchy.	Administer topical or systemic antifungal agents as prescribed. Infected pet is common source of infection. Teach patient prevention measures: avoid heat, moisture, and friction; keep skin areas, especially folds, dry; use clean towel and washcloth daily; wear cotton clothing, especially on hot, humid days.

TABLE 54.4   FUNGAL INFECTIONS—cont'd

Type	Description	Treatment/Nursing Care
Tinea Cruris (Ringworm of Groin, Jock Itch) Tinea cruris (ringworm of groin, jock itch).	Infection of groin, inner thighs, and buttocks area; may occur with tinea pedis; often in obese people who are participate in athletics. Lesion first appears as a small red scaly patch and then progresses to a sharply demarcated plaque with elevated scaly or vesicular borders; itching can range from minimal to severe.	Topical antifungals are prescribed; apply in a thin layer to rash and a few centimeters beyond border. Unresponsive cases may require oral antifungal agent. Teach patient prevention measures: bathe daily and change to clean underwear. Avoid tight clothing. Do not share personal items. Treat tinea pedis to prevent spread.
Tinea Unguium (Ringworm of Nails, Onychomycosis) Tinea unguium (ringworm of nails, **onychomycosis**).	Chronic fungal infection of nails, usually the toenails; a lifelong disease. There is yellow thickening of nail plate; it is friable and lusterless. Eventually crumbly debris accumulates under free edge of the nail and causes nail plate to become separated; over time, the nail may become thickened, painful, and destroyed.	Systemic antifungals are rarely given for toenail involvement but may be prescribed for fingernail involvement. Topical antifungals are usually ineffective because they do not penetrate nails. Nail may have to be surgically removed (nail avulsion). Keep nails neatly trimmed and buffed flat; gently scrape out any nail debris.
Candidiasis/Thrush Candidiasis/thrush. *From Taber's 22e.*	Oral candidiasis is called thrush. Infection of skin or mucous membranes with *Candida.* Grows in warm moist areas such as under breasts, in groin, vagina, or oral mucous membranes. Appears as white patches in mouth, white vaginal discharge, or red irritated areas in skinfolds. May occur as a result of antibiotic therapy because normal flora that usually keep *Candida* in check are destroyed, or with corticosteroid therapy.	Administer oral or topical antifungal agents as ordered. Examples include nystatin "swish and swallow" or lozenges for oral thrush, nystatin powder or ointment for skin infection, or vaginal suppositories or creams. Teach patient to keep skin clean and dry, especially in skinfold areas. Treatment is important to prevent systemic infection.

• **WORD** • **BUILDING** •

onychomycosis: onycho—fingernail or toenail + myco—fungus + osis—condition

Outlining the affected area with a marker can also help monitor progress but may be difficult if the borders are not clear.

Acne Vulgaris

Pathophysiology and Etiology

Acne vulgaris is a common skin disorder of the sebaceous glands and their hair follicles that usually occurs on the face, chest, upper back, and shoulders. The etiology is multifocal. The most common cause is hormonal changes during puberty.

The sebaceous glands are under endocrine control, especially the androgens. Stimulation of androgens (e.g., during adolescence or the menstrual cycle) in turn stimulates the sebaceous glands to increase sebum production. This, along with gradual obstruction of the pilosebaceous ducts with accumulated debris, ruptures the sebaceous glands, which causes an inflammatory reaction that may lead to papules, pustules, nodules, and cysts. Acne occurs when the ducts through which this sebum flows become plugged.

Other factors that influence the occurrence and severity of acne include a hereditary tendency, stress, and external irritants such as strong soaps or cosmetics. Acne is not related to diet, chocolate, sexual activity, or uncleanliness.

Prevention

Acne vulgaris occurs regardless of interventions; however, certain interventions can lessen the severity or prevent complications. Avoidance of "picking" pimples prevents further inflammation and scarring. The patient should avoid excessive washing, irritants, and abrasives.

Signs and Symptoms

The initial lesions are called comedones (singular: **comedo**). Closed comedones, or whiteheads, are small white papules with tiny follicular openings. These may eventually become open comedones, or blackheads. The color is not caused by dirt but by lipids and melanin pigment. Scarring occurs as a result of significant skin inflammation; picking can worsen inflammation and lead to further scarring. The resulting inflammation can lead to papules, pustules, nodules (Fig. 54.6), cysts, or abscesses.

Therapeutic Measures

Medical treatment helps prevent new lesions and helps control current lesions. Effective topical agents include benzoyl peroxide (Desquam-X, Benzagel), which is an antibacterial agent that may help prevent pore plugging; antibiotics (erythromycin,

tetracycline) to kill bacteria in follicles; and vitamin A acid (Retin-A, tretinoin) to loosen pore plugs and prevent occurrence of new comedones. Topical agents may be used alone or in combination. It may take 3 to 6 weeks before improvement is seen.

All topical agents should be applied with clean hands to acne-prone areas, not just where the acne occurs. They must be applied to dry skin. Medications should not be applied near eyes, nasolabial folds, or the corners of the mouth because of the potential for irritation. If the patient is ordered a combination of topical agents, unless contraindicated, the tretinoin is used at night and the others in the morning or afternoon. Tretinoin can be neutralized if mixed directly with other agents. The patient must be careful with sun or sunlamp exposure while using tretinoin. Also, remind the patient that it may be necessary to continue treatment even after the skin clears.

Systemic antibiotics (long term, low dose) and isotretinoin (Accutane) are usually reserved for severe cases of acne; the patient must be closely monitored for side effects. Estrogen therapy (oral contraceptives) may also be prescribed for young women; however, the risks often outweigh the benefits. Women should be aware that some antibiotics reduce the effectiveness of oral contraceptives.

Other medical treatments include comedone extraction, cryosurgery (freezing with liquid nitrogen), mild peeling (UV light, carbon dioxide, liquid nitrogen, mild acid), dermabrasion (deep chemical peel), excision of scars, and injection of fibrin or collagen below the scars. These treatments depend on the severity, age, condition, and physician and patient preference.

NURSING CARE TIP

Topical benzoyl peroxide may bleach colored fabrics. Have the patient wear a white cotton T-shirt under clothing if benzoyl peroxide is used on the back, and use an old or white pillowcase at night.

Nursing Process for the Patient With a Skin Infection

Data Collection

Subjective data collection regarding a skin infection can begin with the **WHAT'S UP?** acronym.

- **W**here is the skin infection located?
- **H**ow does it feel? Does it itch, burn, or hurt?
- What **A**ggravates or **A**lleviates the symptoms?
- **T**iming: How long has it been present?
- How **S**evere is it?
- **U**seful other data: Is there swelling, drainage, or fever?
- **P**atient's **P**erception: What does the patient think caused the infection?

FIGURE 54.6 Acne vulgaris. *From Taber's 22e, p. 33.*

Collection of objective data includes observing the affected area and describing the infection in terms of type and configuration of lesions, color, size, and presence of drainage. Also observe for swelling, and check for elevated temperature. If the patient has cellulitis of an extremity, measure and document the circumference of the extremity daily and as needed (prn).

Determine the patient's understanding of the cause of the infection, and of infection control measures.

Nursing Diagnoses, Planning, and Implementation
Risk for Infection (spread to surrounding or other areas)
EXPECTED OUTCOME: The infected area will not spread to other areas on patient or to other individuals.

- Monitor and document size and location of infected area daily and prn. *Careful monitoring can identify improvement or new spread of infection.*
- Monitor temperature every 8 hours and prn. *An increasing temperature can indicate worsening or systemic infection.*
- Monitor for signs and symptoms of systemic spread of infection, such as hypotension, tachycardia, and increasing temperature. *Systemic infection must be reported and treated promptly to prevent complications, including sepsis.*
- Use standard precautions, including careful hand hygiene, when providing patient care *to prevent transmission to yourself or to others.*
- Implement appropriate isolation precautions for the patient with a contagious infection. Contact precautions are usually sufficient, although airborne precautions may be necessary if immunocompromised individuals are present. *Isolation reduces spread of infection.*
- Instruct the patient on wound care, appropriate hand hygiene, and disposal of soiled dressings. *The patient must follow precautions to protect self and others.*
- Instruct patient on use of prescribed anti-infective agents, including the importance of taking it exactly as directed *to prevent development of a resistant infection.*
- For the patient with acne, advise keeping hands away from the face and avoiding touching or squeezing pimples. Keep hair clean and off the face. *These measures help prevent spread, secondary infection, and scarring.*

Acute Pain related to inflammation as evidenced by patient rating on appropriate pain scale
EXPECTED OUTCOME: The patient will state that pain is controlled at an acceptable level.

- Monitor pain (if present) using a pain scale. *Pain assessment provides a basis for nursing intervention.*
- Administer analgesics as ordered, especially before dressing changes or treatments. *Analgesics relieve pain and help prevent pain during dressing changes.*
- For the patient with shingles:
  - Apply cool, moist compresses to painful or itching lesions to help cleanse and dry lesions and reduce itching.
  - Apply firm dressings such as wraps, stockings, or a snug T-shirt to reduce pain from post-herpetic neuralgia.

- For the patient with cellulitis:
  - Elevate affected extremity as ordered to reduce swelling and increase comfort.

Evaluation
If interventions have been effective, the skin lesions will improve and will not spread to new areas or to others. The patient will state that pain is manageable.

PARASITIC SKIN DISORDERS

Pediculosis
Pathophysiology and Etiology
Pediculosis is an infestation by lice. There are three basic types: pediculosis capitis (head lice), pediculosis corporis (body lice), and pediculosis pubis (pubic, or crab, lice). Generally, the lice bite the skin and feed on human blood, leaving their eggs and excrement, which can cause intense itching. The lice are oval and are approximately 2 mm in length.

In pediculosis capitis, the female louse lays eggs (nits) close to the scalp, where the nits become firmly attached to hair shafts. The most common areas of infestation are the back of the scalp and behind the ears. The nits are about 1 to 3 mm in length and appear silvery white and glistening. Transmission is by direct contact or contact with infested objects, such as combs, brushes, wigs, hats, and bedding. It is most common in children and people with long hair.

Pediculosis corporis is caused by body lice that lay eggs in the seams of clothing and then pierce the skin. Areas of the skin usually involved are the neck, trunk, and thighs.

Pediculosis pubis is caused by crab lice. It is generally localized in the genital region, but it can also be seen on hairs of the chest, axillae, eyelashes, and beard. The lice are about 2 mm in length and have a crablike appearance. It is chiefly transmitted through sexual contact or, to a lesser degree, by infested bed linens.

Prevention
Prevention involves avoidance of contact with an infected person or object. Brushes, combs, hats, and other personal items should not be shared. Good personal hygiene and routine clothes washing are other preventive measures; however, even someone with meticulous hygiene can develop an infestation if there is contact with the organism.

Signs and Symptoms
Pediculosis capitis can result in no itching or intense itching and scratching, especially at the back of the head. Nits may be noticeably attached to hair. A papular rash may be seen.

Pediculosis corporis may appear as tiny hemorrhagic points. Excoriations may be noted on the back, shoulders, abdomen, and extremities. It may also cause intense itching.

Pediculosis pubis results in mild to severe itching, especially at night. Black or reddish brown dots (lice excreta) may be noted at the base of hairs or in underclothing. Gray-blue macules may also be noted on the trunk, thighs, and axillae; this is the result of the insects' saliva mixing with bilirubin.

Complications

Secondary bacterial infections can occur with pediculosis capitis, resulting in impetigo, furuncles, pustules, crusts, and matted hair. Complications of pediculosis corporis include secondary infection and hyperpigmentation. Most important, body lice may be vectors for rickettsial or other systemic disease. Complications with pediculosis pubis include dermatitis and the coexistence of other sexually transmitted infections.

Diagnostic Tests

Diagnosis is made through history and physical examination. The patient may also be tested for other sexually transmitted infections if pediculosis pubis is present.

Therapeutic Measures

Medical treatment is aimed at killing the parasites and mechanically removing nits. Over-the-counter (OTC) pediculicides containing pyrethrins or permethrin are the most commonly recommended compounds. These agents should kill the lice and nits, although some lice develop pesticide resistance, making mechanical removal necessary. Permethrin (Nix) remains active for about a week, killing the adult lice immediately and the nits when they hatch days later. Pyrethrins (RID, A-200 Pyrinate) must be reapplied in 1 week to kill newly hatched lice. Prescription treatments include benzyl alcohol lotion (Ulesfia), ivermectin lotion (Sklice), malathion lotion (Ovide), and spinosad (Natroba).

If initial treatment is not effective, lindane may be prescribed. Lindane is a controversial, highly toxic topical medication that is only used as a second-line agent.

Complications are treated, as appropriate, with antipruritics, topical corticosteroids, and systemic antibiotics. Physostigmine ophthalmic ointment is applied to affected eyebrows and eyelashes. Other medications should not be applied to eyebrows or eyelashes.

Patient Education

Reassure the patient and family that head lice can happen to anyone and that it is not a sign of uncleanliness. Lice infestations are treated on an outpatient basis, so patient education is important. Package instructions should be followed for correct usage of all medications.

Instruct the patient to bathe with soap and water and to disinfect combs and brushes in hot, medicated soapy water. A fine-toothed comb dipped in vinegar can be used to remove nits from hairy areas. Nits can be removed from eyebrows and eyelashes with a cotton-tipped applicator after treatment. Clothing, linens, and towels should be laundered in hot water and detergent; unwashable clothing should be dry cleaned or sealed in a plastic bag for 10 days. Treatment should be started immediately to prevent rapid spread. Family members and close contacts (sexual contacts with pediculosis pubis) should be examined for infestation and should put on clean clothing.

Shampoos and lotions kill nits, but they do not remove them. To loosen nits from the scalp, the hair may be soaked in a solution of equal parts vinegar and water and a shower cap worn for 15 minutes. Then comb the hair with a fine-toothed comb and thoroughly rinse or shampoo to mechanically remove the nits. Children may return to school after adequate medical treatment, even if dead nits are still present.

 NURSING CARE TIP

It is not possible to dry clean or wash all infected items, such as mattresses and upholstered furniture. Teach patients to thoroughly vacuum upholstered furniture. The lice die in 3 to 4 days without human contact.

Scabies

Pathophysiology and Etiology

Scabies is a contagious skin disease caused by the mite *Sarcoptes scabiei*. It results from intimate or prolonged skin contact or prolonged contact with infected clothing, bedding, or animals (e.g., dogs, cats, other small animals). The parasite burrows into the superficial layer of the skin (Fig. 54.7). These burrows appear as short, wavy, brownish black lines. The patient is asymptomatic while the organism multiplies, but it is most contagious at this time. Symptoms do not occur until almost 4 weeks after the time of contact.

Prevention

All persons (and animals) in intimate contact with an infected patient should be treated at the same time to eliminate the mites. The mites survive less than 24 hours without human contact. Therefore, bed linens, clothes, and towels should be washed in hot water and dried at high heat, but furnishings need not be cleaned. Clean clothing and linens should be applied.

Signs and Symptoms

The major complaints are itching and rash. Itching can be intense, especially at night. Itching begins about 1 month after infestation and may persist for days to weeks after treatment. The rash appears as small, scattered erythematous papules, concentrated in finger webs, axillae, wrist folds, umbilicus, groin, and genitals. Crusts and scales may be present. Male patients may have excoriated papules on the penis and groin area.

FIGURE 54.7 *Scabies. From Taber's 22e, p. 2082.*

Complications

Hypersensitivity reactions to the mite can result in crusted lesions, vesicles, pustules, excoriations, and bacterial superinfections.

Diagnostic Tests

Diagnosis is confirmed by a superficial shaving of a lesion and microscopic evaluation for adult mites, eggs, or feces.

Therapeutic Measures

Topical scabicides (permethrin/Elimite, crotamiton/Crotan) are used for chemical disinfection. Usually, the cream or lotion is applied in a thin layer to the entire body from neck to feet (including genitals, umbilicus, and skinfold areas), is left on overnight (8–12 hours), and is washed off in the morning; however, package instructions should be referred to for each medication. One or two applications are usually curative, depending on the agent prescribed. Antipruritics may be prescribed for itching.

Patient Education

A warm soapy bath or shower removes scales and skin debris. Advise the patient to apply the topical medication as ordered, not to use scabicides repeatedly because they can increase itching and cause further skin irritation, to follow medication directions, to treat family members and close contacts simultaneously to eliminate mites, to wear clean clothing, and to use clean linens. Remind the patient that itching may continue for up to 2 weeks after treatment until the allergic reaction subsides. (Dead mites remain in the epidermis until exfoliated.)

NURSING CARE TIP

Animals infested with scabies should be treated by a veterinarian, so they won't infect humans.

PEMPHIGUS

Pathophysiology and Etiology

Pemphigus is an acute or chronic, serious skin disease characterized by the appearance of bullae (large fluid-filled blisters) of various sizes on otherwise normal skin and mucous membranes. The etiology is unclear, but it is known to be an autoimmune disorder. Sun exposure, genetic predisposition, and certain foods and drugs (e.g., penicillamine, captopril, and enalapril) may trigger the disorder. It usually occurs in patients from middle to older age. One type of pemphigus is associated with malignancy.

The autoimmune response that occurs in pemphigus causes a patient's own antibodies to attack the skin and mucous membranes and destroy the protein "glue" that holds the cells together. The result is skin that separates from itself, causing the characteristic blisters.

Signs and Symptoms

Successive crops of bullae suddenly appear on skin or mucous membranes. The bullae are fragile and flaccid. They enlarge, rupture, and form painful, raw, eroded, partial-thickness wounds that bleed, ooze, and form crusts. Pemphigus usually originates in the oral mucosa and then spreads to the trunk. Large areas of the body become involved.

Besides the appearance of the blisters, the patient experiences pain, burning, and itching. The lesions have a foul smell. Involvement of the oral mucosa can interfere with chewing, swallowing, and talking. The patient is in constant misery.

Complications

The major complication is a secondary bacterial infection. This disease has high associated morbidity and mortality rates.

Diagnostic Tests

A positive Nikolsky's sign is a characteristic finding. This occurs when there is sloughing or blistering of normal skin when minimal pressure is applied. A biopsy of a blister reveals acantholysis, or separation of epidermal cells from one another.

Therapeutic Measures

Treatment is aimed at controlling the disease, healing the skin, and preventing complications. Corticosteroids in large doses and immunosuppressants are prescribed to control the disease and bring about remission. Biological therapy (rituximab/Rituxan) targets the offending white blood cells. Medicated mouthwashes may be prescribed for mouth lesions. Antibiotic and antifungal agents are prescribed as needed for secondary infections. Analgesics and antipruritics are prescribed according to the patient's specific signs and symptoms. Because of fluid, blood, and protein losses through the partial-thickness skin injuries, a high-protein, high-calorie diet is recommended, along with appropriate fluid replacement therapy. Generalized pemphigus lesions may be treated in the hospital with a therapeutic plasmapheresis to remove antibodies. Some cases clear up completely. Others require ongoing treatment.

Nursing Care

Monitor fluid balance with regular intake and output, body weight, and blood pressure measurement. Encourage the patient to maintain adequate fluid intake. Offer cool drinks often to lessen discomfort.

Tepid wet dressings or baths help lessen secondary infection, cleanse the area, decrease odor, and increase comfort. Potassium permanganate baths may decrease infection and clean and deodorize the area. Always thoroughly dissolve potassium permanganate crystals in a small container before adding to tub water. Undissolved crystals may further damage and burn the skin. Dry the patient thoroughly after the bath. Do not use tape on the patient because this may cause further blistering. Talcum powder may be used to keep the skin from sticking to clothing and bed linens.

• WORD • BUILDING •
pemphigus: pemphix—blister

Teach the patient to maintain meticulous oral hygiene. Explain the effects and side effects of medications. Teach the importance of avoiding sun exposure or other triggers. Spicy or acidic foods may exacerbate oral lesions. Even dentures and contact lenses can irritate tissues in some patients. Provide appropriate psychosocial support because of the length of illness, the chronic nature of the condition, and the physical appearance of lesions. Find additional information at www.pemphigus.org.

SKIN LESIONS

Skin lesions can be either benign (noncancerous) or malignant. Benign lesions are described in Table 54.5. Malignant lesions are discussed next. Also see "Cultural Considerations."

Malignant Skin Lesions

Pathophysiology and Etiology

The most common skin malignancies include basal cell carcinoma, squamous cell carcinoma, and malignant melanoma. The major cause of skin malignancies is overexposure to ultraviolet rays, most commonly sunlight. Other factors include being fair skinned and blue eyed, genetic tendencies, history of x-ray therapy, exposure to certain chemical agents (e.g., arsenic, paraffin, coal tar), burn scars, chronic osteomyelitis, and immunosuppressive therapy.

Basal cell carcinoma arises from the basal cell layer of the epidermis. It is the most common type of skin cancer. This tumor is mainly seen on sun-exposed areas of the body. The lesion appears as a small pearly or translucent papule with a rolled, waxy edge, depressed center, telangiectasia (lesion formed by dilation of vessels), crusting, and ulceration (Fig. 54.8). Metastasis is rare, although it may be locally invasive.

Squamous cell carcinoma arises from the epidermis. It can occur on sun-exposed areas of the skin and mucous membranes and is mainly seen on the lower lip, neck, tongue, head, and dorsal surfaces of the hands. It can occur on normal skin or on a preexisting lesion (actinic keratosis). The lesion appears as a single, crusted, scaled, eroded papule, nodule, or plaque (Fig. 54.9). A neglected lesion appears more rough, scaly, and darker colored. The lesion is fragile and prone to oozing and bleeding. Untreated squamous cell carcinoma can metastasize to distant areas of the body.

Malignant melanoma, as the name implies, is a malignant growth of pigment cells (melanocytes, Fig. 54.10). It is highly metastatic, with a higher mortality rate than basal or squamous cell carcinomas. This tumor can occur anywhere on the body; about half arise from preexisting nevi or moles. There are three general types: lentigo maligna, superficial spreading, and nodular.

Lentigo maligna melanoma appears as a slow-growing dark macule on exposed skin surfaces (especially the face) of older adults (Fig. 54.11). The lesion has irregular borders and brown, tan, and black coloring. Prognosis is good if treated in the early stage.

Superficial spreading melanoma is the most common melanoma. It can occur anywhere on the body and is usually seen in middle-aged persons. The lesion appears as a slightly elevated plaque with an irregular border. The coloring of the lesion varies in combinations of black, brown, and pink. The fragile surface may bleed or ooze. Eventually the plaque develops into a nodule. The cure rate is excellent when it is in the plaque phase; prognosis is poor in the nodular phase.

Nodular melanoma occurs suddenly as a spherical papule or nodule on the skin or in a mole. Coloration is blue-black, blue-gray, or reddish blue color that may have a rim of inflammation. The lesion is fragile and bleeds easily. Metastasis occurs rapidly. This type of melanoma has the least favorable prognosis. Early diagnosis and treatment is imperative.

Prevention

Risk of most types of skin cancer can be reduced by limiting or avoiding direct exposure to UV rays (sun, tanning booths). If exposure to the sun is necessary, exposure should be avoided during its highest intensity (between 1000 and 1600).

Cultural Considerations

- Darker skinned people have a tendency toward an overgrowth of connective tissue components concerned with the protection against infection and repair after injury. Keloid formation is one example of this tendency toward overgrowth of connective tissue. Lymphoma and systemic lupus erythematosus may occur due to this overgrowth of connective tissue.
- Some African American men have facial hair that is kinky, curls back on itself, and penetrates the skin, which can result in pustules and small keloids. Many use depilatories or electric razors to prevent nicking the skin, which can also cause keloids.
- Darker skinned people have an increased incidence of birthmarks and Mongolian spots compared with lighter skinned people. Mongolian spots disappear over time. The nurse must be cautious not to mistake these spots for bruising, which can indicate injury or abuse.
- For people with light skin, such as those of German, Polish, and Irish descent, prolonged exposure to the sun may increase the incidence of skin cancer. Teach patients to protect themselves from sun exposure to reduce their risk of skin cancer. Nevi (freckles and skin discolorations) occur more often in lighter skinned individuals. They are most common in European Americans, followed by Asians, and then darker skinned African Americans.

TABLE 54.5 BENIGN SKIN LESIONS

Type	Description	Treatment
Cyst	A saclike growth with a defined wall that may contain liquid, semifluid, or solid material. An epidermoid cyst is the most common type of cyst. It results from proliferation of epidermal cells in the dermis. Rarely, it is associated with carcinoma development. Epidermoid cyst.	Not all cysts need to be treated. Treatments include intralesional steroid therapy and antibiotics, if indicated. If excision is done, the entire cyst wall is removed to prevent recurrence.
Seborrheic Keratosis	A benign skin lesion with pigmented light tan to dark brown patches. The plaques or papules have a "stuck-on" appearance caused by the proliferation of epidermal cells and keratin piled on the skin surface. Cause is unknown, but it tends to occur in middle-aged to older patients, most commonly on the trunk, scalp, face, and extremities. Seborrheic keratosis.	Treatment is cosmetic only, or if lesion becomes irritated from friction. Topical agents may be used to reduce lesion size or height. Liquid nitrogen cryotherapy or light curettage may be performed if necessary for removal.

Continued

TABLE 54.5 BENIGN SKIN LESIONS—cont'd

Type	Description	Treatment
Keloid Keloid. *From Taber's 22e, p. 1321.*	A benign growth of fibrous tissue (scar formation) at the site of trauma or surgical incision; occurs in various sizes. Growth of tissue is out of proportion to what is needed for normal healing. The lesion extends beyond the original injury and occurs mainly in middle-aged and older adult clients and darker skinned patients.	Treatment varies and is not always successful; a larger scar may ensue. Some treatment options include compression therapy, corticosteroid injections into lesions, excision, and laser therapy.
Pigmented Nevus (mole)	A benign, flesh-colored to dark brown macule or papule located randomly over the entire skin surface of the body. Can be inherited or acquired and occurs mostly in light-skinned patients. Usually begin to appear between 1 and 4 years of age, increasing in number into adulthood. Some contain a few hairs. There are many variations. Rate of transformation to a malignant melanoma is higher in congenital moles and larger lesions. Clinical signs of melanoma include change in color or size; inflammation of surrounding skin; irregular or spreading borders; variegated colors, especially a bluish pigmentation; bleeding; and oozing, crusting, and itching. Usually nevi larger than 1 cm should be carefully examined. Dermal mole.	Treatment is indicated for risk of melanoma, unsightly nevi (cosmetic), repeated irritation (rubbing from belt, bra), trauma, large moles, and client report of a change in the mole. Surgical removal can include excision (preferred) or surgical shave. All excised moles should be sent for histological examination.

TABLE 54.5 BENIGN SKIN LESIONS—cont'd

Type	Description	Treatment
Wart	Small, common, benign growth of the skin resulting from the hypertrophy of the papillae and epidermis; caused by a virus. Common warts, often seen on hands and fingers, appear as raised, flesh-colored papules that have a rough surface. May crack, fissure, bleed, and be painful to lateral pinching and direct, firm pressure. Plantar warts occur on the sole of the foot. They may appear granular, pitted, or protuberant, with a callous of surrounding normal skin. Incubation period can be several weeks to months. Virus is spread by direct contact.	Patient should be cautioned not to spread lesions by picking or biting them. Treatment is indicated for symptomatic warts and for cosmetic purposes. General treatments include keratolytic agents (e.g., salicylic acid plasters) to soften and reduce keratin; cryotherapy (liquid nitrogen); and light electrodesiccation and curettage (requires local anesthesia).

Warts.

Type	Description	Treatment
Hemangioma (Angioma)	Benign vascular tumor of dilated blood vessels that can have varied clinical manifestations Nevus flammeus involves mature capillaries on the face and neck. It is a congenital neoplasm that appears as a pink-red to bluish purple macular patch. Port-wine stains or port-wine angiomas appear as violet-red macular patches, usually singular lesions, growing proportionately as the child grows. These lesions can persist indefinitely. Cherry hemangiomas are commonly seen in older adults. They appear as small round papules that can vary in color from red to purple.	Nevus flammeus is usually treated for cosmetic reasons. Port-wine stains, if large enough, may be treated surgically or with pulse-dye laser therapy. Cosmetics to camouflage the affected area are also available. Treatment for cherry hemangiomas is usually not prescribed, except for cosmetic purposes.

The patient should use a protective sunscreen with sun protection factor (SPF) of 15 or more, and wear sun-protective clothing such as hats and long sleeves. The patient should seek medical advice if there is a change in color, size, shape, sensation, or character of a lesion or mole.

Diagnostic Tests

A preliminary diagnosis can be based on the appearance of the lesion. A definitive diagnosis is made by biopsy. Other tests are performed based on the results of the pathological examination.

Therapeutic Measures

Medical treatment depends on the type, thickness, and location of the lesion; the stage of the disease; and the age and general health of the patient. Generally, lesions are surgically excised with a 1- to 2-cm margin to make sure no cancer cells remain. Regional node dissection varies; it may be advised if the nodes in the area drain to one group. Grafting may be necessary for closure or repair. Chemotherapy may be used for metastasis. Radiation therapy may be used as adjunct treatment or may be

FIGURE 54.8 Basal cell carcinoma. Note pearly, flesh-colored papule with depressed center and rolled edge. From Goldsmith, L. A., Lazarus, G. S., & Tharp, M. D. (1997). *Adult and pediatric dermatology*. Philadelphia: F.A. Davis, p. 158, with permission.

FIGURE 54.10 Malignant melanoma. From Goldsmith, L. A., Lazarus, G. S., & Tharp, M. D. (1997). *Adult and pediatric dermatology*. Philadelphia: F.A. Davis, p. 137, with permission.

FIGURE 54.9 Squamous cell carcinoma. Surface is fragile and bleeds easily. From Goldsmith, L. A., Lazarus, G. S., & Tharp, M. D. (1997). *Adult and pediatric dermatology*. Philadelphia: F.A. Davis, p. 237, with permission.

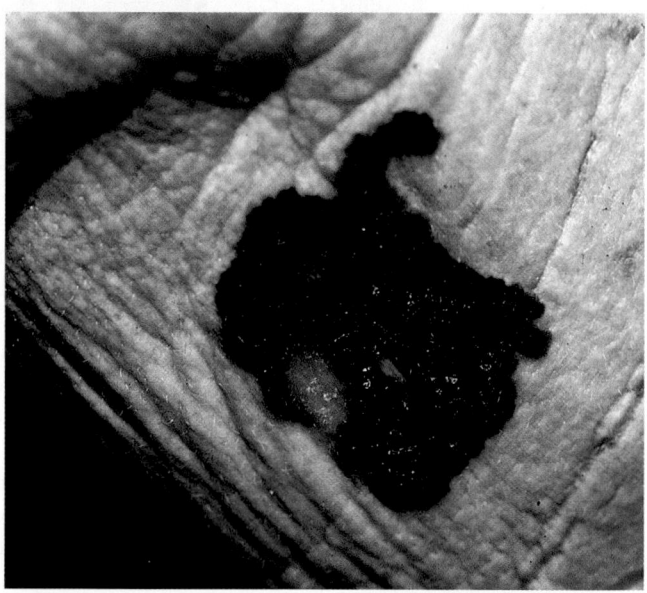

FIGURE 54.11 Lentigo maligna. From Goldsmith, L. A., Lazarus, G. S., & Tharp, M. D. (1997). *Adult and pediatric dermatology*. Philadelphia: F.A. Davis, p. 55, with permission.

recommended for patients with a deeply invasive tumor or those who are poor surgical risks. Other therapies include cryosurgery or curettage and electrodesiccation.

Nursing Care

Perform a complete skin examination. Palpate lesions to determine texture, size, and firmness. Document size, location, color, surface characteristics, pain, discomfort, itching, and bleeding. Note when the patient first discovered the lesion.

Nursing care of the patient with cancer is documented in Chapter 11. Specific nursing care related to cryosurgery includes preparing the patient for the procedure. Explain that minor discomfort can be expected with little or no local anesthesia. Expect swelling, local tenderness, and hemorrhagic

blister formation 1 to 2 days after the procedure. After the procedure, the area is cleansed as ordered and prescribed ointments are applied.

Specific nursing care for curettage and electrodesiccation includes preparing the patient for the procedure. After local anesthesia, a dermal curette is used to scrape away the lesion, followed by electrodesiccation of the remaining wound; the wound heals by secondary intention, usually with minimal scarring. After the procedure, the wound is cleansed and dressed as prescribed.

NURSING CARE TIP

To help patients find melanomas as early as possible, encourage them to examine their skin regularly and report any lesions that fit this profile:

- Asymmetrical shape
- Irregular or poorly defined border
- Variable color
- Diameter larger than that of a pencil eraser
- Changing appearance

DERMATOLOGICAL SURGERY

Plastic or reconstructive surgery is performed to correct certain defects, scars, and malformations and to restore function or prevent further loss of function. This type of surgery is usually an elective procedure; it may be prescribed by the HCP, or it may be the wish of the patient hoping to improve body image. Common types of plastic surgical procedures are listed in Table 54.6. Care of the surgical patient is covered in Chapter 12.

TABLE 54.6 COMMON PLASTIC SURGICAL PROCEDURES

Operation	Description	Purpose	Possible Complications	Postoperative Nursing Care Considerations
Rhinoplasty (Nose)	Removal of excessive nasal cartilage, tissue, or bone; reshaping of nose	Correct congenital or acquired septal defects; improve cosmetic shape of nose	Hemorrhage, hematoma; temporary ecchymosis and edema; infection, septal perforation	Monitor dressing and packing for bright-red bleeding; monitor vital signs and level of consciousness; maintain semi-Fowler's position to minimize edema.
Blepharoplasty (Eyelid)	Incisions on upper and lower lids with excision of fat and skin and primary closure	Removal of bags under eyes and wrinkles and bulges	Corneal injury; hematoma; ectropion; rarely visual loss and wound infection	Administer antibiotic ointment as ordered; maintain eye dressings; maintain semi-Fowler's position to minimize edema.
Rhytidoplasty (Face lift)	Incision anterior to ear with removal of excessive skin and tissue; the subcutaneous tissue and fascia are folded and stretched	Removal of excessive wrinkling or sagging skin	Hemorrhage; hematoma; ecchymosis, and edema (temporary); wound infection, facial nerve damage	Surgical improvement lasts from 5 to 10 years; apply antibiotic ointment to suture line; maintain semi-Fowler's position to minimize edema.
Otoplasty (Ear)	Incision of ear for correction of defect	Correct congenital defects; correct deformities; improve cosmetic shape of ear	Hemorrhage; hematoma; edema; wound infection	Maintain ear dressing for about 1 week; protect ear at times of sleep for about 3 weeks.

Home Health Hints

- A wound-measuring device that will not be misplaced is your hand. Measure your hand, such as the nailbed of a particular finger or the space between joints. Use these as a guide to determine wound measurements.
- Sanitary pads make great cushions for bony prominences. You can also place them in a cotton sock for better molding.
- A handheld shower head is useful for debriding some leg ulcers. Do not use it if it is too painful.
- To relieve pruritus (itchy skin), oatmeal baths are sometimes prescribed. An inexpensive way to do this is to place a half cup of quick-cooking oatmeal in a cotton sock. Put it under the faucet as you fill the tub and ring out the sock.
- Instruct patients to prevent red, dried, cracked skin on hands by wearing gloves outside in the cold or windy weather to prevent chapping, avoiding overheating the house, using a humidifier to keep the air moist, applying hand lotion two or three times a day and after each hand washing, using soaps with added oil and avoiding those with deodorants, using sunscreen with an SPF factor of at least 15, and stopping smoking (smoking reduces blood flow to the skin).
- If necessary, a specialty bed or mattress can be obtained to use in a patient's home.
- Instruct patients who are confined to a wheelchair to rise up briefly, using their armrests, and shift weight every 15 minutes to prevent pressure ulcers.
- Instruct patients with dressings to keep them clean and dry. Unless the patient or caregiver has been instructed on how to perform the dressing change, inform him or her to contact the home care agency if the dressing falls off.
- A patient can wear a cast shoe over a dressing on the foot. This will help protect the dressing and provide additional support for the patient while ambulating.
- Surgi-net, or a similar stretchy cover, can be used to cover dressings for patients with tape sensitivities. They are also good for additional support to prevent a dressing from falling off.

SUGGESTED ANSWERS TO

CRITICAL THINKING

■ *Mr. Russ*

1. Perform a Braden Scale assessment. A specialty pressure-relieving bed may be appropriate for Mr. Russ.
   - Change Mr. Russ's position at least every 2 hours if not more frequently. Keep his heels off of the bed at all times by propping them on pillows.
   - Request a dietary consult because the body cannot meet the increased healing demands if there is an albumin deficiency. Mr. Russ may need increased protein (contraindicated in renal failure). He may also needs fats, carbohydrates, vitamins, and minerals for wound healing. A dietitian can help determine the amounts of calories and types of foods for the best prevention and/or healing.
   - If Mr. Russ is able to sit up in a chair, provide a chair cushion to prevent skin breakdown and have him shift his weight every 15 minutes.
   - Mr. Russ is wearing a brace, so examine the underlying tissue for pressure areas. Braces and splints must be padded to avoid skin breakdown.

2. Involve the physician, dietitian, wound nurse, RN, physical therapist, and nursing assistant. The nursing assistant is one of the most important members of this team because he or she is often responsible for bathing and turning patients. Ask to be called to examine Mr. Russ's skin during bathing, and teach the assistant warning signs to report.

■ *Mrs. Long*

Ask how long she is leaving the shampoo in her hair. For medicated scalp shampoos to work properly, they must remain on the scalp for several minutes. Package instructions should be carefully checked for each product because they vary from product to product.

REVIEW QUESTIONS

1. The nurse notes scratch marks on a patient with psoriasis. What are interventions that will decrease itching and protect the skin that the nurse can teach the patient? **Select all that apply.**
   1. Apply pressure to the itchy area with a clean cloth.
   2. Encourage use of gloves at night.
   3. Bathe daily in a hot soapy bath.
   4. Consider taking an antihistamine at bedtime.
   5. Use a room humidifier.

2. What information is most important for the nurse to teach patients about avoiding malignant skin lesions?
   1. Shower or bathe daily.
   2. Avoid contact with allergens and irritants
   3. Avoid overexposure to ultraviolet rays
   4. Avoid others with malignant lesions

3. The nurse notes a pressure wound on a newly admitted patient's ischial tuberosity, with a thick, tough black center. Which intervention is most appropriate **first**?
   1. Coat the ulcer with antibiotic ointment.
   2. Snip away the black tissue with sterile scissors.
   3. Flush the wound with sterile saline.
   4. Talk to the HCP about débridement.

4. A patient develops wounds on the sacrum and buttocks despite being turned and repositioned regularly. Which factors may have contributed to the patient's skin breakdown? **Select all that apply.**
   1. The patient is 20 pounds overweight.
   2. The patient commonly slides down in the chair.
   3. Staff use a lift sheet to move the patient in bed.
   4. The patient sits in a chair most of the day.
   5. The patient is often diaphoretic.
   6. The patient is incontinent of urine and stool.

5. Which instruction should the nurse provide to the patient being treated for scabies?
   1. "Dry clean all linens, towels, and clothes."
   2. "Wash linens, towels, and clothes."
   3. "Discard infested mattresses."
   4. "Remove infested pets from the home."

6. A patient diagnosed with impetigo contagiosa wants to know when the disease will no longer be contagious. Which response by the nurse is correct?
   1. One week after treatment is started
   2. After spread of lesions has stopped
   3. After all the lesions crust over
   4. When all lesions are healed

Answers can be found in Appendix C.

References

National Pressure Ulcer Advisory Panel. (2007). *Pressure ulcer stages revised by NPUAP.* Retrieved May 24, 2010, from www.npuap.org/pr2.htm

Vig, S., Dowsett, C., Berg, L., Caravaggi, C., Rome, P., Birke-Sorensen, H., . . . Runkel N., and the International Expert Panel on Negative Pressure Wound Therapy. (2011). Evidence-based recommendations for the use of negative pressure wound therapy in chronic wounds: Steps towards an international consensus. *Journal of Tissue Viability, 20,* S1–S18.

 For additional resources and information visit **davispl.us/medsurg5**

55

Nursing Care of Patients With Burns

KEY TERMS

autograft (AW-toh-graft)
epithelialization (ep-ih-THEE-lee-al-eye-ZAY-shun)
escharotomy (ess-kar-AHT-oh-mee)
hemochromogen (HEEM-oh-KROH-moh-jen)

LEARNING OUTCOMES

1. Explain the pathophysiology of burns.
2. Describe current therapeutic measures used for burns.
3. List data to collect when caring for patients with burns.
4. Plan nursing care for patients with burns.
5. Explain how you will know if your nursing interventions have been effective.

Many people are hospitalized each year for burns. Burns affect not only the skin but also every major body system. Smoke inhalation and wound infections complicate care of the patient who has been burned.

PATHOPHYSIOLOGY AND SIGNS AND SYMPTOMS

Burns are wounds caused by an energy transfer from a heat source to the body, heating the tissue enough to cause damage. Locally, the heat denatures cellular protein and interrupts the blood supply. The three zones of tissue damage that occur with burns are described in Figure 55.1.

The amount of skin damage is related to (1) the temperature of the burning agent, (2) the burning agent itself, (3) the duration of exposure, (4) the conductivity of tissue, and (5) the thickness of the involved dermal structures.

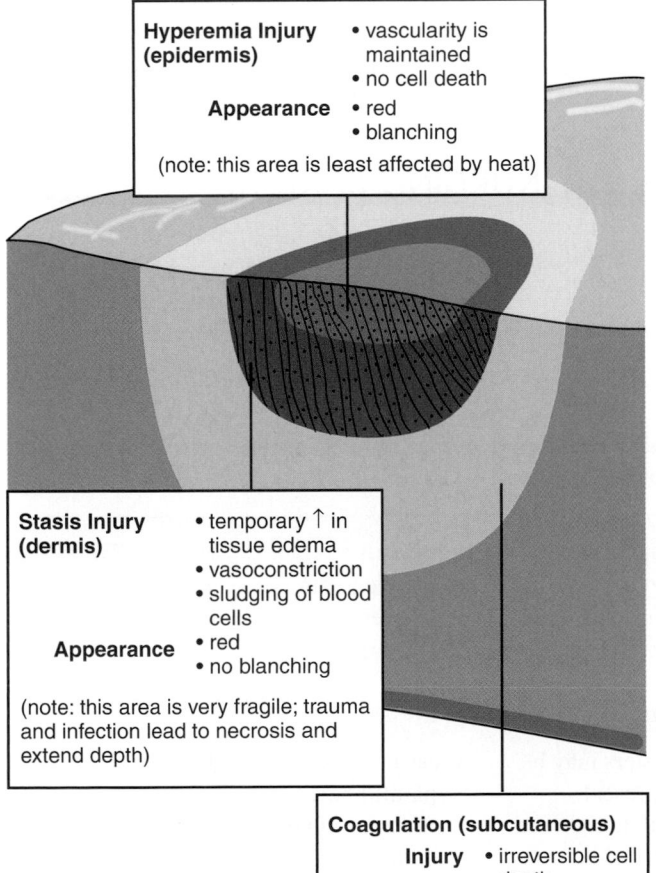

| Hyperemia Injury (epidermis) | • vascularity is maintained • no cell death |
| Appearance | • red • blanching |

(note: this area is least affected by heat)

| Stasis Injury (dermis) | • temporary ↑ in tissue edema • vasoconstriction • sludging of blood cells |
| Appearance | • red • no blanching |

(note: this area is very fragile; trauma and infection lead to necrosis and extend depth)

Coagulation (subcutaneous)	
Injury	• irreversible cell death
Appearance	• white or gray • no blanching

FIGURE 55.1 Three zones of tissue damage. Modified from Ruppert, S. D., Kernick, J. G., & Dolan, J. T. [1996]. *Dolan's critical care nursing*. Philadelphia: F.A. Davis, p. 942, with permission.

Alterations in normal skin function resulting from a major burn injury include loss of protective functions, impaired ability to regulate temperature, increased risk of infection, changes in sensory function, loss of fluids, impaired skin regeneration, and impaired secretory and excretory functions.

Systemic Responses

Alterations in the functional capacity of the skin in response to a burn affect virtually all major body systems.

Fluid Balance

Following a major burn, increased capillary permeability leads to the leakage of plasma and proteins into the tissue, resulting in the formation of edema and loss of intravascular volume. There is also water loss by evaporation through the burned tissue that can be 4 to 15 times normal. Increased metabolism leads to further water loss through the respiratory system.

Cardiac Function

A burn is followed by an initial decrease in cardiac output, which is further compromised by the loss of circulating plasma volume. Severe hematologic changes resulting from tissue damage and vascular changes occur in patients with major burns. Plasma moves into the interstitial space because of increased capillary permeability. In the first 48 hours after a burn, fluid shifts lead to hypovolemia and, if untreated, hypovolemic shock. Loss of intravascular fluid causes a relative increase in hematocrit, and red blood cells are destroyed. The intense heat decreases platelet function and half-life. Leukocyte and platelet aggregation may progress to thrombosis.

Metabolic Changes

Metabolic demands are very high in patients with burns. A high metabolic rate proportional to the severity of the burn is usually maintained until wound closure. This hypermetabolism is further compromised by associated injuries, surgical interventions, and the stress response. Severe catabolism also begins early and is associated with a negative nitrogen balance, weight loss, and decreased wound healing. Elevated catecholamine (epinephrine, norepinephrine) levels are triggered by the stress response. This, along with elevated glucagon levels, can stimulate hyperglycemia.

Gastrointestinal Problems

A few of the gastrointestinal (GI) problems that can develop with a major burn include gastric dilation, peptic ulcers, and paralytic ileus. Most of these problems occur in response to fluid shifting, dehydration, opioid analgesics, immobility, depressed gastric motility, and the stress response.

Renal Function

Acute renal insufficiency can occur as a result of hypovolemia and decreased cardiac output. Fluid loss and inadequate fluid replacement can lead to decreased renal blood flow and glomerular filtration rate. Extensive burns can cause destruction of muscle, creating myoglobin casts that can block renal tubules and lead to renal failure.

Pulmonary Effects

Pulmonary effects are mostly related to smoke inhalation. However, hyperventilation may occur with any moderate to major burn injury, usually proportional to the severity of the burn. Oxygen consumption increases because of the hypermetabolic state, fear, anxiety, and pain.

BE SAFE!

BE VIGILANT! It is not uncommon to administer massive volumes of intravenous (IV) fluids to severely burned patients. The patient must be closely monitored with hemodynamic monitoring to avoid fluid overload.

Immune Function

With the skin destroyed, the body loses its first line of defense against infection. Major burns also depress immunoglobulins (Ig)A, IgG, and IgM.

BE SAFE!

BE VIGILANT! You must be vigilant in monitoring for infection, as infection is a real and life-threatening risk to severely burned patients.

Evaluation of Burn Injuries

The severity of a burn injury is determined by the depth of tissue destruction (Table 55.1 and Fig. 55.2), percentage of body surface area injured, cause of the burn, age of the patient, additional injuries, medical history (e.g., heart disease, diabetes), and location of the burn wound.

The size of a burn wound is estimated based on parts of the body affected. A quick and common method is the Rule of Nines. This method divides the body into segments whose areas are either 9% or multiples of 9% of the total body surface, with the perineum being counted as 1% (Fig. 55.3). This formula is easy, but it is not as accurate when assessing children. A more accurate method uses a table with a relative anatomical scale or diagram that estimates total burned area by ages and by smaller anatomical areas of the body.

NURSING CARE TIP

For a quick estimation of percentage of burn injury, using the Rule of Nines on an adult burn patient, the palm of your hand is about 1%.

TABLE 55.1   CLASSIFICATION OF BURN DEPTH

Classification	Formerly	Areas Involved	Appearance	Sensitivity	Healing Time
Partial thickness (superficial)	First to second degree	Epidermis Papillae of dermis	Bright red to pink Blanches to touch Serum-filled blisters Glistening, moist	Sensitive to air, temperature, and touch	7–10 days
Partial thickness (deep)	Second degree	Epidermis, half to seven-eighths of dermis	Blisters may be present. Pink to light red to white. Soft and pliable. Blanching present.	Pressure may be painful because of exposed nerve endings.	14–21 days; may need grafting to decrease scarring
Full thickness	Third to fourth degree	Epidermis Dermis Tissue Muscle Bone	Snowy white, gray, or brown Texture is firm and leathery Inelastic	No pain because nerve endings are destroyed, unless surrounded by areas of partial-thickness burns	Grafting necessary to complete healing

Source: Trofino, R. B. (1996). Nursing management of the patient with burns. In S. Ruppert, J. Kernick, & J. Dolan (Eds.), *Dolan's critical care nursing.* Philadelphia: F.A. Davis, p. 943.

FIGURE 55.2 (A) Partial-thickness burn. (B) Partial-thickness burn. (C) Full-thickness burn. From Trofino, R. B. (1991). *Nursing care of the burn-injured patient*. Philadelphia: F.A. Davis, plates 1–3, with permission.

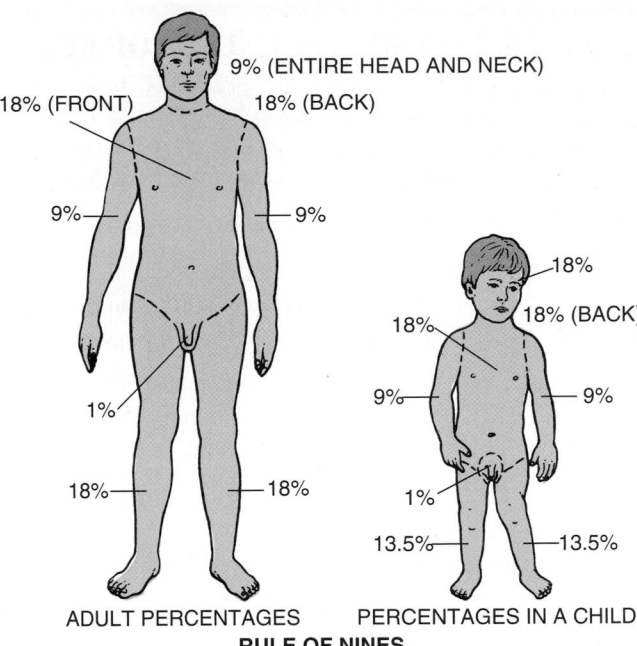

FIGURE 55.3 Estimation of extent of burn injury. From Venes, D. (Ed.). (2009). *Taber's cyclopedic medical dictionary* (21st ed.) Philadelphia: F.A. Davis, p. 2057, with permission. Beth Anne Willert, MS, dictionary illustrator.

 BE SAFE!

BE VIGILANT! Prevention should focus on fire safety, especially in relation to smoking, starting brush fires, cooking, as well as scald prevention, especially in relation to baths, showers, and water temperature (Greenhalgh, 2013).

 Gerontological Issues

Burn Injury and the Older Adult

According to the Centers for Disease Control and Prevention (2009), unintentional injuries from fires and burns are the fifth most common cause of death in the United States. Older adults are among the six risk groups.

Research by Burton et al (2009) found that "patients who die from burns tend to be older, present in the hospital during the winter months, and suffer more acute burns to the torso or multiple body regions." Older age was also associated with increased length of hospital stay. A small burn can lead to the inability to be independent and may require care in a skilled facility (Greenhalgh, 2013).

Prevention measures should consider visual and auditory changes as well as mobility impairments the older adult needs to overcome. Individuals must be able to evacuate in case of a fire and seek help if a burn injury occurs. Nurses should target prevention measures toward the most common activities that can lead to fire or burn injury: smoking and cooking.

CRITICAL THINKING

Mr. Weinberg

■ Mr. Weinberg is admitted to the hospital with superficial and deep partial-thickness burns. His wife asks how long it will take for the burns to heal. What should you tell her?

Suggested answers are at the end of the chapter.

 ETIOLOGY

Burn injuries have many causes. The most common causes include flames, contact burns, scalding, and chemical, electrical, and radiation burns. Table 55.2 summarizes common causes; see also "Gerontological Issues."

TABLE 55.2   COMMON CAUSES OF BURNS

Flame	House fire is a common cause. Usually associated with an inhalation injury. Flash injury occurs from a sudden ignition or explosion.
Contact	Hot tar, hot metals, or hot grease produce a full-thickness injury on contact.
Scald	A burn from hot liquid. More common in children younger than age 5 and adults older than age 65. With an immersion scald, there are usually no splash marks; usually involves lower regions of body.
Chemical	Usually occurs in an industrial setting. Extent and depth of injury are directly proportional to concentration and quantity of agent, duration of contact, and chemical activity and penetrability of agent.
Electrical	One of the most serious types of burn injury; can be full thickness with possible loss of limbs, as well as cause internal injuries. Entry wound is usually ischemic, charred, and depressed. Exit wound may have an explosive appearance. Extent of injury depends on voltage, resistance of body, type of current, amperage, pathway of current, and duration of contact. Bones offer greatest resistance to the current; resulting in great damage. Tissue fluid, blood, and nerves offer least resistance; therefore, the current travels this path.
Radiation	Can occur in an industrial setting, as a result of treatment of disease, or from ultraviolet light (sun or tanning salons). Severity depends on type of radiation, duration of exposure, depth of penetration, distance from source, and absorbed dose.

BE SAFE!

BE VIGILANT! Keep temperature of hot water heater at 120 degrees F—a safe bathing temperature. If water needs to be kept at 140 degrees, be sure to install a temperature-regulating device on taps.

COMPLICATIONS

A major complication that can occur with a flame burn in an enclosed space is inhalation injury. An inhalation injury is a major cause of morbidity and mortality associated with burn injuries. Treatment of an inhalation injury takes precedence over other injuries. (Remember your ABCs? Airway always comes first.) Infection is another common complication with a major burn. The incidence of infection increases with the size of the burn wound because the skin is the first line of defense against microorganisms.

Neurovascular compromise can also occur with a major burn. Eschar formation creates pressure and contributes to decreasing blood flow to areas distal to the burned area. Other systemic complications were reviewed in the "Systemic Responses" section earlier in this chapter.

CRITICAL THINKING

Mrs. Rivera

■ Mrs. Rivera is admitted to the emergency department after sustaining injuries from a house fire. Both arms and hands are burned, she has a right leg fracture and a possible neck fracture, her lips are swollen, her face is sooty, and she is spitting up grayish, blackish sputum.

1. What is your priority concern with all of these injuries?
2. An IV is ordered at 1 L over 6 hours. How many milliliters per hour should be set on the controller?
3. Approximately what percent of her body is burned?
4. What members of the health team will collaborate on Mrs. Rivera's care?

Suggested answers are at the end of the chapter.

DIAGNOSTIC TESTS

Burns are diagnosed by physical assessment. Various diagnostic tests are performed for systemic reactions, infection, and other complications. Common laboratory tests include complete blood cell count (CBC) and differential, blood urea nitrogen (BUN), serum glucose and electrolytes, serum protein and albumin levels, urinalysis, urine cultures, and clotting studies. If an inhalation injury is suspected, arterial blood gases, bronchoscopy, and carboxyhemoglobin levels are done. X-rays, electrocardiogram, and wound cultures are completed if indicated.

 THERAPEUTIC MEASURES

Therapeutic interventions vary according to the severity of the burn and the stage the patient is in. Treatment is managed over three overlapping stages (Table 55.3).

Emergent Stage

At the time of injury, the burning process must be stopped. The clothes are removed, and the wound is cooled with tepid water and covered with clean sheets to decrease shivering and contamination. The burn wound itself is a lower priority than the ABCs (airway, breathing, circulation) of trauma resuscitation. Emergency rescuers at the scene will stabilize the victim by establishing an airway, ensuring oxygenation, inserting an IV line, and stabilizing fractures, hemorrhage, and spinal and other injuries. Inhalation injury is suspected if the patient sustained a burn from a fire in an enclosed space or was exposed to smoldering materials, if the face and neck were burned, if there are vocal changes, or if the patient is coughing up carbon particles. IV fluids are given to prevent and treat hypovolemic shock. The patient is treated for pain with appropriate IV opioid analgesics.

An accurate history of the injury is obtained to determine severity, potential complications, and any associated trauma. The patient's medical history is also obtained. Admission to the facility and burn care treatment are explained to the patient and family.

TABLE 55.3 STAGES OF BURN CARE

Stage	Duration
I (Emergent)	From onset of injury to completion of fluid resuscitation
II (Acute)	From start of diuresis to near completion of wound closure
III (Rehabilitation)	From wound closure to return of optimal level of physical and psychosocial function

Source: Trofino, R. B. (1996). Nursing management of the patient with burns. In S. Ruppert, J. Kernick, & J. Dolan (Eds.), *Dolan's critical care nursing.* Philadelphia: F.A. Davis, p. 948.

 NURSING CARE TIP

If the patient is unable to communicate effectively, interview all involved family witnesses to determine the cause of the injury, as well as past and current medical history and medications the patient is taking. Getting a full description of the cause of the injury may lead to the detection of other injuries that may not be readily visible.

Acute Stage

If the patient is in a facility with a special burn unit, multidisciplinary care from a burn team is provided during the acute stage. Management goals include wound closure with no infection, minimum scarring, maximum function, maintenance of comfort as much as possible, adequate nutritional support, and maintenance of fluid, electrolyte, and acid–base balance. The patient continues to be medicated for pain as needed, especially before painful treatments. Patient-controlled analgesia (PCA) is very effective. Nutritional support may be maintained via nasogastric feeding tube (see "Nutrition Notes").

 Nutrition Notes

Burns

The goals of nutritional support in burned patients are to (1) meet metabolic needs, (2) promote wound healing, (3) promote resistance to infection, and (4) reduce protein loss (severely burned patients can lose nearly one-half pound of skeletal muscle per day).

Early (within 6–12 hours of injury) aggressive enteral feeding into the duodenum or jejunum improves outcomes. Because carbohydrates rather than fats are the best sources of energy after burn injury, formulas may contain 82% carbohydrate, 15% protein, and 3% fat. Protein needs are at least 1.5 to 2 grams/kilogram of body weight/day. Compared with omega-6 fatty acids, omega-3 fatty acids have been associated with an improved inflammatory response. Multivitamin/multimineral supplements are normally included.

Other nutrients and components that might be considered as supplements are the following:
- Vitamin C, up to 20 times the recommended dietary allowance, for collagen synthesis
- Vitamin A for wound healing and epithelial growth
- Zinc for wound healing and lymphocyte function
- The amino acid glutamine to improve visceral protein levels and decrease incidence of infections

Continued

When oral intake is possible, supplemental overnight enteral feeding may be used if intake is inadequate. Because of infection risks, parenteral nutrition is reserved for those who cannot tolerate enteral feeding.

Jeschke, M. G., Finnerty, C. C., Harrison, R. A., & Herndon, D. N. (2012). Nutrition in burn injury. In Ross, A. C., Caballero, B., Cousins, R. J., Ziegler, T. R., & Tucker, K. L. (Eds.), *Modern nutrition in health and disease* (11th ed.). Philadelphia: Lippincott Williams & Wilkins.

NURSING CARE TIP

Remember to provide adequate padding of the bed before an escharotomy because this procedure can be accompanied by copious amounts of drainage. Provide for appropriate disposal of the drainage. For an extremity escharotomy, monitor the patient for return of distal pulses.

The wound is cleansed and débrided daily to promote healing, prevent infection, and provide a clean bed for grafting. Wound cleansing is achieved by showering using a shower trolley or shower chair and bedside care.

Débridement, or the removal of nonviable tissue (eschar), can be mechanical, chemical, surgical, or a combination of these methods. Mechanical débridement can involve the use of scissors and forceps to manually excise loose, nonviable tissue, or the use of wet-to-moist or wet-to-dry fine-mesh gauze dressings (see Chapter 54). Chemical débridement involves the use of a proteolytic enzymatic debriding agent that digests necrotic tissue. Surgical débridement is the excision of full-thickness and deep partial-thickness burns. This method is followed by application of a skin graft.

If the patient has a circumferential burn (one that surrounds an extremity or area), an increase in tissue pressure secondary to tissue edema occurs. The burn then acts like a tourniquet, impeding arterial and venous flow and impairing distal pulses. Common sites for these burns are the extremities, trunk, and chest. If this occurs on the chest and trunk, respiratory insufficiency can occur as a result of restricted chest expansion. An **escharotomy** may be immediately needed to relieve pressure. An escharotomy is a linear excision through the eschar to the superficial fat that allows for expansion of the skin and return of blood flow or chest expansion (Fig. 55.4).

After the area is cleaned, the burn dressing and topical treatment are prescribed. The type of dressing and topical agent chosen depend on the area involved, the extent and depth of injury, and physician preference. Several common topical agents are listed in Table 55.4.

Dressings may be open, closed, biological, synthetic, or a combination. The open method is the use of a topical agent without any dressing. The closed method involves the use of an occlusive dressing over the wound. General principles for dressings include the following:

1. Limit the bulk of the dressing to facilitate range of motion.
2. Never wrap skin-to-skin surfaces (e.g., wrap fingers or toes separately; place a donut gauze dressing around the ear).
3. Base dressings on the size of wounds, absorption, protection, and type of débridement.
4. Wrap extremities from distal to proximal to promote venous return.
5. Do not wrap dressings too tightly. Check peripheral pulses often.
6. Elevate affected extremities.

The term *biological dressing* refers to a dressing that uses tissue from living or deceased humans (cadaver skin) or deceased animals (e.g., pigskin) or to cellular dressings that may use animal tissue, human tissue, or synthetics. Biological dressings assist with wound healing and stimulate **epithelialization**. These dressings may be used as donor site dressings, to manage a partial-thickness burn and to cover the clean, excised wound before autografting. Some cellular wound dressings have varied layers that form a matrix onto which the patient's own cells migrate over a few weeks to form a new dermis. A very thin layer of the person's own skin is then grafted onto this new dermis.

Synthetic dressings are used in the management of partial-thickness burns and donor sites. Synthetic dressings are more readily available, less costly, and easier to store than biological dressings. They are made from a variety of materials and come in many sizes and shapes. Most of these dressings contain no antimicrobial agents.

FIGURE 55.4 Escharotomy. From Trofino, R. B. (1991). *Nursing care of the burn-injured patient*. Philadelphia: F.A. Davis, plate 16, with permission.

• WORD • BUILDING •
escharotomy: eschara—scab + otomy—incision
epithelialization: epi—over + thele—nipple + ization—condition

TABLE 55.4 COMMON TOPICAL BROAD-SPECTRUM ANTIBIOTIC AGENTS

Examples	Nursing Implications
silver sulfadiazine 1% cream (Silvadene)	Intermediate penetration of eschar. Butter on in thick layer. Cover with light dressings once or twice a day.
mafenide acetate (Sulfamylon)	Premedicate for pain. Butter on. Open exposure method. Apply three to four times daily. Keeps eschar soft for easier débridement.
silver nitrate solution 0.5%	Poor penetration of eschar. Ineffective on established wound infections. Apply with wet dressings, change twice daily. Soak every 2 hours.
bacitracin	Poor penetration of eschar. Butter on. Reapply every 4–6 hours.
Gentamicin (Garamycin)	Painful on application. Apply gently three to four times daily.
mupirocin (Bactroban)	May cause burning, itching, and pain on application. Apply three times daily.
neomycin/bacitracin/polymyxin (Neosporin)	Apply one to three times daily.

Biological and synthetic dressings are used as temporary wound coverings over clean partial- and full-thickness injuries. They act as skin substitutes to help maintain the wound surface until healing occurs, a donor site becomes available, or the wound is ready for autografting.

Skin Grafts

AUTOGRAFT. An **autograft** is a skin graft from the patient's unburned skin that is placed on the clean excised burn. The two common types of autografts are the split-thickness skin graft (STSG), which includes the epidermis and part of the dermis, and the full-thickness skin graft (FTSG), which includes the epidermis and entire dermal layer.

SPLIT THICKNESS SKIN GRAFT. An STSG (0.006–0.016 inch or 0.15–0.41 mm may be applied as a sheet graft or a meshed graft. A sheet graft is used for cosmetic effect, such as for a face, neck, upper chest, breast, or hand burn. It is placed on the area as a full sheet. A meshed graft is passed through a mesher that produces tiny splits in the skin, similar to a fishnet, with openings in the shape of diamonds (Fig. 55.5), to permit the skin to expand one and a half to nine times its original size. The meshing allows for coverage of a large burn area with a small piece of skin by stretching it and securing it with sutures or staples. A mesh graft is especially useful when a patient's burns are extensive, resulting in few available donor sites. Graft "take," or vascularization, is complete in about 3 to 5 days.

FIGURE 55.5 Meshed graft. From Trofino, R. B. (1991). *Nursing care of the burn-injured patient.* Philadelphia: F.A. Davis, plate 17, with permission.

FULL THICKNESS SKIN GRAFT. FTSGs (0.035–0.040 inch or 0.9–1.02 mm) can be sheet grafts or pedicle flaps. They are used over areas of muscle mass, soft tissue loss, hands, feet, and eyelids. They are not used for extensive wounds

• **WORD** • **BUILDING** •
autograft: auto—self + graft—tissue transplant

because the donor sites usually require an STSG for closure, or closure from the wound edges. A pedicle graft or flap is a skin flap and subcutaneous tissue that is still attached at one corner by a "pedicle" to a blood supply (artery and vein); it is then attached to an adjacent area in need of grafting. Once the distal part of the graft takes, it remains in place and the flap is divided, with the remainder returning to the original site. Pedicle flaps are not as popular as free skin flaps because they require more than one surgery and take longer for the graft site and donor site to heal. Table 55.5 provides a comparison of split-thickness and full-thickness grafts.

Donor sites are considered partial-thickness wounds. Donor sites usually heal in 10 to 14 days, but this depends on the thickness and method of grafting and the general health of the patient. Treatment for the donor site varies with the individual patient, the area of the body, and physician preference. Considerations for care include promoting comfort and preventing trauma and infection. Use of semiocclusive, transparent dressings such as Op-Site, Biobrane, or Tegaderm, allows for a moist healing environment and is associated with reduced risk of infection. The donor site is very painful. Appropriate pain medications are provided, along with nonpharmacologic measures (e.g., back rubs or distraction).

With any type of graft, the patient must keep the graft site immobilized until the graft takes, to prevent movement or slippage of the grafted skin. Dressings may be bulky to assist in immobilization. These dressings must not be disturbed. The involved area requires frequent circulatory checks, including assessment of color, warmth, sensation, pulses, and capillary refill. Any involved extremities must be elevated to maintain circulation. Table 55.6 describes factors that affect graft viability. A graft has been successful if there is good adherence of the graft to the wound with no evidence of necrosis or infection.

TABLE 55.6 FACTORS AFFECTING GRAFT VIABILITY

Factors That Inhibit Graft Viability	Factors That Promote Graft Viability
Infection	Adequate hemostasis
Necrotic skin (tissue)	Anatomical location of graft
Anatomic location of graft:	Smooth contour
Perineum	Nonjoint areas
Axillae	Graft secured well
Buttocks	Immobilization of graft area
Poor-quality donor skin	Good nutritional status
Poor nutritional status	
Bleeding	
Mechanical trauma	
Shock	

Source: Konop, D. (1991). General local treatment. In R. Trofino (Ed.), *Nursing care of the burn-injured patient.* Philadelphia: F.A. Davis, p. 62.

Rehabilitation Stage

The therapy started during the acute phase continues in the rehabilitation phase. There is wound closure, and the goal is to return the patient to an optimum level of physical and psychosocial function. This may take months to years to accomplish, depending on the extent of the injury. Reconstructive surgeries may be ongoing for many years.

Two things to keep in mind when caring for the patient with a major burn are that (1) the most comfortable position (flexion) is the position of contracture, and (2) the burn wound will shorten until it meets an opposing force. Have you ever seen a contracture? They are uncomfortable and debilitating. To avoid contractures (Fig. 55.6), a specific

TABLE 55.5 COMPARISON OF SPLIT-THICKNESS AND FULL-THICKNESS SKIN GRAFTS

	Split-Thickness Graft	Full-Thickness Graft
Layers	Epidermis Partial layer of dermis	Epidermis. Entire dermal layer.
Advantages	Donor site may be reused. Healing of donor site is more rapid, results in good "take."	Allows more elasticity over joints. Can reconstruct cosmetic defects. Soft, pliable. Gives full appearance. Provides good color match. Less hyperpigmentation. May allow hair growth.
Disadvantages	Prone to chronic breakdown. Likely to hypertrophy. More likely to contract.	Donor site takes longer to heal. Requires split-thickness graft to heal or closure from wound edges.

Source: Konop, D. (1991). General local treatment. In R. Trofino (Ed.), *Nursing care of the burn-injured patient.* Philadelphia: F.A. Davis, p. 61.

FIGURE 55.6 Burn deformity: contracture. From Trofino, R. B. (1991). *Nursing care of the burn-injured patient.* Philadelphia: F.A. Davis, plate 36, with permission.

exercise program is begun 24 to 48 hours after injury, along with the use of splinting devices to maintain proper positioning and stretching. Hypertrophic scarring, or a proliferation of scar tissue, can be minimized or prevented through the use of a pressure garment (Fig. 55.7).

As the burn heals, itching may occur and may be intense at times. It is important to control itching, because scratching can impair healing and increase risk of infection (see "Evidence-Based Practice").

Psychosocial Effects of Burn Injury

A burn affects the patient's psychosocial status in many ways. The magnitude of these effects are related to the age of the patient, location of the burn (e.g., face, hands), recovery from injury, cause of the injury (especially if related to negligence or a deliberate act), and ability to continue at the preburn level of normal daily activities. The patient may experience a disruption of role function and general health and coping ability. Treatment involves the patient and significant others. Referrals to support groups, counselors, and psychiatrists are important during this stage.

FIGURE 55.7 Full-body pressure garment. From Trofino, R. B. (1991). *Nursing care of the burn-injured patient.* Philadelphia: F.A. Davis, plate 39, with permission.

EVIDENCE-BASED PRACTICE

Clinical Question
What interventions are helpful for treating itching in a healing burn?

Evidence
Itching (pruritis) can interfere with activities of daily living. Treatment of itching can include pharmacologic and nonpharmacologic approaches. Some treatments shown to be helpful include cimetidine (an oral antihistamine), colloidal oatmeal baths, and pulsed dye laser therapy (Bell & Gabriel, 2009; UT Southwestern Medical Center, 2009). Nonpharmacologic techniques include massage and application of cold (Kagan et al, 2013).

Implications for Nursing Practice
Postburn itching affects about 87% of patients. Pruritus can increase pain and cause insomnia. It can range from mild to severe. Be sure to assess the presence and severity of itching on a 0-to-10 scale and advocate for appropriate orders.

REFERENCES

Bell, P. L., & Gabriel, V. (2009). Evidence based review for the treatment of post-burn pruritus. *Journal of Burn Care & Research, 30,* 455–461.

Kagan, R. J., Peck, M. D., Ahrenholz, D. H., Hickerson, W. L., Holmes, J., Korefager, R., . . . Kotoski, G. (2013). Surgical management of the burn wound and use of skin substitutes: An expert panel white paper. *Journal of Burn Care & Research, 34,* 60–79.

UT Southwestern Medical Center. (2009). *Burn rehabilitation experts outline best treatments for post-burn itching.* Retrieved August 30, 2009, from www.utsouthwestern .edu/utsw/cda/dept353744/files/518898.html

CRITICAL THINKING

Mrs. Potter

■ Mrs. Potter is recovering from partial-thickness burns and skin grafts. She mentions that she and her family will be going on a much-needed vacation to the shore. What concerns do you have?

Suggested answers are at end of the chapter.

NURSING CARE TIP

Use caution with heating pads, water temperature, and electrical equipment when working with your patients. Burns are considered serious

Continued

reportable events because they can be prevented, and thus hospitals will not be paid by Medicare for treating burns acquired during hospitalization.

 NURSING PROCESS FOR A PATIENT WITH A BURN INJURY

Data Collection

A major burn is painful and frightening for the patient and frightening for the family. Obtain information from the patient, family, and rescuers. If the injury occurred in an enclosed space with flames or smoldering materials, suspect an inhalation injury. If an electrical injury has occurred, ask about voltage, duration of contact, host susceptibility (wet or dry skin), entry and exit sites, and associated falls. With chemical burns, determine type of agent and duration of exposure.

General information to collect for all burns (in addition to normally collected data, such as medical history, allergies, and current medications) includes extent, depth, type, and location of the burn; burn agent; duration of contact with the burning agent; severity and location of pain; and associated injuries. Determine the immediate first aid treatment provided at the scene. Obtain psychosocial information: other people injured, additional losses (home, pets), whether the patient was at fault, and how this injury affects the patient's role function.

Nursing Diagnoses, Planning, Implementation, and Evaluation

See the "Nursing Care Plan for the Patient with a Burn Injury," and Table 55.7, "Burn Summary." For more information on burns, go to the American Burn Association Web site at www.ameriburn.org.

TABLE 55.7 BURN SUMMARY

Signs and Symptoms	Pain Superficial partial thickness: pink to red skin, blisters Deep partial thickness: pink to light red or white skin, blisters, blanching Full thickness: white, gray, or brown color, firm and leathery
Diagnostic Tests	Wound cultures Complete blood count, blood urea nitrogen, glucose, electrolytes, urine studies
Therapeutic Measures	IV fluid replacement Antibiotic/antimicrobial agents Analgesics
Complications	Shock Wound infection
Priority Nursing Diagnoses	*Impaired Gas Exchange* *Impaired Skin Integrity* *Deficient Fluid Volume* *Pain* related to burns or graft donor sites *Impaired Physical Mobility* *Ineffective Peripheral Tissue Perfusion* *Risk for Infection*

NURSING CARE PLAN for the Patient With a Burn Injury

Nursing Diagnosis: *Impaired Gas Exchange* related to upper airway edema, carbon monoxide poisoning, edema of alveolar capillary membranes, as evidenced by abnormal blood gases, elevated CO level

Expected Outcomes: The patient's gas exchange will be improved as evidenced by patent airway, CO level less than 10%, clear lung sounds, Pao_2 80–100 mm Hg, $PaCO_2$ 35–45 mm Hg, Spo_2 ≥95%, responsiveness, and awareness.

Evaluation of Outcomes: Are oxygenation levels improved? Do the lungs sound clear on auscultation? Is patient aware of surroundings? Are there signs of respiratory distress absent (e.g., retractions, nasal flaring, use of accessory muscles)?

Intervention Assess respiratory status: auscultate breath sounds every 15 minutes or as needed. Note any adventitious breath sounds. Observe for chest excursion. Monitor ability to cough. **Rationale** Assessment detects changes in pulmonary function for planning care. **Evaluation** What is patient's respiratory status? Are any adventitious lung sounds noted?

NURSING CARE PLAN for the Patient With a Burn Injury—cont'd

Intervention Monitor arterial blood gases, SpO_2 and CO levels. **Rationale** Assesses level of oxygenation and helps guide oxygen therapy. **Evaluation** Is oxygenation adequate?

Intervention Monitor for nasal flaring, retractions, wheezing, and stridor. **Rationale** Stridor may signal upper airway involvement. Nasal flaring, retractions, and wheezing may indicate lower airway involvement. **Evaluation** Does patient exhibit signs of upper or lower airway involvement?

Intervention Administer humidified 100% oxygen by tight-fitting facemask as ordered. **Rationale** Provides oxygen for adequate gas exchange. **Evaluation** Is oxygen administered appropriately? Are blood gases improving?

Intervention Elevate head of bed (if no cervical spine injuries or no history of multiple trauma). **Rationale** Decreases swelling of face and neck. Increases ability to expand lungs. **Evaluation** Is head of bed elevated? Is there any change in facial or neck swelling?

Intervention Provide appropriate pulmonary care: turn, cough, deep breathe every 2–4 hours. **Rationale** Mobilizes secretions and promotes lung expansion. **Evaluation** Is patient receiving vigorous pulmonary care? Is it affecting outcomes?

Intervention Provide incentive spirometer every 2–4 hours.

Intervention Suction frequently as needed.

Intervention Obtain sputum cultures as ordered. Note amount, color, and consistency of pulmonary secretions. **Rationale** Carbonaceous sputum is diagnostic for smoke inhalation injury. Infection changes color, amount, and consistency of sputum. Culture and sensitivity (C&S) assists in selection of appropriate antibiotic. **Evaluation** Is patient coughing up any sputum? Has character of sputum been reported and documented?

Intervention Administer bronchodilators and antibiotics as prescribed. **Rationale** Bronchodilators decrease bronchospasms and edema. Antibiotics fight infection. **Evaluation** Are medications given appropriately? Are they effective?

Nursing Diagnosis: *Impaired Skin Integrity* related to thermal injury as evidenced by presence of burn lesions

Expected Outcomes: The patient's skin integrity will be improved as evidenced by stopping of burning process and healing of burned areas with no infection present.

Evaluation of Outcomes: Did burning process stop? Is burned area healed and free from infection?

Intervention Obtain history of burning agent. **Rationale** Provides information related to depth, duration of contact, and resistance of tissues. If fire scenario, consider possible inhalation injury. **Evaluation** What caused this thermal injury? How long was patient in contact with agent?

Intervention Assess burning process. If heat is felt on wound, cool with tepid tap water or sterile water. **Rationale** Depth of injury increases with length of exposure to burning agent. **Evaluation** Is heat felt over wounds? Has burn process been effectively stopped?

Intervention Remove clothing and jewelry. **Rationale** These items can retain heat and thermal agent, therefore increasing depth of injury. Jewelry can be constrictive when edema develops. **Evaluation** Are clothing and jewelry removed and constriction avoided?

Intervention Do not apply ice. **Rationale** Ice causes vasoconstriction, further increasing skin damage. Ice also causes a decrease in core body temperature, which may promote shock. **Evaluation** Is burning stopped without the use of ice?

Continued

NURSING CARE PLAN for the Patient With a Burn Injury—cont'd

Intervention Cover patient with clean sheet or blanket. **Rationale** Prevents excessive heat loss. Decreases pain from air exposure. Protects patient from environmental contamination. **Evaluation** Is patient covered?

Intervention For all chemical burns, initiate immediate copious tepid water lavage for 20 minutes along with simultaneous removal of contaminated clothing. Do not neutralize chemical because this takes too much time and resulting reaction may generate heat and cause further skin injury. **Rationale** Dilution and removal of chemical agent halts burning process. Lavage dissipates heat. **Evaluation** Has lavage been initiated?

Intervention Brush off dry chemicals before lavage. **Rationale** To prevent further burn damage due to reaction of dry chemical with water. **Evaluation** Are dry chemicals removed?

Intervention Use heavy rubber gloves or thick gauze for removal of clothing. **Rationale** Protects health care workers from injury. **Evaluation** Do health care workers remain safe?

Intervention Cleanse wound at bedside or via showering. **Rationale** Promotes healing and helps decrease infection. **Evaluation** Is burn wound clean and free of wound debris?

Intervention Assist registered nurse (RN) or HCP to assess the burn area for extent (percentage) and depth (partial thickness, full thickness) of injury. **Rationale** Provides basis for triage of care. Important for calculating resuscitation fluid therapy. **Evaluation** What is the estimation of percentage of burn injury? What is depth of injury?

Intervention Assist RN or physician with debriding wound via surgical, chemical, or mechanical means. Apply topical agent as prescribed. **Rationale** Promotes healing and healthy granulation bed. Most agents prevent infection and promote healing. **Evaluation** Is eschar present? Is wound free of wound debris? Is agent applied as directed?

Intervention Apply dressing as prescribed. **Rationale** Dressing types vary and are influenced by area, extent, and depth of injury, as well as by topical agent used. Dressing protects burn area and promotes healing. **Evaluation** Is dressing applied appropriately?

Intervention Do not wrap skin surface to skin surface (e.g., wrap fingers and toes separately; donut bandage around ears). **Rationale** Wrapping separately prevents webbing and contractures. **Evaluation** Are skin surfaces separated? Are webbing and contractures avoided?

Intervention Limit bulk of dressings. **Rationale** Mobility is enhanced with less bulky dressing. **Evaluation** Is patient's mobility maximized?

Intervention Wrap extremities from distal to proximal. **Rationale** Circulation is increased when extremities are wrapped distal to proximal. **Evaluation** Is wrapping done correctly? Is edema of distal extremity avoided?

Nursing Diagnosis: *Deficient Fluid Volume* related to evaporative losses from wound, capillary leak, and decreased fluid intake as evidenced by urine output less than 50 mL per hour, hypotension, tachycardia, weight loss

Expected Outcomes: The (adult) patient will maintain adequate circulating volume as evidenced by urine output of 50 mL/hr, blood pressure within normal limits, heart rate between 60 and 100 beats per minute, and stabilized body weight.

Evaluation of Outcomes: Is urine output maintained at least at 50 mL/hr? Are the blood pressure and heart rate within normal limits? Is patient's weight stable?

Intervention Obtain admission weight and monitor weight daily. **Rationale** Helps measure fluid loss or gain. **Evaluation** Is patient's weight documented? Is it stable?

Intervention Record intake and output (I&O) hourly. **Rationale** Serves as guide for fluid loss and replacement. **Evaluation** Is urine output adequate?

NURSING CARE PLAN for the Patient With a Burn Injury—cont'd

Intervention Examine for signs and symptoms of hypovolemia (hypotension, tachycardia, tachypnea, extreme thirst, restlessness, disorientation). **Rationale** Fluid volume loss is multifocal (e.g., through increased capillary permeability, insensible loss). **Evaluation** Does patient exhibit any signs or symptoms of hypovolemia?

Intervention Monitor electrolytes, complete blood count (CBC) and report abnormal results to HCP. **Rationale** Serves as guide for electrolyte replacement and blood product replacement. **Evaluation** What are patient's lab values? Are abnormal results reported?

Intervention Administer or monitor IV fluids as ordered via large-bore IV catheter. **Rationale** Fluid replacement begins immediately to prevent hypovolemia. Large vessels are needed for rapid delivery of fluids. **Evaluation** Is patient's fluid replacement adequate? Is catheter patent?

Intervention Insert indwelling urinary catheter. **Rationale** Accurate urine output measurement is essential for fluid replacement calculation. **Evaluation** Is catheter patent and output recorded?

Intervention Monitor urine for amount, specific gravity, and **hemochromogens**. **Rationale** Specific gravity helps predict volume replacement. Hemochromogens can cause renal tubular damage. **Evaluation** What are patient's urine values?

Intervention Administer osmotic diuretics as ordered; monitor response to therapy. **Rationale** Decreased urine output can be caused by decreased renal flow (due to myoglobin in urine). **Evaluation** What is urine output? Has it changed due to therapy?

Intervention Assess gastrointestinal function for absence of bowel sounds. Maintain nasogastric tube as ordered. **Rationale** Splanchnic constriction due to hypovolemia can cause a paralytic ileus. **Evaluation** Are patient's bowel sounds within normal limits? Is nasogastric tube patent?

Nursing Diagnosis: *Pain* related to burns or graft donor sites as evidenced by patient's rating on appropriate pain scale, restlessness, sleeplessness

Expected Outcomes: The patient will experience pain control as evidenced by pain rating acceptable to patient and nonverbal cues, such as less restlessness and ability to rest or sleep.

Evaluation of Outcomes: Does patient verbalize pain control? How many hours of rest/sleep does patient have in 24 hours? Does patient state she or he feels rested?

Intervention Assess pain using **WHAT'S UP?** mnemonic. Rate pain on appropriate pain scale. **Rationale** Provides baseline to monitor response to therapy. **Evaluation** Is patient's individual response to pain documented?

Intervention Observe for varied responses to acute pain: increase in blood pressure, pulse, respirations; increased restlessness and irritability; increased muscle tension; facial grimaces; guarding. **Rationale** Responses to pain are variable. These parameters change in response to pain. **Evaluation** What are patient's responses to pain? Do responses change with treatment?

Intervention Acknowledge presence of pain. Explain causes of pain. **Rationale** Encourages trust and understanding. **Evaluation** Is patient more trusting of the nurse and the treatments?

Intervention Administer opioids as ordered. Use patient-controlled analgesia (PCA) as appropriate. **Rationale** Opioids are needed for severe burn pain. PCA allows patient more control. **Evaluation** Is patient being medicated for pain appropriately?

Continued

• WORD • BUILDING •
hemochromogen: heme—iron + chrom—color + gen—to produce

NURSING CARE PLAN for the Patient With a Burn Injury—cont'd

Intervention Offer diversional activities (e.g., music, TV, books, games, relaxation techniques). **Rationale** Helps patient focus on something other than pain. **Evaluation** Does patient use diversional activities? Do they help?

Intervention Position patient for comfort in good body alignment. **Rationale** Increases comfort. **Evaluation** Is patient positioned as comfortably as possible?

Intervention Elevate burned extremities. **Rationale** Elevation decreases edema and pain. **Evaluation** Are extremities elevated? Is pain reduced?

Intervention Maintain comfortable environment (e.g., bed cradle; comfortable environmental temperature, 86–91.4°F [30–33°C]; quiet environment). **Rationale** Pressure from bed linens may cause discomfort; with loss of integument, body cannot self-regulate temperature. **Evaluation** Does patient verbalize comfort of environment?

Nursing Diagnosis: *Impaired Physical Mobility* related to burn healing, pain, and contractures

Expected Outcomes: The patient will maintain adequate physical mobility as evidenced by ability to ambulate, move in bed, and tolerate activity.

Evaluation of Outcomes: Is the patient able to sit? Is the patient able to get out of bed? Is the patient able to walk with or without assistance?

Intervention Encourage ambulation as able. **Rationale** Helps prevent atelectasis and pneumonia. **Evaluation** Is patient optimally mobilized?

Intervention Perform active and passive range of motion exercises on affected areas. **Rationale** Prevents contractures and hypertrophic scarring. **Evaluation** Do affected areas remain mobile?

Intervention Provide support above and below affected joints. Apply splints and functional devices as ordered. **Rationale** Maintains functional position of extremities. **Evaluation** Are immobilized joints in a functional position?

Intervention For lower extremity burns, apply bandages and elastic bandages before patient is in upright position. **Rationale** Promotes venous return and minimizes edema formation. **Evaluation** Does patient tolerate being upright? Is edema minimized?

Nursing Diagnosis: *Ineffective Peripheral Tissue Perfusion* related to circumferential burns, blood loss, and decreased cardiac output as evidenced by weak pulses, cool extremities, limited movement and sensation

Expected Outcomes: The patient will maintain adequate tissue perfusion as evidenced by presence of peripheral pulses, minimal edema, intact sensation and motion, and warm extremities.

Evaluation of Outcomes: Are peripheral pulses present? Are extremities warm, with adequate sensation, movement, and circulation? Is edema decreased?

Intervention Assess pulses on burned extremities every 15 minutes until stable, then every hour. **Rationale** If pulses diminish, an escharotomy may be indicated. **Evaluation** Are pulses present and documented?

Intervention Use Doppler as needed to detect weak pulses. Assess capillary refill, sensation, color, swelling, and movement. **Rationale** Assesses peripheral perfusion. **Evaluation** Is the extremity warm, with adequate color, sensation, movement, and capillary refill?

Intervention Monitor for numbness, tingling, and increased pain in burned extremity. **Rationale** Can be indicative of increased pressure from edema. **Evaluation** Does patient report numbness, tingling, or pain?

NURSING CARE PLAN for the Patient With a Burn Injury—cont'd

Intervention Measure circumference of burned extremities. **Rationale** Monitors edema formation. **Evaluation** Is there evidence of edema? Is it getting better or worse?

Intervention Report changes in assessment promptly. **Rationale** Emergency intervention may be indicated. **Evaluation** Does patient require an emergency intervention?

Intervention Elevate burned extremity above level of the heart. **Rationale** Enhances venous return and decreases edema formation. **Evaluation** Are all burned extremities elevated above heart level? Is edema decreasing?

Intervention Apply burn dressing loosely. **Rationale** Prevents constriction and allows for expansion as edema forms. **Evaluation** Is dressing limiting circulation?

Intervention Assist with muscle compartment pressure measurement. **Rationale** Helps determine need for escharotomy (if pressure exceeds 25 mm Hg). **Evaluation** What is patient's pressure?

Intervention Assist with escharotomy as needed. **Rationale** If indicated, removal of eschar allows for edema expansion and permits peripheral perfusion. **Evaluation** Does patient require an escharotomy? Is edema relieved?

Nursing Diagnosis: *Risk for Infection*

Expected Outcome: The patient will not develop a wound infection or sepsis.

Evaluation of Outcome: Is there healthy granulation tissue on unhealed areas with no evidence of infection? Are donor sites free of infection? Have skin grafts taken? Is there absence of clinical manifestation of infection (temperature 98.6°F [37°C], normal white blood cell [WBC] count)?

Intervention Use sterile technique with wound care. **Rationale** The unhealed burn wound is an excellent culture medium for bacterial growth. **Evaluation** Is sterile technique used for all wound care?

Intervention Maintain protective isolation with careful hand hygiene. **Rationale** Prevents spread of bacteria from patient to patient or nurse to patient. **Evaluation** Do all persons in contact with patient maintain proper precautions?

Intervention Administer immunosupportive medications as prescribed: tetanus and gamma globulin. **Rationale** Immunoglobulins are depressed at time of severe burn injury. **Evaluation** Have medications been administered if indicated?

Intervention Perform wound care as prescribed, which may include the following: Inspect and débride wounds daily; culture wound three times a week or at sign of infection; shave hair at least 1 inch around burn areas if necessary (excluding eyebrows); inspect invasive line sites for inflammation (especially if line is through a burn area). **Rationale** Provides quick identification of bacterial wound invasion and decreases incidence of infection. Presence of hair increases medium for bacterial growth. **Evaluation** What does wound look like? Is it débrided? What are culture results? Does hair present a risk for infection?

Intervention Continually assess for and report signs and symptoms of sepsis: temperature elevation, change in sensorium, changes in vital signs and bowel sounds, decreased output, positive blood and wound cultures. **Rationale** The burn patient is at risk for sepsis until wound is healed. **Evaluation** Does patient exhibit any signs or symptoms of sepsis?

Intervention Administer systemic antibiotics and topical agents as prescribed. **Rationale** Antibiotics prevent or treat infection. **Evaluation** Does patient require systemic antibiotics? Are topical agents applied appropriately? Is wound healing?

SUGGESTED ANSWERS TO

CRITICAL THINKING

■ *Mr. Weinberg*

Superficial partial-thickness burns usually heal in 7 to 10 days. Deep partial-thickness burns may take up to 3 weeks. All of this depends on the location of the injury, the health of the patient, and if he remains infection free.

■ *Mrs. Rivera*

1. Mrs. Rivera has an inhalation injury. This takes precedence over the burn and other injuries.
2.

$$\frac{1 \text{ L}}{6 \text{ hr}} \quad \frac{1000 \text{ mL}}{1 \text{ L}} = 167 \text{ mL/hr}$$

3. Approximately 18%.
4. Burn care requires a true interdisciplinary approach. She has a major burn, so the burn nurse will collaborate with a burn physician, plastic surgeon, pulmonary physician, orthopedic surgeon, physician assistant or nurse practitioner, physical therapist, occupational therapist and dietitian.

■ *Mrs. Potter*

The burned and graft areas will be sensitive to sunlight for up to 1 year. These areas should be covered, and she needs to use sunscreen anytime she is out in the sun. Her physician should offer guidance as to whether any exposure is safe, and if so, what type of sunscreen agent is recommended. In addition, if any areas are not completely healed, she will be at risk for infection.

REVIEW QUESTIONS

1. A patient is brought to the emergency department after a house fire. The patient has extensive trunk and lower extremity burns, and is diagnosed with a deep partial thickness burn. What assessment findings does the nurse expect?
   1. Snowy white, painless lesions
   2. Blistered, pinkish white, painful lesions
   3. Blackened, painful lesions
   4. Bright red, moist lesions

2. Which of the following actions is appropriate initial treatment of a chemical burn?
   1. Lavage with water.
   2. Neutralize the chemical.
   3. Apply the prescribed topical agent.
   4. Wrap the patient in sterile sheets.

3. A patient is admitted to the emergency department with flame burns to the entire chest, abdomen, back, and upper extremities. Using the Rule of Nines, what approximate percentage of burns should the nurse document?
   1. 36%
   2. 45%
   3. 54%
   4. 64%

4. Which nursing interventions are appropriate for a patient with a circumferential burn to an extremity? **Select all that apply.**
   1. Apply compression bandages starting at the distal end of the extremity.
   2. Administer analgesics if numbness or tingling occur.
   3. Check neurovascular status hourly.
   4. Assist with escharotomy if indicated.
   5. Elevate the extremity.

5. How will the nurse know if interventions for impaired gas exchange related to smoke inhalation have been effective?
   1. $PaCO_2$ is greater than 45 mm Hg.
   2. Spo_2 is less than 90%.
   3. pH is 7.34.
   4. Pao_2 is 88 mm Hg.

Answers can be found in Appendix C.

References

Burton, K. R., Sharma, V. K., Robertson, H., & Lindsay, R. (2009). A population-based study of the epidemiology of acute adult burn injuries in the Calgary Health Region and factors associated with mortality and hospital length of stay from 1995 to 2004. *Burns, 35,* 572–579.

Centers for Disease Control and Prevention. (2009). *Fire deaths and injuries: Fact sheet.* Retrieved August 28, 2009, from www.cdc.gov/HomeandRecreationalSafety/Fire-Prevention /fires-factsheet.html

Greenhalgh, D. G. (2013). Focus on geriatric trauma/burn prevention. *American Burn Association Fire & Burn Prevention News, 9,* 8.

Kagan, R. J., Peck, M. D., Ahrenholz, D. H., Hickerson, W. L., Holmes, J., Koretager, R., Kotoski, G. (2013). Surgical management of the burn wound and use of skin substitutes: An expert panel white paper. *Journal of Burn Care & Research, 34,* 60–79. doi: 10.1097.BCR.0613e31827039a6.

 DavisPlus. | For additional resources and information visit **davispl.us/medsurg5**

unit SIXTEEN

Understanding Mental Health Care

56

Mental Health Function, Assessment, and Therapeutic Measures

MARINA MARTINEZ-KRATZ

KEY TERMS

adaptation (ad-dap-TAY-shun)
affect (AF-fekt)
anxiety (ang-ZY-uh-tee)
behavior management (be-HAYV-yer MAN-ij-ment)
cognitive (KOG-nih-tiv)
coping (KOH-ping)
electroconvulsive therapy (ee-LEK-troh kun-VUL-siv THER-uh-pee)
imagery (IM-ij-ree)
insight (IN-syte)
mental health (MEN-tuhl HELTH)
mental illness (MEN-tuhl ILL-ness)
milieu (meel-YOO)
orientation (OR-ee-en-TAY-shun)
psychoanalysis (SY-koh-uh-NAL-ih-siss)
psychopharmacology (SY-koh-FAR-mah-KAWL-luh-jee)
psychotherapy (SY-koh-THER-uh-pee)
stress (STRESS)
stressor (STRESS-ur)

LEARNING OUTCOMES

1. Define mental health and mental illness.
2. Describe the components of a mental health status assessment.
3. Describe the *Diagnostic and Statistical Manual of Mental Disorders* (5th ed., *DSM-5*) as a tool to diagnose mental illness.
4. Identify common ego defense mechanisms.
5. Describe characteristics of a therapeutic milieu.
6. Explain how psychoanalysis, behavior management, cognitive behavioral therapy, counseling, group therapy, electroconvulsive therapy, and relaxation therapy are carried out.
7. Describe the role of the licensed practical nurse/licensed vocational nurse (LPN/LVN) in mental health nursing.

REVIEW OF NEUROLOGICAL ANATOMY AND PHYSIOLOGY

When studying mental illnesses, it is important to review and understand the anatomy and physiology of the brain and central nervous system (CNS). The brain is involved in thinking, decision making, speaking, emotion, memory, motor and sensory activity, and the basic functions of temperature regulation and breathing, as well as many other functions. Refer to Chapter 47 to review the nerves, structure of neurons, synapses, neurotransmitters, and the autonomic nervous system, as well as the structure and function of the brain. Also see Table 56.1 for the hypothesized roles of CNS neurotransmitters in mental illness.

MENTAL HEALTH AND MENTAL ILLNESS

Opinions within the mental health community differ as to what **mental health** and **mental illness** are. *Mental health* has been defined in many ways. These definitions include the ability to do the following:

• Be flexible.
• Take responsibility for own actions.
• Form close relationships.
• Make appropriate judgments.
• Solve problems.
• Cope with daily **stress**.
• Have a positive sense of self.

TABLE 56.1 NEUROTRANSMITTERS IN THE CNS

Neurotransmitter	Location/Function	Possible Implications for Mental Health
Cholinergics Acetylcholine	Autonomic nervous system (ANS): sympathetic and parasympathetic presynaptic nerve terminals; parasympathetic postsynaptic nerve terminals Central nervous system (CNS): cerebral cortex, hippocampus, limbic structures, and basal ganglia *Functions:* sleep, arousal, pain perception, movement, memory	*Decreased levels:* Alzheimer's disease, Huntington's disease, Parkinson's disease *Increased levels:* depression
Monoamines Norepinephrine	ANS: sympathetic postsynaptic nerve terminals CNS: thalamus, hypothalamus, limbic system, hippocampus, cerebellum, cerebral cortex *Functions:* mood, cognition, perception, locomotion, cardiovascular functioning, and sleep and arousal	*Decreased levels:* depression *Increased levels:* mania, anxiety states, schizophrenia
Dopamine	Frontal cortex, limbic system, basal ganglia, thalamus, posterior pituitary, and spinal cord *Functions:* movement and coordination, emotions, voluntary judgment, release of prolactin	*Decreased levels:* Parkinson's disease, depression *Increased levels:* mania, schizophrenia
Serotonin	Hypothalamus, thalamus, limbic system, cerebral cortex, cerebellum, spinal cord *Functions:* sleep and arousal, libido, appetite, mood, aggression, pain perception, coordination, judgment	*Decreased levels:* depression *Increased levels:* anxiety states

Continued

TABLE 56.1   NEUROTRANSMITTERS IN THE CNS—cont'd

Neurotransmitter	Location/Function	Possible Implications for Mental Health
Histamine	Hypothalamus	*Decreased levels:* depression
Amino Acids		
Gamma-amino-butyric acid (GABA)	Hypothalamus, hippocampus, cortex, cerebellum, basal ganglia, spinal cord, retina *Functions:* slowdown of body activity	*Decreased levels:* Huntington's disease, anxiety disorders, schizophrenia, and various forms of epilepsy
Glycine	Spinal cord and brainstem *Functions:* recurrent inhibition of motor neurons	*Toxic levels:* "glycine encephalopathy"; decreased levels are correlated with spastic motor movement
Glutamate and aspartate	Pyramidal cells of the cortex, cerebellum, and the primary sensory afferent systems; hippocampus, thalamus, hypothalamus, spinal cord *Functions:* relay of sensory information and in the regulation of various motor and spinal reflexes	*Increased levels:* Huntington's disease, temporal lobe epilepsy, spinal cerebellar degeneration
Neuropeptides		
Endorphins and enkephalins	Hypothalamus, thalamus, limbic structures, midbrain, and brainstem; enkephalins are also found in the gastrointestinal tract *Functions:* modulation of pain and reduced peristalsis (enkephalins)	Modulation of dopamine activity by opioid peptides may indicate some link to the symptoms of schizophrenia
Substance P	Hypothalamus, limbic structures, midbrain, brainstem, thalamus, basal ganglia, and spinal cord; also found in gastrointestinal tract and salivary glands *Function:* regulation of pain	*Decreased levels:* Huntington's disease and Alzheimer's disease *Increased levels:* depression
Somatostatin	Cerebral cortex, hippocampus, thalamus, basal ganglia, brain stem, and spinal cord *Function:* inhibits release of norepinephrine; stimulates release of serotonin, dopamine, and acetylcholine	*Decreased levels:* Alzheimer's disease *Increased levels:* Huntington's disease

ANS = autonomic nervous system; CNS = central nervous system.

Source: Townsend, M. C. (2012). *Psychiatric mental health nursing: Concepts of care in evidence-based practice* (7th ed.). Philadelphia: F.A. Davis, pp. 62–63.

Mental illness can be defined as experiencing the following:

- Impaired ability to think
- Impaired ability to feel
- Impaired ability to make sound judgments
- Impaired ability to adapt
- Difficulty in **coping** or inability to cope with reality
- Difficulty in forming or inability to form strong personal relationships.

It is important to remember that mental health and mental illness exist on a continuum. It is natural for emotions to ebb and flow from day to day in response to the degree of stress experienced. People who remain mentally healthy are able to cope with and keep their stress in perspective. Others are not able to do so and over time may develop physical or emotional illnesses as a result of present and past life stresses.

Picture the seesaw that children play on. Mental health and mental illness are like a seesaw. When children of approximately equal weight get on each end of the seesaw, they can balance each other and keep the seesaw even. Mentally healthy people can stay in a state of emotional balance. Sometimes one child weighs just a little more than the other and the seesaw tips just a little to one side. Mentally healthy people can cope with this fluctuation. Sometimes another child gets on or one child greatly outweighs the other, and the seesaw gets out of balance completely; one end goes way up while the other goes way down, and it stays there until someone alters the balance. When a person's moods are way down or way up, he or she is not in emotional *homeostasis* (balance).

Etiologies

The line between the causes of mental illnesses and other brain or neurological disorders is being erased as we learn more about how the brain functions. As scientists study the brains of people who have mental illnesses, they are concluding that mental illness has a biological basis. Changes in the brain's structure, chemistry, and function are associated with expressions of mental illness. However, it is important to note that while mental illnesses can be categorized as brain diseases, not all brain diseases are mental illnesses.

Explanations of mental illness in this unit include concepts from the psychological and the psychobiological (or biological) theories. When pertinent, other theories (e.g., behavioral, environmental) are also presented. Most mental illnesses have no identifiable cause. Some etiological theories have stronger positive correlations to illnesses than others. When appropriate, this unit gives the most current or most widely accepted view of an etiology.

Social and Cultural Environments

Many professionals in the field of behavioral health believe that social and cultural environments have a great influence on the way people develop and process life experiences. Some behavioral health clinicians believe that some cultural traditions and beliefs cause disturbances in personal relationships, which can lead to forms of emotional disturbance. It is part of the nurse's role to take time to learn about traits that are common among people and traits that differ. Although understanding that each person is a unique individual, it is important to have an understanding of broad customs and beliefs to avoid unrealistic expectations of patients.

Spirituality and Religion

Spirituality and religion are extremely important to some patients and unimportant to others. A person's success in recuperating from physical or emotional illness may be deeply tied to spirituality. It is necessary to be comfortable talking to the patient about spiritual needs while being careful

not to impose personal values on the patient. If you are not comfortable in these situations, you should offer to call the spiritual or religious leader of the patient's choice.

For more information about mental health and illness, visit the National Institute of Mental Health at www.nimh.nih.gov, the American Psychiatric Association at www.psych.org, the American Psychological Association at www.apa.org, the American Psychiatric Nurses Association at www.apna.org, or the International Society of Psychiatric-Mental Health Nurses at www.ispn-psych.org.

NURSING ASSESSMENT OF MENTAL HEALTH

During the assessment phase of the nursing process, a mental status examination is performed. This is a series of questions, activities, and observations that evaluate eight areas:

- Appearance and behavior
- Level of awareness and reality **orientation**
- Thinking/content of thought
- Memory
- Speech and ability to communicate
- Mood and **affect**
- Judgment
- Perception

A number of tools of varying names, lengths, and formats are used to evaluate mental capabilities. See Table 56.2 for a sample mental status examination.

After data have been collected, the LPN/LVN collaborates with the registered nurse (RN) to develop nursing diagnoses (Box 56-1).

DIAGNOSTIC TESTS

Physicians use a variety of diagnostic criteria to diagnose mental illness. It is important to rule out physical illness as a cause of symptoms. A primary care provider may choose to refer a patient to a psychiatrist or other mental health professional for further testing and diagnosis.

The diagnostic tool that is used most widely by psychiatrists and other mental health professionals is the *Diagnostic and Statistical Manual of Mental Disorders, Fifth Edition,* or *DSM-5* (American Psychiatric Association, 2013). The *DSM-5* groups illnesses into categories of clinical disorders. This is a complex diagnostic tool. Although as an LPN you will not be responsible for completing the assessment or making a diagnosis, you can contribute valuable information.

There are also batteries of psychological tests that can be administered and interpreted by psychiatrists, psychologists, social workers, or advanced practice nurses. Age, hand tremors, vision, language barriers, educational background, and the interpretation of the health care provider are some factors that can influence the results of these tests.

TABLE 56.2 SAMPLE MENTAL STATUS EXAMINATION

Area to Be Examined	Type of Examination	Normal Parameters	Alterations from Normal
Appearance and behavior	Observations about dress, hygiene, posture, and appearance and about the patient's actions and reactions to health care personnel.	Clean, combed hair. Clothing intact and appropriate to weather or situation. Teeth/dentures in good repair. Posture erect. Cooperates with health care personnel.	Displays either unusual apathy or concern about appearance. Displays uncooperative, hostile, or suspicious behaviors toward health care personnel.
Level of awareness and orientation	Subjective and objective assessment of patient's degree of alertness (wakefulness) and degree of patient's knowledge of self.	Awareness is measured on a continuum that ranges from unconscious to manic. "Normal alertness" is the desired behavior. Facilities may provide a standard format for this assessment, but observations can be documented as well if the patient is not able to stay awake for even short intervals or if the patient is overly active and has difficulty staying in one place. Orientation is assessed by asking the patient questions relating to person, place, and time, such as "Who is this sitting next to you?" "Where are you right now?" or "What year is it?"	Outcome is not considered within accepted normal limits if the patient is difficult to arouse and keep awake or if the patient has difficulty feeling calm. Abnormal results of orientation are the patient's inability to correctly answer orientation questions or inability to answer commonly known questions, such as "Who is the president?"
Thinking/content of thought	Subjective assessment of what the patient is thinking and the process the patient uses in his or her thinking.	Formal testing may be done by a psychologist or psychiatrist to determine the patient's general thought content and pattern. Nurses may contribute to the assessment of thought by documenting statements the patient makes regarding daily care and routines.	Abnormal behaviors include flight of ideas, loose associations, phobias, delusions, and obsessions.
Memory	Subjective assessment of the mind's ability to recall recent and remote (long-term) information.	Recent memory: recall of events that are immediately past or within 2 weeks before the assessment, such as a recent news event. One measurement technique is to ask the patient what they had for breakfast that day or what they did yesterday afternoon. *Remote memory:* recall of events of the past beyond 2 weeks before assessment. Patients may be asked where they were born, where they went to grade school, etc.	Inability to accurately perform recent or remote (long-term) recall exercises within parameters. May indicate symptom of delirium or dementia.

TABLE 56.2   SAMPLE MENTAL STATUS EXAMINATION—cont'd

Area to Be Examined	Type of Examination	Normal Parameters	Alterations from Normal
Speech and ability to communicate	Objective and subjective assessment of how the patient uses verbal and nonverbal communication. Stuttering, repetition of words, and words that the patient makes up (neologisms) are also assessed.	Patient can coherently produce words appropriate to age, education, and life experience. Rate of speech reflects other psychomotor activity (e.g., faster if the patient is agitated). Volume is not too soft or too loud. Speech is fluid and appropriate.	Limited speech production. Rate of speech is inconsistent with other psychomotor activity. Volume is not appropriate to situation (speaks louder or softer than appropriate). Presence of stuttering, word repetition, or neologisms may indicate physical or psychological illness.
Mood and affect	Objective and subjective assessment of the patient's stated feelings and emotions. Affect measures the outward expression of those feelings.	Mood is the stated emotional condition of the patient and should reflect situations as they occur. Facial expression and body language (affect) should match (be congruent with) the stated mood. Affect should change to fluctuate with the changes in mood.	Mood and affect do not match (e.g., facial expression does not appear sad while the patient is expressing sad feelings).
Judgment	Subjective assessment of a patient's ability to make appropriate decisions about his or her situation or to understand concepts.	When given a proverb or situation to solve, such as "You can't teach an old dog new tricks," the patient should be able to give some sort of acceptable interpretation, such as, "Old habits are hard to break" or "It is hard to learn something new."	Patient cannot interpret the sayings or complete problem-solving questions appropriately. The patient might answer very literally, "Dogs can't learn anything when they get old."
Perception	Assessment of the way a person experiences reality. Observation of the patient's statements about his or her environment and the behaviors expressed in association with those statements. Assessment of the patient's insight into his or her condition.	All five senses are monitored for the patient's perception of reality. Perceptions of environment are accurate. Insight into condition is appropriate.	Hallucinations may occur with schizophrenia. Hallucinations are false sensory perceptions. Illusions are misperceptions of reality. Patient unable to state understanding of the origin of the illness; associated behaviors inappropriate. Many people with schizophrenia or mania have poor insight because of impairment of prefrontal cortex functioning during psychosis.

Box 56-1 Nursing Diagnoses Commonly Used to Address Mental Health Problems

Anxiety (mild to panic)
Chronic Sorrow
Compromised Family Coping
Compromised Human Dignity, Risk for
Compromised Resilience
Readiness for enhanced hope
Readiness for enhanced spiritual well-being
Readiness for enhanced decision-making
Decisional conflict
Deficient Community Health
Defensive Coping
Disabled Family Coping
Disturbed Body Image
Disturbed Personal Identity
Disturbed Sensory Perception, Risk for
Disturbed Sleep Pattern
Dysfunctional Family Processes
Fear
Grieving
Complicated Grieving, Risk for
Impaired Individual Resilience
Readiness for Enhanced Resilience
Risk for Compromised Resilience
Impaired Religiosity
Readiness for enhanced religiosity
Risk for impaired religiosity
Ineffective Coping
Ineffective Denial
Ineffective Impulse Control
Ineffective Relationship, Risk for
Ineffective Role Performance
Ineffective Self Health Management
Injury, Risk for
Chronic Low Self-Esteem
Risk for Low Self-Esteem (Chronic or Situational)
Moral Distress
Noncompliance Posttrauma Syndrome, Risk for
Rape-Trauma Syndrome
Powerlessness
Risk for Powerlessness
Readiness for enhanced power
Relocation Stress Syndrome, Risk for
Risk for Violence (Self-Directed or Other-Directed)
Risk-prone health behavior
Self-Care Deficit (specify)
Self-Mutilation
Sexual Dysfunction
Social Isolation
Stress Overload
Suicide, Risk for

Distinguishing Physical Versus Mental Health Disorders

Some physical disorders can mimic mental health disorders, so diagnostic tests may be performed to either confirm or rule out a diagnosis of a mental illness:

- *Laboratory tests* can rule out problems such as electrolyte imbalances, hypothyroidism, infections, dehydration, drug toxicity, or pregnancy.
- *Computed tomography (CT) scans or magnetic resonance imaging (MRI)* can rule out tumors, lesions, or other physical problems.
- *Positron emission tomography (PET) scans* can identify how the parts of the brain are functioning by showing chemical activity or metabolism.

 ## COPING AND EGO DEFENSE MECHANISMS

"Oh, just learn to cope with it." "Get a grip." "Don't make a mountain out of a molehill." These are pieces of advice that people may have heard or given at some point. But what do they mean? What is coping? Coping is the way one adapts psychologically, physically, and behaviorally to a **stressor**. People have different methods of coping or dealing with their stressors. Culture, religion, individual belief systems, experience, and personal choice influence a person's responses to stress. It is not the value of a behavior that we assess as nurses; it is the desired outcome that is important. What is an effective coping skill? Is it healthy? Does it work? How do we as nurses observe and measure it?

Effective Coping Skills

Effective coping skills offer healthy choices for dealing with stressors. Effective coping skills are also conscious mechanisms. Hospitalization is stressful for patients and families. Many things are unknown and unfamiliar. The patient may not understand the illness or the implications of the treatment plan. It is common for patients to use coping mechanisms during hospitalization. The process of effective coping is sometimes called **adaptation**. Allowing the patient to practice new coping techniques will give him or her confidence and will decrease the stress that can accompany change.

Often the dividing line between effective and ineffective coping is the frequency of its use. For instance, mild **anxiety** can be positive. Generally, when there is a little anxiety, people are more alert and ready to respond. The *fight-or-flight mechanism* can actually help one adapt to a new situation. However, too much anxiety begins to cloud the consciousness and interfere with the ability to make appropriate choices and to recall new adaptive tools that have been learned. One of the most helpful roles you can perform is to listen to the patient's thoughts and feelings about the stressor, assist him or her in identifying precipitating factors and patterns to the patient's stress, encourage the patient to problem solve, and provide assistance to develop alternative solutions to a problem.

CRITICAL THINKING

Mr. Joseph

■ Mr. Joseph is noted wailing loudly and continuously after the death of his wife. It is disturbing the other patients on the hospital wing, and one of the nurses comments, "He is a real nut case. Get him out of here."

What is an appropriate response to this nurse? To the husband? How would you document his behavior?

Suggested answers are at the end of the chapter.

CRITICAL THINKING

Mrs. Beison

■ Mrs. Beison, a 44-year-old mother of three teenagers, is diagnosed with breast cancer. She is refusing treatment because she does not believe she has cancer. She says if anything is really wrong, her vitamins will take care of it.

What ego defense mechanism is Mrs. Beison using? Is it effective or ineffective? Why? How can you help? Are there other health care providers (HCPs) who could provide assistance?

Suggested answers are at the end of the chapter.

Ineffective Coping Skills

Sometimes coping behaviors are ineffective. When conscious techniques are not successful, people may unconsciously fall into habits that give the illusion of coping. These habits are called *ego defense mechanisms* (or coping or mental mechanisms). Ego defense mechanisms act as mental pressure valves. The purpose of ego defense mechanisms is to reduce or eliminate anxiety. They give the impression that they are helping alleviate the stress level. When used in very small doses, ego defense mechanisms can be helpful. When they are overused or are the only means used to deal with anxiety, they can become ineffective and unhealthy. People are not born with these coping behaviors; they are learned as responses to stress. Many times they develop by age 10. They may appear to be conscious, but they are, for the most part, unconscious mechanisms. Some commonly used ego defense mechanisms are listed in Table 56.3.

 THERAPEUTIC MEASURES

People who experience alterations in their mental health have special treatment needs. When emotional health is threatened, many other daily activities can be altered as well. **Cognitive** ability (the ability to think rationally and to process thoughts) can be impaired. Emotional responses can be decreased or even absent in some conditions. This can be extremely frightening and can lead to a worsening of the mental disorder or even the development of another disorder. This section provides an overview of selected therapies to help patients deal with alterations in mental health.

TABLE 56.3   EGO DEFENSE MECHANISMS

Mechanism	Description	Examples
Denial	Usually the first defense learned and used. Unconscious refusal to see reality; not conscious lying.	The alcoholic states, "I can quit any time I want to."
Repression (stuffing)	An unconscious "burying" or "forgetting" mechanism. Excludes or withholds from consciousness events or situations that are unbearable.	A step deeper than "denial." A patient may "forget" about an appointment he or she does not want to keep.
Rationalization	Using a logical-sounding excuse to cover up true thoughts and feelings. The most frequently used defense mechanism.	1. "I made a medication error because the doctor's orders were confusing." 2. "I failed the test because the teacher wasn't clear about what would be on it."
Compensation	Making up for something perceived as an inadequacy by developing some other desirable trait.	1. The small boy who wants to be a basketball center instead becomes an honor roll student. 2. The physically unattractive person who wants to model instead becomes a famous designer.

Continued

TABLE 56.3 EGO DEFENSE MECHANISMS—cont'd

Mechanism	Description	Examples
Reaction formation (overcompensation)	Similar to compensation, except the person usually develops the exact opposite trait.	1. The small boy who wants to be a basketball center becomes a political voice to decrease the emphasis on sports in the elementary grades. 2. The physically unattractive person who wants to be a model speaks out for eliminating beauty pageants.
Regression	Emotionally returning to an earlier time in life when the patient experienced far less stress. Commonly seen in patients while hospitalized. *NOTE:* People do not go back to the same developmental age. This is highly individualized.	1. Children who are toilet trained begin to wet the bed after the birth of a younger sibling. 2. Adults start crying and have a "temper tantrum."
Projection	Ascribing one's own unacceptable qualities or feelings to someone else. May lead to scapegoating.	1. A patient might state: "My sister is so jealous of me," when actually the patient is jealous of her sister. 2. An anxious patient may say to the nurse, "Why do I make you so nervous?"
Displacement (transference)	"Kick-the-dog syndrome." Transferring anger and hostility to another person or object that is perceived to be less powerful than oneself.	Parent loses job without notice; goes home and verbally abuses spouse, who unjustly punishes child, who slaps the dog.
Restitution (undoing)	Make amends for a behavior one thinks is unacceptable. Makes an attempt at reducing guilt.	1. A person gives a treat to a child who is being punished for a wrongdoing. 2. The person who sees someone lose a wallet with a large amount of cash does not return the wallet, but puts extra in the collection plate at the next church service.
Conversion reaction	Anxiety is channeled into physical symptoms. Often the symptoms disappear soon after the threat is over.	Nausea develops the night before a major exam, causing the person to miss the exam. Nausea may disappear soon after the scheduled test is finished.
Avoidance	Unconsciously staying away from events or situations that might cause feelings of aggression or anxiety.	"I can't go to the class reunion tonight. I'm just so tired, I have to sleep."

Therapeutic Communication

Many people take communication for granted. In the mental health setting, communication is a tool used to relate therapeutically with patients. It is important to be intentional about the messages we communicate to patients. Therapeutic communication is accomplished through the deliberate use of verbal and nonverbal techniques. Other areas to consider when communicating are the patient's personal values, attitudes, beliefs, culture, religion, social status, gender, and age or developmental level.

Verbal therapeutic communication techniques can help facilitate an interpersonal interaction. For instance, if you ask a patient to explain something to you in more detail, you are using the therapeutic communication technique of *exploring*. Verbal communication is also influenced by the tone, pitch, speed, and volume of speech. Some commonly used therapeutic communication techniques are listed in Table 56.4.

TABLE 56.4 THERAPEUTIC COMMUNICATION TECHNIQUES

Technique	Description	Examples
Encouraging descriptions of perceptions	Asking the patient what he or she is seeing or hearing	"Tell me what the voices are saying to you."
Encouraging comparison	Asking the patient to compare similarities or differences	"How is this medication working for you compared to the last time you used it?"
Exploring	Looking deeper into a subject, idea, or experience	"Tell me more about the last time you were depressed."
Focusing	Concentrating on a single idea or event	"Tell me more about how your divorce made you feel."
Formulating a plan of action	Assisting the patient to come up with a plan to cope with stress	"When this happens in the future, how could you handle it more constructively?"
Giving broad openings	Allowing the patient to steer the interaction	"What would you like to work on today?"
Giving recognition	Acknowledging or showing awareness	"I see you went to your therapy group today."
Making observations	Verbalizing what is observed	"I notice you seemed upset after your visit."
Offering self	Extending one's presence	"I am available to talk whenever you would like."
Offering general leads	Giving the patient encouragement to continue	"I see. . ." "Go on. . ."
Placing event in time or sequence	Clarification of events in time	"Was this before or after your first hospitalization?"
Presenting reality	Defining reality in simple terms	"The voices may seem real to you, but they are a symptom of your illness."
Restating	Repeating the main idea of what the patient has verbalized	"It sounds as if you are feeling frustrated."
Reflecting	Statements, questions, or feelings are referred back to the patient	"What do you think you should do?"
Seeking clarification	Searching for understanding of what was said	"Tell me if this is what you meant when you said. . ."
Verbalizing the implied	Putting into words what the patient has implied or said indirectly	"You must be feeling very sad right now."
Using silence	Gives both the nurse and the patient a chance to collect their thoughts and organize what they are going to say	

Components of *nonverbal communication* include physical appearance, dress, body movement and posture, touch, facial expression, and eye contact. It is believed that most communication takes place nonverbally, so it is possible that while you are saying one thing to a patient, your body language could be saying something else.

There are also barriers to effective communication that are commonly called *communication blocks*. A nurse who tells a patient "Don't worry, everything will be all right" has just given the patient false reassurance. This barrier communicates to the patient that his or her concerns are not being taken seriously. Some common communication blocks are listed in Table 56.5.

TABLE 56.5 COMMUNICATION BLOCKS

Mechanism	Description	Examples
Agreeing/disagreeing	Implies that the patient's ideas or feelings are somehow right or wrong	"That is right on target. I agree 100%."
Asking "why" questions	Asking why implies that the patient knows the reason for his or her behavior and feelings	"Why were you feeling so angry?"
Changing the subject	Changing the subject takes control of the conversation away from the patient	Patient: "I am feeling so hopeless." Nurse: "Did you go to group therapy today?"
Giving advice	Telling the patient what to do implies that the nurse knows what is best	"I think you should. . ."
Giving approval or disapproval	Passes judgment on the patient's ideas or opinions	"That's right."
Giving false reassurance	Devalues the patient's feelings	"Everything will be all right."
Self-focusing behavior	The nurse focuses on his or her own feelings at the expense of the patient's.	"That happened to me once. . . let me tell you about it."
Double-bind messages	When the nonverbal message doesn't match the verbal message	"I'm listening," as the nurse fidgets in her chair, doesn't make eye contact, and then coughs.

Milieu

One area over which you can have some control is the therapeutic environment. In the mental health setting, this therapeutic environment is called the **milieu** or therapeutic milieu. It is believed that environment has an effect on behavior. Milieu therapy is the systematic management of the social environment as a treatment modality.

A therapeutic milieu is an environment that provides containment, support, structure, involvement, and validation during the patient's stay. The goals of milieu therapy are resocialization, ego development, and prevention of regression. Resocialization occurs when patients help govern the running of the unit and attend regular meetings to set rules and assign tasks. Ego development is fostered with structured activities that are provided to assist the patient to learn coping and social skills. Regression is discouraged when patients help with washing dishes or other small jobs that foster independence. Common milieu interventions include role modeling, positive reinforcement, a schedule of events, consistent expectations and rules for behavior, and unit meetings. Milieu therapy is difficult in this era of managed care because of shorter hospital stays.

Psychopharmacology

Psychopharmacology is the use of medications to treat psychological disorders. Since the introduction of the phenothiazine class of drugs in the 1950s (e.g., chlorpromazine), the number of medications available for treating mental health disorders has increased greatly, with newer medications having fewer side effects. The reason for using medications is twofold: First, the medications manage the symptoms, helping the patient feel more comfortable emotionally. Second, the patient is generally more receptive and able to focus on other types of therapy if medications are effective. More information on psychoactive drugs is provided in Chapter 57.

Psychotherapies

Psychotherapy is the term used to describe the form of treatment chosen by the psychologist, psychiatrist, social worker, or advanced practice mental health nurse. The goals of psychotherapy include the following:

• Reduce the patient's emotional discomfort.
• Increase the level of the patient's social functioning.
• Increase the ability of the patient to behave or perform in a manner appropriate to the situation.

Several specific types of therapy that are typically used are described next.

• WORD • BUILDING •

psychopharmacology: psycho—soul or mind + pharmaco—drug or medicine + ology—study of
psychotherapy: psycho—soul or mind + therapy—treatment

Psychodynamic Therapy

Psychodynamic therapy is based on **psychoanalysis** and consists of clarifying the meaning of events, feelings, and behavior and thereby gaining **insight** into them. Psychoanalysis was developed from Sigmund Freud's psychoanalytic theory. Freud believed that anxiety was the primary motivation for behavior and therefore all behavior had meaning. The role of the patient is to provide the therapist with clues to the unconscious source of problems and to try to develop insights into behavior. The role of the therapist is to uncover these unconscious experiences and interpret their meanings to the patient. Some believe that psychodynamic therapies will lose popularity as we gain a better understanding of the role of the brain, neurotransmitters, and genetics in mental health.

Behavior Management

Behavior management (also called behavior modification) is a treatment method that stems from the studies of behavioral theorists such as Skinner and Pavlov. It is a common treatment modality used in long-term care facilities, with children and adolescents, and with individuals who have a low level of cognitive functioning.

According to behavior management theory, all behavior is learned, so it can be unlearned. The belief is that behavior can be changed by either positive or negative reinforcement. *Positive reinforcement* is the act of rewarding the patient with something pleasant when the desired behavior has been performed. For instance, if a patient has the habit of using foul language in an attempt to have a need met, the desired behavior change might be to come to a staff member and ask appropriately for what he or she needs. If this patient loves to be outside but is not allowed out except at supervised times, then a suitable positive reinforcement for her might be to allow 15 more minutes outdoors when the desired behavior is exhibited.

Negative reinforcement is the act of responding to the undesired behavior by taking away a privilege or adding a responsibility. Negative reinforcement can be misinterpreted as punishment. Parents who "ground" their children for unacceptable behavior are using negative reinforcement; requiring the child to perform extra household tasks for a stated period is reinforcing the fact that the behavior has consequences. The child may not repeat the undesired behavior after negative reinforcement has been used. It is necessary to be careful to avoid violating the Patient's Bill of Rights when performing behavior management with patients. A signed consent from the patient is advised when using this form of therapy.

The patient must understand the consequences of the behavior to be changed and the purpose for the type of consequence that is chosen. If the person is not capable of understanding the situation or is not able to remember the consequences, behavior management may not be the best form of treatment.

Cognitive Behavioral Therapy

Jean Piaget and Aaron T. Beck are cognitive theorists who have greatly contributed to modern cognitive behavioral therapy. Cognitive behavioral therapists believe that people experience mental illness due to cognitive distortions about their situations.

Cognitive behavioral therapy stresses ways of rethinking situations. The therapist confronts the patient with certain distortions of thinking and then works out ways of thinking about them differently. This type of treatment is used frequently for affective or mood disorders.

Feeling sad about an unpleasant experience (such as the death of a loved one) is acceptable and normal, but long-term depression about the death is an extreme emotion and therefore considered to be unhealthy. In this situation, the patient might be helped to see the death as a sad loss. Behavioral techniques are also often used with phobias or panic disorders, in which fear may interfere with reasoning.

Cognitive therapies are gaining in popularity because they are usually significantly shorter term than other types of therapy and therefore less costly to the patient. Patients are given "homework" that is specific to their needs; they practice their assignments between sessions. Cognitive behavioral therapy in combination with medications can provide effective treatment for depression.

EVIDENCE-BASED PRACTICE

Clinical Question
Does a nurse-administered minimal psychological intervention affect diabetes-specific quality of life and glycemic control?

Evidence
A randomized controlled trial was carried out comparing the intervention with usual care among 208 primary care patients, 60 years or older with type 2 diabetes and co-occurring minor to moderate depression (Lamers, Jonkers, Bosma, Knottnerus, & van Eijk, 2011). The intervention was a nurse-administered, minimal psychological intervention, consisting of elements of cognitive behavioral therapy and self-management. The short nurse-administered psychological intervention for depression positively influenced diabetes-specific quality of life and glycemic control.

Implications for Nursing Practice
Nurses can potentially play an important role in the emotional and physiological well-being of older persons with diabetes.

REFERENCE
Lamers, F., Jonkers, C. C., Bosma, H., Knottnerus, J. A, & van Eijk, J. T. (2011). Treating depression in diabetes patients: Does a nurse-administered minimal psychological intervention affect diabetes-specific quality of life and glycaemic control? A randomized controlled trial. *Journal of Advanced Nursing, 67,* 788–799. doi:10.1111/j.1365-2648.2010.05540.x.

• WORD • BUILDING •

psychoanalysis: psycho—soul or mind + analysis—dissolving

Counseling

Counseling is the provision of help or guidance by a health care professional. The profession of counseling is licensed and regulated differently by state and sometimes also by municipality. Nurses prepared at an LPN/LVN level or at an RN level, in some areas and with special advanced education, can practice some forms of counseling.

You may be asked or expected to accompany patients to counseling sessions or even to facilitate a group discussion. Remember that these are confidential sessions, even if they are group oriented. Patients are there to work; others are there by invitation for special reasons.

Group Therapy

Therapy groups are formed for many reasons; they can be ongoing or short term depending on the needs of the patients or the type of disorder. Group therapy is a cost-effective means of providing treatment. For example, Alcoholics Anonymous (AA) and similar 12-step self-help groups are well-established, ongoing groups formed around treatment of a specific problem. Family counseling sessions may occur with individual therapists with a specialty in the problem area for that family. Marriage counseling may be done in a group with other couples. Many times, peer counselors are used.

Therapists and counselors are tools, or facilitators, in the therapeutic process. Patients must take the suggestions given by the therapist, try them, and see what works for them. You can help by reinforcing the good work patients do to learn to stay mentally healthy and develop more effective life skills.

Electroconvulsive Therapy

Electroconvulsive therapy (ECT) is a form of treatment that is used for severely depressed patients who have not responded to psychotropic medications. ECT passes an electric current through the brain to produce a tonic-clonic (grand mal) seizure. Most mental health professionals believe ECT stimulates an increase in circulating levels of the neurotransmitters serotonin, norepinephrine, and dopamine in the brain. In essence, ECT affects neurotransmitter activity much like antidepressant medications. ECT may be frightening to patients; it is important for the nurse to provide education and information to the patient and family. Many changes have been made in this form of therapy since the 1940s, and ECT is currently a safe and effective treatment for resistant depression.

Procedure

ECT often takes place in the recovery room of an operating suite, where there is ready access to emergency equipment. Informed consent must be obtained by the physician. About 30 minutes before the procedure, the patient is given a medication to dry secretions and counteract stimulation of the vagus nerve, which can cause bradycardia and syncope. Patients are given a short-acting anesthetic before the treatment and a smooth muscle relaxant to minimize injury. Before giving the muscle relaxant, a blood pressure cuff is placed on one of the patient's lower limbs and inflated. This is to ensure that the seizure

activity can be visually monitored in this limb. Blood pressure and pulse are carefully monitored before and after the treatment. The patient is oxygenated with pure oxygen during and after the seizure until spontaneous respirations return. During treatment, an electrical stimulus is delivered to the brain via unilateral or bilateral electrodes. The amount of electrical energy used is individualized to the patient. The seizure must last at least 30 seconds to be effective. The seizure activity is monitored with an electroencephalogram (EEG) and also in the cuffed limb.

Side Effects

Side effects of ECT can be unpleasant but are usually temporary. The patient may feel confused and forgetful immediately after the treatment. This can be from a combination of the ECT itself and the medication that was used before the treatment. If the seizure was severe, the patient may have some muscle soreness.

ECT is not used indiscriminately. It is used when other therapies have not been helpful and is usually reserved for treatment-resistant depression (see "Patient-Centered Care").

Patient Perspective

A Daughter's Thoughts on ECT

My mom is 83 years old and has had a total of 35 ECT treatments for severe depression in her lifetime. If you met her, you'd never know; you'd find her delightful. She's a sweet little plump German lady with a big heart. I am a nurse, and when I tell fellow nurses about my mom, they often ask me why I didn't get her on antidepressants. I want to scream, "How dumb do you think I am?!" Of course Mom is on antidepressants. But at intervals they don't work and she sinks into severe depression. My choice then is to help her have ECT or let her stay depressed and miserable and put her in a nursing home. And she would soon die because when she is depressed, she refuses to move, doesn't sleep, and is horribly miserable.

The first time my mom was scheduled for ECT, one of the nurses in our local community hospital told her to refuse it, that no one should have to go through that. It was a cruel thing to do. My mom doesn't do well in counseling—she doesn't believe in it. In her mind you don't talk about your "dirty linen." My mom was in an abusive relationship with my father for 47 years, and she hid all the problems away and doesn't talk about them to this day. I'm so grateful to have my mom doing okay and grateful that ECT treatments exist. With ECT my mother is doing well and enjoying life. Without treatment, she would be gone. Please understand that there are times when ECT treatments are the best thing for severely depressed people, when other treatments have been ineffective.

Nursing Care

The patient should receive nothing by mouth (NPO) for at least 4 hours before a treatment. Remind the patient to empty his or her bladder and to remove dentures, contact lenses, hairpins, and other items on the body. Following ECT, carefully monitor vital signs and document the patient's subjective and objective responses to the treatment. Stay with the patient until he or she is oriented and able to care for him or herself. Withhold oral medications and food until the gag reflex returns. Ensure that the patient is kept safe after ECT therapy.

Relaxation Therapy

A variety of relaxation techniques can be taught to help patients manage their responses to stress. Relaxation exercises such as deep, rhythmic breathing can increase oxygenation and provide distraction from stressors. Breathing exercises may be coupled with progressive muscle relaxation exercises. For this technique, patients are taught to start at the head and neck and systematically tense and then relax muscle groups as they progress toward the lower extremities. Soft music may enhance the patient's ability to fully relax.

Imagery is the use of the imagination to promote relaxation. For this technique, the patient is taught to imagine a pleasurable experience from his or her past, such as lying on a beach or soaking in a warm bath. Use of all senses is encouraged—for a beach image, the patient might see a beach, feel the warm sun, smell salt air, and hear waves crashing against the shore. The patient might also be taught to visualize being successful in a problem situation.

Relaxation techniques may be used individually, but they are often used in combination with each other or with other therapies for maximum effect. See Chapter 5 for more information on relaxation and imagery.

Home Health Hints

Assess the patient and the patient's home for safety issues:
- Risk of falls (especially if the patient is experiencing orthostatic hypotension from medications)
- Suicide ideation, plan, and means or access to pill stashes, weapons, or other dangerous items
- Ability to access medications, missed doses, or overdoses
- Need for additional services for activities of daily living (ADLs), such as housekeeping, medication assistance, or safety rails

SUGGESTED ANSWERS TO

CRITICAL THINKING

■ Mr. Joseph

Different people cope in different ways. This may be a healthy way to cope in this grieving husband's culture. Gently guide him to a room where he can express his emotions without disturbing others. Ask if he would like you to contact someone to come help support him. Document objectively: "Patient's husband weeping loudly; guided to consultation room for privacy."

As an LPN, your best course of action may be to report the RN's comment objectively to your supervisor.

■ Mrs. Beison

Mrs. Beison is overusing the ego defense mechanism *denial* to cope with her cancer diagnosis. Although at times denial can be an effective coping mechanism, if Mrs. Beison continues to deny her disease and refuse treatment, her life will be in danger. You can help Mrs. Beison verbalize her fears about cancer and cancer treatment and can provide accurate information to help her make wise choices. If needed, a psychiatric evaluation can be requested. If she is found to be mentally competent, then her wishes must be respected.

REVIEW QUESTIONS

1. Which patient behavior requires additional mental health assessment?
   1. Patient is always happy and smiling.
   2. Patient can verbalize emotions.
   3. Patient is able to cope with bad news.
   4. Patient maintains some close, personal relationships.

2. Which data are important to collect during a mental health assessment? **Select all that apply.**
   1. Orientation to reality
   2. Mobility
   3. Ability to communicate clearly
   4. Heart sounds
   5. Memory
   6. Appearance

3. A patient being evaluated for depression asks why blood must be drawn. Which response by the nurse is best?
   1. "Your physical illnesses must be under control before your depression can be treated effectively."
   2. "The clinician needs to rule out physical causes for your symptoms."
   3. "Many mental health disorders can be identified with blood tests."
   4. "If your lab work is out of balance, then correcting the imbalance will reverse your depression."

4. The nurse recognizes that the patient who always seems to be making excuses is displaying which ego defense mechanism?
   1. Denial
   2. Fantasy
   3. Rationalization
   4. Transference

5. Which of the following milieus would be most therapeutic for a patient experiencing severe anxiety?
   1. An environment that provides for all the patient's physical and emotional needs
   2. An environment that is locked and supervised at all times
   3. An environment that is structured to reduce stress and encourage coping behaviors
   4. An environment that eliminates all anxiety-producing stimuli

6. Which explanation of psychopharmacology by the nurse is best for the patient starting on medication for a mental health disorder?
   1. "Medication can potentially cure a mental illness."
   2. "Medication will help you control your behavior."
   3. "Medication is used to block emotional responses in your brain."
   4. "Medication can reduce your symptoms so you can focus on other therapies."

7. Which statement by the patient with a substance abuse disorder indicates that interventions have been effective?
   1. "I know I have a problem, and I have a lot of work to do to get better."
   2. "If I don't think about my problem, eventually it will fade from my memory."
   3. "I no longer have a substance abuse problem. My treatment has been effective."
   4. "Now that I know that my family is the cause of my problem, I can move on."

8. A patient shares some very traumatic life experiences with the LPN. What is the best response by the LPN?
   1. Assure the patient that the staff will not allow such experiences to happen to the patient again.
   2. Ask probing questions about the patient's emotional responses to the experiences.
   3. Encourage the patient to forget the experiences and move on with life.
   4. Listen attentively to the patient and show empathy.

Answers can be found in Appendix C.

Reference

American Psychiatric Association. (2013). *Diagnostic and statistical manual of mental disorders.* (5th ed.). Arlington, VA: American Psychiatric Association.

 For additional resources and information visit **davispl.us/medsurg5**

Nursing Care of Patients With Mental Health Disorders

MARINA MARTINEZ-KRATZ

LEARNING OUTCOMES

1. Identify etiological theories for common mental health disorders.
2. Describe signs and symptoms of common mental health disorders.
3. Describe therapeutic management for each of the disorders.
4. Identify actions, side effects, and nursing considerations for selected classifications of psychoactive medications.
5. Plan nursing interventions for patients with mental health disorders.
6. Discuss the role of the LPN/LVN in the care of patients with mental health disorders.

KEY TERMS

abuse (uh-BYOOS)
addiction (ah-DIK-shun)
alogia (ah-LOH-jee-uh)
anhedonia (AN-heh-DOH-nee-uh)
avolition (A-voh-LISH-un)
bipolar (bye-POH-lur)
codependence (KOH-dee-PEN-dense)
compulsion (kum-PUHL-shun)
delirium tremens (dee-LEER-ee-um TREE-menz)
delusions (dee-LOO-zhuns)
dependence (dee-PEN-dense)
displacement (diss-PLAYSS-ment)
dysfunctional (diss-FUNK-shun-uhl)
eustress (YOO-stress)
hallucinations (hah-LOO-sih-NAY-shuns)
illusions (ih-LOO-zhuns)
mania (MAY-nee-ah)
obsession (ob-SESH-un)
phobia (FOH-bee-ah)
tolerance (TALL-ler-ense)
withdrawal (with-DRAW-ul)

As we saw in the last chapter, people with mental health problems may experience impaired ability to think, feel, make sound judgments, adapt to changes, cope with stressors, and form strong relationships with others. This chapter covers some of the more common mental health disorders you will see in medical, surgical, and long-term care settings. Patients with mental health disorders may need modified care planning to help them manage both mental and physiological illnesses.

ANXIETY DISORDERS, OBSESSIVE-COMPULSIVE AND RELATED DISORDERS, AND TRAUMA- AND STRESSOR-RELATED DISORDERS

Anxiety Disorders

Do you ever feel stressed? How does it make you feel? Is it possible to live a completely stress-free existence? Stress is everywhere in our society. Stress produces anxiety. Most often, stress is associated with negative situations, but the good things that happen to us, such as weddings and job promotions, also produce stress. The stress from positive experiences is called **eustress**. Eustress can produce just as much anxiety as negative stressors. A *stressor* is any person or situation that produces an anxiety response. Stress and stressors are different for each person; therefore, it is important to ask patients what their personal stress producers are.

Anxiety is the uncomfortable feeling of dread that occurs in response to extreme or prolonged periods of stress. It is commonly ranked as mild, moderate, severe, or panic. It is believed that a mild amount of anxiety is a normal part of being human and that mild anxiety is necessary to change and develop new ways of coping with stress.

Anxiety may also be influenced by one's culture. It may be acceptable for some people to acknowledge and discuss stress, but others may believe that discussing personal problems with others is inappropriate. This cultural behavior can be a challenge for the nurse when attempting to collect assessment data.

Anxiety is usually referred to as either *free-floating anxiety* or *signal anxiety*. Free-floating anxiety is described as a general feeling of impending doom. The person cannot pinpoint the cause but might say something like "I just know something bad is going to happen if I go on vacation." Signal anxiety, on the other hand, is an uncomfortable response to a known stressor ("Finals are only a week away, and I've got that nausea again.") Both types of anxiety are involved in the various anxiety disorders.

Etiological Theories

Psychoanalytical theorists believe that anxiety is a conflict between the *id* (the "all for me" part of the personality) and the *superego* (the conscience), which is repressed in early development but emerges again in adulthood.

Biological theorists view anxiety differently. One biological theory points to the sympathoadrenal (fight-or-flight) responses to stress to explain signs and symptoms of anxiety and observes that the blood vessels constrict because epinephrine and norepinephrine have been released, causing blood pressure to rise. Another biological theory implicates a lack of the neurotransmitter gamma-aminobutyric acid (GABA) in the etiology of anxiety. GABA is an inhibitory neurotransmitter that prevents post-synaptic excitation.

If the body adapts to the stress, hormone levels adjust, and body functions return to a homeostatic state. If the body does not adapt to the stress, the immune system is challenged and risk for physical illness increases.

You may observe psychological responses to physical illness. It is important to recognize the relationship between physical and emotional responses to stress. Some examples of medical conditions that occur because of the body's response to stress are shown in Table 57.1.

• **WORD** • **BUILDING** •

eustress: eu—normal or good + stress

TABLE 57.1 RESPONSES TO STRESS

Stress-Related Medical Condition	Pathophysiology	Outcome of Stress on the Body
Lowered immunity	Interferes with effectiveness of antibodies. Possibly related to interactions among the hypothalamus, pituitary gland, adrenal glands, and immune system.	Increased susceptibility to colds and other viruses and illnesses
Burnout	Stress or work-related emotional exhaustion and depression.	Emotional detachment
Migraine, cluster, and tension headaches	Tightening of skeletal muscles. Dilating of cranial arteries.	Nausea, vomiting, tight feeling in or around head and shoulders, tinnitus, inability to tolerate light, weakness of a limb
Hypertension	Role of stress not positively known. Thought to contribute to hypertension by negatively interacting with kidneys,	Resistance to blood flow through the cardiovascular system, causing pressure on the arteries

TABLE 57.1   RESPONSES TO STRESS—cont'd

Stress-Related Medical Condition	Pathophysiology	Outcome of Stress on the Body
	autonomic nervous system, and endocrine system.	Can lead to stroke, heart attack, and kidney failure
Coronary artery disease	Not fully understood. Stress may be associated with behavioral factors such as overeating, physical inactivity, and obesity.	Hypertension, hypercholesterolemia, atherosclerosis, diabetes
Cancer	Stress lowers the immune response.	Lowered immunity may allow for overcolonization of opportunistic cancer cells.
Asthma	Autonomic (parasympathetic) nervous system stimulates mucus, increases blood flow, and constricts airways. May be associated with other stress-related conditions such as allergy and viral infection.	Wheezing, coughing, dyspnea, apprehension May lead to respiratory infections, respiratory failure, or pneumothorax

Diagnosis

Because there are so many symptoms associated with anxiety disorders, it is important for people to have a complete physical examination before diagnosing an anxiety disorder. Some medical disorders, such as hyperthyroidism, can mimic anxiety; hypothyroidism can mimic depression.

Types of Anxiety

SPECIFIC PHOBIA. Specific **phobias** are the most common of the anxiety disorders. There are more than 700 documented phobias. Specific phobias are defined as irrational fears of distinct objects or situations such as snakes, bridges, or flying. The person is very aware of the fear and even the fact that it is irrational but is unable to gain control over the stressor and the fear continues.

The psychoanalytic view implies that it really is not the object that is the source of the fear but rather that the fear is a result of a defense mechanism called **displacement**. For example, the person with a phobia of snakes may have seen a frightening movie in which someone died from a snakebite. The stated object of the phobia would be interpreted as a symbol for the underlying cause of the fear, such as fear of dying.

SOCIAL ANXIETY DISORDER (SOCIAL PHOBIA). Social anxiety disorder is a social phobia characterized by a persistent fear of behaving or performing in a way that will be humiliating or embarrassing to the individual, such as public speaking, eating in front of others, or using public restrooms. The fear or anxiety is out of proportion to the situation.

PANIC DISORDER. Panic is a state of extreme fear that cannot be controlled; it may be referred to as a panic attack. Panic episodes are recurrent and occur unpredictably. Patients may present themselves at the emergency room because they believe they are having a heart attack or other significant physical illness. Patients must exhibit several episodes within a specified time frame to be given the diagnosis of panic disorder. Some of the symptoms associated with panic disorder include the following:

- Fear (usually of dying, losing control of self, or "going crazy")
- Feelings of impending doom
- Dissociation (feeling that it is happening to someone else or not happening at all)
- Nausea
- Diaphoresis
- Chest pain
- Palpitations
- Shaking.

GENERALIZED ANXIETY DISORDER. In generalized anxiety disorder (GAD), the anxiety itself (also referred to as excessive worry or severe stress) is the expressed symptom. Patients with GAD worry about everything. Symptoms that may be present in GAD include the following:

- Restlessness or feeling "on edge"
- Shaking
- Palpitations
- Dry mouth
- Nausea, vomiting
- Easy frightening
- Hot flashes
- Chills
- Muscle aches
- Hypervigilance (excessive attention to stimuli)

• Polyuria
• Difficulty swallowing.

Nursing care of patients with anxiety is discussed after "Trauma- and Stressor-Related Disorders."

Obsessive-Compulsive and Related Disorders

The *Diagnostic and Statistical Manual of Mental Disorders* (5th ed., *DSM-5*) (American Psychiatric Association, 2013) groups obsessive-compulsive and related disorders together in a distinct category separate from the anxiety disorders. Disorders grouped in this new category have common features such as an obsessive preoccupation and repetitive behaviors. The disorders included in this new grouping include obsessive-compulsive disorder, body dysmorphic disorder and trichotillomania (hair-pulling disorder), as well as two new disorders: hoarding disorder and excoriation (skin-picking) disorder.

Obsessive-Compulsive Disorder

Obsessive-compulsive disorder (OCD) occurs in 2% to 5% of the population and is the fourth most common psychiatric diagnosis. It consists of two parts: the **obsession** (repetitive thought, urge, or images) and the **compulsion** (an excessive or unrealistic repetitive act that the individual feels driven to perform in response to the obsession. An example of OCD is the need to check that the doors are locked numerous times before one is able to sleep or leave the house. This need to repetitively check the locks may prevent the person from sleeping or leaving the house at all. Some individuals wash their hands compulsively to the point of having raw and bleeding hands. Behaviors become ritualistic. The person with OCD is unable to stop the thought or the action. Performing the action (such as checking the locks or hand washing) is the mechanism that reduces the anxiety. Although as the nurse you should not interfere with these repetitive acts, OCD patients can be helped by therapeutic interventions such as cognitive-behavioral therapy or medications (such as fluoxetine). Nursing care of patients with OCD is discussed after "Trauma- and Stressor-Related Disorders."

Trauma- and Stressor-Related Disorders

The *DSM-5* (American Psychiatric Association, 2013) created a category to group trauma and stressor-related disorders. Patients diagnosed with these disorders have experienced exposure to a traumatic or stressful event such as war or natural disasters and experience specific symptoms. The disorders included in this new category include posttraumatic stress disorder as well as reactive attachment disorder, disinhibited social engagement disorder, acute stress disorder, and adjustment disorders.

Posttraumatic Stress Disorder

Posttraumatic stress disorder (PTSD) develops in response to some unexpected emotional or physical trauma when there was the *real threat of death or harm* and the patient was helpless to do anything about it. People who have fought in wars, been raped, or survived violent storms or acts (such as terrorist acts) are examples of those who are susceptible to suffering from this disorder.

A condition that is associated with PTSD is *survivor guilt,* which is the feeling of guilt expressed by those who have survived a tragedy. A survivor of an airline crash may say, "Why me? Why did I make it? I should have died too!" This is especially true if a loved one died in the crash.

Symptoms may appear immediately or may not appear until years later. A key symptom of PTSD is *flashbacks* in which the person may relive the traumatic event as if it were happening at that moment. Sounds and smells associated with the trauma may trigger the flashback.

Signs and symptoms of PTSD include the following:

• Flashbacks or dissociative reactions
• Recurrent intrusive memories of the traumatic event
• Recurrent intrusive dreams/nightmares related to the traumatic event
• Intense psychological distress at exposure to internal or external cues that resemble an aspect of the traumatic event
• Marked physical reaction to internal or external cues that resemble an aspect of the traumatic event
• Persistent avoidance of stimuli associated with the traumatic events
• Social withdrawal
• Feelings of low self-esteem
• Changes in relationships with significant others
• Difficulty forming new relationships
• Hypervigilance
• Irritability and outbursts of anger seemingly for no obvious reason
• Depression
• Chemical dependency.

Therapeutic Measures for Patients With Anxiety, Obsessive-Compulsive, or Trauma-Related Disorders

Treatment for these disorders is individualized and may include one or more of the following: medications (psychopharmacology), individual psychotherapy, group therapy, systematic desensitization, hypnosis, imagery, relaxation exercises, and biofeedback.

Psychopharmacology may involve benzodiazepines, an antianxiety classification of medications. Alprazolam (Xanax) or lorazepam (Ativan) are commonly used and are effective in most cases. Benzodiazepines are used for short-term treatment because of the strong potential for chemical dependency. Individuals who need longer term therapy for anxiety or who have chemical dependency tendencies may be treated with buspirone (BuSpar), the selective serotonin reuptake inhibitors (SSRIs) paroxetine (Paxil) or sertraline (Zoloft), the antihistamine hydroxyzine hydrochloride (Atarax), or the antihypertensive agent clonidine (Catapres). See Table 57.2 for a review of medications.

In *systematic desensitization,* the patient is exposed gradually (rating the fear on a scale from 1 to 10) to the object that causes the anxiety. *Hypnosis* places the patient in a subconscious state and then helps the patient recall

TABLE 57.2   MEDICATIONS USED FOR ALTERATIONS IN MENTAL HEALTH

Medication Class/Action	Examples	Route	Side Effects	Nursing Implications
Typical Antipsychotics Block mainly D$_2$ dopamine receptors (used less often because of serious extrapyramidal side effects).	chlorpromazine (Thorazine) haloperidol (Haldol) fluphenazine (Prolixin) thioridazine (Mellaril) thiothixene (Navane) trifluoperazine (Trilafon) trifluoperazine (Stelazine)	PO, IM PO, IM, long-acting IM PO, IM, long-acting IM PO PO, IM PO, IM PO, IM	Extrapyramidal side effects (EPSEs): pseudo-parkinsonism, akathisia, dystonia, tardive dyskinesia, photosensitivity, orthostatic hypotension, gynecomastia, neuroleptic malignant syndrome, anticholinergic effects	For short-term use because of side effects. Monitor for EPSEs. Have patient rise slowly to counter orthostatic hypotension. Offer ice chips, gum, or hard candy for dry mouth. Monitor urinary and bowel elimination. Avoid use if patient is in first trimester of pregnancy. Do not use/take with alcohol or other CNS depressants. *Patient teaching:* Use sunscreen when outside.
Atypical Antipsychotics Block multiple dopamine and serotonin receptors.	asenapine (Saphris) clozapine (Clozaril) lurasidone (Latuda) risperidone (Risperdal) olanzapine (Zyprexa) quetiapine (Seroquel) ziprasidone (Geodon) aripiprazole (Abilify) paliperidone (Invega)	SL PO PO PO, SL, IM, long-acting IM PO, fast-dissolving tablets PO PO, IM	Agranulocytosis (Clozaril); weight gain; type 2 diabetes; dose-related EPSE (especially with Risperdal and in older adults); lowers seizure threshold; caution with cardiac patients	Monitor CBC (Clozaril). Monitor weight gain. Monitor glucose level for onset of type 2 diabetes. Take Latuda with food. Sublingual forms can dissolve in hands; make sure hands are dry, and take immediately. Do not eat or drink for 10 minutes.

Continued

TABLE **57.2** **MEDICATIONS USED FOR ALTERATIONS IN MENTAL HEALTH—cont'd**

Medication Class/Action	Examples	Route	Side Effects	Nursing Implications
Antidepressants **Selective Serotonin Reuptake Inhibitor (SSRIs)** Block the reuptake of serotonin at the presynaptic receptor.	fluoxetine (Prozac) sertraline (Zoloft) paroxetine (Paxil) escitalopram (Lexapro) citalopram (Celexa) fluvoxamine (Luvox)	PO, once-weekly dosing PO	Excitation, nausea and vomiting, decreased libido, anorexia and weight loss, increased suicide risk the first few weeks of therapy	Allow time for side effects to subside. Do not administer after 1500 to keep excitation from affecting sleep. *Patient teaching:* It will take 6–8 weeks for therapeutic effects to occur. Do not stop drug abruptly. Do not take with other serotonin-type medications including St. John's wort and SAMe.
Tricyclic Antidepressants Partially block the reuptake of serotonin and norepinephrine at the presynaptic receptor (used infrequently because of side effects).	amitriptyline (Elavil) nortriptyline (Pamelor) imipramine (Tofranil)	PO	Anticholinergic effects, sedation, weight gain, orthostatic hypotension, dysrhythmias, increased suicide risk the first few weeks of therapy	Decreases effects of antihypertensives. Lowers seizure threshold. Will affect oral contraceptives. *Patient teaching:* It will take 6–8 weeks for therapeutic effects to occur. Do not stop drug abruptly. Overdose can cause fatal dysrhythmias.
Selective Serotonin Norepinephrine Reuptake Inhibitors (SNRIs)	venlafaxine (Effexor, Effexor XR) duloxetine (Cymbalta) desvenlafaxine (Pristiq)	PO	Anxiety, abnormal dreams, dizziness, nervousness	Monitor blood pressure for systolic hypertension.

TABLE 57.2 MEDICATIONS USED FOR ALTERATIONS IN MENTAL HEALTH—cont'd

Medication Class/Action	Examples	Route	Side Effects	Nursing Implications
				Patient teaching: Do not take with other serotonin-type medications, including St. John's wort and SAMe. Do not stop drug abruptly.
Monoamine Oxidase Inhibitors (MAOIs) Block the action of monamine oxidase.	phenelzine (Nardil) tranylcypromine (Parnate) isocarboxazid (Marplan)	PO	Anticholinergic effects, orthostatic hypotension, will interact with foods containing tyramine and cause hypertensive crisis, headache	Rarely used because of side effects and interactions. Interacts with many prescribed and over-the-counter medications. Serious fatal reactions with SSRIs or SNRIs. *Patient teaching:* Follow tyramine-free diet. Do not stop drug abruptly.
Tetracyclic Antidepressants Blocks multiple serotonin and histamine receptors; adrenoreceptor antagonist.	mirtazapine (Remeron) maprotiline (Ludiomil)	PO	Anticholinergic effects, possible increase in blood pressure, sedation, confusion, orthostatic hypotension, increased appetite, and weight gain	Administer at bedtime to counteract sedating effects. *Patient teaching:* Do not take with alcohol or other CNS depressants.
Antianxiety Agents **Benzodiazepines** Potentiate effects of GABA, which causes a calming effect.	alprazolam (Xanax) diazepam (Valium) lorazepam (Ativan) clonazepam (Klonopin)	PO PO, IM, IV, rectal PO, IM, IV, SL PO	Sedation, hang-over, ataxia, confusion, dizziness, anticholinergic effects	Short-term use only. Addictive. Use cautiously in older adults. Do not use in pregnant patients.

Continued

TABLE 57.2 MEDICATIONS USED FOR ALTERATIONS IN MENTAL HEALTH—cont'd

Medication Class/Action	Examples	Route	Side Effects	Nursing Implications
				Patient teaching: Do not operate heavy machinery. Do not stop drug abruptly.
BuSpar Action is unknown.	buspirone (BuSpar)	PO	Headaches, dizziness, GI upset, light-headedness	Non–habit forming with little sedating effect. *Patient teaching:* It will take 3–6 weeks for drug to work.
Anticonvulsant Mood Stabilizers Antikindling effect, affect GABA receptors.	carbamazepine (Tegretol) lamotrigine (Lamictal) valproic acid (Depakote)	PO	Dizziness, ataxia, drowsiness, blurred vision, nausea, vomiting, headache, weight gain, blood dyscrasias, photosensitivity, rash, Stevens-Johnson syndrome	Loading dose may be ordered for acute mania. Monitor for bleeding. Use cautiously in older adults and in patients with liver or renal disease. Do not use in pregnant or breastfeeding patients. Advise patient to use sunscreen, and report any signs of rash immediately.
Antimanic Agents ***Lithium*** Decreases postsynaptic receptor sensitivity.	lithium carbonate (Eskalith)	PO	Thirst, nausea and vomiting, weight gain, tremors, skin rash (acne), hair loss, hypothyroidism	Narrow therapeutic range increases risk of toxicity. Monitor blood levels. Do not use in cardiac or renal disease. Do not use with diuretics.

TABLE 57.2 MEDICATIONS USED FOR ALTERATIONS IN MENTAL HEALTH—cont'd

Medication Class/Action	Examples	Route	Side Effects	Nursing Implications
				Do not use in pregnant patients. Check interactions with other medications.
Antiparkinsonian Agents Restore the natural balance of acetylcholine and dopamine in the CNS to manage extrapyramidal side effects.	benztropine (Cogentin) trihexyphenidyl (Artane) diphenhydramine (Benadryl)	PO, IM	Anticholinergic effects, nausea, GI upset, sedation, dizziness, orthostatic hypotension	Caution in patients with hypersensitivity, glaucoma, history of urine retention.

CBC = complete blood count; CNS = central nervous system; EPSE = extrapyramidal side effects; GABA = gamma-aminobutyric acid; GI = gastrointestinal; IM = intramuscular; IV = intravenous; PO = by mouth; SAMe = S-adenosylmethionine; SL = sublingual.

events that may be producing anxiety so they can be dealt with. Additional therapies are discussed in Chapter 56.

Nursing Process for the Patient With Anxiety, Obsessive-Compulsive, or Trauma-Related Disorders

DATA COLLECTION. Observe the patient's anxiety level and level of functioning. Ask about triggers of anxiety and coping mechanisms that have been successful or unsuccessful in the past. Stay alert for physical symptoms, such as changes in vital signs, diaphoresis, or tremor. Assess for the presence of suicidal thoughts and observe for suicidal behavior. It is important to identify anxiety and intervene at lower levels, before escalation to severe and panic anxiety levels.

NURSING DIAGNOSES, PLANNING, AND IMPLEMENTATION.
Anxiety related to response to stressors
EXPECTED OUTCOME: The patient will verbalize that anxiety is controlled. The patient will identify precipitants and patterns for anxiety and demonstrate techniques to control anxiety. Physical signs of anxiety, such as tremors or changes in vital signs, will be absent.

- Assist the patient to identify precipitants and patterns to anxiety. *Recognition of patterns can help guide care and allow the patient to initiate measures to stop anxiety from progressing.*
- Maintain a calm milieu and manner. *A chaotic environment can increase the patient's anxiety. Anxiety is contagious and may be transmitted from staff to patient.*
- Maintain open communication. Encourage the patient to verbalize thoughts and feelings. Observe nonverbal communication. *Honesty in dealing with patients helps them learn to trust others and enhances their self-esteem.*
- Encourage the patient to use positive self-talk, such as "I can do this. Anxiety can't kill me." *This helps the patient replace negative anxious thoughts with positive statements to reduce anxiety.*
- Report and document any changes in behavior, such as positive or negative alterations in the way a patient responds to the nursing staff, to the treatment plan, or to other people and situations. *Any change can be significant to the patient's care.*
- Encourage activities but avoid placing the patient in a competitive situation. *Activities that are enjoyable and nonstressful provide diversion and give staff members an opportunity to provide positive feedback about the progress the patient is making. Competitive situations can produce anxiety.*
- Encourage problem solving and assist to develop alternative solutions. Help the patient to identify what has worked in the past. *This can help the patient focus on strategies that were effective in the past and eliminate those that are not effective.*
- Stay with a patient during acute severe or panic levels of anxiety. *Feelings of being abandoned can increase anxiety. The nurse's presence provides a feeling of safety for the patient.*
- Implement suicide precautions if indicated. *The patient may need to be protected from self-harm until treatment is effective.*
- Assess your own level of anxiety. *An anxious nurse may make the patient more anxious.*

EVALUATION. Is the patient able to implement strategies to control anxiety? Does the patient recognize triggers of anxiety? Does the patient state he or she feels less anxious? Are physical signs, such as tremors or changes in vital signs, improved (see Table 57.3)?

EVIDENCE-BASED PRACTICE

Clinical Question
Is the use of music or nature sounds a useful nursing intervention for anxiety?

Evidence
In a randomized controlled study of day surgery patients, patients who listened to music had significantly lower levels of preoperative anxiety than those who did not (Ni, Tsai, Lee, Kao, & Chen, 2012).

Another study looked at the effect of nature-based sounds to reduce agitation, anxiety level, and physiologic signs of stress in patients under mechanical ventilator support (Saadatmand et al, 2013). The experimental group had significantly lower systolic blood pressure, diastolic blood pressure, anxiety, and agitation levels than the control group.

Implications for Nursing Practice
The use of music or nature-based sounds incorporated into nursing care may help reduce anxiety.

REFERENCE
Ni, C., Tsai, W., Lee, L., Kao, C., & Chen, Y. (2012). Minimising preoperative anxiety with music for day surgery patients—a randomised clinical trial. *Journal of Clinical Nursing, 21,* 620–625. doi:10.1111/j.1365-2702.2010.03466.x

Saadatmand, V., Rejeh, N., Heravi-Karimooi, M., Tadrisi, S., Zayeri, F., Vaismoradi, M., & Jasper, M. (2013). Effect of nature-based sounds intervention on agitation, anxiety, and stress in patients under mechanical ventilator support: A randomised controlled trial. *International Journal of Nursing Studies, 50,* 895–904. doi:10.1016/j.ijnurstu.2012.11.018

CRITICAL THINKING

Tommy

■ Tommy has come to the clinic with numerous cracks on his hands. They are bleeding and very sore. Tommy tells you that he has to wash his hands all the time. His mother says he washes for 2 to 3 hours at a time, and he will not stop when she tells him to. The doctor has diagnosed Tommy with obsessive-compulsive disorder and has explained the illness to Tommy and his mother. When the doctor leaves the room, Tommy's mother begins to cry.

TABLE 57.3 ANXIETY SUMMARY

Signs and Symptoms	*Phobia:* irrational fear of object or situation *Panic disorder:* extreme fear, feelings of impending doom, palpitations *Generalized anxiety disorder:* worry, restlessness, palpitations
Diagnosis	History of symptoms; physical causes for symptoms must be ruled out first
Therapeutic Measures	Antianxiety medication Selective serotonin reuptake inhibitors Systematic desensitization Psychotherapy Relaxation exercises
Nursing Diagnosis	Anxiety

"What did he just say? What am I supposed to do? What did I do wrong that Tommy got this illness?"

1. How can you respond therapeutically?
2. What team member would you use as a resource?

Suggested answers are at the end of the chapter.

 MOOD DISORDERS

Mood disorders (also called affective disorders) are disorders in which the major symptom is extreme changes in mood (emotions) and affect (the outward expression of the mood). Moods involving both highs and lows are bipolar disorders; low moods without any highs are described as depressive disorders. Mood disorders are diagnosed when symptoms begin to interfere with normal day-to-day functioning. People of all age groups and all ethnic and socioeconomic groups can develop mood disorders.

Etiological Theories

Psychoanalytic theory explains that people who have suffered loss in their lives are at risk for developing depression. Depression is also associated with unresolved anger and has been described as "anger turned inward." In other words, people who cannot or do not deal appropriately with situations that anger them may repress the anger (turn it inside) and become depressed.

Cognitive theorists believe that the way people perceive events and situations may lead to depression. Instead of thinking about failing an examination as being unfortunate and disappointing, some people with tendencies toward depression may exaggerate the emotion and turn the situation into something much deeper, such as thoughts of "I'm stupid" or "I'll never get anywhere."

Biological theories offer genetic links and neurotransmitter dysfunctions as two etiologies. Serotonin, norepinephrine, and dopamine have an effect on mood; if these neurotransmitters are elevated, mood is elevated; if they are low, mood is low. Some biological theorists also believe that there is a connection between these neurotransmitters and female hormones.

Differential Diagnosis

Symptoms of depression may occur in conjunction with other disorders, such as schizophrenia or drug side effects or overuse. Heart failure, nutritional deficiencies, drug toxicity, thyroid disease, fluid and electrolyte imbalances, infections, and diabetes can be associated with depression.

Types of Mood Disorders
Major (Unipolar) Depression

Major depression is an episodic condition, and symptoms interfere with the person's usual social or occupational functioning. Depressed people view the world through "gray-tinted glasses." The *DSM-5* (American Psychiatric Association, 2013) specifies that symptoms of major depression include either a depressed mood or **anhedonia** (the loss of pleasure in things that are usually pleasurable) along with at least five of the following symptoms:

• Significant weight loss or gain—more than 5% in a month
• Increase or decrease in appetite
• Sleep pattern disturbances—insomnia or hypersomnia
• Increased fatigue or loss of energy
• Increased agitation or psychomotor retardation
• Decreased ability to think, remember, or concentrate
• Feelings of guilt or hopelessness
• Indecisiveness
• Suicidal ideation.

Bipolar Disorder

About 2 million people in the United States have **bipolar** disorder. Formerly called manic depressive illness, bipolar disorder is a mood disorder in which patients experience the mood states of both **mania** (extreme elation or agitation) and extreme depression. Bipolar disorder is more severe than major depression. Affected people stay depressed longer, relapse more often, display more depressive symptoms, have more delusions and hallucinations, commit suicide more often, require more hospitalizations, and overall experience more incapacitation.

Affected people can cycle slowly (over weeks, months, or even years), or they can be "rapid cyclers" who can change moods several times in an hour. Recent research indicates that individuals with bipolar disorder do not experience periods of normal mood alternating with periods of abnormal mood as previously believed. Instead,

bipolar illness is characterized by frequent mood lability, with both manic and depressive symptoms, that are sometimes milder and sometimes more severe (Beddes, 2013).

Common signs of depression were covered in the preceding section. Common signs of mania include the following:

• Excessive high (euphoric) moods lasting at least 1 week
• Increased energy, activity, restlessness
• Decreased need for sleep
• Grandiosity (unrealistic belief in one's abilities or powers)
• Extreme irritability and distractibility
• Uncharacteristically poor judgment
• Pressured and rapid speech
• Flight of ideas or subjective experience that one's thoughts are racing
• Increase in goal-directed behavior
• Excessive involvement in pleasurable activities that have a high potential for unpleasant consequences, such as sex, substance **abuse**, or shopping sprees
• Obnoxious, provocative, or intrusive behavior.

Therapeutic Measures for Patients With Mood Disorders.

About 80% of people with major depression respond to treatment. Bipolar disorder is more difficult to treat. Some common medical treatments for *all* mood disorders include the following:

• Antidepressant medications
• Mood stabilizers
• Psychotherapy
• Electroconvulsive therapy (ECT).

Lithium was once the drug of choice for treating bipolar disorder. Lithium is an antimanic medication with a very narrow therapeutic range, which means that toxic drug levels can easily develop. Blood must be drawn regularly to assess that serum lithium levels are in the therapeutic range.

Mood stabilizers such as the anticonvulsants valproic acid (Depakote) and lamotrigine (Lamictal) are now more commonly used than lithium to treat bipolar disorder. Atypical antipsychotics are also commonly used with a mood stabilizer when the patient is in an acute manic state. Antidepressant agents, if used, should be monitored carefully because they can induce a manic episode. See Table 57.2 for a summary of medications. Also see "Nutrition Notes."

Nursing Process for the Patient With a Mood Disorder

See the "Nursing Care Plan for the Patient With Depression." Also see Table 57.4.

• **WORD • BUILDING** •
anhedonia: an—not + hedonia—pleasure

Nutrition Notes

Food-Drug Interactions in Patients With Mental Health Disorders

Monoamine Oxidase Inhibitors

When a patient taking a monoamine oxidase inhibitor (MAOI) consumes foods high in tyramine (an intermediate product in the conversion of the amino acid tyrosine to epinephrine), the drug prevents the normal breakdown of tyramine, leading to excessive epinephrine levels. Hypertension results, sometimes severe enough to cause intracranial hemorrhage.

All food groups except breads and cereals have some items with sufficient tyramine to cause problems for patients taking MAOIs. The amount of tyramine varies even in different samples of a particular food. Because this interaction can be life threatening, the best advice is to avoid all foods capable of causing problems, even though a small amount of the food, or a given batch of a product, might be safe. Even after the MAOI has been discontinued, its effects and its interactions with foods may persist for 2 weeks. Examples of common foods to be avoided are bananas, raspberries, sauerkraut, aged cheese, sour cream, yogurt, bologna, salami, pepperoni, summer sausage, chocolate, beer, and wine. Some anti-infectives, an antineoplastic, and anti-Parkinson agents also interact with high-tyramine foods.

Lithium Carbonate

Lithium carbonate, used to treat bipolar disorder, is absorbed, distributed, and excreted alongside sodium. Fluctuations in sodium intake affect lithium metabolism:

- Decreased sodium intake with decreased fluid intake may lead to retention of lithium and overmedication.
- Increased sodium intake from food or medications and increased fluid intake may hasten excretion of lithium, resulting in worsening signs and symptoms of mania.

Psychotherapy for the patient and family may be helpful for any type of mood disorder. It can help the patient understand the illness and learn problem solving and other new adaptive coping behaviors. For young children, play therapy is the most common and effective form of therapy. ECT is an option for individuals with rapid-cycling bipolar disorder or major depression that is not responsive to conventional treatment.

BE SAFE!

BE VIGILANT! When collecting data from your patient, be sure to ask about herbal supplements and over-the-counter (OTC) medications the patient may use in addition to prescription medications. Many people take St. John's wort, an OTC herbal supplement, for depression. Although it may be

effective for some people with mild depression, it can interact with many prescribed medications that influence serotonin levels. If combined with prescription serotonin-type antidepressants, it can cause serotonin syndrome, an excess of serotonin resulting in agitation, confusion, diarrhea, muscle spasms, and even death (Lamoure & Stovel, 2011).

CRITICAL THINKING

Mr. Zenz

■ Mr. Zenz is the manager of a busy office. His usual behavior is rather sullen, and he comes across as quiet or sad to various members of the staff. He is in his 40s and married, with three children, ages 4, 5, and 7. He speaks of them proudly but always comments that they "take after their mother." His management style in the office is to let people do their jobs; he rarely interferes, although his door is always open and staff members are told they are welcome any time. Recently, however, staff members have noticed a change in Mr. Zenz. He moves quickly, speaks quickly, and has set unrealistic goals for the staff. He frequently says he has called the president of the company to tell him of his new ideas. He says he has not slept in several days and he feels terrific. He has changed his wardrobe and has begun pointing out specific performance issues to staff. He jokes with staff. Staff members are made aware that he has bipolar disorder and has quit taking his medications. His wife has asked for the staff's help. Remember: He is your boss.

1. How do you respond to Mrs. Zenz?
2. How do you approach Mr. Zenz?

Suggested answers are at the end of the chapter.

TABLE 57.4   DEPRESSION SUMMARY

Signs and Symptoms	*Unipolar:* depressed mood, weight changes, anhedonia, sleep disturbance, social withdrawal *Bipolar:* signs and symptoms of depression cycling with euphoria; delusions, hallucinations
Diagnosis	History; physiological causes must be ruled out
Therapeutic Measures	Antidepressant medication, mood stabilizers (anticonvulsants), psychotherapy, electroconvulsive therapy
Nursing Diagnoses	*Risk for Suicide* *Ineffective Coping* *Powerlessness*

NURSING CARE PLAN for the Patient With Depression

Nursing Diagnosis: *Ineffective Coping*

Expected Outcomes: The patient will cope effectively as evidenced by verbalizing the ability to cope and asking for help when needed and by demonstrating new effective coping strategies.

Evaluation of Outcomes: Does the patient exhibit increased ability to problem solve and cope with stressors?

Intervention Use therapeutic communication techniques to allow the patient to verbalize feelings.
Rationale Verbalization of feelings in a supportive environment can assist patient to work through issues.
Evaluation Does the patient verbalize feelings to nursing staff?

Intervention Assist the patient to describe stressors and identify his or her existing coping skills and knowledge.
Rationale Providing validation of actual stress and available coping resources and strategies aids in positive adaptation to stress. **Evaluation** Is the patient able to identify stressors? Does the patient have some effective coping skills on which to draw?

Intervention Help the patient set realistic goals. **Rationale** Achievement of small steps toward a goal can help the patient feel empowered. **Evaluation** Does the patient set realistic goals?

Intervention Encourage the patient to make choices and participate in care. **Rationale** Active involvement in care increases the possibility of positive adjustment. **Evaluation** Is the patient actively involved in care?

Nursing Diagnosis: *Powerlessness*

Expected Outcomes: The patient will have reduced feelings of powerlessness as evidenced by verbal expression of having control over life, situation, or care and by participation in care or decision making when opportunities are provided.

Evaluation of Outcomes: Does patient identify feelings of powerlessness? Does patient identify factors that are controllable and actively participate in care?

Intervention Assess for factors contributing to powerlessness. **Rationale** Correct identification of actual or perceived problems is essential to providing appropriate support. **Evaluation** Is the patient able to identify factors contributing to powerlessness?

Intervention Help the patient to identify factors that are or are not under his or her control. **Rationale** Identifying factors within the patient's control encourages the patient to take some control over the situation. **Evaluation** Is the patient able to identify what is controllable and what is not controllable in his or her life?

Intervention Allow ventilation of powerless feelings. **Rationale** Sharing feelings in groups can lead to the realization that similar feelings are experienced by others and reduce feelings of powerlessness. **Evaluation** Is the patient sharing feelings with nursing staff and in therapeutic groups?

Intervention Encourage the patient to actively participate in care with goal-directed activities. **Rationale** Goal-directed behavior increases self-efficacy and empowerment. **Evaluation** Does the patient set realistic goals daily and achieve them daily?

Nursing Diagnosis: *Risk for Suicide*

Expected Outcome: The patient will not harm himself or herself.

Evaluation of Outcome: Did the patient remain free from self-harm during hospitalization? Does patient have ongoing support following discharge?

Continued

NURSING CARE PLAN for the Patient With Depression—cont'd

Intervention Ask patient directly about suicidal ideations each shift. **Rationale** Ongoing assessment of suicidal risk is essential to patient safety. **Evaluation** Is the patient verbalizing warning signs of suicide?

Intervention Create a safe environment for the patient. **Rationale** Patient safety is a nursing priority. **Evaluation** Are means of harming self kept from patient?

Intervention Initiate suicide precautions according to agency protocol. **Rationale** The patient must be protected until risk is reduced. **Evaluation** Is increased surveillance of patient implemented and communicated to all staff?

Intervention Encourage the patient to seek out nursing staff when experiencing suicidal thoughts. **Rationale** Active listening and therapeutic communication by staff provide the patient with empathy and alternatives to acting on suicidal thoughts. **Evaluation** Does the patient seek out nursing staff when experiencing suicidal thoughts?

SCHIZOPHRENIA

Schizophrenia is becoming more widely viewed as a group of illnesses rather than a single condition. The term *schizophrenia* (which means "split mind") was first used by a Swiss psychiatrist, Eugene Bleuler (1911). Schizophrenia is a serious disorder of thought and association and is characterized by inability to distinguish between what is real and what is not and also by hallucinations, delusions, and limited socialization. People who have schizophrenia may not be able to differentiate between what is "theirs" and what is "everybody else's" in relation to social functioning. Poor self-esteem may be present. It is difficult for them to focus on one topic for any length of time. Schizophrenia is not the same as dissociative identity disorder (once called multiple personality disorder). Schizophrenia has an insidious onset and often begins during adolescence or young adulthood. It develops over time, and symptoms may go unnoticed for a time before diagnosis. There are four phases of schizophrenia:

1. *Schizoid personality.* Those in this phase are perceived as being indifferent, cold, and aloof. They are often described as loners and don't seem to enjoy close relationships with others. In an adolescent, these behaviors may be dismissed as normal for age. Not all individuals with schizoid personality go on to develop schizophrenia.
2. *Prodromal phase.* Affected people continue to be socially withdrawn and begin to show behavior that is peculiar or eccentric. Role functioning is impaired, personal hygiene is neglected, and disturbances are evident in communication, ideation, and perception.
3. *Schizophrenia.* This is the third and active phase of the disorder. Psychotic symptoms are prominent and include delusions, hallucinations, and impairment in work, social relations, and self-care.
4. *Residual phase.* Symptoms are similar to the prodromal phase, with flat affect and impairment in role functioning.

Positive and Negative Symptoms

Positive symptoms of schizophrenia can be thought of as those symptoms that reflect an "excess" or distortion of normal functioning. Positive symptoms include hallucinations, delusions, disorganized thinking, and disorganized behavior. **Delusions** are fixed, false beliefs that cannot be changed by logic or factual proof. Typically, patients exhibit delusions of grandeur, persecution, or guilt. **Hallucinations** are false sensory perceptions. They can affect any of the five senses; auditory and visual delusions are most common. For example, a person might see a person no one else sees or hear voices that no one else hears. In contrast, **illusions** are mistaken perceptions of reality. For example, a person may see a glowing sunset and think the horizon is on fire. Both typical and atypical antipsychotic medications work well to manage the positive symptoms of schizophrenia.

Negative symptoms of schizophrenia can be thought of as a loss of normal functioning. Negative symptoms include affective blunting or flattening, **alogia**, **avolition**, apathy, anhedonia, and social isolation. It is thought that these are the most debilitating symptoms of schizophrenia because they keep the individual from living a normal life. These symptoms respond to atypical antipsychotic medications but not the typical antipsychotic agents.

Pathophysiology and Etiology

The causes of schizophrenia are widely believed to be a combination of neurobiological and environmental factors. Psychological factors as the cause of schizophrenia are no longer considered valid because most researchers and clinicians consider schizophrenia to be a brain disease.

The role of genetics in schizophrenia (neurobiological or nature theory) has been examined in twin studies, family studies, and adoption studies for more than 75 years. Studies of

---

• WORD • BUILDING •

alogia: a—not + logia—(able to) speak

avolition: a—not + volition—energy or initiative to do something identical twins show that if one twin has schizophrenia, the other has about a 50% chance of developing it. In fraternal twins, the percentage drops to about 10%. It is believed that the more genes twins or family members have in common, the greater the probability of the second twin developing schizophrenia. Additional support for the role of genetics is demonstrated by adoption studies. Research indicates that children born to mothers with schizophrenia are more likely to develop the disorder even when raised in adoptive families.

Other studies have examined brain structure and the relationship between neurotransmitters and schizophrenia. Patients with a diagnosis of schizophrenia typically have elevated dopamine levels or a brain that overreacts to the amount of dopamine present. Glutamate is an excitatory neurotransmitter that also appears to be related to schizophrenia. The glutamate theory proposes that there is an underactivity of glutamate of the brain (Patil et al, 2007). The brains of patients with a diagnosis of schizophrenia show a significant loss of gray matter, enlarged ventricles, and diminished prefrontal cortex functioning. Today, schizophrenia is primarily thought of as a series of brain disorders characterized by brain abnormalities and neurotransmitter dysfunction.

Environmental factors that increase risk of schizophrenia include such things as central nervous system damage during childbirth, some infections, and substance abuse.

Symptoms

Patients with paranoid symptoms tend to exhibit unusual suspicions and fears. The person may also be hostile and aggressive or have delusions of persecution or grandeur. Those with persecutory delusions may state that they feel tormented or followed by people. Patients often integrate people around them into their delusions. They may feel that nursing staff, relatives, or announcers on the radio or television are trying to harm them. In delusions of grandeur, patients might state that they are God or the president of the United States.

Hallucinations often accompany delusions and can affect any of the five senses. The most common hallucinations are auditory, followed by visual. Patients diagnosed with schizophrenia talk about hearing voices. These voices are frightening and derogatory to the patient and are responsible for many of the actions performed by people with paranoid schizophrenia. Patients experience increased fear, anxiety, and suicidal ideation as a result of the voices. You may see or hear patients arguing with what at first appears to be themselves. Actually the patient is arguing with the voices. Describing the voices is difficult, but imagine that you are in a room with six televisions on different stations at the same time. This example comes close to what some patients have described.

Therapeutic Measures for the Patient With Schizophrenia

Medications, social skills training, and individual and family psychotherapy are indicated for patients with schizophrenia. Among the classifications of medications that may be prescribed are the typical and atypical antipsychotics, which block dopamine action in the brain. There are different dopamine tracts in the brain, and typical antipsychotics have a greater effect on the motor function tract, resulting in extrapyramidal side effects such as parkinsonism (see medications in Table 57.2). Anticholinergic medications such as benztropine (Cogentin) or trihexyphenidyl (Artane) are used to combat the extrapyramidal side effects of the typical antipsychotics by helping return balance between dopamine, acetylcholine, and other neurotransmitters. Newer, atypical antipsychotic medications such as clozapine (Clozaril) and risperidone (Risperdal) have fewer extrapyramidal side effects but have other side effects. They are effective in treating both the positive and negative symptoms of schizophrenia.

Psychotherapy can include individual, group, and family therapy. ECT is used in some severe cases or in cases that are difficult to treat; ECT is not usually used until other methods of therapy have been exhausted. Referral of the patient and family to organizations such as the National Alliance on Mental Illness provides helpful education and support www.nami.org.

Nursing Process for the Patient With Schizophrenia

DATA COLLECTION. Observe the patient with schizophrenia for positive and negative symptoms, including hallucinations, delusions, and illusions. Observe interactions with others. Monitor the patient for response to medications, including side effects. Determine the person's ability to function and manage activities of daily living (ADLs).

NURSING DIAGNOSES, PLANNING, AND IMPLEMENTATION.
Disturbed Sensory Perception related to abnormalities in neurotransmitter function
EXPECTED OUTCOME: The patient will be able to determine what is real and what is not and be able to manage medications, perform ADLs, and function in a community.

- Develop trust. Be honest and consistent in all areas of the patient's treatment plan. *Trust is essential to a therapeutic relationship.*
- Allow the patient to verbalize thoughts and feelings when appropriate to the time and place. *Verbalizing feelings can help the patient clarify concerns and feel supported.*
- Whenever possible, maintain consistent staff assignments *to ensure the best possible continuity of care and to promote the development of a trusting relationship.*
- Never whisper or laugh when the patient cannot hear the whole conversation. Face the patient when having a conversation. *Whispering or turning away may be interpreted as rejection; secretive behaviors can reinforce paranoia and suspiciousness.*
- Avoid placing the patient in situations of competition or embarrassment. *These situations can be threatening to the patient.*
- Never reinforce hallucinations, delusions, or illusions. Orient to reality as needed. *The patient needs to know what is real and what is not.*
- Use distraction to deal with the hallucinations (see Table 57.5). Help to connect the delusions and

TABLE 57.5 SUGGESTED INTERVENTIONS FOR PATIENTS WITH SCHIZOPHRENIA WHO ARE HALLUCINATING

Suggested Action	Rationale
1. "Mr. R., I don't see any snakes. It is time for lunch. I will walk to the dining room with you."	1. Lets the patient know you heard him, but brings him immediately into the reality of time of day and need to go to the dining room.
2. "I see a crack in the wall, Mr. R. It is harmless; you are safe. Susan is here to take you down to occupational therapy now."	2. This is in response to a probable illusion. It lets the patient know that you see something. It validates his fear, but it tells him what you see and then moves him into the here and now.
3. "I know that your thoughts seem very real to you, Ms. C., but they do not seem logical to me. I would like for you to come to your room and get dressed now, please."	3. Again, you are validating the patient's concern without exploring and focusing on the delusion.
4. "Ms. C, it appears to me that you are listening to someone. Are you hearing voices other than mine?"	4. This is a method of validating your impression of what you see. This is as far as you will go into exploring what she may be hearing.
5. "Thank you, Ms. C. I want to help you focus away from the other voices. I am real; they are not. Please come with me to the reading room."	5. Responds to her in the present and reinforces her response to you. Attempts to redirect her thinking.

hallucinations to times of increased anxiety. *This models strategies for the patient to use during times of anxiety.*
- Provide a calm and therapeutic milieu *to help reduce anxiety.*
- Provide written instructions and information boards *to help promote reality and self-responsible behavior.*
- Monitor medication use and check the patient's mouth for unswallowed medication as needed. *Patients may have difficulty maintaining a medication schedule or choose to not take medications as prescribed due to paranoia or a lack of insight.*
- Keep communication simple. Be brief and clear with all directions. State what is acceptable, giving the rationale and consequences at the same time. State information in positive rather than negative terms: "Eat your food calmly" rather than "Do not throw your food!" *Patients are more likely to process and respond to simple, direct communication.*
- Use touch cautiously. *Perceptions and distortions of reality may cause patients to misconstrue touch.*

EVALUATION. Is the patient oriented to reality? Is he or she able to manage medications, or is there a plan in place to make sure medications are administered? Is the patient able to manage ADLs and live in a community (see Table 57.6)?

▮ PERSONALITY DISORDERS

How many times have you heard, "She has such a good personality"? What is it that determines an individual's

CRITICAL THINKING

Anne

▪ While preparing to invite Anne, a young woman receiving chemotherapy on your oncology unit, to a movie in the day room, you observe her standing in the corner of her room trembling. You ask her what's wrong, and she responds that she's talking to the woman in the wall. Your first instinct is to giggle, but you ask her, "What woman?" She tells you that you wouldn't understand and says, "You helped put her there, and you told me that it is my job to be sure she can't get out." You report this to the charge nurse, who calls the physician. Tests are run, and it is determined that Anne is not experiencing side effects from the chemotherapy. Further workup delivers the diagnosis of schizophrenia for Anne.

1. What therapeutic responses are appropriate for this situation?
2. What special needs might Anne now experience relating to her chemotherapy, if any?
3. How will you get Anne to the movie or to participate in other care activities?
4. What actions can team members take to promote trust with Anne?

Suggested answers are at the end of the chapter.

TABLE 57.6 SCHIZOPHRENIA SUMMARY

Signs and Symptoms	Disorganized speech and behavior Ineffective thinking and decision making Trouble functioning at school and work; self-care deficits Positive symptoms: hallucinations, delusions Negative symptoms: apathy, flat affect, anhedonia
Diagnosis	History Psychiatric evaluation DSM-5 criteria
Therapeutic Measures	Antipsychotic medications Anticholinergic agents to control side effects Psychotherapy Family education
Nursing Diagnoses	Social skills training and therapy *Disturbed Sensory Perception* *Social Isolation* *Impaired Communication*

personality? Personality is composed of enduring patterns or traits that determine how an individual perceives, relates to, and thinks about the environment and self. An individual's personality develops as the person adjusts to their physical, emotional, social, and spiritual environments. Personality traits or patterns are reflected in how individuals cope with feelings and impulses, see themselves and others, respond to their surroundings, and find meaning in relationships.

Etiology

The causes of personality disorders are unknown. Genetic and family environmental factors are thought to play a role as well as neurobiological and other social factors.

Diagnosis

Personality disorders are diagnosed when the personality patterns or traits are inflexible, enduring, pervasive, maladaptive, and cause significant functional impairment or subjective distress. In the United States, 9.1% of the population has been diagnosed with a personality disorder (National Institute of Mental Health, 2010).

Personality disorders are characterized by the following:

- *Behavioral Manifestations:* Dysfunctional patterns of day-to-day behavior and impulse control
- *Affective Manifestations:* Inappropriate range, intensity, mood lability, and emotional response
- *Cognitive Manifestations:* Inaccurate interpretation of self, others, and events
- *Sociocultural Manifestations:* Ineffective interpersonal functioning

Patients with personality disorders exhibit common problem behaviors that create difficulty in daily living. *Manipulation* is a control behavior that uses and exploits others for personal gain. *Narcissism* is self-centered behavior in which the individual feels entitled to special favors or feels justified in not obeying authority and rules. *Impulsive behavior* creates difficulties for those patients who act without considering the consequences of their own behavior.

The *DSM-5* lists 10 personality disorders that are organized into three diagnostic clusters, Cluster A: Odd and Eccentric, Cluster B: Dramatic and Erratic, and Cluster C: Anxious and Fearful. This text covers two of the more common personality disorders in Cluster B: borderline personality disorder (BPD) and antisocial personality disorder (ASPD).

Borderline Personality Disorder

Individuals with BPD display a pattern of instability of interpersonal relationships, self-image, and affect. There is marked impulsivity. The personality pattern is present by early adulthood and occurs across a variety of situations and contexts. Other symptoms may include intense fear of abandonment, anger and irritability, chronic feelings of emptiness, and transient paranoia or dissociative symptoms. Patients with BPD often engage in idealization and devaluation of others, alternating between high positive regard and great disappointment. This is a defense mechanism referred to as *splitting*. Self-mutilation and recurrent suicidal behavior, gestures, and threats are common.

Antisocial Personality Disorder

ASPD is characterized by a pervasive pattern of disregard for and violation of the rights of others that begins in childhood or early adolescence and continues into adulthood. These individuals have a lack of empathy and/or remorse for their actions. There is a failure to conform to social norms, which often leads to a history of legal problems or criminal behavior. Behavior can be impulsive and aggressive, with a reckless disregard for the safety of self or others. Deceitfulness and consistent irresponsibility is common.

Therapeutic Measures for Patients With Personality Disorders

Psychotherapy

Psychotherapy is the primary way to treat personality disorders. Using the insight and knowledge gained in psychotherapy, patients can learn healthy ways to manage their illness. Types of psychotherapy used to treat personality disorders include cognitive behavioral therapy and psychoeducation. Cognitive behavioral therapy helps patients identify unhealthy, negative beliefs and behaviors and replace them with healthy, positive ones. *Dialectical behavior therapy* is a type of cognitive behavioral therapy that teaches behavioral skills to help patients tolerate stress, regulate their emotions and improve their relationships with others. *Psychodynamic psychotherapy* focuses on increasing the patient's awareness of unconscious thoughts and behaviors, developing new insights and motivations, and resolving conflicts.

Psychoeducation teaches the patient and significant others about their illness, including treatments, coping strategies, and problem-solving skills.

There are no medications specifically approved to treat personality disorders. However, several types of psychiatric medications may help with various common symptoms. Antidepressant medications are used to treat depressed mood, anger, impulsivity, irritability, or hopelessness. Mood-stabilizing medications are used to help even out mood swings or reduce irritability, impulsivity, and aggression. Antianxiety medications can address anxiety, agitation, or insomnia. Antipsychotic medications can help with paranoia, aggression, anger, and impulsiveness.

Nursing Process for the Patient With Personality Disorders

DATA COLLECTION. A priority nursing action is assessment of suicidal or homicidal ideation. Mood and affect should also be assessed as a depressed, angry, or labile mood can indicate a higher risk for self-injury. Assess for paranoia, manipulative behaviors, and impulsiveness. Assess for history of violence. It will also be necessary to obtain a medical history, psychiatric history, developmental history, and information about sociocultural background.

NURSING DIAGNOSIS, PLANNING, AND IMPLEMENTATION.
Risk for Other-Directed Violence related to impulsivity, impaired judgment and disregard for the rights of others
EXPECTED OUTCOME: Patient will not harm self or others. Patient will discuss feelings with staff instead of acting on them. Patient will verbalize adaptive coping strategies for use when hostile or suicidal feelings occur.

- Monitor client's behavior frequently. *Close monitoring is required so that intervention can occur if required to ensure safety.*
- Remove all dangerous objects from client's environment (e.g., sharp items, belts, ties, straps, breakable items, smoking materials). *Safety is a nursing priority.*
- Redirect violent behavior by means of physical outlets for client's anxiety (e.g., exercise machines, walking). *Physical activity can be an effective way of relieving tension and stress.*
- Maintain and convey a calm attitude toward client. *Anxiety is contagious and can be transmitted from staff members to client.*
- Encourage appropriate verbal expression of emotions. *Verbalization of feelings in a nonthreatening environment may assist the patient to develop insight into the situation.*

EVALUATION. Has the patient been able to discuss anger with staff? Has the patient engaged in physical activity to cope with

tension? Is the patient responsive to calm interactions? Are the patient and others safe from harm? Has environmental safety been maintained?

 AUTISM SPECTRUM DISORDER

Autism spectrum disorders (ASDs) are lifelong neurodevelopmental disabilities that are typically recognized during the second year of life. ASD prevalence is believed to occur in about 1% of the population in the United States. ASDs are diagnosed four times more in males than in females.

Etiology

Autism spectrum disorders are characterized by abnormal brain development and function. Although the specific causes are unknown, ASD is likely to have multiple etiologies including genetic factors. A range of studies have found in 10% to 37% of cases there may be an associated medical condition such as tuberous sclerosis, fragile X syndrome, maternal rubella, or Angelman's syndrome. Current research is also showing that the frontal lobe and amygdala appear to have abnormal growth patterns in patients with ASD. A recent study showed that the amygdala, which controls emotions, undergoes disproportionate enlargement by 37 months of age in ASD (Nordahl et al, 2012). Hereditary estimates range from 37% to higher than 90% based on twin studies. Environmental risk factors include advanced parental age, low birth weight, and fetal exposure to valproate, an anticonvulsant medication.

Signs and Symptoms

ASD is characterized by:

- deficits in social communication and social interaction and
- restricted repetitive behaviors, interests, and activities (RRBs).

Patients with ASD tend to have communication deficits, such as responding inappropriately in conversations, misreading nonverbal cues, or having difficulty building friendships appropriate to their age. Patients with ASD may desire friendship and interaction with others, but their inability to understand the emotions, motivations, and perspectives of others thwarts efforts toward developing relationships. In addition, ASD patients may be overly dependent on routines, highly sensitive to changes in their environment, or intensely focused on inappropriate items.

Therapeutic Measures for Patients With ASD

Early intervention services can greatly improve a child's development and can help children from birth to 3 years learn important skills. Such services include therapy to help the child talk, walk, and interact with others.

The various types of treatments are targeted toward addressing deficits in communication, social interaction, and behaviors. Applied behavior analysis (ABA) is a notable treatment approach for people with an ASD. ABA has become widely accepted among health care professionals and is used in many schools and treatment clinics. ABA encourages positive behaviors and discourages negative behaviors to improve a variety of skills.

Occupational therapy teaches skills that help the ASD patient with activities of daily living such as dressing, eating, bathing, and relating to people. Sensory integration therapy helps the ASD patient cope with sensory information, like sights, sounds, and smells. Sensory integration therapy may help a patient who cannot tolerate certain sounds or physical touch. Speech therapy helps to improve the person's communication skills either verbally or by using sign language, gestures, or picture boards. The Picture Exchange Communication System uses picture symbols to teach communication skills.

Medications are not a cure for ASD patients and do not address the key symptoms. Some medications can help people with ASD function better by managing high energy levels, inability to focus, depression, or seizures. The U.S. Food and Drug Administration has approved the use of the antipsychotic medications risperidone and aripiprazole to treat ASD patients who exhibit behavioral problems such as tantrums, aggression, and self-injurious behaviors. Referral of the patient and family to organizations such as the Autism Education Network www.autismeducation.net or Autism Speaks www.autismspeaks.org/family-services/resource-guide can provide helpful education and support.

Nursing Process for the Patient With ASD

DATA COLLECTION. Assess the patient for developmental spurts or lags, uneven development, or loss of previously acquired skills. Observe the caregiver–patient relationship for bonding, anxiety, tension, and difficult fit. Discuss the patient's social, communication, and behavioral strengths and limitations with the caregiver. Assess the ASD patient for communication style and verbal and nonverbal skills. Assess for risk of injury to self and others, and be alert for the potential for abuse.

NURSING DIAGNOSIS, PLANNING, AND IMPLEMENTATION.
Impaired Social Interaction related to neurological alterations
EXPECTED OUTCOME: Patient will interact appropriately with at least one staff member. Patient will develop trusting relationship with at least one staff member. Patient will function appropriately in the inpatient milieu.

- Assign consistent staff to the patient. *This is essential to the development of trust.*
- Provide positive reinforcement for patient's voluntary interactions with others. *Positive reinforcement enhances self-esteem and encourages repetition of desirable behaviors.*
- Provide direct feedback about patient's interactions with others in a nonjudgmental manner. *Direct feedback from a trusted individual may help to alter behaviors in a positive manner.*
- Help client learn how to respond more appropriately in interactions with others. Practice new skills through role-play. *Practicing skills in role-play facilitates their use in real situations.*

- Give positive feedback when eye contact is used. *Positive reinforcement enhances self-esteem and encourages repetition of desirable behaviors.*

EVALUATION. Has the patient been able to establish trust with at least one staff member? Has the patient engaged in voluntary interaction with others? Is the patient responsive to feedback regarding interactions? Is the patient responsive to role-plays? Does the patient make eye contact?

SUBSTANCE-RELATED AND ADDICTIVE DISORDERS

Alcohol and drug use disorders are serious conditions. People start using alcohol and drugs for many reasons, but often it is to feel accepted by a peer group or to feel comfortable and reduce anxiety in a social situation. People mistake the temporary high as a stimulant. In reality, alcohol is a depressant. Any chemical can be potentially dangerous.

It is important to understand the following terms and their definitions:

- **Addiction**—repeated compulsive use of a substance that continues despite negative consequences (physical, social, legal).
- **Tolerance**—a condition in which increased amounts of a substance are needed over time to achieve the same effect as that previously obtained with smaller doses.
- Physical **withdrawal** syndrome—a physiological response to the abrupt stopping or reduction of a substance used (usually) for a long time. Withdrawal symptoms are specific to the substance used.

The substance-related and addictive disorders are conditions in which the patient:

- Takes more of the substance or over a longer period of time than intended
- Has a persistent desire to or unsuccessful efforts to cut down or control use
- Experiences strong craving for the substance
- Is unable to fulfill major role obligations at home, work, or school
- Needs more of the substance and at more frequent intervals to achieve the same "high," or desired effect of the substance (tolerance)
- Spends significant time obtaining the substance
- Gives up important social or professional functions to use the substance
- Has tried at least once to quit but still obsesses about the substance
- Experiences difficulty with job, family, or social activities because of use or withdrawal symptoms
- Uses the substance regardless of the problems it causes
- Experiences the substance-specific withdrawal syndrome
- Uses the substance to avoid withdrawal symptoms

Nurses need to be informed about chemical dependency for several reasons. First, many patients on medical-surgical units are chemically dependent. This affects their healing and the effect of their medications. Second, as part of the human experience, your chance of being in a close personal relationship with a person who is chemically dependent is great. Third, and perhaps most important, you are part of a profession whose members are statistically high users and abusers of drugs and alcohol (see "Ethical Considerations" on DavisPlus). According to the National Council of State Boards of Nursing (2011), between 6% and 15% of nurses in the United States are chemically impaired.

Substance abuse is not a one-person illness; it affects personal and professional relationships with people who are associated with the user. The term **dysfunctional** is often used to refer to the relationships in an alcoholic family or work environment. Dishonesty and inability to discuss the situation are strong components of the disease. Many times, people who live or work in the dysfunctional group begin to cover up for the user's behaviors and lack of responsibility. Family members or significant others may take sides, begin to be dishonest with each other, and erode the bond within that group. Eventually this leads to a condition called **codependence**, which can be as serious as the use and abuse of the substance. Codependent members of a family group begin to lose their own sense of identity and purpose and exist solely for the abuser. Their actions take away the opportunity for the user to take responsibility for his or her own actions. This is called *enabling*.

Etiological Theories

Why do some people become addicted or dependent and others do not? Can it be the chemical, or is it the person? Some theorists believe in the existence of an addictive personality, which may begin to explain addictions to food, sex, and gambling, as well as alcohol, chemicals, and other dependencies.

Psychoanalytical theorists believe that people who develop addictions to alcohol or other substances are people who failed to successfully pass through the "oral" stage of development.

Biological theories include numerous studies that imply some sort of genetic metabolic disorder. Many of these studies were done on twins born to an alcoholic parent or parents and who were separated from the parents at birth or shortly after birth. The number of twins who were born of alcoholic parents but raised by nonalcoholic adoptive or foster parents and yet developed alcoholism was consistently elevated.

Cognitive-behavioral theorists suggest the way in which a person perceives being high may influence the act of becoming high. It can be an innocent beginning: obtaining relief from valid prescription medications can, according to cognitive theory, leave people perceiving that the drugs offer a miracle cure. It becomes appealing to want that kind of relief again, and soon a pattern is formed, and other substances may be added.

Differential Diagnosis

A patient with a chemical dependency may be admitted to the hospital for medical problems associated with the substance use (dehydration, liver failure) or for unrelated problems (cancer, diabetes). Nursing assessment, unexplained tolerance to pain medication, or symptoms of withdrawal may lead you

or the physician to pursue the possibility of chemical dependency. Laboratory tests can rule out physiological problems. Drug levels of alcohol or drugs can also be measured. A patient who is uncommonly anxious for early discharge should also be further assessed.

Alcohol Use Disorders

Use and abuse of alcohol is present in all walks of life, at all economic levels, and in both genders. Sometimes a fine line exists between a person who is a social drinker and a person who has an abuse condition. One factor used to make that differentiation is the degree of need or compulsion to drink. There is a high incidence of alcohol use and abuse among older adults, teenagers, and even younger children. Alcoholism either directly or indirectly decreases a person's life expectancy by an average of 10 to 12 years.

Denial is a common ego defense mechanism used by people who are substance abusers. The person who is alcohol dependent often uses statements such as "I can quit anytime I want to" or "I just need a little bump to loosen me up."

Characteristics of substance use disorders were described earlier. In addition, patients with alcohol use disorders may experience:

- Binges usually lasting 2 days or more
- Blackouts (unable to recall what happened during a period of drinking)
- Vomiting and dehydration
- Disorientation
- Increased vulnerability to infections, accidents, and other injuries

Sometimes patients who are actively using drugs or alcohol when admitted to an inpatient setting, or who are cut off from sedatives or alcohol abruptly, experience a condition called **delirium tremens** (DTs). The DTs develop when alcohol intake is significantly reduced and the neurotransmitters previously suppressed by alcohol are no longer suppressed. They rebound, resulting in a phenomenon known as brain hyperexcitability. Hyperexcitability can cause visual hallucinations, tremors, and possibly tonic-clonic seizures. Elevated blood pressure and pulse and cardiac dysrhythmias also may occur. Symptoms of withdrawal begin within 4 to 12 hours after the patient has stopped drinking and will peak in 24 to 48 hours. Hospitalization is needed to maintain the patient's safety.

Therapeutic Measures

Treatment for and recovery from alcohol use disorders is a slow process. With few exceptions, a person who has an alcohol dependency and who is recovering cannot ever have another drink, or he or she will risk the chance of returning to previous abusive patterns. Some treatment options are described next. Several forms of treatment may be used together.

SUPPORT GROUPS. A common and effective treatment for alcoholism is involvement in Alcoholics Anonymous (AA). AA

• WORD • BUILDING •
dysfunctional: dys—bad or difficult + functional—performance

is a 12-step program that offers support through others who have stopped drinking. For more information on AA, go to www.alcoholics-anonymous.org. Another program for women only is called Women for Sobriety www.womenforsobriety.org.

COGNITIVE-BEHAVIORAL THERAPY. Cognitive behavioral therapy is used as an adjunct therapy for control of substance abuse. Cognitive behavioral therapy advocates believe that with homework and practice, a person can learn to think differently about the event that led to the drinking. When the person changes the belief system about the activating event and the drinking, the consequences of drinking will be less powerful.

PSYCHOTHERAPY Psychotherapy provides one-on-one therapy. Because substance use affects an entire family, family therapy is important in reinstating honest communications. A commitment to stop drinking is required, and therapy will only help with some of the issues resulting from years of drinking.

MEDICATIONS. In the United States, aversion and anticraving medications have been approved to treat alcohol use disorders. If a comorbid anxiety or depressive disorder accompanies the alcohol abuse, other medications may be prescribed. Antidepressant or nonaddictive antianxiety drugs are most often prescribed.

Disulfiram (Antabuse) is an aversion medication that is sometimes prescribed as a deterrent to using alcohol. Disulfiram should never be administered without the patient's full informed consent. If a patient taking disulfiram ingests alcohol, a severe reaction causes chest pain, nausea, vomiting, confusion, and other symptoms. Those taking disulfiram also can be adversely affected if they use products that contain alcohol, such as cologne mouthwash, aftershave, or cough syrup. The effects of disulfiram last 2 to 3 weeks after the last dose.

Acamprosate (Campral) is a newer drug that is thought to work by helping to restore GABA-glutamate equilibrium. Campral is used to combat cravings and is specifically indicated for maintenance of abstinence from alcohol in patients who have stopped drinking.

Naltrexone (ReVia) may reduce craving, which is the urge or desire to drink. Naltrexone helps patients remain abstinent and can interfere with the tendency to want to drink more if a recovering patient relapses and ingests alcohol.

Use of benzodiazepines such as diazepam (Valium) and lorazepam (Ativan) can help prevent symptoms of DTs during acute withdrawal by neurotransmitter action but are not used long term because of risk for **dependence**.

HOSPITALIZATION. Therapy may range from in-house hospitalizations to halfway houses to eventual independence, usually with attendance at AA meetings. It is common for patients to seek treatment multiple times. This should not be interpreted as a weakness in the patient or the treatment program. It is only a sign that the person is learning more about the disorder and the need to help himself or herself. People with all kinds of chronic diseases experience relapse at times.

Nursing Process for the Patient With Alcohol Use Disorders

DATA COLLECTION. A common screening tool to determine if a patient has a drinking problem is the CAGE questionnaire (Ewing, 1984):

• Have you ever felt you should *Cut down* on your drinking?
• Have people *Annoyed* you by criticizing your drinking?
• Have you ever felt bad or *Guilty* about your drinking?
• Have you ever had a drink first thing in the morning (as an "*Eye opener*") to steady your nerves or get rid of a hangover?

A "yes" answer to two or more questions suggests a drinking problem.

Alcohol also can have many physiological effects. See Chapter 32 for assessment of patients with liver disorders.

NURSING DIAGNOSES, PLANNING, AND IMPLEMENTATION. *Ineffective Coping related to lack of effective coping mechanisms as evidenced by abuse of alcohol*

EXPECTED OUTCOME: The patient will accept responsibility for her or his behavior, verbalize acceptance of the relationship between substance abuse and personal problems, and identify effects of alcohol on the body.

• Help patient to identify recent behavior while under the influence of alcohol. *Patients need to see the relationship between their substance abuse and their personal problems.*
• Expect sobriety. *This establishes sobriety as the norm.*
• Teach about the physical impact of drugs and alcohol on the body. *Many patients lack accurate information about the effects of substance abuse on the body.*
• Be honest; be aware of your own thoughts and feelings about addictions. *Effective communication is essential for a therapeutic relationship.*
• Provide group support such as a 12-step program. Many chemical dependency units provide group support meetings. *Peer support is an effective treatment that is often more acceptable to patients than other treatments.*
• Confront the patient immediately if projection, rationalization, or denial behaviors are noted. *Projection, rationalization, and denial are ego defense mechanisms that discourage the patient from accepting responsibility for behavior.*
• Use positive reinforcement. *Positive reinforcement for successes is important when helping a person with an addiction. Every step is a big one in this field; every step taken is a new one.*
• Provide a safe environment. *Patients who are chemically addicted may become suicidal or display other bizarre behavior, especially during withdrawal. A patient under the influence of alcohol or another chemical may have poor impulse control or judgment. Maintaining a safe milieu and calm demeanor will help the patient through this difficult time.*
• Remain alert to the possibility that the patient may be using a substance even in the hospital. Express suspicions honestly and nonjudgmentally to the patient. Report and document all findings and behaviors that may be potential

safety hazards for the patient. *The fact that a patient is hospitalized does not guarantee that he or she has no access to the chemical or way of using it in your presence. Unfortunately, family members or friends sometimes smuggle drugs or alcohol in to patients.*

• Practice "tough love." "Doing for" patients may be tempting, but it is not in the patient's best interest most of the time. *This encourages patients to be responsible for their own healing.*

EVALUATION. Does the patient verbalize acceptance of responsibility for own behavior? Does the patient understand the relationship between personal problems and substance abuse? Does the patient understand the effects of substance abuse on the body?

For additional information, visit the National Institute for Alcohol Abuse and Alcoholism at www.niaaa.nih.gov.

Other Substance Use Disorders

Many substances other than alcohol can be addictive. Caffeine and nicotine are two that are readily available. Coffee, tea, soda, and cigarettes are everywhere in our society and are very addicting. Many experts believe that the single most difficult addiction to overcome is to nicotine.

Illegal substances such as marijuana (in some states), cocaine, crack, phencyclidine (more commonly known as PCP), and prescription medications for pain and mental health treatment are also potentially addictive. Methamphetamine (meth) has led to a substantial substance abuse problem affecting families and society. Inhalants such as lighter fluid, paint, paint thinners, and gasoline also can be used to get high; in the United States, these substances are mainly used by teenagers. The term for their use is *huffing*. These are highly neurotoxic substances, potentially lethal, and usually available in the house or garage.

Signs and Symptoms

The signs and symptoms of drug abuse and dependence can be similar to those of alcohol abuse. Additional signs of drug abuse include the following:

• Red, watery eyes
• Runny nose
• Hostile behavior
• Paranoia
• Needle tracks on arms or legs

Therapeutic Measures

Therapeutic measures for patients with drug abuse and dependence include the following:

• Narcotics Anonymous
• Group therapy
• Psychotherapy
• Methadone programs

Methadone acts as a sort of "step down" for people addicted to certain opioid drugs. Methadone can be legally prescribed and dispensed. It, too, is potentially addicting, and its critics believe it is only a substitute for heroin. It is typically given once a day. Psychotherapy is also provided for patients in methadone programs.

Nursing Care

Nursing care for people who are drug dependent is essentially the same as for those who are alcohol dependent. It is important to remember that nurses and physicians cannot "fix" the patient who is chemically dependent. The desire to be chemically free must come from the person who is addicted (see Table 57.7 for a Substance Abuse Summary).

CRITICAL THINKING

Maria

■ You are a school nurse in your local high school. You notice that Maria, a 17-year-old student, is behaving oddly. She has always been rather loud and even has been referred to as "obnoxious" by several of her peers. Lately you have observed her sitting alone, as if waiting for someone, but when you approach her, she barely greets you and then moves away.

1. What are your concerns about Maria?
2. What are some of the possibilities that might be affecting her?
3. How can you approach her more effectively the next time you see her?

Suggested answers are at the end of the chapter.

TABLE 57.7   SUBSTANCE ABUSE SUMMARY

Signs and Symptoms	Inability to fulfill obligations at work, school, or home Recurrent legal or interpersonal problems Continued use despite social and interpersonal problems Participation in physically hazardous situations while impaired
Diagnosis	History Liver function studies Serum drug or alcohol levels Evaluate for other coexisting disorders (bipolar disorder)
Therapeutic Measures	12-step programs Cognitive behavioral therapy Psychotherapy Disulfiram (Antabuse) Acamprosate (Campral) Naltrexone (ReVia) Benzodiazepines for acute withdrawal
Nursing Diagnoses	*Ineffective Coping* *Ineffective Denial*

■ MENTAL ILLNESS AND THE OLDER ADULT

It is not uncommon for older adults to be admitted to the hospital with a tentative diagnosis of "change in mental status." It is important to distinguish between physical and mental disorders in these circumstances. Some neurocognitive disorders that affect older adults' mental status are as follows.

- *Major Neurocognitive Disorder* is an impairment of mental functioning that interferes with daily activities and relationships. Causes of major neurocognitive disorder include Alzheimer's disease, Lewy body disease, vascular disease, Huntington's disease, HIV infection, and others.
- *Delirium* is an acute change in mental status needing immediate evaluation and treatment. This is often due to a physiological condition such as an infection and can be reversed if recognized and the underlying cause is removed. Read more about dementia and delirium in Chapter 48.
- *Pseudodementia* is a condition in which the patient appears to have a major neurocognitive disorder but is really experiencing depression. Treating the depression can help reverse the mental status changes.
- *Depression* in older adults should not be viewed as a normal part of aging; it should be diagnosed and treated. Older adults may be dealing with physical and mental decline, loss of function, isolation, and loss of a marriage partner and friends; they may express their depression through bodily symptoms such as pain. If not evaluated and treated, depression can lead to suicide (see "Gerontological Issues"). Be sure to review Chapter 15, "Nursing Care of Older Adult Patients."

- Set the plan into action (i.e., bought a gun, has a full bottle of pills in the bedside table)

Any older adult who has a plan to end his or her life and has the ability or resources to do so must be immediately referred for psychological evaluation. Never leave a person with suicidal thoughts alone.

Crisis Intervention for a Suicidal Older Adult

- Remove any items that the older adult could use to inflict an injury or end his or her life, such as razors, jewelry with pins or sharp points, and mirrors.
- Make arrangements for direct supervision and observation that are reliable, considering personnel and family resources. Often, hospital admission is the most appropriate intervention for a person at a high risk for suicide.
- Help the older adult talk about the crisis or life event that has devastated his or her desire to live. For example, encourage reminiscence about the patient's spouse, or allow the older person to express the frustration of being unable to physically meet the daily demands of life.
- Develop a "do no harm" or suicide contract with the older adult. Outline a short-term, structured plan to keep the older adult safe. Focus on decreasing social isolation by requiring personal social contacts (e.g., stay at daughter's home for a weekend; go to the senior center for lunch; call a specific person who is willing and wants to listen to feelings and concerns; exercise; take a walk outside; volunteer services at a nursing home, hospital, or school).

Older adults often need assistance to develop or enhance skills required to cope with life events. Self-care and personal independence in care choices can be encouraged.

Gerontological Issues

Suicide and the Older Adult

Older adults are not immune to suicidal thoughts. In North America, white men older than age 75 have an especially high suicide rate. Comments by any older adult referring to hopelessness or desire to die must be explored to assess suicide risk. The following comments could be a reflection of suicide potential in an older adult who is depressed:

- "Living is harder than dying could ever be."
- "I am a used-up old man who is a burden for everyone."
- "I am useless. I can't do anything anymore."
- "I don't know why God won't take me."

   To adequately assess suicide potential, ask questions that establish whether the older adult has done the following:

- Thought about ending his or her life
- Attempted to end his or her life in the past
- Developed a plan to end his or her life
- Has started to give away as "gifts" his/her personal prized objects

Home Health Hints

- Help patients and families identify pharmacies that will deliver medications to the home.
- Set up medications using a system the patient can easily follow.
- Maintain communication with and act as a liaison between the psychiatrist and primary care provider as needed.
- Assist the patient and family to identify community resources such as support groups and respite care.
- Assess family members for evidence of caregiver role strain.
- Provide education for family/caregivers related to the patient's illness, medications, and symptom management.

SUGGESTED ANSWERS TO
CRITICAL THINKING

■ *Tommy*

You can reassure Tommy's mother that his OCD is not her fault. Tommy can learn to control his illness with medications and therapy. The family must be part of the therapy, for both Tommy's and the family's sake. Positive communication between Tommy and his family is encouraged. Tommy's mother can also be encouraged to attend a support group herself. Suggest to Tommy's mother that she meet with a counselor or behavioral therapist to learn more about the causes and treatment of the disorder.

■ *Mr. Zenz*

It is important to be supportive of Mrs. Zenz while maintaining her husband's confidentiality and privacy. Encouraging Mrs. Zenz to talk to Mr. Zenz's physician is appropriate. Showing empathy with statements such as "It must be confusing and difficult to watch your husband change moods so quickly" are good tools to use. It may be a bit more challenging to approach him as your boss. You may certainly ask him if you can speak frankly and share specific observations. You may share your concern, such as "Mr. Zenz, you are a wonderful boss, but I am frightened when you become loud and boisterous." This may help him to reflect. Chances are, however, that if he is in a manic stage, he will not hear your concern. It may require a delicate conversation with the next person up in the corporate chain of command, being careful to objectively report behavior but not share assumptions. This is a tough one. Good luck!

■ *Anne*

Appropriate communication skills include being positive, reassuring, and not reinforcing the hallucinations. "I don't see or hear a woman, Anne. It is time for the movie. I'd like you to come with me for a while at least" is an example of an appropriate verbal interaction. Reinforcing expectations is also appropriate; you might say "Anne, part of your care plan includes attending one unit activity each day. This is the last opportunity for you to meet your care plan objective for today." At all times, nurses need to be aware of drug interactions. Anne will most likely be medicated for her schizophrenia, and those medications can interact unfavorably with her chemotherapy. If she is receiving oral medications, it may be necessary to check her mouth to ensure she is swallowing them. Work with team members to provide a therapeutic and low stimulus environment for Anne. Good nursing data collection skills are essential.

■ *Maria*

A number of options may explain Maria's behavior, including depression, drug use, schizophrenia, or an eating disorder. Next time you see Maria, you might try constructively confronting her behavior by saying something like "Maria, you used to be much more outgoing. We always were friendly, and now you leave when I'm near. That change in you concerns me. I'm here if you want to talk." Or "Maria, I see your behavior is changing. You are loud one moment and very quiet the next. That is unusual for you. What's happening?"

REVIEW QUESTIONS

1. Which statement by a depressed patient causes the LPN to contact the RN or HCP immediately?
   1. "Everyone is out to get me."
   2. "I have tried to kill myself three times."
   3. "I feel so hopeless."
   4. "My friend is bringing me a gun."

2. A patient states, "My doctor says I have obsessive-compulsive disorder. What does that mean?" Which response by the nurse is best?
   1. "It means that you have experienced a major life stress and will need therapy to help you manage the symptoms."
   2. "You can expect to experience periods of high energy and anxiety, alternating with periods of feeling very low."
   3. "You may experience involuntary, intrusive thoughts, and feel compelled to respond with seemingly meaningless actions."
   4. "People with obsessive-compulsive disorder are very organized. This is a good disorder to have."

3. A patient is experiencing extrapyramidal side effects while taking antipsychotic medication. Which medication on the patient's orders will help reduce these effects?
   1. benztropine (Cogentin)
   2. chlorpromazine (Thorazine)
   3. haloperidol (Haldol)
   4. lithium (Eskalith)

4. A patient who is a veteran of the Gulf War hears the hospital fire alarm go off during a drill and cries, "There are people hiding behind the pillars! They have guns! Be careful!" What action should the nurse take first?
   1. Tell the patient that his behavior is inappropriate and that he is frightening the other patients.
   2. Administer an as-needed (prn) antipsychotic medication as ordered.
   3. Ask him if he is afraid of the guns.
   4. Stay with the patient while calmly reorienting him.

5. A patient is being treated on the mental health unit for an anxiety disorder. The patient approaches the nurse and reports feeling dizzy and weak, with a sensation of a racing heart. The nursing care plan includes interventions of imagery exercises and prn lorazepam (Ativan) for symptoms of anxiety. What should the nurse do first?
   1. Instruct the patient to sit and breathe deeply.
   2. Give the patient the prescribed prn lorazepam.
   3. Obtain the patient's vital signs.
   4. Instruct the patient in an imagery exercise.

6. A patient reports seeing children playing on the floor in the hallway of the mental health unit. There are no children anywhere on the unit. Which response by the nurse is best?
   1. "The children are fine there; they are just playing."
   2. "I don't see any children, and there haven't been any children on the unit today. Would you like to walk with me?"
   3. "Children are not allowed on this unit. I will ask them to leave."
   4. "You know there are no children here. It must be time for your medication."

Answers can be found in Appendix C.

References

American Psychiatric Association. (2013). *Diagnostic and statistical manual of mental disorders* (5th ed.). Arlington, VA: Author.

Beddes, J. R. (2013, May). The future of bipolar disorder: genetics, diagnosis, and treatment. *Program and abstracts of the 2013 American Psychiatric Association Annual Meeting,* San Francisco, CA (Symposium 78).

Bleuler, E. (1911). *Dementia praecox or the group of schizophrenias* (p. 26). New York: International Universities Press.

Ewing, J. A. (1984). Detecting alcoholism: The CAGE questionnaire. *Journal of the American Medical Association, 252,* 1905–1907.

Lamoure, J., & Stovel, J. (2011). Serotonin syndrome: A perfect storm. How to prevent, recognize and manage serotonin syndrome. *Pharmacy Practice, 27,* 22–26, 30–31.

National Council of State Boards of Nursing. (2011). Substance use disorder in nursing. Retrieved January 3, 2014, from www.ncsbn.org/SUDN_10.pdf

National Institute of Mental Health. (2010). Statistics: Any personality disorder. Retrieved December 2011 from www.nimh.nih.gov/statistics/1ANYPERS.shtml

Nordahl, C., Scholz, R., Yang, X., Buonocore, M. H., Simon, T., Rogers, S., & Amaral, D. G. (2012). Increased rate of amygdala growth in children aged 2 to 4 years with autism spectrum disorders: A longitudinal study. *Arch Gen Psychiatry, 69,* 53–61. doi:10.1001/archgenpsychiatry.2011.145.

Patil, S. T., Zhang, L., Martenyi, F., Lowe, S. L., Jackson, K. A., Andreev, B. V., . . . Schoepp, D. D. (2007). Activation of mGlu2/3 receptors as a new approach to treat schizophrenia: A randomized phase 2 clinical trial. *Nature Medicine, 13,* 1102–1107.

 DavisPlus | For additional resources and information visit **davispl.us/medsurg5**

Diagnostic Tests

This is intended to be a quick reference only. Please check a diagnostic test reference manual for comprehensive information.

GENERAL CONSIDERATIONS FOR ALL TESTS:

- Ensure that an informed consent form is signed before any invasive procedure.
- Check orders for need to withhold food or fluids before test.
- Preparation if contrast media will be used: (1) assess for and report allergies to iodine or contrast media; (2) report elevated creatinine/blood urea nitrogen (BUN) levels because dye is nephrotoxic and excreted by the kidneys; (3) consider patient risk factors for contrast-induced nephropathy and discuss with health care provider (HCP) prophylaxis orders such as holding nephrotoxic medications (nonsteroidal anti-inflammatories, aminoglycoside antibiotics, cisplatin, cyclosporin A, amphotericin B) 24 hours or more before the test, and providing intravenous (IV) hydration; (4) if patient is taking metformin, obtain order to hold it before and 48 hours after test to prevent risk for lactic acidosis; (5) encourage fluids after test to promote excretion of dye; and (6) teach that the patient may experience a feeling of warmth or experience a salty or metallic taste when the dye is injected.
- Reinforce patient education for test.

Test or Procedure	Description	Reasons Done	Preprocedure Nursing Considerations	Postprocedure Nursing Considerations
Angiography • abdominal • adrenal • carotid • coronary • pulmonary • renal	Contrast media is injected through a catheter, usually via femoral artery or vein, and then radiographs are taken at intervals to view vasculature.	To view patency and distribution of blood vessels.	Report history of bleeding/clotting disorders. Medications that interfere with clotting are stopped about 1 week before examination. Ensure patent IV is in place.	Monitor vital signs and circulatory status as ordered. Maintain pressure on insertion site as ordered. Ensure hydration (oral or IV) to help excretion of dye. Report bleeding or hematoma formation.
Biopsy	Removal of tissue for microscopic examination. May be done with needle, punch, incision, or endoscopically.	To diagnose cancerous or other lesions	Premedicate for pain.	Monitor vital signs and biopsy site as ordered.
Computed axial tomography (CAT), computed tomography (CT)	Multiple x-ray beams provide three-dimensional cross section visualization of internal structures. Contrast media may be used.	To visualize abnormal structures or masses	Assess for claustrophobia (depending on scanner); patient will be in scanner for up to 1 hour. Premedicate anxious or claustrophobic patients as ordered.	Encourage hydration if contrast media was used.
Electrocardiography (ECG, EKG)	Electrodes provide a graphic display of the electrical current during the cardiac cycle.	To evaluate electrical function of the heart; diagnose dysrhythmias.	Explain test to patient.	None specific.

Test or Procedure	Description	Reasons Done	Preprocedure Nursing Considerations	Postprocedure Nursing Considerations
Electroencephalography (EEG)	Electrodes on scalp evaluate electrical activity of the brain.	To evaluate brain activity, lesions, seizures.	Ensure patient's hair is clean and dry. Check orders for drugs such as sedatives or stimulants that may need to be weaned or withheld before test.	Wash adhesive from hair before it hardens and becomes difficult to remove. Oil or witch hazel may make removal easier. Instruct patient about resuming medications as ordered.
Endoscopy • bronchoscopy • colonoscopy • colposcopy • gastroscopy • sigmoidoscopy	A flexible fiber-optic tube and camera are inserted into a body cavity to observe structures.	To observe for abnormalities, remove polyps, obtain biopsy specimens, suction secretions, coagulate bleeding sites, and more.	Check orders for preparation such as NPO (non per os), laxatives, enemas. Premedicate as ordered.	Check for swallow and gag reflexes after upper endoscopy before offering food or fluids.
Lumbar puncture (spinal tap)	A small needle is used to withdraw cerebrospinal fluid for examination. The needle is typically inserted between the L3–4 or L4–5 vertebrae.	To diagnose infection, central nervous system disease, or cancers. Sometimes used to inject medication.	Premedicate as ordered. Assist patient to sit leaning forward or lay curled up on side according to HCP preference. Be prepared to assist with procedure.	Label specimens and take to laboratory. Monitor site. Implement activity restrictions if ordered. Encourage fluids.
Magnetic resonance imaging (MRI)	Magnetic field and radiofrequency energy are used to obtain a detailed image of tissues. Contrast media may be used.	To visualize structural abnormalities in organs and tissues.	Because powerful magnets are used, question patient about metallic foreign bodies, pacemakers (some new models are MRI compatible), or tattoos with metal-based inks, which are contraindications for this test. Assess for claustrophobia; patient will be in scanner for up to 1 hour. Consider open MRI availability. Request order for sedative or analgesic to be given 1 hour before test if necessary.	Encourage hydration if contrast media used.

Continued

Test or Procedure	Description	Reasons Done	Preprocedure Nursing Considerations	Postprocedure Nursing Considerations
			Explain that patient must lie still in an enclosed area for prolonged period. Remove all jewelry. Teach patient to expect loud knocking sounds during test (headphones with music may be requested). Teach relaxation and deep-breathing exercises.	
Myelography	Contrast media is injected into cerebrospinal space following lumbar puncture. Radiographs are then taken to outline the vertebrae.	Identifies spinal column abnormalities.	Same as lumbar puncture.	Maintain bedrest with head elevated less than 30 degrees. Monitor for seizures. Encourage hydration to promote excretion of contrast media.
Nuclear scan • heart • lungs • CNS • thyroid • bone • other	Radioactive substances are administered (orally, inhaled, or IV), then a special scanner observes where the substance is distributed.	To show both structure and function abnormalities.	Check HCP orders for preparation, which may differ for each scan type. Teach patient that the amount of radioactive material is very small, and no special precautions are needed.	Encourage hydration to promote excretion of radioactive material.
Radiograph (X-ray)	X-ray beams identify internal structures, especially high-density structures such as bone. Contrast media may be used with some tests.	To identify differences in tissue densities. Can help diagnose a variety of structural or other disorders.	Have patient remove jewelry from area to be x-rayed. Laxatives or enemas may be ordered before some gastrointestinal x-rays.	If barium has been used as contrast media to outline the bowel, administer laxative as ordered and increase fluid intake to help evacuate barium before it hardens.
Ultrasonography Endoscopic ultrasound— transesophageal echocardiogram, transrectal ultrasound, transvaginal	High-frequency sound waves are passed through soft tissues to outline tissues and masses. Gel is used on skin and transducer to improve conduction of sound waves.	To identify alterations in soft tissues and organs.	Check orders for preparation if ultrasound will be done endoscopically.	None specific.

Normal Adult Reference Laboratory Values

BLOOD, PLASMA, OR SERUM VALUES

	Reference Range	
Determination	*Conventional*	*SI*
Aldolase	Less than 7.4 units/L	
Ammonia	12–55 μmol/L	12–55 μmol/L
Amylase	30–110 units/mL	
Atrial natriuretic peptide	20–77 pg/mL	20–77 ng/L

	BNP	**Pro-BNP (N-Terminal)**
Male	Less than 100 pg/mL	60 pg/mL
Female	Less than 100 pg/mL	12–150 pg/mL

Bilirubin (total)	0.3–1.2 mg/dL	5–21 μmol/L
Calcium	8.2–10.2 mg/dL	2.05–2.55 mmol/L
Carbon dioxide content	23–29 mEq/L	23–29 mmol/L
Chloride	97–107 mEq/L	97–107 mmol/L
Creatine kinase (CK)	*Female:* 26–140 units/L *Male:* 38–174 units/L	
CK isoenzymes 　CK-BB 　CK-MB 　CK-MM 　CK-MB by immunoassay	 Absent 4%–6% 94%–96% 10 ng/mL	
Creatinine 　Male 　Female	 0.6–1.2 mg/dL 53–106 μmol/L 0.5–1.1 mg/dL 44–97 μmol/L	
d-Dimer	*Semiquantitative:* No fragments detected. *Quantitative:* Less than 250 ng/mL	
Erythrocyte sedimentation rate (ESR) (Westergren method) 　Male 　Female	 *Under age 50:* Less than 15 mm/hr *Over age 50:* Less than 20 mm/hr *Under age 50:* Less than 20 mm/hr *Over age 50:* Less than 30 mm/hr	
Glucose	Fasting: 70–100 mg/dL	3.9–5.5 mmol/L

Continued

BLOOD, PLASMA, OR SERUM VALUES—cont'd

	Reference Range	
Iron		
Male	65–175 µg/dL	11.6–31.3 µmol/L
Female	50–170 µg/dL	9–30.4 µmol/L
Iron-binding capacity	250–350 µg/dL	45–63 µmol/L
Lactic dehydrogenase	90–176 units/L	
Lipase	0–160 units/L	
Lipids (desirable)		
Cholesterol	Less than 200 mg/dL	Less than 5.18 mmol/L
Low-density lipoprotein	Less than 100 mg/dL	Less than 2.59 mmol/L
High-density lipoprotein	Greater than 60 mg/dL	Greater than 1.56 mmol/L
Triglycerides	Less than 150 mg/dL	Less than 1.70 mmol/L
Magnesium	1.6–2.6 mg/dL	0.62–0.91 mmol/L
Myoglobin	0–85 ng/mL	
Osmolality	275–295 mOsm/kg	275–295 mmol/kg
Oxygen saturation (arterial)	95–100%	
PCO_2	35–45 mm Hg	4.66–5.98 kPa
pH	7.35–7.45	Same
PO_2	80–95 mm Hg	10.6–12.6 kPa
Phosphatase (prostatic acid)	Less than 2.5 ng/mL	
Phosphatase (alkaline)		
Male	35–142 units/L	
Female	25–125 units/L	
Phosphorus (blood)	2.5–4.5 mg/dL	0.8–1.4 mmol/L
Potassium	3.5–5.0 mEq/L	3.5–5.0 mmol/L
Protein: Total	6.0–8.0 g/dL	60–80 g/L
Albumin	3.4–4.8 g/dL	34–48 g/L
Sodium	135–145 mEq/L	135–145 mmol/L
Transaminase, alanine aminotransferase (ALT)		
Male	10–40 units/L	
Female	7–35 units/L	
Transaminase, aspartate aminotransferase (AST)		
Male	15–40 units/L	
Female	13–35 units/L	
Troponin I	<0.35 ng/mL	
Troponin T	<0.20 µg/L	
Urea nitrogen (BUN)	8–21 mg/dL	2.9–7.5 mmol/L

BLOOD, PLASMA, OR SERUM VALUES—cont'd

Reference Range

Uric acid		
Male	4.4–7.6 mg/dL	0.26–0.45 mmol/L
Female	2.3–6.6 mg/dL	0.14–0.39 mmol/L

URINALYSIS REFERENCE VALUES

Dipstick pH	5.0–9.0
Protein	Less than 20 mg/dL
Glucose	Negative
Ketones	Negative
Hemoglobin	Negative
Bilirubin	Negative
Urobilinogen	Up to 1 mg/dL
Nitrite	Negative
Leukocyte esterase	Negative
Microscopic examination	
Red blood cells	Less than 5/hpf
White blood cells	Less than 5/hpf
Renal cells	None seen
Transitional cells	None seen
Squamous cells	Rare; usually no clinical significance
Casts	Rare hyaline; otherwise, none seen
Crystals in acid urine	Uric acid, calcium oxalate, amorphous urates
Crystals in alkaline urine	Triple phosphate, calcium phosphate, ammonium biurate, calcium carbonate, amorphous phosphates
Bacteria, yeast, parasites	None seen

HEMATOLOGIC VALUES

Determination	Conventional	SI
Coagulation screening tests		
Bleeding time (template)	2.5–10 min	
Prothrombin time	11–13.5 sec	
International normalized ratio (INR)	Less than 2.0 if no anticoagulation therapy	
	2.0 to 3.0 with treatment for venous thrombosis, pulmonary embolism, or valvular heart disease	
	2.5 to 3.5 with mechanical heart valves or treatment for recurrent systemic embolism	

Continued

HEMATOLOGIC VALUES—cont'd

Partial thromboplastin time (activated)	25–38 sec	25–38 sec
Complete blood count (CBC)		
Hematocrit		
Male	43–49	0.43–0.49
Female	38–44	0.38–0.44
Hemoglobin		
Male	13.2–17.3 g/dL	132–173 mmol/L
Female	11.7–15.5 g/dL	117–155 mmol/L
Erythrocyte count		
Male	4.71–5.14 million cells/mm^3	4.71–5.14 × 10^{12} cells/L
Female	4.20–4.87 million cells/mm^3	4.20–4.87 × 10^{12} cells/L

Red Blood Cell (RBC) Indices	Mean Corpuscular Volume (fl)	Mean Corpuscular Hemoglobin (pg/cell)	Mean Corpuscular Hemoglobin Concentration (g/dL)	RBC Distribution Width Index
Male	85–95	28–32	33–35	11.6–14.8
Female	85–95	28–32	33–35	11.6–14.8

Platelet count	150–450 × 10^3/μL/mm^3	181–521 × 10^9/L

White Blood Cell (WBC) Count and Differential	SI Units WBC × 10^3/mm^3 or cells/mL	Neutrophils Total (Absolute and %)	Lymphocytes Bands (Absolute and %)	Monocytes Segments (Absolute and %)	Eosinophils (Absolute and %)	Basophils (Absolute and %)
Adult	4.5–11.0	1.8–7.7 59%	0–0.7 3.0%	1.8–7.0 56%	1.0–4.8 34%	0–0.8 4.0%

THERAPEUTIC DRUG LEVELS

	Reference Range	
Determination	*Conventional*	*SI*
Carbamazepine	4.0–12.0 mg/mL	17–51 μmol/L
Digoxin	0.5–2.0 ng/mL	0.6–2.6 nmol/L
Ethanol	0 mg/dL	0 mmol/L
Lithium	0.6–1.4 mEq/L	0.6–1.4 mmol/L
Phenobarbital	15–40 mcg/mL	65–172 μmol/L
Phenytoin (Dilantin)	10–20 mcg/mL	40–79 μmol/L
Salicylate	15–20 mg/dL	1.1–1.4 mmol/L

MISCELLANEOUS VALUES

Determination	*Conventional*	*SI*
Carcinoembryonic antigen (CEA)	0–2.5 ng/mL	0–2.5 mcg/L
Gastrin	25–90 pg/mL	25–90 ng/L
Immunological tests:		
Alpha-1-antitrypsin	126–226 mg/dL	1.26–2.26 g/L
Antinuclear antibodies	Negative at a 1:8 dilution of serum	

Reference range values may differ from one institution to another. BNP = brain natriuretic peptide; hpf = high-power field; SI = International System of Units.

Most data from Van Leeuwen, A. M., & Poelhuis-Leth, D. J. (2013). *Davis's comprehensive handbook of laboratory and diagnostic tests with nursing implications* (5th ed.). Philadelphia: F.A. Davis.

Appendix C

Answers to Review Questions

Chapter 1

1. 2. Critical thinking is use of cognitive skills or strategies that increase the probability of a desirable outcome.
2. 4. Asking a question shows humility. The nurse does not "know it all."
3. 1. A respiratory rate of 28 is observable. Selections 2, 3, and 4 are patient perceptions.
4. 4. Selections 1, 2, and 3 all include the nurse's perceptions.
5. 3. Shortness of breath is a physiological need and should be addressed first.
6. 3, 1, 4, 5, 2. These are the steps of the nursing process.
7. 1. The LPN implements interventions and assists the RN with the other steps.
8. 4. *Acute Pain* is a nursing diagnosis. The others are medical diagnoses.
9. 3. The patient who has a specific plan is most likely to be successful.

Chapter 2

1. 4. Providing an explanation of why something is done promotes the understanding for why it is important to be done and therefore will more likely be done.
2. 4. Evidence-based nursing care provides the best and safest patient care.
3. 1. Joanna Briggs best practices guideline identifies valid nursing evidence.
4. 3. The proposed change will need to go through the policy and procedure committee for evaluation.
5. 3. Systematic reviews of randomized controlled trials are the best place to look for evidence.
6. 2. A soft toothbrush/fluoride toothpaste is needed to remove plaque from the teeth.

Chapter 3

1. 2. The older adult population is growing and will require more complex health care.
2. 1, 2, 3, 4. Assessment of conditions present on admission and all care and education to prevent complications, including patient refusal to participate, must be documented during hospitalization.
3. 3. All but ambulating a patient are outside the LPN scope of practice.
4. 2. Autocratic leaders do not seek input to make decisions.
5. 1. LPNs consult with RNs in caring for their patients.
6. 4. Acting on fidelity, because the patient is an adult, the nurse protects the patient's personal health information. Therefore, the nurse does not provide false information but tells the mother to talk to her daughter, who decides how to answer her mother's questions.
7. 3. When patients refuse treatment, it can be a dilemma related to life and death. However, if patients are given correct information and understand the consequences of actions, it is their choice to refuse treatment. It is never OK to coerce patients with fear or make them feel badly about their decision.
8. 1. If the patient has a valid advance directive and the health care provider (HCP) uses a deontological perspective (i.e., Do what's right) and supports autonomy (i.e., The patient's wishes), then a feeding tube will not be inserted. This does not necessarily mean that the advance directive stated do not resuscitate (DNR).

9. 2. Utilitarianism supports decisions based on the best outcome for the greatest number of the people (Butts & Rich, 2013).
10. 2. A patient who is asking to die may be feeling depressed, especially if he or she is missing family. It is a good idea to try to understand more about how the patient is feeling. While getting such patients involved in activities may be helpful, it is not a good idea to minimize their feelings. In addition, although empathizing with feelings can help, option "d" is not therapeutic because the nurse is not in the same situation as the patient. It is never OK to medicate the patient to "numb" these feelings.
11. 1, 3, 5. Institutional policies outline the proper manner for performing certain tasks and procedures for employees who must comply with them; state nurse practice laws outline the scope of practice in a given state that nurses must abide by when practicing under license in that state; local nursing standards of care identify the degree of prudence and caution required for proper nursing practice.
12. 1, 4, 5. See Box 3-3.
13. 2. The Health Insurance Portability and Accountability Act (HIPAA) requires protection for the privacy of personal health information.

Chapter 4

1. 2. Ethnocentrism is thinking one's own ways are the only right and proper ways.
2. 4. Allowing parents to stay and pray in the child's room meets the needs of both parents and child.
3. 1. American Indians may interpret eye contact as rude; they also tend to be comfortable with silences.
4. 3. Islamic Arabs may avoid pork.
5. 1. Nonharmful cultural practices should be allowed.

Chapter 5

1. 3. "Complement" means "something added."
2. 3. Allopathy, or Western medicine such as is practiced in the United States, is based on scientific research.
3. 4. Ginger, as with all herbs, can interact with other medications.
4. 1, 3, and 5 all use some form of relaxation.
5. 2. It is essential that health care providers are aware of patient use of complementary and alternative medicine to evaluate their safety with conventional therapies and medications.

Chapter 6

1. 1, 5. Sodium is the major cation in the blood and helps maintain serum osmolarity. Sodium is also important for cell function, especially in the central nervous system.
2. 2. Dehydration is associated with poor skin turgor because of loss of water in the tissues and with disorientation because of loss of blood volume in the brain.
3. 4. The older adults have reduced kidney function and may not be able to handle excess fluids.
4. 3. Daily weights are the best way to monitor fluid imbalances. They are easier to monitor accurately than intake and output.
5. 1. Elevating the head of the bed will provide more room for lung expansion and provide the quickest relief for shortness of breath.
6. 1. Daily or every-other-day weights are easy to keep track of at home.

7. 4. Hypokalemia is associated with muscle weakness.
8. 2, 3, 4. Potatoes, tomatoes, and bananas are highest in potassium.
9. 2. Retained carbon dioxide leads to acidosis.
10. 1. 7.26 is below 7.35 and is acidotic.

Chapter 7

1. 2. Policies may vary slightly by institution. Always use the policies provided by your workplace.
2. 1 (a man with dehydration requires fluids), 2 (a woman with an eating disorder will benefit from parenteral nutrition), 3 (intravenous [IV] antibiotics may be effective if oral antibiotics have failed), 4 (prolonged vomiting causes fluid and electrolyte loss and requires replacement), 6 (IV diuretics will work the fastest on fluid overload).
3. 1. Site selection should move from distal to proximal on the arm.
4. 2, 5, 6, 1, 3, 8, 9, 4, 7. See Table 7.1.
5. 3. The multiple tourniquet technique will best help visualize veins for cannulation.
6. 2. The patient has signs of an air embolism. The cracked tubing must be clamped, and oxygen will support oxygenation until the registered nurse or physician arrives.
7. 4. Blood products must be administered with sodium chloride to avoid complications
8. 3. The catheter that is palpable under the skin is the tunneled portion of the catheter.
9. 33.

$$\frac{100 \text{ mL}}{1 \text{ hour}} \left| \frac{1 \text{ hour}}{60 \text{ minutes}} \right| \frac{20 \text{ gtt}}{1 \text{ mL}} = 33 \text{ gtt/minute}$$

10. 83

$$\frac{1000 \text{ mL}}{12 \text{ hours}} = 83 \text{ mL/hour}$$

Chapter 8

1. 5, 2, 3, 1, 6, 4. This is the order in the chain of events leading to an infection (Fig. 8.1).
2. 3. Hand hygiene is essential to help prevent infections.
3. 2. Applying lotion to skin, the first line of defense, prevents dryness and cracking.
4. 3. An elevated low-grade temperature when immunocompromised (neutropenia) can be very significant.
5. 1. All patient allergies must be checked to help prevent an allergic reaction.
6. 4. Maintaining a closed urinary drainage system is essential to prevent contamination.
7. 3. Take all medication as ordered to help prevent relapse and development of bacterial resistance.

Chapter 9

1. 3. The sympathetic nervous system (fight or flight) is stimulated to compensate for shock symptoms.
2. 1, 5, 6. Wheezing, urticaria, and bronchospasm are seen specifically in anaphylactic shock.
3. 4. Cerebral hypoxia depresses the central nervous system.
4. 1, 3, 5. When teaching the geriatric patient, include others to reinforce learning, have visible materials in large print, and speak slowly and lower tone to increase understanding of spoken words.
5. 4. Increasing blood pressure indicates the shock is improving.
6. 2. Ineffective tissue perfusion occurs due to shock.
7. Restlessness and confusion indicate a need for oxygen, which is started immediately while other treatment is prepared.
8. 4. These vital signs indicate progressive shock and require immediate intervention.
9. 3. A normal blood pressure would indicate effective treatment for shock.
10. 2, 3, 1. As shock progresses from compensated to decompensated, systolic blood pressure decreases.

Chapter 10

1. 2. Pain is whatever the patient says it is, whenever the patient says it is.
2. 4. Distraction is an effective method when used with medication for pain control.
3. 3. Tolerance is the need for more medication to achieve the same effect. There is no ceiling effect for opioids, so if the patient is still in pain, the dose may need to be increased.
4. 2. Surgery would cause acute nociceptive pain, which will be most appropriately treated with an opioid.
5. 1. Neuropathic pain is most commonly described as shooting, tingling, or shocklike.
6. 3. A valid assessment scale is the best way to quantify pain.
7. 1, 4, 5. According to the World Health Organization ladder, adjuvants are always appropriate in addition to analgesics. They are not intended to substitute for analgesics.
8. 3. The patient will experience the best pain relief with the combination of an opioid and nonopioid.
9. 4. Meperidine should be avoided in older adult patients.
10. 2. Gabapentin must be taken continuously to be effective. Chronic neuropathic pain is not likely to go away, so treatment will be ongoing.
11. 4. A placebo should not be administered except in research studies. The supervisor should be involved in educating the physician.
12. 0.7 mL.

$$\frac{10 \text{ mg}}{} \left| \frac{\text{grain}}{60 \text{ mg}} \right| \frac{1/4 \text{ grain}}{1 \text{ mL}} = 0.7 \text{ mL}$$

Chapter 11

1. 1, 5, 6. Malignant tumors are invasive, lack contact inhibition, and have defective communication.
2. 1. The blood cell counts, including the white cell count, will be decreased at the nadir.
3. 4. Choosing a wig before hair loss will make adaptation easier once it occurs.
4. 4. Nonpharmacological methods should be used with, not instead of, medication.
5. 3. Patients with bone cancer are at risk for spinal cord compression, which can cause difficulty walking.
6. 3. The real goal is intact skin. Selections 1, 2, and 4 are interventions.
7. 1. Only patients with 6 months or less to live, who are no longer treating their cancer, are eligible for hospice care.
8. 3. Teach the patient the reason for the isolation. Having a nurse, family member, or another patient in the room would place them at risk for radiation exposure.

Chapter 12

1. 1, 3, 4, 5, 6. All except 2, which can contribute to increasing anxiety and fear, will calm the patient, place the patient in a healthier state, or teach the patient ways to promote recovery.
2. 1. Assisting in data collection is an LPN function; selections 2 and 4 are the physician's role, and selection 3 is the RN's role.
3. 4, 5, 6. The LPN may refer questions to the surgeon, read the consent to a patient, and witness the signature of a patient who is informed.
4. 2. Large black-on-white printed materials are most easily seen by the older adult.
5. 1, 5, 6. Controlling pain allows the patient to cough and deep breathe more comfortably, which expands the lungs, as does ambulation.
6. 3. Clear lung sounds indicate that the lungs are functioning normally.
7. 1. Tachycardia is a compensatory sign to maintain cardiac output for fluid volume loss, as in hemorrhage.

8. 4. Nausea and vomiting must be controlled before discharge. Pain at a tolerable level is expected in the immediate postoperative period.
9. The home health nurse's role is to assist the patient's recovery.

Chapter 13

1. 1, 2, 3, 5. ABCD and vital signs are part of the primary survey, not chronic illness or deformity, which is part of the secondary survey.
2. 1. Hemorrhaging is controlled by applying pressure at the site.
3. 2. Singed nasal hairs indicate possible inhalation injury from a fire, so the nurse should be alert to possible respiratory complications.
4. 3. The immediate need is to remove the patient from the hot environment to allow other interventions to be effective.
5. 1, 5, 6. Inhaled chlorine is irritating to the respiratory tract, which can cause airway obstruction, dyspnea, and pulmonary edema.
6. 2. Being respectful will gain trust, whereas the other choices will not.
7. 4. The goal is to treat the most critically injured person with the best potential for survival first, which is 4, because patient 3 is unlikely to survive and patients 1 and 2 are not critical and will survive.
8. 3. Airway obstruction can occur in anaphylaxis, which is the most important in ABCs.
9. 3. Shock is a condition of progressively decreasing blood pressure.
10. 1.25 mL

$$\frac{500,000 \text{ units}}{} \left| \frac{1 \text{ mL}}{400,000 \text{ units}} \right. = 1.25 \text{ mL}$$

Chapter 14

1. 3. Integrity versus despair is the developmental stage for those over age 65. Role changes and coping with these losses are typically experienced in this stage.
2. 4. Spiritual distress often occurs with chronic illnesses, along with hopelessness, isolation, and powerlessness.
3. 1. The caregiver is exhibiting behaviors indicating *Caregiver Role Strain.* Because behaviors have been exhibited, it is past the risk stage.
4. 2. Providing education on the chronic illnesses is most essential for the patient to be able to understand and deal with the illness and achieve a higher level of wellness.
5. 2, 3, 6. Nursing care for a patient who is chronically ill should include encouraging family visits, inclusion of family in teaching, and seeking patient input for plan of care. Education should be increased, patients should set their own goals as able, and socialization with friends should be encouraged.
6. 2, 3, 5, 6. The nurse wants to encourage the patient to verbalize feelings of sorrow by having time to listen, actively listening, sharing relevant information to foster coping, and encouraging hope.
7. 2. The statement "Maybe tomorrow will be a better day" indicates the patient is hopeful and looking to the future, which is a goal for resolving chronic sorrow.

Chapter 15

1. 3. Aging is a maturational process, not a disease, creating the need for individual adaptation because of physical and psychological declines that occur during a lifetime, not a specific age.
2. 4. Shortening in height is caused by water loss in the intervertebral disks of the spinal column with aging.
3. 1, 3, 4. Assessment identifies potential problems for prompt intervention. Gentle bathing preserves skin integrity by, for example, reducing friction during drying and using warm not hot water, which is drying to the skin. Massage stimulates circulation for healthy skin.

4. 2. Offering explanations and active participation with the use of reminders encourages self-care and supports independence for older patients in adhering to a prescribed medication routine.
5. 2. Ischemia from unrelieved pressure can begin to develop in 20 to 40 minutes.
6. 3. Decreased gag reflex and relaxation of lower esophageal sphincter, increasing the risk of aspiration.
7. 1, 3, 4, 5. Adequate fiber and water intake and exercise, including participation in activities of daily living, promote bowel evacuation, whereas some drugs can contribute to constipation.

Chapter 16

1. 4. Wald established the Henry Street Settlement in New York City, which laid the groundwork for establishing home care as a nursing specialty.
2. 1, 2, 3, 4, 6. All are team members except a lawyer.
3. 4. The performance of the skills related to the purpose of the visit must be documented for reimbursement.
4. 2. Organizing the night before a visit will instill confidence in the nurse and the patient during the visit.
5. 1. Infection control is an important function of the home health nurse, and disinfecting the home health bag is important.

Chapter 17

1. 3. Difficulty swallowing and weight loss are evidence that the patient is near death.
2. 4. A durable power of attorney is a person who can make decisions for a patient when the patient is no longer able to. A living will is the document that outlines a patient's wishes.
3. 1. A good death is possible if the patient's wishes are followed and the patient is comfortable.
4. 4. There is no one "right" thing to say to a grieving person. Listening is important.
5. 2, 4. Scopolamine and morphine both have anticholinergic properties that will dry secretions.
6. 1, 2, 4, 5. Positioning, comfort measures, and being present are appropriate. Treatments to cure disease or prolong life are inappropriate.
7. 3. Clean the patient and make him presentable for the family. Paperwork can be done later.
8. 3. Spending a few minutes with the wife is the most caring; eventually the bed must be cleaned for the next patient.
9. 1. A patient can change his mind at any time.

Chapter 18

1. 4. Artificially acquired active immunity is provided by a vaccine.
2. 1. Older adults should receive an influenza vaccine.
3. 1. A splenectomy may reduce immune function.
4. 3. Painful enlarged lymph nodes are associated with inflammation and infection.
5. 2. For positive ELISA results, which may indicate HIV infection, results must be confirmed by another test, usually the Western blot.
6. 8 mL

$$\frac{200 \text{ mg}}{} \left| \frac{5 \text{ mL}}{125 \text{ mg}} \right. = 8 \text{ mL}$$

Chapter 19

1. 3. Viral illnesses and exposure to various chemicals and environmental substances can alter the immune system and its response to previously benign stimuli.
2. 1. It is a chronic progressive inflammatory disease of large peripheral joints.
3. 1. Glossitis is a sign of pernicious anemia.
4. 3. A Schilling test requires 24-hour collection of urine.
5. 1, 2, 3, 4, 6. All are used for allergic rhinitis except anticholinergics.

6. 2. It is important to document the appearance of any skin lesions to note healing over time.

7. 4. In an autoimmune disorder, immune cells cannot distinguish "self" from "not self."

8. 3, 4, 5, 6. Selection 1 is not done because the patient may have difficulty swallowing, and for selection 2, an IV is needed for medication administration.

9. 2. Sun exposure should be avoided and long sleeves, pants, a hat, and sunscreen worn due to photosensitivity.

10. 1. A classic symptom of systemic lupus erythematosus is a red rash across bridge of nose that resembles a butterfly.

Chapter 20

1. 4. HIV is transmitted from human to human only through infected blood, through sexual secretions, and from an infected mother to her unborn baby or to her infant via breast milk.

2. 2, 3, 1. ELISA detects antibodies to the HIV antigen. If positive, the test is repeated. If positive again, the Western blot test detects antibodies to four major HIV antigens and is positive if two antibodies are present.

3. 3. HIV is a chronically managed disease with treatment.

4. 2, 3, 5, 6. Ways to prevent HIV infection include abstinence, avoiding injection drug use, autologous (self) blood transfusion, and testing for HIV at the time of labor to begin treatment.

5. 1, 2, 5. Preventing infection risk is done with good hygiene (hand washing, toothbrush washing, not reusing dishes, not sharing grooming items), avoiding deli foods that may harbor bacteria, and promptly reporting infection signs.

6. 3. HIV causes decreased CD4+ T lymphocytes, so the goal of antiretroviral therapy is to control the virus so CD4+ T lymphocytes will increase.

7. 1. Flulike symptoms indicate a reaction to abacavir sulfate (Ziagen) can be occurring.

Chapter 21

1. 4. Tobacco use can be modified through smoking cessation.

2. 1. Decreased arterial flow to the extremity is reflected in a slower capillary refill.

3. 2. A gait or walking belt should be used for patients who risk falling, which someone with orthostatic hypotension could be.

4. 4. On bedrest, edema will be found in dependent areas such as the sacrum.

5. 1, 4, 5, 6. *Patient education:* Types of allergies are asked because a dye is used that causes a flushing sensation; firm pressure is applied afterward to prevent bleeding, and therefore ambulation and flexion are not allowed for several hours.

6. 2. Fiber helps prevent constipation and straining during bowel movements, which reduces cardiac workload.

7. 3. Warfarin (Coumadin) affects clotting and is usually stopped before surgery to prevent bleeding issues.

Chapter 22

1. 1, 3, 5. There is no known cause for primary hypertension as there is for secondary.

2. 1. Reducing weight can help control blood pressure.

3. 2. Elevated blood pressure.

4. 4, 5, 6. A healthy diet can control blood pressure and includes eating fresh or frozen fruits and vegetables, reading food labels to make healthy choices, and being aware of safe salt substitutes.

5. 3. Prehypertension is 120–139/80–89 mm Hg and should be followed up in 1 year.

6. 2. The patient needs immediate treatment for a blood pressure that elevated, so the nurse calls 911.

7. 2, 5. Distended jugular veins in semi-Fowler's position and ankle edema are signs of HF.

8. 1. To prevent falls from orthostatic blood pressure when on diuretics, the patient rises slowly.

9. 3. Blood pressure within normal range indicates effective treatment.

Chapter 23

1. 3. Angina indicates cardiac ischemia and requires prompt intervention.

2. 2. Symptoms are often not present in MVP.

3. 1. In commissurotomy, the valve flaps that have adhered to each other and closed the opening between them, known as the commissure, are separated to enlarge the valve opening.

4. 4. Mechanical valves require lifelong anticoagulation to prevent emboli, unlike biological valves, which are less likely to create emboli.

5. 1. A streptococcal infection is a bacterial infection treated with the antibacterial agent penicillin.

6. 2. Dyspnea can indicate heart failure, which is a complication of cardiomyopathy.

7. 1, 4, 5, 6 indicate a blood clot. Selections b and c are seen with heart failure.

8. 3. INR is checked to determine if it is safe to give warfarin (Coumadin).

Chapter 24

1. 2. Hypertension is a modifiable risk factor for cardiovascular disease, whereas the others are nonmodifiable.

2. 1. Fatigue is an atypical symptom in the absence of chest pain.

3. 2. Coronary artery bypass grafting is done to increase blood flow to the myocardium.

4. 4. Place one tablet under the tongue, and if after 5 minutes pain is not relieved in presence of MI symptoms, don't wait—call 911 because nitroglycerine alone will not treat an MI.

5. 3. Intermittent claudication (calf pain with exertion) occurs with peripheral arterial occlusive disease.

6. 3. Pentoxifylline (Trental) relieves claudication by decreasing blood viscosity, which increases blood flow in the extremities.

7. 3. The patient should keep legs down to promote arterial blood flow to distal extremities.

Chapter 25

1. 2, 5, 1, 3, 4. The SA node is the primary pacemaker and fires the impulse, which then travels across the atria, to the AV node, bundle of HIS, and Purkinje fibers.

2. 1. With a systematic method, it is more difficult to miss abnormalities.

3. 3. Defibrillation is used for initial treatment of pulseless ventricular tachycardia to reset the heart's rhythm.

4. 3. Teaching for pacemaker care includes avoiding strong electromagnetic devices that could interfere with the pacemaker settings.

5. 2. The patient should be assisted onto a gurney (stretcher) to reduce cardiac workload, promote safety, and quickly begin treatment.

6. 4. Bradycardia is the term for a pulse of 59 beats per minute or less.

7. Two tablets should be given per dose.

Chapter 26

1. 2. In heart failure, the heart cannot pump enough blood to meet the body's oxygen needs.

2. 1. Hypertension contributes to left-sided heart failure because the left ventricle must pump against increased pressure in the aorta from the hypertension.

3. 1. A diuretic should be taken in the morning to prevent interference with sleep at night.

4. 3. Bumetanide should be given as scheduled because it is working effectively to control the edema.

5. 1. Daily weights reflect fluid volume changes as weight gain or loss.

6. 454.5 mg per dose. $160/2.2 = 72.72 \times 12.5 = 909/2 = 454.5$

Chapter 27

1. 2. This is a low platelet count; platelets are essential to the clotting process.
2. 1. New-onset petechiae are associated with bleeding or clotting disorders.
3. 2. Indicates more teaching is needed. The space between the fingers or toes, not the groin, is used for lymphangiography.
4. 1, 2, 4. Matching the blood to the order and the patient is essential. Baseline vital signs help identify reactions.
5. 4. Fever and chills could signify a febrile or a hemolytic reaction. For either, the unit should be stopped immediately and the physician contacted.

Chapter 28

1. 2. Anemia means less hemoglobin to carry oxygen to tissues, causing dyspnea.
2. 3. Strenuous activity increases oxygen demand, which can cause cells to sickle.
3. 4. Disseminated intravascular coagulation uses up clotting factors, which leaves the patient at risk for bleeding.
4. 1. A patient with hemophilia should avoid injury; contact sports are too dangerous.
5. 4. A patient with leukemia has poor immune function and should not be around someone with a runny nose.
6. 1. Multiple myeloma causes bone destruction. A fall increases risk of fracture.
7. 1, 4, 6. Intramuscular injections, aspirin, nonsteroidal anti-inflammatory drugs, and walking without shoes or slippers all increase the risk of injury or bleeding in a patient with thrombocytopenia.
8. 1715
9. 1. Neutropenia reduces ability to fight infection; temperature will help detect infection.
10. 4. A high abdominal incision makes deep breathing and coughing difficult, increasing the risk of respiratory complications.

Chapter 29

1. 4. 2.5 packs per day × 10 years = 25 pack-years.
2. 2. Wheezes are violin-like sounds made by narrowed airways.
3. 4. A normal SpO_2 is 95% to 100%. An SpO_2 less than 90% is cause for concern.
4. 3, 5, 2, 1, 4.
5. 2. This delivers the most medication to the lungs.
6. 3. Repositioning the mask can redirect the air, while keeping the continuous positive airway pressure (CPAP) intact.

Chapter 30

1. 2. Influenza is caused by a virus. Antibiotics are not effective against viruses.
2. 1. Airway is always a priority, especially after surgery that affects the airway.
3. 4. Antiviral agents are only effective if they are started within 48 hours of symptom onset.
4. 4. Sitting and leaning forward allows the nurse to observe the amount of blood and prevents aspirating or swallowing of blood.
5. 1, 2, and 5 all help reduce transmission of influenza.
6. 1. The patient with a laryngectomy will suffocate if a finger is placed over the stoma.

Chapter 31

1. 3. LTBI is a latent, not active, infection.
2. 2. Damaged alveoli and air trapping cause diminished breath sounds.

3. 4. Biopsy is always the most definitive test for cancer.
4. 3. Pleurodesis is painful; a pain medication should be administered.
5. 3. Wheezes and crackles can signify sputum that needs to be coughed up.
6. 1. Hypoxia can cause confusion and agitation.
7. 2. Diaphragmatic breathing can help make the breathing pattern more effective.
8. 1. SpO_2 is the best measure of gas exchange.

Chapter 32

1. 2. Pain from a ruptured appendix is located in the right lower quadrant.
2. 4. Increasing dietary fiber will help regulate normal bowel function.
3. 1. Bowel sounds heard at an irregular rate every 5 to 15 seconds are normal.
4. 3. Lightly depress the abdomen, not more than 0.5 to 1.0 inch.
5. 2. Dehydration must be prevented to avoid a barium impaction.
6. 2, 3, 4. Salem nasogastric tubes are larger bore tubes that are not used for feeding or longer term use.
7. 3. A chest x-ray is the only accurate way to verify correct placement of the feeding tube.
8. 4. Hyperglycemia may occur due to the high dextrose concentration in parenteral nutrition.

Chapter 33

1. 2. The priority is to provide nourishment and correct electrolyte imbalance, which can be life threatening.
2. 3. A body mass index of 31 is defined as obese.
3. 4. Topical tetracycline can aid healing canker sores.
4. 1. A symptom of gastritis is bloody diarrhea.
5. 3. *Helicobacter pylori,* a bacterium, is the most common cause of peptic ulcers.
6. 4. H_2 antagonists inhibit secretion of gastric acid.
7. 3. To protect the airway, the patient must be placed onto his or her side.
8. 2. Fluid and fat intake promote rapid gastric emptying.
9. 25.

Chapter 34

1. 1. Report findings because symptoms of dehydration are present along with elevated vital signs.
2. 2. Laxatives should be used only occasionally to prevent dependence and complications.
3. 1, 2, 4, 5. Control pain and promote lung expansion with activity or coughing and deep breathing.
4. 1. Fresh fruit is high in fiber and would promote diarrhea.
5. 4. Coughing is contraindicated to prevent damaging the repair, but deep breathing should be done.
6. 3. This is the only selection that does not contain a type of grain that must be avoided.
7. 1, 2, 3, 4. All but edema are a priority to detect pain, dehydration, infection, or shock.
8. 1. Check vital signs for stability as the black tarry stool indicates bleeding above or within the small bowel.
9. 1. A high-fat, low-fiber intake increases the risk of colon cancer.
10. 1. A dusky color indicates impaired circulation and requires immediate medical treatment to restore blood flow.
11. 2. 10 mL

Chapter 35

1. 2. Vitamin K is needed for blood clotting, so a low level increases the risk of bleeding.
2. 3. Sedatives are potentially toxic to the cirrhosis patient due to impaired hepatic metabolism of these medications.
3. 3. Headache, nausea, and flulike symptoms are symptoms of hepatitis A infection.

4. 4. The serum amylase level is elevated in chronic pancreatitis.

5. 4. A low serum albumin level indicates malnutrition.

6. 1. Because pancreatitis is very painful, patient satisfaction with pain control is a priority.

7. 3. Bile duct obstruction can result in jaundice and dark, amber-colored urine due to bile blockage.

8. 1. Roast chicken, rice, and gelatin dessert is a low-fat meal.

9. 2, 3, 5. Pain relief allows comfortable breathing, preventing shallow respirations and guarding. Splinting makes coughing more comfortable, encouraging coughing and deep breathing to keep lungs clear.

10. 0.25 mL

$$\frac{12.5 \text{ mg}}{50 \text{ mg}} \mid \frac{1 \text{ mL}}{} = 0.25 \text{ mL}$$

Chapter 36

1. 3. Provide a nightlight in the bathroom to prevent falls.

2. 2. Daily weight reflects changes in fluid status.

3. 4. To help prevent contamination, women should keep the labia separated while voiding.

4. 2, 4. Encourage fluids to flush dye from the kidneys, and monitor urine output to detect problems.

5. 4. Kegel exercises strengthen the perineal muscles.

6. 3. Maintaining a closed catheter system prevents contamination.

7. 912 mL.

8. 1, 4, 5. Indicate infection in the urinary tract.

Chapter 37

1. 1, 5. These will help prevent urinary tract infections, but the others do not.

2. 2. All urine is strained to detect passage of a stone.

3. 1. Tobacco use is a risk factor for bladder cancer.

4. 2. Continue changing the pouch because this is normal.

5. 1. Fluid intake is increased to flush the kidneys.

6. 4. The creatinine level must be reported because it is elevated, and the nephrotoxic gentamicin is held until the physician is notified.

7. 2, 3, 4. Bananas are high in potassium and avoided; the other options can be given.

8. 4. Patency is assessed with palpation for a thrill and auscultation of a bruit over the fistula site.

9. 3. Applying pressure to a bleeding site is the first action the nurse takes to control the bleeding.

10. 1600/400 = 4

Chapter 38

1. 1, 5. Antidiuretic hormone and oxytocin are synthesized in the hypothalamus and secreted by the posterior pituitary.

2. 4. T_4 and T_3 regulate metabolic rate and energy production.

3. 3. "Calcitonin tones it down" in the blood and into the bones.

4. 1. Excess cortisol (Cushing's syndrome) is associated with moon face and buffalo hump.

5. 2. A thyroid scan involves injection of radioactive iodine.

Chapter 39

1. 3. Excess cortisol, whether endogenous or exogenous, causes Cushing's syndrome.

2. 3. Antidiuretic hormone causes water retention without sodium or potassium retention.

3. 2, 5, 6. Diabetes insipidus is caused by lack of antidiuretic hormone, which results in excess urination, thirst, and dehydration.

4. 1. Thyroid hormone is essential to survival. If the thyroid gland has been removed, exogenous hormone replacement is required for life.

5. 4. Elevated vital signs can signal the onset of thyrotoxic crisis.

6. 1. Routine neurologic assessments are important to detect complications after surgery involving the central nervous system.

7. 1. A patient with hypothyroidism typically is fatigued; returning energy is a sign of effective therapy.

Chapter 40

1. 1. Insulin is not available in pill form at this time. The patient needs additional education.

2. 126.

3. 2. Frequent urination can be a sign of diabetes.

4. 4. Extra socks are the safest way to warm feet that are at risk for injury.

5. 3. Tight control of blood glucose levels is the best way to prevent complications. Selections 1, 2, and 4 are also helpful, but are not the best way.

6. 4. Includes a balance of complex carbohydrates, fats, and protein. Selection 1 is high fat, low carbohydrate. Selections 2 and 3 have minimal fat or protein.

7. 1. 48 is below normal and is considered hypoglycemia.

8. 1. Sliding scale insulin may be needed during times of stress or illness.

9. 2. Small, frequent, low-carbohydrate meals will help prevent fluctuations in blood glucose.

Chapter 41

1. 2. Young men are at risk for testicular cancer, and so should be taught testicular self-examination.

2. 3. Lying flat will reduce discomfort from the carbon dioxide used for insufflation.

3. 1. The National Institutes of Health recommends 1200 mg calcium and 600 international units vitamin D for women ages 51 to 70.

4. 4. Gravida 4 = fourth pregnancy, Para 2 = 2 births, and A1 = 1 abortion (spontaneous)

5. 3. The LPN/LVN typically would not perform a genital assessment but would prepare the patient and be present during the examination.

Chapter 42

1. 3. Mastalgia can be broken down as mast—breast + algia—pain.

2. 3. Bleeding again after menopause is always cause for concern.

3. 4. Bradycardia and falling blood pressure are signs that the vagus nerve has been stimulated.

4. 1, 3. Atropine is an anticholinergic agent that will reverse the cholinergic response initiated by vagal stimulation. Epinephrine is an adrenergic agonist that will raise heart rate and blood pressure.

5. 2. Relaxation exercises and warm compresses can help relax the patient and reduce the perception of pain, when used with medication.

6. 3. Because of compromised circulation in the affected arm, needlesticks and blood pressure measurements should be avoided.

7. 2. Because the ovaries are removed in a BSO, the patient should expect to experience menopause.

8. 240. The patient should eliminate at least 30 mL per hour times 8 hours = 240 mL.

9. 1. Douching is ineffective because sperm may already be out of reach. It also may push sperm further upward.

Chapter 43

1. 3. Benign prostatic hyperplasia is not cancer, but it must be treated. Telling a patient not to worry is inappropriate.

2. 3. Viagra (sildenafil) is a vasodilator and can cause priapism.

3. 1. A B&O suppository will reduce bladder spasms, which often cause pain after TURP.

4. 2. Cleaning is important but be sure to replace the foreskin afterward to prevent paraphimosis.

5. 2. Herbal remedies should never be tried without consulting the HCP. The patient needs additional education.

6. 1. Reflecting back and asking the patient if he would like to talk more will identify if there is a concern that should be followed up by a physician or care provider.

7. 1, 4. Varicocele is like a varicose vein in the scrotum. It can cause pain and infertility.
8. 4. Nicotine and alcohol use can interfere with male fertility.

Chapter 44

1. 1, 2, 3, 4, 5, 6. All symptoms can occur with sexually transmitted diseases and should be assessed.
2. 3. Having a sexual relationship with someone is the epidemiological equivalent of engaging in sexual activity with all of that person's previous partners.
3. 4. An analgesic is necessary. Wart removal is very painful.
4. 3. The man's statement indicates that he would like to talk. Selection 3 is a therapeutic response that gives the man permission to talk further.
5. 1. Alcohol can cloud judgment.

Chapter 45

1. 3, 5, 6. Exercise and diet are important to maintain bone health. Collecting data about them is the first step in planning interventions for the disease.
2. 4. Pallor of an extremity is not a normal finding and may indicate circulatory problems so the HCP is notified.
3. 1. Ask if there is any metal or a pacemaker in the patient's body to allow the HCP to determine if it is safe to do an MRI.
4. 2. Notify the surgeon because circulation in the extremity may be compromised and require immediate treatment.
5. 2, 5 The patient usually is nil per os (NPO) after midnight the night before surgery in the morning. Patients having general anesthesia are taught coughing and deep-breathing exercises to promote lung expansion and prevent lung complications before surgery so they understand them when prompted to do them after surgery. (1) No food is eaten close to surgery time. (2, 4) are responsibilities of the physician. (6) Straight-leg raises are not taught if surgical repair is performed because activity restrictions may be ordered.

Chapter 46

1. 4, 1, 3, 5, 2. Transfer and positioning cast to prevent pressure points by palming the cast while moving it, placing it on a pillow and leaving it uncovered to air dry is the initial priority; next data collection of circulation, sensation, and mobility status to detect problems with extremity or cast that require prompt action; and then vital signs before analgesic administration to determine stability.
2. 2. Agency protocol specifies pin care.
3. 1, 5. Hand hygiene and wearing sterile gloves to apply a new dressing is essential.
4. 3. Exercise can help prevent osteoporosis.
5. 1. Pain is a classic symptom of Paget's disease. (Remember, P = P).
6. 3. Excessive uric acid is formed in gout.
7. 2. Maintaining ideal body weight will reduce wear and tear on the knee.
8. 2. Maintain legs in abduction to prevent dislocation of the hip.
9. 3. Stump dressings should be monitored for bleeding.
10. 4. An absent left pedal pulse may be due to circulatory impairment caused by the fracture and requires immediate treatment.
11. 4. Notify the HCP because the patient may be developing compartment syndrome, an emergency condition.
12. 0.5 mL

Chapter 47

1. 1, 2, 3, 4. 5, verbal response, is part of the Glasgow coma scale.
2. 4. The trigeminal nerve is a sensory nerve supplying the face.

3. 2. Decreasing level of consciousness may be caused by increasing intracranial pressure or other serious complications, and should always be reported immediately.
4. 2, 3, 4, and 6 arc all normal effects of aging.
5. 4. An angiogram uses x-ray or other imaging following injection of dye.
6. 2. Fluids help the kidneys excrete the dye.
7. 3. High-top tennis shoes keep the feet in functional positions.

Chapter 48

1. 1. A sore throat is caused by a virus or bacterium, which can spread to cause meningitis.
2. 2. Darkening the room will help relieve photophobia, and analgesics reduce pain.
3. 4. A headache diary provides the best data for diagnosis.
4. 3. The patient will be in a deep postictal sleep and can eat when awake.
5. 3, 1, 4, 2. The patient should be assisted to lie down before the seizure starts; safety should be maintained; the patient will sleep after the seizure; document last.
6. 2, 3, 4. Fever and headache could indicate encephalitis or meningitis. Craniectomy and brain tumor can be associated with brain swelling.
7. 2. Elevating the head of the bed can reduce intracranial pressure.
8. 3. This could be a sign of autonomic dysreflexia.
9. 1. Tucking the chin may help guide the food into the esophagus.
10. 2. This validates her feeling of loneliness in a nonthreatening way.

Chapter 49

1. 3, 5, 6. Diabetes, high cholesterol, and obesity are all treatable to reduce the risk of stroke.
2. 1, 2, 4 can all help reduce aspiration. Straws and placing food on the affected side (where the patient may not be aware of it) increase risk.
3. 4. Thrombolytic therapy must be given within 4.5 hours to reverse stroke symptoms and reduce the risk of complications.
4. 4. Receptive aphasia is difficulty receiving, or understanding, language, so use of gestures may help with communication needs.
5. 1. The patient may be experiencing unilateral neglect or visual deficits. Turning the plate and observing can help identify the problem.
6. 3. Call for help immediately. The patient could be experiencing an extension of the bleed or ischemic area.

Chapter 50

1. 3. Anticonvulsants help relieve nerve pain.
2. 4. Amyotrophic lateral sclerosis causes weak muscles. If the respiratory muscles are affected, breathing (and singing) may be compromised.
3. 1. Advance directives will allow the patient to have his wishes recorded.
4. 3. Assessment and maintenance of respiratory function is a nursing priority.
5. 1, 2, 4, and 5 help with symptoms related to paralysis. Selections 3 and 6 are interventions for trigeminal neuralgia.
6. 2. Soft foods are easier to chew and less tiring.
7. 4. Ability to perform activities of daily living and effective breathing are signs that muscle strength is adequate.

Chapter 51

1. 2, 1, 3, 4: cornea, aqueous humor, lens, vitreous humor.
2. 4. Comparing the patient's visual fields with your own assesses visual fields.

3. 2. Those with a hearing loss are often irritable or sensitive during interpersonal relations because of their inability to hear and interact with others.

4. 3. Having regular hearing evaluations helps ensure ear health.

5. 1. Ensuring patient safety to prevent injury is essential.

6. 4. Aspirin can be toxic to the ears is true, which shows understanding of teaching.

7. 1, 2, 3. Gloves, gown, goggles (if splashing is anticipated) are used in contact isolation for this nonsterile procedure, whereas a mask is used for respiratory isolation.

8. 3. Tinnitus occurs with aspirin toxicity.

Chapter 52

1. 3. Otosclerosis is hardening of the stapes from new bone growth.

2. 2. A refractory error requires corrective lenses to see clearly.

3. 1. Pain is experienced with an external ear infection.

4. 1. Because the pupils are dilated, the eyes must be protected from bright light.

5. 2. After pneumatic retinopexy, the patient is educated on positions to keep the air bubble in place.

6. 3, 5. Atropine and hydroxyzine are mydriatics, which are contraindicated in acute angle-closure glaucoma to prevent increasing eye pressure.

7. 1. Furosemide (Lasix) can cause hearing loss.

8. 4. Loss of central vision occurs with macular degeneration.

9. 3. Ménière's disease can cause vertigo, which could result in injury.

10. 2. With presbycusis, there is an inability to decipher high-frequency sounds, so a lower voice pitch is helpful.

11. 4. Mydriatics such as anticholinergics and antihistamines (diphenhydramine) are contraindicated in acute angle-closure glaucoma.

Chapter 53

1. 3. Ointments and creams should be applied to clean, moist skin, so after a bath is an appropriate time.

2. 2, 3, 5. Skin is protected in a warm, not hot bath, using gentle soap or prescribed agent. A warm room prevents chilling

3. 3. A vesicle is a fluid-filled lesion.

4. 1. A severe allergic reaction may require resuscitation.

5. 2. Occlusive dressings must be removed 12 of every 24 hours to prevent skin atrophy, folliculitis, or systemic absorption of medication.

Chapter 54

1. 1, 2, 4, and 5 can all help itching and reduce scratching. Tepid, not hot, baths with oatmeal are encouraged.

2. 3. Exposure to ultraviolet rays is the major cause of skin malignancies.

3. 4. The black tissue is eschar. The eschar must be removed to allow granulation to occur. Mechanical débridement is not in the LPN/LVN's scope of practice.

4. 2, 4, 5, 6 can all increase risk of breakdown. Slight overweight and lift sheets can be protective.

5. 2. Washing linens should be sufficient because mites only survive 24 hours without human contact.

6. 4. Impetigo is contagious until all lesions are healed.

Chapter 55

1. 2. Deep partial-thickness burns are associated with pink to light red or white skin, blisters, and pain.

2. 1. Lavage with water for 20 minutes for all chemical burns, along with simultaneous removal of contaminated clothing. Neutralizing a chemical takes too much time.

3. 3. The trunk is 18% front, 18% back, and each arm is 9%.

4. 3, 4, 5. Circulation must be monitored. Escharotomy may be indicated. Elevation promotes venous return.

5. 4. Pao$_2$ 88 mm Hg is the only normal value listed.

Chapter 56

1. 1. No one is happy and smiling all the time. It is not an expected behavior and follow-up is indicated.

2. 1, 3, 5, and 6 can all reflect level of mental health.

3. 2. Physical causes of symptoms should always be ruled out before making a mental health diagnosis.

4. 3. Rationalization is using logical-sounding excuses to cover up true thoughts.

5. 3. A therapeutic milieu is an environment that provides containment, support, structure, involvement, and validation.

6. 4. Medications can help manage symptoms so patients can engage in therapies.

7. 1. Honest communication is a productive behavior. Selections 2, 3, and 4 reflect defense mechanisms.

8. 4. This selection demonstrates therapeutic communication and active listening.

Chapter 57

1. 4. A depressed patient is at risk for suicide and must be kept safe.

2. 3. Obsessions are repetitive thoughts, and compulsions are related actions.

3. 1. Anticholinergic agents help restore the balance of neurotransmitters to prevent extrapyramidal side effects.

4. 4. The patient has posttraumatic stress disorder and needs calm reorientation until the episode is over.

5. 3. Checking vital signs verifies whether there is a real physical cause for the symptoms and also reassures the patient.

6. 2. Orients the patient to reality, then redirects to another activity.

Appendix D

Medical Abbreviations

Although it is still important to know medical abbreviations, many can increase risk of errors. Check www.jointcommision.org for a list of abbreviations to avoid.

Abbr.	Meaning	Abbr.	Meaning	Abbr.	Meaning
ABG	arterial blood gas	g, gm	gram	PCO_2	carbon dioxide pressure
ac	before a meal	GERD	gastroesophageal reflux disease	PERRLA	pupils equal, regular, react to light and accommodation
AD	advance directive	GI	gastrointestinal		
ad lib	freely; as desired	gr	grain	pH	hydrogen ion concentration
ALT	alanine aminotransferase	gt	drop		
AM	morning	gtt	drops	PM	afternoon/evening
A-P	anterior-posterior	GYN	gynecology	PMI	point of maximal impulse
AST	aspartate aminotransferase	h, hr	hour		
AV	atrioventricular	Hgb	hemoglobin	post	posterior
bid	twice a day	hor som, hs	bedtime	pr	through the rectum
BM	bowel movement	IM	intramuscular	prn	as needed
BP	blood pressure	IUD	intrauterine device	qhr	every hour
BUN	blood urea nitrogen	IV	intravenous	q2hr	every 2 hours
c̄	with	IVP	intravenous pyelogram	q3hr	every 3 hours
cap	a capsule	J	joule	qid	four times a day
CBC	complete blood count	kg	kilogram	qs	as much as is needed
cc	cubic centimeter	KUB	kidney, ureter, and bladder	RBC	red blood cell; red blood count
cm	centimeter				
CNS	central nervous system	L	liter	s̄	without
CSF	cerebrospinal fluid	lb	pound	SA	sinoatrial
CV	cardiovascular	lmp	last menstrual period	SC, sc	subcutaneous(ly)
D & C	dilatation and curettage	mEq	milliequivalent	SOB	shortness of breath
dc	discontinue	mg	milligram	s.o.s.	if necessary
dL	deciliter	mL	milliliter	sq	subcutaneous(ly)
DNR	do not resuscitate	mm	millimeter	STAT	immediately
DOA	dead on arrival	MRI	magnetic resonance imaging	STI	sexually transmitted infection
dr	dram				
Dx	diagnosis	MS	mitral stenosis; multiple sclerosis	T	temperature
ECF	extracellular fluid			tab	medicated tablet
ECG	electrocardiogram	μEq	microequivalent	temp	temperature
ECT	electroconvulsive therapy	μg	microgram	tid	three times a day
		npo	nothing by mouth	top	topically
ED	emergency department	NSAID	nonsteroidal anti-inflammatory drug	URI	upper respiratory infection
EEG	electroencephalogram				
EMG	electromyogram	NSR	normal sinus rhythm	USP	United States Pharmacopeia
EMS	emergency medical service	OB	obstetrics		
		O.C.	oral contraceptive	UTI	urinary tract infection
ENT	ear, nose, and throat	O.D.	right eye	WBC	white blood cell; white blood count
EOM	extraocular muscles	O.S.	left eye		
ER	emergency room	O.U.	both eyes	WF/BF	white female/black female
ESR	erythrocyte sedimentation rate	oz	ounce		
		p̄	after	WM/BM	white male/black male
F	Fahrenheit	pc	after meals	wt.	weight

Adapted from Thomas, C. L. (2013), *Taber's cyclopedic medical dictionary* (22nd ed., p. 2581). Philadelphia: F.A. Davis.

Prefixes, Suffixes, and Combining Forms

a-, an-. Without; away from; not
ab-, abs-. From; away from; absent
abdomin-, abdomino-. Abdomen
-ad. Toward; in the direction of
aden-, adeno-. Gland
adip-, adipo-. Fat
-aemia. Blood
aer-, aero-. Air
-algesia, -algia. Suffering; pain
andro-. Man; male; masculine
angi-, angio-. Blood or lymph vessels
aniso-. Unequal; asymmetrical; dissimilar
ankyl-, ankylo-. Crooked; bent; fusion or growing together of parts
ant-, anti-. Against
ante-. Before
antero-. Anterior; front; before
arteri-, arterio-. Artery
arthr-, arthro-. Joint
-ase. Enzyme
-asis, esis, -iasis, -isis, -sis. Condition; pathological state
aut-, auto-. Self
axo-. Axis; axon
bacteri-, bacterio-. Bacteria; bacterium
bi-, bis-. Two; double; twice
bili-. Bile
bio-. Life
blast-, -blast. Germ; bud; embryonic state of development
blephar-, blepharo-. Eyelid
brady-. Slow
bronch-, bronchi-, broncho-. Airway
cardi-, cardio-. Heart
cat-, cata-, cath-, kat-, kata-. Down; downward; destructive; against; according to
cent-. Hundred
cephal-, cephalo-. Head
cervic-, cervice-. Head; the neck of an organ
chrom-, chromo-. Color
-cide. Causing death
contra-. Against; opposite
crani-, cranio-. Skull; cranium
cry-, cryo-. Cold
cyan-, cyano-. Blue
cyst-, cysto-, -cyst. Cyst; urinary bladder
cyt-, cyto-, -cyte. Cell
derm-, derma-, dermato-, dermo-. Skin
di-. Double; twice; two; apart from
dors-, dorsi-, dorso-. Back
-dynia. Pain
dys-. Difficult; bad; painful
ec-, ecto-. Out; on the outside
-ectomy. Excision
ef-, es-, ex-, exo-. Out
electr-, electro-. Electricity
-emesis. Vomiting
-emia. Blood

en-. In; into
end-, endo-. Within
ent-, ento-. Within; inside
enter-, entero-. Intestine
ep-, epi-. Upon; over; at; in addition to; after
erythr-, erythro-. Red
eury-. Broad
ex-. Out; away from; completely
exo-. Out; outside of; without
extra-. Outside of; in addition; beyond
-facient. Causing; making happen
-ferous. Producing
ferri-, ferro-. Iron
fluo-. Flow
fore-. Before; in front of
-form. Form
-fuge. To expel; to drive away; fleeing
gaster-, gastero-, gastr-, gastro-. Stomach
gen-. Producing; forming
-gen, -gene, -genesis, -genetic, -genic. Producing; forming
glosso-. Tongue
gluc-, gluco-, glyc-, glyco-. Sugar; glycerol or similar substance
gyn-, gyne-, gyneco-, gyno-. Woman; female
hem-, hema-, hemato-, hemo-. Blood
hemi-. Half
hepat-, hepato-. Liver
heter-, hetero-. Other; different
histo-. Tissue
homo-. Same; likeness
hydra-, hydro, hydr-. Water
hyp-, hyph-, hypo-. Less than; below; under
hyper-. Above; excessive; beyond
hyster-, hystero-. Uterus
-ia. Condition, esp. an abnormal state
-iasis. SEE -asis
-iatric. Medicine; medical profession; physicians
in-. In; inside; within; intensive action; negative
infra-. Below; under; beneath; inferior to; after
inter-. Between; in the midst
intra-, intro-. Within; in; into
ipsi-. Same
irid-, irido-. Iris
-ism. Condition; theory
iso-. Equal
-itis. Inflammation of
kera-, kerato-. Horny substance; cornea
kolp-, kolpo, colp-, colpo-. Vagina
kypho-. Humped
leuk-, leuko-. White; colorless; rel. to a leukocyte
lip-, lipo-. Fat
-lite, -lith, lith-, litho-. Stone; calculus

-logia, -logy. Science of; study of
lumbo-. Loins
-lysis. 1. Setting free; disintegration; 2. In medicine, reduction of; relief from
macr-, macro-. Large; long
mal-. Ill; bad; poor
med-, medi-, medio-. Middle
mega-, megal-, megalo-. Large; of great size
-megalia, -megaly. Enlargement of a body part
melan-, melano-. Black
mening-, meningo-. Meninges
-meter. Measure
metr-, metra-, metro-. Uterus
micr-, micro-. Small
mon-, mono-. Single; one
muc-, muci-, muco-, myxa-, myxo-. Mucus
multi-. Many; much
musculo-, my-, myo-. Muscle
my-, myo-. SEE *musculo-*
myel-, myelo-. Spinal cord; bone marrow
naso-. Nose
necr-, necro-. Death; necrosis
neo-. New; recent
nephr-, nephra-, nephro-. Kidney
neur-, neuri-, neuro-. Nerve; nervous system
non-. No
normo-. Normal; usual
oculo-. Eye
-ode, -oid. Form; shape; resemblance
-odynia, odyno-. Pain
olig-, oligo-. Few; small
-ology. Science of; study of
-oma. Tumor
onco-. Tumor; swelling; mass
oo-, ovi-, ovo-. Egg; ovum
oophor-, oophoro-, oophoron-. Ovary
ophthalm-, ophthalmo-. Eye
-opia. Vision
optico-, opto-. Eye; vision
orchi-, orchid-, orchido-. Testicle
orth-, ortho-. Straight; correct; normal; in proper order
os-. Mouth; bone
-osis. Condition; status, process; abnormal increase
oste-, osteo-. Bone
ostomosis, -ostomy, -stomosis, -stomy. A created mouth or outlet
ot-, oto-. Ear
-otomy. Cutting
-ous. 1. Possessing; full of; 2. Pertaining to
pan-. All; entire
para-, -para. 1. Prefix: near; alongside of; departure from normal; 2. Suffix: Bearing offspring

path-, patho-, -path, -pathic, -pathy. Disease; suffering

ped-, pedi-, pedo-. Foot

-penia. Decrease from normal; deficiency

peri-. Around; about

perineo-. Perineum

phaco-. Lens of the eye

phag-, phago-. Eating; ingestion; devouring

-phil, -philia, -philic. Love for; tendency toward; craving for

phlebo-. Vein

-phobia. Abnormal fear or aversion

photo-. Light

phren-, phreno-, -phrenia. Mind; diaphragm

-phylaxis. Protection

-plasia. Growth; cellular proliferation

plasm-, -plasm. 1. Prefix: Living substance or tissue; 2. Suffix: To mold

-plastic. Molded; indicates restoration of lost or badly formed features

-plegia. Paralysis; stroke

pneo-. Breath; breathing

pneum-, pneuma-, pneumato-. Air; gas; respiration

-poiesis, -poietic. Production; formation

poly-. Much; many

post-. After

pre-. Before; in front of

presby-. Old age

pro-. Before; in behalf of

proct-, procto-. Anus; rectum

pseud-, pseudo-. False

psych-, psycho-. Mind; mental processes

pulmo-. Lung

py-, pyo-. Pus

pyro-. Heat; fire

ren-, reno-. Kidneys

retro-. Backward; back; behind

rheo-, -(r)rhea. Current; stream; to flow; to discharge

rhino-. Nose

-(r)rhage, -(r)rhagia. Rupture; profuse fluid discharge

-(r)rhaphy. A suturing or stitching

salping-, salpingo-. Auditory tube; fallopian tube

sclero-. Hard; relating to the sclera

-scopy. Examination

semi-. Half

sero-. Serum

somat-, somato-. Body

sperma-, spermat-, spermato-. Sperm; spermatozoa

steno-. Narrow; short

-stomosis, -stomy. SEE *-ostomosis*

sub-. Under; beneath; in small quantity; less than normal

super-. Above; beyond; superior

supra-. Above; beyond; on top

tachy-. Swift; rapid

tel-, tele-. 1. End; 2. Distant; far

tendo-, teno-. Tendon

thorac-, thoraci-, thoraco-. Chest; chest wall

thrombo-. Blood clot; thrombus

thyro-. Thyroid gland; oblong; shield

-tomy. Cutting operation; excision

top-, topo-. Place; locale

tox-, toxi-,toxico-, toxo-, -toxic. Toxin; poison; toxic

tracheo-. Trachea; windpipe

trans-. Across; over; beyond; through

-tropin. Stimulation of a target organ by a substance, esp. a hormone

tympano-. Eardrum; tympanum

ultra-. Beyond; excess

-uria. Urine

uter-, utero-. Uterus

vaso-. Vessel (e.g., blood vessel)

veno-. Vein

ventro-, ventr-, ventri-. Abdomen; anterior surface of the body

vertebro-. Vertebra; vertebrae

vesico-. Bladder; vesicle

Adapted from Thomas, C. L. (2013). *Taber's cyclopedic medical dictionary* (22nd ed., pp. 2576–2590). Philadelphia: F.A. Davis.

Glossary

ablation: (uh-BLAY-shun) Removal of part, pathway, or function by surgery, chemical electrocautery, or radio-frequency.

abrasion: (ah-BRAY-zhun) A scraping away of skin or mucous membrane as a result of injury or by mechanical means.

abuse: (uh-BYOOS) Misuse; excessive or improper use. May refer to substances or individuals.

accommodation: (uh-KOM-uh-DAY-shun) A reflex action of the eye for focusing.

acidosis: (as-ih-DOH-siss) An actual or relative increase in the acidity of blood caused by an accumulation of acid or a loss of base.

acquired immunodeficiency syndrome (AIDS): (uh-KWHY-erd IM-yoo-noh-de-FISH-en-see SIN-drohm) Suppression or deficiency of the cellular immune response, acquired by exposure to human immunodeficiency virus (HIV).

active immunity: (AK-tiv im-YOO-nih-tee) Acquired immunity attributable to the presence of antibodies or of immune lymphoid cells formed in response to antigenic stimulus.

activities of daily living (ADLs): (ack-TIV-ih-tees of DAY-lee LIH-ving) Those activities and behaviors that are performed in the care and maintenance of self (e.g., bathing, dressing, eating).

acupuncture: (ak-yoo-PUNGK-chur) Technique using needles inserted at specific points to create anesthesia or treat certain conditions.

acute coronary syndromes: (ah-KEWT KOR-un-nah-ree sin-DROMES) Group of conditions, including unstable angina, non-Q-wave myocardial infarction, and ST segment elevation myocardial infarction, caused by a lack of oxygen to the heart muscle.

acute pulmonary hypertension: (ah-KEWT PULL-muh-NAIR-ee HIGH-purr-TEN-shun) An excessive buildup of pressure in the pulmonary arteries caused by sudden obstruction of the pulmonary artery.

adaptation: (ad-dap-TAY-shun) Adjustment to changes in internal or external conditions or circumstances; coping.

addiction: (uh-DIK-shun) Psychological dependence characterized by drug seeking and craving for an opioid or other substance for effects other than the intended purpose of the substance.

adjunct: (ADD-junkt) An addition to the principal procedure or course of therapy.

adjuvant: (ad-JOO-vant) Something that assists something else, such as a second form of treatment added to treat a disease.

administrative laws: (ad-MIN-ih-STRAY-tiv LAWZ) Establish the licensing authority of the state to create, license, and regulate the practice of nursing.

adnexa: (ad-NECK-sah) Appendages or accessory organs.

advance medical directive: (ad-VANS MED-ik-uhl dur-EK-tiv) A set of documents (living will and durable medical power of attorney) that explain a person's end-of-life wishes and direct care when the patient is no longer able to do so.

adventitious: (ad-ven-TI-shus) Abnormal or extra; often refers to extra breath sounds, such as wheezes or crackles.

advocate: (ADD-vuh-kut) Someone who makes sure a person's wishes are adhered to; someone who represents the best interests of the patient.

aerobic: (air-OH-bick) Living only in the presence of oxygen.

affect: (AF-feckt) Emotional tone.

afterload: (AFF-ter-lohd) The forces impeding the blood flow out of the heart (vascular pressure, aortic compliance, blood mass, and viscosity).

agenesis: (ay-JEN-uh-siss) Failure of an organ or part to develop or grow.

agonist: (AG-un-ist) A type of opioid that binds to opioid receptors in the central nervous system to relieve pain.

akinesia: (ah-kih-NEE-zee-ah) Absence or loss of the power of voluntary movement.

alkalosis: (al-ka-LOH-siss) An actual or relative decrease in the acidity of blood caused by loss of acid or accumulation of base.

allopathic: (AL-oh-PATH-ik) Method of treating disease with remedies that produce effects different from those caused by the disease.

alopecia: (AL-oh-PEE-she-ah) The loss of hair from the body and the scalp.

amenorrhea: (ay-MEN-uh-REE-ah) The absence or suppression of menstruation. Amenorrhea is normal before puberty, after menopause, and during pregnancy and lactation.

amputation: (am-pew-TAY-shun) The removal of a limb or other appendage or outgrowth of the body.

anaerobic: (AN-air-ROH-bik) Able to live without oxygen.

analgesic: (AN-uhl-JEE-zik) A drug that relieves pain.

anaphylactic shock: (AN-uh-fuh-LAK-tik SHAWK) Systemic reaction that produces life-threatening changes in the circulation and bronchioles.

anaphylaxis: (AN-uh-fuh-LAK-siss) A sudden severe allergic reaction to an allergen.

anastomose: (uh-NAS-tuh-MOS) To surgically connect two parts.

anemia: (uh-NEE-mee-yah) A condition in which there is reduced delivery of oxygen to the tissues as a result of reduced numbers of red cells or hemoglobin.

anergy: (AN-er-jee) Diminished ability of the immune system to react to an antigen.

anesthesia: (AN-es-THEE-zee-uh) Lack of feeling or sensation; artificially induced loss of ability to feel pain.

anesthesiologist: (an-es-THEE-zee-aw-lah-just) A physician who specializes in anesthesiology.

aneurysm: (AN-yur-izm) A sac formed by the localized dilation of the wall of an artery, a vein, or the heart.

angina pectoris: (an-JY-nah PEK-tuh-riss) Severe pain and pressure in the chest caused by insufficient supply of blood and oxygenation to the heart.

angioedema: (AN-gee-oh-eh-DEE-mah) A localized edematous reaction of the deep dermis or subcutaneous or submucosal tissues appearing as giant wheals.

anion: (AN-eye-on) Electrolyte that carries a negative electrical charge.

anisocoria: (an-ih-soh-KOH-ree-ah) Inequality in size of the pupils of the eyes.

ankylosing spondylitis: (ANG-kih-LOH-sing SPON-da-LEYE-tiss) Inflammatory disease of the spine causing stiffness and pain.

annuloplasty: (AN-yoo-loh-PLAS-tee) Repair of a cardiac valve.

anorexia: (AN-uh-REK-see-ah) Absence or loss of appetite for food. Seen in depression, with illness, and as a side effect of some medications.

anorexia nervosa: (AN-uh-REK-see-ah ner-VOH-sah) Refusal to maintain body weight over a minimal normal weight for age and height.

antagonist: (an-TAG-on-ist) Medication used to counteract the effects of an opioid (e.g., naloxone).

anteflexion: (AN-tee-FLEK-shun) The abnormal bending forward of part of an organ.

anteversion: (AN-tee-VER-zhun) A tipping forward of an organ as a whole, without bending.

1399

anthrax: (AN-thrax) A disease caused by the spore-forming bacterium *Bacillus anthracis* that has three clinical forms in humans: inhalational, cutaneous, and gastrointestinal. It can be used as a biological weapon.

antibodies: (AN-tih-baw-dees) An immunoglobulin molecule having a specific amino acid sequence that gives each antibody the ability to adhere to and interact only with the antigen that induced the synthesis.

anticholinesterase: (AN-tih-KOH-lin-ESS-ter-ays) A substance that breaks down acetylcholinesterase.

antidiuretic: (AN-tih-DYE-yoo-RET-ik) Lessening urine excretion.

antigen: (AN-tih-jen) A protein marker on the surface of cells that identifies the type of cell.

antitussive: (an-tee-TUSS-iv) An agent that prevents or relieves cough.

anuria: (an-YOO-ree-ah) Complete suppression of urine formation by the kidney.

anxiety: (ang-ZYE-uh-tee) The uncomfortable feeling of apprehension or dread that occurs in response to a known or unknown threat.

aphasia: (ah-FAY-zee-ah) Defect or loss of the power of expression by speech, writing, or signs, or of comprehension of spoken or written language, caused by disease or injury of the brain centers, such as stroke syndrome.

aphthous stomatitis: (AF-thus STOH-mah-TYE-tis) Small, white, painful ulcers (also known as canker sores) that appear on the inner cheeks, lips, gums, tongue, palate, and pharynx. They tend to recur.

apnea: (APP-nee-ah) Temporary absence of breathing.

appendicitis: (uh-PEN-dih-SYE-tiss) Inflammation of the vermiform appendix.

arcus senilus: (AR-kus seh-NILL-us) A benign white or gray opaque ring in the corneal margin of the eye.

arrhythmia: (uh-RITH-mee-yah) Irregular rhythm, especially heartbeat.

arteriosclerosis: (ar-TEER-ee-oh-skle-ROH-siss) Term applied to a number of pathological conditions in which there is gradual thickening, hardening, and loss of elasticity of the walls of the arteries.

arthritis: (are-THRYE-tiss) Inflammation of a joint.

arthrocentesis: (ar-THROW-sen-tee-sis) Puncture of a joint space with a needle to remove fluid accumulated in the joint.

arthroplasty: (AR-throw-PLAS-te) Repair of a joint. Also called joint replacement.

arthroscopy: (are-THROSS-scop-ee) Examination of the interior of a joint with an arthroscope.

articular: (ar-TIK-yoo-lar) Pertaining to a joint.

artificial feeding: (ART-ih-FISH-uhl FEE-ding) Feeding via a tube into the stomach or intestine when a person is unable to take oral nutrition.

artificial hydration: (ART-ih-FISH-uhl hy-DRAY-shun) Administration of water via intravenous (IV) or gastric tube when a person is unable to take oral fluids.

ascites: (a-SYE-teez) Abnormal accumulation of fluid in the peritoneal cavity.

asepsis: (ah-SEP-sis) A condition free from germs, infection, and any form of life.

aseptic: (ah-SEP-tik) Free of pathogenic organisms; asepsis.

asphyxia: (as-FIX-ee-ah) A condition in which there is a deficiency of oxygen in the blood and an increase in carbon dioxide in the blood and tissues.

aspiration: (AS-pih-RAY-shun) Accidental drawing in of foreign substances into the throat or lungs during inspiration.

assessment: (ah-SESS-ment) An appraisal or evaluation of a patient's condition.

asterixis: (AS-tur-ICK-siss) Hand flapping tremor and involuntary movements of tongue and feet; may be present in hepatic encephalopathy.

astigmatism: (uh-STIG-mah-TIZM) An error of refraction in which a ray of light is not sharply focused on the retina but is spread over a more or less diffuse area.

ataxia: (ah-TAK-see-ah) Failure of muscular coordination; irregularity of muscular action.

atelectasis: (AT-eh-LEK-tah-siss) Collapsed or airless condition of the lung or portion of lung, caused by obstruction or hypoventilation.

atheroma: (ATH-er-OH-mah) Fatty deterioration or thickening of the walls of the larger arteries occurring in atherosclerosis.

atherosclerosis: (ATH-er-oh-skle-ROH-siss) A form of arteriosclerosis characterized by accumulation of plaque, blood, and blood products lining the wall of the artery, causing partial or complete blockage of an artery.

atrial depolarization: (AY-tree-uhl DE-poh-lahr-ih-ZAY-shun) Electrical activation of the atria.

atrial systole: (AY-tree-uhl SISS-tuh-lee) The contraction of the atria.

atrioventricular node: (AY-tree-oh-ven-TRIK-yoo-lar NOHD) Located in lower right atrium; receives an impulse from the sinoatrial (SA) node and relays it to the ventricles.

atrophy: (AT-ruh-fee) Without nourishment; wasting.

atypical: (ay-TIP-ih-kuhl) Deviating from normal.

augmentation: (AWG-men-TAY-shun) The act or process of increasing in size, quantity, degree, or severity.

auscultation: (AWS-kul-TAY-shun) Process of listening for sounds within the body, usually sounds of thoracic or abdominal viscera, to detect an abnormality.

autoimmune: (AW-toh-im-YOON) A condition in which the body does not recognize itself and the immune system attacks normal cells.

Ayurvedic: (EYE-ur-VAY-dik) An ancient Hindu system of medicine that improves health by harmonizing mind and body.

azotemia: (AY-zoh-TEE-me-ah) An increase in nitrogenous bodies in the blood, especially urea, as measured by the serum blood urea nitrogen (BUN) level.

bacteria: (back-TEER-ee-ah) One-celled organisms that can reproduce but need a host for food and supportive environment. Bacteria can be harmless, normal flora, or disease-producing pathogens.

balanitis: (BAL-uh-NYE-tis) Inflammation of the skin covering the glans penis.

bariatric: (BEAR-ee-AT-trick) Branch of medicine that deals with the prevention, control, and treatment of obesity.

basal cell secretion test: (BAY-zuhl SELL see-KREE-shun TEST) Part of a gastric analysis; measures the amount of gastric acid produced in 1 hour.

behavior management: (be-HAYV-yer MAN-ij-ment) Treatment method that uses positive and negative reinforcement to alter behavior.

belief: (bee-LEEF) Something accepted as true. Does not have to be proven.

beneficence: (buh-NEF-ih-sens) To provide good care; to do good for patients. One of the oldest requirements for health care providers.

benign: (bee-NINE) Not progressive; for example, a tumor that is not cancerous.

beta-hemolytic streptococci: (BAY-tuh-HEE-moh-LIT-ick STREP-toh-KOCK-sigh) Gram-positive bacteria that, when grown on blood-agar plates, completely hemolyze the blood and produce a clear zone around the bacteria colony. Group A beta-hemolytic streptococci cause disease in humans.

bigeminy: (bye-JEM-ih-nee) Occurring every second beat, as in bigeminal premature ventricular contractions.

bilateral salpingo-oophorectomy: (by-LAT-ur-uhl sal-PINJ-oh-ah-fuh-RECK-tuh-mee) Surgical removal of both fallopian tubes and ovaries.

bimanual: (by-MAN-yoo-uhl) With both hands.

biofeedback: (BYE-oh-FEED-bak) A form of therapy that uses provision of visual or auditory evidence to a person of the status of an autonomic body function such as heart rate, blood pressure, or respiratory rate.

biopsy: (BY-awp-see) A sample of tissue removed for examination.

bioterrorism: (BYE-oh-TEAR-uh-RIZ-um) Biological agent use or threat of use with a pathological organism for terrorist purposes.

bipolar: (bye-POH-lur) Having two poles or pertaining to both poles. Bipolar disorder is characterized by episodes of manic and depressive behavior.

blanch: (BLANCH) To lose color.

bleb: (BLEB) An irregularly shaped elevation of the skin, such as a blister. May also occur in lung tissue.

blepharitis: (BLEF-uh-RYE-tiss) Inflammation of the glands and lash follicles along the margin of the eyelids.

blindness: (BLYND-ness) Lack or loss of ability to see.

bolus: (BOH-lus) A dose of intravenous (IV) medication injected all at once.

bone: (BOWN) The hard, rigid form of connective tissue constituting most of the skeleton of vertebrates, composed chiefly of calcium salts.

botulism: (BOTCH-uh-liz-um) A paralytic illness caused by a potent neurotoxin produced by Clostridium botulinum, an anaerobic, spore-forming bacterium. It can be used as a biological weapon.

bowel sounds: (BOW'L SOWNDS) Gurgling and clicking sounds heard over the abdomen caused by air and fluid movement from peristaltic action. Normal bowel sounds occur every 5 to 15 seconds at a rate of 5 to 35 sounds per minute. Absent—no bowel sounds heard after 5 minutes of listening in each quadrant. Hyperactive—bowel sounds that are frequent, high pitched, and loud. Hypoactive—bowel sounds that occur at a rate of one every minute or longer.

bradycardia: (BRAY-dih-KAR-dee-yah) A slow heartbeat characterized by a pulse rate below 60 beats per minute.

bradykinesia: (BRAY-dih-kih-NEE-zee-ah) Abnormal slowness of movement; sluggishness.

breakthrough pain: (BRAYK-throo) Pain that occurs while medicated with long-acting analgesics.

bronchiectasis: (BRONG-key-EK-tah-siss) Chronic dilation of a bronchus or bronchi, usually associated with secondary infection and excessive sputum production.

bronchitis: (brong-KYE-tiss) Inflammation of the mucous membrane of the bronchial airways; may be viral or bacterial.

bronchodilator: (BRONG-koh-DYE-lay-tur) A drug that expands the bronchial tubes by relaxing bronchial smooth muscle.

bronchospasm: (BRONG-koh-spazm) Spasm of the bronchial smooth muscle resulting in narrowing of the airways; associated with asthma and bronchitis.

bruit: (BROO-EE) A humming heard when auscultating a blood vessel that is caused by turbulent blood flow through the vessel.

bulimia nervosa: (buh-LEE-mee-ah ner-VOH-sah) Recurrent episodes of binge eating and self-induced vomiting.

bulla: (BUHL-ah) A large blister or skin lesion filled with fluid. May also occur in lung tissue.

bundle of His: (BUN-duhl of HISS) A bundle of fibers of the impulse-conducting system of the heart. Originates in the atrioventricular (AV) node.

bursae: (BURR-sah) A small fluid-filled sac or saclike cavity situated in tissues such as joints where friction would otherwise occur.

calculi: (KAL-kyoo-lye) An abnormal concentration, usually composed of mineral salts, occurring within the body, chiefly in the hollow organs or their passages. Also called stones, as in kidney stones and gallstones.

cancer: (KAN-sir) A general name for more than 100 diseases in which abnormal cells grow out of control; a malignant tumor.

cannula: (KAN-yoo-lah) A flexible tube that can be inserted into the body guided by a stiff, pointed rod. For example, an intravenous (IV) cannula is guided by a metal needle.

capillary permeability: (KAP-ih-lar-ee PER-mee-ah-BILL-ih-tee) The ability of substances to diffuse through capillary walls into tissue spaces.

capillary refill: (KAP-ih-lar-ee RE-fill) The amount of time required for color to return to the nailbed after having been compressed, normally 3 seconds or less. Indicator of peripheral circulation.

caput medusae: (KAP-ut mih-DOO-see) Dilated veins around the umbilicus, associated with cirrhosis of the liver.

carbuncle: (KAR-bung-kull) A necrotizing infection of skin and subcutaneous tissue composed of a cluster of boils.

carcinoembryonic antigens (CEA): (KAR-sin-oh-EM-bree-aw-nik AN-tih-jens) A class of antigens normally present in fetal cells; CEA level is elevated in many cancers and is measured to guide cancer treatment.

carcinogen: (kar-SIN-oh-jen) Specific agent known to promote the cancer process.

cardiac output: (KAR-dee-yak OWT-put) A measure of the pumping ability of the heart; amount of blood pumped by the heart per minute.

cardiac tamponade: (KAR-dee-yak TAM-pon-AID) The life-threatening compression of the heart by the fluid accumulating in the pericardial sac surrounding the heart.

cardiogenic shock: (KAR-dee-oh-JEN-ick SHAWK) Occurs when the heart muscle is unhealthy and contractility is impaired.

cardiomegaly: (KAR-dee-oh-MEH-gah-lee) Enlargement of the heart.

cardiomyopathy: (KAR-dee-oh-my-AW-pah-thee) A group of diseases that affect the myocardium's (heart muscle's) structure or function.

cardioplegia: (KAR-dee-oh-PLEE-jee-ah) Arrest of myocardial contraction, as by use of chemical compounds or cold temperatures in cardiac surgery.

cardioversion: (KAR-dee-oh-VER-zhun) An elective procedure in which a synchronized shock is delivered to attempt to restore the heart to a normal sinus rhythm.

cataract: (KAT-uh-rakt) Opacity of the lens of the eye.

cation: (KAT-eye-on) Electrolyte that carries a positive electrical charge.

ceiling effect: (SEE-ling e-FEKT) The dose of medication at which the maximum therapeutic effect is achieved. Increasing the dose beyond the therapeutic dose will not result in increased relief and may result in undesirable side effects.

cell-mediated immunity: (SELL ME-dee-ay-ted im-YOO-nih-tee) Production of lymphocytes by thymus in response to antigen exposure.

cellulitis: (sell-yoo-LYE-tiss) Inflammation of cellular or connective tissue.

cerebrovascular: (sir-EE-broh-VAS-kyoo-lur) Pertaining to the blood vessels of the cerebrum or brain.

chalazion: (kah-LAY-zee-on) A small eyelid mass resulting from chronic inflammation of a meibomian gland.

chancre: (SHANK-er) A hard, syphilitic primary ulcer, the first sign of syphilis, appearing approximately 2 to 3 weeks after infection.

chemotherapy: (KEE-moh-THER-uh-pee) The treatment of disease with medication; often refers to cancer therapy.

chiropractic: (ky-RUH-prak-tik) Treatment modality that uses manual adjustment of the vertebral column and extremities to remove interference with nerve function.

cholecystitis: (KOH-lee-sis-TYE-tis) Inflammation of the gallbladder.

choledocholithiasis: (koh-LED-oh-koh-lih-THYE-ah-siss) Gallstones in the common bile duct.

choledochoscopy: (KOH-LED-oh-KOS-koh-pee) An endoscopic test of the gallbladder and common bile duct.

cholelithiasis: (KOH-lee-lih-THYE-ah-sis) Gallstones in the gallbladder.

chorea: (kor-REE-ah) A nervous system condition marked by involuntary muscular twitching of the limbs or facial muscles.

chronic illness: (KRAW-nick ILL-ness) An illness that is long lasting or recurring and usually interferes with a person's ability to perform activities of daily living. Medical care and hospitalization are often required on an ongoing basis.

circumcise: (SIR-kuhm-size) Surgical removal of the foreskin covering the head of the penis.

cirrhosis: (sih-ROH-siss) Chronic disease of the liver, associated with fat infiltration and development of fibrotic tissue.

civil law: (SIV-il LAW) Provides the rules by which individuals seek to protect their personal and property rights.

claudication: (KLAW-di-KAY-shun) Severe pain in the calf muscle from inadequate blood supply.

clubbing: (KLUB-ing) A condition in which the ends of the fingers and toes appear bulbous and shiny, most often the result of lung disease.

cochlear implant: (KOK-lee-er IM-plant) A device consisting of a microphone, signal processor, external transmitter, and implanted receiver to aid hearing.

code of ethics: (KOHD of ETH-icks) A traditional compilation of ideal behaviors of a professional group.

codependence: (KOH-de-PEN-dense) A situation in which the significant others in a family group begin to lose their own sense of identity and purpose and exist solely for the abuser.

cognitive: (KAHG-nih-tiv). The ability to think rationally and to process thoughts.

colectomy: (koh-LEK-tuh-me) Excision of the colon or a portion of it.

colic: (KAH-lick) Spasm of a hollow organ or duct, causing pain.

colitis: (kuh-LYE-tiss) Inflammation of the colon.

collateral circulation: (kuh-LA-tur-ul SIR-kew-LAY-shun) Small branches off of larger blood vessels that will increase in size and capacity next to a main blood vessel that is obstructed.

colonization: (CAW-lin-ih-ZAY-shun) The presence of pathogenic microbes in the body, without development of a symptomatic infection.

colonoscopy: (KOH-lun-AWS-kuh-pee) Examination of the upper portion of the rectum with a colonoscope.

colostomy: (koh-LAH-stuh-me) An artificial opening (stoma) created in the large intestine and brought to the surface of the abdomen for evacuating the bowels.

colporrhaphy: (kohl-POOR-ah-fee) Surgical repair of the vagina.

colposcopy: (kul-POS-koh-pee) Examination of the vulva, vagina, and cervix by means of a magnifying lens and a bright light.

comedone: (KOH-me-doh) Skin lesion that occurs in acne vulgaris (closed form: whitehead; open form: blackhead).

commissurotomy: (KOM-ih-shur-AW-toh-mee) Surgical incision of any commissure as in cardiac valves to increase the size of the orifice.

compliance: (kom-PLYE-ens) The ability to alter size or shape in response to an outside force; the ability of the lungs to distend.

compulsion: (kum-PUHL-shun) A recurrent, unwanted, and distressing urge to perform an act.

conductive hearing loss: (kon-DUK-tiv HEER-ing LOSS) Impaired transmission of sound waves through the external ear canal to the bones of the middle ear.

condylomata acuminata: (KON-dih-LOH-mah-tah ah-KYOOM-in-AH-tah) Warts in the genital region caused by the human papillomavirus (HPV); a contagious sexually transmitted infection.

condylomatous: (KON-dih-LOH-mah-tuss) Pertaining to a condyloma.

confidentiality: (KON-fih-den-she-AL-ih-tee) Maintaining privacy of patient information. The patient and his or her care can be discussed only in the professional setting.

congestive heart failure: (kon-JESS-tive HART FAIL-yur) Results from inability of heart to pump sufficient amounts of blood because of impaired pumping function and sodium and water retention. Congestion refers to the buildup of fluid that ranges from mild to life threatening (pulmonary edema). With left-sided heart failure, the fluid buildup occurs in the lungs and, if severe, immediate treatment is required or death can occur. With right-sided heart failure, the fluid buildup is seen systemically (lower legs/feet, sacral area in bedridden persons, jugular veins, liver, spleen).

conization: (KOH-nih-ZAY-shun) The removal of a cone of tissue, as in partial excision of the cervix uteri.

conjunctivitis: (kon-JUNK-tih-VYE-tiss) Inflammation of the conjunctiva of the eye.

consensual response: (kon-SEN-shoo-uhl ree-SPONS) Reaction of both pupils when one eye is exposed to greater intensity of light than the other.

constipation: (KON-stih-PAY-shun) A condition of sluggish or difficult bowel action/evacuation.

contraceptive: (KON-truh-SEP-tiv) Any process, device, or method that prevents conception.

contracture: (kon-TRACK-chur) Abnormal accumulation of fibrosis connective tissue in skin, muscle, or joint capsule that prevents normal mobility at that site.

contralateral: (KON-truh-LAT-ur-uhl) Originating in or affecting the opposite side of the body.

conversion disorder: (kon-VER-zhun dis-OR-der) An illness that emerges from overuse of the conversion reaction defense mechanism, in which there is impaired physical functioning that appears to be neurologic, but no organic disease can be identified.

coping: (KOH-ping) The process of contending with the stresses of daily life in an effort to overcome or work through them.

cor pulmonale: (KOR PUL-mah-NAH-lee) Hypertrophy or failure of the right ventricle from disorders of the chest wall, lungs, and pulmonary vessels, as with increased pulmonary pressure caused by chronic obstructive pulmonary disease (COPD).

coronary artery disease: (KOR-uh-nah-ree AR-tuh-ree dih-ZEEZ) Narrowing of the coronary arteries sufficient to prevent adequate blood supply to the myocardium.

craniectomy: (KRAY-nee-EK-tuh-mee) Excision of a segment of the skull.

cranioplasty: (KRAY-nee-oh-plas-tee) Any plastic repair operation on the skull.

craniotomy: (KRAY-nee-AWT-oh-mee) Any incision through the cranium.

crepitation: (crep-ih-TAY-shun) A crackling sound such as that heard in the chest with pneumonia or other lung diseases or with grating of the ends of a fractured bone.

crepitus: (KREP-ih-tuss) See crepitation.

criminal law: (KRIM-ih-nuhl LAW) Regulates behaviors for citizens within a country.

critical thinking: (KRIT-ih-kuhl THING-king) Use of knowledge and skills to make the best decisions possible in client care situations.

cryotherapy: (KRY-oh-THER-uh-pee) The therapeutic use of cold.

cryptorchidism: (kript-OR-kih-dizm) A birth condition in which one or both of the testicles has or have not descended into the scrotum.

culdocentesis: (KUL-doh-sen-TEE-siss) The procedure for obtaining material from the posterior vaginal cul-de-sac by aspiration or surgical incision through the vaginal wall, performed for therapeutic or diagnostic reasons.

culdoscopy: (kul-DOS-koh-pee) Direct visual examination of the female viscera through an endoscope introduced into the pelvic cavity through the posterior vaginal fornix.

culdotomy: (KUL-DOT-uh-mee) Incision or needle puncture of the cul-de-sac of Douglas through the vagina.

cultural awareness: (KUL-chur-uhl a-WARE-ness) Being aware of history and ancestry and having an appreciation of and attention to the crafts, arts, music, foods, and clothing of various cultures.

cultural competence: (KUL-chur-uhl KOM-peh-tens) Having an awareness of one's own culture and not letting it have an undue influence over another person's culture. Having the knowledge and skills about a culture that are required to provide care.

cultural diversity: (KUL-chur-uhl dih-VER-sih-tee) Representing two or more cultures; the differences among cultures. For example, the United States includes people from many countries.

cultural sensitivity: (KUL-chur-uhl SEN-sih-TIV-ih-tee) Being aware of and sensitive to cultural differences. Avoiding behavior or language that may be offensive to another person's cultural beliefs.

culture: (KUL-chur) The socially transmitted behavior patterns, beliefs, values, customs, arts, and all other characteristics of people that guide their worldview.

curet: (kyoo-RET) A loop, ring, or spoon-shaped instrument, attached to a handle and having sharp or blunt edges; used to scrape tissue from a surface.

custom: (KUS-tum) A custom is the usual way of acting in a given circumstance or something that an individual or group does out of habit. For example, many people in the United States eat turkey on Thanksgiving.

cyanosis: (SYE-uh-NOH-siss) Slightly bluish, grayish, or dark purple discoloration of the skin caused by the presence of abnormal amounts of reduced hemoglobin in the blood.

cystic: (SISS-tik) Pertaining to cysts or the urinary bladder.

cystitis: (siss-TYE-tiss) Inflammation of the urinary bladder.

cystocele: (SISS-toh-seel) A bladder hernia that protrudes into the vagina.

cystoscopy: (siss-TAWS-koh-pee) A diagnostic procedure using an instrument (cystoscope) via the urethra to view the bladder.

cytomegalovirus: (sye-TOW-meg-ul-low-vigh-russ) Species-specific herpesvirus; usually harmless to those with functional immune systems. May cause fatal pneumonia in those who are immunocompromised. Affects retina and may cause blindness in those with acquired immunodeficiency syndrome.

cytotoxic: (SYE-toh-TOCK-sick) Destructive to cells.

data: (DAY-tuh) A group of facts or statistics.

data, objective: See objective data.

data, subjective: See subjective data.

débridement: (day-breed-MAHNT) The removal of foreign material and contaminated and devitalized tissues from or adjacent to a traumatic or infected area until surrounding healthy tissue is exposed.

decerebrate: (dee-SER-eh-brayt) Abnormal extension posture indicating brainstem damage.

decorticate: (dee-KOR-tih-kayt) Abnormal flexion posture indicating cerebral damage.

defibrillation: (dee-FIB-rih-lay-shun) Use of an electrical device that applies countershock to the heart through electrodes placed on the chest wall to stop fibrillation of the heart.

degeneration: (deh-jen-er-AY-shun) Deterioration.

dehiscence: (deh-HISS-ents) A splitting open (i.e., rupture) of an incision.

dehydration: (DEE-high-DRAY-shun) A condition resulting from excessive loss of body fluid that occurs when fluid output exceeds intake.

delirium: (deh-LEER-ee-um) Acute, reversible state of disorientation and confusion without drowsiness, difficulty focusing attention, inability to sleep, and hyperactivity due to an underlying cause. A fairly common acute condition in older hospitalized adults.

delirium tremens: (deh-LEER-ee-uhm TREE-menz) An acute alcohol withdrawal syndrome marked by acute, transient disturbance of consciousness.

delusions: (dih-LOO-zhuns) False beliefs that are firmly maintained despite incontrovertible proof to the contrary.

dementia: (deh-MEN-cha) A broad term that refers to cognitive deficit, including memory impairment.

demyelination: (dee-MY-uh-lin-AY-shun) Loss of myelin from neurons.

deontology: (DAY-on-TOL-oh-gee) The study of moral obligations and commitments, including medical ethics.

dependence: (dih-PEN-dens) A state of reliance on something. Psychological craving for a drug that may or may not be accompanied by a physiological need.

depression: (dih-PRESS-shun) A mental disorder marked by altered mood with loss of interest.

dermatitis: (DER-mah-TYE-tiss) Inflammation of the skin.

dermatophytosis: (DER-mah-toh-fye-TOH-siss) A fungal infection of the skin.

dermoid: (DER-moyd) Resembling the skin.

developmental stage: (DEE-vell-up-MEN-tal STAYJ) An age-defined period with specific psychological tasks that need to be accomplished to maintain ego as proposed by Erik Erikson, a psychoanalyst.

diabetes mellitus: (DYE-ah-BEE-tis mel-LYE-tus) A chronic disease characterized by impaired production or use of insulin and high blood glucose levels.

diarrhea: (DYE-uh-REE-ah) Passage of fluid or unformed stools.

diastolic blood pressure: (dye-ah-STAH-lik BLUHD PREH-shure) The amount of pressure exerted on the wall of the arteries when the ventricles are at rest. The bottom number in a blood pressure reading.

diffusion: (dih-FEW-zhun) The tendency of molecules of a substance (gaseous, liquid, or solid) to move from a region of high concentration to one of lower concentration.

dilation and curettage: (die-LAY-shun and kyoor-e-TAHZH) A surgical procedure that expands the cervical canal of the uterus (dilation) so that the surface lining of the uterine wall can be scraped (curettage).

diplopia: (dip-LOH-pee-ah) Double vision.

displacement: (dis-PLAYSS-ment) Transference of emotion from the original idea with which it was associated to a different idea, allowing the client to avoid acknowledging the original source.

disseminated intravascular coagulation: (dih-SEH-mih-nay-ted IN-trah-VAS-kyoo-lar koh-AG-yoo-LAY-shun) A pathological form of coagulation that is diffuse (widespread) rather than localized, as would be the case in normal coagulation. Clotting factors are consumed to such an extent that generalized bleeding may occur.

distributive shock: (dis-TRIB-yoo-tiv SHAWK) Excessive dilation of the venules and arterioles, leading to decreased distribution of blood, resulting in shock.

diverticulitis: (DYE-ver-tik-yoo-LYE-tiss) Inflammation of a diverticulum (a sac or pouch in the walls of a canal or organ, usually the colon), especially inflammation involving diverticula of the colon.

diverticulosis: (DYE-ver-tik-yoo-LOH-siss) The presence of diverticula in the absence of inflammation.

do not resuscitate (DNR): (DOO not re-SUSS-ih-TATE) An order not to do CPR (cardiopulmonary resuscitation) at the end of life.

dormant: (DOOR-mant) Condition of greatly reduced metabolic activity permitting long-term survival and possible reactivation of bacterial endospores, protozoan cysts, larval stages of worm parasites, and viruses.

Dressler's syndrome: (DRESS-lers SIN-drohm) Postmyocardial infarction syndrome; pericarditis.

durable power of attorney: (DUR-uh-buhl POW-ur uv uh-TUR-nee) Person legally designated to speak for a patient when the patient is no longer able to speak for himself or herself.

dysarthria: (diss-AR-three-ah) Imperfect articulation of speech caused by disturbances of muscular control resulting from central or peripheral nervous system damage.

dysfunctional: (dis-FUNCK-shun-uhl) Family or work environment that does not function effectively, sometimes because of other problems of members.

dysmenorrhea: (DIS-men-oh-REE-ah) Pain in association with menstruation.

dyspareunia: (DIS-puh-ROO-nee-ah) Occurrence of pain in the labia, vagina, or pelvis during or after sexual intercourse.

dysphagia: (dis-FAYJ-ee-ah) Inability to swallow or difficulty swallowing.

dysplasia: (dis-PLAY-zee-ah) Abnormal development of tissue.

dyspnea: (DISP-nee-ah) Subjective sense of labored breathing that occurs because of insufficient oxygenation.

dysreflexia: (DIS-re-FLEK-see-ah) State in which an individual with a spinal cord injury at or above T6 experiences an uninhibited sympathetic response to a noxious stimulus.

dysrhythmia: (dis-RITH-mee-yah) Abnormal, disordered, or disturbed cardiac rhythm.

dysuria: (dis-YOO-ree-ah) Difficult or painful urination.

ecchymoses: (ECK-uh-MOH-siss) A bruise of varying size, the color of which may be blue-black, changing to greenish yellow or yellow with time.

ectasia: (ek-TAY-zee-ah) Replacement of normal tissue with fibrous tissue.

ectopic: (eck-TOP-ick) Out of normal position. Example, ectopic hormones are secreted from sites other than the gland where they would normally be found.

edema: (uh-DEE-muh) Collection of excess fluid in body tissues.

ejaculation: (ee-JAK-yoo-LAY-shun) The release of semen from the male urethra.

electrocardiogram: (ee-LEK-troh-KAR-dee-oh-GRAM) A recording of the electrical activity of the heart.

electrocautery: (ee-LEK-troh-CAW-tur-ee) Cauterization using platinum wires heated to red or white heat by an electric current, either direct or alternating.

electrocoagulated: (ee-LEK-troh-coh-AG-yoo-LAY-ted) Coagulation of tissue by means of a high-frequency electric current.

electroconvulsive therapy (ECT): (ee-LEK-troh-kun-VUL-siv THER-uh-pee) A type of somatic therapy in which an electric current is used to produce convulsions to treat such conditions as depression.

electroencephalogram: (ee-LEK-troh-en-SEFF-uh-loh-gram) A record produced by electroencephalography; tracing of the electrical impulses of the brain.

electrolyte: (ee-LEK-troh-lite) A substance that when dissolved in water can conduct electricity.

electronic medical record: (e-leck-tronick med-ick-ul wreck-ord) Digital form of patient's entire health record.

electroretinography: (ee-LEK-troh-RET-in-AWG-ruh-fee) Measurement of the electrical response of the retina to light stimulation.

emboli: (EM-boh-lie) Solid, liquid, or gaseous masses of undissolved matter traveling with the fluid current in a blood or lymphatic vessel.

embolism: (EM-buh-lizm) Foreign substance or blood clot that travels through the circulatory system until it obstructs a vessel.

emphysema: (EM-fih-SEE-mah) Distention of interstitial tissue by gas or air; chronic pulmonary disease marked by terminal bronchiole and alveolar destruction and air trapping.

empyema: (EM-pye-EE-mah) Pus in a body cavity, especially the pleural space.

encephalitis: (EN-seff-uh-LYE-tiss) Inflammation of the brain.

encephalopathy: (en-SEFF-uh-LAWP-ah-thee) Dysfunction of the brain.

endarterectomy: (end-AR-tur-EK-tuh-mee) Excision of thickened atheromatous areas of the innermost coat of an artery.

endogenous: (en-DAH-jen-us) Produced or originating from within a cell or organism.

endometritis: (EN-doh-meh-TRY-tiss) Inflammation of the endometrium of the uterus.

endorphins: (en-DOR-fins) Naturally occurring opioids in the body, many times more potent than analgesic medications.

endoscope: (EN-doh-skohp) A device consisting of a tube and optical system for observing the inside of a hollow organ or cavity. Can be flexible or rigid.

enkephalins: (en-KEF-eh-lins) One type of endorphin.

enteritis: (en-ter-EYE-tiss) Inflammation of the intestines, particularly of the mucosa and submucosa of the small intestine.

enucleation: (ee-NEW-klee-AY-shun) Removal of an organ or other mass intact from its supporting tissues, as of the eyeball from the orbit.

epidemiological: (EP-ih-DEE-me-ah-LAHJ-ih-kuhl) The study of the distribution and determinants of health-related states and events in populations and the application of this study to the control of health problems.

epididymitis: (EP-ih-DID-ih-MY-tiss) Inflammation or infection of the epididymis.

epidural: (EP-ih-DUHR-uhl) Situated on or outside the dura mater.

epinephrine: (EP-ih-NEFF-rin) A hormone secreted by the adrenal medulla in response to stimulation of the sympathetic nervous system.

epispadias: (EP-ih-SPAY-dee-ahz) A congenital male defect in which the opening of the urethra is on the dorsum of the penis, instead of the tip.

epistaxis: (EP-iss-TAX-iss) Nosebleed.

epithelialization: (ep-ih-THEE-lee-al-eye-ZAY-shun) The growth of skin over a wound.

equianalgesic: (EE-kwee-AN-uhl-JEE-zik) Drugs having equal pain-killing effect. The same degree of pain relief may require different doses when different medications are given or medications are given by different routes.

erectile dysfunction: (eh-REK-tile dis-FUNCK-shun) Inability to have an erection sufficient for sexual intercourse.

erection: (eh-REK-shun) Enlargement and hardening of the penis caused by engorgement of blood.

erythema: (ER-ih-THEE-mah) Diffuse redness over the skin.

eschar: (ESS-kar) Hard scab or dry crust that results from necrotic tissue.

escharotomy: (ess-kar-AWT-oh-mee) Removal of a slough or scab formed on the skin and underlying tissue of severely burned skin.

esophagogastroduodenoscopy: (eh-SOFF-ah-go-GAS-troh-doo-AW-den-AWS-kuh-pee) An endoscopic procedure that allows the physician to view the esophagus, stomach, and duodenum.

esophagoscopy: (eh-soff-ah-GAWS-kuh-pee) Examination of the esophagus using an endoscope.

esotropia: (ESS-oh-TROH-pee-ah) Strabismus in which there is deviation of the visual axis of one eye toward that of the other eye, resulting in diplopia. Also called cross-eyed.

essential hypertension: (eh-SEN-shul HYE-per-TEN-shun) Chronic elevation of blood pressure resulting from an unknown cause.

ethical: (ETH-ih-kuhl) Describes behavior guided by a system of moral principles or standards.

ethics: (ETH-icks) Branch of philosophy that answers questions about morality such as good, bad or right, wrong.

ethnic: (ETH-nick) Pertaining to a religious, racial, national, or cultural group. For example, individuals may identify with the Jewish, Catholic, or Islamic religions.

ethnocentrism: (ETH-noh-SEN-trizm) The tendency to think that one's own ways of thinking, believing, and acting are the only right ways. People who are different are seen as strange or bizarre. An example is one who believes that his or her religious beliefs are the only right beliefs and other religions are wrong.

eustress: (YOO-stress) Stress from positive experiences.

euthyroid: (yoo-THY-royd) Normal thyroid function.

evaluation: (ee-VAL-yoo-AY-shun) The judgment of something.

evisceration: (eh-VIS-sir-ay-shun) Extrusion of viscera outside the body, especially through a surgical excision.

exacerbation: (egg-sass-sir-BAY-shun) Aggravation of symptoms.

exophthalmos: (ECKS-off-THAL-muss) Abnormal protrusion of the eyeball.

exotropia: (EKS-oh-TROH-pee-ah) Abnormal turning outward of one or both eyes; divergent strabismus.

expectorant: (ek-SPEK-tuh-rant) Agent that promotes removal of pulmonary secretions.

expectorate: (ek-SPECK-tuh-RAYT) The act or process of coughing up materials from the air passageways leading to the lungs.

external otitis: (eks-TER-nuhl oh-TYE-tis) Inflammation of the external ear.

extracardiac: (EX-trah-KAR-dee-ack) Outside the heart.

extracellular: (EX-trah-SELL-yoo-ler) Outside the cell.

extracorporeal shock wave lithotripsy (ESWL): (EKS-trah-koar-POR-ee-uhl SHAWK WAYV LITH-oh-TRIP-see) Noninvasive treatment using shock waves to break up gallstones or kidney stones.

extravasation: (eks-TRAH-vah-ZAY-shun) The escape of fluids into surrounding tissue.

extrinsic factors: (eks-TRIN-sik FAK-ters) External variables.

exudate: (EKS-yoo-dayt) Accumulated fluid in a cavity; oozing of pus or serum; often the result of inflammation.

fasciculation: (fah-SIK-yoo-LAY-shun) Twitching.

fasciotomy: (fash-ee-OTT-oh-mee) Incision of fascia.

fetor hepaticus: (FEE-tor he-PAT-ih-kus) Foul breath associated with liver disease.

fibrocystic: (FYE-broh-SISS-tik) Consisting of fibrocysts, which are fibrous tumors that have undergone cystic degeneration or accumulated fluid.

fidelity: (Fah-dell-eh-tee) Obligation to be faithful to commitments made to self and others.

filtration: (fill-TRAY-shun) The process of removing particles from a solution by allowing the liquid portion to pass through a membrane or other partial barrier.

fissure: (FISH-er) A narrow slit or cleft, especially one of the deeper or more

constant furrows separating the gyri of the brain.

fistula: (FIST-yoo-lah) Any abnormal, tubelike passage within body tissue, usually between two internal organs, or leading from an internal organ to the body surface.

flaccid: (FLAH-sid) Weak, lax, soft muscles.

flail chest: (FLAY-ul CHEST) Condition of the chest wall caused by two or more fractures on each affected rib resulting in a segment of rib that is not attached on either end; the flail portion moves paradoxically in with inspiration and out with expiration.

fluoroscope: (FLOOR-uh-skohp) A device consisting of a fluorescent screen suitably mounted, either separately or in conjunction with an x-ray tube, by means of which the shadows of objects interposed between the tube and the screen are made visible.

fluoroscopy: (fluh-RAWS-kuh-pee) The use of a fluoroscope for medical diagnosis or for testing various materials by roentgen rays.

full-thickness burn: (FUL-THICK-ness BERN) Burn in which all of the epithelializing elements and those lining the sweat glands, hair follicles, and sebaceous glands are destroyed.

fungi: (FUNG-guy) A general term for a group of eukaryotic organisms (e.g., mushrooms, yeasts, molds).

furuncle: (FYOOR-ung-kull) An acute circumscribed inflammation of the subcutaneous layers of the skin or of a gland or hair follicle.

gastrectomy: (gas-TREK-tuh-mee) Any surgery that involves partial or total removal of the stomach.

gastric acid stimulation test: (GAS-trik AS-id STIM-yoo-LAY-shun TEST) A test that measures the amount of gastric acid for 1 hour after subcutaneous injection of a drug that stimulates gastric acid secretion.

gastric analysis: (GAS-trik ah-NAL-ih-siss) A test performed to measure secretions of hydrochloric acid and pepsin in the stomach.

gastric lavage: (GAS-trik la-VAHJ) Washing out of the stomach; used to empty the stomach when the contents are irritating.

gastritis: (gas-TRY-tiss) Acute—The inflammation of the stomach mucosa; also known as heartburn or indigestion. Chronic—Gastritis that is recurrent; classified as type A (asymptomatic) or type B (symptomatic).

gastroduodenostomy: (GAS-troh-DOO-oh-den-AWS-toh-mee) Excision of the pylorus of the stomach with anastomosis of the upper portion of the stomach to the duodenum.

gastroepiploic: (GAS-troh-EP-ih-PLOH-ick) Pertaining to the stomach and greater omentum.

gastrojejunostomy: (GAS-troh-JAY-joo-NAWS-toh-mee) Subtotal excision of the stomach with closure of the proximal end of the duodenum and side-to-side anastomosis of the jejunum to the remaining portion of the stomach.

gastroparesis: (GAS-troh-puh-REE-sis) Paralysis of the stomach, resulting in poor emptying.

gastroplasty: (GAS-troh-PLAS-tee) Plastic surgery of the stomach. Used to decrease the size of the stomach to treat morbid obesity.

gastroscopy: (gas-TRAHS-kuh-pee) Examination of the stomach and abdominal cavity by use of a gastroscope.

gastrostomy: (gas-TRAWS-toh-mee) Surgical creation of a gastric fistula through the abdominal wall.

gavage: (gah-VAZH) Feeding with a stomach tube or with a tube passed through the nares, pharynx, and esophagus into the stomach. The food is in liquid or semiliquid form at room temperature.

generalization: (JEN-er-al-ih-ZAY-shun) An assumption about a group or an individual item or person that leads to seeking additional information to determine if the generalization fits the individual. Whereas generalizations are true for the group, they may not be true for the individual.

glaucoma: (glaw-KOH-mah) A group of eye diseases characterized by increased intraocular pressure.

glomerulonephritis: (gloh-MER-yoo-loh-ne-FRY-tiss) A form of nephritis in which the lesions involve primarily the glomeruli.

glossitis: (glaw-SYE-tiss) An inflammation of the tongue.

glycosuria: (GLY-kos-YOO-ree-ah) Abnormal amount of glucose in the urine, often associated with diabetes mellitus.

goitrogens: (GOY-troh-jenz) Foods or medications that cause a goiter.

gout: (GOWT) A common group of arthritic disorders marked by deposition of monosodium urate crystals in joints and other tissues.

gravida: (GRAV-id-ah) Number of times a woman has been pregnant.

gummas: (GUM-ahs) A soft granulomatous tumor of the tissues characteristic of the tertiary stage of syphilis.

gynecomastia: (JIN-eh-koh-MASS-tee-ah) Excessive breast tissue on a male.

hallucinations: (huh-LOO-sih-NAY-shuns) False perceptions having no relation to reality and not accounted for by any exterior stimuli.

hand hygiene: (HAND HY-jeen) Cleansing of the hands with hand washing as defined by the Centers for Disease

Control and Prevention or an alcohol-based hand sanitizer solution.

health: (HELLTH) A condition in which all functions of the body and mind are normally active.

hearing aid: (HEER-ing AYD) An instrument to amplify sounds for those with hearing loss.

heatstroke: (HEET-strohk) An acute and dangerous reaction to heat exposure, characterized by high body temperature, usually higher than 105°F (40.5°C).

Helicobacter pylori: (HEH-lick-co-back-tur PIE-lori) Bacterium that causes some peptic ulcers.

hemarthrosis: (HEEM-ar-THROH-siss) Bleeding into a joint.

hematochezia: (HEM-uh-toh-KEE-zee-uh) Blood in the feces.

hematoma: (HEE-muh-TOH-mah) A localized collection of extravasated blood, usually clotted, in an organ, space, or tissue.

hematuria: (HEM-uh-TYOOR-ee-ah) Blood in the urine.

hemiparesis: (hem-ee-puh-REE-sis) Weakness affecting one side of the body.

hemipelvectomy: (hem-ee-pell-VEC-toe-me) The surgical removal of half of the pelvis and the leg.

hemiplegia: (hem-ee-PLEE-jee-ah) Paralysis of only one side of the body.

hemodialysis: (HEE-moh-dye-AL-ih-siss) A method for replacing the function of the kidneys by circulating blood through tubes made of semipermeable membranes.

hemolysis: (he-MAHL-eh-siss) The destruction of the membrane of red blood cells with the liberation of hemoglobin, which diffuses into the surrounding fluid.

hemophilia: (HEE-moh-FILL-ee-ah) A hereditary blood disease marked by greatly prolonged coagulation time, with consequent failure of the blood to clot and abnormal bleeding.

hemoptysis: (hee-MOP-tih-siss) Coughing up of blood from the respiratory tract.

hemorrhoids: (HEM-uh-royds) A mass of dilated, tortuous veins in the anorectum involving the venous plexuses of that area.

hemothorax: (HEE-moh-THAW-raks) Blood in the pleural space; may be associated with trauma, tuberculosis, or pneumonia.

hepatitis: (HEP-uh-TYE-tiss) Inflammation of the liver, most often viral.

hepatomegaly: (HEP-uh-toh-MEG-ah-lee) Enlargement of the liver.

hepatorenal syndrome: (hep-PAT-oh-REE-nuhl SIN-drohm) A deadly kidney failure that sometimes accompanies liver disease.

hepatosplenomegaly: (heh-PA-toh-SPLE-noh-MEG-ah-lee) Enlargement of the liver and spleen.

hernia: (HER-nee-uh) The protrusion or projection of an organ or a part of an organ through the wall of the cavity that normally contains it.

herpetic: (her-PET-ick) Pertaining to herpes.

hiatal hernia: (high-AY-tuhl HER-nee-ah) A condition in which part of the stomach protrudes through and above the diaphragm.

high-density lipoprotein (HDL): (HYE DEN-sih-tee LIP-oh-PROH-teen) Plasma lipids bound to albumin consisting of lipoproteins. It has been found that those with high levels of HDL have less chance of having coronary artery disease.

histamine: (HISS-tah-mean) A substance produced in the body that increases gastric secretion, increases capillary permeability, and contracts the bronchial smooth muscle. Plays a role in allergic reaction.

holistic: (hole-ISS-tik) The view that people and other organisms function as complete units that cannot be reduced to the sum of their parts. In health care, holistic care encompasses the person's body, mind, and spirit along with the environment and society in which the person lives.

Homans' sign: (HOH-manz SIGHN) An assessment for venous thrombosis in which calf pain with dorsiflexion occurs if thrombosis is present.

homeopathy: (HO-mee-AW-pa-thee) System of medicine based on the theory that "like cures like" and uses tiny doses of a substance that create the symptoms of disease.

homeostasis: (HOH-mee-oh-STAY-siss) Maintaining a constant balance, especially whenever a change occurs.

hopelessness: (HOHP-less-ness) Subjective state in which a person sees limited or unavailable alternatives; lacking energy.

hordeolum: (hor-DEE-oh-lum) Sty.

hospice: (HOS-piss) A service provided to patients and their families in the last 6 months of life to manage pain and provide emotional support.

host: (HOE-st) The organism from which a parasite obtains its nourishment.

human immunodeficiency virus (HIV): (HYOO-man im-YOO-noh-dee-FISH-en-see VIGH-russ) A retrovirus that causes acquired immunodeficiency syndrome (AIDS).

humoral: (HYOO-mohr-uhl) Pertaining to body fluids or substances contained in them.

hydrocele: (HYE-droh-seel) A collection of fluid in the scrotal sack.

hydrocephalus: (HYE-droh-SEF-uh-luhs) A condition caused by enlargement of the cranium caused by abnormal accumulation of cerebrospinal fluid within the cerebral ventricular system.

hydronephrosis: (HYE-droh-ne-FROH-sis) Abnormal dilation of kidneys caused by obstruction of urine flow.

hydrostatic: (HYE-droh-STAT-ik) Pertaining to the pressure of liquids in equilibrium and to the pressure exerted by liquids.

hypercalcemia: (HYE-per-kal-SEE-mee-ah) An excessive amount of calcium in the blood.

hyperglycemia: (HYE-per-glye-SEE-mee-ah) Excess glucose in the blood.

hyperkalemia: (HYE-per-kuh-LEE-mee-ah) An excessive amount of potassium in the blood.

hyperlipidemia: (HYE-per-LIP-ih-DEE-mee-ah) Excessive quantity of fat in the blood.

hypermagnesemia: (HYE-per-MAG-nuh-ZEE-mee-ah) Excess magnesium in the blood.

hypernatremia: (HYE-per-nuh-TREE-mee-ah) Excess sodium in the blood.

hyperopia: (HYE-per-OH-pee-ah) Farsightedness.

hyperplasia: (HYE-per-PLAY-zee-ah) Excessive increase in the number of normal cells.

hypertension: (HYE-per-TEN-shun) Abnormally elevated blood pressure.

hypertensive emergency: (HYE-per-TEN-siv) Systolic blood pressure above 180 mm Hg and diastolic blood pressure above 120 to 130 mm Hg.

hypertonic: (HYE-per-TAWN-ik) Exerts greater osmotic pressure than blood.

hypertrophy: (hye-PER-truh-fee) An increase in the size of an organ or structure, or of the body, owing to growth rather than tumor formation.

hyperuricemia: (HYE-per-yoor-ah-SEE-me-ah) An excess of uric acid or urates in the blood.

hyperventilation: (HYE-per-VEN-tih-LAY-shun) Increased ventilation that results in a lowered carbon dioxide (CO_2) level (hypocapnia).

hypervolemia: (HIYE-per-voh-LEE-mee-ah) An abnormal increase in the volume of circulating blood.

hypocalcemia: (HYE-poh-kal-SEE-mee-ah) Reduced amount of calcium in the blood.

hypoglycemia: (HYE-poh-glye-SEE-mee-ah) Below-normal amount of glucose in the blood.

hypokalemia: (HYE-poh-kuh-LEE-mee-ah) Reduced amount of potassium in the blood.

hypomagnesemia: (HYE-poh-MAG-nuh-ZEE-mee-ah) Reduced amount of magnesium in the blood.

hyponatremia: (HYE-poh-nuh-TREE-mee-ah) Reduced amount of sodium in the blood.

hypoperfusion: (HYE-poh-pur-FEW-shun) Low blood flow that occurs when the circulatory system cannot deliver adequate oxygenated blood to the organs and tissues, as in shock.

hypophysectomy: (HYE-paw-fih-SECK-tuh-mee) Surgical removal of the pituitary gland.

hypoplasia: (HYE-poh-PLAY-zee-ah) Underdevelopment of a tissue organ or body.

hypospadias: (HYE-poh-SPAY-dee-ahz) A congenital male defect in which the opening of the urethra is on the underside of the penis, instead of the tip.

hypostatic: (HYE-poh-STA-tik) Hypostatic pneumonia occurs from congestion in the lungs associated with lack of activity.

hypotension: (HYE-poh-TEN-shun) Abnormally low blood pressure below 90 mm Hg systolic.

hypothermia: (HYE-poh-THUR-mee-ah) Body temperature below 95°F (35°C).

hypotonic: (HYE-poh-TAWN-ik) Pertaining to defective muscular tone or tension; having a lower concentration of solute than intracellular or extracellular fluid.

hypotropia: (HYE-poh-TROH-pee-ah) Downward deviation of the eye away from the visual axis.

hypovolemia: (HYE-poh-voh-LEE-mee-ah) The most common form of dehydration resulting from the loss of fluid from the body; results in decreased blood volume.

hypovolemic: (HYE-poh-voh-LEEM-ick) Low volume of blood in the circulatory system.

hypovolemic shock: (HYE-poh-voh-LEEM-ick SHAWK) Shock that occurs when blood or plasma is lost in such quantities that the remaining blood cannot fill the circulatory system despite constriction of the blood vessels.

hypoxemia: (HYE-pock-SEE-mee-ah) Deficient oxygenation of the blood.

hypoxia: (hye-POCK-see-ah) Diminished availability of oxygen to the body tissues.

hysterectomy: (HISS-tuh-RECK-tuh-mee) Surgical removal of the uterus through the abdominal wall or vagina.

hysterosalpingogram: (HISS-tur-oh-SAL-pinj-oh-gram) Radiograph of the uterus and fallopian tubes.

hysteroscopy: (HISS-tur-AWS-koh-pee) Endoscopic direct visual examination of the canal of the uterine cervix and the cavity of the uterus.

hysterotomy: (HISS-tuh-RAW-tuh-mee) Incision of the uterus.

icterus: (ICK-ter-uss) Yellowing of the skin and the sclera of the eye.

idiopathic thrombocytopenic purpura: (IH-dee-oh-PATH-ik THROM-boh-SYE-toh-PEE-nik PUR-pew-rah) The total number of circulating platelets is greatly diminished, even though platelet production in the bone marrow is normal, resulting in slowed blood clotting.

ileostomy: (ILL-ee-AW-stuh-me) An artificial opening (stoma) created in the small intestine (ileum) and brought to the surface of the abdomen for the purpose of evacuating feces.

illness: (ILL-ness) The state of being sick.

illusions: (ih-LOO-zhuns) Mistaken perceptions of reality.

imagery: (IM-ij-ree) The use of the imagination to promote relaxation.

immunocompromised: (IM-yoo-noh-KAWM-prah-mized) Having an immune system that is not capable of reacting to a pathogen or tissue damage.

impaction: (im-PAK-shun) An immovable accumulation of feces in the bowels.

imperforate: (im-PER-foh-rate) Without an opening.

in situ: (in-SIT-yoo) Localized, not invading surrounding tissue.

in vitro fertilization: (in VEE-troh FER-tih-lih-ZAY-shun) Fertilization in a test tube.

induction: (in-DUCK-shun) The process or act of causing to occur, as in anesthesia induction.

induration: (IN-dyoo-RAY-shun) Area of hardened tissue.

infective endocarditis: (in-FECK-tive EN-doh-kar-DYE-tiss) Inflammation of the heart lining caused by microorganisms.

infiltration: (in-fil-TRAY-shun) The accumulation of an external substance (such as IV fluids) within tissues.

informatics (in-for-mat-icks) The study of information.

inspection: (in-SPEK-shun) Use of observation skills to systematically gather data that can be seen.

insufficiency: (IN-suh-FISH-en-see) The condition of being inadequate for a given purpose, such as heart valves that do not close properly.

insufflation: (in-suff-LAY-shun) Used to inflate the abdomen during laparoscopic or endoscopic procedures to enhance visualization of structures.

intermittent claudication: (IN-ter-MIT-ent KLAW-di-KAY-shun) A symptom associated with arterial occlusive disease. It refers to pain in the calf of a lower extremity, usually brought on by activity or exercise, and ceases with rest.

international normalized ratio: (IN-ter-NASH-uh-nul NOR-muh-lized RAY-she-oh) The World Health Organization's standard for reporting the prothrombin time assay test when the thromboplastin reagent developed by the first International Reference Preparation is used. The reagent was developed to prevent variability in prothrombin time testing results and provide uniformity in monitoring therapeutic levels for coagulation during oral anticoagulation therapy.

interstitial: (IN-ter-STISH-uhl) Fluid between tissues.

intervention: (in-ter-VEN-shun) One or more actions taken in order to modify an effect.

intracellular: (IN-trah-SELL-yoo-ler) Fluids located within the blood cell.

intracranial: (IN-trah-KRAY-nee-uhl) Within the cranium or skull.

intraoperative: (IN-trah-AWP-er-uh-tiv) Occurring during a surgical procedure.

intravascular: (IN-trah-VAS-kyoo-lar) Fluids located within the blood vessels.

intravenous: (IN-trah-VEE-nus) Within or into a vein.

intrinsic factors: (in-TRIN-sik FAK-ters) Internal variables.

intussusception: (IN-tuh-suh-SEP-shun) The slipping of one part of an intestine into another adjacent to it.

ipsilateral: (IP-sih-LAT-ur-uhl) On the same side; affecting the same side of the body.

ischemia: (iss-KEY-me-ah) Condition of inadequate blood supply.

isoelectric line: (EYE-so-ee-LEK-trick LINE) The period when the electrical tracing is at zero and is neither positive nor negative.

isolated systolic hypertension: (EYE-suh-lay-ted siss-TAW-lik hye-per-TEN-shun) The systolic pressure is 160 mm Hg or more, but the diastolic pressure is lower than 95 mm Hg.

isotonic: (EYE-so-TAWN-ik) A fluid that has the same osmolarity as the blood.

jaundice: (JAWN-diss) Yellowing of the skin and the sclera of the eye.

joint: (JOYNT) An articulation. The point of juncture between two bones.

Kaposi's sarcoma: (ka-POE-sees sar-CO-mah) A vascular malignancy that is often first apparent in the skin or mucous membranes but may involve the viscera.

ketoacidosis: (KEE-toh-as-ih-DOH-siss) A condition in which fat breakdown produces ketones, which cause an acidic state in the body; may be associated with weight loss or diabetes mellitus.

Kussmaul's respirations: (KOOS-mahlz RES-pih-RAY-shuns) Term describing deep respirations of an individual with ketoacidosis.

laceration: (la-sir-A-shun) A wound or irregular tear of the flesh.

lactic acid: (LAK-tik AS-id) By-product of anaerobic metabolism.

laminectomy: (LAM-ih-NEK-toh-mee) The excision of a vertebral posterior arch, usually to remove a lesion or herniated disk.

laparoscopy: (LAP-uh-raw-SKOP-ee) Exploration of the abdomen with an endoscope.

laparotomy: (LAP-uh-RAW-tuh-mee) The surgical opening of the abdomen; an abdominal operation.

laryngeal edema: (lah-RIN-jee-uhl uh-DEE-muh) Sudden swelling of the larynx occurring with severe allergic reactions.

laryngectomy: (lar-in-JEK-tah-mee) Surgical removal of the larynx.

laryngitis: (lare-in-JYE-tiss) Inflammation of the larynx.

laser ablation: (LAY-zer uh-BLAY-shun) Therapeutic destruction of a growth or part of a growth by laser treatment.

lavage: (lah-VAZH) Washing out of a cavity.

law: (LAW) The further formalization of moral considerations.

leadership: (LEE-der-ship) The process of socially influencing others to obtain their assistance and support to accomplish a common task.

leiomyoma: (LYE-oh-my-OH-ma) A myoma consisting principally of smooth muscle tissue.

leukemia: (loo-KEE-mee-ah) A malignancy of the blood-forming cells in the bone marrow.

leukocytosis: (LOO-koh-sye-TOH-siss) An increase in the number of leukocytes in the blood, generally caused by the presence of infection and usually transient.

leukopenia: (LOO-koh-PEE-nee-yah) Abnormal decrease of white blood cells, usually below 5000/mm^3.

liability: (LYE-uh-BIL-ih-tee) The level of responsibility that society places on individuals for their actions.

libido: (lih-BEE-doh) Sexual drive, conscious or unconscious.

lichenified: (lye-KEN-ih-fyed) Thickened or hardened from continued irritation.

limitation of liability: (lim-ih-TAY-shun OF LYE-uh-BIL-ih-tee) Steps that health care professionals can take to limit their liability.

living will: (LIV-ing WIL) A document instructing health care workers about a patient's preferences when he or she is no longer able to communicate. Implementation of living wills varies by state.

lobectomy: (loh-BEK-tuh-mee) Surgical removal of a lobe of any organ or gland.

low-density lipoprotein (LDL): (LOH DEN-sih-tee LIH-poh-PROH-teen) A lipoprotein that transports cholesterol and triglycerides from the liver to peripheral tissues. LDL allows fats and cholesterol to move within the water-based solution of the blood. Increased LDL cholesterol is associated with cardiovascular disease, so it is often referred to as "bad cholesterol."

lower gastrointestinal (lower GI) series: (LOH-er GAS-troh-in-TESS-tih-nuhl SEER-ees) The use of barium sulfate as an enema to facilitate x-ray and fluoroscopic examination of the colon.

lymphadenopathy: (lim-FAD-eh-NAH-puh-thee) Any disorder of the lymph nodes.

lymphangitis: (lim-FAN-je-EYE-tiss) Inflammation of lymphatic channels or vessels.

lymphedema: (LIMPF-uh-DEE-mah) An abnormal accumulation of tissue fluid (potential lymph) in the interstitial space.

lymphocytes: (LIM-foh-sites) Cells present in the blood and lymphatic tissue that provide the main means of immunity for the body; white blood cells.

lymphoma: (lim-FOH-mah) A usually malignant lymphoid neoplasm.

macrodrop: (MAK-roh-DROP) A large drop (typically 15–20 drops per mL). In intravenous (IV) therapy, may refer to an administration device used to deliver large drops of IV solution.

macular degeneration: (MACK-you-lar dee-JEN-uh-RAY-shun) Age-related breakdown of the macular area of the retina of the eye.

maleficence: (ma-LEF-i-cence) Committing harm or evil.

malignant: (muh-LIG-nunt) Growing, resisting treatment; used to describe a tumor of cancerous cells.

malpractice: (mal-PRAK-tiss) A breach of duty arising out of the relationship that exists between the patient and the health care worker.

mammography: (mah-MOG-rah-fee) Use of radiography of the breast to diagnose breast cancer.

mammoplasty: (MAAM-oh-PLAS-tee) Plastic surgery of the breast.

mania: (MAY-nee-ah) Mental disorder characterized by excessive excitement.

marsupialization: (mar-SOO-pee-al-ih-ZAY-shun) Process of raising the borders of an evacuated tumor sac to the edges of the abdominal wound and stitching them there to form a pouch.

mastalgia: (mass-TAL-jee-ah) Pain in the breast.

mastectomy: (mass-TECK-tuh-mee) Excision of the breast.

mastitis: (mass-TYE-tis) Inflammation of the breast.

mastopexy: (MAS-toh-PEKS-ee) Correction of a pendulous breast by surgical fixation and plastic surgery.

mediastinum: (MEE-dee-ah-STYE-num) A septum or cavity between two principal portions of an organ.

megacolon: (MEG-ah-KOH-lun) Extremely dilated colon.

melena: (muh-LEE-nah) Black, tarry feces caused by action of intestinal secretions on free blood.

menarche: (meh-NAR-kee) The initial menstrual period, normally occurring between the ninth and 17th year.

Ménière's disease: (meh-NEARS di-ZEEZ) A recurrent and usually progressive group of symptoms including progressive deafness, ringing in the ears, dizziness, and a sensation of fullness or pressure in the ears.

meningitis: (men-in-JYE-tis) Inflammation of the membranes of the spinal cord and brain.

menopause: (MEN-oh-pawz) The period that marks the permanent cessation of menstrual activity, usually occurring between the ages of 35 and 58.

mental health: (MEN-tuhl HELLTH) State of being adjusted to life; able to be flexible, successful, maintain close relationships, solve problems, make appropriate judgments, and cope with daily stresses.

mental illness: (MEN-tuhl ILL-ness) Any illness that affects the mind or behavior.

metastasis: (muh-TASS-tuh-siss) Movement of bacteria or body cells (especially cancer cells) from one part of the body to another.

microbiota: (MIKE-row-bye-ott-a) Microorganisms inhabiting a bodily organ or part such as the gut.

microdrop: (MIKE-roh-DROP) A small drop (60 drops per mL). In intravenous (IV) therapy, may refer to an administration device used to deliver small drops of IV solution.

milieu: (me-LYU) Environment.

miotic: (my-AW-tik) An agent that causes the pupil to contract.

moral distress: (moh-Ral DIS-tress) Distress experienced when the right thing to do cannot be carried out because of institutional constraints.

morality: (muh-RAL-ih-tee) A social barometer that dictates what is good or bad in a society.

morbidity: (more-BID-ih-tee) State of being diseased.

mortality: (more-TAL-ih-tee) Condition of being mortal; number of deaths in a population.

mucolytic: (MYOO-koh-LIT-ik) Agent that liquefies sputum.

mucopurulent cervicitis: (MYOO-koh-PYOOR-uh-lent SIR-vih-SYE-tiss) Inflammation of the cervix producing mucus and purulent discharge.

mucositis: (MYOO-koh-SYE-tiss) Inflammation of a mucous membrane.

multifocal: (MUHL-tee-FOH-kuhl) Many foci (areas) or sites.

murmur: (MUR-mur) An abnormal sound heard on auscultation of the heart and adjacent large blood vessels.

muscle: (MUSS-uhl) A bundle of long slender cells or fibers that have the power to contract and hence to produce movement.

myalgia: (my-AL-jee-ah) Muscle pain or tenderness.

myectomy: (my-EK-tuh-mee) Surgical removal of a hypertrophied muscle.

myelogram: (MY-eh-loh-gram) The film produced by radiography of the spinal cord after injection of a contrast medium into the subarachnoid space.

myocardial infarction: (MY-oh-KAR-dee-yuhl in-FARK-shun) Death of cells of an area of the heart muscle, myocardium, as a result of oxygen deprivation, which in turn is caused by obstruction of the blood supply. Commonly referred to as a heart attack.

myocarditis: (MY-oh-kar-DYE-tiss) The inflammatory process that causes nodules to form in the myocardial tissue; the nodules become scar tissue over time. Inflammation of the heart muscle.

myocardium: (MY-oh-KAR-dee-um) Heart muscle.

myomectomy: (my-oh-MECK-tuh-mee) Removal of a portion of muscle or muscular tissue.

myopia: (my-OH-pee-ah) The error of refraction in which rays of light entering the eye parallel to the optic axis are brought to a focus in front of the retina; nearsightedness.

myringoplasty: (mir-IN-goh-PLASS-tee) Surgical reconstruction of the tympanic membrane.

myringotomy: (MIR-in-GOT-uh-mee) Incision of the tympanic membrane, usually performed to relieve pressure and allow for drainage of either serous or purulent fluid in the middle ear behind the tympanic membrane.

myxedema: (MICK-suh-DEE-mah) Condition resulting from hypofunction of the thyroid gland.

nasoseptoplasty: (NAY-zoh-SEP-toh-plass-tee) Surgical correction of the nasal septum.

naturopathy: (NAY-chur-AW-pa-thee) System of medicine that uses natural therapies such as nutrition, herbs, hydrotherapy, counseling, physical medicine, and homeopathy to treat disease, promote healing, and prevent illness.

negligence: (NEG-li-jense) An unintentional tort.

neoplasm: (NEE-oh-PLAZ-uhm) New abnormal tissue growth, as in a tumor.

nephrectomy: (neh-FREK-tuh-mee) Surgical removal of a kidney.

nephrogenic: (NEFF-roh-JEN-ick) Caused by the kidneys.

nephrolithotomy: (NEFF-roh-lih-THOT-uh-mee) Incision of a kidney for removal of kidney stones.

nephropathy: (neh-FROP-uh-thee) Any disease of the kidney.

nephrosclerosis: (NEFF-roh-skle-ROH-siss) Hardening of the kidney associated with hypertension and disease of the renal arterioles.

nephrostomy: (neh-FRAWS-toh-mee) Creation of a permanent opening into the renal pelvis.

nephrotoxin: (NEFF-roh-TOCK-sin) A toxin having a specific destructive effect on kidney tissue.

neuralgia: (new-RAL-jee-ah) Nerve pain.

neurogenic: (NEW-roh-JEN-ik) Originating in the nervous system.

neuropathic pain: (NEW-roh-PATH-ik PAYN) Pain resulting from peripheral nerve injury.

neuropathy: (new-RAW-puh-thee) A general term denoting functional disturbances and pathological changes in the peripheral nervous system.

neutrophils: (NEW-troh-fils) Granular leukocytes (white blood cells) having a nucleus with three to five lobes connected by threads of chromatin and cytoplasm containing very fine granules.

nociceptive: (NOH-see-SEP-tiv) Pain sensitive.

nocturia: (nock-TOO-ree-ah) Excessive urination at night.

nodal or junctional rhythm: (NOHD-uhl or JUNGK-shun-uhl RITH-uhm) A cardiac rhythm with its origin at the atrioventricular (AV) node.

nonmaleficence: (NON-muh-LEF-ih-sens) The requirement that health care providers do no harm to their patients, either intentionally or unintentionally.

norepinephrine: (NOR-ep-ih-NEFF-rin) A hormone produced by the adrenal medulla, similar in chemical and pharmacological properties to epinephrine, but chiefly a vasoconstrictor with little effect on cardiac output.

normoglycemia: (NOR-moh-glye-SEE-mee-ah) Normal blood glucose.

normotensive: (nor-moh-TEN-siv) Normal blood pressure.

nosocomial infection: (no-zoh-KOH-mee-uhl in-FECK-shun) Infection acquired in a health care agency.

nuchal rigidity: (NEW-kuhl rih-JID-ih-tee) Rigidity of the nape, or back, of the neck.

nursing diagnosis: (NER-sing DYE-ag-NOH-siss) A standardized label placed on a patient's problem to make it understandable to all nurses.

nursing process: (NER-sing PRAH-sess) An orderly, logical approach to administering nursing care so that the patient's needs for such care are met comprehensively and effectively.

nystagmus: (nih-STAG-muss) Involuntary, cyclical, rapid movement of the eyes in response to vertical, horizontal, or rotary movement.

obesity: (oh-BEE-sih-tee) Abnormal amount of fat on the body ranging from 20% to 30% above average weight for age, sex, and height.

objective data: (ob-JEK-tiv DAY-tuh) Factual data obtained through physical examination and diagnostic tests; objective data are observable or knowable through the five senses.

obsession: (ub-SESH-un) Repetitive thought, urge, or emotion.

obstipation: (OB-stih-PAY-shun) Intractable constipation.

obstructive shock: (ub-STRUCK-tive SHAWK) Shock caused by indirect pump failure.

occult blood test: (ah-KULT BLUHD TEST) A chemical test or microscopic examination for blood, especially in feces, that is not apparent on visual inspection.

oliguria: (AWH-lih-GYOO-ree-ah) Diminished urination.

oncology: (on-CAW-luh-jee) The study of cancer and cancer treatment.

oncovirus: (ON-koh-VYE-russ) Viruses linked to cancer in humans.

onychomycosis: (ON-ih-koh-my-KOH-siss) Disease of the nails caused by fungus.

ophthalmia neonatorum: (ahf-THAL-mee-ah NEE-oh-nuh-TOR-uhm) Conjunctivitis in the newborn resulting from exposure to infectious or chemical agents.

ophthalmologist: (AHF-thal-MAW-luh-jist) A physician who specializes in the treatment of disorders of the eye.

ophthalmoscope: (ahf-THAL-muh-skohp) An instrument used for examining the interior of the eye, especially the retina.

opioid: (OHP-ee-OYD) A narcotic drug with morphine-like effects. True opioids are derived from opium.

optician: (ahp-TISH-uhn) One who specializes in filling prescriptions for corrective lenses for eyeglasses and contact lenses.

optimum level of functioning: (OP-teh-mum LEV-uhl of FUNK-shun-ing) Highest level of patient activity considering the patient's condition.

optometrist: (ahp-TOM-uh-trist) A doctor of optometry who diagnoses and treats conditions and diseases of the eye per state laws.

orchiectomy: (or-key-EK-toh-mee) Removal of one or both testicles; a treatment for prostate cancer.

orchitis: (or-KYE-tiss) Inflammation of a testis.

orgasm: (OR-gazm) Pleasurable physical release sensation related to physical, sexual, and psychological stimulation.

orientation: (OR-ee-en-TAY-shun) The ability to comprehend and to adjust oneself in an environment with regard to time, location, and identity of persons.

orthopnea: (or-THOP-knee-a) Labored breathing that occurs when lying flat; relieved when sitting up; associated with left ventricular heart failure.

osmolality: (ahs-moh-LAL-ih-tee) Osmotic concentration; ionic concentration of the dissolved substances per unit of solvent.

osmosis: (ahs-MOH-sis) The passage of solvent through a semipermeable membrane that separates solutions of different concentrations.

osteomyelitis: (AHS-tee-oh-my-LEYE-tiss) Inflammation of bone, especially the marrow, caused by a pathogenic organism.

osteopathy: (AHS-tee-aw-PATH-ee) System of medicine emphasizing the interrelationship of the body's nerves, muscles, bones, and organs; involves treating the whole person, and stresses the importance of diet, exercise, and fitness, with a focus on prevention.

osteoporosis: (AHS-tee-oh-por-OH-siss) A condition in which there is a reduction in the mass of bone per unit volume.

osteosarcoma: (AHS-tee-oh-sar-KOH-mah) A malignant sarcoma of a bone.

otalgia: (oh-TAL-jee-ah) Pain in the ear.

otorrhea: (OH-toh-REE-ah) Inflammation of the ear with purulent discharge.

otosclerosis: (OH-toh-skle-ROH-siss) A condition characterized by chronic, progressive deafness, especially for low tones.

ototoxic: (OH-toh-TOK-sik) Having a detrimental effect on the eighth cranial nerve or the organs of hearing.

pain: (PAYN) An unpleasant sensory and emotional experience associated with actual or potential tissue damage, or described in terms of such damage. Pain is whatever the patient says it is whenever the patient says it occurs.

palliation: (pal-ee-AY-shun) The relief of symptoms without the intent to cure disease.

palpation: (pal-PAY-shun) Use of the fingers or hands to feel something.

pancreatectomy: (PAN-kree-uh-TECK-tuh-mee) Removal of all or part of the pancreas.

pancreatitis: (PAN-kree-uh-TYE-tiss) Inflammation of the pancreas.

pancytopenia: (PAN-sye-toh-PEE-nee-ah) Abnormal depression of all of the cellular elements of the blood.

panhysterectomy: (PAN-hiss-tuh-REK-tuh-mee) Excision of the entire uterus, including the cervix uteri.

panmyelosis: (PAN-my-eh-LOH-siss) Increased level of all bone marrow components, red blood cells, white blood cells, and platelets.

para: (PAR-ah) Number of deliveries a woman has had from pregnancies after 20 weeks' gestation.

paradoxical respirations: (PAR-uh-DOK-si-kuhl RES-pih-RAY-shuns) Chest movement on respiration that is opposite to that expected.

paranoia: (PAR-uh-NOY-uh) Behavior that is marked by delusions of persecution or delusional jealousy.

paraparesis: (PAR-ah-pah-REE-siss) Partial paralysis of the lower extremities.

paraphimosis: (PAR-uh-fye-MOH-siss) Uncircumcised foreskin that has swollen and stuck behind the head of the penis.

paraplegia: (PAR-ah-PLEE-jah) Paralysis of the lower body, including both legs, resulting from a spinal cord lesion.

parenteral: (pah-REN-tur-ul) A medication delivery route that is "beside" rather than in the intestine, such as intramuscular, intravenous (IV), or subcutaneous.

paresis: (puh-REE-siss) Weakness; incomplete paralysis.

paresthesia: (PAR-es-THEE-zee-ah) A heightened sensation, such as burning, prickling, or tingling.

paroxysmal nocturnal dyspnea: (PEAR-ox-IS-mall knock-TURN-al DISP-knee-ah) Sudden attacks of shortness of breath that usually occur during sleep. Person wakes gasping for breath and sits up to relieve symptoms; associated with left ventricular heart failure.

partial-thickness burn: (PAR-shul THICK-ness BERN) Burn in which the epithelializing elements remain intact.

passive immunity: (PASS-iv im-YOO-nih-tee) Reinforcement of the immune system with immune serum for such conditions as tetanus, diphtheria, and venomous snake bite.

paternalism: (puh-TER-nuhl-izm) A unilateral and sometimes unreasonable decision by health care providers that implies they know what is best, regardless of the patient's wishes.

pathogen: (PATH-oh-jen) A microorganism or substance capable of producing a disease.

pathological fracture: (PATH-uh-LAW-jik-uhl FRAHK-chur) Fracture resulting from weakening of the bone structure by pathological processes such as neoplasia or osteomalacia.

patient-controlled analgesia (PCA): (PAY-shent kon-TROHLD an-uhl-JEE-zee-ah) An apparatus that delivers an intravenous (IV) analgesic to relieve pain, which is controlled by the patient.

pedicle: (PED-ih-kuhl) The stem that attaches a new growth.

pediculosis: (peh-DIK-yoo-LOH-siss) Infestation with lice.

pemphigus: (PEM-fih-gus) Acute or chronic serious skin disease characterized by the appearance of bullae (blisters) of various sizes on normal skin and mucous membranes.

penumbra: (puh-NUM-bra) An area of brain tissue surrounding damage from a stroke that may be revived if the brain is reperfused quickly.

peptic ulcer disease: (PEP-tick UL-sir di-ZEEZ) A condition in which the lining of the esophagus, stomach, or duodenum is eroded.

perception: (per-SEP-shun) A unique impression of events by an individual. These impressions are strongly influenced by personality, cultural orientation, attitudes, and life experiences.

percussion: (per-KUSH-un) A tapping technique used by physicians and advanced practice nurses to determine the consistency of underlying tissues.

percutaneous: (PER-kyoo-TAY-nee-us) Through the skin; may refer to an injection, a medication application, or a biopsy.

perfusion: (per-FEW-zhun) Supplying an organ or tissue with blood.

pericardial effusion: (PEAR-ih-KAR-dee-uhl ee-FYOO-zhun) A buildup of fluid in the pericardial space.

pericardial friction rub: (PEAR-ih-KAR-dee-uhl FRICK-shun RUB) Friction sound heard over the fourth left intercostal space near the sternum; a classic sign of pericarditis.

pericardial tamponade: (PEAR-ih-KAR-dee-uhl TAM-pon-AID) Compression of the heart by an abnormal filling of the pericardial sac with blood.

pericardiectomy: (PEAR-ih-kar-dee-EK-tuh-mee) Excision of part or all of the pericardium.

pericardiocentesis: (PEAR-ih-KAR-dee-oh-sen-TEE-sis) Surgical perforation of the pericardium.

pericardiotomy: (PEAR-ih-KAR-dee-AH-tah-mee) Incision of the pericardium.

pericarditis: (PEAR-ih-kar-DYE-tis) Inflammation of the pericardium.

perimenopausal: (PEAR-ee-MEN-oh-PAWS-uhl) The phase before the onset of menopause, during which the cycle of a woman with regular menses changes, perhaps abruptly, to a pattern of irregular cycles and increased periods of amenorrhea.

perinatal: (PEAR-ee-NAY-tuhl) Concerning the period beginning after the 28th week of pregnancy and ending 28 days after birth.

perioperative: (PEAR-ee-AW-per-uh-tiv) Occurring in the period immediately before, during, and after surgery.

peripheral arterial disease: (puh-RIFF-uh-ruhl ar-TEER-ee-uhl di-ZEEZ) Disease of the peripheral arteries that interferes with adequate flow of blood.

peripheral parenteral nutrition: (puh-RIFF-uh-ruhl pah-REN-ter-ruhl new-TRISH-un) Nutrition by peripheral IV injection.

peripheral vascular resistance: (puh-RIFF-uh-ruhl VAS-kyoo-lar ree-ZISS-tense) Opposition to blood flow through the vessels.

peristalsis: (par-is-TALL-siss) Progressive, wavelike movement that occurs involuntarily in hollow tubes of the body such as the alimentary (digestive) canal; causes contents of tube to be moved onward.

peristomal: (PER-ih-STOH-muhl) Area around a stoma.

peritoneal dialysis: (PER-ih-toh-NEE-uhl dye-AL-ih-siss) The employment of the peritoneum surrounding the abdominal cavity as a dialyzing membrane for the purpose of removing waste products or toxins accumulated as a result of renal failure.

peritonitis: (PEAR-ih-tun-NYE-tiss) Inflammation of the peritoneum.

personal protective equipment: (PUR-sun-al proh-TEK-tiv ih-KWIP-mant) Items worn to protect oneself and one's patients from direct transmission of organisms that includes gloves, surgical masks, goggles, gowns, and shoe booties based on the task to be performed and the type of isolation precautions in use.

petechiae: (peh-TEE-kee-ee, puh-TEE-kee-eye) Small, purplish, hemorrhagic spots on the skin that appear in certain illnesses and bleeding disorders.

phagocytosis: (fay-go-sye-TOH-siss) Ingestion and digestion of bacteria and particles by phagocytes, cells that have the ability to ingest and destroy particulate substances such as bacteria, protozoa, and cell debris.

pharyngitis: (fair-in-JIGH-tiss) Inflammation of the mucous membranes and lymph tissues of the pharynx, usually caused by infection.

pheochromocytoma: (FEE-oh-KROH-moh-sigh-TOH-mah) Rare tumor of the adrenal system that secretes catecholamines.

phimosis: (figh-MOH-siss) Uncircumcised foreskin that cannot be moved down from the head of the penis.

phlebitis: (fla-BYE-tiss) Inflammation of a vein; may be due to irritating intravenous fluids or thrombosis.

phlebotomy: (fleh-BAW-tuh-mee) Entry into a vein for the removal or withdrawal of blood.

phobia: (FOH-bee-ah) A persistent, irrational, intense fear of a specific object, activity, or situation.

photophobia: (FOH-toh-FOH-bee-ah) Abnormal visual intolerance to light.

physical dependence: (FIZ-ik-uhl dee-PEN-dens) A pharmacological phenomenon characterized by signs and symptoms of withdrawal when medication is withdrawn.

phytoestrogens: (FYE-toh-ESS-troh-jens) Naturally occurring plant sterols that have an estrogen-like effect.

pinocytosis: (PIE-noh-sye-TOH-siss) Reabsorption of small proteins from renal filtrate by attachment to the membranes of the tubule cells and then engulfment and digestion.

plague: (PLAYG) A severe febrile illness caused by the Gram-negative cocco-bacillus *Yersinia pestis* that is usually transmitted by the bite of an infectious flea. It can also be used as a biological weapon in which primary pneumonic plague would likely occur.

plaque: (PLAK) A deposit of fatty material on the lining of an artery.

plasmapheresis: (PLAS-mah-fer-EE-siss) Removal of blood to separate cells from plasma.

pleurodesis: (PLOO-roh-DEE-siss) Creation of adhesions between the parietal and visceral pleura to treat recurrent pneumothorax.

Pneumocystis carinii pneumonia: (new-moh-SIS-tiss cah-RIN-ee-eye new-MOAN-yah) An acute pneumonia caused by *Pneumocystis carinii,* a fungus. It occurs in immunodeficient adults and is a defining opportunistic infection of AIDS.

pneumonectomy: (NEW-moh-NEK-tuh-mee) Surgical removal of all or part of a lung.

pneumothorax: (NEW-moh-THORE-raks) Air in the pleural space.

poikilothermy: (POY-kih-loh-THER-mee) The absence of sufficient arterial blood flow, causing the extremity to become the temperature of the environment.

point of maximal impulse: (POYNT of MAKS-ih-muhl IM-puls) The area of the chest where the greatest force can be felt with the palm of the hand when the heart contracts or beats. Usually at the fourth to fifth intercostal space in the midclavicular line.

polycythemia: (PAW-lee-sye-THEE-mee-ah) Excessive red cells in the blood.

polydipsia: (PAW-lee-DIP-see-ah) Excessive thirst.

polyneuropathy: (PAW-lee-new-RAW-puh-thee) A disease involving multiple nerves.

polyphagia: (PAW-lee-FAY-jee-ah) Excessive eating.

polyuria: (PAW-lee-YOOR-ee-ah) Excessive urination.

portal hypertension: (POR-tuhl HYE-per-TEN-shun) Persistent blood pressure elevation in the portal circulation of the abdomen.

postcoital: (pohst-KOH-ih-tal) After sexual intercourse.

postictal: (pohst-IK-tuhl) Occurring after a sudden attack, such as an epileptic seizure.

postmortem care: (pohst-MOR-tum KARE) Care after death.

postoperative: (pohst-AWP-er-uh-tiv) Following a surgical operation.

postprandial: (POHST-PRAN-dee-uhl) After a meal.

powerlessness: (POW-ur-less-ness) Perceived lack of control over a situation.

preload: (PREE-lohd) End-diastolic stretch of cardiac muscle fibers; equals end-diastolic volume.

preoperative: (pre-AWP-er-uh-tiv) Preceding an operation.

preprandial: (PREE-PRAN-dee-uhl) Before a meal.

presbycusis: (PRESS-by-KYOO-siss) Progressive, bilaterally symmetrical perceptive hearing loss occurring with age; usually occurs after age 50 and is caused by structural changes in the organs of hearing.

presbyopia: (PREZ-by-OH-pee-ah) Diminution of accommodation of the lens of the eye occurring normally with aging, and usually resulting in hyperopia, or farsightedness.

pressure ulcer: (PRESS-sure ULL-sir) An open sore or lesion of the skin that develops because of prolonged pressure against an area.

priapism: (PRY-uh-pizm) Erection that lasts too long.

primary hypertension: (PRY-mare-ee HYE-per-TEN-shun) Abnormally elevated blood pressure of unknown cause. Also called essential hypertension.

probiotics: (proh-bye-AWT-iks) Supplements of live bacteria or yeast that assist the body's naturally occurring gut microbiota. Often recommended after antibiotic therapy to reestablish the normal microbiota.

proctitis: (prock-TYE-tiss) Inflammation of the rectum and anus.

proctosigmoidoscopy: (PROK-toh-SIG-moy-DAWS-kuh-pee) Visual examination of the rectum and sigmoid colon by use of a sigmoidoscope.

prodrome: (PROH-drohm) A symptom indicating the onset of a disease.

prostaglandins: (PRAWS-tah-GLAND-ins) Chemical neurotransmitters usually associated with pain at the site of an injury, periphery.

prostatectomy: (PRAWS-tuh-TEK-tuh-mee) Removal of the prostate gland.

prostatitis: (PRAWS-tuh-TYE-tiss) Inflammation or infection of the prostate gland.

protozoa: (pro-tow-ZOH-ah) Single-celled parasitic organisms that can move and live mainly in the soil.

pruritus: (proo-RYE-tiss) Severe itching.

pseudoaddiction: (soo-doh-ad-DIK-shun) Syndrome in which behaviors similar to addiction appear as a result of inadequate pain control and patients fear not receiving adequate pain medications and pain relief.

psoriasis: (suh RYE-ah-siss) Chronic inflammatory skin disorder in which epidermal cells proliferate abnormally fast.

psychoanalysis: (SYE-koh-uh-NAL-ih-siss) Form of therapy based on the theories of Sigmund Freud, regarding the dynamics of the unconscious.

psychogenic: (SYE-koh-JEN-ick) Of mental origin.

psychological dependence: (SYE-koh-LAW-jick-al dee-PEN-dens) Obsession of obtaining drugs for use other than medicinal; addiction.

psychopharmacology: (SYE-koh-FAR-meh-KAWL-uh-jee) The study of the action of drugs on psychological functions and mental states.

psychosomatic: (SYE-koh-soh-MAT-ik) Having bodily symptoms of psychological, emotional, or mental origin; illness traceable to an emotional cause.

psychotherapy: (SYE-koh-THER-uh-pee) A method of treating disease (especially mental illness) by mental rather than pharmacological means.

ptosis: (TOH-sis) Drooping of eyelid.

puerperal: (pyoo-ER-per-uhl) Concerning the puerperium, or period of 42 days after childbirth.

pulmonary edema: (PULL-muh-NAIR-ee uh-DEE-muh) Acute heart failure in which there is severe fluid congestion in the alveoli of the lungs; life threatening.

pulse deficit: (PULS DEF-ih-sit) A condition in which the number of pulse beats counted at the radial artery is less than those counted in the same period of time at the apical heart rate.

purpura: (PUR-pur-uh) Hemorrhage into the skin, mucous membranes, internal organs, and other tissues.

purulent: (PURE-u-lent) Fluid that contains pus.

pyelogram: (PIE-eh-loh-GRAM) A diagnostic procedure involving x-ray of the kidneys; may be done after injection of a dye into the bloodstream or directly into the kidneys.

pyelonephritis: (PYE-eh-loh-neh-FRY-tiss) Inflammation of the kidney and renal pelvis.

pyoderma: (PYE-oh-DER-mah) Any acute, inflammatory, purulent bacterial dermatitis.

QSEN project: Quality and Safety Education for Nurses project; focuses on nursing education that promotes the continual improvement of quality and safety in patient care.

quadriparesis: (kwah-drih-par-EE-siss) Weakness involving all four limbs caused by spinal cord injury.

quadriplegia: (KWAH-drih-PLEE-jah) Paralysis of all four limbs caused by spinal cord injury.

radiation therapy: (RAY-dee-AY-shun THER-uh-pee) Cancer treatment with ionizing radiation.

range of motion (ROM): (RANJE of MOH-shun) The range of movement of a body joint.

Raynaud's disease: (rah-NOHZ di-ZEEZ) A primary or idiopathic vasospastic disorder characterized by bilateral and symmetrical pallor and cyanosis of the fingers.

reality orientation: (ree-AL-ih-tee OR-ee-en-TAY-shun) A process to orient a person to facts such as names, dates, and time, through the use of verbal and nonverbal repeating messages.

rectocele: (RECK-toh-seel) Protrusion or herniation of the posterior vaginal wall with the anterior wall of the rectum through the vagina.

Red blood cells: Erythrocytes; circulating blood cells that contain hemoglobin and carry oxygen to tissues.

regurgitation: (ree-GUR-jih-TAY-shun) A backward flowing, as in the backflow of blood through a defective heart valve.

reminiscence therapy: (rem-uh-NIH-sens THER-uh-pee) Use of life reflection with a therapist to resolve conflicts or bring closure to life events.

remyelination: (ree-MY-uh-lin-AY-shun) Replacement of myelin or neurons.

replantation: (re-plan-TAY-shun) The replacement of an organ or other structure, such as a digit, limb, or tooth, to the site from which it was previously lost or removed.

reservoir: (REZ-er-VWAR) A person, animal, arthropod, plant, soil, or substance in which an infectious agent normally lives and multiplies, on which it depends for survival.

resorption: (ree-SORP-shun) To absorb again, as in removal of bone tissue by absorption.

respiratory excursion: (RES-pih-rah-TOR-ee eks-KUR-zhun) Downward movement of the diaphragm with inspiration.

respite care: (RESS-pit CARE) Short-term, intermittent care for the chronically ill; provides rest for the family members or caregivers from the stress of sustained caregiving.

respondeat superior: (ress-POND-ee-et sue-PEER-ee-or) An institution that employs a worker may be liable for the acts or omissions of its employees.

retinopathy: (RET-ih-NAW-puh-thee) Disease of the retina of the eye.

retroflexion: (RET-roh-FLECK-shun) A bending or flexing backward.

retrograde: (RET-roh-grayd) Moving backward; degenerating from a better to a worse state.

retrograde cholangiopancreatography: (RET-roh-grayd koh-LAN-jee-oh-PAN-kree-ah-TOG-rah-fee) An endoscopic

procedure that permits the physician to visualize the liver, gallbladder, and pancreas using an endoscope, dye, and x-ray examinations.

retroversion: (RET-roh-VER-zhun) A turning, or a state of being turned back; the tipping of an entire organ.

rhabdomyolysis: (wrab-DOE-my-o-LEYE-sis) Rapid skeletal muscle tissue break down that releases damaged cell contents, such as myoglobin, into the bloodstream, which are harmful to the kidneys and can lead to kidney damage.

rheumatic carditis: (roo-MAT-ick kar-DYE-tiss) Serious complication of rheumatic fever in which all layers of the heart become inflamed.

rheumatic fever: (roo-MAT-ick FEE-vur) A hypersensitivity reaction to antigens of group A beta-hemolytic streptococci.

rhinitis: (rye-NIGH-tiss) Inflammation of the nasal mucosa, usually associated with congestion, itching, sneezing, and nasal discharge.

rhinoplasty: (RYE-noh-plass-tee) Plastic surgery of the nose.

Rickettsia: (rih-KET-see-ah) A genus of bacteria of the tribe Rickettsiae that multiply only in host cells.

Rinne test: (RIN-nee TEST) A test of hearing made with tuning forks.

Romberg's test: (RAHM-bergs TEST) A test to determine if a person has the ability to maintain body balance when the eyes are shut and the feet are close together.

Roux-en-Y: (roo-ehn-WHY) Gastric bypass surgery. A small stomach pouch the size of a thumb is created with staples, then a Y-shaped section of the small intestine is attached to the pouch to allow food to bypass the lower stomach and duodenum.

rule of nines: (ROOL of NYNES) A formula for estimating percentage of body surface area, particularly helpful in judging the percentage of skin that has been burned.

sacral radiculopathy: (SAY-krul rah-DIK-yoo-LAW-puh-thee) Pathology of sacral nerve roots.

salpingitis: (SAL-pin-JIGH-tiss) Inflammation of a fallopian tube.

salpingoscopy: (SAL-ping-AWS-koh-pee) Endoscopic visualization of the fallopian tubes.

scleroderma: (SKLER-ah-DER-ma) A chronic manifestation of progressive systemic sclerosis in which the skin is taut, firm, and edematous, limiting movement.

sclerosis: (skle-ROH-siss) A hardening or induration of an organ or tissue, especially from excessive growth of fibrous tissue.

seborrhea: (SEB-oh-REE-ah) Disease of the sebaceous glands marked by increase in the amount and often alteration of the quality of sebaceous secretions.

secondary hypertension: (SEK-un-DAR-ee HYE-per-TEN-shun) High blood pressure that is a symptom of a specific cause, such as a kidney abnormality.

semipermeable: (SEM-ee-PER-mee-uh-buhl) Partly permeable; said of a membrane that will allow fluids but not the dissolved substance to pass through it.

sensorineural: (SEN-soh-ree-NEW-ruhl) Hearing loss caused by impairment of a sensory nerve.

sensory deprivation: (SEN-suh-ree DEP-rih-VAY-shun) No or minimal stimulation of the senses that creates the potential for maladaptive coping.

sensory overload: (SEN-suh-ree OH-ver-lohd) Excessive stimulation of the senses that creates the potential for maladaptive coping.

sepsis: (SEP-siss) Systematic infection caused by microorganisms in the bloodstream.

serologic: (SEAR-uh-LAW-jick) Study of substances present in blood serum.

serosanguineous: (SEER-oh-SANG-gwin-ee-uss) Fluid consisting of serum and blood.

serotonin: (SARE-ah-TOH-nin) A chemical neurotransmitter important in sleep/wake cycles. Reduced serotonin levels are associated with depression.

shock: (SHAWK) A clinical syndrome in which the peripheral blood flow is inadequate to return sufficient blood to the heart for normal function, particularly transport of oxygen to all organs and tissues.

sinoatrial node: (SYE-noh-AY-tree-al NOHD) Node at the junction of the superior vena cava and right atrium, regarded as the starting point of the heartbeat.

sinusitis: (SINE-u-SYE-tiss) Inflammation of the sinuses; may be due to viral or bacterial infection, or to allergies.

smallpox: (SMALL-pox) A disease characterized by high fever and a rash caused by variola virus, an orthopoxvirus unique to humans that has a 30% fatality rate.

Snellen's chart: (SNEL-ens CHART) A chart imprinted with lines of black letters graduating in size from smallest on the bottom to largest on top; used for testing visual acuity.

somatoform: (soh-MAT-uh-form) Denoting psychogenic symptoms resembling those of physical disease; psychosomatic.

spider angioma: (SPY-dur an-jee-OH-mah) Thin reddish-purple vein lines close to the skin surface.

spirituality: (SPEER-ih-chu-AL-ih-tee) Sense of connectedness with all of life and the universe.

splenectomy: (spleh-NEK-tuh-mee) Excision of the spleen.

splenomegaly: (SPLEE-noh-MEG-ah-lee) Enlargement of the spleen.

standard of best interest: (STAN-derd OF BEST IN-trest) A type of decision made about patients' health care when they are unable to make an informed decision about their own care.

standard precautions: (STAN-derd pre-KAW-shuns) Guidelines recommended by the Centers for Disease Control and Prevention to reduce the risk of the spread of infection.

stapedectomy: (stay-pee-DEK-toh-mee) Excision of the stapes to improve hearing, especially in cases of otosclerosis.

Staphylococcus: (STAFF-il-oh-KOCK-uss) A genus of Gram-positive bacteria; they are constantly present on the skin and in the upper respiratory tract and are the most common cause of localized suppurating infections.

status asthmaticus: (STAT-us az-MAT-ih-kus) Prolonged period of unrelieved asthma symptoms.

steatorrhea: (STEE-ah-toh-REE-ah) Fat in the stools; may be associated with pancreatic disease.

stenosis: (steh-NOH-siss) The constriction or narrowing of a passage or orifice, such as a cardiac valve.

stent: (STENT) Any mold or device used to hold tissue in place or to provide a support, graft, or anastomosis while healing is taking place.

stereotype: (STER-ee-oh-TIGHP) An opinion or belief about an individual or group that may not be true.

sternotomy: (stir-NAW-tuh-mee) The operation of cutting through the sternum.

stoma: (STOH-mah) A mouth, small opening, or pore.

stomatitis: (STOH-mah-TYE-tiss) Inflammation of the mouth.

stress: (STRESS) The physical (gravity, mechanical, pathogenic, injury) and psychological (fear, anxiety, crisis, joy) forces that are experienced by individuals.

stressor: (STRESS-ur) Any person or situation that produces an anxiety response.

striae: (STRYE-ee) A line or band of elevated or depressed tissue; may differ in color or texture from surrounding tissue.

subarachnoid: (SUB-uh-RAK-noyd) Below or under the arachnoid membrane and the pia mater of the covering of the brain and spinal cord.

subdural: (sub-DUHR-uhl) Beneath the dura mater.

subjective data: (sub-JEK-tiv DAY-tuh) Information that is provided verbally by the patient.

suffering: (SUFF-ur-ing) A state of severe distress associated with events that threaten the intactness of the person. Emotional pain associated with real or potential tissue damage.

summons: (SUM-muns) A notice of suit.

suprapubic: (SOO-pruh-PEW-bik) Bone of the groin (or region) located above the pubic arch.

surgeon: (SURGE-un) A medical practitioner who specializes in surgery.

synovitis: (sin-oh-VYE-tiss) Inflammation of the synovial membrane that may be the result of an aseptic wound, a subcutaneous injury, irritation, or exposure to cold and dampness.

systolic blood pressure: (sis-TALL-ik BLUHD PRESH-ur) Maximal pressure exerted on the arteries during contraction of the left ventricle of the heart. The top number of a blood pressure reading.

tachycardia: (TAK-ih-KAR-dee-yah) An abnormal rapidity of heart action, usually defined as a heart rate greater than 100 beats per minute in adults.

tachydysrhythmia: (TAK-ee-diss-RITH-mee-yah) An abnormal heart rhythm with rate greater than 100 beats per minute in an adult.

tachypnea: (TAK-ip-NEE-ah) Abnormally rapid respiratory rate.

tamponade: (TAM-pon-AYD) Compression of a part.

telenursing: (TEL-a-NURS-ing) Delivering nursing care from a distance with the use of telecommunications.

tension pneumothorax: (TEN-shun NEW-moh-THOR-raks) Abnormal accumulation of air with buildup of pressure in the pleural space.

teratoma: (tare-uh-TOH-muh) A congenital tumor containing one or more of the three primary embryonic germ layers.

terminal illness: (TERM-in-ul ILL-ness) An illness that will probably cause death in 6 months or less.

tetanus: (TET-nus) A highly fatal disease caused by the bacillus *Clostridium tetani* and characterized by muscle spasm and convulsions.

tetany: (TET-uh-nee) Muscle spasms, numbness, and tingling caused by changes in pH and low serum calcium.

therapeutic privilege: (Ther-uh-PU-tik PRIV-ug lej) Limitation for veracity used by HCPs when telling patients the truth would cause them greater harm.

thoracentesis: (THOR-uh-sen-TEE-siss) Insertion of a large-bore needle into the pleural space to remove fluid.

thoracotomy: (THOR-rah-KAW-tah-mee) Surgical incision into the chest wall.

thrill: (THRILL) Palpation of a vibration on the surface of the skin. Can be caused by turbulent blood flow through a blood vessel (as with a fistula or graft) or cardiac abnormalities.

thrombi: (THROM-bye) Blood clots.

thrombocytopenia: (THROM-boh-SYE-toh-PEE-nee-uh) Abnormal decrease in the number of blood platelets.

thrombolytic: (throm-boh-LIT-ik) Agent that dissolves or splits up a thrombus, an aggregation of blood factors.

thrombophlebitis: (THROM-boh-fleh-BYE-tiss) The formation of a clot and inflammation within a vein.

thrombosis: (throm-BOH-siss) Formation, development, or presence of a thrombus, an aggregation of blood factors.

tidaling: (TYE-dah-ling) Rise and fall; may refer to water in water-seal chamber of a chest drainage system.

titration: (tye-TRAY-shun) Adjustment of medication up or down to meet patient needs.

tolerance: (TALL-er-ens) The response of the body to medication that requires increased medication administration to achieve the same effect. Often refers to opioids.

torts: (TORTS) Lawsuits involving civil wrongs.

toxemia: (tock-SEE-me-ah) Spread of the poisonous products of bacteria throughout the body.

tracheostomy: (TRAY-key-AWS-tuh-me) A surgical opening in the neck into the trachea to provide an airway when the trachea is obstructed.

tracheotomy: (TRAY-key-AW-tuh-me) An opening in the neck into the trachea.

traditions: (trah-DISH-uns) Practices and customs handed down through the generations, often by word of mouth.

transcellular: (trans-SELL-yoo-lar) Across cell membranes.

transdermal: (trans-DUR-mal) Entering through the dermis, or skin, as in administration of a drug applied to the skin in ointment or patch form.

transillumination: (TRANS-ih-loo-mih-NAY-shun) The passage of strong light through a body structure to permit inspection of an observer on the opposite side.

transjugular intrahepatic portosystemic shunt (TIPS): (TRANZ-jug-yoo-lur in-tra-heh-PAT-ik POR-toh-siss-TEM-ik SHUNT) Shunt that sidetracks venous blood around the liver to the vena cava for treatment of ascites.

transmyocardial: (TRANS-my-oh-KAR-dee-yah) Across all layers of the heart.

trauma: (TRAW-mah) Physical injury caused by an external force.

Trendelenburg's position: (tren-DELL-en-bergz PUH-si-shun) A position in which the patient's head is low and the body and legs are on an elevated and inclined plane.

triage: (TREE-ahj) The assignment of degrees of urgency to wounds or illnesses to decide the order of treatment of patients or casualties.

trichinosis: (trick-in-OH-siss) A disease caused by the roundworm *Trichinella spiralis,* which is spread by eating raw or undercooked meat from pigs or wild animals that contains *Trichinella* larvae.

trigeminy: (try-JEM-ih-nee) Occurring every third beat, as in trigeminal premature ventricular contractions.

tropia: (TROH-pee-ah) A manifest deviation of an eye from the normal position when both eyes are open and uncovered.

T-tube: (TEE-toob) A T-shaped tube in the bile duct that allows drainage of bile following gallbladder surgery.

tumor: (TOO-mur) An abnormal growth of cells or tissues; tumors may be benign or malignant.

turbid: (TER-bid) Cloudy.

turgor: (TER-gur) The resistance of the skin to being grasped between the fingers. Dehydration causes poor skin turgor.

unifocal: (YOO-nih-FOH-kuhl) Coming or originating from one site or focus.

upper gastrointestinal (upper GI, UGI) series: (UH-per GAS-troh-in-TES-tih-nuhl SEER-ees) X-ray and fluoroscopic examinations of the stomach and duodenum after the ingestion of a contrast medium.

uremia: (yoo-REE-mee-ah) An excess in the blood of urea, creatinine, and other nitrogenous end products of protein and amino acid metabolism.

urethritis: (YOOR-eh-THRYE-tiss) Inflammation of the urethra.

urethroplasty: (yoo-REE-throh-PLAS-tee) Plastic repair of the urethra.

urinary incontinence: (YOOR-ih-NAR-ee in-KON-tih-nents) Inability to control urine excretion creating accidental urinary leakage.

urodynamic: (YOO-roh-dye-NAM-ik) The study of the holding or storage of urine in the bladder, the facility with which it empties, and the rate of movement of urine out of the bladder during urination.

urosepsis: (YOO-roh-SEP-siss) Septicemia resulting from urinary tract infection.

urticaria: (UR-tih-CARE-ee-ah) Hives signifying an allergic reaction.

utilitarian: (yoo-TILL-ih-TAR-ee-en) Consequences or outcomes of a dilemma are the most important element.

vaginosis: (VAJ-ih-NOH-siss) Inflammation of the vagina caused by *Gardnerella vaginalis.*

values: (VAL-use) Ideals or concepts that give meaning to an individual's life.

valvotomy: (val-VAW-tuh-mee) Cutting through a valve.

valvuloplasty: (VAL-vyoo-loh-PLAS-tee) Plastic or restorative surgery on a valve, especially a cardiac valve.

varices: (VAR-ih-seez) Dilated veins.

varicocele: (VAR-ih-koh-seel) Varicose veins of the scrotum; can lead to infertility.

varicose veins: (VAR-ih-kohs VAINS) Swollen, distended, and knotted veins, usually in the subcutaneous tissue of the leg.

vasculitis: (VAS-kue-LYE-tiss) Inflammation of a vessel.

vasectomy: (vah-SEK-tuh-mee) Surgically cutting and sealing the vas deferens to prevent sperm from getting outside the body. Used as a birth control method for men.

vector: (VEK-tur) Living organism that transmits disease.

venous stasis ulcers: (VEE-nus STAY-siss UL-sers) Poorly healing ulcers that result from inadequate venous drainage.

ventricular diastole: (ven-TRIK-yoo-lar dye-AS-tuh-lee) The period of relaxation of the two ventricles.

ventricular escape rhythm: (ven-TRIK-yoo-lar es-KAYP RITH-uhm) The naturally occurring rhythm of the ventricles when the rest of the cardiac conduction system fails.

ventricular repolarization: (ven-TRIK-yoo-lar REE-pol-lahr-ih-ZAY-shun) Reestablishment of the polarized state of the muscle after contraction.

ventricular systole: (ven-TRIK-yoo-lar SISS-tuh-lee) The contraction of the two ventricles.

ventricular tachycardia: (ven-TRIK-yoo-lar TAK-ih-KAR-dee-yah) A series of at least three beats arising from a ventricular focus at a rate greater than 100 beats per minute.

veracity: (VER-ah-sit-tee) Truthfulness

verrucous: (ve-ROO-kus) Wartlike, with raised portions.

vertebrae: (VER-teh-bray) Any of the 33 bony segments of the spinal column: 7 cervical, 12 thoracic, 5 lumbar, 5 sacral, and 4 coccygeal vertebrae.

vesicant: (VESS-ih-kant) Agent that causes blistering of tissue.

vesicular: (ve-SIK-yoo-lur) Pertaining to vesicles or small blisters.

virulence: (VEER-you-lence) The power of an organism to cause disease.

virus: (VYE-rus) The smallest organism identified by use of electron microscopy; intracellular parasites that may cause disease.

viscosity: (vis-KAW-sih-tee) Thickness, as of the blood.

volvulus: (VOL-view-lus) A twisting of the bowel on itself, causing obstruction.

vulvovaginitis: (VUL-voh-VAJ-I-NYE-tiss) Inflammation of the vulva and vagina.

Weber test: (VAY-ber TEST) A test for unilateral deafness.

white blood cells: (WIGHT BLUHD SELLS) Leukocytes; the body's primary defense against infection.

withdrawal: (with-DRAWL) Symptoms caused by cessation of administration of a drug, especially a narcotic or alcohol, to which the individual has become either physiologically or psychologically addicted.

worldview: (WERLD-vyoo) The way individuals look on the world to form values and beliefs about life and the world around them.

xerostomia: (ZEE-roh-STOH-mee-ah) Dry mouth caused by reduction in secretions.

Index